Facial Plastic, Reconstructive, and Trauma Surgery

Facial Plastic, Reconstructive, and Trauma Surgery

edited by

Robert W. Dolan

Lahey Clinic
Burlington, Massachusetts, U.S.A.

MARCEL DEKKER, INC. NEW YORK • BASEL

Library of Congress Cataloging-in-Publication Data
A catalog record for this book is available from the Library of Congress.

ISBN: 0-8247-4595-7

This book is printed on acid-free paper.

Headquarters
Marcel Dekker, Inc., 270 Madison Avenue, New York, NY 10016, U.S.A.
tel: 212-696-9000; fax: 212-685-4540

Distribution and Customer Service
Marcel Dekker, Inc., Cimarron Road, Monticello, New York 12701, U.S.A.
tel: 800-228-1160; fax: 845-796-1772

Eastern Hemisphere Distribution
Marcel Dekker AG, Hutgasse 4, Postfach 812, CH-4001 Basel, Switzerland
tel: 41-61-260-6300; fax: 41-61-260-6333

World Wide Web
http://www.dekker.com

The publisher offers discounts on this book when ordered in bulk quantities. For more information, write to Special Sales/Professional Marketing at the headquarters address above.

Current printing (last digit):

10 9 8 7 6 5 4 3 2 1

PRINTED IN THE UNITED STATES OF AMERICA

Preface

The purpose of this book is to provide an educational resource for residents and practicing physicians to use in preparing for board examinations and patient care. The book was written to provide a comprehensive yet practical review of all aspects of facial plastic surgery, including basic knowledge; reconstructive surgery for congenital, traumatic, and postsurgical facial and neck defects; evaluation and management of the traumatized patient; and facial cosmetic surgery. Each chapter begins with a basic review of knowledge and builds upon this knowledge base to present more comprehensive information and advanced concepts. Each chapter is thoroughly referenced and multiple figures are provided to add to the understanding of the text. The chapters are written by a variety of colleagues from within the specialties of otolaryngology–head and neck surgery, oculoplastic surgery, plastic surgery, oral and maxillofacial surgery, dermatology, and facial prosthetics. The chapters have been thoroughly edited and referenced to meet the goals of the book in a consistent presentation.

This book began as an attempt to impart relevant basic and advanced information on subjects in facial plastic and reconstructive surgery to otolaryngology–head and neck surgery residents in training. Many of these residents felt that an organized text to study facial plastic surgery that included all aspects of this specialty including cosmetic, reconstructive, and trauma surgery was needed. Indeed, I have spoken to and assisted in the training of residents from all the specialties in facial plastic surgery and they have voiced this same need. An inclusive text avoids redundancy and has consistent organization and presentation. Since facial plastic surgery encompasses an enormous volume of knowledge and expertise, many authors from a variety of specialties have made significant contributions. I have made every effort to edit the text to eliminate irrelevant information and include basic information to orient the reader to the subject. This book is not intended to be a surgical atlas, but multiple figures, tables, and glossaries are included to add to the understanding of the text.

Special thanks goes to my illustrators: Dennis James Martin and George Barile. Dennis provided a few figures initially before his untimely death. He was a good friend and his photorealistic drawings were shown in galleries across the country. His drawings are flawless, incredibly detailed, and consummate in beauty. I was without an illustrator for several months until I found George, who graciously and enthusiastically took the torch. His excellent work is displayed throughout the book. My sincere thanks and gratitude go to him and his staff. I gratefully acknowledge the assistance of Kathy Jacobs and Lajuana King in helping sort through the mountain of paperwork and revisions. I'm indebted to my contributing authors. Of course, I am forever grateful for the inspiration and support from my mentor, Dr. Sebastian Arena. Thanks go to my colleagues who have supported me in this endeavor, especially Dr. Jesus Medina, who continues to provide me with insight and guidance. Finally, this endeavor, as others, would be meaningless without my wife, Janemarie, and my children, Alexander, Benjamin, and Kathryn.

Robert W. Dolan

Contents

Contributors

Brad Andrews, M.D. Resident Physician, Department of Otolaryngology–Head and Neck Surgery, University of Colorado Health Sciences Center, Denver, Colorado, U.S.A.

Gregory Antoine, M.D., F.A.C.S. Associate Professor and Chairman, Department of Plastic Surgery, Plastic and Reconstructive Surgery and Otolaryngology, Head and Neck Surgery, Boston University School of Medicine, Boston, Massachusetts, U.S.A.

Valentina R. Bradley, M.D. Private Practice, Affiliated Dermatology, Dublin, Ohio, U.S.A.

Matthew D. Byers, M.D. Medical Director, Premier Facial and Plastic Reconstructive Surgery Center, Silverstein Institute, and Active Staff, Sarasota Memorial Hospital, Sarasota, Florida, U.S.A.

Joseph R. Cain, D.D.S., MS Professor and Director, Maxillofacial Prosthetics, College of Dentistry, University of Oklahoma, Oklahoma City, Oklahoma, U.S.A.

Khal Chowdhury, M.D., MBA, FRCSC Associate Professor, University of Colorado Health Sciences Center, Center for Craniofacial and Skull-Base Surgery, Denver, Colorado, U.S.A.

Robert E. Clark, M.D., PhD. Medical Director, Cary Skin Center, Cary, North Carolina, U.S.A.

J. Andrew Colgan, D.D.S. Chief Resident, Department of Oral and Maxillofacial Surgery, Health Sciences Center, University of Oklahoma, Oklahoma City, Oklahoma, U.S.A.

Raffi Der Sarkissian, M.D. Director, Richard C. Webster Division of Facial Plastic Surgery, and Assistant Professor, Department of Otolaryngology, Boston University School of Medicine, and Boston Medical Center, Boston, Massachusetts, U.S.A.

Robert W. Dolan, M.D., F.A.C.S. Senior Staff, Facial Plastic, and Reconstructive Surgery, Department of Otolaryngology, Lahey Clinic, Burlington, and Associate Professor, Boston Medical Center, Boston, Massachusetts, U.S.A.

Timothy Egan, M.D. Chief Resident, Department of Otolaryngology, Head and Neck Surgery, Boston Medical Center, Boston, Massachusetts, U.S.A.

Jose N. Fayad, M.D. House Ear Institute, Los Angeles, California, U.S.A.

Joseph G. Feghali, M.D. Clinical Professor, Otolaryngology and Neurological Surgery, Albert Einstein College of Medicine, New York, New York, U.S.A.

Paul Francel, M.D., PhD. Associate Professor, Neurosurgery, Oklahoma University Health Sciences Center, Oklahoma City, Oklahoma, U.S.A.

Carlos Garcia, M.D. Director, Dermatologic Surgery and Cutaneous Oncology, Oklahoma University Health Science Center, Oklahoma City, Oklahoma, U.S.A.

Juan Carlos Giachino Jr., M.D. Private Practice, Plastic Surgery Associates, Stuart, Florida, U.S.A.

Darlene Skow Johnson, M.D. Director and Staff Physician, Dermatologic Surgery Unit, Lahey Clinic Medical Center, Burlington, Massachusetts, U.S.A.

Joshua L. Kessler, M.D. Senior Resident, Department of Otolaryngology, Boston Medical Center, Boston, Massachusetts, U.S.A.

Keith A. LaFerriere, M.D., F.A.C.S. Clinical Professor, Division of Otolaryngology, Department of Surgery, University of Missouri, Columbia, and Private Practice, Facial Plastic Surgery Center, Springfield, Missouri, U.S.A.

Robert E. Lincoln, D.M.D. Oral and Maxillofacial Surgeon, Private Practice, Quincy, and Associate Clinical Professor, Department of Oral Maxillofacial Surgery, Boston Medical Center, Boston, Massachusetts, U.S.A.

Brian P. Maloney, M.D., F.A.C.S. President, Maloney Center, Atlanta, Georgia, U.S.A.

Laurence Milgrim, M.D. Private Practice, Trumbull, Connecticut, U.S.A.

Donald L. Mitchell, D.D.S., MS Professor and Chair, Oral Implantology, College of Dentistry, University of Oklahoma, Oklahoma City, Oklahoma, U.S.A.

Mark R. Murphy, M.D. Department of Otolaryngology, New York Presbyterian Hospital, New York, New York, U.S.A.

Jayesh Panchal, M.D., MBA, CPE Associate Professor, Plastic Surgery, Oklahoma University Health Sciences Center, Oklahoma City, Oklahoma, U.S.A.

Christine M. Puig, M.D. Private Practice, Ear, Nose, and Throat Plastic Surgery Associates, Auburn, Washington, U.S.A.

John H. Romanow, M.D. Senior Staff, Department of Otolaryngology, Lahey Clinic Medical Center, Burlington, Massachusetts, U.S.A.

Guy J. Sciortino, M.D. Anesthesiologist, Department of Anesthesiology, Lahey Clinic Medical Center, Burlington, and Associate Professor of Anesthesiology, Tufts University Medical Center, Boston, Massachusetts, U.S.A.

Jeffrey H. Spiegel, M.D., F.A.C.S. Assistant Professor, Division of Facial Plastic and Reconstructive Surgery, Department of Otolaryngology–Head and Neck Surgery, School of Medicine, Boston University, Boston, Massachusetts, U.S.A.

Steven M. Sullivan, D.D.S. Professor and Chairman, Department of Oral and Maxillofacial Surgery, University of Oklahoma, Oklahoma City, Oklahoma, U.S.A.

Susan M. Tucker, M.D., F.A.C.S. Senior Staff, Department of Ophthalmology, Lahey Clinic Medical Center, Burlington, and Assistant Professor, Oculoplastic and Reconstruction Surgery, New England Medical Center, Boston, Massachusetts, U.S.A.

Facial Plastic, Reconstructive, and Trauma Surgery

1
Facial and Skin Surface Analysis

Robert W. Dolan
Lahey Clinic Medical Center, Burlington, Massachusetts, U.S.A.

BASIC AESTHETIC PHOTOGRAPHY

Equipment Guidelines

The basic equipment for portable aesthetic photography includes a 35 mm single lens reflex (SLR) camera body. A macro lens with a fixed focal length between 90 and 110 mm is widely used (see below). The flash may be handheld or camera-mounted approximately 12 inches above the plane of the lens; if the flash is too close to the camera body, the skin's surface landmarks tend to wash out and red eye becomes more of a problem. Ring flashes are probably best avoided for these reasons. A variety of film types may be used and prints or slides are acceptable. Color film developed by the E-6 process or kodachrome slides developed by Kodak (providing somewhat finer grain and less fading) are satisfactory.

For color pictures, the background elements should include a light blue nondistracting fabric or screen; for black and white photography, a white background provides good contrast with skin tones. Keeping the patient a fixed distance of approximately 4 feet from the background is essential in obtaining uniform pre- and postoperative photographs.

Consistent image magnification is a concern and is calculated for 35 mm film oriented vertically as follows: measure (in cm) the top of the viewed object to the bottom of the viewed object and divide by 3.6 cm; this value is the denominator of the ratio of magnification given as 1: [value]. A magnification ratio of 1:9 is the accepted magnification for the adult head (using a 105 mm lens); 1:9 corresponds to a distance of 3.8 feet from the lens to the subject.

Digital Photography

Digital photography begins with choosing a digital camera and computer interface. This method has several differences from conventional SLR-based photography. The advantages of digital photography over conventional methods include instantaneous results and quick archiving, the ability to enhance picture quality, and the ability to change facial features (morphing) to assess the effects of the proposed surgery. The major drawback of digital photography and conventional photography is lack of image resolution and clarity. A digital image is composed of pixels or tiny dots of information expressed as the pixel resolution: width × height. Therefore, an image with a resolution of 1024 × 768 will be 14.2″ × 10.7″ on a monitor at 72 dots/inch, and 1.4″ × 1.1″ on a printed page at 720 dots/inch. The pixel resolution of a digital camera indicates the density of the image sensors in the camera chip. This chip is very expensive and so the price of a good-quality digital camera is high. At the present time, digital cameras are available that can deliver adequate resolution (e.g., 1024 × 768) for under $1000. However, most of these systems lack the versatility of a standard SLR camera with respect to lenses, control over the depth of field, and lighting capabilities. These digital cameras are essentially point-and-shoot devices, although lens attachments for close-up photography are available. Digital chip inserts in place of conventional film in an SLR camera may be available in the near future.

Once the images are recorded digitally, they must be downloaded into a software program that can archive images seamlessly with the camera and, if desired, a morphing program. A standard Pentium-based computer with at least 64 megabytes of random-access memory will suffice. The digital images are usually received into the computer as bitmaps and can be several megabytes in size. Archiving these images would quickly deplete the hard drive's storage space. An alternative is to save them as compressed images of a few hundred kilobytes, and the most popular mechanism is Joint Photographic Experts Group (JPEG) compression, named after the original committee that wrote the standard. Some image quality is lost after compression but this is not a serious problem with this type of imaging application.

Another method to digitize images is to scan negatives, 35 mm transparencies, or photographs directly into the archiving and morphing software. The advantage of this method is that the scanner's resolution can be much greater (e.g., 2700 dots/inch) than a comparably priced digital camera, and a good-quality hard copy of the original image is retained.

Digital photography and image manipulation may enhance a cosmetic surgical practice by improving doctor–patient communication, resident education and training, and reducing overhead costs for conventional film processing and storage. Despite these potential advantages, misuse of this tool can lead to significant exposure to malpractice claims of implied contract and failure to instruct (1). Although no cases directly related to computer imaging have arisen over the last 10 years, cases resulting from preoperative consent issues are applicable to this technique. Courts have found surgeons liable for specific statements regarding postoperative results. Failure to achieve these results may provoke a claim of malpractice by failure to honor an implied contract. A simple waiver stating that the physician does not guarantee a particular result does not insulate the physician from litigation if specific statements regarding postoperative results were made. Failure-to-instruct claims may arise from allegations that preoperative imaging failed to reveal an undesirable or unexpected surgical outcome. This is analogous to describing only the benefits of a surgical procedure without disclosing the risks.

To avoid litigation related to computer imaging, the rules of informed consent must apply. Computer imaging should be combined with a signed consent outlining the risks of and alternatives to the procedure. Try to convey the average result or less favorable outcomes in the computer images presented to the patient. In the consent form, a statement should be added regarding computer imaging and expected surgical results, since most courts do not question the validity of the signed consent form. In addition, these computer images should be date-stamped or signed by the patient and considered part of the medical record and should not be destroyed or discarded: to do so creates a presumption of harm in malpractice claims.

MACROPHOTOGRAPHY

Macrophotography is the act of taking close-up pictures with a camera lens designed to focus at very short distances with up to life-size magnification of the image.

Lens Options

The choice of lens depends upon the desired final picture quality and the anticipated distance from the object. The standard lens is a 50 mm lens that allows an infinity setting to focus on objects over 20 feet away. It is designed to reproduce an image of similar scale and size to what the human eye sees. This setting encompasses much of the surroundings as well as the object of interest, unless the object is very large. For a lens with a 50 mm focal length, the nodal point of the optics will be 50 mm from the plane of the film near the back of the camera body. As the object moves closer, the lens must be adjusted away from the plane of the film to focus, resulting in a nodal point slightly more than 50 mm. The lens is actually casting an image circle larger than the 24 $\times$ 36 mm frame, and some of the light is lost and bounces around inside the camera. As the object comes even closer, this effect becomes more of a problem, resulting in some loss of contrast. In fact, the normal 50 mm lens cannot focus down to much more than 1:6, a ratio indicating the relative size of the object to the size of the image. A fixed stack of optical lenses is not available that can form sharp images at so many different distances. However, a 1:6 ratio does fall into the range of acceptable magnification for medical photography of the human adult head (1:9). However, the focused distance requires a lens-to-film plane distance that results in an image that lacks some contrast. Sharper imagery required in the preoperative assessment of blepharoplasty or rhinoplasty patients will compound the problems of contrast and light dilution. In addition to the loss of light and contrast, there is a significant loss of depth of field because the f-stop is more open to allow more light in (higher f-stops allow less light in but greater depth of field). An image requiring a lens setting of f/16 at infinity would require a lens setting of about f/8 at 1:1.

Seeing Things Close-up

A magnifying glass helps our eyes to see things close up, and a magnifying lens can be placed over the existing lens to perform close-up photography. These so-called supplementary lenses are in expensive and they do not require skill beyond screwing them onto the end of the existing lens. The main problem with these magnifying lenses is that to focus on objects in the distance again, the existing lens cannot compensate for the magnification and the magnifying lens must be removed. In addition, picture quality may be compromised; high-quality lenses are usually two-element lenses and even these may distort an image to some extent.

Macro Lens

These are not so-called macro zoom lenses. Macro lenses have much greater potential lens-to-film (helical) lengths, but use floating optical lens elements to allow sharper close-up images (1:2/1:1), while still allowing long focused distance imaging (without the need to change lenses). Still, light is reduced and exposure is affected. Manually compensating for ambient light and f-stops requires charts, expertise, and lots of bracketing. The closer the image is to 1:1, the smaller the *effective* aperture, despite the nominal reading of, for example, f/22 on the lens. Charts are available for cross-reference, but for the f/22 at 1:1, the effective f-stop is f/45. That is a small hole to let light in, and the result is increased diffraction and reduced image quality. One solution is to set the f-stop manually on the lens to f/11, despite the light meter calling for an f-stop of f/22. Another solution is to use through-the-lens light metering that automatically corrects for the reduced effective aperture. The effective aperture is actually displayed under the viewfinder in the modern Nikon SLR units. Many medical media departments will use a f/16 fixed f-stop at 1:1 to allow adequate depth of field for focusing and then bracket up to f/22 and down to f/8.

Depth of field is limited and approximates 1 mm at 1:1. Precise distances are paramount to success and tripod setups are often inadequate. Macro focusing rails are helpful since they are able to move the camera precisely up and down. The brand of macro lens makes little difference. Nikon, Canon, Tamron, or Sigma models are all excellent choices.

If macro refers to close-up shots, what is micro? Microphotography refers to when the scale is beyond 1:1. It takes an object and magnifies it, which is the opposite of what a typical lens does. It is a complex process, but involves moving the film away from the lens and using a reversing ring to make a small object appear large.

Subject Positioning

Subject positioning is important: keeping the Frankfort Line at the true horizontal for all frontal, lateral, and oblique views. The Frankfort Line extends from the top of the tragus (easily identified in photos) to the junction of the orbital rim (not so easily identified). To duplicate the true horizontal, have the patient stare into their own eyes using a mirror placed 4 feet in front of them and have them maintain this position for frontal, lateral, and oblique views. Pick consistent landmarks for oblique views. A useful rule is to align the nasal tip to the margin of the cheek. Positions are dependent on the proposed procedure. The guidelines shown in Table 1 are standard using a 105 mm macro lens.

GENERAL FACIAL ANALYSES

Facial Balance

A common standard cited for overall facial aesthetics is the so-called golden proportion based on pythagorean mathematics, yielding the basic ratio: 1:1.618 (2). Phidias applied this in ancient Greek art most notably and this ratio is called phi in his honor. This divine proportion is duplicated in nature and represents a union of geometry and mathematics. A three-point compass dubbed the golden divider maintains

Table 1 Guidelines for Photography using a 105-mm Macro Lens

Procedure	Position
Facial (rhytidectomy)	
4′ Frontal	In repose/smiling/grimacing
4′ Lateral	Left/right
4′ Oblique	Left/right
3′ Malar view (optional)	
Nasal (rhinoplasty)	
3′ Frontal view	
3′ Lateral view	Left/right
3′ Oblique view	Left/right
2.5′ Base view	
3′ Lateral view/smiling	Left/right
2′ Sky view (optional)	
Periorbital (blepharoplasty)	
3′ Frontal view	
2.5′ Frontal view	Eyes open/eyes closed
2.5′ Lateral view	Left/right
2.5′ Oblique view	Left/right
Auricular (otoplasty)	
4′ Frontal view	
4′ Lateral view	Left/right
4′ Posterior view	
1.5′ Close-up view	Left/right
4′ Oblique view (optional)	Left/right
1.5′ Oblique view (optional)	Left/right
Scalp	
4′ Frontal view	
4′ Posterior view	
4′ Head down	Hair combed away from area
4′ Head down	Hair combed to camouflage area

this constant ratio upon expansion. As the compass is expanded, its points align with the following:

Upper lip vermilion show (1) to lower lip vermilion show (1.618)
Total vermilion show (1.618) to mucocutaneous junction–columellar base (1)
Mentum–columellar base (1.618) to columellar base–medial canthus (1)

These ratios also apply on the frontal view, especially relating to intercanthal distances.

Our current concepts of facial balance and proportion are rooted in ancient times from the Egyptians, Greeks, and Romans. Modern facial analysis began with the mathematical formulations of the human face by Leonardo da Vinci, most notably from his *Anatomical Notebooks*. Albrecht Durer, a German artist influenced by Leonardo, wrote the treatise *The Human Figure* containing many careful facial analyses of realistic (not necessarily aesthetic) facial proportions. Several neoclassical canons from this era help to define facial proportion including

Leonardo's facial thirds: forehead height (trichion–glabella) = nose length (nasion–subnasale) = lower face height (subnasale–gnathion)
Nose length (glabella–subnasion) = auricle height (supra-aurale–subaurale)
Interocular distance (endocanthion [medial canthus]–endocanthion) = nose width (ala–ala)
Ocular fissure width (exocanthion [lateral canthus]–exocanthion) = interocular distance
Mouth width (cheilion–cheilion) = 1.5 times the nose width
Nose width = 0.25 times the face width (zygion–zygion)
Nasal bridge inclination parallels ear inclination (along the longitudinal axis)

Modern anthropometric measurements allow us to check these canons against several populations. Based on these data, the canons tend not to reflect the most common composite measurements, even for North American White populations (3). The neoclassical canons also do not perform well in defining aesthetic proportions. In a study of people considered attractive by independent observation, the neoclassical canons failed to differentiate this subset from the overall population (4). Anthropometric measurements of heterogeneous populations have exposed the fallacy of attempting to define a single standard of facial form. Multiple variables affect aesthetic facial analysis including gender, race, and even cultural attitudes. For example, African-Americans tend to have wider and shorter noses as well as wider faces and mouths than North American Whites (5).

The technique of modern facial analysis attempts to reflect the aesthetic ideal, not the anthropometric average. Although beauty is subjective, what we consider beautiful often relates to an underlying symmetry that can be measured objectively. Several proportion-based measurements correlate with the aesthetic ideal; most involve the relationships of the nose to the chin and the face. Proportion-based measurements should be gender- and population-specific, although most correspond to the aesthetic standards of a North American White population. An important first step in any facial analysis is learning the vernacular of soft tissue cephalometrics.

Soft-Tissue Cephalometry

With regard to facial aesthetics, cephalometry is simply a tool to define the anatomical elements of the face for proportional analyses. Hard-tissue reference points form the basis of the soft-tissue reference points outlined below. Cephalometry is useful for preoperative and postoperative objective measurements and for defining certain aesthetic ideals according to the technique used. Facial analyses often begin with simple proportion and balance determinations using the neoclassical canons as guides despite their shortcomings. More specific cephalometric or advanced proportion analyses may be appropriate based on the planned procedure.

Hard-tissue cephalometry uses a basic reference line for analyses called the Frankfurt Horizontal (a line that extends from the superior bony external auditory canal to the inferior border of the infraorbital rim). This is difficult to discern on a photograph, so having the patient assume what is termed the natural head position approximates this true horizontal line. The natural head position was defined by

Table 2 Individual Cephalometric Points

Points	Description
Cervical point (C)	Junction between the submental area and the neck
Tragion (T)	Most anterior portion of the supratragal notch
Trichion (Tr)	Hairline at midsagittal plane
Glabella (G)	Most prominent portion in midsagittal plane of forehead
Nasion (N)	Midpoint of frontonasal suture
Rhinion (R)	Junction of bony and cartilaginous dorsum (bony landmark)
Subnasale (Sn)	Junction of the columella with the upper cutaneous lip
Supratip (ST)	Point cephalic to dome
Tip (T)	Most anterior projection of nose
Columella Point (CM)	Most anterior part of columella
Superior sulcus (SS)	Depth of convexity of upper lip
Labrale superiorus (LS)	Mucocutaneous junction of upper lip
Labrale inferius (LI)	Mucocutaneous junction of lower lip
Mentolabial sulcus (SI)	Most posterior point between lip and chin
Pogonion (PG)	Most anterior point of soft tissue chin
Menton (ME)	Lowest point on contour of soft tissue chin
Horizontal plane (HP)	Line perpendicular to true vertical through tragion
Upper vermilion (Vu)	Upper vermilion lip-skin border
Lower vermilion (Vl)	Lower vermilion lip–skin border
Superior vermilion (Vs)	Vermilion (anteriormost border)
Inferior vermilion (Vi)	Inferior vermilion (anterior-most border)

Broca in 1862 and is achieved by having the patient peer into a mirror in primary gaze placed 4 feet away. The individual cephalometric points are as shown in Table 2 (see also Figure 1).

PROCEDURE-SPECIFIC ANALYSES

Rhinoplasty

The aesthetic proportion-based measurements include the following (Figs. 2–4):

From the basal view, columellar length twice the length of the lobule.
A transverse line across mid-nostril on basal view should be equidistant from the nasal tip and alar crease.
From the lateral view, 2–4 mm of columellar show (the amount of columella visualized on lateral view)
A nasolabial angle of approximately 90° in men and 110° in the women.
The presence of a supratip depression in women (an area cephalic to the point where the lobule meets the dorsum).
The presence of a double break: this describes the aesthetic phenomenon of the division of the lobule–dorsum angle into two angles defined by lines following the columella, dorsum, and lobule at the nasal tip.
From the frontal view, a gentle curve from the supraorbital rim to the tip (6).

Although tip projection and the perceived size of the nose depend on other facial features and the person's height and weight (7), two methods of measurement for tip

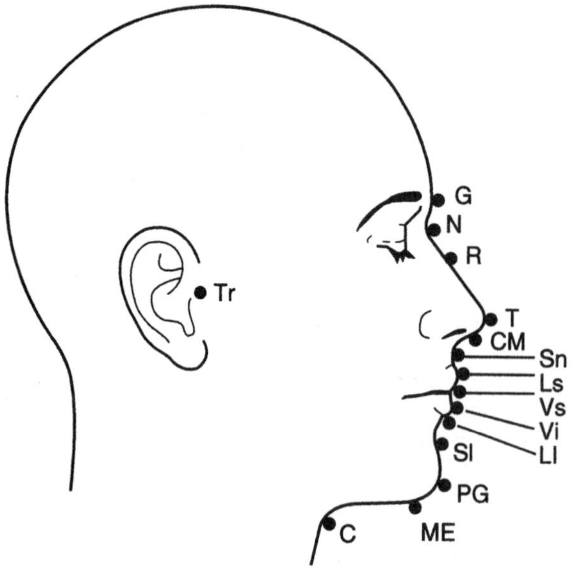

Figure 1 Common soft tissue cephalometric points: G – glabella; N – nasion; R – rhinion; T – tip; CM – columella; Sn – subnasale; LS – labrale superius; Vs – superior vermilion; Vi – inferior vermilion; LI – labrale inferius; SI – mentolabial sulcus; PG – pagonion; ME – menton; C – cervical point.

projection are commonly used: the Upper Vermilion–subnasale Sn) distance should equal the Sn–nasal tip distance (8); and Crumley's method of superimposing a right-angled triangle based at the alar groove with vertices at the nasion and nasal tip whose sides have 3:4:5 proportions (9) (Fig. 5).

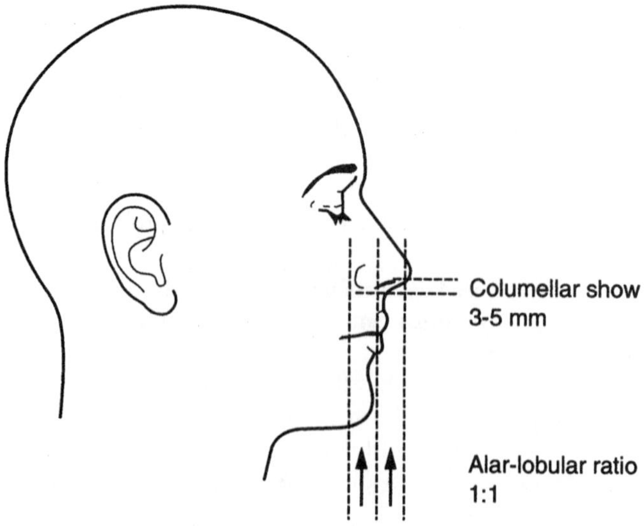

Figure 2 Normative values for columellar show and the alar–lobular ratio.

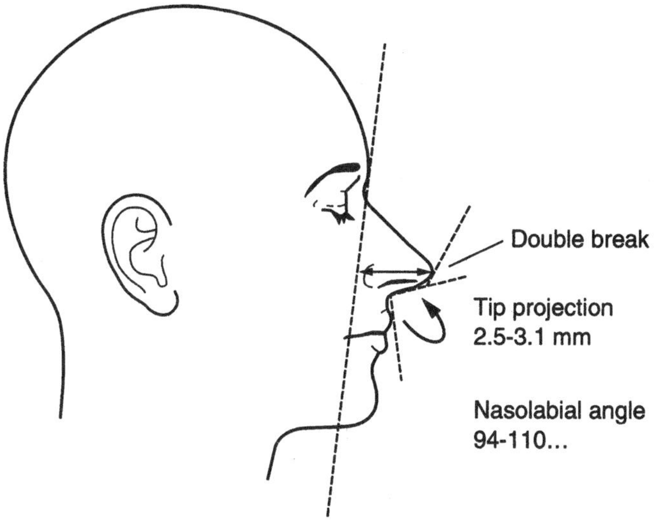

Figure 3 Double break and normative values for tip projection and the nasolabial angle.

Important relationships exist with the rest of the face and chin. The width of the nose (ala-to-ala) should equal the distance between the medial canthi (a neoclassical canon that accurately reflects the aesthetic ideal). Also, the aesthetic triangle of Powell and Humphries (10) (the base of the triangle is a line connecting the nasion and pogonion and its apex is at the nasal tip) (Fig. 6). The ideal values are: nasofrontal angle = 120°; nasofacial angle = 36°; nasomental angle = 130°; mentocervical angle = 85°.

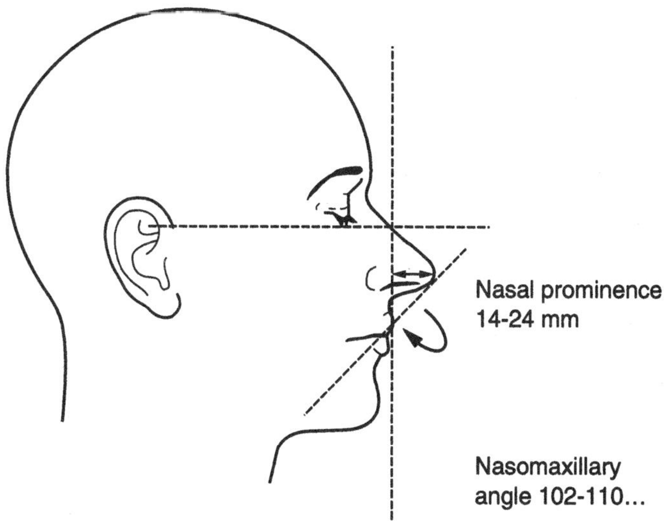

Figure 4 Normative values for nasal prominence and the nasomaxillary angle.

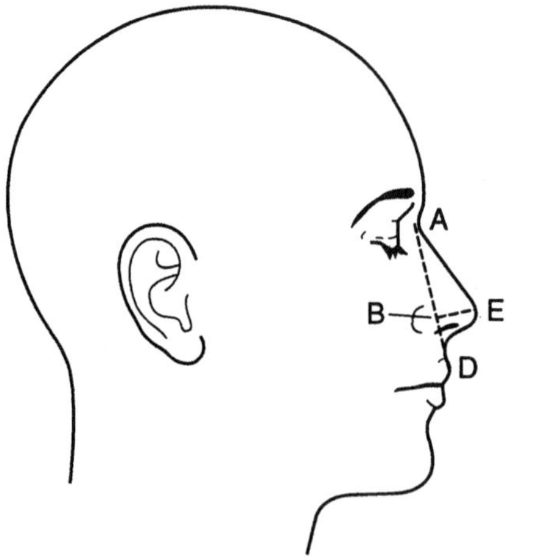

Figure 5 Crumley's method of assessing tip projection drawing. The BE:AD ratio should be approximately 0.2833.

Genioplasty

The visual relationship between the nose and the chin is so intimate that to change the size and shape of one influences the apparent size and shape of the other. Prior to evaluation of the position of the chin, the dental occlusion should be documented. Angle's classification (1899) is widely used and is based on the anteroposterior relationship of the maxillary and mandibular first permanent molars:

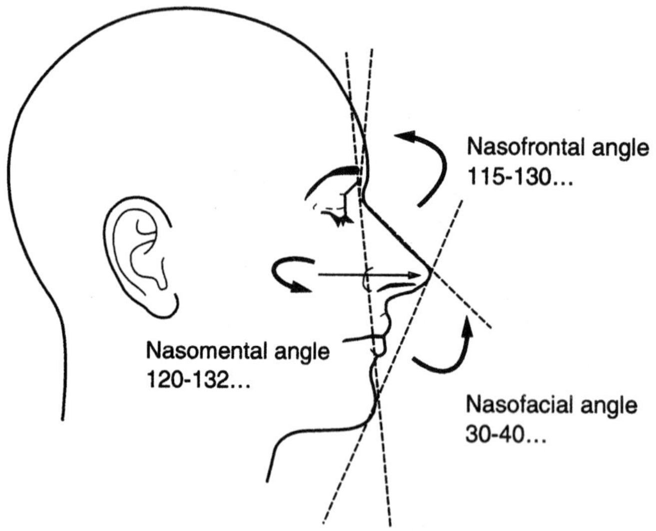

Figure 6 The aesthetic triangle of Powell and Humphries characterized by the nasofrontal angle, nasomental angle, and nasofacial angle.

Class I (neutroclusion). The first molars contact normally.
Class II (distoclusion). The mandibular first molar is displaced posteriorly with respect to the maxillary first molar.
Division 1. In addition to distoclusion, the upper maxillary arch is narrow and the incisors incline in a buccal direction.
Division 2. Distoclusion and the upper incisors incline in a lingual direction.
Class III (mesioclusion). The mandibular first molar is displaced anteriorly with respect to the maxillary first molar.

Patients with malocclusion usually have an abnormal profile and chin position irregularities. A class II malocclusion may result in a receding chin, and a class III deformity may result in a protruding chin. Surgical repair of malocclusions will affect the profile; therefore, patients with malocclusion should be offered orthognathic surgery prior to consideration of genioplasty. Angle's classification system is inadequate to describe chin position completely since malocclusion is only an indirect measure of the potential position of the chin.

Inadequate chin protrusion is usually the clinical finding in potential genioplasty candidates; it may be due to micrognathia, retrognathia, or microgenia. Micrognathia refers to a hypoplastic mandible in which both the ramus and body are underdeveloped, usually associated with neutroclusion or a class II malocclusion. Retrognathia refers to a mandible with an underdeveloped ramus, a normal body, and usually a class II malocclusion. Microgenia refers to a mandible with an isolated underdeveloped chin (normal body and ramus). Microgenia results in a chin that is both retruded and deficient by palpation, unlike micrognathic and retrognathic chins that are retruded but normal by palpation. Micrognathia or retrognathia associated with malocclusion requires more extensive surgical intervention than pure genioplasty, including sagittal osteotomies and mandibular advancements that are beyond the scope of a purely cosmetic procedure. Patients not desiring orthognathic work or those with microgenia are candidates for genioplasty involving augmentation (or retrusion in the case of chin overprotrusion or macrognathia) of the mandibular symphysis.

There are essentially three anatomical abnormalities often associated with a recessive chin: a recessive and procumbent lower lip, a deep labiomental fold, and diminished to normal lower facial height. Therefore, preoperative analysis must include an assessment of these components in both the anteroposterior and vertical planes (Fig. 7). A perpendicular line is dropped from the Frankfort Horizontal (soft tissue cephalometric radiograph) or from the true horizontal line with the patient in the natural head position (photograph) through the subnasale (reference point). Measurements are taken from the vertical line to the lip vermilion and pogonion: Sn-vermilion (Vu) $= 0 \pm 2$ mm, Sn-lower vermilion (Vl) $= -2 \pm 2$ mm, and Sn-Pogonion (Pg) $= (-4 \pm 2$ mm). The vertical chin position is determined by comparing the glabella–Sn distance to the Sn–menton distance: these should be equal (11). Two other methods for determining chin position are also widely used:

A line through superior vermilion and Vi should be tangent to the pogonion.
A line dropped perpendicular to Frankfort's line from the nasion should be tangent to the pogonion (12).

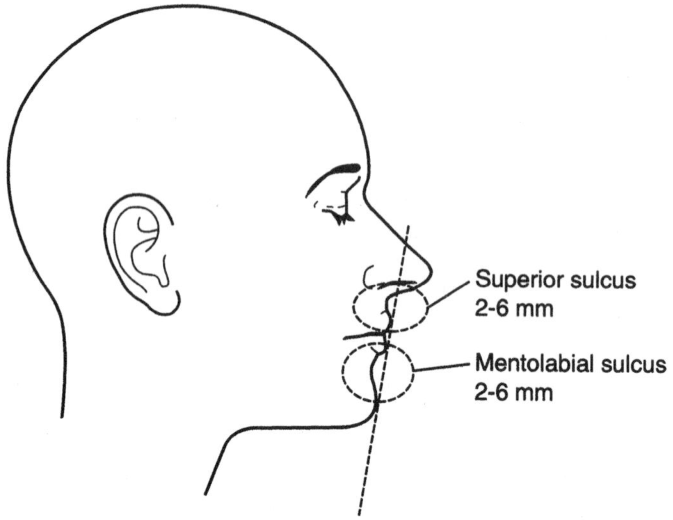

Figure 7 Normative values for the superior sulcus and the mentolabial sulcus.

Facialplasty

Preoperative analysis should address three distinct areas of the face: forehead and brows, cheeks and jowls, and neck and submentum. Surgical correction of deformities in these areas often requires different techniques that may be combined in a single surgical encounter for an optimal outcome.

Evaluation of the forehead begins with a description of the horizontal and vertically oriented rhytids. Horizontal rhytids are formed by the action of the frontalis muscle. The corrugator supercilii muscles form vertical glabellar rhytids, and horizontal rhytids at the root of the nose are formed by the action of the procerus muscle. In women, the aesthetic forehead and glabella complex is smooth with few rhytids; in men some furrowing and rhytids are acceptable. The next step in analysis is evaluation of eyebrow and glabella position. The aesthetic guide to eyebrow position in men is that the brow should lie on the supraorbital rim, while in women the brow should follow or lie slightly above the rim and arch at the lateral limbus of the pupil (13). Brow ptosis or descent bunches the skin over the upper eyelid creating a hooding effect (Fig. 8). This must be appreciated during the preoperative evaluation for blepharoplasty. In women, glabellar and medial brow ptosis disrupts the aesthetically pleasing gently curving line formed along the nasal sidewall and eyebrow.

Analysis of the cheeks and jowls for a traditional rhytidectomy includes an evaluation of the melolabial folds and the position of the sideburns. No exact geometric method is used clinically to describe the position or depth of the melolabial fold. The position of the sideburns, especially in men, should be documented and used in planning preauricular incisions; however, usually no normative relationship is applied. The sideburn should extend below the level of the root of the helix and this relationship should be maintained in treatment planning. The jowls are also assessed qualitatively.

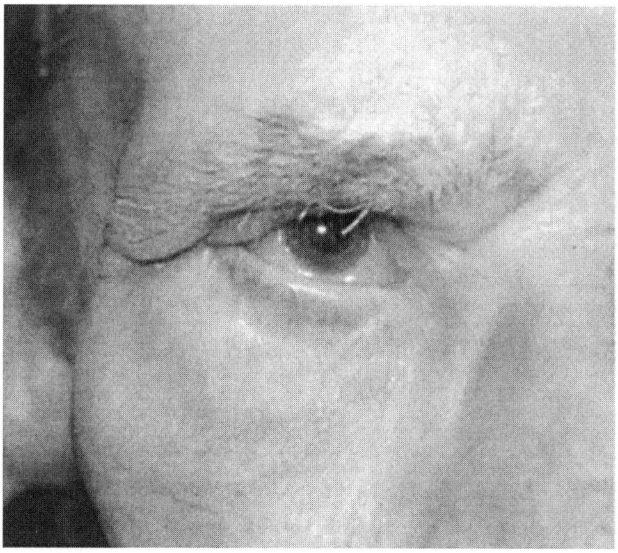

Figure 8 Typical ptotic eyebrow lying well below the superior bony rim.

The ideal mentocervical angle is between 80 and 95 degrees (14) (Fig. 9). Qualitatively, in an anterior–posterior view, the pogonion should clearly delineate the chin from the underlying neck; a weak chin gives the illusion of a short neck. On lateral view, the submentum should be flat and end abruptly at a highly placed hyoid bone. Platysmal banding, resulting from the loss of tone and medial migration of the platysmal muscle (the actual cause is controversial), is a prominence of the medial

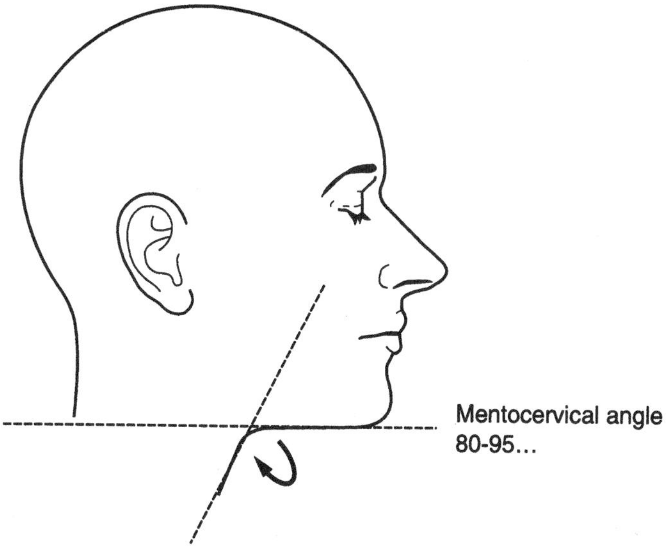

Figure 9 The mentocervical angle.

border of the platysmal muscle causing unattractive vertical lines in the midline of the neck. There may also be senile ptosis of the submandibular glands from laxity of the supporting fascia. A useful classification system for neck/submentum analysis is Dedo's classification of cervical abnormalities (15). The classes are as follows (Fig. 10):

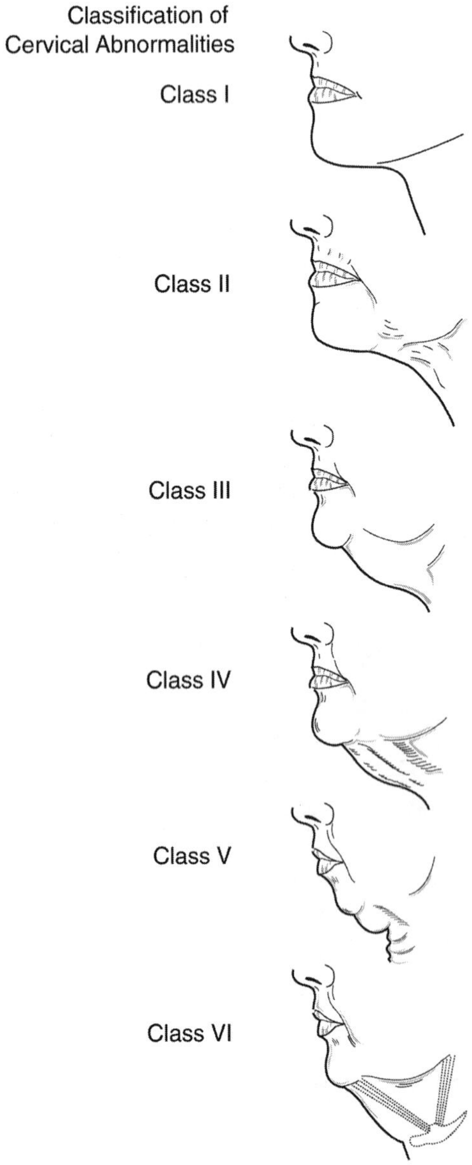

Figure 10 Dedo's classification system of cervical abnormalities. (Adapted from Dedo DD. "How I do it"—plastic surgery. Practical suggestions on facial plastic surgery. A preoperative classification of the neck for cervicofacial rhytidectomy. *Laryngoscope* 1980;90:1894–6).

I. Minimal deformity with an acute cervicomental angle, good platysmal tone, and little accumulation of fat
II. Lax cervical skin
III. Fat accumulation
IV. Platysmal banding
V. Congenital or acquired retrognathia
VI. Low hyoid

Blepharoplasty

Preoperative analysis for blepharoplasty should begin with an evaluation of ocular function including visual acuity, intraocular pressure, tear production, preseptal and intraocular slitlamp examination, funduscopy, and extraocular movement (16). Brow position should be assessed next to determine the contribution of brow ptosis to upper eyelid skin redundancy.

Measurements and evaluation of symmetry of the vertical eyelid fissures are performed to detect congenital or acquired blepharoptosis or vertical eyelid retraction. This is done by measuring the distance between the upper eyelid margin and the lower eyelid margin in primary gaze. The range of normal in men is 8–10 mm, and 9–13 mm in women. Measurements below these ranges indicate blepharoptosis, while measurements in excess of these norms indicate vertical eyelid retraction. Incomplete closure of the eyelids with relaxed effort indicates lagophthalmos. Both the upper and lower eyelid margins normally overlap the corneal limbus in primary gaze; if the lower eyelid margin falls below the limbus some sclera will be exposed: this is termed scleral show. The lateral canthus is positioned above the medial canthus and should be in the same plane, or slightly above, the midpupillary line. Evaluation of lower eyelid laxity is commonly performed by assessing how far the lower eyelid can be pulled away from the globe (>10 mm indicates laxity) and observing its ability to spring back. Significant laxity may indicate a tendency toward postoperative ectropion and the need for a lid-shortening procedure.

The position of the superior palpebral eyelid crease is assessed in the midpupil vertical axis from the lid margin, determined by having the patient slowly look upward from maximal downgaze. The position of the crease varies for different populations and according to gender. Normative values for Whites are 8–10 mm in men and 10–13 mm in women (Fig. 11). Asian patients may have no or very low eyelid creases.

Analysis of the prolapsing fat and redundant skin in the lower eyelid is performed with the patient in primary gaze and in downgaze, although the removal of fat during blepharoplasty is highly individualized and subjective. Dermatochalasis refers to an acquired excess skin laxity due to aging. The amount of excess skin in the lower eyelid can be measured by grasping the putative redundant skin between forceps as the patient gazes upward: production of scleral show or ectropion with this maneuver indicates that a more conservative removal of skin is necessary. Bulging of orbital fat should be documented according to the underlying compartmentalization of the fat in the upper (central and medial) and lower (medial, central, and lateral) eyelids. Lateral hooding in the upper eyelid often indicates a prolapsed lacrimal gland. Concentric folds inferior to the lower lid that may overlap indicate redundant orbicularis oculi muscle and possibly fat; these folds are known as festoons. Festoons

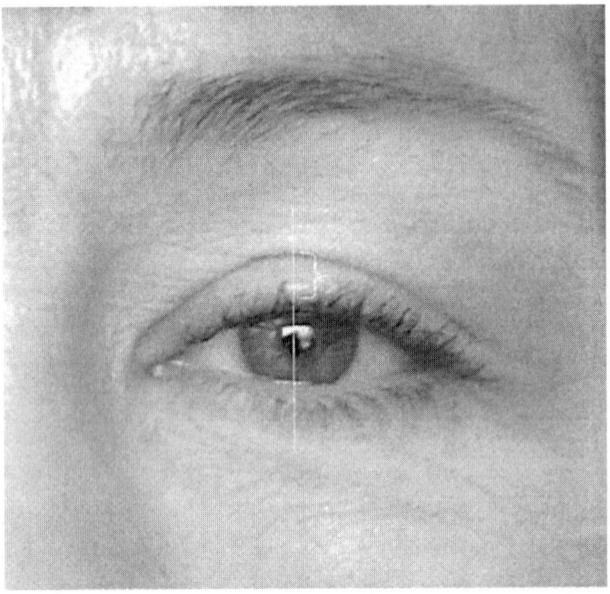

Figure 11 The position and height of the eyelid crease in a White woman. The vertical line corresponds to the midpupillary axis.

may be related to the presence of hypothyroidism (found in 2.6% of patients presenting for aesthetic blepharoplasty) (17). Malar bags form over the superior part of the malar prominence and may be due to dependent edema and fibrosis.

SKIN SURFACE ANALYSIS

Skin surface analysis is often tailored to the goals of restorative surgery or nonsurgical treatments. Patients undergoing scar revisions require analyses to include the resting skin tension lines. In the patient undergoing nasal reconstructive surgery after Mohs' resection, an analysis of the topographical units of the face is important. If cutaneous resurfacing is planned, an analysis of skin type and reaction to solar damage are also needed. Koebner's phenomenon is also an important consideration. This phenomenon describes the tendency for some skin diseases such as psoriasis, lichen planus, discoid lupus erythematosus, and herpes simplex to localize to areas of recent surgery or scars.

Histological Findings

Epidermis

The epidermis is approximately 100 μm thick and is divided into four layers. The basal cell layer or stratum germinativum is a single cell layer giving rise to subsequent layers and interspersed with melanocytes in varying numbers, depending on the part of the body. The prickle cell layer or stratum spinosum is three or four cell layers thick, containing intracellular preformed keratin (named prickle cells

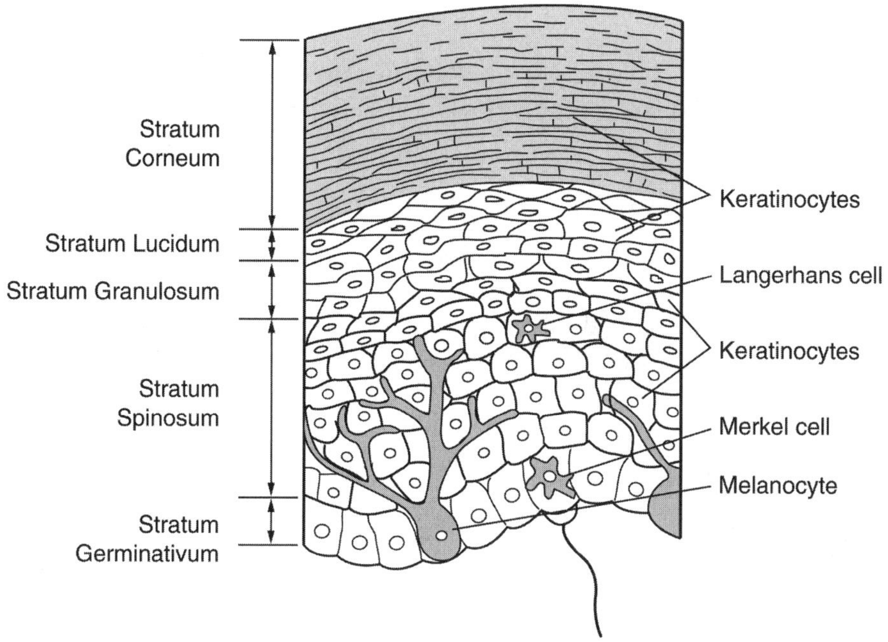

Figure 12 Microanatomy of the epidermis.

based on the desmosomes appearing as small spines coming from the cells). The granular cell layer or stratum granulosum is one to four cell layers thick, containing intracellular preformed keratin granules. A cornified layer or stratum corneum, is several layers thick and is formed by coalescence of the granules in the third layer (Fig. 12).

The epidermis contains four major cell types including keratinocytes (80%), melanocytes, Langerhans' cells, and Merkel's cells. Merkel's cells are found in the basal cell layer of the epidermis and are part of the amine precursor uptake decarboxylation (APUD) system. Their function is unknown; however, Merkel cell tumors may arise from these cells. The melanocytes are also found within the basal cell layer and produce melanin pigment. In blacks, these melanocytes are very active, in areas of vitiligo they are absent, and in those with albinism they are present but lack the enzyme tyrosinase (for tyrosine-to-melanin conversion).

Basement membrane

The basement membrane is a well-defined multilayered structure between the epidermis and dermis that serves two functions: as a barrier to cells and chemicals, and to support and attach the epidermis to the dermis. The membrane consists of several layers visualized on electron microscopy including (18) the following:

Attachment plaque with tonafilaments and hemidesmosomes
The lamina lucida under the attachment plaque with anchoring filaments
The lamina densa under the lamina lucida with anchoring dermal microfibril bundles (type VII collagen)

Rete Ridges

The rete ridges are projections of the epidermis into the dermis, which increase the surface area of contact and help to anchor these two structures through the interface of the basement membrane. The corresponding upward projections of the dermis are termed the dermal papillae. With aging, the length of the rete ridges decreases; in scars, the ridges are lost (19).

Dermis

The dermis is divided into two layers: papillary and reticular (Fig. 13). The thin papillary dermis is just below the basement membrane and contains loose collagen and fibrocytes. The reticular dermis is relatively thick and contains compact collagen and a few fibrocytes. The reticular dermis includes the origins of the epidermal appendages. Collagen is synthesized by fibrocytes, mainly in the papillary dermis. Skin collagen decreases by 1% per year as patients age (20). Reticulin fibers are found throughout the dermis and are probably immature collagen fibers. Elastic fibers are eosinophilic fibers that extend from the basement membrane into the reticular dermis. Sun damage causes the elastic fibers to thicken and collect in the papillary dermis; these elastic fibers are then referred to as elastotic fibers. Aging causes a disappearance of elastic fibers in the papillary dermis (21).

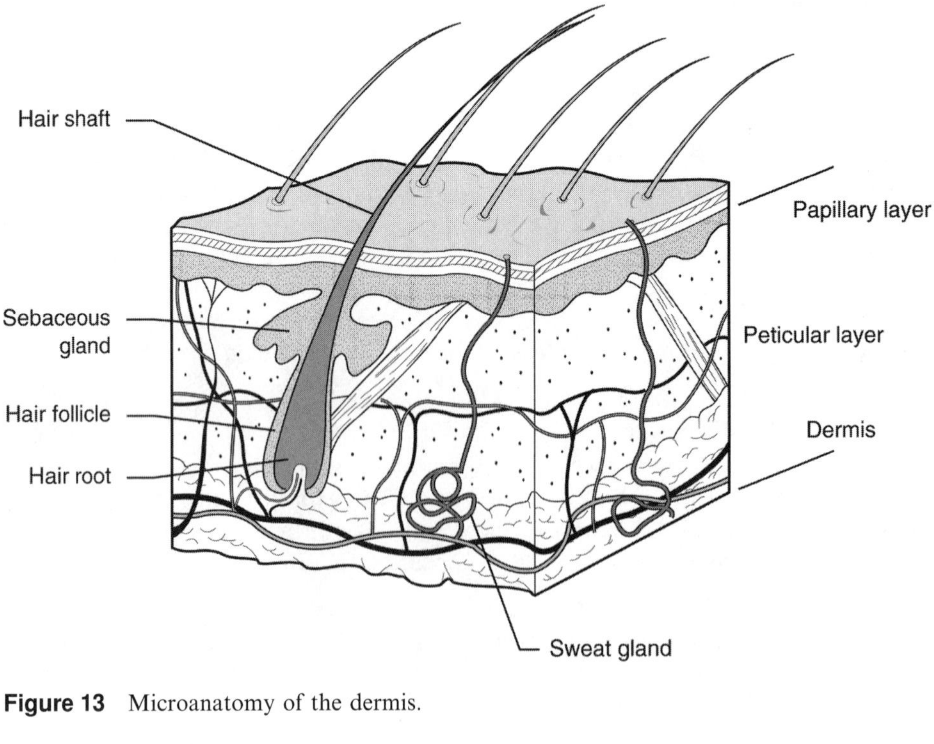

Figure 13 Microanatomy of the dermis.

Lymphatics

The lymphatics begin in the superficial papillary dermis as blind-ended vessels. The more proximal lymphatics have thicker walls and valves.

Pilosebaceous Unit

Pilosebaceous units contain sebaceous glands, sensory end organs, arrector pili muscle, hair, and the hair follicle. Thick hair, such as on the scalp, is terminal hair; fine, nearly imperceptible hair, is vellus hair. Depending on the part of the body, the sebaceous unit may be predominant (e.g., nose). The hair follicle has three named portions (from the skin to the base): the infundibulum (to the sebaceous gland duct), the isthmus (from the duct to the arrector pili muscle insertion), and the inferior portion (below the pili muscle insertion). Hair arises from the base of the hair follicle (the hair bulb). In the hair bulb are cells that make the hair along with melanocytes incorporated into the growing hairs. The hair bulb surrounds a dermal structure called the hair papilla. This papilla regulates the hair bulb activity. The mature hair has a ringlike configuration of several distinct layers (from outer to inner): vitreous membrane, outer root sheath, Henle's layer, Huxley's layer, inner root sheath cuticle, hair cuticle, cortex, and medulla (Fig. 14). Hair growth occurs in stages termed anagen, catagen, and telogen. The anagen stage is the growth phase. The catagen phase is an involutional stage in which the inferior portion ascends to the isthmus. The telogen phase is the resting phase during which the inferior portion of the follicle is absent. Gray hair, seen with advancing age, is caused by reduced hair pigmentation with melanocytes containing large cytoplasmic vacuoles (22).

Resting Skin Tension Lines

The resting skin tension lines (RSTLs) are skin furrows formed when the skin is relaxed (23). They radiate circumferentially outside the melolabial folds; inside the

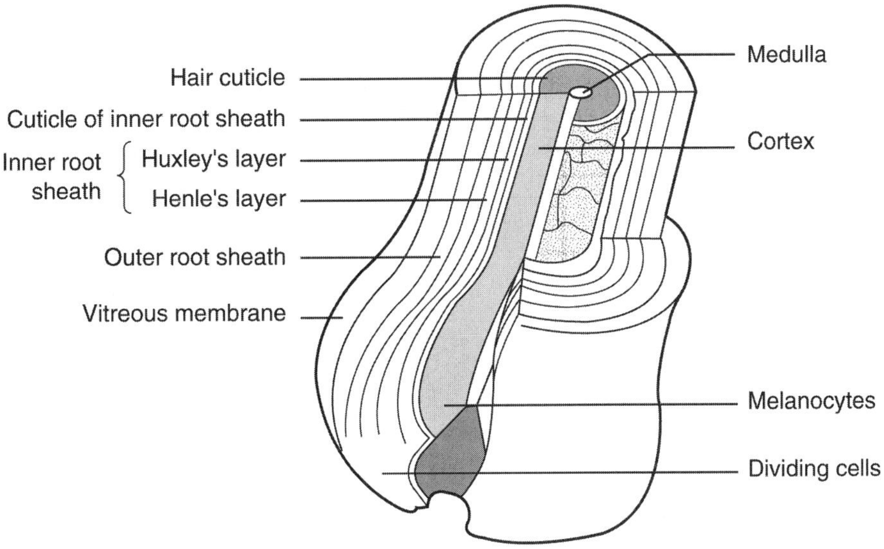

Figure 14 Microanatomy of a hair follicle.

melolabial folds, they are vertically oriented to the pogonion where the lines cross at right angles. The RSTLs should be differentiated from wrinkle lines and Langer's lines. Under the general heading "On the Anatomy and Physiology of the Skin," Langer published a series of four articles involving the study of the dynamic properties of incised skin (24). It was from this collection that the term Langer's lines originated. He attempted to explain the properties of skin elasticity and tension. He studied the skin's directional variations by incising circles and squares and observing the resulting deformation. Under a variety of circumstances (cadaveric skin at rest and cadaveric skin placed on tension from movement of an underlying joint), he recorded a series of cleavage lines (Langer's lines). The cleavage lines followed the long axis of the deformed circle and corresponded to the lines of tension. Incising along the cleavage line was considered desirable to minimize wound gaping and scar contracture.

> ...While the incision is being made parallel to the cleavage lines the knife cuts readily and the skin does not wrinkle and fold under the knife; this, however, occurs when making the cut at right angles to the cleavage lines even with the sharpest well-greased knife and the incision can only be made slowly and with continued pressure. (24–25).

Langer found that the "the skin of the face has less inbuilt tension than the skin of most other parts of the body." The facial cleavage (Langer's) lines correspond poorly to the lines of tension found in living tissue.

The RSTLs represent lines of skin tension in living tissue that are clinically useful in planning incisions that minimize wound separation and scar width. They are not easily visible but are found along the fine skin furrows that form when the skin is relaxed or gathered. The RSTLs are an inherent property of skin unrelated to muscular action. They are formed during embryological development and correspond to the direction of pull in relaxed skin determined by the static elements under the skin including bone, cartilage, and soft tissue bulk, and they are the same in all persons (26).

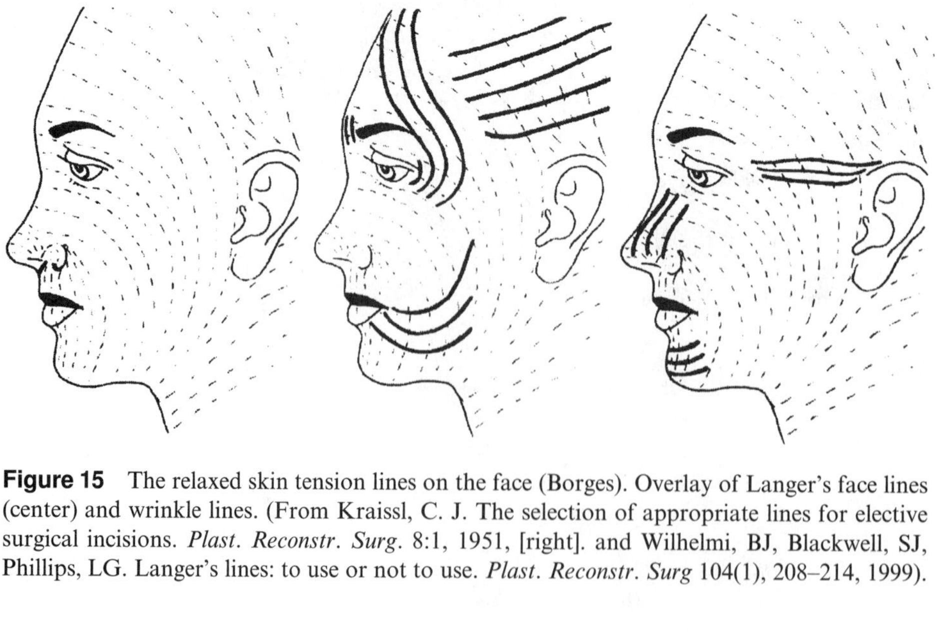

Figure 15 The relaxed skin tension lines on the face (Borges). Overlay of Langer's face lines (center) and wrinkle lines. (From Kraissl, C. J. The selection of appropriate lines for elective surgical incisions. *Plast. Reconstr. Surg*. 8:1, 1951, [right]. and Wilhelmi, BJ, Blackwell, SJ, Phillips, LG. Langer's lines: to use or not to use. *Plast. Reconstr. Surg* 104(1), 208–214, 1999).

Wrinkles may cross the RSTLs, especially in the glabellar region and chin. Over the glabella, wrinkles are vertical, yet the RSTLs are horizontal, and (over the chin) the melolabial sulcus is perpendicular to the RSTLs. Langer's lines represent the skin tension in rigor mortis and have only a loose correlation with the RSTLs (24–25). An incision or scar exactly on an RSTL is ideal, and within 30 degrees is acceptable (Fig. 15).

Facial Topographical Units

Replacing soft tissue defects of the face with identically sized flaps or grafts often produces an obviously patched area. Gonzalez-Ulloa et al. (27) realized that, in the face, there are definite regions in which skin differs in color, texture, mobility, and thickness. The boundaries of these regions represent natural transition zones where incisions and flap or graft borders can escape notice. Therefore, more satisfactory results can be obtained through regional restoration than with local repairs. Gonzalez-Ulloa et al. outlined the patterns of the shape of seven facial regions on cadavers as templates for flaps and grafts.

The borders of the regional facial units present favorable sites of scar placement, while incisions and scars through the borders tend to be unsightly. Reconstructing an entire unit allows the placement of incisions at the unit borders, and scar contracture and depressions become less noticeable. Even trapdoor scarring and bunching of the flap are less noticeable and may result in a net aesthetic improvement in areas that are naturally bulbous (e.g., the nasal alae). Millard's teachings include conforming reconstructive plans to the unit principle. If a large part of a unit is missing, then it is appropriate to extend the defect to include the entire unit and reconstruct it as a whole. Millard's seagull midline forehead flap represents the application of this principle to nasal reconstruction.

The nose, considered a single topographical (aesthetic) unit by Gonzalez-Ulloa et al., can be further divided into aesthetic subunits with borders that fall into natural visual rifts created by subtle shadows, concavities, and convexities (28). They include the dorsum, tip, alae, sidewalls, and soft triangles (Fig. 16). Although the subunits are not exactly the same nose to nose, the general shapes are consistent. The supratip depression divides the dorsum from the tip; this division may be somewhat variable depending upon ethnicity (29). The soft triangle represents a shadowy depression between the start of the cephalic bend on the caudal lower lateral cartilage and the nasal rim. Notching in this area is a problem after reconstructive surgery if the flap tissue extends to the vestibular skin. However, if one respects the superior margin of the soft triangle and sutures flap tissue to this border, the problems of notching give way to depressions in the soft triangle that provide good camouflage. Loss of greater than 50% of a subunit justifies its total replacement. However, removing normal structures to attain a more aesthetic result carries additional risk and requires a motivated and informed patient.

The facial regions (topographical units) and subunits do not necessarily correspond to the RSTLs. If incisions are within a topographical unit, attention to the RSTLs is important to maximize camouflage and to attain the thinnest scar possible by following the natural skin tension lines. An area of obvious disagreement between the unit concept and the RSTLs is around the chin. The RSTLs of the chin are vertical and perpendicular to the melolabial sulcus, while the chin unit follows the

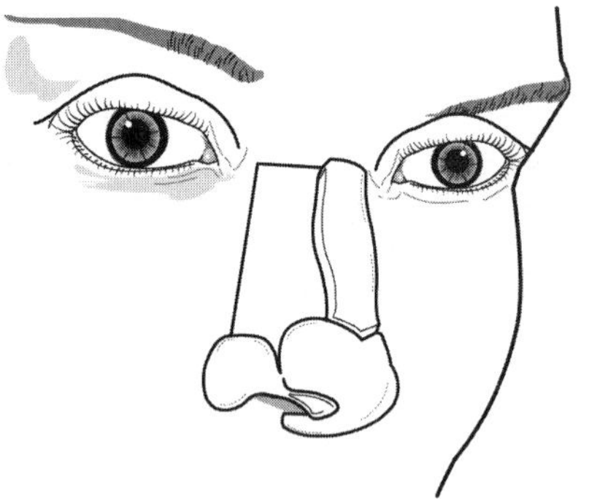

Figure 16 The topographical units of the nose.

melolabial sulcus extending circumferentially around the mentum. Another area of disagreement is along the nasal sidewalls where the RSTLs and the subunit borders are again perpendicular. In most cases, the unit principle will take precedence, especially along the nasal sidewall. Following the chin's unit border may result in a significant widened trapdoor scar and irregular bulging of the chin. However, vertical incisions are obvious due to scar depressions and contour irregularities. A possible solution applicable to similar dilemmas may be to follow the unit borders by placing incisions using techniques that allow the majority of the incision to be within 30 degrees of the RSTLs (e.g., W-plasty).

Skin Typing

Skin typing is helpful in predicting the response of different types of skin to chemical peeling or laser resurfacing. Grading the skin content of melanin is important to assess the risk of postinflammatory hyperpigmentation. The Fitzpatric classification (30) of skin types defines them as I: white skin; always burns (first summer exposure), never tans; II: white skin, usually burns; III: white skin, sometimes burns; IV: moderate brown skin, rarely burns; V: dark brown, very rarely burns; VI: black, never burns.

Skin types IV–VI are most susceptible to postinflammatory hyperpigmentation.

Intrinsic skin aging involves the following factors:

- Atrophy of the subdermal adipose tissue and dermis
- Fine wrinkling
- Irregularly shaped epidermal cells
- Loss of orderly progression of cells from basal cell layer to granular cell layer
- Pseudothinning of the epidermis: the epidermis is not actually thinner but appears so because of underlying dermal changes
- Increases in epidermal turnover rate (usually 2–4 weeks)

Exogenous factors (primarily actinic) involve the formation of coarse rhytids and inelastic skin due to pathological changes to the elastin in the papillary dermis, a process termed photoaging (31). Lymphohistiocytic perivenular infiltrates with many mast cells are a consequence of photodamage that is termed heliodermatitis (32).

In addition, there is a collagen fiber homogenization (with basophilia) and an accumulation of glycosaminoglycan and proteoglycan complexes within the dermis (33). The density of melanocytes is twofold higher in sun-exposed areas for patients of all ages. However, melanocyte density declines approximately 6–8% in the surviving population per decade in exposed and non-sun-exposed sites (22). Grading the skin for actinic damage and scarring is important in documenting and selecting suitable candidates for superficial-to-deep chemical peels. Glogau's classification (34) defines the groups as follows:

I. Mild: no keratoses, little wrinkling, no acne scarring, wears no makeup
II. Moderate: early keratoses, slight yellow skin discoloration, early rhytids, mild scarring, wears some makeup
III. Advanced: actinic keratoses, obvious yellowing with telangiectasia, rhytids, moderate scarring, always wears makeup
IV. Severe: actinic skin cancers, many rhytids, much cutis laxa, severe acne scarring, cakes on makeup

Groups I and II are the most appropriate candidates for superficial peels. Deeper peels are necessary with groups III and IV, and the expected result should be diminished in proportion to the severity of the preoperative changes in those and other groups.

REFERENCES

1. Chavez AE, Dagum P, Koch RJ, Newman JP. Legal issues of computer imaging in plastic surgery: a primer. Plast Reconstr Surg 1997; 100:1601–1608.
2. Ricketts RM. Divine proportion in facial esthetics. Clin Plast Surg 1982; 9:401–422.
3. Farkas LG, Hreczko TA, Kolar JC, Munro IR. Vertical and horizontal proportions of the face in young adult North American Caucasians: revision of neoclassical canons. Plast Reconstr Surg 1985; 75:328–338.
4. Farkas LG, Kolar JC. Anthropometrics and art in the aesthetics of women's faces. Clin Plast Surg 1987; 14:599–616.
5. Jeffries JM, DiBernardo B, Rauscher GE. Computer analysis of the African-American face. Ann Plast Surg 1995; 34:318–321.
6. Sheen JH. Aesthetic Rhinoplasty. St. Louis: C.V. Mosby Co., 1978.
7. Larrabee WF, Jr. Facial analysis for rhinoplasty. [Review] [25 refs]. Otolaryngol Clin North Am 1987; 20:653–674.
8. Webster RC, Davidson TM, Rubin FF, Smith RC. Nasal tip projection changes related to cheeks and lip. Arch Otolaryngol 1978; 104:16–21.
9. Crumley RL, Lanser M. Quantitative analysis of nasal tip projection. Laryngoscope 1988; 98:202–208.
10. Powell N, Humphries B. Proportions of the Aesthetic Face. New York: Thieme-Stratton, 1984.
11. Rosen HM. Aesthetic guidelines in genioplasty: the role of facial disproportion. Plast Reconstr Surg 1995; 95:463–469.
12. Gonzales-Ulloa M. Planning the integral correction of the human profile. J Int Coll Surg 1961; 36:364.
13. Rafaty FM, Brennan HG. Current concepts of browpexy. Arch Otolaryngol 1983; 109:152–154.
14. Legan HL, Burstone CJ. Soft tissue cephalometric analysis for orthognathic surgery. J Oral Surg 1980; 38:744–751.

15. Dedo DD. "How I do it"–plastic surgery. Practical suggestions on facial plastic surgery. A preoperative classification of the neck for cervicofacial rhytidectomy. Laryngoscope 1980; 90:1894–1896.
16. Wolfley D. Blepharoplasty. In: Krause CJ, Mangat DS, Pastorek N, eds. Aesthetic Facial Surgery, Philadelphia: J.B.Lippincott, 1991:571–599.
17. Klatsky SA, Manson PN. Thyroid disorders masquerading as aging changes. Ann Plast Surg 1992; 28:420–426.
18. Briggaman RA, Wheeler CE, Jr.. The epidermal-dermal junction. J Invest Dermatol 1975; 65:71–84.
19. Montagna W, Carlisle K. Structural changes in aging human skin. J Invest Dermatol 1979; 73:47–53.
20. Shuster S, Black MM, McVitie E. The influence of age and sex on skin thickness, skin collagen and density. Br J Dermatol 1975; 93:639–643.
21. Frances C, Robert L. Elastin and elastic fibers in normal and pathologic skin. [Review]. Int J Dermatol 1984; 23:166–179.
22. Gilchrest BA, Blog FB, Szabo G. Effects of aging and chronic sun exposure on melanocytes in human skin. J Invest Dermatol 1979; 73:141–143.
23. Borges AF, Alexander JE. Relaxed skin tension lines, Z-plasties on scars,and fusiform excision of lesions. Br J Plast Surg 1962; 15:242.
24. Langer K. On the anatomy and physiology of the skin. II. Skin tension Presented at the meeting of 27th November 1861. Br J Plast Surg 1978; 31:93–106.
25. Anonymous. On the anatomy and physiology of the skin. I. The cleavability of the cutis. (Translated from Langer, K. (1861). Zur Anatomie und Physiologie der Haut. I. Uber die Spaltbarkeit der Cutis. Sitzungsbericht der Mathematisch-naturwissenschaftlichen Classe der Kaiserlichen Academie der Wissenschaften, 44, 19.). Br J Plast Surg 1978; 31:3–8.
26. Borges AF. Preoperative planning for better incisional scars. In: Thomas JR, Holt GR, eds. Facial scars: Incision, revision, and camouflage, St. Louis: Mosby, 1989:41–56.
27. Gonzales-Ulloa M. Preliminary study of the total restoration of the facial skin. Plast Reconst Surg 1954; 13:151.
28. Burget GC, Menick FJ. The subunit principle in nasal reconstruction. Plast Reconst Surg 1985; 76:239–247.
29. Milgrim LM, Lawson W, Cohen AF. Anthropometric analysis of the female Latino nose. Revised aesthetic concepts and their surgical implications. Arch Otolaryngol Head Neck Surg 1996; 122:1079–1086.
30. Fitzpatrick TB. The validity and practicality of sun-reactive skin types I through VI. Arch Dermatol 1988; 124:869–871.
31. Gilchrest BA. Skin aging and photoaging: an overview. [Review]. J Am Acad Dermatol 1989; 21:610–613.
32. Lavker RM, Kligman AM. Chronic heliodermatitis: a morphologic evaluation of chronic actinic dermal damage with emphasis on the role of mast cells. J Invest Dermatol 1988; 90:325–330.
33. Uitto J, Fazio MJ, Olsen DR. Molecular mechanisms of cutaneous aging. Age-associated connective tissue alterations in the dermis. [Review]. J Am Acad Dermatol 1989; 21: 614–622.
34. Lawrence N, Coleman WP. Superficial Chemical Peeling. In: Coleman WP, Lawrence N, eds. Skin Resurfacing, Baltimore: Williams & Wilkins, 1998:45–56.

2
Anesthetic Issues in Facial Plastic Surgery

John H. Romanow and Guy J. Sciortino
Lahey Clinic Medical Center, Burlington, Massachusetts, U.S.A.

INTRODUCTION

Anesthesia for facial plastic surgery is a broad subject encompassing many issues including use of specific anesthetic drugs, preoperative assessment and preparation, perioperative care, and personnel and facility issues. Although there have been significant advances and changes in the practice of anesthesia over the last 20 years, perhaps the most significant of these is the steadily increasing proportion of ambulatory surgical cases. Approximately 70% of all operations performed in the United States are done as outpatient procedures. Consequently, the number of ambulatory surgery centers (ASC) has increased dramatically. In addition, primarily due to convenience and economic factors, office-based surgery has also increased dramatically. Office-based surgery is unique in that few state regulations exist and the quality of care varies widely among facilities. Nevertheless, this venue will continue to remain a popular choice and every practicing facial plastic surgeon should be familiar with the advantages and disadvantages of such a choice.

ANESTHETIC METHODS

After an appropriate preoperative assessment, the surgeon must consider the various options available with the goal of providing safe, comfortable anesthesia in a relaxed patient. The various options include local anesthesia, regional anesthesia, monitored anesthesia care (MAC), and general anesthesia. The choice depends on many factors including the nature of the procedure, overall health of the patient, the patient's wishes, and the availability of an appropriate facility and equipment. Many minor facial plastic surgery procedures can be performed with local infiltrative anesthesia alone with or without an oral anxiolytic (benzodiazapam). The majority of facial plastic surgery procedures including otoplasty, rhytidectomy, liposuction, and rhinoplasty are routinely performed under MAC. MAC anesthesia is a specific form of anesthesia in which local or regional infiltrative anesthesia is given in conjunction with titrated intravenous anesthetic agents under the guidance of an anesthesiologist. Patients receiving MAC anesthesia have fewer anesthetic-related problems postoperatively (such as disorientation, nausea, and vomiting) than patients receiving general anesthesia.

SETTINGS FOR PLASTIC SURGERY

Once the method of anesthesia is chosen it must be delivered in the appropriate setting. Patients undergoing facial plastic surgery rarely require an overnight stay. Most procedures are performed in an accredited ambulatory care center or in an office-based facility. Only low-risk surgical procedures should be performed in an office setting. Categorization of surgical procedures based on their complexity and requirements for anesthesia is one method to stratify risk. The Board of Medicine classifies surgeries as level I, II, and III. Level I surgery is considered minor and is performed using topical or local infiltrative anesthesia with or without a mild tranquilizer. Level II surgery may involve a minor or relatively superficial procedure that is performed with intravenous consciousness-altering medication. Monitoring of vital signs is required and supplemental oxygen is often needed. Level III surgery entails a moderate-to-complex surgical procedure usually performed under general anesthesia. Of course, all level III surgeries should be performed at an accredited ASC or hospital. Level I surgery can be safely performed in an office setting. The appropriate venue for level II surgeries is the subject of controversy. In the 1990s, several procedure-related deaths in office-based facilities in Florida resulted in a moratorium on all level II and III office-based surgeries. Shortly after this, the American Society of Anesthesiologists published position statements and guidelines for "Nonoperating Room Anesthetizing Locations (1994)" and "Office-Based Anesthesia (1999)." Nevertheless, states have been slow to adopt uniform standards. In 2002, the American Society of Plastics Surgeons convened a task force to look into patient safety in office-based surgery facilities. A variety of criteria were developed to assist the surgeon in determining whether patient or procedure-related risks justified performing the procedure in an ASC or hospital setting (1). There is clearly a need for states to step forward and provide guidelines in this area. For now, only level I surgeries should be performed in an unaccredited office-based facility.

Four organizations accredit ambulatory surgery centers including office-based facilities: Medicare, The Joint Commission on Accreditation of Healthcare Organizations (JCAHO), the Accreditation Association for Ambulatory Health Care (AAAHC), and the American Association for Accreditation of Ambulatory Surgical Facilities (AAAASF). Accreditation by Medicare and JCAHO is most important. Each organization has unique criteria for granting accreditation, but they share a set of basic concerns including:

- Staff credentials
- Types of surgical cases
- Administration
- Staff competency
- Ancillary services
- Emergency contingency plans
- Information management including clinical records, policies, and procedures

- Quality improvement
- Space and equipment

In general, a physician should not perform a surgical procedure in an office-based facility that he or she is not credentialed to perform in their affiliated hospital. There should be adequate administration for basic upkeep of the facility, overview, restocking, and equipment management. Sufficient ancillary services should exist including respiratory therapy and phlebotomy. An office-based facility must be in close proximity to a hospital should an emergency transfer be required. All physician and nursing staff should have at least basic knowledge in life support and at least one staff member should have training in advanced life support measures. A "code cart" should be available and stocked with emergency medications and airway equipment. Accurate medical and anesthesia records are needed. The facility/operating room must be of sufficient size to accommodate needed equipment and supplies. There must be a reliable wall oxygen source in addition to canisters and adequate wall suction. Clean and dirty utility areas should be designated.

LOCAL AGENTS

Local anesthetics are pharmacological agents (Table 1) that cause temporary loss of sensation by inhibiting conduction along nerve fibers. Local anesthetics work at the nerve cell membrane by blocking sodium channels, resulting in inhibition of the development and propagation of an action potential. All local anesthetics are made water-soluble by being placed in an acidic solution. After injection, the physiologic pH of body tissues causes protonization of the ammonia structure and affects the drug's ability to cross the cell wall. The number of anesthetic molecules delivered to the nerve determines both the onset and the intensity of the block. The duration of the block is inversely dependent on the rate of disappearance of local anesthetic molecules from the nerve. Systemic toxicity is more likely after inadvertent intravascular injection. Factors that decrease the vascular uptake of local anesthetics will

Table 1 Pharmacological Properties of Commonly used Local Anesthetics

Class	Agent	Onset	Duration (min)	Maximum single dose for Infiltration (adults; mg)
Amide	Lidocaine	Fast	90–200	300
	Mepivicaine	Fast	120–240	300
	Bupivicaine	Moderate	180–600	175
	Etidocaine	Fast	180–600	300
	Prilocaine	Fast	120–240	400
Esters	Procaine	Slow	60–90	500
	Chlorprocaine	Fast	30–60	600
	Tetracaine	Slow	60–180	20
	Cocaine (topical)	Fast	30–60	200

Source: From Ehlert, T.K. Arnold, D.E., Local anethesia for soft tissue surgery. *Otolaryngol Clin North Am* 1990; 23(5): 835.

increase the duration of the block as well as protect against toxic overdosage through diffusion. The addition of a vasoconstrictor (usually epinephrine) to the injected solution will increase the duration of the block by one-half and increases the safe total dose by about one-third. Inflamed or infected tissue is acidic and impairs the ability of the local anesthetic to cross the cell wall and become active. The effectiveness of the local anesthetic is further diminished by the increased vascularity of an inflammatory process, which may also increase the risk for systemic toxicity due to enhanced diffusion and absorption.

Local anesthetics are classified into two groups based on their structure: amino amides and amino esters. Compounds containing the amide linkage are metabolized in the liver. Most of the ester compounds are metabolized at the site of injection or in the bloodstream by the plasma esterases. Lidocaine, mepivacaine, bupivacaine, dibucaine, and prilocaine are examples of amino amides. Cocaine, procaine (the first derivative of cocaine developed in 1898), and benzocaine are examples of amino esters. As a memory aid, note that the am*i*no esters all have one letter "i" (e.g., proca*i*ne) while the am*i*no am*i*des have two "i's" (e.g., l*i*docai*i*ne). The amino esters were developed first but only cocaine and benzocaine are in common use today, and usually only topically. Procaine (Novocain) was commonly used in dentistry but it is highly allergenic and has a short duration of action. Allergy to amino amide compounds is rare and many have favorable characteristics for infiltrative anesthesia.

Lidocaine is an anesthetic with vasodilator properties (relaxes smooth muscle). The maximum recommended dosage is 3–4 mg/kg when used alone or 6–8 mg/kg when used with a vasoconstrictor (epinephrine). Unlike other local anesthetics, it has the unique property of stabilizing the heart at moderate dosage. Because of its stability, predictability, and high therapeutic index, lidocaine is the most frequently used local anesthetic.

Mepivacaine is similar to lidocaine but lacks its vasodilator and antiarrhythmic effects.

Bupivacaine's initial anesthetic effect is slightly delayed compared to lidocaine; however, its duration of activity is significantly longer. Bupivacaine has been noted to have a greater potential for central nervous system and cardiovascular toxicity (ventricular fibrillation, asystole).

Prilocaine is also similar to lidocaine except that it does not have a vasodilator effect. It has a significantly decreased potential for systemic toxicity due to its rapid rate of clearance. The major deterrent to more widespread use is its metabolism to orthotoluidine: an oxidizing agent capable of converting hemoglobin to methemoglobin.

There are many techniques for administering local anesthetics. Buffering the anesthetic with bicarbonate has been advocated to reduce the discomfort of injection (2). This must be done immediately before injection because the local anesthetic is less soluble in a neutral solution. Frequently aspirating the syringe to confirm that the needle is in the extravascular compartment reduces the risk of a systemic complication since inadvertent intravascular injection is the most common cause of systemic toxicity. A tumescent technique for local anesthesia is a relatively new means of achieving a local block with tissue tumescence over a large surface area (3). This has been especially useful for liposuction. The tumescent technique involves instilling a large volume of dilute lidocaine and epinephrine into the subcutaneous tissues. A tumescent anesthetic may contain a 5–20-fold dilution of the standard commercially available 1% lidocaine with 1:100,000 epinephrine. The subcutaneous infiltration causes the targeted tissue to become swollen, firm, and profoundly vasoconstricted, which may reduce the incidence of systemic toxicity while allowing the surgeon to work in an extended area with little blood loss.

Topicals

Cocaine is an ester and a vasoconstrictor. It is used for topical anesthesia only with a recommended maximal safe dosage of 3 mg/kg. It should be noted that an absolute toxic dose of cocaine has not been determined. Cocaine blocks the uptake of epinephrine and norepinephrine from tissues, causing a relative excess of catecholamines locally. It is most useful for topical anesthesia and vasoconstriction on the mucous membranes of the nose.

Benzocaine used topically is useful for skin and mucous membrane anesthesia. It is most commonly used for pharyngeal anesthesia prior to endoscopic procedures. Its principle advantage is its relatively long duration of action (greater than lidocaine, mepivacaine, and tetracaine). Benzocaine is administered commonly as a spray (Hurricane, Beutlich LP Pharmaceuticals, Waukegan, IL) and each 1 spray delivers approximately 60 mg. The estimated toxic dose is over 200 mg but one of the most common dreaded complications of this medication (methemoglobinemia) occurs with doses well within the putatively safe dosage range. Therefore, the recommended initial dose of benzocaine spray is 30 mg or 0.5 s spray.

A new topical anesthetic consists of a eutectic mixture of local anesthetics (EMLA, AstraZeneca) consisting of a water in oil emulsion of lidocaine and prilocaine (lidocaine 2.5% and prilocaine 2.5% cream). The cream formulation is applied to the skin under an occlusive bandage, but requires at least 45 min to achieve anesthesia. It is most commonly used in pediatric patients, although recent literature is exploring expanding its indications in cosmetic surgery (4).

Although not an anesthetic, phenylephrine hydrochloride (Neosynephrine) deserves mention for its systemic effects and interaction with beta-blockers. Neosynephrine drops are commonly used to control bleeding and decongest nasal tissues. Occasionally, it will cause significant increases in blood pressure and administration of a beta-blocker may be given to counteract this effect. This is a potentially dangerous combination because decreased cardiac output, pulmonary edema, and death may result due to the unopposed alpha-adrenergic effect of the phenylephrine, especially in children (5). If a beta-blocker is inadvertently used, glucagon has been shown to counteract the loss of cardiac contractility. Calcium channel blockers have also been associated with this effect when combined with phenylephrine. The initial dose of phenylephrine solution should be limited to 0.5 mg (4 drops of a 25% solution). If elevation of blood pressure occurs with phenylephrine, then avoiding further application and allowing more time is usually all that is needed. Oxymetazoline (Afrin) has not been associated with this side effect.

Complications

Adverse reactions to local anesthesia include excitement, toxic overdose, and allergic reaction. The excitement reaction is characterized by a nervous, jittery feeling by the

Table 2 Signs of Lidocaine Toxicity

	Central nervous system (CNS)	Cardiovascular system
Early:	Headache Anxiety Restlessness Light-headedness Tinnitus Circumoral paresthesia Cutaneous flush	Hypertension and tachycardia secondary to CNS stimulation (more often due to epinephrine excess)
Intermediate:	Confusion Hyperexcitabiilty Blurred vision Slurred speech Nausea and vomiting Twitching and tremor Nystagmus Lethargy Convulsions	Myocardial depression Mild hypotension Diminished cardiac output
Late:	Respiratory arrest Coma	Severe hypotension Profound peripheral vasodilation Bradycardia Conduction defects Dyshrythmias Circulatory collapse

Source: From Ref. 2.

patient subsequent to being injected with a solution containing epinephrine. A transient tachycardia and hypertension may be observed. These episodes are usually self-limited and resolve spontaneously. If the symptoms are severe or persistent, treatment with alpha-or beta-blocking drugs may be necessary. However, concomitant use of cocaine and a beta-blocker has been associated with decreased coronary artery blood flow and angina. Toxic overdose is usually avoidable if the dosing is kept within the guidelines for body weight and intravenous injection is avoided. Table 2 reviews the early, intermediate, and late signs of systemic lidocaine toxicity. Diazepam has been shown to protect against seizure activity from local anesthetics. In the late stages of toxic overdose, full cardiorespiratory support may be required until the effects of the anesthesia have subsided.

True allergic reactions are uncommon and ester local anesthetics are primarily responsible. The offending allergen is usually para-amino benzoic acid (PABA), a breakdown product after enzymatic degradation of the local anesthetic in plasma. In rare cases, amides may elicit an allergic reaction. Methylparaben, another derivative of PABA, is used as a preservative in multidose vials of amide local anesthetics and may provoke an allergic response. The allergic response may range from urticaria to anaphylaxis.

Methemoglobinemia is an interesting adverse effect of some local anesthetics including benzocaine, lidocaine, and prilocaine that occurs even when these medications are used within their typical therapeutic doses (6). Benzocaine is the most common offending agent among the three (7). Other medications and toxic chemicals cause methemoglobinemia including nitroglycerin, sulfonamides, chloroquine, and dapsone. Concomitant administration of these drugs with the offending local anesthetic may predispose the patient to methemoglobinemia. Hemoglobin normally contains iron in the ferrous form (Fe^{2+}). Oxidation results in transformation of the ferrous iron into ferric iron (Fe^{3+}). Offending drugs and chemicals result in the oxidation of Fe^{2+} and creation of methemoglobin. Methemoglobin cannot bind oxygen and results in reduced oxygen-carrying capacity of blood. A certain degree of methemoglobinemia is well tolerated, especially in healthy young adults. Ten percent methemoglobinemia results in cyanosis but no clinically significant symptoms. Greater than 30% methemoglobinemia will usually produce symptoms of air hunger and reduced consciousness. Cardiopulmonary complications are more common in infants and the elderly, especially those with pre-existing cardiopulmonary disease (8).

The diagnosis of methemoglobinemia is based on clinical signs of hypoxemia and oximetry. Despite significant methemoglobinemia, the partial oxygen tension (PO_2) remains close to normal but the oxygen-carrying capacity of the blood is radically reduced. Standard pulse oximetry may be only slightly abnormal despite obvious signs of profound organ ischemia. A typical pulse oximeter measures the relative absorbance of two wavelengths corresponding to oxy and deoxyhemoglobin. Methemoglobin also absorbs light at these wavelengths so even in the presence of overwhelming methemoglobinemia the pulse oximeter may only show mildly abnormal values (80s).

Co-oximetry should be requested and will give accurate readings regarding the concentration of methemoglobin in the blood. It is a spectrophotometer capable of measuring the unique absorbance of methemoglobin. The mainstay of treatment for methemoglobinemia is intravenous methylene blue (1–2 mg/kg). This drug potentiates NADPH reductase, providing an alternative pathway for reduction of methemoglobin. Other therapies include hyperbaric oxygen and exchange transfusion (8).

REGIONAL BLOCKS

Regional anesthesia is defined here as direct injection into or around the nerves supplying a specific anatomical or surgical site. Regional anesthesia in the head and neck follows many of the principles discussed in the previous sections. A full preoperative evaluation should be completed. In a cooperative patient, regional anesthesia with or without supplemental sedation and analgesia will often provide excellent anesthesia. The procedure needs to be relatively short, because although the duration of the block may be fairly long, it is often difficult for even a sedated patient to remain cooperative and comfortable for an extended length of time. Depending on the extent and site of surgery, restriction of oral intake prior to the procedure is recommended according to the guidelines for MAC and general anesthesia. Deeper sedation or even general anesthesia may be required if the regional block and light sedation are inadequate.

The local anesthetics used in regional anesthesia have already been discussed. Care should be taken not to exceed the recommended dosages. Large volumes of

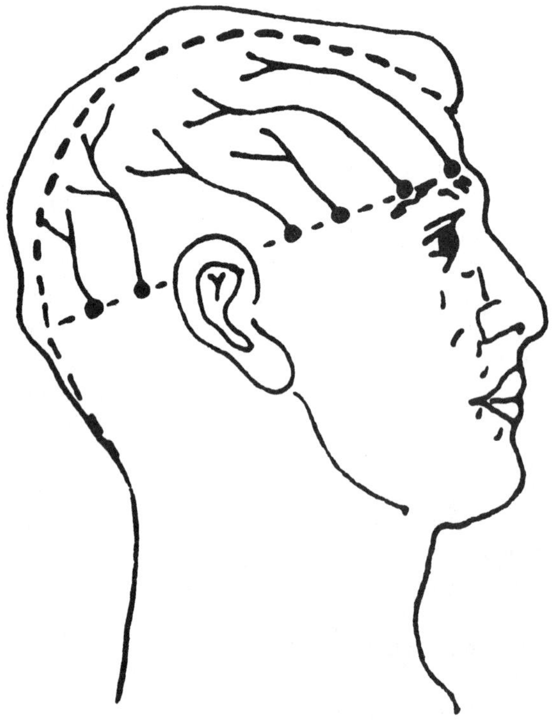

Figure 1 Distribution of sensory nerves of the scalp as they become subfascial. (From Ref. 9.)

the injection may occasionally be required for the institution of large field blocks and it may be necessary to dilute the concentration of the anesthetic. In a field block, it may be necessary to supplement the anesthetic with epinephrine to achieve an adequate duration of anesthesia and hemostasis.

The general complications of local anesthesia have been described and only complications limited to the specific technique will be discussed here. Many of these blocks can be achieved by a variety of techniques. The most common methods of achieving the blocks will be discussed according to site.

Scalp

The primary sensory innervation of the scalp is by the cervical nerves and the trigeminal nerve. The supraorbital, supratrochlear, and zygomaticotemporal nerves supply the forehead and occiput. The temporomandibular and the auriculotemporal branches of the trigeminal nerve innervate the temporal regions. The greater and lesser occipital nerves, which are distal branches of the cervical nerves, innervate the occipital and parietal regions. These nerves originate deep and enter a subfascial plane on a line encircling the head that passes above the ear and through the occiput and glabella (Fig. 1). The regional block is accomplished by subcutaneous injection of a large volume of (usually) diluted lidocaine with epinephrine. This infiltration will anesthetize the skin, fascia, and pericranium. Anesthesia is obtained in a skull cap distribution (Fig. 2).

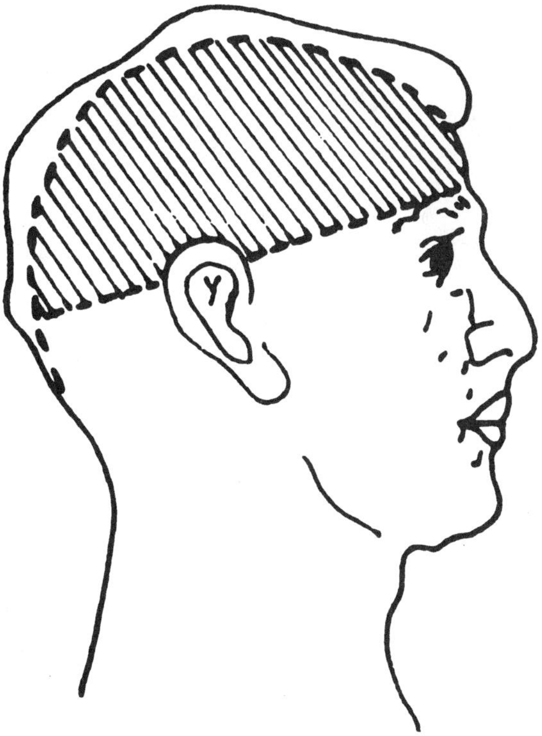

Figure 2 Region of anesthesia in a regional scalp block. (From Ref. 9.)

Forehead

The face and anterior scalp are innervated by the trigeminal nerve. Cervical nerves innervate posterior portions of the scalp as well as the neck and lower portions of the jaw. Operations on the forehead and scalp are possible using blocks of the supratrochlear and supraorbital nerves. These nerves are located in the supraorbital ridge/foramen of the frontal bone (Fig. 3). One to two milliliters of local anesthesia is injected in the region. It is sometimes difficult to locate the supraorbital foramen but it is helpful to note that the supraorbital, infraorbital, and mental foramina all lie in a straight line approximately 2.5 cm from the midline of the face. In neutral gaze, the pupils will also lie in this line. When large or midline lesions are to be excised, a bilateral block may be performed.

Possible complications include unusual swelling and ecchymoses around the orbit. This is usually secondary to either a large volume of anesthesia being injected or hemorrhage from the supraorbital vessels. It is usually self-limited and requires no specific treatment.

Infraorbital Nerve

An infraorbital nerve block can facilitate operations upon the lower eyelid, lateral aspect of the nose, the mucous membranes around the upper incisors, and the cuspid

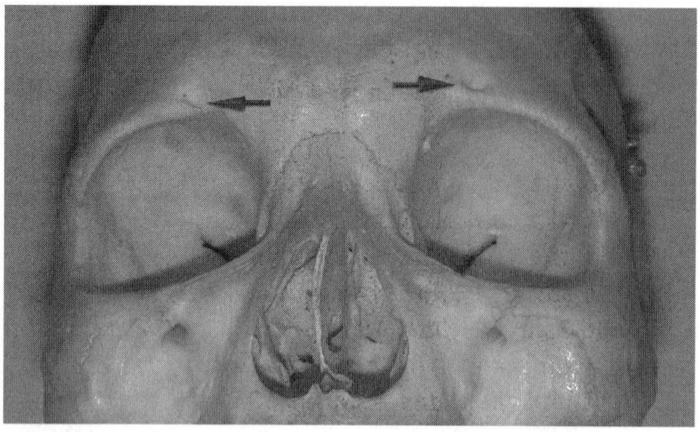

Figure 3 Location of supraorbital notch/foramen.

teeth. The infraorbital nerve emerges from the infraorbital foramen and divides into the inferior palpebral nerve, the external nasal nerve, the internal nasal nerve, and the superior labial nerve. The infraorbital nerve lies 2.5 cm from the midline of the face in the frontal process of the maxillary bone (Fig. 4). It is usually numbed with the injection of 2.5 ml of 1% lidocaine. This can be accomplished via either a sublabial injection or direct percutaneous injection. Care should be taken not to inject in the orbital cavity because hemorrhage may occur. Bilateral blocks may be required for lesions near the midline.

Mentum/Lip

The lower lip and mandible between the mental foramen and the midline, as well as the central incisor teeth, can be anesthetized by a mental nerve block. The nerve is the terminal branch of the inferior alveolar nerve. The position of the mental nerve is important to this block and varies with the age of the patient (9). In a young child, the foramen lies close to the inferior border of the mandible. In the adult, the foramen lies midway in the mandible. In an elderly patient, there is usually some atrophy of the mandible, and the foramen lies near the upper margin (Fig. 5). Usually, 1 ml of 1% lidocaine is injected at the root of the second bicuspid through an intraoral

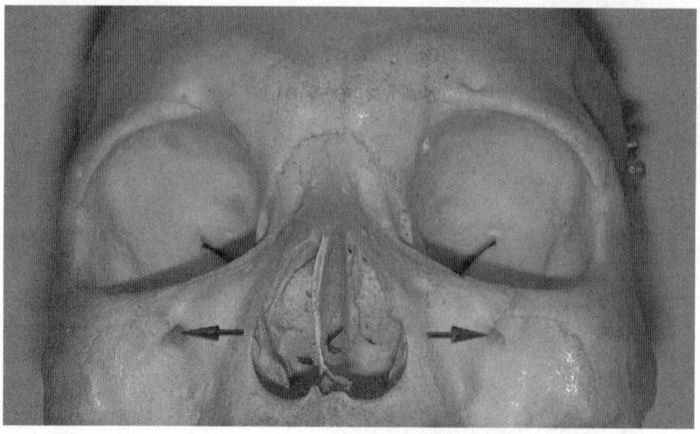

Figure 4 Location of infraorbital foramen.

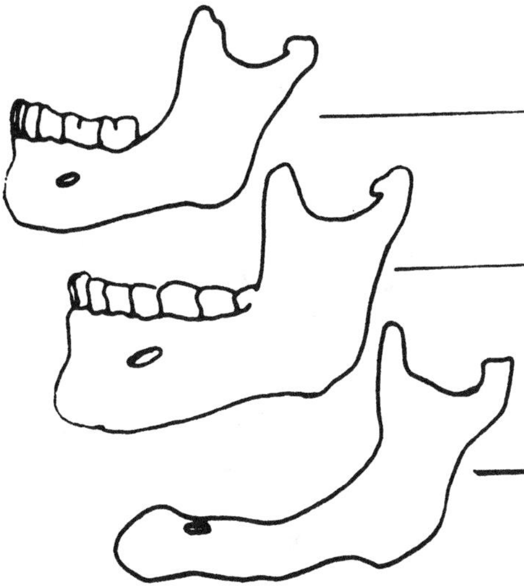

Figure 5 Location of Mental Nerve, based on age. (From Ref. 9.)

injection. As mentioned, if difficulty is encountered in locating the foramen, remember that it is in line with the supraorbital and infraorbital foramina. It is important to aspirate periodically prior to injection of the anesthetic since both intravenous and intra-arterial injections are more likely in this region.

Mandibular Nerve

The mandibular nerve is the third branch of the trigeminal nerve and contains both sensory and motor fibers. After exiting the foramen ovale it divides into anterior (primarily motor; only buccal branch is sensory) and posterior (primarily sensory) divisions. The largest constituent of the posterior division is the inferior alveolar nerve. A successful mandibular nerve block will anesthetize the inferior alveolar nerve, the mental nerve, and frequently the lingual nerve. This causes anesthesia in the mandibular teeth to the midline, the mucous membranes, and anterior two-thirds of the tongue. In addition to anesthesia, this block may be helpful in relaxing spasm of the masseter muscle and relieving trismus.

The mandibular nerve is most easily approached in the infratemporal fossa posterior to the pterygoid plate and between the pterygoid muscles. The needle is placed intraorally, beginning just lateral to the pterygomandibular raphe. The needle is advanced between the ramus and the muscles covering the internal surface of the mandible (Fig. 6). One to 2 ml of a 1% lidocaine solution is injected after a negative aspiration. Complications are rare, but hematoma at the injection site is seen and will usually resolve spontaneously.

Maxillary Nerve

Blocking the maxillary nerve produces profound anesthesia in the hemimaxilla, cheek, and upper jaw. The maxillary nerve is the second division of the trigeminal

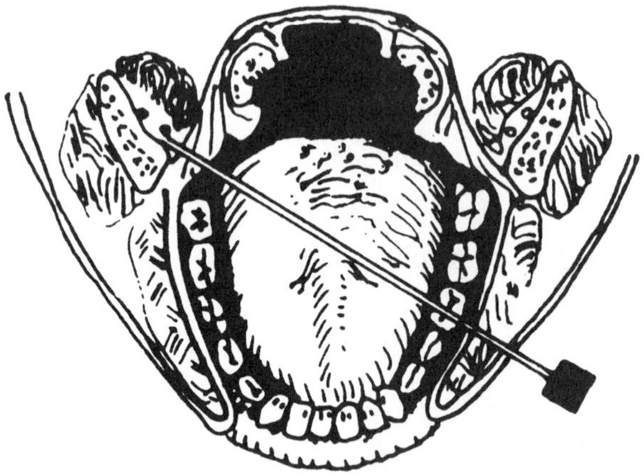

Figure 6 Intraoral block of the branches of the mandibular nerve. (From Ref. 9.)

nerve and exits through the foramen rotundum. It crosses the pterygopalatine fossa and subsequently becomes the infraorbital nerve. The nerve can be approached by a lateral or anterior approach.

The lateral approach requires palpation of the sigmoid notch on the zygoma. With the patient's jaw relaxed, a long needle is inserted inferior to the sigmoid notch and directed anteriorly until the lateral pterygoid plate is felt. The needle is then withdrawn and reintroduced in a more anterior and superior direction, anterior to the pterygoid plate and into the sphenomaxillary fossa (Fig. 7). Parasthesias will usually be encountered and 2 to 3 ml of 1% lidocaine are injected.

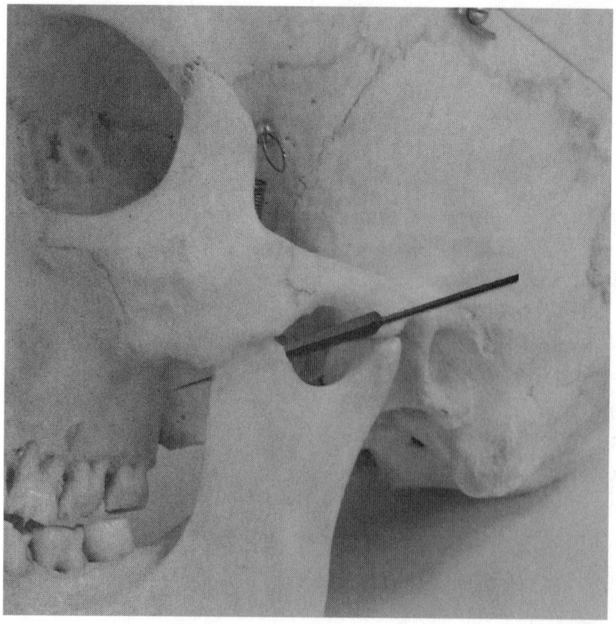

Figure 7 Lateral approach to the maxillary nerve block.

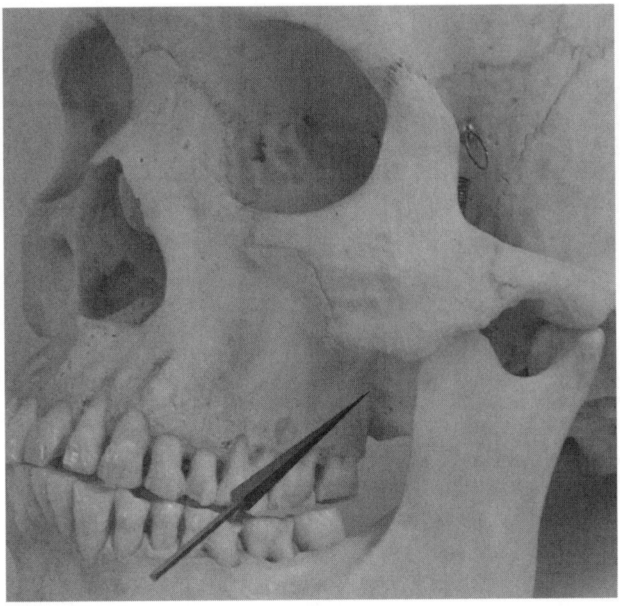

Figure 8 Anterior approach to the maxillary nerve block.

The anterior approach requires locating the anterior border of the coronoid process and the inferior margin of the zygoma. A long needle is inserted perpendicular to the skin until the maxilla is felt. The needle is then withdrawn and directed superior and posterior to enter the sphenomaxillary fossa (Fig. 8). There are no specific complications of this technique. If air is encountered during aspiration, it usually means that the pharyngeal space has been entered and the needle must be repositioned.

Nose

Sensory innervation of the nose is derived principally from the infratrochlear, infraorbital, nasopalatine, and external nasal nerves. Branches of the anterior ethmoidal and sphenopalatine ganglion supply the anterior aspect of the nose. Intranasal blocks are usually obtained by placement of intranasal topical cocaine in the region of the middle meatus, sphenopalatine ganglion, and the dorsal root of the nose. An external block can be performed with the injection of local anesthetic in the manner of a rhinoplasty block, with care taken to anesthetize the infratrochlear, infraorbital, and external nasal nerves (Fig. 9). There are no specific complications of this technique, but care should be taken to use cocaine appropriately.

Ear

The auriculotemporal nerve, mastoid branch of the occipital nerve, and the occipital nerve provide the sensory innervation to the external ear (Fig. 10). These nerves are readily anesthetized using a circular field block technique. There are no unique complications of this technique.

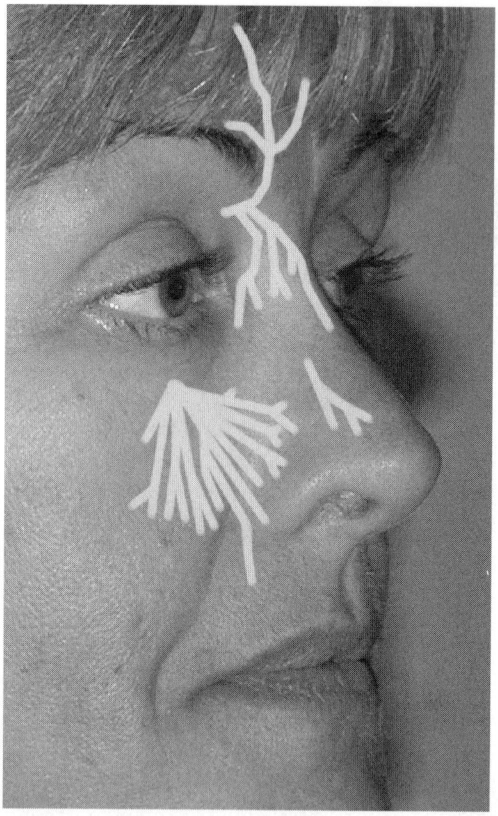

Figure 9 Sensory innervation of the nose: infratrochlear nerve, external nasal nerve, and infraorbital nerve.

GENERAL ANESTHESIA

Preoperative Considerations

Health Assessment

The American Society of Anesthesiology (ASA) uses a classification system to help assess a patient's risk for general anesthesia. This system considers a patient's overall health, activity level, and disease status to help determine the likelihood of morbidity or death from general anesthesia. The ASA status is reported as grades I–V. An ASA I patient is in excellent health with no limitations on activity while an ASA V patient is moribund, incapacitated, and expected to die within the next 24 h (10). In practice, the ASA level is considered only a convenient method to report a patient's overall health status and is not very useful in determining whether a patient will have a poor outcome after a general anesthetic. Nevertheless, Wolters et al. found that ASA class IV and V patients were more likely to experience intraoperative and postoperative problems including greater intraoperative blood loss, longer intensive care unit stays, and higher mortality rates (11). An organ-specific classification is more likely to be useful in predicting morbidity strictly from administration of a general anesthetic.

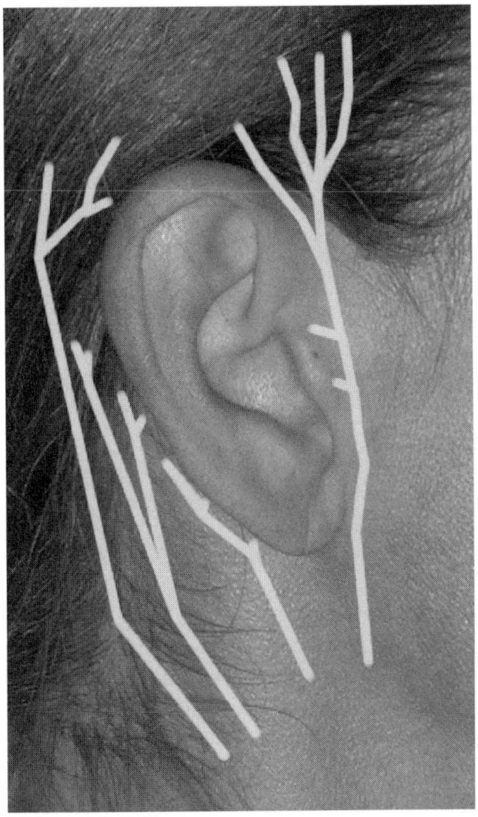

Figure 10 Sensory innervation of the external ear: occipital nerve, mastoid branch of the occipital nerve, greater auricular nerve, and auriculotemporal nerve.

Fasting Guidelines

Fasting is necessary before monitored anesthesia care (MAC) and general anesthesia to reduce the risk of pulmonary aspiration. Guidelines for fasting have changed over the last several years. Recently, a report from the ASA chaired by Dr. Mark Warner outlined the Society's specific recommendations for preoperative fasting:

- Clear liquids (water, fruit juices without pulp, carbonated beverages, clear tea, and black coffee [no cream]) may be taken up to 2 h before surgery in healthy, nontrauma patients
- Light meals and milk products may be ingested up to 6 h before surgery
- A period of no less than 8 h should elapse between the ingestion of fried or fatty foods and surgery

Premedication

Premedication is the use of sedatives, hypnotics, narcotics, or belladonna alkaloids to make the patient drowsy, cooperative, and comfortable perioperatively. Premedication can be used to provide a comfortable preoperative environment and smooth out the operative anesthetic technique. Certainly, many of these drugs have side

Table 3 Types of Premedication

Class	Drug	Dose (mg)	Route of delivery
Barbiturates	Secobarbital	50–150	PO, IM
	Pentobarbital	50–150	PO, IM
Narcotics	Morphine	5–15	IM
	Meperidine	50–100	IM
Tranquilizers or sedatives	Diazepam	5–10	PO
	Midazolam	1–4	IV, IM
	Droperidol	2.5–5	IM
	Hydroxyzine	50–150	IM
	Promethazine	25–50	IM
Anticholinergic	Atropine	0.3–0.6	IM
	Scopolamine	0.3–0.5	IM
	Glycopyrrolate	0.2–0.4	IM
Antacids	Cimetidine	300	PO, IM, IV

PO, orally; IM, intramuscularly, IV, intravenously
Source: From Pratt JM. Analgesics and sedation in plastic surgery. *Clin Plast Surg* 1985; 12(1): 74.

effects and care must be taken not to oversedate the patient. A disadvantage of some of the premedication agents is their long duration of action, which may prolong recovery. Midazolam and fentanyl are primarily used today; these medications have a relatively short duration and are unlikely to prolong recovery.

The appropriate drug used for any patient should be individualized based on the preoperative evaluation. On occasion, it may be inadvisable to use premedication.

Table 4 Classes of Premedication: Advantages and Disadvantages

Class	Advantage	Disadvantage
Barbiturates	Good sedation	No analgesia
	Minimal respiratory or circulatory collapse	Occasional disorientation
		Don't use with porphyria
Narcotics	Sedative and anxiolytic	Respiratory depression
	Analgesia	Orthostatic hypotension
	Reduce the amount of other anesthetics	Nausea and vomiting
		Smooth muscle contraction
	Readily reversible with naloxone	Occasional dystonic reaction
Tranquilizers, or Sedatives	Anxiolytic with minimal cardiorespiratory depression	Possible depressants
		Prolonged duration of action
	Droperidol: Anxiolytic and antiemetic	Dystonia, possible hypotension
		Don't use in Parkinson's disease
	Hydroxyzine: Sedative, antiemetic, and antihistamine	
Anticholinergic	Antisialogogues	
	Amnesia and sedation	
	Prevents reflex bradycardia	

Source: From Pratt JM., Analgesics and sedation in plastic surgery. *Clin Plast Surg* 1985; 12(1): 74.

Examples of this include some geriatric patients, patients with pulmonary disease, or patients who are very sensitive to medications. In general, premedications are classified as barbiturates, narcotics, tranquilizers and sedatives, and anticholinergics (Tables 3, 4). If a significant amount of insomnia and anxiety is expected the night before surgery, either a mild tranquilizer or sleep medication may be prescribed. On the day of surgery, a narcotic and a tranquilizer may be administered orally 2–4 h prior to surgery.

Airway Issues

The ability to obtain and maintain a reliable airway is a critical factor in the administration of both MAC and general anesthesia. Although MAC does not usually involve endolaryngeal or endotracheal intubation, due to the loss of pharyngeal tone, airway compromise is sometimes encountered and the anesthesiologist must be prepared to intubate the airway. It is sometimes difficult to determine whether intubation will be difficult and special measures or techniques are needed. The anesthesia record, if it is available, can be reviewed if the patient has had general anesthesia in the past. In addition, a history of pharyngeal or laryngeal masses or abnormalities should alert the anesthesiologist to a difficult airway. Although no preoperative assessment will identify a difficult airway with absolute certainty, the facial plastic surgeon should be aware of the Mallampati classification. The Mallampati classification is based on the fact that the base of the tongue is a key anatomical element with regard to ease of laryngeal visualization and intubation using an intubating laryngoscope (12). It is assessed by having the patient open his or her mouth maximally with tongue protrusion in the sitting position and is classified as follows:

- Class I: the soft palate, tonsillar pillars, and uvula are visualized.
- Class II: visualization of the uvula is obscured by the base of the tongue.
- Class III: only the upper soft palate is seen.
- Class IV: only the hard palate is seen.

If a difficult airway is found or expected, a variety of techniques can be used to obtain a safe airway. Of course, the preoperative evaluation is critical and fiberoptic visualization of the larynx may be needed for planning. Emergent or awake tracheotomy will be needed in some cases. Many newer techniques are now available to deal with the difficult airway that obviate the need for tracheotomy.

A light wand is a method of establishing an endotracheal airway without actually visualizing the larynx. It can be utilized effectively in patients with retrognathia and occasionally in cases of trauma. A laryngeal mask airway is a common method of providing general anesthesia without actually intubating the glottis. It can be used in either pediatric or adult patients. One advantage is that it does not enter either the glottis or the respiratory tract and may decrease the incidence of postoperative laryngeal edema or bronchoconstriction. It should be used with caution in patients with gastroesophageal reflux disease or significant bleeding in the oropharynx to avoid aspiration. A safe technique in a cooperative patient is an awake fiberoptic intubation. This provides the reassurance of obtaining an airway in an awake patient who has not had his or her respiratory drive diminished with medication. Adjunctive techniques such as retrograde intubation placed over a guidewire inserted through a percutaneous cricothyroid puncture are rarely necessary but may be lifesaving.

Aside from obtaining an airway, the apparatus must be placed in a manner that it will not interfere with the surgical field. Nasal intubation can be utilized to provide maximal exposure to the oral cavity. Taping and draping techniques should be used to minimize the interference of the airway apparatus with the surgical field. Depending on the proposed surgical method, there may be specialized instrumentation designed to maximize safety, especially when a laser is in use.

Monitored Anesthesia Care

The traditional technique for facial plastic surgery has been local anesthesia supplemented by sedation. This technique requires selection of appropriate sedative drugs administered in proper dosages to a cooperative patient according to the patient's needs. An anesthesiologist or nurse anesthetist titrates the sedative medications and is responsible for monitoring the patient. This will allow a separation of duties, with the surgeon and the anesthetist each concentrating on their area of expertise. Monitoring for local anesthesia with intravenous sedation is very similar to that used for general anesthesia. Patients undergoing surgery with MAC usually experience less postoperative nausea, vomiting, and disorientation than those undergoing general anesthesia. As the newer general anesthetic drugs improve, these differences may become less apparent. MAC may offer some cost savings to patients undergoing cosmetic surgery.

Sedation/analgesia is available in oral, intramuscular, intravenous, and inhalant forms. The latter consists of a dental-type nitrous oxide machine that may be used in a fail-safe mode (13). This has become popular as an aid to injecting local anesthesia or for such procedures as chemical/laser peeling, hair transplantation, and other dermatological surgeries. Each patient's response to sedation/analgesia is unique and techniques must be adapted to the type and length of the surgical procedure, the preoperative assessment, and the postoperative care arrangements. The drugs in Table 5 are commonly used for sedation and analgesia.

These medications are usually administered intermittently throughout the procedure to titrate the drug level to the level of consciousness and cooperation and, most importantly, to preserve the patient's ability to maintain a patent airway. An infusion pump may be used to provide a continuous infusion of drugs. Sedation is begun prior to the injection of local anesthetics. Since many of these drugs depress the respiratory drive, supplemental oxygen is usually used and the airway is carefully maintained. Once adequate local anesthesia has been obtained, the level of anesthesia is often lightened. Propofol is often used along with short-acting narcotics such as fentanyl and alfentanil.

General Anesthesia

As with MAC anesthesia, a full preoperative assessment is performed. A qualified anesthetist always administers general anesthesia. Extensive monitoring and intravenous access are required. The choice of general anesthetic agents depends on various factors evaluated in the preoperative assessment. There are two major classifications of general anesthetic agents: inhalational and intravenous. Many of the other agents discussed in previous sections can be utilized in an effort to produce what is termed a balanced technique. This allows adequate anesthesia to be obtained with

Table 5 Uses, Administration, and Properties of Common Sedatives

Generic drug (Trade name)	Uses	Dosage	Onset	Duration	Effects	Comments
Alfentanil (Alfenta)	Pain, sedation, anesthesia	Initially 130–240 μg/kg, then increments 3–5 μg/kg IV	Immediate	Incremental: 30 min; infusion 45 min	Narcotic	Chest wall rigidity, hypotension, bradycardia
Butorphanol (Stadol)	Pain, sedation	Dosage individualized; IV: 0.05–2.0 mg IM: 1.0–4.0 mg	IV: rapid IM:10–30 min	Variable	Analgesia, CNS depression, narcotic antagonism	May cause hypotension, nausea, vomiting, dizziness, respiratory symptoms; narcotic antagonist
Diazepam (Valium)	Anxiety, agitation, convulsions, sedation	IV 0.03–0.10 mg/kg	IV: rapid PO: 30–60 min	IV: 15 min to 3 h; active metabolites, 2–8 days	CNS depression, amnesia, increase in seizure threshold	May cause hypotension; idiosyncratic increase in anxiety, psychosis, mild respiratory depression; thrombophlebitis.Tissue irritant: IV, IM injections painful; frequent dosing may result in accumulation of active metabolites
Diphenhydramine (Benadryl)	Allergic reactions, drug-induced extrapyramidal reactions, sedation	IV/IM: 10–50 mg PO: 25–50 mg	IV: rapid PO	15–30 min	Antagonism of histamine action of H_1 receptors; anticholinergic effect on CNS	May cause hypotension (IV), tachycardia, dizziness, or seizures
Droperidol (Inapsine)	Nausea, vomiting, agitation, sedation, adjunct to neuroleptic anesthesia	IV: 0.625–10 mg	IV: 5–8 min	3–6 h.	Psychic indifference to environment, antipsychotic effect; antiemetic	May cause anxiety, extra pyramidal reactions; hypotension from moderate alpha-adrenergic and dopaminergic antagonism

Continued

Table 5 (Continued)

Generic drug (Trade name)	Uses	Dosage	Onset	Duration	Effects	Comments
Fentanyl (Sublimaze)	Pain, induction of general anesthesia	IV: 10–100 μg (in increments)	IV: 2 min IM: 7–15 min	Variable	Narcotic similar to morphine	Chest wall rigidity, accumulation with frequent dosing
Flurazepam (Dalmane)	Insomnia, sedation	PO: 15–30 mg	PO: 15–45 min	7–8 h	CNS depression	May cause idiosyncratic excitement, abnormal liver function, nausea, vomiting
Hydroxyzine (Vistaril, Atarax)	Anxiety, nausea, vomiting, allergies, sedation	IM/PO: 25–100 mg. *not approved for IV use*	PO: 15–20 min	PO: 4–6 h	Antagonism of histamine action on H_1 receptors, CNS depression, antiemetic	May cause dry mouth, minimal cardiorespiratory depression, IV injection may cause thrombosis, arterial injection may cause gangrene
Ketamine (Ketalar, Ketaject)	Induction of general anesthesia	IV LD: 1–3 mg/kg, MD 1/3–1/2 LD as necessary (usually every 5–30 min); IM LD: 5–10 mg/kg	IV: rapid IM: 3–5 min	IV: 5–10 min IM: 10–20 min	Somatic analgesia with poor visceral analgesia, block of cerebral association	Usually preserves and exaggerates airway reflexes; may cause transient, modest hypertension and tachycardia; regurgitation; salivation; lacrimation; diaphoresis; increase in intraocular pressure; bronchodilation; dreams and hallucinations
Meperidine (Demerol)	Pain, sedation	IV/IM: 0.5–1.0 mg/kg	IV: 5 min IM: 10 min	Variable	Similar to morphine, mild vagolytic effect	Similar to morphine, may cause tachycardia; mild negative inotropic effect; metabolic products can cause CNS excitement in high doses; avoid concurrent use of monoamine oxidase inhibitors

Methohexital (Brevital)	Induction of general anesthesia	IV: 1–2 mg/kg	Rapid	5 min	CNS depression	May cause hiccoughs, respiratory depression, mild cardiovascular depression, muscle tremors, pain along injection site
Midazolam (Versed)	Sedation, hypnotic adjunct to balanced anesthesia, induction of general anesthesia	IV: 0.07–0.08 mg/kg in 1–2 mg increments; IM: 0.07–0.08 mg/kg	IV: 1–3 min IM: 15–30 mg	IV: 2–6 h IM: 1–2 h	CNS depression, amnesia, increased seizure threshold	Water-soluble, predictable uptake. *Doses should be reduced by 25% in the elderly and when used in combination with narcotics*
Morphine	Pain, sedation	IV/IM: 0.1 mg/kg	IV: 5–10 min IM: 30–60 min	Variable	Analgesia, CNS depression, euphoria	May cause respiratory depression, bronchospasm, hypotension, nausea, vomiting, dysphoria, diaphoresis, allergic reactions, histamine release, increase in biliary pressure, decrease in gastrointestinal and genitourinary motility
Nalbuphine (Nubain)	Pain, sedation	IV/IM: 0.14 mg/kg; 10 mg similar to morphone 10 mg	IV: 2–3 min IM: 15 min	Variable	Similar to butorphanol	Similar to butorphanol
Naloxone (Narcan)	Reversal of narcotic effects	IV: 0.1–0.4 mg titrated to patient response	IV: 1–2 min	IV: 1 h	Antagonism of narcotic effects	May cause reversal of analgesia, hypertension, arrhythmias, pulmonary edema, delirium, or withdrawal syndrome (in addicts)
Pentobarbital (Nembutal)	Sedation	IV: 1 mg/kg slowly IM: 100–200 mg	IV: 1 min	IV: 15 min; half-life, 20–50 h	CNS depressant, anticonvulsant	May cause hypotension, hiccoughs, laryngospasm, or respiratory depression; may antagonize oral anticoagulants

Continued

Table 5 (Continued)

Generic drug (Trade name)	Uses	Dosage	Onset	Duration	Effects	Comments
Physostigmine (Antilirium)	Post operative delirium, tricyclic antidepressant overdose, reversal of CNS effects of anticholinergic	IV: 0.5–2 mg	IV: 3–8 min	30 min–5 h	Inhibition of cholinesterase	May cause bradycardia, tremor, hallucinations, CNS depression, mild ganglionic blockade, or cholinergic crises
Prochlorperazine (Compazine)	Nausea and vomiting	IV: 5–10 mg IM: 5–10 mg	IV: rapid IM: 10–20 min	3–4 h	Antiemetic effects	May cause hypotension, extrapyramidal reactions
Promethazine (Phenergan)	Nausea, vomiting, allergies, sedation	IV/IM: 12.5–50 mg	IV: 3–5 min IM: 20 min	IM: 4–6 h	Antagonism of histamine action on H_1 receptors, CNS depression, amnesia	May cause mild hypotension or mild anticholinergic effects; may interfere with blood grouping; intra-arterial injection can cause gangrene; relatively free of extrapyramidal effects

Propofol (Dipravan)	Anesthesia	IV: 0.1–0.2 mg/kg/min	Immediate	2–3–mn; IV bolus	Anesthetic induction	Anesthetic may cause hypotension in elderly, debilitated patients
Sufetanil (Sufenta)	Pain, induction of general anesthesia	IV: 0.2–0.8–μg/kg	< 1 min	Variable, half-life, 3 h	Similar to morphine, but with minimal cardiovascular depression	Dose-related muscle rigidity and bradycardia, respiratory rate depression
Thiopental (Pentothal)	Induction of general anesthesia	IV: 1–4 mg/kg	Rapid	10–15 min	CNS depression, decrease in cerebral blood flow	May cause hypotension (from myocardial depression and peripheral vasodilation), tachycardia, congestive heart failure, respiratory depression; intra-arterial injection can cause gangrene; exacerbates porphyria

Source: Mannino M.J. Uses, administration and properties of common sedatives. Clin Plast Surg 1991; 18(4): 870–872.
PO, orally; IV, intravenously; IM, intramuscularly.

the advantage of minimizing the complications of any one specific agent, thereby increasing overall safety.

Intravenous Agents

The intravenous agents include barbiturates, narcotics, benzodiazepines, and muscle relaxants.

Thiopental (4 mg/kg) is a short-acting barbiturate that can be used for speedy induction or maintenance of general anesthesia. Thiopental acts by suppressing short synaptic pathways in the central reticular formation of the brainstem. Although it has no analgesic properties, its effects range from mild sedation to profound coma. It decreases cardiac contractility as well as cardiac output. Pain and sloughing of tissue have been associated with improper injection. Thiopental should be avoided in patients with asthma or porphyrias.

Etomidate is a newer intravenous agent for the induction of general anesthesia. Induction with etomidate (0.3 mg/kg) is more rapid than thiopental. It is a respiratory depressant but has little or no effect on the circulatory system. There are few systemic side effects observed with etomidate.

Propofol is an intravenous sedative–hypnotic agent for use in the induction and the maintenance of anesthesia or sedation. Cardiorespiratory depression may occur at higher drug levels due to arterial hypotension without a change in heart rate. Propofol is suspended in a soybean oil emulsion and there is risk of bacterial contamination: care must be taken to use aseptic technique. There is often pain with intravenous injection but this may be diminished with the administration of intravenous lidocaine prior to injection. The induction dosage is 2.0–2.5 mg/kg in an adult and 2.5–3.5 mg/kg in a child. Anesthesia may be maintained on a continuous infusion basis or with so-called bumps. Propofol is contraindicated in pregnant or nursing women because it crosses the placenta and is found in breast milk. Propofol is contraindicated in patients allergic to soybean oil or eggs. Propofol has egg lecithin (found in egg yolk); most patients who are egg-allergic have more severe reactions to egg white.

The muscle relaxants succinylcholine, vecuronium, rocuronium, and pancuronium are used when paralysis is required. They may be used with either the induction or maintenance of anesthesia. Succinylcholine (0.6–1 mg/kg) is an ultra-short-acting depolarizing skeletal muscle relaxant for intravenous administration. It binds at the cholinergic receptor of the motor end plate to produce depolarization, resulting in flaccid motor paralysis less than 1 min after intravenous administration. Succinylcholine is contraindicated in patients at risk for malignant hyperthermia, patients with hyperkalemia, patients with skeletal muscle myopathies, and in patients who have sustained major injuries (e.g., trauma or burns). Prolonged neuromuscular blockade may be noted in patients with pseudocholinesterase deficiency. Vecuronium is a nondepolarizing neuromuscular blocking agent that acts by competing for cholinergic receptors at the motor end plate. The initial dosage is about 0.1 mg/kg, producing initial paralysis after about 1 min and lasting between 30 and 45 min. There are no clinically significant hemodynamic effects. Rocuronium is another nondepolarizing neuromuscular agent. It has an initial dosage of 0.6 mg/kg and will usually produce paralysis in 1–2 minutes lasting about 30 min. Pancuronium was one of the first nondepolarizing neuromuscular agents. It is used less frequently today due to its relatively long onset of action and duration.

Inhalational Agents

Inhalational anesthetics make up the other major class of general anesthetics. These agents are typically used for the maintenance of anesthesia rather than induction. Induction with an inhalational anesthetic is usually reserved for infants and children in whom intravenous access may be limited.

Nitrous oxide is a frequently administered anesthetic agent. It can be used as a single agent. At 60–75%, in conjunction with other agents, it provides adequate analgesia. It is a mild myocardial depressant and will diffuse into all air-containing cavities of the body, which may represent a major deterrent to its use in certain circumstances.

Halothane is one of the earliest halogenated hydrocarbon inhalational anesthetics. It is used less frequently today due to its slow uptake and emergence and there is an association with hepatic necrosis (1 : 35,000 cases). It is a potent bronchodilator and an excellent choice for patients with asthma. Inhalational induction with halothane is well tolerated in children due to its weak potency.

Enflurane was introduced into clinical practice in 1972. It is a stable anesthetic, but also a potent respiratory and cardiovascular depressant. Therefore, the patient's ventilation either needs to be assisted or controlled during its use. Use of this agent can be associated with a profound drop in blood pressure, especially with initiation. Its minimum anesthetic concentration is 1.7%. Fluoride ions are a major byproduct of the metabolism of enflurane (and sevoflurane) and may worsen renal function in patients with chronic renal disease. Enflurane should probably not be used in patients with chronic renal failure.

Isoflurane was introduced into clinical practice in 1981. It is a respiratory depressant, but seems to maintain cardiac output. A decrease in blood pressure associated with a drop in peripheral vascular resistance may be noted. Its minimum anesthetic concentration is about 1.2%. It has excellent muscle relaxant qualities. It has a very pungent odor that limits its use as an induction agent.

Desflurane is a volatile liquid inhalational anesthetic biotransformed in the liver. During desflurane anesthesia, systemic vascular resistance and mean arterial blood pressure decrease, while cardiac index, heart rate, and stroke volume increase. Its minimum anesthetic concentration is about 7.5%. It is not recommended for the induction of general anesthesia in the pediatric population because it has a high incidence of laryngospasm, coughing, breath holding, and excess salivation. Due to its physical properties, desflurane requires a heated vaporizer.

Sevoflurane is very similar to desflurane. It has a weak pungent odor and may be used successfully as an inhalational induction agent, especially in children. Its minimum anesthetic concentration varies between 1.5 and 3.0%, depending on age and whether nitrous oxide is used. Its cardiovascular effects are similar to desflurane, except the tachycardia is not observed.

Complications

There are a variety of complications from general anesthesia, ranging from clinically insignificant to cardiorespiratory arrest and death. It is not the intention of this chapter to discuss all of these. Probably the single most dreaded complication unique to general anesthesia is malignant hyperthermia, a hypermetabolic crisis that can be triggered by several anesthetic agents. It is invariably fatal if untreated. Male patients are affected more than female patients. The genetics favor an autosomal dominant transmission but penetrance is variable. Even with increased awareness, the present mortality rate is about 50% (9). It occurs most often with the administration of halothane and succinylcholine; however, it has been reported with other forms of general anesthesia. Diagnosis is imprecise but the clinical signs include high fever, tachycardia, cardiac arrhythmias, cyanosis, and rigidity. There occurs a severe metabolic acidosis and elevated levels of serum potassium, lactate, magnesium, and myoglobin. Dantrolene, a direct-acting skeletal muscle relaxant and the only known therapy, should be administered as soon as possible once the clinical signs are recognized (Table 6). This medication is given intravenously (IV) 1–10 mg/kg, then 4–8 mg/kg/day orally divided in four daily doses for 1–3 days. Dantrolene may also be used prophylactically in its oral form 1–2 days preoperatively. A qualified anesthesiologist appropriately manages patients recognized to be at risk preoperatively: succinylcholine and inhalation agents are avoided.

Pseudocholinesterase deficiency is an uncommon disorder that is most notable for prolonged paralysis after even a nominal dose of succinylcholine (14). In addition to succinylcholine, enzyme deficiency results in prolonged metabolism of several common anesthetic medications including cocaine, procaine, and mivacurium. The enzyme deficiency may be minor resulting in only slightly prolonged paralysis after administration of succinylcholine or major leading to paralysis lasting several hours after a single injection. Plasma cholinesterase activity must be reduced to 75% of normal before clinically significant effects are seen. The enzyme deficiency follows an autosomal recessive mode of inheritance and only about 1 : 25 people is heterozygous for a defective allele (of which there are multiple types producing enzymes of variable activity) (15). Even if a person is homozygous for defective alleles he or she is asymptomatic unless medications metabolized by the enzyme are given. In addition, depending on the severity of the defect, clinical manifestations vary widely. Enzyme deficiency is most common in peoples of European descent. Aside from genetic causes, chronic wasting disease and some medications are associated with mild pseudocholinesterase deficiency. The diagnosis of an enzyme deficiency is made by a plasma assay. The treatment for patients exhibiting prolonged paralysis is mechanical ventilatory support until the paralysis spontaneously resolves.

SPECIAL CONSIDERATIONS

Anesthesia for infants and children is a distinctively different entity. Children often metabolize drugs differently and have less reserve in terms of blood volume and ability to tolerate untoward events. Psychologically and socially, the pediatric patient and their families will have a great deal of apprehension concerning the upcoming surgical procedure and frequently they are most apprehensive about the anesthesia. Children must be dealt with in an appropriate age-specific manner, and the preoperative visit can do much to allay the patient's and family's concerns. Elective surgery should be postponed in a child with an upper respiratory infection because a more serious pulmonary infection may occur after general anesthesia. Premature infants requiring surgery within the first few months of life should be observed overnight. Infants less than 44 weeks of gestational age have a susceptibility to retrolental

Table 6 Treatment of Malignant Hyperthermia

1. Discontinue anesthetic agents.
2. Hyperventilate with 100% oxygen
3. Administer dantrolene (Dantrium), 1–2 mg/kg intravenously; repeat every 5–10 min to a total dosage of 10 mg/kg or until temperature starts to decrease.
4. Administer procainamide, 1 mg/kg/min intravenously for muscle hypertonus or arrhythmias. Total dosage not to exceed 7 mg/kg.
5. Cool the patient with alcohol baths, cold towels, cooling blankets, lavage of body cavities with cold crystalloid solutions. Stop when temperature reaches 38° C.
6. Correct metabolic acid/base abnormalities with sodium bicarbonate.
7. Treat hyperkalemia.
8. Give diuretics (mannitol, 0.5 g/kg, and furosemide, 2 mg/kg), and fluids to maintain good urine output: greater than 2 ml/kg/h.

Source: Stromberg, B.V. Treatment of malignant hyperthermia. Clin Plast Surg 1985; 12(1): 92.

fibroplasia, and if the surgery cannot be delayed, a minimal concentration of oxygen should be used (16). In children less than 10–12 years of age, induction can be accomplished with an inhalational anesthetic and an intravenous line can be placed following induction. Intubation is usually accomplished using an uncuffed tube to minimize the risk of subglottic injury. Intravenous fluids need to be replaced aggressively because children experience a greater percentage of loss of body water when fasting. In addition, body temperature should be closely monitored because children lose body heat faster than adults do and hypothermia increases the risk of anesthetic complications.

Facial trauma usually presents as part of multiple organ system trauma. To administer safe anesthesia, the associated injuries must be diagnosed, monitored, and treated in the resuscitative and operative phases. There is a high association between facial trauma and either intracranial or cervical spine injuries (17). Care should be taken in the movement and positioning of the patient. In cases of multiple facial fractures, a difficult airway is often present and early consideration should be given to tracheotomy.

REFERENCES

1. Iverson RE. Patient safety in office-based surgery facilities: I. Procedures in the office-based surgery setting. Plast Reconstr Surg 2002; 110:1337–1342.
2. Marten TJ. Physician-administered office anesthesia. Clin Plast Surg 1991; 18:877–889.
3. Klein JA. Tumescent technique chronicles. Local anesthesia, liposuction, and beyond. Dermatol Surg 1995; 21:449–457.
4. Cesany P. Local anaesthesia in cosmetic surgery. Acta Chir Plast 1991; 33:151–154.
5. Groudine SB, Hollinger I, Jones J, DeBouno BA. New York State guidelines on the topical use of phenylephrine in the operating room. The Phenylephrine Advisory Committee. Anesthesiology 2000; 92:859–864.
6. Karim A, Ahmed S, Siddiqui R, Mattana J. Methemoglobinemia complicating topical lidocaine used during endoscopic procedures. Am J Med 2001; 111:150–153.

7. Abdallah HY, Shah SA. Methemoglobinemia induced by topical benzocaine: a warning for the endoscopist. Endoscopy 2002; 34:730–734.
8. Rehman HU. Methemoglobinemia. West J Med 2001; 175:193–196.
9. Stromberg BV. Regional anesthesia in head and neck surgery. Clin Plast Surg 1985; 12:123–136.
10. Owens WD, Felts JA, Spitznagel EL, Jr.. ASA physical status classifications: a study of consistency of ratings. Anesthesiology 1978; 49:239–243.
11. Wolters U, Wolf T, Stutzer H, Schroder T. ASA classification and perioperative variables as predictors of postoperative outcome. Br J Anaesth 1996; 77:217–222.
12. Mallampati SR, Gatt SP, Gugino LD, Desai SP, Waraksa B, Freiberger D et. al. A clinical sign to predict difficult tracheal intubation: a prospective study. Can Anaesth Soc J 1985; 32:429–434.
13. Chrisman BB, Watson MA, Macdonald DE. Outpatient anesthesia. J Dermatol Surg Oncol 1988; 14:939–946.
14. Jensen FS, Viby-Mogensen J. Plasma cholinesterase and abnormal reaction to succinylcholine: twenty years' experience with the Danish Cholinesterase Research Unit. Acta Anaesthesiol Scand 1995; 39:150–156.
15. Behrman RE, Vaughan VC, Nelson WE. Nelson textbook of pediatrics, 13th ed. Philadelphia: WB Saunders, 1987.
16. Wallace CT. Anesthesia for plastic surgery in the pediatric patient. Clin Plast Surg 1985; 12:43–50.
17. Manson PN, Saunders JR, Jr. Anesthesia in head and neck surgery. Head and neck cancer surgery and maxillofacial trauma. Clin Plast Surg 1985; 12:115–122.

3

Principles of Wound Healing and Bioimplantable Materials

Joshua L. Kessler
Boston Medical Center, Boston, Massachusetts, U.S.A.

Matthew D. Byers
Sarasota Memorial Hospital, Sarasota, Florida, U.S.A.

INTRODUCTION

Wound repair is a complex process involving both humoral and cellular elements. While it is incumbent upon all surgeons to understand the basic processes involved, the facial plastic surgeon is particularly interested in the factors that promote optimal wound repair to achieve the best functional and aesthetic result possible. This knowledge will provide the conditions necessary to optimize wound healing and, perhaps as importantly, provide the tools necessary to manage nonhealing wounds more effectively.

Another important aspect in wound healing involves the use of bioimplantable materials. Research in the field of plastic and reconstructive surgery has continued to broaden the spectrum of materials available for implantation and augmentation. Each material has advantages and disadvantages based on its molecular structure and inflammatory response. This chapter will focus on the mechanisms of surgical wound healing and address the various materials available to the plastic surgeon for implantation.

BASIC PRINCIPLES OF WOUND HEALING

Any type of injury to the skin or soft tissues triggers a well-organized and complex cascade of cellular and biochemical events that ultimately lead to a healed wound. This sequence of events is organized into three separate but overlapping phases known as the *inflammatory*, *proliferative*, and *remodeling phases*. The information in the following section on the basic principles of wound healing is a summary of several classic and modern texts (1–7).

The Inflammatory Phase

The inflammatory phase is characterized by initiation of the clotting cascade, increased vascular permeability by the release of cytokines and other chemical mediators, and chemotaxis of cells and their subsequent activation. The initial event after injury is the activation of the coagulation cascade that results from the exposure of platelets to exposed subendothelial collagen from injured vessels (8). This recruitment and aggregation of platelets not only result in formation of a clot but also trigger the release of various cytokines and growth factors through the process of platelet degranulation (9). These mediators include platelet-derived growth factor (PDGF), transforming growth factor-beta (TGF-β), platelet-activating factor (PAF), fibronectin, serotonin, prostaglandins, thromboxanes, leukotreines, and proteases. The release of these substances into the wound milieu is chemotactic for neutrophils, macrophages, lymphocytes, fibroblasts, and endothelial cells. These cells are then activated and release their own specific mediators (Fig. 1).

Fibronectin forms cross-links within the clot and provides a scaffold for migrating keratinocytes, endothelial cells, and fibroblasts (10,11). It has been demonstrated experimentally in animals that in the absence of fibrinogen, clot formation fails and wound repair is significantly hindered.

Neutrophils are the first inflammatory cells to arrive at the injured site (Fig. 2). They gain access to the wound via increased vascular permeability and are recruited and activated by a concentration gradient of chemotactic substances such as

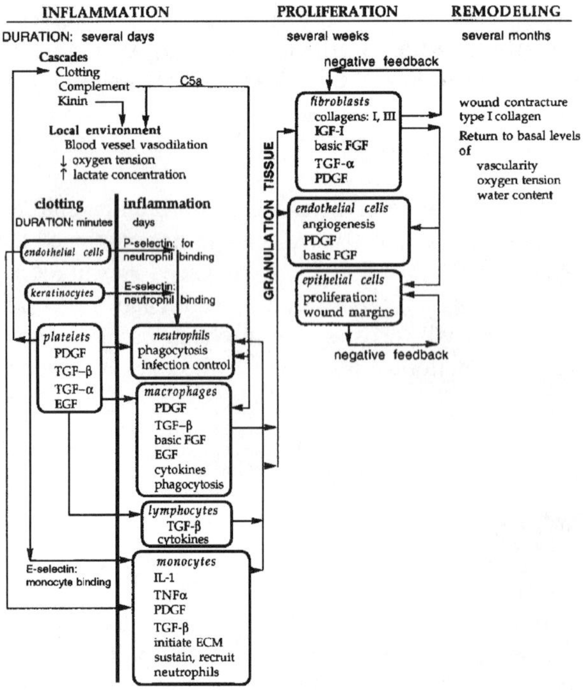

Figure 1 The phases of soft tissue wound repair and cellular and mediator interaction. (*From* Wong ME, Hollinger JO, Pinero GJ. Integrated processes responsible for soft tissue healing. *Oral Surg Oral Med Oral Pathol* 1996;82:475–92.)

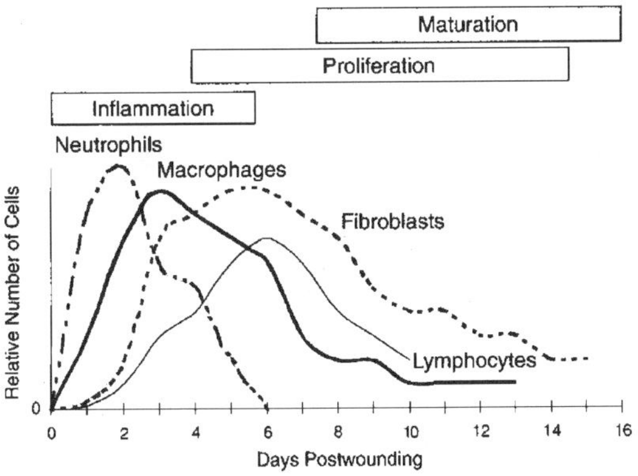

Figure 2 The chronology of cellular migration into the wound. (From Ref. 7.)

prostaglandins, complement factors, interleukin (IL)-1, tumor necrosis factor (TNF)-alpha, TGF-β, and bacterial products. The number of neutrophils in the wound is at its greatest concentration 2 days after the initial injury. Cell surface receptors also play an important role in neutrophil migration. Specific receptors found on the endothelial cells (selectins) and on the neutrophil cell surface (integrins) assist in adherence to the endothelium and the extracellular matrix, respectively. The primary role of neutrophils is to provide an antibacterial defense.

Macrophages are involved in the second wave of inflammatory cell migration. Studies have shown that macrophages are the most important cellular component in the process of wound healing (12). It is well documented that normal wound healing can occur in the presence of neutropenia but cannot occur in the absence of macrophages. Chemotactic agents released during platelet degranulation recruit macrophages to the wound.

Upon arrival at the site of injury, macrophages are activated by cytokines and growth factors released by platelets. This activation signals the release of specific cytokines and growth factors by macrophages that are important in mediating four major processes (Fig. 3). These include (1) angiogenesis through the release of fibroblastic growth factor (FGF) (and vascular endothelial growth factor (VEGF); (2) regulation of matrix synthesis through the release of TGF, PDGF, TNF-α, interferon (IFN), IL-1, and prostaglandins; (3) phagocytosis/antimicrobial function and wound debridement through production of free radicals and enzymes; and (4) cellular recruitment and activation of fibroblasts. This multifactorial role of macrophages is instrumental in directing the future course of wound healing.

The recruitment and activation of lymphocytes occur late in the inflammatory phase (days 5–10). The function of lymphocytes is not completely clear but they may play a role in augmenting macrophage expression and fibroblast accumulation and proliferation through the release of IFN, IL-2 and macrophage-activating factor. T lymphocytes appear to have some regulatory role in mediating macrophage function.

The Proliferative Phase

The proliferative phase entails neoangiogenesis, autolytic debridement of dead tissue, wound matrix formation, and re-epithelialization of the wound by migrating

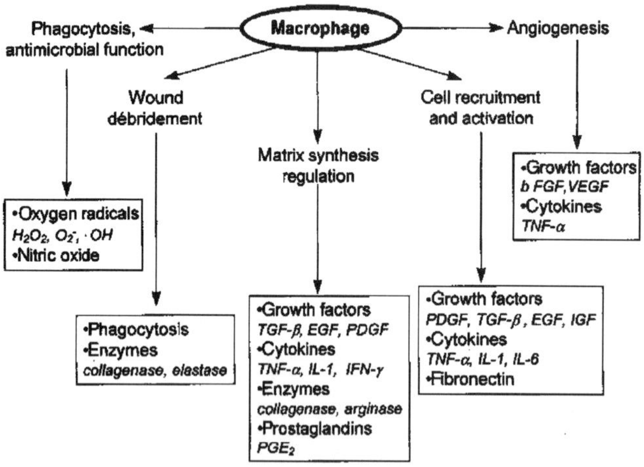

Figure 3 The macrophage is a key actor in the initial phases of wound repair. The myriad functions of the macrophage within the wound are shown. (From Ref. 7.)

keratinocytes. The recruitment and proliferation of fibroblasts are the hallmark events in the beginning of the proliferative phase. This begins around day 4 and continues for an additional 10 days. The activation of fibroblasts is influenced by many growth factors including FGF, epidermal growth factor (EGF), and PDGF, all of which are released by platelets and macrophages.

Neoangiogenesis occurs through the migration and proliferation of endothelial cells from intact adjacent venules surrounding the wound. This process is heavily mediated by chemotactic growth factors (principally FGF, TNF-α, and EGF) and degrading proteases released previously by macrophages.

The formation of the wound matrix predominately takes place during the proliferative phase and is mediated primarily by fibroblasts (13). The matrix is mainly comprised of fibrin, glycosaminoglycans, laminins, and fibronectin, and provides a scaffold for new migrating cells.

Keratinocyte proliferation also occurs during the proliferative phase and plays a role in establishing a protective barrier against matrix fluid losses and infection. These cells migrate from the free edges of the wound as well as from skin appendages. Keratinocytic growth factor (KGF), (FGF-7), PDGF, EGF, and TGF-β influence their activation. As a result of keratinocyte proliferation and migration, most wounds are re-epithelialized within 7–10 days.

Although extensive research has been devoted to exploring the mediators involved in turning on the proliferative phase, little is known about the signals that downregulate this phase and herald the remodeling and maturation phase.

The Remodeling and Maturation Phase

The main features involved in the remodeling and maturation phase are the removal of the matrix by proteolytic enzymes and the deposition of collagen from fibroblasts. This phase begins around the eighth day following injury and can continue for up to 2 years during which time collagen is continually degraded and synthesized in a balanced manner.

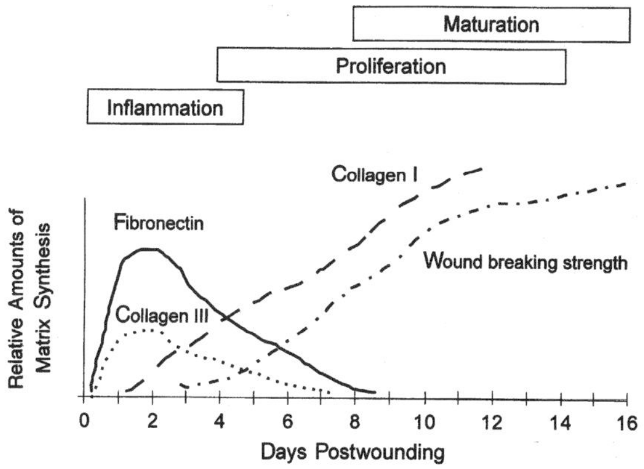

Figure 4 Chronology of wound matrix composition and wound breaking strength throughout the phases of wound healing. (From Ref. 7.)

The production and deposition of collagen occur either at the end of the proliferative phase or at the beginning of the remodeling phase. Type III collagen production predominates early, peaks at day 2, and is gone by day 7. Type I collagen predominates later and is present throughout the remodeling and maturation phase for at least 4–6 weeks (Fig. 4) (14). The collagen initially involved in the formation of a scar is thin and arranged parallel to the skin. These fibers gradually thicken and will organize along the stress line of the wound. This transformation is accompanied by increased scar strength. These collagen fibers have been shown to differ biochemically from nonscar collagen with greater hydroxylation and glycosylation of lysine (15). Although the scar undergoes remodeling for up to 2 years, it never becomes as organized or exhibits the tensile strength when compared to uninjured skin.

The tensile strength of the wound increases with time. After 1 week, the scar has 3% tensile strength. After 3 weeks, the wound has a tensile strength of 20% of its initial strength. After 3 months, the scar exhibits approximately 80% of tensile strength and no further increase will occur thereafter.

The mature scar is comprised mainly of type I collagen (80–90%) with some interspersed type III collagen. As mentioned, type III collagen predominates during the proliferative phase and is involved in the production of granulation tissue. Its production tapers off later during this phase. The actual role of type III collagen is unknown. Evidence suggests that it does not contribute to the strength of the wound but may play a causal role in the production and deposition of type I collagen because its presence coincides with the appearance of fibronectin.

Another important aspect of wound healing is the process of wound contraction. The degree of contraction varies depending on whether the wound is closed primarily or allowed to heal by secondary intention. Although the exact mechanism of wound contracture is not clear, two theories have been proposed. The prevailing theory involves the activation of myofibroblasts. After 4 weeks, cells from the proliferative phase are believed to undergo apoptosis. This process transforms the wound milieu from a cell-rich environment into a scar that is almost completely acellular. The summation of all remaining contracting myofibroblasts then brings the wound edges closer together (16). The second theory maintains that the rearrangement of fibroblasts leads to a reorganization of the matrix and subsequent contraction.

Factors That Influence Wound Healing

An extensive search for a means to promote wound healing through the use of artificial and natural products has been underway for many years. One area of focus is the potential clinical use of natural or recombinant growth factors. A multitude of growth factors have been identified and studied clinically. Growth factors in general have chemotactic properties that attract inflammatory cells and fibroblasts, are mitogenic and stimulate cellular proliferation, stimulate angiogenesis, have a profound effect on the production and degradation of the extracellular matrix, and influence the synthesis of cytokines.

Growth Factors

The target cells, major effects, and sources of several of the commonly known growth factors are outlined in Table 1. PDGF is a product of platelets and macrophages. It is chemotactic for fibroblasts, smooth muscle cells, and neutrophils and is also a mitogen for smooth muscle cells and fibroblasts (17). It is noteworthy that VEGF is also in the same family as PDGF and is a potent angiogenic factor. FGF is a mitogen for fibroblasts but also has angiogenic activities (18,19). TGF-β 1 is a very potent stimulator for collagen deposition and inhibits collagen breakdown. It has also been found to be an important downregulator of the inflammatory response and inhibits scar formation. EGF stimulates the proliferation and migration of all types of epithelial cells (20,21). All of the previously mentioned factors have also been shown to promote protein synthesis through the mediation of growth hormones (22).

Most of these growth factors have either been studied alone or in combination in animals and clinical trials on acute and chronic wounds (23). They have been found to improve healing in almost every type of wound (24,25). In clinical trials, they have been shown to augment repair in patients with diabetes, malnutrition, infection, hypoxia, and those undergoing treatment with chemotherapy, steroids, and radiation. Angiogenic factors have also been used experimentally in pigs to increase the survival of skin flaps by enhancing the ingrowth of blood vessels. Recent clinical studies have demonstrated that several growth factors including PDGF, FGF, EGF, and TGF-β enhance healing in patients with chronic wounds (28,26,27,28). Steed et al. recently published the results of a multicenter study suggesting that diabetic ulcers healed twice as fast when treated with PDGF as with placebo (29).

Topical Antiseptics

The utilization of topical antiseptics as surgical disinfectants is a common practice for many operative procedures (30). It is important to note that some of these agents have been found to affect wound healing adversely. Many studies have identified the direct deleterious effects of hydrogen peroxide, chlorhexidine, and providone–iodine

Table 1 Multiple Growth Factors, Their Major Cell Source, and Known Effects

Cytokine	Major source	Target cells and major effects
Epidermal growth factor family		Epidermal and mesenchymal regeneration
Epidermal growth factor	Platelets	Pleiotropic cell motility and proliferation
Transforming growth factor α	Macrophages, epidermal cells	Pleiotropic cell motility and proliferation
Heparin-binding epidermal growth factor	Macrophages	Pleiotropic cell motility and proliferation
Fibroblast growth factor family		Wound vascularization
Basic fibroblast growth factor	Macrophages, endothelial cells	Angiogenesis and fibroblast proliferation
Acidic fibroblast growth factor	Macrophages, endothelial cells	Angiogenesis and fibroblast proliferation
Keratinocyte growth factor	Fibroblasts	Epidermal cell motility and proliferation
Transforming growth factor β family		Fibrosis and increased tensile strength
Transforming growth factors $\beta 1$ and $\beta 2$	Platelets, macrophages	Epidermal cell motility, chemotaxis of macrophages and fibroblasts, extracellular matrix synthesis and remodeling
Transforming growth factor $\beta 3$	Macrophages	Antiscarring effects
Other		
Platelet-derived growth factor	Platelets, macrophages, epidermal cells	Fibroblast proliferation and chemoattraction, macrophage chemoattraction and activation
Vascular endothelial growth factor	Epidermal cells, macrophages	Angiogenesis and increased vascular permeability
Tumor necrosis factor α	Neutrophils	Pleiotropic expression of growth factors
Interleukin-1	Neutrophils	Pleiotropic expression of growth factors
Insulin-like growth factor 1	Fibroblasts, epidermal cells	Reepithelialization and granulation tissue formation
Colony-stimulating factor 1	Multiple cells	Macrophage activation and granulation tissue formation

Several of the growth factors have multiple (pleiotropic) effects.
Source: From Singer AJ, Clark RA. Cutaneous wound healing. *N Engl J Med* 1999;341:738–746.

on fibroblasts, keratinocytes, and endothelial cells (31–33). A study by Goldenheim compared iodine scrub to iodine solution and found that the iodine scrub adversely affected wound repair (34). The detergent in the scrub preparation was determined to be the component responsible for impairing wound healing.

Systemic Conditions

Many systemic conditions can adversely affect the process of wound healing. Some of the more common conditions include poor nutritional status, immunodeficiency, hypoxia, diabetes mellitus, and the presence of endogenous or exogenous steroids (Table 2) (35).

Malnutrition

The negative impact of malnutrition on healing is well known. The degree of protein deficiency required to affect wound repair is usually quite severe and typically only seen in cases of chronic alcohol abuse or patients with advanced malignancies. Clinical studies have shown that the levels of albumin, prealbumin, transferrin, and total lymphocyte counts are sensitive indicators of malnutrition.

Albumin is an excellent predictor of chronic malnutrition. Because its half-life is 20 days, it is a good measure of long-term malnutrition. Levels less than 2.5 mg/dl

Table 2 Common Disease States Associated with Poor Wound Healing

Disease states	Local factors
Hereditary	Ischemia
Coagulation disorders	Infection
Ehlers-Danlos/Marfan syndrome	Tissue trauma
Prolidase deficiency	Retained foreign body
Werner syndrome	Desiccation
Vascular disorders	
Congestive heart failure	Medications
Atherosclerosis	Glucocorticoids
Hypertension	Anticoagulants
Vasculitis	Antineoplastic agents
Venous stasis	Colchicine
Lymphedema	Penicillamine
Metabolic	Vitamin E
Chronic renal failure	Salicylates (high-dose)
Diabetes mellitus	Nonsteroidals (high-dose)
Malnutrition	Zinc sulfate (high-dose)
Cushing's syndrome	Vitamin A (high-dose)
Hyperthyroidism	
Immunological deficiency states	
Others	
Chronic pulmonary disease	
Liver failure	
Malignancy	

Source: From Singer AJ, Clark RA. Cutaneous wound healing. *N Engl J Med* 1999;341:738–746.

indicate severe malnutrition. Prealbumin has a half-life of 2–3 days, rendering it an accurate indicator of acute protein deficiency.

Transferrin is the most sensitive indicator of rapid changes in protein stores. It has a half-life of 8–10 days and levels less than 100 mg/dl indicate severe protein depletion, which has been shown to increase the risk of complications from surgery by two and a half times.

Total lymphocyte count is another commonly monitored nutritional marker. Similar to albumin, it is a better indicator of chronic malnutrition. Levels below 1200 cells/ml indicate severe malnutrition and have been shown to increase the risk of infection by 50 percent.

Weight loss is also a good indicator of a patient's nutritional reserves. Losses up to 20% below ideal body weight increase surgical wound complications by up to 20–30%, whereas weight loss of greater than 50% has been shown to increase mortality rate by up to 50%.

Nitrogen balance is an excellent means of assessing the adequacy of nutritional supplementation. In patients with chronic protein depletion, a positive nitrogen balance of a least 4–6 g/day is required in order to replete protein stores.

Vitamins and minerals play a pivotal role in wound repair. Specifically, vitamin A, vitamin C, zinc, and iron have all proven to be vital cofactors involved in the wound healing process. Vitamin A has been shown to increase the rate of epithelial turnover, increase collagen synthesis rates, and promote cross-linking of collagen. Preoperative treatment with Retin A is now standard for most surgeons performing any resurfacing procedure because it has been shown to increase rates of re-epithelialization. Vitamin C plays a crucial role in wound repair by providing the hydroxylation of lysine and prolene during collagen synthesis. Vitamin C is also important in neutrophil function and serves as a reducing agent in superoxide radical formation. Vitamin E is an oxygen radical scavenger but it is not routinely administered because it inhibits collagen production and may reduce the tensile strength of scars. Due to these properties, however, it is commonly used as a topical preparation to soften the appearance of scars postoperatively.

Zinc and iron represent the most important trace elements in wound repair. Their importance is in mediating the expression of growth factors and collagen synthesis and also in enhancing the immune system.

Diabetes Mellitus

Diabetes mellitus is one of the more common systemic illnesses affecting wound healing. The prolonged elevated levels of blood glucose render an irreversible angiopathy that predominantly involves small vessels. This microangiopathy diminishes blood flow, causing a decrease in oxygen delivery and the supply of vital nutrients and inflammatory cells required for healing. Furthermore, diabetes adversely affects the immune system. The elevated blood glucose levels directly alter leukocyte function that is important in the early phase of wound healing.

Treatment is aimed at controlling elevated blood glucose. There is also evidence that the use of supplemental vitamin A (25,000 units/day) appears to offset the effects of hyperglycemia and improve wound healing. Some physicians also advocate the routine administration of vitamin C prior to and after surgery, since hyperglycemia has been shown to block its absorption.

Radiation Therapy

Patients who have received therapeutic or supratherapeutic doses of radiation are at risk for poor wound healing. Radiation has a direct effect on arterioles and the supportive tissue surrounding the vasculature resulting in obliterative endarteritis similar to the microangiopathy seen in diabetics. The administration of vitamin A and hyperbaric oxygen has been shown to promote healing in irradiated tissue.

Systemic Glucocorticosteroids and Other Medications

The adverse effects of prolonged use of exogenous or the presence of excessive levels of endogenous steroids on wound healing are well documented. Steroids directly alter the inflammatory phase of wound repair and decrease collagen synthesis and wound contraction. It has also been shown that steroids can decrease levels of TGF-β, which is a potent stimulator of collagen production and deposition. Vitamin A has been found to reverse temporarily many of the adverse effects of steroids and restore levels of TGF-β back to normal. In addition to glucocorticosteroids, many other medications have been implicated in altering wound healing (36,37).

Hypoxemia

Hypoxemia resulting from infection, hematoma, anemia, vasculitis, or poor surgical technique can severely affect wound healing. Oxygen is consumed in large amounts in a healing wound and many important functions are inhibited with its depletion. However, not all phases of wound healing are adversely affected by low oxygen tension. In fact, low O_2 tension in the early phase of healing actually promotes chemotaxis of inflammatory cells and expression of growth factors, angiogenesis, and epithelial migration. The phase most adversely affected by low O_2 tension is the proliferative phase, because fibroblasts are dependent on adequate levels of oxygen to proliferate and produce collagen. The critical level of oxygen tension required for normal healing to ensue is 30–40 mmHg.

The delivery of supernormal levels of oxygen to wounds, as occurs in hyperbaric oxygen treatment, has been shown to enhance the rate of re-epithelialization, fibroblast proliferation, and deposition of collagen. However, hyperbaric oxygen's impact on improving chronic nonhealing wounds remains controversial.

Congenital Abnormalities

Many congenital abnormalities are important to recognize preoperatively. These include Ehlers-Danlos syndrome, cutis laxa, pseudoxanthoma elasticum, osteogenesis imperfecta, and progeria. A common factor in these disorders appears to be that congenital errors in the metabolism of collagen invariably result in poor wound healing. Elective surgery in patients with these conditions should be avoided.

HYPERTROPHIC SCARS AND KELOIDS

The emphasis up to this point has been on conditions that downregulate the phases of wound healing, resulting in poor wound repair. An overactivation of the wound healing process can also occur, as evidenced by the formation of hypertrophic scars and keloids. These two conditions share an excessive production and deposition of collagen without the equivalent balance of degradation and remodeling. They also appear to occur more frequently in areas that are under increased skin tension or constant motion; earlobes appear to be an exception to this rule. The major difference between these two conditions is that while hypertrophic scars tend to remain within the original tissue injury site and will eventually regress over time, keloids grow beyond the boundaries of the injured site and do not regress.

Keloids and hypertrophic scars also differ histopathologically. Keloids contain abundant mucin and large, thick bundles of collagen that lie haphazardly within the dermis. They are also quite vascular. The keloid extracellular matrix is composed primarily of glycoproteins and water. In contrast, hypertrophic scars contain well-organized fibrillar collagen, contain no mucin, are less vascular, and contain abundant myofibroblasts (38).

It is unclear whether the pathogenesis of keloids is secondary to the overproduction of collagen or a defect in collagen degradation (39). Various theories propose a deficiency or defect in collagenase, a disproportionate level of collagenase inhibitors, or an abnormal growth regulation of fibroblasts mediated through TGF-β (40,41). It is well documented that the metabolic activity in keloids is much greater than in hypertrophic scars. A variety of cytokines and growth factors have been implicated in the regulation of this metabolic activity (42). TGF-β and IL-1 have been shown to increase collagen gene expression in vitro. Studies have demonstrated that inhibiting TGF-β leads to reduced scar formation.

Two cytokines that appear to be major factors in downregulating collagen production and reducing scar formation are IFN-γ and IFN-α. Clinical trials using intralesional injections of IFN-γ and IFN-α have demonstrated significant decreases in keloid and hypertrophic scar formation. Some authors have suggested that the formation of keloids is the result of a cell-mediated response to sebum released from sebaceous glands following incision. The specific mechanism involved in the development of keloids is still unknown and remains an area of active research.

The treatment of keloids is challenging and controversial. Treatment is aimed at reducing the metabolic activity within the keloid and ultimately suppressing the production of collagen. The goal in the treatment of both hypertrophic scars and keloids is to improve their appearance by decreasing the volume of collagen and extracellular matrix. While intralesional injection of steroids continues to be the mainstay of treatment, there have been a number of clinical trials supporting alternative methods of therapy for keloids (43). These include, but are not limited to, re-excision of the keloid followed by low-dose radiation therapy (1500–2000 cGY), laser excision, interferon injection, treatment with adrenocorticotropic hormone (ACTH), vitamin A, retinoic acid, compressive devices, and the use of silicone sheeting (44,45).

WOUND HEALING IN OTHER TISSUES

The phases of wound healing in cutaneous injury generally reflect the same principles during healing in other tissues. However, in certain types of tissues the processes occurring within each phase of healing can be quite different. This section will focus specifically on the sequence of wound repair as it applies to the healing of bone fractures, free and revascularized bone grafts, and the processes involved in what is termed the 'take' of skin grafts.

Bone

Bone is a complex tissue containing osteoblasts, osteoclasts, and bone matrix. Osteoblasts are mononuclear cells derived from mesenchymal precursors and are predominantly surrounded by bone matrix. Their primary role is in bone formation. Osteoclasts are multinuclear cells derived from the macrophage–monocyte cell line and are responsible for bone resorption. Bone matrix is the noncellular component of bone and is comprised of an inorganic and an organic portion. The organic portion contains collagen (95% type I), glycoproteins, and proteoglycans, and has similar microscopic components to those of dermal skin. The inorganic component of bone matrix consists of calcium salts, predominantly hydroxyapatite.

Vital to the survival of these bone constituents is the blood supply. Bone is a highly vascularized tissue and receives its blood supply from the periosteum, endosteum, and surrounding soft tissues. For this reason, it is important for the surgeon to preserve as much periosteum and soft tissue as possible during the management of facial fractures and the harvesting of osteomyocutaneous free flaps.

Bone is a highly dynamic tissue that continuously undergoes remodeling throughout adult life. This remodeling is a fine balance of the resorptive properties of osteoclasts coupled with bone formation by osteoblasts, allowing for continued metabolic changes to occur without net bone gain or loss.

The healing process that occurs from an injury to bone, either from traumatic fracture or surgical osteotomy, follows the same principles during the early phases of wound healing as does healing in other tissues. Healing in the later phase is quite different and unique to bone (46,47). Initial injury to bone results in disruption of the blood supply and subsequent recruitment of platelets and fibrinogen to form a hematoma. Platelet aggregation and degranulation provide the initial release of cytokines and growth factors and trigger the onset of the inflammatory phase. The resulting ischemia and release of lysosomal enzymes from dying osteocytes leads to further propagation of the inflammatory phase.

The mediators of the inflammatory phase consist of neutrophils, macrophages, and mast cells that originate from the marrow, endosteum, and periosteum. These cells enter the fracture site early to begin debriding the wound of devitalized tissue. The release of cytokines and growth factors from this initial phase sets up the proliferative phase characterized by the migration of precursor mesenchymal and osteoprogenitor cells from the marrow, endosteum, periosteum, and surrounding muscle. Activation of these cells, in combination with neovascularization, initiates bone formation. Later in the process, undifferentiated mononuclear cells differentiate into fibroblasts, chondroblasts, and osteoblasts that produce collagen, lay down cartilage, and form new bone, respectively. The aggregation of fibrous tissue, cartilage, and loosely woven bone forms what is termed a soft callus around the fracture. The primary component of the soft callus is unmineralized cartilage.

At about 6 weeks, the soft callus is slowly transformed into bone by the process of endochondral ossification. Type II collagen is degraded and replaced by type I (48). The organic matrix is converted to calcium hydroxyapatite and mature osteoblasts lay down woven bone to create a hard callus or bony union. The fracture site at this stage can withstand weight loading.

Once the hard callus has been formed, remodeling takes place to restore normal architecture and re-establish the marrow cavity. A balance of osteoclastic and osteoblastic activity within the hard callus replaces the woven bone with layers of mature lamellar bone. The end result is a healed bone that is virtually indistinguishable from intact bone. An important factor unique to wound healing in bone is the presence of mechanical shearing and torsional forces during repair. These forces have been found to be essential in the development of a strong bony union (49,50). In fact, rigid fixation of mandibular fractures through the use of large reconstruction plates can prevent these vital forces from occurring, leading to a less than optimal bony union. This process is known as 'stress-shielding' (51).

The utilization of bone grafts is common in facial plastic surgery. Bone grafts are primarily used in the management of extensive facial trauma and reconstruction following oncological resections, in which bone replacement is the goal. Bone graft healing generally follows the same principles of wound healing in bone fractures. One of the most important factors in optimizing bone graft survival is placement of the graft in a recipient bed with adequate vascularity. Free bone grafts placed in a previously irradiated field or an actively infected area will invariably fail (52).

Bone graft healing involves three separate but overlapping processes: osteoinduction, osteoproduction, and osteoconduction. Osteoinduction involves the transformation and activation of mesenchymal cells in the recipient bed into osteoclasts and osteoblasts that act to debride devitalized bone and build new bone. Mesenchymal differentiation is induced by bone morphogenetic proteins (BMPs), which are inherently present in the bone graft (53). Osteoproduction is the process by which surviving osteoblasts within the graft produce new bone. Osteoconduction is the process of vascular and cellular ingrowth into the grafted bone and is mediated by growth factors. The existing architecture of the bone graft provides a scaffold for the formation and deposition of new bone. Of note, osteoinduction and osteoconduction are the two processes primarily involved in the acceptance and healing of nonvascularized bone grafts, whereas osteoproduction contributes more to the healing of free vascularized bone grafts.

Upon placement of a bone graft into the recipient site, an inflammatory response ensues leading to cellular proliferation, migration, and differentiation(54). Devitalized bone is removed by osteoclastic activity. Neovascularization provides revascularization of the graft. Osteoblasts within the bone are either induced from undifferentiated mesenchymal cells or carried into the bone during vascular ingrowth. The final result leads to a variable degree of preserved graft as well as new bone formation.

Nonvascularized bone grafts consist of cancellous bone, cortical bone, or a combination of the two. Their properties are very different, but the overall healing process is much the same. Cancellous bone is medullary bone and has a highly cellular component consisting mainly of osteoblasts. It has the highest percentage of viable transplanted cells per surface area, allowing it to become revascularized as early as 2 weeks. The presence of haversian canals allows for this rapid revascularization. Most studies have shown that the amount of retained graft after implantation is up to 80–90%. Due to the highly cellular properties of cancellous bone, it is used most commonly as a packing material into areas of bone loss, as in mandible fractures or in nonunion fractures. When the process is complete, cancellous bone grafts are completely replaced by new bone.

Cortical bone, on the other hand, is lamellar bone. Its predominant cell type transferred is the osteocyte. This graft initially is much stronger and is commonly used as a strut to bridge larger areas of bone loss. However, the percentage of graft take for free cortical bone is much less than with cancellous bone. This decreased viability is due to the death of osteocytes resulting from the prolonged period of time required for revascularization. Membranous cortical bone, such as calvarial bone, has been shown to exhibit greater take rates (up to 90% in some studies) than endochondral bone (55,56). Cortical bone grafts transferred with a cancellous component, such as calvarial or iliac grafts, have a much greater chance of survival, as do grafts transferred with retained periosteum.

Skin Grafts

Perhaps the most versatile of all reconstructive options, skin grafts are also one of the most common procedures performed by the facial plastic surgeon. Skin grafts will be discussed in greater detail elsewhere, but a brief overview of their physiology in relation to wound healing is warranted here.

Skin grafts can be harvested as either full-thickness grafts containing an intact epidermis and dermis or as partial-thickness grafts containing an intact epidermis and a partially intact dermis. Graft survival initially depends on the diffusion of nutrients and oxygen through the vascularized recipient bed in a process known as imbibition. Later in the process, the graft receives nutrients through inosculation, which is the connection of vascular channels in the graft to blood vessels in the wound bed. This process is complete by 3–4 days. However, the graft acquires a more permanent means of sustaining survival through direct vascular ingrowth.

After the graft has established its blood supply, healing at the interface ensues. The remodeling and maturation phase is the most clinically significant phase of skin graft healing. During this phase, an immature scar will form at the junction between the graft and the recipient. This leads to two different types of contraction: scar contraction and wound bed contraction. Scar contraction occurs predominantly around the periphery of the graft and is dependent on the degree of extracellular matrix in the dermis. Split-thickness grafts are less affected by this type of contraction because they contain fewer dermal elastic fibers and matrix elements. Full-thickness grafts, on the other hand, contract significantly more because the entire dermal matrix is present.

Wound bed contraction, as the name implies, refers to contraction that occurs between the base of the wound and the dermal interface of the graft. The degree of contraction is dependent on the thickness of the dermal matrix in the skin graft. Studies have shown that the thickness of the dermis correlates well with the suppression of wound bed myofibroblasts and ultimately contraction (57). Split-thickness grafts exhibit the greatest degree of wound bed contraction (up to 50% reduction in the surface area) due to the paucity of dermal elements present to suppress myofibroblasts and resist contractile forces adequately (58).

It is important for the surgeon to be aware of these inherent physiological skin graft mechanisms because choosing the wrong type of graft for a particular situation can have potentially devastating aesthetic and functional consequences. Other important factors in ensuring graft survival are good surgical technique and postoperative care to prevent infection, seroma, or hematoma.

OCCLUSIVE DRESSINGS

The basic observation that blisters heal much faster when left intact than when ruptured demonstrates the mechanism by which occlusive dressings enhance the healing and re-epithelialization of wounds. Winter (1960) showed that occlusion of wounds with a polyethylene film more than doubled wound epithelialization in animals (59). This discovery ushered in the production and utilization of a variety of occlusive dressings for the treatment of acute and chronic wounds.

The theory of treating wounds with occlusive or semiocclusive dressings is also based on the fact that desiccated, crusted wounds heal more slowly than those that are kept in a moist environment. Dressings promote the healing of wounds by providing a moist, humid environment by the entrapment of exudate (60). This environment has been shown experimentally to enhance the function and migration of epithelial cells. The exudate is also rich in growth factors that further promote epidermal migration and activation of fibroblasts. Numerous studies have shown that occlusive or semiocclusive dressings can accelerate re-epithelialization and wound closure up to 40–50% (61,62). This moisture-rich environment also enhances the autolytic debridement of wounds and provides bacteriostatic properties. A summary of the advantages and disadvantages of occlusive dressings is shown in Table 3.

There are a number of different types of dressings available. Most contain hydrocolloids, hydrogels, polymer films, perforated plastic films, or petrolatum-based products. The choice of dressing has been based on certain properties inherent in the material. Favorable properties include a high degree of absorbency, low adherence, transparency, pain reduction, and ease of application. A dressing should also be gas-permeable, allowing for the introduction of oxygen into the wound as well as the elimination of carbon dioxide (63).

Occlusive and semiocclusive dressings have gained tremendous popularity in the field of facial plastic surgery for the postoperative management of skin resurfacing procedures such as laser resurfacing and chemical peels. At one point, sheeting materials (Saran Wrap, Vigilon) were commonly used postoperatively after resurfacing. These materials have been generally abandoned due to difficulty with application and adherence and the potential of causing more extensive injury by allowing

Table 3 Advantages and Disadvantages of Occlusive Dressings

Advantages	Disadvantages
Rapid healing	Accumulation of pus
Reduced pain	Hematoma or seroma
Fewer dressing changes	Silent infections
Exclusion of micro-organisms	Folliculitis
Better cosmetic results	Need for healthy borders
	Trauma to adjacent skin
	Adherence to new tissue
	Allergy
	Fear of infection
	Retarding gain in tensile strength

Source: From Ref. 64.

chemical peels to penetrate deeper. The dressings of choice that have been accepted by most surgeons are petroleum-based topical products such as Vaseline and Aquafor. These agents have become popular due to their ease of application, their transparent properties enabling one to monitor the status of the wound easily, low cost, and the rapid acceleration of re-epithelialization. Eaglstein studied the relative rate of wound healing with the application of a number of different topical agents (64). Geronemus et al. found that Silvadene and Neosporin increased the relative rate of wound healing by a factor of 25, while Furacin decreased it by factor of 24 (65). Use of Neosporin as a topical dressing after skin resurfacing has been abandoned by most practitioners due to reports of hypersensitivity reactions.

NEW HORIZONS IN WOUND HEALING

One of the most promising areas of wound healing research involves the clinical use of the growth factors PDGF and KGF (or FGF-7). PDGF can either be derived from harvested human platelets or generated from recombinant DNA. Multiple studies have shown that the topical application of PDGF to wounds accelerates neoangiogenesis and re-epithelialization. Harvest Technologies Corp. (Norwell, MA) recently developed SmartPReP, an autologous platelet gel, which contains not only PDGF but also other growth factors such as TGF-β, VEGF, and EGF. Its beneficial properties include decreased bleeding and hematomas, reduced swelling and bruising, no need for postoperative drains or compression dressings, and an accelerated healing process. Other products such as TISSEEL and FLOSEAL have also emerged. These products are similar to fibrin glue and their benefits are similar to platelet gel. Clinical trials are presently underway to determine their efficacy in facial plastic procedures.

KGF (or FGF-7) is one of the more recently discovered FGFs. It is produced by dermal fibroblasts, exerts most of its action on epithelial cells, and is found to have a profound effect on inducing epithelialization (64). It is also indirectly involved in inducing angiogenesis, granulation tissue, matrix deposition, and collagen synthesis. Numerous small studies have confirmed the effects of KGF on wound epithelialization but larger clinical studies are needed.

Bioimplantable Materials

Another important aspect of wound healing pertains to the widespread use of alloplastic material for facial implantation. There are many different types of materials, all of which may be categorized into a subset of groups based on their inherent properties and the body's reaction to the material. The remainder of this chapter will focus on both historical and popular materials for facial implantation, their applications and shortcomings, as well as the histological changes observed subsequent to their implantation.

The most important biological events in response to the implant material occur in the inflammatory phase. All implants trigger a dense inflammatory response within the host that usually results in capsule formation. The characteristics of this capsule, when formed, dictate the clinical outcome of the surgery depending on the location of implantation and the desired physical properties of the implant after surgery.

Metals and Alloys

The strength and rigid properties of metals render them excellent implant materials for the repair and augmentation of skeletal defects. Stainless steel, vitallium, and titanium are all examples of metals that have been used for implantation. Stainless steel was likely the first modern implant used in facial plastic surgery dating to the era before World War II; it was introduced in the 1920s. Another popular metal for implantation, vitallium is a cobalt–chromium alloy introduced in the 1930s that is composed of 60% cobalt, 30% chromium, and 10% nickel. Titanium is implanted in almost pure elemental form and is currently the most commonly used metal for implantation.

The major disadvantage of metal implantation is the inevitable corrosion of the implant material (66). Although stainless steel is highly susceptible to corrosion, vitallium and titanium are highly resistant to corrosion because of their natural tendency to form an oxide film. This film both prevents local corrosion of the implant and decreases the host inflammatory response. Sutow and Pollack cited the fact that only a minimal localized reaction is observed in bone and periosteum after the implantation of titanium and vitallium (66). Titanium-osseointegrated implants, used commonly in oral surgery procedures, produce a minimal response that allows them to have an intimate connection to surrounding bone and maintain integrity to support the forces of mastication (67). Titanium is the metal implant material of choice in modern plastic surgery because of its strength, high resistance to corrosion, resilience, and light weight.

Roussett first described gold for facial implantation in 1828. Because of its high degree of malleability, it lacks the structural support necessary for most facial plastic surgical procedures. However, its use as a weight for eye closure in facial nerve paralysis is well documented (68,69). It is ideal in this application because of its heavy atomic weight and the minimal tissue reaction observed on supratarsal implantation.

Polymers

Commonly referred to as plastic material, polymers have arguably made the most significant impact on the science of implantation. Polymerization refers to the process by which carbon links are chained together in a repeating monomeric unit. The physical attributes of polymeric material are dictated by the degree of polymerization, cross-linking, the size of the repeating unit, and the position of the repeating unit in the chain (70). Polymers are classified into several groups based on their physical characteristics: solid, porous, woven, or injectable. In general, the lower the molecular weight of the material and the less cross-linking, the more fluid the polymer.

Solid polymers include solid silicones and polymethylmethacrylate. Silicones have been used in a variety of procedures in facial plastic surgery. Silicones have a repeating unit of dimethylsiloxane that dictates the viscosity of the material (71). This may vary from a liquid injectable form to sheets of solid silicone manufactured under the name of Sialastic (Dow Corning, Midland, Michigan). When solid silicone is implanted, a thin fibrous capsule is formed around the material. There is minimal to no ingrowth of host tissues into the implant. This minimal inflammatory response occurs only under the optimal conditions of small implants that have been well stabilized (72). In implants subject to migration, a dense reaction is noted resulting in a much thicker capsule. For silicone rubber and Sialastic, rare instances of resorption have been reported (73). Although the Food and Drug Administration (FDA) does not approve of injectable silicone, preformed silicone implants are used for malar, mental, nasal, and mandible augmentation. The use of silicone in nasal augmentation has fallen out of common use because of a relatively high degree of extrusion (74).

Polymethylmethacrylate is an acrylic polymer that possesses the advantages of great strength and rigidity and may be sculpted in the operating room during surgery. The polymer is supplied in a powder form that is mixed with a monomer liquid to form the final product. This process is highly exothermic and may reach temperatures in excess of 100° C. These high temperatures have rarely resulted in intraoperative complications (75). Such reactions are exceedingly rare and have never been reported in facial plastic procedures. The inflammatory response to implantation of polymethylmethacrylate has been described as intense and characterized by a multinucleated giant cell reaction (76). Because of its many potential advantages, it remains a viable choice for cranioplasty in neurosurgical procedures and in selected cases of orbital reconstruction.

The porous polymers include high-density porous polyethylene (HDPE) (Medpore, Marlex) and polytetrafluorethylene. HDPE exhibits a minimal inflammatory response with the ingrowth of tissue into the porous implant (77). It is composed of chains of ethylene units with a high degree of side-chain branching. The size of the pores within the HDPE dictates the amount of fibrous ingrowth with the pore size of 150 μm being ideal.

Polytetrafluorethylene (PTFE; Proplast II, Vitek, Houston, TX) is also highly porous; the size of the pores range from 200 to 500 μm and the pore volume makes up to 90% of the total volume of the implant (78). Implantation has been shown to have few complications and a high degree of reliability. Within the implant, a dense inflammatory cell response with granulation occurs (79). Another advantage of Proplast II is its relative ease of sculpture and it has been used successfully in orbital, malar, nasal, mandibular, and ossicular chain reconstruction.

Gore-Tex (W.L. Gore, Flagstaff, AZ), a fibrillated polytetrafluorethylene, has been more recently introduced and met with wide success. It is produced as a soft tissue augmentation patch in thicknesses of 1, 2, and 4 mm and is easily cut and shaped. It has been used commonly for nasal, malar, lip, and brow augmentation (80). A pore size of 30 μm may delay the ingrowth of fibrous tissue; however, the inflammatory response is similar to that seen in Proplast. In general, it is a reliable and stable implant.

The meshed polymers include polyamide mesh (Nylamid Mesh, S. Jackson Inc, Mineapolis, MN), HDPE mesh (Marlex Mesh), polypropylene polymer mesh (Prolene, Ethicon, Inc, Somerville, NJ), and polyethylene terephthalate (Dacron, Merceline, Ethicon). The major advantages of mesh include its malleability and stability with implantation due to ingrowth of surrounding tissue. It may be folded, sutured, cut, and shaped with ease. The material can be problematic, however, if infected and removal is difficult due to its adhesion to surrounding tissue. Polymer mesh was initially thought to be chemically inert and highly resistant to breakdown. Due to evidence of structural breakdown and loss of material, meshes are now used infrequently for facial implantation (81). Several authors have found Mersiline mesh to be helpful in malar and chin augmentation, but by far the most common use of mesh polymers is in abdominal wall repair (82–84). Silver and Maas suggest in previously unpublished data that Mersiline also undergoes significant resorption and loss of structural support after several years of implantation and question its use in facial augmentation (76). As expected, a dense inflammatory response with multinucleated giant cells is seen surrounding the implanted mesh (85).

Injectable polymers include silicone and PTFE paste, and while initially promising, these materials have shown various problems in clinical use. Injectable silicone was widely used in facial augmentation when first released, however, major problems with migration and extrusion were noted. Case reports of systemic and severe local allergic and inflammatory reactions were published. As a result, injectable silicone is not approved for facial augmentation and is not widely used. PTFE paste (Polytef paste) has been used successfully in vocal cord augmentation, however, its use in facial augmentation is limited due to foreign body reaction and difficulties in injection due to its high viscosity. Injectable collagen and Alloderm have generally replaced injectable polymers in facial plastic surgery.

Ceramics

Ceramics have been used extensively in facial implantation. These are silicate-based materials that have recently become more popular due to the development and extensive use of hydroxyapatite. The implant's chemical similarity to osseous bone and teeth allows the implant to become easily integrated into bony tissue and promote replacement of bony tissue when placed next to bone (82,83,86). Its uses include genioplasty, alveolar ridge augmentation, orbital floor and roof repair, and tegmen repair in middle ear surgery (87,88). It is easily shaped and contoured as a cement form and has been shown to be relatively resistant to infection (89).

Acellular Human Dermis and Mammalian-derived Implant Materials

In contrast to the synthetic materials previously described, several bioimplantable materials are derived from mammalian tissues, especially from human cadavers. Injectable collagen is derived from bovine tissue and is comprised mainly of type I collagen. While it has been used extensively in lip, malar, and chin augmentation, it typically resorbs in 3–9 months. Minimal tissue reaction is seen in most forms. A concern when using collagen for implantation is its relatively high propensity for allergic reaction. As such, skin testing is recommended prior to the implantation of large amounts of collagen.

With the availability of acellular human dermis (Alloderm, Lifecell Corp., The Woodlands, TX), the field of tissue implantation has rapidly expanded (90). Acellular human dermis is processed from cadaveric human dermis and rendered acellular through a process of detergent treatment that rids the tissue of antigenic cellular material while maintaining the structural integrity of the extracellular matrix. This matrix is composed of glycosaminoglycans, collagens, and growth factors. Further treatment with amorphous ice crystals maintains the structure of the matrix for storage and subsequent reconstitution in normal saline in the operating room. Animal studies and human clinical trials have revealed no evidence of allergic response (50).

Over time, the implant is repopulated with the recipient's own cells and revascularized.

Many aesthetic procedures have been performed with acellular human dermis. It has been used in lip augmentation; sheets or rolls of the material are placed in a tunnel superficial to the orbicularis oris. Nasolabial sulcus augmentation with the material is performed in a similar fashion through carefully placed nasal sill incisions. Sheets of acellular human dermis have been placed for glabellar, malar, submalar, and chin augmentation. In rhinoplasty, it is often useful in tip and dorsum contouring, especially in patients with very thin or traumatized skin. Another use is in the augmentation of depressed scars and in acne pit repair. Although Alloderm is commonly used to augment various areas of the face, it is prone to at least partial resorption, especially if the graft is placed in an area subject to movement such as the nasal tip. For example, Alloderm should not be used to repair a saddle nose deformity because the deformity may recur due to implant resorption.

An injectable form of Alloderm (Cymetra) has been successfully used in vocal cord augmentation and in applications previously reserved for injectable collagen. Other similar materials, such as acellular porcine small intestine submucosa (Surgisis, Cook Surgical, Bloomington, IL), have met with similar success to Alloderm in experimental models.

CONCLUSIONS

The intrinsic complex molecular mechanisms involved in wound healing, the external factors that augment or impede healing, and the effect of the implantation of material for augmentation all play important roles in the final appearance of facial surgical procedures. Extensive knowledge of these factors is imperative when considering the surgical management of facial defects. Many materials are available to the surgeon and the appropriate selection may make the difference between an acceptable result and an exceptional result. Newer implantable materials and treatments to promote organized wound healing promise improved aesthetic results in the hands of skilled surgeons. Only through further basic science and clinical research will this vital aspect of plastic surgery continue to advance at a rapid pace.

REFERENCES

1. Goslen JB. Wound healing for dematologic surgeons. J Dermatol Surg Oncol 1988; 14(4):959–972.
2. Kanzler MH, Gorsulowsky DE, Swanson NA. Basic mechanisms in the healing cutaneous wound. J Dermatol Surg Oncol 1986; 12:1156–1164.
3. Kirsner RS, Eaglstein WH. The wound healing process. Dermatol Clin 1993; 11(4):629–640.
4. Pollack SV. Wound healing, a review, the biology of wound healing. J Dermatol Surg Oncol 1979; 5:389–393.
5. Schaffer CJ, Narrey LB. Cell biology of wound healing. Int Rev Cytol 1996; 169:151–181.
6. Wahl LM, Wahl SM. Inflammation. In: Cohen IK, Diegelman RF, Lindblad WJ, ed. Wound Healing Biochemistry and Clinical Aspects. Philadelphia: WB Saunders, 1992.

7. Witte MB, Barbul A. General principles of wound healing. Surg Clin North Am 1997; 77:509–552.
8. Santaro SA. Identification of a 160,000 dalton platelet membrane protein that mediates the divalent cation-dependent adhesion of platelets to collagen. Cell 1986; 46:913–920.
9. Lawrence WT, Diegelmann RF. Cytokines and antagonist wound healing. In: Sugarman HJ, Demaria EJ, eds. Cytokines in Trauma Hemorrhage, Austin, TX: RG Landers Co., 1997.
10. Grinnell F. Fibronectin and wound healing. Am J Dermatopathol 1982; 4:185.
11. Wikner NE, Persichitte KA, Baskin JB et al. Transforming growth factor-beta stimulates the expression of fibronectin by human keratinocytes. J Invest Dermatol 1988; 91(3):207–212.
12. Diegelmann RF, Cohen IK, Kaplan AM. The role of macrophages in wound repair: a review. Plast Reconstr Surg 1981; 68(1):107–113.
13. Van Winkle W, Hastings JC, Barker E, et al. Role of the fibroblast in controlling rate and extent of repair in wounds of various tissues. In: Kulonen E, Pikkarainen J, eds. Biology of Fibroblast, New York: Academic Press, 1973.
14. Ross R, Bendit EP. Wound healing and collagen formation I, Sequential changes in components in guinea pig skin wounds observed in the electron microscope. J Biophys Biochem Cytol 1961; 11:677.
15. Bailey AJ, Bazin S, Delawney A. Changes in the nature of collagen during development and resorption of granulation tissue. Biochem Biophys Acta 1973; 328:383–390.
16. Mayno G. The story of myofibroblasts. Am J Surg Pathol 1979; 3:535.
17. Pierce GF, Mustoe TA, Altrach BW, et al. Role of platelet-derived growth factor in wound healing. J Cell Biochem 1991; 45:319–326.
18. Finch PW, Rubin JS, Miki T, et al. Human KGF is FGF-related with properties of a paracrine effector of epithelial cell growth. Science 1989; 245(4919):752–755.
19. O'Keefe EJ, Chiu ML. Stimulation of thymidine incorporation in keratinocytes by insulin, epidermal growth factor, and placental extract: comparison with cell number to assess growth. J Invest Dermatol 1988; 90(1):2–7.
20. Eisinger M, Sadan S, Silver IA, et al. Growth regulation of skin cells by epidermal cell-derived factors: implications for wound healing. Proc Natl Acad Sci USA 1988; 85(6):1937–1941.
21. Laato M, Niinikoski, Lundberg C et al. Effect of epidermal growth factor (EGF) on experimental granulation tissue. J Surg Res 1986; 41(3):252–255.
22. Grottendorst GR. Chemoattractants and growth factors. Choen IK, Diegelmann RF, Lindblad WJ, ed. Wound Healing: Biochemical and Clinical Aspects. Philadelphia: WB Saunders, 1992.
23. Bennett NT, Schultz GS. Growth factors and wound healing: part II, role in normal and chronic wound healing. Am J Surg 1993; 166:74–81.
24. Greenhalgh DG. Role of growth factors in wound healing. J Trauma 1996; 41:159–167.
25. Kiritsy CP, Lynch AB, Lynch SE. Role of growth factors in cutaneous healing: a review. Crit Rev Ora Biol Med 1993; 4:729–760.
26. Knighton DR, Ciresi K, Fiegel VD. Stimulation of repair in chronic non-healing cutaneous ulcers using platelet-derived wound healing formula. Surg Gynecol Obstet 1990; 170:56–60.
27. Lynch SE, Nixon JC, Colvin RB et al. Role of platelet-derived growth factor in wound healing: synergistic effects with other growth factors. Proc Natl Acad Sci USA 1987; 84(21):7696–7700.
28. Varga J, Jiminez SA. Stimulation of normal human fibroblast collagen production and processing by transforming growth factor-beta. Biochem Biophys Res Commun 1986; 138:974–980.
29. Steed DL. Role of growth factors in wound healing. Surg Clin North Am 1997; 77:577–585.

30. Dzubow LM, Halpern AC, Leyden JJ, Grossman D, McGinley KJ. Comparison of preoperative skin preparations for the face. J Am Acad Dermatol 1988; Oct; 19(4) 737–741.
31. Branemark PI, Ekholm R. Tissue injury caused by wound disinfectants. J Bone Joint Surg Am 1967; 49(1):48–62.
32. Brennan SS, Leaper DJ. The effect of antiseptics on the healing wound: a study using the rabbit ear chamber. Br J Surg 1985; 72(10):780–782.
33. Custer J. Studies in the management of contaminated wounds: an assessment of the effectiveness of pHisohex and betadine surgical scrub solution. Am J Surg 1971; 121: 572–575.
34. Goldenheim PD. An appraisal of povidine–iodine and wound healing. Postgrad Med J 1993; 69Suppl(3):97–105.
35. Chvapil M, Koopmann CF. Age and other factors regulating wound healing. Otolaryngol Clin North Am 1982; 15(2):259–270.
36. Ferguson MK. The effect of antineoplastic agents on wound healing. Surg Gynecol Obstet 1982; 154(3):421–429.
37. Pollack SV. Wound healing: a review IV, systemic medications affecting wound healing. J Dermatol Surg Oncol 1982; 8(8):667–672.
38. Bailey AJ, Bazin S, Sims TJ et al. Characterization of the collagen of human hypertrophic and normal scars. Biochem Biophys Acta 1975; 405(2):412–421.
39. Murray JC, Pollack SV, Pinnell SR. Keloids: a review. J Am Acad Dermatol 1981; 4(4):461–470.
40. Kischer CW, Shetlar MR, Chvapil M. Hypertrophic scars and keloids: a review and new concept concerning their origin. Scan Electron Microsc 1982; (pt 4):1699–1713.
41. Savage K, Swann DA. A comparison of glycosaminoglycan synthesis by human fibroblasts from normal skin, normal scar, and hypertrophic scar. J Invest Dermatol 1985; 84(6):521–526.
42. Abergel RP, Pizzuro D, Meeker CA, et al. Biochemical composition of the connective tissue in keloids and analysis of collagen metabolism in keloid fibroblast cultures. J Invest Dermatol 1985; 84(5):384–390.
43. Berman B, Bieley HC. Adjunct therapy to surgical management of keloids. Dermatol Surg 1996; 22:126–130.
44. Ahn ST, Monafo WW, Mustoe TA. Topical silicone gel for the prevention and treatment of hypertrophic scar. Arch Surg 1991; 126:499–504.
45. Lawrence WT. In search of the optimal treatment of keloids: report of a series and a review of the literature. Ann Plast Surg 1991; 27:164–178.
46. Szahowicz EH. Facial bone wound healing, an overview. Otolaryngol Clin North Am 1995; 28:865–880.
47. White AA 3rd, Panjabi MM, Southwick WO et al. The four biomechanical stages of fracture repair. J Bone Joint Surg Am 1977; 59(2):188–192.
48. Sandberg M, Aro H, Multimaki P, et al. In situ localization of collagen production by chondrocytes and osteoblasts in fracture callus. J Bone Joint Surg 1989; 71A:69–77.
49. Ashurst DE. The influence of mechanical conditions on the healing of experimental fractures in the rabbit: a microscopic study. Trans R Soc Lond B 1986; 313:271–302.
50. Livesy S, Herndon D, Hollyoak M, et al. Transplanted acellular allograft dermal matrix: Potential as a template for the reconstruction of viable dermis. Transplantation 1995; 60:1–9.
51. LaTrenta GS, McCarthy JG, Breitbart AS, et al. The role of rigid skeletal fixation in bone-graft augmentation of the craniofacial skelton. Plast Reconstr Surg 1989; 84(4):578–588.
52. Hobar PC. Implantation: bone, cartilage, and allografts. Sel Read Plast Surg 1992; 7: 1–2.

53. Kirker-Head CA, Herhart TN, Schelling SH, et al. Long term healing of bone using recombinant human bone morphogenetic protein 2. Clin Orthop 1995; 318:222–230.
54. Zins JE, Kisiak JF, Whitaker LA, et al. The influence of recipient site on bone grafts to the face. Plast Reconstr Surg 1984; 73:371–379.
55. Smith JF, Abramson M. Membranous vs. endochondral bone autografts. Arch Otolaryngol 1974; 99:203–205.
56. Zins JE, Whitaker LA. Membranous versus endochondrial bone: implications for craniofacial reconstruction. Plast Reconstr Surg 1983; 72:778–785.
57. Kobayashi K, Agarwal K, Jackson IT, et al. The effect of insulin-like growth factor 1 on craniofacial bone healing. Plast Reconstr Surg 1996; 97:1129–1135.
58. Rudolph R. Inhibition of myofibroblasts by skin grafts. Plast Reconstr Surg 1979; 63:473–480.
59. Winter GD. Formation of the scab and the rate of epithelialization of superficial wounds in the skin of the young domestic pig. Nature 1962; 193:293.
60. Brown CD, Zitelli JA. Choice of wound dressings and ointments. Otolaryngol Clin North Am 1995; 28:1081–1091.
61. Hanna JR, Giacopelli JA. A review of wound healing and wound dressing products. J Foot Ankle Surg 1997; 36(1):2–14.
62. Lotti T, Gasperini S, Rodofili C. Should we use occlusive dressings in the treatment of acute wounds. Int J Dermatol 1997; 36:97–99.
63. Hinman CD, Maibach H. Effect of air exposure and occlusion on experimental human skin wounds. Nature 1963; 200:377.
64. Eaglstein WH. Experiences with biosynthetic dressings. J Am Acad Dermatol 1985; 12(2):434–440.
65. Geronemus RG, Mertz PM, Eaglstein WH. Wound healing: the effects of topical antimicrobial agents. Arch Dermatol 1979; 115(11):1311–1314.
66. Sutow EJ, Pollack SR. The biocompatability of certain stainless steels. In Williams DF, ed. Biocompatability of clinical implant materials, vol 1. Boca Raton, Fla: CRC Press, 1981.
67. Fuleihan NS. Facial implants. In: Cummings CW, Fredrickson JM, Harker LA et al, eds. Otolaryngology Head and Neck Surgery. St. Louis: Mosby, 1998.
68. Kartush JM, Linstrom CJ, McCann PM et al. Early gold weight eyelid implantation for facial paralysis. Otolaryngol Head Neck Surg 1990; 103(6):1016–1023.
69. May M. Gold weight and wire spring implants as an alternative to tarsorrhaphy. Arch Otolaryngol Head Neck Surg 1987; 113(6):656–660.
70. Quatela, VC. Synthetic Implants. In Papel ID, Nachlas NE, eds. Facial Plastic and Reconstructive Surgery. St Louis: Mosbys-Year Book 1992.
71. Rees TD, Balantyne DL Jr, Hawthorne GA. Silicone fluid research: a follow-up summary. Plast Reconstr Surg 1970; 46(1):50–56.
72. Lin KY, Barlett SP, Yaremchuk MJ et al. The effect of rigid fixation on the survival of onlay bone grafts: an experimental study. Plast Reconstr Surg 1990; 86:449–459.
73. Frisch EE, Langley NR. Biodurability of medical-grade high performance silicone elastomer. In: Fraker AC, Griffin CD, eds. Corrosion and degradation of implant materials: Second symposium ASTM, STP859, Philadelphia, 1985, American Society for Testing and Materials.
74. Davis PK, Jones SM. The complications of sialastic implants: experience with 137 cases. Br J Plast Surg 1971; 24(4):405–411.
75. Schultz RC. Reconstruction of facial deformities using silicones and acrylics. Rubin LR, ed. 1 ed. Biomaterials in reconstructive surgery. St Louis: CV Mosby Co, 1983.
76. Silver FH, Maas CS. Biology of synthetic facial implant materials. Facial Plast Surg Clin North Am 1994; 2(3):241–253.

77. Romo T, Foster CA, Korovin GS. Aesthetic reconstruction of the platyrrhine nose. 1 ed. Plastic and Reconstructive Surgery of the Head and Neck. Philadelphia: BC Decker, 1991.
78. Kent JN, Misiek DJ. Biomaterials for cranial, facial, mandibular, amd TMJ reconstruction. In Fonesca RJ, Walker RV, ed. Oral and maxillofacial trauma. Philadelphia: WB Saunders, 1991.
79. Kasperbauer JL, Kern EB, Neel HB. Grafts and implants in rhinologic surgery: laboratory findings and clinical considerations. Facial Plast Surg 1983; 3:125.
80. Owsley TG, Taylor CO. The use of Gortex for nasal reconstruction: a retrospective study using 106 patients. Plast Reconstr Surg 1994; 94(2):241–248.
81. Beekhuis GJ. Augmentation mentoplasty with polyamide mesh: update. Arch Otolaryngol 1984; 110(6):364–367.
82. Beekhuis GJ, Colton JJ. Nasal tip support. Arch Otolaryngol Head Neck Surg 1986; 112(7):726–728.
83. Grower MF. Bone inductive potential of biodegradable ceramic Millipore filter chambers. J Dent Res 1978; 57:108.
84. Byrd HS, Hobar PC, Shewmake K. Augmentation of the craniofacial skelton with porous hydroxyapatite granules. Plast Reconstr Surg 1993; 91(1):15–22.
85. McCollough EG, Weil C. Augmentation of facial defects using Mersiline mesh implants. Otolaryngol Head Neck Surg 1979; 87(4):515–521.
86. Adams BJS, Feurstein SS. Looking under the epidermis: a histologic study of implants. In plastic and reconstructive surgery of the head and neck. St Louis: CV Mosby, 1984.
87. Ohgushi H, Okumura M, Yoshikawa T et al. Bone formation process in porous calcium carbonate and hydroxyapatite. J Biomed Mater Res 1992; 26(7):885–895.
88. Cranin AN, Sher J, Shpuntoff R. Reconstruction of the endentulous mandible with a lower border graft and subperiosteal implant. J Oral Maxillofacial Surg 1988; 46(4): 264–268.
89. Kent JN, Quinn JH, Zide MF, et al. Correction of alveolar ridge deficiencies with nonresorbable hydroxylapatite. J Am Dent Assoc 1982; 105(6):993–1001.
90. Costantino PD, Freidman CD, Lane A. Synthetic biomaterial in facial plasticsurgery. Facial Plast Surg 1993; 9(1):1–15.
91. Terino EO. Alloderm acellular dermal graft: applications in aesthetic soft-tissue augmentation. Clin Plast Surg 2001; 28(1):83–99.

4
Management of Skin Neoplasms

Carlos Garcia
Oklahoma University Health Science Center, Oklahoma City, Oklahoma, U.S.A.

Robert E. Clark
Cary Skin Center, Cary, North Carolina, U.S.A.

This chapter provides the cutaneous surgeon with an up-to-date, practical approach to skin neoplasms to encourage organized thinking from the time of initial contact with the patient to the selection and execution of the most appropriate therapy. This is not a exhaustive review. Many entities for which surgery is not indicated have not been included (i.e., cutaneous lymphomas) and from each group of neoplasms only the most frequent were selected. Both benign and malignant tumors will be described, but emphasis is placed in those most likely to be found in clinical practice. Rare tumors are only briefly mentioned for the sake of completeness.

BENIGN TUMORS OF THE SKIN

Benign tumors (Table 1) are extremely common but an accurate estimate of their true incidence is impossible because most patients seek medical attention only after symptoms appear, or when a long-standing lesion undergoes noticeable change in size or color. The majority of benign cutaneous tumors present nonspecifically and preoperative diagnosis is difficult. Lesions may appear as papules, nodules, or plaques varying in size from a few millimeters to several centimeters. They can be single or multiple and may involve any body part. Color ranges from various tones of red, pink, or blue to skin-colored. Genetic influences must be suspected when tumors are multiple and symmetrically distributed on the face, scalp or trunk.

Treatment of benign skin tumors is usually requested for cosmetic reasons, fear of having a skin cancer, or, less frequently, because a concerned parent or spouse brings the patient for evaluation. Diagnosis of benign skin neoplasias is based on clinical identification and histological confirmation. Scaling, ulceration, and hyperkeratosis indicate epidermal involvement. Dermal tumors are characterized by induration and plaque formation. Some tumors may be painful on pressure, the most characteristic of these being leiomyoma, endometrioma, neuroma, dermatofibroma, angiolipoma, neurilemmoma, eccrine spiradenoma, granular cell tumor, and glomus tumor (the mnemonic is LEND AN EGG) (1).

Table 1 Benign Tumors of the Skin

- Nevi
  1. Melanocytic Nevi
     - Junctional
     - Compound
     - Intradermal
     - Atypical
     - Congenital Melanocytic
     - Halo
     - Nevus Spilus
     - Blue
     - Mongolian blue spot
     - Nevus of Ota and Ito
     - Spitz
  2. Nevus verrucosus
  3. Becker's nevus
  4. Sebaceous nevus
  5. Comedo nevus
  6. Nevus lipomatosous superficialis
  7. Connective tissue nevus
- Skin tags
- Seborrheic keratoses
- Actinic keratoses
- Dermatofibromas
- Keloid scars
- Adnexal tumors
  1. Hair differentiation
     - Trichoepithelioma
     - Trichofolliculoma
     - Trichillemoma
     - Pilomatrixoma
  2. Eccrine differentiation
     - Eccrine hidrocystoma
     - Syringoma
     - Eccrine poroma
     - Eccrine spiradenoma
     - Clear cell hidradenoma
     - Chondroid syringoma
  3. Apocrine differentiation
     - Apocrine hidrocystoma
     - Syringocystadenoma papilliferum
     - Hidradenoma papilliferum
     - Cylindroma
  4. Sebaceous differentiation
     - Sebaceous hyperplasia
     - Sebaceous adenoma
- Cutaneous cysts
  - Epidermoid
  - Milia

(Continued)

Table 1 (Continued)

Pilar
Dermoid
Steatocystoma Multiplex
Oral Mucous
Mucous cyst of the Fingers
Bronchogenic and Thyroglossal duct cysts
Vascular tumors
1. Congenital hemangiomas
Nevus flammeus
Capillary hemangioma
Cavernous hemangioma
2. Angiokeratomas
Angiokeratoma circumscriptum
Angiokeratoma Mibelli
3. Pyogenic granuloma
4. Glomus tumor
5. Lymphangioma
Lipoma
Neurofibroma
Granular cell tumor
Leiomyoma

Benign neoplasms are recognized by their nonaggressive clinical behavior and lack of local tissue destruction. On histological examination they are identifiable by architectural order in the arrangement of cellular nuclei, uniformity in size and shape of nuclei, a controlled ratio of growth, a low number of normal mitoses, and absence of metastases (2).

For most tumors, the initial diagnostic biopsy is also therapeutic. To ensure suitable specimens consisting of epidermal and dermal elements along with subcutaneous fat, we recommend excisional biopsies over shave biopsies because the latter are too superficial. This is particularly relevant in cases of pigmented lesions when melanoma is part of the differential diagnosis. However, if the lesion is larger than 2 cm or is located on the face, genitals, or digits, an incisional or punch biopsy is advisable to document the diagnosis prior to therapeutic excision.

Nevi

Nevi are lesions usually present at birth and are composed of mature or nearly mature structures. The term is more often applied in the literature to melanocytic nevi, which are benign proliferations of nevomelanocytes. Hamartoma is the appropriate term to describe nevi without nevus cells.

Melanocytic Nevi

Melanocytic nevi are benign collections of nevus cells, which are identical to melanocytes but arranged in clusters or nests. They present clinically as flat, pedunculated, dome-shaped, or papillomatous lesions with variable pigmentation. These tumors are extremely common and everyone has such blemishes, sometimes in profusion. They are commonly referred to as moles, usually develop during infancy and adolescence, and tend to disappear in middle age.

On histological examination, nevus cells have a variable appearance and sometimes the diagnosis is based on the observation of their gathering in clusters. Individual cells are cuboidal or oval, with homogeneous cytoplasm and a large or oval nucleus. Frequently they contain melanin. Deeper into the dermis, nevus cells resemble fibroblasts since they are elongated and posses a spindle-shaped nucleus.

Junctional nevi represent the earliest stage of development. The clusters of nevus cells are localized to the lower epidermis. On clinical examination they are either flat or slightly raised, and have a single color or are two-toned. In contrast to malignant melanoma, the pigment within the lesion is uniform. The surface is usually smooth and the skin creases preserved. The shape is oval or round, and size is variable but usually ranges from 6 to 10 mm.

Compound nevi represent a later stage of development with the nevus cells distributed in both the lower epidermis and superficial dermis. They are slightly to moderately raised, round, smooth or warty, sharply defined, and two-toned (Fig. 1). Some may grow coarse hairs on the surface.

Intradermal nevi tend to be flesh-colored because most cells containing pigment are situated deep in the dermis. Lesions are dome-shaped and may have telangiectasias on the surface. On histological examination the junctional component is lost, which leaves an entirely intradermal lesion. Nevus cells become progressively

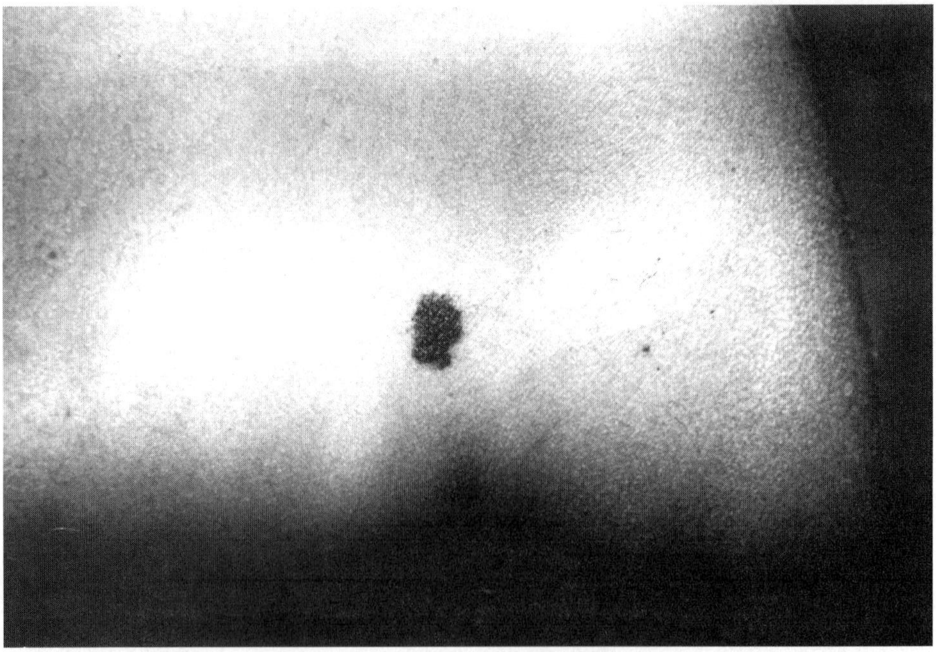

Figure 1 Compound melanocytic nevus of the lower midback. Lesion is small, slightly elevated, with well-demarcated borders and even pigmentation.

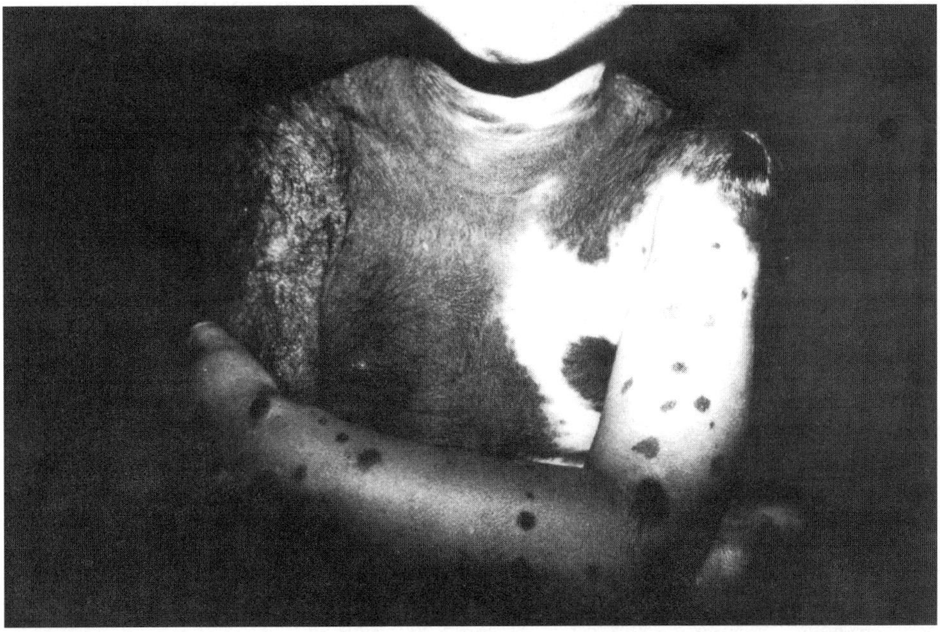

Figure 2 Giant bathing trunk nevus with extensive involvement of trunk and extremities. This variety of compund melanocytic nevus carries a significant risk for melanoma during infancy.

smaller with darkly staining nuclei and little cytoplasm. They may adopt a spindle cell form and frequently show what are termed neural features.

Atypical nevi or dysplastic nevi (3) are larger than their normal acquired melanocytic counterparts, ranging in size from 5 to 15 mm. They show various tones of tan, brown, black, and pink and characteristically there is a central palpable elevation. Atypical nevi continue to appear throughout life and are considered a marker and a risk factor for malignant melanoma. On histological examination these are compound nevi with atypical individual cells and nests.

Congenital melanocytic nevi (CMN) are present at birth. They affect approximately 1% of newborns and persist throughout life (4). They are usually larger than 1 cm, round to oval in shape, and elevated from surrounding skin. The surface may be smooth or warty and frequently hairy. Color ranges from light tan to dark brown with the darker portion located in the center of the lesion. The so-called giant bathing trunk nevus is a CMN covering one or several body segments (Fig. 2). On histological examination, CMN are either compound or intradermal nevi but extend deeper into the dermis and subcutaneous fat. The nevus cells involve sebaceous glands, hair follicles, arrector pili muscles, and eccrine glands. In general, CMN smaller than 10 cm have a 1% chance of malignant transformation, whereas lesions larger than 10 cm have a 6% chance.

Halo nevus (Sutton's nevus) is a melanocytic nevus surrounded by an area of complete depigmentation (5). It is thought to be an autoimmune phenomenon because patients have detectable antibodies against melanocytes (Fig. 3). Lesions are single or multiple and are completely benign. There is an association with other

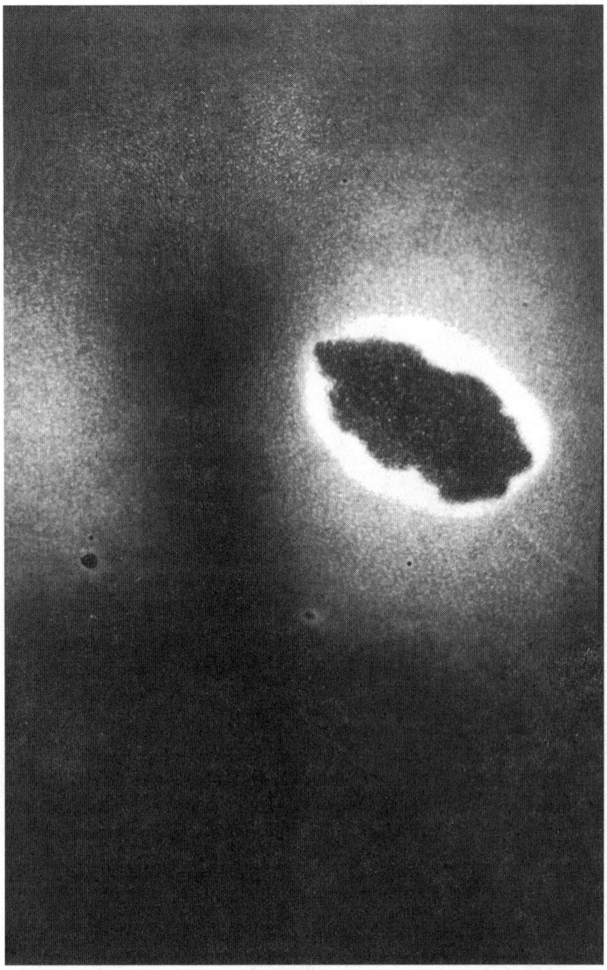

Figure 3 Halo nevus consists of a characteristic depigmented ring around a congenital melanocytic nevus.

autoimmune disorders, particularly vitiligo. On histological examination, halo nevi represent compound melanocytic nevi. There is a marked inflammatory infiltrate surrounding the lesion with progressive destruction of pigmented cells.

Nevus spilus (6) is an acquired lesion characterized by a macular background with a raised and darker component within it. It has been associated with neurofibromatosis. On histological examination the lesion is characterized by epidermal lentiginous hyperplasia in association with a junctional or compound nevus.

Blue nevus (7) represents a failure of melanocytes migrating from the neural crest to arrive at the dermal–epidermal junction. Lesions appear as round to oval blue papules with a smooth surface. The melanocytes are found in the lower dermis and the refraction of light at this level results in the blue appearance (Tyndall's effect). On histological examination there are heavily pigmented spindle-shaped melanocytes arranged in fascicles in the dermis.

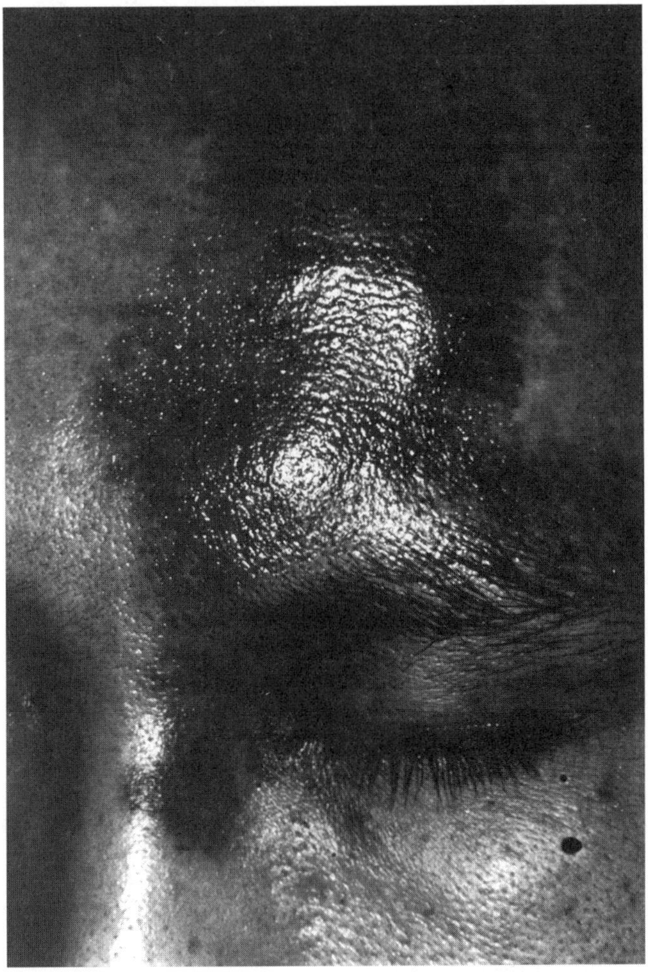

Figure 4 Nevus of Ota involving the left forehead, eyebrow, eyelid, and inner canthus. The lesion is blue, congenital, and permanent.

Mongolian blue spots (8) also represent a migratory arrest of melanocytes. They appear as extensive blue macules over the buttocks and sacrum. Asian, Latin American, and African-American newborns are more susceptible. Lesions tend to disappear with time and there is no risk of malignant transformation. There are elongated dendrytic melanocytes in the reticular dermis on histological examination.

Nevus of Ota and Ito (9) is a permanent blue macule indistinguishable from the Mongolian blue spot. Nevus of Ota occurs in the face on the area supplied by the ophthalmic and maxillary divisions of the trigeminal nerve (Fig. 4). Nevus of Ito affects the shoulder in an area supplied by the posterior supraclavicular and lateral brachial cutaneous nerves. Both are more frequent in Japanese patients. They are identical histologically to the Mongolian blue spot.

Spitz nevi (juvenile melanoma) are uncommon but important because they may create confusion with malignant melanoma (10). The lesions are usually solitary smooth-papules or nodules that often involve the face. They are dome-shaped and red to brown in color. Their size is variable but usually less than 1 cm. In contrast to melanoma, Spitz nevi typically affect children and adolescents. On histological examination the cells are epithelioid or, more commonly, spindle-shaped with abundant eosinophilic cytoplasm and large but typically uniform nuclei. Mononuclear and multinucleate giant cells may be present. The deeper aspect of the lesion shows evidence of maturation, as would be expected in a benign compound nevus. In approximately 60% of cases there are eosinophilic globules in the epidermis (Kamino bodies). In addition, the lack of atypical mitoses, and the evident maturation towards deeper parts of the tumor, help to differentiate a Spitz nevus from melanoma.

Management of Melanocytic Nevi

Junctional, compound, and intradermal nevi have negligible malignant potential and surgical excision is indicated only for cosmetic or diagnostic reasons. Congenital melanocytic nevi larger than 10 cm must be excised because they have a 6% chance of malignant transformation. Dysplastic nevi must be excised to rule out melanoma. Nevus of Ota is best treated with lasers (11). Both the alexandrite (755 nm) and Q-switched ruby laser (694 nm) are effective but require multiple sessions given 8 weeks apart.

Other Cutaneous Nevi or Hamartomas

Nevus Verrucosus (12) appears at birth as a well-defined, raised, and verrucous plaque (Fig. 5). It may be unilateral (nevus unis lateralis) or bilateral, extensive, and

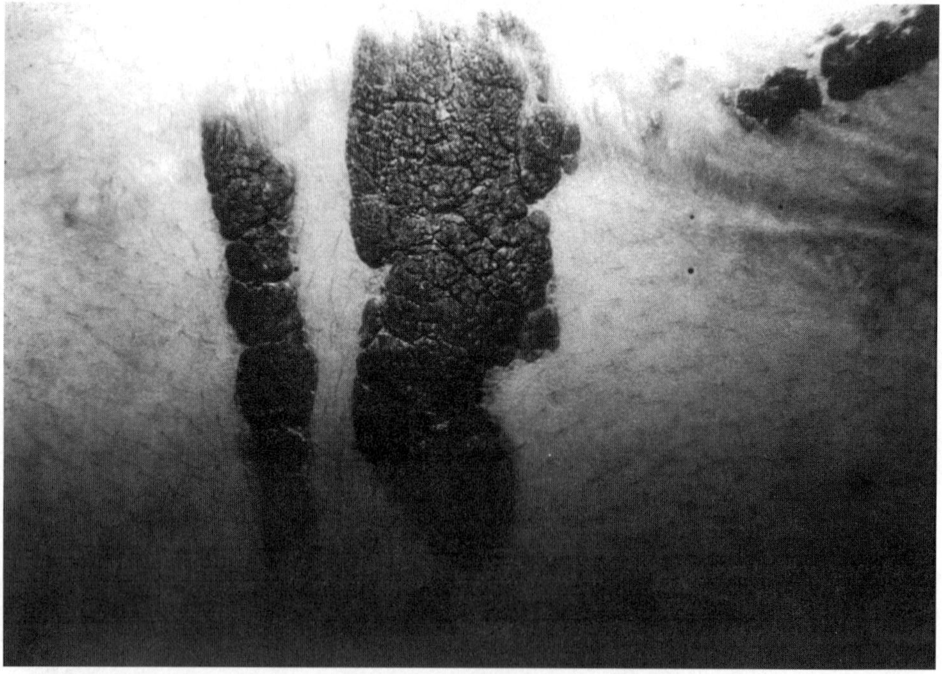

Figure 5 Nevus verrucosus of the midanterior trunk. The lesion is a congenital, verrucous, and hyperpigmented plaque with linear arrangement.

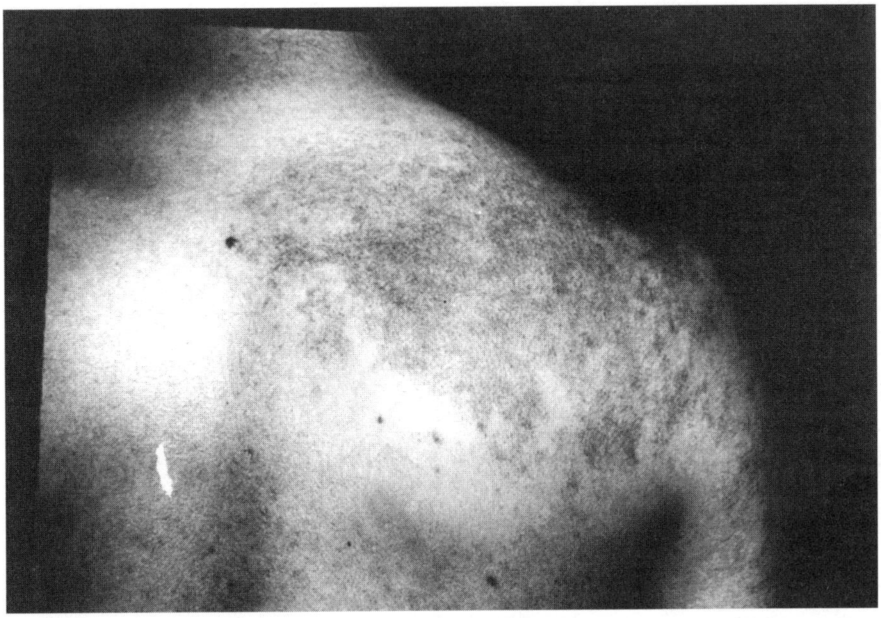

Figure 6 Becker's nevus of the right shoulder. The lesion is hyperpigmented, appears during adolescence, and may become thick and hairy.

frequently associated with skeletal or central nervous system (CNS) abnormalities (ichthyosis hystrix). Occasionally, an inflammatory component may be present in association with linear epidermal nevi (inflammatory linear verrucous epidermal nevus [ILVEN]. The histological appearance is characterized by squamous papillomata showing hyperkeratosis, papillomatosis, and acanthosis.

Becker's nevus (BN) appears during adolescence, is flat initially, but may become raised (13). It is pigmented and subsequently grows thick, coarse hairs. BN is more common in male patients and although the chest, shoulder, and upper arms are the usual sites of involvement, it may arise anywhere (Fig. 6). An association with other developmental abnormalities (spina bifida), multiple lesions, and familial cases have been noted. Histological examination shows mild hyperkeratosis, focal acanthosis, and a slight increase in the granular cell layer. There is a marked pigmentation of the basal layer associated with increased number of melanocytes and pigmentary incontinence. A common finding is the presence of abundant smooth muscle bundles in the dermis.

Sebaceous nevus is a congenital lesion that originates in the sebaceous glands. The tumor is a hairless yellowish plaque of variable size and warty surface. Most commonly, it affects the scalp as a solitary lesion. Sebaceous nevus is an androgen-dependent tumor, which enlarges at puberty synchronous with the rest of the sebaceous glands. It is medically important because a significant number of cases may transform into syringocystadenoma papilliferum (14) or basal cell carcinoma. On histological examination the tumor is characterized by acanthosis and papillomatosis. Sebaceous glands are increased in numbers and are situated abnormally high in the dermis. There may be abundant cysts and the hair follicles are reduced in number or absent.

Comedo nevus (15) presents as numerous keratin-filled pits (blackheads). Most commonly, the lesion develops during childhood, although some cases may be present at birth. The most frequent location is the face but it can occur on the neck, extremities, or trunk. Tumors are single or multiple, and may be arranged in linear fashion. Histological examination shows an atrophic epidermis with numerous cystically dilated hair follicles.

Nevus lipomatosus superficialis is characterized by dermal deposits of mature fatty tissue. The lesions are soft cerebriform papules and plaques, usually located on the thighs, back, or buttocks of children. Nevus lipomatosus superficialis can be present at birth or develop during the first two decades of life. Histological examination shows mature fat cells within the superficial dermis.

Connective tissue nevus (16) is a benign collection of dermal collagen and elastic fibers. The lesions are firm, smooth nodules and plaques located on the back, thighs, and buttocks. They are skin-colored and of various sizes. Tumors appear during the second decade of life and may be associated with hypertension and cardiomyopathy. Connective tissue nevi may also be present in patients with tuberous sclerosis (angiofibromas of the nose, mental retardation, seizures) and the Buschke-Ollendorf syndrome (asymptomatic, irregular, radiopaque lesions situated especially in the long bones, pelvis, hands, and feet). The characteristic histopathological change is a marked increase in dermal collagen.

Management of Nonmelanocytic Nevi

The nevi may be surgically excised for diagnostic or cosmetic purposes.

Skin Tags

Skin tags are small, pedunculated, soft papules with variable pigmentation. They usually affect the neck, groin, and axillae, and tend to increase in number with advancing age. On histopathological examination, there is a mature keratinizing squamous epithelium, which overlies a fibrovascular core.

Skin tags are usually excised for cosmetic reasons. Scissor excision is adequate for most lesions. Cryotherapy or electrodesiccation is a valid alternative.

Seborrheic Keratoses

Seborrheic keratoses (SK) are benign proliferations of epidermal cells. They are extremely common in the elderly and consist of well-defined, raised papules or plaques with rough warty surface. A characteristic feature of SK is that they seem to be stuck onto the skin (Fig. 7). Color varies from skin-colored to brown or black. Dermatosis papulosa nigra is a variant that occurs in African-Americans, mostly on the face. Lesions are small, black, and multiple. On histological examination, there is hyperkeratosis, acanthosis, papillomatosis, and cyst formation.

Cryotherapy with liquid nitrogen is highly effective (17). Inflammation and redness are evident immediately, and the lesion sloughs off in approximately 2 weeks.

Curettage and electrodesiccation are also effective but require local anesthesia.

Laser therapy (Ultrapulse CO_2 or erbium) is an elegant but expensive modality to treat multiple SK.

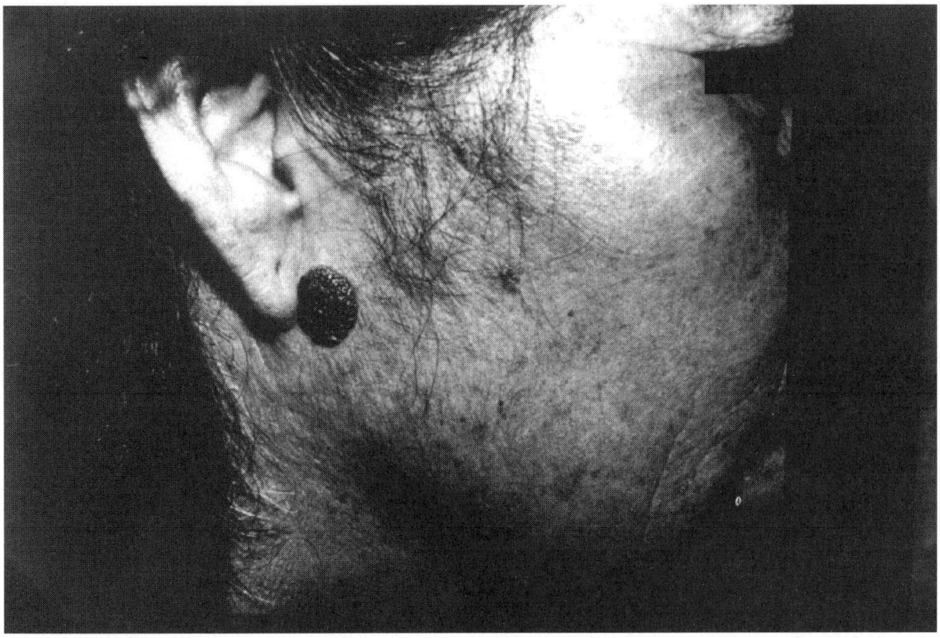

Figure 7 Seborrheic keratosis shows a verrucous hyperpigmented surface with characteristic stuck-on appearance.

Actinic Keratoses

Actinic keratoses (AK) are premalignant skin lesions occurring in sun-damaged skin. They appear clinically as erythematous papules with a rough scaly surface (18). Early lesions may be felt more than seen. Most commonly, AK affect the exposed skin of the face and upper extremities. The cheeks, forehead, and dorsum of hands are frequent locations (Fig. 8). The lower lip (actinic cheilitis) and, in balding men, the scalp are also involved. Lesions are multiple and develop gradually over the years. Most tend to become thicker (hypertrophic AK). The rate of malignant transformation for each individual AK is approximately 5%, but in patients with multiple lesions the risk is over 20%. On histopathological examination the most characteristic findings are variable degrees of focal epidermal displasia with overlying parakeratosis and crowding of basal cells. The dermis shows solar elastosis.

Cryotherapy with liquid nitrogen may be the treatment of choice. It is effective, quick, inexpensive, and widely available (19). Two freezing cycles of 10 s each are usually sufficient for each lesion, although, hypertrophic AKs require longer cycles.

Topical 5-fluorouracil (5-FU) (an antimetabolite that blocks the incorporation of thymidine into DNA) is also effective. The usual regimen involves twice-daily applications and a topical steroid is prescribed to decrease the inflammatory reaction, which in some patients is quite severe. Another option involves application of topical 5-FU in the morning and night in combination with topical tretinoin (Retin A) at midday for 4 weeks.

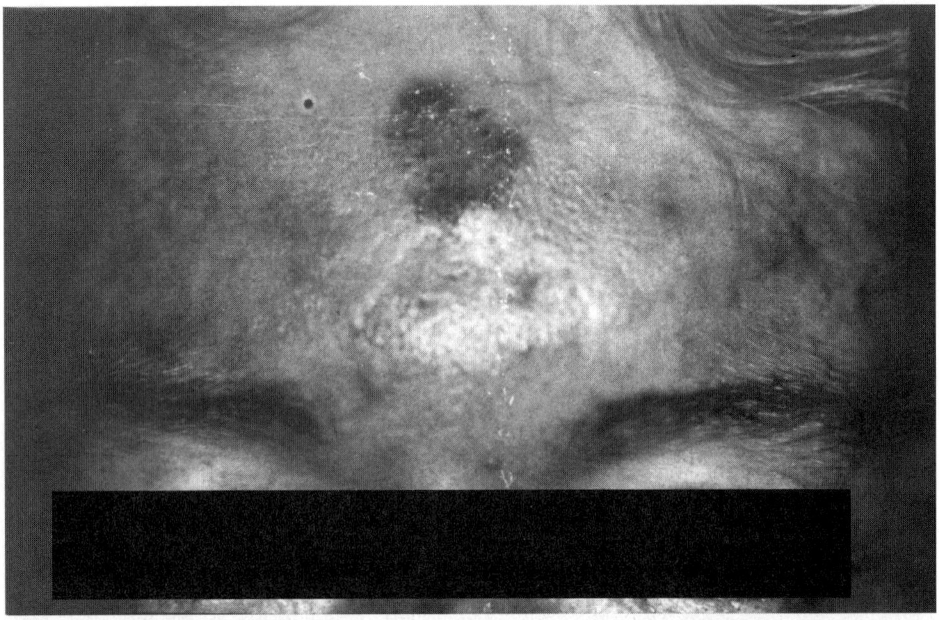

Figure 8 Actinic keratoses on the forehead of an albino female patient. The lesions are red with a rough scaly surface.

Medium-depth chemical peel is indicated for multiple lesions and extensive solar damage. We prefer glycolic acid 70% for 2 min followed by trichloroacetic acid (TCA) 30% until mild frosting; or Jessner's solution (resorcinol 14 g, salicylic acid 14 g, lactic acid 14 g) followed by TCA 35%. Treatment is done under local anesthesia, peeling occurs at 4 days, and complete recovery is usually seen at 7 days.

Dermabrasion and ultrapulse CO_2 laser therapy yield similar results to chemical peel. The latter is the treatment of choice for actinic cheilitis.

Curettage and electrodesiccation are the preferred modalities for hypertrophic AKs because these are the only modalities that provide a histological specimen to allow one to rule out squamous cell carcinoma.

Dermatofibroma

Dermatofibroma (DF) is a reactive proliferation of fibroblasts, histiocytes, and endothelial cells, probably occurring in response to a remote insect bite (20). Lesions are firm, round to oval, from 3 mm to 3 cm, hyperpigmented, and with a smooth surface (Fig. 9). DF may be single or multiple and affect any body site, although the leg is the most frequent location. Pain is a variable feature. Histological examination shows interlacing fascicles of spindle cells, foamy histiocytes, and variable multinucleated giant cells. An important feature that differentiates DF from malignant fusiform tumors is the lack of nuclear pleomorphism, necrosis, or mitotic activity.

DF has no malignant potential, therefore, treatment is not necessary (21). Surgical excision is the treatment of choice for painful tumors, for cosmetic reasons, or to rule out malignant melanoma.

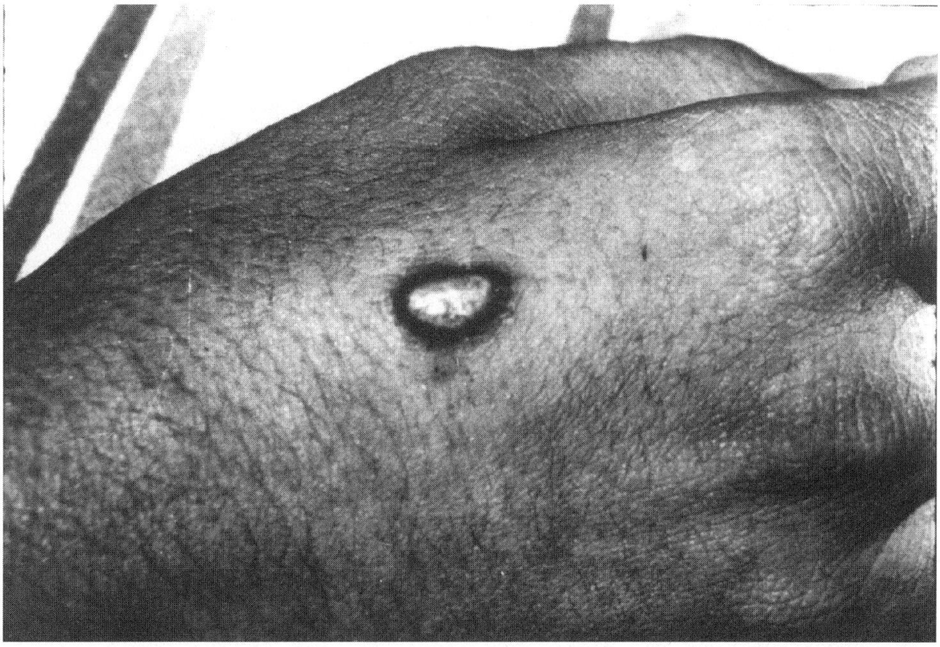

Figure 9 Dermatofibroma of the right hand dorsum. The lesion is firm, smooth, and hyperpigmented.

Keloid Scars

Keloid scars represent a hyperproliferative response of connective tissue to trauma (22). Known stimuli include burns, inflammatory acne, surgery, and ear piercing. The tendency to form keloids is inherited, although a precise mode of transmission has not been defined. There is a racial predisposition, and African-American people are more susceptible. The most frequent locations are the chin, earlobe, neck, shoulders, upper back, and sternum, probably in relation to skin tension and mobility. The posterior scalp may also be involved (acne keloidalis nuchae). By definition, keloids spread beyond the area of initial trauma. Lesions are firm, thick, hyperpigmented papules, nodules, or plaques. They have a characteristic shiny surface and may be confluent. Histological examination shows dense fibrous tissue composed of thick collagen bundles and variable inflammatory infiltrates.

Surgery followed by radiation therapy has a 75% response rate (23–25). However, keloids larger than 2 cm and those that have failed to respond to previous therapy are likely to recur.

Surgical excision alone has been disappointing. Essentially 100% of keloids recur within 4 years. At least 50% regrow even when flaps or grafts are used.

Intralesional triamcinolone (10–40 mg/ml every month alone or in combination with surgery) is moderately effective. When given as an adjunct to surgery, the triamcinolone is injected at the time of excision, at 2 weeks, and monthly thereafter for several months. Adverse effects include skin atrophy, telangiectasias, necrosis, and Cushingoid features.

Compression therapy can be combined with surgery and steroids. Results are good, although recurrences occur after the pressure is released. Best results are obtained in earlobe keloids.

Cryotherapy with liquid nitrogen alone or in combination with intralesional steroids is moderately effective. Injections are maintained for several months to prevent recurrences.

Electrosurgery in combination with intralesional steroids shows results similar to other therapies.

Silicone patch occlusive therapy is moderately effective for some keloids. Studies show favorable results when the patch is used at least 12 h daily for 8–12 weeks.

Benign Adnexal Tumors

The pluripotential cells that give rise to these tumors may differentiate into four basic groups: hair follicle, eccrine gland, apocrine gland, and sebaceous gland (26,27). The degree of differentiation is established according to the resemblance of the tumor cells to the normal structures. Hyperplasias are composed of mature elements, almost identical to normal tissue, but increased in number. Adenomas are less differentiated but mature glandular or follicular structures are identified. In epitheliomas, the degree of differentiation is even less, and it is hard to identify the type of structures that the tumor is forming. Sweat gland origin is suggested by positive immunohistochemical (IHC) stains to carcinoembrionic antigen (CEA), epithelial membrane antigen (EMA), cytokeratins (CK), and gross cystic disease fluid protein (GCDFP-15).

Tumors with Hair Follicle Differentiation

Trichoepithelioma is an autosomal dominant condition characterized by multiple, small, skin-colored papules on the central face, trunk, or proximal extremities (28–31). The cheeks, nose, and nasolabial folds are favorite sites (Fig. 10). Lesions have surface telangiectasias and pearly border and resemble small basal cell carcinomas clinically. Histopathological examination shows islands of small basophilic cells with central keratin cyst formation. Abortive hair germs may be present and peripheral palisading is variable.

Trichofolliculoma (32) presents as a skin-colored, dome-shaped papule on the face and neck. A characteristic feature in some lesions is a central pore containing delicate hairs. On histological examination there is a cystic cavity lined by keratinizing squamous epithelium from which multiple primordial hair follicles arise.

Trichilemmoma presents as a small, warty, flesh-colored papule on the face of an elderly patient. The lesion is solitary and the most frequent location is the nose. When multiple lesions occur, the diagnosis of Cowden's disease is likely, and a search for breast cancer is indicated. This disorder is inherited as an autosomal dominant trait. On histopathological examination there are small uniform cells with round or vesicular nuclei that show peripheral palisading.

Pilomatrixoma (calcifying epithelioma) is common in children of both genders. It predominates on the head and neck areas, where more than 70% of the lesions occur. The lesions tend to be round to oval, dome-shaped, or multilobulated. Size ranges from 0.5 to 5 cm in diameter. Color is usually erythematous, skin-colored,

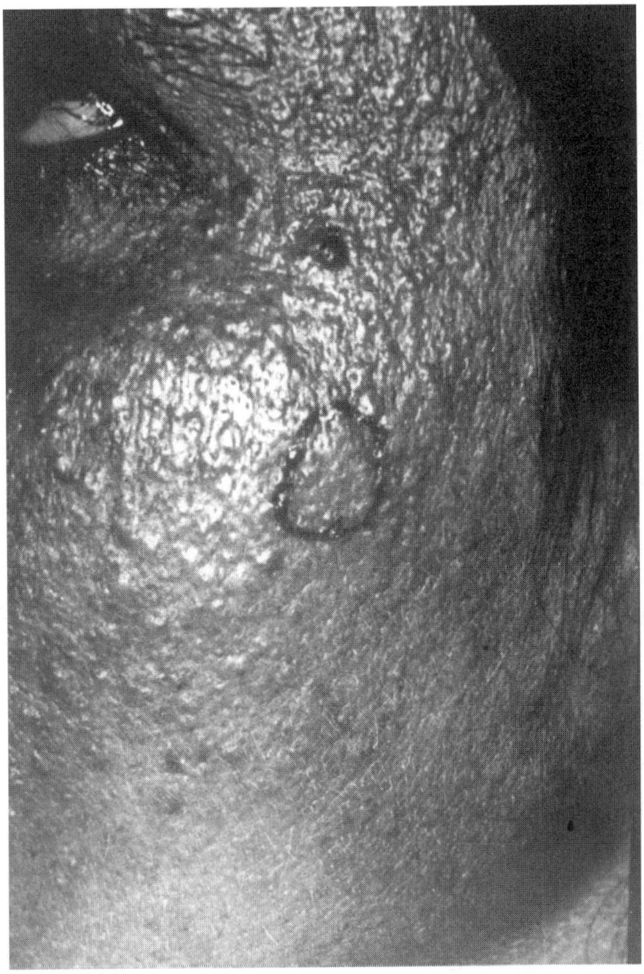

Figure 10 Multiple trichoepitheliomas appearing as innumerable skin-colored papules on the face of a young woman. The area to be biopsied was marked with ink.

or yellowish. Individual lesions are firm in consistency and many calcify. On histological examination the tumor is in the lower dermis where a characteristic dual population of basophilic and so-called shadow cells is observed.

Tumors with Eccrine Differentiation

Eccrine hidrocystoma is bluish in color and cystic in consistency (33–35) (Fig. 11). The most common location is around the eyelids of middle-aged women. Some tumors may show an increase in size during summer when sweat production is increased. Histopathological examination demonstrates a cystic cavity lined with a double layer of cuboidal epithelial cells with eosinophilic cytoplasm.

Syringoma (36) usually presents as multiple, bilateral, skin-colored papules around the eyelids (Fig. 12) but chest, neck, and distal extremities may also be involved. Women are more frequently affected than men and familial aggregation

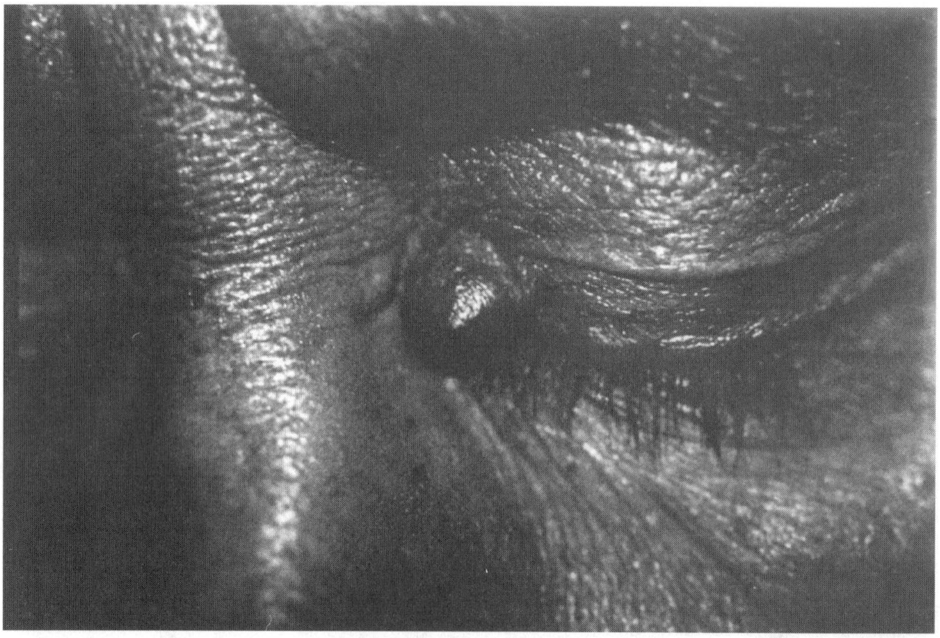

Figure 11 Cystic bluish papule on the eyelid corresponds to an eccrine hidrocystoma.

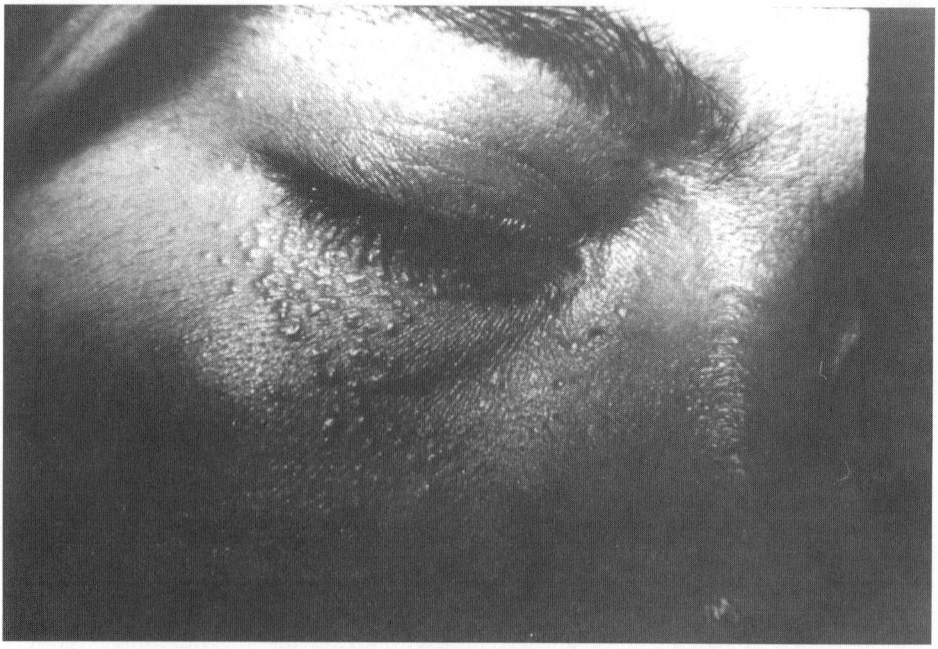

Figure 12 Syringomas presenting as multiple skin-colored papules on the eyelids of a young woman. Her mother and brother have similar lesions.

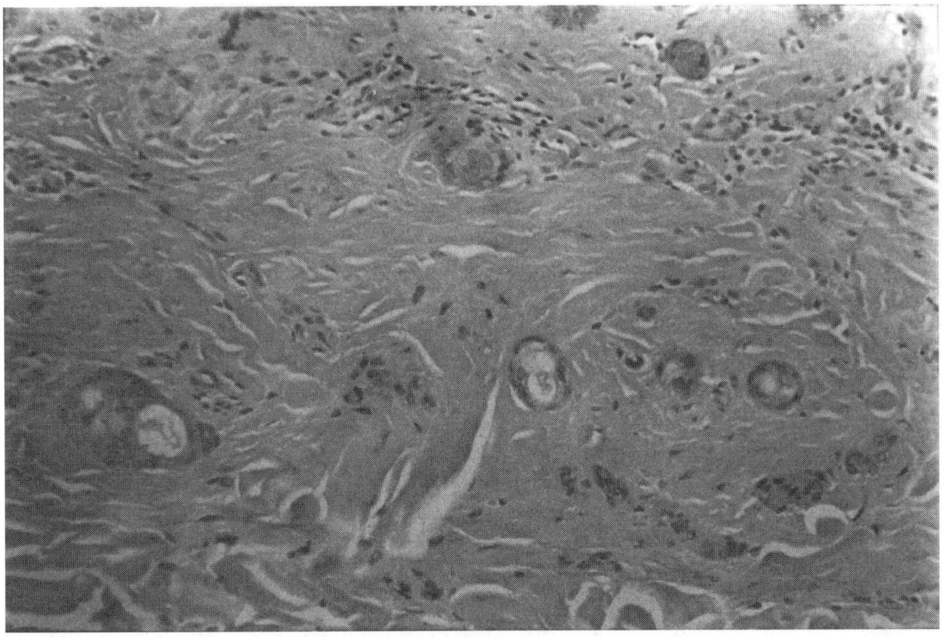

Figure 13 Histopathological examination of syringomas shows dermal glandular structures with characteristic tadpole-like appearance.

is possible. On histological examination there are multiple small, irregular, cleftlike glandular spaces within the dermis (Fig. 13). The spaces are lined with a double layer of epithelium and tangential cutting gives the characteristic tadpole-like appearance.

Eccrine poroma (37) is usually single and affects the palms or soles. The lesions are pink or red, sessile or pedunculated nodules with a surrounding moat (Fig. 14). On histopathological examination there are broad anastomosing bands of small and uniform cells replacing the epidermis and forming ductlike structures.

Eccrine spiradenoma (38) usually affects young adults of both genders in any location. It presents as a solitary intradermal nodule measuring 1–2 cm in diameter. Lesions may be tender or painful. Histopathological examination demonstrates well-demarcated, sometimes encapsulated dermal lobules with two types of cells. Cells in the periphery have small dark nuclei and represent undifferentiated cells. Central cells have a large pale nucleus and are located around small lumina.

Clear cell hidradenoma appears as a cyst or intradermal nodule measuring between 0.5 and 2.0 cm. Both men and women are affected equally. Location is variable. On histological examination the tumor consists of lobular masses composed of cells with clear cytoplasm. Cystic spaces and lumina lined by cuboidal or columnar secretory cells are present.

Chondroid syringoma (39,40) is rare, usually solitary, and occurs predominantly on the head and neck. It is a firm, intradermal, or subcutaneous nodule. Histopathological examination shows tubular lumina embedded in abundant mucoid stroma containing fibroblasts and chondrocytes.

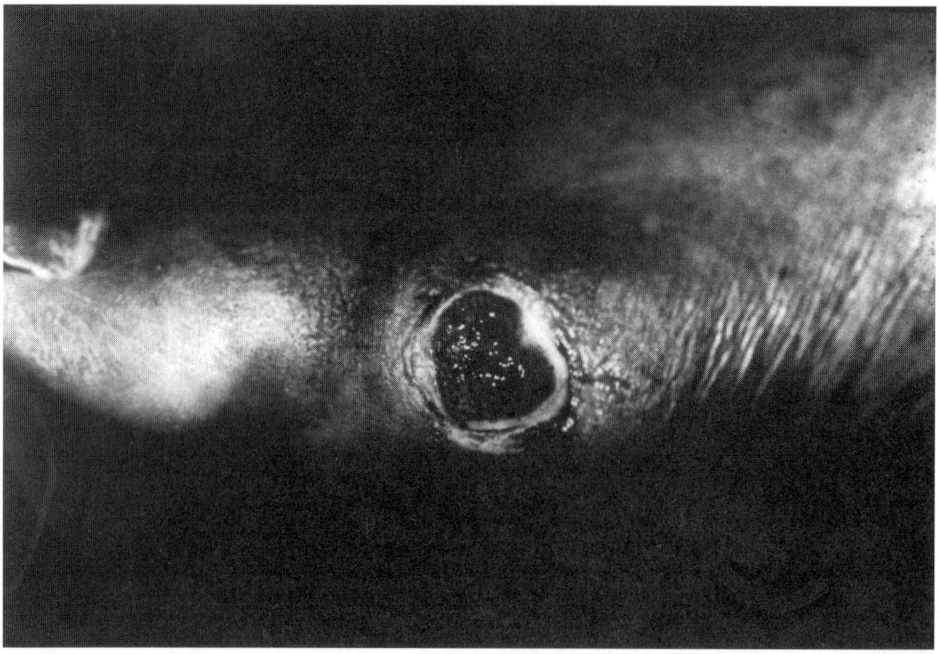

Figure 14 Eccrine poroma of the foot. The lesion is an erythematous sessile nodule with surrounding moat.

Tumors with Apocrine Differentiation

Apocrine hidrocystoma (41–34) is less common than its eccrine counterpart. It appears clinically as a cystic bluish nodule on the face. On histopathological examination there are dermal cystic spaces lined by a double layer of epithelium. The inner layer cells are tall, with eosinophilic cytoplasm, and show decapitation secretion typical of apocrine glands.

Syringocystadenoma papilliferum presents either as a solitary plaque on the scalp or a solitary nodule on the shoulder. The scalp lesion is present at birth and resembles a sebaceous nevus: lesions are devoid of hair and become nodular or verrucous after puberty. The nodular variant of the shoulder arises at puberty and presents as multiple lesions with a crusted surface. Histological examination shows papillae lined with two layers of epithelium communicating with ducts.

Hidradenoma papilliferum (44,45) occurs only in women, affecting the labia majora or the perianal region. Lesions are solitary, small, nonspecific papules. Histopathological examination shows large cystic spaces with numerous papillary projections into the cystic lumen. Lumina are lined with a single layer of columnar cells with decapitation secretion.

Cylindroma (46) affects adults and is more common in women than in men. The most frequent location is the scalp. Clinical appearance is quite characteristic: tumors resemble a tomato. Sporadic cylindroma presents as a solitary, red, firm, dermal tumor with overlying telangiectasias. Familial cylindromas are multiple and may cover the scalp resembling a turban. The condition is inherited as an autosomal dominant trait. Histological examination shows irregular islands surrounded by a hyaline sheath. The islands fit together like pieces of a jigsaw puzzle. Epithelial structures are mixed with glandular lumina showing decapitation secretion.

Tumors with Sebaceous Differentiation (47)

Sebaceous hyperplasia (48) is a well-differentiated collection of mature sebaceous glands. It appears clinically as a yellowish papule with a central depression and surface telangiectasias. Sebaceous hyperplasia is more common in elderly men but begins to appear after age 30. Lesions are multiple and predominate on the face. The cheeks and forehead are favorite locations. Histopathological examination reveals mature sebaceous glands communicating with the epidermis through a dilated duct.

Sebaceous adenoma appears as multiple skin-colored, small, noncharacteristic papules over the face, neck, and trunk. The tumor is rare and its diagnosis must raise the possibility of Muir-Torre syndrome (49). The latter is an autosomal dominant condition characterized by multiple sebaceous tumors in association with multiple internal neoplasias. Several keratoacanthomas, basal cell, and squamous cell carcinomas have also been reported. Sebaceous tumors include sebaceous adenomas and sebaceous hyperplasias. Internal malignancies are usually low-grade carcinomas of the larynx, stomach, duodenum, colon, prostate, endometrium, lung, and kidney. On histopathological examination, there are incompletely differentiated sebaceous lobules sharply demarcated from the surrounding tissue.

Adnexal tumors are best treated with surgical excision. Multiple small trichoepitheliomas may be managed with dermabrasion or resurfacing lasers but recurrence is common. Sebaceous hyperplasias can be eradicated with electrodesiccation or cryotherapy. Multiple cylindromas are difficult to manage because recurrence is the rule.

Cutaneous Cysts

Epidermoid cyst (50,51) is a common cutaneous tumor derived from squamous epithelium. It is skin-colored or yellowish, dome-shaped, smooth, mobile, and ranges in size from 0.5 to 5 cm in diameter. Many lesions have a characteristic central punctum from which a cheeselike material can be expressed. They usually appear on the face or trunk. Epidermoid cysts develop in patients with acne conglobata or by implantation of squamous epithelium into the dermis secondary to sharp injury or trauma. Lesions are often inflamed or infected. The presence of multiple cysts is suggestive of Gardner's syndrome, which incorporates intestinal fibromatosis, jaw osteomas, and colonic polyps. Histological examination shows a cystic cavity lined by keratinizing squamous epithelium with intact granulosa, and the cavity is filled with well-defined keratin lamellae.

Milia cysts (52) are white or cream in color and are known as white heads. They frequently appear in patients with acne, after application of occlusive ointments following resurfacing procedures, in patients with certain blistering diseases such as porphyria or bullous pemphigoid, and as a manifestation of chronic solar damage. On histological examination milia cysts are identical to epidermoid cysts.

Pilar cyst (trichilemmal cyst) is similar to its epidermoid counterpart but much less frequent (ratio 3:1). It affects the scalp (90%) and is frequently multiple (30%). On histological examination the cyst wall shows peripheral palisading of clear cells,

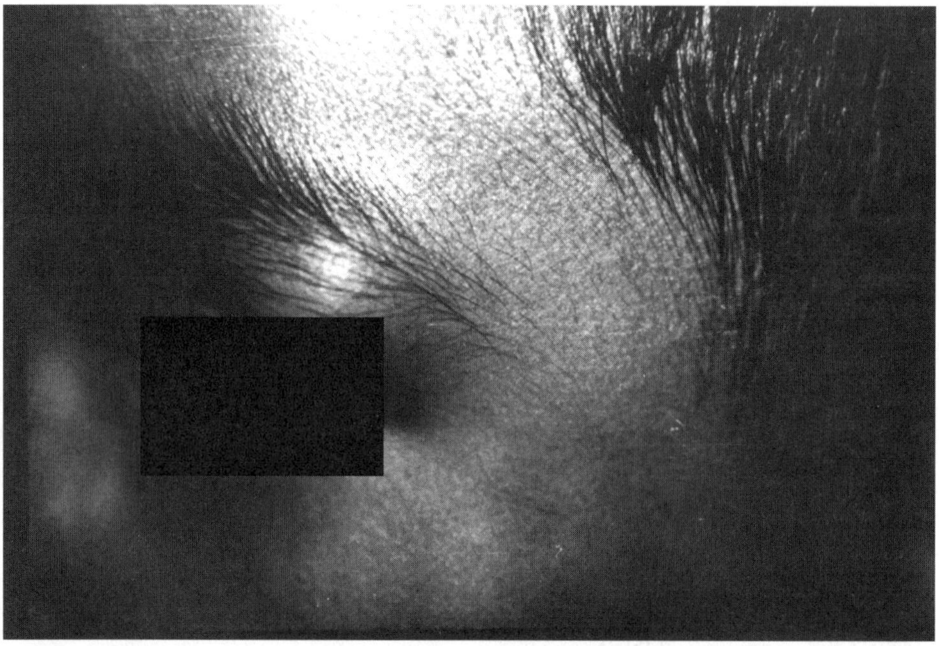

Figure 15 Dermoid cysts occur along lines of embryonic fusion. Location on the eyebrow region is characteristic.

has no granular layer, and the cystic cavity is filled with homogeneous horny material, not lamellae.

Dermoid cysts result from the sequestration of skin along lines of embryonic fusion. They are present at birth, usually around the eyes or nose (Fig. 15). Histological examination shows a cystic cavity lined by epidermis containing various skin appendages (hair, sebaceous and sweat glands).

Steatocystoma multiplex (53) is a true sebaceous cyst that occurs during adolescence as an autosomal dominant condition. Tumors are multiple, smooth, yellowish, or skin-colored, measuring from 0.3 to 3 cm in diameter, and with surface telangiectasias. The most common locations are the scrotum, axillae, chest, or neck. On histological examination these cysts are considered a variant of dermoid cysts because the wall contains multiple sebaceous glands.

Oral mucous cyst (mucocele) develops after the rupture of an obstructed salivary duct (54). On clinical examination the tumor is soft, approximately 1 cm or less in diameter, cystic in consistency, and fluctuant. Lesions affect the lower lip, are asymptomatic, and red or blue. On histopathological examination there are multiple cystic spaces filled with sialomucin surrounded by granulation tissue.

Mucous cyst of the finger represents either an overproduction of hyaluronic acid or a leakage of hyaluronic acid from the interphalangeal joint. Lesions are firm, skin-colored, well circumscribed, and located on the dorsal aspect of the distant phalanx of fingers. On histological examination there is a cystic cavity filled with mucin.

Bronchogenic cysts (55) are small, subcutaneous, solitary lesions located in the area of the sternal notch. They appear at birth and may have a draining sinus.

Thyroglossal duct cysts are clinically identical to bronchogenic cysts but located on the anterior aspect of the neck. On histological examination bronchogenic cysts are lined by pseudostratified columnar epithelium. Thyroglossal duct cysts lack muscle tissue but contain thyroid follicles.

Cysts have no malignant potential. Surgical excision is the treatment of choice for diagnostic or cosmetic reasons.

Vascular Tumors

Congenital Hemangiomas

Nevus flammeus (56,57) is most commonly referred to as port-wine stain (Fig. 16). It is characterized clinically by a vascular, dull red, or bluish-red plaque that usually affects the lateral and medial face. Lesions tend to thicken and become nodular with time. They do not show spontaneous regression. Histological examination shows abundant, mature, dilated capillaries lined by a single layer of endothelial cells. The Sturge-Weber syndrome (58) is the association of a port-wine stain of the face with leptomeningeal and ocular angiomatosis. Approximately 80% of patients have epilepsy and cerebral calcifications. In the Klippel-Trenaunay syndrome, there is a nevus flammeus on a limb with hypertrophy of the soft tissues and bones of the same extremity.

The flashlamp-pumped pulsed dye laser is the treatment of choice (59,60). This laser system emits yellow light with a wavelength of 585 nm and pulse duration

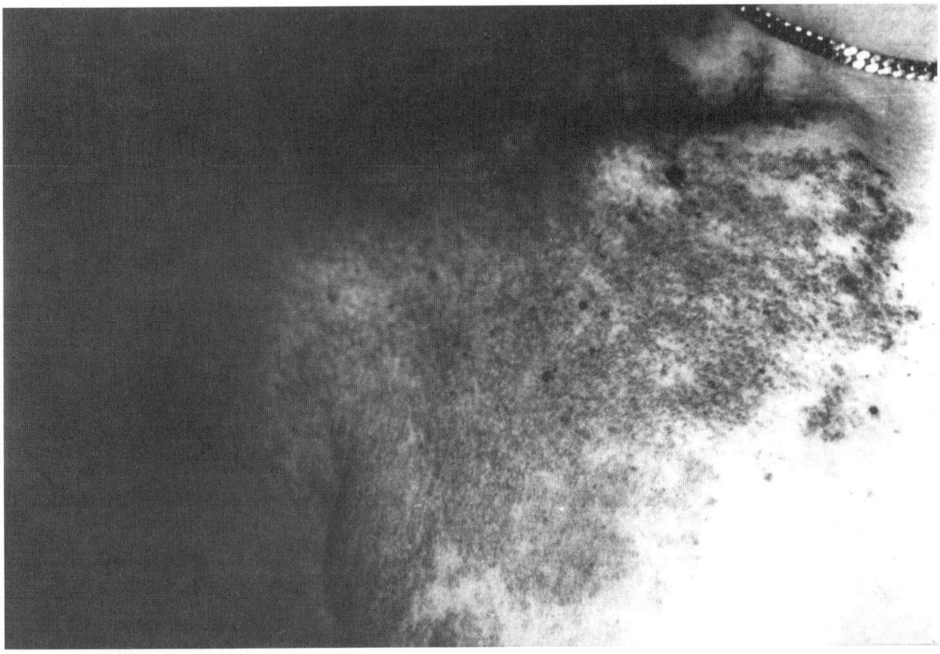

Figure 16 An extensive port-wine stain of the right chest, shoulder, and arm. Initially, the lesion is bright-red and flat but it becomes thicker and purple over time.

of 450 μs. Results are excellent and there is minimal risk of scarring. Treatment with this laser requires multiple sessions given 6–8 weeks apart until resolution. The major disadvantage is immediate purpura in the treated sites lasting 10–12 days.

Capillary hemangiomas are rapidly growing, benign vascular tumors appearing shortly after birth. Lesions are sharply circumscribed, dome-shaped, bright red or purple, and with a smooth or lobulated surface. The clinical evolution is characteristic. The hemagiomas appear within the first months of life, grow rapidly until a significant size is reached, and then slowly involute leaving an atrophic scar. Occasionally, the tumors become ulcerated and bleed. Large lesions may obstruct the airway, interfere with feeding, or with binocular vision. In rare cases a large hemangioma sequestrates and destroys platelets, leading to marked thrombocytopenia and consumption coagulopathy, the so-called Kasabach-Merritt syndrome. On histopathological examination, there is considerable proliferation of endothelial cells and numerous capillary lumina.

Treatment is not necessary for uncomplicated lesions located on the trunk or other noncosmetic areas because lesions will resolve spontaneously. Therapy is indicated for hemangiomas located on functional or cosmetic areas of the face, distal extremities, and genitalia; ulcerated and bleeding lesions; and lesions occurring as part of the Kasabach-Merritt syndrome.

Effective therapies include oral prednisone (2–4 mg/kg/day for 2 weeks), surgical excision, or flashlamp-pumped pulsed dye laser. In cases of Kasabach-Merritt syndrome, platelets and blood transfusions are indicated.

Cavernous hemangiomas are true vascular malformations and therefore do not resolve spontaneously. They are deep, subcutaneous, compressible nodules of various sizes that can occur at birth, in infancy, or adulthood. Histological examination shows dermal and subcutaneous vascular spaces lined by endothelial cells and containing blood. The blue rubber-bleb syndrome consists of multiple congenital cavernous hemangiomas associated with intestinal and visceral angiomas. Patients experience chronic gastrointestinal bleeding and anemia or acute bleeding episodes. Maffucci's syndrome is the association of cavernous hemangiomas with dyschondroplasia (defective calcification and deformities of bone) and osteochondromas. The latter may transform into chondrosarcomas.

Vascular and magnetic resonance imaging (MRI) studies are indicated prior to surgical excision. Lasers are not effective treatment for such large and deep structures.

Other Vascular Tumors

Angiokeratoma circumscriptum (64) is usually present at birth and is characterized by multiple, keratotic, vascular papules, that may appear individually or forming larger plaques. The lesions are bluish, with a verrucous surface, and may show linear arrangement (Fig. 17). Histopathological examination shows hyperkeratosis, papillomatosis, and irregular acanthosis. Multiple vascular spaces filled with blood are evident in the papillary dermis.

Angiokeratoma Mibelli is an autosomal dominant condition characterized by multiple keratotic vascular papules of the distal extremities in association with cold intolerance. Lesions appear in infancy, predominantly on acral sites, such as fingers and toes. There is a slight predominance in female patients. Histological examination

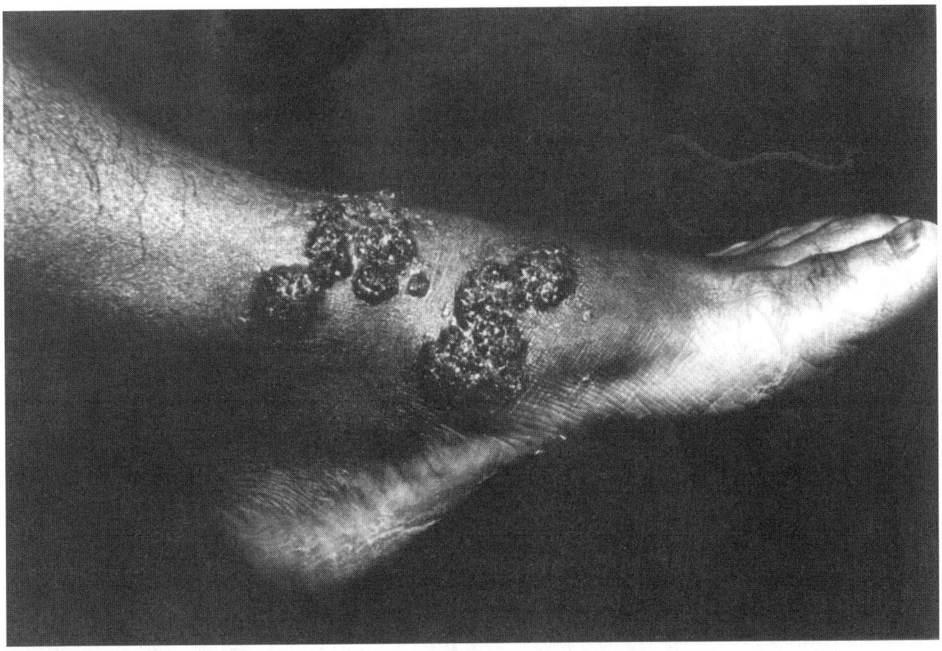

Figure 17 Angiokeratomas are congenital vascular papules or nodules with keratotic surface. Acral lesions of the foot may be associated with cold intolerance.

shows, ectatic blood vessels in the papillary dermis, with an overlying keratotic epidermis.

Pyogenic granuloma (65) is a confusing term that defines a proliferation of granulation tissue secondary to trauma. The lesions appear at any age and in patients of both genders. The tumor appears clinically as a red- to- purple vascular nodule of variable size. Common sites include the fingers, toes, lips, oral mucosa, and trunk. Lesions are usually single and bleed easily. On histological examination there is a proliferation of dermal blood vessels in a gelatinous stroma, surrounded by fibroblasts, neutrophils, and mast cells. The epidermis forms a collarette at the base of the lesion.

Glomus tumor (66) presents as a single bluish nodule on acral sites. Frequently it is subungual and tender. There are some familial cases inherited in autosomal dominant fashion. Histological examination shows dermal vascular spaces and glomus cells arranged around endothelial cells. Glomus cells are cuboidal and have a central rounded nucleus.

Lymphangioma (67) is noted at birth or immediately after. It presents as a collection of small, deep vesicles resembling frog spawn. Favorite locations include the trunk, axillae, shoulders, neck, extremities, and oral mucosa. On histological examination, there are dilated lymphatic channels lined by normal lymphatic endothelium.

Vascular tumors are best treated with surgical excision. Small lesions may be treated with the flashlamp-pumped pulsed dye laser. Pyogenic granuloma and glomus tumors may respond to curettage and electrodesiccation or cryotherapy.

Lipoma (68)

Lipomas are benign tumors composed of mature fat cells. They are subcutaneous nodules with a soft consistency. Lesions may be multilobulated and range in size from 1 to 10 cm. Common locations include the upper extremities, trunk, and neck. Histological examination shows lobules of mature fat cells enclosed in a fibrous capsule.

Surgical excision is the treatment of choice for symptomatic lesions or for cosmetic reasons. An alternative is liposuction using tumescent anesthesia. This method may result in better cosmesis with less evident scars.

Neural Tumors

Neurofibroma is a skin-colored papule or nodule with a soft consistency that occurs anywhere in the body. Multiple lesions occur in the neurofibromatosis syndrome or Von Recklinghausen's disease (69). Histological examination shows interlacing fascicles of Schwann's cells with irregular elongated nuclei. Variable amounts of mucopolysaccharides and collagen are present.

Granular cell tumor (GCT) affects people between 30 and 50 years of age, with a mean of 39 years. The tumor is more common in women than in men (3:1) and in African-Americans than Whites (5:1). The majority of cases (23–35%) occur on the tongue. Lesions are usually asymptomatic but may become painful. Histopathological examination shows a tumor composed of polygonal epithelioid cells with granular eosinophilic cytoplasm. There is a characteristic pseudoepitheliomatous hyperplasia of the overlying epidermis. IHC stains show S-100, vimentin, neuron-specific enolase, and myelin basic protein.

Leiomyoma

Leiomyoma (70) is derived from the arrector pili muscle of hair follicles or from muscle fibers present in the wall of blood vessels. In the multiple familial type, lesions are distributed over neck and limbs. Onset is in childhood and tumors are red, pink, or brown. A characteristic feature is that pain can be elicited by pressure or low temperature. Also, lesions may shrink when the skin is chilled. The solitary leiomyoma occurs anywhere in the body including the nipple and areola. It is also painful. On histopathological examination there are interlacing fascicles of smooth muscle cells with elongated, blunt, cigar-shaped nuclei.

Surgical excision is the treatment of choice for these tumors.

MALIGNANT TUMORS OF THE SKIN

Basal Cell Carcinoma

Basal cell carcinoma (BCC) is the most common of human cancers (Table 2). It develops from the epidermis at the level of the bulge region of hair follicles. Most studies favor unicentric origin. Multiple risk factors are recognized, including ultraviolet (UV) and ionizing radiation, arsenic, chronic wounds, immunosuppression, and reduced DNA-repair mechanisms. The most significant is chronic exposure to

Table 2 Malignant Tumors of the Skin

Basal cell carcinoma
  Superfical multicentric
  Nodular
  Morpheaform
  Fibroepithelioma of Pinkus
Squamous cell carcinoma
  1. In situ
    Bowen's disease
    Erythroplasia of Queyrat
  2. Invasive
  3. Verrucous
    Buschke- Lowenstein tumor
    Oral florid papillomatosis
    Carcinoma cuniculatum
Keratoacanthoma
  Common solitary keratoacanthoma
  Giant keratoacanthoma
  Keratoacanthoma centrifugum marginatum
  Multiple self-Healing keratoacanthoma (Ferguson-Smith syndrome)
  Eruptive keratoacanthoma of the Gryzbowski type
Malignant melanoma
  Superficial spreading melanoma
  Nodular melanoma
  Lentigo maligna melanoma
  Acral lentiginous melanoma
  Amelanotic melanoma
  Desmoplastic neurotrophic
Adnexal carcinomas
  1. Hair follicles: Pilomatrix carcinoma
  2. Sweat Glands
    Microcystic adnexal carcinoma
    Malignant eccrine spiradenoma
    Malignant chondroid syringoma
    Eccrine porocarcinoma
    Malignant clear cell hidradenoma
    Eccrine mucinous carcinoma
    Primary cutaneous adenoid cystic carcinoma
    Malignant cylindroma
    Paget's disease of the nipple
    Extramammary Paget's disease
    Malignant hidradenoma papilliferum
    Apocrine carcinoma
  3. Sebaceous glands: Sebaceous Gland Carcinoma
Merkel cell carcinoma
Sarcomas
  1. Fibrous tissue
    Fibrosarcoma
    Dermatofibrosarcoma protuberans

(Continued)

Table 2 (Continued)

Atypical fibroxanthoma
Malignant fibrous histiocytoma
2. Vascular tissue
Angiosarcoma
Kaposi's sarcoma
Hemangiopericytoma
3. Muscular tissue
Leiomyosarcoma
Cutaneous rhabdomyosarcoma
4. Neural tissue
Malignant peripheral nerve sheath tumor
Malignant granular cell tumor
5. Liposarcoma
6. Epithelioid sarcoma
Cancer metastatic to the skin

UV radiation in individuals with fair skin, blue eyes, blond hair, and poor tanning ability. Estimates in the Unites States indicate approximately 700,000 new BCCs every year (71). The tumor occurs most frequently in individuals 60 years of age and older and predominates in men. BCC is more common in Whites in whom it forms 70% of skin cancers, compared to 24% in Japanese, and 8% in African-Americans. Approximately 80% of tumors involve the head and neck regions, with almost 30% affecting the nose. Up to 13% of cases present with multiple BCCs, and patients with only one lesion have a cumulative 5 year risk of 45% of showing another BCC (72). The nevoid basal cell carcinoma syndrome (Gorlin's syndrome) is characterized by innumerable BCCs, jaw cysts, palmar and plantar pits, skeletal abnormalities, and calcification of the falx cerebri (73).

Nodular BCC is a translucent pearly papule or nodule with telangiectasias (Fig. 18). It frequently ulcerates, hence the term rodent ulcer. Approximately 70% of tumors belong to this variety, with 7% showing hyperpigmentation due to melanin (pigmented BCC).

Superficial BCC appears as an erythematous scaly patch of variable size. It may contain some areas of atrophy, hypopigmentation and scarring. It resembles tinea, psoriasis, or eczema clinically.

Morpheaform BCC is an indistinct white-to-yellow plaque with marked induration and surface telangiectasias. It is also termed desmoplastic or sclerosing BCC (Fig. 19).

Fibroepithelioma of Pinkus resembles a benign fibroma: the lesion is a smooth, pedunculated, erythematous nodule occurring on the back (Fig. 20).

On histological examination BCC shows islands of basaloid cells with peripheral palisading and tumor–stromal separation artifact (Fig. 21). Occasionally, the cells show features of both BCC and squamous cell carcinoma and the term basosquamous carcinoma is applied (74). Overall, there are four main histological patterns:

Nodular BCC: Approximately 70% of tumors show basaloid nodules as described above, some with cystic degeneration.

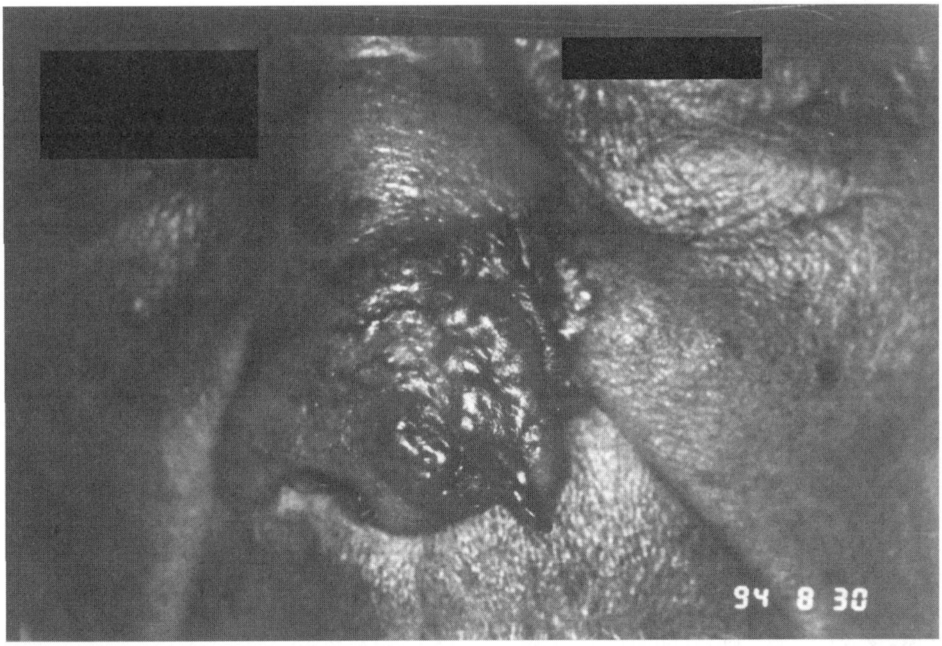

Figure 18 Nodular basal cell carcinoma of the nose. This lesion shows characteristic pearly border and surface telangiectasias.

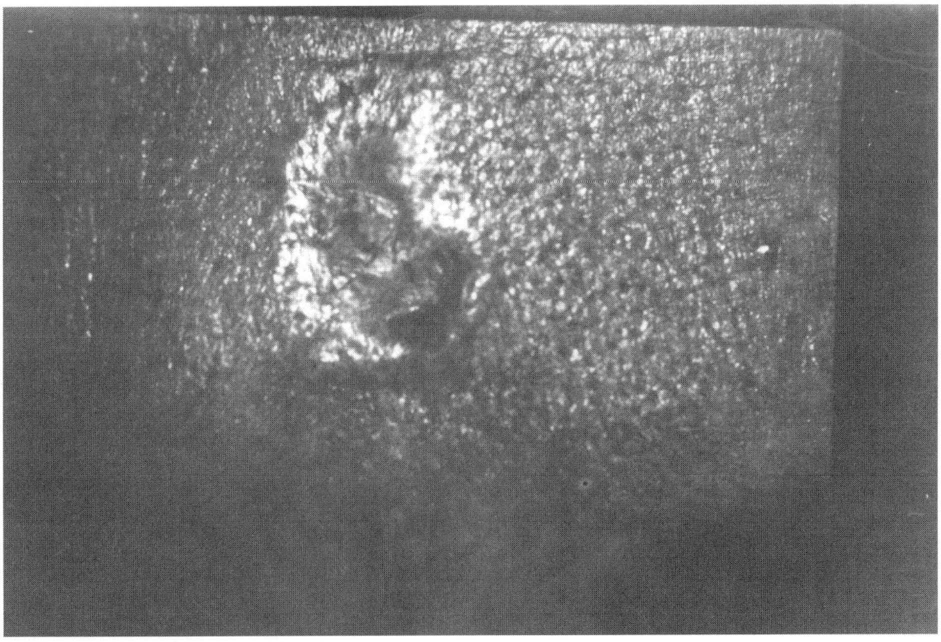

Figure 19 Morpheaform basal cell carcinoma on the midcentral forehead. The plaque is slightly depressed, indurated, and hypopigmented. This variety of basal cell carcinoma is characterized by extensive subclinical extension and aggressive histologic characteristics.

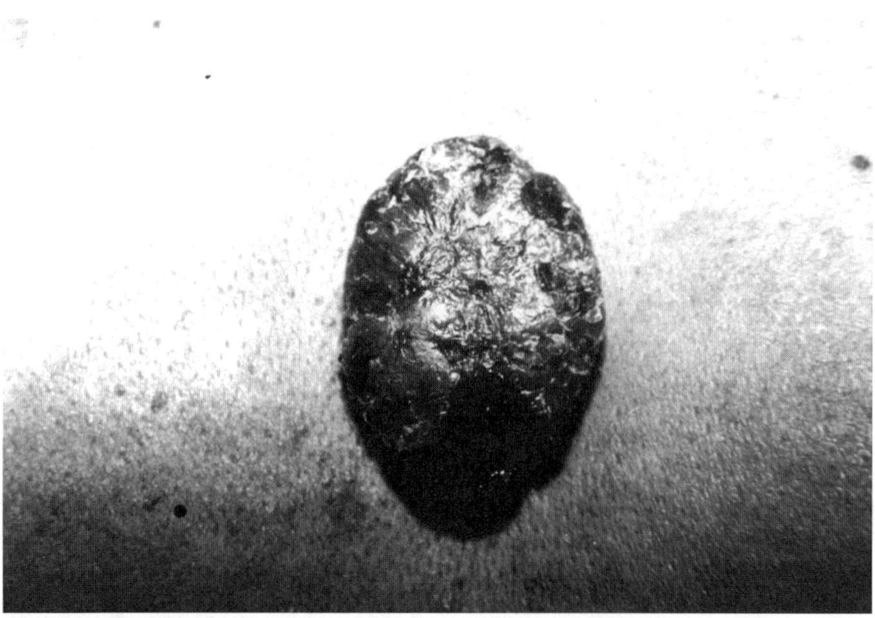

Figure 20 Fibroepithelioma of Pinkus is a basal cell carcinoma that resembles a benign fibroma. Lesions tend to be larger than 1 cm and usually affect the trunk.

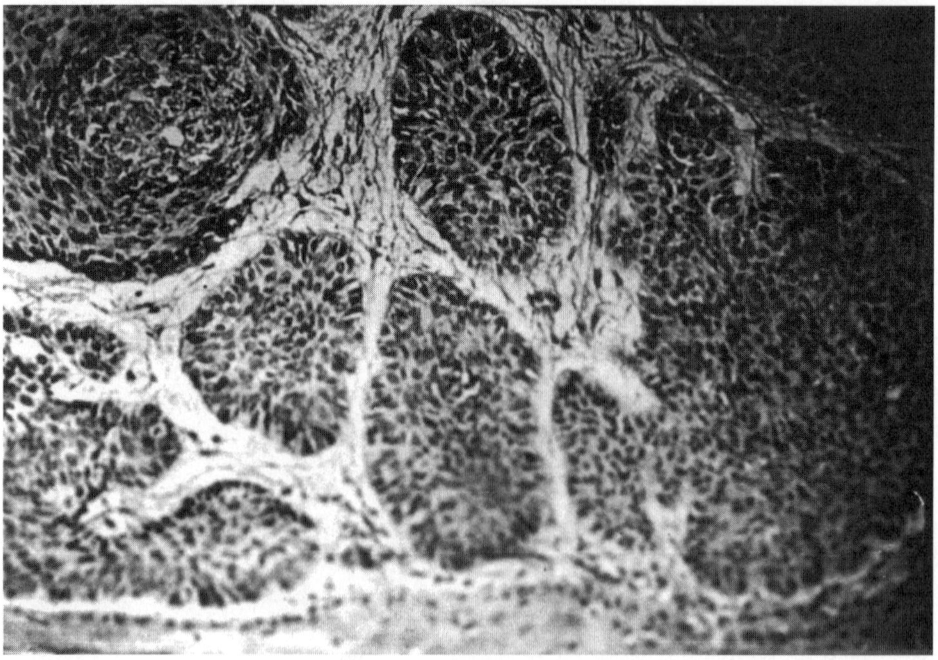

Figure 21 Typical nodular basal cell carcinoma shows multiple nodules of basophilic epithelial cells with peripheral palisading.

Superficial BCC: Ten percent of tumors show small buds of basaloid cells arising from the epidermis. It is difficult to delineate lateral margins.

Micronodular BCC: Smaller round lobules or buds with marked subclinical extension.

Aggressive growth BCC: Nearly 10%–15% of cases comprise this group. The morpheaform or sclerosing variety is characterized by small spiky islands in a markedly sclerotic stroma. The infiltrative type shows, in addition, a variable nodular component.

Management of Primary BCC

Overall, 90% of tumors can be completely eradicated with simple techniques, but recurrences are likely if therapy is not optimal (75). Recurrent lesions are larger, more aggressive and difficult to treat, and may appear only after several years have elapsed, therefore, the first treatment session is the most important and must be definitive. To ensure an adequate therapeutic plan, the pathologist's report should include not only the histological diagnosis of BCC and the adequacy of surgical margins but also the architectural variety of the tumor.

Curettage and electrodesiccation (C&E) is an excellent treatment for primary, well-defined, nodular BCC in areas of low risk for recurrence such as the neck, trunk, and extremities. It is relatively contraindicated in morpheaform BCC; infiltrative BCC; recurrent tumors (the fibrous stroma does not allow the detection of the difference in consistency between BCC and healthy skin); and tumors extending deeply into fat, or areas with a high risk for recurrence, including the central face, periocular, and perioral regions (due to the high content of pilosebaceous units harboring tumor cells in the hair follicles). Overall cure rates are 90–98% for primary nodular tumors in low-risk areas. Recently, reports have shown similar cure rates for high-risk areas if tumors are smaller than 6 mm (76,77).

Surgical excision with 4 mm margins results in 90–100% cure rates for primary BCC in low-risk locations (78). Recurrence is as low as 3.2% for primary tumors less than 6 mm in diameter, but BCCs of the ear, nasolabial fold, scalp, and forehead are difficult to eradicate. Recurrence rates for these locations are 42%, 20%, 14.7%, and 8.4%, respectively (79). The advantages of surgical excision include rapid healing, good cosmesis, histological verification of margins, and suitability for all BCC types. Disadvantages are the sacrifice of normal skin and lower cure rates for high-risk areas and recurrent tumors. Incompletely excised BCC recurs in at least 35% of cases, and the recurrence rate for recurrent BCC treated with surgery alone is 17.4%. Recently, the combination of C&E with surgical excision using 4 mm margins for recurrent tumors has resulted in recurrence rate of only 2.4% at 2 years (80).

Mohs' Micrographic Surgery (MMS) involves intraoperative examination of horizontal frozen sections, with verification of 100% of surgical margins, as compared to less than 1% when using traditional vertical bread-loafing methods. Both the surgical procedure and the histopathological examination and mapping are done by the Mohs' surgeon (see diagram 1). MMS is the treatment of choice for BCCs with a high probability of recurrence, such as those located on high-risk areas (nose, ears, perioral, periocular, nasolabial folds), recurrent and incompletely excised tumors, tumors larger than 2 cm in diameter, and BCC with aggressive histological characteristics (morpheaform, infiltrative, micronodular). This method allows preservation of normal tissue in cosmetically or functionally important areas such as digits, genitalia, and face. Reported 5 year cure rates are 99% for primary and 94% for recurrent BCC (81,82). Disadvantages include the need for special equipment and training and the fact that the technique is time-consuming.

Cryosurgery with liquid nitrogen is indicated for primary and recurrent BCC of the trunk, extremities, and face (even in high-risk areas if the tumors are well delineated); small and large tumors; and those fixed to cartilage or bone. It is extremely useful for patients with coagulopathies or pacemakers, to reduce tumor bulk in combinational approaches, and for palliation of inoperable tumors. Cryosurgery is not a good option for BCCs with significant subclinical extension and fibrosis (indistinct margins, morpheaform, and infiltrative subtypes), deeply invasive tumors, or tumors located on highly cosmetic areas of the face (a white scar is produced). It is contraindicated for patients with Raynaud's phenomenon, connective tissue diseases, cold intolerance, or cryoglobulinemia.

Reported 5 year cure rates are 98–99% for primary and 87–95% for recurrent BCC (83,84). Cosmesis is similar to other modalities. The technique is particularly advantageous for treatment of tumors of the ear and nose because cartilage is relatively resistant and overall architecture is preserved. It is also adequate for preservation of lacrimal structures. Complications include edema, hypertrophic scarring, neuropathy, infection during healing, delayed hemorrhage, ectropion, and hypopigmentation.

Radiation therapy is effective for BCC when used in dosages of 3000–5000 cGy in 6–20 fractions (200–500 cGy each). Five-year cure rates of 97–99% have been reported for primary tumors less than 2 cm in diameter (85). Response rates are less impressive for recurrent BCC (85%) and larger tumors (92% for BCC 2–5 cm in diameter, and 60% for BCC larger than 5 cm) (86).

Radiotherapy is indicated for elderly and debilitated patients, individuals with multiple medical conditions or who are taking anticoagulants (who are poor surgical candidates); those who refuse surgery for any reason; incompletely excised BCC; and tumors with perineural invasion (which have a high risk for recurrence). It is an excellent adjuvant modality for large, recurrent BCC tumors, or in cases with perineural extension, in which surgery or radiotherapy alone results in 30% and 67% cure rates, respectively.

Radiation is contraindicated in tumors with abundant fibrotic tissue such as morpheaform and infiltrative BCC; tumors that recurred after initial radiotherapy; and in patients younger than 50 years (due to poor cosmesis after 10 years).

Photodynamic therapy (PDT) involves the topical or systemic administration of a photosensitizer that is selectively taken up by tumor cells. The photosensitizer is then activated by visible light to produce singlet oxygen. This reaction leads to oxidation of proteins and lipids with subsequent cell death and tumor elimination. Use of topical aminolevulinic acid (ALA) results in 98% cure rate of superficial BCCs but only 82% of nodular tumors (87). Systemic photophrin (1 mg/kg with 630 nm light doses of 72–288 J/cm^2) achieves cure in up to 94% of superficial and nodular tumors (88% complete and 12% partial response) (88). Other studies show a 10% recurrence at 2 years for morpheaform BCC and tumors located on the nose. PDT retreatment of therapeutic failures is successful in 73% of cases.

Topical 5-FU is an antimetabolite that blocks the incorporation of thymidine into DNA, leading to death of neoplastic cells. This agent (in 5% and 20%

concentrations, twice a day for 3–4 weeks) has resulted in 88% cure rates for superficial BCC tumors (89). Results are comparable to surgery and radiotherapy but with better cosmetic results. Nodular tumors respond in only 50% of cases and this therapy is not recommended (90). Recent attempts to improve the results include the addition of light curettage prior to the application of 5-FU 25% under occlusion for 3 weeks. Response rate was 94% at 5 year follow-up; further validation of these results is awaited (91). Topical 5-FU is useful preoperatively to reduce the size of superficial tumors and to delineate further the lateral margins.

Retinoids are vitamin A analogues that inhibit cell proliferation and malignant transformation. Despite encouraging initial case reports, topical Retin A is not effective for BCC tumors and is not recommended. Systemic oral isotretinoin (in dosages up to 4.5 mg/kg/day) has resulted in only 10% cure rates for nodular tumors. However, dosages as low as 0.5–1.0 mg/kg/day have prevented the development of new lesions in patients with multiple BCCs (92,93). This beneficial effect is transient and new BCCs occur after therapy is suspended.

Interferons (IFN) are proteins with immunomodulatory, antiviral, antiproliferative, and antineoplastic effects. They are produced by leukocytes (IFN alpha), fibroblasts (IFN β), and lymphocytes (IFN γ). Interferon alpha 2b (1.5 M units subcutaneously [SQ], three times per week for 3 weeks) achieved 100% cure rate for superficial BCC tumors (94). Multicenter trials with varying dosages, however, yielded poorer results, with only 24–81% complete responses. For nodular tumors of the central face, the response may be 80%, but much higher and toxic doses (13.5–27 M units) are needed (95). Common side effects include flu-like symptoms (arthralgias, fever, headache, malaise, weakness), bone marrow suppression, cardiovascular toxicity, and CNS toxicity. IFN therapy is contraindicated in patients with significant heart/ kidney/ liver disease, in patients who have received transplants, and in patients with connective tissue disease.

Treatment of Metastatic BCC

Metastases occur in fever than 0.55% of cases. These patients are immunosuppressed or debilitated, have multiply recurrent and aggressive tumors, or have predisposing conditions such as the nevoid basal cell carcinoma syndrome. Approximately 50% of cases disseminate via lymphatics into regional nodes. The other 50% spread hematogenously into lungs or bones. Survival is 20% at 1 year, and 10% at 5 years (96,97). Surgery is performed for treatment of the primary site and for removal of affected lymph nodes. Postoperative radiation is indicated in all cases. Chemotherapy is used in nonsurgically treated cases and for palliation of symptoms. Its role as an adjuvant to surgery has been explored in case reports for a single node larger than 3 cm, and for multiple nodes (98).

Squamous Cell Carcinoma

Squamous cell carcinoma (SCC) is a true invasive carcinoma of the surface epidermis. It affects people over 50 years of age with fair skin, blue eyes, blond hair, and poor tanning ability. Contributing factors include chronic solar damage, ionizing radiation, chronic wounds or ulcers, human papilloma virus infection (serotypes 5, 8, 16 and 18), exposure to chemical carcinogens (arsenic, polycyclic aromatic hydrocarbons, and topical nitrogen mustard), immunosuppression (patients who

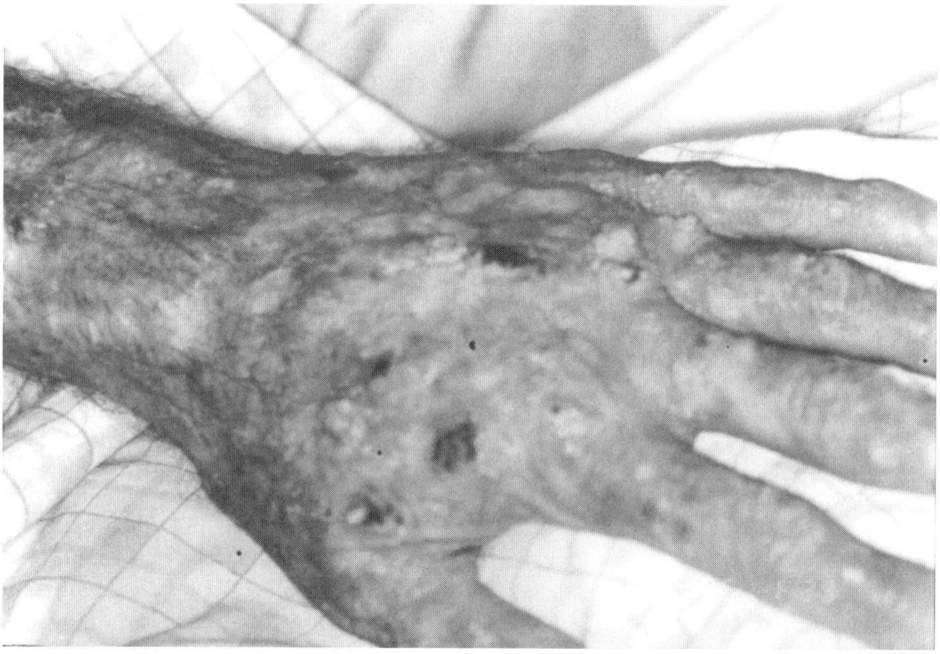

Figure 22 Multiple keratotic lesions on the hand of a patient who underwent renal transplantation. Some lesions correspond to hypertrophic actinic keratoses but others have evolved towards invasive squamous cell carcinoma.

have received transplants), chronic inflammatory disorders (epidermolysis bullosa), and genetic syndromes characterized by poor DNA repair mechanisms (xeroderma pigmentosum) (99). The highest incidences are reported from Texas and Queensland, Australia (100).

SCC arises de novo in sun-damaged skin or from precursor lesions such as actinic keratoses (Fig. 22). The latter are erythematous, scaly, or keratotic papules of sun-exposed skin of the face, neck, arms and hands, and carry a collective 20% overall risk of malignant transformation (101).

Bowen's disease presents as erythematous scaly patches of variable size (Fig. 23). It resembles tinea, psoriasis, eczema, or superficial BCC (102). The lesions enlarge slowly over time, are asymptomatic or slightly pruritic, and affect glabrous skin. Some cases evolve into invasive SCC. Human papilloma viruses (HPV) 16, 18, 31, 32, 39, 51, 52, 53, 54 are of causative importance (103). The relationship with visceral neoplasia is controversial and probably related to arsenic ingestion.

Queyrat's erythroplasia is identical to Bowen's disease but located on the glans penis. Approximately 40% of cases develop invasive SCC.

Invasive SCC presents as an indurated nodule of variable size. The surface may be keratotic, ulcerated, or exophytic (Fig. 24). Most commonly, the lesions affect the head and neck or extremities (104). The lower lip is a frequent site in smokers, with 95% of cases occurring in men.

Verrucous carcinoma (105) is a variety of SCC with low metastatic potential. Lesions appear clinically as are exophytic (cauliflower-like), asymptomatic, and

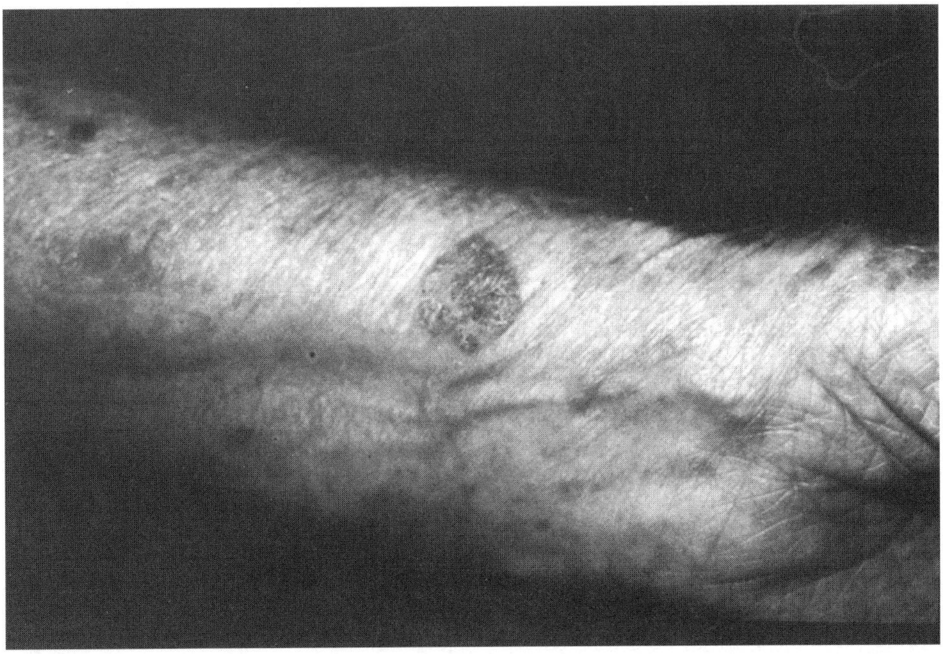

Figure 23 Bowen's disease of the left inner forearm. The lesion is a round, erythematous, scaly patch that resembles psoriasis, tinea, or eczema.

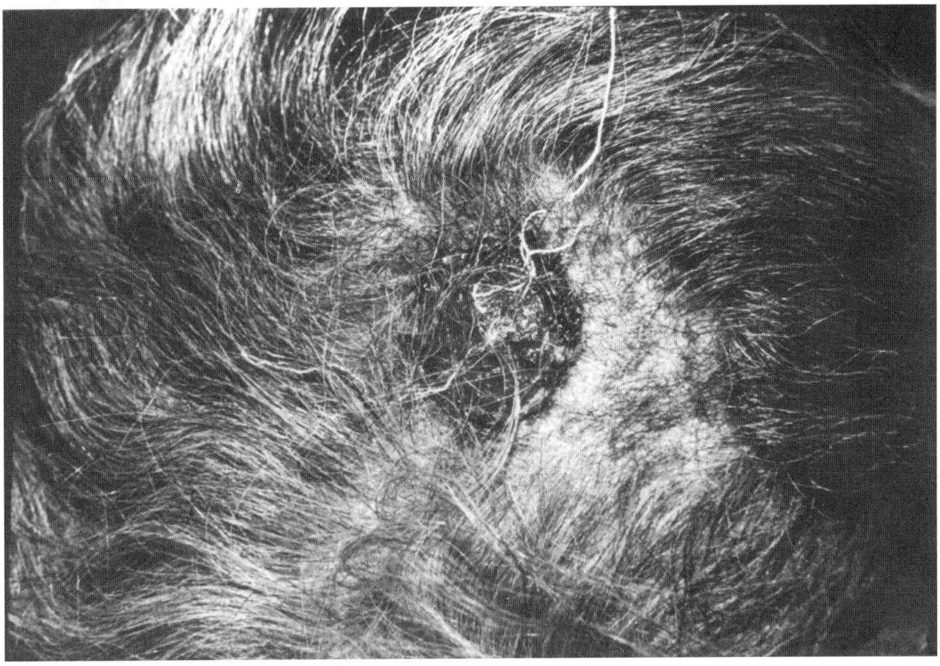

Figure 24 A large ulcerated squamous cell carcinoma of the scalp. The lesion starts as a keratotic papule or nodule that bleeds with minimal trauma.

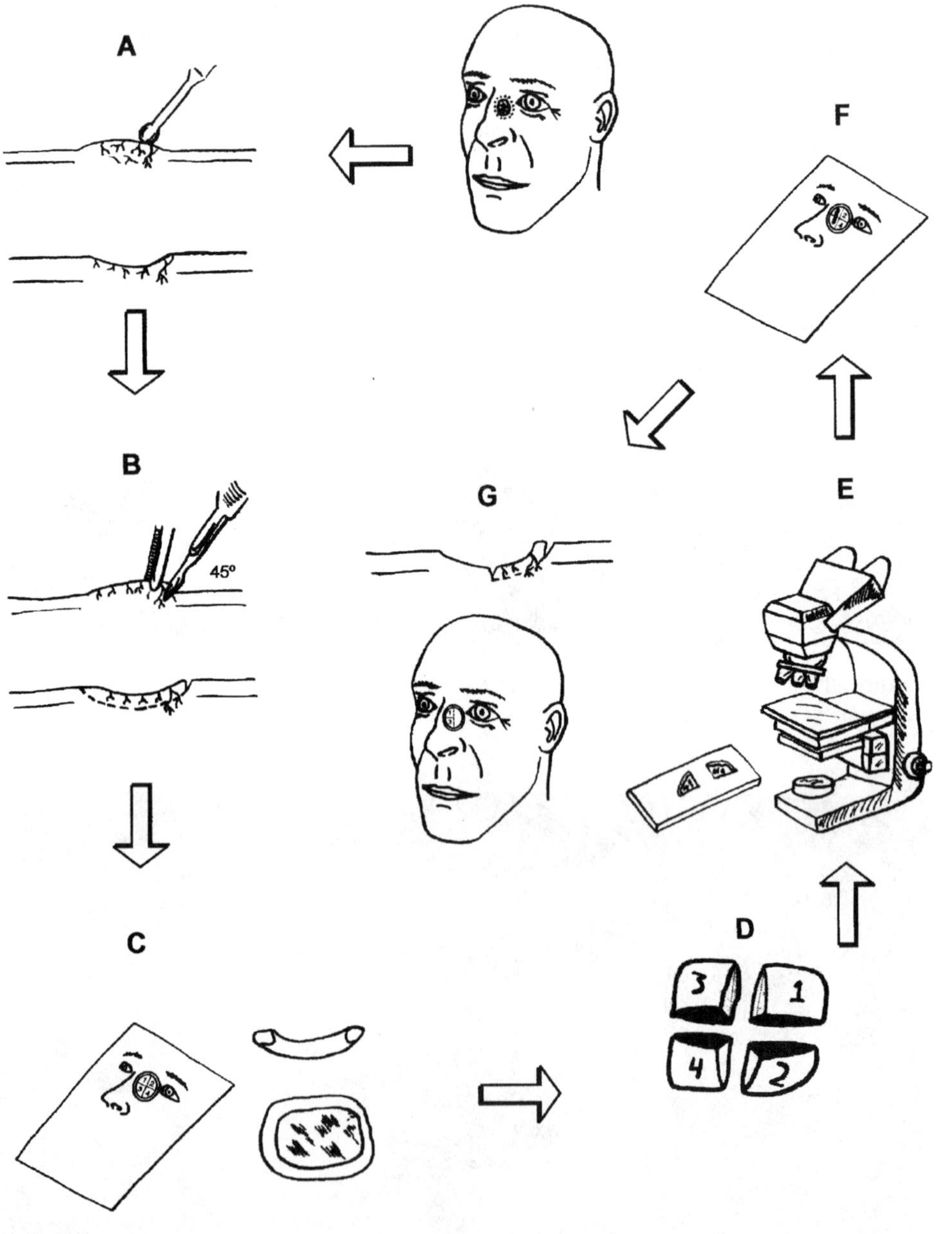

Diagram 1 Mohs' Surgery Procedure. A. A map is drawn depicting the anatomical location and approximate size of the tumor. Debulking is then performed under local anesthesia using a small curette. B. The resultant debulked defect and any area suspicious for tumor is excised using 2–3 mm margins. The incision is made at a 30–45-degree angle to create a disk-like specimen that will allow easier processing of the lateral margins. Identifying marks such as skin nicks are made on the patient and specimen to identify proper orientation. C. The specimen is divided and each section is properly marked on the diagram. D. Sections are color-coded with ink, embedded in a chuck with embedding medium, and quick frozen in liquid nitrogen. The blocks are then sectioned at 4–10 μm in the cryostat, starting from the deepest portion of the specimen and with the deepest margin at the same level than the lateral epidermal borders.

slowly growing. There are three types depending on location: florid oral papillomatosis, carcinoma cuniculatum of the foot, and Buschke-Lowenstein tumor of the genitalia. Histological examination shows variable degrees of keratinocytic atypia (nuclear enlargement, hyperchromatism, prominent nucleoli, increased nuclear-cytoplasm ratio, abnormal intra- or extracellular keratin production) (106). Bowen's disease and Queyrat's erythroplasia are in situ carcinomas with full-thickness keratinocytic atypia and frequent mitotic figures. The loss of polarity gives the epidermis a characteristic windblown appearance (107). In invasive SCC, the bands of atypical cells penetrate the dermis and there are variable atypical mitoses.

Four grades of severity are recognized for SCC according to the proportion of differentiated cells present in the tumor (Broders' classification). In this system, differentiation equals keratinization (108,109). In grade 1, more than 75% of cells are differentiated (multiple horn pearls); in grade 2, more than 50% (several horn pearls); in grade 3, more than 25% (many atypical cells, horn pearls absent); and in grade 4, less than 25% (only spindle cells).

Verrucous carcinoma (110) shows a proliferation of well-differentiated keratinocytes with minimal atypia and a bulbous pushing base that is characteristic. There is epidermal hyperplasia, papillomatosis, and hyperkeratosis.

Management of Primary SCC

Treatment of SCC varies depending on its cause, anatomical site, growth rate, previous treatment, size, depth of invasion, differentiation, patient's immune status, and perineural invasion. It is important to encourage microstaging as in melanoma using depth and Clark's level.

Surgical excision is the preferred modality for treatment of SCC. Approximately 95% of tumors less than 2 cm in diameter can be excised with 4 mm margins, whereas those larger than 2 cm require 6 mm margins (111). Surgical excision achieves 5 year cure rates of 92%, with overall recurrence rate of 8% (112). Recurrence rates, however, vary according to size, location, previous treatment, and histological factors. Higher rates are reported for tumors larger than 2 cm (15%), deeper than 4 mm (17%), with perineural invasion (50%), poorly differentiated (28%), or for recurrent tumors (23%). Tumors of the ear and lip have a recurrence rate of 18% and 10% respectively.

Mohs' micrographic surgery (See diagram 1) should be considered for SCC with high probability of recurrence or metastasis, including those located on high-risk areas (nose, ears, lips, eyelids, scalp, nasolabial folds); recurrent and incompletely excised tumors; tumors larger than 2 cm in diameter or deeper than 4 mm; SCC with aggressive histological appearance (poorly differentiated, perineural involvement); tumors arising on irradiated skin or chronic ulcers; and SCC in immunosuppressed patients (renal transplant). It is recommended for tissue preservation in cosmetically or functionally important areas such as digits, genitalia, and the face.

Representative cuts are placed on slides and stained with hematoxylin and eosin. E. The slides are interpreted by the Mohs' surgeon. F. If residual tumor is observed, the location of tumor is noted in the map. G. Re-excision is performed in the affected areas only and a map of the excision is created. The entire cycle is repeated until the whole tumor is excised.

Overall cure rates with MMS are 96% for primary and 92% for recurrent SCC (113). Nevertheless, recurrences are higher for leg tumors in patients under 39 years of age, lesions greater than 5 cm in diameter, retroauricular tumors, or those requiring more than four Mohs layers for excision (114). Adjuvant radiotherapy must be considered under these circumstances and in patients with perineural involvement.

C&E results in cure rates of 95% for well-differentiated, small (< 2 cm), and superficial (< 4 mm deep) tumors (115). C&E is also a good option for Bowen's disease of the trunk or extremities. It is not indicated for recurrent tumors (50% failure), or for lip and ear tumors (curettage is technically difficult to perform). A disadvantage of the technique is the lack of verification of surgical margins.

Cryosurgery with liquid nitrogen is an excellent modality for well-delineated and well-differentiated SCCs of any size and location. It is extremely useful for patients with coagulopathies to reduce tumor bulk in combination approaches, and for palliation of inoperable tumors. Relative contraindications include poor tumor margins, recurrent SCC, tumors deeper than 4 mm, and poorly differentiated neoplasms. Cryosurgery is contraindicated in patients with cryoglobulinemia, Raynaud's syndrome, and cold intolerance. The reported 5 year cure rate for suitable SCCs is 96–98% (116). Cosmesis is similar to other modalities. The technique is particularly advantageous for tumors of the ear and nose because cartilage is relatively resistant and lacrimal architecture is preserved. It is also adequate for preservation of lacrimal structures. Complications include edema, hypertrophic scarring, neuropathy, infection during healing, delayed hemorrhage, ectropion, and hypopigmentation.

Radiation therapy is indicated for treatment of large or inoperable tumors, those in high-risk areas (central face, nasolabial, ear, nose), and for multiple lesions (117). It is also useful as an adjuvant to surgery for nodal involvement and in aggressive or recurrent SCCs. For example, tumors involving cartilage or bone have a recurrence rate of 53% for surgery alone, but this can be reduced to 12.5% with adjuvant radiotherapy (118).

Doses range from 4,000 to 6,000 cGy in multiple fractions of 200–300 cGy each, and with 2.0 cm margins. Control rates are 99% for tumors smaller than 2 cm, 92% for tumors between 2 and 5 cm, and 60% for those larger than 5 cm in diameter (119).

Side effects include erythema, desquamation, and hair loss. Late effects occur months to years after radiotherapy in approximately 5% of individuals. Serious effects include skin, bone, or cartilage necrosis; telangiectasias and atrophy; alopecia; and local carcinogenesis.

PDT involves the topical or systemic administration of a photosensitizer that is selectively taken up by tumor cells. The photosensitizer is then activated by visible light to produce singlet oxygen. This reaction leads to oxidation of proteins and lipids with subsequent cell death and tumor elimination. PDT is a good option for Bowen's disease (BD) or for treatment of multiple lesions in patients with xeroderma pigmentosum. It is also useful for debulking large tumors that would otherwise require disfiguring surgery or in patients who are poor surgical candidates (120).

Systemic PDT with photofrin has resulted in 100% elimination of Bowen's disease. Topical 20% ALA under occlusion for 4 h or overnight cures 85–92% of cases. The response rate for invasive SCC is approximately 45% and PDT is not considered a first-line therapy (121). The major disadvantage with the use of photofrin is cutaneous photosensitivity lasting 4–6 weeks. Topical PDT is not associated with photosensitivity.

Topical 5-FU is an antimetabolite that blocks the incorporation of thymidine into DNA leading to death of neoplastic cells. The thymine deficiency leads to arrest of the cell cycle and the cells undergo apoptosis with release of inflammatory mediators. Treatment of SCC with topical 5-FU 5% twice a day for 6 weeks has resulted in cure rates between 70 and 98% (122). Best results are obtained for carcinoma in situ. Five recent trials have shown that invasive SCC does not respond to this therapy.

Retinoids are vitamin A analogues that inhibit cell proliferation and malignant transformation. Complete and partial responses have been documented for oral isotretinoin (1 mg/kg/day) in large, recurrent, or metastatic SCC (123). Responses, however, are maintained only while the patient is taking the medication, and tumors recur after stopping treatment. Isotretinoin is best indicated to prevent the development of new SCC's in susceptible individuals. An important limiting factor is toxicity, both acute and chronic, and some side effects are severe enough to preclude further therapy. Frequent acute side effects include cheilitis, dry skin, hair loss, elevated liver enzyme levels, and hypertriglyceridemia. Chronic toxicity is manifested as skeletal changes, cheilitis, dry skin, and aggravation of underlying disorder. Etretinate, another oral retinoid, is also effective for chemoprevention of SCC when used in dosages of at least 30–50 mg/day.

Interferon-alpha yields the best results when used in dosages of 3 M units/day SQ. Cure rates of 96–100% have been reported for SCC in situ, but the cure rate for invasive SCC is negligible (124). Even when IFN-α is combined with interleukin-2, the response rate is 18%, and toxic side effects are frequent (125).

Combination therapy with IFN-α (3 M units/day SQ) and isotretinoin (1 mg/kg/day for at least 2 months) results in a 93% response rate of locally advanced tumors. Yet multiple side effects occur including fatigue (78%), dry skin and mucosa (86%), and hypertriglyceridemia (50%).

Management of Distant Metastatic SCC

Overall, SCC metastasizes in 0.3–3.6% of cases. Higher figures are reported for recurrent tumors (23–30%), tumors on the lip (11%), ear (14%), or those developing in chronic ulcers (40–60%). The risk for metastatic spread is greater for lesions larger than 2 cm or deeper than 4 mm, recurrent tumors, tumors with invasion of bone or cartilage, and those with perineural involvement. Usual route of spread is via lymphatics into regional nodes or hematogenously to liver, lung, or bones. Approximately 95% of metastases are evident within 2 years. The reported 5 year survival for metastatic SCC is 25% (126).

Chemotherapy is indicated for treatment of distant metastatic disease and for preoperative debulking of large SCCs. Response rates are variable but are usually 19–54% (127). The most frequent agents are cisplatin, 5-FU, doxorubicin, and bleomycin. Surgery and/or radiation therapy is useful for palliation.

Management of the Neck in Patients with Invasive SCC of the Head and Neck

Management depends on the presence or absence of clinical nodal disease. For patients without clinically evident nodes, a conservative approach (observation) is reasonable. However, tumors with at least a 20% chance of metastasis (large, undifferentiated, recurrent) require surgical treatment of the primary site and neck. Suprahyoid neck dissection(128) is as effective as radical neck dissection or radiotherapy, but results in less morbidity. This surgical intervention removes nodal levels I (submandibular), II (high cervical), and III (midcervical). If nodes are negative, the possibility of positive nodal disease in level IV (lower neck) or V (posterior neck) is minimal and observation is recommended. Should any of the nodes be positive for tumor, a modified radical neck dissection is performed. Radiotherapy is added if further examination reveals multiple positive nodes or extracapsular invasion (129).

For clinically positive nodes smaller than 3 cm, a radical neck dissection is indicated (130). Adjuvant radiotherapy is provided for multiple nodes, nodes larger than 3 cm, or with extracapsular involvement. The management of parotid nodes or gland disease also includes surgery and radiation (131).

Keratoacanthoma

Keratoacanthoma (KA) is a tumor derived from hair follicle epithelium and associated with HPV 9, 16, 19, 25, and 37. It is a rapidly growing neoplasm that resembles SCC. Whites are more commonly affected than other racial groups and the tumors present in sun-exposed areas of the extremities, head, and neck. KA affects all age groups (occurring most often in the middle-aged and elderly) and it has a 3:1 predominance in men. Sun exposure is the main predisposing factor, but immunosuppression and exposure to tar are also important (132). The five clinical variants are described here.

Common solitary KA starts as a keratotic papule or nodule that reaches 1–3 cm in size. The tumor is erythematous, firm, and has a keratin-filled crater. There is spontaneous involution in a few weeks leaving an atrophic scar.

Giant KA (Fig. 25) is clinically similar to the common variant but grows up to 10 cm in diameter.

KA Centrifugum marginatum is a keratotic erythematous enlarging plaque.

Multiple self-healing KA (Ferguson-Smith type) involves multiple lesions, autosomal dominant inheritance, and a positive family history.

Eruptive KA (Gryzbowski type) is characterized by innumerable, disseminated, 2–3 mm lesions with mucosal involvement and severe pruritus.

The majority of KAs have a benign course. The risk for malignant transformation seems minimal and, when it occurs, the possibility of misdiagnosed SCC should be considered. Many authors believe that malignant transformation from KA into SCC is frequent, although this is controversial. We think of KA as having a continuous spectrum of manifestations, from the most benign to the locally invasive, to those that can rarely metastasize.

On histological examination KA is a flask-shaped lesion with well-developed lateral borders (so-called collarette) and a central keratin-filled epithelial invagination. The epithelium is well differentiated, shows marked keratinization, and has a ground-glass appearance (133).

KA should be treated because clinical differentiation with SCC is not always possible. Treatment is also provided to hasten resolution for cosmetic reasons, to reduce recurrences, and because treatment is simple and effective in most cases.

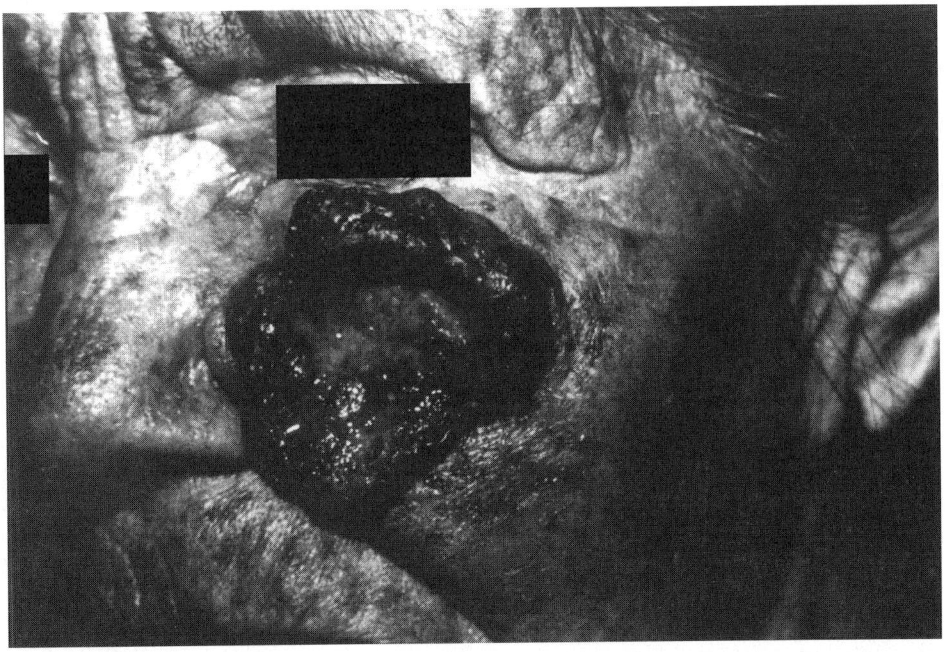

Figure 25 A large, asymptomatic, ulcerated nodule on the left cheek of an elderly woman with extensive solar damage. The lesion corresponds to a giant keratoacanthoma but differentiation from invasive squamous cell carcinoma cannot be done on clinical grounds; a biopsy is always indicated.

Surgical excision is the treatment of choice. The recurrence rate is 4–6% but higher figures are reported for lesions on lips, hands, and fingers, and for giant KA (134).

Mohs' micrographic surgery is indicated for tumors with a greater probability of recurrence, such as giant KA, and tumors located on digits or lip. It is also recommended for tissue preservation in cosmetically or functionally relevant areas (135).

Curettage and electrodesiccation are also effective therapy for KA. A drawback is the hypopigmented residual scar (136).

Radiation therapy is indicated for poor surgical candidates, patients who refuse surgery, and for inoperable tumors (137).

Chemotherapy with intralesional bleomycin or 5-FU is indicated for inoperable tumors, multiple tumors, and to reduce the size of giant KA lesions (138). Therapy is convenient, relatively inexpensive, and produces minimal side effects. Weekly doses of oral methotrexate have proven effective for speeding the resolution of large lesions that are not amenable to surgical treatment (139).

Oral retinoids (isotretinoin and etretinate 1 mg/ kg/ day) have proven effective for the treatment and prevention of KA. Common, giant, eruptive, and recurrent lesions have all been treated successfully (140).

Malignant Melanoma

Melanoma (MM) is a malignant and potentially fatal neoplasm derived from melanocytes. It may arise de novo or from precursor lesions, and is more common in fair-skinned individuals with poor tanning ability. Acute intermittent sun exposure and number of childhood sunburn episodes are more important than chronic sun exposure. The association with tanning bed use is more controversial. Estrogen, oral contraceptives, and pregnancy are no longer considered risk factors (141).

Risk for MM ranges from 1.8 to 13% in congenital melanocytic nevi (estimates are 6.3% risk for giant lesions) (142). The risk is less for common acquired nevi, but there is a significant association in patients with more than 100 lesions. Dysplastic nevi (DN) occur in 2–18% of whites. All studies have demonstrated an increased risk for melanoma in patients with these nevi (143). In the familial melanoma/dysplastic nevus syndrome, several members present with DN and/or a history of MM. Approximately 50% of individuals carry the trait. MM risk approaches 100% over the course of a lifetime. There is a 56% risk between the ages of 20 and 59. Studies have identified two sites for melanoma genes: chromosomes 1p and 9p (144).

The clinical identification of MM is based on the ABCDE of pigmented lesions: *a*symmetry, *b*order irregularity, *c*olor variegation, *d*iameter >6 mm, and elevation (145). Once diagnosed, MM is better thought of in terms of its growth pattern. Lesions with vertical growth are capable of metastasis, while those with only radial growth are confined to the skin. The most common locations are the trunk, head, and neck in men; and the lower extremities in women.

Superficial spreading melanoma (SSM) occurs in 70% of cases. It presents as a pigmented plaque with different shades of brown/black, and a notched border. Sometimes there is erythema or ulceration (Fig. 26). Differential diagnoses includes dysplastic nevus, Spitz nevus, pigmented BCC, seborrheic keratosis, and common nevus.

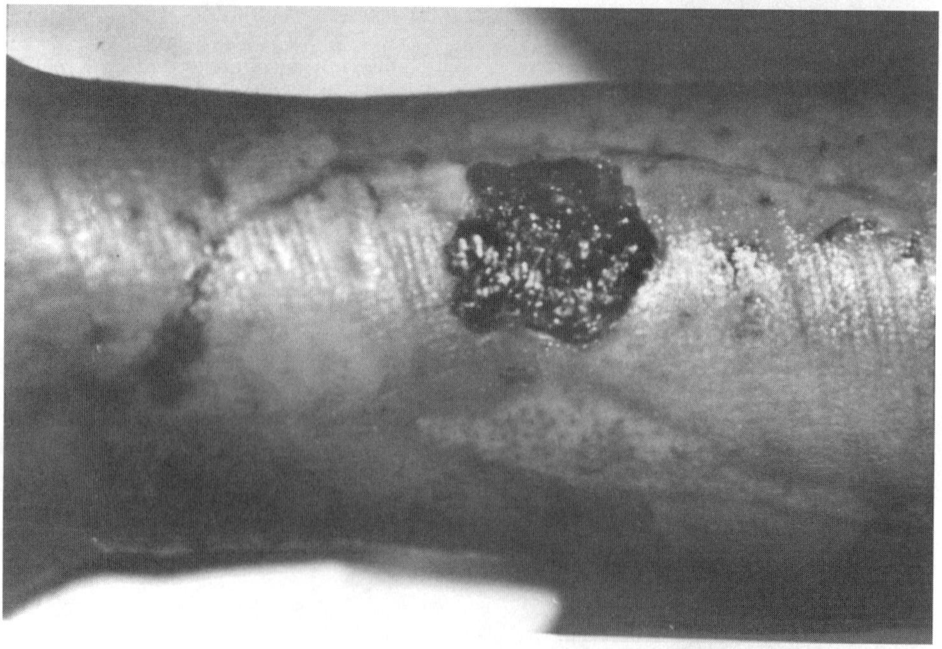

Figure 26 Recurrent superficial spreading melanoma of the leg along a surgical scar. As evident in this case, operative margins in melanoma do not correlate with prognosis. The lesion was treated initially using 5 cm margins.

Lentigo maligna melanoma (LMM) occurs in 5% of cases. It develops from a precursor lesion called lentigo maligna, which is a hyperpigmented flat patch occurring on the face of elderly individuals. Malignant transformation (progress from a radial to vertical growth phase) occurs in 20–50% of cases.

Nodular melanoma (NM) occurs in 15% of cases. It has no radial growth phase and presents as a growing dark nodule with color variation (Fig. 27). The differential diagnosis includes thrombosed skin tag, hemangioma, pigmented BCC, common nevus, blue nevus, and seborrheic keratosis.

Acral lentiginous melanoma (ALM) occurs in 8% of cases. It is the most common MM in dark-skinned persons and presents as an irregular pigmented patch with notched border and color variation (Fig. 28). The most common locations are the volar surfaces of the hands and feet, and subungual. Differential diagnosis includes melanocytic nevi, hematoma, and paronychia. A pigmented nail streak with pigmentation of surrounding skin constitutes Hutchinson's sign.

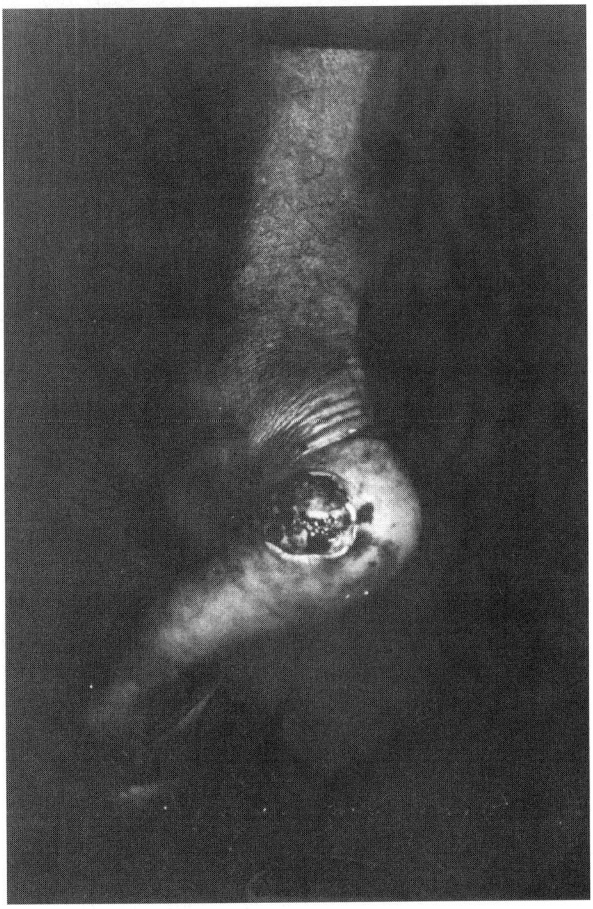

Figure 27 Nodular melanoma of the left foot. This melanoma is characterized histologically by a vertical growth phase and clinically by aggressive behavior.

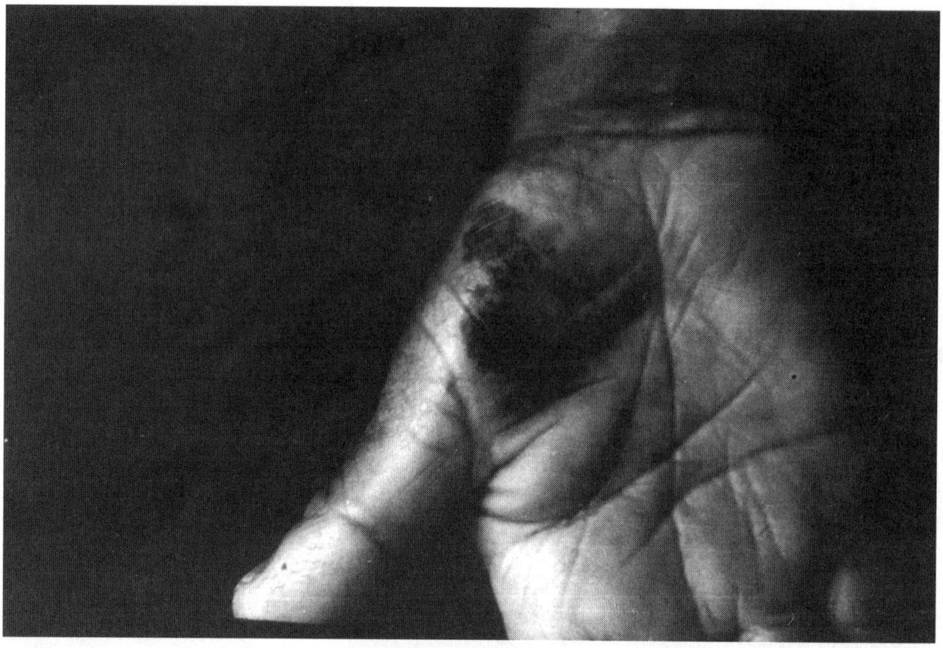

Figure 28 Acral lentiginous melanoma is the most frequent form of melanoma in dark-skinned individuals. This large patch shows various tones of black and brown and has ill-defined borders.

Desmoplastic neurotrophic melanoma presents as a nonpigmented scar without history of previous trauma. Preoperative diagnosis is difficult since it resembles keloid scar, morpheaform BCC, or dermatofibroma.

Amelanotic melanoma does not produce pigment. It presents as erythematous or skin-colored papules, nodules, or plaques. It resembles insect bite, folliculitis, BCC, adnexal tumor, or sarcoma.

Mucosal lentiginous melanoma presents in the oral cavity as a pigmented area showing the ABCDE changes. It resembles a nevus or a venous lake.

On histological examination, MM is identified by the presence of highly atypical melanocytes (Fig. 29). A pagetoid pattern refers to scattering of individual melanocytes and nests throughout all layers of epidermis. This pattern is seen in SSM. A lentiginous pattern is characterized by proliferation of atypical cells in the basal layer of epidermis with involvement of skin appendages. This pattern is seen in LMM and ALM. Amelanotic melanoma makes up 1.8% of most series. MM cells stain positive for S-100 and HMB-45.

The prognosis and management of melanoma are based on the histological findings; therefore, the pathologist's report should include:

1. Breslow depth: Thickness in millimeters measured from the granular layer to greatest depth. If ulcerated, from surface of ulcer to greatest depth.
2. Clark's level of invasion: I, cells localized to epidermis; II, through dermoepidermal junction into papillary dermis; III, filling papillary dermis; IV, reticular dermis; V, subcutaneous fat.

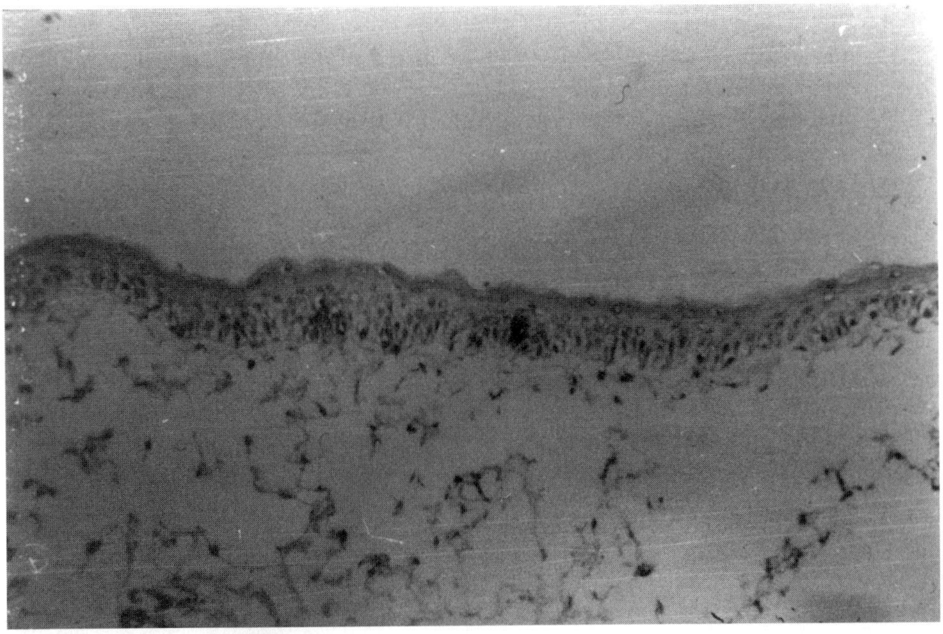

Figure 29 Characteristic lentiginous proliferation of neoplastic melanocytes in malignant melanoma. The darker areas show positive immunostaining reaction with S-100 monoclonal antibodies.

3. Radial vs. vertical growth phase.
4. Pagetoid vs. lentiginous pattern.
5. Mitotic rate (number of mitoses per mm^2) and prognostic index (mitotic rate × thickness in mm)
6. Presence or absence of ulceration, desmoplasia, neurotropism, regression, and satellite lesions (focus of MM larger than 0.5 mm, located on reticular dermis, and separated from main tumor by normal tissue)
7. Surgical margins

Staging of Melanoma According to the American Joint Commission for Cancer (AJCC).

				%Survival	
Stage	Tumor	Nodes	Metastases	5 years	10 years
0	Tis	N0	M0	100	99
1	T1-2	N0	M0	97	93
2	T3-4	N0	MO	77	68
3	Any T	N1-2	M0	48	40
4	Any T	Any N	M1	0	0

Tis = in situ/Clark I; T1 = < 0.75 mm/Clark II; T2 = 0.76–1.49 mm/Clark III; T3 = 1.5–3.99 mm/Clark IV; T4 = > 4.0 mm/Clark V; N1 = Nodes < 3 cm; N2 = Nodes > 3 cm; M1 = Distant metastases

Indicators of a bad prognosis include the following findings:

Breslow's thickness: The 5 year survival rate is 99% for melanomas <1 mm; 80–90% for 1–3 mm; 58% for 3–4 mm; and 30% for >4 mm.
Clark's level: The 5 year survival rate is 100% for levels I and II; 90% for level III; 66% for level IV; and 15–25% for level V.
Male gender
Ulceration
Mitotic rate $>5/mm^2$
Axial location (trunk, arm)
Age >50 years
Tumor size >2 cm
Satellitosis
Tumor volume $>200\,mm^3$

Management of Malignant Melanoma Localized to the Skin (Stage I and II)

Surgical excision is the treatment of choice. Wide margins of 5–10 cm were traditionally recommended but it is clear now that the margins of resection have no effect on prognosis. Zitelli gathered important information from more than 500 cases of MM treated with Mohs' surgery. He found that 83% of MM were completely excised with 6 mm margins, and 97% with 1.2 cm margins (146). This author also reported his findings in 50 cases of recurrent MM. Approximately 84% of tumors were cleared with <1 cm margins, and the remaining 16% with margins ranging from 1 to 2.1 cm.

In the recent past, several prospective studies have validated the use of conservative margins according to Breslow's depth (147–152). The NIH consensus was that in situ melanoma required 5 mm margins, <1 mm required 1 cm margins, and >1 mm required 2–3 cm margins. Veronesi recommended that melanomas <2 mm deep could be treated with 1 cm margins. Balch recommended 2 cm for melanomas with Breslow's depth of 1–4 mm.

Based on these data, the following conservative margins are widely accepted:

0.5 mm for MM in situ
1.0 cm for MM 1–2 mm
2.0 cm for MM 2–4 mm
3.0 cm for MM >4 mm

Treatment of MM with Mohs surgery is controversial. The detection of atypical melanocytes in frozen sections from MMS is difficult and highly correlated with experience (153). Yet, Zitelli reported 100% sensitivity and 90% specificity, while Cohen reported 73% and 68% respectively. The 5 year recurrence rate after Mohs surgery has been 0.5–1.2% and survival is similar to conventional surgical techniques. The use of IHC stains for S-100 and HMB-45 improves detection. Current indications for MMS in melanoma include:

Recurrent lesions
MM located on the head and neck, digits, and genitalia, where cosmesis and maximum preservation of tissue are essential
Lesions >2 cm in diameter
Ill-defined tumors

Treatment of metastic MM is difficult. The preferred approach to limb MM involves hyperthermic infusion of melphalan. Retrospective data suggest an improved survival for early MM (83% vs. 44%). A prospective study by Ghussen showed decreased recurrence and improved survival (92% vs. 61%) in patients with MM > 1.5 mm localized to the extremities (154). Further validation is awaited.

Approximately 20% of stage I and II melanomas will metastasize to regional lymph nodes within 3 years. Nevertheless, the risk is variable according to Breslow's-depth. Elective lymph node dissection (ELND) is not recommended for melanomas 1.5 mm or thinner because the risk for nodal disease is very low. Delayed therapeutic nodal dissection performed at the time of detection of clinical nodes is effective. ELND is likewise not recommended for lesions thicker than 4 mm. Distantmetastasis, with or without nodal involvement, occurs in 60% of these patients. Intermediate-thickness melanoma (1.5–4.0 mm) has a 38% risk for nodal involvement. Initial retrospective studies reported beneficial effects of ELND in patients with intermediate-thickness melanoma; however, further prospective experience has failed to validate the approach. At least three different prospective trials (WHO, Mayo Clinic, National Intergroup Melanoma Surgical Trial) have reported no benefit in survival (155,156).

Recent emphasis has been placed on the detection of so-called sentinel nodes: the first nodes to drain the area where the melanoma is located. Both blue dye injection and lymphoscintigraphy are employed singly and in combination (157,158). If microscopic disease is discovered in sentinel nodes, then a regional lymph node dissection is performed. If the sentinel node is free of tumor, it is assumed that the rest of the nodes are also negative. Results have been impressive and suggest that metastases in melanoma occur in stepwise fashion, with an identifiable first node of dissemination. The negative predictive value of sentinel node biopsy is approximately 99%. In other words, the risk for having MM in other lymph nodes when the sentinel node is negative is only 1%. In 95% of positive cases, the sentinel node is the only node affected.

Management of Lentigo Maligna and Lentigo Maligna Melanoma in situ

Cryotherapy with liquid nitrogen using 60 s freezing times and double freeze–thaw cycles results in 6.6% recurrence rate at 3 year follow-up (159,160).

Radiation therapy is indicated for large tumors that would necessitate disfiguring surgery and for poor surgical candidates. Conventional fractionated radiation results in 89% cure rate, with excellent cosmesis in 90%. Surgical salvage is always possible with reported 100% cure rates.

Curettage and electrodesiccation result in 23% recurrence rates, probably because the technique does not allow elimination of MM cells in hair follicles. It is not a preferred modality.

Topical 5-FU twice a day for 13 weeks has been successful in some patients, but Retin A and azelaic acid have been ineffective. Topical therapy is only indicated for LM after confirmatory biopsy.

Surgical excision is superior to destructive modalities. Reported cure rates have been 91% for surgery and 45% for other therapies but treatment is not always feasible due to extensive lesions requiring mutilating surgery.

Management of Nodal Disease (MM Stage III)

The 5 year survival for patients with nodal disease is 25–45%. The number of affected nodes and tumor penetration through the capsule are the most important factors. The treatment of choice is surgical excision of the primary site with therapeutic lymph node dissection. Overall survival, however, is 35% at 5 years.

Adjuvant interferon alpha 2b is the first and only agent to show a beneficial effect on recurrence and survival for these patients (161). The recommended regimen is 20 M units/m^2/day intravenously, 5 days a week for 4 weeks. This is followed by 10 M units SQ daily for 11 months. Shorter periods and lower dosages have not been effective. Unfortunately, side effects are common and 75% of patients require a change of dosage. The most frequent side effects are fever, chills, flu-like symptoms, fatigue, depression, and abnormal liver function tests. Interferon alpha cannot be used in the elderly or in patients with heart or liver disease.

Other options currently being investigated include adjuvant radiation (162) and hyperthermic limb perfusion with melphalan in combination with tumor necrosis factor. Results have been variable.

Management of Distant Metastatic Disease (MM Stage IV)

Mean survival for stage IV melanoma is 6 months. The majority of advanced melanoma cases either do not respond or have marginal responses to treatment. However, several clinical trials using chemotherapy and interleukin-2 (IL-2) have demonstrated lasting complete responses in a small number of patients. Some patients with metastases do relatively well, including some with solitary metastases to brain, lung, or skin.

Dimethyl triazeno imidazole cartoxamide (DTIC) is the best single chemotherapeutic agent for stage IV melanoma, with a 20–30% response rate (163,164). Temozolamide is a new chemotherapeutic agent with activity similar to DTIC (165). It is less emetic, has better CNS penetration, and can be taken orally. Other agents, single and in combination, are not superior to DTIC. The initial 55% response rate reported for the so-called Dartmouth Regimen (Carmustin, DTIC, cisplatin, tamoxifen) has not been reproduced. Furthermore, tamoxifen itself has minimal activity against MM.

High-dosage interferon alpha has resulted in 50% transient response rate, but with significant toxicity (166). Low-dosage IFN is ineffective.

High-dosage IL-2 has a 15– 25% response rate (167). The combination of IL-2 with IF is ineffective and toxicity is significant. The combination of Dartmouth regimen + IF + IL-2 shows response in 15–30% of cases.

External beam radiation therapy provides excellent palliation and symptomatic relief. It also helps to preserve neurological function (168).

Experimental therapies (169) include vaccines, monoclonal antibodies, and gene manipulation.

Work-up for Melanoma Stage I and II

Distant metastatic disease is incurable; therefore, its detection is not the main purpose of follow-up for patients with early melanoma. Recurrence rate is 1% for MM < 0.76 mm; 5.7% for 0.76–1.5 mm; 18% for 1.51– 4.0 mm; and 33% for > 4.0 mm (170). Approximately 94% of recurrences are detected by patients, 68% by history, 26% by physical examination, 11% by abnormal results of tests, and 6% by x-rays. More than 65% of recurrences happen within the first 24 months, and 81% are manifest within 36 months. The overall metastatic rate for MM is 2–8%. More than 50% of metastases are to regional nodes, but nodal spread is rare in melanomas thinner than 0.75 mm. Hematogenous spread involves lungs (18–36%), liver (14–20%), brain (12–20%), and bones (11–17%). Based on the above information, the initial work-up for MM stage I and II should include lactic dehydrogenase (LDH) levels and chest x-rays exclusively. Imaging techniques (computed tomographic [CT] scan, MRI) are not indicated. Follow-up visits are scheduled every 3 months for 2 years; every 6 months for 3 years; and yearly thereafter. The major benefit is detection of additional melanomas.

Work-up for Melanoma Stage III and IV

Prognosis is usually poor for these patients. Clinically evident nodes must be confirmed histologically. Screening should be limited to LDH levels and chest x-rays. Further evaluation should be guided by symptoms, including CT scan of the head and neck, chest, abdomen, and regional nodes; liver function tests; and MRI of the brain.

Malignant Adnexal Tumors

Hair Follicle Differentiation

Pilomatrix carcinoma (PC) is a rare tumor that originates in the hair cortex. Most lesions arise de novo and not from pre-existing benign pilomatrixoma. The tumor presents in the fourth and fifth decade of life and predominates in men (ratio 3:1). Approximately 57% of cases affect the head and neck (Fig. 30) followed by the chest

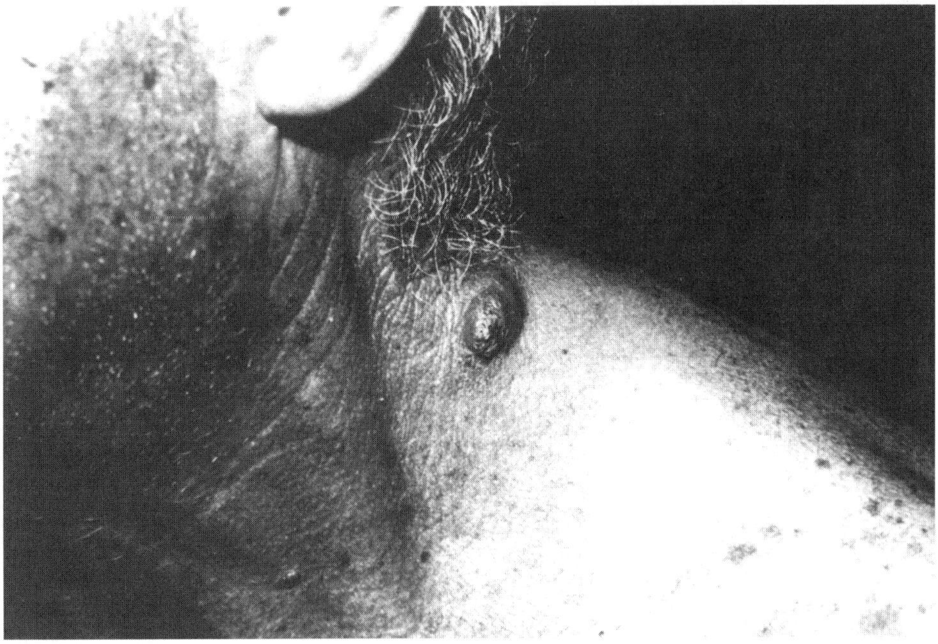

Figure 30 Pilomatrix carcinoma in the neck of an elderly man. The lesion started as a small subcutaneous nodule that later increased in size. The keratotic surface indicates epidermal involvement. It is worth remembering that various malignant adnexal tumors may present in such a noncharacteristic fashion.

(13%), back (11%), and upper (11%) and lower extremities (9%). Metastases occur in only 9% of patients, usually to lungs, bone, and lymph nodes (171). Histopathological examination shows infiltrating sheets and islands of basaloid cells extending deep into dermis and subcutaneous tissue. Two populations of cells are clearly identified: basophilic cells with indistinct borders and ghost cells with a well-defined border and nonstaining nuclei.

PC is difficult to cure using traditional surgical excision. Recurrence rates are 26% for conservative excision and 23% for wide excision (172). Only three reported cases were treated with surgery followed by radiation. One developed distant metastases. Mohs' micrographic surgery has not been employed but may prove useful.

Sweat Gland Differentiation

Microcystic adnexal carcinoma (MAC) shows dual differentiation into sebaceous gland and sweat gland structures. There are no known causative factors, although in some cases there is history of ionizing radiation exposure. The incidence in men and women is approximately equal and the median age at presentation is 65 years (range, 11–82). MAC presents clinically as a nodule, plaque, or cyst that grows slowly over years (173). The lesion is markedly indurated and has surface telangiectasias. It rarely undergoes ulceration. The main clinical differential diagnosis is morpheaform BCC, SCC, dermatofibrosarcoma protuberans (DFSP), and other adnexal tumors. MAC metastasizes to lymph nodes only occasionally but may directly invade bone in advanced cases. On histological examination there is a desmoplastic stroma, nests and cords of basaloid cells with ductal structures, and keratin-filled cysts. MAC is a dermal tumor, the epidermis is rarely involved, and there is perineural involvement in 80% of cases. IHC stains show CEA, S-100, and CF-1. MAC is difficult to eradicate due to marked subclinical extension and perineural involvement. The recurrence rate is 47% after surgical excision with margins up to 5 cm. Current recommendations include preoperative CT scan and MRI assessment of extension followed by Mohs' micrographic surgery (174).

Malignant eccrine spiradenoma (MES) shows differentiation toward eccrine intradermal ductal cells or secretory cells and affects people 50 years and older. It presents clinically as a sudden change in color or size of a pre-existing benign eccrine spiradenoma. Ulceration may also occur. Approximately 40% of cases are located on the upper extremities. Metastases occur only in lesions larger than 2 cm in diameter, usually to lymph nodes or lungs. Histological examination shows cords of basophilic cells with compact nuclei. Lobules are surrounded by a hyaline fibrous capsule (175). IHC stains show CEA, EMA, CK, and S-100. Surgical excision with 1–2 cm margins is the treatment of choice (176). Elective lymph node dissection should be considered. For clinically positive nodal disease, a therapeutic lymph node dissection is performed. Radiation therapy was not effective in two case reports.

Eccrine porocarcinoma (EPC) derives from the intraepidermal portion of the eccrine duct or acrosyringium. There are no known causative factors. Some 30–50% of cases originate from malignant transformation of pre-existing benign eccrine poromas. PC affects people older than 50 years and there is a slight predominance in women. The tumor is more frequent in whites (85%) than in Japanese (14%). The most frequent location is the lower extremities (50%), legs (25%), foot (14%), and thigh (12%). Malignant transformation of a benign poroma is manifested by ulceration, bleeding, or sudden growth (177). Metastases occur in 20% of cases, usually with tumors larger than 1 cm in diameter. Metastases involve the lymph nodes, lungs, retroperitoneum, bone, and liver. Mortality is approximately 68%. On histopathological examination, there are intraepidermal nests of basaloid cells, absent keratinization, and small clefts within tumor islands. IHC stains show positive reaction to CEA, EMA, and CK. Both surgical excision and Mohs' micrographic surgery offer cure rates of 85% (178). The latter is preferred for recurrent lesions. If PC spreads to lymph nodes, cure is difficult. Therapeutic lymph node dissection is successful in only 17% of cases, with 83% developing distant metastases. There are no data on ELND. Chemotherapy has variable response rate for distant metastatic disease.

Malignant clear cell hidradenoma (MCCH) is considered to be the malignant counterpart of eccrine acrospiroma. It is a rare tumor, accounting for only 6% of malignant eccrine neoplasms. There are no known risk factors. The tumor has an equal gender distribution, and patients have an average age of 52 years. MCCH presents as a nonspecific nodule or plaque, usually 3 cm in diameter or smaller. The lesion is red with surface telangiectasias. Ulceration is rare. At least 49% occur on the scalp or face, followed by acral sites in 28%, and trunk 23% (179). On histological examination, there are lobules with two cell populations. Centrally located are clear cells containing glycogen; basophilic spindle cells are found at the periphery. A characteristic feature is the presence of prominent squamous proliferation. Like most eccrine tumors, IHC staining shows EMA, CEA and CK positivity. MCCH tends to recur in 50% of cases due to extensive subclinical extension and perineural involvement (180). Radiation therapy should be avoided because it has been associated with more aggressive behavior. Metastases involve lymph nodes (40%) or distant sites. Recurrent tumors or MCCH with nodal involvement is best approached with Mohs' surgery followed by chemotherapy (doxorubicin, 5-FU, cisplatin). Distant metastatic disease is uniformly fatal despite chemotherapy.

Eccrine mucinous carcinoma (EMC) is derived from the eccrine secretory coil. It is a rare tumor that predominates in Whites (65%) and men (66%). Patient's median age is 63 years, ranging from 50 to 70. The lesion is usually single and asymptomatic. Approximately 75% of cases affect the eye, face, or scalp. It presents as a clinically translucent papule or nodule with a red or blue hue (181) resembling BCC or pyogenic granuloma. Most EMCs follow an indolent course, but metastases may occur in 10% of cases (3% of eye tumors but 38% of truncal lesions). Metastatic spread is to regional lymph nodes with only occasional reports of distant metastases. Histopathological examination reveals basaloid cells within mucinous stroma. Cells are uniform in size and shape with few mitotic figures. IHC stains are positive for EMA, CEA, and CK. Traditional surgical excision with 2 cm margins has a 28% recurrence rate (182). Mohs' surgery may offer a better control rate, especially for eyelid tumors and recurrent cases. Regional nodal disease is treated with therapeutic lymph node dissection. The role of ELND is unknown. Distant metastases fail to respond to both radiation therapy and chemotherapy.

Malignant chondroid syringoma (MCS) originates from apocrine structures. It differentiates into sweat gland and chondroid elements. Most lesions develop de novo and not from benign counterparts. At least two-thirds of cases occur in women (183). Age ranges from 13 to 89, with an average of 52 years. The most frequent location is the lower extremity (35%) followed by the upper extremity (20%), head and neck (25%), and trunk (15%). MCS presents clinically as firm nodules that may ulcerate. Approximately 80% are painful. Histological examination shows lobules containing epithelial and mesenchymal elements (chondrocytes) with variable pseudocapsule. Wide local excision results in a 50% recurrence rate and 45% metastases to lymph nodes. Mohs' surgery is probably useful. ELND and adjuvant radiation should be considered (184). Nodal disease is best approached with surgical excision of the primary site and therapeutic lymph node dissection. Chemotherapy is not effective.

Primary cutaneous adenoid cystic carcinoma (PCACC) is a rare tumor with eccrine/apocrine origin (185). It affects both men and women at a mean age of 59 years (range, 14–90 years). The most common location is the scalp, followed by the trunk and extremities. Tumors resemble furuncles or larger erythematous nodules. Metastases occur in 11% of cases, mostly to the lungs. On histological examination, PCACC is indistinguishable from adenoid cystic carcinoma of salivary glands. There are uniform basaloid cells with oval nuclei, solitary nucleoli, and rare mitotic figures. Two patterns exist: a cribiform pattern with pseudolumina resembling Swiss cheese and a tubular pattern with multiple ductlike structures. The tumor is deep dermal and has no connection to the epidermis. There is frequent perineural involvement. IHC stains are positive for EMA, CEA, and CK. Surgical excision results in a 64% recurrence rate. Larger size and perineural involvement are risk factors. Mohs' micrographic surgery has been successfully attempted in at least two cases but the follow-up has been too short for definitive results (186). One case treated with radiation recurred after 15 months. Recurrent tumors are best approached with Mohs' surgery. It is impossible to make recommendations regarding metastatic disease due to the scarcity of reported cases.

Malignant cylindroma may arise de novo or from pre-existing benign cylindromas. Risk factors for malignant transformation of cylindroma include chronic irritation and trauma, incomplete excision, and ionizing radiation. Approximately 90% of cases involve the scalp and women are more commonly affected. Malignant cylindroma affects the elderly (average age, 72) and latency from onset of benign tumor to malignant transformation is 27 years (187). Cylindromas are red, firm nodules of various sizes. Malignant transformation is manifested by rapid growth or ulceration. It is more likely in multiple tumors (64%) than in single neoplasms (36%). Regional metastases occur in 44% of cases. Distant metastases are possible to liver, lungs, or bone. Histopathological examination shows multiple irregular islands of uniform cells surrounded by a hyaline sheath. There are small cells with dark nuclei at the periphery and large, pale cells at the center. IHC stains are positive for CEA, EMA, and CK. Surgical excision results in a 36% recurrence rate. Mohs' surgery may be useful. Radiation is not recommended. Regional disease is approached with therapeutic lymph node dissection. Distant metastatic disease is incurable (188).

Paget's disease of the nipple originates in luminal lactiferous ducts of breast tissue. It affects women in the fifth decade of life (a decade older than most breast cancer patients) and is frequently associated with an underlying intraductal carcinoma. Paget's disease presents clinically as an erythematous scaly patch that, in contrast to benign eczema, is indurated and well-demarcated (189). Mammography shows changes in only 50–70% of cases. On histological examination there is a pagetoid distribution of large, pale, round cells in all layers of the epidermis. IHC staining is positive for CEA, EMA, and CK. Mastectomy is the treatment of choice.

Approximately 50% of patients have no associated intraductal carcinoma, and their survival is 100%. For those with underlying carcinoma, survival is 43% at 5 years. There is limited experience with conservative surgery in combination with radiotherapy (190). If nodes are positive, survival drops to 10% even after therapeutic lymph node dissection.

Extramammary Paget's disease (EMPD) differentiates into both eccrine and apocrine elements. The tumor presents as an erythematous scaly patch of variable size and indistinct border (Fig. 31). It resembles tinea, psoriasis, eczema, Bowen's disease, or superficial BCC. EMPD is usually located on the anogenital area, axillae head, or neck. It is more common in Whites and women during the sixth to ninth decades of life. Approximately 24% of patients have an underlying adnexal carcinoma and 12% of cases are associated with an internal malignancy of the gastrointestinal (GI) or genitourinary tract (191). Histopathological examination shows large pale epithelial cells in what is termed a buckshot distribution (Fig. 32). Some nests show glandular array. Dermal invasion signals the presence of adnexal carcinoma. IHC stains are positive for CEA, EMA, and GCDFP-15 (apocrine glands). EMPD is negative for S-100, HMB-45 (MM), or CK (SCC). Surgical excision or Mohs' surgery is the treatment of choice (192). IHC are useful to define surgical margins. Topical 5-FU is used preoperatively to delineate subclinical extension, and postoperatively to detect recurrences (193). Therapeutic lymph node dissection is indicated for nodal disease. Radical vulvectomy with bilateral groin lymphadenectomy is recommended for invasive cases. Mohs' surgery is the treatment of choice for

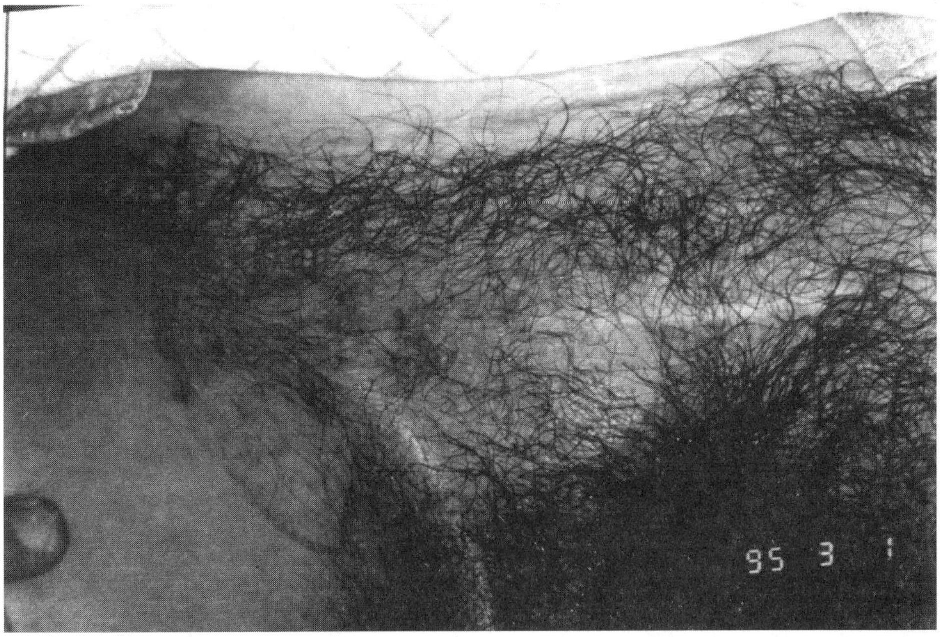

Figure 31 Long-standing erythematous scaly patch on the pubic area that was repeatedly treated as tinea and eczema without response. A diagnostic biopsy specimen showed extramammary Paget's disease. A short course of topical 5-FU was used to delineate subclinical extension prior to treatment with Mohs' surgery.

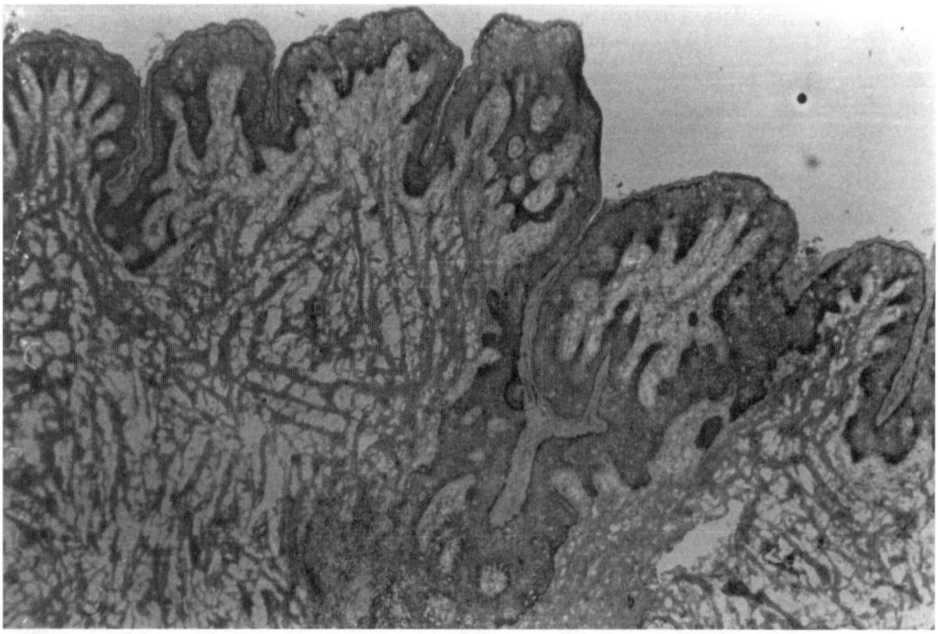

Figure 32 Histopathological examination in Paget's disease shows characteristic proliferation of large pale cells in a buckshot distribution. Some glandular-like nests are evident at the level of the hair follicle. Such pagetoid proliferation is seen also in malignant melanoma and squamous cell carcinoma, and differentiation is established with the help of immunohistochemical stains.

recurrent tumors (194). Radiation therapy and chemotherapy are not curative but may be useful as palliation in advanced cases. The initial work-up should include physical and rectal examination, sigmoidoscopy, and cystoscopy. For women, mammography and colposcopy are also indicated. Mortality is 18% but increases to 46% if associated with adnexal or visceral neoplasia.

Malignant hidradenoma papilliferum (MHP) arises from pre-existing benign hidradenoma papilliferum (HP). There are no other known risk factors. MHP and HP present clinically as nonspecific dermal nodules with normal overlying skin. The tumor affects women more than men, and Whites more than other races. The most common location is the anogenital area. Although HP affects prepubertal patients, MHP is usually seen in middle-aged women (195). Histopathological examination shows an encapsulated dermal tumor without connection to the epidermis. There are tubular and cystic structures with papillary projections. Active decapitation secretion is a characteristic feature common to apocrine neoplasms. IHC stains are positive for CK, CEA, S-100, and GCDFP-15. Surgical excision with 2 cm margins is the treatment of choice (196). Mohs' surgery is a valid alternative.

Apocrine carcinoma (AC) is a rare tumor that accounts for 0.005% of surgical specimens. The tumor usually affects areas rich in apocrine glands such as the axilla, anogenital area, external auditory canal (EAC), Moll's glands in the eyelid, and mammary glands. Peak incidence is during the fifth to sixth decade without gender predominance (197). The only risk factor may be ionizing radiation. AC presents non-characteristically as a firm or cystic, nontender dermal nodule of variable size. Lesions are single, mobile, and red, blue, or skin-colored. On histological examination, AC shows glandular nests and cords of polygonal eosinophilic cells forming lumina (ductopapillary variety). Signs of malignancy include atypia, nuclear pleomorphism, necrosis, vascular or perineural invasion, and poor delimitation. IHC staining is positive for CEA, EMA, CK, and GCDFP-15. Wide surgical excision is the treatment of choice but 80% recurrence rates have been reported. Metastases occur in 30%, mostly to lymph nodes, but also to lungs, liver, and bone. Mohs' surgery may improve cure rates (198). It is currently indicated for cosmetic areas, tissue preservation, and recurrent tumors. Therapeutic lymph node dissection is performed for nodal disease. Consider sentinel node biopsy (see section on malignant melanoma). Metastatic disease is treated with chemotherapy. Radiation therapy is ineffective.

Sebaceous Gland Differentiaton

Sebaceous carcinoma arises from meibomian (51%) and Zeis glands (10%) of the eyelid. The tumor is not caused by ultraviolet (UV) radiation but certain HPVs and ionizing radiation are contributing factors. Chronic chalazion is also a predisposing factor due to inflammation and production of oleic acid. Sebaceous carcinoma may occur singly or in association with keratoacanthomas and internal (GI tract) malignancies as part of the Muir-Torre syndrome (199). Sebaceous carcinoma affects women more than men, usually in the sixth or seventh decade of life. It predominates in Asians. Approximately 25% of cases are extraocular, mostly from the parotid gland (20%). A multicentric origin is reported in 12% of cases. Clinically, the lesions present as yellowish nodules of variable size. Histopathological examination shows lobules and cords of neoplastic cells with sebaceous differentiation. Cells have a foamy cytoplasm, nuclear pleomorphism, and mitotic figures. A pagetoid pattern is observed in 40–80% of cases. IHC stains are positive for EMA, but are negative for CEA, breast carcinoma antigen, S-100, or GCDFP-15. Stains for lipids are useful, including Sudan IV and oil red 0. Surgical excision is the treatment of choice but the recurrence rate is 30%. Mohs' surgery is indicated for tissue preservation and better margin control (200). Recurrence rates are lower but the pagetoid pattern and multicentric origin impair the effectiveness of the Mohs' technique. Metastases occur in 14–25% of cases, mostly to lymph nodes, liver, lungs, bones, and brain. Nodal disease is treated with surgical excision of the primary site, lymph node dissection, and radiation therapy. Distant metastatic disease is managed with surgery, radiation and chemotherapy.

Initial work-up includes physical examination, rectal and breast examination, ophthalmological evaluation, stool guaiac, complete blood count (CBC), chest x-ray, mammography, and colonoscopy. Follow-up is done at 1 and 3 months after surgery; every 3 months for 2 years; and yearly thereafter.

Merkel Cell Carcinoma

Merkel cell carcinoma originates in Merkel cells (cutaneous mechanoreceptors that provide a template for nerve arborization during neural development). It is an infrequent tumor with unknown incidence. Men and women are equally affected and patients' mean age is 69 years. UV radiation, immunosuppression, and glucocorticosteroids are relevant contributing factors. Merkel cell carcinoma (MCC) presents as an asymptomatic, erythematous–violaceous nodule with telangiectasias (Fig. 33). It may resemble BCC, SCC, or MM, and is usually less than 2 cm in diameter. Approximately 50% of lesions affect the head and neck followed by the extremities in 35% of cases (201). Histological examination shows monotonous small cells with round nuclei, marked mitotic activity, and prominent nucleoli. Histologically, MCC resembles undifferentiated small-cell carcinoma. IHC staining is positive for neuron-specific enolase, neurofilament and CK. Localized disease is best approached with surgical excision using 3 cm margins or Mohs' micrographic surgery (202). Overall, cure rates are 60–90% for primary and 50% for recurrent lesions. Primary tumors of the head and neck, however, have a recurrence rate of 20–100% after surgery alone, and various centers advocate adjuvant external beam radiation therapy. This approach reduces recurrence rates to 10–40%. Initial work-up should include physical examination with detailed node evaluation, CBC, LFT's, and chest radiographs. CT scans of the chest, neck, abdomen, and pelvis are also

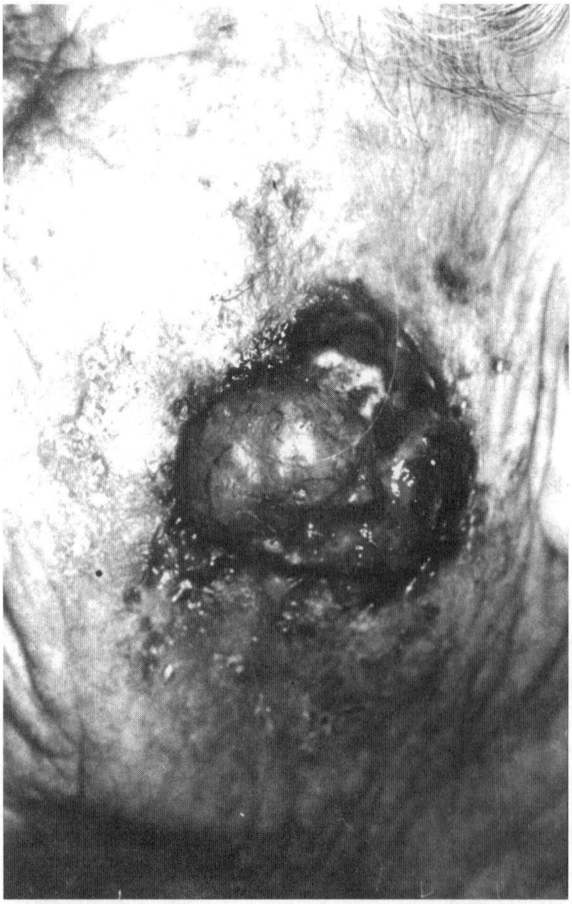

Figure 33 Large, nonspecific, ulcerated nodule on the cheek of an elderly women. The biopsy showed Merkel cell carcinoma and the patient was treated with Mohs' surgery.

indicated. Nodal disease occurs in approximately 50% of patients; therefore, a sentinel node biopsy is recommended for most lesions. Survival is only 48% after surgical excision, therapeutic node dissection, and radiotherapy (203). Distant metastatic disease may involve the skin, lungs, liver, and brain. Combination chemotherapy is palliative and all patients eventually die from their disease within 6 months.

Sarcomas

Sarcomas are soft tissue tumors with variable malignant potential. Tumors are classified as benign, intermediate (locally invasive and tend to recur) or malignant (locally aggressive with potential for metastases). Their development is related to genetic factors, trauma, radiation, immunosuppression, carcinogens, and/or viruses. Histological grading, although subjective, plays an important role in classification and management. Aggressive sarcomas are usually poorly differentiated and tend to metastasize early. Nodal involvement is unusual but its presence constitutes a poor prognostic sign. It has also been recognized that biopsies, drains and sutures, along with postoperative fluid collection, are risk factors for tumor implantation and recurrence.

Sarcomas of Fibrous Tissue

Fibrosarcoma is a rare malignant tumor from deep tissues such as fascia or tendons. Well-established causative factors include ionizing radiation (204), chronic scars, and certain chromosomal aberrations. Fibrosarcoma affects all ages but is more common during the fourth to sixth decade of life. Tumors present clinically as subcutaneous masses with intact overlying skin. Ulceration indicates aggressive growth. Pain is present in 50% of cases. Approximately 50% of lesions occur on the lower extremity with marked predominance of the thigh (205). On histopathological examination, there are masses of spindle cells with variable differentiation, storiform pattern, and myxoid changes. IHC stains are positive for CD34 and vimentin, but not for epithelial, muscular, neural, melanocytic, or vascular markers (see below). Treatment is similar for all soft tissue sarcomas. Wide local excision with or without amputation is the usual approach. Adjuvant radiation therapy is indicated for aggressive or invasive cases. Recurrence rates are unknown but 5 year survival is 50%. Current protocols also include chemotherapy with doxorubicin but the survival rate has not been modified (206).

Dermatofibrosarcoma protuberans (DFSP) is an uncommon soft tissue tumor accounting for fewer than 0.1% of all malignancies and 1% of soft tissue sarcomas. This tumor arises in the dermis and invades the surrounding tissue by radial and vertical extension through the pre-existing collagen bundles and along connective tissue septa. Fifty percent of these neoplasms arise on the trunk, 35% involve the extremities, and 15% occur on the head and neck. DFSP has been reported in all races with a slight predominance in men (207). Most cases occur in patients between ages 20 and 50 years. Twenty percent of all patients report antecedent trauma. This tumor has also been reported to arise in surgical scars, vaccination scars, and burn scars. Tumors may appear as a plaque or nodular growth. The initial presentation is usually a dusky, indurated plaque that may go unrecognized for an extended period of time. The color of the plaque may vary from brown to bluish-red with a blue or reddish hue of the surrounding skin. The plaque is usually flat and in some cases

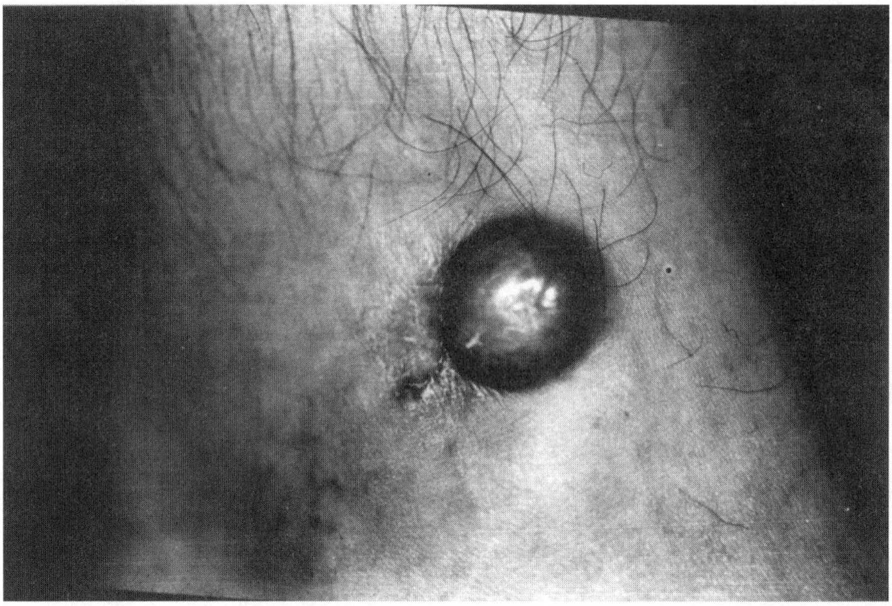

Figure 34 Dermatofibrosarcoma protuberans on the ankle of a young man. The lesion is firm, brown, and well-demarcated. DFSP lesions may be clinically identical to keloid scars or dermatofibromas.

depressed, resembling morphea, and over time the plaque becomes larger with the gradual development of a nodular component within the sclerotic area. The nodular component may become quite large in advanced tumors and vary in color from flesh-colored to dusky red or red-brown (Fig. 34). Five percent of DFSPs may present as a rare variant known as a Bednar tumor. This pigmented form occurs predominantly in black patients and contains melanin. Histologically, DFSP is composed predominantly of cells with large, spindle-shaped nuclei embedded in varying amounts of collagen. The cells are arranged in irregular, intertwining bands producing a storiform or matlike pattern (Fig. 35). IHC staining is positive for CD-34 (208). Surgical excision is the treatment of choice. Recurrences are common because the infiltrating growth pattern often extends well beyond the perceived clinical margins. Reported rates of recurrence vary from 11 to 54% following treatment with conventional surgical excision (209). Mohs' micrographic surgery along with rapid immunohistochemical staining for CD-34 antigens is useful in the surgical management of DFSP. More than 200 cases have been treated to date with only seven recurrences (3.3% recurrence rate) (210). Radiation therapy is indicated for inoperable tumors and as an adjunct to surgical removal. However, it should be used cautiously because fibrosarcomatous changes within DFSP have been reported following irradiation. Chemotherapy plays no role in the treatment of DFSP. DFSP metastasizes in fewer than 4% of cases. Metastatic cases almost always are recurrent tumors with a considerable time elapsed between diagnosis, multiple recurrences, and metastasis. Favored metastatic locations include lung, brain, bone, and, rarely, lymph nodes.

Atypical fibroxanthoma (AFX) is a fairly common tumor that presents predominantly on the sun-exposed areas of the head and neck regions of elderly

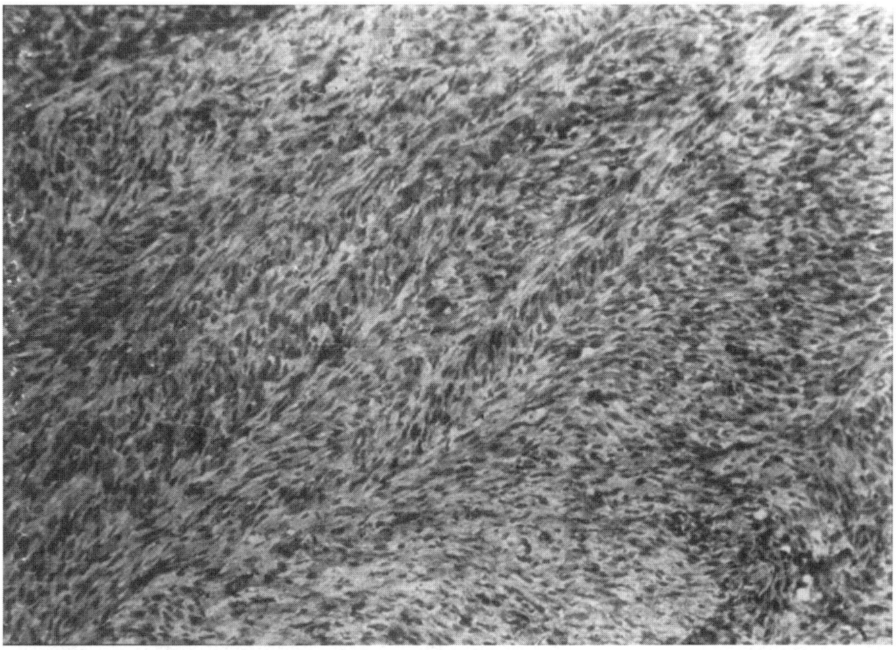

Figure 35 Characteristic storiform arrangement of spindle cells in dermatofibrosarcoma protuberans. A rare variant containing large amounts of melanin is known as the Bednar tumor.

patients. The most common locations are the nose, cheek, and ear with occasional occurrences on the trunk and limbs. This tumor usually presents as an asymptomatic solitary nodule or ulcerating nodule 2 cm in diameter or smaller. Clinically, AFX may resemble squamous cell carcinoma, basal cell carcinoma, epidermal inclusion cyst, or an ulcerated pyogenic granuloma. UV radiation appears to play an etiologic role since many of these tumors occur on severely actinically damaged skin in elderly individuals. Radiation therapy is also thought to be a contributing factor (211). AFX is often considered a superficial form of malignant fibrous histiocytoma. Due to its superficial location within the skin and its relatively small size, the tumor usually pursues a benign course. It has rarely been reported to metastasize to regional lymph nodes and parotid gland. On histological examination, AFX is composed of cells with pleomorphic, often hyperchromatic, nuclei in an irregular arrangement. Cells may appear spindle-shaped and lie in small bundles resembling fibroblasts. Other cells may appear polygonal and have foamy vacuolated cytoplasm and thus resemble histiocytes. Most AFX tumors will have large, bizarre, multinucleated giant cells showing marked nuclear atypicality. Recommended treatment for cutaneous AFX is surgical excision with margin control. Mohs' micrographic surgery has been used to treat AFX with excellent clinical results (212). Nodal disease is approached with surgical excision of the primary site and lymph node dissection. Adjuvant radiation therapy has been successfully employed in some cases.

Malignant fibrous histiocytoma (MFH) is a pleomorphic sarcoma representing the most common soft tissue sarcoma of middle and late adult life. It is an aggressive soft tissue sarcoma that has been subclassified into superficial and deep tumor types. Superficial tumors originate in the subcutaneous tissue and attach to the underlying fascia. In rare cases these tumors may invade the overlying dermis, resulting in ulceration. The deep tumor variety may originate in the subcutaneous tissue and extend through the underlying fascia into the muscle, or may originate within the muscle itself. The deep tumor variety appears to be twice as common as the superficial type, with poorer survival. Metastases occur in regional lymph nodes and the lungs and are the usual cause of death (213). On histological examination, MFH is a highly cellular tumor made up of fibroblastic, histiocytic, and bizarre-appearing cells. Fibroblastic cells have elongated-to-spindle-shaped nuclei and are arranged in storiform patterns. Histiocytic cells have a polygonal structure with irregularly shaped nuclei and cytoplasm that may be eosinophilic or vacuolated. Multinucleated giant cells with bizarre, hyperchromatic nuclei can be noted. IHC stains are positive for vimentin (mesenchymal); lysozyme, alpha-1 antitrypsin, and CD-68 (histiocytes); and collagen- and fibroblast-associated antigen (fibroblasts). Surgical excision with or without regional lymph node dissection is the treatment of choice. Reported recurrence rates are 30–47% even after amputation. Adjuvant radiation lowers the recurrence rate to 19% (214). Mohs' micrographic surgery can be used for the superficial type of MFH. A retrospective study involving 17 patients demonstrated a single recurrence after an average of 3 years' follow-up. Overall 5 year survival is 70% (215). The metastatic rate is variable depending on the depth of invasion. MFH confined to the subcutaneous tissue metastasizes in fewer than 10% of cases; those involving the subcutaneous and fascial planes have a metastatic rate of 27%. Deep-seated tumors involving skeletal muscle metastasize in 43% of cases. The 5 year survival rate is approximately 60%.

Sarcomas of Vascular Tissue

Angiosarcoma (AS) is a malignant tumor that originates from vascular endothelium and accounts for 1–4% of soft tissue sarcomas. The only known predisposing factors are ionizing radiation and chronic lymphedema. It is classified into cutaneous (60%) and deep angiosarcoma (40%) but we will review the former only (216).

AS associated with lymphedema presents in areas of chronic lymphedema occurring after radical mastectomy for treatment of breast cancer. However, fewer than 1% of patients with breast cancer develop it. Patients are usually in the seventh decade of life and AS presents an average of 10 years after surgery. Lesions are single or multiple, red to violaceous nodules. The most common location is the arm.

Cutaneous AS of the face and scalp accounts for 50% of tumors. Typically, the lesions present on the head, neck, or scalp of elderly men. Mean age at presentation is 67–74 years and whites are most frequently affected. The tumors are purple–red nodules and plaques that tend to ulcerate during the course of the disease. Multiple lesions occur in 60% of patients.

Primary AS of the breast is a variant that makes up 0.4% of breast tumors. It usually occurs in young women between the ages of 30 and 40. Lesions are painless red or blue nodules and plaques.

Post-irradiation AS occurs in 0.1% of cancer patients who survive more than 5 years. Latency period from irradiation to tumor is 2 to 50 years. Median age is 63 and the ratio of women to men is 2:1.

On histological examination, the angiomatous pattern represents the best-differentiated form of AS. There are multiple vascular channels lined by neoplastic endothelial cells with hyperchromatic nuclei and increased mitotic activity. The projection of cells into vascular lumina is pathognomonic. The spindle-cell variant corresponds to an intermediate grade of differentiation. The cells are fusiform and placed around vascular spaces. Undifferentiated AS is indistinguishable from other sarcomas. There are polygonal epithelioid cells with prominent nucleoli arranged in sheets. IHC stains show vascular markers such as factor VIII, UEA-1, and CD-31.

AS associated with lymphedema responds poorly to conservative surgery (217). Amputation leads to fewer recurrences and improves survival. The overall prognosis is dismal, with patients surviving up to 36 months. Most develop distant metastases to lungs, bones, or liver.

Cutaneous AS of the face and scalp is associated with nodal involvement in 13% of cases and has an 80% recurrence rate after conventional surgery. Multicentric origin and subclinical extension account for the poor results. Mohs' micrographic surgery offers better margin control, and sentinel node biopsy is emerging as a useful approach. Current treatment of choice is surgery in combination with adjuvant high-energy electron beam radiation. The reported 5 year cure rate is 54% compared to 19% with traditional therapy (218). Radiation therapy alone has not been effective and chemotherapy has not been adequately investigated. In contrast to other sarcomas, histological grading bears little relationship with prognosis, but survival varies inversely with size. There is 100% mortality for tumors larger than 10 cm compared with 67% in smaller lesions. The prognosis is also poor for recurrent tumors: only 8% can be rendered disease-free. At least 50% of patients develop metastases to lungs, liver or spleen. Lymph node involvement occurs in 15% of patients. Average survival is 10–20 months and reported 5 year survival rate is 25–33%.

Mammary AS is treated with mastectomy, but without axillary lymph node dissection, since the tumor rarely invades the regional nodes (219). Adjuvant chemotherapy yields significant beneficial results in patients with well-differentiated tumors (survival: 91%) but most others die of their disease. Metastases occur to lungs, liver, and spleen. Radiation-induced AS is treated according to clinical presentation.

Kaposi's sarcoma (KS) occurs in 15% of human immunodeficiency virus (HIV)-positive homosexual male patients. Human herpes virus type 8, and to a lesser degree HPV 16, has been identified as an causative cofactor. Recent evidence suggests that HIV per se can induce KS via production of gene products and cytokines. The typical clinical presentation includes macules, papules, nodules, or plaques that are symmetrically distributed over skin and oral mucosa (220). Lesions are pink to red or purple. Differential diagnosis must include purpura, hemangiomas, bacillary angiomatosis, lymphoma, and syphilis. Histological examination shows a dermal tumor. The earliest change is a subtle proliferation of blood vessels occurring in clinically unaffected skin. Next is the development of the patch stage, characterized clinically by pinkish macules and evident histologically as increased numbers of dilated slit-like vascular spaces lined by flat endothelial cells. The plaque stage is recognizable by abundant slit-like vascular spaces and scattered extravasated erythrocytes and siderophages. The nodular stage is characterized by cellular proliferation of spindle cells. Atypia is prominent and there is marked pleomorphism and multiple mitotic figures. IHC stains are positive for factor VIII, UEA-1, CD-31, and CD-34. Treatment of uncomplicated KS of the skin is done for cosmetic reasons. Options include cryotherapy with liquid nitrogen and intralesional vinblastin or interferon alpha 2b (221). Life-threatening disseminated KS is best managed with systemic high-dosage interferon alpha (8 M units/day), which is very effective if the CD-4 counts are higher than 200 cells/mm^3. Promising therapies include liposomally encapsulated doxorubicin and daunorubicin (90% response) and topical photodynamic therapy in combination with interferon alpha 2b.

Hemangiopericytoma (HPC) originates in the pericyte, a spindle cell found around capillaries and venules that may be involved in regulation of vessel caliber. No specific causative factors have been implicated but multiple chromosomal abnormalities, including translocations of chromosome 29, have been identified. Mean age at presentation is 38–58 years, ranging from infancy to 92 years. Men and women are equally affected. HPC involves the lower extremities in approximately 35% of cases, followed by the pelvis and retroperitoneum in 25%, and head/neck in 17% (222). Meningeal HPC accounts for fewer than 1% of tumors. Like other sarcomas, HPC presents as an asymptomatic, slowly growing mass. Size is variable but may reach 35 cm. Color is gray, tan, pink, or purple. Subclinical extension is revealed by CT scans and MRI. Angiography demonstrates the vascular nature of the tumor with many small corkscrew vessels. On histological examination, HPC is characterized by multiple vascular channels in a so-called stag-horn distribution. There are spindle cells with ill-defined cytoplasm, mitoses, and anaplasia. IHC staining is positive for vimentin and factor VIII. Differentiation from malignant fibrous histiocytoma is almost impossible. Surgical excision is the treatment of choice. Massive bleeding is common and preoperative embolization is now routine. Radiation may be used as primary or adjuvant therapy. Cure rates of 90% have been reported (223). Chemotherapy is not effective.

Sarcomas of Muscular Tissue

Cutaneous leiomyosarcoma (LMS) is a rare tumor that accounts for 7% of soft tissue sarcomas. It arises from the arrector pili muscle of hair follicles or muscles associated with sweat glands. Subcutaneous LMS develops from vascular smooth muscle. There are no known causative factors. A relationship with irradiation, trauma, and malignant transformation of pre-existing leiomyoma is anecdotal. Median age at presentation is 40–70 years. There is no gender or racial predominance. The most frequent location is the thigh (Fig. 36). The tumor presents as a slowly growing, solitary mass that is red or blue. Ulceration and pain are variable. Histological examination shows typical muscular spindle cells arranged in bundles (224). Mitotic figures and nuclear atypia are common. Blunt-edged, cigar-shaped nuclei are characteristic (Fig. 37). IHC staining is positive for desmin, actin and vimentin. The current recommendation is surgical excision with 2 cm margins. Recurrent rates are as high as 40–60% (225). Mohs' surgery offers better margin control and tissue preservation. Adjuvant radiation therapy is indicated for tumors with high-grade histological characteristics, larger than 5 cm, or recurrent. Chemotherapy has been used only in the context of clinical trials. Nodal disease is best treated with a lymph node dissection. Metastases, although rare in cutaneous LMS, are treated with surgery in combination with chemotherapy. The response rate varies between 15 and 30%.

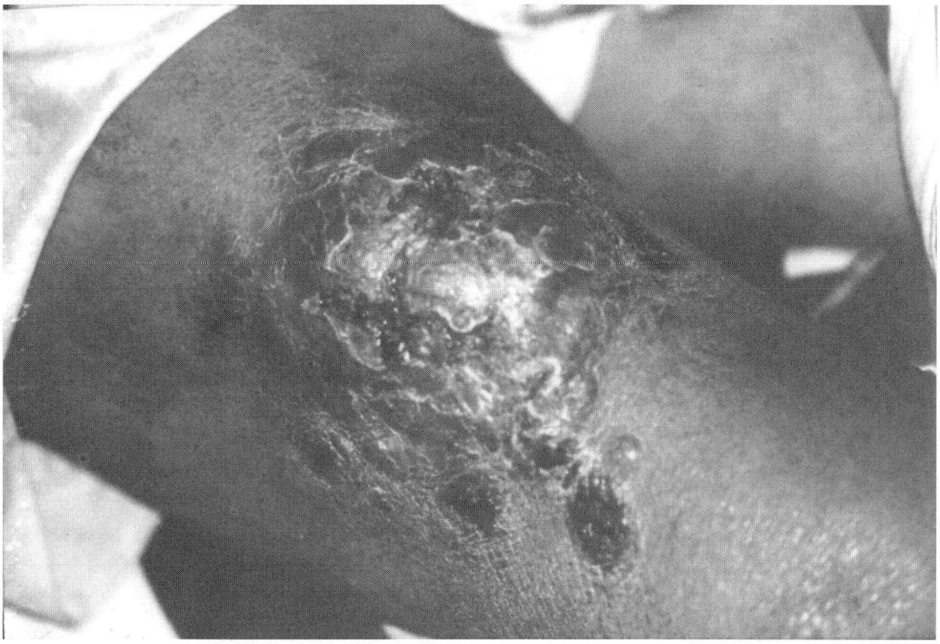

Figure 36 Large leiomyosarcoma of the thigh. Lesion is firm, hyperpigmented, and fixed to deep tissues.

Cutaneous rhabdomyosarcoma (RMS) is the most common soft tissue sarcoma in children and adolescents. Purely cutaneous RMS is exceedingly rare. It arises from primitive undifferentiated mesenchymal tissue, not from mature skeletal muscle as the name may suggest. The only predisposing factors are genetic, with familial aggregation and association with neurofibromatosis and retinoblastoma. Mean age at presentation is 10 years and the tumor predominates in males (226). The lesion presents nonspecifically as a subcutaneous nodule that grows slowly. Head and neck lesions account for 70% of cases, with the remaining tumors affecting the trunk (20%) and extremities (10%). Histological examination shows ill-defined aggregates of poorly differentiated round or oval cells. Hyaline fibrous septa and giant cells are characteristic. IHC stains are positive for desmin, actin, myoglobin, vimentin, and myosin. RMS requires a multidisciplinary approach for treatment. The current recommendation is surgical excision in combination with radiation and multiagent chemotherapy. The overall 5 year survival is 63% (227). Prognosis for localized, fully resected disease is excellent, with an 80–85% 5 year survival rate. Survival is lower for patients with incompletely excised tumors (65%) or metastatic disease (20%). Metastatic spread occurs to lung, bone marrow, and lymph nodes.

Sarcomas of Neural Tissue

Malignant peripheral nerve sheath tumor (MPNST) is rare and accounts for 10% of soft tissue sarcomas. Ionizing radiation is the only known causative factor, however, it is present in only a minority of patients. The tumor usually manifests as a sudden

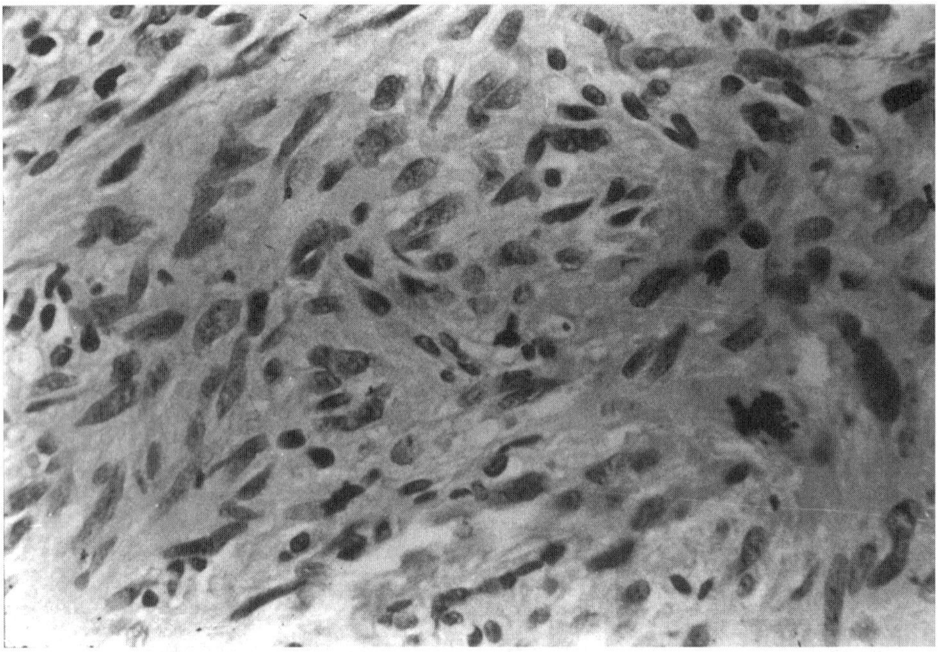

Figure 37 Typical blunt-edged nuclei in neoplastic cells of leiomyosarcoma. Malignancy is suggested by prominent hyperchromatism, nuclear atypia and abnormal mitotic figures.

growth of a pre-existing neurofibroma in patients with neurofibromatosis (228). The neoplasia is commonly associated with a nerve plexus and many patients have evidence of neuropathy or pain. Histological examination demonstrates spindle cells arranged in interlacing fascicles. Nuclear atypia and hyperchromasia are present. IHC stains are positive for S-100, vimentin, myelin basic protein, and neuron-specific enolase. Currently available therapy is disappointing. Wide surgical excision results in recurrence rates higher than 50% (229). The tumor is not responsive to either chemotherapy or radiation. Metastases are documented in 50% of deep-seated lesions.

Malignant granular cell tumor (MGCT) is a rare tumor. Mean age at presentation is 48 years. Lesions tend to be large (4–10 cm), grow rapidly, and become ulcerated. The most frequent location is the tongue. Histological examination shows polygonal epithelioid cells with granular eosinophilic cytoplasm. A characteristic pseudoepitheliomatous hyperplasia of the overlying epidermis is frequent (230). These changes are similar to those of benign granular cell tumors, but there is more pleomorphism, hyperchromatism, spindle cells, and necrosis. IHC stains do not differentiate between benign and malignant tumors. There is positive staining for vimentin, S-100, neuron-specific enolase, and myelin basic protein. The treatment of choice is wide surgical excision with regional lymph node dissection (231). Adjuvant radiation is provided for aggressive tumors, positive nodal disease, and palliation for metastatic lesions. The value of chemotherapy is controversial but doxorubicin may be useful. Most series report 65% mortality at 3 years. Poor prognostic signs include older age, female gender, midline location, larger size, and evidence of necrosis. Metastases occur via lymphatics to regional nodes and via blood to lungs, liver, and bones.

Liposarcoma

Liposarcoma (LS) originates in the lipoblast, which is similar to a mature lipocyte but is larger size and has a more pleomorphic nucleus. There appears to be an association with neurofibromatosis, asbestos, and ionizing radiation. The development from benign lipomas is controversial. LS is the most common soft tissue sarcoma of the lower extremities. It occurs in any age group but most frequently in patients between 45 and 55 years (232). There is a slight male predominance. The most common location is the thigh followed by the retroperitoneum. LS presents as an asymptomatic mass that grows slowly over time. Retroperitoneal tumors manifest as a palpable abdominal mass. Pain is a variable feature. On histological examination, approximately 50% of LS tumors show lipoblasts included in a myxoid stroma, variable hyperchromasia, and pleomorphism. In the sclerosing variant, there are dense collagenous septa. Pleomorphic LS accounts for 10–30% of cases. It is characterized by marked anaplasia and pleomorphism, and variable bizarre multinucleated giant cells. Lipoblasts show hyperchromatic scalloped nuclei with multiple vacuoles. Round cell LS makes up less than 10% of cases and shows poorly differentiated, small, round lipoblasts with minimal intracellular lipid. IHC stains are positive for S-100 and vimentin.

Local disease is treated with wide surgical excision. Amputation is recommended only for aggressive tumors invading muscle or bone. Local recurrence ranges from 45 to 75%, with the highest recurrence rate (78%) for retroperitoneal LS. Better results may be obtained with a combination of surgery and radiation (233). Prognosis is better for children with an overall survival of 70–90%.

Metastases occur in 15–45% of cases, with a higher incidence for pleomorphic, poorly differentiated, and round cell variants. The most common site for metastases is the lung, followed by bone and liver. Lymph node disease is extremely uncommon. Metastatic disease is best approached with surgery and adjuvant radiation therapy but most patients eventually die of their disease. Radiation therapy can provide effective palliation.

Epithelioid Sarcoma

Epithelioid sarcoma (ES) is derived from pluripotential mesenchymal cells or histiocytes. It accounts for 1% of soft tissue sarcomas. ES affects young people with a median age of 23 years. It predominates in men (1.8:1). The most frequent location is the upper extremity (58–68% of cases) followed by the lower extremity (27%). Favored locations are the hands and feet (234). ES presents as a firm, slowly growing, subcutaneous mass that shows ulceration or sinus formation. Only 20% are painful. Differential diagnosis must include fibrous histiocytoma, fasciitis, fibromatoses, other sarcomas, and granular cell tumor. Histopathological examination shows nodules of eosinophilic epithelioid and spindle cells. The characteristic pattern of growth shows epithelioid cells surrounding central necrotic or acellular areas. IHC staining is positive for CK and EMA (epithelial markers) and vimentin (mesenchymal marker).

Wide surgical excision with margin control is as effective as amputation (235). However, metastases occur in 45–50% of cases. Prognosis is dismal because lesions are resistant to radiation and chemotherapy. Frequent metastatic sites include the lymph nodes (48%), lungs (25%), scalp (10%), and skin (6%). Survival ranges from months to years but at least 90% of patients eventually die from this tumor. Poor prognosis is associated with proximal location, male gender, advanced age, size larger than 5 cm, deep local invasion, vascular or perineural involvement, necrosis, hemorrhage, high mitotic rate, and nodal involvement.

Cancer Metastatic to the Skin

Metastases to the skin from an internal neoplasia are rare (236). Reported incidence varies from 0.7 to 9% but the most realistic figure is approximately 1.3%. Skin involvement as the presenting sign of visceral cancer is even less frequent, occurring in 0.8% of cases. In general, a metastatic event must be viewed as a multistep process that involves detachment from the primary site, intravasation (penetration to blood-/lymphatic vessels), circulation (survival of cells by homotypic aggregation), stasis, and extravasation with tissue invasion. The biological basis for site-specific metastases is complex and not well understood, but the following factors may be involved: cellular adhesion molecules, ability to invade tissue by producing proteases, and ability of tumor cells to induce angiogenesis.

The most common sites of origin for cutaneous metastases are the breast, lung, and colon. Clinically, metastatic lesions present as any of the following:

Intradermal or subcutaneous nodules of variable size that range from skin-colored to red or violaceous. Should the metastatic lesions be located on the umbilical area, they are known as Sister Mary Joseph's nodules (tumors from the GI and GU tract). Sometimes the lesions show a characteristic dermatomal or zosteriform distribution.

Inflammatory metastases are red, indurated plaques resembling erysipelas.

Cicatricial metastases resemble scars.

Carcinoma en cuirass implies extensive and confluent disease, conveying the impression that the patient is encased in armor (cuirasse).

Breast Carcinoma

Approximately 6.3% of patients with breast carcinoma experience cutaneous involvement, but in only 3.5% of cases is this the initial presentation. More than 50% of metastatic lesions occur as direct extension from the tumor mass in the form of Paget's disease or as nodular–ulcerative lesions. Other common presentations are inflammatory carcinoma and carcinoma en cuirass.

IHC stains may aid in the diagnosis of highly undifferentiated tumors (adenocarcinomas): GCDFP-15 antigen is highly specific for breast carcinoma.

Lung Carcinoma

It has been reported that approximately 5.7% of patients with cutaneous metastases have an underlying lung carcinoma, but the true incidence of skin involvement with this tumor is unknown. Lesions present clinically as nonspecific nodules, zosteriform metastases, or inflammatory carcinoma.

Colon and Ovarian Carcinoma

Colon and ovarian carcinoma may present as abdominal subcutaneous nodules, extramammary Paget's disease of the anogenital area, carcinoma en cuirass, or inflammatory carcinoma. Diagnosis must be established by histological examination and, in difficult cases, by IHC stains. GI adenocarcinoma stains for EMA, CK, and CEA. Ovarian carcinoma shows positive staining with CEA, CA-125, and CA-19-9.

Treatment of cutaneous metastases is difficult (237). Radiotherapy usually provides only temporary improvement and many metastatic neoplasms are resistant to chemotherapy. In general, surgical excision of individual lesions is considered palliative. Only modest results have been achieved with innovative immunotherapeutic regimens.

Cutaneous metastatic disease carries a dismal prognosis. Survival is approximately 31 months for breast carcinoma, 18 months for colon carcinoma, 16 months for melanoma, and 5 months for lung carcinoma.

REFERENCES

1. Naversen DN, Trask DM, Watson FH, Burket JM. Painful tumors of the skin: "LEND AN EGG". J Am Acad Dermatol 1993; 28(2 Pt 2):298–300.
2. Pariser RJ. Benign neoplasms of the skin. Med Clin North Am. 1998; 82(6):1285–1307.
3. Lefkowitz A, Schwartz RA, Janniger CK. Melanoma precursors in children. Cutis 1999; 63(6):321–324.
4. Lawrence CM. Treatment options for giant congenital naevi. Clin Exp Dermatol. 2000; 25(1):7–11.
5. Zeff RA, Freitag A, Grin CM, Grant-Kels JM. The immune response in halo nevi. J Am Acad Dermatol. 1997; 37(4):620–624.
6. Langenbach N, Pfau A, Landthaler M, Stolz W. Naevi spili, Cafe-au-lait spots and melanocytic naevi aggregated alongside Blaschko's lines, with a review of segmental melanocytic lesions. Acta Derm Venereol. 1998; 78(5):378–380.
7. Knoell KA, Nelson KC, Patterson JW. Familial multiple blue nevi. J Am Acad Dermatol. 1998; 39(2 Pt 2):322–325.
8. Park KD, Choi GS, Lee KH. Extensive aberrant Mongolian spot. J Dermatol. 1995; 22(5):330–333.
9. Stanford DG, Georgouras KE. Dermal melanocytosis: a clinical spectrum. Australas J Dermatol. 1996; 37(1):19 25.
10. Helm KF, Schwartz RA, Janniger CK. Juvenile melanoma (Spitz nevus). Cutis. 1996; 58(1):35–39.
11. Carpo BG, Grevelink JM, Grevelink SV. Laser treatment of pigmented lesions in children. Semin Cutan Med Surg. 1999; 18(3):233–243.
12. Losee JE, Serletti JM, Pennino RP. Epidermal nevus syndrome: a review and case report. Ann Plast Surg. 1999; 43(2):211–214.
13. Brown TJ, Friedman J, Levy ML. The diagnosis and treatment of common birthmarks. Clin Plast Surg. 1998; 25(4):509–525.
14. Shapiro M, Johnson B Jr, Witmer W, Elenitsas R. Spiradenoma arising in a nevus sebaceous of Jadassohn: case report and literature review. Am J Dermatopathol. 1999; 21(5):462–467.
15. Patrizi A, Neri I, Fiorentini C, Marzaduri S. Nevus comedonicus syndrome: a new pediatric case. Pediatr Dermatol. 1998; 15(4):304–306.
16. Toussaint S, Salcedo E, Kamino H. Benign epidermal proliferations. Adv Dermatol. 1999; 14:307–357.
17. Wetmore SJ. Cryosurgery for common skin lesions. Treatment in family physicians' offices. Can Fam Physician. 1999; 45:964–974.
18. Schwartz RA. The actinic keratosis. A perspective and update. Dermatol Surg. 1997; 23(11):1009–1019.

19. Barnaby JW, Styles AR, Cockerell CJ. Actinic keratoses. Differential diagnosis and treatment. Drugs Aging. 1997; 11(3):186–205.
20. Nestle FO, Nickoloff BJ, Burg G. Dermatofibroma: an abortive immunoreactive process mediated by dermal dendritic cells? Dermatology 1995; 190(4): 265–268.
21. Jacobs IA, Chevinsky A. Angiomatoid fibrous histiocytoma: a case report and review of the literature. Dermatol Surg. 2000; 26(5):491–492.
22. Niessen FB, Spauwen PH, Schalkwijk J, Kon M. On the nature of hypertrophic scars and keloids: a review. Plast Reconstr Surg. 1999; 104(5):1435–1458.
23. Berman B, Flores F. The treatment of hypertrophic scars and keloids. Eur J Dermatol. 1998; 8(8):591–595.
24. Ellitsgaard V, Ellitsgaard N. Hypertrophic scars and keloids: a recurrent problem revisited. Acta Chir Plast. 1997; 39(3):69–77.
25. Poston J. The use of silicone gel sheeting in the management of hypertrophic and keloid scars. J Wound Care. 2000; 9(1):10–16.
26. Cook TF, Fosko SW. Unusual cutaneous malignancies. Semin Cutan Med Surg. 1998; 17(2):114–132.
27. Smith KJ, Skelton HG, Holland TT. Recent advances and controversies concerning adnexal neoplasms. Dermatol Clin. 1992; 10(1):117–160.
28. Rosen LB. A review and proposed new classification of benign acquired neoplasms with hair follicle differentiation. Am J Dermatopathol. 1990; 12(5): 496–516.
29. Massa MC, Medenica M. Cutaneous adnexal tumors and cysts: a review. Part I. Tumors with hair follicular and sebaceous glandular differentiation and cysts related to different parts of the hair follicle. Pathol Annu. 1985; 20 Pt 2:189–233.
30. Kolenik SA 3rd, Bolognia JL, Castiglione FM Jr, Longley BJ. Multiple tumors of the follicular infundibulum. Int J Dermatol. 1996; 35(4):282–284.
31. Waibel M, Blume U, Anhuth D, Almond-Roesler B, Orfanos CE. Tumors of the pilosebaceous unit. Skin Pharmacol. 1994; 7(1-2):90–93.
32. Mizutani H, Senga K, Ueda M. Trichofolliculoma of the upper lip: report of a case. Int J Oral Maxillofac Surg. 1999; 28(2):135–136.
33. Cooper PH. Carcinomas of sweat glands. Pathol Annu 1987; 22(part1):83–124.
34. Wick MR, Swanson PE. Sweat gland neoplasms. Cutaneous adnexal tumors. A guide to pathologic diagnosis. Chicago: ASCP, 1991, 1–77.
35. Santa Cruz DJ. Tumors of sweat gland differentiation. In: Farmer ER, Hood AF, eds. Pathology of the skin, Norwalk: Appleton & Lange, 1990:624–662.
36. Murphy GF, Elder DE. Benign tumors with eccrine differentiation. Atlas of tumor pathology. Nonmelanocytic tumors of the skin. Third series. Washington, DC: AFIP, 1991, 64–89.
37. Abenoza P, Ackerman AB. Neoplasms with eccrine differentiation. Philadelphia: Lea and Febiger, 1990, 442–456.
38. Berke A, Grant-Kels JM. Eccrine sweat gland disorders: Part I—neoplasms. Int J Dermatol. 1994; 33(2):79–85.
39. Dominguez Iglesias F, Fresno Forcellado F, Soler Sanchez T. Chondroid syringoma: a histological and immunohistochemical study of 15 cases. Histopathology 1990; 17:311–317.
40. Nasser NA, Dodd SM. Chondroid syringoma. Int J Oral Maxillofac Surg 1987; 16:521–523.
41. Massa MC, Medenica M. Cutaneous adnexal tumors and cysts: a review. Part II—Tumors with apocrine and eccrine glandular differentiation and miscellaneous cutaneous cysts. Pathol Annu. 1987; 22 Pt 1:225–276.
42. Warkel RL. Selected apocrine neoplasms. J Cutan Pathol. 1984; 11(5):437–449.

43. Fukuda M, Kato H, Hamada T. Apocrine hidrocystoma—a report of five cases and review of the Japanese literature. J Dermatol. 1989; 16(4):315–320.
44. Santa Cruz JD, Priloleau PG, Smith ME. Hidradenoma papilliferum of the eyelid. Arch Dermatol 1981; 117:55–56.
45. Goette DK. Hidradenoma papilliferum. J Am Acad Dermatol 1988; 19:133–135.
46. Cotton DW, Braye SG. Dermal cylindromas originated from the eccrine sweat gland. British J Dermatol 1984; 11:53–61.
47. Prioleau PG, Santa Cruz DJ. Sebaceous gland neoplasia. J Cutan Pathol. 1984; 11(5):396–414.
48. Dent CD, Hunter WE, Svirsky JA. Sebaceous gland hyperplasia: case report and literature review. J Oral Maxillofac Surg. 1995; 53(8):936–938.
49. Schwartz RA, Torre DP. The Muir-Torre syndrome: a 25-year retrospect. J Am Acad Dermatol 1995; 33(1):90–104.
50. Tumors and Cysts of the Epidermis. In: Lever WF, Schaumburg-Lever, eds. Histopathology of the skin, Philadelphia: Lippincott Company, 1983:472–521.
51. Vicente J, Vazquez-Doval FJ. Proliferations of the epidermoid cyst wall. Int J Dermatol. 1998; 37(3):181–185.
52. Langley RG, Walsh NM, Ross JB. Multiple eruptive milia: report of a case, review of the literature, and a classification. J Am Acad Dermatol. 1997; 37(2 Pt 2):353–356.
53. Requena L, Martin L, Renedo G, Arias D, Espinel ML, de Castro A. A facial variant of steatocystoma multiplex. Cutis. 1993; 51(6):449–452.
54. Yamasoba T, Tayama N, Syoji M, Fukuta M. Clinicostatistical study of lower lip mucoceles. Head Neck. 1990; 12(4):316–320.
55. Zvulunov A, Amichai B, Grunwald MH, Avinoach I, Halevy S. Cutaneous bronchogenic cyst: delineation of a poorly recognized lesion. Pediatr Dermatol. 1998; 15(4):277–281.
56. Requena L, Sangueza OP. Cutaneous vascular anomalies. Part I. Hamartomas, malformations, and dilation of preexisting vessels. J Am Acad Dermatol. 1997; 37(4):523–549.
57. Powell J. Update on hemangiomas and vascular malformations. Curr Opin Pediatr 1999; 11(5):457–463.
58. Kihiczak NI, Schwartz RA, Jozwiak S, Silver RJ, Janniger CK. Sturge-Weber syndrome. Cutis. 2000; 65(3):133–136.
59. Dover JS. New approaches to the laser treatment of vascular lesions. Australas J Dermatol. 2000; 41(1):14–18.
60. Dover JS, Arndt KA. New approaches to the treatment of vascular lesions. Lasers Surg Med. 2000; 26(2):158–163.
61. Reischle S, Schuller-Petrovic S. Treatment of capillary hemangiomas of early childhood with a new method of cryosurgery. J Am Acad Dermatol. 2000; 42(5 Pt 1):809–813.
62. Burstein FD, Simms C, Cohen SR, Williams JK, Paschal M. Intralesional laser therapy of extensive hemangiomas in 100 consecutive pediatric patients. Ann Plast Surg. 2000; 44(2):188–194.
63. Hastings MM, Milot J, Barsoum-Homsy M, Hershon L, Dubois J, Leclerc JM. Recombinant interferon alfa-2b in the treatment of vision-threatening capillary hemangiomas in childhood. J AAPOS 1997; 1(4):226–230.
64. Schiller PI, Itin PH. Angiokeratomas: an update. Dermatology. 1996; 193(4):275–282.
65. Kirschner RE, Low DW. Treatment of pyogenic granuloma by shave excision and laser photocoagulation. Plast Reconstr Surg. 1999; 104(5):1346–1349.
66. Moor EV, Goldberg I, Westreich M. Multiple glomus tumor: a case report and review of the literature. Ann Plast Surg. 1999; 43(4):436–438.
67. Orvidas LJ, Kasperbauer JL. Pediatric lymphangiomas of the head and neck. Ann Otol Rhinol Laryngol. 2000; 109(4):411–421.

68. Christenson L, Patterson J, Davis D. Surgical pearl: use of the cutaneous punch for the removal of lipomas. J Am Acad Dermatol. 2000; 42(4):675–676.
69. North KN. Neurofibromatosis 1 in childhood. Semin Pediatr Neurol. 1998; 5(4):231–242.
70. Spencer JM, Amonette RA. Tumors with smooth muscle differentiation. Dermatol Surg. 1996; 22(9):761–768.
71. Cancer statistics. CA 1989; 39:9–20.
72. Kaldor J, Shugg D, Young B. Non-melanoma skin cancer: ten years of cancer-registry based surveillance. Int J Dermatol 1993; 53:886–891.
73. Gorlin R. Nevoid basal cell carcinoma syndrome. Dermatol Clin 1995; 131:113–125.
74. Sexton M, Jones DB, Maloney ME. Histologic pattern analysis of basal cell carcinoma. Study of a series of 1039 consecutive neoplasms. J Am Acad Dermatol 1990; 23:1118–1126.
75. Rowe DE, Carroll RJ, Day C. Long term recurrence rate in previously untreated (primary) basal cell carcinoma: Implication for patients follow-up. J Dermatol Surg Oncol 1989; 15:315–328.
76. Silverman MK, Kopf AW, Grin CM. Recurrence rates of treated basal cell carcinomas. Part 2: Curettage–electrodesiccation. J Dermatol Surg Oncol 1991; 17:720–726.
77. Diwan R, Skouge JW. Basal cell carcinoma. Curr Probl Dermatol 1990; 2:70–91.
78. Wolf DJ, Zitelli JA. Surgical margins for basal cell carcinoma. Arch Dermatol 1987; 123:340–344.
79. Silverman MK, Kopf AW, Bart RS, Grin CM. Recurrence rates of treated basal cell carcinomas. Part 3: Surgical excision. J Dermatol Surg Oncol 1992; 18:471–476.
80. Johnson TM, Tromovitch TA, Swanson NA. Combined curettage and excision: a treatment method for primary basal cell carcinoma. J Am Acad Dermatol 1991; 24:613–617.
81. Ratner D, Grande DJ. Mohs micrographic surgery: an overview. Derm Nursing 1994; 6:269–273.
82. Drake KA, Dinehart SM, Goltz TW. Guidelines of care for Mohs micrographic surgery. Dermatol World 1994; (suppl):17–23.
83. Kuflik EG. Cryosurgery updated. J Am Acad Dermatol 1994; 31:925–944.
84. Kuflik EG, Gage AA. Cryosurgical treatment for skin cancer, New York: Igaku-Shoin, 1990:35–51.
85. Cox JD. 7th. Moss' radiation oncology: rationale, technique, results, Philadelphia: CV Mosby, 1994:99–118.
86. Lovett RD, Perez CA, Shapiro SJ, Garcia DM. External irradiation of epithelial skin cancer. Int J Radiat Oncol Biol Phys 1990; 19:235–242.
87. Svanberg K, Andersson T, Killander D. Photodynamic therapy of nonmelanoma malignant tumors of the skin using topical aminolevulenic acid sensitization and laser irradiation. Br J Dermatol 1994; 130:743–751.
88. Oseroff AR, Wilson BD, Shanler SD. Clinical studies with topical 5-aminolevulinic acid (ALA) and photofrin: results and mechanisms. Laser Surg Med 1994; 14:43.
89. Klein E, Stoll HL, Milgrom H. Tumors of the skin. VI. Study on effects of local administration of 5-fluorouracil in basal cell carcinoma. J Invest Dermatol 1966; 47 22–26.
90. Stoll HL, Klein E, Case R. Tumors of the skin. VII. Effects of varying the concentration of locally administered 5-fluorouracil on basal cell carcinoma. J Invest Dermatol 1967; 49:219–224.
91. Epstein E. Fluorouracil paste treatment of thin basal cell carcinomas. Arch Dermatol 1985; 121:207–213.
92. Brenner S, Wolf R, Dascalu DI. Topical tretinoin treatment in basal cell carcinoma. J Dermatol Surg Oncol 1993; 19:264–266.

93. Kraemer KH, DiGiovanna JJ, Peck GL. Chemoprevention of skin cancer in xeroderma pigmentosum. J Dermatol 1992; 19:715–718.
94. Greenway HT, Cornell RC, Tanner DJ. Treatment of basal cell carcinoma with intralesional interferon. J Am Acad Dermatol 1986; 15:437–443.
95. Edwards L, Tucker SB. The effect of an intralesional sustained release formulation of interferon alfa 2-b on basal cell carcinoma. Arch Dermatol 1990; 126:1029.
96. Scanlon EF, Volkmer DD, Oviedo MM. Metastatic basal cell carcinoma. J Surg Oncol 1980; 15:171–180.
97. Hartman R, Hartman S, Green N. Long-term survival following metastases from basal cell carcinoma. Arch Dermatol 1986; 122:912–914.
98. Bason MM, Grant-Kels JM, Govil M. Metastatic basal cell carcinoma: response to chemotherapy. J Am Acad Dermatol 1990; 22:905–908.
99. Gallagher RP, Hill GB, Bajdik CD. Sunlight exposure, pigmentation factors, and risk of nonmelanocytic skin cancers. Arch Dermatol 1995; 131:164–169.
100. Graham GG, Marks R, Foley P. Incidence of non-melanocytic skin cancer treated in Australia. Br J Med 1988; 296:13–16.
101. Bernstein D. Squamous cell carcinoma. J Derm Surg 1996; 22:243–254.
102. Kossard S, Rosen R. Cutaneous Bowen's disease. J Am Acad Dermatol 1992; 27: 406–410.
103. Eliezri YD. Occurrence of human papillomavirus type 16 DNA in cutaneous squamous and basal cell neoplasms. J Am Acad Dermatol 1990; 23:836.
104. Kwa RE, Campana K, Moy RL. Biology of cutaneous squamous cell carcinoma. J Am Acad Dermatol 1992; 26:1–26.
105. Klima M, Kurtis B, Jordan PH. Verrucous carcinoma of the skin. J Cutan Pathol 1980; 7:88–98.
106. Marks R, Rennie G, Selwood T. The relationship of basal cell carcinomas and squamous cell carcinomas to solar keratoses. Arch Dermatol 1988; 124:1039–1042.
107. Ragi G, Turner MS, Klein LE, Stoll HL. Pigmented Bowen's disease and review of 420 Bowen's disease lesions. J Dermatol Surg Oncol 1988; 14:765–769.
108. McGibbon DH. Malignant epidermal tumors. J Cutan Pathol 1985; 12:224–238.
109. Broders AC. Squamous cell epithelioma of the skin. Ann Surg 1921; 73:141–160.
110. Brodin MB, Mehregan AH. Verrucous carcinoma. Arch Dermatol 1980; 116:987.
111. Brodland DG, Zitelli JA. Surgical margins for excision of primary cutaneous squamous cell carcinoma. J Am Acad Dermatol 1992; 27:241–248.
112. Johnson TM, Rowe DE,Nelson BR, Swanson NA. Squamous cell carcinoma of the skin (excluding lip and oral mucosa). J Am Acad Dermatol 1992; 26:467–484.
113. Roenigk RK. Mohs micrographic surgery. Mayo Clin Proc 1988; 63:175–183.
114. Rowe DE, Carrol RJ, Day CL. Prognostic factors for local recurrence, metastasis, and survival rates in squamous cell carcinoma of the skin, ear, and lip. J Am Acad Dermatol 1992; 26:976–990.
115. Salasche SJ. Status of curettage and electrodesiccation in the treatment of primary basal cell carcinoma. J Am Acad Dermatol 1983; 8:496.
116. Zacarian SA. Cryosurgery of cutaneous carcinomas: an 18-year study of 3,022 patients with 4,228 carcinomas. J Am Acad Dermatol 1983; 9:947–956.
117. Fitzpatrick PJ, Thompson GA, Easterbrook WM. Basal and squamous cell carcinoma of the eyelids and their treatment by radiotherapy. Int J Radiat Oncol Biol Phys 1984; 10:449–454.
118. Mendenhall NP, Million RR, Cassisi NJ. Parotid area lymph node metastases from carcinomas of the skin. Int J Radiat Oncol Biol Phys 1985; 11:707–714.
119. Fishbach AJ, Sause WT, Plenk HP. Radiation therapy for skin cancer. West J Med 1980; 133:379–382.

120. Jones CM, Mang T, Cooper M. Photodynamic therapy in the treatment of Bowen's disease. J Am Acad Dermatol 1992; 27:979–982.
121. Wenig BL, Kurtzman DM, Grossweiner LI. Photodynamic therapy in the treatment of squamous cell carcinoma of the head and neck. Arch Otolaryngol Head Neck Surg 1990; 116:1267–1270.
122. Maxson BB, Scott RF, Headington JT. Management of oral squamous cell carcinoma in situ with topical 5-fluorouracil and laser surgery. Oral Surg Oral Med Oral Pathol 1989; 68:44–48.
123. Rook AH, Jaworsky C, Nguyen T. Beneficial effect of low-dose systemic retinoid in combination with topical tretinoin for the treatment and prophylaxis of premalignant and malignant skin lesions in renal transplant recipients. Transplantation 1995; 59: 714–719.
124. Edwards L, Berman B, Rapini RP. Treatment of cutaneous squamous cell carcinomas by intralesional interferon alfa-2b therapy. Arch Dermatol 1992; 128:1486–1489.
125. Lippman SM, Parkinson DR, Itri LM. 1 3-cis-retinoic acid and interferon alfa 2a: effective combination therapy for advanced squamous cell carcinoma of the skin. J Natl Cancer Inst 1992; 84:235–241.
126. Haydon RC. Cutaneous squamous cell carcinoma and related lesions. Otolaryngol Clin North Am 1993; 26:57–71.
127. Sadek H, Azli N, Wendling JL. Treatment of advanced squamous cell carcinoma of the skin with cisplatin, 5-fluorouracil, and bleomycin. Cancer 1990; 66:1692–1695.
128. Kowalski LP, Magrin J, Waksman G. Supraomohyoid neck dissection in the treatment of head and neck tumors. Arch Otolaryngol Head Neck Surg 1993; 119:958–962.
129. Olsen KD, Caruso M, Foote RL. Primary head and neck cancer. Histopathologic predictors of recurrence after neck dissection in patients with lymph node involvement. Arch Otolaryngol Head Neck Surg 1994; 120:1370–1374.
130. Medina JE. A rationale classification of neck dissections. Otolaryngol Head Neck Surg 1989; 100:169–176.
131. Taylor BW, Brant TA, Mendenhall NP. Carcinoma of the skin metastatic to parotid area lymph nodes. Head and neck 1991; 13:427–433.
132. Straka BF, Grant-Kels JM. Keratoacanthoma. Fruedman RJ, Rigel DS, Kof AW, ed. Cancer of the skin. Philadelphia: WB Saunders, 1991, 390–407.
133. Kern WH, McCray MK. The histopathologic differentiation of keratoacanthoma and squamous cell carcinoma of the skin. J Cutan Pathol 1980; 7:318–325.
134. Pagani WA, Lorenzi G, Lorusso D. Surgical treatment for aggressive giant keratoacanthoma of the face. J Dermatol Surg Oncol 1986; 12:282–284.
135. Larson PO. Keratoacanthomas treated with Mohs' micrographic surgery (chemosurgery): a review of forty-three cases. J Am Acad Dermatol 1987; 16:1040–1044.
136. Reymann F. Treatment of keratoacanthomas with curettage. Dermatologica 1977; 155:90–96.
137. Donahue B, Cooper JS, Rush S. Treatment of aggressive keratoacanthomas by radiotherapy. J Am Acad Dermatol 1990; 23:489–493.
138. Parker CM, Hanke CW. Large keratoacanthomas in different locations treated with intralesional 5-fluorouracil. J Am Acad Dermatol 1986; 14:770–777.
139. Kestel JL, Shelton Blair D. Keratoacanthoma treated with methotrexate. Arch Dermatol 1973; 108:723.
140. Shaw JC, White CR. Treatment of multiple keratoacanthomas with oral isotretinoin. J Am Acad Dermatol 1986; 15:1079.
141. Duncan LM, Travers RL, Koerner FC. Estrogen and progesterone receptor analysis in pregnancy-associated melanoma: absence of immunohistochemically detectable hormone receptors. Human Pathol 1994; 25:36–41.

142. Rhodes AR. Congenital nevomelanocytic nevi. Histologic patterns in the first year of life and evolution during childhood. Arch Dermatol 1986; 122:1257–1262.
143. Greene MH, Clark WH Jr, Tucker MA. High risk of malignant melanoma in melanoma-prone families with dysplastic nevi. Ann Int Med 1985; 102: 458–465.
144. Cannon-Albright LA, Goldgar DE, Meyer LJ. Assignment of a locus for familial melanoma, MLM, to chromosome 9p13-p22. Science 1992; 258:1148–1152.
145. Fitzpatrick TB, Milton GW, Balch CM. Clinical characteristics. In: Balch CM, Houghton AN, Milton GW, eds. 2nd. Cutaneous melanoma, Philadelphia: JB Lippincott, 1992:228–229.
146. Zitelli JA, Moy RL, Abell E. The reliability of frozen sections in the evaluation of surgical margins for melanoma. J Am Acad Dermatol 1991; 24:102–106.
147. Aitken DR, Clausen K, Klein JP. The extent of primary melanoma excision. A re-evaluation: how wide is wide? Ann Surg 1983; 198:634–641.
148. Goldman LI, Byrd R. Narrowing resection margins for patients with low-risk melanoma. Am J Surg 1988; 155:242–244.
149. Cascinelli N, van der Esch EP, Breslow A. Stage I melanoma of the skin: the problem of resection margins. Eur J Cancer 1980; 16:1079–1085.
150. Veronesi U, Cascinelli N. Narrow excision (1-cm margin): a safe procedure for thin cutaneous melanoma. Arch Surg 1991; 126:438–441.
151. Banzet P, Thomas A, Vuillemin E. Wide vs. narrow surgical excision in thin (< 2mm) stage I primary cutaneous melanoma: long term results of a French multicentric prospective randomized trial on 319 patients. Proc Am Soc Clin Oncol 1993; 12:387, A1320.
152. Balch CM, Urist MM, Karakousis CP. Efficacy of 2-cm surgical margins for intermediate-thickness melanomas (1 to 4 mm): results of a multi-institutional randomized surgical trial. Ann Surg 1993; 218:262–267.
153. Cohen LM, McCal MW, Hodge SJ. Successful treatment of lentigo maligna melanoma with Mohs micrographic surgery aided by rush permanent sections. Cancer 1994; 73:2964–2970.
154. Ghussen F, Nagel K, Groth W. A prospective randomized study of regional extremity perfusion in patients with malignant melanoma. Ann Surg 1984; 200:764–768.
155. Sim FH, Taylor WF, Pritchard DJ. Lymphadenectomy in the management of stage I malignant melanoma: a prospective randomized study. Mayo Clin Proc 1986; 61: 697–705.
156. Balch CM, Soong SJ, Urist MM. A prospective surgical trial of 742 melanoma patients comparing the efficacy of elective (immediate) lymph node dissection vs. observation. American Surgical Association, Program of the 116th Annual Meeting 1996; 22–23.
157. Albertini JJ, Cruse CW, Rapaport D. Intraoperative radiolymphoscintigraphy improves sentinel lymph node identification for patients with melanoma. Ann Surg 1996; 223:217–224.
158. Morton DL, Wen DR, Foshag LJ. Intraoperative lymphatic mapping and selective lymphadenectomy for early-stage melanomas of the head and neck. J Clin Oncol 1993; 11:1751–1756.
159. Robinson JK. Margin control for lentigo maligna. J Am Acad Dermatol 1994; 31: 79–85.
160. Cockerell CJ. A rational method of management of maligna melanoma in situ on sun-damaged skin. Am J Dermatopathol 1985; 7(suppl):191–192.
161. Kirkwood JM, Strawderman MH, Ernstoff MS, Smith TJ, Borden EC, Blum RH. Interferon alfa-2b adjuvant therapy of high-risk resected cutaneous melanoma: the Eastern Cooperative Oncology Group Trial EST1684. J Clin Oncol 1996; 14: 7–17.

162. Burmeister BH, Smithers BM, Poulsen M. Radiation therapy for nodal disease in malignant melanoma. World J Surg 1995; 19:369–371.
163. Hill GJ, Krementz ET, Hill MZ. Dimethyl triazeno imidazole carboxamide and combination therapy for melanoma. Cancer 1984; 53:1299–1305.
164. Cocconi G, Bella M, Calabresi F. Treatment of metastatic malignant melanoma with dacarbazine plus tamoxifen. N Engl J Med 1992; 327:516–523.
165. Bleehen NM, Newlands ES, Lee S. Cancer research campaign phase II trial of temozolomide in metastatic melanoma. J Clin Oncol 1995; 13:910–913.
166. Quesada JR, Talpaz M, Rios A, Kurzrock R, Gutterman JV. Clinical toxicity of interferons in cancer patients: a review. J Clin Oncol 1986; 4:234–243.
167. Whittington R, Fauld D. Interleukin-2. A review of its pharmacological properties and therapeutic use in patients with cancer. Drugs 1993; 46:446–514.
168. Sause WT, Cooper JS, Rush S. Fraction size in external beam radiation therapy in the treatment of melanoma. Int J Radiat Oncol Biol Phys 1991; 20:429–432.
169. Mittelman A, Chen Z, Yang H. Treatment with antiidiotypic monoclonal antibodies of stage IV patients with malignant melanoma. Proc Am Soc Clin Oncol 1991; 10:1036.
170. Khansur T, Sanders J, Das SK. Evaluation of staging work-up in malignant melanoma. Arch Surg 1989; 124:847–849.
171. Sau P, Lupton GP, Grahma JH. Pilomatrix carcinoma. Cancer 1993; 71:2491–2498.
172. Green DE, Sanusi D, Fowler MR. Pilomatrix carcinoma. J Am Acad Dermatol 1987; 17:264–270.
173. Goldstein DJ, Barr RJ, Santacruz DJ. Microcystic adnexal carcinoma: a distinct clinicopathologic entity. Cancer 1982; 50:566–572.
174. Cooper PH, Mills SE. Microcystic adnexal carcinoma. J Am Acad Dermatol 1984; 10:908–914.
175. Mambo NC. Eccrine spiradenoma: clinical and pathologic study of 49 tumors. J Cutan Pathol 1983; 10:312–320.
176. Zamboni AC, Zamboni WA, Ross DS. Malignant eccrine spiradenoma of the hand. J Surg Oncol 1990; 43:131–133.
177. Shaw M, McKee P, Lowe D, Black M. Malignant eccrine poroma: a study of 27 cases. Br J Dermatol 1982; 107:675–680.
178. Mikhail GR. Mohs micrographic surgery. Philadelphia: WB Saunders, 1991, 124–128.
179. Wong TY, Suster S, Nogita T, Duncan LM, Dickersin RG, Mihm MC. Clear cell eccrine carcinomas of the skin: a clinicopathologic study of nine patients. Cancer 1994; 73:1631–1643.
180. Dzubow LM, Grossman DJ, Johnson B. Chemosurgical report: Eccrine adenocarcinoma—report of a case, treatment with Mohs surgery. J Dermatol Surg Oncol 1986; 12(10):1049–1053.
181. Fukamizu H, Tomita K, Inoue K, Takigawa M. Primary mucinous carcinoma of the skin. J Dermatol Surg Oncol 1993; 19:625–628.
182. Snow SN, Reizner G. Mucinous eccrine carcinoma of the eyelid. Case report and review of the literature. Cancer 1992; 70:2099–2104.
183. Ishimura E, Iwamoto H, Kobashi Y. Malignant chondroid syringoma. Cancer 1983; 52:1966–1973.
184. Hong JJ, Elmore JF, Drachenberg CI, Jacobs MC, Salazar OM. Role of radiation therapy in the management of malignant chondroid syringoma. Dermatol Surg 1995; 21:781–785.
185. Salzman MJ, Eades E. Primary cutaneous adenoid cystic carcinoma: a case report and review of the literature. Plast Reconst Surg 1991; 88:140–144.
186. Lang PG, Metcalf JS, Maize JC. Recurrent adenoid cystic carcinoma of the skin managed by microscopically controlled surgery (Mohs surgery). J Dermatol Surg Oncol 1986; 12:395–398.

187. Hammond DC, Grant KF, Simpson WD. Malignant degeneration of dermal cylindroma. Ann Plast Surg 1990; 24:176–178.
188. Lo JS, Peschen M, Snow SN. Malignant cylindroma of the scalp. J Dermatol Surg Oncol 1991; 17:897–901.
189. Dixon AR, Galea MH, Ellis IO. Paget's disease of the nipple. Br J Surg 1991; 78–722.
190. El-Sharkawi A, Walters JS. The place for conservative treatment in the management of Paget's disease of the nipple. Eur J Surg Oncol 1992; 18:301.
191. Chanda JJ. Extramammary Paget's disease: prognosis and relationship to internal malignancy. J Am Acad Dermatol 1985; 13:1009–1014.
192. Pug JC, Tung KH, Wong YE. Extramammary Paget's disease: a report of three cases and a review of the literature. Ann Acad Med 1995; 24:636–639.
193. Eliezri YD, Silvers DN, Horan DB. Role of preoperative topical 5-fluorouracil in preparation for Mohs micrographic surgery of extramammary Paget's disease. J Am Acad Dermatol 1987; 17:497–505.
194. Harris DWS, Kist DA, Bloom K, Zachary CB. Rapid staining with carcinoembryonic antigen aids limited excision of extramammary Paget's disease treated by Mohs surgery. J Dermatol Surg Oncol 1994; 20:260–264.
195. Pelosi G, Martignoni G, Bonetti F. Intraductal carcinoma of mammary-type apocrine epithelium arising within a papillary hidradenoma of the vulva. Report of a case and review of the literature. Arch Pathol Lab Med 1991; 115:1249–1254.
196. van-der-Putte SC. Mammary-like glands of the vulva and their disorders. Int J Gynecol Pathol 1994; 13:150–160.
197. Lambert WC, Brodkin RH, Schwartz RA. Apocrine carcinoma developing within a longstanding apocrine hidrocystoma. Proc Ann Mtg Am Soc Dermatopathol 1986; 111.
198. Dhawan SS, Nanda VS, Grekin S, Rabinovitz H. Apocrine adenocarcinoma: case report and review of the literature. J Dermatol Surg Oncol 1990; 16:486–490.
199. Cohen PR, Kohn SR, Davis DA, Kurzrock R. Muir-Torre syndrome. Dermatol Clin 1995; 13:79–89.
200. Nelson BR, Hamlet KR, Gillard M. sebaceous carcinoma. J Am Acad Dermatol 1995; 33:1–15.
201. Shaw JH, Rumball E. merkel cell tumour: clinicalbehaviour treatment.Review. Br J Surg 1991; 78:138–142.
202. Ratner D, Nelson BR, Brown MD, Johnson TM. Merkel cell carcinoma. J Am Acad Dermatol 1993; 29:143–156.
203. Boyle F, Pendlebury S, Bell D. Further insights into the natural history and management of primary cutaneous neuroendocrine (Merkel cell) carcinoma. Int J Radiat Oncol Biol Phys 1995; 31:315–323.
204. Bloechle C, Peiper M, Schwarz R. Post-irradiation soft tissue sarcoma. Eur J Cancer 1995; 31A:31–34.
205. Enzinger FM, Weiss SW. 3rd Soft tissue tumors.. St. Louis: CV Mosby, 1995.
206. Engel CJ, Eilber FR, Rosen G. Preoperative chemotherapy for soft tissue sarcomas of the extremities: the experience at the University of California, Los Angeles. Cancer Treat Res 1993; 67:135–141.
207. Bendix-Hansen K, Myhre-Jensen O, Kaae S. Dermatofibrosarcoma protuberans. A clinico-pathological study of nineteen cases and review of world literature. Scan J Plast Reconstr Surg 1983; 17:247–252.
208. Jimenez FJ, Grichnik JM, Buchanan MD, Clark RE. Immunohistochemical margin control applied to Mohs micrographic surgical excision of dermatofibrosarcoma protuberans. J Dermatol Surg Oncol 1994; 20:687–689.
209. Gloster HM, Harris KR, Roenigk RK. A comparison between Mohs micrographic surgery and wide surgical excision for the treatment of dermatofibrosarcoma protuberans. J Am Acad Dermatol 1996; 35:82–87.

210. Ratner D, Thomas C, Johnson T, et al. Mohs micrographic surgery for the treatment of dermatofibrosarcoma protuberans. Results of a multi-institutional series and analysis of the extent of microscopic spread. J Am Acad Dermatol 1997; 37:600–613.
211. Helwig EB, Fretzin DF. Atypical fibroxanthoma of the skin. A clinicopathologic study of 140 cases. Cancer 1973; 31:1541.
212. Davis JL, Randle HW, Zalla MJ. A comparison of Mohs micrographic surgery wide excision for the treatment of atypical fibroxanthoma. Dermatol Surg 1997; 23:1223–1224.
213. Pezzi CM, Rawlings MS Jr, Esgro JJ. Prognostic factors in 227 patients with malignant fibrous histiocytoma. Cancer 1991; 69:2098–2103.
214. Zagers GK, Mullen JR, Pollack A. Malignant fibrous histiocytoma: outcome and prognostic factors following conservative surgery and radiotherapy. Int J Radiol Oncol Biol Phys 1996; 34:983–994.
215. Brown MD, Swanson NA. Treatment of malignant fibrous histiocytoma and atypical fibrous xanthomas with micrographic surgery. J Dermatol Surg Oncol 1989; 15: 1287–1292.
216. Maddox U, Evans H. Angiosarcoma of skin and soft tissues. Cancer 1981; 48: 1907–1921.
217. Sordillo P, Chapman R, Hajdu S. Lymphangiosarcoma. Cancer 1981; 48:1674–1679.
218. Holden C, Spittle M, Jones E. Angiosarcoma of the face an scalp, prognosis and treatment. Cancer 1987; 59:1046–1057.
219. Buatti, Harari P, Leigh B, Cassady R. Radiation-induced sarcoma of the breast. Am J Clin Oncol 1994; 17:444–447.
220. Friedman-Kien AE, Saltzman BR. clinical manifestations of classical endemic African, epidemic AIDS-associated Kaposi's sarcoma. J Am Acad Dermatol 1990; 22:1237–1250.
221. Serfing U, Hood AF. Local therapies for cutaneous Kaposi's sarcoma in patients with AIDS. Arch Dermatol 1991; 127:1479–1481.
222. Eisinger FM, Smith BH. Hemangiopericytoma: an analysis of 106 cases. Hum Pathol 1976; 7:61–82.
223. Staples JJ, Robinson RA, Wen BC, Hussey DH. Hemangiopericytoma: the role of radiotherapy. Int J Radiat Biol Phys 1990; 19:445–451.
224. Fields JP, Helwig EB. Leiomyosarcoma of skin and subcutaneous tissue. Cancer 1981; 156–159.
225. Davison LL, Frost ML, Hanke CW. Primary leiomyosarcoma of the skin. J Am Acad Dermatol 1989; 21:1156–1160.
226. Maurer HM, Beltangandy M, Gehan EA. The intergroup rhabdomyosarcoma study I: a final report. Cancer 1988; 61:209–220.
227. Maurer HM, Gehan EA, Beltangandy M. The intergroup rhabdomyosarcoma study II. Cancer 1993; 71:1904–1922.
228. Ducatman BS, Scheithauer BW, Piepgras DG. Malignant peripheral nerve sheath tumors: a clinicopathologic study of 120 cases. Cancer 1986; 57:2006–2021.
229. Dabski C, Reiman HM, Muller SA. Neurofibrosarcoma of skin and subcutaneous tissues. Mayo Clin Proc 1990; 65:164–172.
230. Gokaslan ST, Terzakis JA, Santagada EA. Malignant granular cell tumor. J Cutan Pathol 1994; 21:263–270.
231. Lack EE, Worsham GF, Callihan MD. Granular cell tumor: a clinicopathologic study of 110 patients. J Surg Oncol 1980; 13:301–316.
232. Enzinger FM, Weiss SW. Liposarcoma. 3rd. Soft tissue tumors, St. Louis: CV Mosby, 1995:431–466.
233. Brooks JJ, Connor AM. Atypical lipoma of the extremities and peripheral soft tissues with dedifferentiation: Implications for management. Surg Pathol 1990; 3:169–178.
234. Zanolli MD, Wilmoth G, Shaw J. Epithelioid sarcoma: clinical and histologic characteristics. J Am Acad Dermatol 1992; 26:302–305.

235. Chase DR, Enzinger FM. Epithelioid sarcoma: Diagnosis, prognostic indicators, and treatment. Am J Surg Pathol 1985; 9:241–263.
236. Lookingbill DP, Spangler N, Helm KF. Cutaneous metastasis in patients with metastatic carcinoma: a retrospective study of 4020 patients. J Am Acad Dermatol 1993; 29:228–236.
237. Schildberg FW, Meyer G, Piltz S, Koebe HG. Surgical treatment of tumor metastases: general considerations and results. Surg Today 1995; 25:1–10.

5
Flap Survival and Tissue Augmentation

Robert W. Dolan
Lahey Clinic Medical Center, Burlington, Massachusetts, U.S.A.

FLAP PATHOPHYSIOLOGY

Reperfusion Injury and the No-Reflow Phenomenon

The common basic problem with any failing flap is lack of nutrient blood flow. However, a compromised flap can sustain a paradoxical increase in tissue injury after the re-establishment of nutrient blood flow by a phenomenon known as reperfusion injury. Reperfusion injury occurs within seconds of blood flow being re-established to a compromised flap (Fig. 1). The primary cell responsible for reperfusion injury is the neutrophil, which is attracted to ischemic tissue by cytokines. Neutrophils migrate into the flap parenchyma and release free radicals causing cellular injury (1). Compromised reperfused flaps also exhibit the no-reflow phenomenon; the finding that blood flow does not return immediately to some parts of a flap. This is believed to be due to neutrophil plugging; however, the actual cause is unknown.

Reducing reperfusion injury is beneficial to all types of flaps (2,3) and several experimental and clinical protocols show that oxygen free radical scavengers (3), antineutrophil antibodies (4), and anti-inflammatory drugs are effective. Anti-inflammatory agents including phospholipase A2 inhibitors (steroids) and lipoxygenase inhibitors are effective in reducing ischemia–reperfusion injury (5,6). However, cyclo-oxygenase inhibitors (nonsteroidal anti-inflammatory drugs [NSAIDS]) are not effective in reducing reperfusion injury (7). By inhibiting phospholipase A2, steroids including dexamethasone and hydrocortisone reduce the concentration of arachidonic acid (AA) and the formation of prostaglandins and leukotrienes. Prostaglandins are formed by the action of cyclo-oxygenase on arachidonic acid; however, inhibition of this enzyme is ineffective in reducing reperfusion injury. Leukotrienes are formed by the action of lipoxygenase on arachidonic acid and inhibition of this enzyme is effective in reducing reperfusion injury (5) (Fig. 2). Systemic steroids are probably effective due to a reduction in the concentration the leukotrienes, not prostaglandins. In fact, prostacyclin (a prostaglandin) is protective in several experimental canine models of myocardial ischemia because it inhibits neutrophil activation and accumulation (8). Based on improved flap survival in several animal studies, systemic dexamethasone can improve the survival of random-pattern flaps if it is administered prior to, or shortly after, flap elevation. Steroids may also be beneficial in secondary ischemic events encountered in free flaps.

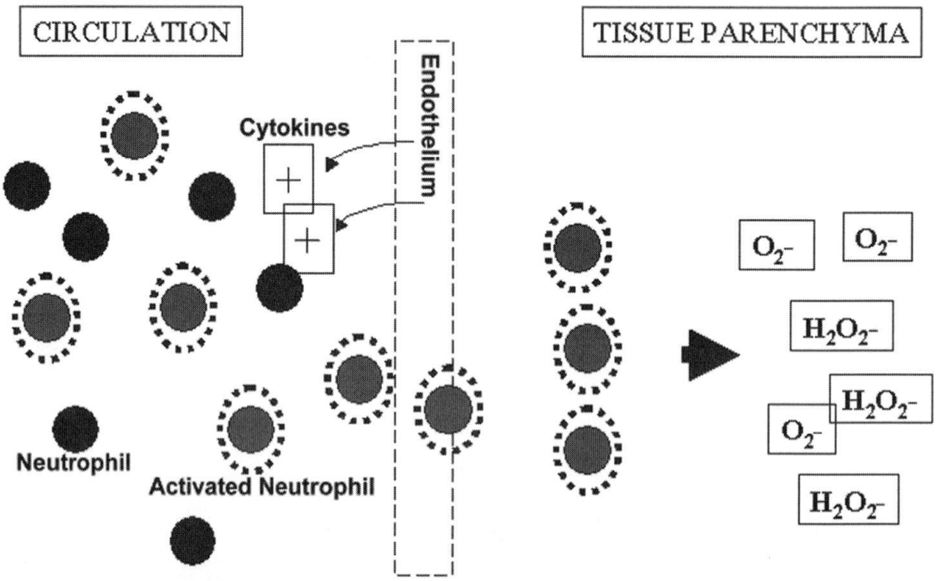

Figure 1 A simplified representation of reperfusion injury. Injured endothelial cells liberate a variety of cytokines. Upon reperfusion, these cytokines attract and activate circulating inflammatory cells including neutrophils. These activated cells (indicated by halos) express receptors on their surfaces that interact with endothelial cell surface receptors allowing attachment and transmigration. The neutrophils release their oxygen free radicals (respiratory burst) leading to parenchymal tissue damage. This process occurs within minutes of reperfusion.

Certain pathophysiological events depend on the type of flap (random, axial, or free) because of the fundamental differences in nutrient blood flow, and in the differing methods of tissue transfer to the recipient site.

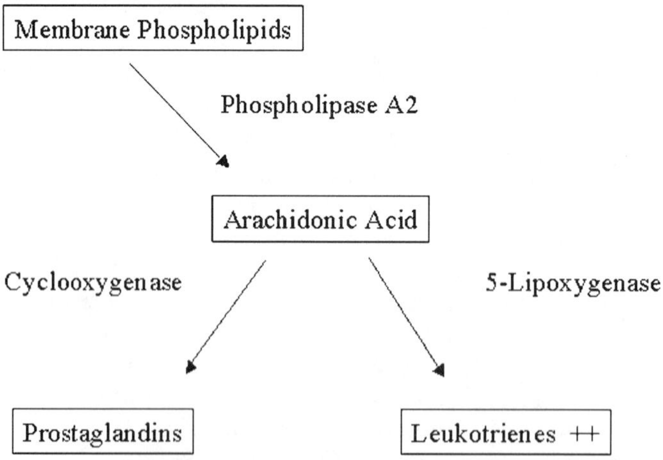

Figure 2 The phospholipase A2 pathway.

Random Flap Pathophysiology

Random flaps undergo necrosis secondary to lack of nutrient blood inflow rather than lack of venous outflow (9). The sympathetic nervous system is primarily responsible for determining the blood flow to the skin. Cutting the skin causes a release of norepinephrine from the severed sympathetic nerves and the release of thromboxane A from platelets, both of which are potent vasoconstrictors. Vasoconstriction may be the underlying factor behind two common theories regarding the pathophysiology of random flap failure: arteriovenous shunting and arterial insufficiency. Arteriovenous shunting is a lack of nutrient blood flow to the distal part of a flap through pathological arteriovenous shunts. Closure of these shunts either pharmacologically or spontaneously (theoretically) will lead to an improvement in survival of the distal portion of the flap (10). Kerrigan (11) disputes arteriovenous shunting as the cause of random flap failure and reports arterial insufficiency alone as the cause for distal flap failure. She found that during flap harvest there is a proximal to distal decrease in blood flow despite patent vascular channels and an increased intravascular hematocrit and pooling of red blood cells.

The clinical factors associated with ischemic necrosis in random flaps include the following:

Excessive tension along the wound edges from taut sutures.

Compressive dressings.

Infection which incites an inflammatory reaction in flap tissues with recruitment of neutrophils and similar cytotoxic cells. Flap adhesion to the wound bed and general healing are also delayed, often leading to flap dehiscence.

Hematoma: clot releases oxygen free radicals (12), increases the tension on flap edges, prevents adhesion to the bed, and produces a medium for bacteria to proliferate leading to a wound infection. Medications that affect blood coagulation (NSAIDS, wartanin) should be discontinued. Salicylates irreversibly block platelet function and should be discontinued at least 1 week prior to surgery. Acetaminophen does not affect blood coagulation.

Subcutaneous epinephrine (e.g., 1/200,000) if used in the area of a random-pattern nondelayed flap has no effect on tissue survival. However, it significantly reduces tissue survival in random-pattern delayed and expanded flaps (10).

Smoking.

The effect of smoking on random flap necrosis correlates with the amount the patient smokes (13). Smokers using more than one pack per day experience random flap necrosis at three times the rate of lower-level and nonsmokers. Lower-level, former, and nonsmokers have similar risk profiles. If the patient can discontinue smoking 48 h prior to and 7 days after surgery, flap survival is greatly improved (13). Two mechanisms are involved in smoking-related random flap necrosis: vasoconstriction by nicotine and tissue hypoxia due to carbon monoxide competing with oxygen for hemoglobin-binding sites (14).

Despite fixed length-to-width ratio rules for random flaps, widening of the pedicle will not always improve vascularity in the distal parts of the flap. However, a thicker flap may improve distal vascularity by including deeper plexuses containing larger-caliber vessels (15).

Therapeutic Interventions for Random Pattern Skin Flaps

Therapeutic interventions directed towards improving the nutrient blood flow and reducing random flap necrosis include the following:

Direct vasodilators (e.g., histamine): several vasodilators have been studied that show sporadic benefit in flap survival including phenethylamines (alpha and beta- adrenergic receptor antagonists) (16), calcium channel blockers (17), and topical nitroglycerin (18).

Adrenergic bockade: several vasodilating agents may have a beneficial effect on flap survival including isoflurane, which is a sympatholytic vasodilator (Compared with nitrous oxide, which is a vasoconstrictor) (19).

Growth factors: topical endothelial cell growth factor improved random flap survival in rabbits (20).

Rheological agents: pentoxifylline (increases red blood cell deformability and decreases platelet aggregability) improves random skin flap survival in pigs (21). Agents that lower blood viscosity have mixed results (22).

Hyperbaric oxygen administered within 48 h before or 4 h after surgery is beneficial to random flap survival in rats (23).

Decreasing temperature is aimed at reducing the metabolic demands of tissue, effectively increasing the ischemic tolerance of free tissue transplants. However, an improvement in survival of pedicled flap tissue is not seen (24).

Tissue expansion: blood flow and survival in expanded tissue that has undergone even an accelerated, brief expansion over a period of 5 days, were found to be greater than in flaps overlying a noninflated expander in a porcine model (25), similar to the enhanced survival seen after delaying a flap.

Flap delay: a compromised flap recognized during the primary surgery should be replaced in its bed and delayed for at least 1 week.

Axial Flap Pathophysiology

The best-studied axial flap is the pectoralis musculocutaneous flap. The factors associated with necrosis of this flap help to illustrate the potential problems with all axial flaps used for head and neck reconstruction. However, unique problems attend some flaps such as the latissimus dorsi (seroma at the donor site, pedicle kinking), and lower island trapezius (flap loss due to previous neck dissection). For a full discussion of the unique disadvantages of the axial flaps, refer to Chapter 8.

The pectoralis flap undergoes complete necrosis in 2–3% of cases (26,27). Marginal distal necrosis occurs in 20–30% of cases, more often in smokers, patients with a higher tumor stage, musculocutaneous flaps (compared with muscle alone), and in patients with poor nutrition (as measured by serum albumin levels) (26). In addition, Mehta et al. (27) found that female gender, prior chemotherapy, and the presence of diabetes were significant factors in flap loss. However, Kroll et al. did not find that gender affected flap outcome (26). Patients with a higher tumor stage required larger flaps, thus increasing the potential for distal necrosis. Muscle-alone flaps experienced less necrosis, illustrating the point that the skin's vascular supply (by indirect musculocutaneous perforators) may be somewhat tenuous.

Free Flap Pathophysiology

The immediate pathophysiological cause in the majority of free flap failures is lack of nutrient blood flow secondary to anastomotic problems. Venous occlusion, either directly from anastomotic thrombus or vessel kinking, is the most common cause. The maximum tolerable arterial ischemia time for a skin flap is approximately 8 h (6). However, tissue tolerance to venous occlusion is less than 4 h (28). Flap survival is usually an all-or-none phenomenon because these composite tissues predominantly encompass a single angiosome (see section on flap delay below) (29). However, vascular salvage efforts may result in a partially viable flap with only partial necrosis (30).

The International Microvascular Research Group (31) participated in a prospective survey of microvascular free flap practices and found only two factors associated with flap loss: reconstruction of an irradiated site and use of a skin grafted muscle. The overall flap loss rate was 4.1%. The elapsed time from irradiation to free flap reconstruction correlates with the degree of risk to the free flap (32). The use of skin-grafted muscle interferes with postoperative monitoring, resulting in the lack of early detection of perfusion abnormalities.

The International Research Group also found that venous thrombosis is the most common underlying pathophysiology of flap loss. Although the study did not correlate chronic wounds or the use of vein grafts with higher flap-loss rates, these two conditions were correlated with increased rates of thrombosis. Lower rates of thrombosis are found with certain flaps (especially the rectus abdominis free flap) and when subcutaneous heparin is used postoperatively. The salvage rate of compromised flaps is approximately 70% (32,33).

Factors found not be related to free flap loss include: tobacco use, recipient site (head and neck vs. extremities), indications for surgery (trauma vs. cancer), use in diabetic patients, age of the patient, type of anastomosis (end-to-side vs. end-to-end or running suture vs. interrupted sutures), use of heparin in the vessel irrigating solution, and a wide spectrum of postoperative antithrombotic therapies (dextran or systemic heparin).

Special Topics in Therapeutic Flap Management

Postoperative Monitoring of Microvascular Free Flaps

Monitoring vascular patency and flap perfusion is an essential component of the postoperative care of patients undergoing free tissue transfer. Postoperative compromise of arterial inflow or venous outflow results in the lack of nutrient blood flow to flap tissue and inevitable flap loss without therapeutic intervention. Approximately 10% of flaps will have a detectable perfusion abnormality in the immediate postoperative period. Most of these flaps are salvageable; however, an effective postoperative monitoring method is essential if salvage interventions are to be initiated in a timely fashion. There are no currently available monitoring techniques that can provide flawless objective and continuous flap evaluations in the postoperative period. An international review of practices in microvascular surgery (1991) reported that postoperative monitoring of tissue viability was performed, at least in part, by clinical methods in 75% of respondents (34). In addition to direct observation of tissue, clinical observation involves the use of exteriorized monitoring segments when the useful portion of the flap is buried. Exteriorized segments brought to the skin surface allow for monitoring and should ideally reflect perfusion abnormalities in the main flap (Fig. 3). The cutaneous portion of the free flap is monitored by observing the capillary refill: a pale flap with no capillary refill indicates a problem with inflow or arterial thrombosis; skin with a blue hue and very rapid refill indicates a problem with outflow, usually venous kinking or thrombosis. The presence of bright red blood on pinprick is a sign of a healthy flap; no blood may indicate an inflow problem and dark blood may indicate an outflow problem. Timing of these evaluations varies; however, a commonly used protocol is every hour for the first 24 h postoperatively; every 2 h for the next 24–48 h; and every 3 h thereafter until postoperative day 5.

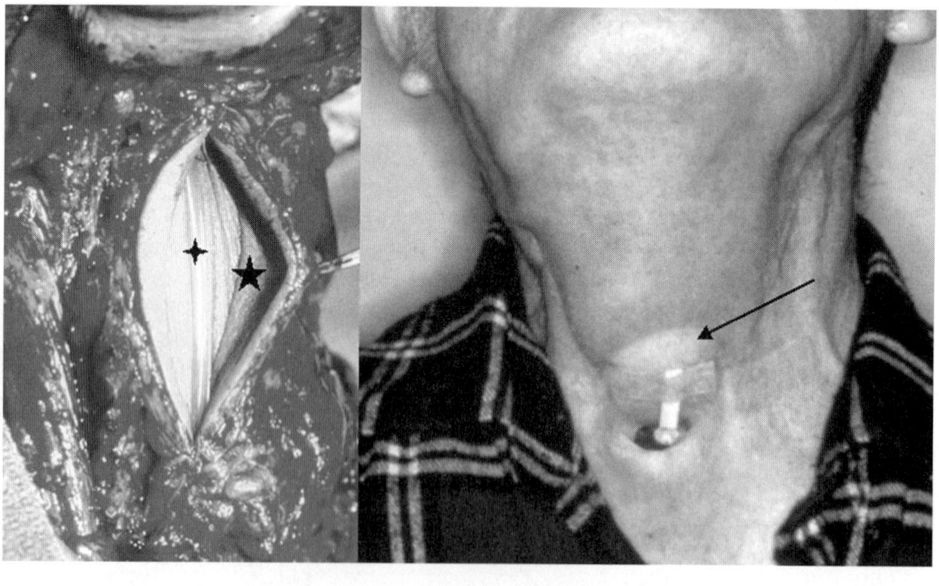

Figure 3 An example of an exteriorized monitor segment. Depicted on the left is a partially tubed lateral thigh free flap. Once the tubing is complete and the neck flaps replaced, the flap will be buried and unavailable for monitoring effectively. A subcutaneous-based skin paddle was created at the time of flap harvest and brought out to be incorporated into the neck incision (right). This allows effective monitoring of the main flap, since the health of this exteriorized monitoring segment reflects the health of the buried flap. The four-pointed star marks the nasogastric tube, five-pointed star marks the interior of the neopharynx and main flap, and the arrow indicates the exteriorized marking segment. (Photos courtesy of John Gooey, M.D.)

The most reliable method of monitoring skin circulation is through the use of radioactive microspheres; obviously, this method is limited to the laboratory. Although clinical observation is the most common method of monitoring the health of free flaps postoperatively, several other methods are available and relied upon in some institutions.

Laser Doppler Flowmetry

The laser Doppler apparatus consists of a probe that is surface-mounted to the cutaneous portion of a free flap.The probe is connected to a portable monitor displaying continuous variations in flow. The laser Doppler measures the frequency shift of light rather than the sound waves used in standard ultrasound Doppler. The reflected light has very limited penetration and surface measurements only capture the movement of red blood cells in the cutaneous microcirculation. It is unable to differentiate between venous and arterial flow. Significant perfusion abnormalities leading to flap compromise can go undetected using this system (35). However, it is probably the most accurate of the commonly used systems for monitoring. The accuracy of this method may be improved if the Doppler flowmeter is linked to a computerized data acquisition system (36) that can process and detect more subtle signal abnormalities.

Thermocouple Probe

The thermocouple probe is based on the physical finding that when two different metals are in contact, a change in temperature causes proportional changes in the rate of electron transport. Placement of probes distal and proximal to an anastomosis allows differential temperature measurements. Clot or static blood cool is cooler and causes a difference in the readings of the probes, indicating a perfusion problem. This technique is invasive and is prone to errors in probe placement as well as to iatrogenic vascular trauma.

Temperature Probe

The temperature probe is placed on the skin to provide continuous measurement of skin temperature. Due to the poor correlation of blood flow to surface temperature, this method is unreliable.

Pulse Oximetry

Pulse oximetry is commonly used for continuously monitoring digital pulse and oxygen saturation by measuring the difference between wavelengths of light absorbed by reduced and oxygenated hemoglobin. It has been used successfully for digit replants by monitoring differences between the replanted digit and a normal digit.

Fluorescein Dye

Fluorescein dye is administered systemically and is detectable in nonpigmented skin in 20 min by Wood's lamp. The fluorescein is deposited in the extracellular space and is cleared slowly, requiring several hours between observations. It may be useful for determining the initial viability of flaps, including pedicled flaps (37). More frequent observations are possible using a quantitative fluorometer probe that allows detection of smaller amounts of dye (38).

Doppler Ultrasonography

Doppler ultrasound converts sound waves reflected by a moving column of blood into an audible signal or wave form. The probe can be placed directly on the vessel or used on the skin surface. Different output is obtained for arterial vs. venous flow. When used on the skin surface, the probe may detect a vessel in the vicinity of the vessel in question, resulting in false-positive readings. This may be circumvented by placing the probe on an area of skin overlying the vascular pedicle that is well away from other vascular structures (e.g., in the midline of the neck). Venous flow problems may go undetected for several hours because of the persistence of arterial pulsations in the flap pedicle. Implantable probes are sutured to the vessel adventia and are prone to malalignment and iatrogenic injury to the vessel wall.

Leech Therapy

Leeches are hermaphroditic ectoparasites of the class Hirudinea. There are several species of leech, but the most commonly used medicinal leech is *Hirudo medicinalis*. Leech therapy is indicated for relief of venous congestion in a failing flap. Improved tissue blood flow in leech-treated venous compromised flaps has been demonstrated (39). Leech therapy has also been used to treat a variety of other conditions including soft tissue swelling, periorbital hematoma, cauliflower ears, ecchymoses, and purpura fulminans (40). Leech therapy should be reserved for cases that are not amenable to surgical correction. The leeches are applied to the skin surface of the flap and

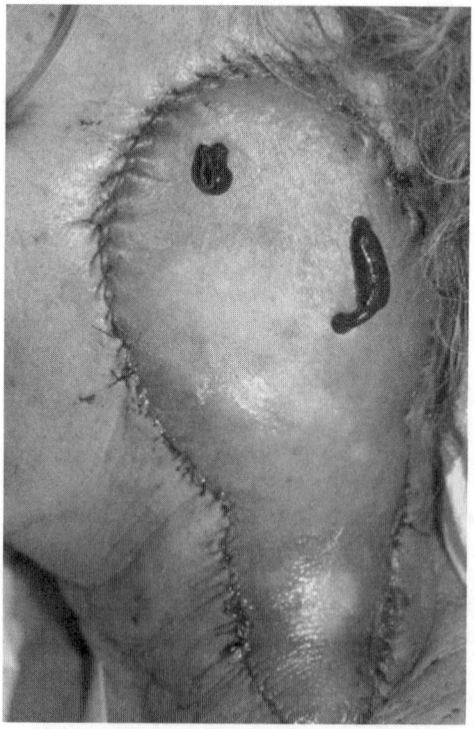

Figure 4 Leeches applied to pedicled latissimus dorsi flap to relieve venous stasis.

allowed to feed until they fall off (15–120 min) (Fig. 4). The wound continues to ooze due to the action of several substances present in the leech saliva including hirudin, vasodilators, and hyaluronidase. Hirudin is the most potent natural inhibitor of thrombin known (41). The leech can ingest up to 8–10 ml blood, and the wound can continue to ooze another 50 ml blood from the bite site. Leech therapy is successful in 70–80% of cases (40).

The leech has a large posterior sucker for attachment and crawling and a smaller anterior sucker (the head) for feeding. The posterior end is sometimes mistaken for the head because it also leaves a bite mark. Placing a drop of blood at the desired site of attachment can facilitate application of the leech. Migration can occur so the leech must be closely supervised and the site should be encircled with surgical towels.

Complications associated with leech therapy include wound infection and bleeding requiring blood transfusion. Wound infection is most commonly caused by *Aeromonas hydrophila,* a facultative gram-negative rod that is part of the normal flora in the leech gut. Prophylactic antibiotics should be administered to cover this organism: *Aeromonas hydrophila* is sensitive to third-generation cephalosporins, ciprofloxacin, aminoglycosides, sulfa drugs, and tetracycline (41) (ceftriaxone is commonly used). The success of leech therapy drops to less than 30% in the presence of a clinically significant infection (40). Immunosuppression or arterial in sufficiency in the flap predisposes the patient to infection and are contraindications to leech therapy.

FLAP AND TISSUE AUGMENTATION

Flap Delay

Skin flap delay is a technique to increase the vascular territory of a flap prior to its definitive transfer to a recipient site. The surviving length of a flap can be increased by at least 100%. Surgical flap delay involves incising the flap margins, extensive flap undermining at the donor site, or ligation of distal source vessels along the long axis of the flap. Pharmacological flap delay involves the use of medications to increase the vascular territory of a flap without surgical intervention. Surgical flap delay is the most effective method to augment flap circulation.

The principle behind surgical skin flap delay is interruption of the neurovascular supply to the distal parts of a flap prior to definitive flap transfer. After a delay of up to 3 weeks, the flap is harvested and transferred to the recipient site. The technique is dependent upon the underlying vascular anatomy at the donor site. In areas of mobile skin such as the scalp and forehead, the neurovascular structures tend to course longitudinally in the subcutaneous plexus and can be interrupted by simply incising three sides of the flap without undermining (the flap edges are then resutured during the delay period). Limited undermining (below the subdermal plexus) may be necessary to interrupt the blood supply if the distal part of the flap is supplied by perforating vessels. The extent of safe undermining can be determined clinically by verifying that the capillary refill is as rapid in the undermined skin as that in the adjacent unoperated skin. A variety of incisions and extent of undermining is described in the older plastic surgery literature (42).

The delay phenomenon describes the physiological events that result in clinical flap delay. The events are poorly understood and are frequently debated in the literature. There are several hypotheses regarding the mechanisms underlying the delay phenomenon including Reinisch's denervation supersensitivity-arteriovenous [AV] shunt mechanism (10), adrenergic spasm, and vascular collateral development. Reinisch's theory states that the sympathectomy created by surgical delay results in denervation supersensitivity that shuts down AV shunts, thus increasing nutrient blood flow to the distal parts of a flap. The adrenergic spasm hypothesis states that once the sympathetics are cut, the release of norepinephrine and subsequent vasoconstriction are significantly reduced during definitive flap transfer, resulting in improved flap survival (43). The development of vascular collaterals within the flap itself probably best accounts for the physiological events associated with flap delay. The angiosome concept helps to define the events during flap delay based on the dilation of vascular collaterals, especially at the choke vessel zone (44).

In nondelayed flaps, a source vessel can support the survival of its own vascular territory (angiosome) and an adjacent vascular territory or angiosome. The line of necrosis in nondelayed flaps generally corresponds to the choke vessel zone between the adjacent angiosome and the next angiosome along the axis of the flap. Delaying the flap interrupts the adjacent angiosome's neurovascular supply, resulting in dilation of the surrounding arterial choke vessels and increased capillary blood flow. In theory this allows easy through-flow for enhanced vascularity of the distal angiosome. This theory is supported by the histological findings of arterial vascular dilation and decreased vessel thickness, especially at the choke vessel zone, between 48 and 72 h after flap delay, not accompanied by vascular ingrowth or neovascularization (44). Venous valves direct blood flow in adjacent angiosomes away from the primary angiosome. The caliber of these vessels increases with flap delay; they become regurgitant and are bypassed by venous collateral vessels. The indications for surgical flap delay include the following:

- To extend the expected survival of a flap by progressive division of source vessels along its vascular axis (a flap can be delayed several angiosomes beyond the source artery by progressive division of source vessels staged at time intervals of at least 5 days) (44)
- To define the survival length of an uncertain flap
- To improve the circulation of an established flap

Tissue Expansion

In 1957 Neumann was the first to find a practical clinical application for prolonged tissue expansion by using a subcutaneously placed balloon for auricular reconstruction (45). In the 1970s, Radovan (46) and Austed (47) independently studied the principles behind tissue expansion, including the histological changes of expanded skin. The indications for tissue expansion include inadequate adjacent tissue for primary closure, inadequate tissue for repair with a local flap, and for repair of defects that are amenable to repair by a standard flap but only with significant donor or recipient site deformity (48). Disadvantages include the need for at least two separate procedures, that expansion takes several weeks, the expansion creates a significant temporary cosmetic deformity, and the procedure is limited primarily to elective reconstructive procedures.

Prolonged tissue expansion should be differentiated from rapid intraoperative tissue expansion. The latter is a technique introduced by Sasaki in 1987 to gain tissue volume rapidly intraoperatively by acutely expanding the tissue (49). Up to 3 cm tissue can be gained using this technique; less can be gained in areas of thick skin including the scalp, nasal tip, and back (49).

Expander Shape

The three most common shapes of expanders are round, rectangular, and crescent. The shape of the expander should match the shape of the region to be expanded and not the shape of the defect. The most effective surface area gain is with a rectangular expander: approximately 40% of the calculated surface increase of the expander is actually gained in tissue area in vivo. Round expanders gain 25% of calculated surface increase, and crescent expanders gain 30% of calculated surface increase. The expander base should be approximately 2.5 times as large as the defect to be closed for rectangular or crescent shaped expanders. For round expanders, this correction factor is true for the diameter of the expander rather than the area of the base. Custom-fitted expanders may allow more surface area gain. It is difficult to calculate the exact required size of a tissue expander since the ability of the skin to expand varies between sites and even from patient to patient. The age of the patient is also a factor; patients less than 2 years of age show a significantly greater response to skin expansion (45).

Expander Types

There are three types of expanders: a self-inflating expander that is osmotically powered and expands slowly at a constant rate (this is still experimental) (50); an expander with a distant filling valve (the most common type); and an expander with an incorporated filling valve on its surface. Directional expanders that expand more at one end than the other may be useful for correction of male-pattern baldness.

Expanders with distant filling valves come in sizes ranging from 1 to 1000 ml. However, expanders may be inflated up to 15 times over the manufacturers' stated maximum (51). It is more important to select an implant with the correct base size rather than volume. Overinflation leads to leaks at the dome of the injection port, so choosing the proper size expander is important despite the ability to overinflate (48). The filling valve should be placed in a separate subcutaneous pocket through the main access incision away from the main expander.

Expanders with incorporated filling valves have their injection port located at the apex of the expander, and, as in a distant filling port, contain a self-sealing membrane. A 21–25 gauge needle should be used for injections. A steel plate at the base of the filling port prevents an inadvertent deep puncture. A separate tunnel is not needed as in the expander with a distant filling port. Available sizes range from 50 to 1000 ml: miniexpanders are not available due to limits in the design of the attached filling port. There may be some increased risk of expander exposure over the injection port due to its stiffness.

Prolonged (Standard) Tissue Expansion

Prolonged tissue expansion is commonly used for scalp, nasal, and ear reconstruction, and for skin replacement in the forehead, cheek, and neck. Expansion of the

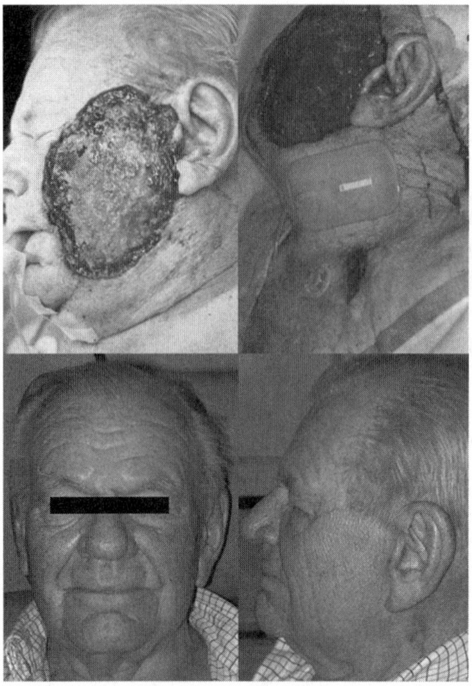

Figure 5 Tissue expansion for a cheek defect.

forehead flap with a rectangular tissue expander (250 ml) allows primary closure of the donor site and additional tissue for near-total or total nasal reconstruction. The expander is placed submuscularly (subgaleal) and is expanded over 8–10 weeks. Expansion of the postauricular skin for microtia repair can be done; however, risk of implant exposure, infection, and thickened flaps is a potential drawback to its use. Tissue expansion for skin replacement in the forehead, cheek, and neck is valuable since the expanded skin is adjacent to the defect and, in most cases, is almost identical to the missing or damaged skin (Fig. 5). Perhaps the most popular application in the head and neck is for defects of the scalp since hair-bearing skin is required (Fig. 6).

Expanded tissue arises from two sources: recruitment from adjacent tissue and altered histological nature of the overlying skin. The histological skin changes result from mechanical creep and biological creep (52). Mechanical creep refers to the ability of skin to stretch beyond its inherent extensibility through water and ground substance displacement, elastic fiber fragmentation, realignment of the collage fibers, and adjacent tissue migration. Biological creep refers to an increase in tissue volume through proliferation of epithelial cells, increased epidermal mitotic activity, expansion of the subdermal vascular network, and increased synthesis of collagen by fibroblasts.

The technique of prolonged tissue expansion involves placement of the expander adjacent to the defect through an incision at the edge of the defect or in a hidden area such as the hairline, except if the defect is covered with a skin graft. However, placement of access incisions at or near the junction of the defect

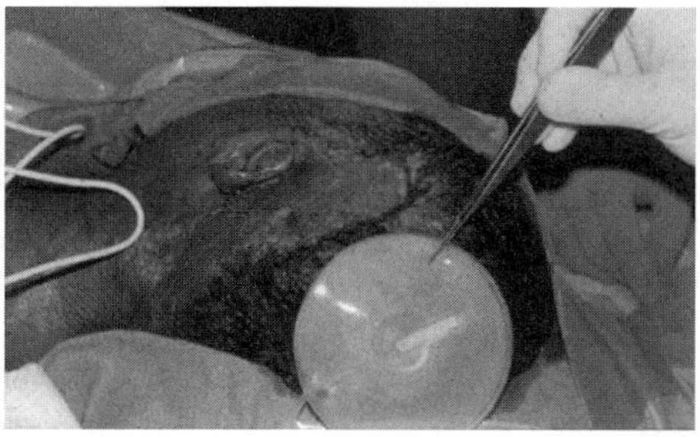

Figure 6 A typical round tissue expander with a remote port for scalp expansion.

and the adjacent skin to be expanded leads to higher rates of expander exposure and premature removal (48). Placement is usually in the subcutaneous plane in the face, under the platysma for neck expansion (avoiding placement over vital vascular structures), or under the galea for scalp expansion. Placement of deep permanent sutures may decrease the incidence of implant exposure (48). Slight initial expansion is helpful to eliminate dead space, but definitive (weekly) expansions should be delayed for at least 2 weeks postoperatively. The amount of saline injected should be gauged by changes in the overlying skin (tension or pallor). The overlying skin should retain capillary refill after expansion. An interval capsulotomy is occasionally necessary if expansion is arrested prematurely due to an overly dense capsule. The expander may leak slightly after placement, however, expansion should proceed if possible.

Histological Changes

The epidermis is the only skin layer to thicken during the expansion process; however, it eventually normalizes in the postexpansion period. Also noted are flattening of the rete pegs and increases in mitotic activity lasting up to 3 months. The dermis undergoes permanent thinning, increased collagen synthesis, realignment of collagen fibers to a more parallel orientation, and a temporary increase in melanin production that causes hyperpigmentation. Hair follicles and sebaceous glands move farther apart without increasing in number. Subcutaneous fat undergoes a decrease in the number of fat cells and a decrease in the size of the remaining cells with some associated fat necrosis. This layer may fully recover after several months (53). Skeletal muscle undergoes the following (54): muscle cells increase in the number of mitochondria, fibers thin and become atrophic with some necrosis, and hyalinization and calcifications develop. There is no change in the number of muscle cells after expansion. Blood vessels undergo dramatic proliferation, as well as arterial and venous elongation with no loss of diameter. The vascular supply to the overlying skin is enhanced. Nervous tissue tolerates expansion without significant demylinization, dysfunction, or necrosis (55).

A double-layered capsule forms by 1 week. The inner layer consists of macrophages and the outer layer is composed primarily of fibroblasts that are active in collage production. It reaches its maximum thickness at 8–10 weeks and is richly vascularized. Although this capsule is often included with the overlying skin after removal of the expander, its preservation does not add to the survival benefit of expanded skin (i.e., capsulectomy has no detrimental effect on skin flap viability, but may serve to thin the flap if required) (56).

Rapid Intraoperative Tissue Expansion

Sasaki (49) originally reported the technique of rapid intraoperative tissue expansion in 1987. The mechanisms involved include mechanical creep (described above) and stress relaxation. Stress relaxation refers to the finding that the load required to maintain the skin in a stretched position decreases with time. There is controversy as to whether there is an actual gain in tissue volume or simply an apparent gain secondary to recruitment of adjacent tissue (45).

Expanders are placed adjacent to the defect by creating a subcutaneous pocket followed by cyclic loading and unloading. To achieve the maximum amount of tissue stretch (approximately 2–3 cm), multiple cycles (every 3 min) of inflation/deflation are necessary resulting in microfragmentation of the elastin fibers. The amount of skin stretching depends on the area being stretched: areas with thick skin including the scalp, nasal tip, and back are less amenable to expansion.

Contraindications

The contraindications to prolonged tissue expansion include the following:

- Prior irradiation, which increases the risk of expander exposure but it is not an absolute contraindication if the expander is used with caution (45)
- Patients with major psychiatric disorders
- Patients who have demonstrated noncompliance with prior therapies

Complications

Complications are most common in the head and neck and lowest for breast expansion. Within the head and neck, the scalp is the area associated with the lowest complication rate. Complications, most commonly implant exposure, occur in less than 10–30% of patients (57). The most common complications include the following:

- Implant or filling port exposure. This more often occurs early in the course of expansion prior to the formation of a dense vascular capsule. Deflating the expander temporarily may help. An exposed filling valve may be well tolerated with no intervention.
- Implant infection. The expander should be removed if this occurs immediately after placement. However, if it occurs after partial expansion, partially deflate expander, administer antibiotics, and observe. Only remove if this regimen does not result in resolution.
- Implant leakage. Some leakage is tolerable and expansion should proceed; excess leakage may require premature implant removal.
- Overlying skin ischemia. Capillary refill should be present after inflation. Usually the patient will complain of pain and the expander should simply be partially deflated.
- Hematoma. Immediate postoperative expansion to eliminate dead space and active wound drains will help prevent seroma and hematoma formation. Light compressive dressings are applied if these measures fail.
- Bone absorption underlying scalp and forehead expanders. Thinning of the outer table may be seen. Full-thickness erosion is extremely rare and

usually occurs with expanders over 400 ml in the presence of infection and an abnormally extended expansion time (48).

Complications using tissue expansion in a pediatric population are more common in patients less than 7 years of age, those with internal expander ports (vs. a remote filling port), and in patients with a history of two or more prior expansions (58). The most common indications for pediatric prolonged tissue expansion are for the treatment of congenital nevi, burns, and soft tissue losses (58). Friedman et al. (58), in a study of tissue expansion in children from 8 months to 15 years of age, found that the major complication rate (resulting in failure of tissue expansion) was 9% and the minor complication rate was also 9%. The major complications include implant exposure, deflation, and wound dehiscence.

Distraction Osteogenesis

Distraction osteogenesis is a process that results in the creation of new bone in an enlarging gap between two bone fragments caused by their gradual separation (59). Originally described by Codivilla (1904) for lengthening lower extremity bones, the process gained wider acceptance after Gavril Ilizarov, a Russian surgeon, studied the mechanics and physiology of limb lengthening in 1954. Dr. Ilizarov continued his work and has contributed much of the current clinical knowledge of the method and biology of distraction osteogenesis (60–62).

Three methods of distraction osteogenesis are described: monofocal, bifocal, and trifocal. Monofocal distraction is the separation of two fragments of bone with one focus of new bone formation between the fragments (e.g., limb lengthening). Bifocal distraction is the movement of a single bone fragment or what is termed a transport disk, cut from the remaining bone stump, across a gap to unite with the opposite native bone (Fig. 7). Trifocal distraction is the movement of two apposing disks across a gap (e.g., advancing osteotomized mandibular body segments for symphyseal reconstruction. (63).

The method of distraction osteogenesis for maxillofacial application is extrapolated largely from the experiences with long bone distraction. First, division of the bone cortex (corticotomy) is required, preserving the medullary blood supply (e.g., inferior alveolar artery) and the periosteum. A latent period of up to 15 days (shorter for younger patients) is required for adequate callus formation and regeneration of central vessels and periosteal tissue. The external distraction device is connected to the underlying bones percutaneously via pins attached to a threaded bar for manual separation. Internalization of the distraction device to avoid cutaneous scarring has recently been studied (64). New bone formation occurs in the distracted mandible by intramembranous ossification. Distraction results in new bone formation induced by the combination of stretching and compressive forces by functional activity, referred to by Ilizarov as the tension-stress effect. The surrounding soft tissue envelope is concurrently expanded. The ideal rate of distraction was determined by Ilizarov in canines to be 1 mm/day in 0.25 mm increments. A slower rate of distraction resulted in premature union, and a faster rate resulted in delayed or nonunions. Osteogenic activity at the callous is greatest with continuous distraction; however, distracting in 0.25 mm increments results in satisfactory new bone formation.

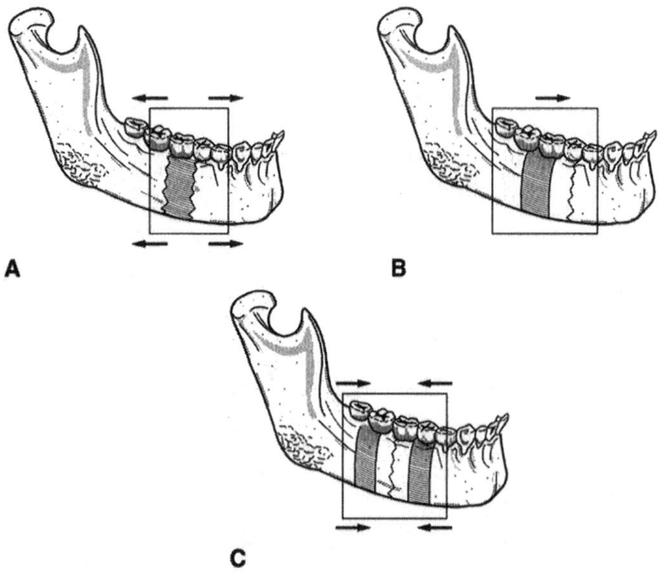

Figure 7 Various tissue distraction techniques including (a) monofocal distraction, (b) bifocal, distraction and (c) trifocal distraction.

Indications for distraction osteogenesis in the maxillofacial region include treatment of the following:

Transverse maxillary deficiency (65) and congenital mandibular hypoplasia (e.g., hemifacial microsomia) (66)
Treacher Collins syndrome for tracheotomy decannulation (67)
Mandibular defects from tumor resection or trauma
Sagittal maxillary deficiency secondary to cleft palate
Craniosynostoses (59)

Potential complications using distraction in the facial region include premature union, nonunion, elongated cutaneous scars, and patient intolerance of the device. Even very minor movement, other than the controlled daily distractions, can lead to fibrous nonunion or cartilage formation. Although the effects of radiation on distraction require further study, Gantous et al. successfully distracted irradiated canine mandibles (68). Neurosensory disturbances in the cheek (infraorbital nerve) after maxillary distraction or in the chin (inferior alveolar nerve) after mandibular distraction can occur early in distraction, but resolve over time (69).

REFERENCES

1. Dolan RW, Kerr DC, Arena S. Improved reflow and viability in reperfused ischemic rat island groin flaps using dexamethasone. Microsurgery 1995; 16:86–89.
2. Angel MF, Ramasastry SS, Swartz WM, Narayanan K, Kuhns DB, Basford RE, et al. The critical relationship between free radicals and degrees of ischemia: evidence for tissue intolerance of marginal perfusion. Plas Reconstr Surg 1988; 81:233–239.

3. Manson PN, Anthenelli RM, Im MJ, Bulkley GB, Hoopes JE. The role of oxygen-free radicals in ischemic tissue injury in island skin flaps. Ann Surg 1983; 198:87–90.
4. Vedder NB, Winn RK, Rice CL, Chi EY, Arfors KE, Harlan JM. A monoclonal antibody to the adherence-promoting leukocyte glycoprotein, CD18, reduces organ injury and improves survival from hemorrhagic shock and resuscitation in rabbits. J Clin Invest 1988; 81:939–944.
5. Dolan R, Hartshorn K, Andry C, McAvoy D. Systemic neutrophil intrinsic 5-lipoxygenase activity and CD18 receptor expression linked to reperfusion injury. Laryngoscope 1998; 108:1386–1389.
6. Dolan RW, Kerr D, Arena S. Reducing ischemia–reperfusion injury in rat island groin flaps by dexamethasone and BW755C. Laryngoscope 1995; 105:1322–1325.
7. Bonow RO, Lipson LC, Sheehan FH, Capurro NL, Isner JM, Roberts WC. Lack of effect of aspirin on myocardial infarct size in the dog. Am J Cardiol 1981; 47:258–264.
8. Simpson PJ. Arachidonic acid metabolites. In: Zelenock GB, ed. Clinical Ischemic Syndomes, St. Louis: CV Mosby Co, 1990:277–285.
9. Roberts AP, Cohen JI, Cook TA. The rat ventral island flap: a comparison of the effects of reduction in arterial inflow and venous outflow. Plast Reconstr Surg 1996; 97:610–615.
10. Reinisch JF. The pathophysiology of skin flap circulation. The delay phenomenon. Plast Reconstr Surg 1974; 54:585–598.
11. Kerrigan CL. Skin flap failure: pathophysiology. Plast Reconstr Surg 1983; 72:766–777.
12. Angel MF, Narayanan K, Swartz WM, Ramasastry SS, Basford RE, Kuhns DB, et al. The etiologic role of free radicals in hematoma-induced flap necrosis. Plast Reconstr Surg 1986; 77:795–803.
13. Goldminz D, Bennett RG. Cigarette smoking and flap and full-thickness graft necrosis. Arch Dermatol 1991; 127:1012–1015.
14. Jensen JA, Goodson WH, Hopf HW, Hunt TK. Cigarette smoking decreases tissue oxygen. Arch Surg 1991; 126:1131–1134.
15. Daniel RK, Kerrigan CL. Skin flaps: an anatomical and hemodynamic approach. Clin Plast Surg 1979; 6:181–200.
16. Neligan P, Pang CY, Nakatsuka T, Lindsay WK, Thomson HG. Pharmacologic action of isoxsuprine in cutaneous and myocutaneous flaps. Plast Reconstr Surg 1985; 75:363–374.
17. Nichter LS, Sobieski MW. Efficacy of verapamil in the salvage of failing random skin flaps. Ann Plast Surg 1988; 21:242–245.
18. Nichter LS, Sobieski MW, Edgerton MT. Efficacy of topical nitroglycerin for random-pattern skin-flap salvage. Plas Reconstr Surg 1985; 75:847–852.
19. Dohar JE, Goding GSJ, Maisel RH. The effects of inhalation anesthetic agents on survival in a pig random skin flap model. Arch Otolaryngol Head Neck Surg 1992; 118:37–40.
20. Hom DB, Assefa G. Effects of endothelial cell growth factor on vascular compromised skin flaps. Arch Otolaryngol Head Neck Surg 1992; 118:624–628.
21. Pratt MF. Edmund Prince Fowler Award thesis. Evaluation of random skin flap survival in a porcine model. Laryngoscope 1996; 106:700–712.
22. Ramasastry SS, Waterman P, Angel MF, Futrell JW. Effect of Fluosol-DA (20%) on skin flap survival in rats. Ann Plast Surg 1985; 15:436–442.
23. Nemiroff PM, Merwin GE, Brant T, Cassisi NJ. Effects of hyperbaric oxygen and irradiation on experimental skin flaps in rats. Otolaryngol Head Neck Surg 1985; 93:485–491.
24. Goding GS, Hom DB. Skin flap physiology. In: Baker SR, Swanson NA, eds. Local Flaps in Facial Reconstruction, St. Louis: Cv Mosby, 1995:15–30.
25. Marks MW, Burney RE, Mackenzie JR, Knight PR. Enhanced capillary blood flow in rapidly expanded random pattern flaps. J Trauma 1986; 26:913–915.

26. Kroll SS, Goepfert H, Jones M, Guillamondegui O, Schusterman M. Analysis of complications in 168 pectoralis major myocutaneous flaps used for head and neck reconstruction. Ann Plast Surg 1990; 25:93–97.
27. Mehta S, Sarkar S, Kavarana N, Bhathena H, Mehta A. Complications of the pectoralis major myocutaneous flap in the oral cavity: a prospective evaluation of 220 cases. Plast Reconstr Surg 1996; 98:31–37.
28. Kerrigan CL, Wizman P, Hjortdal VE, Sampalis J. Global flap ischemia: a comparison of arterial versus venous etiology. Plas Reconstr Surg 1994; 93:1485–1495.
29. Taylor GI, Palmer JH. The vascular territories (angiosomes) of the body: experimental study and clinical applications. Br J Plast Surg 1987; 40:113–141.
30. Weinzweig N, Gonzalez M. Free tissue failure is not an all-or-none phenomenon. Plast Reconstr Surg 1995; 96:648–660.
31. Khouri RK, Cooley BC, Kunselman AR, Landis JR, Yeramian P, Ingram D, et al. A prospective study of microvascular free-flap surgery and outcome. Plast Reconstr Surg 1998; 102:711–721.
32. Bodin IKH, Lind MG, Arnander C. Free radial forearm reconstruction in surgery of the oral cavity and pharynx: surgical complications, impairment in speech and swallowing. Clin Otolaryngol 1994; 19:28–34.
33. Kroll SS, Schusterman MA, Reece GP, Miller MJ, Evans GR, Robb GL. Timing of pedicle thrombosis and flap loss after free-tissue transfer. Plast Reconstr Surg 1996; 98:1230–1233.
34. Salemark L. International survey of current microvascular practices in free tissue transfer and replantation surgery. Microsurgery 1991; 12:308–311.
35. Sloan GM, Sasaki GH. Noninvasive monitoring of tissue viability. [Review]. Clin Plast Surg 1985; 12:185–195.
36. Gross JE, Friedman JD. Soft tissue reconstruction. Monitoring. [Review]. Orthop Clin North Am 1993; 24:531–536.
37. McCraw JB, Myers B, Shanklin KD. The value of fluorescein in predicting the viability of arterialized flaps. Plast Reconstr Surg 1977; 60:710–719.
38. Silverman DG, LaRossa DD, Barlow CH, Bering TG, Popky LM, Smith TC. Quantification of tissue fluorescein delivery and prediction of flap viability with the fiberoptic dermofluorometer. Plast Reconstr Surg 1980; 66:545–553.
39. Hayden RE, Phillips JG, McLear PW. Leeches. Objective monitoring of altered perfusion in congested flaps. Arch Otolaryngol Head Neck Surg 1988; 114:1395–1399.
40. de Chalain TM. Exploring the use of the medicinal leech: a clinical risk-benefit analysis. J Reconstr Microsurg 1996; 12:165–172.
41. Utley DS, Koch RJ, Goode RL. The failing flap in facial plastic and reconstructive surgery: role of the medicinal leech. Laryngoscope 1998; 108:1129–1135.
42. Grabb WC, Smith JW. Basic techniques in plastic surgery. In: Grabb WC, Smith JW, eds. Plastic Surgery, London: J. & A. Churchill Ltd, 1968:54–57.
43. Norberg KA, Palmer B. Improvement of blood circulation in experimental skin flaps by phentolamine. Eur J Pharmacol 1969; 8:36–38.
44. Morris SF, Taylor GI. The time sequence of the delay phenomenon: when is a surgical delay effective? An experimental study. Plast Reconstr Surg 1995; 95:526–533.
45. Swenson RW. Tissue Expansion. In: Papel ID, Nachlas NE, eds. Facial Plastic and Reconstructive Surger, St. Louis: CV Mosby, 1992:56–67.
46. Radovan, C. Adjacent flap development using expandable silastic implants. Presented at the annual meeting of the American Society of Plastic and Reconstructive Surgeons. 1976.
47. Austad ED, Pasyk KA, McClatchey KD, Cherry GW. Histomorphologic evaluation of guinea pig skin and soft tissue after controlled tissue expansion. Plast Reconstr Surg 1982; 70:704–710.

48. Baker SR, Swanson NA. Tissue expansion of the head and neck. Indications, technique, and complications. Arch Otolaryngol Head Neck Surg 1990; 116:1147–1153.
49. Sasaki GH. Intraoperative sustained limited expansion (ISLE) as an immediate reconstructive technique. Clin Plast Surg 1987; 14:563–573.
50. Austad ED, Rose GL. A self-inflating tissue expander. Plast Reconstr Surg 1982; 70:588–594.
51. Hallock GG. Maximum overinflation of tissue expanders. Plast Reconstr Surge 1987; 80:567–569.
52. Gibson T. The physical properties of skin. In: Converse JM, ed. Reconstructive Plastic Surgery, Philadelphia: WB Saunders, 1977.
53. Pasyk KA, Argenta LC, Hassett C. Quantitative analysis of the thickness of human skin and subcutaneous tissue following controlled expansion with a silicone implant. Plas Reconstr Surg 1988; 81:516–523.
54. van Rappard JH, Grubben MJ, Jerusalem C. Histological changes in expanded soft tissue. In: van Rappard JH, ed. Controlled Tissue Expansion of Reconstructive Surgery, Nijmegen, Netherlands, 1988.
55. Hall GD, Van Way CW, Kung FT, Compton-Allen M. Peripheral nerve elongation with tissue expansion techniques. J Trauma 1993; 34:401–405.
56. Morris SF, Pang CY, Mahoney J, Lofchy N, Kaddoura IL, Patterson R. Effect of capsulectomy on the hemodynamics and viability of random-pattern skin flaps raised on expanded skin in the pig. Plast Reconstr Surg 1989; 84:314–322.
57. Antonyshyn O, Gruss JS, Zuker R, Mackinnon SE. Tissue expansion in head and neck reconstruction. Plast Reconstr Surg 1988; 82:58–68.
58. Friedman RM, Ingram AEJ, Rohrich RJ, Byrd HS, Hodges PL, Burns AJ. Risk factors for complications in pediatric tissue expansion. Plast Reconstr Surg 1996; 98:1242–1246.
59. Tavakoli K, Stewart KJ, Poole MD. Distraction osteogenesis in craniofacial surgery: a review. [Review]. Ann Plast Surg 1998; 40:88–99.
60. Ilizarov GA. Clinical application of the tension-stress effect for limb lengthening. [Review]. Clin Orthop Rel Res 1990; 8–26.
61. Ilizarov GA. The tension-stress effect on the genesis and growth of tissues. Part I. The influence of stability of fixation and soft-tissue preservation. Clin Orthop Rel Res 1989; 249–281.
62. Ilizarov GA. The tension-stress effect on the genesis and growth of tissues: Part II. The influence of the rate and frequency of distraction. Clin Orthop Rel Res 1989; 263–285.
63. Annino DJJ, Goguen LA, Karmody CS. Distraction osteogenesis for reconstruction of mandibular symphyseal defects. Arch Otolaryngol Head Neck Surg 1994; 120:911–916.
64. Altuna G, Walker DA, Freeman E. Rapid orthopedic lengthening of the mandible in primates by sagittal split osteotomy and distraction osteogenesis: a pilot study. Int J Adult Orthodont Orthognath Surg 1995; 10:59–64.
65. Basdra EK, Zoller JE, Komposch G. Surgically assisted rapid palatal expansion. J Clin Orthodont 1995; 29:762–766.
66. McCarthy JG, Schreiber J, Karp N, Thorne CH, Grayson BH. Lengthening the human mandible by gradual distraction. Plast Reconstr Surg 1992; 89:1–8.
67. Moore MH, Guzman-Stein G, Proudman TW, Abbott AH, Netherway DJ, David. Mandibular lengthening by distraction for airway obstruction in Treacher-Collins syndrome. J Craniofac Surg 1994; 5:22–25.
68. Gantous A, Phillips JH, Catton P, Holmberg D. Distraction osteogenesis in the irradiated canine mandible. Plast Reconstr Surg 1994; 93:164–168.
69. Karas ND, Boyd SB, Sinn DP. Recovery of neurosensory function following orthognathic surgery. J Oral Maxillofac Surg 1990; 48:124–134.

6
Flap Classification and Local Facial Flaps

Robert W. Dolan
Lahey Clinic Medical Center, Burlington, Massachusetts, U.S.A.

FLAP CLASSIFICATION AND VASCULARITY

Flap classification is based on an evolving paradigm as new uses and new flaps are discovered. The earliest report of a facial flap (the midline forehead flap) is found in the Sushruta Samhita, a Hindu holy book, in 600 BCE (1). Flap development was largely ignored or relegated to the unholy in the period between the emergence of Buddhism in India to the 16th century (2). In the 1500s, Tagliacozzi perfected the arm-pedicled technique of nasal reconstruction that became known as the Italian method. The Hindu method was introduced to English speaking society by "B.L." in a letter to the *Gentleman's Magazine* in London in 1794 (3). This spawned a new era and signaled the rebirth of reconstructive surgery (4).

Flaps for facial reconstruction can be classified into three general categories: local, regional, and distant (free). A local flap is adjacent to the defect, a regional flap is remote (off the face) from the defect, and a distant flap is a flap whose pedicle is completely detached for transfer as a free flap or (rarely) what is termed a walking flap. Further subclassification is based on the nature of the arterial supply to the flap, and, in the case of local facial flaps, the type of tissue movement (e.g., interpolation or advancement). The type of arterial supply varies according to the configuration of the deep-fascia–skin vascular network.

Manchot (1889) (5) introduced the concept that cutaneous arteries have definite vascular territories. Segmental arteries penetrate muscle (musculocutaneous perforators) or bypass the muscular tissue via intermuscular septa [septo/fasciocutaneous perforators (Fig. 1)] and arborize extensively in several distinct cutaneous and subcutaneous plexuses. The plexuses represent the major blood supply to the skin and form in several distinct planes comprising the subfascial, prefascial, subcutaneous, subdermal, dermal, and subepidermal plexuses (Fig. 2). The subepidermal plexus serves primarily a nutritive role while the dermal plexus serves a thermoregulatory role. The subdermal plexus is the primary blood supply to the skin and is responsible for the bleeding noted clinically at a flap or laceration's edge (6). The subcutaneous plexus is better developed on the torso and enhanced flap survival may be achieved when this plexus is included in the flap design (e.g., the deltopectoral flap). The orientation of these vascular territories in the subcutaneous and deep fascial planes form the basis of many of the subsequent so-called axial flaps

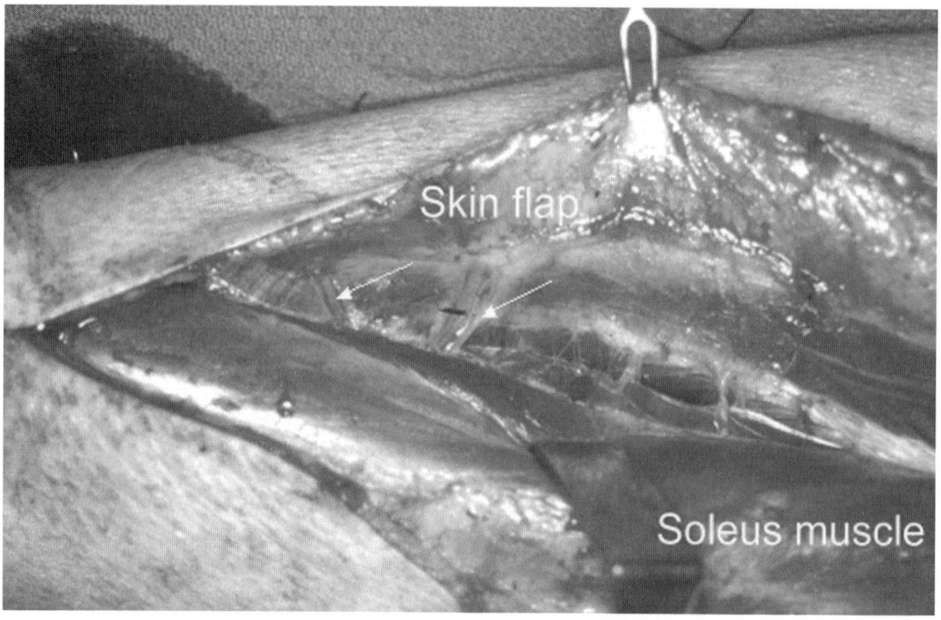

Figure 1 Lateral skin island reflected anteriorly during harvest of a fibular free flap. Note the septocutaneous perforators (arrows).

described in the latter half of the 20th century. McGregor et al. (1973) further defined the terms axial and random in their analysis of the system of arteries in the deltopectoral and groin flaps (7). An axial pattern flap is a single-pedicled flap that has an anatomically recognized arteriovenous system running along its long axis; a random pattern flap lacks any significant bias in its vascular pattern. Flaps with an axial pattern, with or without inclusion of the deep fascial plexus, can have significantly greater length-to-width ratios than a random pattern flap.

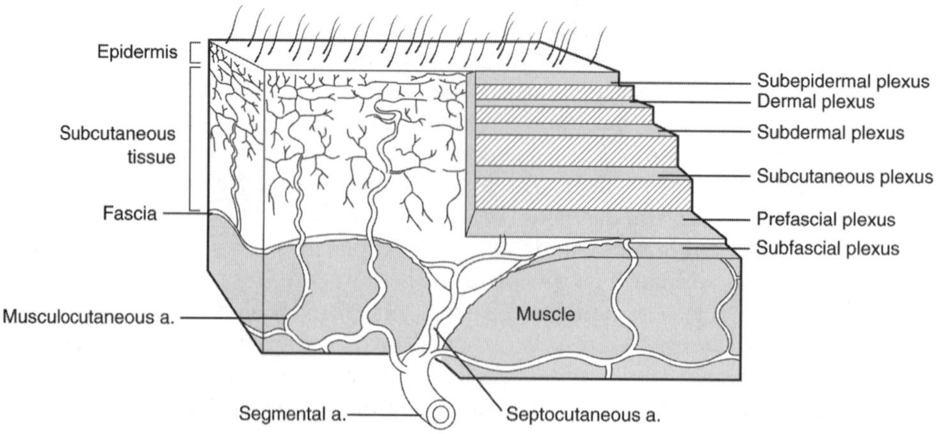

Figure 2 The cutaneous vascular plexuses.

The deep fascial plexus is a newly recognized important component of blood supply to the skin in areas of the body where this fascial network is well developed. This plexus tends to be well developed in the extremities and around the shoulders. Fasciocutaneous flaps from these areas depend upon the axial vascular network coursing within the deep fascial plexus for survival (e.g., the parascapular flap). The source arteries reach the deep fascial plexus via septocutaneous segmental arteries and an axial vascular network is then formed at the deep fascial level. There are two components to the deep fascial plexus: the subfascial plexus and the prefascial plexus. The axial vascular network is mainly concentrated in the prefascial plexus.

A random pattern skin flap may include tissue from the subdermis through the deep fascia. Random skin flaps are the first to be described in detail in the 20th century along with the "rule of ratios" that dictates safe length-to-width ratios based on clinical observations of survival. The ratios range from less than 1:1 for extremity skin flaps to up to 5:1 for flaps on the face. The extended ratios for many facial flaps may actually be an indication of their axial subcutaneous vascular patterns from terminal musculocutaneous vessels (e.g., nasolabial flap) and may be more properly classified as axial skin flaps.

LOCAL FLAPS OVERVIEW

It is helpful to subclassify local flaps based on the type of tissue movement involved in transferring the flap from the donor site to the recipient site (8). The two basic classes of flaps are sliding and lifting. Sliding flaps move tissue by direct advancement, leaving a donor defect adjacent to the newly covered recipient site that is of unequal length and is closed primarily. Included in this class are the subcutaneous pedicle/advancement flaps (cheek, V–Y, island pedicled, O–T/A–T plasty); and rotation flaps (dorsal nasal). Lifting flaps cross normal issue to reach the recipient site and include transposition flaps (bilobe and rhombic flaps); and interpolation flaps (melolabial, midline forehead). A transposition flap is adjacent to the defect and transfers tissue in one stage. An interpolation flap is remote from the defect and transfers tissue in two stages: the second stage is for sectioning of the pedicle after an appropriate period of time (usually 2–3 weeks).

There are several local cutaneous flaps described for limited defects on the face. It is helpful to consider the following in preoperative planning:

1. The desires of the patient: Does the patient value cosmesis over the expediency of a skin graft or healing by secondary intention?
2. Medical comorbidities: Is there a history of radiation therapy, tobacco use, or insulin-dependent diabetes mellitus? All these factors increase the likelihood of ischemic flap loss.
3. Is a skin graft capable of obtaining similar or better results than tissue transposition or advancement? In general, concave areas such as the medial canthal areas and nasal sidewall subunits do very well with full-thickness skin grafts.
4. Is primary closure possible without undue tension or disfigurement?

BASIC LOCAL FLAPS

Some local flaps involve fundamental soft tissue movement and can be considered for general use depending upon the surrounding characteristics of the skin. After skin grafting, these basic local flaps should be considered before more complicated or staged procedures. The basic local flaps include the single/bilateral pedicle advancement (U-plasty/H-plasty), island subcutaneous V–Y advancement, O–T/A–T plasty, rotation, banner, bilobe, and rhombic. If a basic local flap is planned, there is a step-by-step method described by Calhoun et al. (9) to aid in the conceptualization of the process of flap selection. First, the characteristics of the defect are noted including its size, shape, and location. Good and bad lender units adjacent to the defect are outlined. Good lender units supply adjacent tissues with little distortion or tension of surrounding structures that are distortable such as the eye or lip. Second, the characteristics of each available flap must be considered, including:

1. The amount of skin undermining required for tissue movement expressed in diameters of the defect size: if a defect is 2 cm in diameter, an A–T plasty requires two times the defects diameter (2D or 4 cm) of adjacent tissue undermining for adequate advancement. Diameter ratios are listed for the flaps discussed by Calhoun including the rhomboid, bilobed, subcutaneously pedicled, V–Y, and A–T plasty.
2. The arc (in degrees, 90–360) of territory required for skin undermining: the diameters of skin undermining and the arc describe the surface area and direction of dissection required for each flap.
3. The vector of maximum tension after flap inset: this is important in determining if structures in line with the tension vector may be distorted.
4. Final scar orientation with respect to the resting skin tension lines (RSTLs): although most of these flaps have multidirectional scars that inevitably cross the RSTLs.

The vector of maximum tension runs perpendicular to a radial line bisecting the arc (Fig. 3). The flap should be oriented around a defect so as to place its tension vector away from distortable structures such as the lower eyelid and lip vermilion. If this is not possible, another flap should be considered. Finally, the orientation

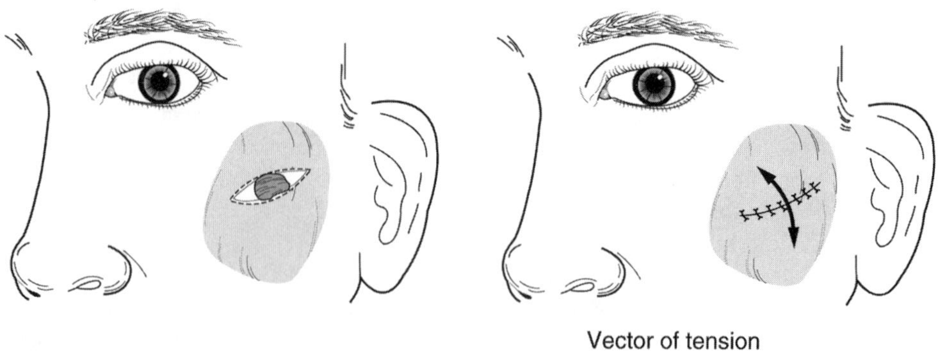

Figure 3 The vector of maximum tension runs perpendicular to a radial line bisecting the arc.

of the scars should be with the RSTLs as much as possible. However, most of the flaps require incisions that will be unfavorable to the RSTLs. Some flaps do have a more linear orientation, including the subcutaneous pedicled and V–Y flaps, and these should be oriented with the RSTLs.

Single/bilateral-Pedicle Advancement (U-plasty/H-plasty)

Description

Single and bilateral pedicle advancement flaps are sliding random pattern flaps that involve advancing skin toward the defect from either one side (single pedicle or U plasty) or opposite sides (bilateral pedicle or H plasty) (Fig. 4). The shape of the flap is rectangular, taking advantage of the extensibility of the skin after wide undermining. These flaps are designed to include the subdermal plexus and the safe length to width ratio is 3:1; however, if the base is situated over a named artery this ratio can be increased. Burow's triangles usually must be excised lateral to the base of the flap to eliminate dog-ears.

Indications

The forehead is an ideal site for using this flap, making use of the horizontally oriented RSTLs. The arc is 90 degrees and the diameter 2D.

Advantages

The primary advantage of this flap is that it will fill smaller defects expeditiously, especially those on the forehead where the RSTLs are ideal for this type of tissue movement.

Disadvantages

There may be a tendency to overstretch the flap to accommodate larger defects, putting the crucial distal part of the flap in danger of ischemic necrosis; bilateral advancements help to overcome this limitation. Another disadvantage is the considerable additional incisions necessary to harvest the flap.

Island Subcutaneous V–Y Advancement

Description

The concept of the subcutaneous island advancement flap was first described by Esser in 1917 (10). This is a random-pattern sliding skin flap freed from its cutaneous

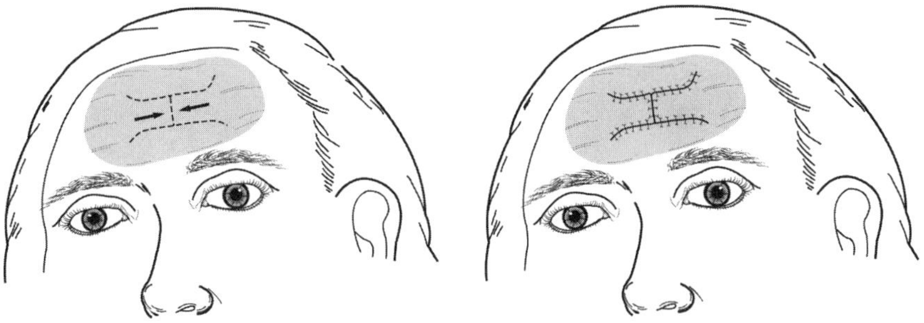

Figure 4 H plasty.

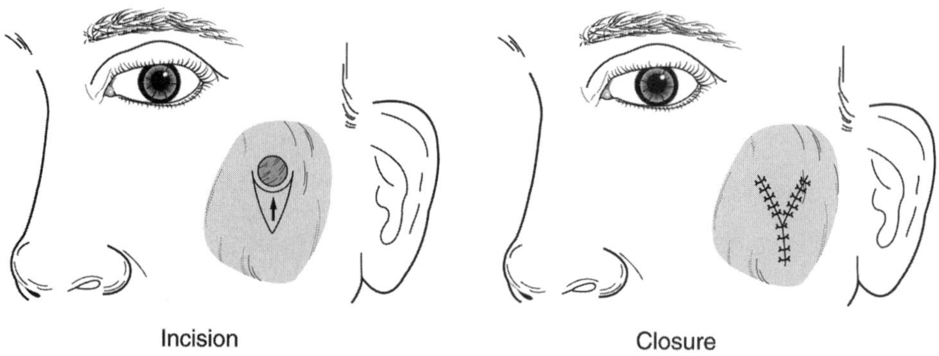

Figure 5 V–Y advancement flap.

connections and advanced into a defect based only on the underlying subcutaneous tissue (Fig. 5). The degree of advancement possible is proportional to the amount and laxity of the underlying subcutaneous tissue. The donor defect is then closed primarily, resulting in a Y-shaped scar. The flap is triangular and should be as wide as the defect, but 1.5–2 times longer (11) (Fig. 6).

Indications

This flap is useful when the subcutaneous tissues in line with the defect are plentiful and lax. Cheek defects along the melolabial fold, especially adjacent to the ala are ideal. It may also be used to lengthen structures such as a shortened columella, or to release contracted scars that may be distorting surrounding structures such as the eyelid or vermilion. Additional indications include upper lip defects using bilateral V–Y plasties, or a single vertically oriented V–Y transposition for lower eyelid defects. The arc is 90 degrees and the diameter 1.5D.

Advantages

For flaps along the melolabial sulcus and lips, the topographical unit borders can camouflage the incisions. Very little tension results, due to the pushing effect on the island of skin from primary closure of the donor site. Skin color and texture match are excellent.

Disadvantages

Adequate subcutaneous tissue must be present to maintain flap vascularity. Therefore in areas with little subcutaneous tissue the flap is either unreliable or of very limited mobility (e.g., nasal tip). Since this flap is based on a vertically oriented blood supply, its application to scalp defects is limited due to the horizontally oriented blood supply in the galea aponeurosis.

O–T/A–T plasty

Description

The T-plasty consists of bilateral random-pattern sliding skin advancements transforming an O-shaped defect (O–T plasty) or an A-shaped defect (A–T plasty) into a final T-shaped scar. A circular defect is converted to an A shape by excising a superior wedge of tissue creating a partial ellipse with a blunt base. The base is closed

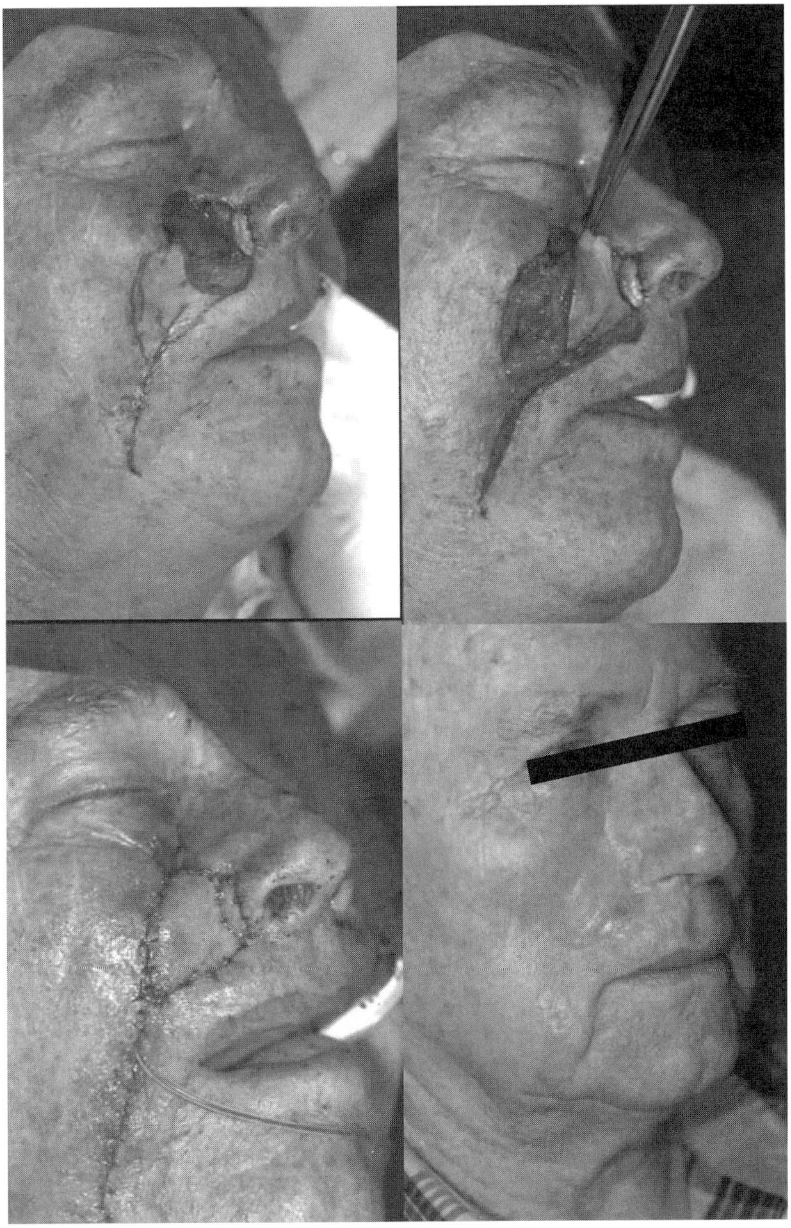

Figure 6 Sequence of a typical nasolabial V–Y advancement flap.

through bilateral tissue advancement with lateral tissue wedges (Burow's triangles) to avoid tissue bunching and dog-ears. An O–T plasty is similar except instead of excising the superior wedge, a tissue-sparing M-plasty is created at the superior margin.

Indications

The A–T plasty is indicated when the final scar base can be placed along a topographical unit border: around the lip or forehead adjacent to the eyebrow where the cross can be placed at the vermilion border or superior eyebrow margin. Another common indication is for defects in the temporal area, where the cross on the T can be placed along the hairline and the forehead and cheek areas can be widely undermined to allow tissue movement. The arc is 180 degrees and the diameter 2D.

Advantages

Using a T-plasty instead of converting the defect into an ellipse saves tissue and can avoid crossing a topographical unit border.

Disadvantages

As in all advancement flaps, incision placement should be with the RSTLs, respecting the topographical unit border. Since this flap results in scars at right angles, it is limited to areas in which the scars can be camouflaged, usually bordering a topographic subunit that can accommodate the cross of the T.

Rotation

Description

Rotation flaps are random-pattern sliding pivotal flaps with a curvilinear design. The flap sweeps into a triangular defect, pivoting at the base of the defect like the hand of a clock. The apex of the triangle is directed toward the base of the flap. After rotation of the skin into the defect, a dog-ear at the base of the flap may be created and can be excised with a Burow's triangle. The length of the curvilinear incision for the flap should be approximately four times the length of the defect (12) to minimize wound closure tension.

Indications

Rotation flaps are well-suited for closure of triangular-shaped defects with one side of the triangle representing the advancing edge of the flap. Extensive areas of the face including the cheek and neck are amenable to rotation flap closure (Fig 7). This is often the method of choice for closure of scalp defects; however, longer flaps are often required because the skin of the scalp is less distensible. More limited defects of the chin may also be closed using this flap. It may be difficult to camouflage a curvilinear incision in the forehead, so rotation flaps have a limited role in this area. The glabellar area is an exception and smaller tissue rotations are acceptable. Because of the large incision, rotation flaps have a very limited role in nasal reconstruction. The arc is 90 degrees and the diameter 3D, depending on the length of the curvilinear incision.

Advantages

The flap is very reliable with a broad base and a very low length-to-width ratio. The scars left after a rotation flap are of a simple curvilinear design and can often be hidden at aesthetic unit borders or directed with the RSTLs. There is virtually no limit to the size of a rotation flap: it can encompass the entire ipsilateral cheek to close large medial cheek–upper lip defects.

Disadvantages

The defect needs to conform to a triangle with its base along the incision for the flap. The incision is very lengthy; if it crosses an aesthetic unit border another local flap should be considered.

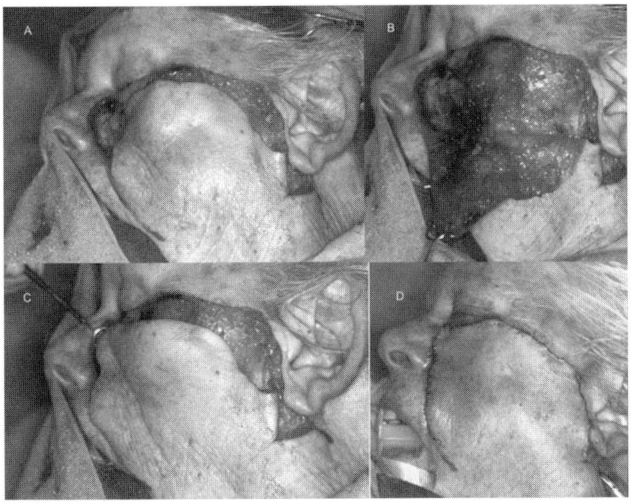

Figure 7 Cervicofacial rotation cheek flap cheek. An elliptical incision is made to follow the zygomatic arch and preauricular area (A) and widely undermined in the subcutaneous plane (B). The flap is advanced (by rotation, C) facilitated by a back cut near the earlobe. Final operative result shown in D.

Banner

Description

Originally named a banner flap because of its triangular shape (13), this flap is a simple transposition of adjacent tissue in the form of an unequal Z-plasty (Fig. 8). The flap is random-pattern and subsists on the subdermal plexus. It is designed to mimic a Z-plasty by considering the long axis through the defect as one limb and placing the remaining two limbs at approximately 60 degree angles to allow the final scar to follow either the border of a topographical subunit or the RSTLs. The flap is significantly longer and somewhat narrower than the diameter of the defect to allow easy primary closure of the donor site.

Indications

The principal indications for the banner flap are defects between 1 and 1.5 cm on the lower two-thirds of the nose.

Advantages

This is a very hardy flap with little risk of distal necrosis.

Disadvantages

Distortion of surrounding structures perpendicular to the long axis of the donor site (e.g., alar retraction). Undue tension may be alleviated by conversion of the banner flap to a bilobe flap.

Bilobe

Description

Originally described by Esser in 1918 for reconstruction of nasal tip defects (14), it consists of two lifting-type random-pattern transposition flaps that pivot into position. The first flap fills the defect and the second flap fills the donor site (Fig. 9).

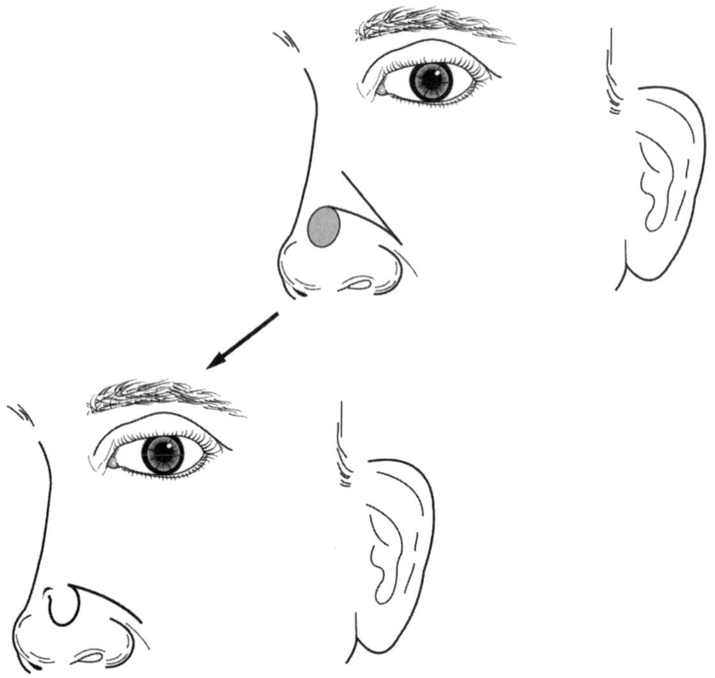

Figure 8 Banner flap.

The release of tension by raising the second flap is analogous to that associated with a Z-plasty. The angles between the defect and each lobe of the flap should be narrow enough to limit the transposition arc to 90 degrees to avoid standing cutaneous and trapdoor deformities common to Esser's original design using an arc of 180 degrees (15). The technique begins by changing a circular defect into a teardrop by excising a Burow's triangle. Arcs are then created centered along the base of the defect; the first arc crosses the outside limit of the defect and the second arc bisects the defect. The first arc marks the height of the primary donor flap, the

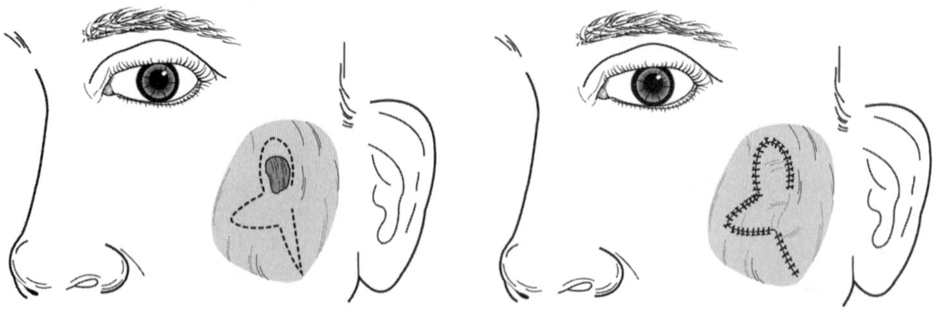

Figure 9 Bilobe flap.

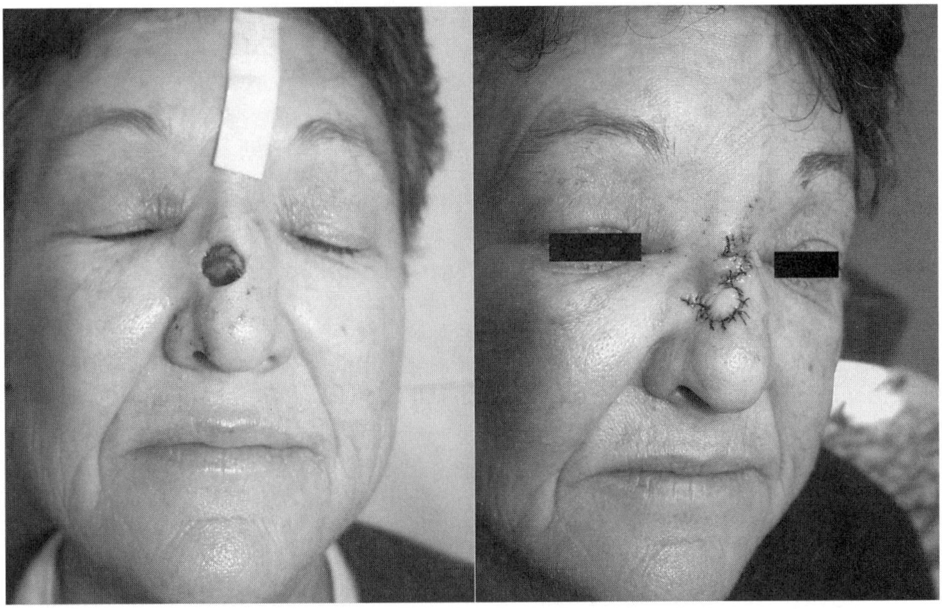

Figure 10 Bilobe flap in a patient with a circular nasal skin defect.

second arc marks the base of both donor flaps. The secondary donor flap is twice the height of the first. Closure begins with the donor site of the secondary flap.

Indications

The bilobed flap is very useful for limited defects (1–1.5 cm) of the nose (Fig. 10). The arc is 90 degress and the diameter 2.5D.

Advantages

It is the flap of choice for limited defects (1–1.5 cm) on the lower two-thirds of the nose. The primary flap is placed with little tension and little tendency to distort surrounding structures such as the alar rim or nasal tip. This flap is ideal for alar-tip defects: the base of the flap can be positioned laterally and primary closure of the secondary defect is accomplished through recruitment of skin lateral to the nasal sidewall subunit.

Disadvantages

As with many of these local flaps, the curvilinear design creates scars that cross the RSTLs.

Rhombic

Description

The nomenclature surrounding this flap is inconsistent. Flaps called rhombic/rhomboid/rhombus all share a common origin with Limberg's original flap described in 1963 (16). These designations do not reflect the shape of the flap but more literally the shape of the defect. A rhombic defect has the shape of a rhombus (an equilateral parallelogram). Limberg's flap is rhombic (i.e., a rhombic flap) with opposing angles of 60 and 120 degrees that is random-pattern and lifting. A rhombic flap is similar to a transposition flap; however, unlike a transposition flap, the rhombic pivots and also advances toward the defect, requiring extensive undermining of skin at the base of the flap. A rhombus-shaped defect can be conceptualized as a typical elliptical defect with opposing 60 degree angles that cannot be closed primarily (17). The design of a rhombic flap involves tracing a line through the opposing 120 degree angles. Outside the rhombus, this line is followed at a distance equal to the length of the defect, and four lines are extended at 60 degree angles parallel to the side of the rhombus. This outlines four possible flaps surrounding the defect (Fig. 11). The appropriate one to use will depend upon the availability of surrounding skin, the placement of incisions, and the maximum tension vector (which is within 20 degrees along the line intersecting the 120 degrees angles) (18). Only two flaps are appropriate based on skin extensibility. The final decision as to which flap to use will be based on minimizing the distortion of surrounding structures. The classic Limberg flap is equal in size to the defect; however, as the rhombus approaches the shape of a square, the transposed flap size is reduced to 40% of the defect size (19).

A rhomboid flap is different from Limberg's rhombic flap and is designed for rhomboid-shaped defects (oblong parallelograms with opposite sides of equal length). Subsequent variations of the Limberg flap are found throughout the literature (17–20).

Indications

Since much of the scar from the rhombic flap does not align with the RSTLs, it is best used in areas that have less prominent skin creases such as the cheek: the fore-

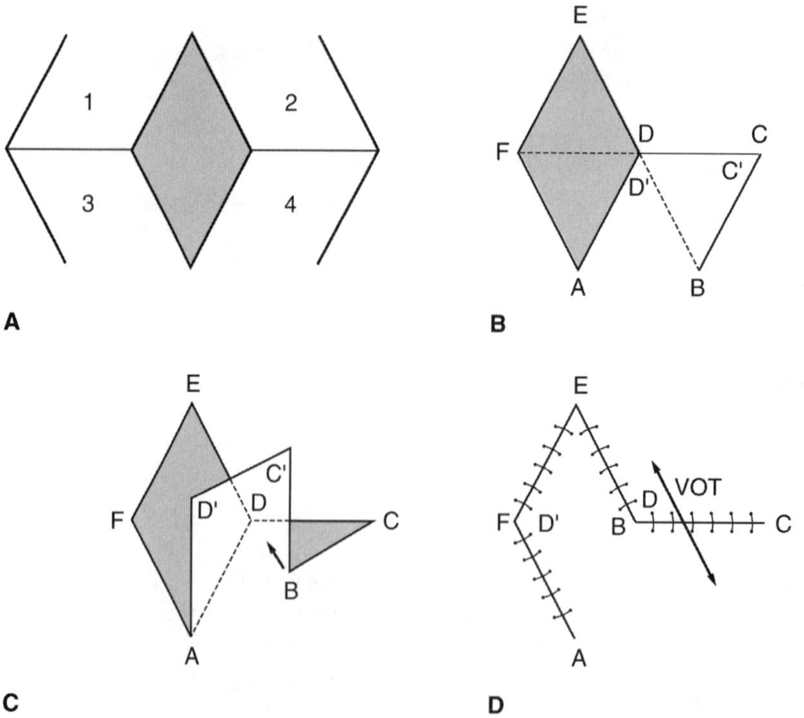

Figure 11 Rhombic flap: four possible flaps to fill the defect.

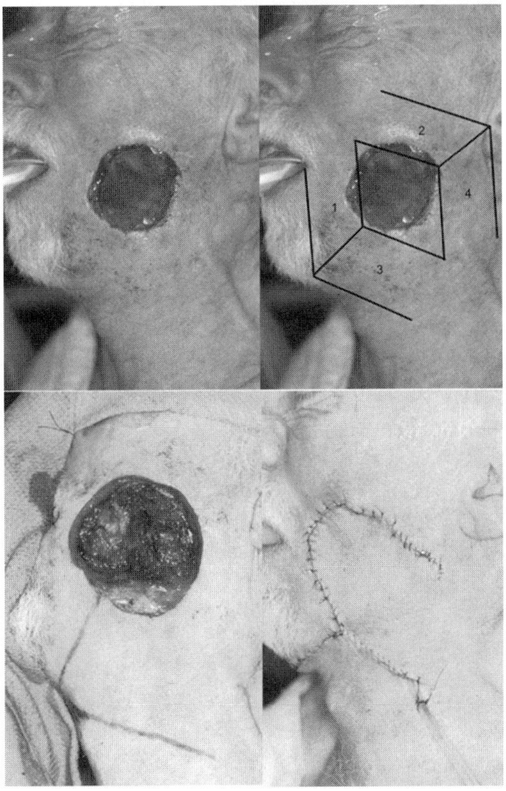

Figure 12 Potential rhombic flaps designed around a lower cheek skin defect. Flap 3 was chosen due to considerations of adjacent structures and the ability to 'borrow skin' from the neck.

head and temple areas are less favorable (17) (Fig. 12). The arc is 90 degrees and the diameters 1.5D.

Advantages

The majority of the resulting skin tension is at the base of the flap, minimizing the danger of tissue ischemia in the distal part of the flap. It combines the benefits of both pivoting and advancing adjacent skin, maximizing adjacent tissue movement.

Disadvantages

This flap may distort surrounding cutaneous structures because of the marked tissue movement involved. The resulting scar is multidirectional and much of it will not fall into good alignment with the RSTLs. This is most important in areas with prominent skin lines such as the forehead.

PERINASAL LOCAL FLAPS

Dorsal nasal (Miter)

Description

The dorsal nasal flap (miter) is a sliding rotation advancement flap that recruits tissue from the glabella and nasal dorsum to cover partial-thickness defects of

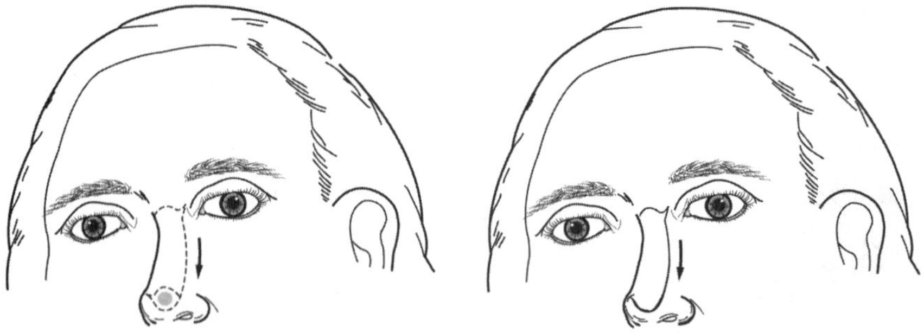

Figure 13 Dorsal nasal flap.

the lower nose (21) (Fig. 13). This is an extension of the sliding glabellar flap described by Gillies (22), which was designed for upper nasal defects. The incisions for the miter flap extend into the glabella from the medial brow and descend medial to the opposite brow along the lateral side of the nose, arching toward the defect respecting the borders of the nasal subunits. Wide subcutaneous undermining over the dorsum of the nose proceeds to the base of the flap near the medial canthus and the flap is transposed into the defect. A V–Y closure of the glabella facilitates flap transposition.

The frontonasal flap is identical to the miter flap except that the vascular pedicle (angular vessel) is dissected and the flap is islanded. This flap is therefore considered axial and provides greater freedom of tissue movement (23).

Indications

The miter flap is designed to reconstruct defects at or near the nasal tip that are less than 2 cm (Fig. 14).

Advantages

The quality of skin is nearly identical to that being replaced and the flap is technically easy to use. The incisions for the flap can be created along the nasal subunit borders.

Disadvantages

The major disadvantage is that the entire skin of the nasal dorsum is put at risk because of the wide undermining required. The nasal tip is elevated due to the limited reach of the flap and in the postoperative period due to scar contracture.

Melolabial (Nasolabial)

Description

The melolabial (nasolabial) flap is a random-pattern local flap based either superiorly or inferiorly along the melolabial sulcus and cheek–nasal sidewall. The type of tissue movement is lifting either by transposition into the defect or by interpolation. If the intervening skin between the melolabial sulcus and the defect remains intact, then a staged interpolation flap may be necessary. The flap is harvested preserving the subdermal plexus distally and is based on a skin–subcutaneous pedicle; the flap may also be created as an island based only on a subcutaneous island in selected circumstances (i.e., a subcutaneous island melolabial flap).

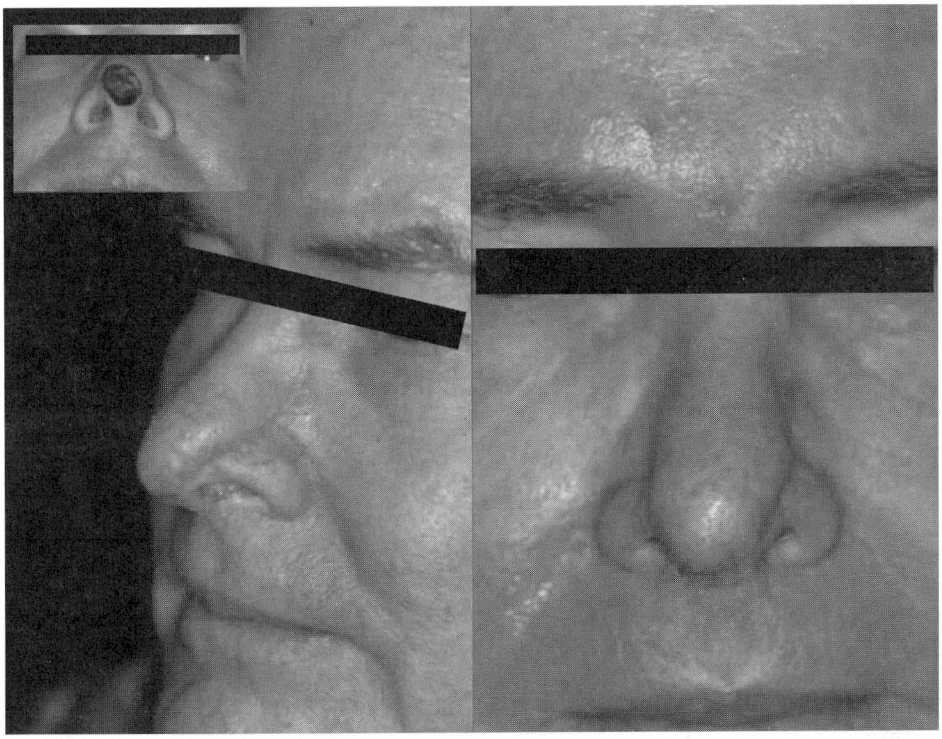

Figure 14 Results of a dorsal nasal flap transposition in a patient with a nasal tip skin defect.

The length-to-width ratio can be as high as 4:1, although flaps over 10 cm have been used augmented by surgical delay. The width of the flap is limited by the ability to close the donor site primarily (usually < 2.5 cm). Harvesting the melolabial flap begins with an incision along the melolabial sulcus from near the corner of the lip to no more than the distal border of the defect. The width of the flap is the same as the width of the defect, and this measurement determines the lateral incision on the cheek outlining the long axis of the flap. This lateral incision will be open-ended to leave a skin–subcutaneous pedicle positioned inferiorly for inferiorly based flaps and superiorly for superiorly based flaps.

Indications

Superiorly based melolabial flaps are indicated for central, lateral, alar, and nasal tip defects, and for defects of the lower eyelid. For more centrally located defects including the nasal tip, interpolation and staging are necessary (Fig. 15). Full-thickness alar defects are ideally reconstructed with a superiorly based flap as a one-stage procedure using the twisted melolabial flap (24) (Figs. 16, 17). Partial-thickness defects may best be reconstructed using an interpolated flap from the lateral cheek (25).

Inferiorly based melolabial flaps are indicated for upper and lower lip, floor of the nose, columellar, and intraoral defects. Columellar defects may require bilateral staged interpolation flaps. A partially de-epithelialized flap may be used for single-staged reconstruction of the alveolar ridge and anterior floor of mouth.

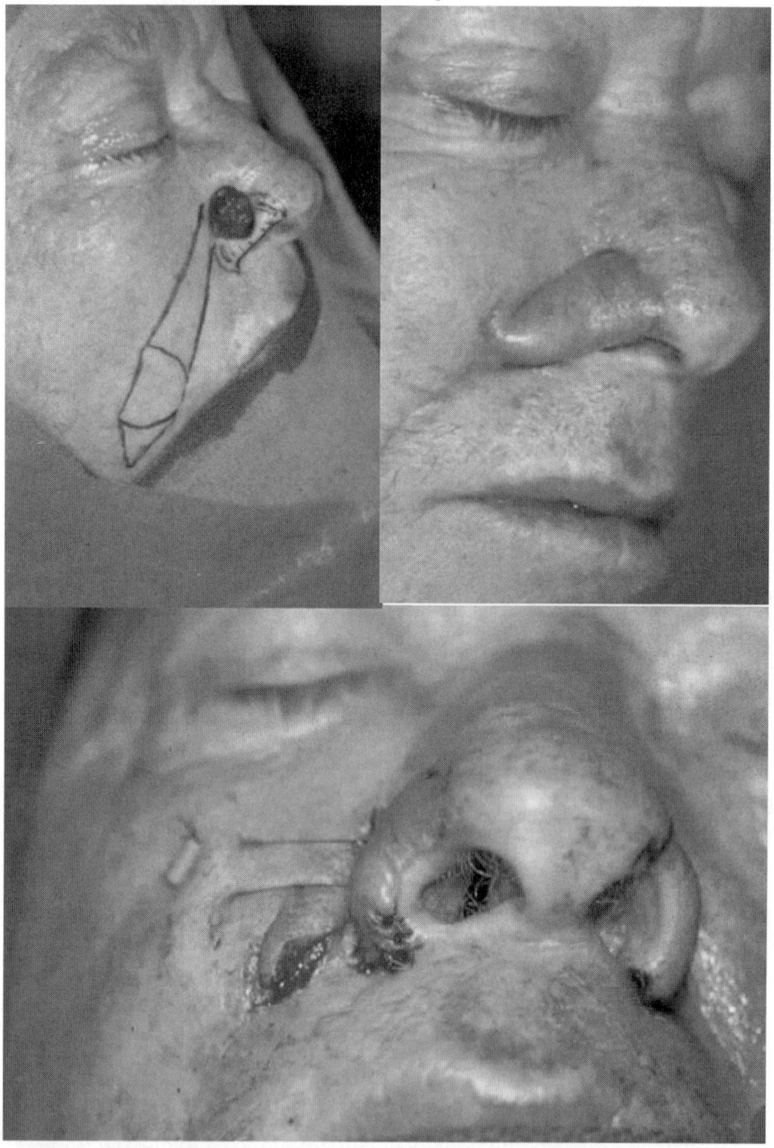

Figure 15 Interpolated nasolabial flap for a partial-thickness defect in the ipsilateral nasal ala. Note in upper right photograph the intermediate stage after initial flap transfer and before final flap division. Lower photograph shows flap inset with shape-retaining suture for the nasal alar flare.

Advantages

The incisions for flap harvest can be hidden in the melolabial fold. There is usually a lot of redundant tissue lateral to the melolabial fold that can be recruited to the flap, especially in older patients. The color match to the skin of the nose is usually very good, second only to the midforehead flap. The melolabial flap accepts cartilage grafts well.

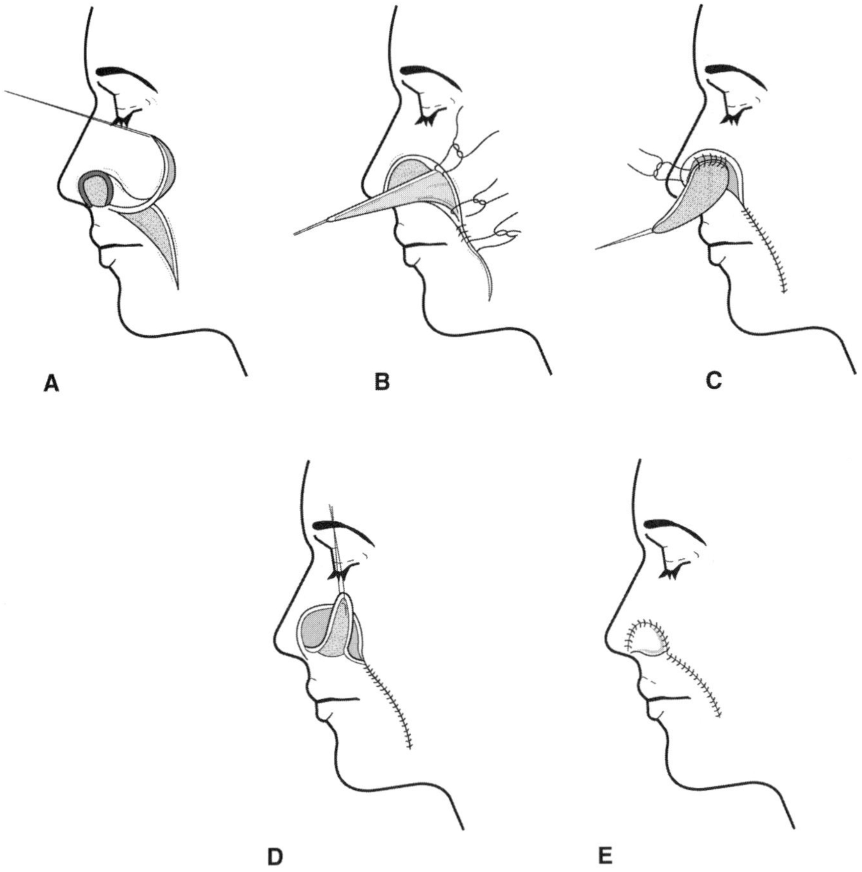

Figure 16 A stepwise depiction of harvesting and insetting a twisted nasolabial flap.

Disadvantages

Blunting and asymmetry of the melolabial fold may require surgical revision. Dissecting below the level of the mimetic musculature will place the medial branches of the facial nerve (especially the buccal branches) at risk. Superiorly based flaps are subject to trapdoor and pincushioning deformities because the scar is oriented in a curvilinear fashion near the nasal sidewall. Blunting of the nasofacial sulcus is common, requiring secondary defatting procedures. Inferiorly based melolabial flaps are also subject to trapdoor deformities of the upper lip.

Midforehead Flap

Description

Midforehead flaps are staged local axial musculocutaneous flaps with a variable distal random-pattern component. Types of midforehead flaps include the precise midline forehead flap, the paramedian forehead flap, and the oblique forehead flap (Fig. 18). The precise midline forehead flap is centered vertically in the forehead and its base is between the eyebrows, encompassing both supratrochlear and angular arteries. The paramedian forehead flap is just off the midline and its base is over

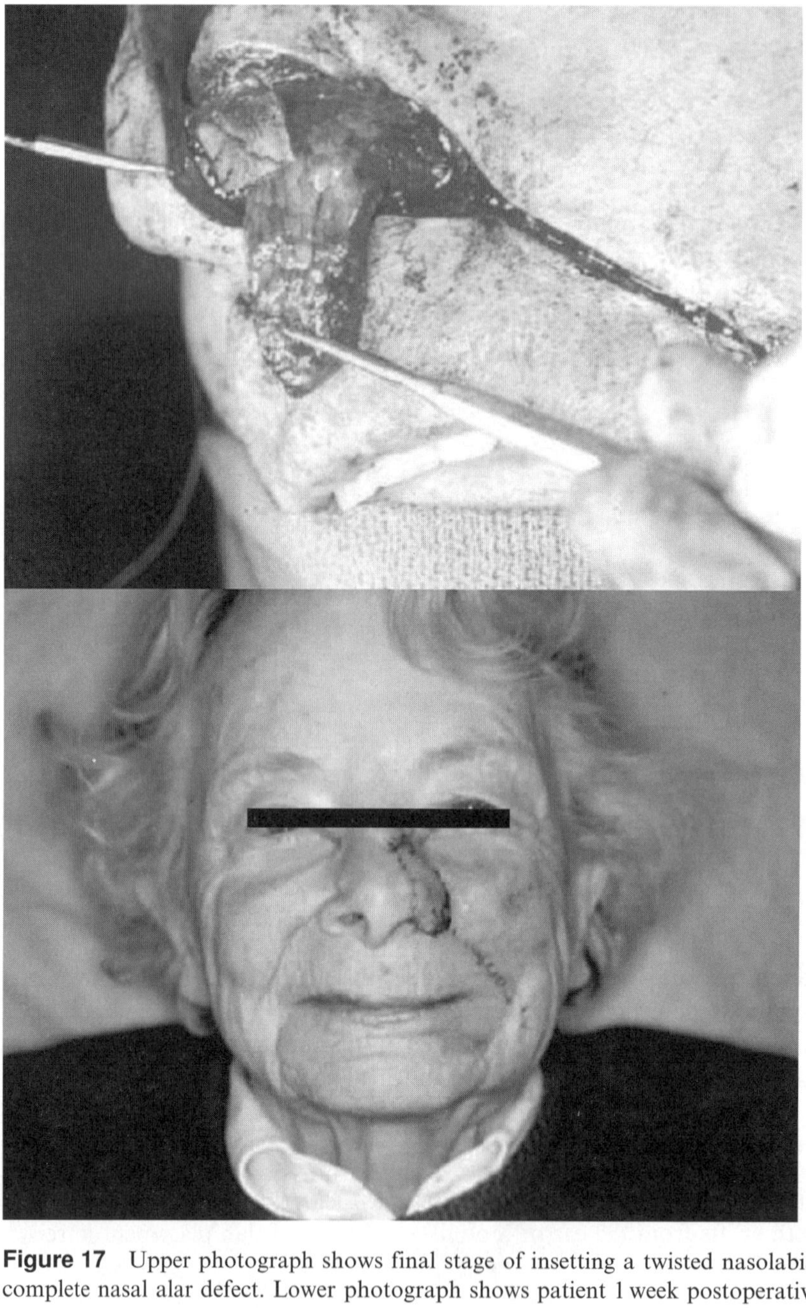

Figure 17 Upper photograph shows final stage of insetting a twisted nasolabial flap for a complete nasal alar defect. Lower photograph shows patient 1 week postoperatively.

the medial eyebrow, over the ipsilateral supratrochlear artery, and extending vertically to the hairline. The oblique flap is a paramedian flap that extends across the midline of the forehead and along the hairline for additional flap length. Modern refinements to the precise midline forehead flap include its being based on only one supratrochlear artery, allowing the pedicle more freedom to achieve greater flap length.

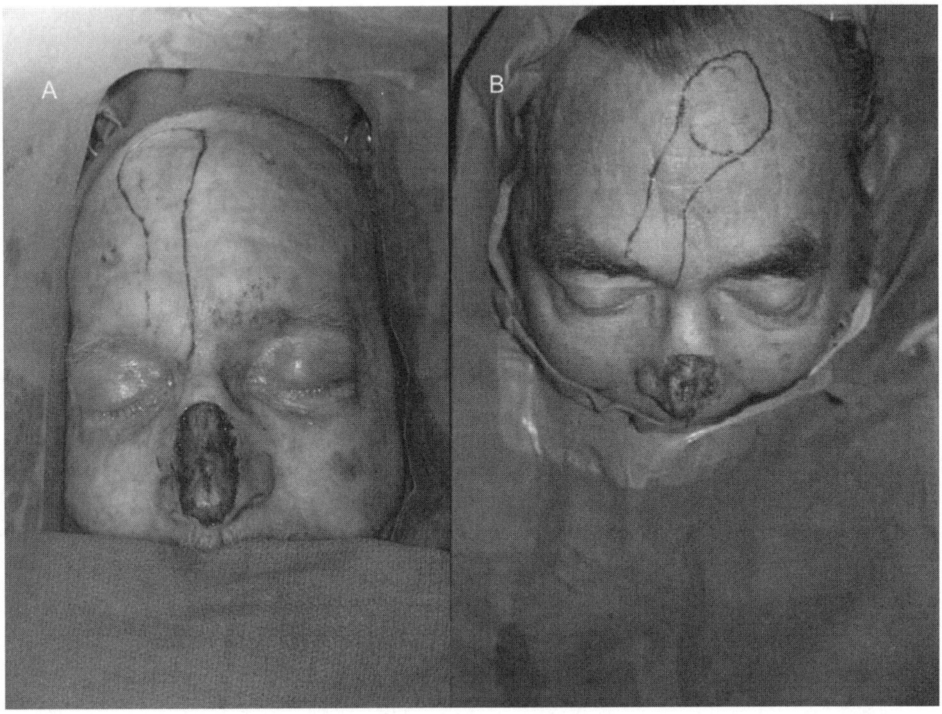

Figure 18 Penned outline of a paramedian (A) and oblique forhead flap (B).

The midforehead flap is transferred in stages. The first stage involves interpolation of the flap to the donor site leaving the pedicle exposed over the intervening tissues (Fig. 19). The second stage involves pedicle division with local anesthesia 2–3 weeks later. Pedicle division can be delayed to a third stage if intermediate aggressive thinning and sculpture are required at the second stage. After the pedicle is divided; the remainder of the unused flap should be trimmed and replaced into the forehead as an inverted V no higher than the level of the arch of the eyebrows; replacing the entire unused flap with extension above this level gives a less aesthetic result.

The design of the flap should be an exact match to the recipient site defect because forehead skin will not contract. The distal portion of the flap can be thinned to the subdermal plexus (2–3 mm thick), while the proximal part of the flap should include the periosteum (and frontalis muscle) to protect the axial vessels against injury while freeing the flap near its base. Missing cartilage framework should be replaced with grafts from the ear or septum at the time of flap placement in reconstruction of nasal defects. Local septal flaps, such as the septal hinge flap based on the anterior ethmoidal vessels, are useful to provide inner nasal lining (25). Inner nasal lining can also be furnished by enfolding the flap and this usually provides good alar and columellar contour if the flap can be sufficiently thinned distally. Middle vault through-and-through defects are best lined with adjacent skin turnover and septal flaps, appropriate cartilage grafts, and forehead skin for coverage (26).

The vertically oriented wound at the donor site is closed, primarily facilitated by extensive undermining in the subgaleal plane. Flaps required for the more extensive nasal defects may leave a donor site that will not close primarily near

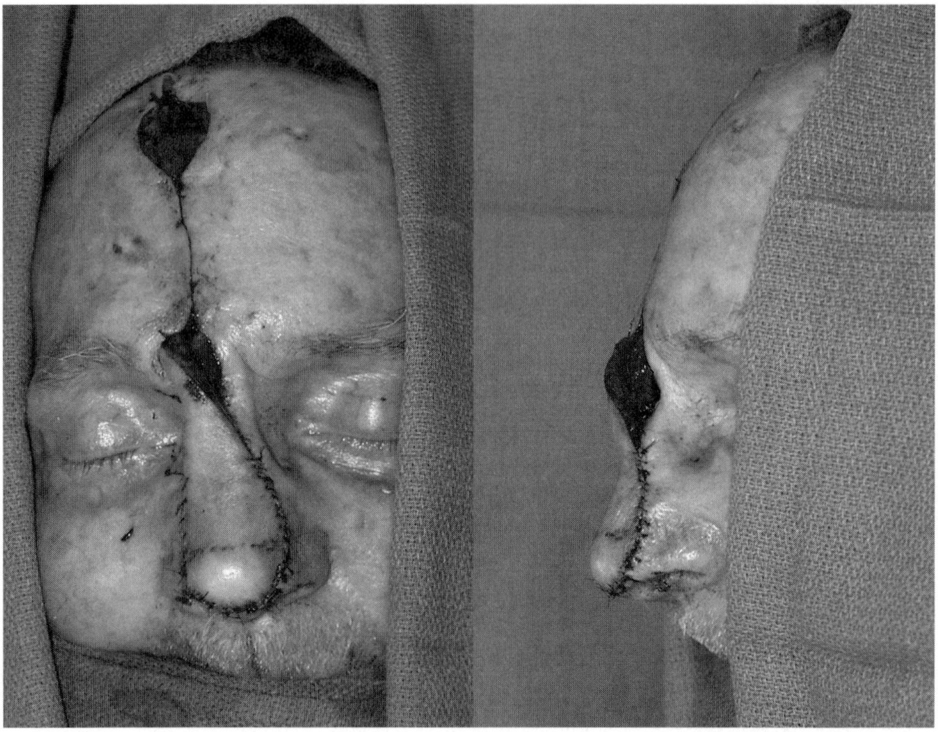

Figure 19 Harvested and transferred paramedian forehead flap in patient A shown in Fig. 18. This is the initial transfer. After 2–3 weeks the flap is divided at the glabella.

the hairline. These wounds can be left open to contract over several weeks, resulting in a very acceptable cosmetic result.

The main vascular supply to this axial flap is the supratrochlear artery; secondary arterial sources include the angular and supraorbital arteries (27).

Indications

Midforehead flaps are used for nasal reconstruction; expanded flaps may reach the lip or cheek but they are rarely used for reconstruction of these areas. The midforehead flap is best reserved for defects of the nose over 2.5 cm in length (28) (Fig. 20).

Advantages

Forehead skin is nearly identical in color and texture to nasal skin. The distal 2 cm of the flap can be aggressively thinned to match the thickness of the skin in the lower nose. Less aggressive thinning is required in smokers to avoid distal flap necrosis.

Disadvantages

The main disadvantage to the midforehead flap is the vertical scar on the forehead. Primary closure is not always possible, leaving an area, usually near the hairline, to heal by secondary intention. The length of the flap is limited somewhat by the hairline, although this can be circumvented to a limited extent by using the oblique midforehead flap, tissue expansion, or extension into the hair-bearing scalp. If the distal flap is overly thinned, distal necrosis is ensured, especially in smokers.

Island-Pedicled Musculocutaneous Nasolabial

Description

The island-pedicled musculocutaneous nasolabial flap incorporates the underlying mimetic musculature at the base (29) (Fig. 21). The flap can then be formed into

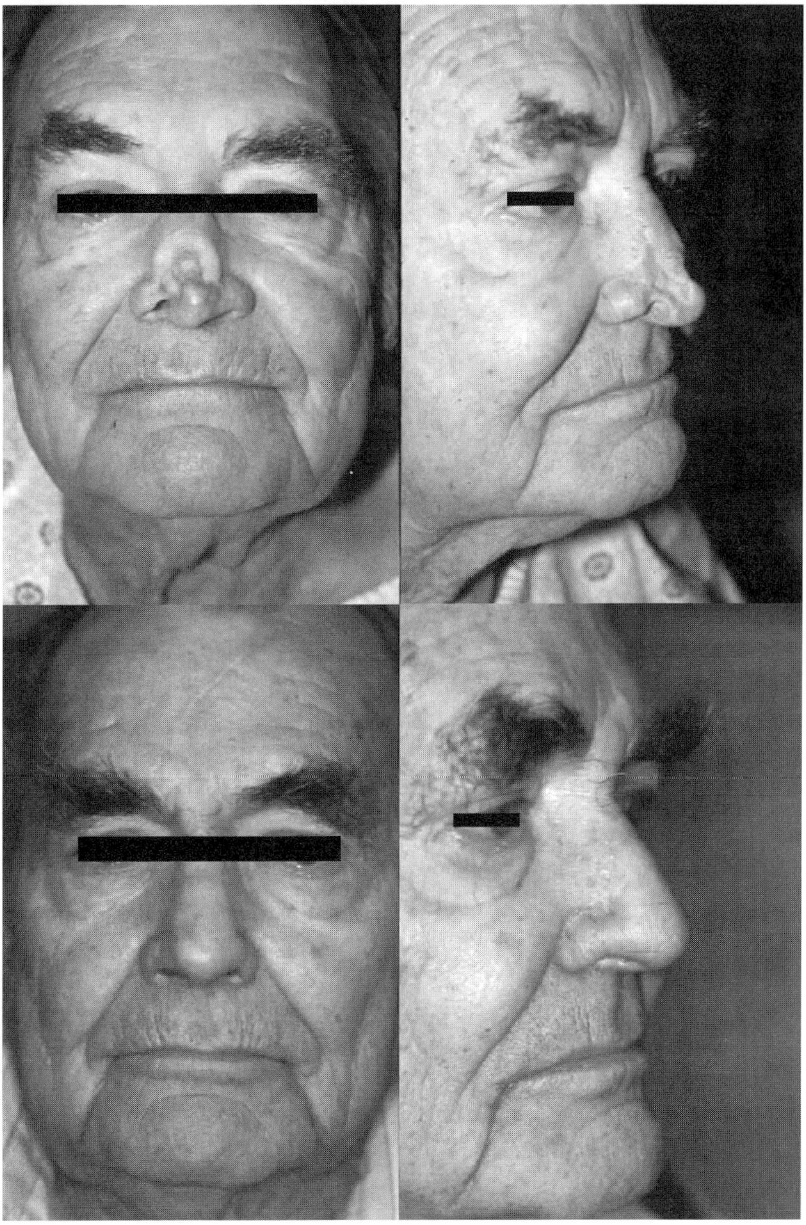

Figure 20 Patient in upper photographs with a deformity of his nasal tip created after cancer was excised and a skin graft applied 15 years earlier. An oblique forehead flap was used to resurface the defect after the skin graft was removed. The result is seen in the lower photographs.

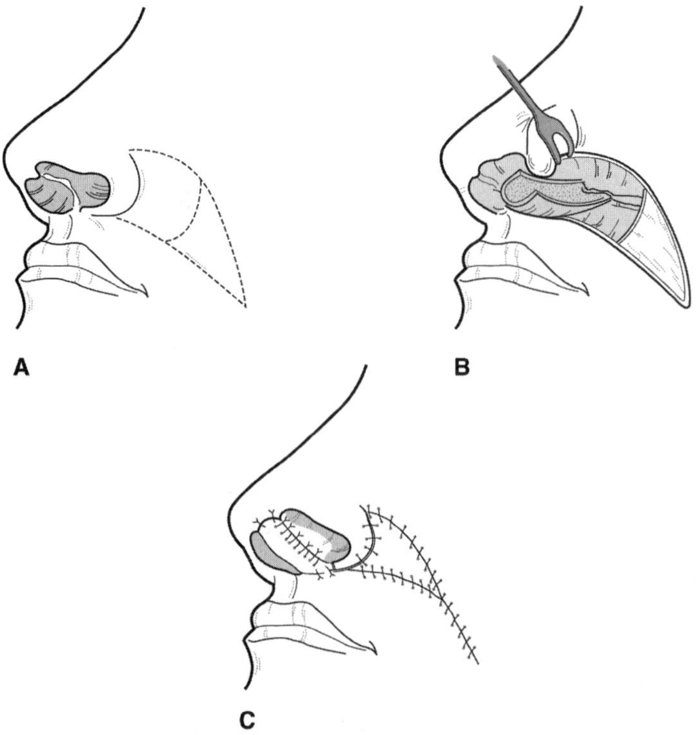

Figure 21 Island-pedicled nasolabial flap for repair of a total columellar defect.

an island based on muscular perforating vessels. This island of nasolabial tissue is much more mobile than traditional subcutaneous-based nasolabial flaps and can be transposed to donor sites up to 5 cm away, thus extending the indications of the nasolabial flap to include the total restoration of midline nasal and septal defects (30).

Perforating vessels (terminal arteries) penetrate the overlying levator labii superioris and nasalis muscles to supply the flap. The location of the donor vessels is adjacent to the piriform aperture, and consists of distal branches of the facial artery distal between the labial and alar arteries and more variable superficial facial veins. After penetrating the muscles, these vessels continue in the subdermal plexus. Mobilization of the flap is accomplished through dissection in the nasolabial fold and freeing of the facial artery and vein (Fig. 22).

Indications

The island-pedicled musculocutaneous nasolabial flap is descri bed for total columellar and caudal septal–columellar defects (Fig. 23).

Advantages

There is minimal donor site distortion and blunting of the alar–cheek junction because the flap is transferred as an island; staging and secondary revisions are minimized. Despite inclusion of muscle at the base of the flap, the vast majority of the tissue is elevated in a much more superficial plane based on the subdermal plexus, resulting in thin and pliable flap tissue. Cartilage grafting for nasal support is well tolerated.

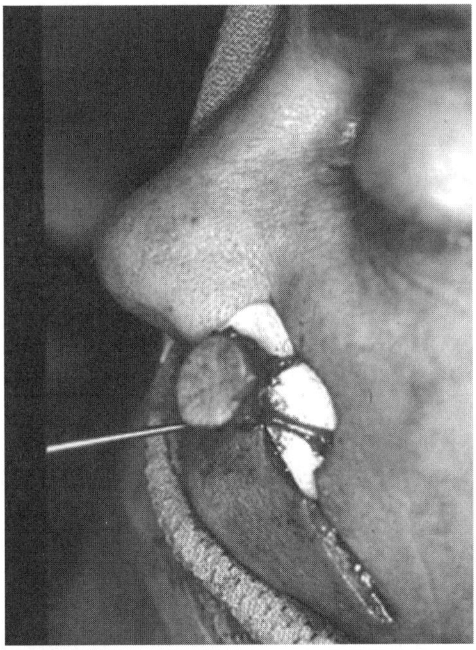

Figure 22 Nasolabial island flap nourished by angular artery and vein.

Disadvantages

Closure of the donor site as a V–Y advancement can result in a noticeable dual scar in the melolabial crease. Injury to the buccal branches of the facial nerve is a potential complication; however, this has not occurred in reported series (29).

Cheek Advancement

Description

This is a laterally based random-pattern sliding skin–subcutaneous flap; several variations are described (31). Wide subcutaneous undermining is necessary, creating a

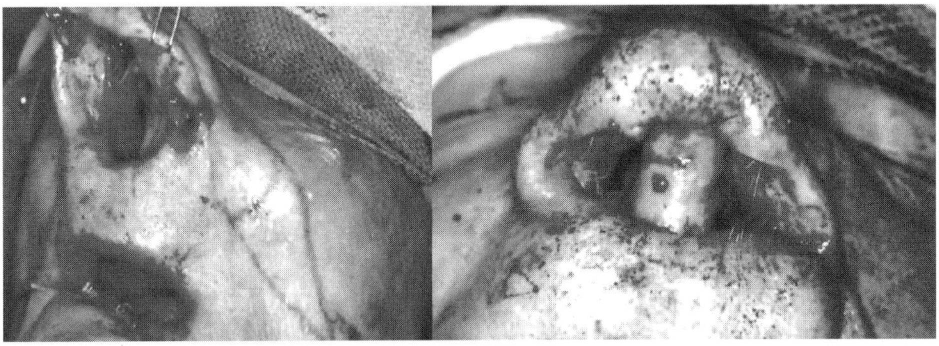

Figure 23 Nasolabial island flap for total columellar reconstruction: intraoperative sequence.

cervicofacial flap that can be advanced into the defect. Incisions should be placed along topographical borders such as the melolabial and preauricular sulci. The elevated cheek flap is heavy and dermal retaining sutures to immovable landmarks such as the malar periosteum can prevent surrounding structures from being distorted, such as the lower eyelid.

Indications

Cheek flaps are applied most often for reconstructing defects medially on the face, near the melolabial fold or nasal sidewall.

Advantages

Cheek advancements take advantage of the large surface area and loose cheek skin–subcutaneous unit. Large defects (2–3 cm) adjacent to the nose are amenable to repair using this flap. No incisions are necessary in the cheek itself, which is very beneficial since these incisions are often obvious.

Disadvantages

Tension medially can blunt the natural nasal–cheek crease. This can be minimized with dermal–periosteal sutures to the nasal sidewall. Inferolaterally based flaps for defects near the lower lid may result in ectropion. This problem may be avoided by using oversized lower eyelid cartilage grafts and subdermal-to-periosteal fixation sutures to lateral canthal area.

INTRAORAL AND MISCELLANEOUS FLAPS

Buccinator Musculomucosal

Description

The buccinator musculomucosal flap (BMF) was originally described for reconstruction of defects of the hard palate. Experience with intraoral tumor extirpations expanded its use for surgical defects of the posterior oral cavity that were too small to justify a regional flap (32). The flap is based on the buccal neurovascular pedicle and includes cheek mucosa and the buccinator muscle (Fig. 24). Cadaveric studies demonstrate the consistent isolation of the buccal artery, and India ink injections demonstrate the generous blood supply from this artery to the overlying cheek mucosa. The buccal nerve is adjacent to the buccal artery and is easily included with the flap to maintain sensation in the overlying mucosa.

The tumor is extirpated by an intraoral approach and the defect sized. Stensen's duct is identified and the superior margin of the flap is outlined, keeping at least 5 mm inferior to the duct papilla. The anterior limit of the flap is one cm behind the oral commissure. The maximal graft size possible is 4 cm in a superior–inferior direction and 7 cm in an anterior–posterior direction. The buccal mucosa and the buccinator muscle are incised to the level of the buccopharyngeal fascia working in an anterior to posterior direction (Fig. 25). A loose areolar plane exists between the buccinator muscle and the buccopharyngeal fascia, facilitating elevation of the flap with blunt dissection. The buccopharyngeal fascia should be preserved for two reasons: to prevent buccal fat pad herniation into the field of dissection and to avoid injury to branches of the facial nerve. Small branches from the facial artery may require ligation as may venous tributaries from the pterygoid

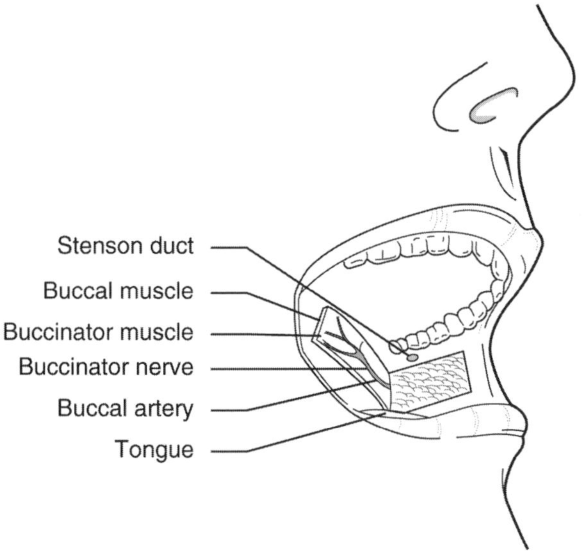

Figure 24 Right buccinator flap reflected to show underlying anatomy.

plexus. The neurovascular pedicle may be isolated to create an island flap to facilitate rotation, but this is not usually necessary. The flap is then transferred into the defect and secured with long-lasting absorbable sutures and the donor site is closed primarily.

Indications

In the past, these flaps were used primarily for reconstruction of cleft palate defects. This versatile local flap should be considered for reconstruction of defects of the floor of mouth, retromolar trigone, and soft palate.

Neurovascular Anatomy

The buccal artery and nerve arise laterally at the posteroinferior aspect of the buccinator muscle. The neurovascular bundle arises between the ramus of the mandible and medial pterygoid muscle.

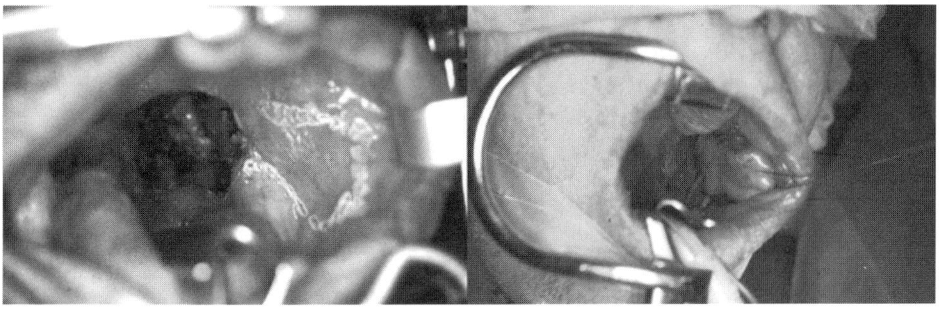

Figure 25 Surgical outline of a left buccinator flap: the flap raised and held out with a suture along its anteriormost margin.

Advantages

The BMF is a reliable, easily harvested local flap, useful for reconstruction of lesions involving the floor of mouth, retromolar trigone, and soft palate. It obviates the need for an intraoral bolster or harvesting of tissue beyond the oral cavity. The BMF is raised within 30 min without the use of magnification, thus minimizing total intraoperative time. There are no adverse affects secondary to harvesting the muscle, particularly with respect to mastication, oral continence, or facial nerve function. When tested over the area of reconstruction in the early postoperative period, patients report fine touch perception, which may be an aid to oral rehabilitation.

The BMF has several advantages over typical alternative reconstructive methods including skin grafts, tongue flaps, and nasolabial flaps. Skin grafts "take" poorly over exposed bone and require placement of a bolster that may be technically difficult in this area. Tongue flaps usually require two stages and speech and swallowing may be adversely affected. The nasolabial flap requires an external excision and may not reach the retromolar trigone. Regional flaps (such as the temporalis muscle flap) or free flaps (such as the radial forearm) involve extensive extraoral dissection and are better reserved for more extensive defects.

Disadvantages

Although this flap can be used in previously irradiated fields, the risk of partial loss may be higher. In addition, external carotid artery resection or thrombosis may also preclude use of this flap.

Palatal (Arena)

Description

The palatal flap (i.e., Arena flap) was originally described in 1977 (33). It is a mucoperiosteal flap that can encompass up to 85% of the palatal mucosal based on a sin-

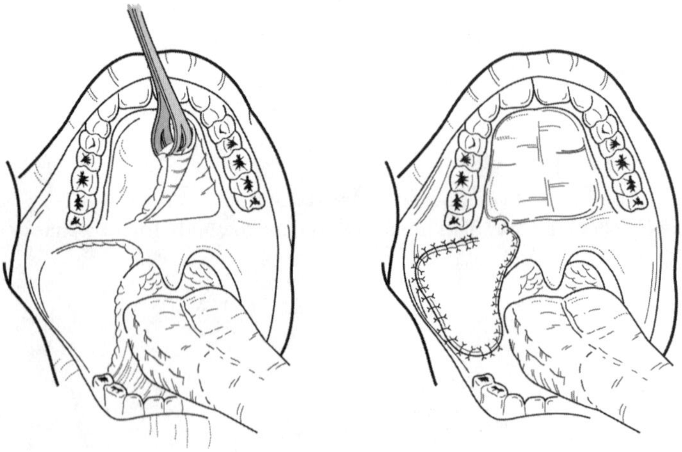

Figure 26 A palatal flap raised based on a single greater palatine artery. The harvest site may be skin-grafted.

gle greater palatine artery (Fig. 26). The flap tissue can be rotated 180 degrees to cover defects in the posterior oral cavity.

Dissection involves incising through the mucoperiosteum along the perimeter of the hard palate and ligating the opposite greater palatine neurovascular bundle. The flap is raised with a periosteal elevating instrument and traverses the multiple fibrous tissue pegs (Sharpey's fibers). When the ipsilateral greater palatine foramen is reached, an additional 1 cm of length on the pedicle can be obtained by fracturing the hook of the hamulus.

Indications

The palatal flap is indicated to resurface defects up to 8 cm^2 involving the lateral soft palate and retromolar trigone. It is useful when a defect is too small for a regional flap but is suitable for a local flap. The flap has been used in the past for closure of oroantral fistulas and in palate-lengthening procedures.

Neurovascular Anatomy

The vascular supply to the flap is the greater palatine artery and vein that emerge from the greater palatine foramen and course anterolaterally to the incisive foramen. There is excellent collateral flow across the midline of the palate, allowing the mucoperiosteum of the entire hard palate to be harvested based upon a single palatine artery.

Advantages

The advantages of the palatal flap include ease of harvest, excellent reliability, local source of tissue, avoidance of a skin graft and intraoral bolster, and minimal contracture over the reconstructed site.

Disadvantages

The major disadvantage in using the palatal flap is the prolonged re-epithelialization of the raw surface of the palate (2–3 months). This flap should not be used in children because of the possibility of altered midface growth.

REFERENCES

1. Wallace AF. From Moses to Mahon (Gillies Memorial lecture 1989). Br J Plast Surg 1990; 43:713–723.
2. Davis JS. The story of plastic surgery. Ann Surg 1941; 113:656.
3. McDowell F. The "B.L." bomb-shell (B. Lucas). Plast Reconstr Surg 1969; 44:67–73.
4. Nichter LS, Morgan RF, Nichter MA. The impact of Indian methods for total nasal reconstruction. Clin Plast Surg 1983; 10:635–647.
5. Manchot C. Die Hautarterien des Menschlichen Koerpers. Leipzig: F.C.W. Bogel, 1889.
6. Ciresi KF, Mathes SJ. The classification of flaps. [Review]. Orthop Clin North Am 1993; 24:383–391.
7. McGregor IA, Morgan G. Axial and random pattern flaps. Br J Plast Surg 1973; 26:202–213.
8. Swanson NA. Classifications, definitions, and concepts in flap surgery. In: Baker SR Swanson NA, eds. Local flaps in facial reconstruction, Mosby, 1995:63–74.
9. Calhoun KH, Seikaly H, Quinn FB. Teaching paradigm for decision making in facial skin defect reconstructions. Arch Otolaryngol Head Neck Surg 1998; 124:60–66.

10. Esser FJS. Island flaps. NY State J Med 1917; 106:264.
11. Zook EG. V–Y advancement flap for facial defects. Plas Reconstr Surg 1980; 65:786.
12. Cook TA, Brownlee RA. Rotation flaps. In: Baker SRSwanson NA, eds. Local Flaps in Facial Reconstruction, St. Louis, CV: Mosby, 1995:75–90.
13. Elliott RA, Jr. Rotation flaps of the nose. Plast Reconstr Surg 1969; 44:147–149.
14. Zitelli JA, Baker SR. Bilobe flaps. In: Baker SR, Swanson NA, eds. Local Flaps in Facial Reconstruction, St. Louis, CV: Mosby, 1995:165–180.
15. McGregor JC, Soutar DS. A critical assessment of the bilobed flap. Br J Plast Surg 1981; 34:197–205.
16. Limberg AA. Modern trends in plastic surgery. Design of local flaps. Modern Trends Plast Surg 1966; 2:38–61.
17. Bray DA. Rhombic flaps. In: Baker SR, Swanson NA, eds. Local Flaps in Facial Reconstruction. St. Louis, CV: Mosby, 1995:151–164.
18. Fee WEJ, Gunter JP, Carder HM. Rhomboid flap principles and common variations. Laryngoscope 1976; 86:1706–1711.
19. Koss N, Bullock JD. A mathematical analysis of the rhomboid flap. Surg Gynecol Obstet 1975; 141:439–442.
20. Roggendorf E. Rhombic and rhomboid Schwenklappen-plasty. In: Strauch B, Vasconez LO, eds. 2 ed. Grabb's Encyclopedia of Flaps, Philadelphia: Lippincott-Raven, 1998:359–364.
21. Rieger RA. A local flap for repair of the nasal tip. Plast Reconstr Surg 1967; 40:147–149.
22. Rieger RA. Lateral nasal (miter) skin flap. In: Strauch B, Vasconez LO, eds. 2 ed. Grabb's Encyclopedia of Flaps, Philadelphia: Lippincott-Raven, 1998:183–185.
23. Marchac D, Toth B. The axial frontonasal flap revisited. Plast Reconstr Surg 1985; 76:686–694.
24. Spear SL, Kroll SS, Romm S. A new twist to the nasolabial flap for reconstruction of lateral alar defects. Plast Reconstr Surg 1987; 79:915–920.
25. Menick FJ. Reconstruction of the nose. In: Baker SR, Swanson NA, eds. Local Flaps in Facial Reconstruction, St. Louis, CV: Mosby, 1995:323–328.
26. Quatela VC, Sherris DA, Rounds MF. Esthetic refinements in forehead flap nasal reconstruction. Arch Otolaryngol Head Neck Surg 1995; 121:1106–1113.
27. Mangold U, Lierse W, Pfeifer G. [The arteries of the forehead as the basis of nasal reconstruction with forehead flaps]. [German]. Acta Anat 1980; 107:18–25.
28. Alford EL, Baker SR, Shumrick KA. Midforehead flaps. In: Baker SR, Swanson NA, eds. Local Flaps in Facial Reconstruction, St. Louis, CV: Mosby, 1995:197–223.
29. Dolan R, Arena S. Clinical applications of the island-pedicled nasolabial musculocutaneous flap. Am J Rhinol 1995; 9:219–224.
30. Dolan R, Arena S. Reconstruction of the total columellar defect. Laryngoscope 1995; 105:1141–1143.
31. Juri J, Juri C. Cheek reconstruction with advancement-rotation flaps. Clin Plast Surg 1981; 8:223–226.
32. Licameli GR, Dolan R. Buccinator musculomucosal flap: applications in intraoral reconstruction. Arch Otolaryngol Head Neck Surg 1998; 124:69–72.
33. Gullane PJ, Arena S. Palatal island flap for reconstruction of oral defects. Arch Otolaryngol 1977; 103:598–599.

7

Specialized Local Facial Flaps for the Eyelids and Lips

Robert W. Dolan and Susan M. Tucker
Lahey Clinic Medical Center, Burlington, Massachusetts, U.S.A.

EYELID RECONSTRUCTION

The goals of eyelid reconstruction are to:

- Restore nonkeritanized internal lining
- Provide form and rigidity to the eyelid margin
- Re-establish fixation at the medial and lateral canthi
- Provide corneal protection
- Restore the thin and supple skin over the eyelids for proper function and cosmesis
- Provide appropriate elevation of the upper eyelid by the action of the levator muscle

Eyelid Anatomy

Knowledge of eyelid anatomy is essential to planning periocular reconstruction. Both anterior and posterior lamellae of the eyelid must be replaced to maximize structural integrity and function. The anterior lamella consists of the skin and orbicularis oculi muscle with its associated vascular elements. The posterior lamella consists of the levator muscle and aponeurosis (upper eyelid), Müller's muscle, tarsus, and conjunctiva. The gray line, visible along the middle of each eyelid margin, denotes the junction of the anterior and posterior lamella of the eyelid (Fig. 1). The openings of the meibomian glands mark the mucocutaneous junction and lie just posterior to the gray line.

The tissue layers in the upper eyelid over the tarsus are skin, pretarsal orbicularis muscle, levator aponeurosis, tarsus, and conjunctiva. Above the tarsus the tissue layers are skin, preseptal orbicularis muscle, orbital septum, orbital fat, levator muscle and aponeurosis, Müller's muscle, and conjunctiva. In the lower eyelid the capsulopalpebral fascia is equivalent to the levator of the upper eyelid and the inferior tarsal (Horner's) muscle is the counterpart of Müller's muscle in the upper eyelid.

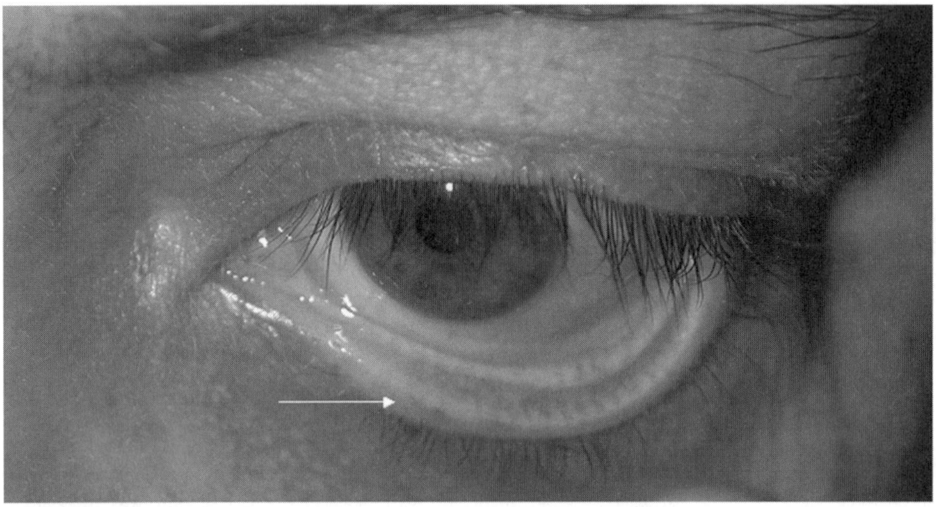

Figure 1 The gray line (arrow). Note meibomian glands posterior to it.

The orbicularis oculi muscle encircles the palpebral aperture and is organized into concentric zones: orbital and palpebral. The palpebral zone is divided into pretarsal and preseptal components. These components possess deep and superficial heads as they pass medially, forming the medial canthal tendon. The superficial head of the medial canthal tendon merges with the superior and inferior tarsal plates and inserts medially onto the frontal process of the maxilla, just anterior to the anterior lacrimal crest. The deep head of the medial canthal tendon inserts posterior to the lacrimal sac on the lacrimal bone (the posterior lacrimal crest). The lateral canthal tendon arises from the periosteum over the lateral orbital rim and also from Whitnall's tubercle located 5 mm behind the lateral rim; medially it splits to merge with the upper and lower eyelid tarsal plates.

The orbital septum is an effective barrier to the spread of infection from the more superficial parts of the eye (preseptal) to the deeper parts of the eye (postseptal). The orbital septum originates at the bony orbital rim as a thickening called the arcus marginalis. The facial periosteum also attaches at this point forming a trifurcation of fascias consisting of the facial fascia, periorbital fascia, and the orbital septum. The septum attaches onto the levator complex 2–4 mm above the tarsal border in whites. In Asians, the septum inserts more inferiorly onto the tarsal border. Beneath the septum lies the orbital fat pads; hence the fullness of the Asian eyelid is a result of the more inferior extension of the septum and underlying fat (see the chapter on Blepharoplasty). In surgery, identification of the orbital fat is an important landmark because just below it lies the levator complex in the upper eyelid and the capsulopalpebral fascia in the lower eyelid.

The levator muscle arises from the roof of the orbit above the superior rectus muscle. It continues forward for about 40 mm where it ends just behind the septum as an aponeurosis. Close to the origin of the aponeurosis the muscle sheath is thickened to form a sleeve referred to as Whitnall's ligament (1) (Fig. 2). This fascial sleeve attaches to the trochlear fascia medially and the fascia of the orbital lobe of

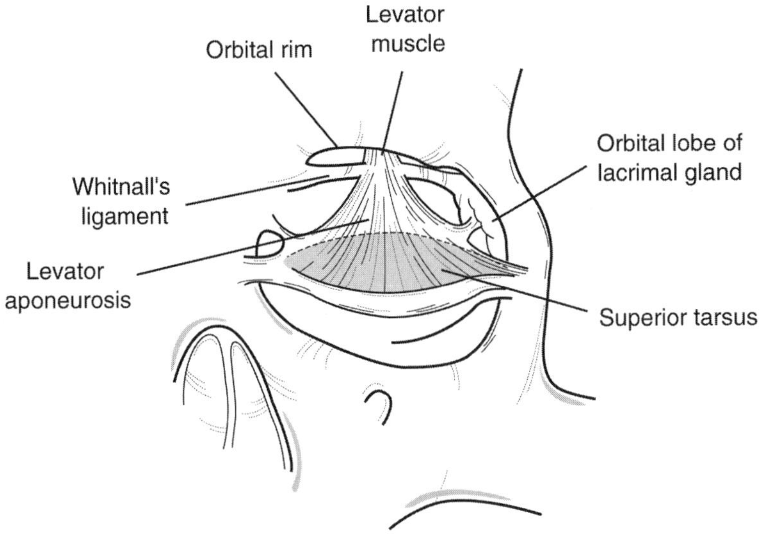

Figure 2 Whitnall's ligament.

the lacrimal gland laterally and acts as a fulcrum for the action of the levator. The aponeurosis inserts onto the lower anterior two-thirds of the tarsal plate and sends fibers to the orbicularis and skin. Müller's muscle is a nonstriated, sympathetically innervated elevator of the upper eyelid that arises from the undersurface of the levator muscle close to the junction of striated muscle and aponeurosis. It descends between the levator aponeurosis and the conjunctiva for 5–20 mm to insert into the superior edge of tarsus. In the lower eyelid, the capsulopalpebral fascia (the levator equivalent) is a fibrous tissue retinaculum, attached to and powered by the inferior rectus muscle that depresses the eyelid in downgaze (2). The inferior tarsal muscle (Muller's muscle equivalent) also arises from the sheath of the inferior rectus muscle and lies between the capsulopalpebral fascia and conjunctiva.

The tarsal plates are fibroelastic structures extending across the margin of each eyelid. The upper tarsus is 10–12 mm in height centrally, tapering to 6 mm laterally and medially extending from the superior punctum to approximately 3 mm from the lateral canthal angle. The lower tarsus is 3–5 mm in height.

Branches of the ophthalmic artery (from the internal carotid artery) give rise to the palpebral vessels: laterally from the lacrimal artery and medially from the terminal branches of the ophthalmic artery (Fig. 3). The peripheral arcade of the upper eyelid courses beneath the levator aponeurosis at the superior border of the tarsus, and the marginal arcade courses 2–4 mm above the lid margin deep to the pretarsal orbicularis oculi muscle. The inferior marginal arcade supplies the lower eyelid and courses 2–3 mm below the lid margin deep to the pretarsal orbicularis oculi muscle. Important contributions from the external carotid system occur via branches of the infraorbital, anterior deep temporal, and superficial temporal arteries (3).

The normal position of the upper eyelid margin in primary gaze is 1–2 mm below the superior limbus. The highest point is just nasal to the center of the pupil in whites, and at the midpoint of the eyelid in Asians. The lower eyelid should

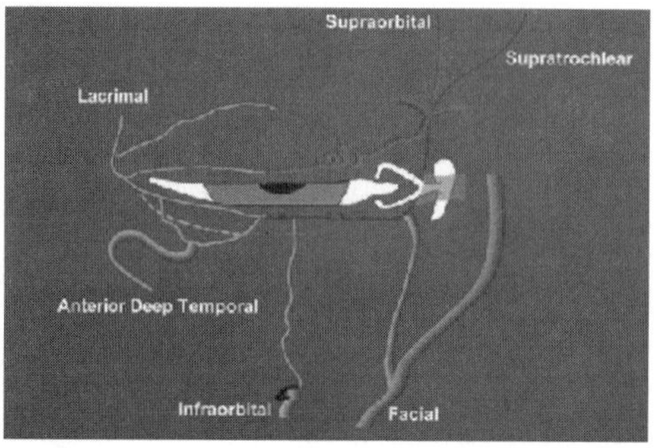

Figure 3 Vascular anatomy of the eyelids. (Courtesy Dr. Susan Tucker, Lahey Clinic Burlington, MA.)

slightly overlap the inferior limbus and the lowest point is just temporal to the pupil. The upper eyelid crease in whites 8–12 mm above the eyelid margin formed by the insertion of fibers from the levator aponeurosis into the orbicularis muscle and skin. The perceived fullness of the Asian eyelid is a result of the more inferior insertion of the orbital septum (onto the tarsus compared with 2–3 mm superior to it), and the low skin crease is due to the low and less prominent subcutaneous insertions of the levator aponeurosis.

Partial-Thickness Lid Defects

Both the anterior and posterior lamellae must be adequately restored, and at least one must be vascularized to support nonvascularized grafts, if needed. Anterior lamellar defects may be reconstructed with a basic local flap or a full-thickness skin graft; split-thickness skin grafts should be avoided due to excess contraction that could lead to ectropion or lagophthalmos. The order of preferred donor sites for full-thickness skin grafts is upper eyelid, retroauricular, and supraclavicular. It is acceptable to orient scars vertically (against the resting skin tension lines [RSTLs]) to avoid displacement of the lid margin in the process of skin recruitment in closing an elliptical defect. Eyelid skin generally heals with minimal cicatrization and post-operative pulling on the eyelid margin in the direction of the scar is minimal. Posterior lamellar defects may be repaired with free autogenous composite grafts (e.g., tarsoconjunctival, septal cartilage–mucosa, hard palate mucosa), advancement or rotational conjunctival flaps, and periosteal strips.

Full-Thickness Lid Defects

The method of closure for full-thickness eyelid defects depends upon the location and shape of the wound. The vast majority of defects from cancer resection will be located on the lower eyelid, most often in the shape of a wedge. Wedged-shaped defects involving up to 50% of the lid margin may be closed primarily in older patients. However, a lateral cantholysis is necessary if the edges of the defect cannot be brought together easily. The edges of the defect must be perpendicular to the lid margin along the full height of the tarsus to avoid notching. Marginal horizontally shaped defects of this extent may be converted into a wedged-shaped defect to facilitate primary closure. Advancing the lateral cheek facilitated by wide undermining and release of the lateral eyelid remnant by cantholysis may close wedged-shaped defects of the lower eyelid involving move than 50% of the lid margin. Flaps for this purpose include the Tenzel and the Mustardé cheek rotation flaps. For marginal horizontally shaped defects of this size, upper eyelid tissue can be used in the form of a full-thickness unipedicle flap, a bipedicled flap, or a Hughes tarsoconjunctival flap. Flaps for extensive defects of the upper eyelid include the Abbé-type full-thickness flap from the lower eyelid (switch flap) and the Cutler-Beard flap.

Periosteal Strips

Description

Strips of deep temporalis fascia and periosteum pedicled near the orbital rim are useful for replacement of the lateral tarsus and conjunctiva (4,5). The strip is oriented at a 45 degree angle from the lateral orbital rim either in a superior direction for lower lid defects or in an inferior direction for upper lid defects. The inner surface of the periosteal strip will re-epithelialize from the bordering conjunctiva. The anterior lamella is reconstructed with musculocutaneous flaps for full-thickness defects.

Indications

Periosteal strips may be used for lateral posterior lamella defects involving up to 60% of the upper or lower lid margin. They may also be used under a semicircular flap (Tenzel) for improved lateral fixation of the eyelid.

Advantages

This is a one-staged reconstruction that uses nonvital, easily harvested tissues. The location of the pedicle provides good lateral support for the reconstructed eyelid. The upper and lower eyelids may be reconstructed simultaneously with properly designed flaps.

Disadvantages

The periosteum is less rigid than the tarsus making eyelid margin malposition and entropion more likely. This is a nonepithelial surface and a foreign body sensation is present until re-epitheliazation occurs (by 1 month postoperatively). Periosteal flaps have insufficient vascularity to nourish full-thickness skin grafts and should be covered with skin flaps.

Semicircular (Tenzel) Flap

Description

A Tenzel flap is a musculocutaneous rotation flap extending from the lateral canthus (Fig. 4). The flap can be marked approximately 22 mm vertically (upwards to reconstruct the lower eyelid and downwards to reconstruct the upper eyelid), and 18 mm in horizontal direction. This should not extend further lateral than the end of the eyebrow. Cantholysis frees the flap to rotate medially, allowing the free eyelid margin to be closed. The new lateral canthus is fixed to the lateral orbital rim with dermal–periosteal sutures.

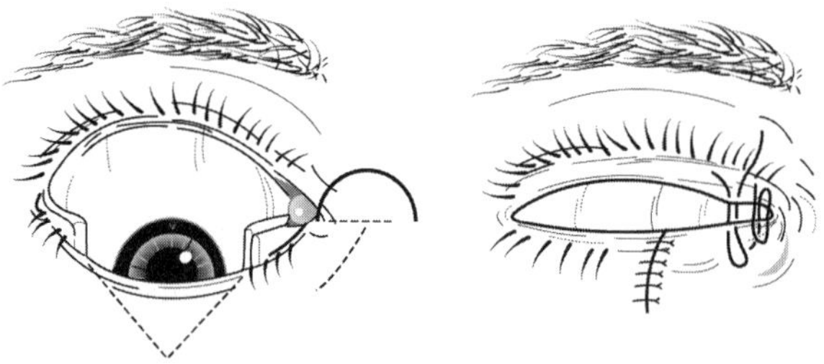

Figure 4 A Tenzel flap used to reconstruct an extensive defect of the medial lower eyelid margin.

Indications

A Tenzel flap is indicated for central or medial defects of the eyelid affecting up to 60% of the eyelid margin. For excessively large defects, the posterior lamella should also be reconstructed to stabilize the eyelid margin (using tarsus, hard palate, nasal septum, ear cartilage, or periosteum).

Advantages

The primary advantage of the Tenzel flap is that it advances normal eyelid tissue to the center of the lid, leaving flap tissue in a less conspicuous area near the lateral canthus.

Disadvantages

If this flap is used to repair excessively large defects, a greater amount of unsupported tissue results in the lateral lid, potentially resulting in eyelid malposition including entropion or ectropion. Eyelid malposition including entropion or ectropion may occur when the posterior lamella is not reconstructed.

Hard Palate Graft

Description

The hard palate is composed of variably keratinized stratified squamous epithelium, a lamina propria made up of densely packed collagen fibers, a submosal layer with adipose and glands, periosteum, and the maxillary and palatine bones. The covering layers are used to replace posterior lamella (Fig. 5). This can be done under local or intravenous sedation. A bite block is used to keep the mouth wide open. The soft palate, midline of the hard palate, and arteries should be avoided (the greater and lesser palatine adjacent to the third molar, and the nasopalatine artery just posterior to the central incisors). The graft is oversized by 30% and prepared by removing fat and thinning the thick submucosa. A clear plastic palate stent custom-fit preoperatively at the dental office or dentures can be used for pain relief. Viscous lidocaine can also help, and soft foods should be eaten for 3 weeks.

Indications

Hard palate grafts are indicated for defects between 60 and 100% of the length of the eyelid of any depth.

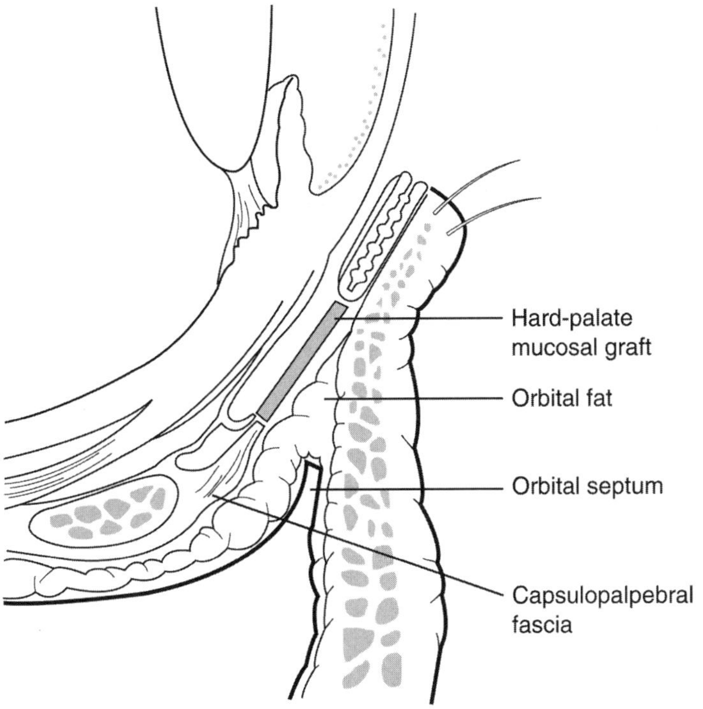

Figure 5 A hard palate graft used to resurface the posterior lamella.

Advantages

The mucosal surface minimizes ocular irritation postoperatively. Hard palate is often rigid enough to support the reconstructed eyelid without the use of cartilage or other rigid grafts (e.g., conchal cartilage). Additional rigidity may be afforded by the use of a composite nasal septal graft consisting of mucoperiosteum and underlying cartilage.

Disadvantages

Because the hard palate is variably keratinized, it may take up to 6 months for metaplasia to nonkeratinized mucosal epithelium causing prolonged ocular irritation, foreign body sensation, and excess lacrimation. In rare cases, keratinization may persist. Postoperative shrinkage between 10 to 60% (mean of 25%) total surface area has been reported, usually by 1 month (6).

Tarsoconjunctival (Hughes) Flap (for Lower Eyelid Repair)

Description

The Hughes tarsoconjunctival flap is a staged lid-sharing procedure that transfers a posterior lamellar flap from the upper eyelid to a lower eyelid defect (Fig. 6). The technique involves everting the upper eyelid and incising through tarsus at least 4 mm above the eyelid margin, equal in width to the lower eyelid defect. Vertical superior cuts are created to allow the flap to reach the inferior edge of the defect in the lower eyelid. The flap is composed of a portion of the height of the superior

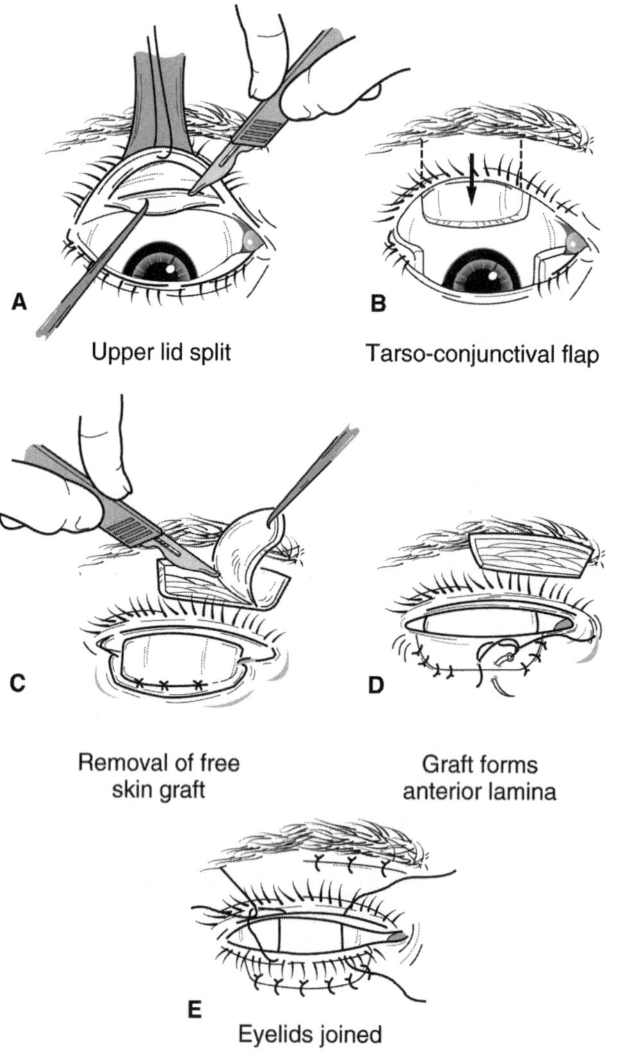

Figure 6 Step by step depiction of a Hughes flap for repair of a lower eyelid margin defect.

tarsus and conjunctiva (a tarsoconjunctival flap). To enhance the blood supply to the flap, Muller's muscle or both Muller's muscle and the levator muscle may be included (7). The flap is composed of conjunctiva, tarsus, Muller's muscle, levator aponeurosis, and orbital septum. The flap is left in place 6–8 weeks for delay and for upward traction to minimize postoperative cicatricial ectropion. The second stage consists of flap division allowing excess conjunctival tissue to drape over the lower lid margin. The anterior lamella must be reconstructed independently using a skin graft or local flap.

Indications

The indication for this flap is for marginal lower eyelid defects involving greater than 60% of the lid margin and limited to 7 mm in height (4).

Advantages

The main advantage to this flap is that it replaces the posterior lamella with similar tissue.

Disadvantages

The main disadvantage to this procedure is that the size of the graft is limited to approximately 5×25 mm and tapered nasally and laterally. It may result in 0.5–1.0 mm upper eyelid retraction. To minimize eyelid retraction, avoid cautery to the surgical area after removing the graft and use corticosteroid drops for 2–3 weeks. Eye irritation can result from the tarsal scar (8,9).

Cutler-Beard

Description

The Cutler-Beard flap is a staged lid-sharing procedure that transfers a full-thickness flap from the lower eyelid to an upper eyelid defect (10) (Fig. 7). The technique involves creating a transcutaneous full-thickness horizontal incision below the level of the marginal vessels in the lower eyelid (4 mm below the lid margin), equal in extent to the upper eyelid defect. Full-thickness vertical inferior cuts are made that create a rectangular flap based inferiorly that is pulled superiorly under the inferior eyelid margin to the upper lid defect. The flap is composed of skin, orbicularis oculi muscle, orbital septum, capsulopalpebral fascia, and conjunctiva. The capsulopalpebral fascia at the leading edge of the flap is sutured to the levator aponeurosis in the upper eyelid as part of a layered closure. The flap is left in place 6–8 weeks for delay and to allow lengthening. The second stage consists of flap division allowing excess conjunctival tissue to drape over the upper lid margin. The lower lid is closed in layers including conjunctiva.

Indications

It can be used for full-thickness upper eyelid defects involving over 75% of the upper eyelid margin. Like the Hughes flap, this flap is contraindicated for patients with ocular disease that require regular examinations or those with very poor or no sight in the opposite eye.

Advantages

The advantages of this flap include replacement of similar tissue from that lost in the upper eyelid and provision of a natural lining for corneal protection.

Disadvantages

Vision is obstructed for a prolonged period of time prior to flap division and inset. Since no tarsus or rigid structure is restored in the upper eyelid margin, entropion may result. Postoperative ectropion in the lower eyelid is also a significant risk. There are no lashes on the reconstructed lid margin.

Switch Flap (for Upper Eyelid Repair)

Description

The switch flap is a two-stage procedure involving transfer of a wedge-shaped full-thickness marginal flap from the lower eyelid to the upper eyelid (11). The

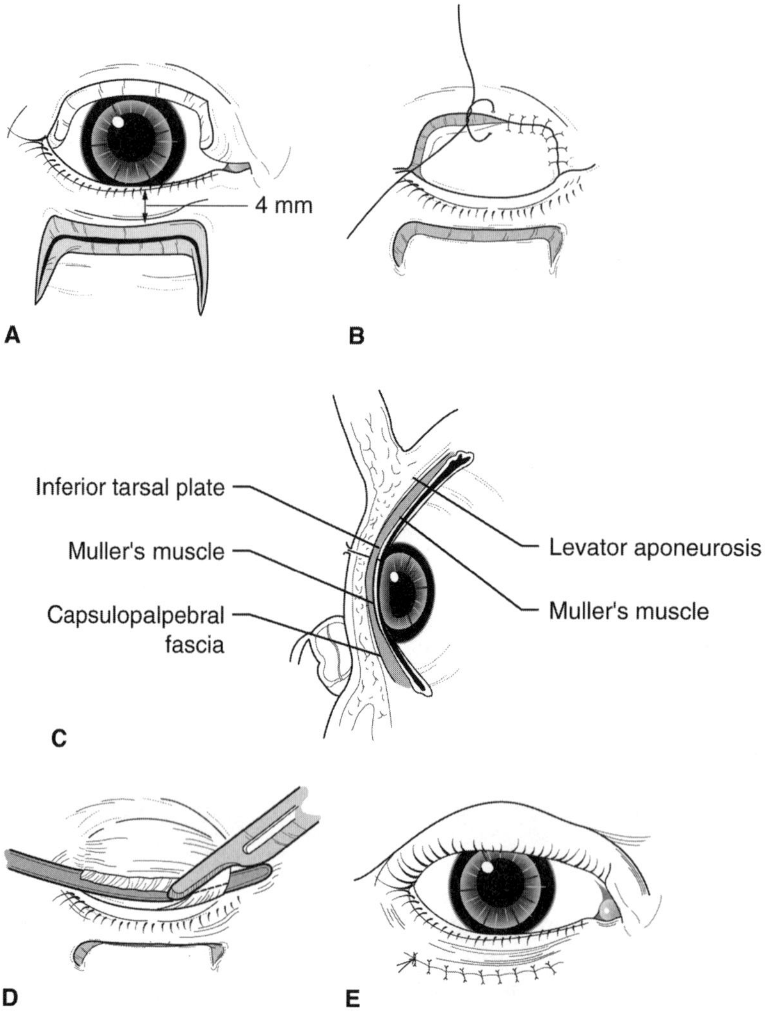

Figure 7 Cutler-Beard flap for upper eyelid reconstruction.

hinge of the flap should lie at the midpoint of the upper lid defect, and the flap is pedicled medially closing the visual axis after transfer to the upper lid. The height of the flap should be at least 4 mm from the lid margin preserving the marginal arcade. At the second stage (2–3 weeks later), the pedicle is divided and the lower eyelid is closed primarily by any appropriate technique as described in this section.

Indications

The main indication for the switch flap is for central marginal upper eyelid defects involving 50% of the lid margin. This technique transfers full-thickness lower eyelid, together with the lashes, into the upper eyelid defect.

Advantages

The major advantage of the switch flap is that it replaces similar tissue to that lost in the upper eyelid, including the eyelashes.

Disadvantages

A disadvantage to this flap is that is requires two stages, and vision in the affected eye is interrupted during the delay period.

Mustardé Cheek Rotation Flap (for Lower Eyelid Repair)

Description

A Mustardé cheek flap is a large rotation flap with its leading edge at the lateral canthus extending laterally and arching like a Tenzel flap (12). The incision is then continued laterally to the preauricular crease toward the level of the earlobe. A wide subcutaneous undermining proceeds, the extent of which is determined by the laxity of the skin and the extent of the defect. The posterior lamella must be reconstituted and Mustardé recommends a composite graft of nasal septal cartilage and mucosa. The mucosa should be harvested in excess to cover the lid margin, and the nasal septal cartilage must be thinned to 1 mm and be oversized with respect to normal tarsus to extend to the lower orbital rim.

Indications

The Mustardé cheek rotation flap is indicated in lower eyelid defects involving over 75% of the lid margin. This flap may best be reserved for patients who cannot undergo a two-staged operation (Hughes tarsoconjunctival flap) or when an extensive lower lid defect extends over 7 mm below the lid margin (13).

Advantages

The advantages to using this flap include the ability to apply it to very extensive and total lower lid defects; use of cheek tissue and sparing of thc upper lid as a donor site; and the use of incisions that are well-hidden following the borders of the cheek topographical unit.

Disadvantages

This flap leaves a large segment of the lid margin with little structural support potentially resulting in eyelid malposition including entropion or ectropion.

Bipedicle

Description

The bipedicled flap transfers tissue from the upper eyelid to the lower eyelid in two stages (Fig. 8). The skin bridges medially and laterally remain intact after the first stage and are divided and discarded during the second stage 2–3 weeks later. The flap may be composed of skin and orbicularis oculi muscle only (Tripier flap) or the full-thickness of the upper eyelid including a portion of the upper tarsus (14). If tarsus is harvested, the marginal arcade must be preserved. Leaving at least 5 mm of upper tarsus will preserve the marginal arcade and the stability of the

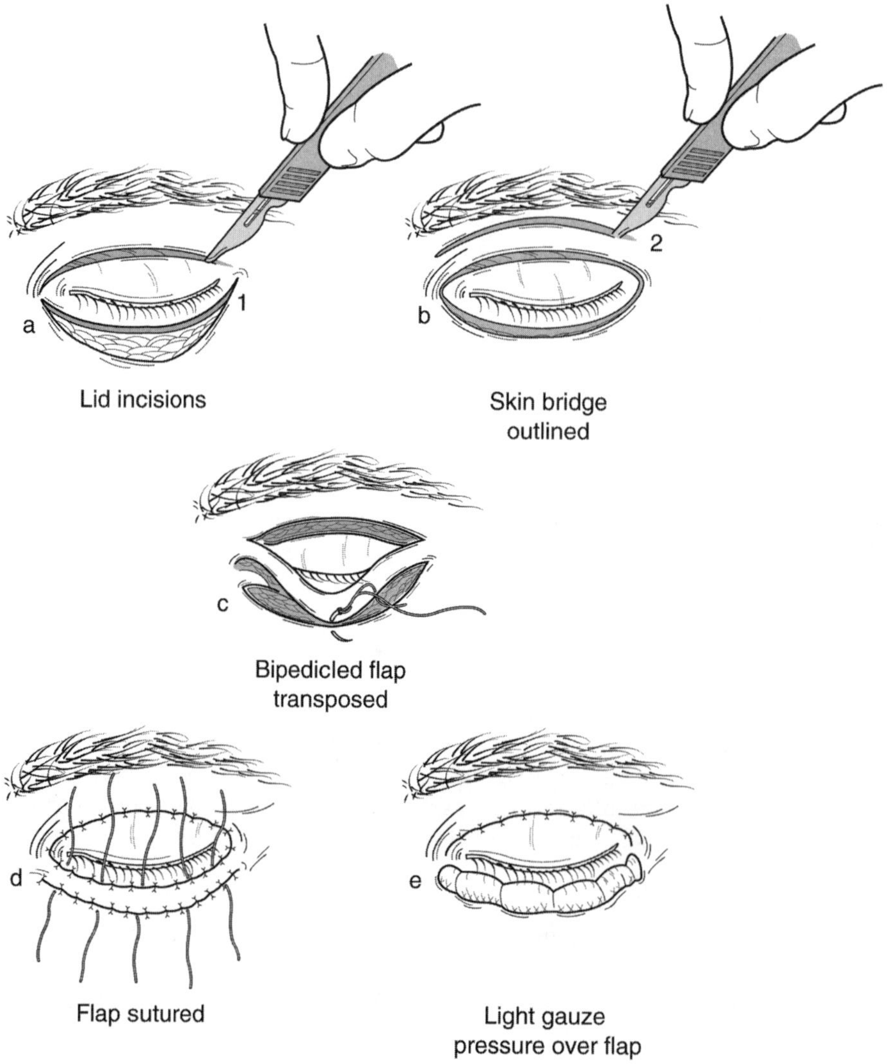

Figure 8 Two-staged bipedicled flap for defect in lower eyelid.

upper eyelid margin. The initial incision for the Tripier flap is oriented along the supratarsal crease and the superior incision is 10–15 mm above and parallel to the inferior incision. The donor site of the partial-thickness Tripier flap is closed primarily as in standard blepharoplasty. The donor site of the full-thickness flap requires a complex layer repair including pushing back or recessing the upper lid retractors and suturing the free conjunctival edge to the upper border of the remaining tarsus. The upper lid retractors are then sutured to the conjunctiva at their recessed position and the skin is closed primarily. A laterally based composite unipedicle flap may be designed for marginal defects of the temporal lower eyelid (4).

Indications

The bipedicled flap is indicated for horizontal lower eyelid defects limited to 10–15 mm in height. Non-marginal anterior lamella defects may be repaired with a partial-thickness flap. Marginal defects, if repaired with a partial-thickness flap, will require an autogenous composite graft (e.g., a nasal septal cartilage–mucosal graft). A full-thickness bipedicled flap will reconstitute both the anterior and posterior lamellae.

Advantages

The advantages of the bipedicled flap are that it provides tissue with excellent texture, color, and thickness. It may be single-staged for total marginal defects using the full-thickness bipedicled flap. The tarsus incorporated into the flap provides support for the lower eyelid margin. The nature of the transposition provides good support laterally and medially to the newly reconstructed lid margin.

Disadvantages

The upper eyelid may be malpositioned or lagophthalmus may result from harvest of the full-thickness flap. The height of the defect that can be repaired is limited to 10–15 mm. No eyelashes are included in the flap for marginal repairs.

LIP RECONSTRUCTION

More than 90% of lip defects involve the lower lip because the majority of lip carcinomas occur in this area. Basic goals in lower lip reconstruction are the prevention of drooling and re-establishment of the continuity of the lips. A variety of local and regional flaps are capable of meeting these goals. However, with the recent advent of several innervated local flaps and modified versions of previously nondynamic and nonsensate flaps, function and cosmesis are now of primary importance. Although not yet within reach, the ideal lip repair results in a completely functional lip demonstrating normal sphincteric and complex motor actions with identical texture and color to the missing lip segment. There should be no donor site morbidity or noticeable scar, and the flap should be reliable, easily harvested, and sensate.

Lip Anatomy

The lips are paired mobile folds covered externally by skin and internally by mucous membrane encompassing a highly muscular inner layer. The upper lip extends to the base of the nose medially and to the nasolabial folds lateral. The lower lip is separated from the chin by the mentolabial sulcus (mental crease) (15). The surface anatomy of the lip consists of the topographical subunits, oral commissures, red-lip margin, inner vermilion line, philtrum, red line, white line, and Cupid's bow (Fig. 9). Burget et al. (16) have organized the upper lip into topographical subunits including two lateral subunits and two medial subunits. The borders of a lateral subunit are the ipsilateral philtral column, nostril sill, alar base, melolabial fold, and inner vermilion line. The borders of a medial subunit are the ipsilateral philtral column, nostril sill, midphiltral trough, and inner vermilion line. The oral commissures demarcate the upper lip aesthetic subunits from the lower lip subunits. When more

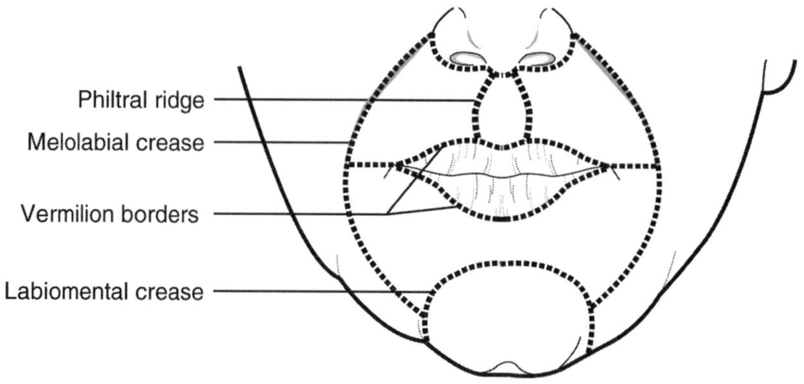

Figure 9 Topographical subunits of the lip.

than 50% of a subunit is missing, superior aesthetic results will be obtained if the entire subunit is replaced. The lower lip includes two lateral subunits and a central subunit. The borders of a lateral subunit are the labiomental crease, mandibular margin, mental crease, and inner vermilion line. The lateral subunits meet in the midline over the mental crease and central subunit. The mental crease defines the central subunit as it courses horizontally under the mid-portion of the lower lip and descends inferolateral to the mandibular margin (17).

The red-lip margin is the vermilion surface external to the occlusal surface of the upper and lower lips (inner vermilion line). It is composed of modified mucosal epithelium devoid of minor salivary glands. The perioral skin meets the deep red color of the vermilion at the red line. Just outside the red line is a raised surface prominence of paler skin that forms the white line. Malalignment or deformity of the white line is very noticeable and careful reapproximation of this line during lip reconstruction is essential. The philtrum, above the midline of the upper lip, is defined by vertical raised skin prominences forming the philtral columns and the portion of the white line inferiorly forming a gentle curve known as Cupid's bow.

The layers of the lip include the vermilion, orbicularis oris muscle, labial glands, and oral mucosa. The orbicularis oris muscle is an oral sphincter but is not simply a sheet of continuous muscle fibers that encircle the mouth. The oral sphincter is a complex composite of muscle fibers including those of the orbicularis oris that radiate from dense fibromuscular masses (the modioli) located approximately 1.25 cm lateral to the oral commissures. The modioli are focal points of transit, insertion, and decussation of several different muscles that together result in the complex movements associated with the lip (Fig. 10). The orbicularis oris muscle fibers radiate from the modioli and converge in the midline of each lip. The muscle fibers that travel under the red-lip margin represent the pars marginalis component of the orbicularis oris muscle. The pars marginalis consists of a single (in some races a double) band of narrow muscle fibers within the red-lip margin. The pars marginalis is unique to higher primates and is essential to normal vocalization and production of some musical tones. The peripheral component of the orbicularis oris muscle is the pars peripheralis; these fibers aggregate into cylindrical bundles that fan out from each modiolus from the white line to the peripheral areas of the upper and

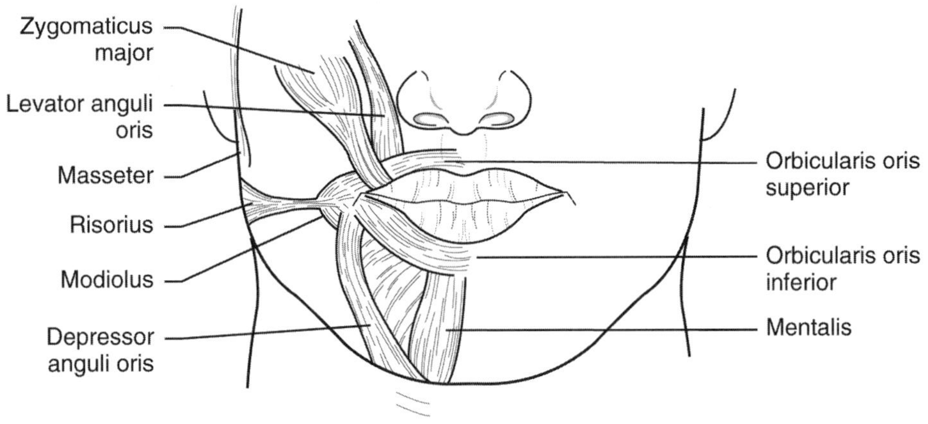

Figure 10 The modioli: note the common insertion of the facial mimetic muscles.

lower lips (Fig. 11). On sagittal section, the pars peripheralis as it approaches the red-lip margin and the pars marginalis are classically described as resembling the shank and curved portions of a hook. The buccinator muscle forms a large part of the oral sphincter, its peripheral fibers passing directly into the upper and lower lips, and its central fibers decussating at the modioli before passing into the lips (18). Superficial to the buccinator muscle course fascicles from the levator anguli oris and depressor anguli oris, inserting and crossing at the modioli. Entering the orbicularis obliquely, the zygomaticus major, levator labii superioris, and depressor labii inferioris contribute other superficial fascicles. The motor supply to all these muscles is from the buccal and mandibular branches of the facial nerve. Sensation is mediated through the infraorbital and mental branches of the trigeminal nerve. The labial arteries are branches of the facial artery that course immediately beneath the labial mucosa deep to the inner vermilion line.

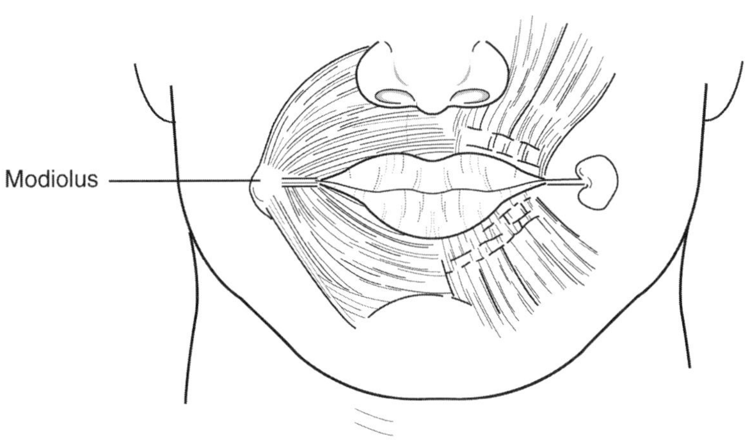

Figure 11 The orbicularis oris (pars peripheralis) inserting into the modiolus (patient's right).

Vermilion Defects

Partial-thickness defects involving the vermilion and white line that can be closed primarily should be repaired in line with the resting skin tension lines (RSTLs); extension beyond the borders of the surrounding topographical subunits (e.g., mental crease) should be avoided. The RSTLs radiate out from the white line and tend to follow the fine rhytids in this area. If the partial-thickness defect involves the underlying orbicularis muscle and superficial repair would leave an adynamic segment of lip, consideration should be given to converting it into a full-thickness defect to allow approximation of the orbicularis oris muscle to maintain oral competence. More extensive partial-thickness vermilion defects may be repaired with a variety of flaps including mucosal advancement from the labial mucosal behind the inner vermilion line, skin grafting with tattooing, and ventral or marginal musculomucosal tongue flaps. Vermilion mucosal defects may be repaired with mucosal advancement; however, if the vermilion defect is thick, involving submucosal tissues, then a more substantial musculomucosal tongue or cheek flap is preferred. Tongue flaps must be designed carefully to ensure their viability. The median raphe separates the vascularity of the tongue in the sagittal plane with very poor collateral circulation. For this reason, tongue flaps should be designed longitudinally along the margin of the tongue, or transversely, across the median raphe, as a bipedicled flap (19). Tongue flaps for vermilion reconstruction should be obtained from the undersurface or margin of the tongue because these surfaces are smooth and resemble vermilion. Underlying tongue muscle should be selectively harvested to provide sufficient bulk to the new vermilion. The undersurface of the tongue can be transferred to the lower lip vermilion surface using staged marginal and ventral bipedicled tongue flaps (Fig. 12). The second stage, usually 3 weeks later, is for flap division and inset; the defect on the undersurface of the tongue can be left to heal by secondary intention. For upper lip defects, the tongue tip may be sutured to the vermilion and severed 3 weeks later.

Full-thickness vermilion-only defects that are limited to one-half the length of the lip may be repaired with unilateral or bilateral full-thickness vermilion advance-

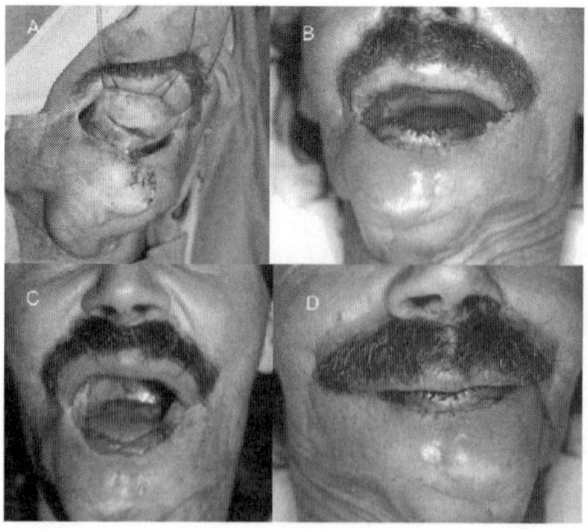

Figure 12 Staged ventral tongue flap for lip vermilion reconstruction. Upper photographs show incision in ventral tongue (A) and intermediate attachment to lower lip (B). Lower photographs (C, D) show lower lip after detachment from the tongue.

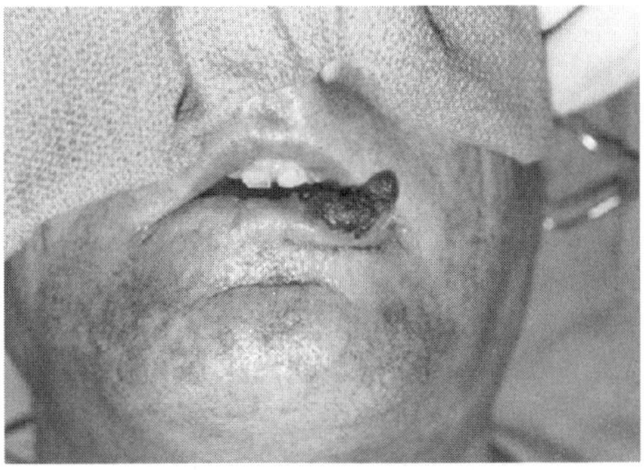

Figure 13 Patient with a verrucous growth of the left lower lip. After resection, this patient

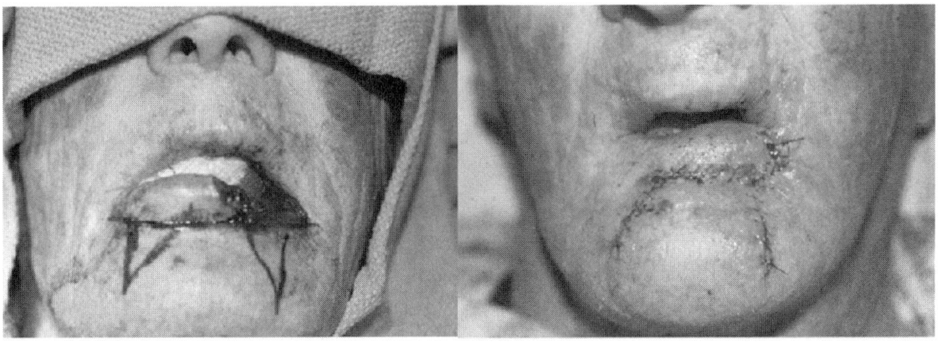

Figure 14 Sliding vermilion advancement flap for repair of a lower lip defect.

ment flaps (Figs. 13, 14). Sliding vermilion advancement flaps for full-thickness vermilion defects of the lower lip take advantage of the elasticity of completely released segment of vermilion. The vermilion is released by full-thickness cuts at the white line to the oral commissure, being careful to angle the cut appropriately to include the labial artery. The flaps are then simply brought together on stretch and all incisions are sutured primarily (20).

Commissure Reconstruction

Some local flaps (e.g., Estlander flap or Karapandzic flap) result in a blunted or rounded commissure that requires secondary revision. Most commonly, revision involves lateral horizontal transection through a point corresponding to the desired location of the buccal angle. Buccal mucosa is advanced anteriorly to form the new red lip. Converse described a method of commissuroplasty that removed a triangular unit of skin and subcutaneous tissue lateral to the blunted region and advancement of the underlying mucosa to form the new redlip (21).

Commissure defects are most commonly secondary to trauma, especially electrical burns. An electrical burn injury affects the lower lip and commissure most severely. The commissure becomes rounded with adjacent cutaneous and subcutaneous scarring that pulls the uninjured surrounding lip and cheek tissues inward, resulting in excessive bulk and anteromedial rotation of the affected commissure. Delayed reconstruction in these cases is preferred in contrast to immediate reconstruction for cases due to cancer resection. The early use of an oral splint may reduce the need for extensive reconstructive surgery in milder cases. A restored commissure should ideally be symmetrical with respect to the opposite side in repose and during mouth opening, with no webbing, and with a normal well-defined vermilion. The lateral extent of the commissures should fall in line with the medial aspect of the cornea. The variety of reconstructive methods described for this injury is evidence for the fact that there is no 'best' technique and the ideal result is seldom achieved. In general, the techniques involve some degree of scar release and excision; formation of a more naturally placed commissure; and mucosal, adjacent vermilion, or tongue flaps to form the new vermilion.

Despite the plethora of available techniques, some basic tenets should be considered. Adequate release of all contracted tissues including mucosa and muscle should be performed initially to reduce the excess bulk by allowing the tissues of the cheek and adjacent lip to retract back to their normal positions. A limited amount of indurated fibrous tissue should be excised. If an excessive amount of scar tissue is removed, the commissure will thicken as cheek and adjacent lip are again pulled into the area postoperatively. The opened commissure is deficient of tissue; therefore, buccal mucosal, adjacent vermilion, or ventral tongue flaps must be recruited. Using adjacent buccal mucosal or vermilion may be counterproductive since they are harvested from a region that is already deficient of tissue. A staged, anteriorly based, ventral tongue flap avoids the use of adjacent tissue and may be the best choice, especially for more significant injuries (22).

Full-Thickness Defects

The factors influencing lip reconstruction are the extent and location of the lip defect, associated bony defects of the anterior arch of the mandible, prior neck dissection, and the quality and quantity of adjacent lip and cheek tissues. Definitive repair at the time of cancer resection is customary because, with the selective use of Mohs' micrographic surgery and frozen section control of surgical margins, the risk of recurrence requiring further surgery is rare.

Defects involving up to one-third of the length of the lip can be closed primarily with a pentagonal wedge excision keeping the edges of the vermilion parallel and wedging out a triangle of skin below the white line (Fig. 15). Primary closure of defects involving up to one-half of the lip is possible in selected patients with significant lip laxity. Two techniques that allow primary lip closure for defects involving one-half the lower lip that cannot undergo simple closure are the staircase technique and bilateral lip advancement flaps. The staircase technique is employed for rectangular defects and involve lateral advancement flaps from the remaining parts of the lower lip and chin prepared by stepwise incisions. Defects can be closed with either unilateral or bilateral flaps. The rectangles are excised below the steps down to the orbicularis oris muscle (originally these were described as full-thickness [23]) to allow the remaining lip segments to advance medially (24). Rectangular defects can be repaired using full-thickness bilateral advancement flaps of the remaining lower lip by extending the horizontal limits of the base of the defect laterally along the mental

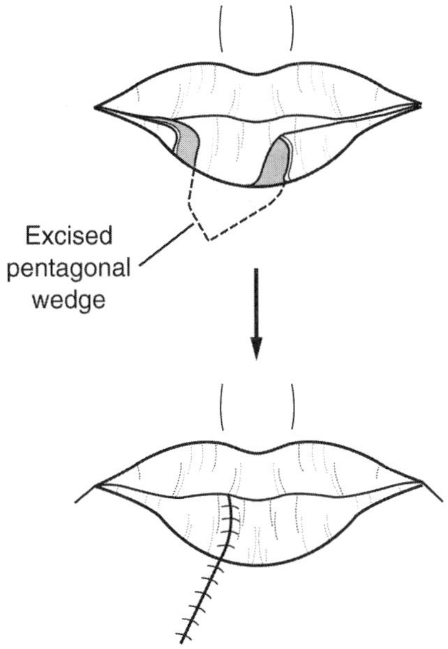

Figure 15 Pentagonal closure of a lip defect. Note the pentagonal wedge of tissue excised to allow closure and accurate alignment of the white line.

creases. After full release of the lateral lip segments they are advanced toward the midline and sutured in layers (Fig. 16).

Defects involving over one-half of the lip require tissue recruitment from the opposite lip (e.g., Karapandzic or cross-lip flap); the perioral area (e.g., steeple, depressor anguli oris, or facial platysmal flap); or the cheek (e.g., modified Bernard or fan flap). These local flaps are functional (sensory and motor) and the resulting scars often fall on the borders of the lip topographical subunits. The steeple flap and cross-lip flaps (Abbé and Estlander) depend upon reinnervation from the

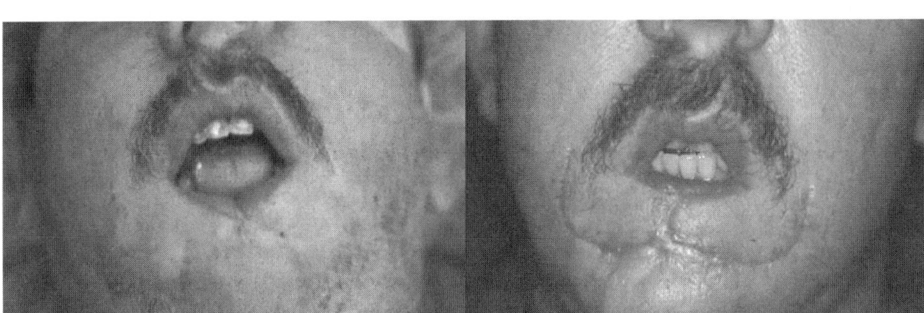

Figure 16 Rectangular lip defects closed with horizontally advanced tissue. This patient had an extensive lower lip/mandible defect. The lip was originally closed primarily after transfer of a composite scapular free flap (left photograph). A second-stage procedure involving horizontal advancement of the adjacent lip and chin soft tissues resulted in improved appearance and function of the lower lip (right photograph).

Table 1 Flap Selection for Lower Lip Reconstruction

Lower lip defect	Repair
Lateral 1/3 to 2/3	Depressor anguli oris flap Innervated facial platysmal flap
Central 1/3 to 2/3	Karapandzic flap Modified Bernard flap
Total	Bilateral depressor anguli oris flap Bilateral innervated platysmal flap

surrounding lip tissue that may be partial and delayed for several months. Tobin (25) has created a useful paradigm for flap selection in lower lip reconstruction to maximize postoperative lip function and cosmesis (Table 1).

Associated bony defects of the anterior arch of the mandible and prior neck dissection may affect the choice of flap for lip repair. Mandibular arch resection for cancer requiring lip resection often results in large lower lip tissue deficiencies that include the depressor anguli oris and facial platysmal, eliminating the use of the perioral flaps that are based on these muscles. The soft tissue component of the free flap may be available for lip reconstruction. However, these tissues are usually excessively thick and nonsensate, with the exception of the osteocutaneous radial forearm flap that is rarely used for mandibular arch defects. Perioral and cheek flaps are still preferred despite underlying bone reconstruction and the availability of the soft tissue component of the free flap. If local tissue is unavailable, concurrent or subsequent transfer of a sensate radial forearm free flap is satisfactory (26,27).

Prior or simultaneous neck dissection should have little bearing on the choice of flap for lip reconstruction unless the marginal mandibular nerve is disrupted, in which case the functional local flaps that depend upon this nerve for movement would be less effective (e.g., depressor anguli oris and facial platysmal). The modified Bernard flap and the Karapandzic flap would also be expected to result in a poorly functioning lip, but may benefit from the remaining buccal branches for orbicularis oris muscle tone and movement. More commonly, the facial artery is divided, jeopardizing the vascular supply to the perioral and cheek flaps. However, retrograde collateral flow through the facial arterial branches from the angular, infraorbital, dorsal nasal, and transverse facial vessels is sufficient to supply the majority of these flaps (28). Nevertheless, the facial artery should be preserved, if possible.

The quality and quantity of adjacent lip and cheek tissue may be diminished, most commonly by the presence of inelastic and fibrotic skin secondary to irradiation or dysplastic changes in the skin of the cheek or opposite lip. When local flaps are unavailable, regional or free tissue transfers must be considered. The most common regional flaps for subtotal or total lower lip reconstruction include the staged paired deltopectoral flap, and the pectoralis flap (29,30). These flaps have several inherent deficiencies including poor color match, no movement, no sensation, multiple stages, marginal distal viability, and excess bulk. Regional flaps for the upper lip include the staged temporal forehead (unipedicled or bipedicled) and staged bipedicled–scalping flap. These flaps can bring hair-bearing skin to the upper lip, and may be satisfactory because limited sphincteric movement and absence of sensation are better tolerated in the upper lip. Scalp flaps used to reconstruct the lips are axial based on the posterior branch of the superficial temporal artery. For full-thickness lip defects, additional flaps or skin grafts must furnish an inner lining. Although these flaps result in adequate lip replacement with hair-bearing potential, they suffer from requiring a staged procedure and significant donor site morbidity. The radial forearm free flap for both total and subtotal upper and lower lip defects is superior to regional flap repair (Figs. 17–19). It is potentially sensate, appropriately thin to

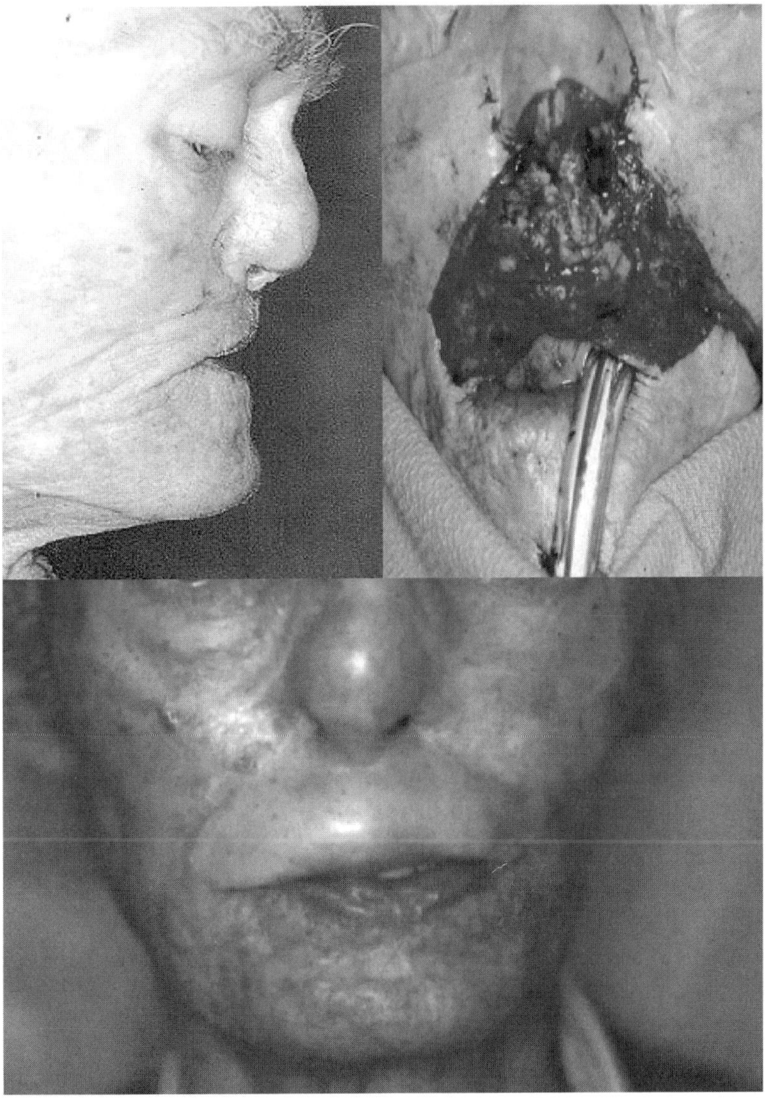

Figure 17 Upper lip defect closed with a radial forearm free flap. This patient received radiation therapy as a teenager to control facial acne. He had multiple skin cancers throughout his face and extensive scarring within his upper lip, causing permanent retraction of this structure (upper left photo). The skin and upper lip were resected within the aesthetic unit (upper right photo) and a radial forearm free flap was fashioned using a template. It was used to repair the missing lip and skin, providing a long-term solution (lower photo).

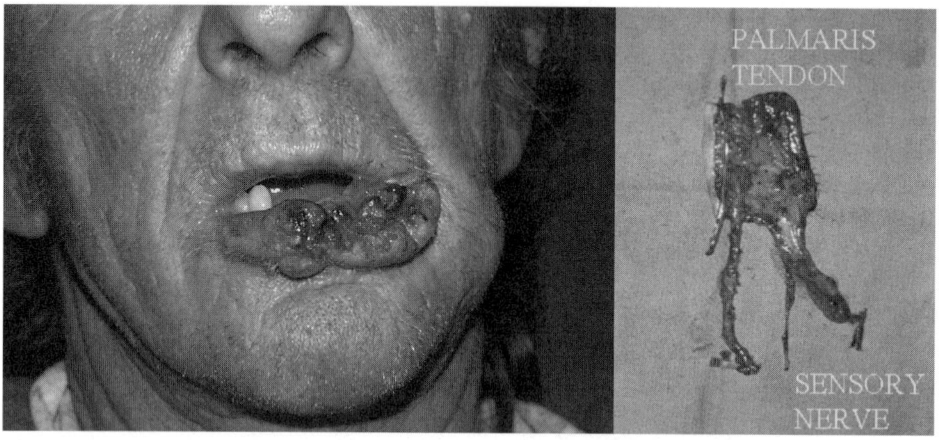

Figure 18 A patient with extensive squamous cell cancer of the lower lip requiring total excision of his lower lip, underlying mucosa, and adjacent chin (left photo). A sensate radial forearm free flap was planned with harvest of the palmaris tendon to support the free edge of the new lip/vermilion.

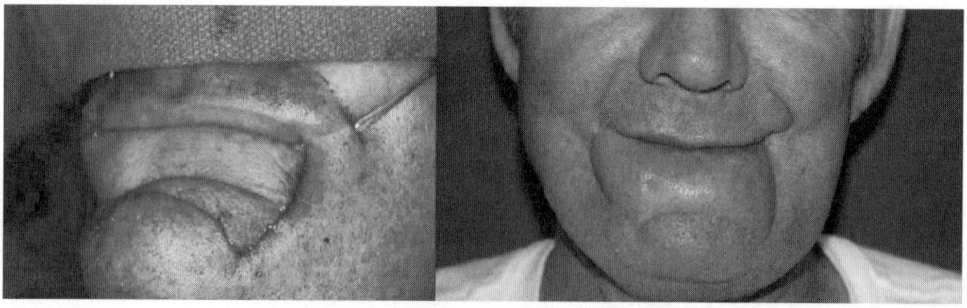

Figure 19 Patient in Figure 18 during (left photo) and after (right photo) flap transfer. Note in left photo the red rubber tube attached to the palmaris tendon. The flap is folded over this tendon, providing extra- and intraoral coverage and the tendon is secured with permanent suture to the modioli. The patient also underwent vermilionplasty using a staged ventral tongue flap.

fold on itself at the free lip margin for interior lip coverage, and can be supported using the palmaris tendon draped under the free lip margin (its ends sutured to the modioli or zygomatic–malar complexes).

Karapandzic Flap

Description

Karapandzic originally described this flap in 1974 as a means of perioral lip advancement that maintains the sensory and motor function of the orbicularis oris muscle and perioral skin (31). The technique consists of bilateral circumoral incisions from the edge of the defect maintaining an equal distance from the white line to a point just medial to the nasolabial fold (i.e., the width of the flap is equal to the height of the

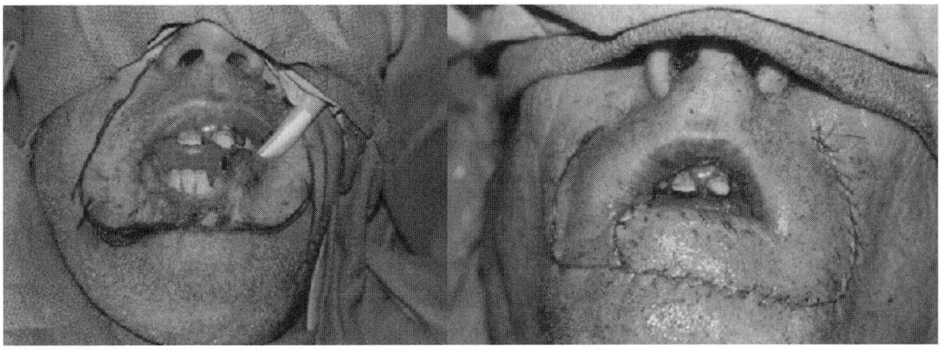

Figure 20 A Karapandzic flap used for repair of a subtotal lower lip defect.

defect) (Fig. 20). The neurovascular structures at the outer edges of the defect and at the corners of the lips are preserved and the orbicularis oris is selectively cut and released around these structures to allow flap rotation. Only the superficial fibers of the orbicularis oris muscle are cut at the commissures to preserve the radiating deeper fibers of the buccinator muscle. To minimize the rounded appearance of the commissures, the distal cut ends of the zygomaticus major muscles may be sutured relative to the new position of the commissures. Limited gingival labial sulcus mucosal incisions are necessary to facilitate movement of the lip tissues toward the defect.

Indications

The procedure may be used in any patient with a full-thickness lip defect involving the vermilion and perioral skin. However, the degree of postoperative microstomia is proportional to the length of the defect. Therefore, the Karapandzic flap is mainly indicated for defects involving up to two-thirds of the lower lip and up to one-half of the upper lip. Rectangular defects are most amenable to this type of repair.

Advantages

The main advantage of the Karapandzic flap is that is maintains a continuous circle of functioning orbicularis oris muscle and sensate perioral skin that results in a functional reconstruction.

Disadvantages

The main disadvantage of the Karapandzic flap is that the oral cavity aperture will be smaller (microstomia), thus impeding oral access, which is especially significant in patients with dentures. The nature of the incisions can result in a clown-like appearance. The location of the modioli is altered and the new commissures often take on a rounded appearance that may require commissuroplasty.

Abbé Flap

Description

The Abbé flap is a two-stage full-thickness lip switch flap based on the labial artery taken from the opposing lip medial to the oral commissure (32). The shape and size of the flap depend upon the dimensions of the defect; however, the height of the flap should be equal to the height of the defect, and the width of the flap should be half the width of the defect. The flap is transposed 180 degrees and after 7–10 days the pedicle is divided and the lips are closed in layers.

Indications

The Abbé flap is indicated for full-thickness central defects involving up to one-half of either lip. This flap may be used to reconstitute a missing philtrum. A unique use of an Abbé flap described by Millard involves transfer from the central lower lip to the central upper lip in patients with a tight upper lip after unilateral cleft lip repair. This relieves the tension on the upper lip and provides a philtrum with the philtral columns corresponding to the vertical scars resulting from flap placement (33).

Advantages

The Abbé flap provides nearly identical tissue to that lost including red lip, orbicularis oris muscle, and intraoral mucosa. The resulting length of the donor lip is proportional to the length of the recipient lip. The new lip segment regains motor innervation within 8 weeks and sensation within several months (34).

Disadvantages

This is a two-stage procedure that requires the placement of a temporary pedicle that partially blocks the oral aperture. Although motor reinnervation occurs, the quality is variable and may result in an adynamic or poorly functioning segment of lip. Return of sensation may take several months, returning in the order of pain, touch, and temperature (cold, then hot). The continuity of the orbicularis oris in the normal lip is disrupted, potentially resulting in muscle denervation and dysfunction. The oral aperture is reduced, and repair of larger defects in some patients may result in significant microstomia. The scar in the recipient lip often results in bunching up of the flap tissue causing a trap door deformity.

Estlander Flap

Description

Estlander (35) described a single-stage full-thickness cross-lip flap based on the labial artery for closure of lower lip defects near the commissure of the mouth. As with the Abbé flap, the width of the flap should be one-half the width of the defect, and the height should equal the height of the defect. The Estlander flap transfers the lateral portions of the opposite lip around the existing commissure to replace the missing lip tissue. Blunting of the commissure is expected and secondary revisions are usually necessary.

Indications

The Estlander flap is indicated for full-thickness lateral defects involving up to one-half of either lip (Fig. 21).

Advantages

The Estlander flap provides nearly identical tissue to that lost including red lip, orbicularis oris muscle, and intraoral mucosa. Balance between the lips is preserved because the resulting length of the donor lip is proportional to the length of the recipient lip. The new lip segment regains motor innervation within 8 weeks (34).

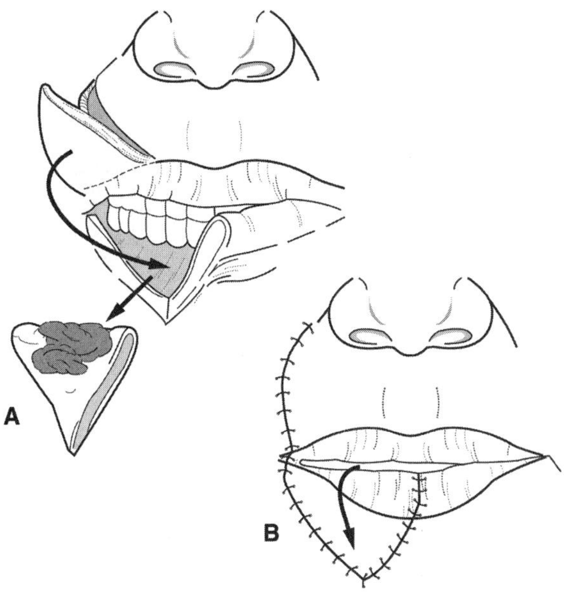

Figure 21 A superiorly based Estlander flap for repair of a lower lateral lip defect. Note how the donor site scar falls within the nasolabial crease.

Disadvantages

The modiolus is disrupted, altering the functionality of the lip elevators and depressors. The Estlander flap blunts the ipsilateral commissure and a secondary commissuroplasty is usually necessary. The return of motor and sensory innervation is variable. Like the Abbé flap, the Estlander flap may result in significant microstomia and trap door scarring.

Bernard–Von Burow Cheek Advancement

Description

Bernard and Von Burow were two 19th century surgeons who described the use of cheek tissue advancement using perioral triangular excisions of redundant tissue to close large full-thickness lip defects (36). To reconstruct large upper lip defects, Burow's triangles are placed lateral to the alae and oral commissures. For lower lip defects, the Burow's triangles are placed at the oral commissures and the defect is excised in the shape of a large 'V' that includes much of the chin tissue inferior to the lip. The mucosa in the depth of the triangles is incised and left pedicled inferiorly; this excess mucosa is draped anteriorly after flap inset to form the new vermilion.

The Webster modification of the Bernard flap was described for lower lip reconstruction (37). It spares the facial musculature, including the orbicularis oris and the neurovascular structures, by excising skin only within the Burow's triangles. The underlying muscles and neurovascular structures are released similarly to the Karapandzic flap. The Burow's triangles are also placed more laterally and their bases tilted slightly superolateral with respect to the oral commissures to fall within

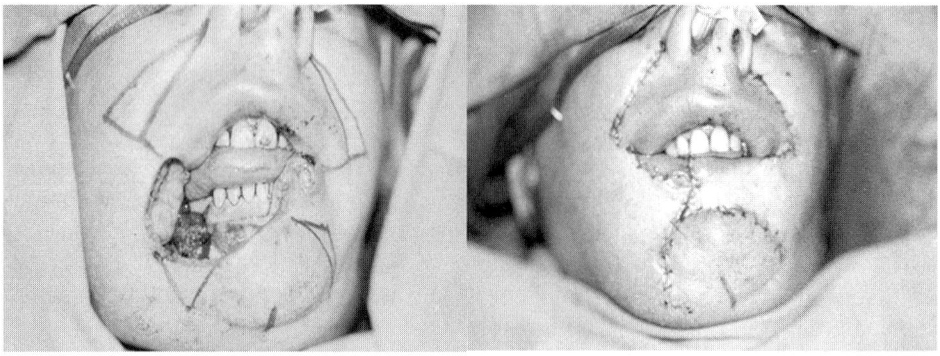

Figure 22 The Webster modification of the Bernard flap for repair of an extensive lower lip and chin defect. See text for details.

the melolabial fold. The requirement of a V-shaped defect is abandoned in favor of a chin-sparing rectangular defect. Two additional Burow's triangles (skin only) are placed opposite the inferior aspect of the defect within the buccolabial folds. Mucosal-only incisions are made under the upper Burow's triangles to create excess mucosa that is pedicled inferiorly to drape over the new lip margin.

Indications

This flap was originally described to reconstruct subtotal and total defects of the upper or lower lip. The Webster cheiloplasty is indicated for lower lip defects, especially subtotal defects of the central lower lip (Fig. 22). Total lower lip reconstruction may be facilitated by a cross-lip Abbé flap to augment the central part of the lower lip, reduce tension on the closure, and reduce the size of the upper lip to more closely match the deficient lower lip (38). Modified Bernard flaps (muscle and nerve sparing) for subtotal or total upper lip defects may also be augmented with a cross-lip flap to the philtrum.

Advantages

The modified Bernard flap preserves the integrity and position of the modioli and creates a functional lip. Limiting its use to subtotal defects of the lip will result in a satisfactory repair. These defects may also be repaired with a Karapandzic flap; however, the Bernard flap will not result in microstomia.

Disadvantages

The original Bernard–von Burow flap resulted in denervation of the orbicularis oris, interruption of the sensory supply to both the upper and lower lips, and disruption of the modioli. These problems are avoided using the modified flaps. A large amount of healthy tissue must be discarded in the nasolabial and mentolabial folds. If defects involving greater than two-thirds of the lip are reconstructed using this technique, a tight lip deficient in tissue often results. Solving this problem by using cross-lip flaps results in a new set of problems inherent in the use of the Abbé flap. Use of a cross-lip flap may be particularly problematic if the donor site is from the upper lip, because this would disrupt the philtrum.

Steeple Flap

Description

The steeple flap is a full-thickness island musculocutaneous flap that is vertically oriented and rectangular (39). The base of the flap extends laterally from the base of a rectangular lateral lower lip defect. The height of the flap should equal the horizontal length of the defect. A triangular excision of tissue over the flap facilitates primary closure of the donor site and gives the flap the appearance of a steeple. For a left-sided defect, if the facial artery enters the flap in its superolateral aspect, the flap is rotated counterclockwise into the defect. If the facial artery enters the flap in its inferolateral aspect, the flap is rotated clockwise into the defect. Excess mucosa should be harvested on the appropriate side of the flap to form the new vermilion. Recovery of sensory and motor innervation is anticipated within several months, similarly to a lip-switch flap.

Indications

The steeple flap is designed for ipsilateral lower lip defects involving up to 60% of the lip. Total lower lip reconstruction can be accomplished with bilateral flaps.

Advantages

The main advantage to the steeple flap is that it can potentially provide a functional reconstruction for extensive lower lip defects. In addition, the skin of the flap matches the skin and texture of remaining perioral areas.

Disadvantages

The muscle fibers are not in exact alignment with the remaining orbicularis oris fibers and surface irregularities may be unmasked during active lip closure. The entrapped scar predisposes to trap door deformity and a patched appearance. Sensory and motor recovery may be incomplete. The resulting donor site scar is in an unnatural location, immediately adjacent to the oral commissure.

Depressor Anguli Oris Flap

Description

The depressor anguli oris flap is a full-thickness musculocutaneous flap that provides functional (both sensory and motor) lower lip and oral sphincter reconstruction (40). Flap dimensions reflect the size of the underlying depressor muscle and are approximately 4 cm long by 2 cm wide. The vascular pedicle is the inferior labial artery off the facial artery entering the flap near the oral commissure. Sensation is derived from the mental nerve (trigeminal) and the motor innervation is from the marginal branch of the facial nerve. These two nerves are dissected independent of the vascular pedicle and are sufficiently released to allow transposition of the flap. The flap is based superiorly with its medial border originating at the modiolus. It extends inferiorly along the buccolabial fold (marionette line) encompassing the underlying depressor anguli oris muscle. The layers of the flap include skin, depressor anguli oris muscle, and mucosa. Harvesting additional tissue laterally from the labial–gingival sulcus can enlarge the mucosal component. The flap pivots into position, bringing the depressor anguli oris muscle into the same orientation as the lost orbicularis oris muscle. The facial artery must occasionally be divided near the inferior aspect of the flap to allow transposition. Mucosal advancement or a ventral tongue flap reconstitutes the vermilion border.

Indications

The depressor anguli oris flap is most favorable for lateral ipsilateral defects involving up to 60% of the lower lip (Fig. 23). Total lower lip reconstruction can be accomplished with bilateral flaps.

Advantages

The upper lip and modioli are undisturbed and the full length of the lower lip is reconstructed, minimizing the problem of postoperative microstomia. The principal advantages to this method are recreation of a sensate lower lip with sufficient motor activity to recreate a functional oral sphincter, avoidance of microstomia, preservation of upper lip structure and function, and provision of all lip elements by a single flap.

Disadvantages

A functional donor deficit of commissure depression is evident in scowling. The commissure also rises excessively during smiling as a consequence of the unopposed action of the lip elevators.

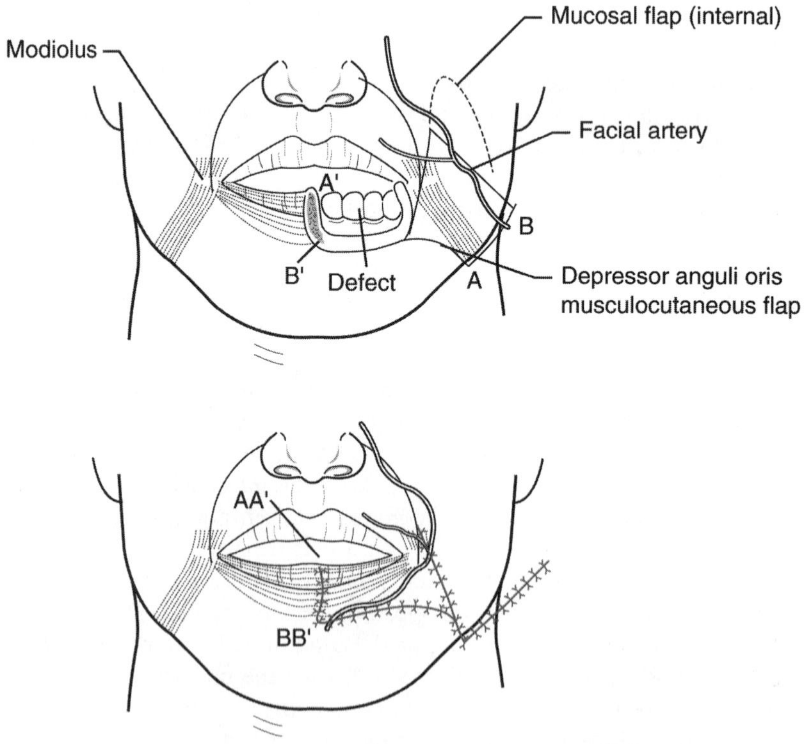

Figure 23 The depressor anguli oris flap for dynamic and sensate repair of a lower lip defect (see text).

Fan Flap

Description

The fan flap, originally described by Gillies in 1954, derived its name from its resemblance to the rotational opening of a handheld fan. The flap is full-thickness including mucosa and is based on the opposing lip's labial artery. In designing the flap, the opposing lip's white line is marked at a point away from the lateral aspect of the defect along the vermilion equal in length to the width of the defect. This mark represents the area on the opposing lip that will become the new commissure after flap inset. Extending out from this mark, along a radiant RSTL, a full-thickness incision is made approximately 1.5 cm in length. The incision is then turned acutely at an angle of approximately 60 degrees to the outer part of the nasolabial fold. The incision then follows the fold and turns acutely toward the defect to match the height and width of the flap to the height and width of the defect. To facilitate flap transfer, an opposing 60 degrees angled incision from the nasolabial fold is made into the cheek, creating a Z-plasty at the base of the flap.

Indications

The fan flap is primarily indicated for full-thickness defects of the central upper or lower lips. The use of bilateral symmetrical flaps results in the most cosmetic reconstruction. Defects involving between one-third and one-half of the lower lip may be repaired with a unilateral fan flap, but an Estlander flap may be more appropriate.

Advantages

The fan flap provides actual lip tissue for replacement of the lost segment of lip.

Disadvantages

The use of a classic fan flap always results in some degree of microstomia. The modiolus is malpositioned and a second stage is required for commissuroplasty. The sensory and motor nerves to the transposed segment of orbicularis oris muscle are divided, resulting in a nonsensate and adynamic repair. The Karapandzic flap attempts to improve on this type of flap design by preserving the sensorimotor components to the transposed lip segment. However, some sensory and motor reinnervation may occur with the fan flap as seen with the Abbé and Estlander flaps, taking up to 2 years for maximal return.

Facial Platysma Flap

Description

The facial platysma flap is a skin–muscle flap based on the pars modiolaris portion of the platysma (41). The pars modiolaris represents the muscle fibers that extend over the mandible to insert on the ipsilateral modiolus, and are located just lateral to the lateral border of the depressor anguli oris muscle. Motor innervation is via the marginal branch of the facial nerve and sensory innervation is from the mental nerve (trigeminal). Vascular supply is via the facial artery as it crosses the mandible. The defect should be triangular or wedge-shaped and the flap is designed just lateral in the shape of an inverted 'V' with identical dimensions; its base is oriented along the border of the mandible. The platysmal fibers are incised, preserving the neurovascular structures to the flap. The flap is rotated toward the defect, leaving a raw inner surface that must be covered with a cheek mucosal flap. Flap rotation results in the reorientation of the platysmal fibers into a more horizontal position. A similar type of flap (the submental artery island flap) harvested from the submental area has been described (42).

Indications

This flap is indicated for lateral defects involving over one-third of the length of the lower lip, where the depressor anguli oris muscle is missing or of no use (Fig. 24). Bilateral flaps must be used for total lip reconstruction.

Advantages

The flap provides a functional reconstruction of the lower lip with local tissues. The color and texture match to the missing segment of lip is excellent.

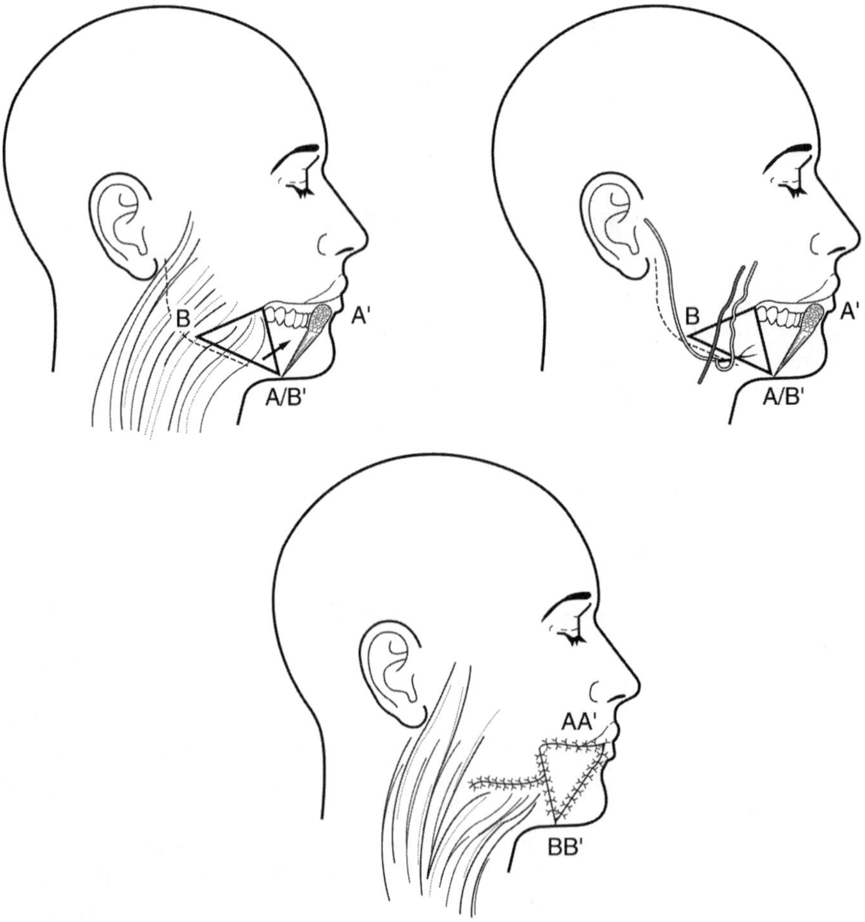

Figure 24 The facial platysmal flap (see text for details).

Disadvantages

This is not a full-thickness flap and mucosal lining must be obtained from the adjacent cheek. The platysmal fibers under the flap may be difficult to identify in some patients due to excessive thinning of the muscle in the perioral area. The marginal branch of the facial nerve is at risk for injury because it must be dissected laterally to free the flap for sufficient rotation. Trap door scarring is common.

REFERENCES

1. Codere F, Tucker NA, Renaldi B. The anatomy of Whitnall ligament. Ophthalmology 1995; 102:2016–2019.
2. Goldberg RA, Lufkin R, Farahani K, Wu JC, Jesmanowicz A, Hyde JS. Physiology of the lower eyelid retractors: tight linkage of the anterior capsulopalpebral fascia demonstrated using dynamic ultrafine surface coil MRI. Ophthal. Plast. Reconstr. Surg. 1994; 10:87–91.
3. Tucker SM, Linberg JV. Vascular anatomy of the eyelids. Ophthalmology 1994; 101:1118–1121.
4. Patel BCK, Flaharty PM, Anderson RL. Reconstruction of the Eyelids. In: Baker SR, Swanson NA, eds. Local Flaps in Facial Reconstruction, Mosby, CV: St. Louis, 1995:275–302.
5. Hurwitz JJ, Corin SM, Tucker SM. The use of free periosteal grafts in extensive lower lid reconstruction. Ophthalm Surg. 1989; 20:415–419.
6. Holck DE, Foster JA, Dutton JJ, Dillon HD. Hard palate mucosal grafts in the treatment of the contracted socket. Ophthal. Plast. Reconstr. Surg. 1999; 15:202–209.
7. Maloof A, Ng S, Leatherbarrow B. The maximal Hughes procedure. Ophthal. Plast. Reconstr. Surg. 2001; 17:96–102.
8. Hawes MJ, Jamell GA. Complications of tarsoconjunctival grafts. Ophthal. Plast. Reconstr. Surg. 1996; 12:45–50.
9. Stephenson CM, Brown BZ. The use of tarsus as a free autogenous graft in eyelid surgery. Ophthal Plast Reconstr Surg 1985; 1:43–50.
10. Cutler NI, Beard CA. Method for partial and total upper lid reconstruction. Am J Ophthalmol 1955; 39:1.
11. Mustarde JC. Reconstruction of the eyelids and eyebrows. In: Grabb WC, Smith JW, eds. Plastic Surgery, London: J & A. Churchill, 1968:393–414.
12. Mustarde JC. Repair and Reconstruction in the Orbital Region. 2 ed. Livingstone: Churchill, 1980.
13. Moy RL, Ashjian AA. Periorbital reconstruction [Review]. J Dermatol Surg Oncol 1991; 17:153–159.
14. Bucko CD. Bipedicle upper eyelid flap (Tripier) for lower eyelid reconstruction. In: Strauch B, Vasconez LO, eds. 2. Grabb's Encyclopedia of Flap, Philadelphia: Lippincott-Raven, 1998:72–74.
15. Woodburne RT. Essentials of Human Anatomy, 7 ed. New York: Oxford University Press, 1983:226–227.
16. Burget GC, Menick FJ. Aesthetic restoration of one-half the upper lip. Plast Reconstr Surg 1986; 78:583–593.
17. Iwahira Y, Maruyama Y, Yoshitake M. A miniunit approach to lip reconstruction. Plas Reconst Surg 1994; 93:1282–1285.
18. Essentials of Human Anatomy. 7 ed.Essentials of Human Anatomy. New York: Oxford University Press Inc, 1983, 202–203.
19. Guerrerosantos J. Tongue mucosal and musculomucosal flap for lip reconstruction. In: Strauch B, Vasconez LO, eds. 2 ed. Grabb's Encyclopedia of Flaps, Philadelphia: Lippincott-Raven, 1998:627–632.

20. Ohtsuka H, Nakaoka H. Bilateral vermilion flaps for lower lip repair. Plast Reconstr Surg 1990; 85:453–456.
21. Converse JM. Surgical Treatment of Facial Injuries. Baltimore: Williams & Wilkins, 1959, 795.
22. Donelan MB. Reconstruction of electrical burns of the oral commissure with a ventral tongue flap. Plast Reconstr Surg 1995; 95:1155–1164.
23. Johanson B, Aspelund E, Breine U, Holmstrom H. Surgical treatment of non-traumatic lower lip lesions with special reference to the step technique. A follow-up on 149 patients. Scand J Plast Reconstr Surg 1974; 8:232–240.
24. Kuttenberger JJ, Hardt N. Results of a modified staircase technique for reconstruction of the lower lip. Cranio-Maxillo-Facial Surg 1997; 25:239–244.
25. Tobin GR. Functional lower lip and oral sphincter reconstruction with innervated depressor anguli oris flaps. In: Strauch B, Vasconez LO, eds. 2 ed. Grabb's Encyclopedia of Flaps, Philadelphia: Lippincott-Raven, 1998:595–599.
26. Serletti JM, Tavin E, Moran SL, Coniglio JU. Total lower lip reconstruction with a sensate composite radial forearm–palmaris longus free flap and a tongue flap. Plast Reconstr Surg 1997; 99:559–561.
27. Serletti JM, Coniglio JU, Tavin E, Bakamjian VY. Simultaneous transfer of free fibula and radial forearm flaps for complex oromandibular reconstruction. J Reconstr Microsurg 1998; 14:297–303.
28. Yotsuyanagi T, Yokoi K, Urushidate S, Sawada Y. Functional and aesthetic reconstruction using a nasolabial orbicularis oris myocutaneous flap for large defects of the upper lip. Plast Reconstr Surg 1998; 101:1624–1629.
29. Baker SR, Krause CJ. Pedicle flaps in reconstruction of the lip. Facial Plast Surg 1984; 1:61–68.
30. Bakamjian VY. A two-staged method for pharyngoesophageal reconstruction with a primary pectoral skin flap. Plast Reconstr Surg 1965; 36:173.
31. Karapandzic M. Reconstruction of lip defects by local arterial flaps. Br J Plast Surg 1974; 27:93–97.
32. Abbe R. A new plastic operation for the relief of deformity due to double harelip. Med Rec 1898; 53:477.
33. Millard DR. Lip-switch Abbe flap for philtrum. In: Strauch B, Vasconez LO, eds. 2 ed. Grabb's Encyclopedia of Flaps, Philadelphia, : Lippincott-Raven, 1998:547–548.
34. Rea JL, Davis WE, Rittenhouse LK. Reinnervation of an Abbe-Estlander and a Gillies fan flap of the lower lip: electromyographic comparison. Arch Otolaryngol 1978; 104:294–295.
35. Estlander JA. Eine methods aus der einen lippe substanzverluste der anderen zu ersetzen. Arch Klin Chir 1872; 14:622.
36. Bernard C. Cancer de la levre inferieure aperee par un procede nouveau. Bull Mem Soc Chir Paris 1853; 3:337–343.
37. Webster R, Coffey RJ, Kellcher RE. Total and partial reconstruction of the lower lip with innervated muscle-bearing flaps. Plast Reconstr Surg 1960; 25:360.
38. Williams EF, Setzen G, Mulvaney MJ. Modified Bernard-Burow cheek advancement and cross-lip flap for total lip reconstruction. Arch Otolaryngol Head Neck Surg 1996; 122:1253–1258.
39. Stranc MF, Robertson GA. Steeple flap reconstruction of the lower lip. Ann Plast Surg 1983; 10:4–11.
40. Tobin GR, O'Daniel TG. Lip reconstruction with motor and sensory innervated composite flaps. Clin Plast Surg 1990; 17:623–632.
41. Moschella F, Cordova A. Platysma muscle cutaneous flap for large defects of the lower lip and mental region. Plast Reconstr Surg 1998; 101:1803–1809.
42. Yilmaz M, Menderes A, Barutcu A. Submental artery island flap for reconstruction of the lower and mid face. Ann Plast Surg 1997; 39:30–35.

8
Regional and Free Flaps

Robert W. Dolan
Lahey Clinic Medical Center, Burlington, Massachusetts, U.S.A.

MUSCULOCUTANEOUS FLAPS

To enhance the survival of extended skin flaps, Owens (1) incorporated underlying muscle and the musculocutaneous vessels. This report led to several applications of musculocutaneous flaps including one of the most useful flaps in head and neck reconstruction: the pectoralis musculocutaneous flap (2).

The skin component of a musculocutaneous flap is supplied via musculocutaneous arterial perforators from a source artery. These perforators may supply the skin either indirectly or directly. Indirect perforators supply the skin through terminal arteries whose main purpose is to supply the underlying muscle. Direct perforators either follow intermuscular septa or pierce muscles en route; their main purpose is to supply the overlying skin (e.g., the deltopectoral flap) (3). Musculocutaneous flaps are categorized by Mathes and Nahai (4) including the following types:

I. Single dominant pedicle as sole blood supply to the flap (e.g., tensor fascia lata)
II. One dominant pedicle and multiple minor pedicles that cannot support the flap if the dominant pedicle is severed (e.g., trapezius)
III. Dual dominant pedicles (e.g., rectus)
IV. Multiple segmental pedicles (e.g., sartorius)
V. One dominant pedicle and several segmental pedicles, either of which is capable of supporting the tissue (e.g., pectoralis major, latissimus)

Axial pattern skin flaps that are supplied at their base by indirect musculocutaneous perforators are considered musculocutaneous flaps, most notably (in the head and neck) the nasolabial musculocutaneous flap (5) and the forehead flap. These local axial pattern flaps may also be considered lifting flaps either of the transposition or interpolation type depending on flap design.

Fasciocutaneous Flaps

The concept of including the deep fascia to extend the length-to-width ratio is described by Ponten (6) and further subclassified by Cormack et al. (7) into four types, each representing a specific pattern of blood supply:

A. Multiple perforators at base (e.g., medial thigh flap)
B. Single vascular perforator (e.g., parascapular flap)
C. Segmental arterial vascular supply (e.g., radial forearm)
D. Type C with bone (e.g., osteoseptocutaneous radial forearm or fibula)

There is controversy over what constitutes a true fasciocutaneous flap. Several cutaneous flaps are harvested with fascia; however, Cormack believes that to be classified as a fasciocutaneous flap the source artery must reach the skin via intermuscular septa, and the skin must be dependent on the underlying deep fascial vascular network to survive (8). The dominant vascularity of fascial flaps is in the prefascial plexus. This deep fascial network is found most prominently around the shoulders and extremities where the skin is tightly adherent to the underlying deep fascia (whereas the subdermal vascular plexuses tend to be dominant in loose-skinned areas such as the torso) (3). Rigorous application of the definition of a fasciocutaneous flap would include only extremity and shoulder girdle skin flaps that derive their blood supply from direct arteries via intermuscular septa.

Some flaps, composed of only skin and fascia, defy classification; they cannot strictly be classified as fasciocutaneous flaps since the level of the dominant vascular plexus is subdermal (e.g., lateral intercostal flap and the deltopectoral flap) (9). The source arteries reach the skin by direct perforators through inter/intramuscular septa. The classification of these skin flaps is unresolved in the literature. Despite the common reference to the deltopectoral flap as a fasciocutaneous flap, it cannot technically be considered a true fasciocutaneous flap because it does not depend on the deep fascial vascular plexus for survival. No resolution to this confusion in nomenclature can be offered based on the modern vernacular of flap classification; however, it is reasonable to refer to these types of flaps as axial skin flaps.

Microvascular Free Flaps

The first reported microsurgical free flap transfer was for esophageal reconstruction using a jejunal segment in 1957. However, this method of flap transfer by tissue transplantation did not become popular until the early 1970s. Today, it has a pre-eminent role in many cases of head and neck reconstruction. Many of the traditionally regional musculocutaneous and fasciocutaneous flaps can be used as free tissue transfers throughout the head and neck (e.g., a free latissimus dorsi transferred to a large scalp defect). During the 1970s and 1980s, flap success continued to increase (to 98% in most large series today). Our increasing understanding of skin flap vascularity has resulted in the discovery of many new potential donor sites. Over the last several years, however, certain donor sites have become preferred based on ease of harvest, quality of the donor vessels, donor site morbidity, and needs at the recipient site. The vast majority of head and neck defects can be reconstructed using only six flaps, including the osteocutaneous fibular flap, fasciocutaneous radial forearm flap, musculocutaneous rectus flap, jejunal flap, osteomusculocutaneous scapular system of flaps (including the latissimus), and osteomusculocutaneous iliac crest flap (10).

The principal indication for microvascular free tissue transfer is immediate reconstruction of complex oncological surgical defects. Typical surgical defects or conditions that mandate free tissue transfer include composite mandibulectomy, pharyngoesophagectomy, partial and total glossectomy, selected cases of facial paralysis, extensive cranial base resections, extensive scalp loss, and total composite maxillectomy.

Future Directions

Further advances in flap classification are on the horizon. The reverse pedicled fasciocutaneous flap for lower limb reconstruction has recently been described (11). The artery is based distally, and the multiple interconnections between the venae comitantes allow the venous effluent to bypass the venular valves. Another flap that will likely gain in popularity and add to our understanding of flap physiology and classification is the venous flap (12,13). A venous flap survives as an island based only on proximal and distal venous connections with no arterial inflow. This research may also reveal new concepts regarding microcirculation.

REGIONAL FLAPS

Latissimus

Description

This type of V flap was first described as a pedicled flap for breast reconstruction in 1896 by Tansini (14) and as a free flap in 1978 by Maxwel et al. (15) (Fig. 1). The latissimus muscle is broad and flat, taking origin from multiple structures including the lumbodorsal fascia, the lower thoracic spinous processes, the posterior iliac crest, the lower four ribs, and the tip of the scapula. It inserts into the intertubercular groove of the posterior humerus. The latissimus serves to help stabilize the shoulder and inwardly rotate and adduct the arm (e.g., important in operating a wheelchair).

Indications

As a regional flap, the latissimus muscle and musculocutaneous flaps are seldom used. The flap has been applied to various defects requiring a relatively large amount of soft tissue, especially over the lateral skull base and neck. The latissimus has infrequently been used for reconstruction of the tongue and floor of mouth. With regard to regional flaps, the pectoralis major is just as useful and easier to harvest. In addition, a latissimus flap is prone to venous congestion because the vascular pedicle is subject to compression as the flap is passed under the axilla. This problem is avoided when the flap is transferred as free tissue.

Neurovascular Anatomy

The blood supply to the latissimus muscle is the thoracodorsal artery (subscapular artery) with its lateral and medial branches. The muscle can be split longitudinally, supplied separately by these branches, if desired. The thoracodorsal vein runs with the artery and is relatively large (2–4 mm) near its origin from the subscapular vein. The sensory nerves originate from intercostal nerve perforators but they are small and exceedingly difficult to incorporate with the flap. The thoracodorsal nerve, however, is large and branches are harvestable that innervate separate segments of muscle.

Advantages

The major advantage of this muscle is its broad shape that is ideal for covering large surface defects (Fig. 2). Primary closure of the donor site is possible, except in cases requiring an exceptionally large skin paddle (over 9 cm depending on the surrounding skin laxity and patient habitus).

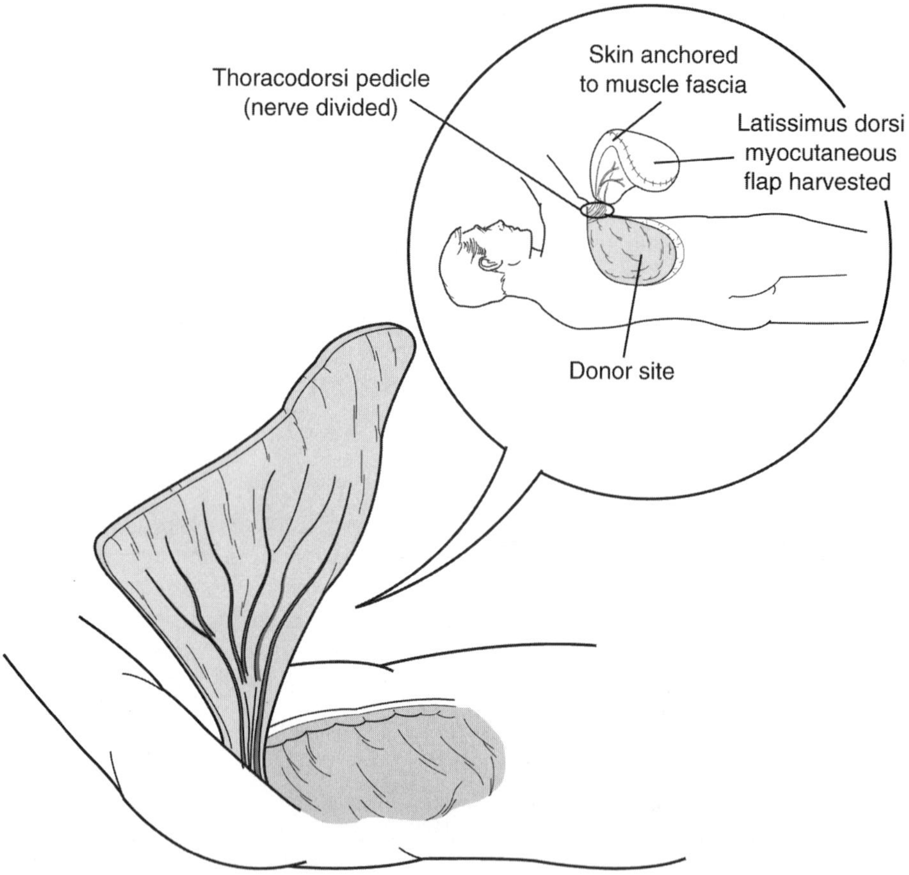

Figure 1 Harvested pedicled latissimus muscle flaps showing large fanlike anatomy. Note the large thoracodorsal pedicle.

Disadvantages

The main disadvantage to using the latissimus flap is the risk of vascular compression and flap loss. The vascular pedicle is subject to compression as it passes under the axilla. The patient must be placed in a lateral decubitus position to harvest the flap and the access incision along the axillary fold is lengthy. The donor site has a propensity to form seromas often requiring prolonged ($>$ 1 week) placement of suction drains. Brachial plexus shearing or stretch injury may occur if precautions are not taken including head flexion and shoulder/axilla support during flap harvest. Loss of the latissimus muscle results in little functional morbidity except in those patients who require the specific actions provided by this muscle including wheelchair users, swimmers, or construction workers.

Sternocleidomastoid

Description

The sternocleidomastoid flap is a type IV musculocutaneous flap that been used in reconstructing oral and cheek defects since 1955 (1). The muscle extends from an

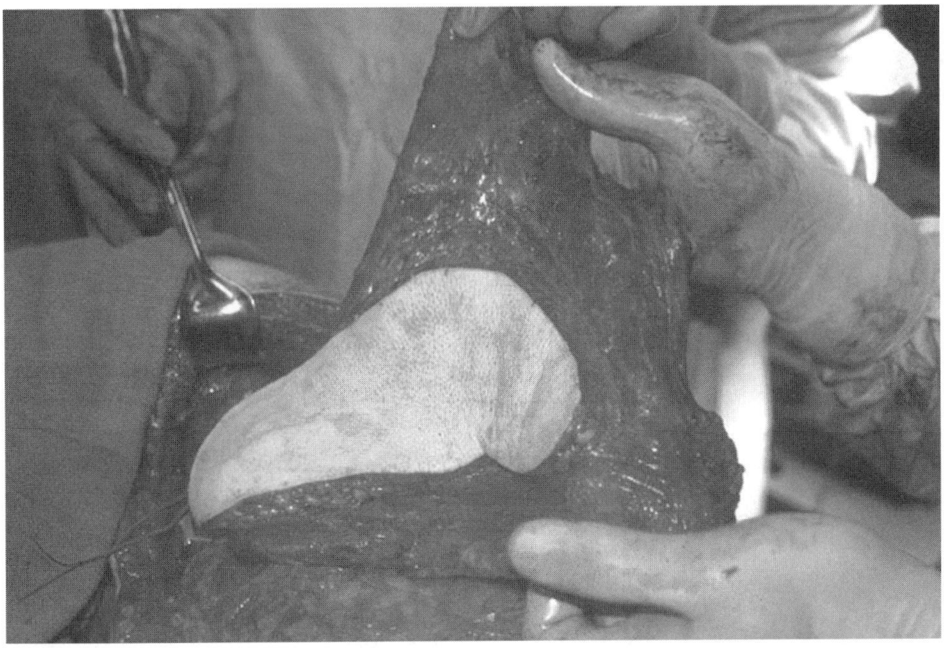

Figure 2 Pedicled latissimus musculocutaneous flap showing large expanse of muscle with a central skin island.

inferomedial attachment to the clavicle and sternum to a superolateral attachment to the mastoid process. The muscle is usually pedicled superiorly for oral defects, taking advantage of its superiorly oriented blood supply.

Indications

This flap is able to reach the ipsilateral cheek, mandible, and intraoral defects extending from the retromolar trigone to the contralateral floor of mouth. The flap will also cover selected cervical defects within its arc of rotation. Because of serious drawbacks listed below, the flap is rarely used.

Neurovascular Anatomy

The blood supply is from branches of the occipital, superior thyroid, and thyrocervical trunk arteries (Fig. 3). Preserving two-thirds of the vascular sources is necessary to ensure viability, especially for musculocutaneous flaps. The nerve supply is from a branch off the spinal accessory nerve. Preservation of the innervation to the muscle is not necessary for the application of this flap.

Advantages

It is local tissue for potential one-staged reconstruction of oropharyngeal defects. The donor site (neck) may be closed primarily.

Disadvantages

The major disadvantage is that its use may interfere with an oncological neck operation. The reliability of this flap is also a major drawback, especially if the neck has been previously irradiated. The arc of rotation is necessarily limited because of the

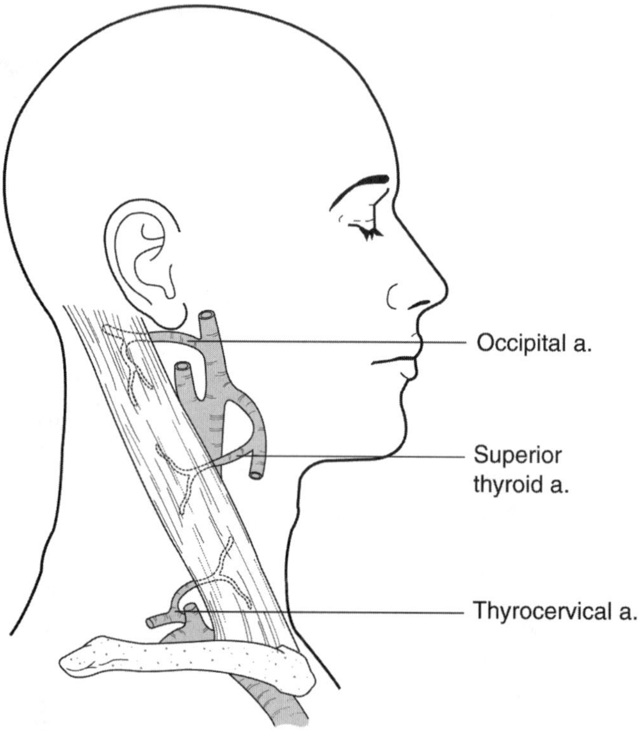

Figure 3 Three arteries principally supply the sternocleidomastoid muscle: (1) occipital, (2) superior thyroid, and (3) thyrocervical. Two of three of these arteries must remain intact to ensure viability of this flap.

blood supply requirements. This flap can only support a small cutaneous island of no more than 3–4 cm.

Pectoralis Major

Description

The pectoralis major is a type V musculocutaneous flap originally reported by Ariyan in 1979 (2). The pectoralis muscle over the anterior chest wall takes origin from the lateral sternum, the second through the sixth ribs, and medial clavicle and inserts into the upper humerus. Underlying rib may be harvested with this flap based on its (tenuous) periosteal blood supply.

The first step in harvesting the pectoralis major flap is to outline on the skin the expected course of the vascular pedicle and the size and configuration of the skin paddle. The course of the vessels under the muscle extends along a line dropped from the midclavicle towards the nipple; the vessels then turn medial on a line from the acromion to the xiphoid process. The design of the skin paddle is usually a simple ellipse oriented along the vascular line medial to the nipple and above the inferior border of the muscle (superior border of the rectus sheath). A variety of skin paddle designs can be harvested as well as separate skin islands over the proximal muscle for separate defects or for inner and outer lining (16,17). An incision is then designed to extend from the superior border of the skin paddle in a superolateral direction to facilitate flap harvest toward the base of the vascular pedicle. The incision should either stop or curve away laterally from the inferior border of a potential deltopectoral flap that may be needed in the future (Fig. 4). The skin paddle–muscle unit is raised distal to proximal by outlining muscular incisions that preserve the vascular pedicle under direct vision. Once the skin paddle–muscular unit is freed to the clavicle, it is passed under the neck–chest skin bridge and over the clavicle to reach the head and neck. The donor site is almost always closed primarily facilitated by widely undermining and advancing the surrounding skin.

Indications

The pectoralis major flap is one of the most common flaps used for head and neck reconstruction. It is used to reconstruct through-and-through oropharyngeal,

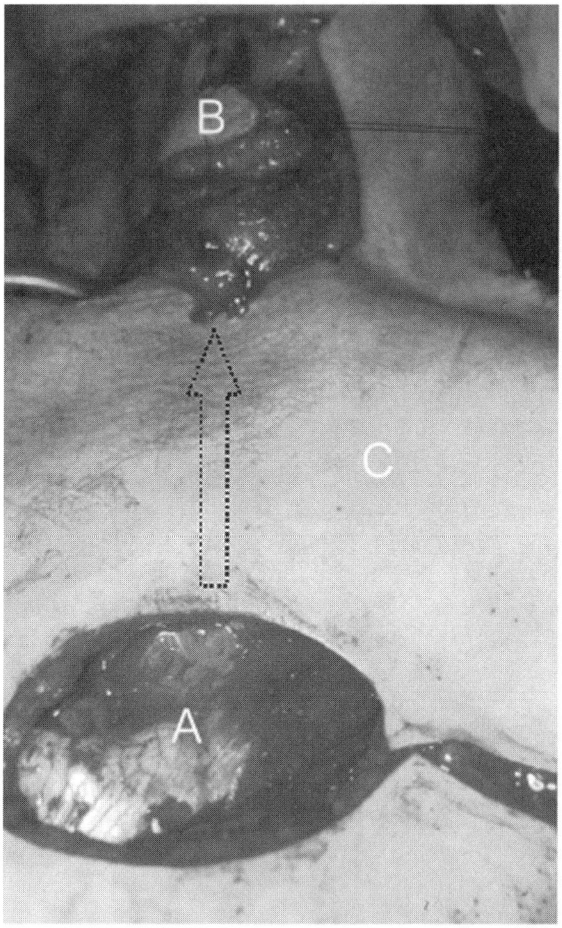

Figure 4 A harvested and transferred pectoralis major musculocutaneous flap. Note the harvest site (A) and the lateral incision for access to the vascular pedicle. The dotted arrow represents the subcutaneous course of the transferred skin paddle (B). Note also that the lateral access incision does not violate the territory of the deltopectoral flap (C), in case this flap is needed in the future.

lateral skull (temporal bone), neck skin, noncircumferential esophageal, and mandibular defects. It may be considered the flap of choice for posterior mandibular composite defects, tongue replacement in total glossectomy–laryngeal defects, significant base of tongue defects, and noncircumferential esophageal defects. The pectoralis flap is not easily formed into a tube, making it unsuitable for circumferential esophageal defect reconstruction. Attempts lead to strictures and intractable dysphagia.

Neurovascular Anatomy

The motor supply comes from the lateral and medial pectoral nerves from the brachial plexus. The medial pectoral nerve supplies and then passes through the pectoralis minor muscle to reach the pectoralis major muscle. This nerve is visualized and cut to free the vascular pedicle completely. The lateral pectoral nerve pierces the costocoracoid membrane to reach the pectoralis muscle, coursing with the vessels. If this nerve is cut, atrophy of the muscle can be expected (and may be desirable in many circumstances). The pectoral branches of thoracoacromial artery (from the axillary artery) supply the muscle after coursing medial to the insertion of the pectoralis minor muscle. The lateral thoracic artery (from the axillary artery) also supplies the muscle after coursing lateral to the insertion of the pectoralis minor muscle. Although the lateral thoracic artery may be more prominent in some patients, especially females, preservation is unnecessary despite some surgeon's admonitions regarding its potential dominant role (16). In addition, preserving the lateral thoracic pedicle significantly limits the rotation and reach of the flap.

Advantages

The donor site can easily be hidden under clothing, and the loss of the muscle is well tolerated. The flap is easy to harvest and reaches the most common areas of the head and neck that require tissue of this quality and quantity. The vascular anatomy is very reliable and the flap is robust.

Disadvantages

The vascular supply to the rib via the periosteum is tenuous and its use for mandibular segmental defects is associated with a high rate of failure. Marginal necrosis of the skin paddle is relatively common, especially if the distal part of the skin paddle extends beyond the underlying muscle (18). The subcutaneous tissue can be bulky, especially in women in whom the incisional scars may be less acceptable. The weight of the flap and the tendency for regional flaps to return to their site of origin result in an inferior migration of flap tissue. This is well tolerated for posteriorly oriented defects; however, reconstruction of anteriorly oriented defects, especially around the mandibular symphysis, may result in neck contracture, jaw contracture, or exposure of underlying plates and bone grafts.

Deltopectoral

Description

The deltopectoral flap, originally reported by Bakamjian, is an axial skin flap supplied by parasternal direct cutaneous perforators (19). The flap is composed of the fascia overlying the pectoralis major, subcutaneous tissue, and skin (Fig. 5). It is based along the parasternal area over the first through the fourth intercostal spaces

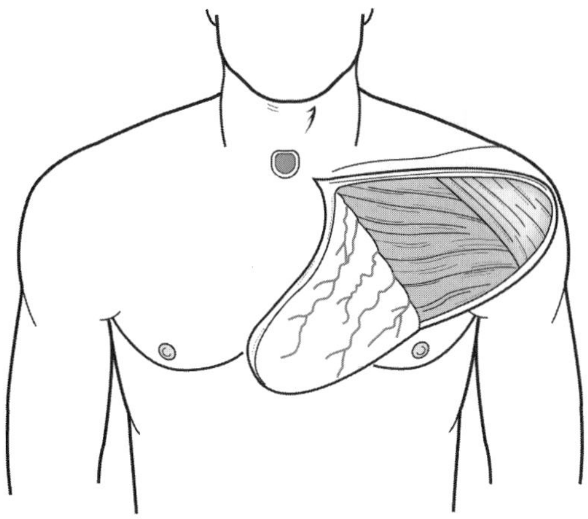

Figure 5 The deltopectoral flap is a medially based flap supplied by the intercostal perforators, predominantly the second intercostal perforator. The flap is raised off the medial aspect of the deltoid muscle and the pectoralis. Extension much beyond the medial aspect of the deltoid muscle places the distal aspect of the flap at risk for necrosis if no delay is used.

and extends laterally with equal width toward the shoulder. The flap is usually transferred as a staged transposition flap, but may also be islanded for single-stage transfer or as a free flap (20). The flap can be extended over the tip of the shoulder; however, this extension will encompass a third angiosome and put this distal part at significant risk of necrosis. Surgical delay is effective in augmenting the flap to capture this third angiosome. The delay may be accomplished by simply ligating the thoracoacromial vessels or partially elevating the flap to sever these vessels. Simply performing the skin incisions alone may be effective without cutting the thoracoacromial vessels (21).

Indications

The original principal indication for the deltopectoral flap was for staged circumferential esophageal reconstruction. This was a significant advance and inspired the development of several subsequent landmark advances in head and neck reconstructive surgery. Today, the deltopectoral flap serves a secondary role in lower neck skin coverage or as a salvage procedure if first-line flaps fail. It may be used as external cover with the pectoralis flap to reconstruct combined cervical esophageal and neck skin defects (Fig. 6). As an island, it is very useful for paratracheal coverage.

Neurovascular Anatomy

The blood supply to the deltopectoral flap is from the first through the fourth perforating vessels from the internal mammary artery. The dominant perforator is usually the second and this vessel supplies the island and free flap (Fig. 7). It is a nonsensate flap.

Advantages

It is a robust flap that can be transferred in its islanded form or as a free flap. The proximal part can be de-epithelialized and left under an intact intervening skin bridge.

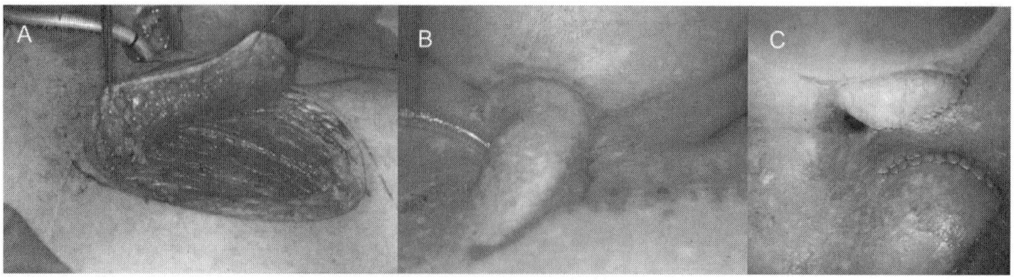

Figure 6 A staged deltopectoral flap used to resurface a recently closed salivary fistula superolateral to the tracheostomy. The fasciocutaneous flap is raised lateral-to-medial directly over the pectoralis muscle (A). The flap is transferred in an intermediate stage (B). After 3 weeks the pedicle is divided, leaving the distal skin intact over the defect (C).

Disadvantages

Extending the flap beyond the deltopectoral groove places the distal portion at risk for necrosis; certainly any part of the flap that extends beyond the tip of the shoulder must be surgically delayed. The donor site requires a skin graft except in cases where a short island flap is uscd. Thc sccond pcrforator is small (1 mm) and may be technically difficult to use as a free flap.

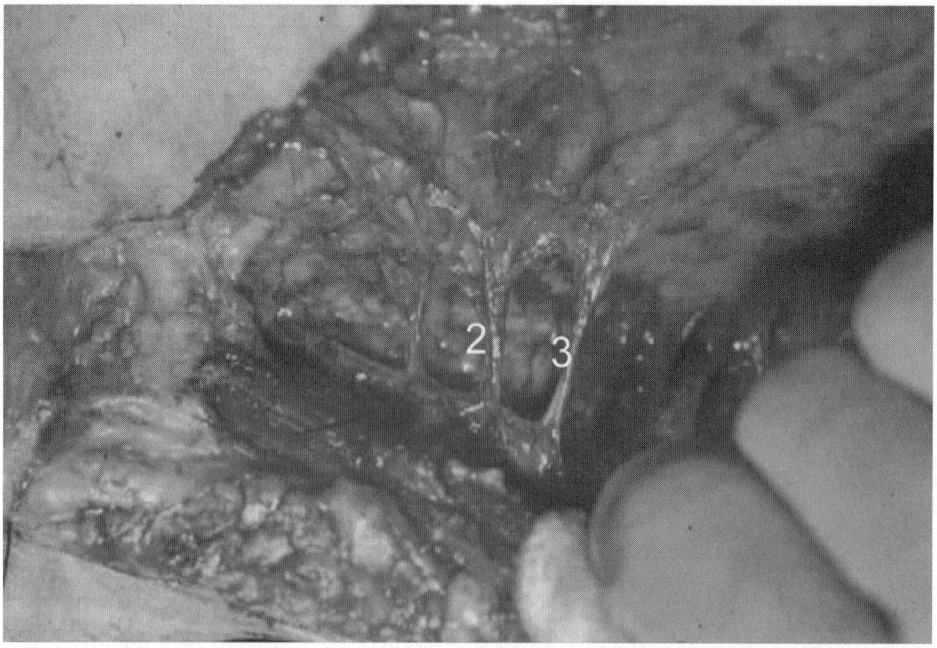

Figure 7 Intercostal perforators from the internal mammary supplying the deltopectoral flap. The second perforator (2) is usually the largest.

Forehead (Temporal)

Description

The forehead flap is a type III musculocutaneous flap encompassing all the layers of the forehead except the periosteum. The flap is based laterally (whereas the midforehead flap is based centrally) and is oriented horizontally across the forehead, often extending beyond the midline (Fig. 8). The flap may be used in one-stage reconstruction as a transposition or turnover flap or in two-stage reconstruction as an interpolation flap (common in nasal reconstruction). The undersurface of the flap may be skin grafted for through-and-through defects of the cheek or nose.

Indications

This flap is mainly of historical interest only. The forehead flap will cover ipsilateral cheek, eye, and nasal defects. It has also been used for reconstruction of defects involving the lateral floor of mouth, inner cheek, retromolar trigone, and the soft palate.

Neurovascular Anatomy

The forehead flap is based on both the parietal and temporal branches of the superficial temporal artery. It is nonsensate.

Advantages

The forehead flap is very similar to the color and texture of normal facial skin. The flap is very robust and provides an abundant amount of tissue for lateral and midface reconstruction.

Disadvantages

The major disadvantage in using the forehead flap is the unsightly skin-grafted donor site.

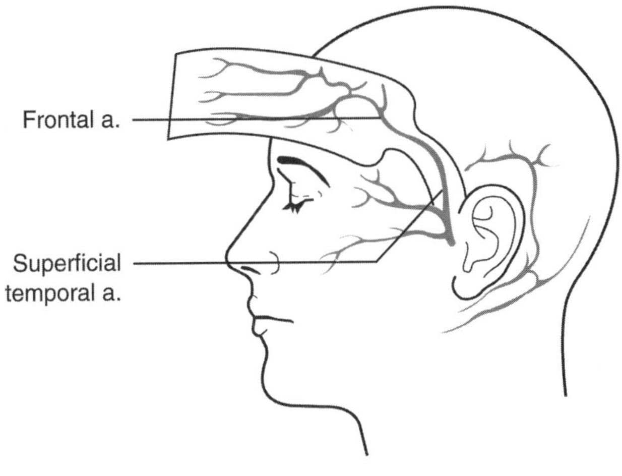

Figure 8 The forehead flap (as opposed to the medial or paramedian forehead flap) is based laterally on the superficial temporal artery. It is seldom used today because of the availability of other flaps and the significant donor site morbidity (primarily cosmetic). It was mainly used for tonsillar and retromolar trigone defects.

Temporalis Muscle

Description

This type III flap was first described by Golovine in 1898 for obliteration of dead space after orbital exenteration (22). The origin of the temporalis muscle is the temporal line and part of the inferior zygomatic arch as the muscle passes under this structure. The muscle is shaped like an inverted triangle and inserts onto the coronoid process and ramus of the mandible. The approach to harvesting the muscle is through a temporal rhytidectomy incision and subperiosteal dissection to protect the neurovascular bundle that travels on the undersurface of the muscle. Dissection superficial to the muscle should proceed under the superficial temporal fascia, preserving this structure. To facilitate the muscle's movement into the oral cavity, a segment of the zygomatic arch and the coronoid are removed, and a tunnel is created bluntly between the temporal fossa, over the masseter muscle, and into the oral cavity. The zygomatic arch may be replaced; however, the muscle itself fills this defect with little residual depression. The available surface area in the oral cavity for coverage is approximately $4 \times 5\,\text{cm}$ (23). A split-thickness skin graft may be placed over the muscle 10–14 days prior to the definitive harvest to reduce secondary healing, granulation tissue, and unwanted adhesions at the recipient site (24). However, this muscle re-epithelializes well in the oral cavity despite a large expanse of uncovered surface. Finally, the temporalis muscle may be harvested with a vascularized periosteal–split calvarial bone graft superior to the temporal line, if needed.

Indications

The primary indications for the temporalis muscle flap are for intraoral, cranial base, and, as originally described, orbital reconstructions (25,26) (Fig. 9). The use of split temporalis muscle as a sling for the lower eyelid and lip in facial paralysis is another common indication: some dynamic movement is possible through the V_3 branch of the trigeminal nerve (Fig. 10). Less common indications are for palate and maxillary reconstructions (27,28).

Neurovascular Anatomy

The arterial supply to the temporalis flap is via the anterior and posterior branches of the deep temporal artery (a branch of the second division of the maxillary artery) and the middle temporal artery (a branch of the superficial temporal artery). The middle temporal artery is sacrificed in most circumstances of flap transfer. The motor supply is the third division of the trigeminal nerve. No sensory component is described.

Advantages

The advantages of the temporalis flap include its proximity to common defects of the head and neck. It is technically easy to harvest and has a robust blood supply. The muscle and fascia are easily draped over defects with little tendency to retract toward the donor site. The nature of the blood supply allows longitudinal splitting of the muscle into segments supplied by the posterior and anterior branches of the deep temporal artery. This allows independent reconstruction of independently functioning units (e.g., floor of mouth and tongue or lip and eye). The function of the mandible after harvest of this mandible is essentially unchanged.

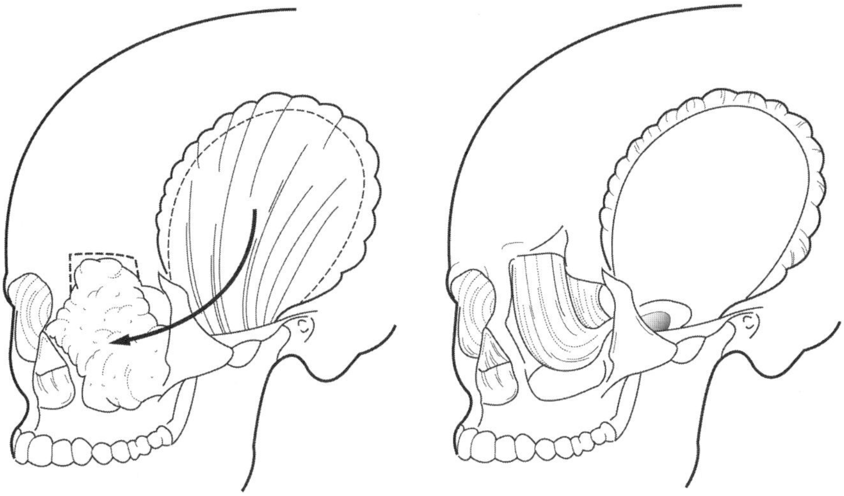

Figure 9 The temporalis muscle flap is useful for obliteration of an exenterated orbit. This is an example of one of the earliest and most useful applications of this flap.

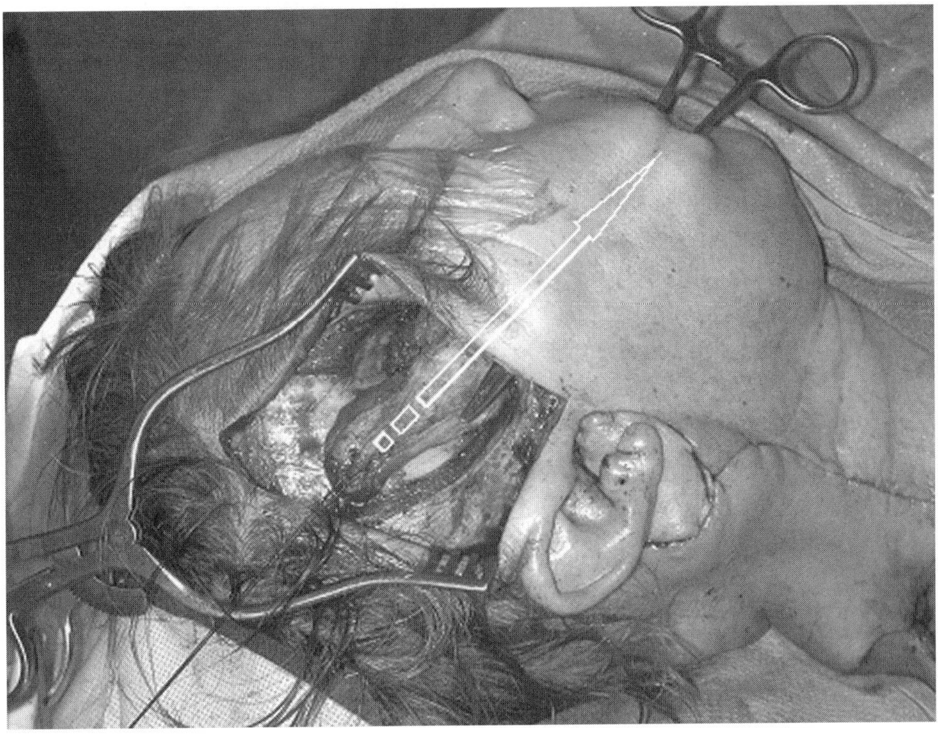

Figure 10 Temporalis sling for lip support. This patient had a radical temporal bone resection with sacrifice of the facial nerve and multiple mimetic muscles. Pictured are a freed temporalis muscle and a subcutaneous tunnel created (clamp) for transposition of the muscle into the modiolus (arrow).

Disadvantages

The most difficult problem with harvest of the temporalis flap is the hollowing of the donor site that can be a significant cosmetic deformity. If only a portion of the flap is used, or if the superficial temporal fascia is preserved, this problem is less noticeable. Immediate reconstitution of bulk in this area is possible through the use of autogenous materials such as split calvarial bone grafts or the transpositioning of galeal flaps (29). Hydroxyapatite-based pastes are also useful in providing bulk to the area (Fig. 11). This material becomes incorporated into the surrounding bone, and eventually transforms into viable bone over time. This is superior to implants such as methylmethacrylate that are encapsulated and never incorporate into the surrounding bone. Another disadvantage to the temporalis muscle flap is that the dissection anteriorly is close to the temporal branch of the facial nerve. Even temporary paralysis is uncommon. However, with overzealous retraction or dissection in the wrong plane, this nerve can be permanently injured. The nerve courses in close proximity to the superficial temporalis fascia and is avoided by dissecting anteriorly under the superficial slip of the deep temporal fascia inferior to the deep temporal fat pad.

Galeal Frontalis

Description

The galeal frontalis is a type B fascial flap similar to temporoparietal flap, and is part of the occipitofrontalis fibromuscular layer of the scalp extending from the eyebrows to the nuchal line. The flap is usually harvested directly off a coronal flap just prior to its transfer to the anterior skull base (Fig. 12). It is placed over the anterior skull base through the inferior margin of the cranial bone flap. Length can be gained posteriorly by harvesting galea–pericranial tissue behind the coronal incision (extended galeal frontalis flap) prior to elevation of the coronal flap in the subperi-

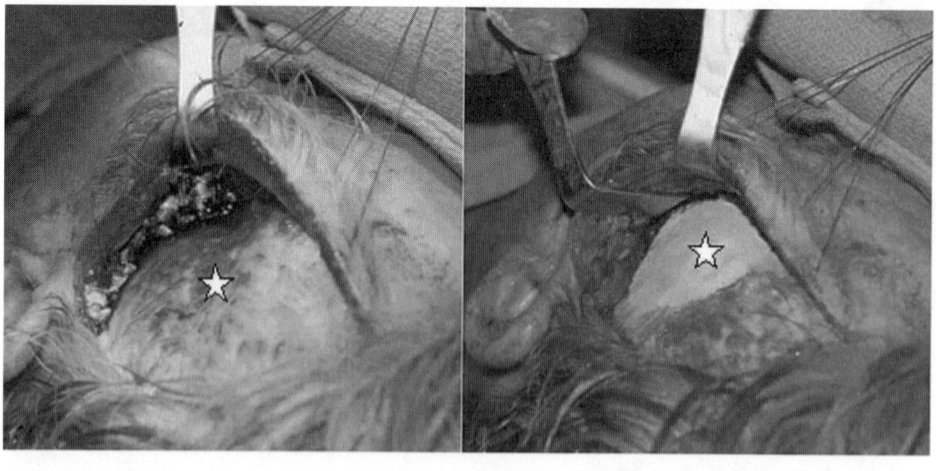

Figure 11 Hydroxyapatite paste placed into the temporalis donor site. After the harvest of the temporalis muscle, a significant volume defect is created in the temporal fossa (left star). Hydroxyapatite will effectively correct this deformity (right star) and prevent the wasted appearance in this area postoperatively.

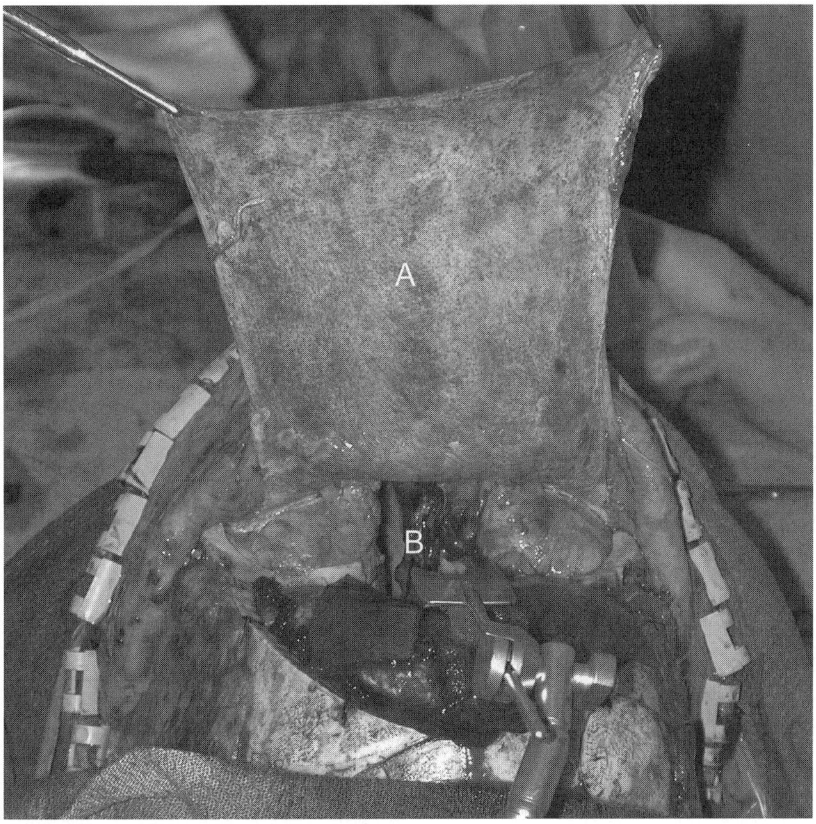

Figure 12 The galeal frontalis flap (A) used to cover an extensive craniofacial defect (B). The flap is folded into the defect to separate the cranial contents from the nose.

cranial plane. Inclusion of the pericranium may enhance flap vascularity (30), especially over the cranial summit. The width of the flap is determined by the size of the defect (between 2 and 10 cm).

Indications

The galeal frontalis flap's primary indication is for defects of the cribriform and anterior skull base. It provides highly vascularized tissue for support of free bone and fascial grafts, and will help seal cerebrospinal fluid leaks from dural dehiscence.

Neurovascular Anatomy

The galeal flap is based anteriorly on a rich vertically oriented vascular network provided by the supratrochlear and supraorbital vessels. The flap may be based unilaterally or bilaterally. The accompanying nerves are sacrificed during flap harvest.

Advantages

The galeal flap is a highly vascular soft tissue flap readily available for cranial base reconstruction after craniofacial surgery. It is technically easy to harvest and effectively isolates the nose from the cranium with hardy tissue.

Disadvantages

Although it provides good nose–anterior cranial fossa separation, it is of limited bulkiness. Therefore, if bulk is required, a free flap should be used such as the rectus myocutaneous flap or the augmented radial forearm flap. Harvest of the flap thins the scalp and may predispose the scalp to radiation-induced ischemia and necrosis. Alopecia from hair follicle injury, loss of ability to wrinkle the forehead, and neurosensory loss over forehead are additional disadvantages of the galeal flap.

Trapezius

Description

This is a type II regional musculocutaneous flap. The trapezius system of flaps includes the superior trapezius flap (31,32), the lateral island trapezius flap (33), and the lower island trapezius flap (34,35). The trapezius muscle originates from the medial one-third of the superior nuchal line and the external occipital protuberance of the occipital bone, the ligamentum nuchae, and the spines of the seventh cervical and all thoracic vertebrae. It inserts into the posterior border of the lateral one-third of the clavicle, the spine of the scapula, and the crest of the spine of the scapula (36). The trapezius muscle functions to suspend the shoulder girdle and to elevate and rotate the shoulder.

The superior trapezius flap is a musculocutaneous flap based superiorly along the nuchal line and paraspinous region. The flap drapes like a scarf to the midline of the neck. This flap should be differentiated from a nape of neck flap (Mutter's flap, 1842) that does not include the underlying trapezius muscle.

The lateral island trapezius flap is based laterally as an island of skin and muscle proximal to the acromion and spine of the scapula. The flap is mobilized along with the vascular pedicle for transfer to the ipsilateral head and neck.

The lower island trapezius flap is based on the inferior aspect of the trapezius muscle between the medial border of the scapula and the spine, often including tissue below the tip of the scapula. This flap is mobilized superiorly to the anterior border of the trapezius muscle without manipulation or mobilization of the vascular pedicle in the posterior triangle of the neck.

Indications

The most useful of the three flaps is the superior trapezius flap. Although this is not a first-line flap, it is extremely hardy and can be used after radical neck dissection. It provides coverage for difficult wounds including persistent orocutaneous fistulas and exposed carotid arteries (Figs. 13, 14).

The lateral and lower island trapezius flaps provide thin pliable tissue for reconstruction of almost any defect in the ipsilateral head and neck (Figs. 15, 16). The lower island flap is most often used for lateral skull base defects since the patient can be placed in the lateral decubitus position for both recipient site extirpation and flap harvest (Figs. 17, 18).

The anatomy of the vascular pedicle in the posterior triangle of the neck is extremely variable, and the artery or, more commonly, the vein will pass under the scalenes or brachial plexus. This limits the mobility of the vascular pedicle, thus severely limiting the use of the lateral island flap.

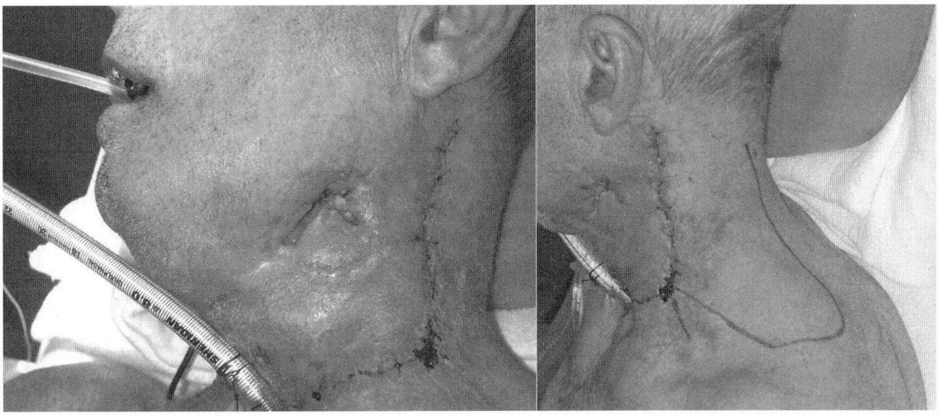

Figure 13 A superior trapezius flap is planned to repair an orocutaneous fistula. Note the penned outline of the superior trapezius flap in the photo on the right.

Neurovascular Anatomy

The motor supply is derived from the spinal accessory nerve but is sacrificed during flap harvest. The main vascular supply to the muscle is the transverse cervical artery. The transverse cervical artery runs a variable course across the posterior triangle: it originates either from the thyrocervical trunk (most commonly), directly from the subclavian artery, or as a branch of the dorsal scapular artery. At the anterior border of the levator scapulae muscle the transverse cervical artery divides into deep and superficial branches. The deep branch may arise separately from the subclavian artery as the dorsal scapular artery. The deep branch travels deep to the levator scapulae muscle and the superficial branch proceeds superficial to the levator scapulae muscle and divides into an ascending and descending branch.

The superior trapezius flap is nourished solely by the paraspinal perforators and, less so, by postauricular descending branches of the occipital artery. The lateral

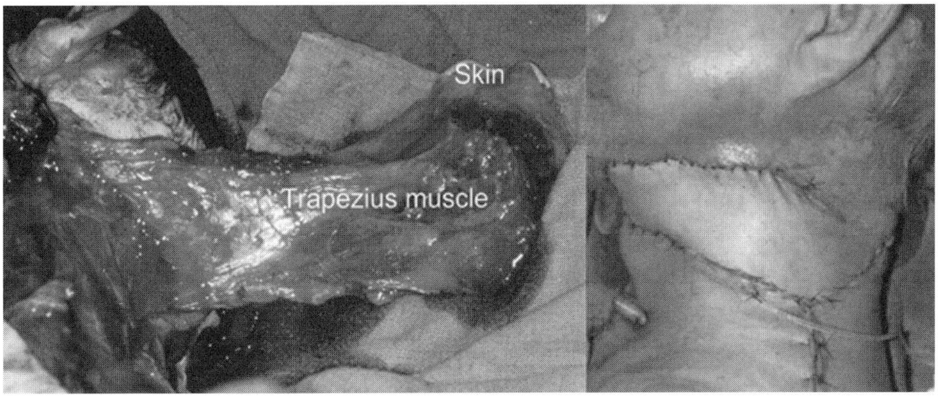

Figure 14 Harvest of the superior trapezius flap involves reflection of the trapezius muscle and overlying skin toward the nape of neck and upper paraspinal area. The flap is then folded around the neck like a scarf to close the defect (photo on right).

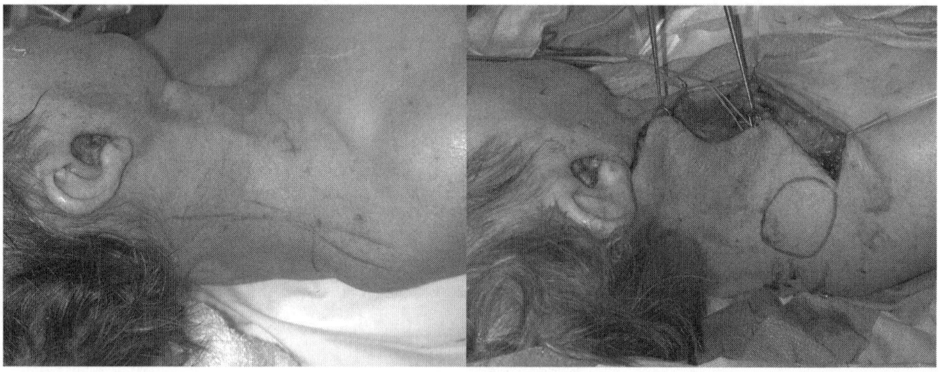

Figure 15 Lateral island trapezius flap used to repair a chronic nonhealing ulcer in a patient who received radical radiation therapy for an ear canal carcinoma. Note on right that the flap is outlined over the trapezius muscle and a skin flap is being raised over the posterior neck to locate the feeding vessels.

island trapezius flap is based on the ascending branch of the superficial transverse cervical artery.

The lower island trapezius flap is based on the descending branch of the superficial transverse cervical artery. The deep transverse cervical artery (dorsal scapular artery) passes under the lesser rhomboid muscle and sends a branch to the inferior portion of the trapezius muscle (Fig. 19). Inclusion of the dorsal scapular artery by harvesting a segment of the lesser rhomboid muscle with the artery may be desirable to ensure adequate vascularity to the distal muscle (37). However, in a large series by Urken et al., no distal flap loss occurred with sacrifice of the dorsal scapular artery if the inferior border of the flap did not extend more than 5 cm below the border of the scapula (38). The primary venous drainage comes from the transverse cervical vein. This vein runs a variable course through the posterior triangle and may not accompany the artery. It empties into either the thyrocervical trunk or into the inferior part of the external jugular vein. To ensure the viability of a lower or

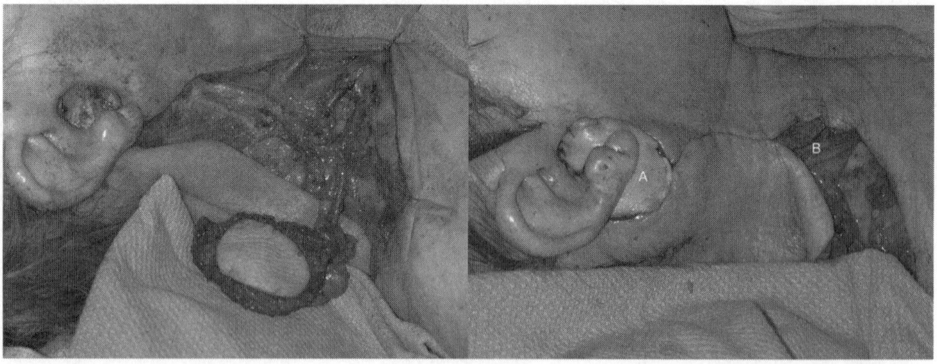

Figure 16 Lateral island trapezius flap pedicled on its feeding vessels (transverse cervical vessels, photo on left). Photo on right shows the flap in place (A) and its feeding vessels (B) under the neck flap.

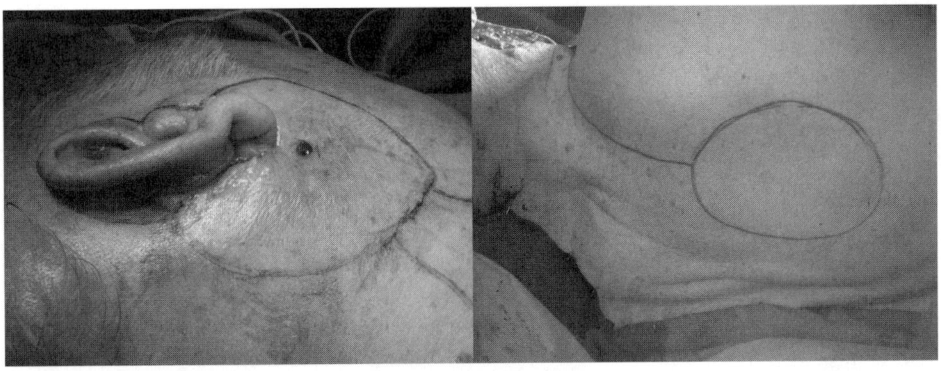

Figure 17 Lower island trapezius flap for repair of a planned temporal bone and postauricular skin excision. Note the outline of the flap (photo on right) over the lower aspect of the trapezius muscle.

lateral island flap, the inferior jugular vein must be preserved if this anatomical configuration exists which is especially important in patients undergoing neck dissection.

Advantages

Prior radical neck dissection has no bearing on the use of the superior trapezius flap; in fact, resection of the transverse cervical artery serves to delay the flap thus improving its distal vascularity (32). This flap is very hardy and will survive in open infected and irradiated wounds, making it very useful for difficult situations where soft tissue coverage is crucial in the lateral and upper neck.

The lower island trapezius flap offers thin, pliable tissue and is unaffected by variations in the anatomy of the transverse cervical artery and vein, unlike the lateral island flap. The donor site can be closed primarily and is the least conspicuous of all the trapezius family of flaps. It also offers the longest arc of rotation.

The lateral island flap also offers thin pliable tissue for a variety of defects in the ipsilateral head and neck and the patient does not have to be placed in the full lateral decubitus position for flap harvest.

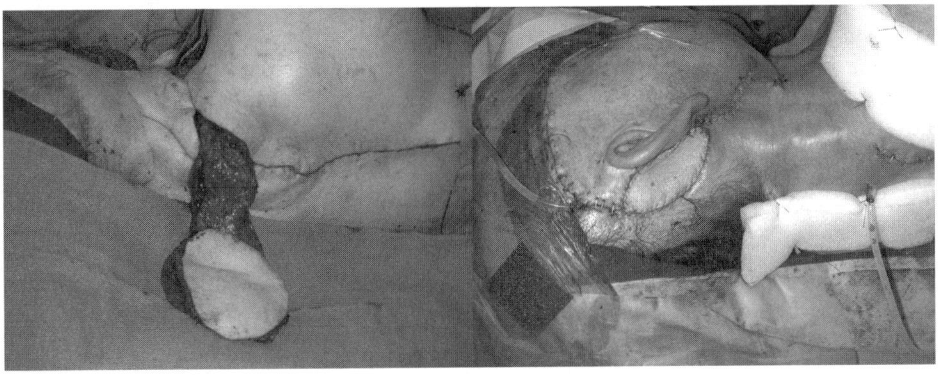

Figure 18 Lower island trapezius flap raised and pedicled before final inset on left. On right, the flap is inset to fill the defect.

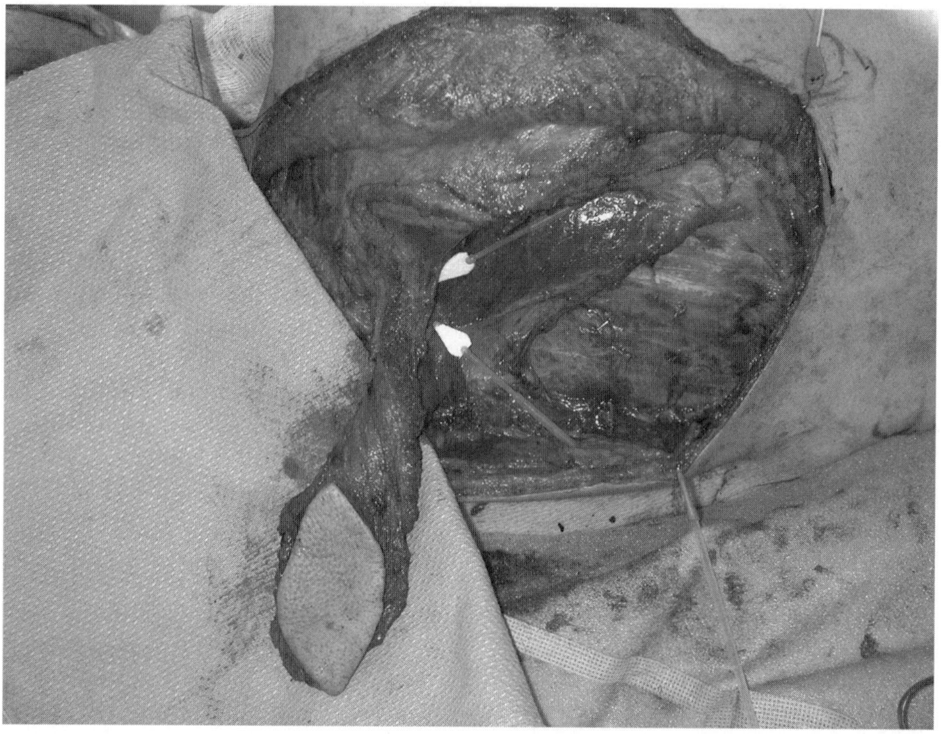

Figure 19 The dorsal scapular arterial supply to the lower island trapezius muscle (arrows).

Disadvantages

The superior trapezius flap is bulky and has a limited arc of rotation (to just above the mandibular border) and limited reach (to midline). The donor site most often needs to be skin grafted.

The lower island trapezius flaps requires the patient to be placed in a full lateral decubitus position for flap harvest. Loss of shoulder function is similar to that occurring in patients who have had their accessory nerve cut during a radical neck dissection.

The lower and lateral island flaps are unreliable in patients who have undergone an ipsilateral neck dissection, due to either venous or arterial insufficiency (38,39). Preoperative angiography is of limited usefulness since it often cannot delineate a patent transverse cervical vein. The lateral island flap is often abandoned intraoperatively due to variations in the anatomy of the transverse cervical vessels.

Temporoparietal Fascia

Description

The temporoparietal fascial flap is a type B fascial flap that is harvested as a fascia-only flap, either pedicled or free. The temporoparietal fascia is the superior extension of the superficial musculoaponeurotic system (SMAS) to the temporal line lying between the subcutaneous fat and a loose areolar plane above the temporalis muscle. The flap is harvested through the temporal extension of a face lift incision. The anterior extent of flap dissection is limited by the location of the frontal branch of the facial nerve. This branch is intimately associated with the flap and anterior flap dissection must stop short of the nerve. The course this branch can be traced by extending a line from just below the tragus to an area extending 2 cm from the lateral brow. The flap is pedicled near the upper tragus: its harvest as a free flap includes a vascular pedicle length around 6 cm.

Indications

The temporoparietal fascial flap is used most commonly to resurface pinna defects as a turndown-lining flap. As a pedicled flap it may also be used for improving facial contour after a parotidectomy, eyelid reconstruction (for which it was originally described in 1898), and resurfacing temporal facial defects providing a vascularized surface for a skin or bone grafts (Fig. 20). As a free flap, it has been used for limited defects of the nose, extremity, and hand. Overlying hair-bearing scalp can be transferred with flap if needed (see the forehead flap).

Neurovascular Anatomy

No sensory component is described. The temporoparietal fascia's blood supply is the superficial temporal artery and vein emanating from the depths of the parotid at the tragus: the vessels lie either on the surface of the fascia or within it. The superficial temporal vessels leave the fascia and enter the subdermal plane approximately 10 cm above the crus helix (40). Above the level of the zygoma, the vessels split into parietal

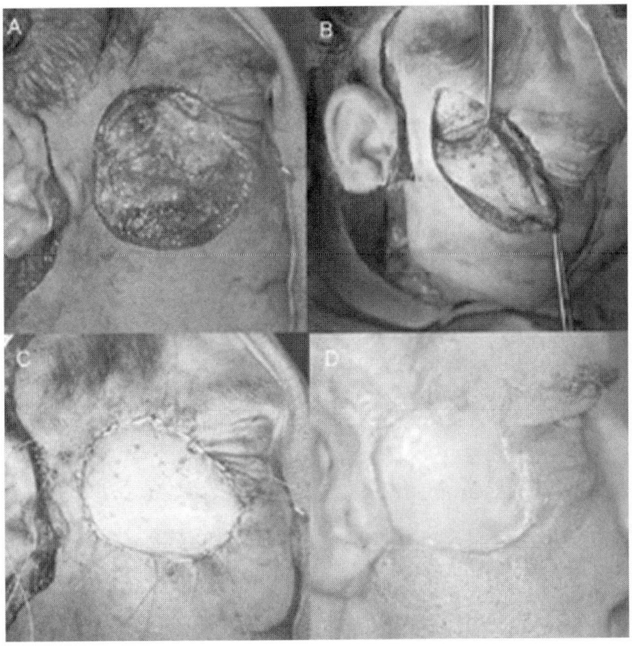

Figure 20 Temporoparietal fascial flap inset over a facial defect, providing a vascularized surface for a split-thickness skin graft. The defect (A) resulted from a wide local excision of a skin cancer; zygomatic bone was exposed. A temporoparietal fascial flap (B) was harvested and transferred over the defect. A skin graft was placed (C) and the final appearance is shown (D).

and temporal branches, allowing the fascia to be split (Fig. 21). In addition, the middle temporal artery branches from the superficial temporal artery just superior to the zygomatic arch to supply the temporalis fascia and underlying muscle. The use of the superficial layer of deep temporalis fascia and the temporoparietal fascia based on the proximal superficial temporal artery is described (41).

Advantages

The temporoparietal flap is very thin and pliable, extremely well vascularized, and able to support soft tissue and osseus grafts. Primary closure of the donor site is always possible and secondary contour defects do not occur as a result of harvesting the flap.

Disadvantages

Injury to the frontal branch of the facial nerve may occur because it is near the temporal branch of the superficial temporal artery. The skin over the flap is harvested in

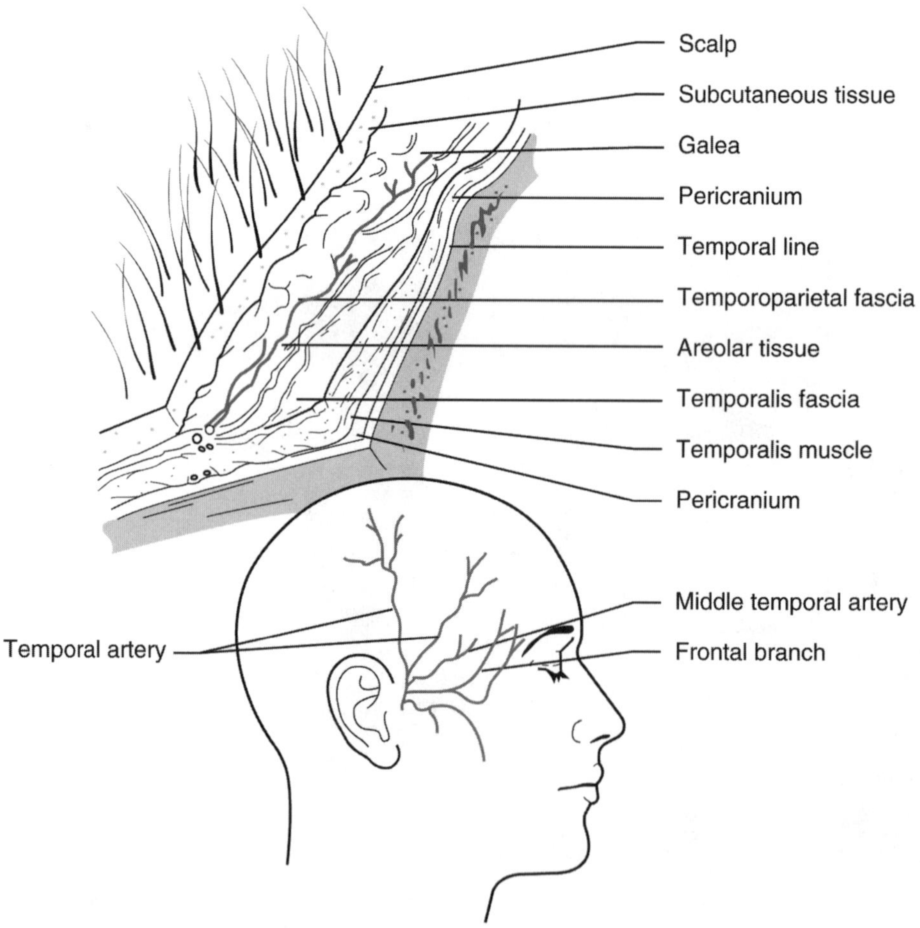

Figure 21 The depth and vascular supply of the temporoparietal fascial flap are demonstrated. Note the parietal and temporal branches of the superficial temporal artery supplying the flap.

an immediate subdermal plane occasionally leading to ischemic necrosis of the skin edges or limited alopecia. Attempts to harvest the flap beyond 12 cm above the crus helix may result in the loss of this distal portion of the flap (40).

DISTANT (FREE) FLAPS

History

Microvascular free tissue transfer has spawned a new era of reconstructive surgery. The variety of regional and free flaps available today is a culmination of work done throughout the 20th century, especially since the introduction of Bakamjian's deltopectoral flap in the late 1960s (19). The modern reconstructive surgeon is able to deliver vast quantities of well-vascularized tissue that allow closure of even the most complex head and neck postsurgical and traumatic wounds.

Prior to the deltopectoral flap, closure of complex head and neck wounds was accomplished by secondary intention or by mobilizing skin from the anterior chest wall through a series of so-called 'delay' procedures. Particularly problematic were pharyngeal wounds that required multiple delay procedures and skin grafts often resulting in a prolonged open and draining wound and several months in hospital. The first reported microsurgical flap transfer was for a cervical esophageal defect reconstructed with a jejunal segment in 1957 by Seidenberg (42). However, microvascular reconstruction was not practiced with any regularity until the early 1970s. During this period, there was more interest in regional tissue transfer and basic flap vascular physiology. In the late 1960s, despite requiring at least two stages, the deltopectoral flap became available and was immediately embraced as a significant advance in pharyngeal reconstruction. During the 1970s, several axial soft tissue and composite flaps were discovered. The most important regional axial flap discovery with regard to head and neck reconstruction was the pectoralis flap (2). Several potential microvascular free tissue flaps were also discovered but microvascular reconstruction remained unpopular due to technical demands and problems with flap viability. Improvements in mandibular plating systems occurred during this same period and many patients received these plates in lieu of the much more involved technique of microvascular bone transfer. Although regional composite flaps were available (e.g., pectoralis–rib), the bone often resorbed and was inadequate. The reconstructive plate restored form and, since patients rarely sought dental rehabilitation even when reconstructed with vascularized bone, this method was arguably adequate and less costly and demanding. Over the years, these plates were covered with a variety of flaps including free and regional (most often the pectoralis flap). This method was popular but suffered a major setback as clinicians began noticing with increasing frequency plate breakage and exposure leading to complete loss of the reconstruction. This was particularly evident when a plate was used to bridge an anterior segmental mandibular defect, with plate exposure or breakage often occurring within months. However, it was reported that vascularized bone placed behind the plate resulted in a hardy and permanent reconstruction. Since only microvascular free tissue provided durable bone of adequate stock, this method became the only reasonable choice for anterior mandibular defects. An increasing awareness of the versatility and viability of microvascular flaps has advanced free tissue transplantation to the forefront of head and neck reconstruction. The success rate of free flap transfer approaches 100% today due to improvements in flap selection, development of precise techniques and instrumentation, and careful postoperative monitoring. In addition, microvascular reconstruction reduces the number and length of hospitalizations and operations, thus lowering health care costs and returning the patient to a more normal routine sooner.

Certain donor sites have become preferred for the head and neck based on their ease of harvest, quality of donor vessels, donor site morbidity, and the specific needs at the recipient site. The majority of head and neck defects can be reconstructed with one of four flaps including the radial forearm, osteocutaneous fibula, rectus musculocutaneous, and jejunal. The iliac osteocutaneous flap, the scapular system of flaps, and the lateral arm flap are also useful in many selected situations.

Merits

1. Microvascular flaps improve wound vascularity and will survive in hostile wound beds that are grossly contaminated with saliva and infection.
2. Repair of complex wounds requires fewer procedures and a shorter hospital stay.
3. Microvascular bone survives completely even in irradiated and saliva-contaminated wounds.
4. Microvascular free tissue transfer is the method of choice to reconstruct anterior mandibular, circumferential cervical esophageal, total and subtotal scalp, extensive cranial base, and large orofacial defects.
5. The combination of a composite microvascular flap, prosthetic device(s), and local flap(s) often produces the best aesthetic and functional outcome.
6. Overall success rates, in terms of flap viability, of over 95% is expected.
7. Donor site morbidity is minimized with proper flap selection.
8. A two-team approach, with separate teams for harvesting the flap and removing the tumor, minimizes operative time.

Overview

Despite the availability of numerous microvascular tissue flaps, only a few are routinely used in the head and neck including the radial forearm, fibula, rectus, scapula, latissimus, jejunum, iliac crest, and gracilis. The radial forearm or so-called ‘Chinese’ flap was first described by Yang et al. in 1981 (43). It provides thin pliable fasciocutaneous tissue from the ventral wrist and forearm based on the radial artery, cephalic vein, and medial and lateral antebrachial cutaneous nerves. The proximal fibrofatty tissue in the forearm can also be harvested for augmentation or coverage in selected cases. The radial forearm flap can also be harvested with a portion of the underlying radial bone. However, pathological fracture of the radial bone is a significant risk despite prolonged cast immobilization. Considering the variety of alternative donor sites for vascularized bone, radial bone harvest is rarely warranted.

The fibula, scapula, and iliac crest are used nearly exclusively for bony defects in the head and neck. The fibular osteocutaneous free flap was originally described for use in mandibular reconstruction by Hidalgo et al. in 1989 (44). The fibula is a tubular, primarily cortical, bone and is the longest available microvascular bone for mandibular reconstruction (26 cm). Since the bone is perfectly straight, several osteotomies are usually required, especially if it is being used to replace the mandibular symphysis. The blood supply to the bone is based on the peroneal artery and vena comitantes. Septocutaneous vascular twigs from the peroneal artery course posterior to the fibular bone and enter the posterior crural intermuscular septum to nourish the skin of the lateral leg. A skin paddle can be harvested with the fibular bone up to 6 cm wide along the entire length of harvested bone. Wider skin paddles leave a donor site that must be reconstructed with a skin graft. Sensory reinnervation is possible if the lateral sural cutaneous nerve is harvested with the skin paddle (45). Donor site morbidity is minimal and full unassisted ambulation is expected within 2–3 weeks postoperatively.

The scapular osteocutaneous flap was originally described by Swartz et al. in 1986 for mandibular reconstruction (46). The lateral border of the scapula provides approximately 16 cm of straight elliptical bone based on the circumflex scapula artery and vena comitantes. Large independent skin paddles can be harvested (transverse and parascapular fasciocutaneous flaps) with or without the underlying bone. The angular artery, a branch of the artery to the serratus muscle, additionally nourishes the distal third of the scapular bone. This artery should be preserved if a distal osteotomy is planned. Although the osteocutaneous scapular flap and the latissimus–serratus flaps can be harvested together based on the subscapular artery, this large flap is rarely needed. The donor site is rarely troublesome.

Taylor described the iliac crest osteocutaneous flap in 1982 for mandibular reconstruction (47). The iliac crest provides vascularized bone up to 16 cm in length that is naturally curved, lessening the need for osteotomies. The bone and overlying skin are based on the deep circumflex iliac artery. The overlying skin receives nourishment from septocutaneous branches, similarly to the osteocutaneous fibular flap. The bone height and cortical:cancellous ratio closely match the native mandible. The skin component of the iliac crest flap is excessively thick when it is used to cover the free edge of the bone intraorally, which is similar to the problems encountered with the skin components of the scapula and fibula flaps. Thick tissue over the neoalveolus impedes the placement of osseointegrated implants and implant-borne dentures. To avoid this problem, it is possible to harvest a portion of the thin internal oblique muscle with the iliac crest bone and skin based on the ascending branch of the deep circumflex iliac artery. The muscle can be draped over the neoalveolus and allowed to re-epithelialize providing improved contour to the neoalveolus that more closely matches the natural alveolus. Although the iliac crest flap is an excellent substitute for native mandible, there is significant donor site morbidity, which is the main drawback to using this flap. Chronic pain and difficulty walking are common, at least for the first several months postoperatively. There is also a risk of hernia and bowel injury. The significant morbidity associated with flap harvest has considerably lessened the initial enthusiasm for its use.

Tansini first described the latissimus musculocutaneous flap as a pedicled flap for breast reconstruction in 1896; Maxwell et al. subsequently described it as a free flap in 1978 (15). The flap is supplied by the thoracodorsal artery and vein and the thoracodorsal motor nerve. The full muscle and overlying skin are more often indicated for extensive traumatic or oncological trunk or extremity wounds. The thoracodorsal nerve may be harvested with a portion of the muscle to maintain bulk and achieve movement. Donor site morbidity is usually minimal; however, the site is prone to delayed healing and seroma formation.

The rectus abdominis musculocutaneous free flap was first described in 1980 for an infraclavicular defect and in 1984 for use in the head and neck (48,49). The flap is based on the deep inferior epigastric artery and vein. The cutaneous component can be bulky with a substantial amount of subcutaneous fat that varies at the recipient site based on the patient's adiposity. Despite the size of the skin paddle, it can be sustained by a single periumbilical vascular perforator. Therefore, this so-called 'perforator flap' can be transferred with almost no underlying muscle except a muscular cuff around the lone vascular perforator. The motor supply is segmental, with short nerve twigs entering the lateral aspect of each rectus muscle. The multiple tendinous inscriptions limit muscle excursion, making it ineffective for facial reanimation. Donor site morbidity is minimal; however, hernia can occur especially if the anterior rectus sheath is not preserved below the arcuate line.

Seidenberg et al. first used the jejunal flap clinically to reconstruct a cervical esophageal defect in 1959. The flap fared well but the patient died of a stroke on postoperative day 5. The jejunal flap consists of a segment of jejunum 3 feet beyond the ligament of Treitz. The vascular supply is based on the mesenteric arterial arcade from the superior mesenteric artery and vein. The jejunal flap may be left intact and used as a conduit or split along its antimesenteric border and used as a patch. The revascularized jejunum actively secretes mucous and this attribute has been espoused for irradiated recipient sites.

Harii et al. introduced the gracilis free flap in 1976 for the surgical treatment of facial paralysis (50). It provides a tubular muscle innervated by multiple neural fascicles from the anterior division of the obturator nerve. The blood supply is from the medial femoral circumflex artery (a branch of the profunda femoris artery). The gracilis muscle, as is the case with all microvascular flaps for facial paralysis, is reserved for patients with absent or nonviable facial musculature. The obturator nerve is anastomosed to a motor nerve in the recipient site, most commonly the hypoglossal nerve or a previously placed cross-facial nerve graft. Cross-facial nerve grafting must precede microvascular flap transfer by several months to allow time for the regenerating axons to reach the recipient site. Although donor site morbidity is negligible regarding the gracilis muscle, sural nerve harvest leaves the patient with permanent numbness and paresthesia over the lateral foot. The diameters of the artery (1–2 mm) and the vein (1–1.5 mm) to the gracilis muscle are relatively small, making the microvascular anastomosis more difficult. A potential complication of flap harvest is paralysis of the adductor muscles of the extremity if the obturator nerve is taken too proximally but this is extremely rare. The latissimus muscle–thoracodorsal nerve flap may obviate the need for two stages by providing a sufficient length of nerve to reach the opposite donor facial nerve without the need for an intervening avascular nerve graft. Early experience with this technique appears promising, with good return of function within 8 months.

Microvascular Technique

Microsurgery describes a surgical procedure performed under the magnification of a surgical microscope. Although the vast majority of vessel anastomoses involving free tissue transfer are performed with the aid of a microscope (6–25×), surgical loupe magnification (2.5–3.5×) may be adequate for larger vessels with diameters over 2.0 mm. The microscope should be configured with dual heads with stereovision to allow an assistant to be seated across the operating table (Fig. 22). Thorough

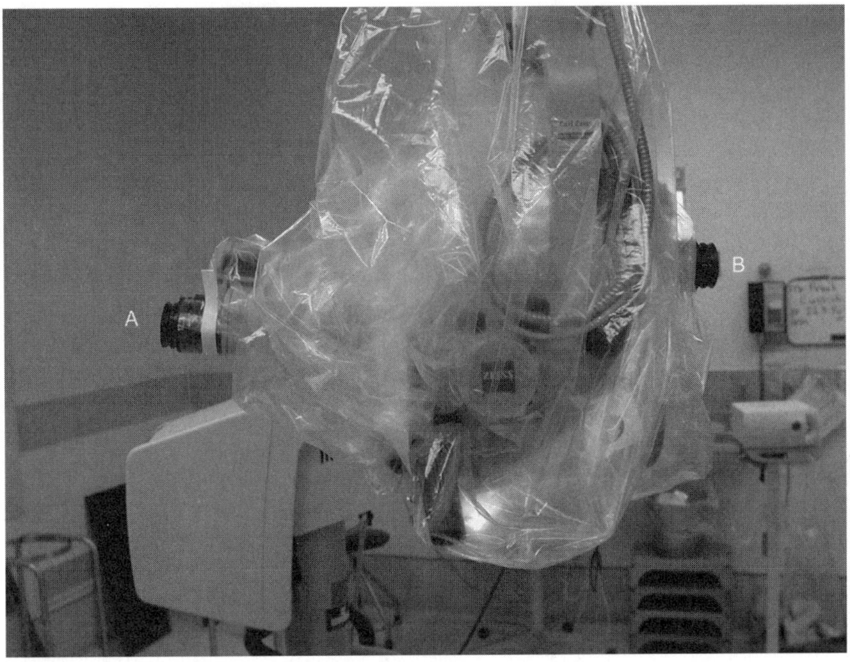

Figure 22 Surgically draped dual-headed microscope for microsurgery. The operator's oculars (A) are oriented 180° from the assistant's oculars (B).

attention to detail and meticulous atraumatic technique are essential components of success in microvascular surgery. Appropriate microvascular instrumentation is essential including straight jewelers forceps, a straight or curved microneedle holder, straight and curved microscissors, a vessel dilator, a clamp applicator, and a microbipolar (Fig. 23). An assortment of microvascular clamps should be available with closing pressures less than 30 g/mm^2. The clinical instruments should be duplicated in a small animal laboratory to facilitate realistic training sessions. The novice microvascular surgeon should first practice microsurgical techniques using synthetic vascular material with diameters between 1 and 2.5 mm. After the basic skills are established, the surgeon should advance to the deep inferior epigastric artery and vein in the rat. Consistent performance resulting in serial patent anastomoses indicates sufficient expertise to proceed into the operating room. The number of laboratory training sessions needed varies but approximates 40.

It makes little difference whether the artery or vein is anastomosed first unless an impediment is created that will present problems with access to the subsequent anastomosis. End-to-end anastomoses are always done on the arterial side but end-to-side anastomoses are often performed on the venous side between the donor vein and the internal jugular vein. It makes no difference at what angle the donor vein connects to the recipient vein unless the vein is kinked or compressed. The novice microvascular surgeon should be familiar with the end-to-end microvascular anastomotic technique.

End-to-end anastomoses begin by meticulous vessel preparation. The vessels are handled using jewelers forceps by grasping only the adventitia. The closing

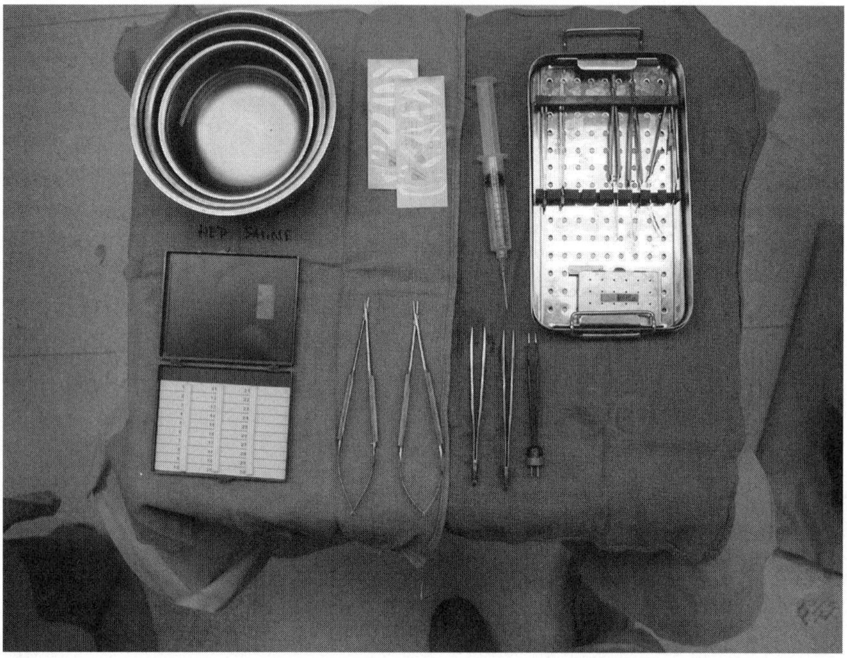

Figure 23 Bird's eye view of a typical microvascular instrument table. It is a comparatively simple set-up with straight and curved microvascular needle holders and pick-ups. A 10 cc syringe is supplied with a 22 gauge angiocatheter for intermittent heparin–saline irrigation. A variety of microvascular temporary occlusion clips are also supplied in the case on the upper right corner of the table.

forces generated by arterial clamps correlate with the extent of intimal injury and thrombogenic potential. Therefore, vascular occlusion clamps are applied with only enough pressure to occlude blood flow. The donor and recipient vessels can be clamped independently or a framed clamp (clamps joined by two parallel bars) may be used to keep the vessel ends in alignment. The adventitia is strongly thrombogenic, so it is removed from around the area of the proposed anastomoses using the curved microvascular scissors. Heparinized saline irrigation (100 U/cc) is applied to each lumen to keep them clear of clots and debris. Papaverine (30–40 mg/cc) or 2% lidocaine can be applied to minimize vessel spasm. The vessel ends are gently dilated with a spatulate dilator forceps. Depending on the diameter of the vessel, an atraumatic nylon suture is chosen between 8-0 and 10-0. Carrell's triangulation method of suture placement is popular. Three stay sutures are placed initially to approximate the vessel ends 120 degrees apart. As the stay sutures (two at a time) are pulled taut, the back wall tends to fall away facilitating accurate placement (Fig. 24). Sutures are placed by continually halving the distance between the apposing sutures to achieve a watertight seal. The needle must pass through the media and intima at a right angle approximately two vessel thicknesses away from the edge. The posterior edge is accessed for suture placement by flipping the vascular clamps 180 degrees. Problems that may lead to thrombosis include inadvertent suture placement through the back wall of the vessel, rough handling, failure to

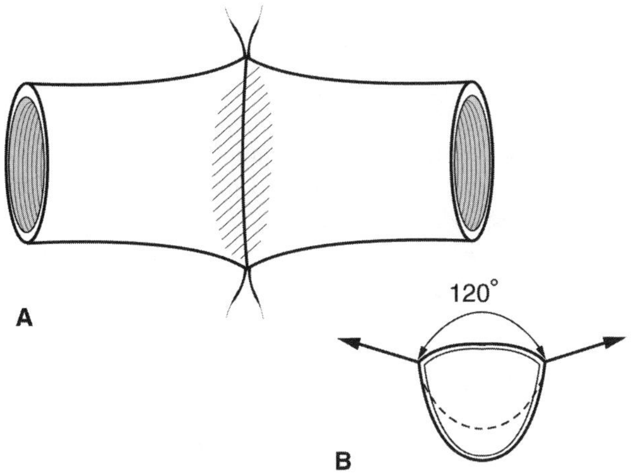

Figure 24 The triangulation method of microvascular suture placement is convenient since the 120 degree offset of the sutures allows the back wall of the vessel to fall away, thereby avoiding inadvertent suture placement through it.

include a slightly separated intima with the stitch, and inclusion of a significant amount of adventitia within the vessel lumen. The venous anastomosis is slightly more difficult than the arterial anastomosis because the walls of the veins are thinner and collapsible; however, fewer sutures are required. The venous clamps are released first. Arterial leakage is common but will usually subside. Brisk bleeding will require the placement of additional sutures. Re-endothelialization along the suture line begins by day 3 and is complete by day 7 in the veins and arteries.

Vessel size mismatch is better tolerated on the venous side where mismatches up to 2:1 are acceptable. Cutting the smaller vein at an angle allows end-to-end approximation but greater mismatches are best handled by an end-to-side anastomosis. The usual problem on the arterial side is that the donor artery is much smaller than most of the branches of the external carotid artery. End-to-side anastomoses are generally not performed on the arterial side because of technical limitations and connecting to the common or internal carotid system is contraindicated because of the risk of thrombosis.

Interrupted sutures are preferred but a continuous suture technique is feasible for both the artery and vein. Continuous suturing is reserved for larger vessels with a diameter of at least 2 mm because the continuous suture narrows the lumen. A continuous suture technique is most applicable to large veins where slight luminal narrow is insignificant and tight approximation is not critical. Interpositional vein grafts can be used to bridge arterial and venous gaps, with comparable success to single anastomoses. Vein grafts must be reversed so that the valves do not obstruct flow.

A useful alternative to suture for the venous anastomosis is a stapling device (e.g., 3M Coupler). The end of each vein is pulled through a plastic ring and spread over protruding prongs that penetrate and secure the veins. The opposing plastic rings are approximated and secured by penetration of the prongs into the opposite ring. These devices are indicated only for the venous anastomosis. Anastomotic time is significantly reduced and animal studies show that patency rates are equivalent to hand-sewn anastomoses.

Neurorrhaphy

Often in microvascular surgery it is necessary to perform neural anastomoses to reconstitute motor or sensory function to the transferred flap tissue. Essentially, a nerve trunk is a collection of axons (nerve fibers) ensheathed in endoneurium, perineurium, and epineurium. Endoneurium surrounds the individual axons, perineurium encases groups of axons, and epineurium surrounds the perineurium and ensheaths the entire nerve trunk (Fig. 25). A nerve fascicle is a group of axons and its perineurium and it is the smallest component of a nerve trunk that can be used for microneural anastomosis. A monofascicular nerve (e.g., facial nerve trunk) consists of a single large fascicle ensheathed by epifascicular epineurium. A polyfascicular nerve (e.g., inferior alveolar nerve and lingual nerve) consists of many small fascicles of varying size with intervening interfascicular perineurium all ensheathed by epifascicular epineurium. In cases of microvascular transplantation of muscle for facial paralysis, fascicular (perineural) repairs are done to match precisely the unique donor motor fascicles to the appropriate division of the facial nerve. For example, the obturator nerve trunk consists of nerve fascicles that innervate discrete areas of the gracilis muscle. The epifascicular epineurium is opened and the individual fascicles are electrically stimulated to define two independent areas of muscular movement and innervation. The fascicle supplying the part of the muscle used for the oral commissure is anastomosed to the lower division of the facial nerve. The fascicle supplying the upper part of the muscle that is used for the eyelids is anastomosed to the upper division of the facial nerve (or cross-facial nerve graft from the upper division of the opposite facial nerve).

Epineurium-to-epineurium microneural anastomosis is sufficient in the majority of cases involving microvascular surgery. Unlike peripheral nerve coaptation after traumatic neurolysis, the topographical precision provided by a perineural repair is not needed when purely sensory or purely motor nerves are being coapted. Cutaneous sensory reinnervation is possible using the radial forearm flap and the fibular osteocutaneous flap. The greatest benefit of sensory reinnervation is found

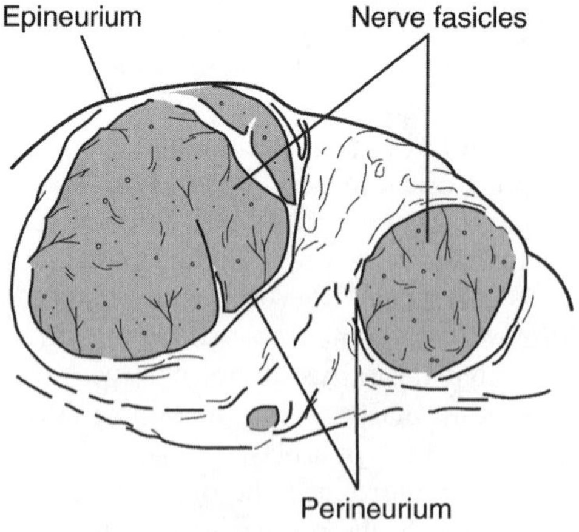

Figure 25 Layers of a typical peripheral nerve. The nerve fascicles are enveloped in perineurium that is in turn enveloped in epineurium. Microneural anastomosis is usually performed at the level of the perineurium.

in the perioral area to prevent drooling. Sensation around the lips and anterior oral cavity improves articulation, oral competence, and food bolus manipulation. Sensory reinnervation using the lingual nerve or inferior alveolar nerve results in the return of all aspects of normal sensation including touch, pressure, temperature, and pain. An interesting finding is that sensory discrimination may actually be improved at the recipient site because of the greater cortical representation of the cranial nerves. Motor reinnervation is possible using the rectus, latissimus, and gracilis muscles. Reinnervation is useful to maintain muscle bulk in cases of tongue reconstruction and to achieve movement in cases of facial paralysis and tongue base reconstruction. The ipsilateral facial nerve or a cross-facial nerve graft is used for cases of microvascular muscle transfer to correct facial paralysis.

The technique of microneurorrhaphy is a precise method of nerve anastomosis ideally resulting in the accurate alignment of nerve sheaths composed of viable Schwann's cells to allow free axonal regrowth across the site of coaptation. A tensionless epineural repair is important because the epineurium will stretch imperceptibly, separating the underlying nerve fascicles. An epineural repair that results in prolapsing fascicles may be too tight and should be loosened to allow the fascicles to lie end to end. Excess nerve fascicles extruding through the suture line should be trimmed so that regenerating nerve fibers are not directed outside the anastomosis. If the individual fascicles are sufficiently large, one or two 10-0 approximating perineural sutures can be used prior to suture coaptation of the epineurium.

Excess adventitia is trimmed from the end of the donor and recipient nerve trunks under the microscope. Two stay sutures (10-0 or 9-0 nylon) are placed 180 degrees apart through the epineurium of each nerve trunk, with care taken not to penetrate the underlying nerve fascicles. Subsequent epineural sutures are placed to allow adequate coaptation. Small nerves may only require four sutures while larger nerve trunks may require up to eight sutures. Factors associated with successful neural anastomosis include optimal nerve coaptation, minimal surgical trauma, and survival of the nerve graft. Survival of the nerve graft is important because viable Schwann cells are needed for axonal propagation along the nerve graft. This is usually not an issue with microvascular transfer since the nerves are revascularized with the rest of the transplant. Schwann cells in nonvascularized nerve grafts depend upon a healthy vascularized bed for survival. A nonvascularized nerve graft undergoes inosculation and ingrowth of blood vessels in a process similar to revascularization of a skin graft. Nonvascularized nerve grafts may not perform well if they are placed on an avascular (e.g., previously irradiated) bed. In these cases, a vascularized nerve graft should be considered to maximize neural regeneration (51).

Planning and Implementation

A typical microsurgical case that will involve an extirpative surgical team and a reconstructive surgical team requires careful planning. Two nursing teams and instrument sets are required to allow the two surgical teams to operate simultaneously. The patient is positioned on the operating room table so that the head and neck is cantilevered away from the base of the table. This usually requires that the patient's head be placed at the foot end of the table. If the position of the patient must be changed during the course of the procedure to allow harvest of the free flap, this should be anticipated by placing the patient on an appropriately conforming mattress (e.g., sand bag). The donor and recipient sites are prepped separately. Once the flap is dissected, it is allowed to remain pedicled by its source artery and vein until needed at the recipient site in the head and neck. Prior to flap release, the donor vessels should be dissected. The free flap is transferred to the head and neck and inset before the microvascular anastomosis. Once the flap is inset, the donor vessels are allowed to drape across the neck in a position that will now be relatively stable. Recipient vessels should be chosen that closely match the size and geometric orientation of the donor vessels, unless an end-to-side anastomosis is planned. The microscope is sterilely draped and brought to the head of table. It makes no difference whether the artery or vein is anastomosed first. An appropriate donor artery or vein is chosen, often the facial or superior thyroid vessels, and the microvascular anastomoses proceed with the aid of the microscope. The microsurgical instruments are arranged on a separate table with the microvascular clamps, irrigation solutions, and extra suture. The irrigating solutions consist of heparin 100 units/cc and papaverine 30–40 mg/cc and are dispensed through 22 gauge intravenous catheters connected to 10 cc syringes. Ischemia time or the elapsed time between removing the flap from the donor site and re-establishment of blood flow is recorded but is rarely an issue. The ischemia time during initial flap transfer is the so-called ‘primary’ ischemia time, while ischemia time during secondary postoperative ischemic events is termed ‘secondary’ ischemia time. Composite microvascular flaps can endure over 8 h of ischemia time without any loss of viability. Intestinal flaps including the jejunum may only tolerate as little as 4 h of primary ischemia time before loss of viability. If a prolonged primary ischemia time is anticipated the flap should kept cool at 45–55°F.

Vessel Selection in the Difficult Neck

The lack of a suitable recipient vessel may jeopardize successful free tissue transfer. Common problems include inadequate pedicle length, a lack of suitable veins, arterial mismatch, poor-quality vessels, or a total lack of a suitable artery or vein. Inadequate pedicle length can be remedied through the use of reversed vein grafts. Vein grafts are most commonly obtained from the cephalic vein, external jugular veins, or from various leg veins. Vein grafts are reversed so that the valves are non functional. Notably, the use of vein grafts is not associated with an increased incidence of flap loss or thrombosis. If a vein is not available for anastomosis within the head and neck, the cephalic vein can be divided distally and turned into the head and neck based on the axillary vein. The cephalic vein is of large caliber and is not typically within prior surgical or radiation fields.

Arterial mismatch is a common problem when the donor artery is small (1–1.5 mm). The majority of the named vessels from the external carotid artery and thyrocervical trunk are much larger with a single exception: the ascending pharyngeal artery. The ascending pharyngeal artery is often neglected because of its posterior location. It originates posteriorly just beyond the carotid bulb and is not easily seen. The great advantage of this artery is that its diameter is much smaller than the other primary branches of the external carotid, yet its flow is very brisk. It is an ideal recipient artery for flaps with smaller donor arteries.

Finally, in some cases, there are no vessels in the neck that are useable. If a flap is to be transferred an artery and vein must be brought into the field. Thoracodorsal vessel transposition provides a practical solution to this problem (52). The thoraco-

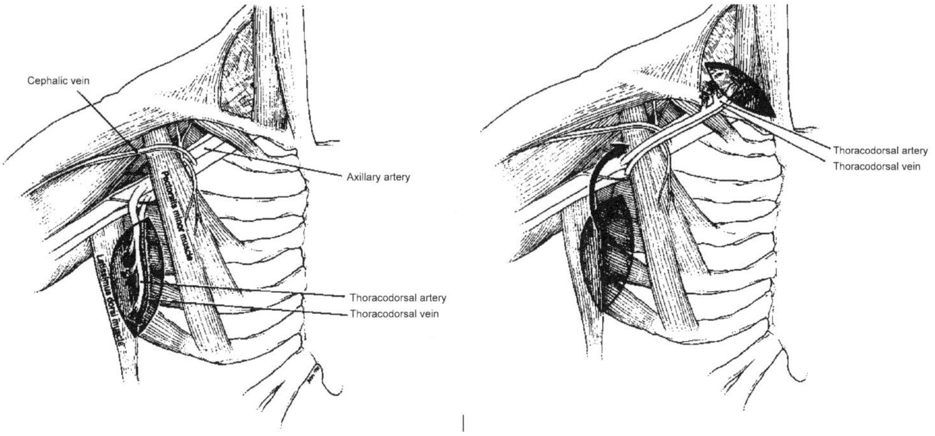

Figure 26 Thoracodorsal transposition to supply virgin large-caliber vessels to the neck to act as recipient vessels for a microvascular free flap. [From Ref. (52).]

dorsal vascular pedicle provides both arterial and venous components of large caliber (3–4 mm for the artery and vein) without manipulation of the carotid system that may be encased in scar (Fig. 26). This technique possesses several advantages: the vessels are not in the typical radiation field for head and neck cancer; they are of sufficient length to reach the lower neck easily; and the necessity for additional anastomoses is eliminated, thus reducing operating time.

The characteristics and relative qualities of each flap are presented in Table 1. A star is placed under each characteristic that is considered a favorable quality of the flap.

Rectus Abdominus

Description

The rectus abdominus is a type III free flap first described for an infraclavicular defect in 1980 and subsequently described for use in the head and neck in 1984 (48,49). The rectus abdominis muscle is approximately 30×6 cm originating from the pubic tubercle and inserting onto the costal cartilages of ribs 5–7 (Fig. 27). The rectus muscles are enclosed in two layers of fascia: the anterior rectus sheath and the posterior rectus sheath. The posterior sheath thins considerably below the arcuate line consisting only of transversalis fascia and is an area predisposed to hernia formation after flap harvest.

Indications

The principal indications for the rectus flap include large-volume defects involving the cranial base, midface, and tongue. It is the flap of choice for extensive anterior skull base defects for its capacity to seal dural defects (Fig. 28). A rectus musculocutaneous flap with multiple paddles is often used for complicated composite radical maxillectomy defects with orbital exenteration (Fig. 29).

Neurovascular Anatomy

The deep inferior epigastric vascular pedicle arises from the external iliac inferior and deep to the inguinal ligament and courses superomedially to enter the lateral aspect

Table 1 Characteristics of Free Flaps

	SimHarvest	PedLength	VDiam	ADiam	EHarvest	DSMorb	Sensory	Motor
Rectus abdominis	⋆	⋆	⋆	⋆	⋆	⋆		⋆
Pectoralis minor	⋆					⋆		⋆
Gracilis	⋆		⋆		⋆	⋆		⋆
Fibular osteocutaneous	⋆		⋆	⋆		⋆	⋆	
Radial forearm	⋆	⋆	⋆	⋆	⋆			
Scapular system of flaps			⋆	⋆			⋆	⋆
Dorsalis pedis	⋆				⋆	⋆		
Iliac osteocutaneous	⋆	⋆	⋆					
Lateral arm	⋆	⋆	⋆		⋆	⋆	⋆	
Lateral thigh	⋆		⋆	⋆		⋆	⋆	
Omental/gastro-omental	⋆	⋆	⋆	⋆		⋆		
Jejunal	⋆	⋆	⋆	⋆				

SimHarvest: The flap can be harvested simultaneously while the head and neck donor site is being prepared or extirpated thereby significantly reducing operative time.

PedLength: Pedicle lengths of over 6 cm are favorable to reach most donor vessels in the head and neck.

VDiam/ADiam: Arterial and venous diameters over 1.5 mm make microvascular anastomoses less technically demanding.

EHarvest: The overall ease of harvest describes whether the patient must be repositioned to harvest the flap or if the dissection is tedious and time-consuming.

DSMorb: Trouble-free donor site with regard to aesthetics and function / low risk of postoperative morbidity.

Sensory: The ability to re-establish sensation via neurorrhaphy.

Motor: A motor nerve is associated with the flap for reinnervation.

of the rectus muscle near the arcuate line (Fig. 30). Within the vascular pedicle lie the inferior epigastric artery and the venae comitantes. The musculocutaneous perforators from the deep inferior epigastric artery tend to follow two vertical parallel lines that course along the midpoint and lateral border of the muscle. They are most numerous at the umbilicus (paraumbilical perforators). A single paraumbilical perforator can supply virtually any size of paramedian or transverse skin paddle (Fig. 31). The smaller superior epigastric vascular pedicle (the continuation of the internal mammary artery) enters the rectus muscle superomedially. Although the flap can be sustained by this pedicle, it is rarely used for microvascular anastomosis because of deficiencies in pedicle size and length. The motor nerve supply is segmental originating from the T7 through T12 intercostal nerves along the muscle's lateral border.

Surgical Highlights

The patient is placed supine. The deep inferior epigastric artery is marked originating superior to the inguinal ligament and entering the deep inferolateral portion of the muscle midway between the umbilicus and pubic symphysis. The lateral extent of the muscle is approximately 10 cm from the midline.

The choice of skin incision depends on whether a muscle-only flap or a musculocutaneous flap is required. A muscle-only flap can be harvested through a paramedian vertical incision or a low transverse Pfannenstiel-type incision. A skin paddle can be oriented along the surface of the muscle (vertically) or transversely across the midline, depending on the needs at the recipient site. For example, one option

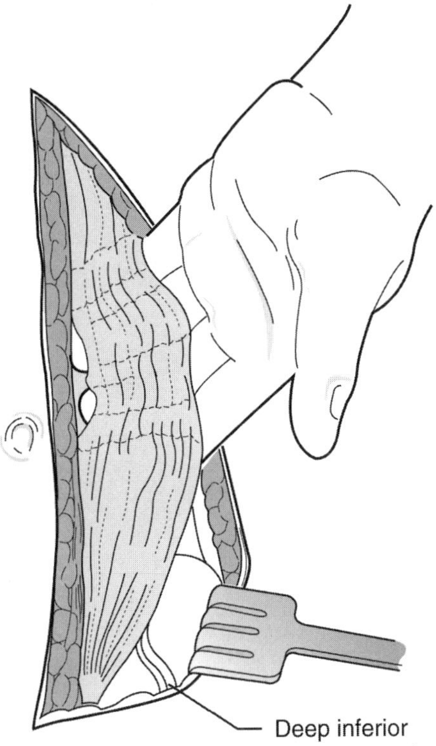

Figure 27 The rectus muscle free flap freed from its tendinous insertions. Note the position of the deep inferior epigastric vessels coursing superomedially inferior to the arcurate line.

for reconstruction of a total tongue defect requires a musculocutaneous rectus flap with an overlying skin paddle oriented vertically along the surface of the muscle. This allows the transversely oriented tendinous inscriptions to be sutured to the mandible for support of the skin paddle. The skin paddle should be based on an ipsilateral periumbilical perforator. If a very long skin paddle is required (> 20 cm) it should be oriented vertically along a line from the lateral border of the muscle to the tip of the scapula (Fig. 32). There is a hardy subdermal plexus along this line that allows the distal paddle to survive.

Harvesting a muscle-only flap does not require sacrifice of the anterior rectus sheath and the risk of postoperative hernia is low. However, skin harvest will require removal of a portion of the anterior rectus sheath and the risk of postoperative hernia formation increases. This is particularly relevant in cases that involve sacrifice of the anterior rectus sheath below the arcuate line where the posterior sheath of the rectus abdominis is deficient. Dehiscence of the anterior rectus sheath is avoided by meticulous dissection around the tendinous inscriptions and sacrificing only the portion of the rectus sheath that immediately surrounds the major perforating arteries. If the anterior rectus sheath is deficient below the arcuate line, a synthetic mesh may be used to reinforce the abdominal wall.

The inferior epigastric artery and its venae comitantes are found along the lateral aspect of the muscle below the arcuate line and dissected inferiorly to their origin

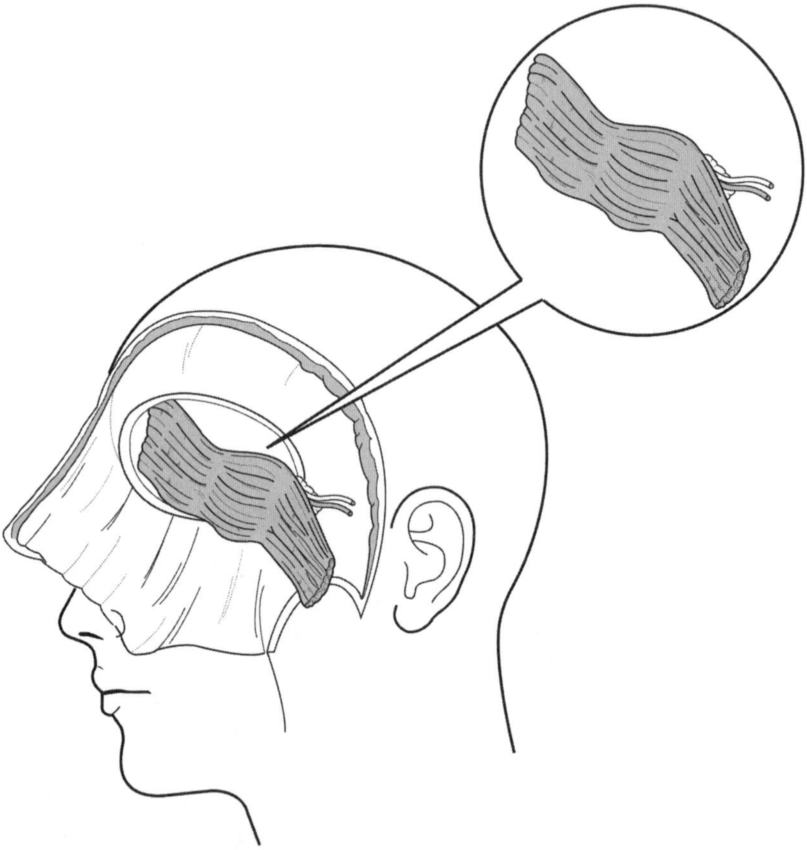

Figure 28 A muscle-only rectus flap is commonly used in skull base surgery to resurface the inferior and inferolateral aspects of the brain, providing separation of the cranial contents from the nose and infratemporal fossa. Typically, the superficial temporal vessels serve to nourish the flap.

at the external iliac vessels. A vascular loop is placed around the vessels and they are divided distal to their origin as a final step in harvesting the flap. A segment of muscle between the tendinous inscriptions may be reanimated by harvesting the intercostal nerve to that segment and connecting it to a motor nerve at the recipient site.

For a muscle-only harvest, the anterior rectus sheet may be split vertically over the middle of the muscle or along its lateral border. The sheath is tightly adherent to the tendinous inscriptions on the muscle and must be sharply divided.

Much of the anterior sheath can be preserved since only the sheath surrounding the perforators need be sacrificed. Only a single perforator is required to support a large skin paddle and only a small portion of the anterior sheath surrounding the perforating vessel need be sacrificed.

Advantages

A two-team approach is possible allowing simultaneous extirpation of a head and neck cancer and harvest of the free flap. The pedicle length is good at 6–8 cm and

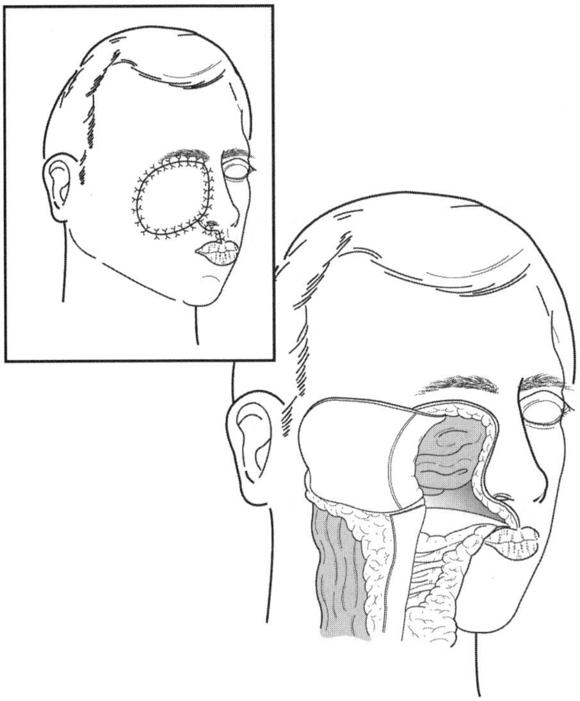

Figure 29 A common use for the musculocutaneous rectus flap is to close extensive complex combined orbit, palate, and maxillary defects. The flap is designed to provide skin coverage over the orbit and cheek, lateral nasal wall, and palate.

the vessel diameters are very large (2–3 mm), making the microvascular portion of the procedure straightforward. In fact, the rectus free flap is the most reliable free tissue transplant in terms of survival. The large adipose component of the musculocutaneous flap can be used for permanent volume replacement because, unlike muscle, revascularized adipose tissue will not atrophy. This is useful if maintenance of bulk is desirable such as in tongue reconstruction. The tendinous inscriptions can be sutured to the mandible to support the neotongue. Although the segmentally oriented motor nerve supply can be used, the minimal movement achieved for tongue reconstruction is probably of no benefit to speech and swallowing.

Disadvantages

The thickness of the skin paddle at the recipient site varies with the patient's habitus. Careless dissection below the arcuate line, resulting in sacrifice of the anterior rectus sheath, can result in abdominal laxity or hernia. The segmental nerve supply and its poor excursion limits it use for a functional muscle transplant. The skin color is a poor match for the head and neck.

Pectoralis Minor

Description

The pectoralis minor muscle free flap was originally described in 1982 for facial reanimation (53). The muscle is flat and thin with several muscular slips taking origin from

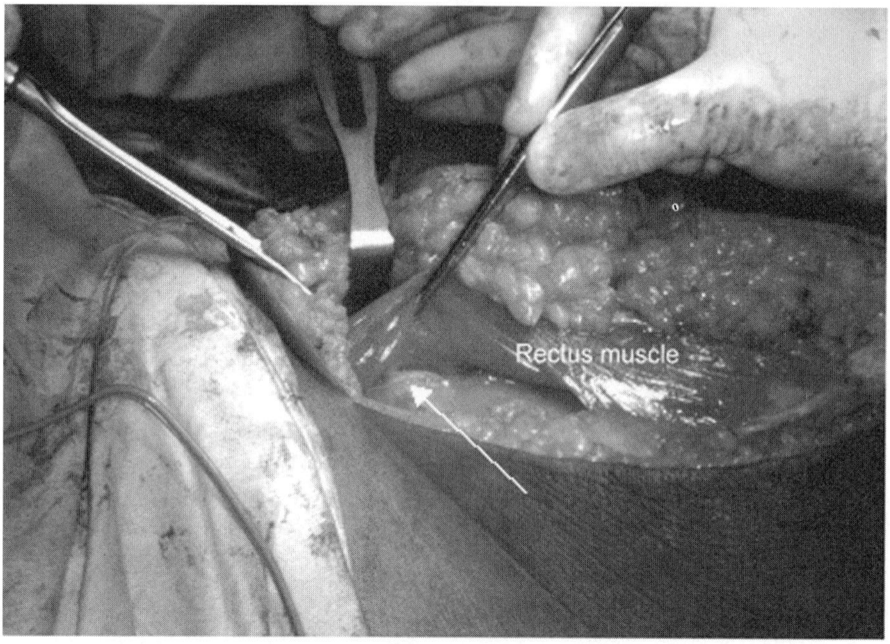

Figure 30 Blood supply to the rectus muscle. Note the deep inferior epigastric vessels (arrow) entering the undersurface of the inferior aspect of the rectus muscle. The lateral aspect of the rectus muscle is slightly retracted to expose the vasculature.

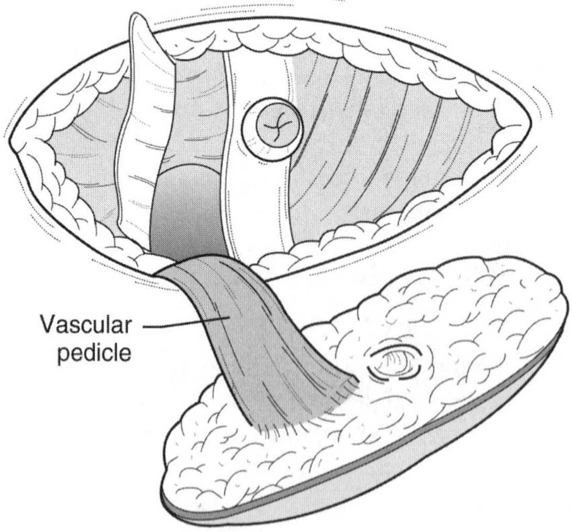

Figure 31 Transverse rectus abdominis flap. Note that the flap is primarily subcutaneous fat and skin. One or two periumbilical perforators supply the entire flap including the large portion extending over the midline. As with all musculocutaneous rectus flaps, only a small segment of the anterior rectus sheath need be sacrificed: just enough to accommodate the vascular perforators.

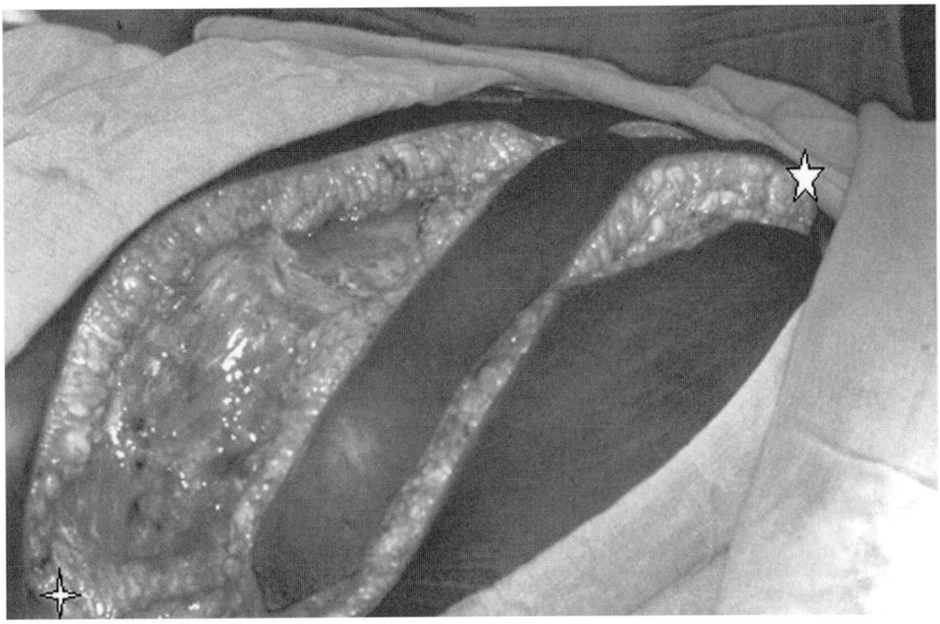

Figure 32 Orientation of long skin paddle for rectus flap. It is oriented vertically along a line from the lateral border of the muscle (five-pointed star) to the tip of the scapula (four-pointed star).

the third through the fifth ribs and converging to insert onto the coracoid process of the scapula. The muscular slips are 10–14 cm long in the adult and 6–10 cm in the child. Cross-facial nerve grafting is usually required several months prior to flap transfer.

Indications

According to its originator, the pectoralis minor muscle is best suited for developmental facial paralysis in young children. Muscle size and length are ideal in a 4- or 5-year-old. The flap is often unsuitably thick in adult patients with well-developed upper torso muscles.

Neurovascular Anatomy

A small branch of the lateral pectoral nerve innervates the upper muscular slip while the medial pectoral nerve supplies the remaining muscular slips. The main trunk of the lateral pectoral nerve passes through the minor muscle to supply the pectoralis major muscle. The blood supply is variable and dual: superomedially from the thoracoacromial artery and vein and inferolaterally from the lateral thoracic artery and vein (Fig. 33). The dominant vascular pedicle is usually the lateral thoracic contribution and the arterial diameter is less than 1 mm. The venous anatomy is variable. A separate suitable vein or the vena comitantes is available for anastomosis.

Surgical Highlights

Since the pectoralis minor muscle is a deep structure, there are no surface landmarks except those relating to the relative position of the pectoralis major muscle and coracoid process. The access incision is placed along the anterior axillary fold. Dissec-

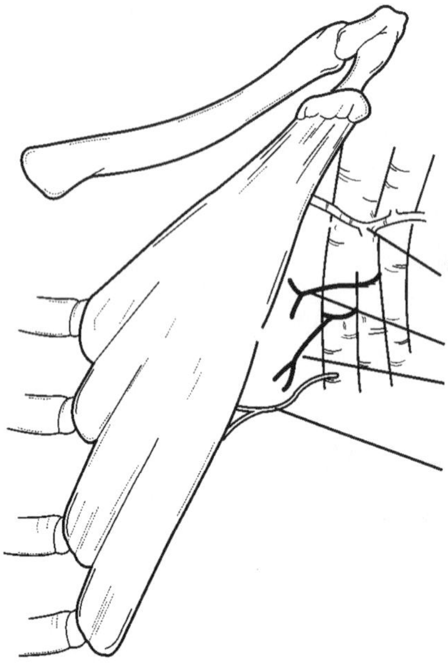

Figure 33 The important neurovascular anatomy of the pectoralis minor muscle flap. Note how a small branch of the lateral pectoral nerve innervates the upper muscular slip, while the medial pectoral nerve supplies the remaining muscular slips. The dominant vascular pedicle is usually the lateral thoracic artery.

tion proceeds to the lateral border of the pectoralis major muscle where the lateral thoracic vascular pedicle is identified. The lateral thoracic pedicle is followed to its branch to the pectoralis minor muscle. The muscle is dissected along its outer and inner surfaces to expose the pectoral nerves, veins, and thoracoacromial vascular pedicle. The dominant vascular structures are noted and preserved. Prior to flap harvest, fine silk sutures are placed in exactly 1 cm increments along the inferior border of the muscle corresponding to the inferior-most muscular slip. These sutures mark the in situ tension of the muscle. The harvested muscle is placed over a template from the face and stretched to approximate the desired resting tension. The template serves to gauge the distances between the body of the zygoma (insertion point of the proximal muscle) and the insertion points for the muscular slips (alar base, nasolabial fold, modiolus, and lower lip). The muscular slips are trimmed as needed. Once the muscle is inset, the microvascular and neural anastomoses can proceed.

Advantages

The pectoralis minor possesses a dual nerve supply allowing independent action of its upper and lower portions. It is possible to have independent eye and mouth movements. Donor site morbidity is minimal both functionally and cosmetically. Since the lateral pectoral nerve is sacrificed there will be some minor atrophy of the pectoralis major muscle.

Disadvantages

This flap should not be used in adult patients with well-developed upper torsos. The diameter of the donor vessels can be small, making the anastomoses quite challenging. There is significant variability in the vascularity of the pectoralis minor muscle. Although the excursion (degree of contraction) is adequate, the gracilis muscle may be better in this regard.

Gracilis

Description

The gracilis is a type II flap first introduced into clinical practice in 1976 by Harii et al. for the treatment of facial paralysis (50). The gracilis muscle lies directly posterior to the great saphenous vein and takes its origin from the pubic tubercle and inserts on the upper tibia. The gracilis muscular and musculocutaneous free flaps have limited application for voluminous defects of the head and neck. They are of primary importance for facial reanimation, due to the muscle's segmental motor supply and excellent contraction characteristics (large excursion). Individual branches of the motor nerve innervate separate territories of the gracilis muscle allowing independent contraction of each territory depending upon the selected neural anastomoses in the recipient bed. The upper inner thigh skin over the gracilis muscle can be harvested for limited defects in the head and neck.

Indications

The principal indication for the gracilis free flap in head and neck reconstruction is for secondary facial reanimation or primary reconstruction of lateral facial defects that include the mimetic musculature (Fig. 34). The motor nerves of the gracilis muscle can be reinnervated through anastomoses with either the facial nerve stump or a previously placed cross-facial nerve graft.

Neurovascular Anatomy

The arterial supply is from the medial femoral circumflex artery (a branch of the profunda femoris artery). The artery courses between the adductor longus and adductor brevis muscles to reach the middle third of the gracilis muscle. The diameter of the artery is between 1 and 2 mm and the diameter of the accompanying vena comitantes

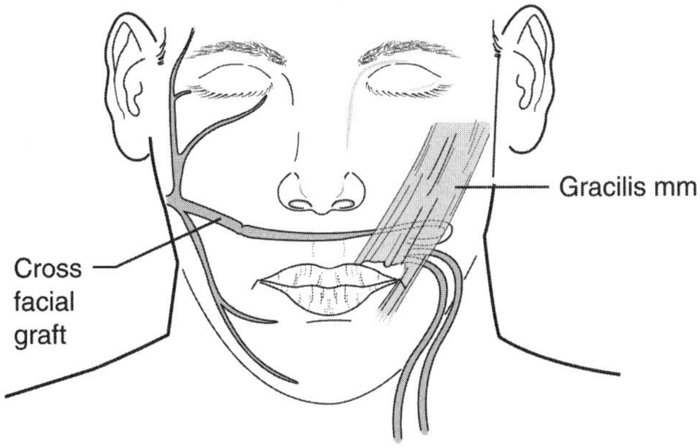

Figure 34 Typical configuration for a free gracilis muscle flap to correct facial palsy. The muscle is anchored along the zygoma and sutured into the modiolus. A cross-facial nerve graft was previously placed and anastomosed with the anterior branch of the obturator nerve.

is between 1 and 1.5 mm. Multiple musculocutaneous perforators supply the overlying skin. No sensory component is described. The motor nerve is derived from the anterior branch of the obturator nerve (Fig. 35). The obturator nerve splits into a posterior branch that passes under the adductor brevis muscle and an anterior branch that passes superficial to this muscle on its way to the gracilis muscle. Prior to entering the muscle, the anterior branch of the obturator nerve divides into several branches that innervate distinct longitudinal segments of gracilis muscle.

Surgical Highlights

The gracilis muscle is easily harvested with the patient in a supine position and the lower limb in a flexed and abducted position exposing the inner thigh. A linear incision is made over the muscle along a line tangent to the pubis and medial condyle of the tibia. The intermuscular septum between the gracilis muscle and adductor longus muscle is identified, and the skin and subcutaneous tissues are dissected off the gracilis. The vascular pedicle (medial femoral circumflex artery and vein) is noted entering the anterior aspect of the gracilis muscle posterior to the adductor longus muscle. The anterior branch of the obturator nerve is also noted along the posterior border of the adductor longus muscle splitting to innervate several longitudinal muscular fascicles separately upon entering the gracilis muscle. If only a single functional unit is needed, only the anterior longitudinal half of the muscle is harvested since the vascular pedicle enters this portion. The neurovascular pedicles are dissected proximally and divided. Prior to release of the muscle distally and proximally, several shallow

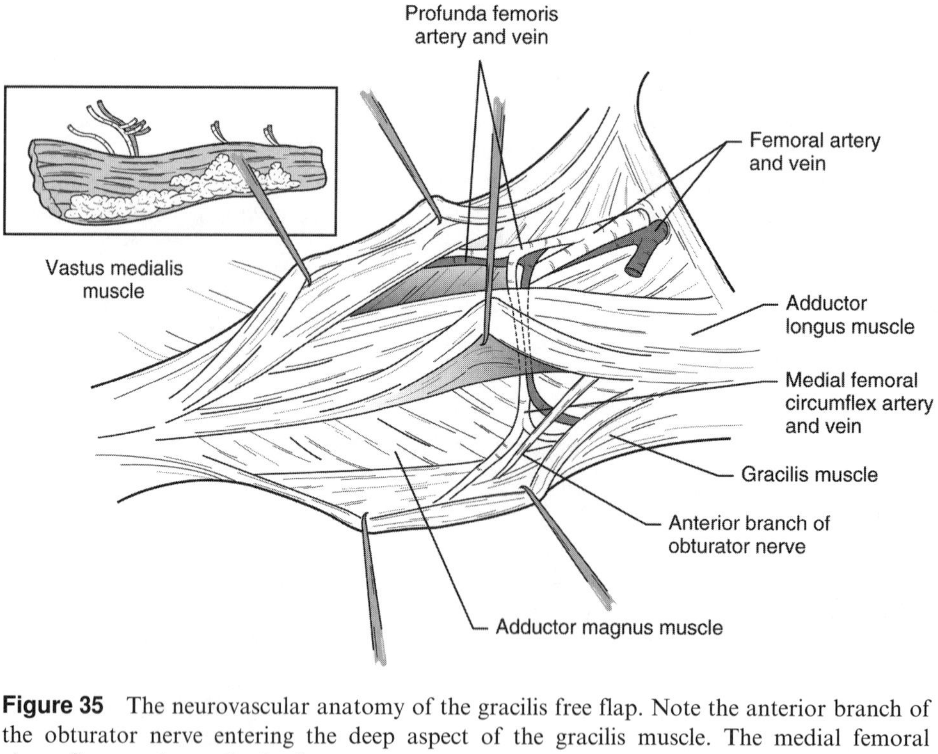

Figure 35 The neurovascular anatomy of the gracilis free flap. Note the anterior branch of the obturator nerve entering the deep aspect of the gracilis muscle. The medial femoral circumflex vessels supply the flap.

sutures are placed through the muscular fascia exactly 1 cm apart to mark the resting tension of the muscle. The muscle is re-expanded in the face during insetting to approximate the resting tension marked by the sutures. Cross-face nerve grafting is usually required several months prior to flap transfer. The hypoglossal nerve can also be used.

Advantages

A two-team approach is possible. If peripheral branches of the facial nerve are available, or if the recipient bed has been prepared with cross-facial grafts, localized facial movements are possible. The vascular pedicle length is between 6 and 8 cm. The donor site morbidity is negligible with a hidden scar.

Disadvantages

The diameters of the artery (1.2–1.8 mm) and the vein (1–1.5 mm) are relatively small. A potential complication is paralysis of the adductor muscles if the obturator nerve is taken too proximally.

Fibula

Description

The fibular osteocutaneous free flap is a type D flap originally described for use in mandibular reconstruction by Hidalgo et al. in 1989 (44). The fibular bone is composed largely of thick cortical bone and is tubular in shape. It is perfectly straight and must be osteotomized to fit most mandibular defects. The skin over the lateral leg can be harvested with the underlying fibular bone as a sensate soft tissue flap. The width of skin available is up to 6 cm (while still allowing primary closure of the donor site), and the length of skin available may be up to 25 cm (Fig. 36).

Indications

The osteocutaneous fibular flap is the most commonly used free flap for mandibular reconstruction and the only microvascular osseous flap that can used to reconstruct the entire mandible (Fig. 37). It can also be used to reconstruct the upper maxillary alveolar ridge and, with the skin paddle, can close large oronasal defects associated with total or subtotal maxillary defects. The skin paddle may be unsuitable for composite tongue defects because its bulkiness and stiffness may impede tongue mobility. To address this problem, some centers have used dual or in-tandem free tissue transfers using the fibular flap and the radial forearm flap.

Neurovascular Anatomy

The peroneal artery and its vena comitans travel along the inner border of the fibula to supply its distal two-thirds. An endosteal branch enters near the midfibula but the bone is supplied primarily through its periosteal attachments. The skin overlying the posterior crural intermuscular septum (PCIM) is supplied by septocutaneous perforators from the peroneal artery that course around the posterior border of the fibula through the PCIM and musculocutaneous perforators from the peroneal artery via the soleus muscle (Fig. 38). The septocutaneous perforators tend to be more numerous in the distal half of the leg. Cuffs of soleus muscle may provide more soft tissue (although closely adherent to the bone) and will aid in the preservation and inclusion of these perforators with the flap. The peroneal artery and vena

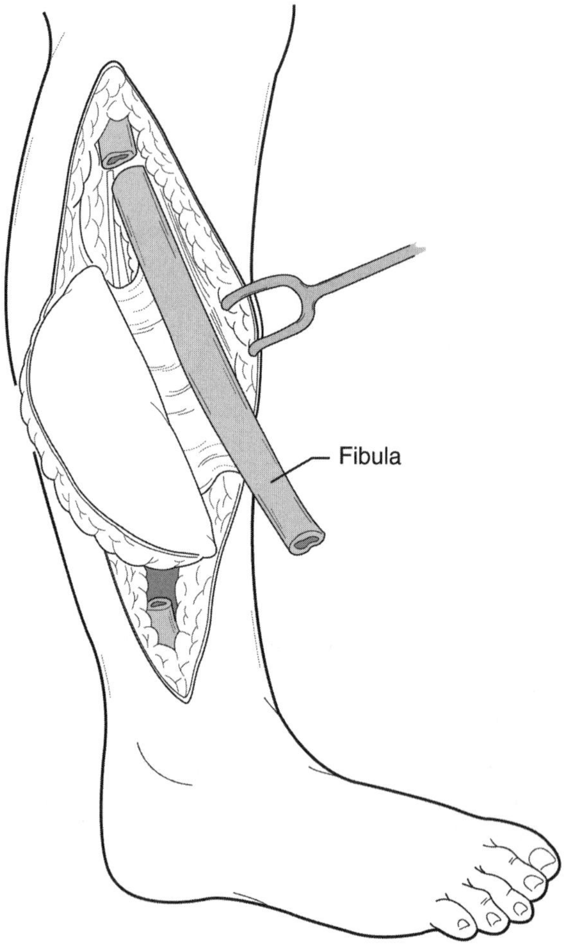

Figure 36 A harvested osteocutaneous fibular free flap temporarily pedicled on the peroneal vessels. Note the close and broad attachment of the skin paddle to the bone.

comitans are relatively large-diameter vessels: the artery is 2–4 mm and the venae comitantes are 2–3 mm each.

The length of the vascular pedicle varies depending on the size of the leg, the level at which the vascular pedicle branches from the posterior tibial artery, the length of bone required, and the segment along the length of bone used for reconstruction. Preoperative vascular studies may be helpful in determining which leg has the longer vascular pedicle. The middle two-thirds of the fibula (preserving 5 cm proximally and 10 cm distally for knee and ankle stability) provides ample bone for most mandibular defects. Excess bone can be discarded proximally by first stripping its periosteum and the overlying tissues and cutting away the unneeded bone, which effectively lengthens the vascular pedicle.

Sadove (1993) first described successful incorporation of a sensory nerve with the osteocutaneous fibula flap for penile reconstruction (54). The lateral sural

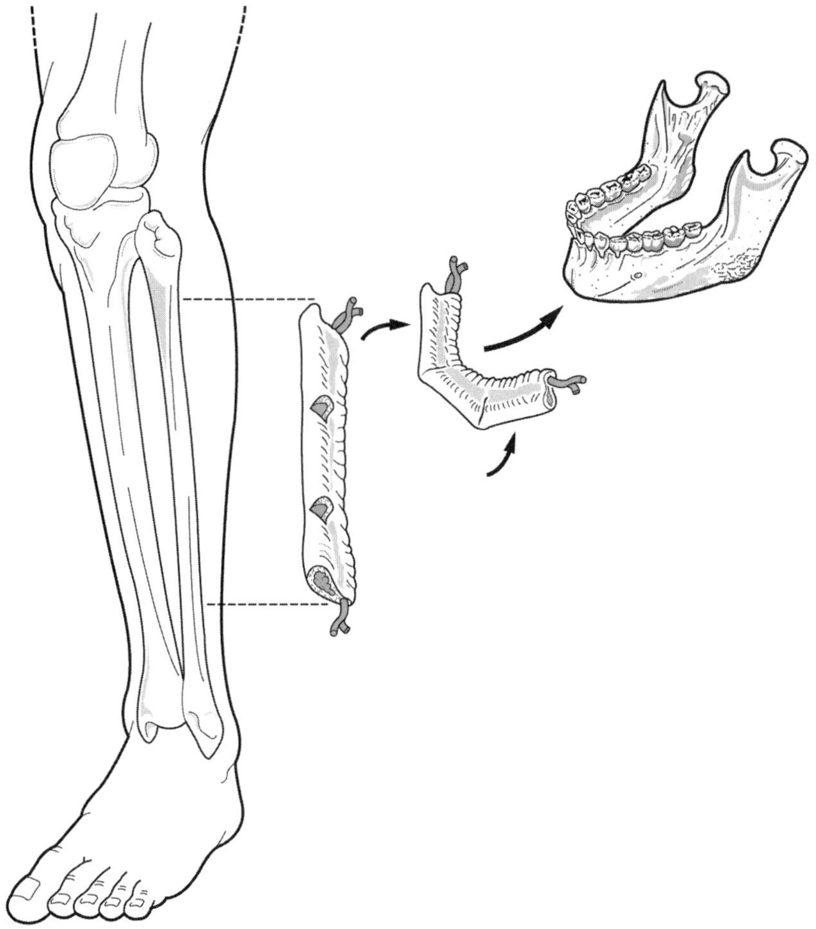

Figure 37 An osseous flap harvested with its proximal vascular pedicle. Note that the vascular "mesentery" is oriented away from the neoalveolar surface. Closed or open osteotomies can be made to shape the bone. Closed osteotomies are demonstrated here.

cutaneous (LSC) nerve is the most consistent and accessible donor sensory nerve in the posterior leg for harvest with the osteocutaneous fibula free flap. Congenital absence of the LSC nerves is rare, occurring in 1.7–22% of legs (45,55). The origin of the common LSC nerve from the peroneal nerve is at or above the head of the fibula (HF). The peroneal nerve is typically identified and traced superiorly to the common LSC nerve. The diameter of the nerve is approximately 3 mm at the HF, making identification and dissection of the nerve straightforward. However, it is approximately 1 cm below the skin surface in the subcutaneous tissues, requiring more dissection than might be anticipated in harvesting a sensory nerve. The common LSC is then followed inferiorly into the posterior calf to its division into the medial LSC and lateral LSC (Fig. 39). The level of the division is inconstant, ranging from 5 cm above to 8 cm below the HF. The medial LSC terminally arborizes approximately in the midleg and the lateral LSC nerve terminally arborizes

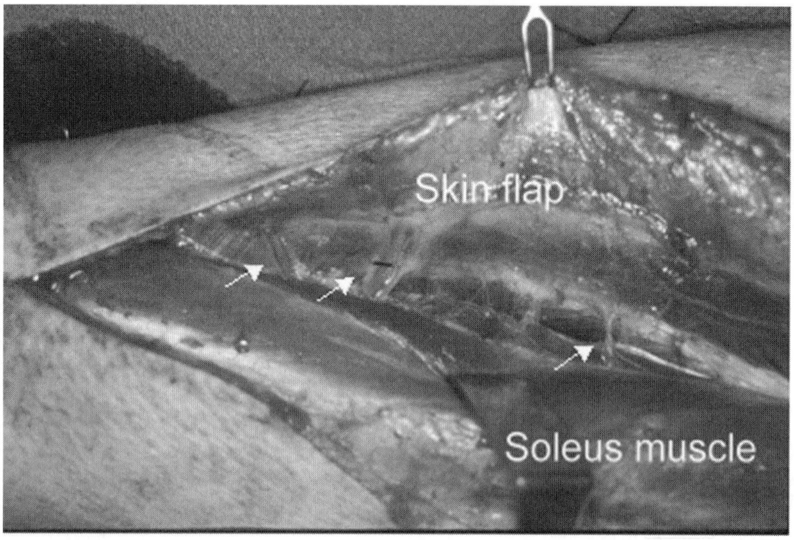

Figure 38 Fibular septocutaneous perforators (arrows).

within 7 cm below the HF. The lateral division is approximately 3 cm medial to the PCIM and must be incorporated into the design of the skin paddle.

Surgical Highlights

The osteocutaneous fibular flap is harvested simultaneously with the ablative portion of the procedure with the patient in the supine position and the knee slightly flexed. A pneumatic tourniquet around the thigh may be used but is not required. The

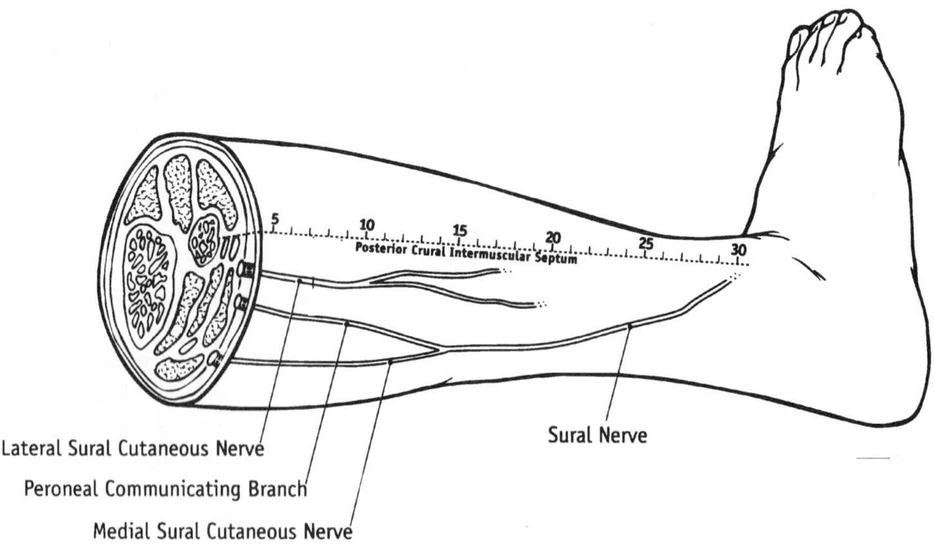

Figure 39 Fibular sensory nerves (see text).

PCIM follows the posterior border of the fibula and is an essential landmark in flap harvest. It is on a line from the fibular head to the lateral malleolus (the process at the lateral side of the lower end of the fibula). The skin paddle is typically 6 cm wide by 6–20 cm long and must lie over the PCIM to accommodate the septocutaneous vascular perforators that supply the skin of the lateral leg (Fig. 40). The need to harvest a very long skin paddle in the hope of capturing a septocutaneous perforator can be obviated by incising the anterior portion of the skin paddle first and dissecting down to the PCIM to look for perforators. Once a perforator is identified, a skin paddle of any size can be designed around it. Prior to dissection of the skin paddle superiorly, the common peroneal nerve should be identified as it courses anteroinferior to the head of the fibula.

After the skin paddle is dissected, the peroneus longus and brevis muscles and the extensor hallucis muscle are retracted anteriorly by carefully incising the longitudinal muscle fibers just outside the periosteum. The anterior tibial vessels and nerve are encountered and must be preserved. Bone cuts are prepared by carefully dissecting a cuff of periosteum around the circumference of the bone at the desired proximal and distal osteotomy sites, preserving at least 5 cm proximal fibula and 10 cm distal fibula. The inferior and superior osteotomies free the bone graft laterally since only the peroneal vessels and interosseus membrane now tether it. The distal peroneal vessels are found immediately behind the inferior osteotomy and divided. In an inferior-to-superior direction, the interosseus septum is divided, greatly freeing the osteocutaneous unit. Remaining muscular attachments including the soleus, flexor hallucis longus, and tibialis posterior are divided. A portion of the soleus and flexor hallucis muscles must be preserved around perforating peroneal musculocutaneous vessels if no purely septocutaneous vessels can be identified to supply the skin paddle. The flap may remain attached to its vascular pedicle in the leg while the ablative team is working (Fig. 41). Shaping osteotomies and application of hardware may also be performed at the donor site. To harvest the flap, the proximal peroneal vascular pedicle is dissected and taken distal to its branching from the posterior tibial artery. Dividing the pedicle intact is desirable since dissecting the vena comitans away from the peroneal artery is tedious and can lead to excessive bleeding.

A suction drain is placed into the wound and the muscles are allowed to fill the wound passively without suture fixation. The skin is closed primarily or covered with

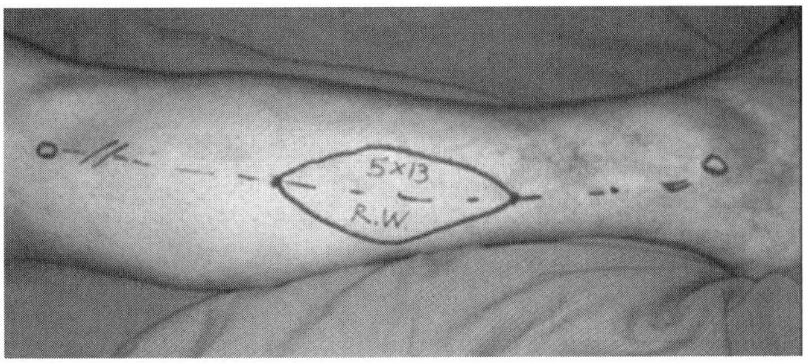

Figure 40 Fibula surface markings in preparation for harvest of an osteocutaneous flap. Note that the skin paddle is designed over the distal half of the lateral leg because the septocutaneous perforators tend to be more numerous in this region.

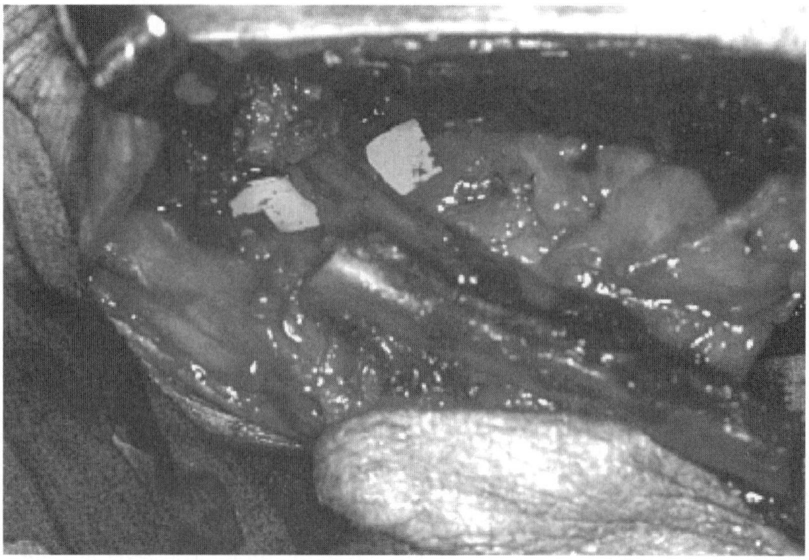

Figure 41 Pedicled osteocutaneous flap at donor site. Note the peroneal vessels over the background material. If desired, shaping osteotomies may be performed while the flap is being perfused.

a skin graft harvested from the lateral thigh (Fig. 42). A below-the-knee plaster splint is placed and the leg is kept elevated on a pillow while the patient is supine. Weight bearing with assistance can be started after 2 days, and full ambulation can begin as early as 1 week postoperatively.

Advantages

The fibular flap provides the greatest stock of bone for mandibular reconstruction of any other free bone flap. Recovery is rapid with full ambulation in 1 week and donor site morbidity is minimal. The skin paddle is reliable with careful dissection and can be sensate via the lateral sural cutaneous nerve.

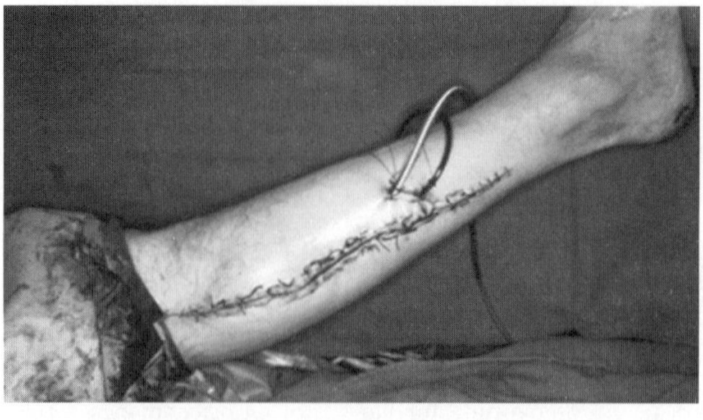

Figure 42 Fibular donor site closed. Primary closure is nearly always possible if the width of the skin flap is kept within 6 cm.

Disadvantages

The common peroneal nerve may be injured with dissection around the head of the fibula, resulting in foot drop. However, the nerve is quite large and inadvertent injury is very uncommon. If the peroneal artery is a significant source of blood supply to the foot (due to developmental anomaly or peripheral vascular disease), ischemic complications to the foot may occur postoperatively. A preoperative angiogram or magnetic resonance angiogram of the leg is obtained to study the vasculature of the lower leg and rule out significant arterial disease or congenital anomalies. Dissection of the sensory nerves can be tedious since their anatomy is inconsistent. The subcutaneous tissue of the lateral leg can be thick, making the skin paddle bulky and nonpliable. The skin paddle must also remain closely attached to the bone due to the nature of its blood supply, further limiting its ability to conform to soft tissue defects at the recipient site. It is not uncommon to observe a few centimeters of skin slough along the midportion of the incision at the donor site where the skin edges are brought together under some tension. However, healing by secondary intention is usually successful in these cases.

The bone often requires several osteotomies to imitate the curvature of a mandibular defect. This results in isolated segments of bone that are at risk for ischemic necrosis. The skin is at risk for ischemic necrosis if septocutaneous perforators are not included at the time of flap dissection or if these perforators are compressed by hardware.

Radial Forearm

Description

The radial forearm or so-called 'Chinese' flap is a type C fasciocutaneous flap first described by Yang et al. in 1981 in China (43) (Fig. 43). The flap is an osteofasciocutaneous free flap but the fasciocutaneous portion is most often transferred

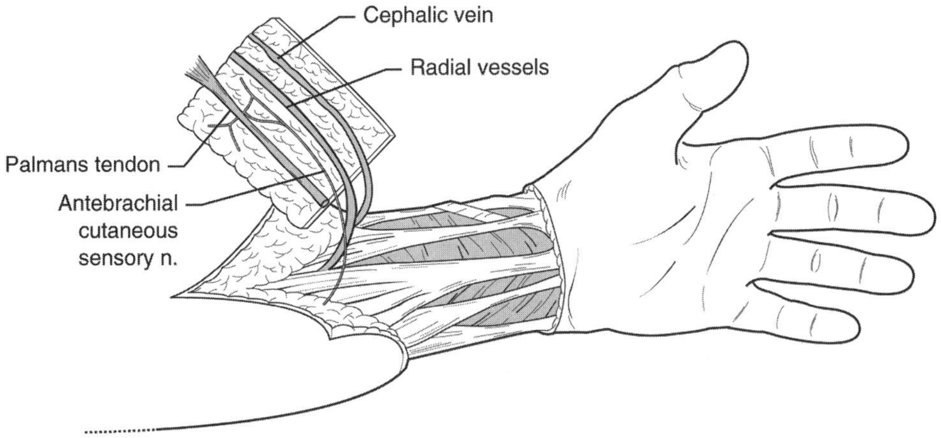

Figure 43 A partially harvested fasciocutaneous radial forearm flap showing its underlying anatomy. Note the cephalic vein, vascular pedicle, palmaris tendon, and antebrachial cutaneous nerve. The tendon is especially useful for lip reconstruction to support the free edge of the flap under the new lip.

without attached bone due to the significant donor site morbidity associated with bone harvest. The fasciocutaneous component may be up to 10 cm in width by 20 cm in length depending on the available surface area of the volar forearm. It is possible to include a portion of the underlying radius bone (up to 40% of the circumference), making this a potential osteocutaneous flap. Harvesting the subcutaneous tissue in the proximal forearm adds significant additional bulk.

Indications

The benefits of using the underlying radial bone rarely justify its use, considering the significant risk of radial bone fracture in the postoperative period. However, the thin, pliable, and potentially sensate skin is an excellent choice for a variety of surface and deep defects. Virtually any defect over the face and neck can be resurfaced with a radial forearm free flap. The flap is commonly used for extensive lip, cheek, and nasal defects. The palmaris tendon can be safely harvested with the flap and is useful in supporting a newly reconstructed lower lip. An augmented flap is useful for voluminous tongue defects, medial cheek defects, or for moderately sized anterior cranial base defects (Fig. 44). A combination of a radial forearm flap and a fibular flap is useful for composite defects of the tongue, floor of mouth, and mandible. In cases that require a completely buried flap (pharyngeal reconstruction), an exteriorized monitor is used. This is simply an island of skin connected via a subcutaneous pedicle with the main flap that is sutured into the neck. The exteriorized segment reflects the vitality of the buried portion of the flap (Fig. 45).

Neurovascular Anatomy

The medial antebrachial and lateral antebrachial cutaneous nerves innervate the skin of the volar forearm and inclusion of either nerve provides a potentially sensate free flap (Fig. 46). A commonly used recipient nerve in oral reconstruction is the lingual

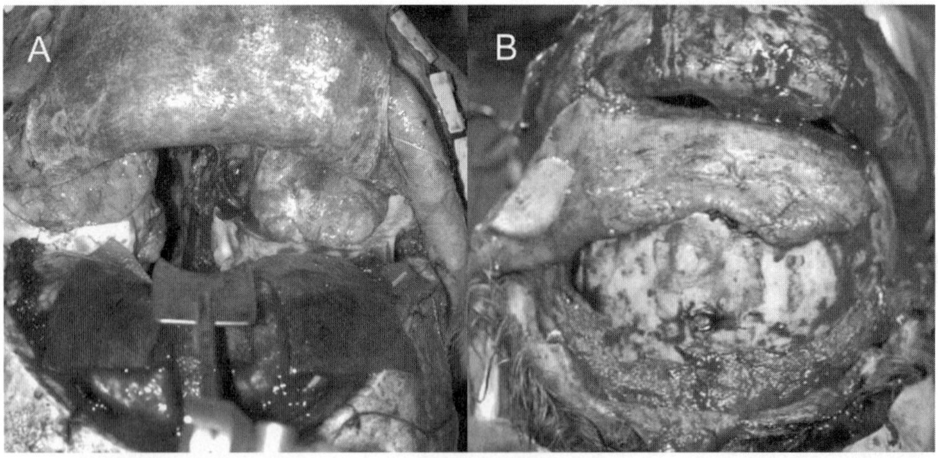

Figure 44 De-epithelialized radial forearm free flap with distal marker segment used for repair of an extensive craniofacial defect. Note the defect with communication of the anterior cranial fossa and the nasal cavity (A). The flap is placed over the defect and secured (B). The distal marker skin segment is incorporated into the scalp incision for monitoring purposes.

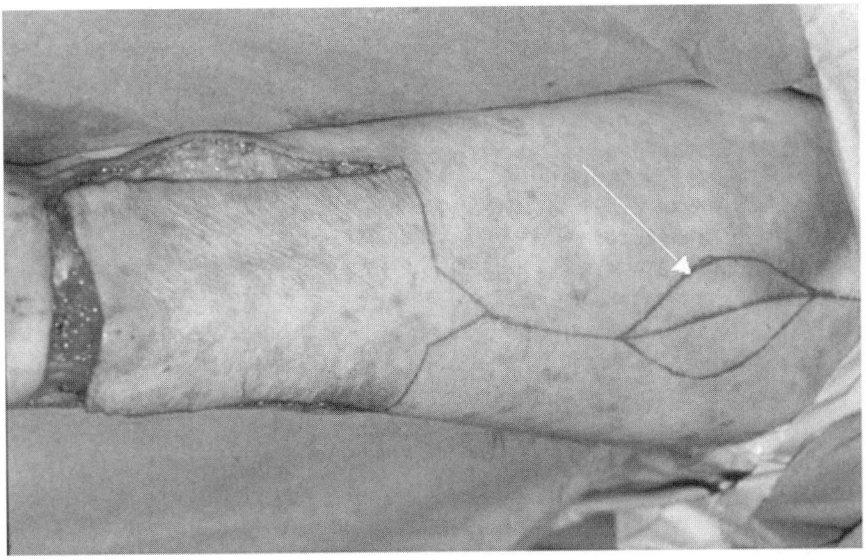

Figure 45 Radial forearm free flap for pharyngeal reconstruction with planned marker segment (arrow) to be incorporated into the neck skin flap.

nerve. The radial artery and venae comitantes are enveloped by fascial extensions from the intermuscular septum. The fascio cutaneous component receives its blood supply from the radial artery via septocutaneous perforators that course through the lateral intermuscular septum between the brachioradialis and flexi carpi radialis.

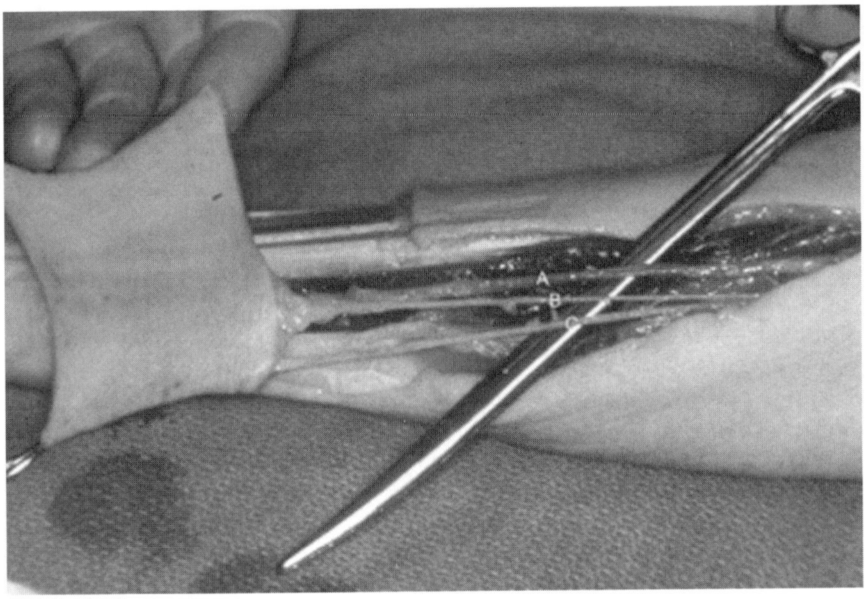

Figure 46 The radial vessels (A), lateral antebrachial cutaneous nerve (B), and cephalic vein (C).

Muscular perforators provide the vascular supply to the underlying periosteum and radial bone. The vascular pedicle (radial artery and vena comitantes) courses toward the antecubital fossa to the brachial artery. Dissection and freeing of the vascular pedicle between the superior flap edge and brachial artery require division of multiple muscular perforators.

The venae comitantes drain a deep venous system that freely communicates with the superficial system of veins. The much larger superficial venous drainage system fully supports venous outflow and can be used in place of or in addition to the venae comitantes. The superficial cephalic vein over the dorsoradial aspect of the wrist is most often incorporated.

The presence of an intact circulation between the deep and superficial palmar arches is important to ensure that the hand is adequately perfused after the radial artery is sacrificed. The lack of a collateral system may be found in as many as 15% of patients, and can be investigated clinically by performing an Allen's test (56). Edgar V. Allen originally described the Allen's test in 1929 as a noninvasive evaluation of the patency of the arterial supply to the hand of patients with thromboangiitis obliterans. In the early 1950s, the Allen's test was modified for use as a test of collateral circulation prior to arterial cannulation (57). With respect to the forearm free flap, the Allen's test is used to test the adequacy of the ulnar artery to supply the hand in the absence of the radial artery. It is performed by elevating the hand in question above the patient's head, manually occluding both the radial and ulnar arteries, dropping the hand to the level of the heart, having the patient open and close the fist several times, releasing the ulnar artery, and timing the return of capillary refill to the radial side of the hand. A positive (normal) test should document the return of capillary refill after release of the ulnar artery within 6 s. An Allen's test is not fail-safe and the adequacy of crossover blood flow between the ulnar and radial arteries should also be assessed in the operating room before the radial artery is harvested by temporary occlusion (58). If inadequate crossover exists, the flap should either be abandoned or the radial artery reconstructed with a saphenous vein graft.

After flap harvest, the donor site is covered with a skin graft. It is important to preserve the fragile tendon fascial sheaths (the peritenon) during flap harvest to provide a vascularized bed for the skin graft.

Surgical Highlights

The design and dimensions of the skin component depend upon the needs at the donor site. A simple rectangular design of appropriate dimensions will suffice in the vast majority of cases. A special design such as a bilobe is useful if a combined floor-of-mouth defect is associated with a hemiglossectomy. If the flap is used for an extensive base of tongue defect, fascia may be harvested in the mid and upper forearm continuous with the proximal aspect of the flap to fold into the defect for increased bulk.

A pneumatic tourniquet around the upper arm may be used but is usually unnecessary. The radial artery should be marked out at the wrist and the flap must be designed to incorporate this vessel. To incorporate the cephalic vein the flap is designed to extend over the dorsoradial aspect of the wrist (Fig. 47). The initial incision should be along the wrist and the radial artery identified. A temporary occlusion clamp or suture is placed around the artery and, with the tourniquet deflated, the

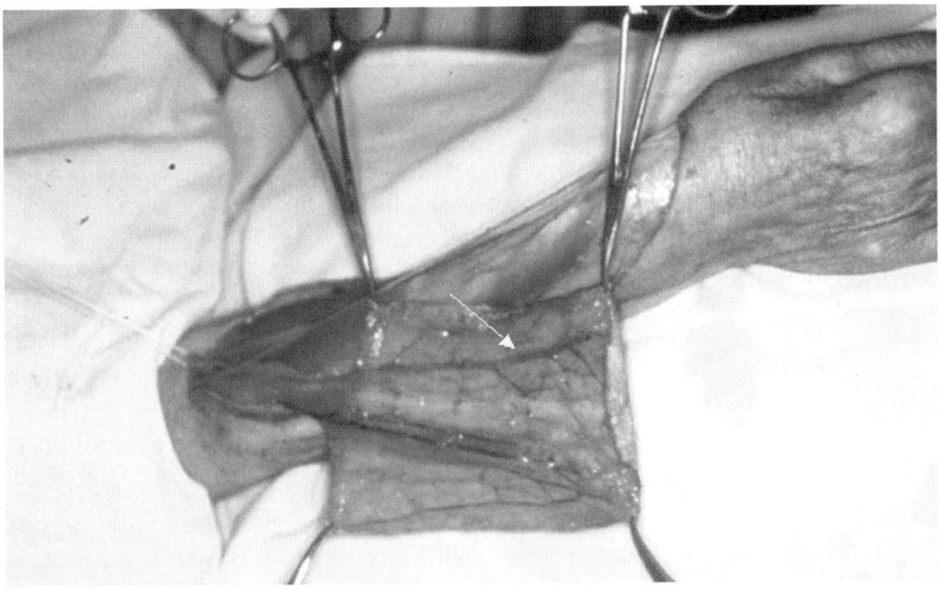

Figure 47 Radial forearm free flap designed and incised to include the cephalic vein (arrow).

Allen's test should be repeated. If the test is positive, the pedicle can be divided between clamps and ligated with sutures. The flap may be harvested from lateral to medial, completely releasing the flap to remain pedicled along its superior border. The superficial branch of the radial nerve is identified and preserved and the distal cephalic vein is divided. If needed, the palmaris tendon is easily included by dividing the tendon near the wrist and keeping the tendon with the flap during the subsequent dissection. As the flap is dissected the fascia should be taken with the flap while preserving the fine peritenon. A 10–12 cm segment of radius bone (up to 40% of the circumference) can be harvested starting from 2 to 3 cm behind the styloid process and proceeding proximally. The bone must be kept attached to the overlying vascular pedicle and skin to maintain the integrity of the muscular and septocutaneous perforators. The proximal and distal bone cuts should be directed at a gentle angle into the bone (not perpendicular) to lessen the risk of fracture. Superior to the midupper edge of the flap a gently curved cutaneous incision is made toward the antecubital fossa. Medial and lateral thin skin flaps are created to expose the underlying subcutaneous tissues and fascia.

The lateral antebrachial cutaneous nerve is very superficial and closely associated with the cephalic vein. The cephalic vein is harvested with a cuff of surrounding fascia to prevent kinking at the recipient site. Within this fascial cuff lies the sensory nerve and it may be freed by careful dissection to allow it to be directed away from the cephalic vein. Dissection of the vascular pedicle commences after the cephalic vein and sensory nerve have been dissected and divided near the antecubital fossa. The vascular pedicle is released superior to the flap within the volar forearm by dividing the numerous muscular perforators. The pedicle is dissected to its junction with the brachial artery, divided between clamps and suture-ligated, and the flap transferred to the recipient site.

Donor site closure is straightforward, involving primary closure of the incision over the volar forearm and placement of a split-thickness skin graft over the site of flap harvest. To prevent desiccation of the superficial radial nerve it should be covered by medial advancement of the lateral skin. During the initial 7 days postoperatively a temporary palmar splint is placed to allow care of the wound and to accommodate the bolster for the skin graft. If bone is harvested, an above-the-elbow cast is placed after removal of the temporary splint and worn for approximately 2 months.

Advantages

A two-team approach is possible, which significantly decreases operative time. The radial forearm flap is thin and pliable and relatively hairless. It can be folded upon itself relatively sharply to imitate the abrupt angles that may be required at the recipient site. It may also be de-epithelialized for both internal and external lining as well as for limited defects of the cranial base. The radial artery is large (2 mm) and the cephalic vein can be included when harvesting the flap, making the microvascular anastomoses straightforward.

Disadvantages

Harvesting the underlying radius bone entails several weeks of postoperative cast immobilization and carries a significant risk of radial bone fracture. The dorsal cutaneous branch of the superficial radial nerve courses over the dorsoradial aspect of the wrist in close association with the cephalic vein. It is at risk when the distal cephalic vein is divided. Injury results in numbness over the anatomical snuff box, the thenar eminence, and the dorsoradial and ulnar aspects of the thumb.

The donor site requires a skin graft and the appearance of the site can be unsightly during healing. Portions of the skin graft will often slough due to movement or loss of peritenon. It takes several weeks for these areas to heal completely. Nevertheless, even if a tendon is exposed, standard wet-to-dry dressings will be sufficient and complete healing is expected. Some patients, especially African-Americans, are prone to hypertrophic scars (Fig. 48). Subcutaneous injection of steroids may be helpful.

Scapula

Description

The scapular system of flaps consists of multiple bone and soft tissue free flaps that can be harvested alone or in combination based on a single vascular pedicle (the subscapular artery). The most popular is the scapular osteocutaneous flap, which is a type B flap originally described by Swartz et al. in 1986 for mandibular reconstruction (46). The circumflex scapular artery and the thoracodorsal artery are the two main tributaries of the subscapular artery. The circumflex scapular territory includes the lateral border of the scapula and a 500 cm^2 area of overlying skin. The thoracodorsal territory includes the latissimus muscle and the lower slips of the serratus anterior muscle.

Up to 14 cm lateral border of the scapula can be harvested in men based on the circumflex scapular artery. Although the entire lateral border of the scapula is supplied by the circumflex scapular artery, the distal third including the tip is additionally supplied by the angular artery from the thoracodorsal system. Preservation of the thoracodorsal contribution allows the harvest of independent bone segments and ensures viability of the bone distal to shaping osteotomies. The lateral border

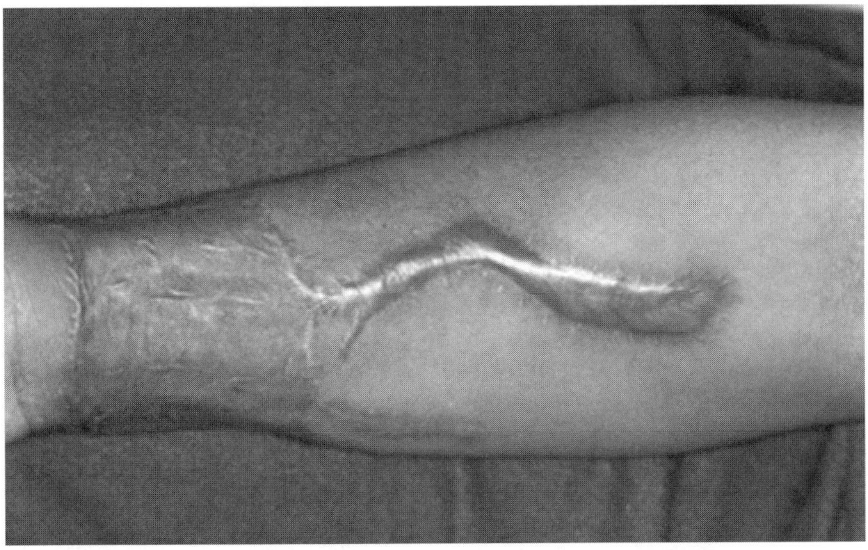

Figure 48 Hypertrophic scarring that developed several weeks after harvest of a radial forearm flap in an African-American woman.

of the scapula provides a cylindrical segment of corticocancellous bone that is able to accommodate osseointegrated implants. The diameter of the bone is relatively small compared to the fibula and iliac crest and it is unable to restore the vertical height of the mandible in most cases. Conforming dentures will not be successful, but implant-borne dentures are usually workable.

The fasciocutaneous territory of the circumflex scapular system is extremely large and nearly all the skin of the upper hemiback can be harvested. However, to provide for primary closure of the donor site, the flaps must be limited in size: 6×15 cm transverse flap and up to 12×20 cm parascapular flap. These flaps can be separated and manipulated independently on their respective arterial vascular pedicles (the transverse and descending branches of the circumflex scapular artery).

The thoracodorsal territory includes the latissimus muscle and overlying skin, and the lower three or four muscular slips of the serratus anterior muscle with the underlying ribs. The latissimus muscle is an extremely broad and thin muscle with the potential for motor reinnervation via the thoracodorsal nerve. The skin is highly dependent upon direct musculocutaneous perforators from the underlying latissimus muscle and only the skin directly over the muscle should be transferred. The serratus anterior muscle originates from the first nine ribs, forming independent bands of muscle that course posterosuperiorly to insert as a broad conjoined tendon onto the medial and inferior borders of the scapula. The lower three or four muscular slips can be transferred as free tissue supplied by branches of the thoracodorsal artery and long thoracic nerve.

Indications

The scapular system of flaps provides a huge amount of tissue with multiple components that can be transferred based on a single vascular pedicle (the subscapular artery). Rarely is such an enormous amount of tissue required. However, such a flap

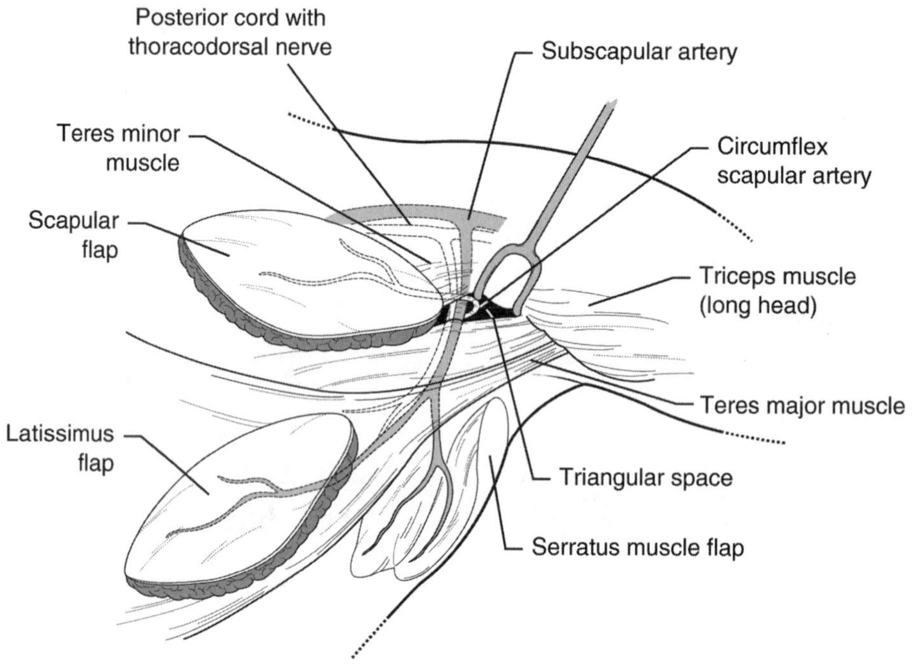

Figure 49 The subscapular system of flaps is extensive with multiple components all based on the subscapular vessels. Although rarely needed, this megaflap includes transverse and parascapular skin paddles, scapular bone, musculocutaneous latissimus flap, and serratus muscle and underlying rib.

is useful for a combined composite defect of the tongue, floor of mouth, mandible, and neck skin. The mega flap would consist of a transverse scapular flap (tongue), a parascapular flap (chin/cheeks), the lateral scapula (mandible), and a musculocutaneous latissimus flap (neck) (Fig. 49).

Most patients require only certain components of the scapular system alone or in combination. The most useful flap within the circumflex scapular system is the osteocutaneous scapular (parascapular) flap consisting of scapular bone and an associated fasciocutaneous flap for composite mandibular defects (Fig. 50). Although the bone is too short for extensive mandibular defects, it is capable of reconstructing anterior or lateral defects up to 14 cm in length. An osteocutaneous flap is also suitable for reconstruction of complex composite midfacial defects (e.g., radical maxillectomy with an overlying cheek defect). The lateral wall of the nasal cavity and facial skin defect is closed with the parascapular and transverse fasciocutaneous flaps while the alveolar ridge and hard palate are reconstructed with the scapular bone. The thinner medial portion of the scapula can also be used for reconstruction of the floor of the orbit.

The fasciocutaneous flaps alone are useful for simple soft tissue coverage, through-and-through defects of the cheeks, or as a filler or barrier in their fascial or de-epithelialized forms. The scapular fasciocutaneous flap is a second-line alternative in covering surface skin defects of the scalp and lateral skull base because of bulk and color problems (Fig. 51). The combination of transverse and parascapular flaps

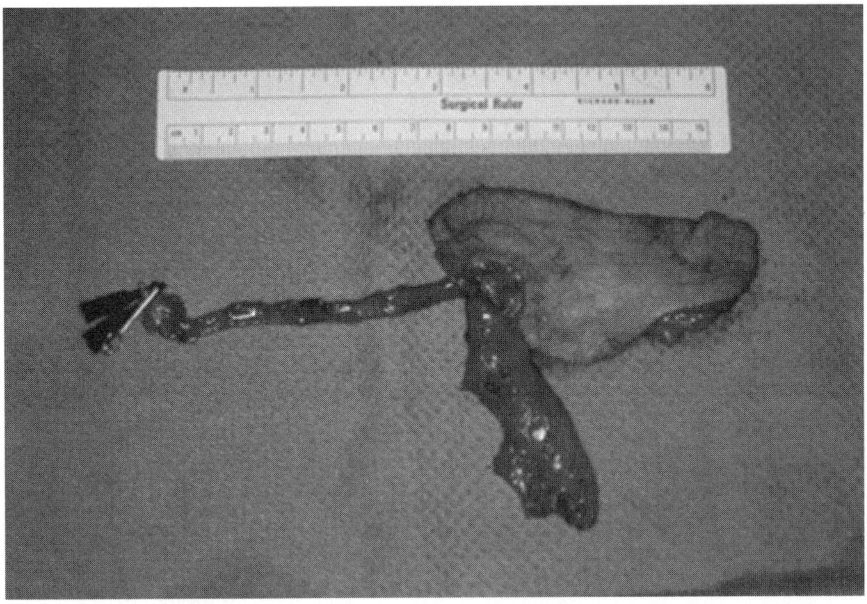

Figure 50 An osteocutaneous scapular flap. The bone is relatively short compared to the fibula and iliac crest.

is useful for through-and-through defects owing to their capacity for complete separation and maneuverability. The de-epithelialized or fascial flap is a first-line alternative for filling subcutaneous deficiencies in the face secondary to trauma or hemifacial microsomia.

The latissimus musculocutaneous flap is useful for extensive hemifacial or cervical cutaneous defects. The latissimus muscle with a split-thickness skin graft is the method of choice for reconstruction of extensive surface defects of the scalp. A musculocutaneous free tissue transplant is described for functional tongue reconstruction after subtotal or total resection (59). The fibers of the latissimus muscle are oriented transversely and secured to the angles of the mandible to create a mound of skin and muscle at the level of the soft palate. The thoracodorsal nerve is anastomosed to the hypoglossal nerve and subsequent movement of the flap towards the soft palate occurs during speech and swallowing. The movement is quite gross but improvements in articulation and swallowing are reported compared to patients reconstructed with nonfunctional tissue.

The latissimus muscle has recently been described as a single-stage method for reanimation of the paralyzed face (60). The thoracodorsal nerve is able to reach the opposite face (and donor facial nerve branches), obviating the need for cross-face nerve grafting. In the report by Harii et al., the muscle acquired functionality at a mean of 7 months postoperatively, which is better than expected based on clinical experience using nonvascularized nerve grafting techniques. The serratus anterior muscle is more typical of free muscle transplants for facial reanimation. The lower three slips of the serratus anterior muscle are useful for facial reanimation. Preservation of the insertions and nerve supply (long thoracic nerve) of the upper muscular slips is important to prevent winging of the scapula. This will

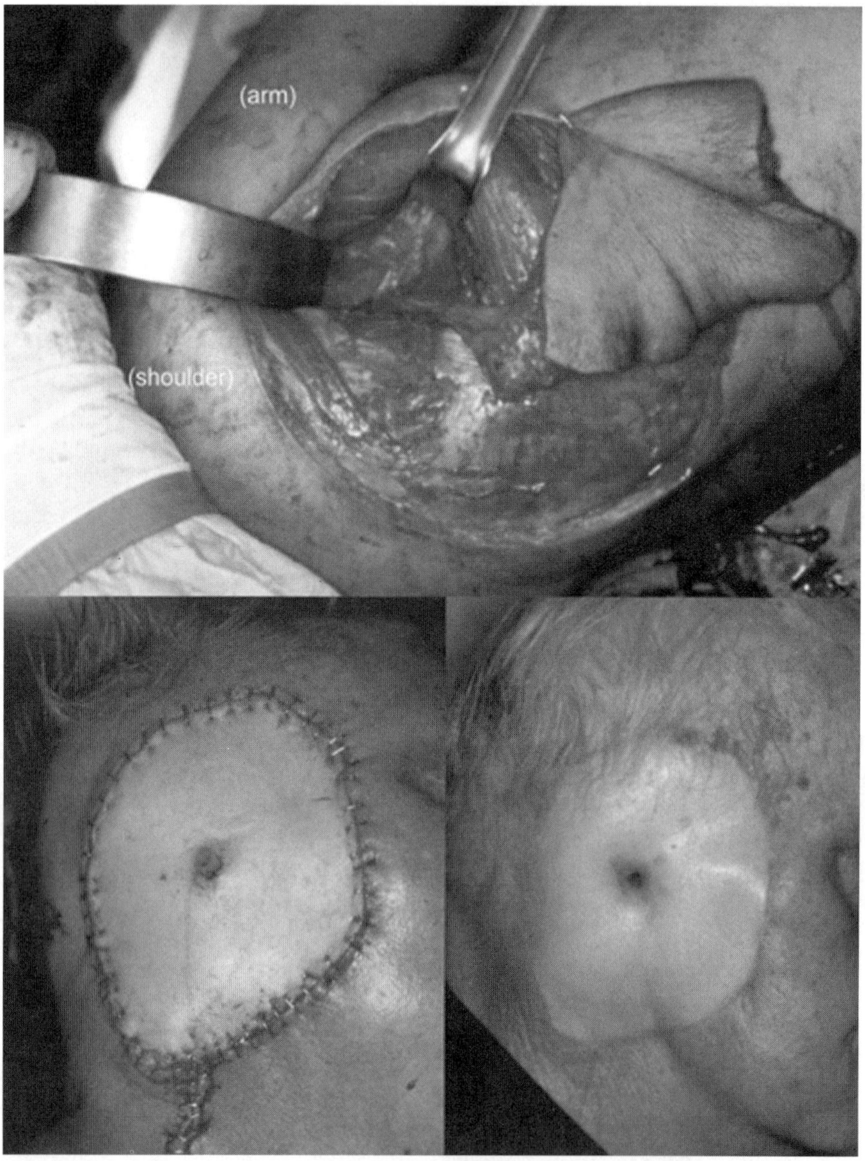

Figure 51 Scapular fasciocutaneous flap used to resurface a lateral skull defect. Note the transverse skin flap pedicled on its feeding vessels coming from deep within the triangular space (upper photo). Intraoperative and postoperative results depicted in lower photos.

result in a relatively short nerve pedicle, but preserving the upper long thoracic nerve must take priority. Cross-face nerve grafting is usually required several months prior to flap transfer.

The serratus anterior is occasionally harvested with the underlying sixth and seventh ribs for composite defects in the head and neck. Combined latissimus muscle (with or without skin) and serratus anterior myo-osseous flaps are described for large composite defects of the mandible and scalp (61). The main benefit of this combination is that the musculocutaneous component can be completely separated and maneuvered independently from the myo-osseous component.

Neurovascular Anatomy

The subscapular artery branches within a few millimeters of its origin from the axial artery into the circumflex scapular artery and the thoracodorsal artery. The triangular space is the essential anatomical landmark for the system of flaps nourished by the circumflex scapular artery. The long head of the triceps, teres minor muscle, and teres major muscle form the boundaries of the space. Deep within the triangular space, the circumflex artery gives off several ascending and descending branches along the lateral border of the scapula to supply the periosteum and underlying bone. As the artery exits the triangle, it divides into transverse and descending branches to supply the transverse and parascapular fasciocutaneous flaps, respectively. The transverse flap tends to be a slightly better color match to the face and neck but the dimensions must be smaller than a parascapular flap to allow primary closure of the donor site. A transverse flap can be up to 6 × 15 cm while a parascapular flap can be much larger depending on the size and habitus of the patient. The length of the vascular pedicle including the subscapular artery ranges from 6 to 8 cm and the individual components (bone and skin flaps) can be freely manipulated based on their respective vascular pedicles.

The thoracodorsal artery does not exit the triangular space but continues inferiorly behind the teres major muscle to travel deep to the latissimus muscle. A branch to the serratus anterior muscle is found at approximately the inferior border of the teres major muscle. The angular artery branches off the artery to the serratus to supply the tip and lower third of the scapula. This portion of the scapula can be harvested with the thoracodorsal system or it can be preserved with the circumflex scapular system. If it is preserved with the circumflex scapular system, the lower third of the scapula will be vascularized despite osteotomies that would otherwise place this segment at risk. The artery to the serratus anterior continues on to supply the lower three or four slips of the serratus anterior. The lateral thoracic artery supplies the upper five slips of the serratus anterior muscle. Injection studies demonstrate that the thoracodorsal artery provides reliable vascularity to the sixth and seventh ribs at the origin of the serratus muscle (62). A twig from the long thoracic nerve and a segmental branch of the artery supply each slip of muscle. The thoracodorsal artery penetrates the deep surface of the latissimus muscle approximately 10 cm from the axillary artery, well inferior to its insertion into the humerus (at the intertubercular groove). After penetrating the latissimus muscle, the thoracodorsal artery splits into a lateral branch that parallels the anterior border of the muscle and a medial branch that courses inferomedially.

No harvestable sensory nerves are described for any component of the scapular system. Most components have two veins accompanying the artery (the venae comitantes) that measure between 1.5 and 3 mm. The venae comitantes usually merge into a single large vein near the subscapular artery.

Surgical Highlights

The Fasciocutaneous Flaps and the Osteocutaneous Scapular Flap. As for all of the scapular flaps, the patient must be placed in the lateral decubitus position for flap harvest. The ipsilateral arm can be gently supported over a sterilely covered Mayo stand with generous cushioning around the elbow. An axillary roll should be placed under the opposite shoulder and axilla to prevent a neuropraxic injury. The key surface landmark is the triangular space bounded by the long head of the triceps, the teres major muscle, and the teres minor muscle (Fig. 52). It is palpated with the thumb as the axilla is grasped and the arm is extended (Fig. 53). The circumflex scapular artery passes through this space to supply the transverse and parascapular fasciocutaneous components. En route through the space, the artery sends periosteal branches to the lateral border of the scapular. The transverse and parascapular fasciocutaneous flaps can be harvested as separate components based on the transverse and descending branches of the circumflex scapular vascular bundle. The lateral aspect of the flap must be placed over the triangular space to capture the circumflex artery as it exits the triangular space. A parascapular flap, due to its oblique orientation on the back, can be designed much larger (up to 12 cm × 20 cm) than its counterpart, the transverse scapular flap, while still allowing primary donor site closure. Dissection begins medially by raising the flap (including its underlying fascia) towards the triangular space. The fasciocutaneous vessels (transverse and descending branches of the circumflex scapular) are visualized on the undersurface of the flap while the thick white deep fascia over the infraspinatus muscle is left undisturbed. Once the vessels are seen diving into the triangular space, the fasciocutaneous flap is raised circumferentially, pedicled only by its vascular supply (Fig. 54). The periosteal branches to the scapular bone are divided and the teres minor and major and triceps muscles are retracted. The circumflex scapular vessels are dissected to their origin from the subscapular artery where they are divided, thereby harvesting the skin flap and its attached vascular pedicle.

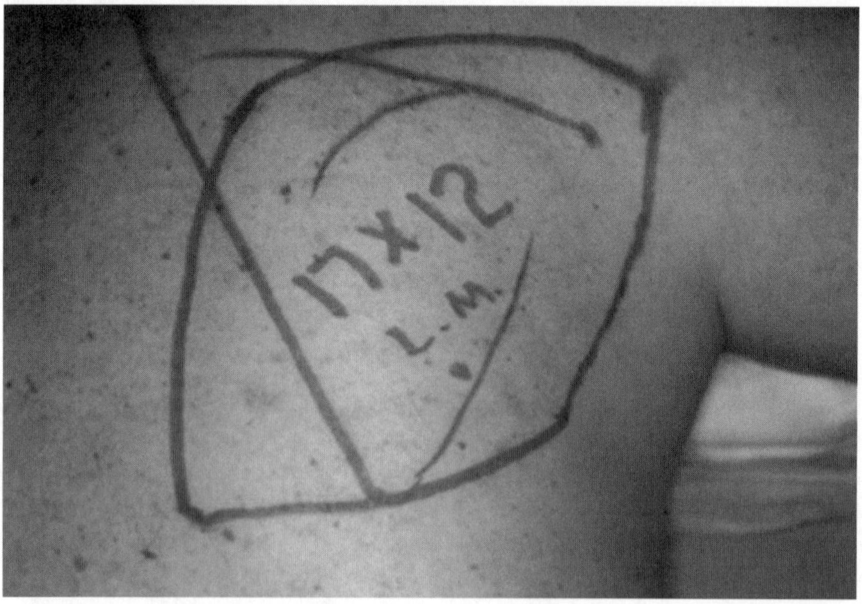

Figure 52 A large parascapular flap marked over the back. The dimensions of a parascapular flap can be much greater than a transverse flap, while still allowing for primary closure of the donor site.

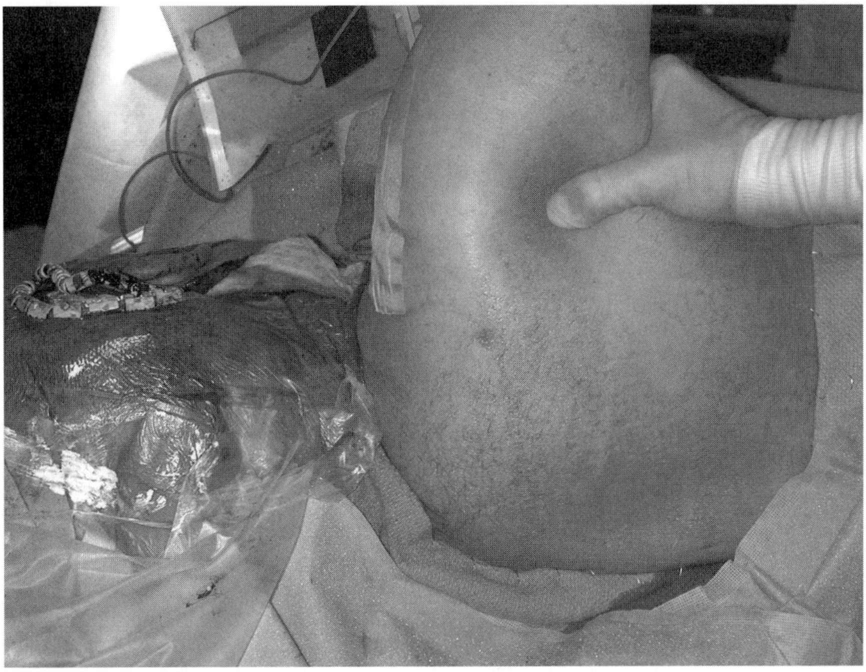

Figure 53 Seeking the triangular space with the thumb. This is the first step to determine the exit point of the feeding vessels. The skin flaps must be harvested to include the skin and subcutaneous tissues over this space.

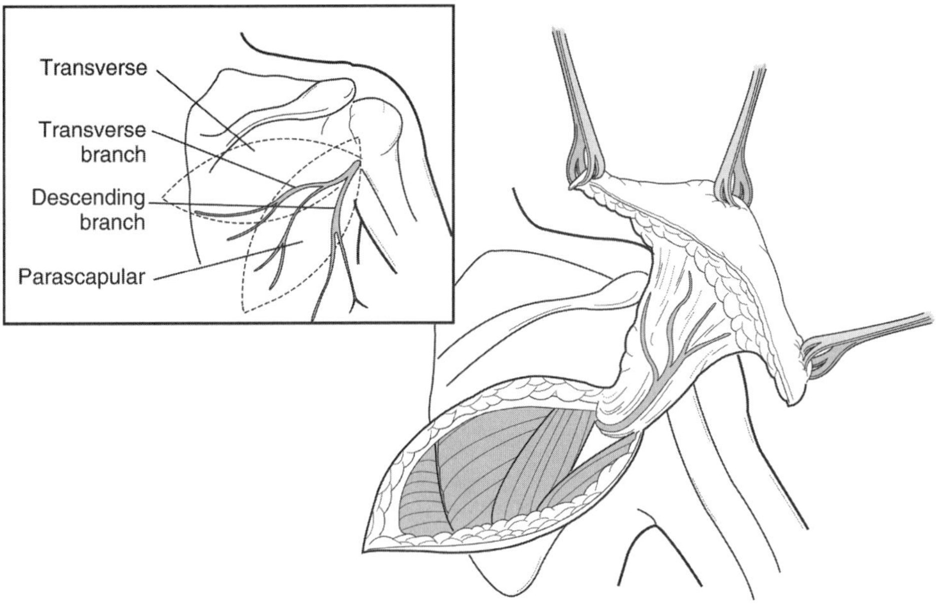

Figure 54 The transverse scapular flap harvested and pedicled on the circumflex scapular vessels. Note the origin of the vessels through the triangular space.

Harvest of an osteocutaneous scapular flap requires that the periosteal branches to the lateral border of the scapula be preserved while the pedicle is being dissected toward the subscapular artery. To harvest the bone, a cautery device is used to incise the teres and infraspinatus muscles sharply along a line approximately 2 cm from the lateral scapular border. The glenoid fossa is palpated and an oscillating saw is used to cut along the line previously outlined by cautery. A transverse osteotomy is made 2 cm below the glenoid fossa, thereby completing the bony cuts. Once the bone is pulled laterally, it will be noted that muscular slips from the serratus anterior and subscapularis must also be divided with cautery. The angular artery enters the tip of the scapula and should be preserved if conforming osteotomies are planned. This artery is a branch from the artery to the serratus anterior muscle (a division of the thoracodorsal artery). The artery to the serratus muscle is divided distal to the take-off of the angular branch (Fig. 55). The osteocutaneous flap is finally freed by dividing the subscapular artery. The circumflex scapular and thoracodorsal arteries should be carefully preserved. After harvesting the flap, the cut teres muscles

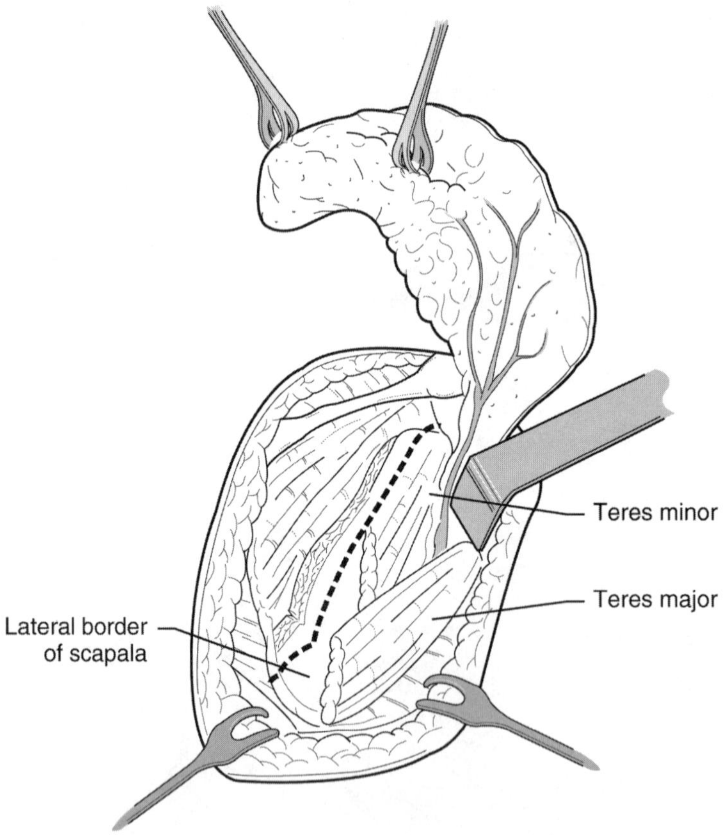

Figure 55 The parascapular skin flap harvested with the scapular bone (osteocutaneous scapular flap). Note that the bone consists of only the lateral border of the scapular bone. The bone along the tip of the scapular is prone to necrosis only if a shaping osteotomy is created that isolates the tip from its vascular supply. To ensure adequate vascularity of this segment of bone in the event of osteotomy, the angular artery should be preserved (see text).

are not sutured together but are left in situ to prevent shoulder stiffness postoperatively. The serratus muscle fibers may be reattached to the inferior aspect of the scapula to stabilize this structure, if needed.

The Latissimus Musculocutaneous Flap. The latissimus muscle is harvested via an access incision along the posterior axillary fold. The extent of the incision depends on the volume of muscle to be harvested and whether a muscle-only or a musculocutaneous flap is planned (Fig. 56). The anterior border of the muscle is retracted and the neurovascular anatomy is exposed (Figs. 57, 58). If a segment of muscle is going to be used for facial reanimation, the thoracodorsal nerve is dissected free and traced superiorly to deep within the axilla near the axillary artery. Additional length on the nerve can be achieved by dissection of the nerve distally toward the muscle and division of small twigs until the main body of the nerve actually penetrates the segment of muscle that will be transferred. The length of nerve that can be harvested is up to 15 cm. The segment of muscle should be 3–4 cm wide by 8–10 cm long, with the direction of the fibers paralleling the long axis. The vascular pedicle is dissected proximally to the subscapular artery and divided. The muscle is inset into the face in the typical manner (see section on gracilis muscle) from the zygoma to the modiolus and inferior lip. The thoracodorsal nerve is placed through a subcutaneous pocket in the upper lip to the preauricular area over the opposite cheek. The thoracodorsal nerve is anastomosed end-to-end with two or three buccal branches of the facial nerve.

When harvesting the latissimus muscle with or without the overlying skin, the thoracodorsal vascular pedicle should be identified first through the upper part of the access incision. This simplifies the dissection because the vascular pedicle enters the muscle well inferior to, and at a variable distance from, its insertion into the upper humerus. A muscle-only flap is harvested by dissecting the subcutaneous tissues of the surface of the latissimus muscle while identifying the entire anterior

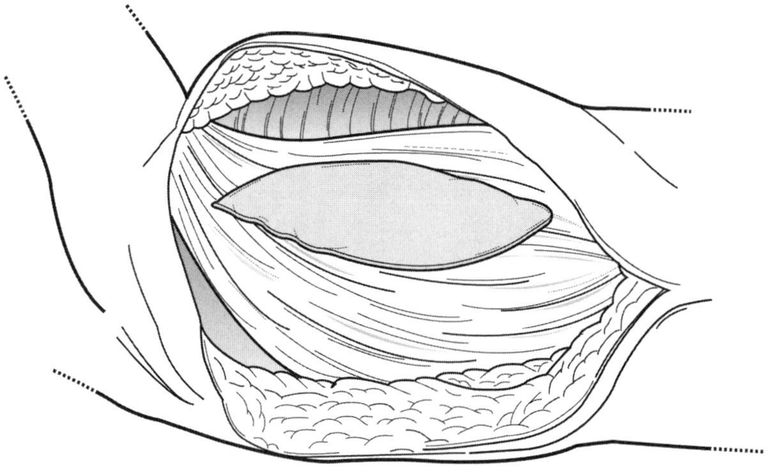

Figure 56 After a lengthy longitudinal incision along the axillary fold corresponding to the anterior border of the latissimus muscle, anterior and posterior subcutaneous flaps are raised over the muscle outside the intended skin paddle. The skin paddle must be of sufficient size to capture the terminal musculocutaneous vessels that nourish it.

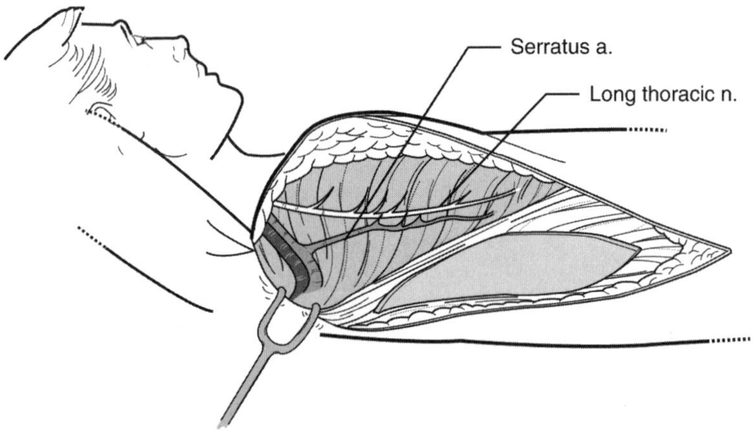

Figure 57 Retraction of the anterior border of the latissimus muscle uncovers the relevant neurovascular anatomy. Note the surface neurovascular structures over the serratus muscle including the long thoracic nerve and serratus vessels. The thoracodorsal vessels supplying the latissimus muscle are large and easily identified.

edge of the muscle. The thoracodorsal pedicle is identified as mentioned by retracting the humeral head of the muscle and a vessel loop is placed around the vascular pedicle. The natural tissue plane between the underlying muscles and fascia including the serratus muscle is bluntly dissected. The vascular pedicle is separated from the thoracodorsal nerve and dissected superiorly to the subscapular artery after the branch to the serratus muscle is divided. The humeral head of the muscle is divided using cautery. The muscle is freed by dividing its inferomedial insertions and, finally, dividing the subscapular artery and thoracodorsal nerve.

To harvest a musculocutaneous flap, a skin island is designed that is completely within the boundary of the latissimus muscle since any portion of the skin that extends beyond the muscle is subject to ischemia and necrosis. The skin paddle should be no less than $25\,cm^2$ to ensure the inclusion of sufficient musculocutaneous perforating vessels. The outline of the skin island is sharply incised to (not through) the underlying muscle. A subcutaneous dissection over the muscle proceeds outside the borders of the skin island. The anterior edge of the latissimus muscle is identified through the posterior axillary incision and the dissection proceeds as in a muscle-only harvest.

Primary closure over one or two large suction drains is typical. The subcutaneous tissues are closed with strong absorbable sutures and the skin is closed with staples supplemented with horizontal mattress nonabsorbable sutures. This harvest site is especially prone to the formation of seromas; therefore, the drains should remain in place for 10 days. Some collection of fluid is to be expected after the drains are removed but the strong closure should prevent dehiscence of the wound.

The Serratus Anterior Muscle for Facial Reanimation. The anterior border of the latissimus muscle is identified through the posterior axillary fold incision. The serratus muscle is exposed by posterior retraction of the latissimus muscle, blunt dissection, and subcutaneous dissection over the muscle itself. The neurovascular components are easily identified since they enter the muscle from its outer surface.

The thoracodorsal vessels are divided distal to the take-off of the serratus branch. The serratus branch supplies only the lower three or four slips of the muscle and these slips of muscle will be harvested. The long thoracic nerve is split with respect to its segmental innervation of each muscular slip with the aid of a nerve stimulator. The muscular slips to be harvested are separated from their site of origin (underlying rib) and insertion (scapula) and freed (Fig. 58). The thoracodorsal nerve is divided proximally and the serratus and thoracodorsal vessels are dissected towards the subscapular artery and divided. Donor site closure is accomplished through simple layered approximation of the subcutaneous and cutaneous tissues over a suction drain.

The slips of the serratus muscle can be used to rehabilitate separate functioning units of the face. Cross-face nerve grafting is usually required several months prior to flap transfer. Immediate anastomosis with the hypoglossal nerve is also described (63).

Advantages

Advantages to the scapular flap include pedicle length, vessel diameter, donor site morbidity, and versatility. Perhaps the most important characteristic of the scapula free flap is the ability to use several composite tissues based on a single vascular pedicle for the reconstruction of very large and complex three-dimensional defects.

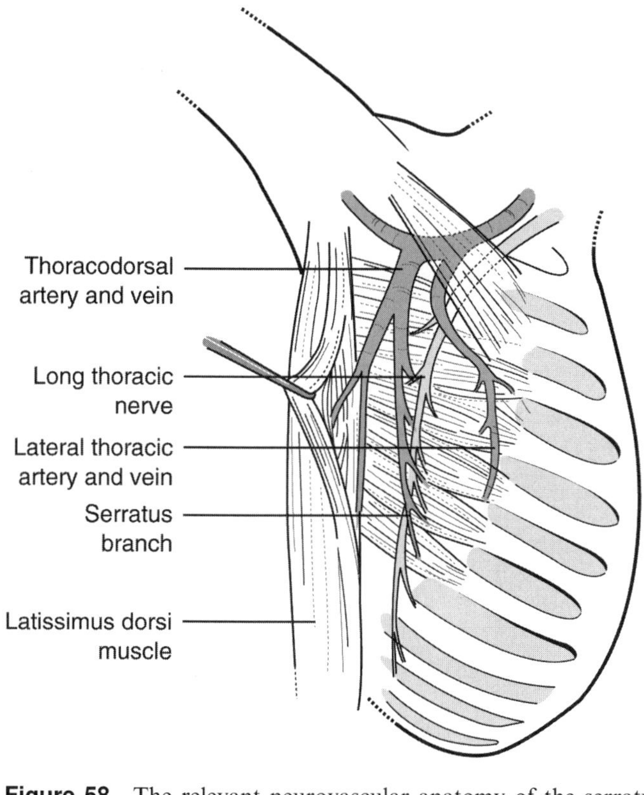

Figure 58 The relevant neurovascular anatomy of the serratus flap. Note that the nerves and vessels enter the muscle from its outer surface. The serratus branch of the thoracodorsal artery supplies only the lower three or four slips of the muscle and these slips of muscle will be harvested.

Disadvantages

Disadvantages include the inability simultaneously to harvest the flap with the extirpative portion of the procedure, lack of sensory reinnervation, thin and short scapular bone (especially in female patients), and often bulky skin paddles. The main disadvantage accounting for the lack of widespread use of this flap is the difficulty in performing this dissection coincidentally with the ablative surgery. In addition, the bone tends to be significantly thinner than the iliac crest and fibula, making osseointegration more tenuous. Bone length also falls well short of that of the fibula and cannot be used to reconstruct anything more that an anterior arch or lateral segmental mandibular defect.

Dorsalis Pedis

Description

The dorsalis pedis flap is an osteomusculocutaneous flap with the cutaneous portion supplied by a direct cutaneous artery passing through the extensor hallucis brevis muscle. The skin component extends from the dorsum of the foot: from the ankle crease to the toe web spaces (64). The dorsalis pedis flap may be harvested as a skin–fascial flap only or may be a composite flap to include tendons, innervated muscle (extensor digitorum brevis), bone (second metatarsal), and whole digits or joints (Fig. 59).

Prior to flap elevation, the dorsalis pedis pulse should be verified by palpation, and the course of the superficial venous system is outlined for incision planning. The presence of a first dorsal metatarsal artery should also be confirmed with Doppler ultrasound—(arteriography is unnecessary). The flap is usually harvested distal to proximal to include the first dorsal metatarsal artery and the dorsalis pedis artery while preserving the superficial venous system. Inclusion of the second metatarsal bone requires that the periosteal blood supply remain intact beneath the artery. The extensor retinaculum is divided proximally and the anterior tibial artery is dissected as needed for pedicle length. Preservation of the fine peritenon is important since the donor site must be closed with a skin graft.

Indications

The dorsalis pedis flap is most often used in hand reconstruction. In the head and neck, intraoral defects requiring thin and mobile skin may be reconstructed with this flap similarly to areas that may be reconstructed with a radial forearm flap. The skin also conforms well to external facial defects including those involving the nose, lip, and orbit. Limited segmental mandibular defects (< 6 cm) may be reconstructed using the second metatarsal bone. This bone may also be used as a cantilevered bone graft for nasal reconstruction. Replacement of the temporomandibular joint with the second metatarsal joint is also described (65). The extensor digitorum brevis muscle may be used for facial reanimation, although other flaps are more useful in this regard.

Neurovascular Anatomy

The dorsalis pedis artery (an extension of the anterior tibial artery under the extensor retinaculum) and, the first dorsal metatarsal branch supply the flap. The venous drainage consists of a deep system (the venae comitantes that accompany the dorsalis pedis artery) and a superficial system in the subcutaneous substance of the flap that coalesce medially to form the long saphenous vein. The sensory supply to the

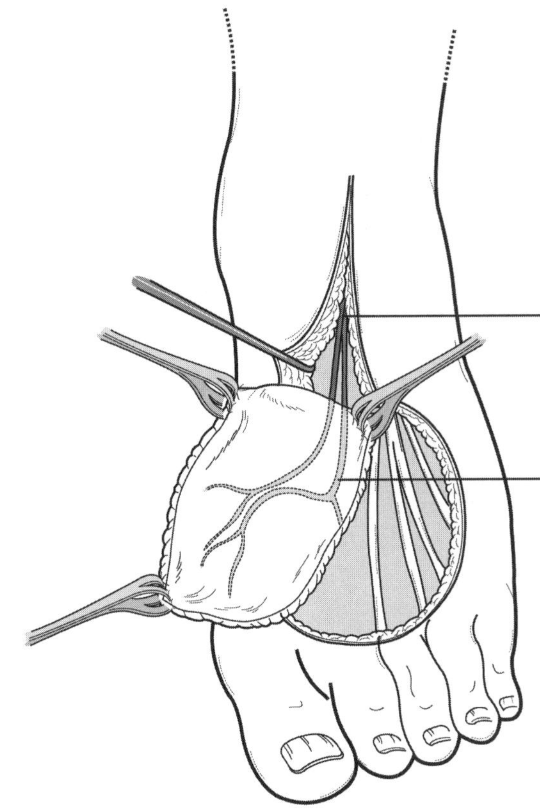

Figure 59 Surgical anatomy of the little-used dorsalis pedis flap. Note the vascular supply of this flap as the dorsalis pedis artery and vein.

skin is from terminal branches of the superficial peroneal nerve proximally and minor branches of the deep peroneal nerve distally. The motor supply to the extensor digitorum brevis is from tributaries of the deep peroneal nerve and its blood supply is from lateral tarsal branches of the dorsalis pedis artery.

Advantages

A two-team approach is possible and significantly reduces operative time. The vascular pedicle is quite long and can be extended if the anterior tibial artery is harvested. The vessel diameters are large (the artery diameter approaches 3 mm). The skin is very thin, pliable, hairless, and potentially sensate.

Disadvantages

The primary disadvantage to the dorsalis pedis flap is donor site morbidity. Delayed wound healing and poor skin graft take are common problems. The flap is contraindicated for patients with poor wound healing potential including diabetic patients or those with peripheral vascular disease. The anatomy of the first dorsal metatarsal artery is variable and may be absent in 14% of patients, putting the survival of the distal part of the flap in jeopardy (66). There is a poor skin color match to the facial skin. The extensor digitorum brevis muscle is weak and is a relatively poor choice for facial reanimation.

Iliac

Description

Taylor first described this type C flap for mandibular reconstruction in 1982 (47). The bone available for harvest includes the anterior iliac spine and wing of the ilium (14–16 cm). The ilium is a curvilinear, thick, bicortical bone. The amount of harvestable bone is 4 cm in height by 14 cm in length, either bicortical or inner cortex only. The skin directly overlying the bone, supplied by septocutaneous perforating vessels closely applied to the bone, may also be harvested (Fig. 60). In addition, based on the ascending branch of the deep circumflex artery, the internal oblique muscle may be harvested for either intra- or extraoral use (67).

Indications

The iliac crest bone is ideally shaped for replacement of a hemimandibular defect. Associated soft tissue defects of the cheek, tongue, or neck may be simultaneously reconstructed using the skin overlying the ilium. The internal oblique muscle may be included with an osseous or osteocutaneous flap (Fig. 61). It can be manipulated independently to drape over vital neck vessels or to cover the bone in the oral cavity. If the muscle is used to drape over the neoalveolus, it can be left to re-epithelialize or skin-grafted to form a thin gingiva-like surface ready for osseointegrated implants.

Neurovascular Anatomy

The deep circumflex iliac artery (DCIA) provides the blood supply to the flap. It originates from a branch of the external iliac artery or femoral artery inferior to the

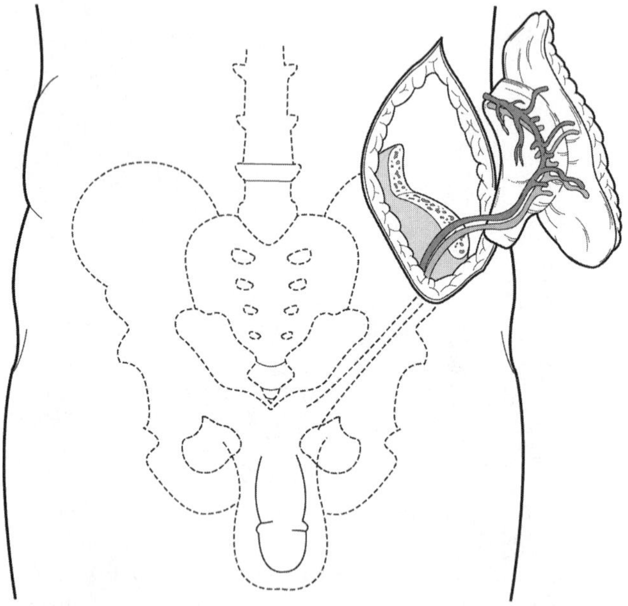

Figure 60 The iliac crest flap is harvested with a closely attached overlying skin paddle based on the deep circumflex iliac artery. This flap can also be harvested with the internal oblique muscle (not shown).

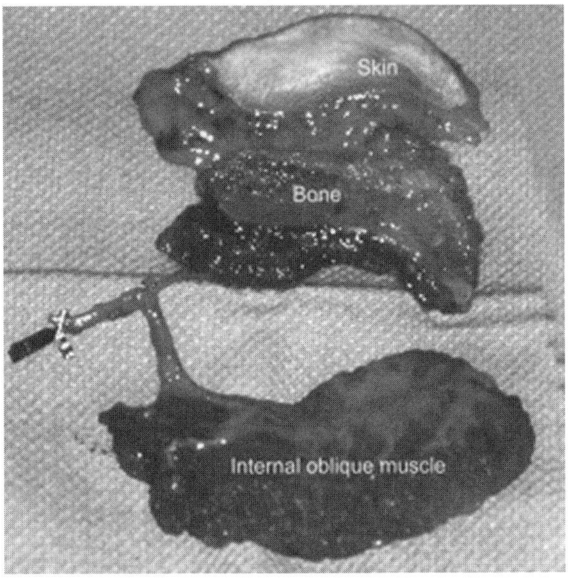

Figure 61 Iliac crest free flap with skin and internal oblique muscle harvested. The muscle is thin and easily draped over the bone to form the neoalveolus.

inguinal ligament. The external diameter of the DCIA near its origin is between 1–2 mm. Venae comitantes accompany the DCIA and join to form a common vein (approximately 4 mm in external diameter) as it nears the external iliac vein. The vascular bundle courses superolaterally, crossed by ilioinguinal and lateral femoral nerves, from behind the inguinal ligament toward the inner aspect of the anterior superior iliac spine (ASIS), resulting in a potential pedicle length of approximately 6 cm. The ascending branch takes off from the DCIA just proximal to the ASIS, coursing between, and supplying, the internal oblique and transversalis muscles. The vascular bundle follows the inner border of the iliac crest and sends several branches into the periosteum to supply the bone and overlying skin.

There is no sensory nerve for reinnervation of the skin paddle. The lateral femoral cutaneous nerve provides sensation to the lateral thigh, and should be preserved as it crosses the vascular pedicle proximal to the ASIS.

Surgical Highlights

The skin paddle is outlined in the form of an ellipse centered over the iliac crest, along a line from the pubic tubercle to the tip of the scapula. The anteriormost portion of the skin paddle is placed over the ASIS, and may be up to 12 cm wide by 25 cm long. The skin paddle must be of sufficient size to capture reliably at least one of the septocutaneous perforators along the iliac crest (Fig. 62).

The lateral femoral cutaneous and ilioinguinal nerves cross the DCIA and should be preserved during the dissection. Occasionally, the lateral femoral cutaneous nerve is so intimately involved with the DCIA that extensive dissection is necessary to separate them. Injury to the nerve is more likely in these cases and the patient should be warned preoperatively that lateral thigh numbness might occur.

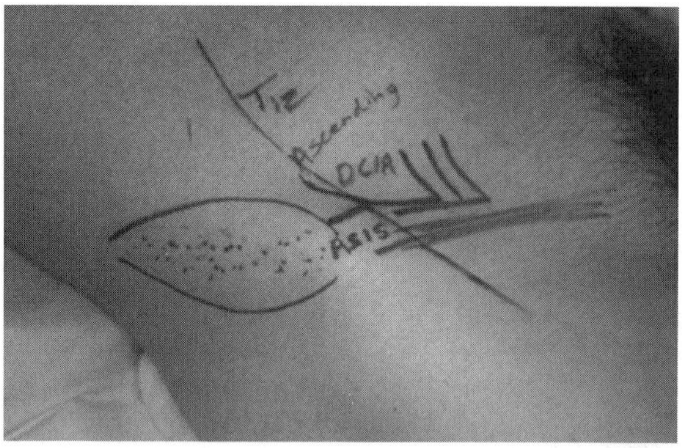

Figure 62 Iliac crest osteocutaneous flap surface landmarks. Prior to flap harvest, the skin paddle is outlined over the iliac crest bone. Also note the position of the feeding vessels (DCIA and ascending branch) and the likely course of the lateral femoral cutaneous nerve (T12).

If the internal oblique muscle is harvested, the ascending branch of the DCIA must be preserved. The ascending branch is found just anterior to the ASIS as a discrete artery in 80% of patients. In the remaining 20%, the internal oblique muscle is supplied by smaller vessels along the DCIA and is therefore not harvestable as a separate component.

In preparation for bone harvest, the iliacus muscle is sharply incised approximately 1 cm inferior to the vascular bundle and the periosteum stripped along the planned cut. The tensor fascia lata and periosteum are stripped from the outer iliac crest, and a reciprocating saw is used to cut the bone from the outer aspect. A hand is placed over the inner cortex to protect the abdominal contents. The use of chisels is discouraged since this may lead to occult fractures and splintering of the bone at the donor site.

The wound is closed in several layers using heavy nonabsorbable suture for the first two layers. The transversalis fascia is sutured to the tensor fascia lata inferior to the iliac crest or to the iliac crest directly with holes drilled through the bone to anchor the suture. The external oblique muscle is sutured to the fascia lata over the iliac crest, followed by routine closure of the subcutaneous tissues and skin. Two large drains are placed medial to the iliac crest and brought out separate stab incisions.

Advantages

The advantages of the iliac crest flap include the ability to harvest the bone simultaneously with the mandibular resection; adequate pedicle length; a large vein for easy anastomosis; a hidden donor site; and provision of bone that matches the shape, contour, and bulk of the mandible more closely than other type of free bone flap.

Disadvantages

Disadvantages include a donor artery that may have a relatively small external diameter; a lengthy and work-intensive harvest; considerable donor site morbidity, including lateral thigh numbness and a prolonged period of painful ambulation; no potential for sensory reinnervation of the donor tissues; bulky skin paddle that is closely adherent to the underlying bone; the potential risk of abdominal herniation. The major problem with using the iliac crest flap is the prolonged pain patients often experience at the donor site. This pain may be unremitting, resulting in a permanent limp.

Lateral Arm

Description

The lateral arm free flap was originally described by Song et al. in 1982 (68). It is a type C fasciocutaneous flap that, as originally described, is harvested from the upper lateral arm between the lateral epicondyle and deltoid muscle convergence (Fig. 63). The potential width of the flap is 6 cm (greater widths are possible but primary closure is not possible, necessitating a skin graft), and the potential length of the flap is 15 cm (69). The flap may be osteocutaneous (partial-thickness humerus, type D); however, the risk of a fractured humerus relegates this well below other favored osseous sites such as the scapula, fibula, or iliac crest.

More recently, a significant variation of this flap has been described that provides for a longer and more substantial vascular pedicle (70). The flap, as originally described, had an important technical problem: the diameter of the feeding artery (radial collateral) was small (1 mm or less), making the microvascular anastomosis difficult. However, a larger donor artery and vein are possible if the dissection of the vascular pedicle is extended posteromedially to the deep brachial artery and, finally, to the main trunk of the brachial artery and vein.

Neurovascular Anatomy

The vascular supply to the lateral arm flap is the posterior radial collateral artery and vein. However, the profunda brachii artery and vein, from which the radial collateral vessels branch, are often used to exploit their greater length and size. The

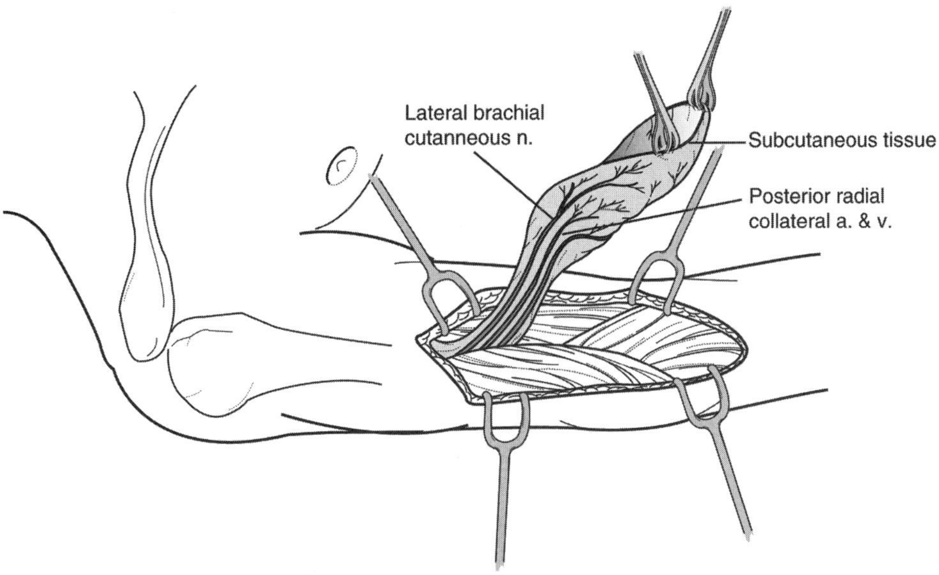

Figure 63 Surgical anatomy demonstrated in a harvested and pedicled lateral arm flap. Note the positions of the lateral brachial cutaneous and posterior radial collateral vessels. A larger donor vessel diameter is possible if the vascular pedicle is further dissected posteromedially to the deep brachial artery. Although two sensory nerves are associated with this flap—the lateral brachial cutaneous nerve and the posterior cutaneous nerve of the forearm—only the former supplies the skin territory of the flap.

profunda brachii artery arises from the posteromedial aspect of the brachial artery, below the lower border of the teres major muscle. Traveling with the radial nerve, the artery passes posteriorly around the humerus between the medial and lateral heads of the triceps muscle. The vascular pedicle is covered by the lateral head of the triceps muscle. On the lateral side of the arm, the artery pierces the lateral intermuscular septum and descends inferiorly between the brachioradialis and brachialis muscles to pass anterior to the lateral epicondyle. The radial collateral artery branches from the profunda brachii artery behind the humerus and descends within the lateral intermuscular septum behind the lateral epicondyle (Fig. 64). The radial collateral artery sends multiple septocutaneous perforating vessels to the lateral arm corresponding to the vascular territory of the lateral arm flap. In addition, the artery sends perforators more inferiorly into the forearm, so the true vascular territory of the artery extends several centimeters beyond the lateral epicondyle (so-called extended lateral arm free flap) (71).

The sensory nerve to the lateral arm flap is the lateral brachial cutaneous nerve. Two sensory nerves are associated with this flap, but only one supplies the skin covering the flap. The posterior cutaneous nerve of the forearm arises from

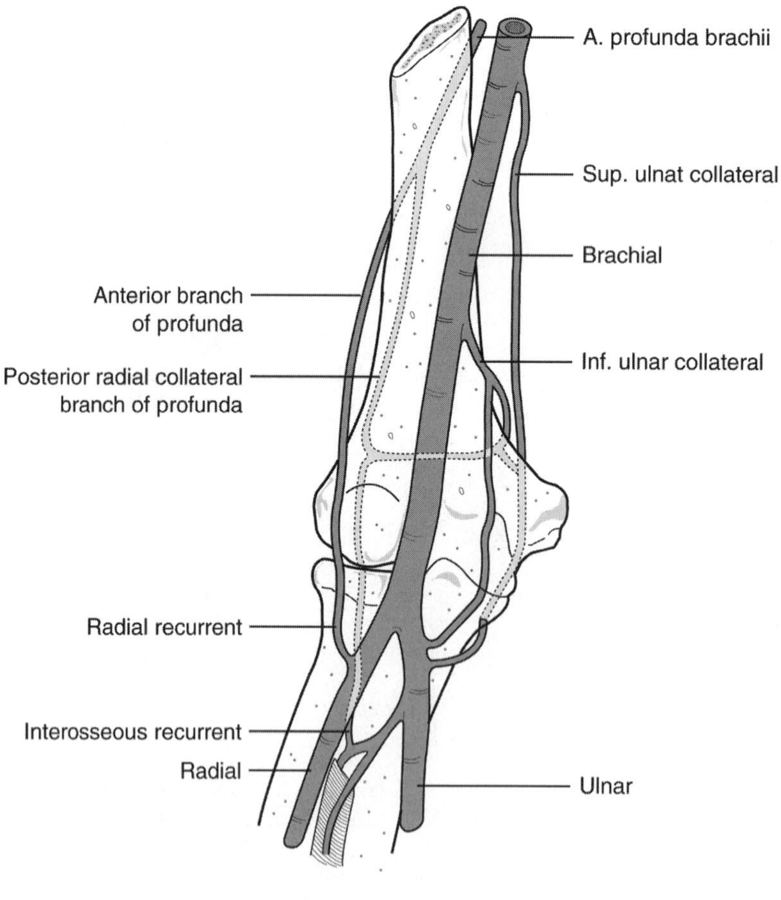

Figure 64 Further posteromedial dissection of the vascular pedicle of the lateral arm flap will uncover and allow harvest of the larger profunda brachii artery and vein.

the lateral septum 2.5–7.5 cm above the epicondyle and continues into the forearm. It does not serve the flap but may be harvested with the flap and used as a vascularized nerve graft (72). The lateral brachial cutaneous nerve follows the posterior border of the deltoid muscle and supplies the skin of the lateral arm, entering the flap near its proximal posterior border. To facilitate its incorporation into the flap, it is useful to identify this nerve early in the dissection. The extended lateral arm flap incorporates skin supplied by the posterior cutaneous nerve of the forearm and so this nerve can be used for reinnervation when the flap territory extends significantly below the lateral epicondyle.

Surgical Highlights

The lateral aspect of the nondominant arm is prepped and draped and the flap is outlined (Fig. 65). The surface landmarks for the lateral intermuscular septum are the lateral epicondyle of the humerus and the deltoid insertion. The skin paddle must be centered on the septum and is generally designed as a simple ellipse to facilitate donor site closure. The skin paddle and the underlying fascia are raised off the underlying muscle posteriorly and anteriorly towards the intermuscular septum. The sensory nerve is found posteriorly on line with the posterior border of the deltoid muscle. It can be dissected and cut proximally early. The vascular pedicle is identified emanating from the lateral intermuscular septum. It is dissected posteriorly along the spiral groove on the posterior aspect of the humerus. Care must

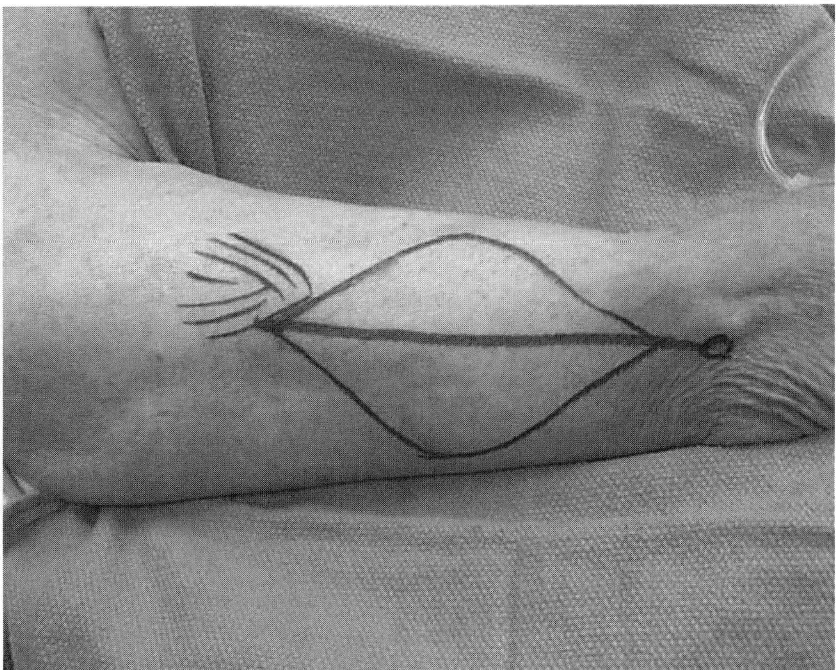

Figure 65 The lateral arm free flap is depicted. The solid line represents the lateral intermuscular septum and the skin flap is centered along this line. The landmarks for the septum are the lateral epicondyle of the humerus and the deltoid insertion.

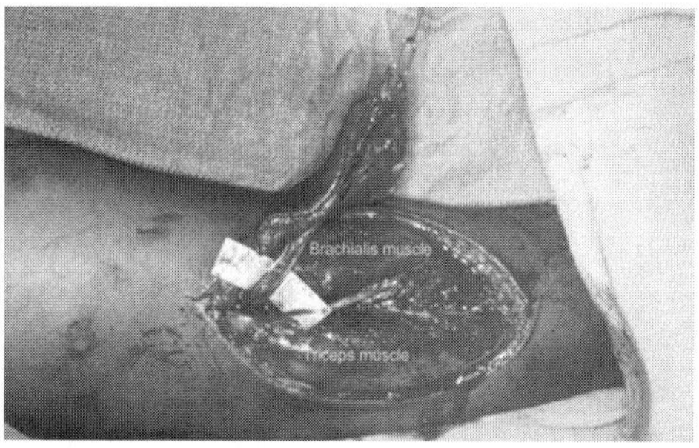

Figure 66 Lateral arm flap pedicled on its feeding vessels: the posterior radial collateral artery and vein.

be taken not to injure the radial nerve since it runs with the vascular pedicle within the groove. An additional skin incision is made from the apex of the skin ellipse to the deltoid insertion to facilitate separation of the musculature and dissection of the pedicle. Further superior extension of the incision along the posterior border of the deltoid allows separation of the lateral head of the triceps and the deltoid muscle (Fig. 66). To gain additional length on the pedicle, the insertion of the lateral head of the triceps is sharply incised and the radial collateral artery is seen joining the profunda brachii artery. The profunda brachii vessels are then dissected to the brachial artery and vein where they are divided to release the flap. Finally, a layered closure of the donor site over a large suction drain is performed.

The extended lateral arm flap includes an ellipse of skin over the lateral epicondyle and upper lateral forearm. The flap is raised in an identical fashion; however, the posterior cutaneous nerve of the forearm, which accompanies the vascular pedicle, can be used for sensory reinnervation of the flap since this nerve inserts into the skin of the upper lateral forearm (71).

Advantages

A two-team approach for simultaneous donor and recipient site dissection is possible. The flap is technically easy to harvest. The scar is inconspicuous in most patients, not requiring a skin graft. The flap is usually hairless and thin (although not as thin as the radial forearm flap). No major vessels need be sacrificed.

Disadvantages

The flap can be bulky in obese individuals. Although the vascular anatomy is fairly constant, in less than 2% of cases, an anomalous dual arterial supply from the profunda brachii artery can occur. These arteries may be smaller than usual. Even with normal arterial anatomy, the artery is small, measuring between 1 and 2 mm; however, this shortcoming can be overcome by dissecting the vascular pedicle to the brachial artery and vein. The donor veins are usually much larger: between 2 and 3 mm. Postoperative anesthesia of the upper lateral forearm is to be expected.

Lateral Thigh

Description

The lateral thigh free flap is a type IV fasciocutaneous flap first described in 1983 by Baek for the resurfacing of cutaneous defects in various anatomic areas (73). The flap includes up to 30 × 15 cm of the skin, subcutaneous tissue, and fascia over the lateral aspect of the thigh. The dominant blood supply is from the third perforator of the deep femoral artery and the flap may be made sensate using the lateral femoral cutaneous nerve. The thickness of the flap varies depending on the patient's adiposity and the area of the flap under consideration. The proximal aspect of the flap is much thicker, especially in patients with significant so-called saddle bag deformities.

Indications

For those with the most experience using the lateral thigh flap, it is usually reserved for reconstruction following total laryngopharyngectomy (74). Nevertheless, the flap can be applied to a variety of defects in the head and neck, especially in cases that require a large thin skin paddle. The proximal fatty portion of the flap has been exploited for glossectomy defects and the large surface area for cervical burn contracture tissue replacement and reconstruction of sizable composite oropharyngeal defects.

Neurovascular Anatomy

The lateral thigh flap is based on the third perforator of the profunda femoris artery. The profunda femoris artery gives off several branches that course in a posterolateral direction to supply the lateral thigh musculature and overlying skin. However, the third perforator is usually the dominant blood supply to the lateral thigh skin encompassed by the flap (Fig. 67). The length of the vascular pedicle (third perforator plus the profunda femoris artery up to the second perforator) may be up to 10 cm while the diameters of the artery and vein may be as large as 4 mm and 5 mm, respectively. Sensation can be restored to the flap via the lateral femoral cutaneous nerve. This nerve passes under the inguinal ligament where it divides into an anterior branch and a posterior branch. The posterior branch pierces the fascia lata and distributes posteriorly in the upper thigh. The anterior branch distributes along the anterolateral thigh within the territory of the lateral thigh flap.

Surgical Highlights

To harvest this flap the knee is flexed and internally rotated to expose the posterolateral aspect of the thigh. The midpoint of the thigh is marked (halfway between the greater trochanter and the lateral femoral condyle) along the intermuscular septum between the vastus lateralis muscle and biceps femoris muscle. The width of the flap can be up to 15 cm while still allowing for primary closure of the donor site. More of the flap should be designed anterior to the intermuscular septum because the skin is thinner in this area. The flap can extend along the entire thigh, if needed. Dissection proceeds from anterior to posterior in a subfascial plane (over the thick iliotibial tract) down to the intermuscular septum. The lateral femoral cutaneous nerve can be included in flap design, if desired. The posterior portion of the flap is dissected to the intermuscular septum as well. The vastus lateralis must be retracted anteriorly to expose the vessels along the septum. The third perforator passes superior, through, or posterior to the short head of the biceps and there is a wide variation in its vertical position along the intermuscular septum, ranging from 8 to 32 cm above the lateral femoral condyle (75). The adductor magnus and the short head of the biceps must be sharply incised to follow the profunda femoris vessels superiorly. The profunda femoris artery and its accompanying venae comitantes are transected just distal to the second perforator. Dividing the profunda femoris artery proximal to the second perforator (usually the largest of the perforators) may cause

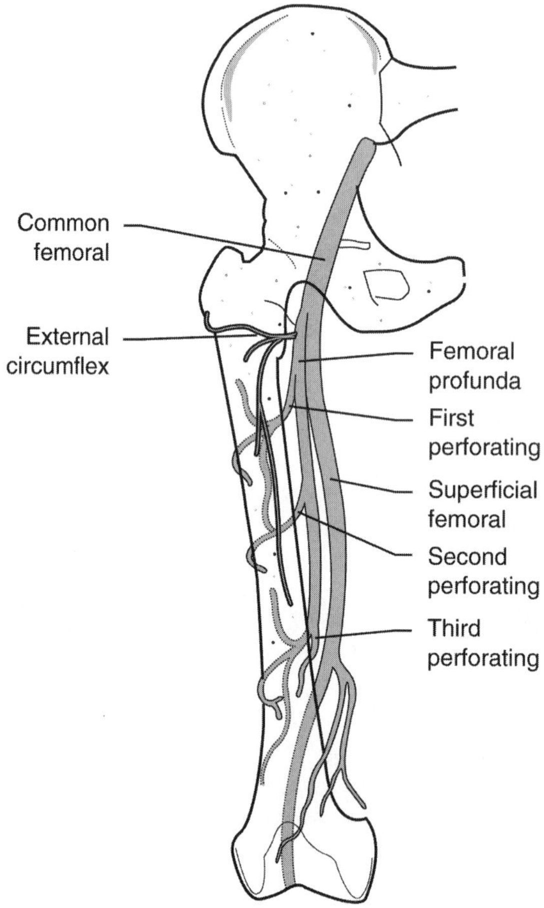

Figure 67 The third perforator of the profunda femoris artery is the dominant blood supply to the lateral thigh free flap.

muscular weakness. The second perforator is identified clinically by noting its close relationship to the insertion of the gluteus and the iliotibial tract (76). The dissection within the intermuscular groove is tedious and difficult. It may be best to leave the posterior portion of the flap attached and if the feeding vessels are transected accidentally the flap can be replaced intact. According to Hayden et al., the most difficult part of the dissection is freeing the third perforator as it exits the hiatus through the origin of the adductor magnus muscle along the posterior border of the femur (74). Multiple branches to the vastus lateralis must be carefully ligated and the hiatus enlarged superiorly and inferiorly. Once this is accomplished, the profunda femoris vessels are uncovered and relatively easily dissected to the second perforator. The flap is release by dividing the artery and vein and a layered closure of the donor site over a large suction drain is performed.

Advantages

In thin individuals, the lateral thigh flap is well suited for a variety of defects in the head and neck. The supplying artery is nonessential to the vascularity of the thigh and the donor site scar is quite acceptable to most patients. Functional morbidity is minimal after harvest. A two-team simultaneous harvest is possible, reducing operative time. The vascular pedicle is relatively lengthy and the vascular pedicle is large in terms of microvascular surgery. There is a potential for sensory innervation. Good-quality tracheoesophageal voicing is possible after routine placement of a speaking valve.

Disadvantages

Contraindications include local obesity (so-called saddle-bag thighs), previous trauma, severe peripheral vascular disease, or prior hip replacement surgery that may have disrupted the perforating vessels. The donor site may leave a slight contour defect with primary closure or require skin grafting when an excessively wide flap is taken. The principal disadvantage is the difficulty in harvesting the flap. It is a tedious and arduous dissection that can take up to 3.5 h to perform. However, an experienced surgeon should take no more than 2–2.5 h to raise the flap. Accidental division of the vascular pedicle, especially as the third perforator passes through the adductor magnus muscle, is a realistic possibility. The flap skin is quite pale in most individuals, making it a poor color match with the cervicofacial region. There is a small risk of wound dehiscence and compartment syndrome, especially if the donor site is closed under excessive tension. When used for pharyngeal reconstruction, stenosis at the distal anastomosis may occur. This is avoided by designing the inferior circumference of the flap with a "V" type extension to break up the scar.

Omental

Description

Free omental flaps, primarily consisting of fat, have long been used for surface reconstruction with skin grafts and for facial contour restoration (77). For contour restoration, the base of the omentum is placed vertically along the preauricular crease and the omental appendages, with their individual vascular arcades, are spread out anteriorly under a face-lift-like skin flap. For surface reconstruction, most commonly scalp, the omentum is simply draped over the area and skin-grafted.

The greater curvature of the stomach may also be harvested (gastro-omental flap) with a varying amount of omentum (78). The amount of the stomach available for transfer is approximately 7 cm wide by 13 cm long. The quantity of harvestable omentum is large: over 25 cm^2.

Indications

In the past, the free omental flap has been used most frequently for facial contour restoration for hemifacial subcutaneous fat deficiency (secondary to Romberg's disease, trauma, or hemifacial microsomia). However, de-epithelialized free tissue transfers (e.g., the parascapular flap) have largely replaced the free omental flap for facial contour restoration. This flap has recently been used for massive scalp defects (with application of a split-thickness skin graft) due to its lengthy vascular pedicle and expansive surface area.

A gastro-omental flap can be used for large pharyngoesophageal defects (Fig. 68). This flap is useful when there are no usable donor vessels in the neck. Due to the long vascular pedicle, the neck vasculature can be bypassed for the unspoiled vessels in the axilla. If the vessels in the neck are workable, then a fasciocutaneous flap should be used. Another alternative, when the neck vessels are inadequate, is to transpose the thoracodorsal vessels from the axilla and over the clavicle to serve as donor vessels for the traditional free flaps (52). The gastro-omental flap, besides reconstructing the pharynx, provides for vascularized coverage of the heavily irradiated neck with omentum. This is advantageous for obvious reasons, especially considering the high incidence of salivary fistulas in this group of patients (79).

Neurovascular Anatomy

The omentum and greater curvature of the stomach are supplied by the right gastroepiploics. The pedicle length for the omentum is approximately 10 cm. The pedicle length for the gastric flap is up to 30 cm if the length of pedicle along the omental–gastric junction is used along the path to the donor vessels. The vessels are large from a microvascular surgery point of view: 2.5 mm for the vein and 2 mm for the artery. The vascular arcades allow longitudinal division of the omentum in viable segments based on a single vascular pedicle.

Surgical Highlights

A laparotomy is usually required to harvest the omental and gastro-omental flaps, although laparoscopic harvest is feasible. To maximize the length of the pedicle (up

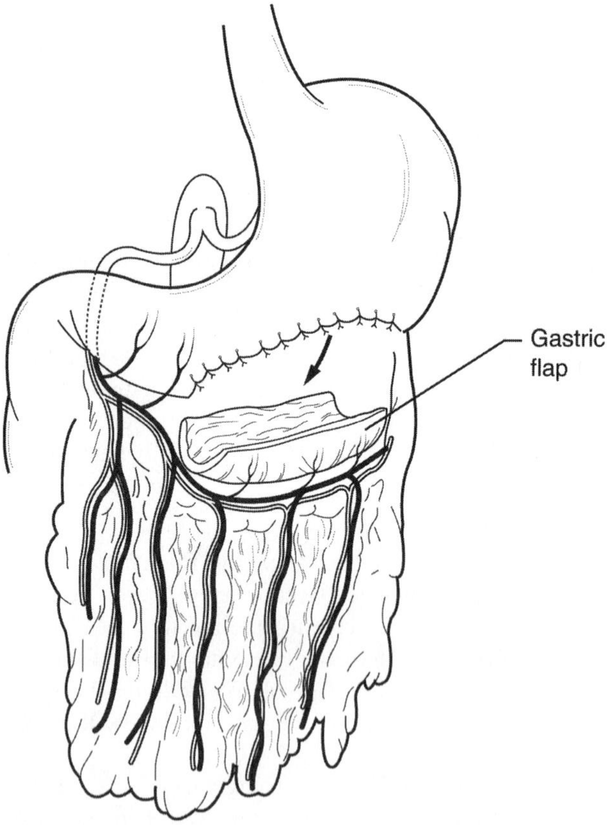

Figure 68 The gastro-omental flap is supplied by the right gastroepiploic vessels. The length of the vascular pedicle is approximately 10 cm for the combined flap and can be up to 30 cm for the gastric flap by exploiting the portion of the vascular pedicle along the greater curvature of the stomach.

to 30 cm for the gastro-omental flap), the most distal part of the stomach based on the right gastroepiploic artery and vein should be harvested.

Advantages

The gastro-omental flap provides a long pedicle able to reach vessels outside the neck (e.g., axilla). Patients with unusable or unavailable neck donor vessels with pharyngoesophageal defects are candidates for this flap.

The omentum possesses several attributes that make it ideal for use in heavily irradiated, ischemic tissues and even septic tissues. It is able to fight infection actively, produce healing granulation tissue, and adhere tenaciously to compromised tissues.

Disadvantages

The major disadvantage to using the omental flaps is the requirement for laparotomy. The major problem with using omentum to correct facial contour is the late occurrence of sagging.

There is a persistent acidic milieu in the reconstructed pharynx after stomach transfer for pharyngoesophageal reconstruction (pH = 5); however, there has been no reports of peptic ulcerations in the esophageal mucosa.

Jejunal

Description

The jejunal free flap was first described in 1959 by Seidenberg et al. (42). The jejunal segment provides an internal diameter of functional (peristaltic and mucus-secreting) intestine that closely matches that of the missing esophagus.

A brief historical review of cervical esophageal reconstruction is helpful to understand how the jejunal flap came into widespread use. Pedicled colon transposition and gastric pull-up are two common methods of esophageal reconstruction. Pedicled colon transposition using the right or left side of the colon has been used sporadically since the early part of the 20th century. Gastric pull-up involves the transposition of the entire stomach, pedicled by the right gastric and gastroepiploic vessels, to the proximal defect (esophagus, hypopharynx, or base of tongue) via blunt posterior mediastinal dissection (80). The colon and stomach transpositions allow for total esophageal reconstruction. Gastric pull-up is still used commonly although colonic transposition is used only rarely. Gastric pull-up, in contrast with colonic transposition, has a more reliable blood supply, is a single-staged procedure, and requires a single intestinal anastomosis that is resistant to stricture formation. With the advent and success of the jejunal free flap, another option became available for a subgroup of patients requiring esophageal replacement. The jejunal flap proved to be just as reliable as the gastric pull-up but could be transferred to the neck as a free flap, obviating the need for an attached pedicle and mediastinal dissection. Therefore, the morbidity of entering the chest was eliminated. Free jejunal transfer was the method of choice for patients requiring esophageal replacement above the thoracic inlet. Most patients who are candidates have undergone a total laryngopharyngectomy. More recently, however, free folded fasciocutaneous flaps have proved to be just as effective at recreating a viable neopharynx. Although the jejunum is still the method of choice for some surgeons, most centers have adopted fasciocutaneous flaps for this role because the morbidity of a laparotomy is avoided.

Indications

The jejunum provides an alternative method of reconstructing combined upper esophageal (above the thoracic inlet) and hypopharyngeal circumferential defects. This method of reconstruction avoids mediastinal dissection and is often favored over the more traditional methods including gastric pull-up and colon transposition.

The jejunal segment may also be split along its antimesenteric border and used as a patch to cover a variety of oral and oropharyngeal defects. The mucus-secreting properties can be exploited for reconstruction of defects in patients with radiation-induced xerostomia. However, the benefit of additional mucus is dubious.

Esophageal defects that extend below the thoracic inlet can be most simply reconstructed using the gastric pull-up and blunt posterior mediastinal dissection. The use of the jejunal free flap would necessitate a thoracotomy; therefore, esophageal defects that extend below the thoracic inlet are generally not considered for jejunal flap transfer.

Patients who have had previous abdominal surgery (not specifically involving the vascular supply or the jejunal segment itself) remain candidates for jejunal flap harvest.

Neurovascular Anatomy

The vascular supply is from the jejunal arteries (branches of the superior mesenteric artery) that form arcades within the mesentery to encompass the jejunal segment (Fig. 69). No usable neural elements accompany the jejunal segment.

Surgical Highlights

A two-team approach is possible, significantly shortening the operative time. Harvest of the jejunal segment may be done via an open abdominal procedure or laparoscopically (81). The jejunal segment is taken 3 feet distal to the ligament of Treitz to facilitate the subsequent enteric anastomosis. The length of the segment should equal the length of the defect plus 3 cm to accommodate the exteriorized monitoring segment (82). The exteriorized monitoring segment is a portion of the flap separated from the main flap along the radiating mesenteric vessels and draped onto the skin through the neck incision. This segment of bowel reflects the health of the main flap and is inspected for mucus production, peristalsis, and color. After approximately 3 days, the base of the monitoring segment is cauterized or suture ligated and removed.

Prior to harvest, the jejunal segment should be marked as to the direction of peristalsis. It should be placed in the neck so that peristalsis is from proximal to distal (antiperistaltic positioning results in dysphagia); it should also be placed on some stretch to eliminate redundancy.

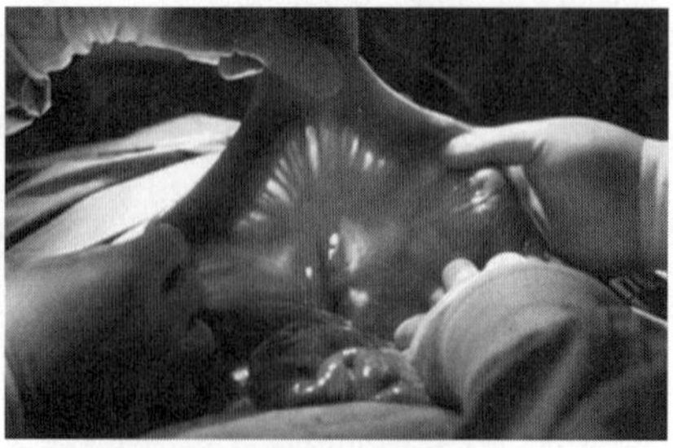

Figure 69 Transilluminated jejunal flap in situ. The vascular supply to the flap is from the jejunal arteries (branches of the superior mesenteric artery). Note the arcades within the mesentery that encompass the jejunal segment.

Postoperative care consists of placement of a nasogastric tube for stomach decompression until bowel sounds resume, at which time feeding through the tube may be slowly advanced. As an alternative, a feeding gastrostomy or jejunostomy tube may be placed during the original harvesting procedure. A jejunostomy tube allows immediate feeding prior to the return of bowel sounds. Oral feeding may commence on day 7–10 after surgery.

Advantages

The jejunal free flap was originally introduced as an alternative to gastric and colon transposition. With the introduction of tubed free fasciocutaneous flaps (e.g., radial forearm or lateral thigh free flaps) for circumferential hypopharyngeal reconstruction, the jejunal flap has lost popularity.

Disadvantages

The major drawback to using the jejunal free flap is the necessity of abdominal surgery. The literature reports a complication rate of over 30%. Distal anastomotic strictures (at the jejunal-proximal esophageal junction) occur as a late complication in approximately 22% (11/50 cases) and esophageal speech is often of poorer quality compared to reconstruction using skin flaps (e.g., radial forearm) (83). Most strictures are due to redundancy and kinking of the bowel at the distal suture line (84,85). Treatment involves surgical resection of the distal suture line and elimination of the redundancy.

The ischemic tolerance of the jejunal segment is significantly less than is found in fasciocutaneous flaps; ischemic periods of over 4 h result in areas of full-thickness necrosis. This is rarely a problem during the initial surgery; however, if subsequent problems with the anastomosis occur that result in ischemia, salvage is less likely (85).

REFERENCES

1. Owens NA. A compound neck pedicle designed for the repair of massive defects: formation, development and application. Plast Reconstr Surg 1955; 15:369.
2. Ariyan S. The pectoralis major myocutaneous flap. A versatile flap for reconstruction in the head and neck. Plast Reconstr Surg 1979; 63:73–81.
3. Taylor GI, Palmer JH. The vascular territories (angiosomes) of the body: experimental study and clinical applications. Br J Plast Surg 1987; 40:113–141.
4. Ciresi KF, Mathes SJ. The classification of flaps [Review]. Orthop Clin North Am 1993; 24:383–391.
5. Dolan R, Arena S. Clinical applications of the island-pedicled nasolabial musculocutaneous flap. Am J Rhinol 1995; 9:219–224.
6. Ponten B. The fasciocutaneous flap: its use in soft tissue defects of the lower leg. Br J Plast Surg 1981; 34:215–220.
7. Cormack GC, Lamberty BG. Fasciocutaneous vessels. Their distribution on the trunk and limbs, and their clinical application in tissue transfer. [Review]. Anat Clin 1984; 6:121–131.
8. Cormack GC, Lamberty BG. Fasciocutaneous flap nomenclature [letter]. Plast Reconstr Surg 1984; 73:996.
9. Gumener R, Montandon D, Marty F, Zbrodowski A. The subcutaneous tissue flap and the misconception of fasciocutaneous flaps. Scand J Plast Reconstr Surg 1986; 20:61–65.
10. Hidalgo DA, Disa JJ, Cordeiro PG, Hu QY. A review of 716 consecutive free flaps for oncologic surgical defects: refinement in donor-site selection and technique. Plast Reconstr Surg 1998; 102:722–732.

11. Donski PK, Fogdestam I. Distally based fasciocutaneous flap from the sural region. A preliminary report. Scand J Plast Reconstr Surg 1983; 17:191–196.
12. Amarante J, Costa H, Reis J, Soares R. Venous skin flaps: an experimental study and report of two clinical distal island flaps. Br J Plast Surg 1988; 41:132–137.
13. Baek SM, Weinberg H, Song Y, Park CG, Biller HF. Experimental studies in the survival of venous island flaps without arterial inflow. Plast Reconstr Surg 1985; 75:88–95.
14. Swartz WM. Latissimus dorsi muscle and musculocutaneous flaps. In: Swartz WM, Banis JC, eds. Head and Neck Microsurgery. Baltimore: Williams & Wilkins, 1991:92–98.
15. Maxwell GP, Stueber K, Hoopes JE. A free latissimus dorsi myocutaneous flap: case report. Plast Reconstr Surg 1978; 62:462–466.
16. Lore JM. An Atlas of Head and Neck Surgery, 3 ed. Philadelphia: W.B. Saunders, 1988, 316–343.
17. Ariyan S. Pectoralis major muscle and musculocutaneous flaps. In: Strauch B, Vasconez LO, eds. 2 ed. Grabb's Encyclopedia of Flaps, Philadelphia: Lippincott-Raven, 1998:470–477.
18. Kroll SS, Goepfert H, Jones M, Guillamondegui O, Schusterman M. Analysis of complications in 168 pectoralis major myocutaneous flaps used for head and neck reconstruction. Ann Plast Surg 1990; 25:93–97.
19. Bakamjian VY. A two-stage method for pharyngoesophageal reconstruction with a primary pectoral skin flap. Plas Reconstr Surg 1965; 36:173.
20. Portnoy WM, Arena S. Deltopectoral island flap. Otolaryngol Head Neck Surg 1994; 111:63–69.
21. Lore JM. 3 ed.An Atlas of Head and Neck Surgery. Philadelphia: W.B. Saunders, 1988, 344–357.
22. Golovine SS. Procede de cloture plastique de l'orbite apres l'exenteration. Arch Ophthalmol 1898; 18:679–680.
23. Huttenbrink KB. Temporalis muscle flap: an alternative in oropharyngeal reconstruction. Laryngoscope 1986; 96:1034–1038.
24. Koranda FC, McMahon MF. The temporalis muscle flap for intraoral reconstruction: technical modifications. Otolaryngol Head Neck Surg 1988; 98:315–318.
25. Bradley P, Brockbank J. The temporalis muscle flap in oral reconstruction. A cadaveric, animal and clinical study. J Maxillofac Surg 1981; 9:139–145.
26. Shagets FW, Panje WR, Shore JW. Use of temporalis muscle flaps in complicated defects of the head and face. Arch Otolaryngol Head Neck Surg 1986; 112:60–65.
27. Campbell HH. Reconstruction of the left maxilla. Plast Reconstr Surg 1948; 3:66.
28. Demas PN, Sotereanos GC. Transmaxillary temporalis transfer for reconstruction of a large palatal defect: report of a case. J Oral Maxillofac Surg 1989; 47:197–202.
29. Cordeiro PG, Wolfe SA. The temporalis muscle flap revisited on its centennial: advantages, newer uses, and disadvantages. Plas Reconstr Surg 1996; 98:980–987.
30. Jackson IT, Potparic Z. Galeal frontalis myofascial flap. In: Strauch B, Vasconez LO, eds. 2 ed.. Grabb's Encyclopedia of Flaps, Philadelphia: Lippincott-Raven, 1998:37–41.
31. Conley J. Use of composite flaps containing bone for major repairs in the head and neck. Plast Reconstr Surg 1972; 49:522–526.
32. Aviv JE, Urken ML, Lawson W, Biller HF. The superior trapezius myocutaneous flap in head and neck reconstruction. Arch Otolaryngol Head Neck Surg 1992; 118:702–706.
33. Panje WR. Myocutaneous trapezius flap. Head Neck Surg 1980; 2:206–212.
34. Baek SM, Biller HF, Krespi YP, Lawson W. The lower trapezius island myocutaneous flap. Ann Plast Surg 1980; 5:108–114.
35. Netterville JL, Wood DE. The lower trapezius flap. Vascular anatomy and surgical technique. Arch Otolaryngol Head Neck Surg 1991; 117:73–76.
36. Woodburne RT. Essentials of Human Anatomy, 7 ed. New York: Oxford University Press, 1983, 49–50.
37. Cummings CW, Eisele DW, Coltrera MD. Lower trapezius myocutaneous island flap. Arch Otolaryngol Head Neck Surg 1989; 115:1181–1185.

38. Urken ML, Naidu RK, Lawson W, Biller HF. The lower trapezius island musculocutaneous flap revisited. Report of 45 cases and a unifying concept of the vascular supply. [Review]. Arch Otolaryngol Head Neck Surg 1991; 117:502–511.
39. Chandrasekhar B, Terz JJ, Kokal WA, Beatty JD, Gottlieb ME. The inferior trapezius musculocutaneous flap in head and neck reconstruction. Ann Plast Surg 1988; 21:201–209.
40. Byrd HS. Temporoparietal (superficial temporal artery) fascial flap. In: Strauch B, Vasconez LO, eds. 2 ed.. Grabb's Encyclopedia of Flaps, Philadelphia: Lippincott-Raven, 1998:26–30.
41. Abul-Hassan HS, von Drasek AG, Acland RD. Surgical anatomy and blood supply of the fascial layers of the temporal region. Plast Reconstr Surg 1986; 77:17–28.
42. Seidenberg B. Immediate reconstruction of the cervical esophagus by a revascularized isolated jejunal segment. Ann Surg 1959; 142:162.
43. Yang G, Chen B, Gao Y. Forearm free skin flap transplantations. Nat Med J China 1981; 61:139.
44. Hidalgo DA. Fibula free flap: a new method of mandible reconstruction. Plast Reconst Surg 1989; 84:71–79.
45. Dolan R, Carr RM, McAvoy D. Operative anatomy of the sensory nerves to the fibula osteoseptocutaneous flap. Arch Facial Plast Surgery 2000.
46. Swartz WM, Banis JC, Newton ED, Ramasastry SS, Jones NF, Acland R. The osteocutaneous scapular flap for mandibular and maxillary reconstruction. Plast Reconstr Surg 1986; 77:530–545.
47. Taylor GI. Reconstruction of the mandible with free composite iliac bone grafts. Ann Plast Surg 1982; 9:361–376.
48. Pennington DG, Pelly AD. The rectus abdominis myocutaneous free flap. Br J Plast Surg 1980; 33:277–282.
49. Taylor GI, Corlett RJ, Boyd JB. The versatile deep inferior epigastric (inferior rectus abdominis) flap. Br J Plast Surg 1984; 37:330–350.
50. Harii K, Ohmori K, Torii S. Free gracilis muscle transplantation, with microneurovascular anastomoses for the treatment of facial paralysis. A preliminary report. Plast Reconstr Surg 1976; 57:133–143.
51. Schultes G, Gaggl A, Karcher H. Reconstruction of accessory nerve defects with vascularized long thoracic vs. non-vascularized thoracodorsal nerve. J Reconstr Microsurg 1999; 15:265–270.
52. Dolan R, Gooey J, Cho YJ, Fuleihan N. Microvascular access in the multiply operated neck: thoracodorsal transposition [published erratum appears in Laryngoscope 1997 Jan;107(1):149]. Laryngoscope 1996; 106:1436–1437.
53. Terzis JK. Pectoralis minor: a unique muscle for correction of facial palsy. Plast Reconstr Surg 1989; 83:767–776.
54. Sadove RC, Luce EA, McGrath PC. Reconstruction of the lower lip and chin with the composite radial forearm-palmaris longus free flap. Plast Reconstr Surg 1991; 88:209–214.
55. Woerdeman LA, Chaplin BJ, Griffioen FM, Bos KE. Sensate osteocutaneous fibula flap: anatomic study of the innervation pattern of the skin flap. Head Neck 1998; 20:310–314.
56. Swartz WM, Banis JC. Head and Neck Microsurgery. Baltimore: Williams & Wilkins, 1992, 43.
57. Fuhrman TM, Pippin WD, Talmage LA, Reilley TE. Evaluation of collateral circulation of the hand. J Clin Monitoring 1992; 8:28–32.
58. Jones BM, O'Brien CJ. Acute ischaemia of the hand resulting from elevation of a radial forearm flap. Br J Plast Surg 1985; 38:396–397.
59. Haughey BH. Tongue reconstruction: concepts and practice. Laryngoscope 1993; 103:1132–1141.
60. Harii K, Asato H, Yoshimura K, Sugawara Y, Nakatsuka T, Ueda K. One-stage transfer of the latissimus dorsi muscle for reanimation of a paralyzed face: a new alternative. Plast Reconstr Surg 1998; 102:941–951.

61. Netscher D, Alford EL, Wigoda P, Cohen V. Free composite myo-osseous flap with serratus anterior and rib: indications in head and neck reconstruction. Head Neck 1998; 20:106–112.
62. Bruck JC, Bier J, Kistler D. The serratus anterior osteocutaneous free flap. J Reconstr Microsurg 1990; 6:209–213.
63. Ueda K, Harii K, Yamada A. Free vascularized double muscle transplantation for the treatment of facial paralysis. Plast Reconstr Surg 1995; 95:1288–1296.
64. McCraw JB, Furlow LT, Jr. The dorsalis pedis arterialized flap. A clinical study. Plast Reconstr Surg 1975; 55:177–185.
65. Zuker RM, Manktelow RT. The dorsalis pedis free flap: technique of elevation, foot closure, and flap application. Plast Reconstr Surg 1986; 77:93–104.
66. Serafin D. The Dorsalis Pedis flap. Philadelphia: W.B. Saunders, 1996, 89–95.
67. Urken ML, Vickery C, Weinberg H, Buchbinder D, Biller HF. The internal oblique-iliac crest osseomyocutaneous microvascular free flap in head and neck reconstruction. J Reconstr Microsurg 1989; 5:203–214.
68. Song R, Song Y, Yu Y. The upper arm free flap. Clin Plast Surg 1982; 9:27–35.
69. Sullivan MJ, Carroll WR, Kuriloff DB. Lateral arm free flap in head and neck reconstruction. Arch Otolaryngol Head Neck Surg 1992; 118:1095–1101.
70. Civantos FJ, Jr., Burkey B, Lu FL, Armstrong W. Lateral arm microvascular flap in head and neck reconstruction. Arch Otolaryngol Head Neck Surg. 1997; 123:830–836.
71. Ross DA, Thomson JG, Restifo R, Tarro JM, Sasaki CT. The extended lateral arm free flap for head and neck reconstruction: the Yale experience. Laryngoscope 1996; 106: 14–18.
72. Culbertson JH, Mutimer K. The reverse lateral upper arm flap for elbow coverage. Ann Plast Surg 1987; 18:62–68.
73. Baek SM. Two new cutaneous free flaps: the medial and lateral thigh flaps. Plast Reconstr Surg 1983; 71:354–365.
74. Hayden RE, Deschler DG. Lateral thigh free flap for head and neck reconstruction. Laryngoscope 1999; 109:1490–1494.
75. Miller MJ, Reece GP, Marchi M, Baldwin BJ. Lateral thigh free flap in head and neck reconstruction. Plast Reconstr Surg 1995; 96:334–340.
76. Truelson JM, Leach JL. Lateral thigh flap reconstruction in the head and neck. Otolaryngol Head Neck Surg 1998; 118:203–210.
77. Harii K. Clinical application of free omental flap transfer. Clin Plast Surg 1978; 5:273–281.
78. Panje WR, Little AG, Moran WJ, Ferguson MK, Scher N. Immediate free gastro-omental flap reconstruction of the mouth and throat. Ann. Otol. Rhinol. Laryngol. 1987; 96:15–21.
79. Carlson GW, Thourani VH, Codner MA, Grist WJ. Free gastro-omental flap reconstruction of the complex, irradiated pharyngeal wound. Head Neck 1997; 19:68–71.
80. Ong GB, Lee TC. Pharyngogastric anastomosis after esophagopharyngectomy for carcinoma of the hypopharynx and cervical esophagus. Br J Surg 1960; 48:193.
81. Gherardini G, Gurlek A, Staley CA, Ross DA, Pazmino BP, Miller MJ. Laparoscopic harvesting of jejunal free flaps for esophageal reconstruction. Plast Reconstr Surg 1998; 102:473–477.
82. Bradford CR, Esclamado RM, Carroll WR. Monitoring of revascularized jejunal autografts. Arch Otolaryngol Head Neck Surg 1992; 118:1042–1044.
83. Schusterman MA, Shestak K, de Vries EJ, Swartz W, Jones N, Johnson J, et al. Reconstruction of the cervical esophagus: free jejunal transfer versus gastric pull-up. Plast Reconstr Surg 1990; 85:16–21.
84. Swartz W, Banis JC. 1 ed Head and Neck Microsurgery. Baltimore: Williams & Wilkins, 1992, 182.
85. Olding M, Jeng JC. Ischemic tolerance of canine jejunal flaps. Plast Reconstr Surg 1994; 94:167–173.

9

Reconstruction of Specialized Tissues: The Mandible, Tongue, Pharynx, and Maxilla

Robert W. Dolan
Lahey Clinic Medical Center, Burlington, Massachusetts, U.S.A.

MANDIBULAR RECONSTRUCTION

The technique of choice for reconstruction of segmental mandibular defects following cancer resection is primary microvascular bone transfer and the favored donor sites are iliac crest, fibula, and scapula. Alternative methods for primary or secondary mandibular reconstruction include the use of mandibular reconstruction plates (MRP), free nonvascularized bone grafts, bone cribs, and pedicled vascularized bone grafts. Segmental mandibular defects that are left to swing freely with no attempt at reconstruction may result in significant aesthetic and functional morbidities depending on the size and location of the defect. Use of pedicled vascularized bone including trapezius–scapular spine, pectoralis major–rib, and latissimus dorsi–rib has been reported but avascular necrosis of the bone segment is frequent, probably due to the tenuous periosteal blood supply from the muscle to the bone (1). The method of choice depends on the condition of the neck and surrounding tissues and the size and location of the mandibular and associated soft tissue defects. The overall health, prognosis, and desires of the patient and the suitability of potential donor sites are also important considerations.

Condition of the Neck and Surrounding Tissues

Prior radiation therapy and salivary contamination are the most important causes of failure of both nonvascularized and vascularized bone grafts. Prior irradiation results in an ischemic tissue bed and pathological changes in blood vessels including endothelial cell dehiscence, vessel wall fibrosis, and intimal fragility. An ischemic tissue bed from radiation therapy is a poor substrate for avascular bone grafts; however, vascularized bone (free osseous microvascular flaps) is unaffected and often results in neovascularization of the surrounding tissues. However, prior radiation therapy is the only factor that has consistently been associated with microvascular flap loss (2). This effect is proportional to the time elapsed between radiation therapy and microvascular flap transfer (3).

Avascular mandibular grafts, including cancellous bone grafts in bone cribs, have very poor success rates (less than 50%) if used in the presence of a through-and-through defect of the oral cavity that results in salivary contamination of the recipient bed (4). Recent work using growth factors including bone morphogenic protein and platelet-rich plasma is promising with regard to enhancing the survival of these avascular bone implants (5). Nevertheless, these grafts are not recommended for use in the primary setting. It is possible, however, to use these grafts in a secondary setting. This requires interim maintenance of mandibular spacing by internal or external fixation to prevent soft tissue contraction and mandibular drift. The graft is then placed through the neck to avoid salivary contamination. This method was the standard until the advent of microvascular free bone transfers. Free vascularized bone is successful in re-establishing an osseous bridge between the cut ends of the mandible in the primary setting in more than 95% of cases. This bone provides adequate stability to resist the forces of mastication and will provide adequate substrate for osseointegrated dental appliances. It is the method of choice for most institutions that regularly treat patients with cancers involving the mandible. Despite wide acceptance, microvascular bone transfer has several drawbacks including potential donor site morbidity; poor height match to the adjacent normal mandible, making dental rehabilitation more difficult; poorer osseointegration than to cancellous cellular bone grafts; and overbulked soft tissue components that require secondary revision to re-establish a workable alveolar ridge.

Size and Location of Mandibular and Soft Tissue Defects

Mandibular segmental defects involving the symphysis and parasymphysis are the most significant in terms of aesthetic and functional morbidity. Failure to reconstruct this part of the mandible results in the Andy Gump deformity and loss of the tongue-anchoring and masticatory platform functions of the anterior arch. The anterior arch also serves to anchor the hyomandibular muscle complex involved in laryngeal elevation and deglutition. Experience with MRPs has revealed an unacceptably high rate (35%) of hardware failure, mainly from plate exposure and breakage due to the pulling forces of the geniohyoid and digastric muscles attached to the remaining soft tissues surrounding the plate (6) (Fig. 1). This effect is compounded by gravity and the use of regional myocutaneous flaps pedicled inferiorly (e.g., the pectoralis flap).

Two common issues with regard to microvascular mandibular replacement are the type of fixation needed to secure the bone graft in place and the method used to size and shape the bone graft accurately to match the resected segment closely. Rigid fixation is required to secure the bone graft to the mandibular stumps. Either simple mandibular plates fixed to either end of the bone graft to the mandibular stumps or a continuous microvascular reconstruction plate can be used. Wire fixation should be avoided as excessive movement may impede osseous union. The mandibular plates are each secured with three screws in the native mandible and two screws in the graft. A continuous microvascular plate is thinner than the typical MRP and the newer plates are locking screw-type with smaller holes and screws. With regard to the sizing and shaping of the bone graft, a microvascular plate can be adapted to the native mandible prior to resection and the bone graft fit to it ex vivo. As an alternative, the resected specimen is inspected and the bone graft is osteotomized and sized to

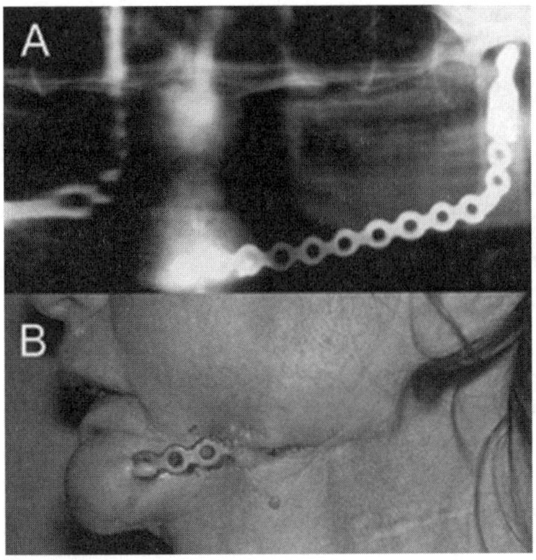

Figure 1 An MRP alone was used to reconstruct an anterior arch defect. This patient experienced both plate breakage (a) and exposure (b) approximately 2 years postoperatively.

approximate the size and shape of the resected bone. If possible, it is helpful to place the patient in temporary maxillary–mandibular fixation during placement of the bone graft and application of hardware. Often the bone graft lacks the height of the native mandible. In these cases, the graft should be aligned with the superior aspect of the native mandible to minimize the required height of osseointegrated implants and to eliminate any step-offs that may interfere with a tissue-borne denture. In some cases, a template-driven method for sizing and shaping the bone graft is lacking and a stereolithographic model may be of use. Using computed tomography (CT) data, a three-dimensional model is created using computer-aided design (CAD) software. This model is then used to create custom reconstruction plates that can be used as a template for the bone graft and to secure the graft into place (Fig. 2).

Central Segmental Mandibular Defects

Microvascular bone transfer has resulted in durable anterior arch replacement in the vast majority of cases, far exceeding the results of prior methods of reconstruction. Isolated anterior arch defects can be reconstructed using any of the available favored donor sites; however, the associated soft tissue defects may require more discernment in choice of the most appropriate flap. Common associated soft tissue defects include those involving the floor of mouth, lower lip, chin and neck, and tongue. The scapula, iliac crest, and fibula each possess unique attached soft tissue components. The soft tissue components of the iliac crest include a closely attached and relatively thick skin paddle and a thin sheetlike muscular component. The fibula possesses a closely attached thin skin paddle that may be made sensate. Although the scapular system has the least substantial bone of the three flaps, it possesses the most substantial and adaptable soft tissue components including the transverse scapular and

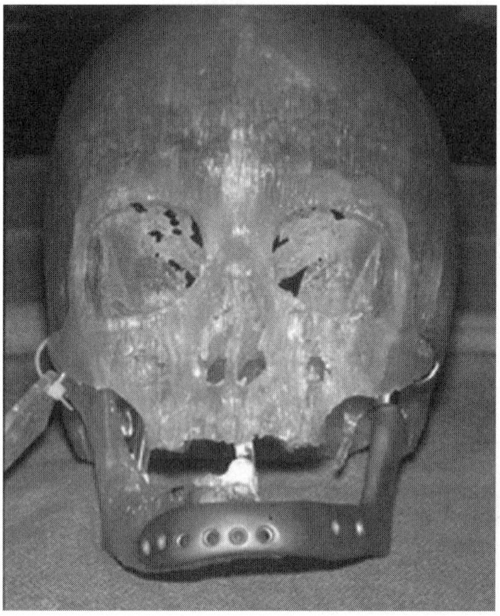

Figure 2 Stereolithographic model used to adapt a reconstruction plate and bone graft accurately into a segmental mandibular defect.

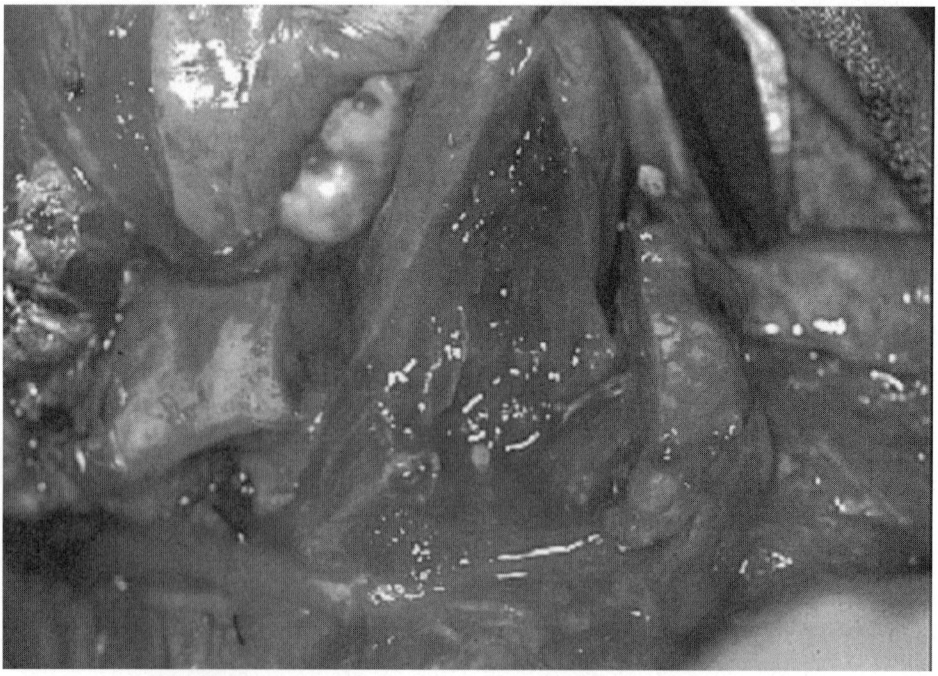

Figure 3 Typical anterior mandibular defect associated with a defect in the anterior floor of mouth.

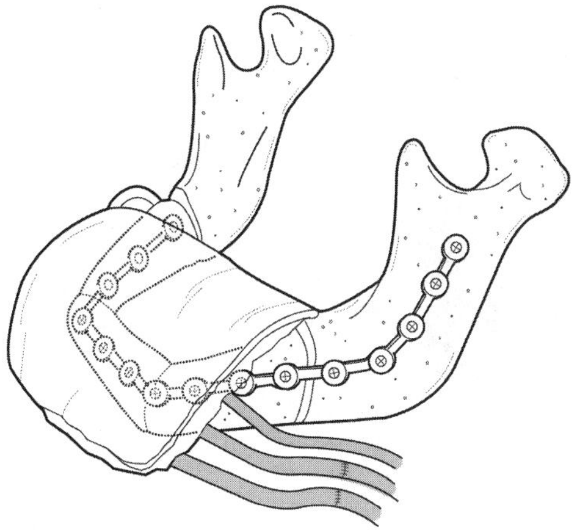

Figure 4 Osteotomized fibular bone with associated skin paddle draping over the neoalveolus and anterior floor of mouth.

parascapular flaps (sometimes thick), latissimus dorsi muscle and overlying skin, and serratus anterior muscle (and underlying ribs).

Most anterior segmental mandibular defects will have an associated defect of the anterior floor of mouth (Fig. 3). Therefore, at least a portion of the soft tissue component of the free flap must be used to resurface the anterior floor of mouth and close the through-and-through defect in this area. It is fortunate that most resections involve this type of defect and the fibular flap performs well with its thin and pliable skin component draped over the neoalveolus and anterior floor of mouth (Fig. 4). The skin component can also be draped over partial defects of the anterior mobile tongue, if needed. The iliac crest also performs well in this situation. The muscular component of this flap is draped over the neoalveolus and anterior floor of mouth and left to resurface with epithelium. The scapular flap is less desirable because its skin component is relatively thick (Fig. 5). Nevertheless, it can be used if the other flaps are unavailable.

Anterior segmental defects associated with even total loss of the lower lip are best approached by considering the lip defect as a totally separate entity from the mandibular and anterior floor of mouth defect. The lip is best reconstructed independently using advancement or transposition flaps from the opposite lip or cheek because no soft tissue components of an osseous free flap will adequately duplicate the appearance of a natural lip (Fig. 6). As an alternative, a radial forearm free flap could be used in addition to the osseous flap to reconstruct the lower lip.

Sometimes the anterior arch defect is associated with a substantial loss of skin over the chin and neck. The fibular flap often proves inadequate to reconstruct the intra- and extraoral soft tissue deficits. However, the iliac crest flap is suitable with its muscular component for the intraoral defect and its skin component for the chin and neck defect (Fig. 7). The fibular flap could be used and the extraoral defect resurfaced with a regional flap (lower island trapezius or pectoralis flap). Although the scapular flap is also suitable, the drawbacks regarding the intraoral reconstruction persist.

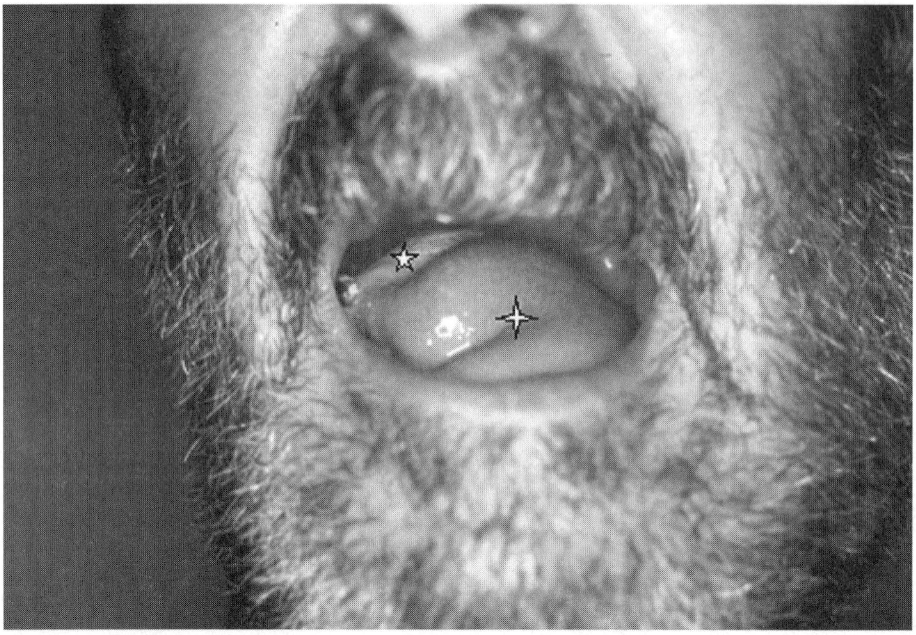

Figure 5 Anterior segmental defect reconstructed with a scapular flap. Note the thick skin flap over the anterior floor of mouth displacing tongue superolaterally. 4-point star = parascapular skin flap; 5-point star = remaining tongue.

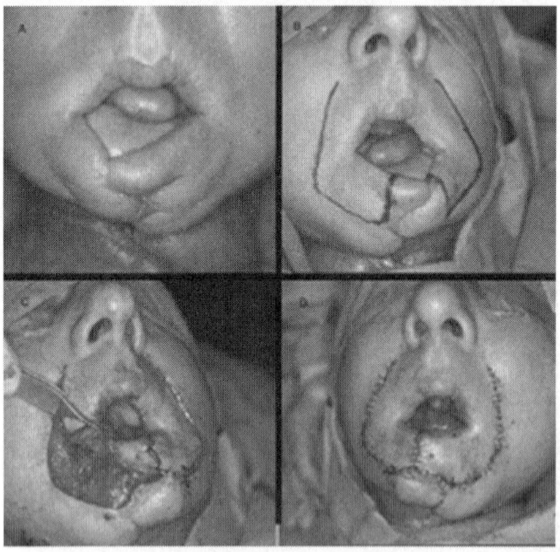

Figure 6 Secondary reconstruction of the lower lip in a patient reconstructed with a fibular flap. The skin component was used to resurface the anterior floor of mouth (a). The lower lip defect was initially closed with a portion of the skin from the free flap, but healing resulted in the deformity shown. Secondary repair of the lip with a Karapandzic advancement was performed (b–d). Use of the skin from the free flap was clearly inadequate and the patient would have been better served by reconstruction of the lip independently during the initial surgery.

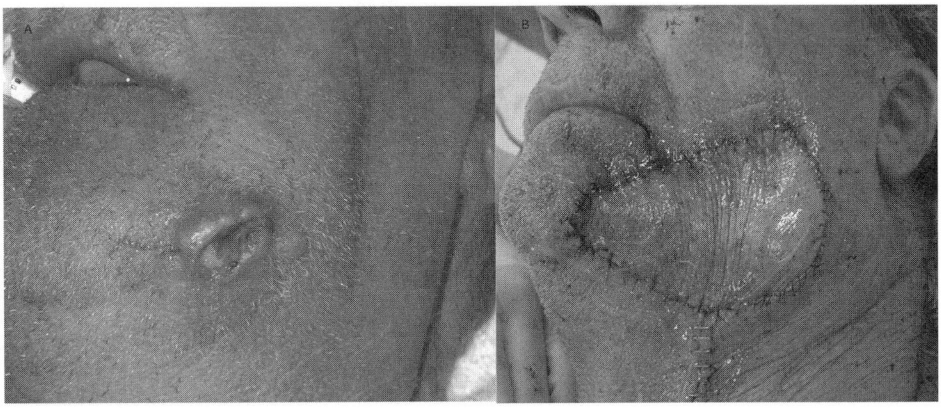

Figure 7 Patient with a squamous cell cancer eroding the central and lateral mandibular segments and skin (a). The patient underwent reconstruction with an iliac crest composite flap (b).

Patients with substantial defects of the tongue combined with chin and neck defects often require multiple regional or free flaps. The scapular system of flaps can be used as an alternative. The parascapular and transverse scapular flaps can be used to reconstruct the tongue (if bulk is needed) and the chin/neck defect. Reconstruction of the floor of the mouth often is obviated by the use of the large skin flap for the tongue. If there is an expansive defect in the neck, the musculocutaneous latissimus component of the scapular system is used.

Lateral Segmental Mandibular Defects

Lateral segmental mandibular defects (posterior to the mental foramen) tend to be less morbid than anterior arch defects in terms of both aesthetics and function. Failure to reconstruct this part of the mandible results in a mild to moderate contour deficiency, mandibular drift toward the side of the defect, and malocclusion. The functional deficits with regard to speech and swallowing are often related more to associated soft tissue deficits and radiation therapy (7).

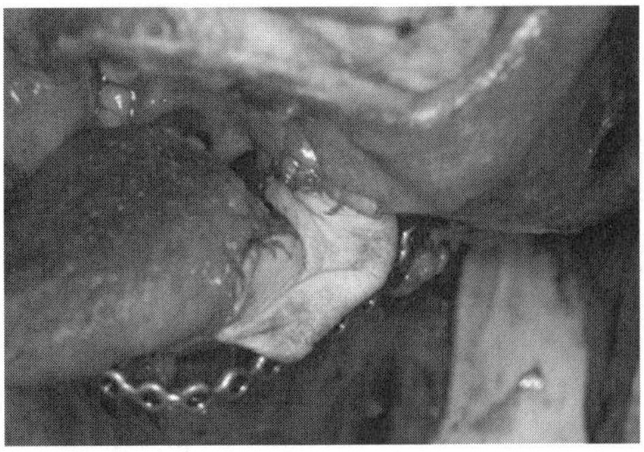

Figure 8 A radial forearm free flap used to cover an MRP to reconstruct a lateral mandibular defect.

The best method to reconstruct lateral segmental defects is controversial. Based on past clinical experience with lateral composite resections, a regional flap (e.g., the pectoralis flap) can function as a mandibular spacer, preventing significant mandibular drift and contour deformities. However, a regional flap may not be ideal for the intraoral soft tissue component of the defect. The remaining choices for primary reconstruction of lateral segmental defects include pedicled vascularized bone, MRPs, and microvascular bone transfers. Pedicled vascularized bone tends to undergo avascular necrosis as previously mentioned. An MRP covered with a regional flap (e.g., pectoralis major) has been shown to have high plate exposure and extrusion rates. This problem was improved by using microvascular free tissue (e.g., radial forearm, parascapular, or rectus abdominis) (Fig. 8), however, problems of plate exposure persist if the associated soft tissue defect is large. Vascularized bone under an MRP or other means of rigid fixation (mandibular plates or wires) demonstrates long-term implant retention and avoids soft tissue contour deformities and plate exposure or breakage (8) (Fig. 9). The iliac crest composite flap is useful for lateral mandibular defects. The height of the bone nearly matches that of native mandible and the internal oblique muscle can be draped over the neoalveolus to provide a very thin gingivalike covering. The ipsilateral hip can be used to reconstruct a lateral mandibular defect to orient the vessels into the posterior neck (Fig. 10). As an alternative, a scapular composite flap is used and the attached skin paddle draped over the neoalveolus and lateral floor of mouth (Fig. 11). An MRP alone may be appropriate in patients who do not desire the potential for full dental restoration, have a very poor prognosis, or are unsuitable candidates for microvascular bone transfer (Fig. 12). If an MRP is used alone, a locking screw-type plate is preferred with a minimum of three screws placed at the proximal and distal ends. This type of plate has several advantages over the older AO stainless steel plates, including less breakage, loosening of screws, and absorption of bone under the plate. However, the problem of plate exposure persists and is the most common complication associated with locking screw-type plates.

Lateral resections that include the condyle represent a special problem since no proximal segment of mandible is available for rigid fixation of plates or grafts. Failure to bring the reconstruction up to the glenoid fossa may result in lateral mandibular instability, drift, and malocclusion. Condylar prostheses connected to plates or

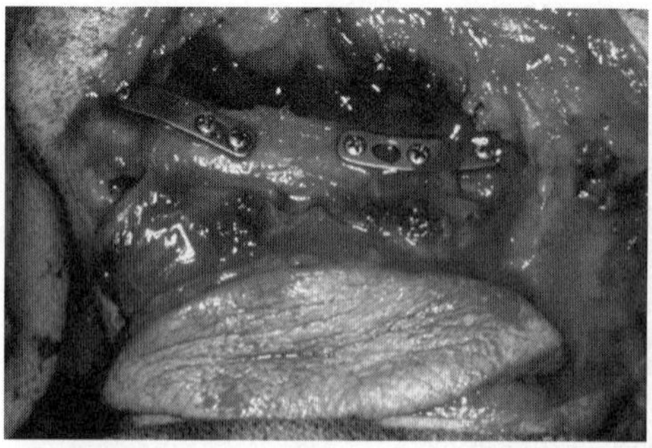

Figure 9 A reconstructed lateral mandibular defect using a composite fibular flap. Note the bone in place with the attached skin island that will be rotated into the oral cavity over the neoalveolus.

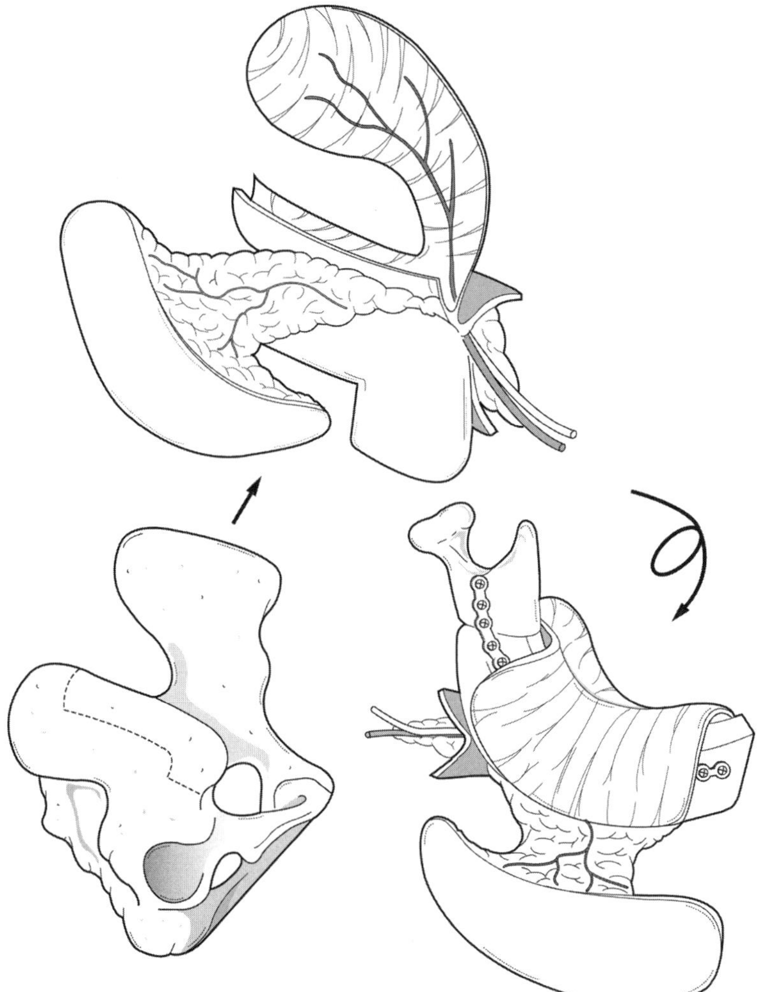

Figure 10 Ipsilateral iliac crest harvest to orient the donor vessels into the ipsilateral neck. The muscle is used to cover the neoalveolus and the skin paddle is used to resurface external chin and neck defects.

grafts have been associated with extrusion and erosion into the middle cranial fossa. A free microvascular graft can be placed near the glenoid fossa with stacked cartilage or fascia; however, the results of this reconstruction are uncertain and joint ankylosis may occur. A viable option is to remove the condyle from the specimen (since it is rarely involved in the malignant process) and rigidly fixate it to the proximal end of free vascularized bone (condylar autotransplantation) (9). This assumes that the malignant process and mandibular resection has extended up the ramus to preclude leaving an adequate length of condyle for plating. Another alternative is to harvest a costochondral graft from the sixth or seventh rib and affix it to the proximal end of the vascularized graft. The costochondral graft is molded into the

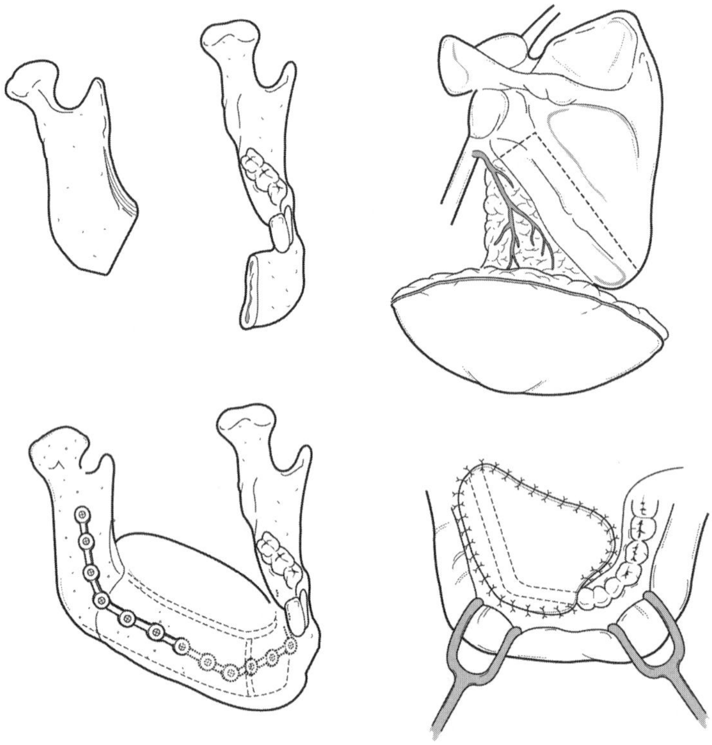

Figure 11 A scapular composite flap for reconstruction of a lateral mandibular defect. The skin component is used to cover the neoalveolus and close the through-and-through defect of the lateral floor of mouth.

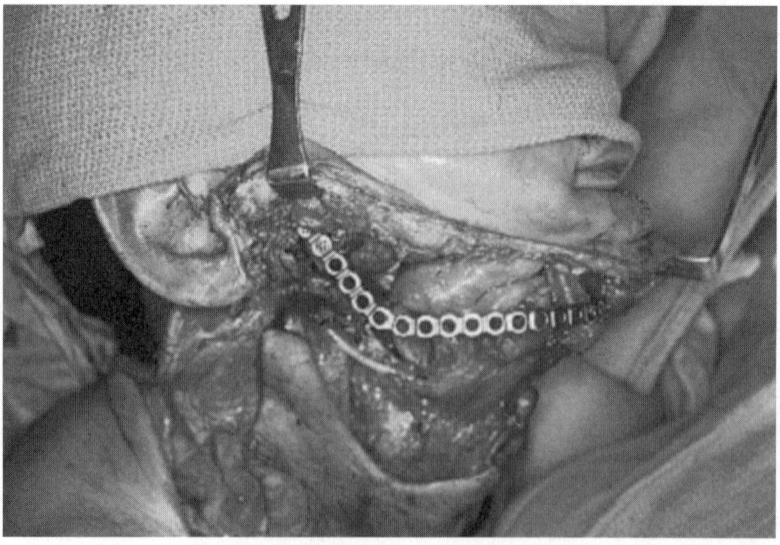

Figure 12 An MRP used to reconstruct a lateral mandibular defect in a patient with a very poor prognosis.

shape of a condyle and seated into the glenoid fossa; intermaxillary fixation for 3–4 weeks facilitates capsule formation around the graft (10). If the condyle is not to be reconstructed, the graft should be left well short of the glenoid fossa to prevent impairment of mouth opening and ankylosis.

TONGUE RECONSTRUCTION

Pertinent Anatomy

The tongue is enveloped by mucosa that contains mucous and serous glands, special taste sensory end organs, as well as general sensory end organs. There are four paired extrinsic tongue muscles: the genioglossus, the hyoglossus, the palatoglossus and the styloglossus. The intrinsic muscles of the tongue consist of an ill-defined network of fiber bundles. Their cooperative movement ensures normal articulation, food bolus manipulation, and swallowing. The nerve supply is from four cranial nerves: the hypoglossal providing motor innervation to all but the palatoglossus, which is supplied by the vagus; the lingual providing taste and sensation to the anterior two-thirds; and the glossopharyngeal (along with a small portion supplied by the superior laryngeal) providing taste and sensation to the posterior third. The specialized tissues of the tongue that control its complex motor and sensory activity make it a far more difficult structure to duplicate than the less specialized and adynamic tissues that surround it, including the floor of mouth, cheek, and mandible.

Reconstruction Overview

The goals of tongue reconstruction are to attain wound closure, minimize complications, and optimize articulation and deglutition. Although wound closure and avoidance of wound complications were major concerns as recently as 15 years ago, modern reconstructive surgery rarely results in failure to attain these basic objectives. However, restoring adequate articulation and deglutition remain serious challenges. Despite the method of reconstruction, the ability of the patient to articulate and swallow seems to be directly proportional to the amount of tongue resected (11,12). There are minor differences in the use of flap tissue or primary closure in patients amenable to these reconstructive modalities. Flap tissue appears to have a detrimental effect on speech and swallowing. This is probably due to the creation of bulk in the oral cavity that is adynamic, resulting in impairment of the function of the remaining tongue. Based on these findings, fundamental objectives in reconstructing the tongue are to close the tongue primarily if possible, minimize the use of flaps placed over the remaining tongue, restore sensation to flap tissue, and preserve the mobility of the remaining tongue. To preserve the mobility of the remaining tongue, the adjacent tissues (floor of mouth, mandible, and retromolar trigone) should be reconstructed as independent units with respect to the tongue. Primary closure of the remaining tongue is preferred and is usually possible in defects involving less than 30% of the oral tongue and tongue base. In cases of larger defects, preserving the function and mobility of the remaining tongue requires a flap that is sufficiently pliable to allow untethered movement.

The importance of maintaining volume is inadequately defined and should not be of major concern except in cases of total and subtotal tongue resections involving the base of tongue. In these circumstances, sufficient tongue bulk in the midline may be helpful in directing food and liquids toward the piriform sinuses. The importance of the tongue base in swallowing is illustrated in McConnell's two-pump theory of swallowing. The first pump is the pistonlike action of the tongue base driving the food bolus through the oropharynx and creating a positive pressure in the upper pharynx. This requires a competent palate, constricting pharyngeal muscles, and an adequate and dynamic tongue base. A deficiency in tongue base volume may be compensated for by an enhanced constriction of the pharyngeal muscles including the superior constrictor. Resection of adjacent structures such as the pharynx, soft palate, or supraglottis, in addition to the tongue base, compounds the problem in this phase of swallowing. These combined resections most often lead to a failure to regain the ability to swallow, leading to total dependence on a stomach tube for nutrition. The second pump is created by elevation of the larynx and opening of the piriforms, causing a negative pressure and suction action in the hypopharynx.

Restoring sensation is an important but controversial consideration. Kapur et al. demonstrated the detrimental effects of regional oral anesthesia on mastication (13). Using sensate flaps for the oral tongue may improve manipulation of the oral bolus; however, the adynamic tissues used in the reconstruction may offset the beneficial effects of reinnervation. Restoring sensation at the tongue base has not been proven to be of benefit to the swallowing reflex.

Primary Closure

McConnell et al. recently reported on a 10 year prospective multi-institution study of speech and swallowing outcomes following reconstruction of limited tongue resections (14). Pairs of patients within the same surgical resection category were matched with respect to the percentage of oral tongue resected, percentage of tongue base resected, and whether postoperative radiotherapy was given. Three reconstructive methods were analyzed: primary closure, distal (regional) flap closure, and free flap closure. The extent of oral (anterior two-thirds) tongue and base of tongue resected was 5–30% and 5–60%, respectively. An implicit assumption in the study was that all the defects in the primary closure vs. distal flap and primary closure vs. free flap groups were amenable to primary closure. The choice of reconstructive method depended upon the participating institution. Those using distal (regional) or free flaps apparently did so to provide sufficient tissue to separate the floor of mouth from the remaining tongue in an effort to minimize tethering. The study indicates that primary closure resulted in equal or better function than the use of flap reconstruction. Swallowing and speech outcomes do not support the theory that skin flaps or skin muscle flaps (distal or free) enhance function.

Although primary closure will inevitably lead to some degree of tethering of the remaining tongue, the use of a flap appears to lead to a greater decrement in speech and swallowing function. Patients with limited tongue defects associated with defects of the floor of mouth may ultimately benefit most by closure of the tongue defect, either primarily or by secondary intention, and reconstruction of the floor of mouth independently using a local, regional, or free flap depending upon the size and adjacent mandibular or pharyngeal defects (Fig. 13). Split-thickness skin grafts provide ample pliable tissue for resurfacing significant defects of the tongue and even combined defects of the mobile tongue and floor of mouth that are not through-and-through to the neck. The sensations of pain, touch, and temperature return in that

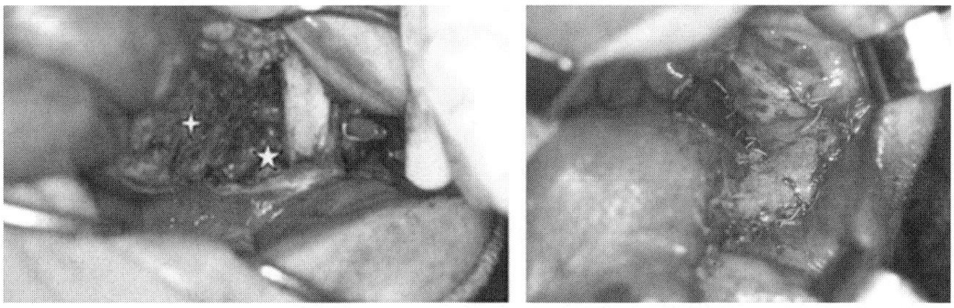

Figure 13 Patient with a significant lateral tongue defect closed primarily with independent reconstruction of the lateral floor of mouth and mandibular ramus (left image: 4-point star denotes lateral tongue defect; 5-point star denotes combined ascending ramus and floor of mouth defects). Image on right shows primary closure of lateral tongue defect with buccinator flap in place over floor and mandibular defects.

order to skin grafts. The sensation to touch returns in most patients; however, in approximately 30% of cases there is no recovery of thermal sensation (15).

Flap Closure

Flaps most commonly used for tongue reconstruction include regional flaps (pectoralis major, lateral and lower island trapezius, latissimus dorsi), and free flaps (rectus abdominus, radial forearm, transverse and parascapular, and lateral arm). Local flaps including the buccinator myomucosal and nasolabial are useful for adjacent defects of the floor of mouth or alveolar ridge. The buccinator flap can be used to reconstruct the lateral and anterior floor of mouth defects, allowing the tongue to be reconstructed independently.

Regional myocutaneous flaps provide reliable vascularized tissue. However, gravitational pull and their inevitable tendency to displace toward their origin often lead to displacement of the flap and remaining tongue. Nevertheless, regional flaps are useful in the patient undergoing total glossectomy when an expedient operation may be required. The muscle-containing flaps (free and regional) used for the tongue are anesthetic, and motor reinnervation only serves to maintain bulk rather than serve any useful reanimation function. In patients who keep their larynx, sensory restoration in the reconstructed portion of the tongue may be an important consideration. In these cases, sensory reinnervation using a thick or augmented fasciocutaneous flap is needed (lateral arm and radial forearm, respectively).

Adjuvant Procedures

Aside from reconstructing the oral cavity, other maneuvers may be useful in enhancing function or preventing complications including: laryngeal suspension, epiglottic laryngoplasty, and inferior alveolar nerve reanastomosis. When the anterior mandible or hyomandibular muscles are disrupted, laryngeal suspension may be useful by statically opening the piriforms and placing the laryngeal inlet in a more infantile and anterior position. Epiglottic laryngoplasty is performed by closing the epiglottic folds over the laryngeal inlet and is useful for patients at great risk for aspiration but in whom preservation of the larynx is anticipated. This procedure is easily reversible and may even be accomplished endoscopically. In cases of hemimandibulectomy, especially for treatment of osteoradionecrosis, the inferior alveolar nerve may be preserved through drill-out or by bridging the gap with a nerve graft. This takes little time and the benefit is a sensate lower lip for improved bolus control and prevention of drooling. For midline mandibulotomies used for surgical access, some surgeons prefer to avoid splitting the lip and instead use a visor flap for mandibular exposure. The visor flap entails sacrifice of the mental nerves; therefore, we prefer a lip-splitting incision and preservation of the mental nerves. The scar may be noticeable but the result is improved function in the lower lip.

Defect Classification

A classification system is important for uniform reporting of results and, to a more limited degree, planning the surgery (16). First, the tongue may be divided along the circumvallate papillae dividing the mobile tongue from the tongue base. To quantify the amount of tissue lost, the tongue is further organized into longitudinal quarters. Although dividing the tongue in this fashion is useful, denervation of the remaining tongue (hypoglossal and lingual nerves) is more important than the actual volume of tongue resected for ultimate functional outcome. Adjacent defects in the floor of the mouth or mandible will affect the reconstructive method as well. However, these areas may be regarded as static and adynamic platforms that should be reconstructed independently from the tongue.

Common Reconstructive Challenges and Their Solutions: Case Studies

One-quarter to One-half Glossectomy of the Anterior Tongue

A 44-year-old patient had a T2N0 squamous cell cancer involving the right lateral tongue. The defect was estimated to be 4 × 4 cm isolated to the right mobile tongue with no associated floor of mouth defect. The goals were to maintain mobility of the remaining oral tongue and to optimize sensibility of the reconstructed segment.

The solution was to close the hemitongue defect primarily. Primary closure is usually possible for isolated defects involving up to 25% of the anterior tongue. Through-and-through defects of the floor of mouth should be reconstructed independently using a local, regional, or free flap. If the floor of mouth defect is not open to the neck, then a local flap or a skin graft should be used.

If primary closure is not possible, a split-thickness skin graft will suffice. If the floor of mouth is also involved associated with a through-and-through defect into the neck, a sensate radial forearm free flap may be used both to reconstruct the floor of the mouth and to resurface the tongue (Fig. 14). This defect combined with a mandibular segmental defect is a difficult reconstructive challenge. The soft tissue components of the osseous free flaps are either too bulky or too tethered to provide independent pliable tissue for the anterior tongue. Repairing posterior mandibular defects with a reconstruction plate may circumvent this. If the cutaneous component of the osseous flap is used, then secondary releasing procedures may be required. One-staged reconstruction can be accomplished with dual free flaps using an osseous free flap combined with a radial forearm flap for the floor of mouth and tongue.

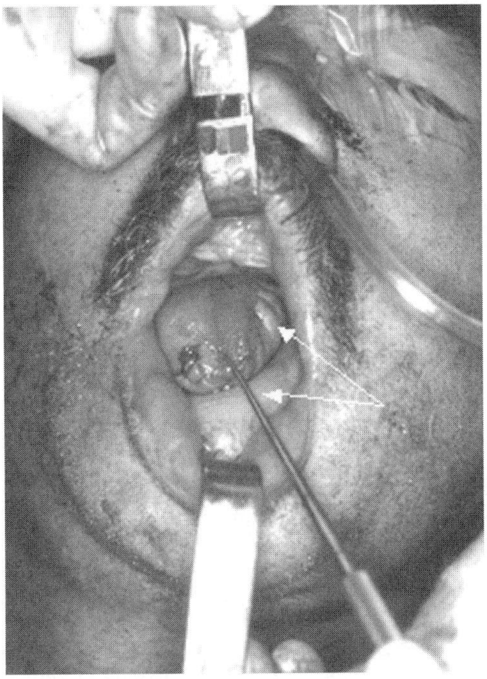

Figure 14 Combined defects of the lateral tongue and floor of mouth reconstructed with a sensate radial forearm free flap. Arrows depict the surface of the flap.

One-quarter to One-half Glossectomy of the Posterior Tongue

A 48-year-old patient had a T2N0 squamous cell cancer involving the right posterior tongue, tonsil, and mandible. This defect was approximately 3×4 cm involving the right base of tongue, tonsillar fossa, and mandibular ramus. The main goal of reconstruction was to provide sufficient bulk so that posterior movement of the tongue would result in contact of this reconstructed segment with the posterior wall and oropharyngeal structures to allow sufficient pumping action during the initial reflex swallow. The benefit of sensory reinnervation was dubious.

The solution was to reconstruct the base of tongue and adjacent tonsillar defect with a pectoralis flap. The posterior mandibular defect was bridged with an MRP (Fig. 15). Posterior tongue defects (behind the circumvallate papilla) that encompass up to 25% of its substance can usually be closed primarily or left to close by secondary intention. Surgical exposure for adequate control of tumor margins and primary closure usually requires that a mandibular split be performed. For defects that also include the lateral pharyngeal wall, a vascularized flap (regional or free) should be used (Fig. 16). The critical mass of tongue base that can be removed while still maintaining an intact and functional swallow is unknown. Many variables play a part in determining the final outcome for these patients including their overall health, physiological age, other coincident abnormalities of the oral cavity or larynx, and the type of reconstruction. Primary closure may not be adequate because it is unlikely that exaggerated pharyngeal constriction will be able to compensate and seal the

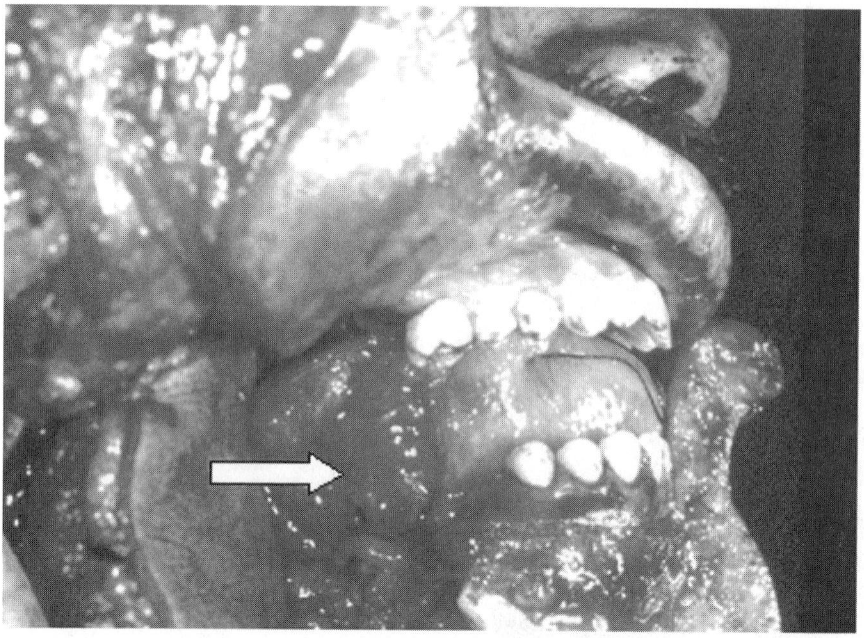

Figure 15 Composite defect of tongue base, tonsillar fossa, and mandibular ramus shown. Base of arrow marks location of the myocutaneous pectoralis flap paddle; tip of arrow indicates the tongue base defect. The flap paddle is subsequently sutured along the margins of the tongue defect both to reconstruct this structure and to close the through-and-through defect.

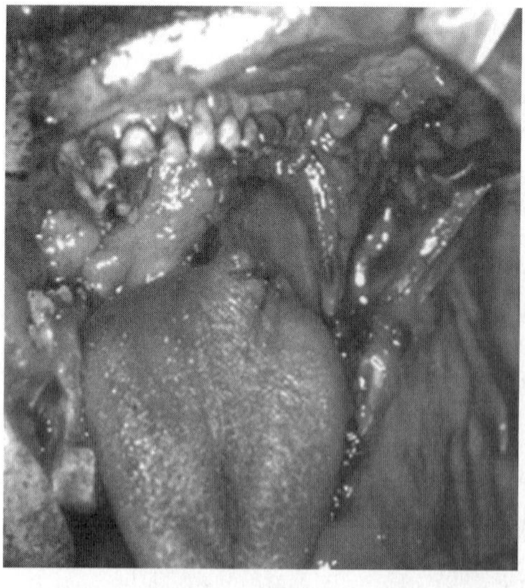

Figure 16 Exposure and primary closure of a 25% loss of the base of tongue performed through a mandibular split approach.

oropharynx. Restoration of bulk, sensation, and coordinated fine motor movement would be ideal. Today, the closest alternative would be an enhanced sensate radial forearm. The forearm flap can be augmented with subcutaneous tissue harvested beyond the skin component in the forearm. This type of reconstruction may help the patient return to a normal diet sooner, especially if the defect extends beyond the base of tongue to involve the epiglottis or pharyngeal wall. A much simpler and effective method for the patient with a substantial base of tongue defect is reconstruction with a pectoralis major flap, as illustrated. Although the flap will have a tendency to migrate inferiorly, this movement will actually increase the bulk and posterior displacement of the tongue without affecting the swallow reflex.

Total Glossectomy with Preservation of the Larynx

A 52 year old patient had extensive squamous cell carcinoma involving the base of the tongue. The total glossectomy defect was devastating to both speech and swallow. Traditional treatment would include removal of the larynx to avoid problems with aspiration, but in selected cases this is unnecessary and laryngeal preservation should be considered. The basic reconstructive challenge was to replace the bulk of the diseased tongue with flap tissue to ensure contact with the hard palate. Duplicat-

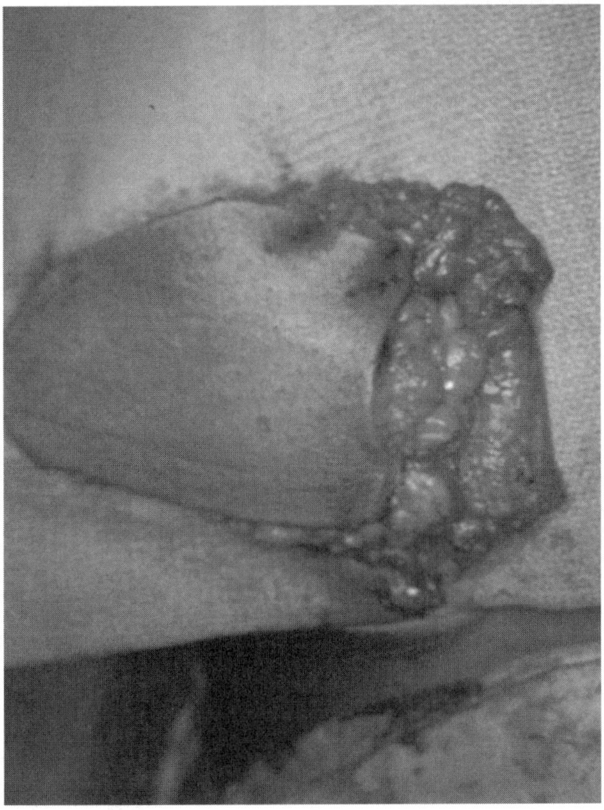

Figure 17 Harvested myocutaneous rectus neotongue flap.

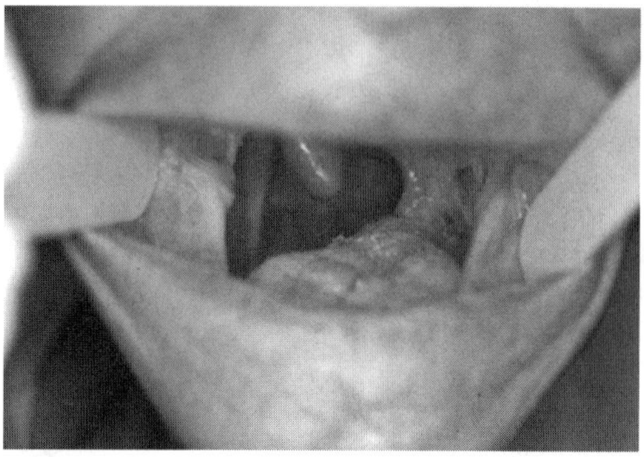

Figure 18 Pectoralis flap used for tongue replacement in a patient who had undergone a total glossectomy and laryngectomy. Note how the neotongue lacks sufficient bulk and height to contact the hard palate. This is due to significant inferior migration and atrophy of the flap.

ing the intricate movement of the native tongue and restoring the patient to near-normal function was unrealistic. The best that can be hoped for is restoration of some degree of intelligible speech and minimal aspiration during a conditioned swallow. Some patients are able to rid themselves of their gastric tubes but advancement to a fully normal diet is seldom attained.

The solution was to reconstruct the total glossectomy defect with a myocutaneous free flap (Fig. 17). Articulation and mastication would be severely compromised independent of the reconstruction technique. With intensive swallow and speech therapy, motivated patients can learn an effective method to initiate deglutition.

This is obviously a devastating defect and the primary goal is to prevent the wholesale delivery of the food bolus to the larynx or pharynx. To achieve this, bulk must be present, and the rule is to ensure contact between the neotongue and the hard palate. This may also improve articulation with the gross movements of the neotongue through its connections to the functioning mandible. The requirement for a sensate flap is not well accepted. However, in cases of laryngeal preservation it may be beneficial to assist in gross localization of the food bolus within the oral cavity. Using a sensate flap in the hope of triggering a normal swallow reflex is too optimistic at this point. Laryngeal preservation should be considered on an individual basis. All of these patients will aspirate to a degree; therefore several factors must be involved in the decision including the patient's physiological age, pulmonary reserve, and motivation. As mentioned previously, adjunctive procedures should be considered such as a tubed laryngoplasty, laryngeal suspension, or near-total laryngectomy.

Regional flaps tend to displace inferiorly and atrophy over time, pulling away from the hard palate (Fig. 18). Despite these problems, however, in patients with coincident total laryngectomies a regional flap will be used because contact with the hard palate is not critical. Free musculocutaneous flaps such as the rectus abdominis and the latissimus dorsi may be sutured directly to the mandible to support the position of the overlying fat and skin. The rectus abdominis also has tendinous inscriptions that may be used with supporting sutures to counteract the weight of the overlying muscle and fat. The fat in these flaps will not atrophy like muscle. It is possible to reinnervate the latissimus dorsi muscle with the hypoglossal nerve stump and attain movement at the base of tongue. This may improve speech and swallow function (17).

Revascularized subcutaneous fat remains essentially unchanged after transfer; therefore, in addition to the free musculocutaneous flaps, sensate flaps with abundant subcutaneous fat would be appropriate. The lateral thigh and lateral arm free flaps fulfill these requirements. The lateral arm flap (introduced by Song in 1982), based on the posterior radial collateral branch of the profunda brachii artery, can be made sensate via its posterior cutaneous nerve. The lateral thigh flap (introduced by Baek in 1983), based on the third perforator of the profunda femoris artery, can be made sensate via its lateral femoral cutaneous nerve. Suspension and maintenance of the position of these flaps in the oral cavity are somewhat more difficult compared to the myocutaneous flaps.

PHARYNGEAL RECONSTRUCTION

When discussing pharyngeal defects it is helpful to define the problem more precisely. The great majority of these defects are created after extirpative cancer surgery. The tissues have commonly been exposed to radical radiation therapy and salivary contamination. It is an oversimplification to consider all pharyngectomy defects together. The main variables to consider with regard to the defect are the anatomical location of the defect within the pharynx, the amount of pharynx that has been resected, and the presence or absence of an intact larynx.

The pharynx is organized anatomically into the nasopharynx, oropharynx, and hypopharynx. Nasopharyngeal extirpation and reconstruction fall more appropriately within the purview of cranial base reconstruction and will not be considered here. The oropharynx includes the soft palate, posterior oropharyngeal mucosa to the level of the hyoid bone, the tonsillar fossae, and the base of the tongue. The hypopharynx includes the piriforms, postcricoid region including the cricopharynx, and the posterior and lateral pharyngeal walls from the hyoid bone to cricopharyngeus. The cervical esophagus begins below the cricopharyngeus and ends at the sternal notch.

Modern reconstruction of the pharynx and cervical esophagus is usually limited simply to providing coverage that can be made sensate. Flaps cannot match the missing tissue exactly but are often successful in duplicating the form of what is missing. The oropharynx and hypopharynx are highly developed and complex anatomical areas that function to prevent aspiration and to allow the food bolus to pass unobstructed to the esophagus. Reconstruction of these areas with inanimate and insensate flap tissue can be inadequate to prevent disabling aspiration. Although form can be provided, function does not necessarily follow. This is illustrated in patients with multiple cranial nerve deficits after skull base surgery who experience crippling aspiration and dysphagia. The sensorimotor deficits caused by dysfunction of cranial nerves 9 and 10 predispose the patient to dysphagia and aspiration despite possessing a perfectly formed pharynx and larynx. For a patient with a significant surgical defect involving the pharynx, even dynamic or sensate flap tissue will lack the coordinated movement required for a normal swallow. In fact, attempts to reform vital areas of the pharynx by simple replacement with various flaps may be futile, and partial or complete obliteration of the affected portion may be more effective in restoring a successful swallow. This is often the case in defects involving the soft palate and piriform sinuses. Intractable aspiration may be inevitable after large or critical areas of the pharynx are resected. In these cases, a total laryngectomy should be planned coincidentally with the pharyngeal resection even if the larynx is uninvolved with tumor.

Soft Palate Resection

The speech and swallow disability experienced after resection of the soft palate is generally proportional to the amount of palate excised. Although important in the production of intelligible speech, the soft palate's main function is to close off the nasopharynx during the pharyngeal phase of swallowing. This obviously prevents the food bolus from entering the nasopharynx but also provides a pumping mechanism to propel the bolus over the epiglottis to enter the piriforms. The ability of the soft palate to seal off the nasopharynx actively is essential. Loss of up to half the soft palate is manageable with flaps or obturation because the remaining palate is dynamic and can provide for the natural valvular function of this structure. Complete loss of the soft palate portends a poor prognosis with respect to nasal and oral function. The valvular function of the soft palate is completely lost and only static obturation remains as a reconstructive option. In this case, there is a trade-off between nasal breathing and sealing the nasopharynx during swallowing. Flaps and obturators will perform the same function: providing for a subtotal static seal.

In cases of total or near-total removal of the soft palate or if the remaining soft palate is dysfunctional, mechanical obturation is preferred to obturation using flap tissue because adjusting the amount of leak is difficult with a soft tissue flap. However, if adequate dynamic soft palate remains then reconstruction with a flap is preferred. The amount of soft palate necessary to effect an adequate seal is usually about half. The palate must be dynamic and of adequate length to reach the posterior oropharyngeal wall and Passavant's ridge. Minor tissue loss at the lateral margin of the soft palate may be amenable to primary closure along the free edges of the palatal and pharyngeal defect margins. More extensive tissue loss will require reconstruction. With regard to flap reconstruction, two choices are available: recreate the form of the soft palate using thin folded tissue, or obliterate the portion of the oropharynx on the side of the defect with no attempt to recreate the form of the soft palate in the area of the defect. Recreating the form of the soft palate with a folded flap may seem logical but can lead to a poor functional outcome. The typical flap used for this purpose is the radial forearm free flap because it is thin and easily folded. Immediately postoperatively, the patient usually experiences minimal problems with nasopharyngeal leak or velopharyngeal incompetence (VPI) and is able to perform an adequate swallow. However, the VPI and swallow function inevitably worsen within weeks as tissue edema subsides and scar contracture occurs. The tissue edema helps to obliterate the space occupied by the flap, thereby reducing VPI. As the edema dissipates, VPI increases because the remaining dynamic soft palate cannot lift the adynamic flap tissue adequately to seal off the nasopharynx. In addition, scar contracture across the reconstructed portion of the soft palate will pull the dynamic portion of the palate forward (clothesline effect), significantly worsening

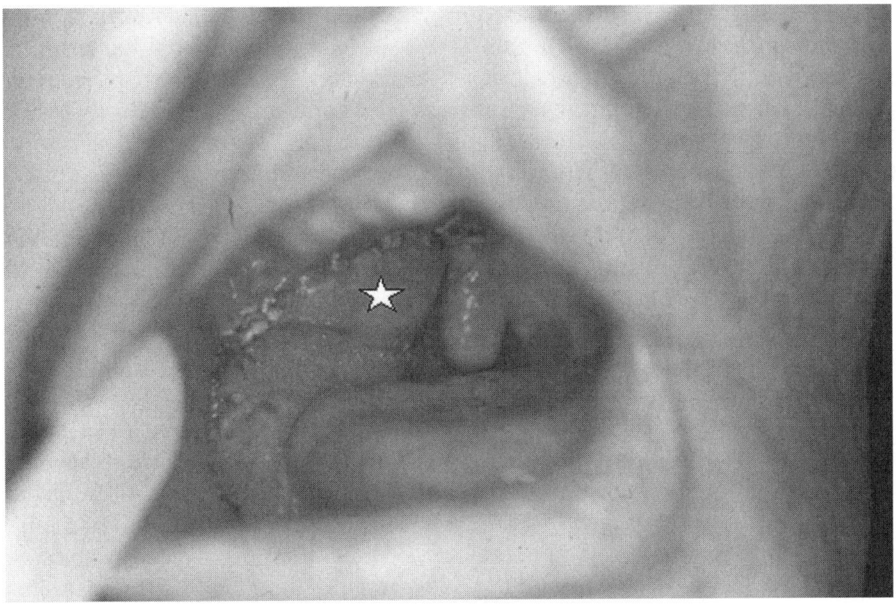

Figure 19 Sensate lateral arm free flap used to obliterate a lateral soft palate defect and reconstruct the lateral oropharyngeal wall. Note the portion of the flap used to obliterate the space behind the palatal defect (star).

VPI. These factors make attempts at recreating the form of the soft palate futile and counterproductive.

In the absence of truly dynamic tissue able to replicate soft palate function exactly, it is best to obliterate the space. This can be accomplished with a variety of soft tissue flaps since their bulk is not an issue unless the excess bulk intrudes on the opposite normal side. The free lateral edge of the soft palate should be approximated to the posterior oropharyngeal wall as much as possible. In patients with significant palatal defects, this will leave deadspace lateral to this closure that can be filled with flap tissue (Fig. 19). Postoperatively, the remaining dynamic palate is able to seal the nasopharynx and this function is minimally affected by scarring within the soft palate or flap tissue.

Hypopharyngectomy

The piriform sinuses play a critically important role in a successful swallow. Their main function is to transmit the food bolus safely into the esophagus without laryngeal penetration or aspiration during the final phase of swallowing. During a normal swallow, the larynx elevates and the piriform sinuses open widely to accept the food bolus passing it through a relaxed cricopharyngeal conduit. This sequence of events is critical to propel the bolus into the cervical esophagus, since residual or regurgitated food or liquid will spill over the aryepiglottic folds (penetration) and be sucked into the trachea (aspiration) after the swallow is complete and the larynx returns to its normal unprotected position. Anything that disrupts this intricate process will often result in disabling dysphagia and aspiration. Even an adynamic upper esophageal segment (within about 3 cm from the cricopharyngeus) will disrupt this process. Therefore, circumferential reconstruction of the esophagus within 3 cm of the cricopharyngeus places the patient at significant risk for aspiration. Even relatively minor resection and primary closure of the lateral piriform sinus often result in aspiration difficulties, but these problems can usually be overcome with intensive swallow therapy. Through this, the patient is taught to turn the head toward the affected side to close off (functionally obliterate) the piriform sinus. This directs the bolus to transit the normal side. The success of this maneuver provides insight into how to prevent aspiration in patients with larger piriform defects. It must be stated, however, that the majority of patients undergoing significant partial resection of their piriform sinus will require a coincidental total laryngectomy since disabling (and life-threatening) aspiration will result if the larynx is left intact. Attempting to reconstruct the piriform sinus, even with a thin sensate flap (e.g., radial forearm), is often ineffective in restoring a normal swallow and preventing intractable aspiration. Like soft palate reconstruction, simply recreating the form is inadequate. Obliteration of the affected piriform holds promise by redirecting the food bolus. Still, the patient will be at significant risk for aspiration and must be warned that total laryngectomy may be required if postoperative rehabilitation to prevent aspiration is unsuccessful. Obliteration of the piriform is accomplished by limited recruiting of adjacent pharyngeal

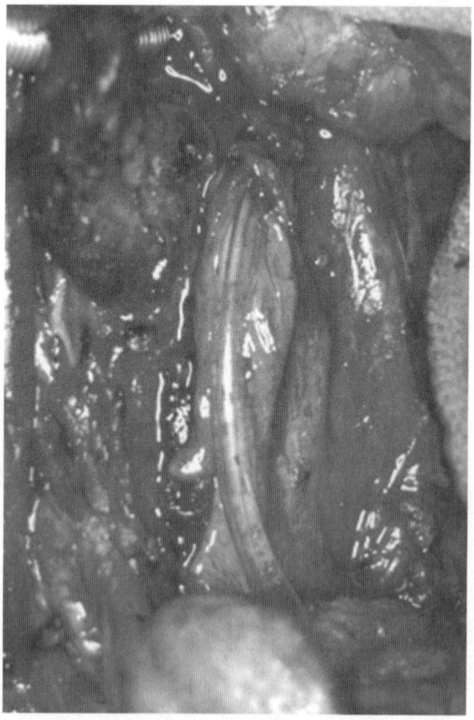

Figure 20 Typical posterior pharyngeal remnant remaining after partial laryngopharyngectomy.

mucosal to allow closure. The piriform is essentially closed as the surrounding mucosa is recruited. A soft tissue flap may be placed over the suture line to further aid in collapsing the sinus. Nevertheless, the success of this operation with regard to the preservation of laryngeal and swallow function is poor. The surgical treatment of defects that extend beyond a single piriform is total laryngopharyngectomy with partial or total pharyngectomy. Coincidental laryngectomy is usually necessary after surgical resection of a piriform sinus neoplasm, especially in older patients, those with pre-existing sensory or pharyngeal motor disturbance, and patients with a history of prior radiation therapy.

Partial Laryngopharyngectomy

Total laryngectomy and partial hypopharyngectomy are common defects most often resulting from resection of a laryngeal tumor that has spread to a piriform sinus. The remaining pharynx usually consists of a vertically oriented remnant extending from the base of tongue (oropharynx) to the cricopharyngeus (Fig. 20). If this posterior hypopharyngeal remnant cannot be closed primarily, pharyngeal reconstruction using flap tissue is needed. An adequate amount of pharyngeal mucosa is characterized by its ability to allow primary closure with a continuous vertically oriented suture line around a #8 endotracheal tube without tension. As with all mucosal

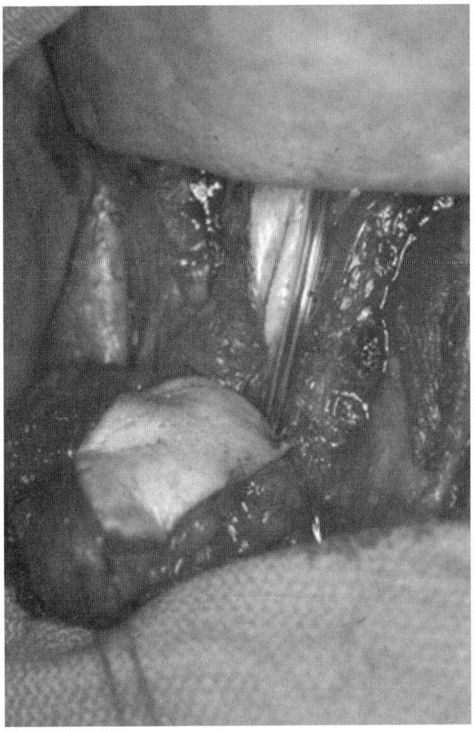

Figure 21 Pectoralis myocutaneous flap being sutured to the posterior pharyngeal remnant to form a complete tube.

suturing techniques in the pharynx, inverting (interrupted) absorbable sutures (Vicryl or polydioxanone suture on a tapering needle) are used to achieve a watertight closure. There is no serosa associated with the pharyngeal mucosa, so a second layer of constrictor muscle over the suture line is useful. If the posterior remnant is deemed inadequate to form a suitable tube for swallowing then a soft tissue flap is needed. The flap of choice in this circumstance is the pectoralis major myocutaneous flap because of its reliability, availability, and ease of harvest. Although the flap does not easily form a tube on itself, it is adequate to create a partial tubular form with the posterior wall consisting of the existing pharyngeal strip (Fig. 21). The posterior remnant provides adequate elasticity for unimpeded food bolus transit to the esophagus. It makes little difference which regional or free cutaneous flap is used, as long as the anterior wall is replaced with well-vascularized skin to achieve a watertight seal. In patients with a hirsute chest or in women an alternative to the pectoralis flap may be chosen.

Total Laryngopharyngectomy

Total laryngopharyngectomy is a relatively common operation characterized by absence of the larynx, pharynx, and upper cervical esophagus. This operation is typically done for treatment of hypopharyngeal or postcricoid cancers. Reconstruction of this defect is deceivingly complex. In a most basic sense, only a simple conduit of adequate diameter is required to allow dependent passage of the food bolus from the upper pharynx to the cervical esophagus. Concerns regarding the intricacies of normal swallowing, especially sensation and coordinated movement, can largely be discarded because the larynx is removed and aspiration is not a risk. The various reconstructive methods have evolved dramatically from Wookey's operation described over 60 years ago to modern techniques utilizing microvascular flap transfers (Table 1).

Historical Perspective

The modern era of pharyngeal reconstructive surgery using flaps began with the now-classic Wookie operation. Wookie (1942) described the use of staged cervical

Table 1 Various Reconstructive Methods, Both Historical and Modern, with Representative Procedures in Each Category

Reconstruction method	Representative procedures
Prosthetic tubes	Salivary bypass tube Plastic and Teflon tubes
Local flaps	Wookey operation (1942)
Local pedicled autografts	Laryngotracheal autograft (1956)
Regional flaps	Deltopectoral flap (1965)
	Lateral trapezius (1980)
	Pectoralis major (1979)
Colon transposition	Transverse/descending colon (1954)
Stomach transposition	Reversed gastric tube (1957)
	Gastric pull-up (1960)
Microvascular visceral transplants	Jejunum (1957)
Microvascular skin transplants	Radial forearm (1985)
	Lateral thigh (1983)

flaps to reconstruct a total laryngopharyngectomy defect. A laterally based subplatysmal cervical flap equal to the vertical height of the defect was raised and transposed to the posterior aspect of the defect, thereby covering the cervical spine. The flap must be raised over the side of the neck dissection; an ipsilateral neck dissection (under the base of the flap) cannot be done because it may compromise the flap's vascularity. The upper and lower free edges of the cervical flaps are sutured to the posterior aspect of the oropharyngeal and esophageal defects, respectively. Temporary pharyngostoma and esophagostoma are created. After several weeks to months, bilateral medially based cervical flaps are elevated and closed to each other in the midline. The raw surfaces left after inward rotation of the skin flaps are covered with a skin graft. This procedure is rarely if ever used today. Multiple problems were associated with this procedure including the need for multiple stages and revisions, frequent partial flap loss, the presence of a salivary fistula that often diverts saliva directly into the tracheostome, frequent pharyngeal stenosis and dysphagia, risk of flap necrosis if bilateral neck dissections are performed, and prolonged hospitalization. Radiation therapy, if instituted after the first stage, makes the remaining cervical flaps unusable.

Subsequent significant developments included the use of more reliable and single-staged procedures. The use of the adjacent larynx (laryngotracheal autograft), especially for small-volume circumferential postcricoid defects, was one of the earliest attempts to utilize flap tissue to achieve one-stage closure of pharyngeal defects (18). Pedicled colonic interposition was described in the early part of the 20th century (Kell). This operation had many variations but eventually the use of the left colon became favored because of its superior reach and vascularity. A sufficient length of colon (to reach the oropharynx) can be obtained by harvesting the full length of intestine between the cecum and sigmoid. The primary blood supply to the middle colon is from several middle colic arteries via the superior mesenteric artery. The distal (sigmoid) colon is transferred into the neck behind the stomach and sternum and suture-anastomosed circumferentially to the oropharynx. The proximal ascending colon is suture-anastomosed to the stomach along the lesser curvature. Colonic transfer is not a first-line reconstructive method, especially for replacement of hypopharyngeal circumferential defects. Because of perfusion problems and bringing contaminated segments of bowel into the neck, this method is prone to postoperative infection and a 45% incidence of significant thoracoabdominal complications. Flap loss from inadequate pedicle length may occur, more commonly with right colon transfers than left, and overall mortality approaches 10%.

Despite the significant morbidity associated with colonic transfer, intestinal transfer is considered to be the closest match to the missing pharyngeal segment available in the body. Microvascular transfer of a free jejunal segment was successfully performed in 1957, and with improvements in microvascular technique this method eventually surpassed all others in popularity in the late 20th century. However, several significant advancements occurred in the interim, including the development of gastric transposition flaps and regional flaps.

Gastric Esophageal Replacement

The reversed gastric tube (1957) and gastric pull-up (1960) seemed to possess many advantages over colonic transfer, including improved vascularity and the requirement of only a single intestinal anastomosis. Although the reversed gastric tube is still used today for primary esophageal replacement, especially in children with benign strictures, it is rarely applied to the typical circumferential hypopharyngeal defect. Gastric pull-up continues to be a useful method for total esophageal replacement. The gastric fundus is able to reach the oropharynx in the majority of cases, making it a viable and useful method for reconstruction of circumferential hypopharyngeal defects.

The gastric pull-up procedure is the modern technique of choice for reconstructing the pharynx when the hypopharyngeal tumor extends significantly into the proximal cervical esophagus. If the planned surgical resection includes the upper cervical esophagus, at or below the sternal notch, then gastric pull-up is the procedure of choice because the proximal esophagus is inaccessible from the neck for an anastomosis. Thoracotomy to access the proximal esophagus is not recommended since an intrathoracic intestinal anastomosis should be avoided. Gastric pull-up is a good solution to this problem because an intrathoracic anastomosis is avoided.

The gastric pull-up operation was first described by Ong and Lee in 1960 but became popular after development of the technique of blunt esophagectomy by Orringer and Sloan in 1978. To mobilize the stomach, the left gastric and short gastric arteries and left gastroepiploic vessels are divided, leaving the stomach supplied by the right gastric and right gastroepiploic arteries. The diaphragmatic hiatus is enlarged, the duodenum is mobilized, and vagotomy and pyloroplasty are performed. The surgical team from below bluntly mobilizes the thoracic esophagus towards the neck while the surgical team in the head and neck pulls the esophagus and stomach into the neck. The esophagus is then divided at the gastroesophageal junction and delivered with the laryngopharyngectomy specimen. The gastroesophageal junction is sewn over and an opening is created in the fundus for anastomosis with the circumferential oropharyngeal defect. Multiple retaining sutures are placed posteriorly from the fascia over the cervical spine to the stomach to support the weight of the stomach and relieve the oropharyngeal anastomosis of excessive tension. Since there is only one suture line, there is a reduced chance of wound breakdown and the suture line is high in the neck where stricture formation is uncommon. The flap has excellent blood supply and allows one-stage reconstruction, even in irradiated patients.

Despite the popularity of this procedure, the associated morbidity and mortality are significant. Major abdominal or thoracic complications occur in 25–50% of patients and stomach necrosis occurs in 3% of cases. Mortality has dropped from 15% to around 7% today. Functional problems include regurgitation of gastric contents, dumping syndrome, and poor-quality tracheoesophageal speech. The advantages include improved distal margins (because the entire esophagus is removed) and better access to the paratracheal lymph nodes. Recovery times are generally rapid, with a return to swallowing usually within 2 weeks. Stenosis is relatively rare because of the absence of a distal suture line. Contraindications include prior gastric surgery, portal hypertension, and advanced cardiopulmonary disease. High lesions where the proximal resection approaches the nasopharynx may not be suitable for pull-up due to insufficient reach of the flap. Larynx-preserving procedures are not possible with gastric pull-ups.

Jejunal Esophageal Replacement

The free jejunal autograft is the most popular transplant for reconstruction of pharyngoesophageal defects. A segment of the second jejunal loop along with its superior

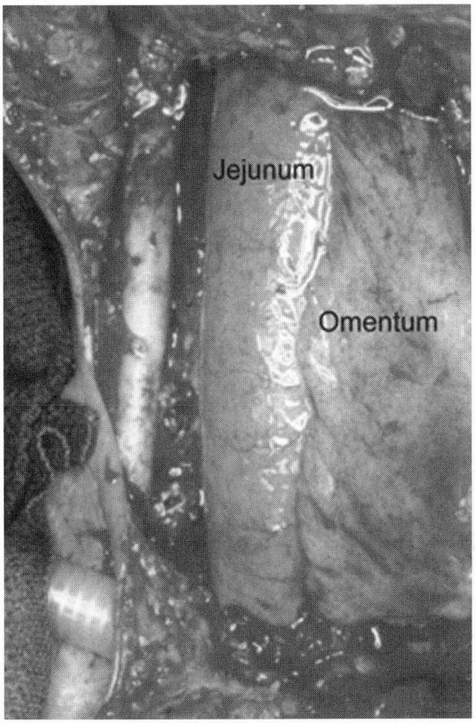

Figure 22 Revascularized jejunal segment in place provides a conduit between the oropharynx and esophagus.

mesenteric arcade of vessels is transplanted into the neck and revascularized using microvascular techniques (Fig. 22). A general surgical team can harvest the flap in less than 1 h. A feeding jejunostomy is performed at the same setting. The flap is carefully placed in an isoperistaltic orientation and both enteric anastomoses are completed prior to revascularization. The marker segment is brought out through the lower medial neck incision (Fig. 23). The distal anastomosis (esophagojejunal) is prone to stricture because of the continuous circumferential suture line. It is best to break up the continuous line of suture by creating a V-plasty. Postoperative radiation is well tolerated with minimal morbidity. Although distal anastomotic stricture is relatively rare, it is obviously more common to this technique than to gastric pull-up. Significant intra-abdominal complications occur infrequently. Voice rehabilitation is on par with gastric pull-up.

Regional Flap Esophageal Replacement

Regional flaps have a limited role in the reconstruction of circumferential pharyngeal defects. However, prior to the common use of microvascular flaps, regional flaps were briefly the flap of choice. The deltopectoral flap (1965) was heralded as a major advance in reliable pharyngoesophageal replacement. The deltopectoral flap was also a significant advance in the understanding of axial flap physiology. This flap

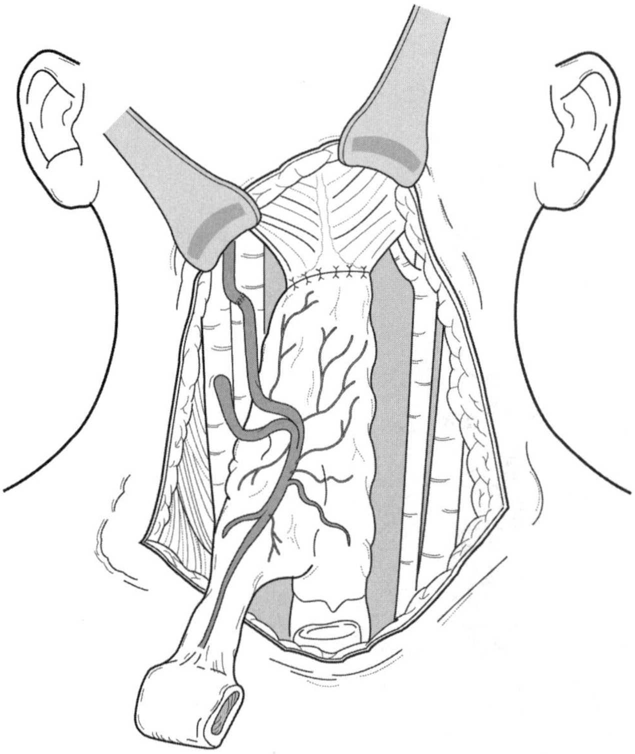

Figure 23 The jejunum is in place with the marker segment extending through the lower neck incision.

was well vascularized and outside the usual neck irradiation portals and it could be transferred easily to the pharynx. However, as with the Wookie procedure, reconstruction required multiple stages. A controlled fistula is created after the initial surgical transfer of the flap. After at least 3 weeks, the pedicle is divided and the esophageal anastomosis is completed, closing the fistula. In practice, multiple procedures are usually required finally to close the fistula and postoperative stricture at the distal anastomosis is common. Time to a successful swallow averages 10 weeks and several months of hospitalization are typical.

The other most commonly used regional flap is the pectoralis major. This flap became the workhorse of head and neck reconstruction including the pharynx shortly after it was introduced in the late 1970s. Early reports of its use by Baek and Withers for circumferential defects included a recommendation to create of a temporary controlled fistula because of the high rate of uncontrolled fistula formation after primary reconstruction. The main problem using the pectoralis flap for circumferential pharyngeal defects is its excessive bulk. Forming a tube with this flap has been likened to trying to form the New York City Yellow Pages into a tube. The suture line is under some tension as a result of this phenomenon, making postoperative fistulization more likely. In addition, the interior of the neopharynx becomes quite tight causing significant dysphagia postopera-

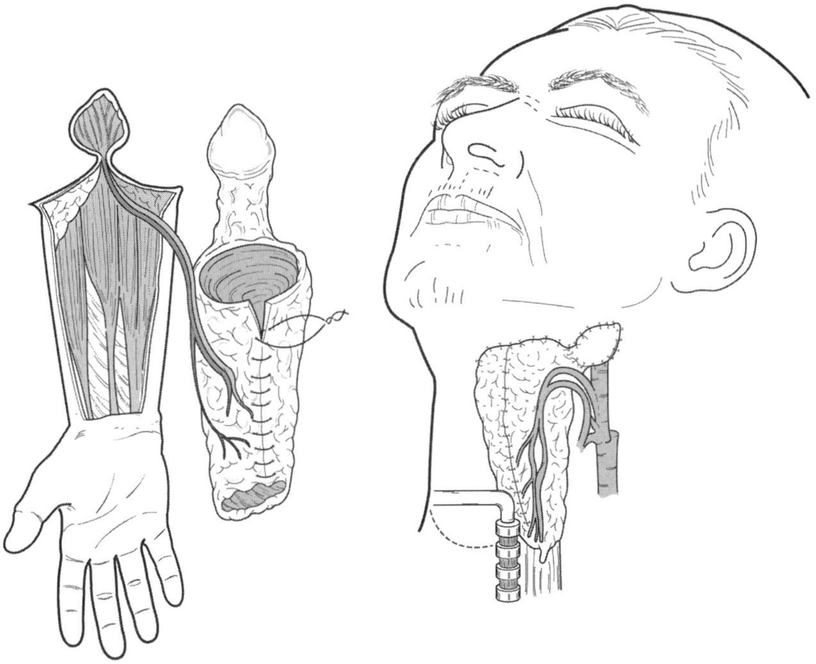

Figure 24 The tubed radial forearm flap is depicted as harvested from the arm with a proximal marker segment. After the flap is inset, the marker segment is incorporated into the cervical flap incision for monitoring purposes.

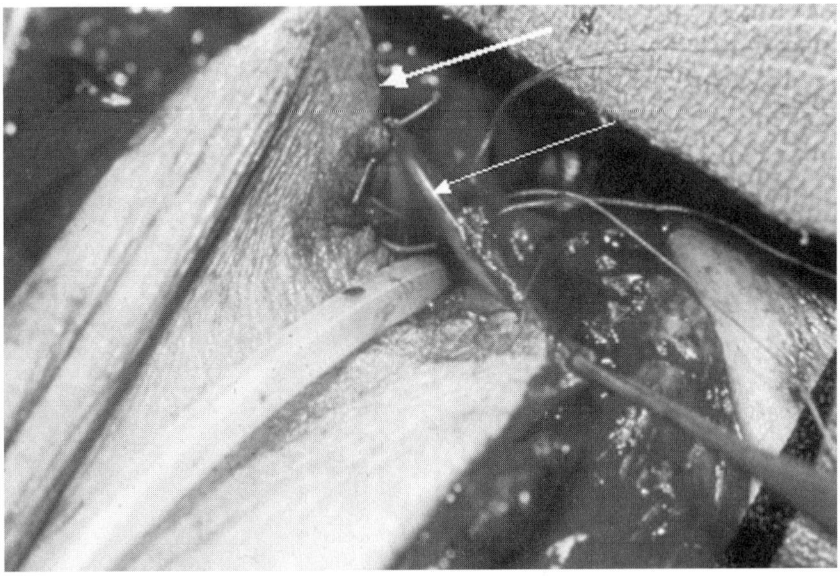

Figure 25 The distal anastomosis is demonstrated (thin arrow:esophagus; thick arrow:flap) and the flap is shown nearly completely tubed.

tively. Today, the pectoralis flap is relegated to repair of only partial pharyngeal defects. Of course, it remains a workhorse for other types of head and neck defects.

Free Fasciocutaneous Flap Esophageal Replacement

Using skin flaps for pharyngeal reconstruction has many advantages. Skin is the most donatable and easily accessible organ in the body; it is relatively ischemia-tolerant; providing it is sufficiently pliable and thin, it can be formed into a tube easily; morbidity associated with harvest can be insignificant; and tracheo-neoesophageal speech is better than that achieved with visceral flaps. The fact that skin flaps do not provide a moist or secreting surface and that they are adynamic appears to make no difference with respect to a functional swallow compared to visceral flaps. The most common microvascular skin flaps used are the radial forearm and lateral thigh. The radial forearm flap is easily tubed and readily available in most patients (Fig. 24). It is rapidly harvested with large donor vessels. The ease, reliability, and functionality of this flap for pharyngeal reconstruction are unsurpassed. A useful alternative is the lateral thigh flap, although its harvest is more difficult (Fig. 25). Harvested from the lateral aspect of the thigh, the donor site can be closed primarily in most instances leaving only a linear scar. As with a radial forearm flap, a two-team approach is possible, reducing operative time. First described by Baek in 1983, the lateral thigh flap is based on the third perforating branch of the profunda femoris artery running in the intermuscular septum between the vastus lateralis and biceps femoris muscles. In selected patients, flap thickness rarely exceeds 5 mm, so forming it into a tube is quite easy (Fig. 26). A V-plasty should be done at the distal anastomosis and a marker segment is attached for remote monitoring (as with the radial forearm) (Fig. 27). Sensory reinnervation is possible but unnecessary. Contraindications include local obesity (saddle-bag thighs), previous trauma, severe peripheral vascular disease, or prior hip replacement surgery that may have disrupted the perforating vessels.

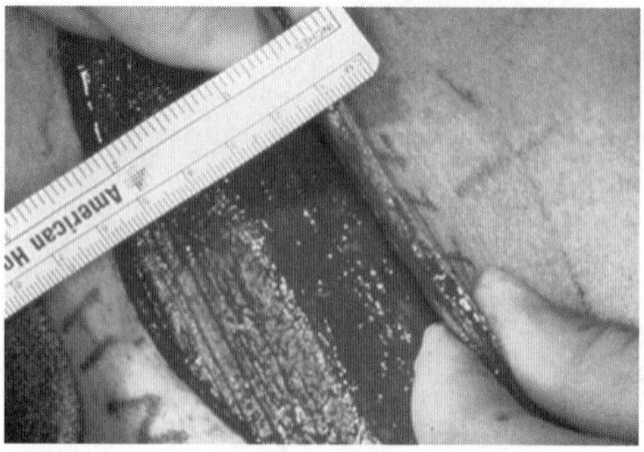

Figure 26 Thickness of the lateral thigh fasciocutaneous flap.

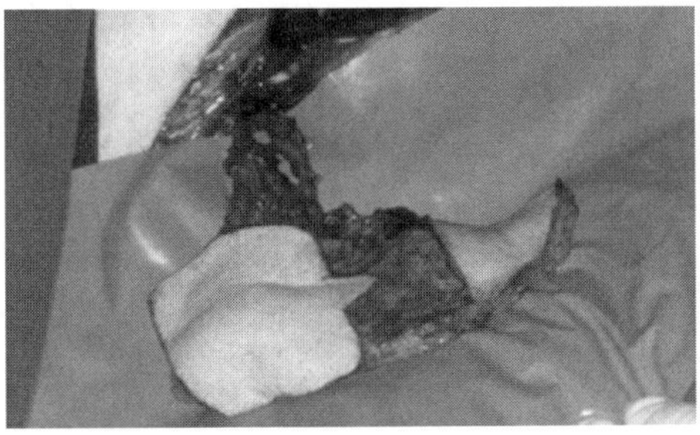

Figure 27 Lateral thigh flap harvested with a "V" incorporated for the distal anastomosis and an island-monitoring segment.

RECONSTRUCTION AFTER MAXILLECTOMY

Introduction

The maxillectomy surgical defect varies widely with respect to size, orientation, and complexity. The traditional radical maxillectomy defect is usually amenable to prosthetic rehabilitation with good success. In fact, traditional teaching favors a prosthetic-only approach because it allows easy inspection of the cavity for tumor surveillance after removal of the prosthetic appliance in the office. Proponents of flap reconstruction for these classic defects argue that leaving the cavity open is worthless because patients with tumor recurrence are most often unresectable anyway. In addition, they cite the fact that maxillary carcinoma carries a poor prognosis and flap reconstruction improves the patient's quality of life because it frees them from having to care for the prosthesis and the large cavity that tends to gather crusts and bits of food. Although these arguments are compelling, flap reconstruction is a more complex and uncertain endeavor than prosthetic rehabilitation. Although reconstructive surgery after maxillectomy is an increasingly popular alternative to prosthetic rehabilitation, the use of prosthetic appliances remains the popular choice.

Although the classic radical maxillectomy defect (maxilla including the hemi-hard palate sparing the orbital rim and globe) is most commonly found after resection of maxillary sinus carcinoma; lesser or greater removal of hard and soft tissues may be needed in selected patients. In general, surgical reconstruction is reserved for maxillectomy defects that are quite small (amenable to local or regional flap coverage) or large (significantly larger than after routine radical maxillectomy). With the advent of microsurgical flaps, the ability to close large complex defects successfully has improved dramatically. In fact, microsurgical flap reconstruction has become the mainstay of treatment in these cases. Local and regional flaps such as the temporalis and various oral transposition flaps (e.g., palatal and buccinator myomucosal) are used rarely and usually reserved for smaller defects.

Goals

The goals of rehabilitation after maxillectomy using a prosthesis or a flap are similar and include restoration of a sealed oral and oropharyngeal cavity and normal speech and swallowing. After routine maxillectomy, a skin graft is used to line the cavity, bolstered with temporary packing supported by an interim (initial) surgical prosthesis. A subsequent prosthesis is fashioned after the skin graft has healed to obturate the cavity and close the oronasal fistula.

Although the functional goals (speech and swallowing) are similar, flap reconstruction of large complex maxillectomy defects also includes obtaining a healed wound, soft and hard tissue obliteration of the surgical cavity, restoration of facial contour, and soft tissue coverage of cheek and orbital defects (19). Both in prosthetic management and flap reconstruction, restoration of an even and stable distribution of occlusal forces is needed for successful mastication.

Pertinent Anatomy

The maxillae are paired structures consisting of hollow pyramids with their apexes situated posteriorly, each supported by three buttresses that resist the forces of mastication. The buttresses include the nasomaxillary, zygomaticomaxillary, and pterygomaxillary. The multiple buttresses help to distribute the forces of mastication evenly. The components of each maxilla include the homolateral hard palate, lateral nasal wall, homolateral alveolus, and the anterior face. Each maxilla has four processes that articulate with surrounding facial bones including the zygomatic, frontal, alveolar, and palatine.

Each maxilla contributes to several important anatomical structures including the medial and inferior bony orbital rim, lacrimal fossa, and floor of the orbit. The nasolacrimal duct and infraorbital vessels and nerve course through the maxilla. The orbital surface of the maxilla is triangular and forms the majority of the floor of the orbit. Resection of the floor of the orbit, sparing the orbital rim, is commonly done in the course of a routine maxillectomy. There is usually no need to replace this bony support since Lockwood's ligament serves to prevent herniation of the orbital contents into the surgical defect.

Prosthetic Management

Prosthetic management of the radical maxillectomy defect is the traditional method of rehabilitation. Clinical experience using prosthetic devices for this purpose is significant and it has become clear that certain factors are favorable with regard to prosthesis retention and function. These include the presence of an intact opposite hemipalate, retention of healthy teeth adjacent to the palatal defect, retention of the majority of the soft palate, and formation of a linear contracted scar around the cheek facilitated by the placement of a skin graft at the time of the extirpative surgery. The size of the defect is proportional to the likelihood of excessive prosthesis movement and failure. The presence of stable teeth, especially next to the defect, significantly improves this relationship. Using a prosthesis after maxillectomy nonselectively will result in several patients experiencing difficulties that include leakage and poor mastication. Approximately 70% of patients describe their swallowing and speech as fair to good. To avoid these complications, certain surgical defects should either be prepared with osseointegrated implants or left for flap reconstruction.

Prosthesis retention and stability are major determinants of successful obturation and mastication. An unstable prosthesis is more likely to leak and be unable to withstand the forces of mastication. Stability and retention are intimately related. In

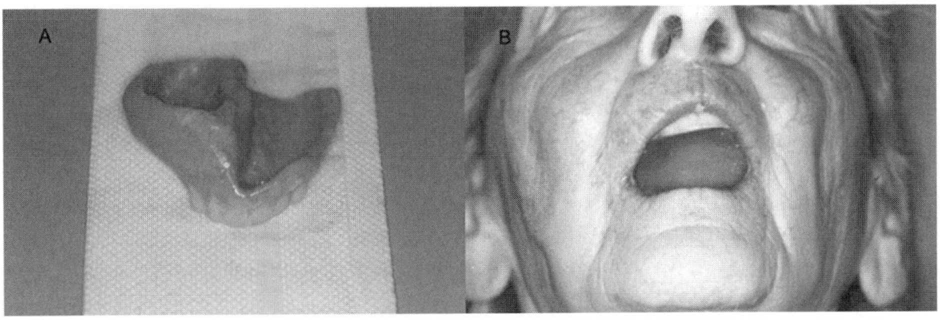

Figure 28 Typical tissue-borne prosthesis consisting of an obturator portion that extends into the maxillary defect and a denture portion that conforms to the remaining hard palate (a). The tissue-borne prosthesis in place (b).

general, stability increases as the size of the opposing hard palate increases. The cantilever effect of vertical prosthesis movement within the cavity secondary to mastication is lessened when the opposite normal palate extends beyond the midline. If there is significant remaining normal hard palate, it is possible that a tissue-borne prosthesis will work (Fig. 28). A tissue-borne prosthesis is one that depends only on the underlying tissues for support, much like a denture. With less remaining hard palate it is possible to extend the obturator into the cavity to engage the bony elements, including the proximal stumps of the buttresses. After engaging these bony surfaces, the prosthesis is retained over the lateral scar band at the junction of the skin graft and oral mucosa. The prosthesis can also be attached to healthy teeth in the remaining alveolus to improve its stability and retention when the hard palate defect extends across the midline. This tooth-borne prosthesis can be quite stable since the teeth assist to retain the prosthesis and to limit the cantilevering effect of mastication. The prosthesis attaches to the teeth with clasps similar to a partial denture. If teeth are not present in the remaining alveolus and the prosthesis is unstable, the patient may be a candidate for osseointegrated implants. These implants are best placed along the remaining alveolus and are essentially tooth substitutes that act to secure a full denture. This implant-borne prosthesis can be snapped out for cavity inspection and cleaning.

Preparation of the surgical cavity to accept a prosthesis is an important aspect of treatment. During resection, healthy teeth in the remaining alveolus should be preserved. The abutment teeth are most important. To ensure the survival of abutting teeth, the osteotomy should be done through the adjacent tooth socket instead of the space between the teeth. This will preserve a stabilizing shelf of bone around the last tooth. The radical maxillectomy cavity is skin-grafted to enhance healing and facilitate the formation of a scar band inferolaterally that will be important to help retain the final prosthesis. An initial (surgical) prosthesis is used to hold the bolster in the cavity against the skin graft. It also facilitates speech and swallowing in the immediate postoperative period and after the bolster is removed. This prosthesis is created preoperatively by the prosthodontist. A new interim prosthesis is created by the prosthodontist after the acute postoperative period that will better fit the defect and minimize leakage. The patient usually uses this prosthesis through radiation therapy. Once the cavity has stabilized, the final prosthesis will be fitted. This prosthesis will be modified as needed to enhance function and comfort.

Prosthetic management of soft palate defects is more difficult because of the mobility and intricate muscular coordination of this structure. A significant defect in the soft palate may leave an orphaned area of soft palate (a band of tissue); this defect is difficult to obturate effectively. Removal of the remaining soft palatal band of tissue may be needed to improve the ability of the obturator to create an effective seal. This is especially true if the posterior band is foreshortened and not able to reach the posterior pharyngeal wall. A notable exception to this is in a patient that has undergone a maxillectomy and a large cavity is created above the level of the hard and soft palates. In such a case, the soft palatal band of tissue will assist in retaining the prosthesis.

Certain size-related and configuration-related factors may be present after maxillectomy that impede the successful use of a prosthesis. Large-volume defects including radical maxillectomy associated with orbital exenteration and/or removal of cheek skin are difficult or impossible to obturate effectively. Facial contour problems arise when the resection approaches the medial zygomatic bone and inferior orbital rim. Due to the limitations of local flap tissue design, periorbital reconstruction including the inferior orbital rim requires the use of nonvascularized bone grafts and titanium mesh. These implants require envelopment in vascularized flap tissue for survival and integration. When the resected palate includes the premaxilla (including the canines and nasal spine), prosthetic rehabilitation is difficult and movement of the prosthesis with mastication is common. Vascularized bone reconstruction is essential to provide a stable base for a prosthesis or osseointegrated implants and to maintain the contour and projection of the upper lip and nasal base.

Commonly Used Flaps

Flaps have traditionally played a small role in the rehabilitation of patients who have undergone routine maxillectomy. However, some maxillectomy defects are difficult to manage prosthetically as outlined above. For example, large-volume defects that include orbital exenteration along with the typical radical maxillectomy. Conventional treatment of this defect is to resurface the bony orbital cavity with a temporalis flap and obturate the maxillary defect. A medial forehead flap has also been used for this purpose. Large-volume defects that include the overlying cheek skin are complex and difficult to reconstruct. The priority with regard to reconstructive surgery shifts away from the maxillectomy defect to the need for extensive facial reconstructive surgery. In the past, regional flaps, including the deltopectoral or lower island trapezius flaps, were used in combination with a skin graft and obturator. The results ranged from dysfunctional to grotesque.

The modern era of reconstructive surgery began with the introduction of free flaps. A free flap consists of components that can be manipulated to reconstruct complex composite maxillary defects without the use of prostheses. Their bony and soft tissue components can be formed into a three-dimensional composite graft that will readily resurface large cheek defects, fill the bony orbit, obliterate the maxillary cavity, and resurface the lateral nasal cavity, while providing vascularized bone to act as a neoalveolus for the acceptance of osseointegrated implants. Still, due to the difficulties encountered in shaping the bone, reconstructing the orbital floor and rim is usually done with nonvascularized bone grafts and mesh. The flap that is most

Table 2 Maxillectomy Classification

Designation	What's removed
Type 1: limited maxillectomy	Anterior and/or medial walls: sometimes the orbital rim w/soft tissues and cheek skin
Type 2: subtotal maxillectomy	Lower five walls including the palate (classic hemimaxillectomy)
Type 3a: total maxillectomy	All six walls w/sparing of orbital contents (radical maxillectomy)
Type 3b: extended maxillectomy	Total maxillectomy w/orbital exenteration
Type 4: orbitomaxillectomy	Upper five walls w/orbital exenteration and sparing of hard palate

Source: From Ref. (22).

appropriate to resurface large-volume defects that include cheek skin while providing vascularized bone is the scapular free flap (subscapular system). Other commonly used free flaps for maxillary reconstructions include the fibular osteocutaneous flap, rectus myocutaneous flap, iliac crest osteocutaneous flap, and radial forearm osteocutaneous flap. There are few reports of prefabrication using osseointegrated implants and skin grafts to mold the free flap at the donor site into the proper configuration prior to definitive transfer (20).

Defect Classification

The nomenclature involving maxillectomy is confusing and arbitrary. A cogent classification system is needed to associate the described maxillary defect better with the appropriate method of rehabilitation and reconstruction. A good place to start is to better define the classic defect or 'so-called' radical maxillectomy. A radical maxillectomy is the most common type of maxillectomy and is usually amenable to management with prostheses. Radical maxillectomy includes the removal of the entire maxilla, including the majority of the orbital floor. This term is also applicable when removal of the maxilla includes the removal of the pterygoid plates, ipsilateral nasal bone, ethmoid labyrinth, and lamina papyracea. Modern vernacular often substitutes the term 'radical' with 'total'. Anything less than a total maxillectomy is designated as 'subtotal' or 'limited'. More extensive removal of surrounding structures is designated as 'extended'. Cordeiro et al. describe a classification schema based on these designations (Table 2).

Surgical Algorithm

Although management of each type of maxillectomy defect may vary somewhat according to the surgeon's preference, consideration of each individual defect according to the aforementioned schema helps to narrow the reconstructive options significantly. Unless a free flap is definitely planned with complete obliteration of the maxillary defect, the prosthodontist should be consulted preoperatively.

Type 1: Limited Maxillectomy

Loss of only the anterior or medial walls of the maxillary sinus is inconsequential and requires no reconstructive or prosthetic management. Occasionally, the orbital rim must be sacrificed along with a variable quantity of cheek skin. These are small-volume but potentially large-surface-area defects that require bone for replacement of the orbital rim. Small cheek defects are best managed with cheek rotation or transposition. Larger defects not amenable to cheek rotation are managed with a radial forearm free flap. The underlying orbital rim defect is managed with a non-vascularized bone graft in any case. The osteocutaneous radial forearm flap should be avoided because of significant potential donor site morbidity.

Type 2: Subtotal Maxillectomy

This classic hemimaxillectomy defect is probably best managed by the traditional prosthetic management protocol. Avoidance of a prosthesis is possible but a free flap is necessary. Obliteration of the maxillary sinus cavity, provision of bone for the neoalveolus and for support and anterior projection of the upper lip, and skin coverage for the neopalate and lateral nasal cavity are needed. An augmented (large subcutaneous extension) radial forearm free flap with a nonvascularized bone graft (e.g., hip) for the neoalveolus will fulfill these requirements. The free flap is designed in an 'L' shape to provide skin coverage for the neopalate and lateral nasal wall. However, a drawback of this method is that if postoperative radiation therapy is planned the nonvascularized bone graft will most likely not survive. Although potentially morbid, an osteocutaneous radial forearm flap is a better choice in this situation. Another option is a fibular osteocutaneous flap. The bone is osteotomized to follow the anterior curvature of the native alveolus and the skin of the lateral leg is used to cover the neopalate and lateral nasal cavity. Significant muscle is left attached to the fibular bone during harvest to assist in obliteration of the maxillary sinus. A third option is a composite scapular flap, but the thickness of the skin paddles often leads to an overly bulky flap that results in nasal obstruction and hangs down into the mouth. Multiple revisions are needed for adequate thinning.

Anterior bilateral subtotal maxillectomies (essentially a total palatectomy) cannot be reconstructed effectively with a prosthesis because of the extensive bony loss and absence of support for a prosthesis. In this type of defect, obliteration of the maxillary antra is often not necessary since only a portion of the floor of each antrum is involved and the majority of each sinus is left intact. The main consideration is replacement of bone to form a new palate with minimal overlying soft tissue. The entire floor of the nose must also be reconstructed. A sandwich flap consisting of bone sandwiched between skin is required. Either a fibular osteocutaneous flap or scapular osteocutaneous flap will suffice. The fibular bone must be osteotomized extensively to follow the natural curve of the anterior and lateral dental alveoli. The skin of the lateral leg is often quite thin and will cover the bone without undue bulkiness. There is no need to osteotomize the scapular bone since a bite of lateral scapular bone can be taken. Its free thick edge is used to reconstruct the anterior and anterolateral neoalveolar ridges and is suitable for osseointegration. The bone is secured with straight titanium miniplates that extend onto the nasomaxillary and zygomaticomaxillary buttresses. The scapular skin paddles are typically relatively thick and, on the palatal side the flap, tend to hang into the oral cavity. Subsequent revision and thinning are necessary.

Total maxillectomy (type 3a, radical maxillectomy) is a similar defect to the classic hemimaxillectomy except that the majority of the orbital floor is removed.

This rarely presents a problem with support of the globe because of the presence of Lockwood's ligament. However, if enophthalmos or vertical dystopia is noted, titanium mesh can be placed as in a typical blow-out fracture. There is no need to cover the plate on the defect side with vascularized tissue.

Type 3b: Extended Maxillectomy

The extended maxillectomy defect is a large-volume defect that includes the orbital contents and/or cheek skin. Aside from the usual requirements of soft tissue and bone after a subtotal maxillectomy, there is a need to cover (or obliterate) the eye socket and to reconstruct the often-extensive cheek defect. The inferior orbital rim is often also removed when the cheek skin is involved.

Patients undergoing maxillectomy with orbital exenteration are candidates for a bone-containing free flap. Only the scapular flap and iliac crest flap possess sufficient soft tissue bulk to close these defects effectively while providing adequate bone substrate for osseointegration. Multiple paddles can be created to close the nasal, palatal, and socket defects independently while completely obliterating the maxilla. The thickness of the flaps can be significant and, although fine for socket obliteration, this excessive bulk will cause nasal obstruction and a large roof-of-mouth mass. The iliac crest flap is a good solution since it provides adequate bone stock for both the neoalveolus and orbital rim, and the internal oblique muscle can be draped over the bone intraorally to provide a relatively thin covering (21). The skin component may be used for obliteration of the socket.

Extended maxillectomy with cheek skin excision (but not orbital exenteration) may be reconstructed with a bone-containing free flap to provide a substrate into which osseointegrated implants are placed for denture retention. Any of the common osseous free flaps are capable of closing this defect. For example, an osteocutaneous scapular flap can be used with the bone secured across the neoalveolus with a straight miniplate (Fig. 29). The skin components are used to cover the lateral nasal wall, cheek, and hard palatal defects. Unfortunately, the osseous free flaps do not have skin components that are a good match in terms of color and texture with natural cheek skin. Patients undergoing maxillectomy, orbital exenteration, and excision of overlying cheek skin are also candidates for a bone-containing free flap. Of the bone-containing free flaps, only the subscapular system and iliac crest osteomyocutaneous flaps possess sufficient tissue volume and plasticity to reconstruct this

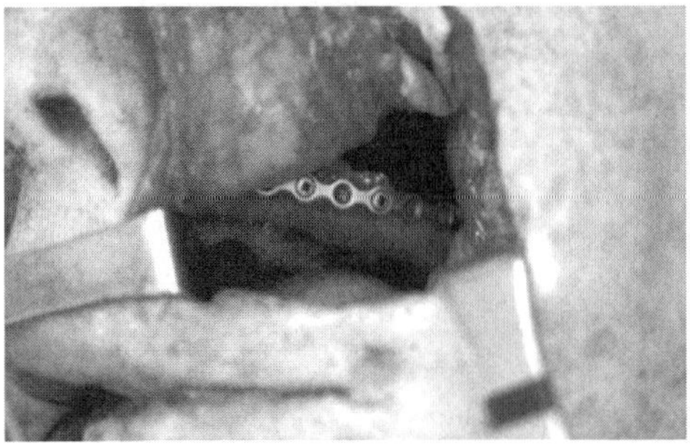

Figure 29 Bone graft secured across the neoalveolus with a lengthy miniplate.

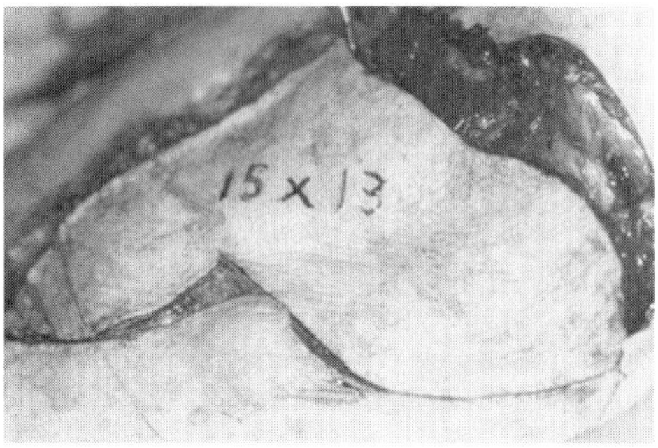

Figure 30 Tripartite myocutaneous rectus flap to reconstruct a complex three-dimensional extended maxillectomy defect.

extensive defect. The drawbacks to using the scapular flap include the need to turn the patient for flap harvest and the problems previously mentioned regarding excess bulk. In fact, the excessive bulk and small bone stock in the oral cavity often impede the placement of osseointegrated implants unless multiple shaping and debulking procedures are performed. The prognosis for these patients is poor and they may not desire or have sufficient survival time to complete the multiple revision procedures necessary for full oral rehabilitation. Palliation in these patients is of utmost concern. For this reason, a more expeditious method with lower potential donor site morbidity is chosen. The flap most often used in this circumstance is the myocutaneous rectus abdominis free flap. It can be fashioned into a tripartite soft tissue flap that is folded to provide skin cover for the lateral nasal wall, hemipalate, cheek, and orbit while obliterating the antrum and socket (Fig. 30). This type of reconstruction is applicable to patients with extensive cheek resections with or without orbital exenterations (Figs. 31, 32).

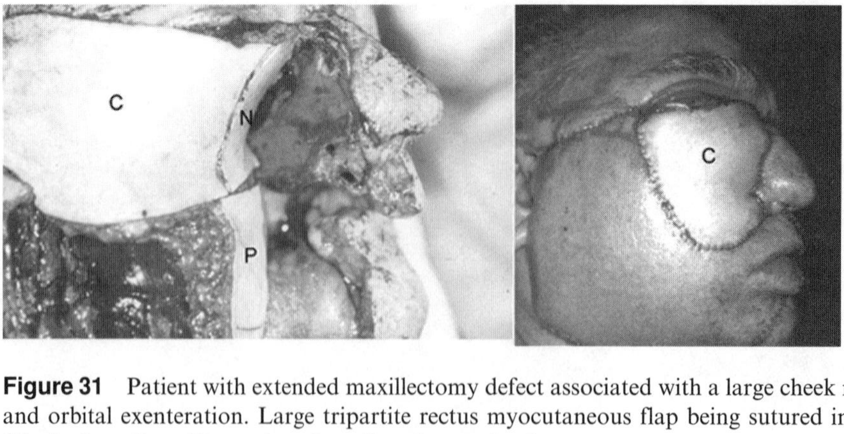

Figure 31 Patient with extended maxillectomy defect associated with a large cheek resection and orbital exenteration. Large tripartite rectus myocutaneous flap being sutured into place (C, cheek surface; N, nasal surface; P, palate surface).

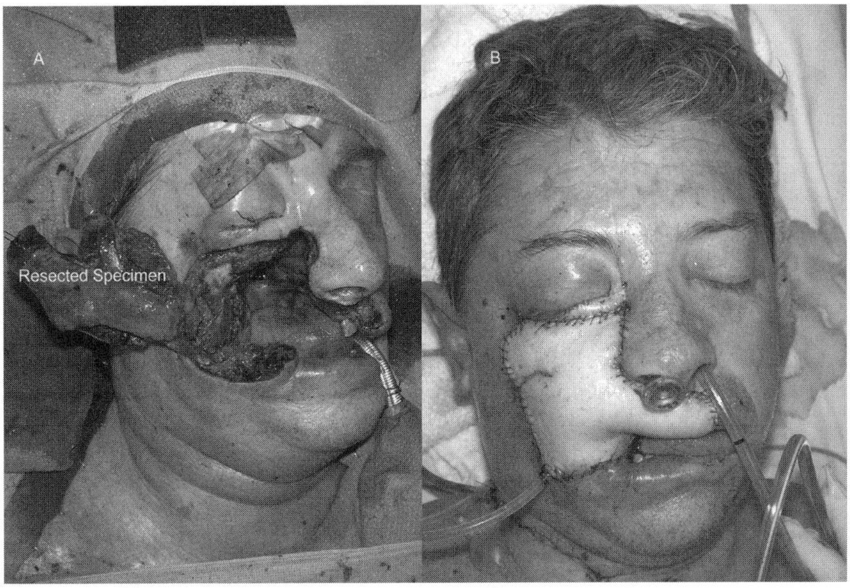

Figure 32 Another patient with a similar defect to that shown in Figure 31: without orbital exenteration but with extension onto the upper lip (a). This patient was also reconstructed with a tripartite rectus flap (b).

Type 4: Orbitomaxillectomy

The orbitomaxillary defect is relatively simple in that the hard palate remains intact. The surgical requirements include obliteration of the antrum and socket with skin coverage over the orbit. Reconstruction of the orbital rim can be done with a nonvascularized bone graft to maintain cheek contour. Although this defect does require free tissue transfer, most of the fasciocutaneous flaps will suffice. The augmented radial forearm flap, lateral arm flap, and rectus flap are sufficient.

Conclusion

An orderly approach to reconstruction after maxillectomy using a simple classification system is helpful. Although the majority of patients undergoing maxillectomy are still good candidates for management with a prosthesis, the use of flap tissue alone or in combination with a prosthesis is sometimes necessary. With the advent of free tissue transfer, reconstruction of even the classic maxillectomy defect is becoming more common. Free flaps have also significantly improved our ability to reconstruct defects that were previously difficult or impossible to obturate effectively.

REFERENCES

1. Mehta S, Sarkar S, Kavarana N, Bhathena H, Mehta A. Complications of the pectoralis major myocutaneous flap in the oral cavity: a prospective evaluation of 220 cases. Plast Reconstr Surg 1996; 98:31–37.

2. Khouri RK, Cooley BC, Kunselman AR, Landis JR, Yeramian P, Ingram D. A prospective study of microvascular free-flap surgery and outcome. Plast Reconstr Surg 1998; 102:711–721.
3. Bodin IKH, Lind MG, Arnander C. Free radial forearm reconstruction in surgery of the oral cavity and pharynx: surgical complications, impairment in speech and swallowing. Clin Otolaryngol 1982; 19:28–34.
4. Lawson W, Loscalzo LJ, Baek SM, Biller HF, Krespi YP. Experience with immediate and delayed mandibular reconstruction. *Laryngoscope* 1982; 92:5–10.
5. Weibrich G, Kleis WK, Hafner G, Hitzler WE. Growth factor levels in platelet-rich plasma and correlations with donor age, sex, and platelet count. *J Craniomaxillofac. Surg*. 2002; 30:97–102.
6. Rustad TJ, Hartshorn DO, Clevens RA, Johnson TM, Baker SR. The subcutaneous pedicle flap in melolabial reconstruction. Arch Otolaryngol Head Neck Surg 1998; 124:1163–1166.
7. Curtis DA, Plesh O, Miller AJ, Curtis TA, Sharma A, Schweitzer R. A comparison of masticatory function in patients with or without reconstruction of the mandible. Head Neck 1997; 19:287–296.
8. Blackwell KE, Buchbinder D, Urken ML. Lateral mandibular reconstruction using soft-tissue free flaps and plates. Arch Otolaryngol Head Neck Surg 1996; 122:672–678.
9. Hidalgo DA. Condyle transplantation in free flap mandible reconstruction. Plast Reconstr Surg 1994; 93:770–781.
10. Hildago DA, Shenaq SM, Larson DL. Mandibular reconstruction in the pediatric patient. Head Neck 1996; 18:359–365.
11. Pauloski BR, Logemann JA, Colangelo LA, Rademaker AW, McConnel FM, Heiser MA. Surgical variables affecting speech in treated patients with oral and oropharyngeal cancer. Laryngoscope 1998; 108:908–916.
12. McConnel FM, Teichgraeber JF, Adler RK. A comparison of three methods of oral reconstruction. Arch Otolaryngol Head Neck Surg 1987; 113:496–500.
13. Kapur KK, Garrett NR, Fischer E. Effects of anaesthesia of human oral structures on masticatory performance and food particle size distribution. Arch Oral Biol 1990; 35:397–403.
14. McConnel FM, Pauloski BR, Logemann JA, Rademaker AW, Colangelo L, Shedd et al. Functional results of primary closure vs flaps in oropharyngeal reconstruction: a prospective study of speech and swallowing. Arch Otolaryngol Head Neck Surg 1998; 124:625–630.
15. Waris T, Astrand K, Hamalainen H, Piironen J, Valtimo J, Jarvilehto T. Regeneration of cold, warmth and heat-pain sensibility in human skin grafts. Br J Plast Surg 1989; 42:576–580.
16. Urken ML, Moscoso JF, Lawson W, Biller HF. A systematic approach to functional reconstruction of the oral cavity following partial and total glossectomy. Arch Otolaryngol Head Neck Surg 1994; 120:589–601.
17. Haughey BH. Tongue reconstruction: concepts and practice. Laryngoscope 1993; 103:1132–1141.
18. Som ML. Laryngopharyngectomy. Primary closure with a laryngotracheal autograft. Arch Otolaryngol Head Neck Surg 1956; 63:474–478.
19. Hoopes JE, Edgerton MT. Surgical rehabilitation after radical maxillectomy and orbital exenteration. MD State Med J 1966; 15:91–97.
20. Vinzenz KG, Holle J, Wuringer E, Kulenkampff KJ. Prefabrication of combined scapula flaps for microsurgical reconstruction in oro-maxillofacial defects: a new method. J Craniomaxillofac Surg 1996; 24:214–223.

21. Brown JS, Jones DC, Summerwill A, Rogers SN, Howell RA, Cawood JI et al. Vascularized iliac crest with internal oblique muscle for immediate reconstruction after maxillectomy. Br. J Oral Maxillofac Surg 2002; 40:183–190.
22. Cordeiro PG, Santamaria E. A classification system and algorithm for reconstruction of maxillectomy and midfacial defects. Plast Reconstr Surg 2000; 105:2331–2346.

10
Cleft Lip and Palate

Timothy Egan
Boston Medical Center, Boston, Massachusetts, U.S.A.

Gregory Antoine
Boston University School of Medicine, Boston, Massachusetts, U.S.A.

INTRODUCTION

Management of patients with craniofacial anomalies is a time-consuming and difficult process for parents and physicians alike. For parents, the birth of a baby with a cleft lip or cleft lip and palate deformity is always an exhausting and emotional time. Many new parents only learn of their child's condition on the day of the birth. Without forewarning, the parents are faced with the fact that their baby is not how they imagined. They may react with shock, fear, grief, disbelief, and worry (1). Parents will want to know what is wrong with their child and what can be done to help.

Because of the depth and breadth of the effects of a cleft lip and palate deformity, these children will require long-term management. To facilitate treatment and ensure continuity of care, most centers have developed a multidisciplinary craniofacial anomalies team. Most teams provide tertiary level medical and surgical care at large medical centers (2). The cleft team should include members of the medical, surgical, and allied health professions who will be involved in the care of patients with cleft lip and palate. The team typically includes a plastic surgeon, nurse, otolaryngologist, geneticist, developmental pediatrician, social worker, pediodontist, orthodontist, oral surgeon, and a speech and language specialist.

The team approach to the treatment of cleft lip and palate was designed to provide comprehensive health care in a setting that is convenient for both parents and health care workers. The parent's life is simplified because they can schedule all of their appointments in one office visit. This limits the amount of time that the parents and child have to spend commuting to and from appointments, which is particularly important in rural areas where families may live considerable distances from the medical center. The team approach also benefits the physicians, who can quickly and easily consult other members of the cleft team, allowing for more timely and convenient medical care and an improved continuity of care. An effective cleft team eliminates the dehumanization that occurs when several specialities are involved in the care of a patient (3).

CAUSES

Cleft lip and palate occur in isolation and as part of various syndromes. Currently, there are over 300 identified syndromes that include facial clefting (4). The genetic cause of many of these syndromes has been elucidated; however, much work remains to be done.

Despite tremendous amounts of research, the cause of nonsyndromic cleft lip and palate remains unknown. Genetic factors are thought to contribute to the development of cleft lip and palate since 20% of patients have a positive family history (5). Nonsyndromic cleft lip and palate is categorized as cleft lip with or without cleft palate (CL±P) and cleft palate only (CPO). This classification is based on the fact that CL±P and CPO are two separate diseases with distinct causes (6).

There is likely a genetic component to CPO and CL±P; however, the details of the inheritance remains unclear. It is currently believed that the causes of CPO and CL±P are multifactorial, with both genetic and environmental contributions. Several genes have been implicated as causative factors in CL±P, specifically loci on chromosome regions 2p, 4q, 6p, 17q, and 19q (5).

Several common environmental influences are thought to be contributing factors in both CL±P and CPO. Several studies have found an association between cigarette smoking and CL±P and CPO. Among its many detrimental effects, maternal cigarette smoking has now been shown to increase the risk of having a child with CL+P and CPO (6). Furthermore, there is a dose–response phenomenon with fetal tobacco exposure: the more cigarettes a woman smokes while pregnant the greater the risk of her having a child with a cleft defect (7).

Other factors including maternal age, alcohol, drug exposure, race, and gender have been studied as contributing factors.

EMBRYOLOGY

Cleft lip and cleft palate result from an error in normal development. To understand the formation and morphology of these defects, one must understand the normal embryology of the lip and palate. Three areas are considered in the discussion of the formation of the upper lip: the centrally located frontonasal process and the two laterally located maxillary prominences. Through an orderly sequence of steps, the frontonasal process develops into the premaxilla. In the fully developed fetus, the premaxilla becomes the central portion of the upper lip, the anterior alveolus, and the primary palate. The two laterally located maxillary prominences grow and develop into the lateral aspects of the lip.

Before considering the detailed steps involved in this process, it is wise to consider an overview of the major events. The centrally located frontonasal process and the two lateral maxillary processes enlarge and fuse to form the intact lip. The maxillary process grows from posterolateral to anteromedial to fuse with the centrally located frontonasal process. If one imagines the upper lip to be an archway, then the frontonasal process is the keystone and the two maxillary processes are the arms of the arch. Failure of fusion can occur on either side of this keystone and therefore cleft lip defects can be unilateral or bilateral.

The upper lip develops during weeks 4–6 of gestation, beginning with the formation of the frontonasal process. Initially, the frontonasal process is a mound of tissue in the center of the developing face. Later, two shallow dimples appear on either side of this mound forming the nasal placodes. Eventually, the nasal placodes deepen to form the nasal cavity and nasopharynx. The depressions formed by the nasal placodes generate ridges on the medial and lateral sides of the nasal placodes. These ridges are the medial and lateral nasal elevations. In total, there are four nasal elevations: two medial and two lateral. In time, the medial nasal elevations fuse and give rise to the premaxilla. These structures form the keystone of the arch. The lateral nasal elevations develop into the nasal alae but they do not contribute to the formation of the lips.

In the 5th week of gestation, the two maxillary arches begin to enlarge and grow towards the midline where they will eventually fuse with the nasal prominences. The maxillary arches are derivatives of the first branchial arch. They begin to develop on either side of the primitive mouth and move towards the center. Eventually, they become sufficiently large to contact either side of the fused medial nasal elevations. To continue the analogy, the two limbs of the arch expand and contact the keystone. Fusion is completed when the groove between the medial nasal prominence and the maxillary prominence is obliterated by mesoderm. Failure of fusion on either side of the medial nasal elevation will result in a cleft lip.

The term cleft lip is misleading since defects may involve more than just the lip. A complete failure of fusion of the lateral maxillary process and median nasal elevations results in a cleft of the upper lip, alveolus, nasal sill, nasal floor, and primary hard palate.

The hard palate is formed of the primary palate and the secondary palate. The primary palate develops into the portion of the hard palate anterior to the incisive foramen and posterior to the section of the alveolar ridge containing the incisors. The formation of the primary palate was discussed above since it develops from the premaxilla. The secondary palate develops into the remainder of the hard palate as well as the soft palate and uvula.

The development of the secondary palate occurs from weeks 6 to 12 of gestation. The process begins with the formation of the lateral palatine processes that develop from the maxillary process. Initially, the palatine processes are oriented vertically on either side of the developing tongue. The tongue is displaced inferiorly as the head grows and the neck straightens. With the path cleared of the obstructing tongue, the lateral palatine processes are freed to grow medially. Eventually, the two lateral palatine processes meet in the midline and fuse. The hard palate fuses from anterior to posterior, beginning at the alveolar ridge and continuing though to the tip of the uvula. Therefore the mildest form of cleft palate is a bifid uvula. Additionally, a cleft of any portion of the palate must also include the remaining posterior aspect of the palate. Fusion is complete and the intact palate is identifiable by the completion of the 12th week of gestation.

SURGICAL ANATOMY

The palate forms a dynamic boundary between the oral cavity and the nasal cavity. It is composed of the hard palate anteriorly and the soft palate posteriorly. The soft palate is a dynamic structure that functions as a valve between the oropharynx and nasopharynx. The intact palate can periodically, selectively, and completely isolate the nasopharynx from the oropharynx. An intact and functioning soft palate is essential for normal speech and feeding.

The hard palate is composed of the bony palate and the overlying mucosa that is firmly adhered to the periosteum. The bony palate is composed of the paired palatine processes of the maxilla and the horizontal portions of the palatine bones. The alveolar ridge of the maxilla defines the anterior and lateral limit of the hard palate. The posterior aspect is known as the free edge since it lacks a bony attachment. From this free edge the soft palate attaches to the hard palate.

Three pairs of foramina mark the surface of the bony palate. The incisive foramen is located immediately posterior to the middle incisors; it transmits the nasopalatine artery and nerve. The greater palatine foramen, located at the posterior lateral border of the bony canal, transmits the greater palatine artery and nerve. The greater palatine artery and nerve leave the greater palatine foramen and head anteriorly to supply the hard palate. The lesser palatine foramen, located immediately posterior and lateral to the greater palatine foramen, transmits the lesser palatine artery and nerves. The lesser palatine artery and nerve supply the soft palate and uvula.

The mucosa of the soft palate attaches to the hard palate anteriorly and to the pharyngeal walls laterally. The posterior margin of the soft palate is free from attachments. The musculature of the soft palate can selectively isolate the nasopharynx from the oropharynx. When breathing, the posterior edge of the soft palate is in an almost vertical position. This allows free communication between the oral and nasal cavities, which thereby facilitates nasal breathing. Conversely, during speech and swallowing the musculature of the soft palate contracts and pulls the soft palate into a more horizontal position where it contacts the posterior pharyngeal wall.

The soft palate is composed of five paired muscles and a central aponeurosis. The paired uvula muscles take origin from the posterior nasal spine and insert on the uvula. The tensor veli palatini takes origin from the lateral wall of eustachian tube. It becomes a narrow tendon that curves laterally around the hamulus before joining the soft palate as a broad triangular tendon. Within the soft palate the fibers of the tensor veli palatini run in a lateral to medial direction. Contraction of this muscle produces a laterally directed force that tenses the soft palate. The tensor veli palatini is the primary opener of the eustachian tube.

The levator veli palatini takes origin from the medial aspect of the eustachian tube and the inferior surface of the temporal bone. It courses anteriorly and inferiorly to insert on the upper surface of the soft palate. Contraction of the levator veli palatini raises the soft palate and occludes the nasopharynx.

The last two pairs of muscles that contribute to the soft palate are the palatoglossus and palatopharyngeus muscles. The palatoglossus together with its overlying mucosa form the anterior tonsillar pillar. The palatoglossus extends from the tongue inferiorly to the soft palate superiorly. The palatoglossus functions as a sphincter to prevent oral regurgitation of food during swallowing. The paired palatopharyngeus muscles run from the lateral pharyngeal wall to the soft palate. The palatopharyngeus together with its overlying mucosa forms the posterior tonsillar pillar. The palatoglossus elevates the larynx during swallowing to help prevent aspiration.

The upper and lower lips form a curtain that demarcates the opening of the oral cavity. The functional unit of the lip is the orbicularis oris muscle, which functions as a sphincter. The fibers of the obricularis oris take origin from the oral commissure and cross the midline to insert onto the contralateral commissure. The lip is composed of a central muscular layer that is covered on its outer surface with skin and on its undersurface with moist oral mucosa. The skin and moist mucosa meet along the free edge of the lip where they form the vermilion border.

An appreciation of the surface anatomy of the lip is essential to understand the planning and execution of a cleft lip repair. The central portion of the upper lip is graced with a crescent-shaped depression known as cupid's bow. From its perch in the center of the upper lip, the two sides of cupid's bow curve superiorly and laterally to their peaks at the base of the philtral ridges. The two philtral ridges begin at the vermilion border and angle vertically and slightly medially towards the base of the columella. The philtral ridges flank a small valley known as the philtrum dimple. Together, the paired philtral ridges and philtrum dimple form the philtrum.

CLASSIFICATION OF THE CLEFT LIP AND CLEFT PALATE

Over the years several classification systems have been proposed for cleft lip and palate; however, none has gained universal acceptance. The fact that no one has been able to derive a simple and convenient classification system for cleft lip and palate speaks for the complexity and variation of this defect. The primary purpose of a classification system is to describe quickly and accurately the nature and extent of a disease process. This is a daunting task since there is great variety in the combination and severity of clefts.

A cleft lip and palate may occur together or either may occur on its own. Furthermore, a cleft lip may be unilateral or bilateral. The lip and palate are formed from the premaxilla and the secondary palate. The premaxilla is the precursor of the central upper lip, anterior alveolus, and the primary palate. A cleft lip defect occurs along the line of fusion between the lateral maxillary processes and the premaxilla. The cleft may include only a section of the line of fusion or may include the entire line of contact between the maxillary process and the premaxilla. A complete cleft lip involves the philtrum of the lip, nasal floor, and anterior alveolus as well as the portion of the hard palate anterior to the incisive foramen. Remember that the premaxilla represents the keystone of the arch that is bounded on either side by the maxillary processes. Since either of the two lines of contact can be involved, a cleft lip may be unilateral or bilateral. In the case of bilateral cleft lip, the two sides are not necessarily affected with equal severity (Fig. 1). Therefore, it is necessary to describe the extent of clefting on both sides separately.

Cleft lip defects are generally broken down into three broad categories: microform, incomplete, and complete. Microform clefts represent the least severe form of cleft lip and involve some degree of scarring along the philtrum with no real separation (Fig. 2). When true separation is apparent the cleft is either described as

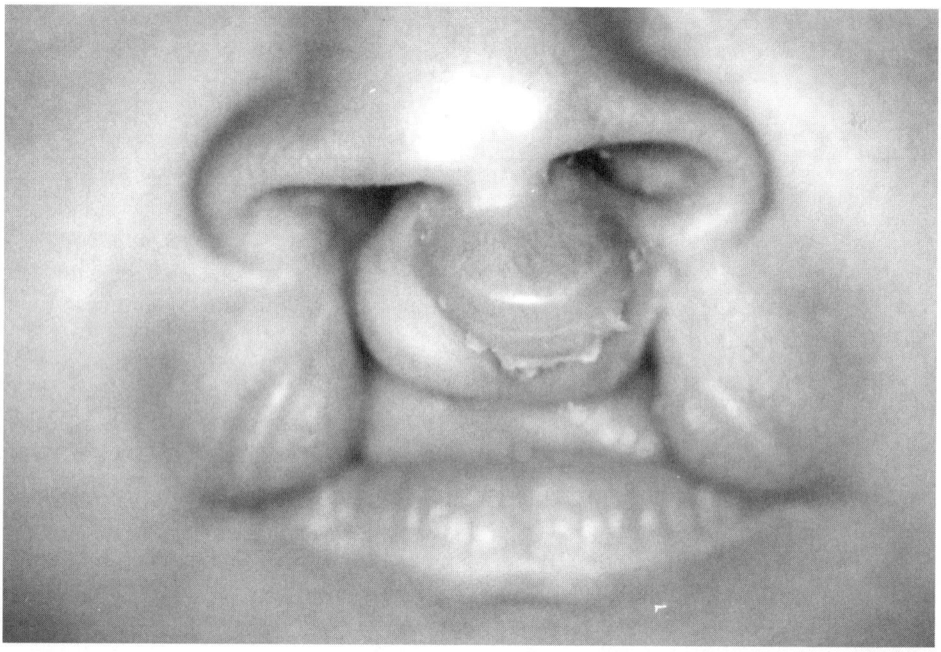

Figure 1 A bilateral cleft lip with a complete cleft on the right side and an incomplete cleft on the left side.

complete or incomplete. An incomplete cleft lip involves separation of the lip but does not involve the floor of the nose. There is an intact band of tissue across the nasal sill known as Simonart's band. A complete cleft involves the floor of the nose and may also involve the alveolus and primary palate. Complete and incomplete cleft lip defects involve a nasal deformity; therefore, a classification system would also have to describe the extent of nasal deformity.

Since there are two lines of fusion between the maxillary segments and the premaxilla, a cleft lip may be bilateral. In a bilateral cleft lip the two sides do not necessarily have similar degrees of clefting. A bilateral cleft may include two complete clefts, two incomplete clefts, or one of each. In the case of a bilateral complete cleft the premaxilla is completely separated from the remainder of the upper lip. The prolabial tissue lacks orbicularis fibers, and the mucosa and skin are underdeveloped. Therefore, repair of bilateral clefts must augment the prolabial segment to get a cosmetically appealing result.

A cleft palate is formed from a failure of fusion of the right and left sides of the secondary palate. As in a cleft lip, the defect may be partial or complete. A complete cleft palate involves the entire secondary palate and extends from the incisive foramen to the tip of the uvula. An incomplete cleft only involves part of the length of the palate. However, since fusion of the palatal shelves always occurs from anterior to posterior, a partial cleft always involves the uvula.

Accurately and completely describing the combination of clefting defects in a patient can be difficult and time-consuming. Dr. Desmond Kernahan, a cleft surgeon, was frustrated by the cumbersome and confusing descriptions in his

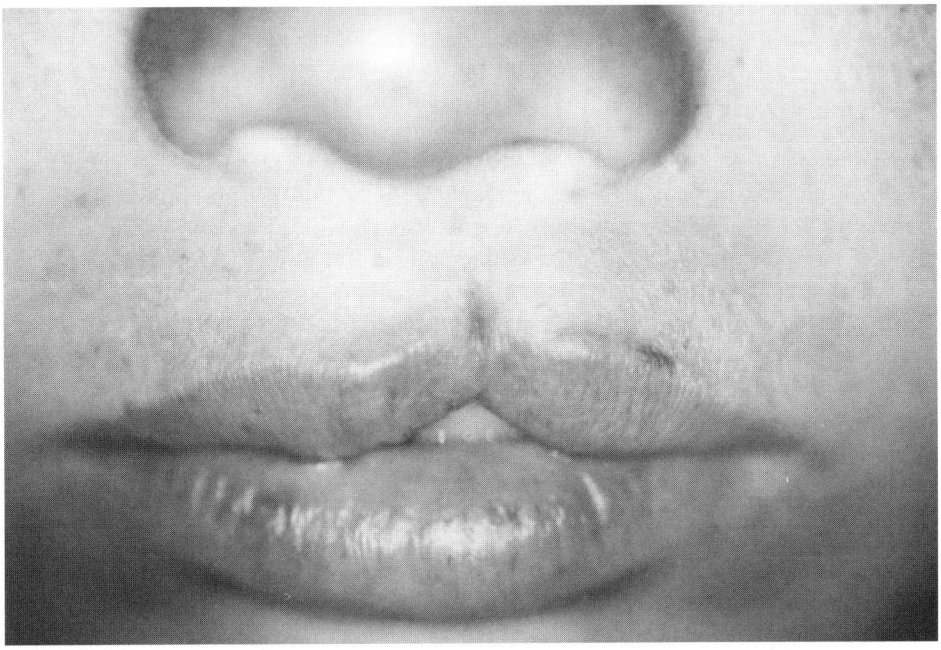

Figure 2 A left microform cleft. Note that there is no true separation of the tissues.

patient's medical records (8). Knowing that a picture is worth a thousand words, Dr. Kernahan used a diagram in the shape of a Y to represent the lines of fusion of the lip, primary palate, and secondary palate. The forked limbs of the Y represent the lines of fusion of the premaxilla and the long arm of the Y represents the line of fusion of the secondary palate. The junction of the three lines is the incisive foramen. The two anterior limbs of the Y are organized into three blocks representing the lip, alveolus, and primary palate. The posterior arm of the Y is also organized into three blocks. The anterior two together form the hard palate and the last block is the soft palate. By shading in the boxes corresponding to the areas involved by the cleft, one can quickly generate a diagrammatic representation of the various combinations of cleft lip and palate defects. Dr. Kernahan's original design has been modified to include nasal deformities as well.

PRENATAL DIAGNOSIS

Cleft lip and palate deformities can now be diagnosed in utero in some patients. Ultrasound examination has become a routine part of prenatal care and increasingly sophisticated technology offers better resolution and more accurate detection of congenital anomalies. The first reported case of an ultrasound diagnosis of a cleft lip was in 1981 by Christ and Meninger (9). Since that time several studies have been conducted to determine the diagnostic and therapeutic value of prenatal diagnosis of cleft lip and palate.

Cleft lip and cleft palate can be diagnosed on routine transabdominal ultrasound; however, there are several limitations. First, in order to diagnose a cleft lip or palate deformity the ultrasonographer must be able to see the face of the fetus. This is often not easy and the test may have to be repeated on several occasions (10). Even with an adequate examination the specificity of transabdominal ultrasound is poor. One large study reported that less than one-third of cleft lip and palate cases were previously diagnosed on ultrasound (10). Detection rate varies depending on the skill of the sonographer, gestational age, presence of other anomalies, and the skill of the radiologists reading the film. A surprising finding is that the sensitivity does not increase by increasing the number of ultrasound examinations a woman had during her pregnancy (11).

The sensitivity increases dramatically when transvaginal ultrasound is performed instead of routine transabdominal ultrasound (12). However, the improved sensitivity of a transvaginal ultrasound comes at a price, since it is more invasive and is not a part of routine prenatal care.

Despite its limited sensitivity, transabdominal ultrasound remains a valuable tool in the diagnosis of cleft lip and palate. Screening transabdominal ultrsound is a routine part of prenatal care so there is no added cost, morbidity, or inconvenience for the patient. Although many patients with cleft lip and palate will not be diagnosed on prenatal examination, for the 30% of women in whom the diagnosis is made prenatally the benefits can be great. Early detection allows the family to prepare ahead of time for the reality that their child will have a cleft. They can meet with members of the cleft team, learn about special feeding requirements, and understand what to expect when the baby is born. In comparison, mothers who receive counseling in the first 2 weeks of life are more likely to feel confused and overwhelmed (10).

Early detection also allows the surgeon to meet with the family before birth in a relaxed atmosphere and discuss the repair options. With adequate time for counseling and planning, it is often possible to perform the repair of a unilateral cleft lip in the first week of life (10).

INITIAL MANAGEMENT

As part of the initial evaluation, all patients with cleft lip and cleft palate should be observed for feeding difficulties. Almost all cleft lip and palate patients will have some difficulty feeding. The amount of difficulty will depend on the type and severity of the cleft. Children with cleft lip have difficulty maintaining a seal around a nipple. If the defect is minor, the infant may do well if given extra time to nurse or bottle-feed. Children with a cleft palate are unable to generate a negative intraoral pressure since there is a constant communication between mouth and nose. Because of this persistent communication they may also have nasal regurgitation. These children have an ineffective suck and require special feeding techniques to ensure adequate caloric intake.

If special techniques are used to feed these children, they can receive adequate nutrition with a bottle. It is rarely necessary to rely on alternative means of enteral feeding to maintain caloric intake. Several techniques are used to increase delivery of formula to the mouth. Enlarging the size of the hole in the nipple decreases the resistance and increases the flow of formula with the same suck. Specialized nipples are made for children with cleft palates, which are longer and larger than normal and are designed to occlude and bypass the cleft. If these techniques do not sufficiently increase the delivery of formula, the parents can try using a specially manufactured squeeze bottle. The bottles are made of soft plastic that can be squeezed in concert with the infant's suck to increase delivery of formula. Some or all of these techniques may be required to deliver adequate calories. Only in exceptional situations is it necessary to place a nasogastric or gastrostomy feeding tube.

To limit the amount of nasal regurgitation, it is helpful to feed the child in the seated position. Children with cleft palate will feed more slowly and swallow more air than a normal child; therefore, they should be allowed more time for feeding and they should be burped frequently.

All children with cleft lip and palate should be monitored closely in their early life to ensure that they are feeding adequately and gaining weight. Weekly weight checks are recommended until the infant has demonstrated an ability to gain weight.

TIMING OF CLEFT LIP AND PALATE REPAIR

The timing and goals of cleft lip and palate surgery are different. Cleft lip is repaired earlier in life and the goal of surgery is to correct the cosmetic deformity. Cleft palate, on the other hand, is repaired at about 1 year of life and the goal of surgery is to restore function to the palate and allow normal speech and feeding. However, there is no consensus as the correct time to perform a palate closure (13).

The timing of cleft lip surgery remains controversial. A cleft lip can be surgically repaired at any time yet there is still debate as to what is the ideal time. Over the years, the trend has been to do surgery at a younger age. The scheduling of a unilateral cleft lip repair was traditionally guided by the "rule of 10s." This rule says that surgery should be delayed until the child weighs 10 pounds, the hemoglobin is 10 grams/deciliter or greater, and the child is at least 10 weeks of age. The rule of 10s is a list of criteria designed to ensure that the child is of adequate size, age, and health to undergo general anesthesia with an acceptable level of risk. Significant advances in pediatric anesthesiology and intensive care medicine have now made it safe for younger and smaller children to undergo cleft lip repair. In fact, some centers are now routinely performing cleft lip repair during the first few weeks of life and have found that, with careful preoperative evaluation, neonatal cleft lip repair involves minimal morbidity (14).

The rule of 10s is now more of an interesting historical footnote than a reliable guide for scheduling cleft lip repair. Cleft lip surgeons now have the ability to repair a cleft lip as early as the first 48 h of life. However, not all patients with cleft lip are good candidates for neonatal repair. The surgeon must examine several factors before deciding when to perform the repair, including the overall health of the patient, severity of the cleft, need for further diagnostic studies, and the wishes of the parents. Under ideal circumstances, the cleft lip repair can be performed during the initial hospitalization. Early repair allows the parents to bring home a new baby who has a single suture line rather than an unsightly cleft lip deformity. This helps the parents to feel more comfortable with their new child. In one center where neonatal cleft lip repairs are performed, members of the team feel strongly that the early repair has a positive effect on the way that parents interact with their child (14). Critics of neonatal cleft lip repair believe that the surgery limits the amount of time for maternal–infant bonding during the first days of life.

The timing of cleft palate repair is also controversial. In the past, cleft palate repair has been performed around 1 year of life, prior to the development of speech. However, as with cleft lip repair, the trend has been to perform cleft palate repair at younger ages. In fact, since 1991 one center has been performing neonatal cleft palate closure with the hope of improving speech development. The rationale for the early repair is that it is not known how prelingual phonation contributes to the normal development of speech. If the cleft palate is repaired early in life, then the child will have a normal palate during the time when he or she begins to make sounds. However, it is too early to determine whether early closure leads to improved speech development (13).

REPAIR OF UNILATERAL CLEFT LIP

Once the decision of when to perform a cleft lip repair is made, the surgeon must decide how to perform the repair. The most common technique used for the repair of a unilateral cleft lip is the rotation advancement technique developed by Ralph Millard, the father of modern cleft lip and palate surgery. This procedure is technically challenging but provides excellent cosmetic results. In the past, cleft lip operations closed the defect but sacrificed the cupid's bow in the process. The results were eye-catching and unsightly. Frustrated by this, Dr. Millard spent countless hours studying pictures of patients with cleft lips trying to develop a repair that could preserve cupid's bow (8). He developed a technique that utilizes a rotation and an advancement flap to close the defect while preserving cupid's bow. His technique repositions the laterally displaced alar base restoring symmetry to the nostril and ala and closing the floor of the nose defect. The results are aesthetically appealing, with an intact cupid's bow and a scar that is vertically oriented and approximates the normal philtral ridge. The Millard repair produces consistent results in the unilateral incomplete cleft lip.

The Millard repair uses four flaps to close the cleft lip and restore the alar base to a more natural position: rotation flap, advancement flap, alar flap, and columellar flap. The rotation flap lowers the medial aspect of the lip to level the cupid's bow and add length to the lip. The advancement flap includes the portion of the lip lateral to the cleft and is used to close the cleft defect by suturing it to the rotation flap. Medialization of the alar flap restores the ala to a more natural position. Suturing the alar flap to the columellar flap closes the cleft in the floor of the nose.

The following is a summary of the technique first described by Millard and still frequently used today. The first and most important step in the Millard repair is identifying the landmarks and marking the key points used in the repair (Fig. 3). This process is time-consuming and tedious; however, patience and attention to detail at this stage will facilitate the rest of the operation and lead to a good cosmetic result. Marking is done with the patient anesthetized and the surgeon in the seated position.

The marking process consists of identifying and measuring 12 points along the upper lip and base of nose (Table 1) (8). The first area of interest is the cupid's bow: a crescent-shaped depression in the center of the upper lip. The low point of the cupid's bow marks the center of the upper lip; (point 1). The high points of the cupid's bow are where the vertical philtral ridges meet the vermilion border of

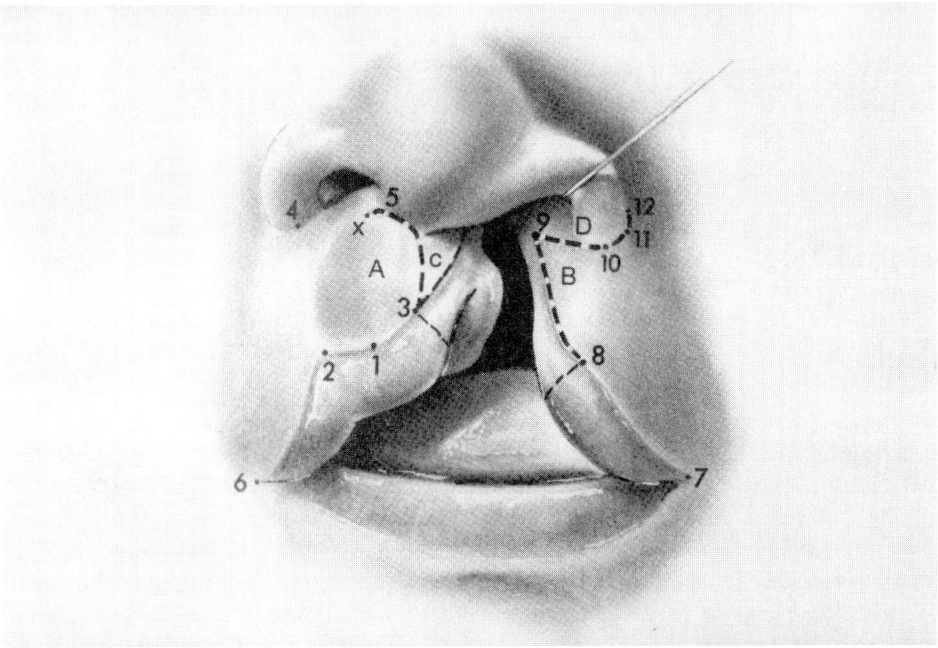

Figure 3 The landmarks of a Millard repair are identified before beginning the procedure. Reprinted with permission from Ref. 8.

the upper lip. The high point on the noncleft side is identified and marked as point 2. Point 3 is the high point on the cleft side. The distance from the high point to the low point on the normal side is measured and this distance is used to calculate the proper location of the high point on the cleft side. This point is identified and marked to correspond to point 3. This point lies on the vermilion border on the medial side of the cleft. Points 1–3 mark the cupid's bow: the first two points are identified and the third is measured such that the distance from point 1 to 2 is equal to the distance from 1 to 3.

Next, the surgeon's attention is turned to the noncleft nasal ala. The alar base on the noncleft side is identified and marked with a 4. Likewise, the columella base on the noncleft side is identified and marked with a 5. This point will correspond to the superior limit of the incision for the rotation flap. If additional rotation is needed to add length to the lip, a 1–2 mm back cut is made from point 5 to point X. Making small cuts and assessing the rotation can help to determine the amount of back cut needed. Adequate rotation has been achieved when the lip segment is easily rotated so that the cupid's bow is leveled in the horizontal plane.

The oral commissures are marked with a 6 on the noncleft side and a 7 on the cleft side. Point 8 represents the measured location of the high point of cupid's bow on the lateral portion of the lip. This is found by measuring the distance from the commissure to the high point of cupid's bow on the normal side: the distance from point 6 to point 2. This distance is measured from the commissure on the cleft side to the point that will represent the high point of the cupid's bow on the cleft side. The distance from point 6 to point 2 must equal the distance from point 7 to point 8

Table 1 12 points of the Millard Repair

Point	Location
Point 1	Low point of cupid's bow
Point 2	High point of cupid's bow on the noncleft side
Point 3	High point of cupid's bow on the cleft side
Point 4	Alar base on the noncleft side
Point 5	Columellar base on the noncleft side
Point 6	Oral commissure on the noncleft side
Point 7	Oral commissure on the cleft side
Point 8	High point of cupid's bow on the lateral lip segment
Point 9	Medial limit of the advancement incision
Point 10	Alar base on the cleft side
Point 11	Intersection of nasolabial fold and alar crease
Point 12	Lateral extent of advancement incision

(Fig. 4). In other words, the distance from the high point of cupid's bow and the commissure on the same side should be equal for the two sides. When the repair is complete point 3, which also represents the high point of cupid's bow, should be approximated with point 8.

The final area to be marked is the alar base on the cleft side. Point 9 marks the medial limit of the advancement flap. When the incisions are closed, point 9 will lie in the triangular defect created by the rotation of the medial lip segment. The total length of the rotational incision, point 3–5–X, will determine the exact location of point 9. The incisions from point 3 to 5 to X must equal the incision from point 8 to 9 since these two segments will be sutured together and must line up evenly. Millard recommended using a malleable piece of wire to measure the length of the rotational incision and then placing point 9 exactly this far from point 8 (Fig. 5).

The circumalar incision is then marked to allow the ala to be advanced medially and assume a more natural position (Fig. 6). The alar base on the cleft side is identified and marked with 10. Point 11 should be placed along the border of the ala at the point where it intersects with the nasal labial fold. Point 12, also along the alar facial crease, represents the most lateral aspect of the advancement flap. The amount of medialization of the ala will determine the final location of this point. Millard taught that the initial location of points 9–12 are estimations and that their final location is determined by what he termed by the cut as you go policy (8). Millard was referring to the fact that the surgeon must make small adjustments throughout the repair to get the best results.

The Millard repair includes two main incisions: a rotation incision medial to the cleft and an advancement incision lateral to the cleft. The rotation incision is a gentle crescent-shaped curve that connects the high point of cupid's bow on the cleft side with the base of the columella on the noncleft side. In other words, the incision connects points 3 and 5 and a small back cut to X if needed. The incision for the advancement flap follows the mucocutaneous junction to connect points 8 and 9. This incision is then extended in the alar facial crease to connect points 9 and 12. These two incisions involve the full thickness of the lip.

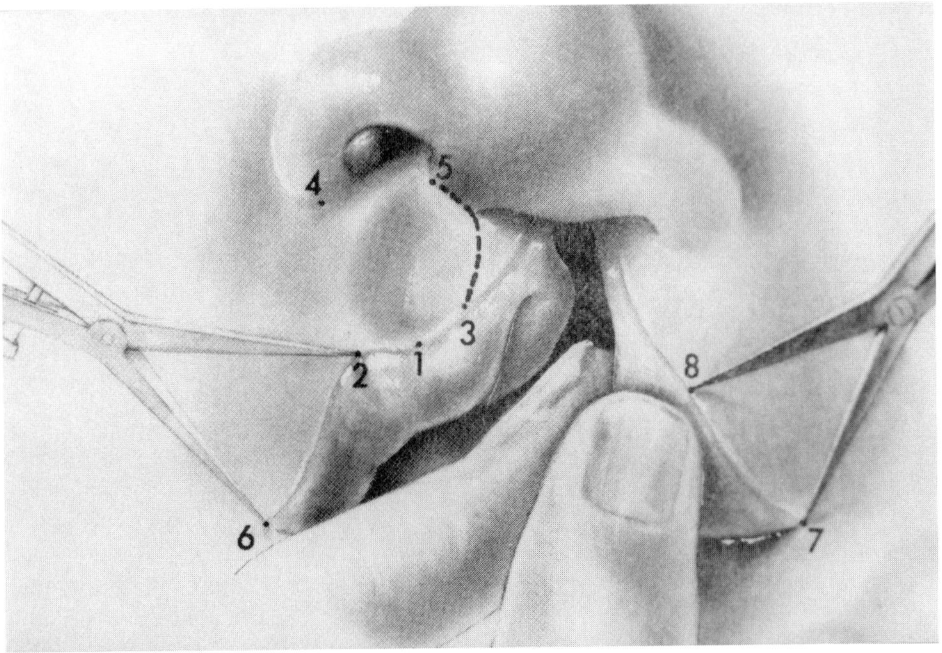

Figure 4 Calipers are used to determine the proper location of cupid's bow. The distance from bow peak to commissure should be the same for the two sides. Reprinted with permission from Ref. 8.

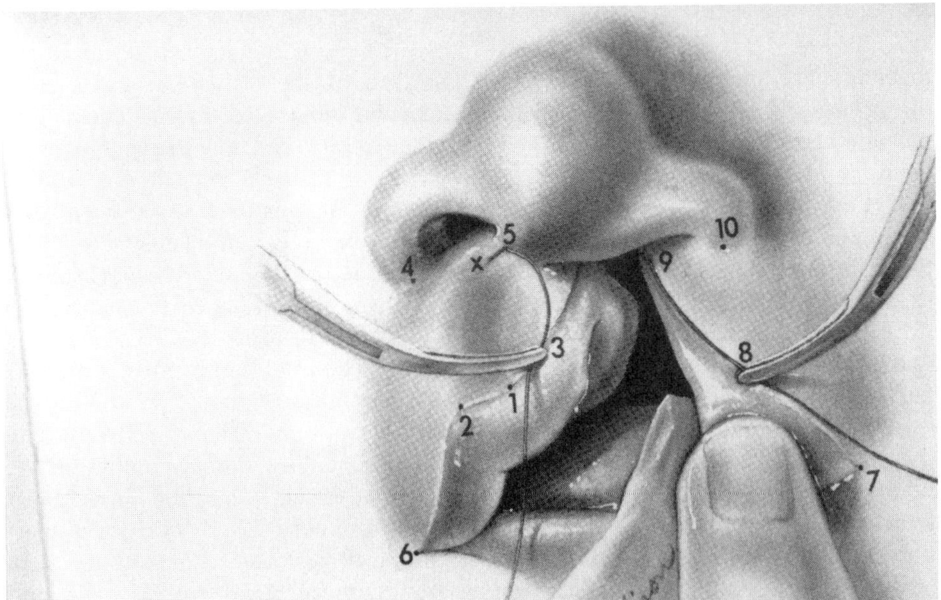

Figure 5 A section of malleable wire is used to measure the length of the rotation and advancement incisions. These two lines must be of equal length to ensure a good result. Reprinted with permission from Ref. 8.

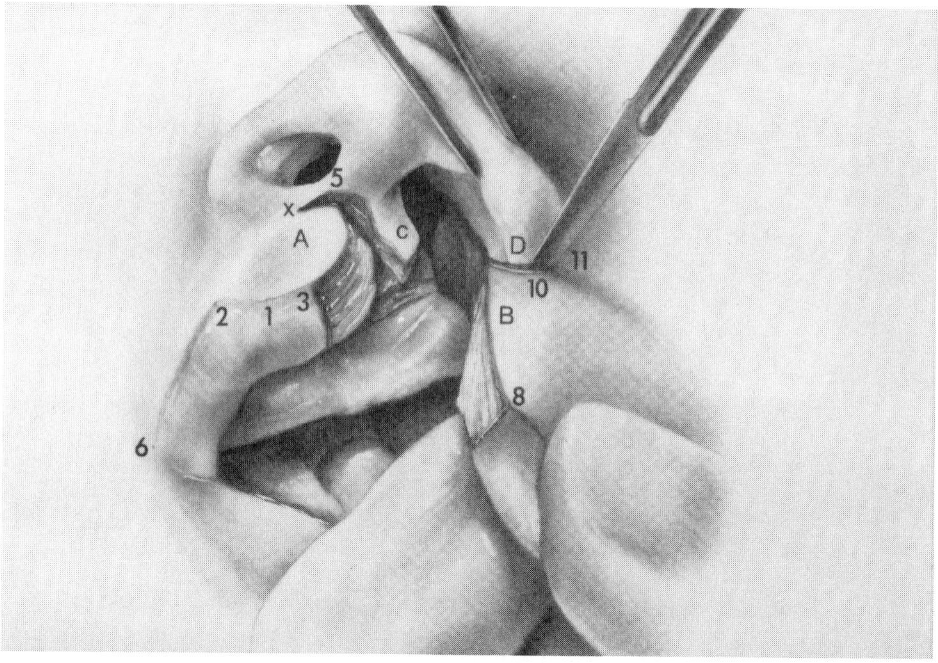

Figure 6 The circumalar incision allows the alar flap and advancement flap to be moved independently. The helps to reposition the nose to a more natural position. Reprinted with permission from Ref. 8.

The borders of the cleft are also incised to provide a fresh edge to suture together. The incised mucosa along the borders of the cleft is dissected from the orbicularis and is left attached to the alveolar ridge. The medial and lateral mucosal flaps are used to line the gingivolabial sulcus and the vestibule, respectively.

Completion of these incisions produces a total of four flaps and two mucosal pairings. The rotation and advancement flaps are on either side of the cleft. These two flaps are full thickness and include skin, mucosa, and the underlying orbicularis oris muscle. The medial and lateral mucosal pairings are attached to the alveolar ridge. The columellar flap is from a flap of skin attached superiorly to the columella that will be rotated to close the floor of the nose. The final flap created is the alar flap consisting of the nasal ala on the cleft side.

Before closing the defect, the rotation and advancement flaps are freed from the nose and maxilla. The rotation and advancement flaps should contain all the fibers of orbicularis oris, including those that inadvertently inserted on adjacent structures. An alotomy is performed to separate the ala from the pyriform aperture. When the lip release and alotomy are properly performed, the rotation flap, advancement flap, and ala should all move freely and independently. The skin and mucosa of the rotation and advancement flaps are undermined to free the orbicularis oris fibers.

The medial and lateral aspects of the cleft are drawn together and sutured in layers. According to Millard, there is a single key stitch that must be placed perfectly

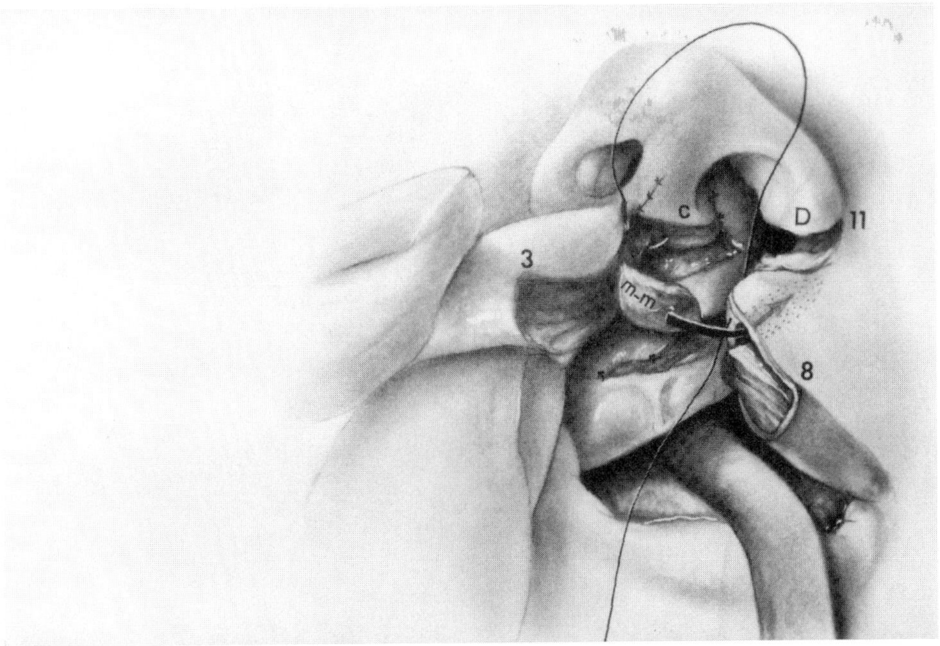

Figure 7 The key stitch is so named because it determines the exact amount of rotation. Correct placement of this stitch is essential to a good outcome. Reprinted with permission from Ref. 8.

to ensure that the wound edges line up properly (Fig. 7). The stitch is placed in the leading edge of the advancement flap and in the depth of the defect in the rotation flap. When this stitch is tied, the advancement flap and rotation flap are fixed into their final position (8). With proper closure, point 8 and point 3, both of which represent the high point of cupid's bow, should come together. The medial aspect of the advancement flap, point 9, should easily reach the point where the back cut was made earlier: point X. The ala flap is rotated medially to meet the columella flap to close the floor of the nose.

The defect is closed in three layers including the mucosa, orbicularis oris, and skin. The suture line and resulting scar approximate the philtral ridge and are well camouflaged (Fig. 8).

There is always some degree of nasal deformity associated with unilateral cleft lip. The nasal deformity is produced both by the embryological error that led to the cleft and by the deforming effects of inappropriately inserted fibers of the orbicularis oris muscle. These actions lead to a laterally displaced ala and displacement of the columella and caudal septum to the noncleft side. By releasing the inappropriately inserted fibers of orbicularis oris and performing the nasal release, the columella and ala can be restored to a more natural position.

Postoperative care focuses on feeding and wound care. Feeding is typically performed using a syringe with a soft catheter attached to deliver formula to the oropharynx. Since sucking requires use of the orbicularis oris and stresses the wound, it is avoided when possible. However, some surgeons permit breastfeeding

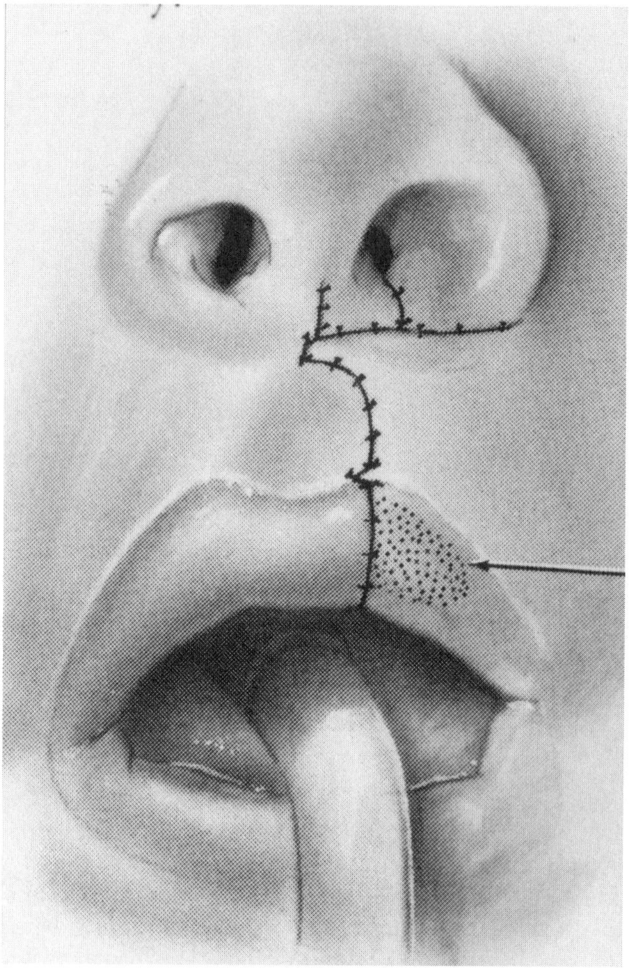

Figure 8 The incision line has a gentle curve that mirrors the natural philtrum of the noncleft side. A small flap of muscle can be used to add volume to the lateral segment of the lip if needed. Reprinted with permission from Ref. 8.

in the early postoperative period. Routine feeding can be resumed 3 weeks postoperatively.

The wound is cleansed several times daily with half-strength hydrogen peroxide and topical antibiotic ointment is applied. Skin sutures are removed on or around postoperative day 5. Although controversial, Logan's bow is sometimes used to reinforce the suture line: an arched metal bar that bridges the two sides of the incision and is attached to both cheeks with adhesive. All children will require the use of Velcro arm restraints to prevent them from manipulating the wound.

In recent years there has been a renewed interest in the primary repair of cleft nasal defect (15). With the Millard repair the nasal floor is closed and the alar base is reapproximated. However, the nasal deformity may also include the nasal septum, lower lateral cartilage, columella, vestibular dome, nasal tip, and nasal pyramid.

Some surgeons have recently been performing primary nasal repair at the time of lip repair. The early nasal repair is typically done at 3 months of age and focuses on the deformed and malpositioned lower lateral cartilage. By rearranging and reshaping the lower lateral cartilage, the surgeon is able to improve nasal tip projection and create a more symmetrical nostril and ala (16).

Even with primary nasal repair, revision nasal surgery is usually needed to correct any remaining distortions. These distortions are slight but are expected in the majority of cases of primary nasal repair (16). Depending on the extent of the nasal deformity, secondary surgery may also include nasal osteotomies and onlay bone grafting to augment the paranasal region.

A complete unilateral cleft lip involves the lip, nose and alveolar ridge. The repairs discussed above do not address the defect in the alveolar ridge. The goal of alveolar bone grafting is to bridge the gap in the alveolus with cancellous bone so that the adult dentition can erupt naturally. The optimal time for alveolar bone grafting is 8 years of age, which is the time when the adult canine teeth typically erupt. Alveolar bone grafting has been one of the major improvements in the treatment of patients with unilateral cleft lip deformity (16).

REPAIR OF CLEFT PALATE

Repair of the cleft palate includes the hard palate posterior to the alveolus and the soft palate. The soft and hard palate should be considered separately since the goals of repair are different in each. The primary goal of the repair of the soft palate is to restore normal function. In repairing the hard palate the surgeon strives to achieve normal facial growth, dentition, and aesthetics (17). In the ideal patient, after repair the soft palate should be able to periodically, voluntarily, and completely isolate the nasopharynx from the oropharynx. Normal soft palate function is essential for speech and feeding. If, after repair, the soft palate is too short to contact the posterior pharyngeal wall, the child will have poor articulation and nasal regurgitation of food and liquid.

Defects in the palate can include the primary and secondary palate or may be isolated to the secondary palate alone. Clefts isolated to the secondary palate, posterior to the incisive foramen, range from complete clefts involving the entire secondary palate to a simple bifid uvula. Defects in the primary palate are always associated with a cleft lip since they share a similar embryological origin. The defect in the primary palate may be unilateral or bilateral.

Closure of the hard palate involves raising mucoperiosteal flaps on the oral and nasal side of the hard palate. Relaxing incisions are often used in order to achieve a tension-free closure. If the mucoperiosteum is not adequately undermined the closure will be under tension and there is an increased risk of fistula formation. Therefore, the surgeon must undermine enough to allow a tension free closure. Conversely, wide undermining of the mucoperiosteum with denuded areas of palatal bone can have adverse effects on facial growth (17). The surgeon is charged with the challenge of undermining just enough mucoperiosteum to achieve tension-free closure while limiting the risk of adverse facial growth (17). It is also important to limit trauma to the soft tissues of the palate since this will limit the amount of postoperative scar tissue formation.

For a complete cleft of the secondary palate with no involvement of the primary palate, a three-flap repair is used. The incisions are made at the anterior extent of the cleft and extended towards the canine teeth on both sides, forming a V. The incisions continue posteriorly along the alveolar ridge to the maxillary tuberosities. Next, the free edges of the cleft mucosal flaps are incised. Mucoperiosteal flaps are raised using a periosteal elevator. At the posterior lateral margin of the bony palate the greater palatine neurovascular bundle is identified and preserved. The nasal mucosa is dissected free from the palatine bones using a right-angle elevator. The nasal mucosa is elevated as far as the nasal sidewalls to ensure adequate tissue for a tension-free closeure. Mucoperiosteal vomer flaps can be raised and used to help close the nasal mucosa.

The nasal mucosa is closed first using interrupted sutures. Next the muscular sling of the soft palate is reapproximated and the mucosa is closed. Because this repair involves relaxing incisions along the alveolar ridges, there remains a section of denuded palatal bone in this area. This should heal well by secondary intention. The hard palate is closed in two layers while the soft palate includes the muscular layer for a total of three layers. It is not necessary to close the defect in the bony palate.

After completion of the repair, the soft palate is assessed to ensure that it has adequate length to function normally. To function properly, the soft palate should be able to touch the posterior pharyngeal wall easily. If the soft palate is too short at this stage, two options are available to the surgeon. First, length can be added to the palate by converting the V-shaped incision at the medial margin of the cleft into a Y. This modification is known as the V-Y pushback technique (4).

A second option is to create a superiorly based flap from the posterior pharyngeal wall that is sutured to the nasal surface of the soft palate. Because the flap is narrow, the primary defect can be closed primarily. This is generally not performed during initial repair of the palate.

A two-flap technique uses similar principles to repair clefts involving the primary and secondary palate whether unilateral or bilateral. The major difference between this repair and the three-flap repair described above is that there is no anterior margin to the cleft since the palate defect is contiguous with a cleft lip. Therefore, instead of creating the V-shaped incision as described above, the incision along the alveolar ridge is continued anteriorly until it reaches the alveolar ridge. As with the three-flap technique, the edges of the cleft are incised and mucosal flaps are raised on the nasal and oral side. The hard palate is closed in two layers and the soft palate in three.

In a bilateral cleft of the primary palate there is inadequate tissue available to close the defect on the nasal side; therefore, bilateral vomer mucoperiosteal flaps are rotated to close the nasal floor.

The musculature of the soft palate is not oriented properly when a cleft is present. The repairs described above close the muscular layer but do not address the problem of improper orientation. In 1978, Leonard Furlow introduced a unique approach to the repair of soft palate. His technique differed from traditional repairs in two dramatic ways. First, it used two opposing Z-plasties to close the defect and reorient the muscular sling of the soft palate. Second, the hard palate is closed without relaxing incisions to prevent adverse effects on facial growth (18). The Furlow repair uses a nasal and an oral Z-plasty flap to close the defect and add length to the soft palate. This repair affords the additional benefit of realigning the muscle fibers of the palatal sling. The nasal and oral Z-plasties consist of an anterior and a posterior flap. The anterior flap of each side includes only mucosa, either oral or nasal. The posterior flap consists of mucosa and the underlying palatal muscle. Transposition of the posterior nasal flap draws the palatal muscular sling across the cleft and reorients the fibers so they run transversely across the palate. Transposition of the posterior oral flap likewise draws the muscle across the cleft and overlies the muscle fibers of the nasal flap. This repair adds length to the palate while improving function of the palatal musculature. A retrospective study of the Furlow palatoplasty compared to the intravelar veloplasty found that the Furlow technique might provide a better functional result; however, further study is needed (19).

CONCLUSION

Cleft lip and palate are congenital disorders that have varied presentations, ranging from barely detectable lesions with no functional impairment to disfiguring defects with major functional impairment. The anatomical defect may be associated with one of many syndromes or it may occur alone. Because of the variability and complexity of cleft lip and palate, caring for these patients is challenging.

The care of a patient with cleft lip and palate is part art and part science. The surgical repair of cleft lip truly is an art. In the last century, tremendous advances have been made in the repair of cleft lip and palate. Through innovative techniques, surgeons are now able to repair major defects with little scarring. While the art of cleft lip repair has made great progress in the last 100 years, there is still much to be learned about the science of cleft lip and palate. We are just now beginning to explore the role of genetics as a causative factor in cleft lip and palate. This is an area of rich scientific investigation and the years to come promise to be fruitful.

REFERENCES

1. Endriga MC, Kapp-simon KA. Psychological issues in craniofacial care: state of the art. Cleft Palate Craniofac J 1999; 36(1):3–9.
2. Day DW. Perspectives on care: the interdisciplinary team approach. Otolaryngol Clin North Am 1981; 14(4):769–775.
3. Strauss RP. The organization and delivery of craniofacial health services: the state of the art. Cleft Palate Craniofac J 1999; 36(3):189–194.
4. Cotton RT, Myer III CM. Practical Pediatric Otolaryngology. New York: Lippincott-Raven Publishers, 1999.
5. Carinci F, Pezzetti F, Scapoli L, Martinelli M, Carinci P, Tognon M. Genetics of nonsyndromic cleft lip and palate: a review of international studies and data regarding the Italian population. Cleft Palate Craniofac J 2000; 37(1):33–40.
6. Romitti P, Lidral AC, Munger RG, Daack-Hirsch S, Burns TL, Murray JC. Candidate genes for nonsyndromic cleft lip and palate and maternal cigarette smoking and alcohol consumption: evaluation of genotype-environment interactions from a population-based case–control study of orofacial clefts. Teratology 1999; 59:39–50.
7. Chung KC, Kowalski CP, Kim HM, Buchman SR. Maternal cigarette smoking during pregnancy and the risk of having a child with cleft lip/palate. Plast Reconstr Surg 2000; 105(2):485–491.

8. Millard DR. Cleft Craft The Evolution of Its Surgery. New York: Little, Brown, 1976.
9. Christ JE, Meininger MG. Ultrasoud diagnosis of cleft lip and cleft palate before birth. Plast Reconstr Surg 1981; 68:854–859.
10. Davalbhakta A, Hall PN. The impact of antenatal diagnosis on the effectiveness and timing of counseling for cleft lip and palate. Br J Plast Surg 2000; 53(4):298–301.
11. Clementi M, Tenconi R, Bianchi F, Stoll C. Euroscan study group. Evaluation of prenatal diagnosis of cleft lip with or without cleft palate by ultrasound: experience from 20 European registries. Prenatal Diagn 2000; 20(11):870–875.
12. Blumenfeld Z, Blumenfeld I, Bronshtein M. The early prenatal diagnosis of cleft lip and the decision-making process. Cleft Palate Craniofac J 1999; 36(2):105–107.
13. Denk MJ, Magee WP Jr. Cleft palate closure in the neonate: preliminary report. Cleft Palate Craniofac J 1996; 33(1):57–60.
14. Freedlander E, Webster MHC, Lewis RB, Blair M, Knight SL, Brown AI. Neonatal cleft lip repair in Ayrshire; a contribution to the debate. Br J Plast Surg 1990; 43:197–202.
15. Schendel SA. Unilateral cleft lip repair. Cleft Palate Craniofac J 2000; 37(4):335–341.
16. Salyer KE. Early and late treatment of unilateral cleft nasal deformity. Cleft Palate Craniofac J 1992; 29(6):556–568.
17. LaRossa D. The state of the art in cleft palate surgery. Cleft Palate Craniofac J 2000; 37(3):225–227.
18. Furlow LT. Cleft palate repair by double opposing Z-plasty. Plast Reconstr Surg 1986; 78(6):724–773.
19. Gunther E, Wisser JR, Cohen MA, Brown AS. Palatoplasy: Furlow's double reversing Z-plasty versus intravelar veloplasty. Cleft Palate Craniofac J 1998; 35(6):546–548.

11
Management of Congenital Craniofacial Anomalies

Jayesh Panchal and Paul Francel
Oklahoma University Health Sciences Center, Oklahoma City, Oklahoma, U.S.A.

CRANIOSYNOSTOSIS

Causes

The calvarium develops by intramembranous ossification. Islands of bone develop within the fibrous membrane, which later ossify. When two osteogenic fronts come in close proximity, a cranial suture develops (1). The sutures are essential to allow continuing expansion of the calvarium with age, especially in the first year of postnatal life when brain growth is rapid. The sutures close physiologically with age. The metopic is first to close in early perinatal life (3–9 months). Although normal fusion is thought to occur secondary to the loss of forces of separation created by the underlying brain, the precise cause of premature fusion is unknown.

Three theories have been purported to explain premature closure. Virchow (2) believed that the suture was abnormal and the cranial base abnormality was secondary to the primary suture fusion. Moss (3) put forth the concept that the cranial base was the site of primary abnormality and the dura transmitted abnormal tensile forces to the suture leading to a premature closure. Recent evidence points to the contrary. Eaton (4), in his elegant study examined the skulls of North Indian tribes who intentionally modified the skull shapes by head binding. Intentional modification of the calvarium produced secondary changes in the cranial base, thus refuting the theory that the cranial base drives the calvarial shape. Finally, Park and Powers (5) have suggested that the defect is in the mesenchymal blastema of both the cranial base and the cranial sutures.

Recently, the focus has shifted to the underlying dura and the growth vectors of the underlying cortex. Longaker (6) examined the posterior frontal cranial suture in rats, which closes physiologically, and the sagittal suture, which does not. They reversed the suture leaving the dura intact and demonstrated that the underlying dura determined the fate of the overlying suture. The dura is responsible for sending abnormal signals through increased levels of transforming growth factor – beta (TGF β) and m-RNA to the overlying suture (7). The reason for the generation of these abnormal signals is unknown but is believed to originate in the central nervous system and mediated through the growth factors. Marsh (8) presented data supporting the concept that the underlying cortex was abnormal. The diminished growth vector provided by the abnormal cortex led to generation of the abnormal signal by the dura to the overlying suture to close prematurely. Significant advances in genomic research are now revealing abnormal genetic expression at site of premature closure. Mutations in fibroblastic growth factor R2 (FGFR2) and FGFR3 were present in all patients with syndromic craniosynostosis and in 74% of children with unclassified so-called non syndromic craniosynostosis (9).

Pathogenesis

The neonatal calvarium is composed of the frontal, parietal, temporal, sphenoid and occipital bones. The metopic suture separates the frontal bones and the coronal separates the frontal and the parietal bones. The squamosal suture lies between the parietal and the squamosal temporal bone. The lambdoid suture lies between the parietal and occipital bones and the sagittal suture separates the two parietal bones. The patent sutures allow continuing separation of the calvarial bones. Virchow suggested that the prematurely fused suture restricts calvarial growth in a direction transverse to the fused suture. The metopic suture is responsible for continuing transverse expansion of the frontal bones. A pathologically closed metopic suture prevents this, leading to a narrow frontal and fronto-orbital region. This anterior narrowing manifests as trigonocephaly and hypotelorism. The coronal suture could close prematurely either unilaterally or bilaterally resulting in unicoronal or bicoronal synostosis, respectively. Unicoronal synostosis results in diminished growth in the ventral–dorsal direction on the ipsilateral side and compensatory growth on the contralateral side. This asymmetry is known as frontal plagiocephaly. The fronto-orbital bar is recessed ipsilaterally and projects further ventrally on the contralateral side. Bilateral closure of the coronal suture produces a diminished growth vector in the ventral–dorsal direction and compensatory growth takes place in the medial–lateral direction. This results in brachycephaly and bilateral recession of the fronto-orbital bar, which, in severe conditions, can result in exorbitsm. Premature closure of the sagittal suture results in continuing growth of the calvarium in the ventral–dorsal direction and diminished growth in the transverse direction. This leads to scaphocephaly. Premature closure of the lambdoid suture leads to occipital plagiocephaly with ipsilateral flattening of the occipital region with contralateral bulging.

The cranial base deforms secondary to the calvarial abnormality. The anterior cranial base deviates towards the fused suture in unicoronal synostosis. The posterior cranial base similarly deviates towards the ipsilateral fused lambdoid suture. Since the face is a template, which is based on the cranial base, uncorrected unicoronal synostosis leads to asymmetry of the face and occlusal plane.

Closure of multiple sutures can limit expansion of the calvarium and therefore of the underlying cortex. The continuing expansile forces provided by the cortex against the fixed volume of the calvarium lead to an increase in the intracranial pressure with its associated sequelae. Two studies have measured the intracranial pressure in children with craniosynostosis and reported that multiple suture synostosis is associated with raised intracranial pressure in 48% of the studied subjects and approximately 18% of subjects with single suture craniosynostosis (10,11). Gault and Renier measured intracranial pressure by an invasive technique overnight to find the trend. Unfortunately the range of intracranial pressures in what are termed normal children is unknown.

The closed suture prevents calvarial expansion and this would lead to decreased intracranial volume. The compensatory growth of the contralateral calvarium may possibly lead to fallacious measurements. Segmental volumes of the cortex and the calvarium and cranial fossa are beginning to be measured with sophisticated software, which may reveal more accurate findings in children with craniosynostosis (12).

Clinical Examination and Diagnosis

Although premature fusion of the sutures is a prenatal event, children with craniosynostosis do not always present in the neonatal period. The passage of the head through the birth canal deforms the head and makes it difficult to ascertain whether the head is normal or abnormal. Either the parent or the pediatrician notices the abnormal shape in early infancy and the child is referred to a craniofacial or a neurosurgeon.

Since calvarial deformation is secondary to the sutural fusion and is characteristic, clinical diagnosis is not very difficult. Clinical history should include the birth events (length of term, birth weight, and complications during and after birth). A detailed history of the perinatal sleeping position is critical in differentiating craniosynostosis from plagiocephaly without synostosis (see below). Syndromic craniosynostosis involve multiple systems and may be associated with other congenital anomalies. Family history of abnormal head shape is crucial in the diagnosis of syndromic craniosynostosis.

Clinical examination should include examination of the head and neck. Measurement of the head circumference aids in ruling out microcephaly and microcephaly with associated hydrocephalus. The calvarial shape is characteristic for each sutural synostosis. An increase in anteroposterior length or scaphocephaly is associated with sagittal synostosis (Fig. 1). Narrowing of the anterior calvarium or trigonocephaly is associated with metopic synostosis (Fig. 2). The distance between the medial canthii of the eyes (intermedial canthus distance) is decreased. The orbital rims may appear hypoplastic. Bicoronal synostosis results in shortening of the skull in the anteroposterior direction and widening at the bitemporal region. The fronto-orbital rim is recessed bilaterally, which leads to exorbitism with its associated complication of exposure keratitis (Fig. 3). Unilateral asymmetry or plagiocephaly can result from coronal or lamdoid synostosis. Unilateral coronal synostosis results in a recessed forehead and fronto-orbital rim. There is contralateral bossing of the forehead and the fronto-orbital rim. The eyebrow on the ipsilateral side is raised and the palpebral fissure is increased in its vertical height. The ocular globe is sometimes raised along with the pupil. (Figs. 4,5). An older child with uncorrected unicoronal synostosis demonstrates asymmetry of the facial skeleton. This is associated with a reduction in the height of the ipsilateral maxilla and mandible, resulting in an oblique occlusal cant. Lamdoid synostosis is rare and has to be differentiated from deformational plagiocephaly or plagiocephaly without synostosis.

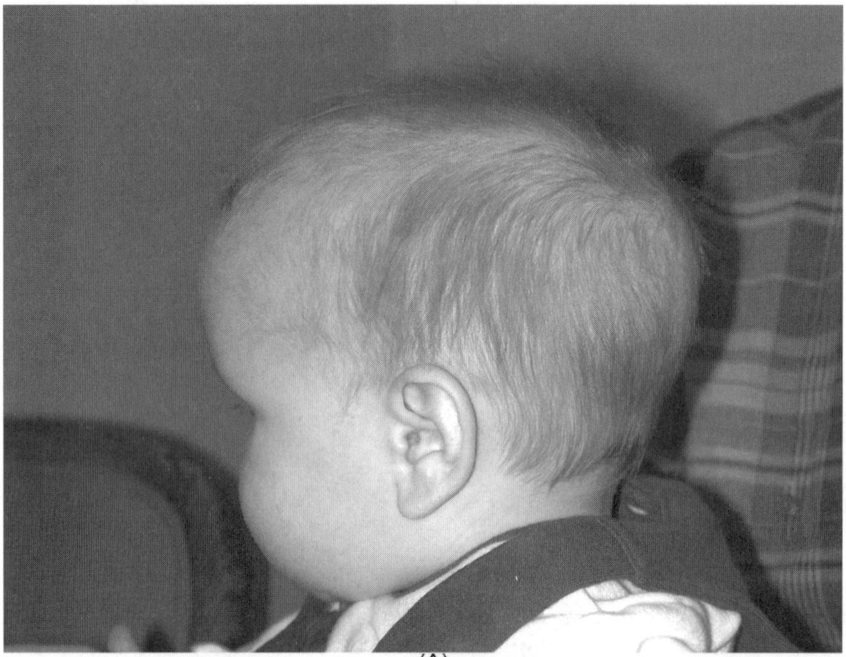

(A)

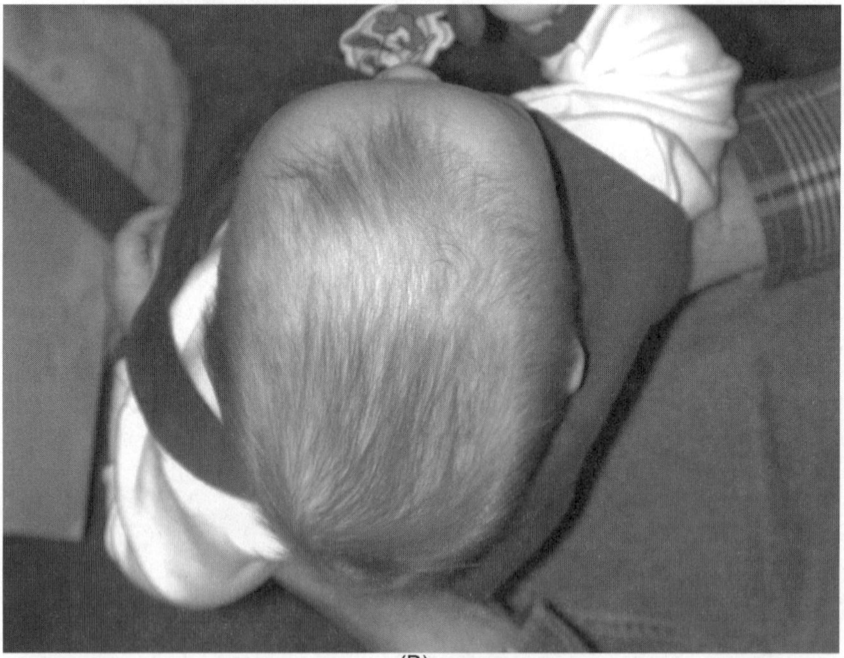

(B)

Figure 1 A. Lateral view of a child with sagittal craniosynostosis demonstrates frontal and occipital bossing and dolichocephaly. B. Superior view demonstrates frontal bossing bilaterally and dolichocephaly.

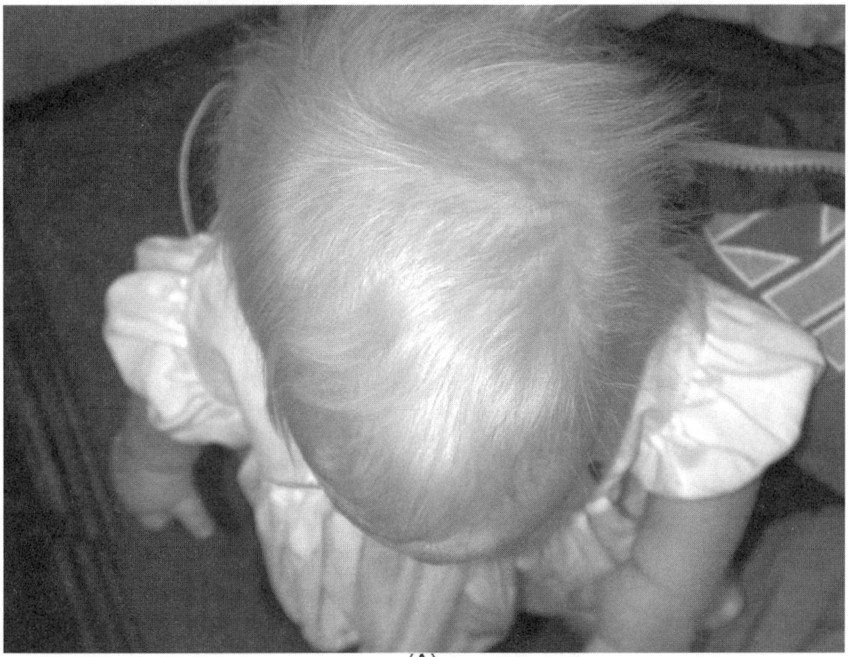

(A)

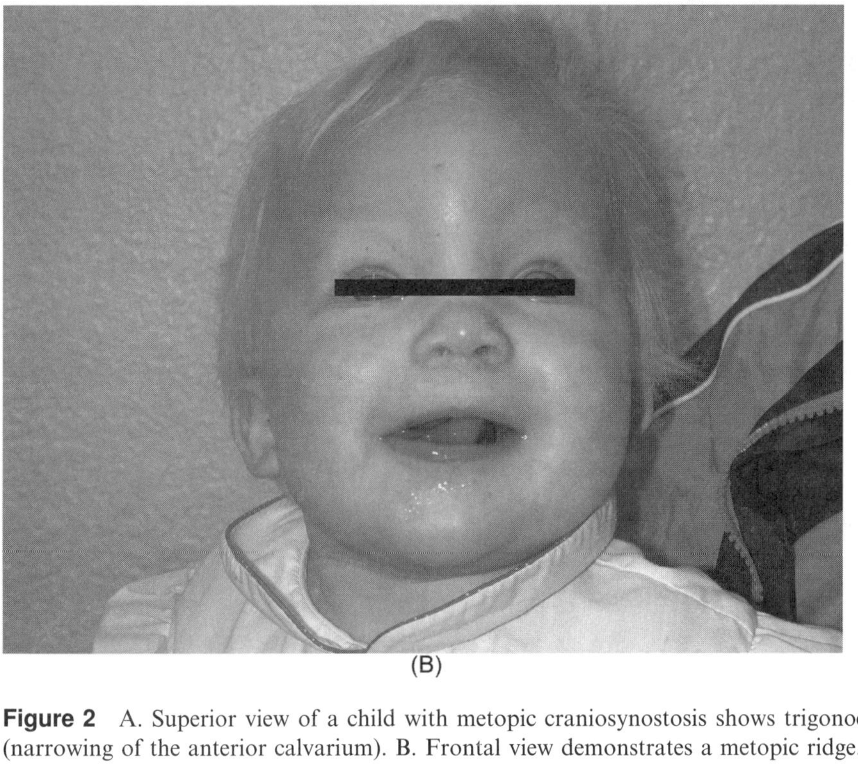

(B)

Figure 2 A. Superior view of a child with metopic craniosynostosis shows trigonocephaly (narrowing of the anterior calvarium). B. Frontal view demonstrates a metopic ridge.

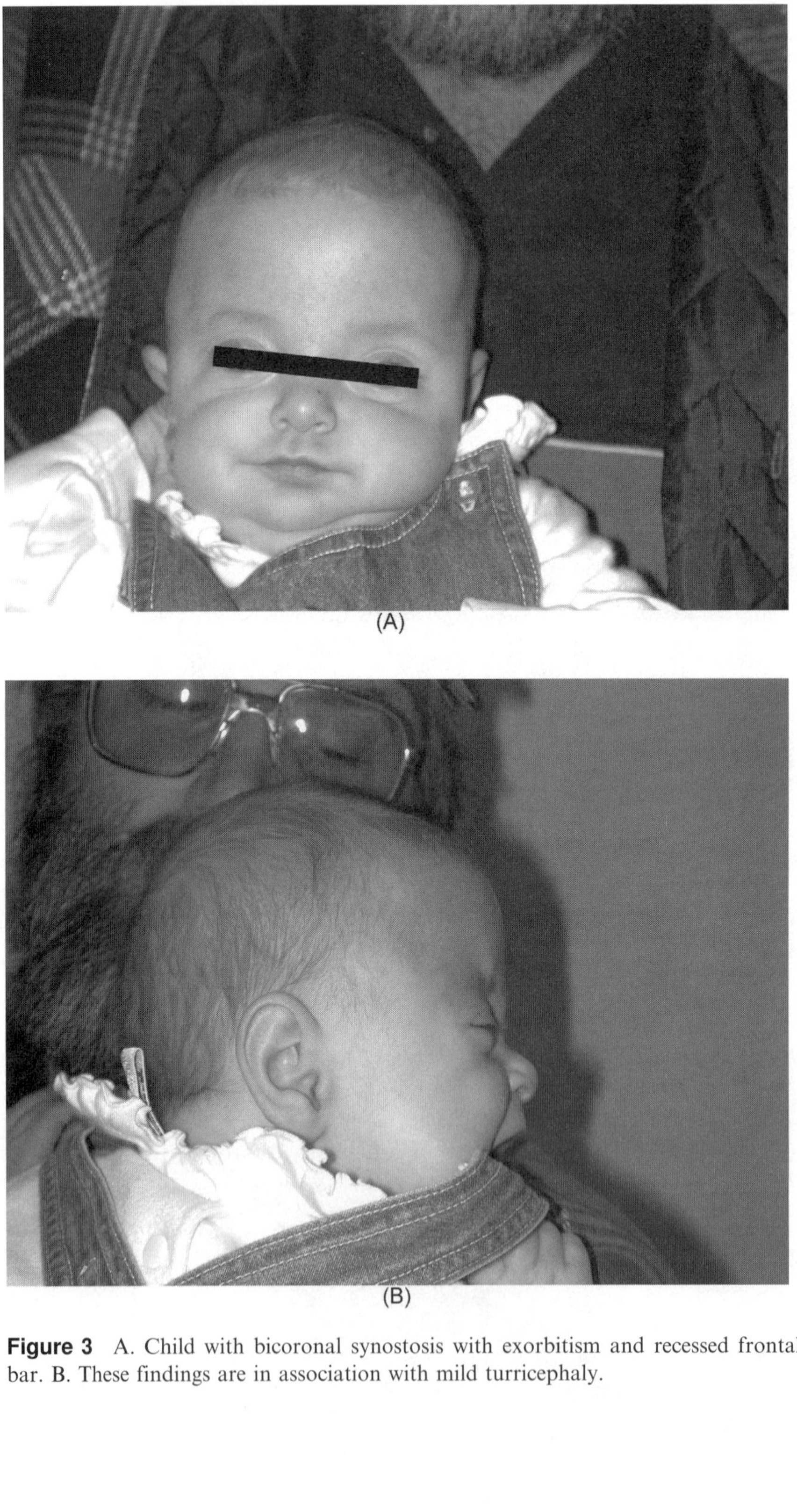

Figure 3 A. Child with bicoronal synostosis with exorbitism and recessed frontal orbital bar. B. These findings are in association with mild turricephaly.

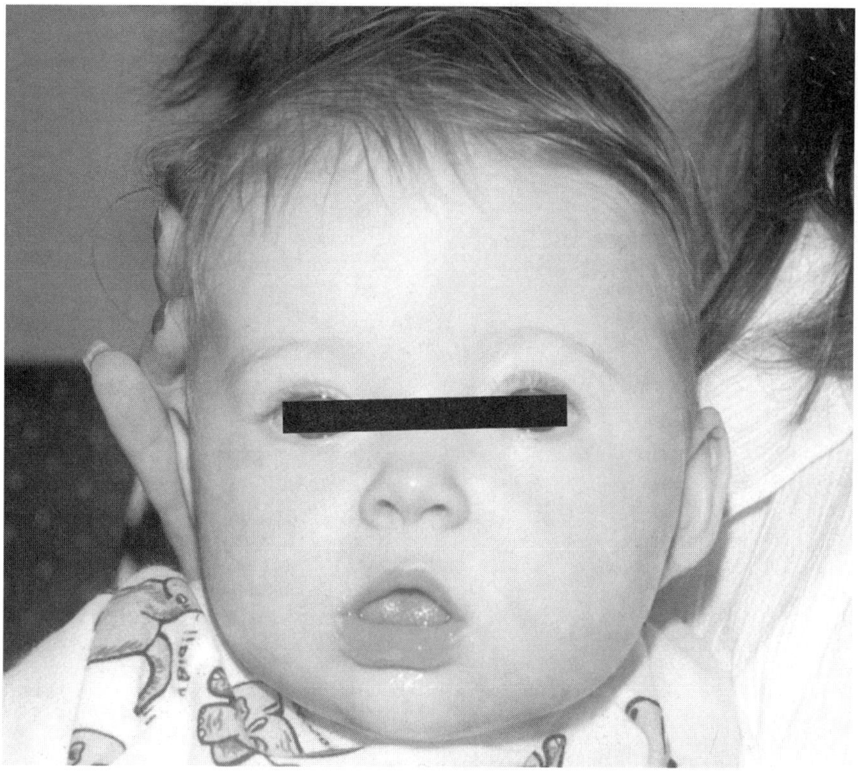

Figure 4 Child with left unicoronal synostosis demonstrates asymmetry of the orbits and widened palpebral fissure on the left in association with superiorly displaced left eyebrow. Notice the asymmetry of the face and deviation of the facial axis to the contralateral side.

Plagiocephaly Without Synostosis or Deformational Plagiocephaly

Plagiocephaly without synostosis or deformational plagiocephaly is a very common cause of an asymmetrical head associated with an ipsilateral occipital flattening. Over the past few years the incidence of asymmetrical head shapes in infants has increased significantly (13). Although asymmetrical heads have been present for many centuries, the recent increase has been associated with the "Back to Sleep" campaign to reduce the incidence of sudden infant death syndrome (SIDS). The skull of a newborn child is soft and easily deforms if left in the same position for a prolonged time. Infants neck muscles are weak and they are unable to move their head in the first few months of life. This may be further complicated by torticollis, in which the tight neck muscles may prevent the infant or the parent from repositioning the head (14). The deforming force flattens the occipital skull and, like a ball inflated with less air, it preferentially tends to lie in that position. The continuing force not only flattens the occipital region but also pushes the forehead and the ear forward and, in extreme cases, the cheekbones, jaw joints, and mandible. This leads to a typical parallelogram-shaped head, referred to as deformational plagiocephaly or

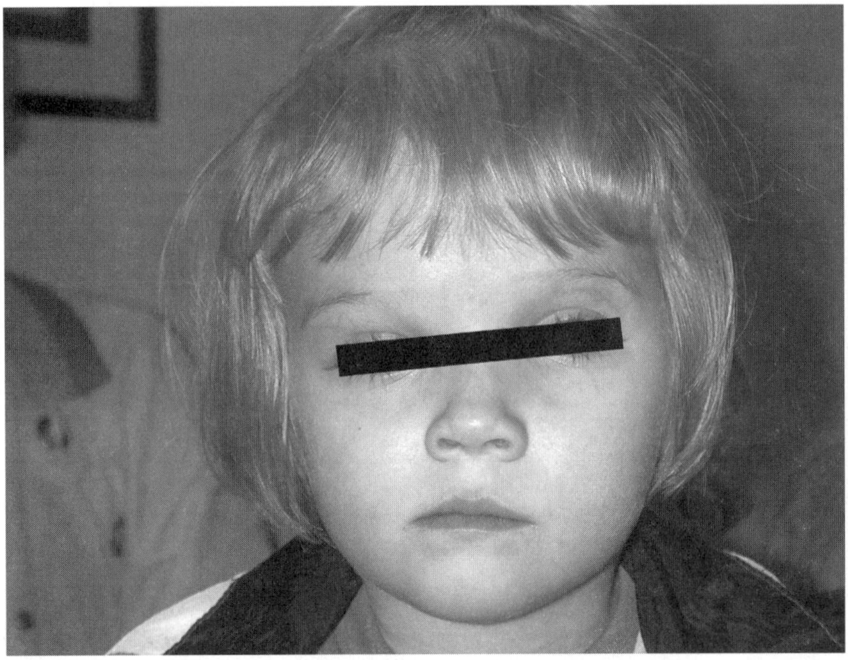

Figure 5 An older child with unicoronal synostosis with asymmetry of the facial axis and progressive deformity of orbital asymmetry.

plagiocephaly without synostosis (15). The use of a customized molding helmet for 23 hours/day until age 1 year is very successful in treating this condition. Helmet therapy needs to start by age 6 months to be effective (Fig. 6).

Investigations

The clinical diagnosis of craniosynostosis or plagiocephaly without synostosis is substantiated by results of radiological investigations.

Skull X-Ray

This preliminary examination helps to visualize whether the sutures are patent or not. The test is simple but its accuracy is not perfect and differentiation between a lamdoid synostosis and plagiocephaly without synostosis is sometimes difficult. Special views are needed to visualize all the sutures (Fig. 7).

Ultrasonography

This noninvasive nonradiological modality has recently been studied to determine whether it is useful in the diagnosis of a patent suture. The ultrasound is more accurate than an x-ray examination but requires a sonographer who is willing to specialize in interpreting the results.

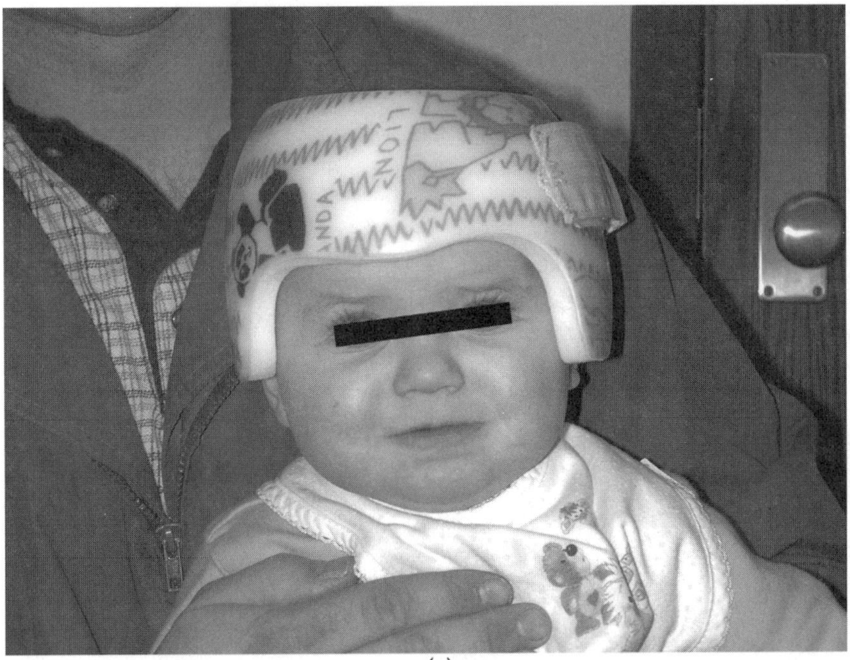

(a)

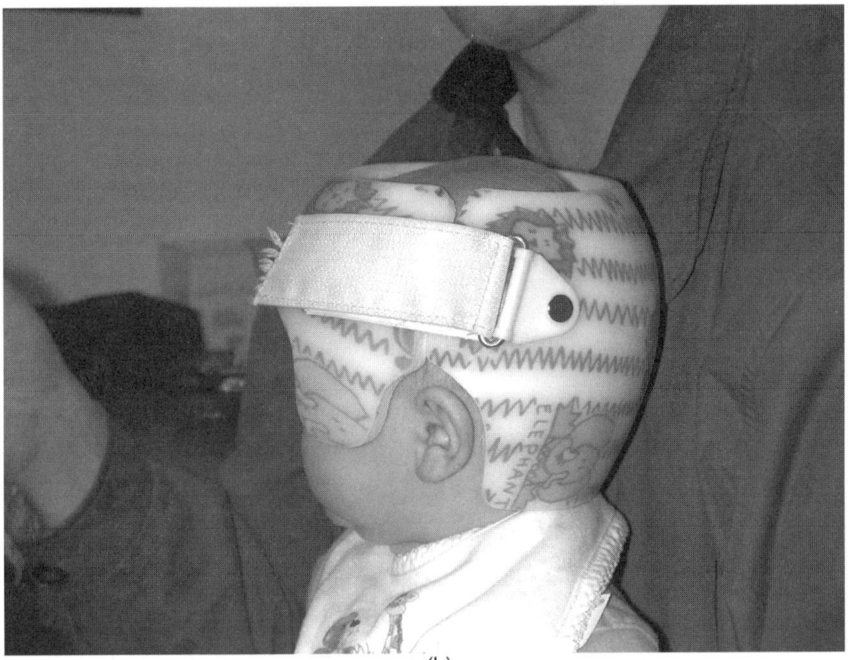

(b)

Figure 6 Customized molding helmet for treatment of deformational plagiocephaly.

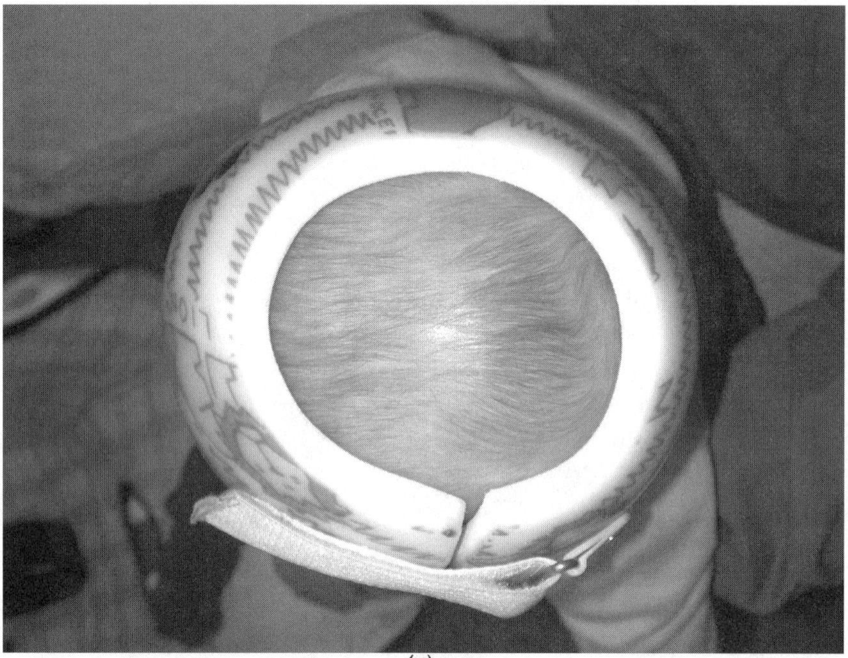

(c)

Figure 6 Continued.

Computed Tomographic Scan

A computed tomographic (CT) scan is the gold standard for determining whether a suture is patent or fused. Two-dimensional views allow direct visualization of each suture but make it difficult to grasp the extent of the associated deformity. This makes preoperative planning very difficult and consistent outcomes unreliable. Three-dimensional CT scans, in contrast, allow complete visualization of the skull and document the extent of the deformity. The windows utilized in reconstruction of the three-dimensional images can sometimes white out the sutures and these may appear as fused when they are not. If one is in doubt about the patency of the suture, it is prudent to look for the associated deformity that accompanies the fused suture and determine whether the suture is patent or not from the two-dimensional views. Specific views (i.e., frontal, posterior [occipital], right and left profile, superior, inferior ectocranial, and endocranial) can be utilized as a protocol to allow comparison among pre-, peri-, and postoperative CT scans. A radiographical scale should be placed by the images for approximate measurements of the various bony landmarks. This aids in preoperative planning and allows a meaningful outcome analysis to be performed. Sophisticated software is available for performing manipulation of the osteotomies on a graphic workstation (16).

Sagittal Synostosis

The sagittal suture is fused (Fig. 8) restricting the transverse growth of the skull resulting in reduction of the transverse diameter at the parietal eminences (biparietal

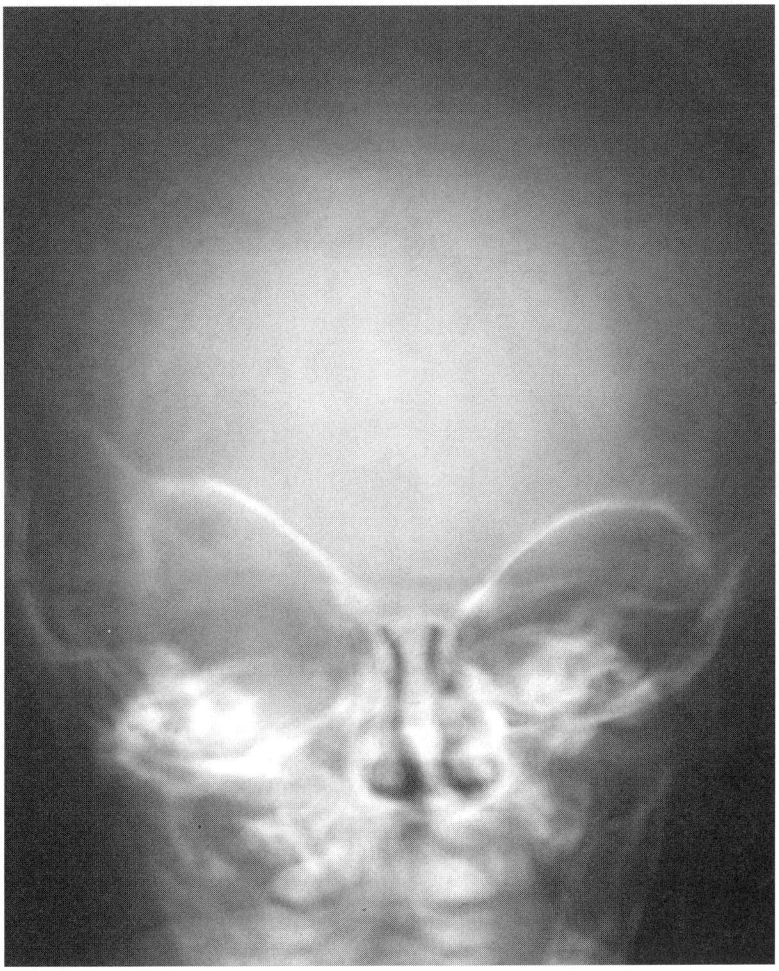

Figure 7 X-ray examination of the skull in a child with unicoronal synostosis demonstrates an elevated sphenoidal wing on the right, asymmetry of the orbits, and of the facial skeleton.

diameter), and an increase in the anteroposterior length of the skull. The cephalic index (maximum transverse width/maximum anteroposterior length) is reduced. Normograms for cephalic indices are available (17) and the severity of the scaphocephaly can be determined. The cranial base is on the midline.

Metopic Synostosis

The metopic suture is fused, restricting the transverse growth of the frontal bones (Fig. 9). This results in narrowing of the anterior cranial fossa and trigonocephaly. The restriction in the transverse direction also results in reduction in the distance between the orbits (interorbital distance). The orbital rims are hypoplastic. The metopic suture is the first suture to close physiologically. Previous studies documented

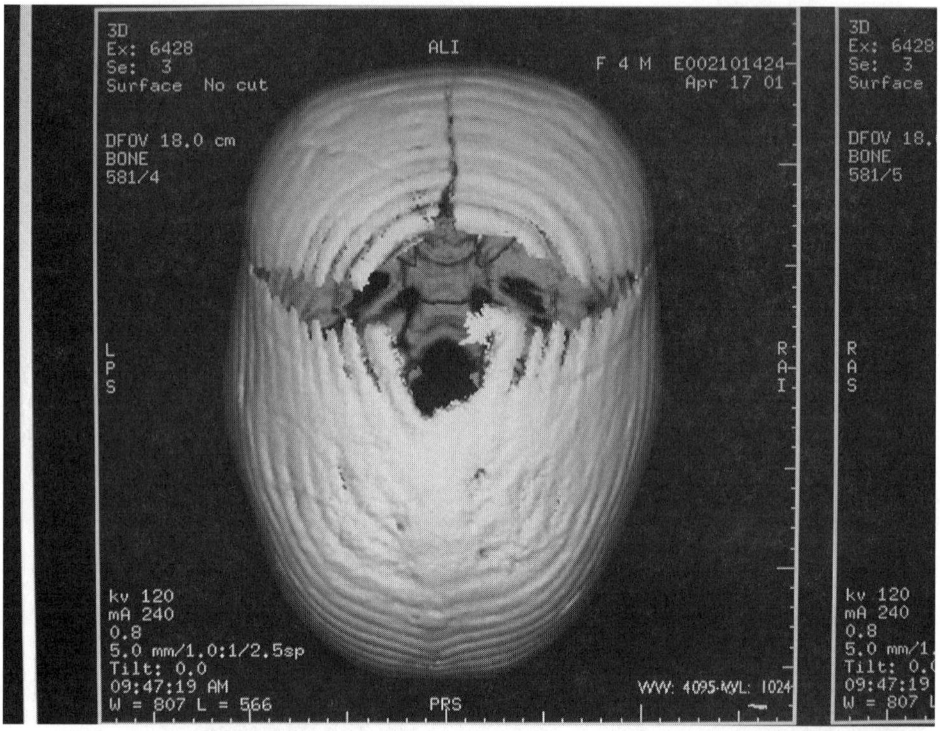

Figure 8 Superior view of a three-dimensional CT scan demonstrates a fused sagittal suture with frontal bossing and patent frontal and coronal sutures.

this closure to be in the first and second year of postnatal life. However with more CT scans being performed in the neonatal period it obvious that the metopic suture closes physiologically at a much earlier age, most likely between 3 and 6 months of postnatal life (18). The interorbital distance should be measured preoperatively and compared to a normogram (19). The ideal distance is documented and intraoperative correction is performed to increase the interorbital distance to normal.

Bicoronal Synostosis

The bicoronal suture is fused restricting the anteroposterior growth of the anterior cranial fossa (Fig. 10). This results in a decreased anteroposterior dimension of the anterior cranial fossa. The bitemporal diameter is increased. The fronto-orbital bar is recessed bilaterally. The supraorbitale (the most prominent point of the fronto-orbital rim) is normally 2 mm ventral to the plane of the cornea. In a child with bicoronal synostosis, the fronto-orbital bar is recessed and the supraorbitale is more dorsal (posterior) to the corneal plane (20). This leads to exorbitsm with its associated complications. The objective of the surgery is therefore to place the fronto-orbital bar 2 mm ventral to the corneal plane.

(A)
(B)
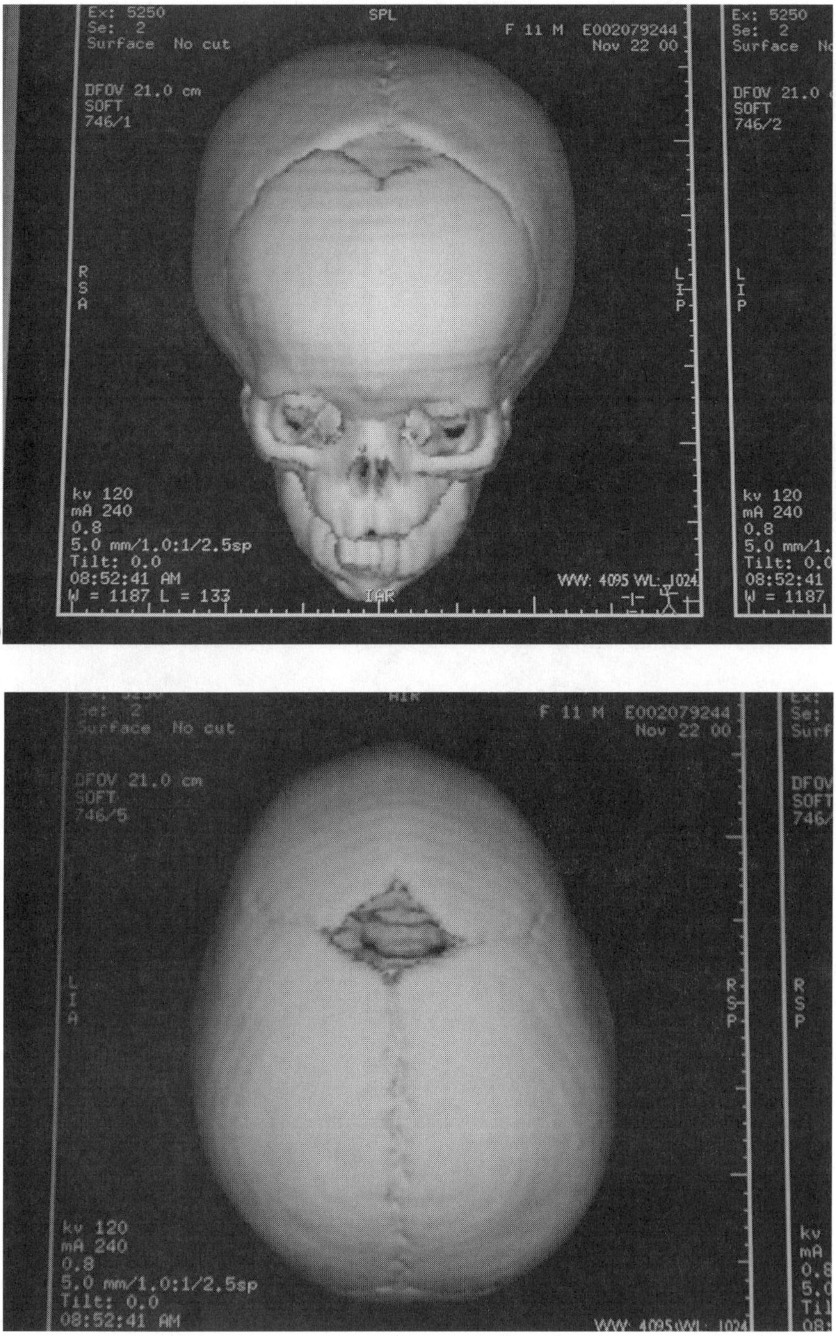

Figure 9 A. A child with metopic craniosynostosis with ridging at the site of the metopic suture and hypoplasia of the orbits. B. Superior view of three-dimensional CT scan of a child with metopic craniosynostosis and patent coronal and sagittal sutures. Note the trigonocephaly.

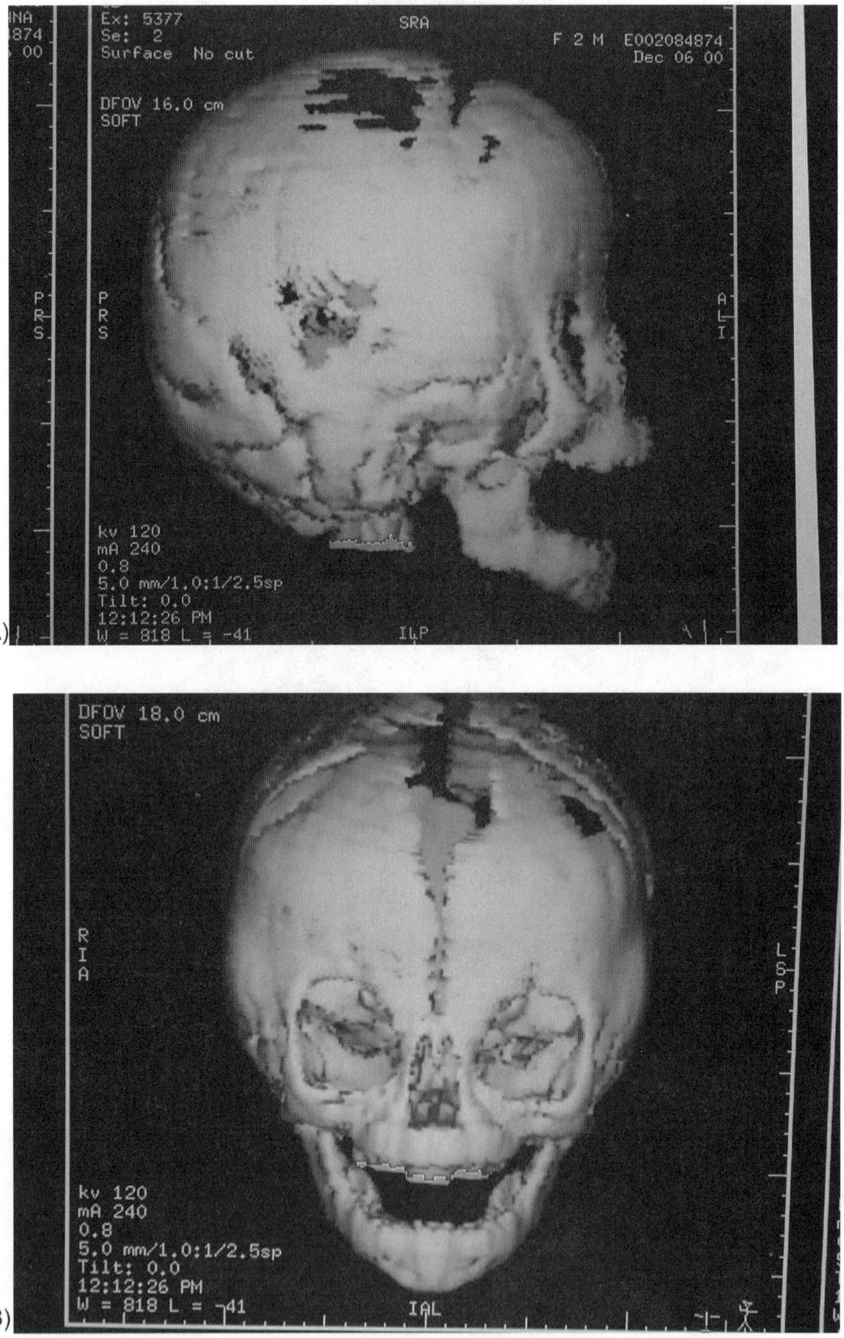

(A)

(B)

Figure 10 A. Lateral view of three-dimensional CT scan of a child with bicoronal synostosis. Note the recession of the frontal orbital bar and turricephaly. B. Frontal view demonstrates turricephaly and recession of the frontal orbital bar. C. Superior view shows bicoronal synostosis with significant recession of the frontal orbital bar and the frontal bones. Both the frontal orbital bar and the frontal bones lie dorsal to the malar eminences and the maxillary anterior nasal spine.

(C)
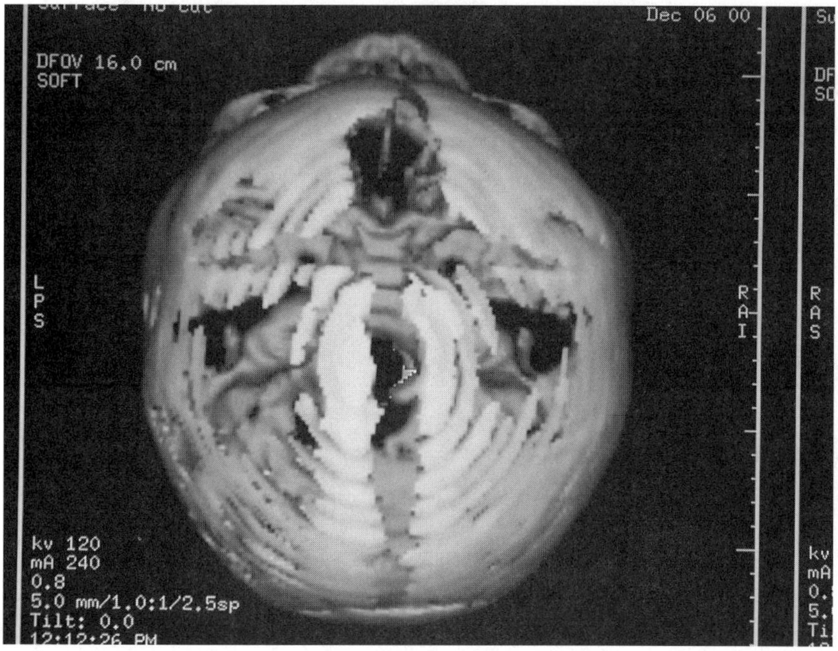

Figure 10 Continued.

Unicoronal Synostosis

A unicoronal synostosis is characterized by a fused coronal suture (Fig. 11). The ipsilateral fronto-orbital bar is recessed and the contralateral fronto-orbital bar and frontal bone are more ventral. This is due to the secondary deforming changes that occur due to the closed suture. Since anteroposterior growth cannot take place across the closed coronal suture, compensatory changes take place along the contralateral suture. This information is critical to understand when correcting unicoronal synostosis: surgery will require correction of ipsilateral and contralateral bones. The fused suture also restricts the growth of sphenoid, resulting in a reduction of the anteroposterior dimension of the anterior cranial fossa. As a consequence, the anterior endocranial base deviates towards the ipsilateral side. The ectocranium is likewise also deviated to the ipsilateral side and, if uncorrected, would lead to deviation of the face and the occlusal cant. The posterior cranial base is unaffected. The roof of the orbit, which is formed by the greater wing of the sphenoid, is raised. The shape of the ipsilateral orbit is more vertical and the contralateral more horizontal (21).

Lamdoid Synostosis

This is characterized by an obliterated ipsilateral lamdoid suture. The anteroposterior dimension of the posterior cranial fossa is reduced. The contralateral suture therefore protrudes. The ipsilateral mastoid process bulges and in many ways is

(A)
(B)

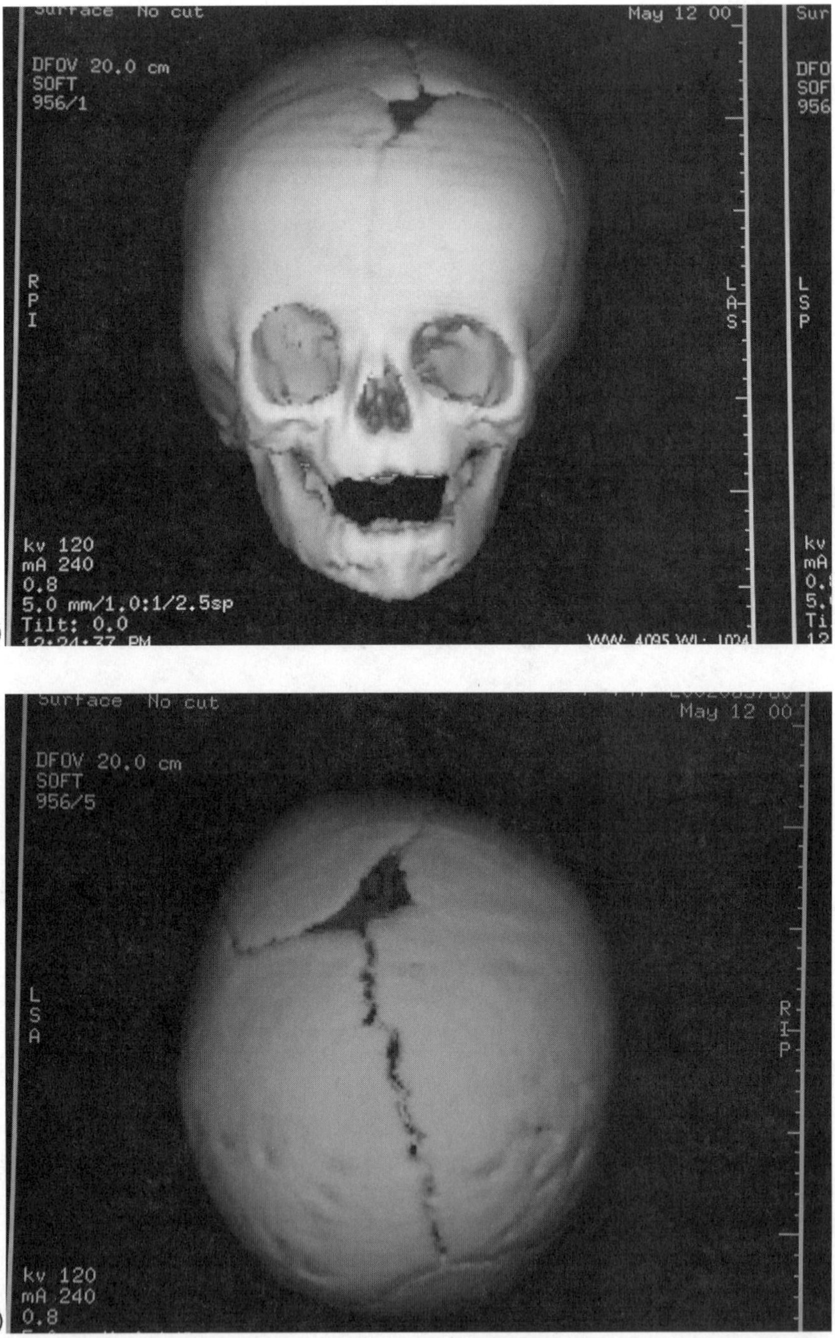

Figure 11 A. Child with right unicoronal synostosis demonstrates asymmetry of the orbits. The right orbit is narrower and taller than the contralateral side and there is mild deviation of the facial axis. B. Three-dimensional CT scan demonstrates right unicoronal synostosis with fused right coronal suture, and patent metopic, left coronal, and sagittal sutures. The right frontal orbital bar and the right frontal bone are more dorsal than the contralateral side, which demonstrates frontal bossing.

characteristic of the lamdoid synostosis. The posterior cranial base is deviated to the ipsilateral side whereas the anterior base is unaffected. The greatest difficulty lies in differentiating between the deformational plagiocephaly or plagiocephaly without synostosis and lamdoid synostosis. Synostosis restricts growth on the ipsilateral side compared to deformational plagiocephaly, which deforms by pushing ventrally. Thus in a lamdoid synostosis the petrous part of the temporal bone is pulled towards the closed lamdoid suture. The external auditory canal is likewise also pulled towards the fused suture. In contrast, the petrous temporal bone and the external auditory canal are pushed anteriorly in deformational plagiocephaly. It is also not uncommon to see ipsilateral frontal bossing in deformational plagiocephaly and almost never in lamdoid synostosis. Thus the diagnosis of deformational plagiocephaly or lamdoid synostosis is made by assessing the secondary changes rather than assessing the suture itself. This eliminates the diagnosis of partial suture closures and lamdoid suture thickening.

Magnetic Resonance Imaging Scan

The magnetic resonance imaging (MRI) scan helps to delineate the pattern of cortical gyrii and sulcii underneath the fused suture. There has been intense debate over whether the abnormal pattern is secondary to the pressure from the overlying fused suture or whether the pattern is a primary event and leads to a fused suture (Fig. 12). Although a simple follow-up study comparing the preoperative MRI scans to the 1 year postoperative scans would allow the question to be answered, it has been very difficult to measure the extent of the flattening of the gyrii and sulcii objectively despite the sophisticated software used at the Natioanl Institutes of Health (NIH). The study is further complicated by a lack of a database of normal MRI scans in children of that age. The MRI scan only allows anatomical delineation of the cortex and does not provide any information about cortical function.

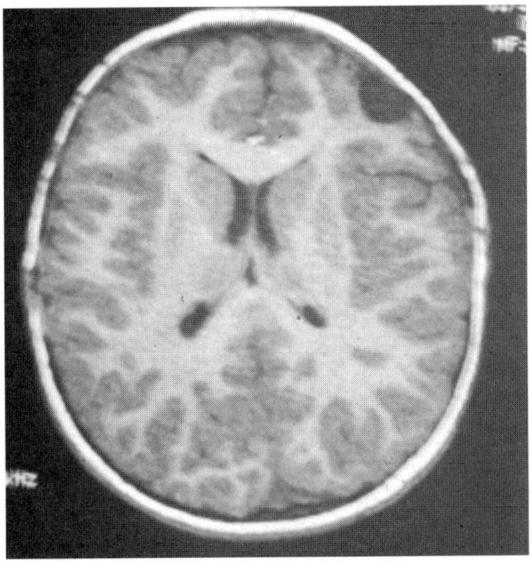

Figure 12 Two-dimensional MRI examination in a child with unicoronal synostosis demonstrates abnormality of the underlying cortex.

Neurodevelopmental Analysis

The purpose of neurodevelopmental testing is to obtain information about cortical functioning prior to and after cranial vault remodeling. Bayley Scales of Infant Development – II (22) are frequently utilized to procure this information. A longitudinal assessment is essential to performance of a meaningful analysis. These tests allow a comparison of the child's mental and psychomotor scales to a normogram and thus help to quantify whether the child is delayed and whether the surgery helps in reducing the severity of the delay. Children with syndromic craniosynostosis characterized by multiple system involvement are often developmentally delayed. This delay can be severe and the child could be classified as mentally retarded. However, children with single-suture craniosynostosis do not have significant delays (23,24,25). A more detailed assessment with more sophisticated analysis is therefore needed (26). Such analyses show that these children have minor delays in learning and speech, which were not previously recognized in this population (27,28). The greatest difficulty with neurodevelopmental testing is the lack of accuracy in measuring cortical function at age 3–6 months.

Positron Emission Tomographic Scan

A positron emission tomographic (PET) scan help to assess and quantify crudely the glucose uptake of the cortex under the involved suture and also allows comparison of pre- and postoperative status. A single study documented that the glucose uptake is reduced under the fused suture and becomes normal after cranial vault reconstruction. The temporal effect of growth on underlying cortex is however unknown. The frontal cortex has only a minimal intake in the first 3–6 months of life and increases dramatically by age 1 year (29). Thus, the surgical intervention could be viewed as beneficial although the improvement in the glucose uptake was physiological. A normal temporal pattern of glucose uptake in an infant has not yet been established.

Need for Surgery

The aim of the surgical intervention is not only to excise the prematurely fused suture but also to correct the associated deformities of the calvarium. Uncorrected synostosis is associated with an increase in intracranial pressure documented in both animal model and in humans (11,12).

If not corrected, the deformity progresses to involve the facial skeleton and is associated with asymmetry of the face and malocclusion. The asymmetry of the orbit leads to ocular dystopia and consequent strabismus. The objective of the surgery is to increase the intracranial volume, especially under the fused suture, and prevent long-term complications. This is achieved by normalizing the calvarial shape.

Timing of Surgery

Surgery is best performed in early infancy for the following reasons:

1. The majority of the growth of the brain takes place in the first year of the life. The deforming vectors of the growing brain result in progression of the deformity with increasing age.

2. Few studies have demonstrated an increase in the intracranial pressure in nonsyndromic single-suture synostosis (11,12).
3. Single photon emission computed tomographic (SPECT)/PET scans have demonstrated a decrease in the cortical blood supply underlying the premature suture, which was normalized following surgery.
4. Osseous defects following surgery undergo reossification more completely before age < 1 year than later. Delay in surgery beyond the first few years of life leads to progressive deformity of the cranial base, which results in abnormal facial growth, as well asasymmetry of the maxilla and the mandible.
5. Surgery performed in early infancy corrects the abnormalities in the cranial base (30).

For these reasons, there is now an increasing consensus among craniofacial surgeons and neurosurgeons that surgery should be performed in early infancy.

SURGERY

Sagittal Craniosynostosis

Sagittal craniosynostosis is characterized by an increase in the anteroposterior direction and a reduction in a transverse direction. The objective of the surgery is not only to excise the fused suture but also to correct the secondary deformational changes due to the sagittal synostosis. In the past, the aim was to excise the fused suture only in the hope that the secondary changes would correct themselves as the underlying brain grew in the first year of postnatal life. This simple objective was achieved by removing the fused suture with a strip craniectomy. The initial strip craniectomies were associated with refusion and various agents were utilized to keep the sutures patent (31). Later modifications included numerous variations of the strip craniectomies (32).

Over the last decade, craniofacial surgeons have become more aggressive in trying to correct the suture as well as the associated deformities of frontal bossing and occipital bullet or bathrocephaly. This procedure of subtotal calvarectomy and cranial vault remodeling involved excision of frontal, parietal, and occipital bones. These were trimmed, reshaped, relocated, and then fixed with absorbable plates. The primary objective of surgery was to release the synostotic constraint to normal calvarial growth and improve the calvarial contour by reduction of anteroposterior length and increase in transverse width.

Abandonment of accepted procedures and adoption of novel ones should be predicated upon outcome assessment. Comparative evaluation among treatment modalities requires identification of the goals of intervention as well as means for assessing those goals. Over the past 25 years, normalization of the shape of the head has been the ill-defined primary goal of craniosynostosis surgery. Whether such normalization can be achieved has only infrequently been reported using standard anthropometric measurements sensitive to cranial width and length (cranial index). A retrospective quantitative analysis (using cephalic index) of

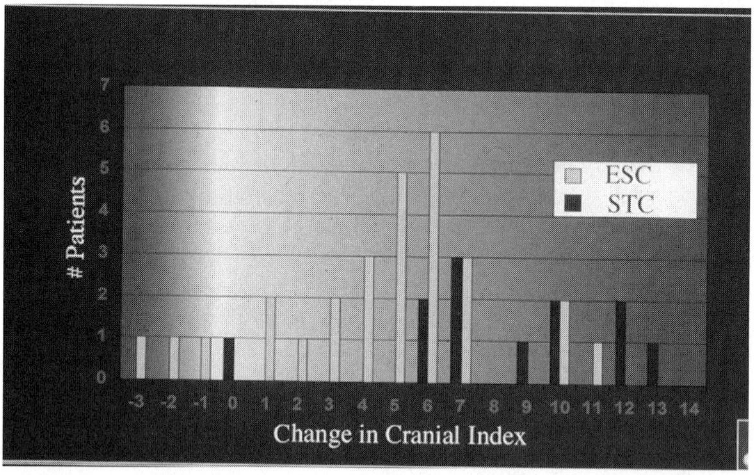

Figure 13 Graphic representation in the extent of improvement/deterioration. A comparison of children who have undergone STC vs. ESC.

40 infants who underwent surgery for sagittal craniosynostosis was therefore, conducted to determine whether any difference in outcome, with respect to cranial index, could be associated with either the age at surgery or extent of the operation.

The cephalic index (CI) was calculated from the three-dimensional CT scan images. The infants underwent either extended strip craniectomies (ESC) or subtotal calvarectomy and cranial vault remodeling (STC). The CI and percentage changes were compared preoperatively, perioperatively, and postoperatively within each group, between two different techniques, and between two age groups. The mean change (preoperative vs. postoperative) in actual CI of infants who underwent ESC was 4 compared to 8 in infants who underwent STC ($p = 0.08$). The mean percentage change of CI (preoperative vs. postoperative) following ESC was 4.6 compared to 8.2 following STC ($p = 0.003$). Following ESC, three patients demonstrated deterioration in CI necessitating a reoperation in one patient. In contrast, none of the patients who underwent STC demonstrated deterioration in CI (Fig. 13). The mean CI of infants following ESC did not reach age-matched norm values and only 29% had cephalic indices within normal range. In contrast, the mean CI in infants who underwent STC reached age-matched norm values and 66% of the patients had cephalic indices within normal range. The percentage change in CI in infants who underwent ESC and whose age at surgery was $\leq$ 4 months compared to $>$ 4 months did not reach statistical significance. Also, the mean cephalic indices in either group (age $\leq$ 4 months and age $>$ 4 months) did not reach age-matched norm values (Fig. 14).

If normalization of cranial shape is the goal of sagittal synostosis surgery, a more extensive operation than an extensive strip craniectomy is necessary and age at surgery between 1 and 13 months does not affect the outcome of infants undergoing ESC (33).

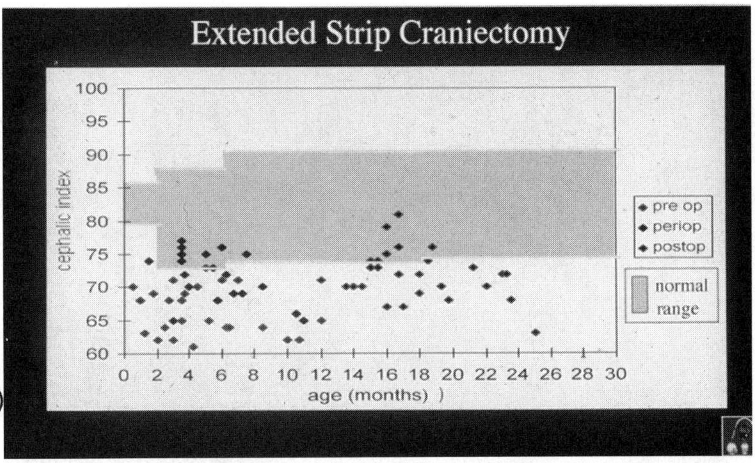

(A)

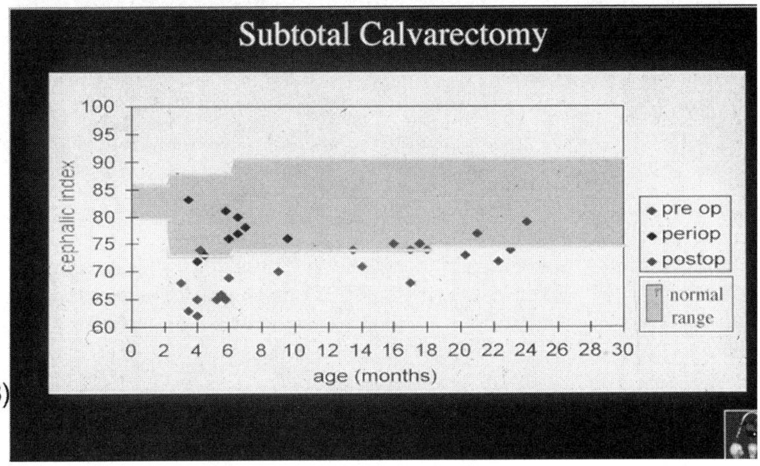

(B)

Figure 14 A. Graphic representation of the normalization of cranial shape in children who have undergone ESC. Only 29% of the postoperative cephalic indexes were within normal range. B. Graphic representation of the cephalic indexes of children who have undergone STC: 66% had postoperative indexes within normal range.

Neurosurgeons have recently been using the endoscope to perform strip craniectomies, followed by use of a molding helmet for 6–8 months postoperatively (34). The technique certainly reduces the morbidity and blood loss but does not allow the surgeon to alter the shape or the cephalic index intraoperatively. The procedure is a strip craniectomy but is performed with an endoscope. In the above-mentioned study the extent of improvement using a strip craniectomy was inferior to the cranial vault remodeling.

The technique adopted by the authors is a more extensive procedure of subtotal calvarectomy and cranial vault remodeling. The technique utilizes a controlled squeeze of the intracranial contents to reduce the anteroposterior dimension of the calvarium and increase the transverse width of the skull.

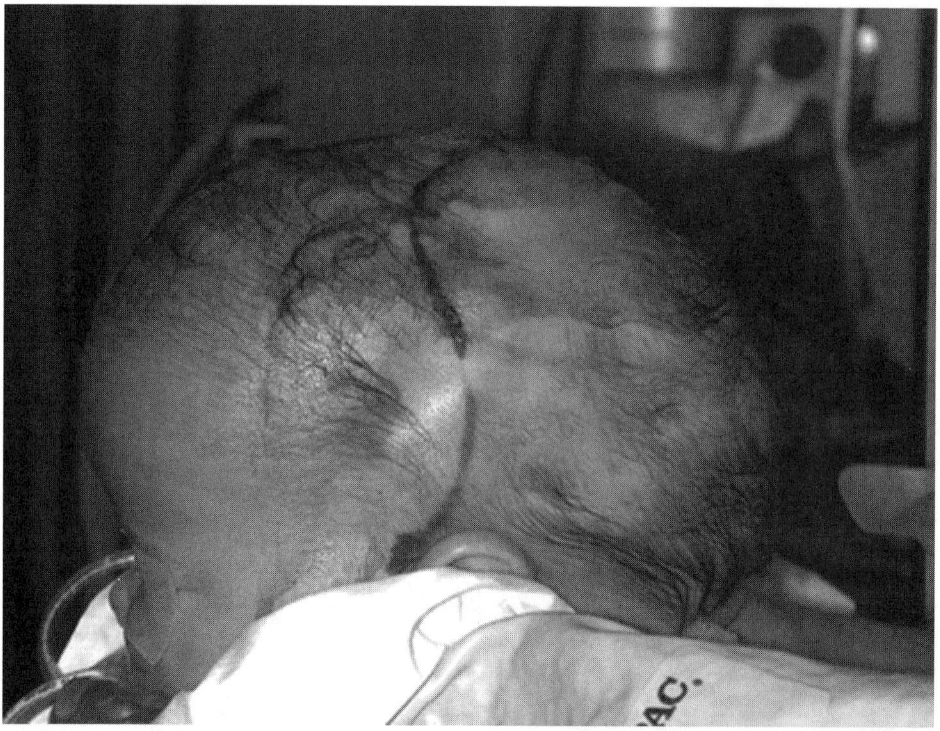

Figure 15 Position of a child with sagittal craniosynostosis. The child is supported on a bean bag in a prone position with the neck held in cervical extension. This position allows access to the anterior and the posterior aspects of the calvarium to allow correction of frontal bossing and occipital bullet.

Technique

The exposure is as described previously. A zigzag incision is utilized as a bicoronal incision across the vertex for cosmetic reasons (Fig. 15). This heals and gives a less visible scar. After extending the incision down to the subgaleal plane, a subgaleal dissection is utilized to elevate the flap both anteriorly and posteriorly. The anterior flap is brought as far as down to the level of the orbital rim. The posterior flap is brought all the way down to 1 or 2 cm above the foramen magnum. After elevation of the scalp flap, two burr holes are created. Each is at the intermedial corner of their respective parietal bones. Then, using a craniotome with a footplate, the two pure parietal bone flaps are elevated with the borders corresponding to their respective sutures: the sagittal suture, the lambdoid suture, the squamosal suture, and the coronal suture.

By opening these two parietal bone flaps, exposure of the remaining bone off the underlying dura can be done under direct vision reducing the potential of an intraoperative tear of a major dural sinus and/or the creation of a cerebrospinal fluid (CSF) leak. We have found that this particular step has increased safety and significantly reduced the time of the craniotomy flap elevation.

After mobilizing the dura, it is important then to obtain dural separation off the sagittal suture. Because the suture is already fused, this is usually quite easy and much simpler than could be done in the nonfused sagittal suture. The craniotome is usually brought across the midposition of the parietal bone, across the sagittal suture, and then carried around to create a biparietal frontal bone flap. There is no need to bring the orbital cut more than 1–1.5 cm above the orbital rim. In trying to bring it lower in this direction, the risk of dural tear in the anterior cranial dura is heightened. However, rising several centimeters usually will not enable enough of the frontal bone to be removed for reconstruction of frequently-accompanying frontal bossing.

The same procedure is repeated for the posterior bone flap in which case a biparietal occipital bone flap is elevated in the same fashion. In this posterior direction one must be particularly careful in bringing the craniotome across not only the sagittal sinus but also the transverse sinuses bilaterally. The best bone exposure extends slightly below the level of the two transverse sinuses. The parietal bones are then brought to the back table for radial osteotomies and recontouring with Tessier bone benders and other craniofacial tools.

First the bifrontal parietal bone flap is replaced followed by the biparieto-occipital bone flap. These are secured to the adjacent margins using absorbable plates. This is only done, however, after creating barrel stave osteotomies in the cranial base bone and in the temporal bone regions where an increase in the width can easily be obtained. There is no need to create barrel staves in the region of the orbital rim, which would also be dangerous. The barrel stave bones are then greenstick fractured to provide the appropriate width increase. This is checked repeatedly after bone flap adjustment to ensure that an appropriate amount of green fracturing has been obtained. The most important area of green fracturing is the sphenoid wing, because patients with sagittal synostosis often have significant temporal narrowing created by the sphenoid wing. If this is brought out laterally, the width will be significantly improved in the patient.

As mentioned, the bifrontal parietal bone flap and the biparieto-occipital bone flap can then be secured to the adjacent cranial border. Finally the midline bone struts that had been left over the sagittal suture can be decreased in length to provide the so-called squeeze technique for anteroposterior (AP) shortening. As mentioned above, this squeeze is usually 10–20 mm. It is done gradually with measurement using rule or calipers, and very slowly so that no real direct compression of the brain structure results. One will often find after the bone has been removed in a subtotal calvarectomy that the brain will easily accommodate this squeeze technique.

All that remains before the final skin closure is replacement of the parietal bone flaps. Because of the reduction in the AP length, the parietal bone flaps will need to be shorted in the AP dimension as well. These will undergo radial osteotomies and remodeling. The bone flaps are then replaced and secured with several absorbable plates and screws. If necessary, a few additional Vicryl sutures can also be utilized to hold these flaps in position.

After the approximation of the skin and a two-layer closure over a drain, the head shape can be visualized and a cephalic index can be measured directly to determine if the appropriate amount of improvement has been obtained. If 10–20 mm of shortening of the AP length is produced, an appropriate improvement in the cephalic index has been attained (Figs. 16,17).

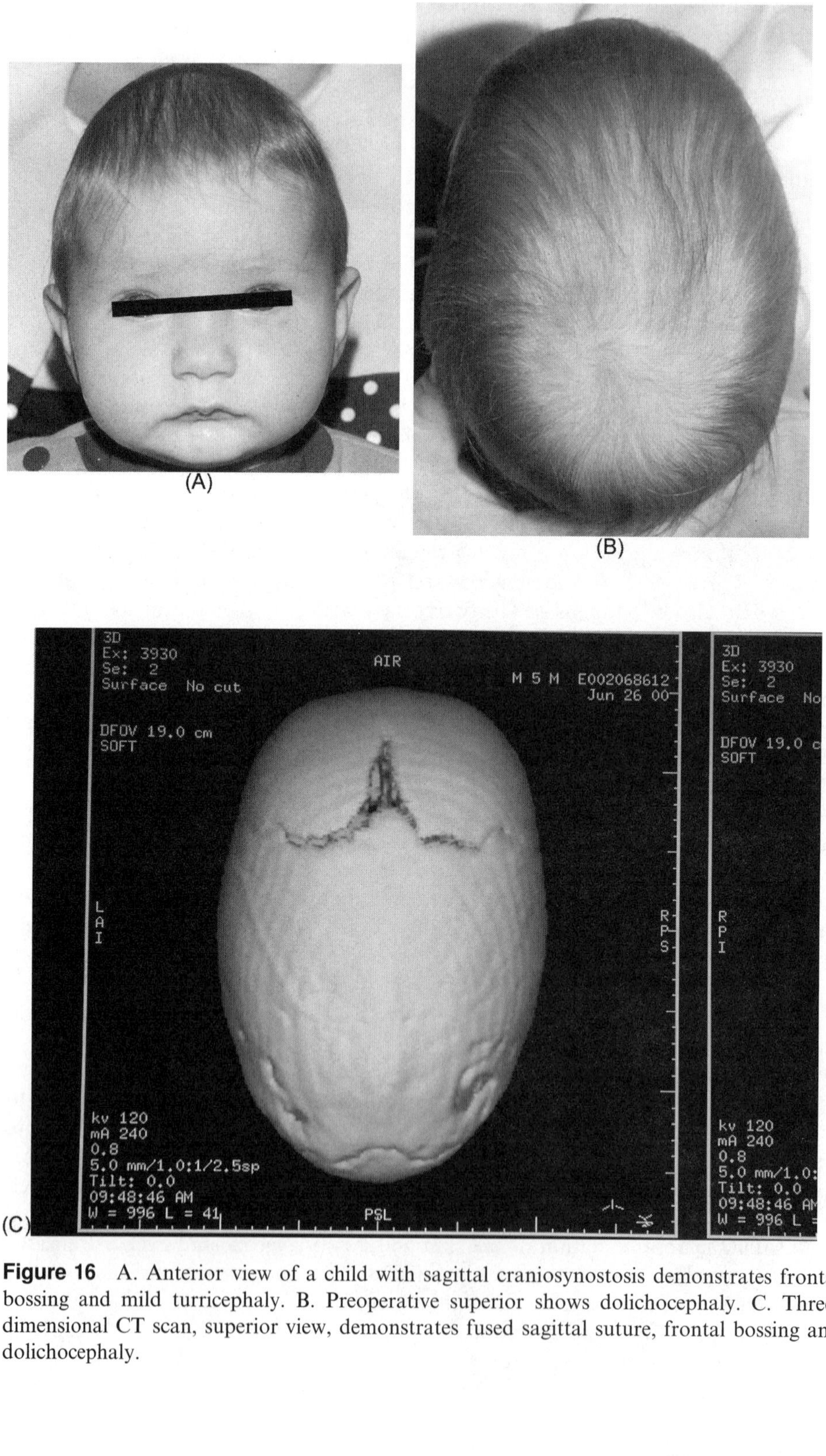

Figure 16 A. Anterior view of a child with sagittal craniosynostosis demonstrates frontal bossing and mild turricephaly. B. Preoperative superior shows dolichocephaly. C. Three-dimensional CT scan, superior view, demonstrates fused sagittal suture, frontal bossing and dolichocephaly.

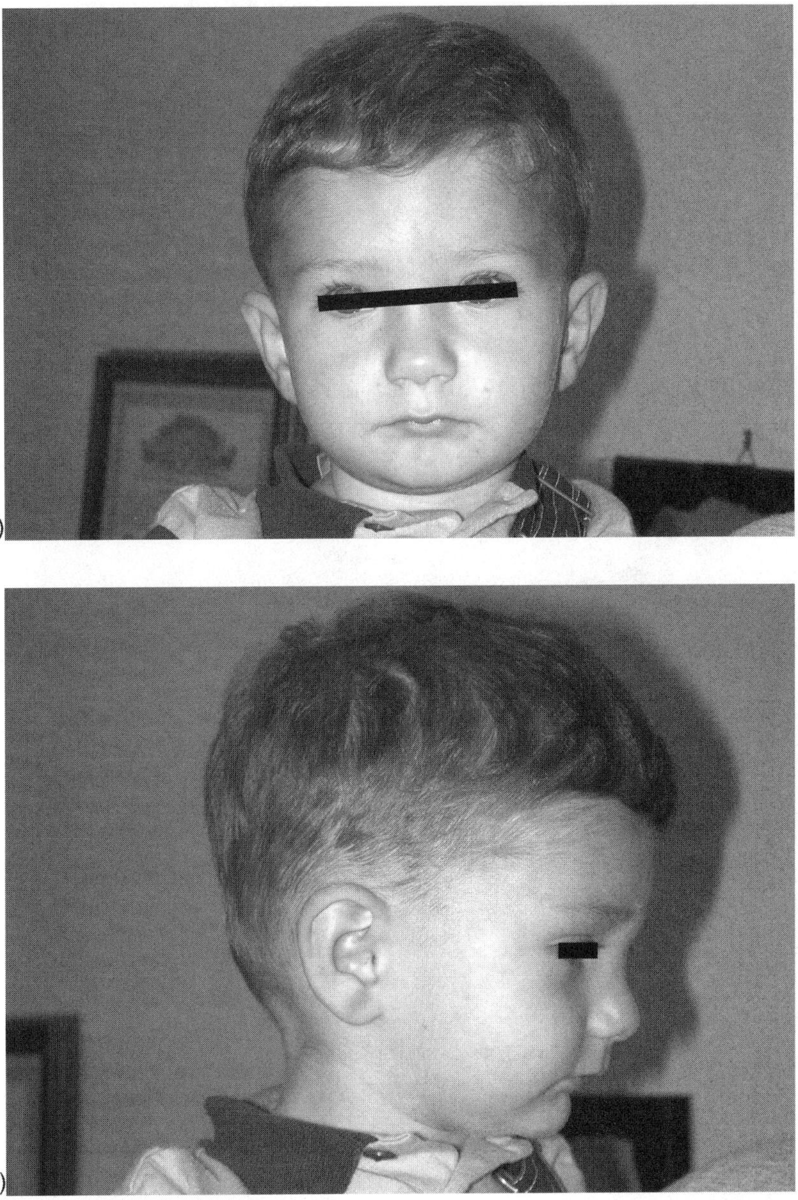

(A)

(B)

Figure 17 A. Postoperative frontal view of the same child 1 year after surgery for correction of sagittal craniosynostosis. B. Postoperative lateral view shows normocephaly and absence of frontal bossing, turricephaly and occipital bullet. C. View of a child with sagittal craniosynostosis who underwent cranial vault remodeling (1 year follow-up). Note normalization of the calvarial shape and no evidence of dolichocephaly. D. Three-dimensional CT scan 1 year following correction of sagittal craniosynostosis demonstrates normalization of the calvarial shape without evidence of dolichocephaly.

(C)
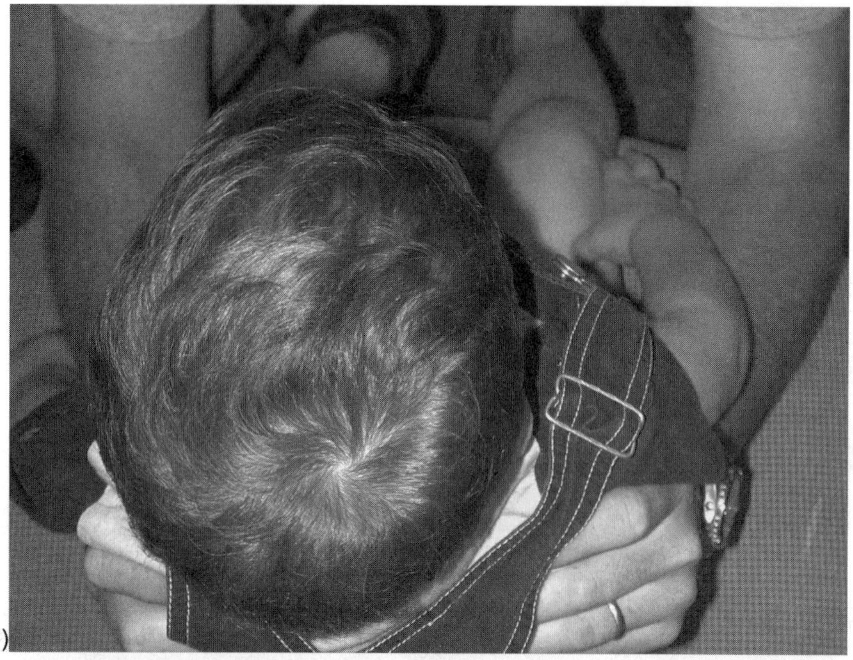

(D)
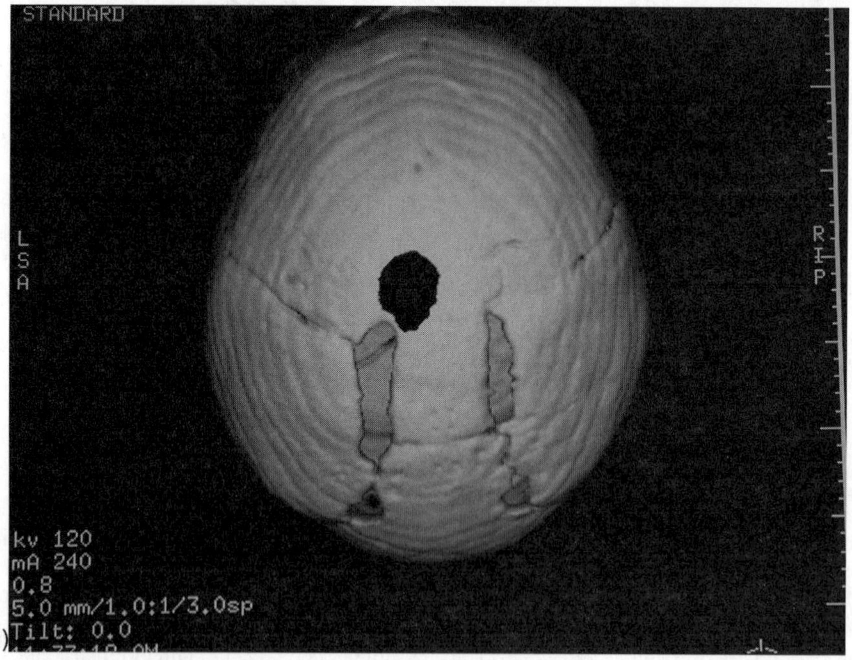

Figure 17 Continued.

Unicoronal Synostosis

Preoperative Planning

Ventral Advancement of the Supraorbital Bar. The ipsilateral supraorbital rim is recessed. A two-dimensional long-axis view along the apex of the orbit and the center of the cornea demonstrates the extent of the recession. The ipsilateral supraorbital rim is dorsal to the plane of the cornea. Normograms have revealed that the supraorbital rim is 2–3 mm ventral to the vertical plane of the cornea. The extent of ventral movement of the supraorbital rim, so as to position it 3 mm ventral to the vertical plane of the cornea, is measured. This varies between 7 and 15 mm, depending on the severity of the unicoronal synostosis.

Correction of the Asymmetry of the Orbits. The ipsilateral roof of the orbit is higher than the contralateral orbit. The contralateral orbit, in contrast, is wider than normal. The height and width of the orbit are determined utilizing normograms and the extent of correction is determined. The height of the ipsilateral orbit is reduced by excising bone at the frontozygomatic and nasomaxillary sutures. The width of the ipsilateral orbit is increased by inserting a cranial bone graft into the supraorbital rim. The height of the contralateral orbit is likewise increased by elevating the supraorbital bar and its width is then reduced by excising a bone segment from the supraorbital bar (Fig. 18).

Preoperative Preparation

As with all craniosynostosis patients, careful examination is essential to rule out other congenital anomalies. Preoperative work-up includes determination of the child's blood group. Parents or relatives are requested to donate two units of blood prior to surgery. Cell Savers are used intraoperatively to aid autotransfusion. A complete blood count (CBC) and cross match are performed intraoperatively. Surgery should be performed with a wide-bore intravenous access, intra-arterial pressure monitoring, and urethral catheterization. Intraoperative antibiotics include gentamycin and nafcillin.

Surgical Technique

After endotracheal intubation (35) the child is positioned supine on the operating table with the head on a well-padded neurosurgical horseshoe. Depending on the preference of the parents, either all the hair or only the hair along the planned incision is shaved. The head and the face to the tip of the nose are prepped and draped. This allows access to the calvarium and the orbits. A zigzag bicoronal incision is marked at midvertex to prevent the hair from parting along a straight line and thereby concealing the scar. The skin is divided with a #15 scalpel. Further dissection is performed in the subgaleal plane utilizing a coagulating cautery. The temporalis fascia is divided laterally close to its insertion and the temporalis muscle is elevated from the parietal bone until the lateral orbital wall is exposed. The dissection continues in the subgaleal plane until a point 10 mm above the supraorbital rim. The periosteum is divided with a cautery and stripped to expose the supraorbital rim. The supraorbital neurovascular bundle is gently teased out of the notch. In rare cases a narrow osteotome is necessary to relieve the neurovascular bundle. Further dissection is continued in the subperiosteal plane to expose the roof of the orbit.

A

B

C

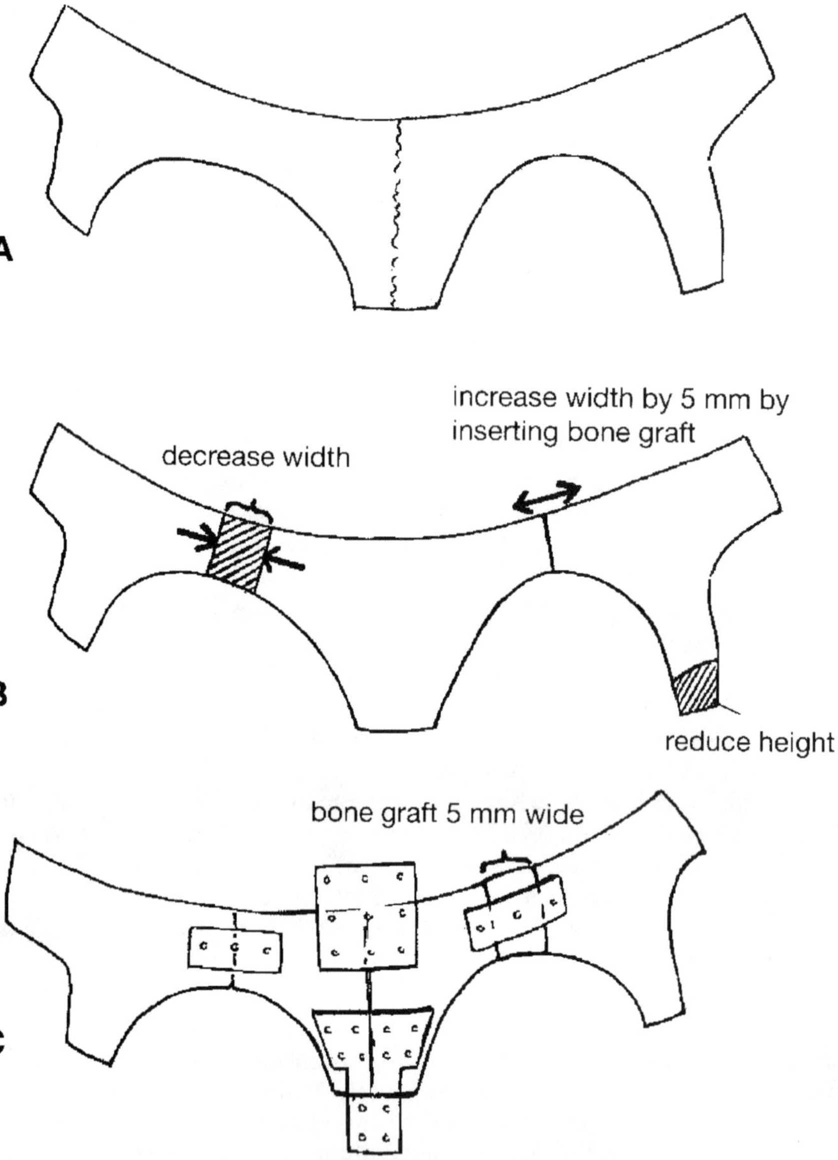

Figure 18 Graphic representation of the method of correction of the orbital asymmetry. A. Right orbit is wider and shorter than the left which is narrower and taller. B. Right orbit is decreased in its width by reducing the width of the frontal orbital bar on the right. The left frontal orbital bar is widened by 5 mm. The height of the left orbit is reduced by 3 mm. C. Corrected position of the right and the left orbit, held in position by Lactosorb plates and screws. Bone graft on the left orbit, which is 5 mm wide, is also fixed by Lactosorb plates and screws.

Care should be taken not to violate the periorbital contents. The orbital roof from the lacrimal crest medially to the frontozygomatic suture laterally is exposed.

The neurosurgeon and the craniofacial surgeon plan osteotomies. The osteotomy is planned anteriorly 12–15 mm above the supraorbital rim. Laterally the osteotomies reach the pterion and extend inferiorly and ventrally to span the lateral orbital wall to reach the frontozygomatic suture. Posteriorly the osteotomies are planned to reach 20–25 mm dorsal to the coronal sutures. Once the surgeons mark the osteotomies, the neurosurgeon creates a burr hole at the intersection of the proposed osteotomy sites. The osteotomies are performed utilizing a Midas-Rex osteotome with a shoe. Once the frontal osteotomies are performed, the dura is separated from the bone using a Penfield dissector. Care is taken to prevent any dural perforation. If any dural lacerations are detected, these are immediately repaired. The frontal bones are excised and delivered to the craniofacial surgeon. The dura from the anterior cranial fossa is dissected from pterion to pterion. Malleable retractors are used to retract the frontal lobes and the periorbital contents. An osteotomy is made in the roof of the orbit using a Midas osteotome. The osteotomy in the anterior cranial fossa is extended medially to reach the crista galli and laterally to reach the pterion. A reciprocating saw is then used to complete the osteotomy from the pterion to the frontozygomatic suture and from the ipsilateral lacrimal crest to the contralateral lacrimal crest across the nasofrontal suture. A 3 mm osteotome is then utilized to complete the osteotomy by gently tapping with a mallet. The supraorbital bar is then excised and delivered to the side assembly table.

The craniofacial surgeon divides the supraorbital bar in the midline. Each superior orbital bar is split at the highest point and either widened or narrowed depending on the preoperative measurements from the three-dimensional CT scan. The supraorbital bar is likewise either located inferiorly or superiorly to reduce or increase the height of the orbit. A T-shaped Lactosorb absorbable is utilized to fix rigidly the two halves of the supraorbital bar. An eight-hole absorbable plate is fixed at the most lateral end of the supraorbital bar. The supraorbital bar is then advanced by 7–15 mm depending on the preoperative CT scan measurements. A tenon and mortise calvarial bone graft is then inserted in the interval at the site of the advancement. The posterior (dorsal) end of the absorbable plate is rigidly fixed using absorbable 1.5 mm screws. This method allows achievement of symmetrical orbits and supraorbital bar irrespective of the severity of the synostosis.

If narrowing is present at the pterion preoperatively, it is corrected by radial osteotomy at the pterion and outfractures of the pterion. Each frontal bone is then shaped by performing multiple radial osteotomies along the inferior and posterior border. Tessier's bone benders are used to correct the frontal bossing by either increasing or decreasing the convexity of the frontal bones. Once both frontal bones appear symmetrical in shape, they are placed over the supraorbital bar and rigidly fixed using absorbable 1.5 mm plates and screws (Fig. 19).

The temporalis muscle is advanced and reattached to the temporal bone utilizing absorbable sutures through holes created in the calvarium. This step is essential to prevent an hourglass deformity of the calvarium. The scalp flap is replaced and symmetry is confirmed. A single 7 mm suction drain is placed underneath the scalp flap and the wound closed in layers using interrupted sutures of 4/0 Vicryl for the

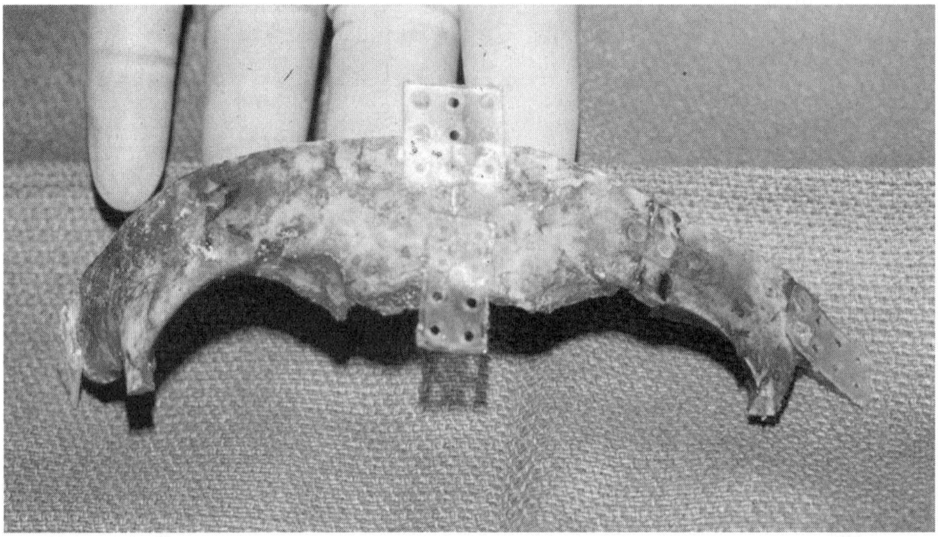

Figure 19 Fronto-orbital bar demonstrates correction as mentioned in Figure 18. Note the presence of an absorbable plate at the lateral aspect of the fronto-orbital bar, which will allow rigid fixation and advancement of the left frontal orbital bar at the pterion.

galea and continuos percutaneous rapidly absorbing Vicryl for the skin. A light dressing and a head bandage complete the procedure. (Figs. 20,21).

Bicoronal Synostosis

The objective of surgery is to increase the anteroposterior dimension of the calvarium by ventrally advancing the frontoparietal bones and the fronto-orbital bar. The latter would increase the projection of the supraorbital rim 2 mm beyond the corneal plane.

Planning

Appropriate software that allows delineation of the bone segments and their advancements can be used. Most such programs are cumbersome and require prolonged duration of manipulation before the appropriate position is obtained. In spite of the most accurate preoperative planning, current software does not allow intraoperative confirmation that the desired position is reached. The recent surge in frameless stereotactic neurosurgery procedures will probably allow accurate confirmation of the desired position intraoperatively.

A two-dimensional sagittal image is used for preoperative calculations. This image traverses the centroid (center of the ocular globe) and the center of the orbital apex. The position of the supraorbitale is confirmed on this view. The corneal plane is developed by passing a line connecting the infraorbitale to the most prominent point of the cornea. The line is extended so that it passes 2 mm ventral to

(A)

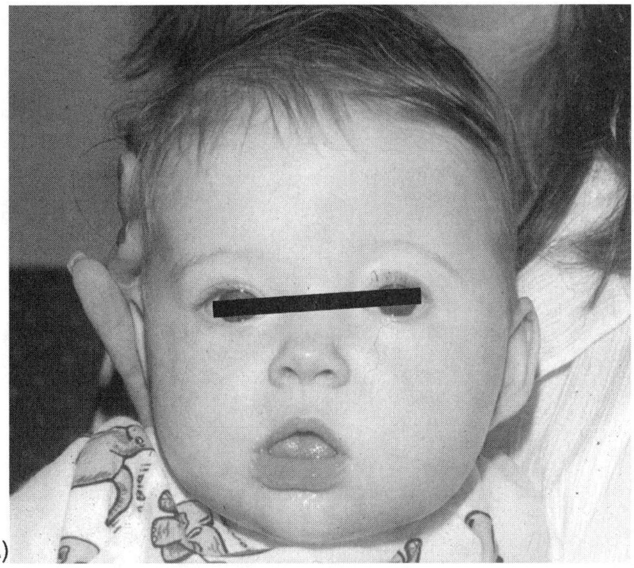

(B)

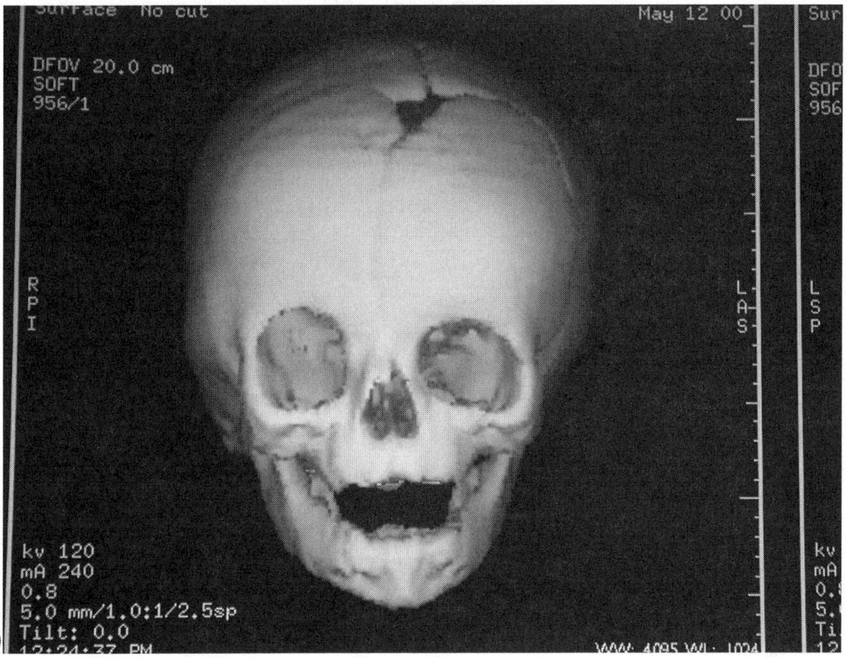

Figure 20 A. A 4-month-old child with unicoronal synostosis with asymmetry of the orbits and mild asymmetry of the facial axis. Note the discrepancy between the size of the palpebral fissures. B. Three-dimensional CT scan demonstrates right unicoronal synostosis. The right orbit is narrower and taller than the contralateral side. Note the deviation in the facial axis. C. Preoperative three-dimensional CT seen from the superior view. Note that the right coronal suture is fused compared to the metopic, left coronal, and sagittal sutures, which are patent. D. Preoperative three-dimensional CT scan endocranial view demonstrates asymmetry of the greater wings of the sphenoid and anterior cranial fossa, with deviation of the facial axis.

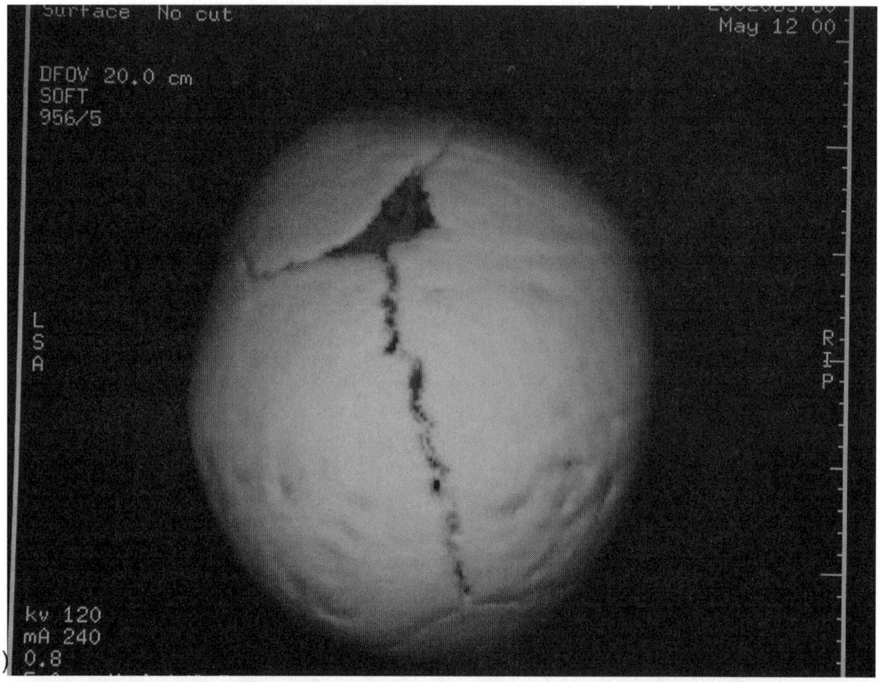

(C)

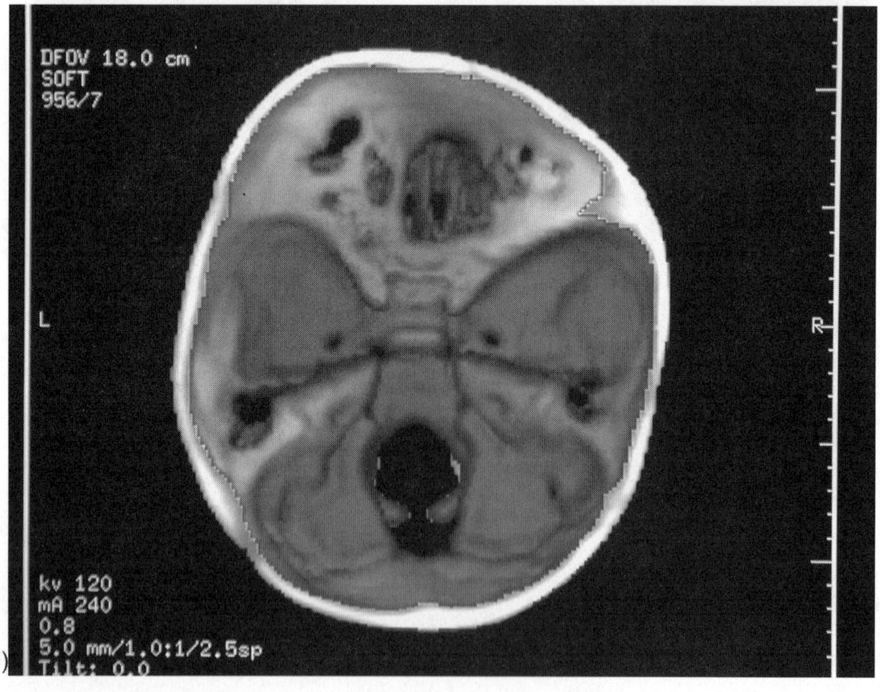

(D)

Figure 20 Continued.

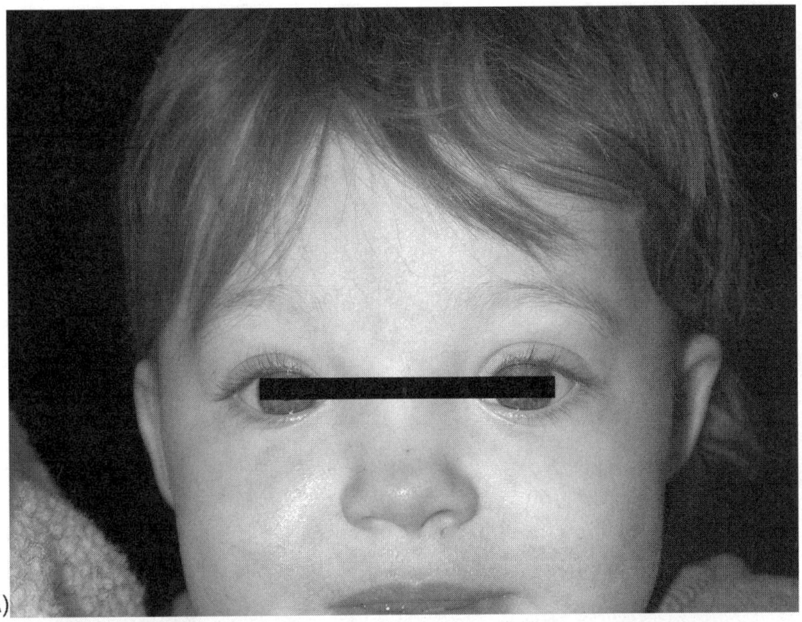

(A)

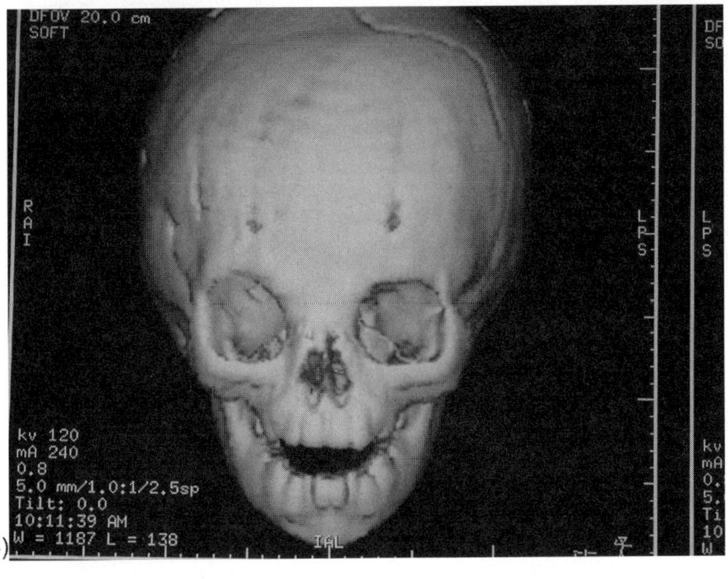

(B)

Figure 21 A. Same child 1 year after surgery. Note significant improvement in the position of the orbit and the palpebral fissure and improvement in the deviation of the facial axis. B. One year postoperative three-dimensional CT scan. Note the improvement in the position of the orbits as well as correction of deviation in the facial axis. C. One year postoperative three-dimensional CT scan also shows perfect symmetry of the calvarium, correction of frontal bossing, and minimal-size osseous defects. D. One year postoperative endocranial view shows significant improvement in the symmetry of the anterior cranial fossa and improvement in deviation of the anterior cranial base.

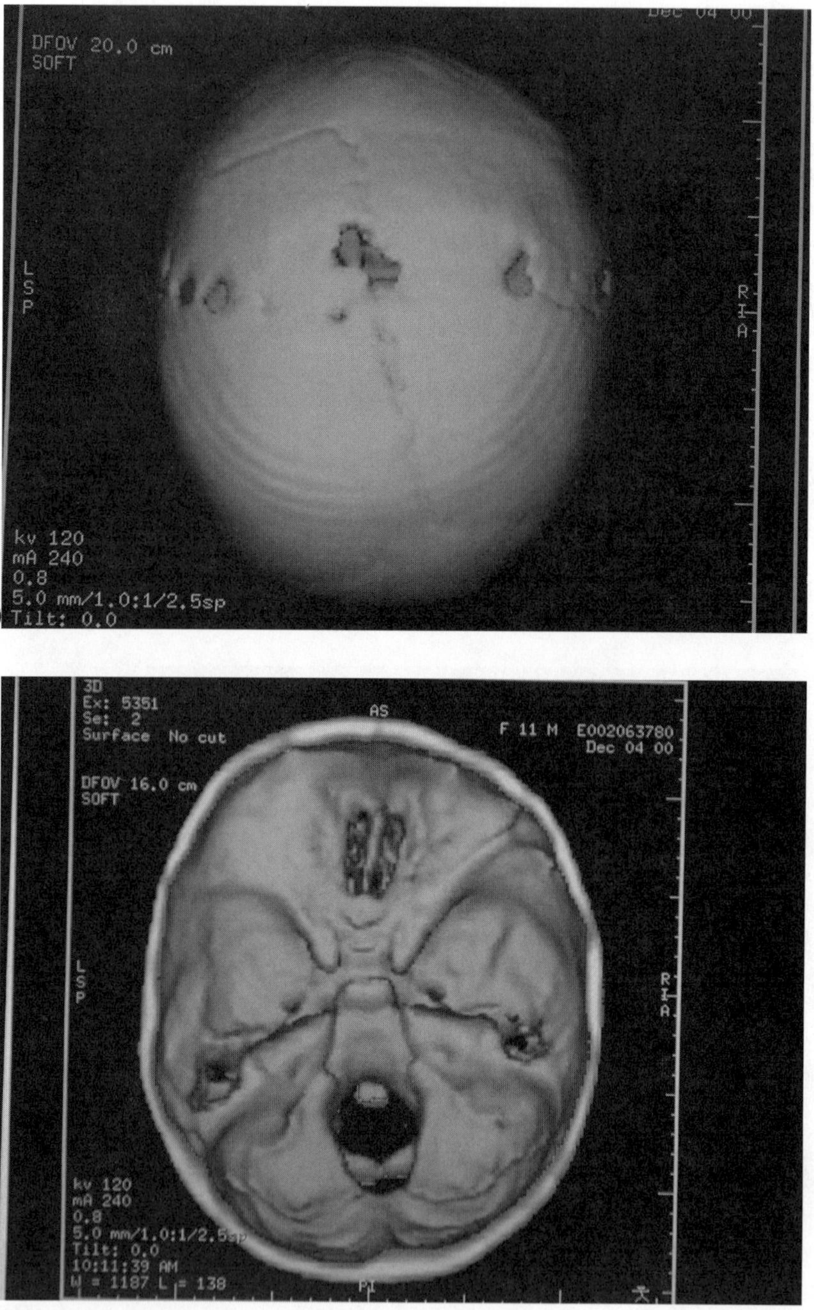

(C)

(D)

Figure 21 Continued.

the cornea. This gives an approximate extent of ventral advancement of the fronto-orbital bar.

Operative details

A frontal and parietal craniotomy is performed and the fronto-orbital area is excised as in unicoronal synostosis. The fronto-parietal bar is then advanced by 7–15 mm so that the supraorbitale is 2 mm ventral to the corneal plane (the precise measurement is calculated preoperatively as discussed above). The fronto-orbital bar is then rigidly fixed at three points: nasion, and bilaterally at the pterion. Rigid fixation especially at the nasion is critical. A study comparing rigid fixation with bone graft and poly-lactic acid suture (Vicryl) revealed a better outcome for rigid fixation at 1 year. While making the osteotomy within the calvarium, it is useful to place it posterior to the bicoronal suture at the maximum transverse biparietal diameter. The site of the cal-varial advancement thereby comes to lie dorsal to the maximum biparietal diameter. As reossification takes place within the osseous defect created by the advancement, it is not uncommon to have a narrowing at this site. If this narrowing is dorsal to the widest part of the calvarium, it not visible and prevents the typical hourglass deformity of the calvarium. (Figs. 22,23).

Metopic Synostosis

The objective of surgery is to increase the volume of the anterior cranial fossa by performing a ventral advancement of the fronto-orbital bar. Since the interorbital distance is reduced, the bifrontal diameter needs to be increased at the pterion to correct the abnormality (Fig. 24).

Operative Details

These are described in detail elsewhere (36) Following the frontoparietal craniotomy, the fronto-orbital bar is excised and transferred to the side assembly table. The bar is split in the midline. A calvarial bone graft is placed between the two halves to correct the reduced interdacryon distance. The width of the bone graft should be equal to the extent of correction necessary to normalize the interdacryon distance. If the bar is thick at the midline, a tenon mortise bone joint is used to increase the stability of the bone graft. A T-shaped absorbable plate is utilized to fix the graft at the junction of the fronto-orbital bar and the nasion. The extent of advancement does not generally exceed 5 mm at the pterion. The fronto-orbital bar is typically V-shaped in metopic synostosis due to the trigonocephaly. It is therefore important to change the shape of the fronto-orbital bar by creating a wedge-shaped cut at the junction of the medial two-thirds and lateral one-third of the fronto-orbital bar. This allows creation of a normal contour of the forehead. The frontal bones are reshaped by making multiple osteotomies. The osteotomies are made with straight Mayo scissors if the child is less than 6–8 months in the older child, one needs to use a side cutting burr or a sagittal saw. The remodeled bone is fixed using absorbable plates. A T-shaped plate is used at the nasion and a 2×4 plate at the pterion (Figs. 25,26).

Postoperative Care and Follow-up

Following extubation the child is transferred to the pediatric intensive care unit for 24–48 h. This allows close monitoring for level of consciousness and hemodynamic

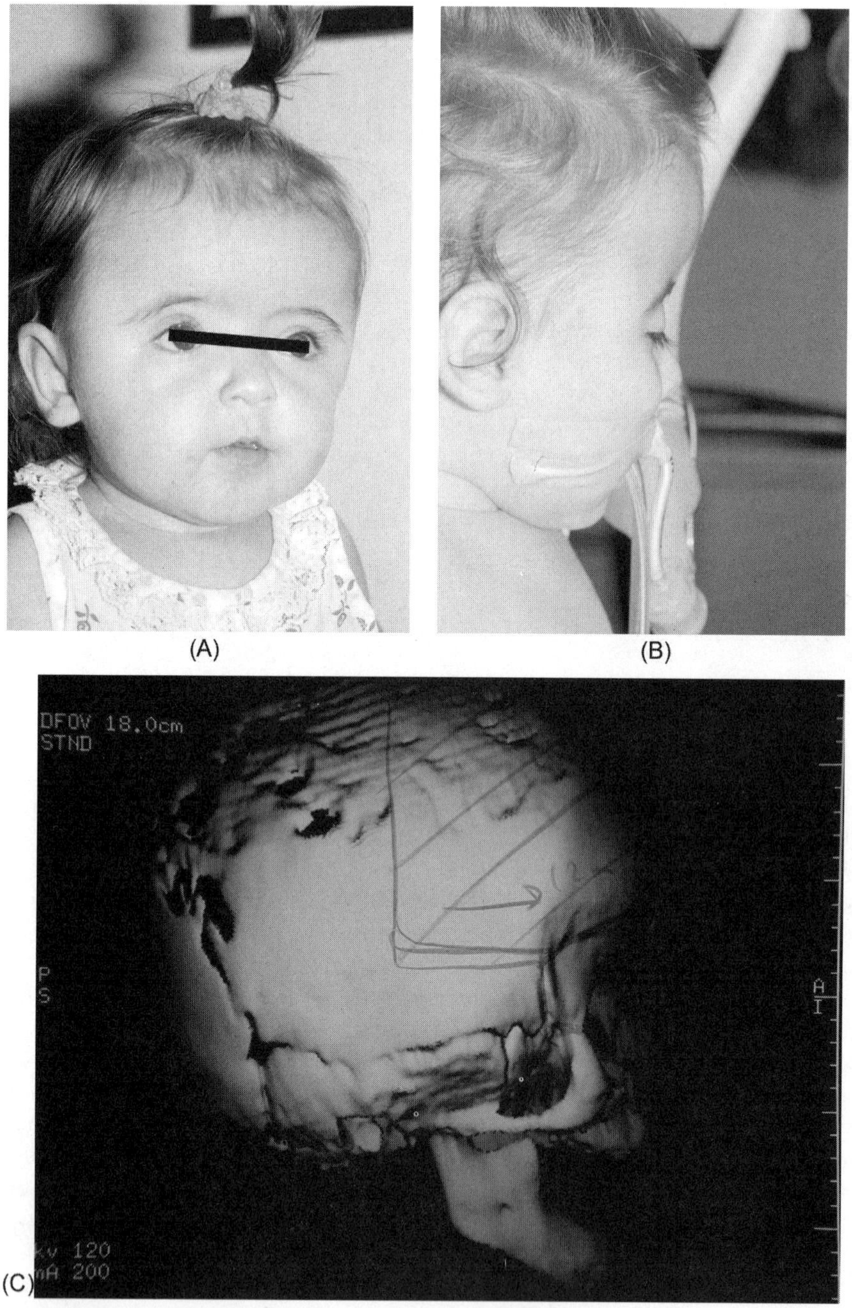

Figure 22 A. Preoperative frontal view photograph of a 6-month-old child with bicoronal synostosis. Note the frontal bossing bilaterally. B. Preoperative lateral photograph shows recession of the frontal orbital bar and exorbitism. C. Preoperative three-dimensional CT scan lateral view demonstrates bicoronal synostosis, recession of frontal orbital bar and hypoplasia of the lateral wall of the right orbit. D. Preoperative three-dimensional CT scan superior view demonstrates bilateral fused coronal sutures with patent sagittal and lambdoid sutures with severe restriction in the anterior/posterior dimension of the anterior cranial fossa.

(D)
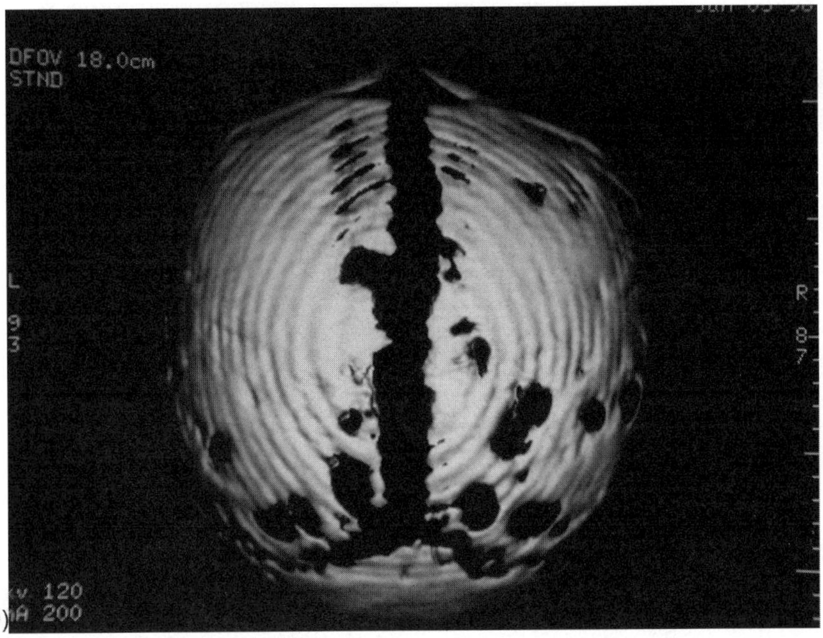

Figure 22 Continued.

stability. Parents are warned that there will be considerable swelling of the scalp and periorbital contents, which diminishes in 3 days. It is not unusual for the child to experience a temperature of 38°C for the first 72 h. Continuing pyrexia and persistent swelling and cellulitis should be a source of concern and investigated.

A three-dimensional CT scan is performed on the fifth postoperative day. This provides an accurate documentation of the sites of osteotomy and allows the surgeons to confirm whether the appropriate symmetry and ventral advancement were achieved intraoperatively. The child is then discharged. Further follow-up is performed at 3 weeks, 6 weeks, 3 months, 6 months, 1 year, an annual visit until age 6, and then once every 2–3 years. Longitudinal follow-up by a craniofacial team allows assessment of the disease and the procedure on the child's neuropsychological development and craniofacial growth.

A three-dimensional CT scan and MRI scan performed 1 year following surgery are helpful in documenting whether the ventral movement and symmetry of the orbits have been maintained. Recently, the authors have started performing a PET scan before and 3 months postoperatively to document changes in metabolism of the cortex underlying the fused suture.

Complications

To reduce mortality and morbidity, this surgery should be performed in a children's hospital with pediatric anesthesiology and pediatric intensive care facilities. Recent series have demonstrated only isolated cases of mortality. The most common cause of mortality is insufficient blood replacement intraoperatively. Blood loss should be minimized and replaced quickly.

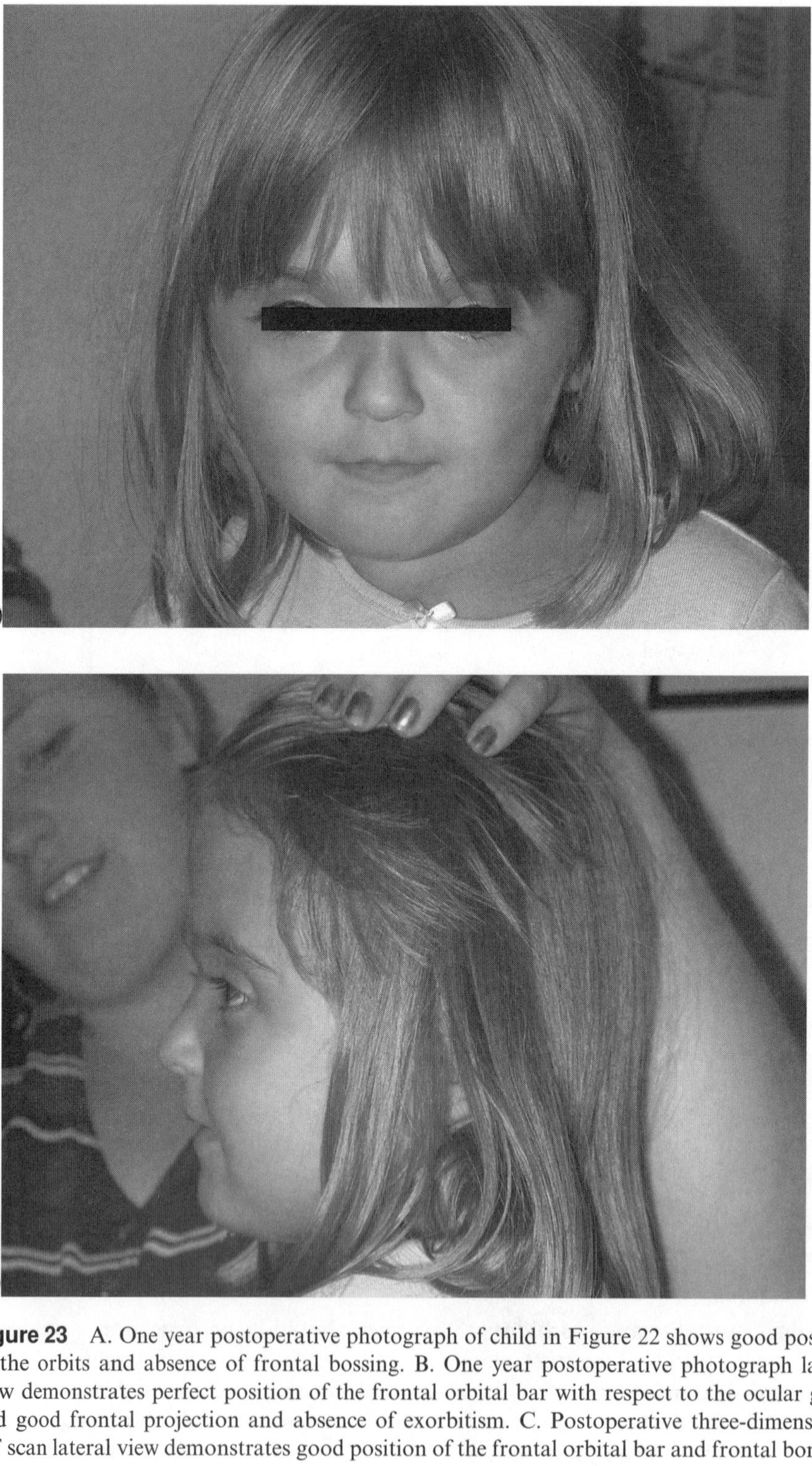

(A) (B)

Figure 23 A. One year postoperative photograph of child in Figure 22 shows good position of the orbits and absence of frontal bossing. B. One year postoperative photograph lateral view demonstrates perfect position of the frontal orbital bar with respect to the ocular globe and good frontal projection and absence of exorbitism. C. Postoperative three-dimensional CT scan lateral view demonstrates good position of the frontal orbital bar and frontal bones in

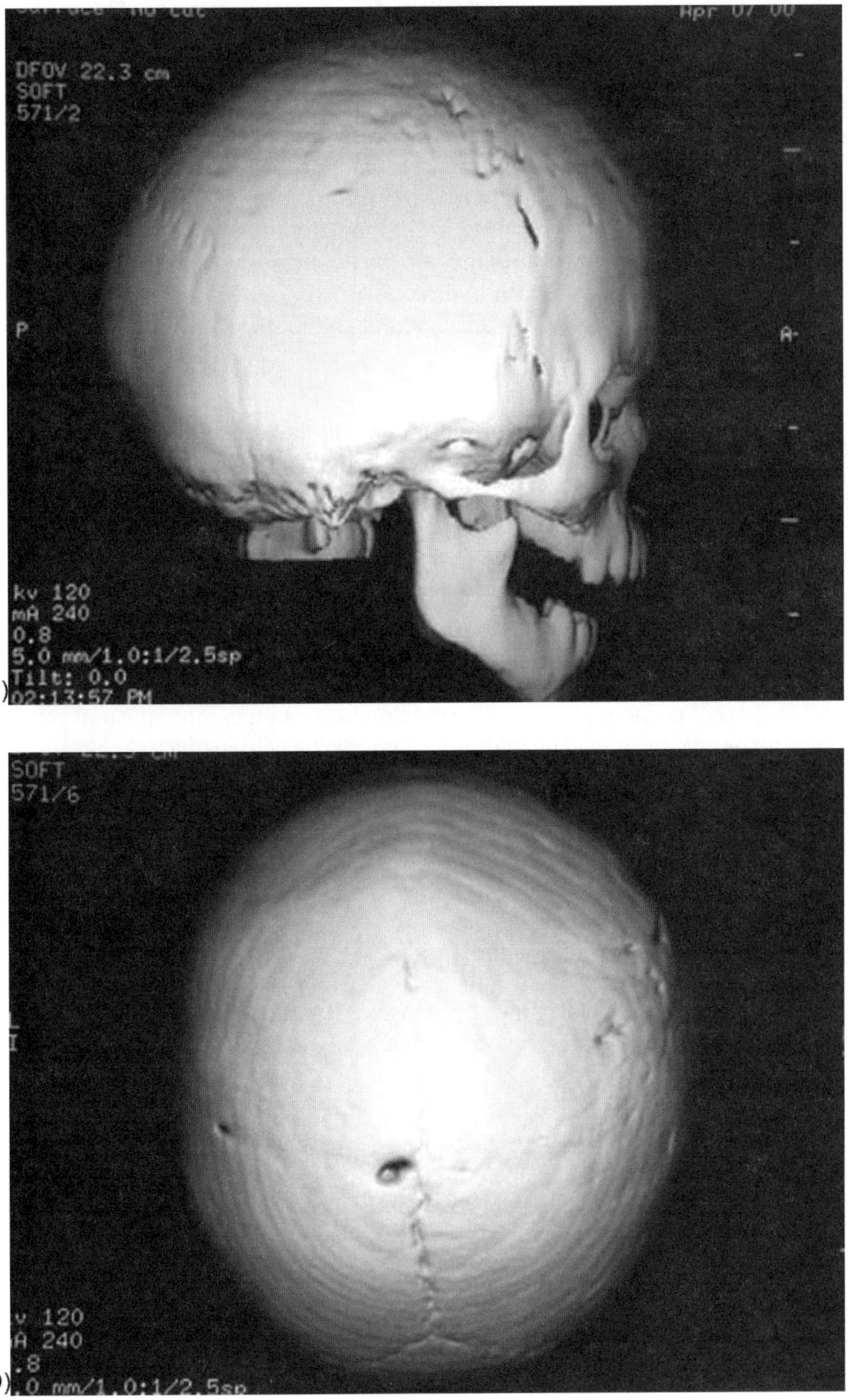

(C)

(D)

Figure 23 (continued) relation to the orbits, and correction of the anterior/posterior dimension of the lateral wall of the right orbit. D. Note perfect symmetry of the right and left frontal bones and good projection of the anterior cranial fossa without osseous bony defects.

The incidence of wound infection and dehiscence is extremely low. Cranial bone graft infection can be minimized significantly by administering a 48 h prophylactic antibiotic regimen consisting of nafcillin and gentamycin. Continuing CSF leakage is extremely rare if adequate precautions are taken to ensure the proper closure of dural tears intraoperatively.

Long-term follow-up may reveal minor asymmetries of the supraorbital bar and forehead. They can be corrected using hydroxyapatite paste. Ossification within the orbit takes place rapidly and is complete in the majority of patients within a year following surgery (38). Persistent areas of incomplete ossification larger than a centimeter in diameter are similarly treated with hydroxyapatite paste. Major asymmetries may require revision osteotomy and readvancement of the supraorbital bar.

Absorbable Plates

Just as titanium plating devices revolutionized maxillofacial fixation ensuring a rigid fixation that resulted in a better outcome, absorbable plating systems have revolutionized pediatric craniofacial surgery.

There was initial enthusiasm for using titanium plating devices in children with growing calvarium. Complications occurred as the resorption of inner table and deposition of new bone on the outer table led to gradual progression of the titanium plates over the calvarium onto the dura, sometimes coming in direct contact with the brain.

At the same time the absorbable plating technology was becoming more dependable (Fig. 27). These plates are manufactured from a combination of polyglycolic acid and polylactic acid. The addition of polylactic acid increases the resorption period of the plate, which varies from 12 to 36 months. Resorption typically occurs by hydrolysis and therefore does not incite a inflammatory reaction. Studies have documented that the rigidity offered by absorbable plating devices is equivalent to that of titanium devices. The absorbable screws, unfortunately, need to be tapped adding time to surgery, but with practice this is negligible.

Use of Hydroxyapatite Bone Substitute

Although hydroxyapatite has been used extensively by orthopedic surgeons for joint implants and by maxillofacial surgeons for chin augmentation, the compound has

Figure 24 A. The frontal orbital bar has been excised and split in the midline. B. Lateral view. A small burr is used to create a tenon and mortise joint reconstruction for stability to widen the frontal orbital bar. C. Small calvarial graft between the two halves of the frontal orbital bar. The tenon and mortise fixation technique is demonstrated. D. The small calvarial bone graft is placed between the right and the left frontal orbital bar and held in position. E. Superior view of the frontal orbital bar demonstrates the calvarial bone graft with the two halves of the frontal orbital bar. F. An absorbable inverted T-shaped plate is used to fix the bone graft to the frontal orbital bar. The vertical element of the T plate will be used to fix the frontal orbital bar at the nasion. G. The greenstick osteotomies are performed at the junction of the medial two-thirds and lateral one-third of the frontal orbital bar on each side to improve the projection of the frontal orbital bars at these sites. H. Superior view of the frontal orbital bar and dura of the underlying cortex. Note the position of the frontal orbital bar, demonstrating an improvement in the widening of the bifrontal diameter and improving projection of the frontal orbital bar.

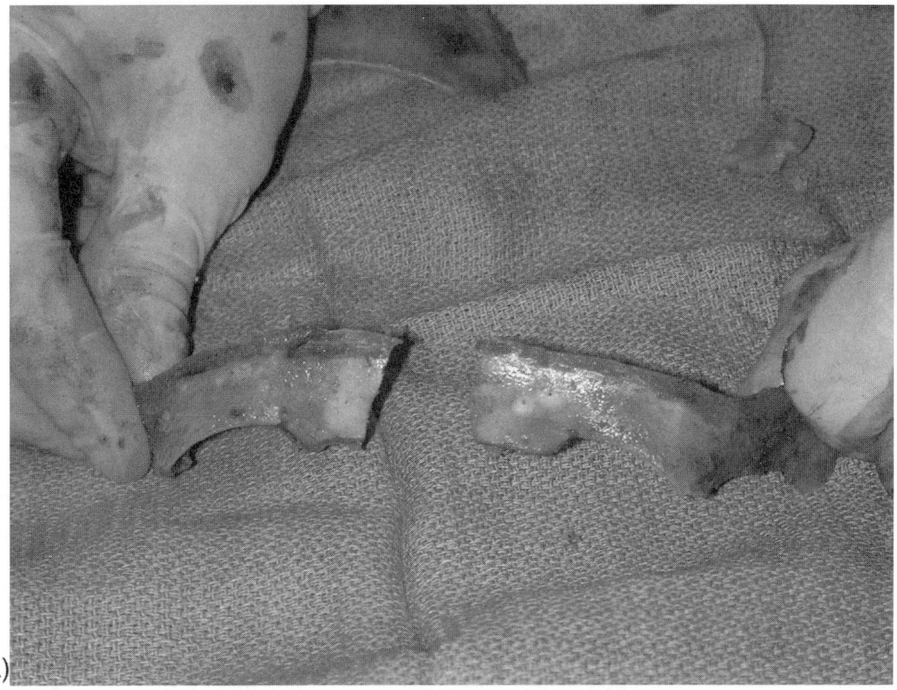

(A)

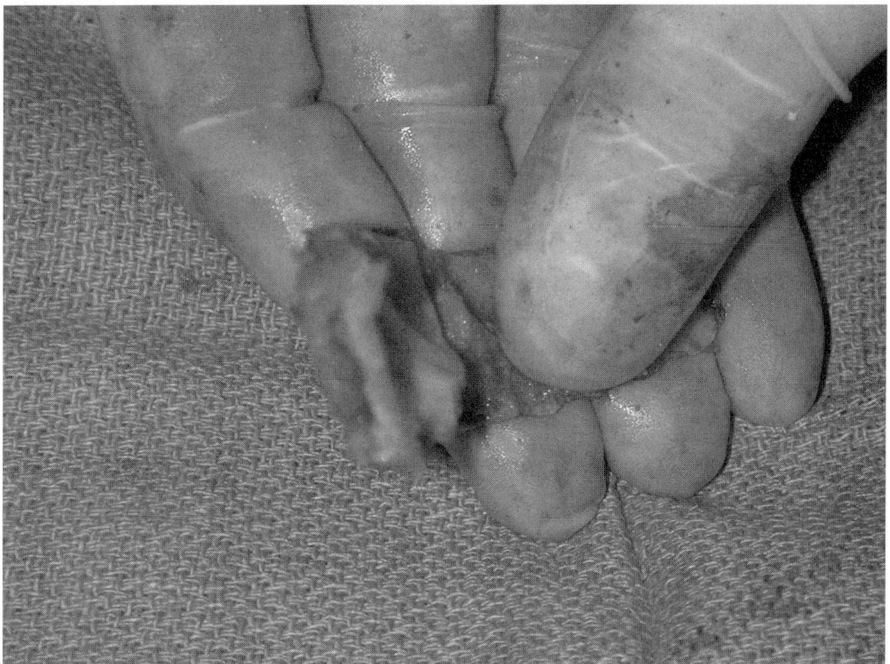

(B)

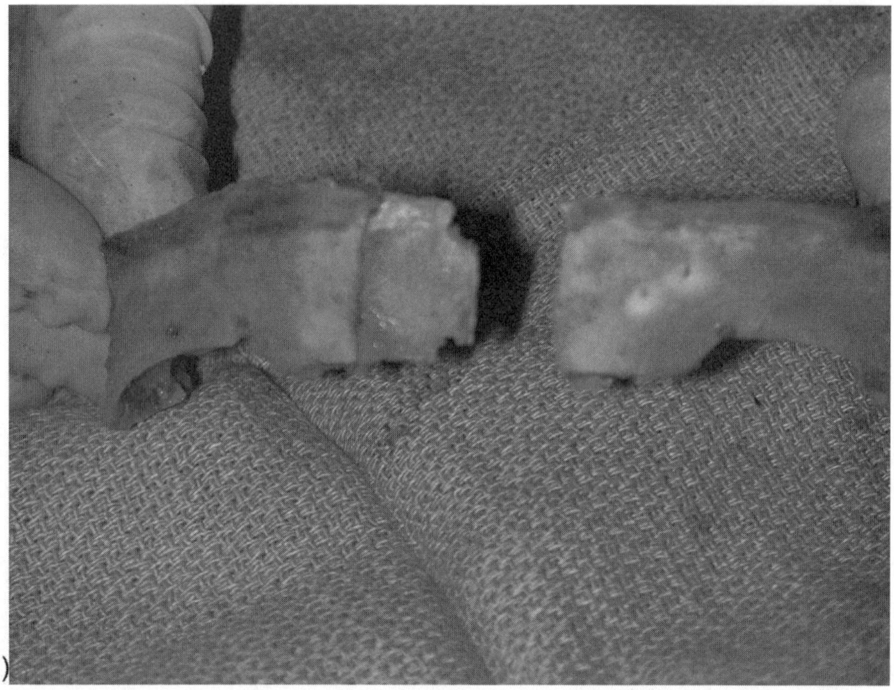

(C)

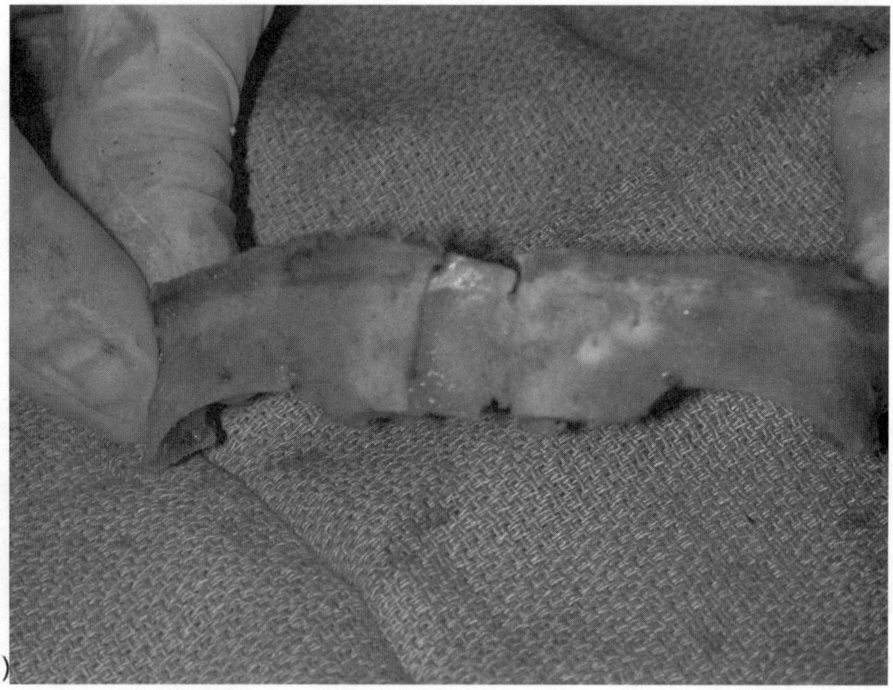

(D)

Figure 24 Continued.

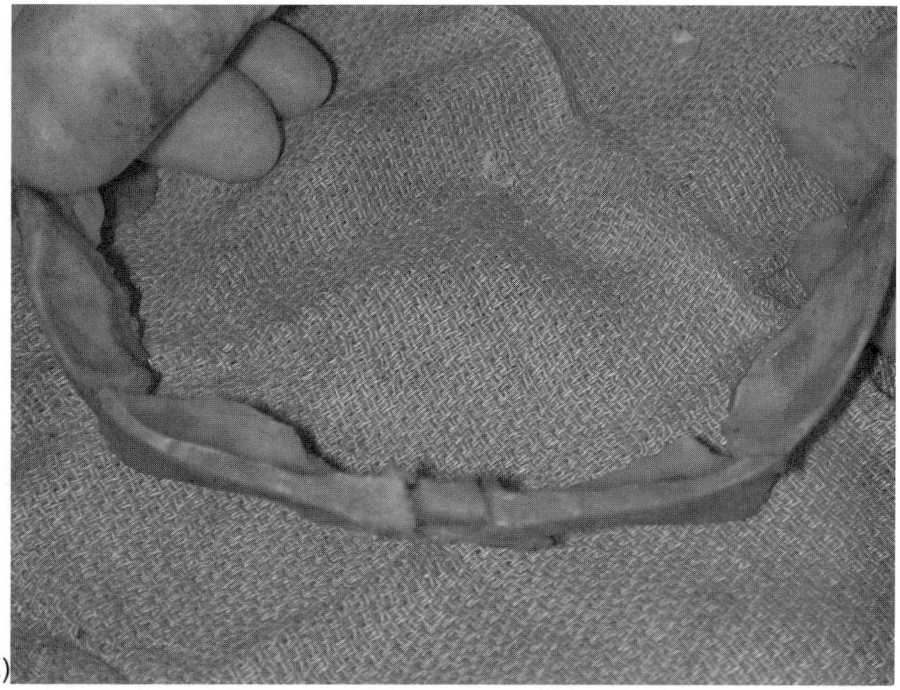

(E)

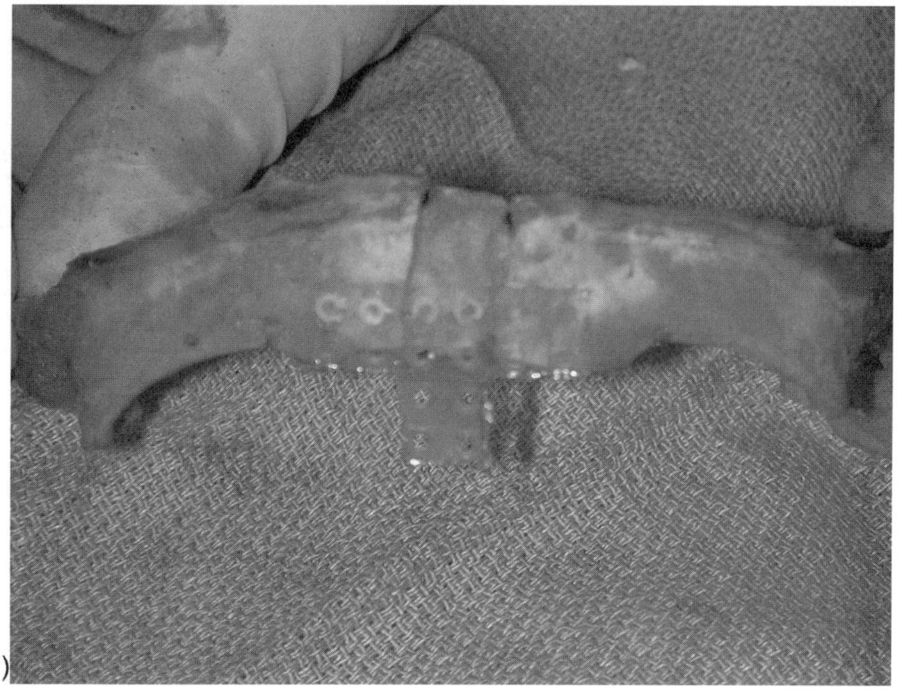

(F)

Figure 24 Continued.

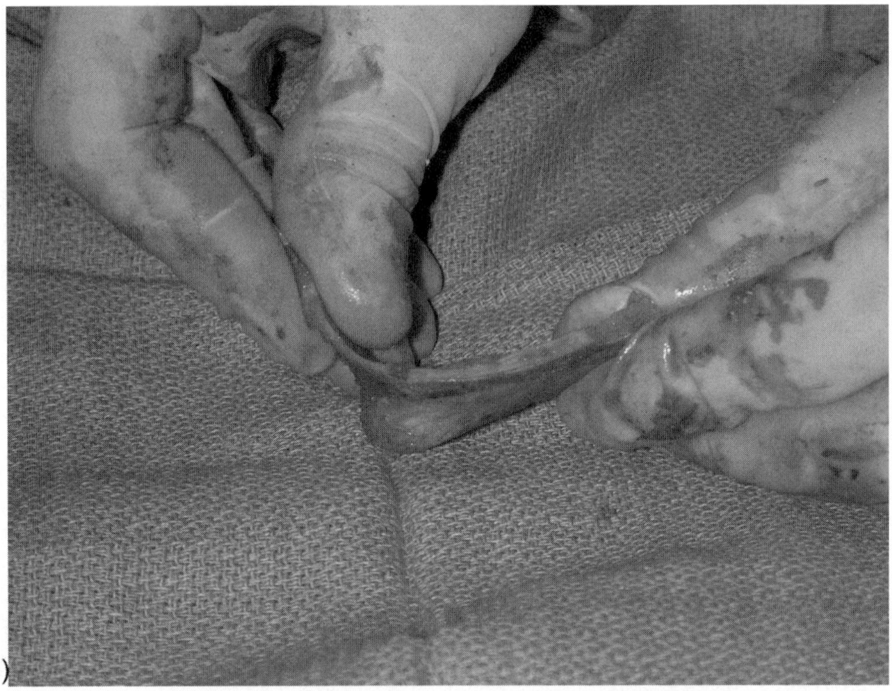

(G)

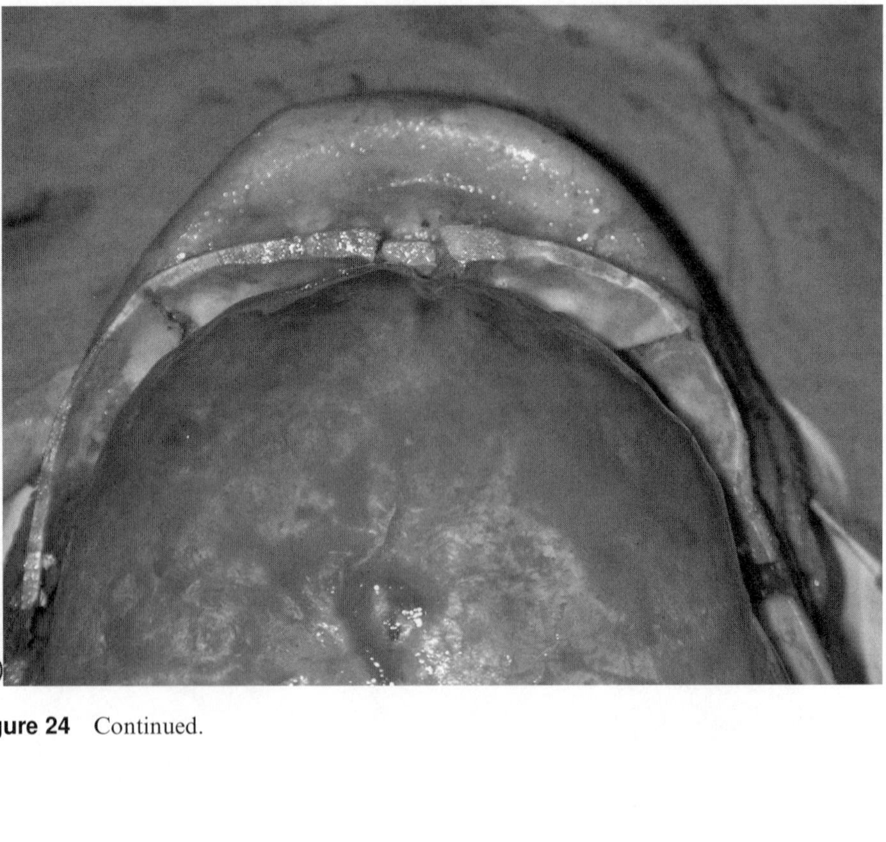

(H)

Figure 24 Continued.

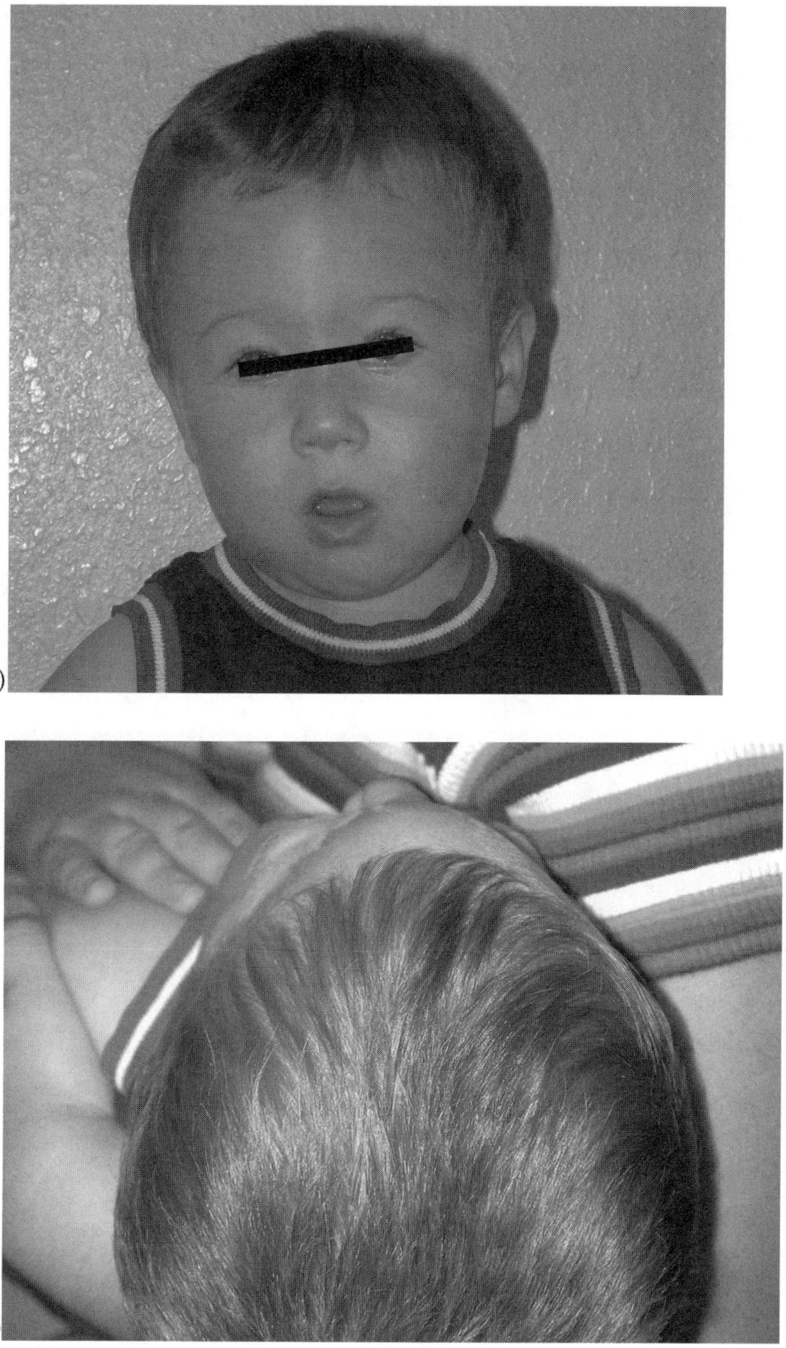

(A)

(B)

Figure 25 A. Preoperative frontal view of a child with metopic craniosynostosis shows a visible metopic ridge. B. Preoperative superior view demonstrates trigonocephaly. C. Preoperative three-dimensional CT scan frontal view demonstrates metopic craniosynostosis. D. Preoperative three-dimensional CT scan superior view demonstrates trigonocephaly and fused metopic suture.

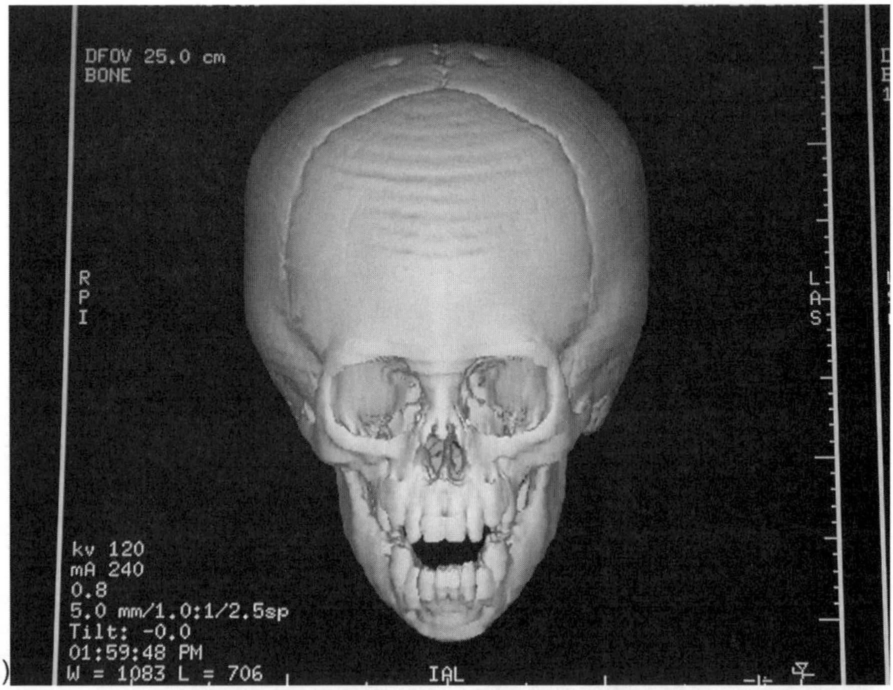

(C)

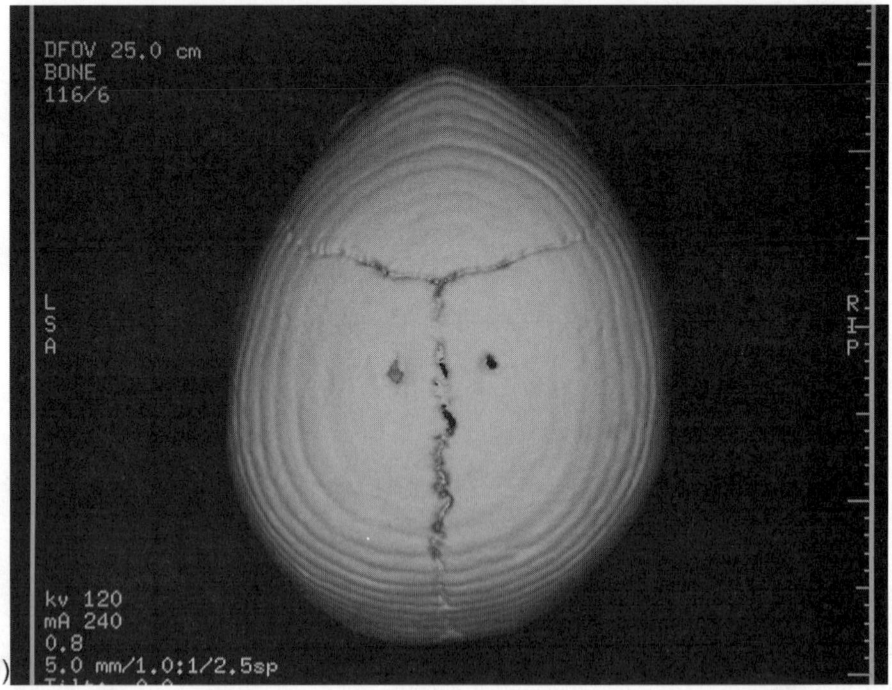

(D)

Figure 25 Continued.

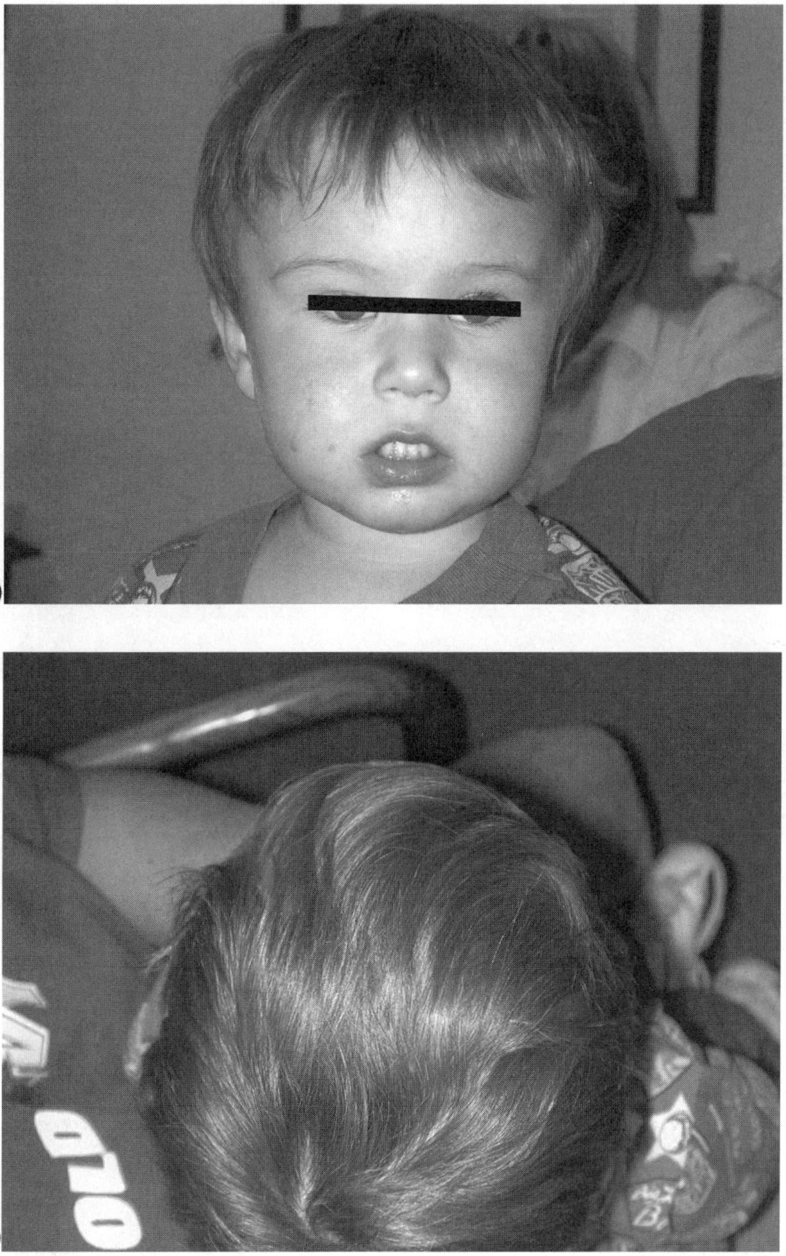

(A)

(B)

Figure 26 A. Postoperative frontal view demonstrates normalization of the trigonocephaly. B. Postoperative superior view demonstrates correction of trigonocephaly. C. Postoperative three-dimensional CT scan frontal view demonstrates correction of trigonocephaly D. Postoperative three-dimensional CT scan superior view demonstrates site of the osteotomy and improvement in the trigonocephaly.

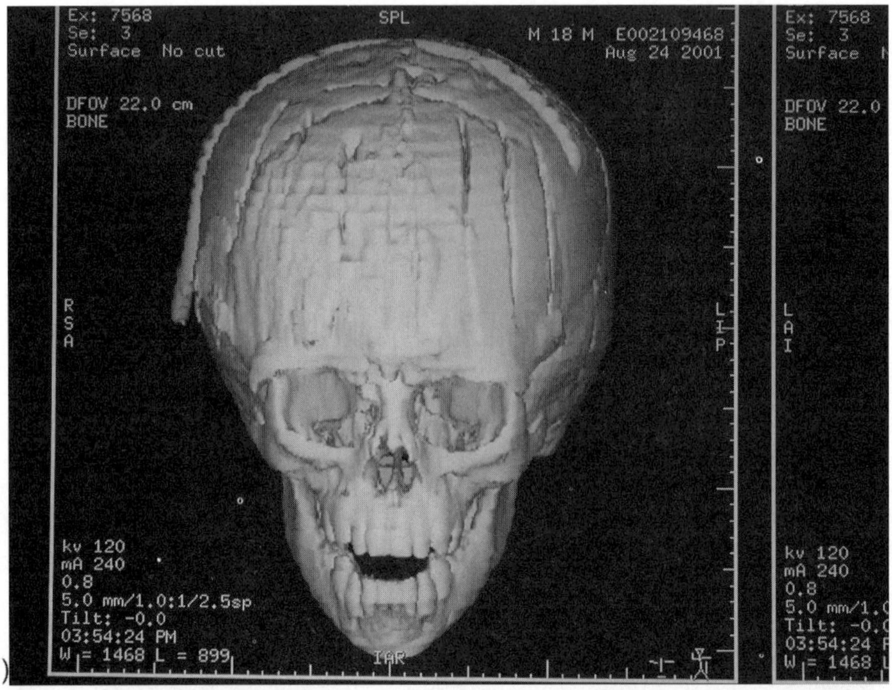

(C)

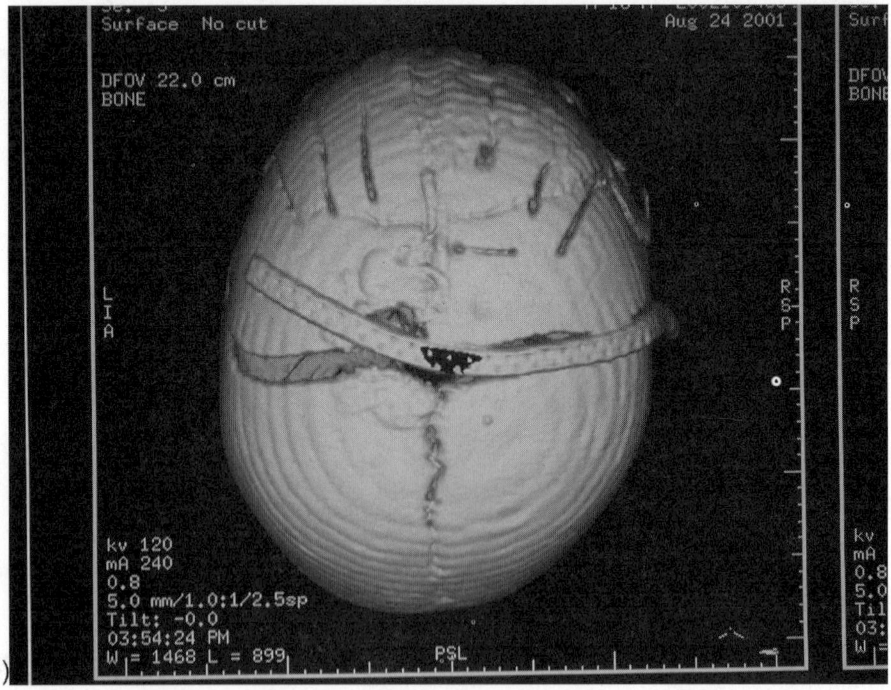

(D)

Figure 26 Continued.

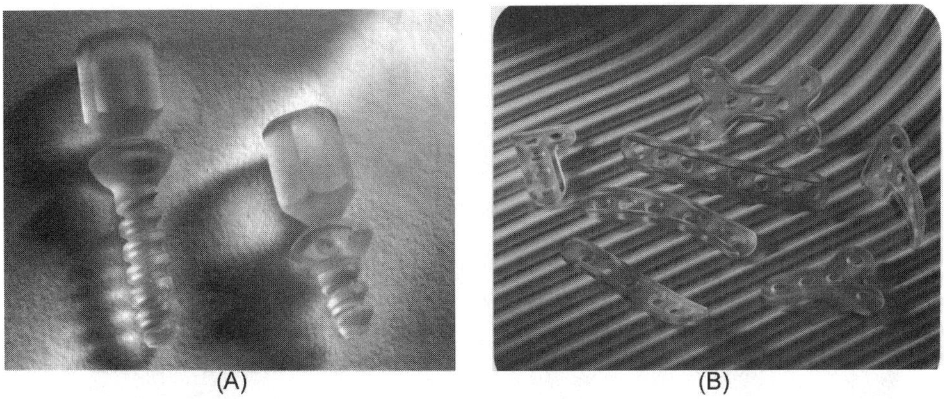

Figure 27 A. Absorbable screw, 1.5 mm diameter, utilized for rigid fixation of the calvarium. B. Various sizes and shapes of 1.5 mm thick absorbable plates utilized for rigid fixation.

been available only as blocks. The material has recently been produced as powder, which is mixed with sodium phosphate. This results in a paste that can be used to fill osseous defects and also augment frontal or temporal bones. Although the first products did not solidify for 24 h, especially in presence of moisture, more recent products solidify in 10 min even in presence of moisture and blood, giving more reliable results. The product is now used extensively by craniofacial surgeons for augmentation of the frontal and the temporal bones after cranial vault remodeling for craniosynostosis for temporal hollowing and minor asymmetries. It is also used for osseous defects that have failed to ossify after cranial vault remodeling (Fig. 28). The authors have extended their indications to malar augmentation successfully (38).

Craniofacial Syndromes

Apert's syndrome is a rare craniofacial syndrome that occurs sporadically in most cases but can be transmitted by an autosomal dominant trait in some families. The syndrome is also known as acrocephalosyndactyly due to the cranial and extremity involvement. The syndrome is characterized by a bicoronal synostosis, turricephaly, severe exorbitism, midface hypoplasia, anterior open bite, and bilateral symmetrical complex syndactyly of the digits and toes. These children also have developmental delays and hyperactivity and often experience obstructive sleep apnea due to the airway restriction caused by midface retrusion (Fig. 29).

Crouzon syndrome or craniofacial dysostosis is a rare syndrome (prevalence 1 : 25000 in the general population). The syndrome, which transmits as an autosomal dominant trait within families, is characterized by exorbitism, midface retrusion, and brachycephaly due to bicoronal synostosis. The midface is characteristically box-shaped and may be associated with hypertelorism. The mandible grows normally but may be secondarily deformed by maxillary retrusion and malposition (Fig. 30).

Pfeiffer syndrome, described in 1964, consists of craniosynostosis, broad thumbs, broad great toes, and occasionally partial soft tissue syndactyly of the hand. The syndrome is inherited as an autosomal dominant trait with complete penetrance (Fig. 31).

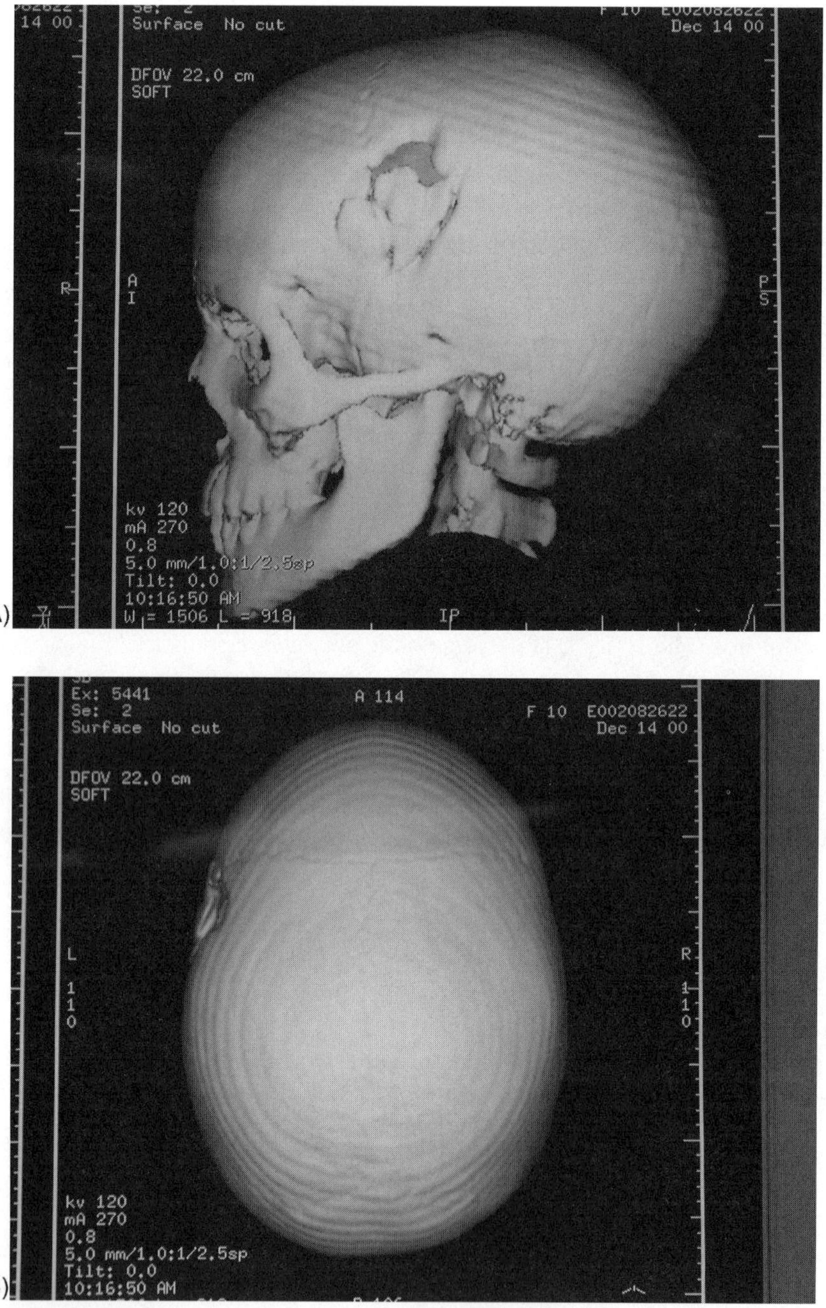

(A) (B)

Figure 28 A. Osseous defect left in the calvarium after compound comminuted fracture due to trauma. B. Three-dimensional CT scans demonstrates abnormality in the contour and osseous defect over the left temporoparietal skull. C. Intraoperative view of the osseous defect with exposed dura. D. Absorbable 0.25 mm Lactosorb mesh used as an intervening surface between the dura and the overlying osseous defect. E. Intraoperative view shows position of the absorbable plate at the dural interface. F. Hydroxyapatite powder is

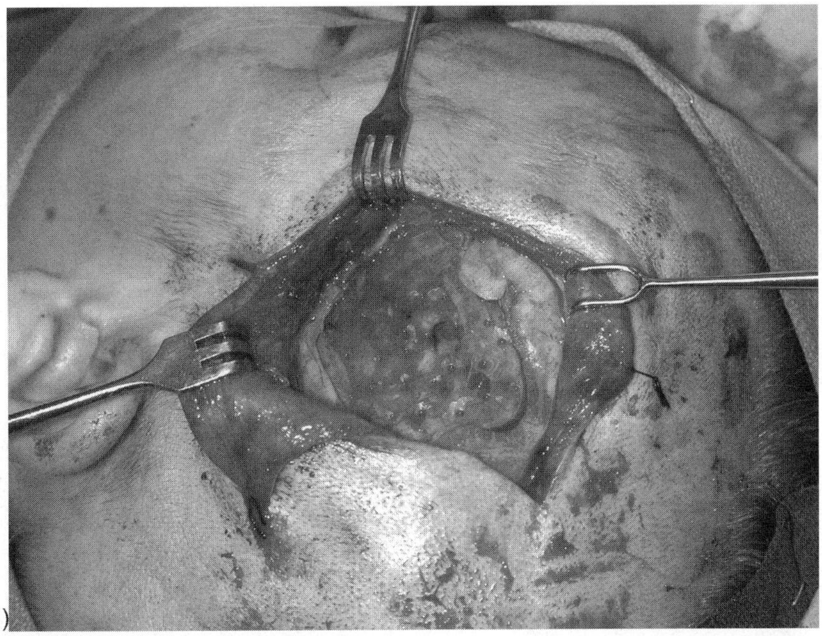

(C)

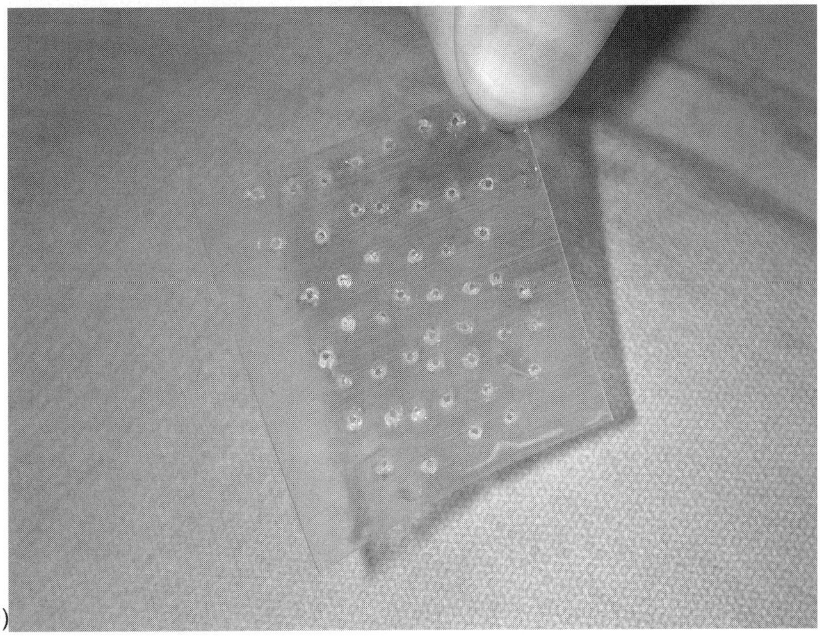

(D)

Figure 28 (continued) transferred to a container in sterile fashion. G. Hydroxyapatite is mixed with sodium phosphate solution to form a paste. H. The paste is applied to the osseous cavity and allowed to set and harden. I. Three-dimensional CT scan after application of the hydroxyapatite into the osseous defect. Note that the osseous defect is completely obliterated. J. Postoperative three-dimensional CT scan superior view demonstrates perfect contour between the right and the left temporoparietal regions following application of hydroxyapatite.

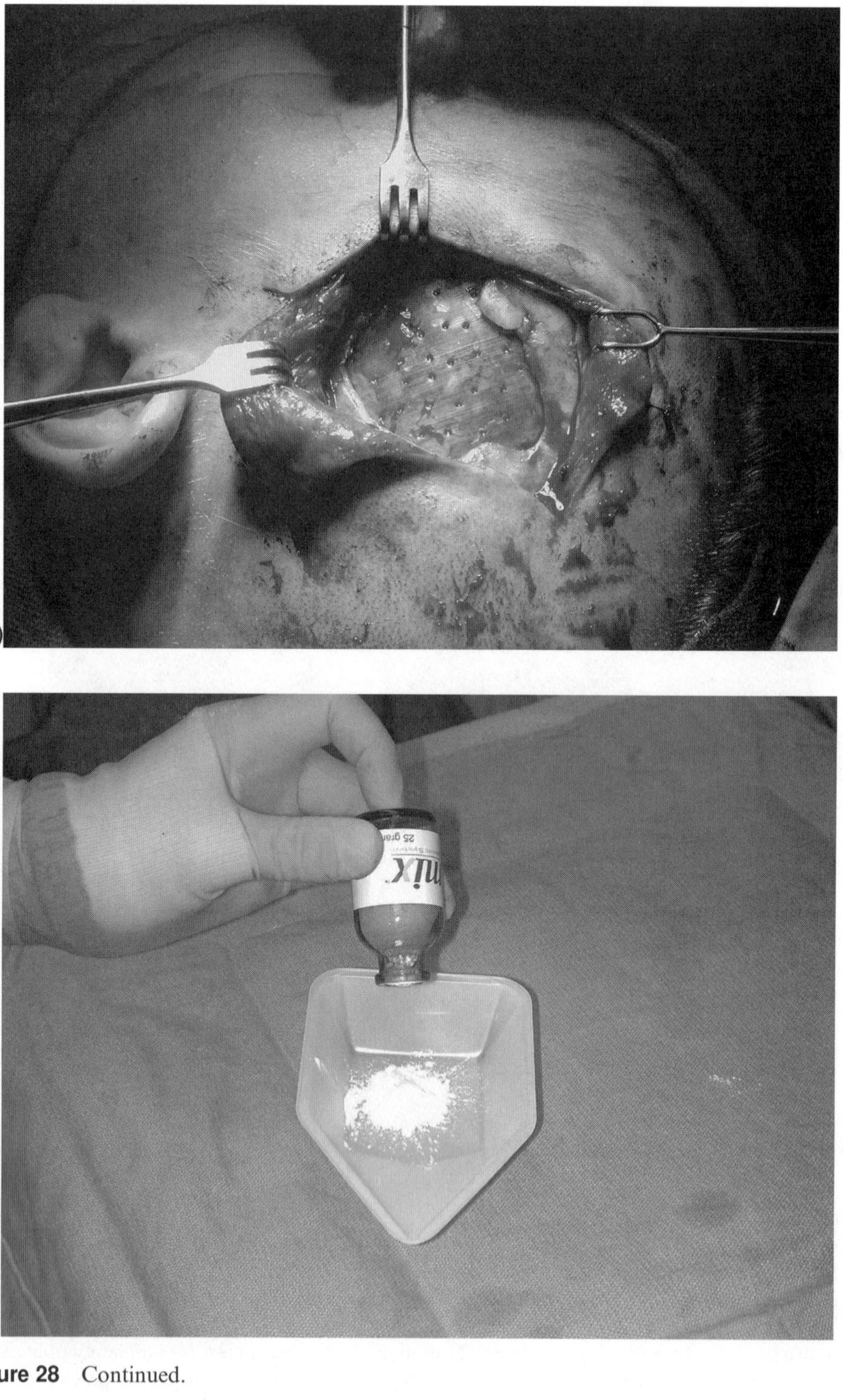

(E)

(F)

Figure 28 Continued.

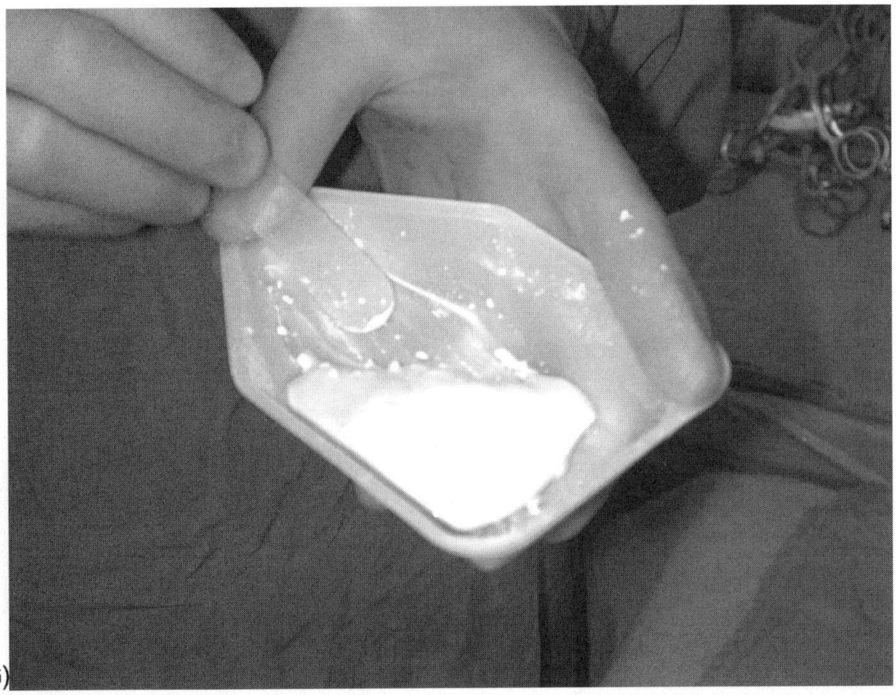

(G)

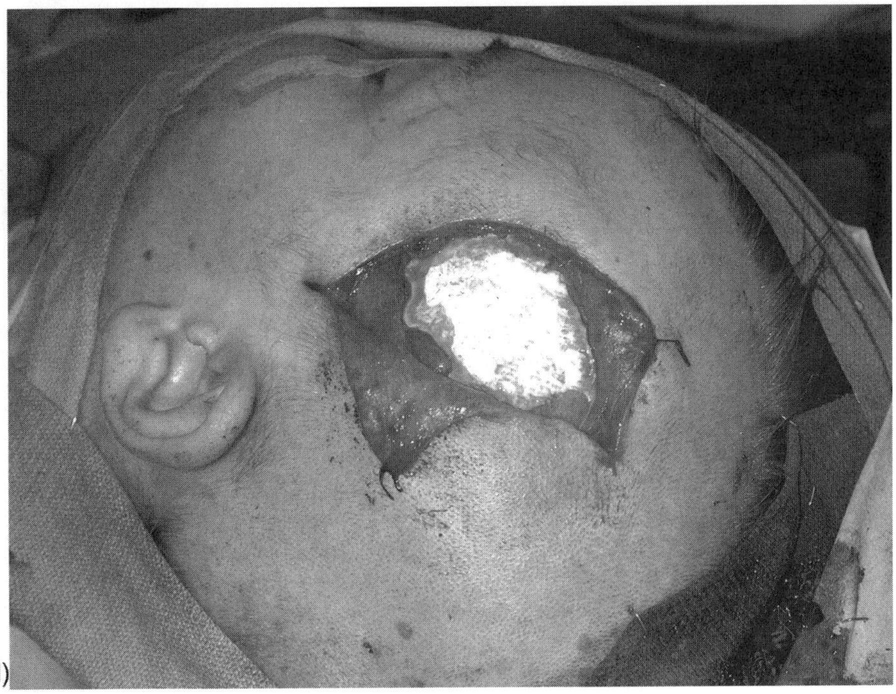

(H)

Figure 28 Continued.

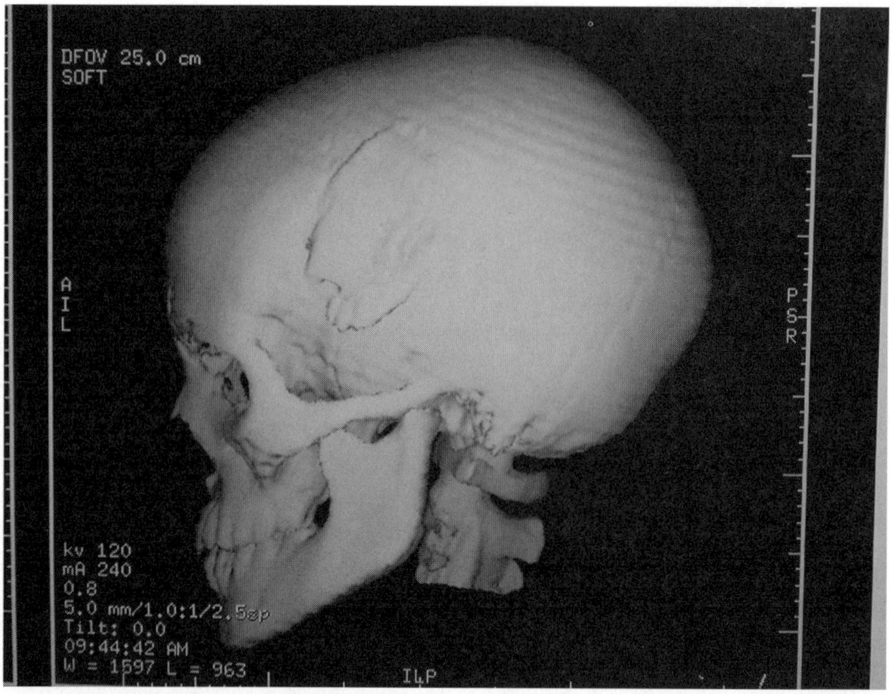

(I)

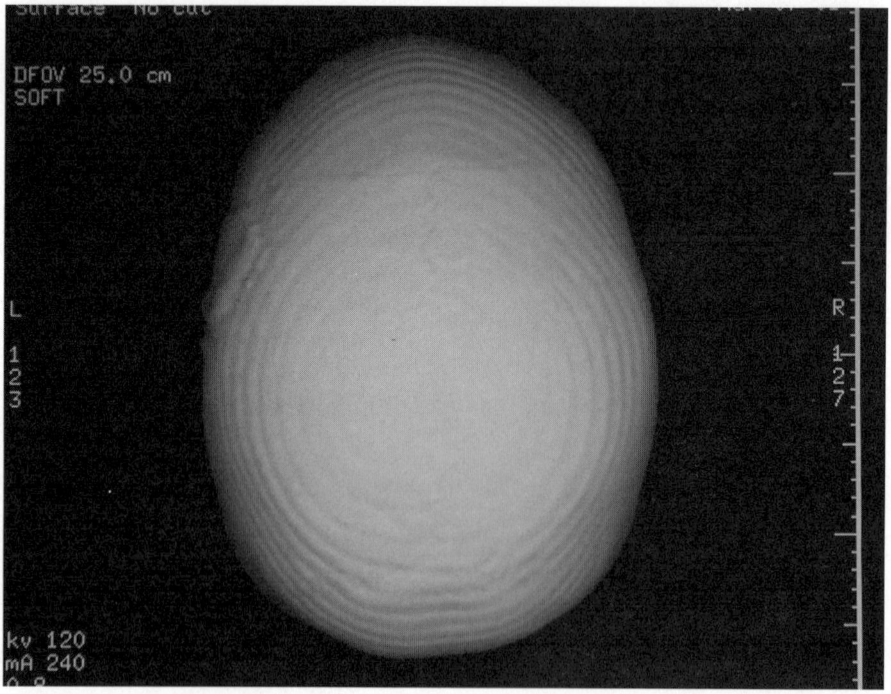

(J)

Figure 28 Continued.

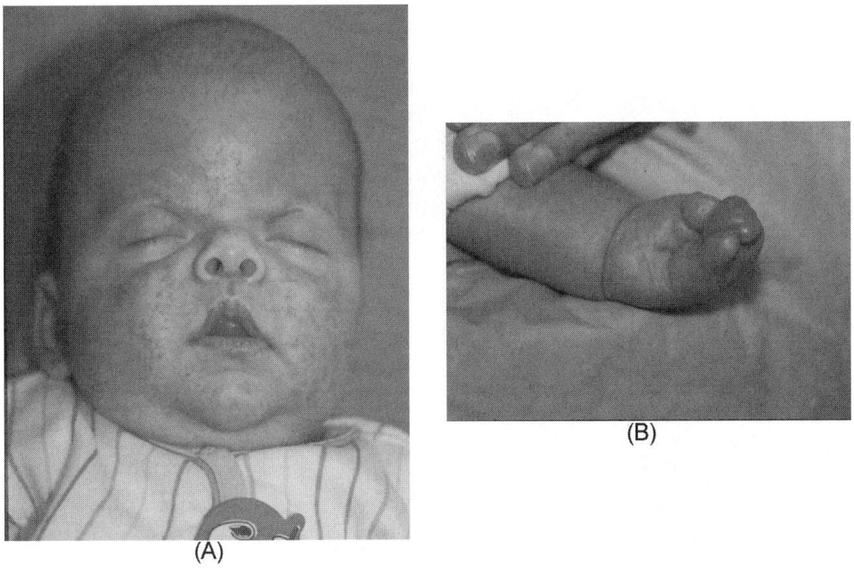

Figure 29 A. 3-month-old child with Apert's syndrome demonstrates turricephaly, frontal bossing, and recessed frontal orbital bar. B. Complex syndactyly of the left hand.

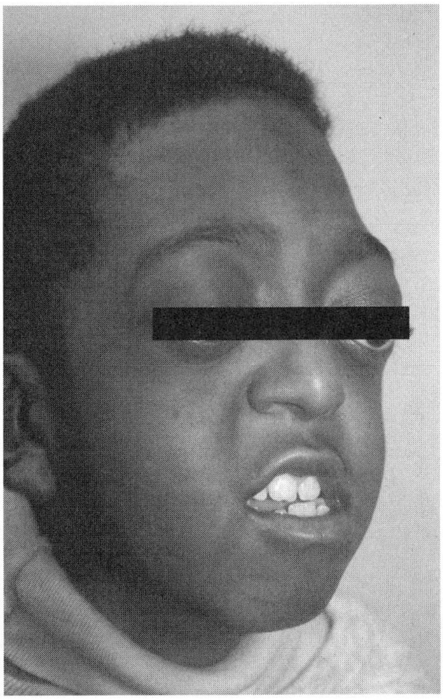

Figure 30 Older child with Crouzon syndrome shows bilateral exorbitism, midface retrusion and class III malocclusion.

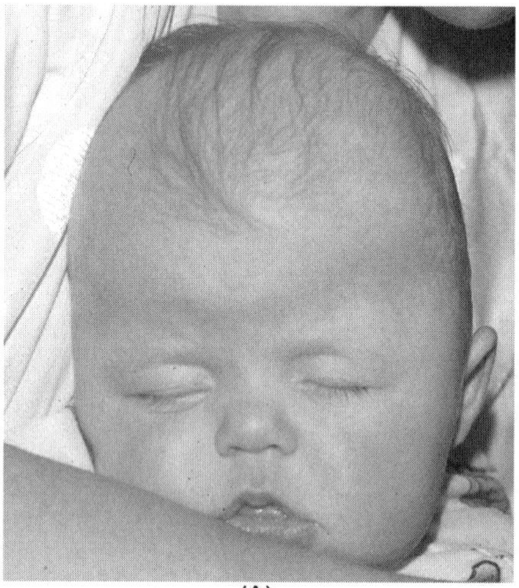

(A)

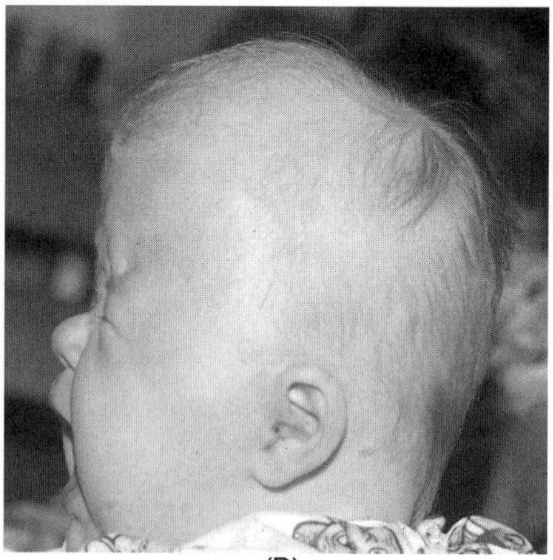

(B)

Figure 31 A. Frontal view of a child with Pfeiffer syndrome. Note the frontal bossing and significant recession of the frontal orbital bar. B. Profile: note the recession of the frontal orbital bar, exorbitism, and turricephaly.

Carpenter syndrome is characterized by craniosynostosis in association with preaxial polysyndactyly of the feet, short fingers with clinodactyly, and variable soft tissue syndactyly. It is transmitted by autosomal recessive inheritance.

Saethre Chotzen syndrome has an autosomal dominant inheritance pattern and is characterized by craniosynostosis, low-set hairline, and ptosis of the upper eyelids, facial asymmetry, brachydactyly, partial cutanoeus syndactyly, and other skeletal anomalies.

Management

The management of these syndromes involves the following:

I: Correct craniosynostosis between the ages of 3–6 months.
II: Correct syndactyly between the ages of 1–2 years.
III: Correct midface retrusion by distraction by age 4–5 years if the child has severe obstructive sleep apnea, severe malocclusion, or severe psychological disturbance.
IV: Correct hypertelorism and turricephaly, if present, at age 4–6 years.
V: Await full maturity and perform Le Fort I or Le Fort III procedure in conjunction with mandibular osteotomy to normalize appearance and correct malocclusion.

CRANIOFACIAL DISTRACTION

Introduction

Distraction as a concept for lengthening was introduced by Codvilla but popularized by Ilizarov (39) who performed gradual distraction of the limbs of dogs at the very slow rate of 1 mm/day. He applied this science to human long bones by performing an incomplete osteotomy of the tibia and applying gradual distraction forces. He was successful in lengthening congenitally short limbs. His technique has been adopted by orthopedic surgeons around the world not only for congenital cases but also for osseous defects following trauma.

In the past, craniofacial surgeons have been disappointed by the outcome of immediate intraoperative lengthening of the mandible and the midface for children with mandibular and maxillary hypoplasia in association with obstructive sleep apnea. Intraoperative advancement was limited by the severely deficient soft tissue and, in spite of rigid fixation, there was recurrence of the deformity.

McCarthy (40) commenced lengthening the mandibles of dogs initially, followed by procedures in humans. He was successful in obtaining significant ventral advancement. The technique was quickly applied to the hypoplastic mandible of children with obstructive sleep apnea. Initial results suggested that the technique was successful in relieving the obstructive sleep apnea and even allowed decannulation. Subsequent studies showed that advancement remained stable and the mandible continued to grow (41). The technique has been widely adopted for mandibular and maxillary advancement (42).

Basic Science

Distraction osteogenesis is defined as creation of new bone at the site of osteotomy/corticotomy by a process of gradual separation of the bony segments. The process of distraction creates a tension stress effect and promotes metabolic activation, vasculogenesis, and eventually new bone formation (43). The new callus being formed is comprised of four zones:

Fibrous central zone akin to the inflammatory response seen following trauma or injury
Transition zone marked by progenitor cells transforming into osteoblasts and creating new bone
Bone remodeling characterized by mature osteoblasts and osteoclasts remodeling the newly created bone
Mature bone zone following a period of consolidation.

Recent studies (44) have focused on the molecular changes that accompany distraction osteogenesis.

Transforming growth factor-beta has been found to be the primary initiator of events. TGF beta initiates vasculogenesis and stabilizes the walls of the new vessels. The presence of vasculogenesis is critical in setting the stage for the next step of osteogenesis. Without the aid of the augmented blood supply, the osteoblasts are incapable of supporting mitosis. The presence of TGB beta upregulates the deposition of type I collagen molecules, eventually leading to membranous ossification of the regenerate. TGF beta may also be responsible for the mineralization of the regenerate by osteocalcin gene expression.

Distraction Osteogenesis

Advantages

These include the following:

- Limits the extent and the morbidity of surgery of ventral advancement.
- Allows significant ventral advancement of the bone segments in spite of soft tissue constraints.
- Produces a stable ventral advancement with minimal or no relapse (41).
- Provides soft tissue augmentation along with the osteogenesis.
- Distraction osteogenesis can be repeated at a later time if necessary.
- Is a successful technique to decannulate children with obstructive sleep apnea (45).
- Can prevent the use of a trachoetomy in neonates with severe mandibular hypoplasia (46).

Disadvantages

These include the following:

- The external pin tracts leave scars that may require revision.
- The devices are socially unacceptable.
- The process of distraction and later consolidation is 6–12 weeks long.
- Accurate planning and distraction vector projection make it difficult to correct malocclusion.

Mandibular Distraction

Indications

These include the following:

- Obstructive sleep apnea secondary to mandibular hypoplasia
- Malocclusion with symptoms
- Psychosocial abnormalities associated with a severe deformity

Investigations and Preoperative Planning

The presence of obstructive apnea is documented by performing a sleep study. This is followed by a nasoendoscopy to rule any other causes of the obstructive apnea. A three-dimensional CT scan is performed to document the anatomy and help plan a vector of distraction. Measurement of occlusal cant is helpful in determining the extent of vertical correction. Computer-aided planning is now available to improve accuracy and outcome (47). The role of the soft tissue constraints in distraction are difficult to predict. The use of multiplanar devices somewhat obviates the need for very accurate planning because of their flexibility. Following completion of distraction and removal of devices, a three-dimensional CT scan is performed to document the extent of correction achieved. A postoperative sleep study is also necessary to confirm correction of the obstructive apnea.

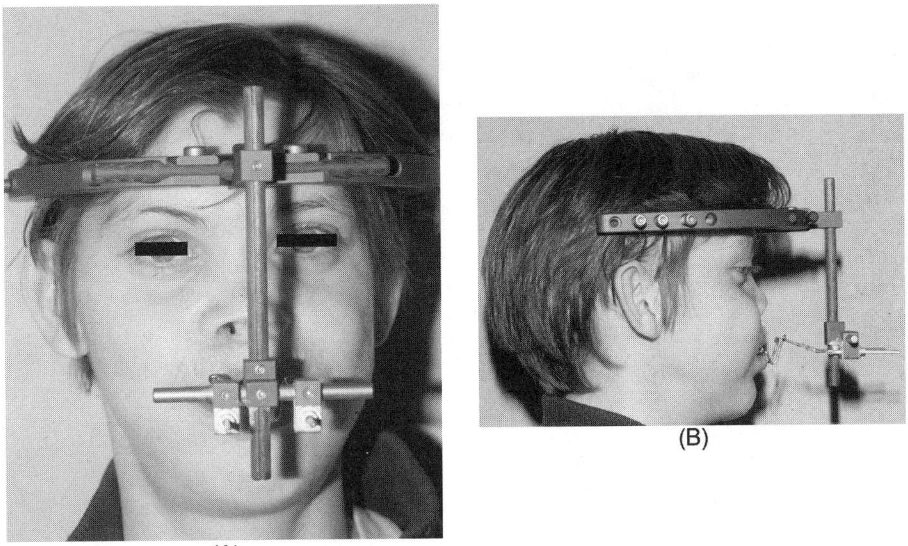

(A) (B)

Figure 32 A. 16-year-old undergoing maxillary distraction utilizing an RED device. The device is fixed to the skull utilizing four superficial pins that penetrate the outer layer of the calvarium. The central bar allows placement of the fixation device on the maxillary alveolus at any location, allowing significant flexibility in the direction of the maxillary distraction. B. Profile view of the RED device.

Procedure

The technique can be performed using either an external or an internal distractor. External distractors allow multiplanar distraction vectors thereby improving the outcome but are cumbersome and sometimes socially unacceptable. Internal distractors are lightweight and not visible but allow uniplanar distraction only and require a second procedure to remove the device.

The technique involves intraoral exposure of the buccal surface of the mandible followed by an osteotomy of the buccal, superior, and inferior surfaces. Two percutaneous pins are inserted proximal to the osteotomy and two distal. The osteotomy over the lingual surface is completed using a narrow osteotome to protect the inferior alveolar nerve. The procedure is repeated on the contralateral side if the deformity is bilateral. The external devices are fitted and the surgical incision is closed. After a latent period of 5–7 days, the process of distraction is commenced at the rate of 0.5 mm twice daily. For multiplanar devices, ventral advancement is commenced first followed by changes in the gonial angle and the transverse dimension of the mandible. The ventral advancement is performed by the parents daily and assessed by the physician on a weekly basis. The process of distraction is continued until the desired outcome is obtained. On completion of the distraction process, a 6 week period of consolidation is recommended to stabilize the bone segments. The distraction devices are then removed, generally under sedation.

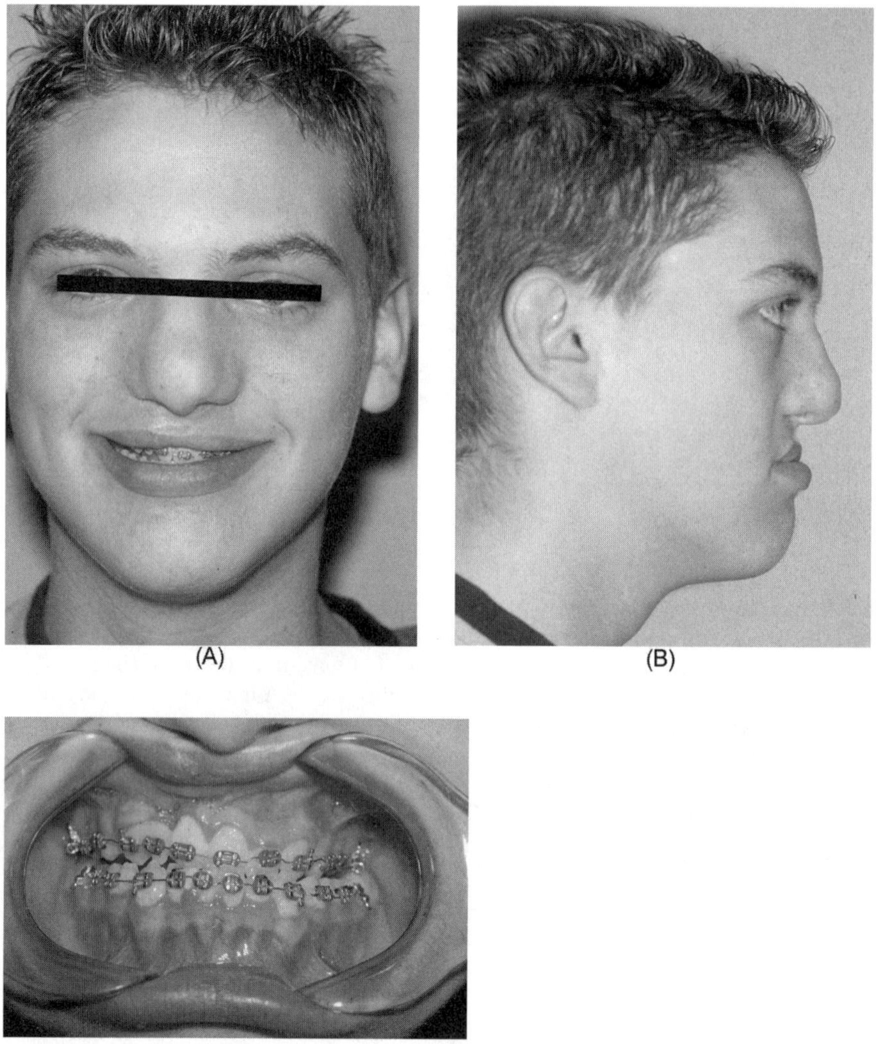

(A) (B)

(C)

Figure 33 A. Frontal view of the teenager in Figure 32: class III malocclusion. B. Appearance after cleft palate surgery with significant class III malocclusion.

Complications

Infection. The presence of percutaneous pins for 6–8 weeks predisposes the sites to infection. Although common, the infection rarely leads to osteomyelitis requiring removal of the pins and the device. The pin tracts need to be kept clean to prevent infection.

Damage to the Inferior Alveolar Nerve. It is nearly impossible to perform a split-ramus osteotomy in a child, especially with a hypoplastic mandible. The nerve

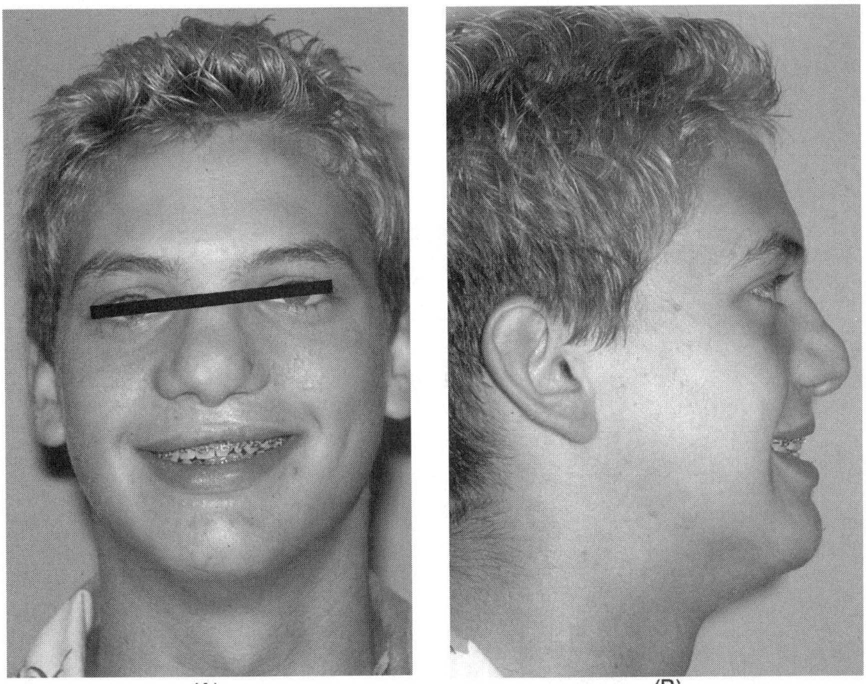

(A) (B)

Figure 34 A. Postoperative view after maxillary distraction using the RED device. B. Profile view.

is within the path of osteotomy. Some surgeons perform an incomplete osteotomy and then continue distraction until the lingual cortex fractures. This is painful in the postoperative period. Other surgeons perform a separate osteotomy of the lingual cortex with a narrow osteotome, which eases the pain during distraction. Although it is difficult to document accurately the effect of distraction of the nerve in a child, no adverse effects have been noted in long-term studies.

Asymmetry of the Mandible. In spite of accurate preoperative planning, it is difficult to achieve a perfectly symmetrical result. The presence of multiplanar device allows for some correction during the distraction period. The patient and the parents need to be warned about this and informed that if the distraction is performed in the prepubertal phase, a final orthognathic surgery may be necessary on cessation of postpubertal growth.

Long-term Growth. Studies have documented that results following distraction have not showed evidence of relapse (41).

Inability to Decannulate Successfully. It is critical to investigate and rule out or treat all other causes of obstructive apnea before contemplating a mandibular osteotomy. If not, it is difficult to decannulate the tracheotomy-dependent child.

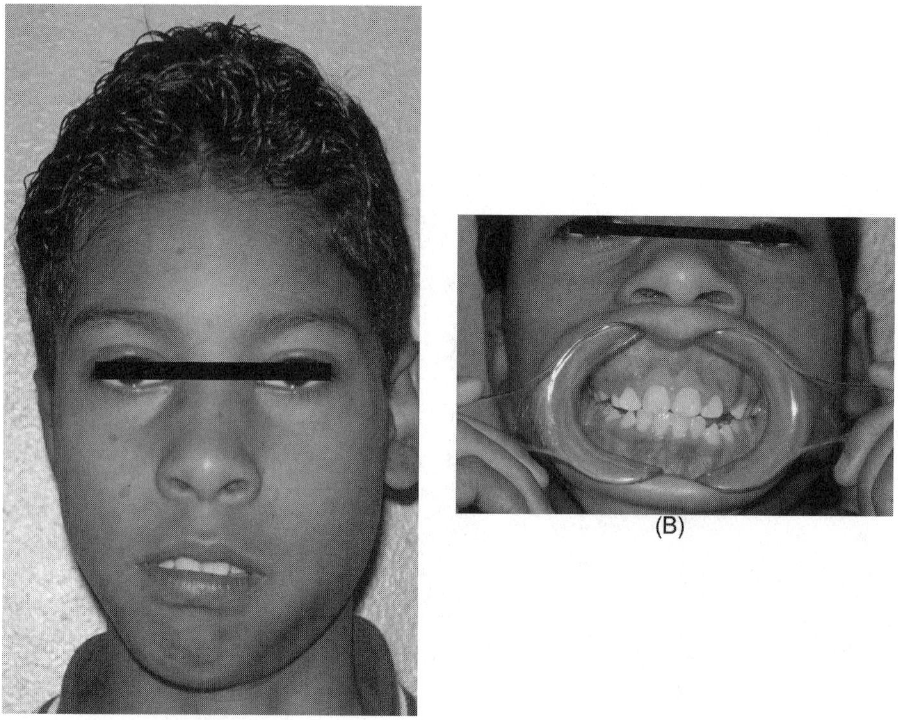

(A) (B)

Figure 35 A. Frontal view of a child with right hemifacial microsomia with asymmetry of the mandible and maxilla. B. Class II malocclusion with deviation of the occlusal cant due to involvement of the right mandible and secondary involvement of the maxilla.

Maxillary Distraction Osteogenesis

It was only natural that the process of distraction be applied next for maxillary distraction. The initial devices were used with Le Fort I level osteotomies but later devices were designed to be used with Le Fort III osteotomies.

Indications

Indications include severe midface deficiency secondary to cleft palate or craniofacial anomalies especially Apert's, Crouzon, and Binder syndromes in association with obstructive sleep apnea and/or exorbitism and/or severe malocclusion. Although surgery has traditionally been performed after postpubertal growth, over the last decade this has been relaxed to include younger children because of the availability of distraction and an earlier recognition of sleep apnea with the use of sophisticated investigative technology. Before the age of 3 years, facial sutures are not fused and distraction forces tend to disrupt the sutures before they produce significant ventral movement.

Technique

Le Fort I Osteotomy and Distraction. Preoperative planning is essential using cephalographs and three-dimensional CT scans. The design of the movement vector

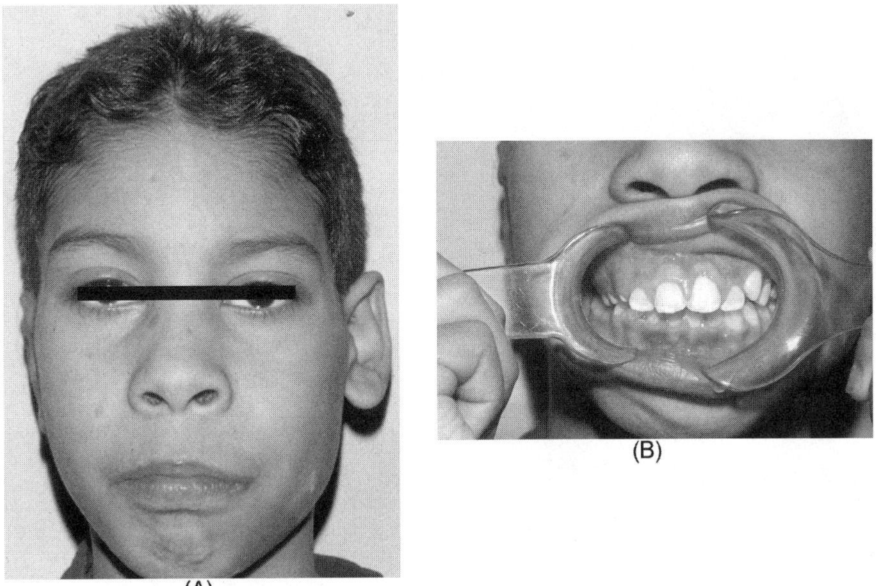

Figure 36 A. Postoperative view following combined distraction of the maxilla and the mandible utilizing a single device: significant improvement in the facial symmetry is noted. B. Postoperative view demonstrates maxillary and mandibular midlines on the midsagittal line following combined distraction.

is important to determine the final position of the maxilla. An acrylic model can be manufactured from data provided by the scan. Surgery can be performed on the model to simplify the process intraoperatively. Dental occlusion is very important and preoperative orthodontic evaluation followed by a postoperative treatment plan helps immensely in correcting malocclusion. In contrast, orthodontic evaluation is not absolutely essential for patients with deciduous dentition.

The most popular system for Le Fort I osteotomy is rigid external distraction (RED) (48). A maxillary splint is made by an orthodontist and fitted preoperatively. The device is fixed as a halo using four scalp screws fixed to the temporal skull. A central rod projects down from the halo. A single central bar is attached horizontally. Two thick wires project from the maxillary splint and are attached to the horizontal rod with a screw. The screw is rotated twice daily until the desired occlusion is reached. Although the device is cumbersome, it offers the advantage of manipulating the Le Fort I maxillary segment until the desired position is reached without difficulty. In contrast, other devices on the market do not allow that flexibility and therefore can be used reliably only for patients with deciduous dentition.

Access to the maxilla is obtained through the gingivobuccal sulcus. The periosteum is stripped from the anterior surface of the maxilla, taking care not to damage the infraorbital nerve. An osteotomy is then made along the anterior surface of the maxillary antrum extending from the anterior nasal spine to the maxillary tuberosity using a reciprocating saw. A curved osteotome is used to perform a pterygomaxillotomy. Rowe's forceps are used to downfracture the maxilla. The appropriate device

(A)

(B)

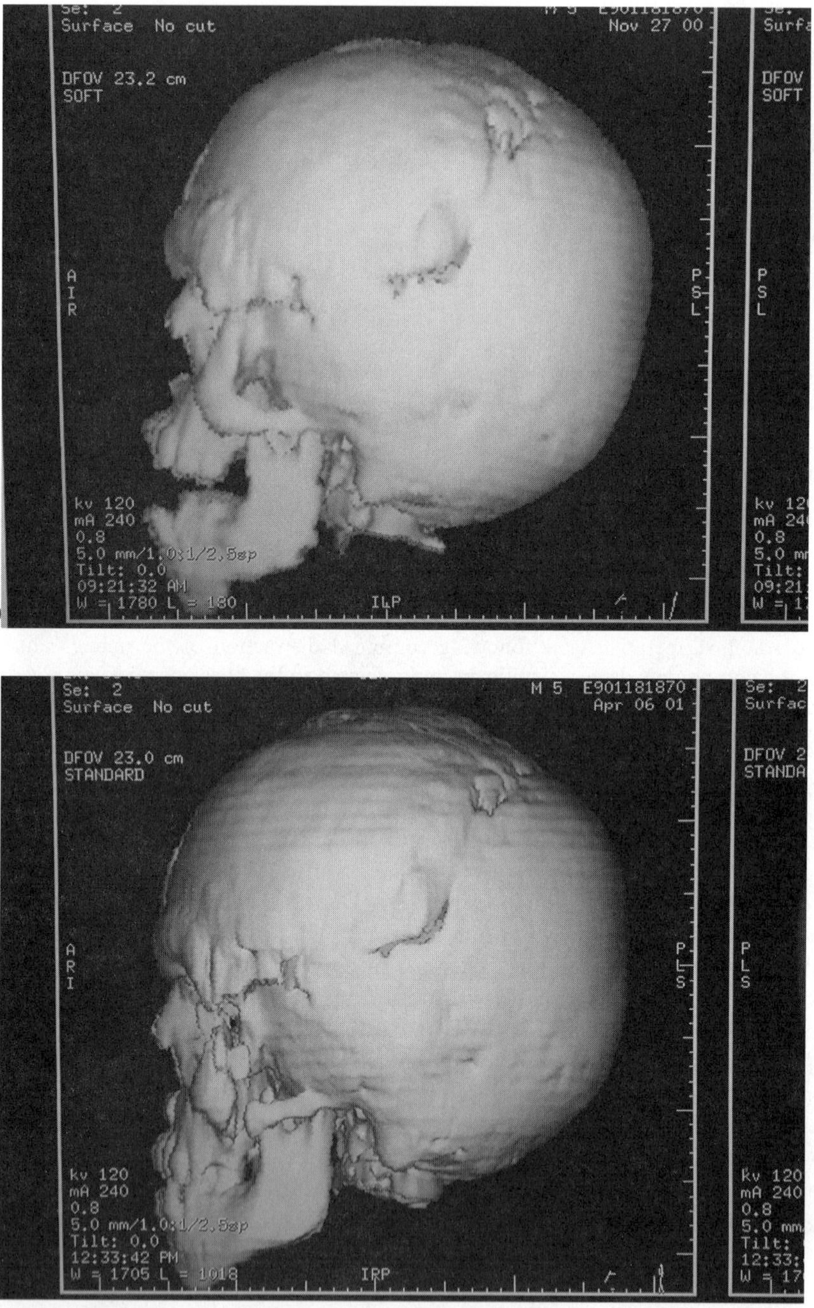

Figure 37 A. Preoperative profile view of a three-dimensional CT scan of a child with Apert's syndrome demonstrates significant maxillary hypoplasia. This child had already undergone frontal orbital bar advancement. B. Three months postoperative profile three-dimensional CT scan demonstrates perfect alignment of the maxilla and the mandible after a LeFort III advancement utilizing a distraction device.

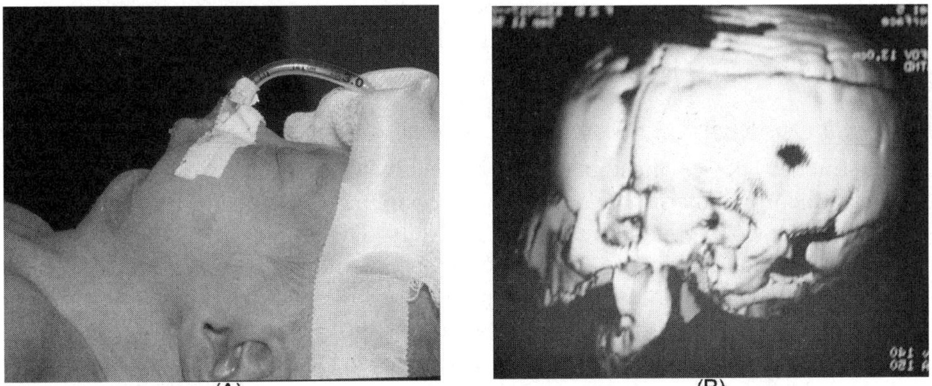

Figure 38 A. Preoperative view of a neonate with significant mandibular hypoplasia and significant obstructive sleep apnea 5 days following birth. B. Preoperative three-dimensional CT scan demonstrates significant hypoplasia of the horizontal ramus of the mandible with a normal height of the vertical ramus.

is used to fix the Le Fort I segment and distraction is commenced on day 5 at a rate of 1 mm/day. After reaching the appropriate position, the regenerate is allowed to ossify for 6 weeks. The device is then taken out (Figs. 32–34).

Complications. The process of distraction is relatively safe for surgeons performing large-volume surgery and who are familiar with the devices. It is possible to have continuing malocclusion and misalignment of the device. The device may disengage at the site of contact with the maxilla. If the device is taken out too early, maxillary relapse is possible. If, however, the regenerate is completely ossified, long-term studies have demonstrated that there is no relapse. This is the greatest advantage to the process of distraction.

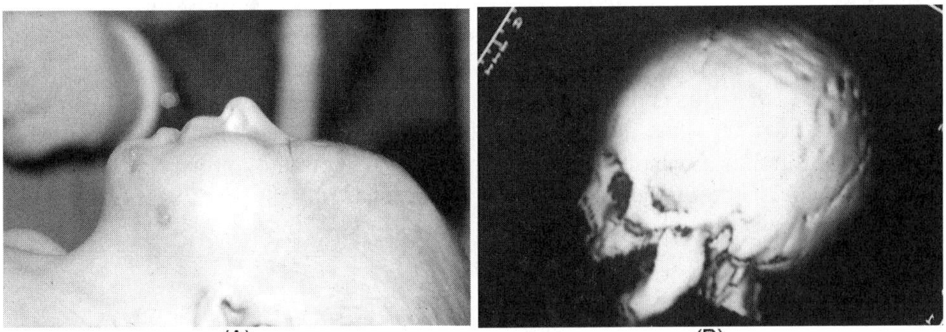

Figure 39 A. Two month postoperative profile view of the child in Figure 38 after undergoing neonatal mandibular distraction at day 5. Note the significant improvement in the position of the chin. B. Postoperative three-dimensional CT scan profile view demonstrates significant improvement in the length of the horizontal ramus of the mandible following distraction.

Combined distraction of maxilla and mandible can be performed to obviate the difficulties faced by correcting the malocclusion secondary to movement of the mandible alone (49) (Figs. 35,36).

Le Fort III Osteotomy and Distraction

The distraction device most commonly used by craniofacial surgeons is placed through a bicoronal incision over the temporoparietal skull dorsally and the zygoma (inferior to the frontozygomatic suture) ventrally. The initial device was completely metallic including the fixation elements on the skull and the zygoma. Recently, with the great success enjoyed by the absorbable plates, the metallic distraction screw is incorporated with the absorbable plates so that removal of the device is very easy.

The subcranial osteotomy is performed following exposure of the temporoparietal skull, lateral orbital wall, nasion, zygomatic arch, and the body. The anterior surface of the maxillary antrum can be approached through the gingivobuccal sulcus. Osteotomies are then made through the frontozygomatic suture, floor of the orbit, and the nasion using a reciprocating saw. A cephalo-osteotome is used to separate the vomer and the ethmoid from the cranial base in the midline. The pterygomaxillary suture is separated either from the bicoronal approach or the gingivobuccal sulcus incision. Once again, Rowe's forceps are used to disimpact the Le Fort III segment. The devices are applied and the procedure completed (Fig. 37).

Distraction has been successful for treatment of obstructive sleep apnea allowing decannulation in most cases. Over the past few years, the author has used mandibular distraction in neonates with mandibular hypoplasia and airway obstruction. This involves performing a mandibular osteotomy a few days following birth in children with severe airway obstruction at birth. Following bilateral osteotomy, an internal distraction device is fixed to the mandible at the angles. The child is left intubated, transferred to the intensive care unit, and distraction is performed at a rapid rate (2 mm/day) until an appropriate maxillary and mandibular occlusion is achieved. The technique is successful in avoiding a tracheotomy and its associated complications (46) (Figs. 38,39).

The second advantage has been to use the technique of distraction for craniosynostosis (50). The technique involves performing a cranial suturectomy through a bicoronal incision. A distraction device is applied to the suture and the process of distraction is continued postoperatively until the desired position is reached. Although the technique is promising, it has several drawbacks. The need for distraction is questionable when a desired position can be reached intraoperatively with minimal additional morbidity. Also, distraction prevents the ability of the surgeon to modify the shape of the bone, which is crucial to obtain an appropriate shape of the calvarium.

REFERENCES

1. Decker JD, Hall SH. Light and electron microscopy of the newborn sagittal suture. Anat Rec 1985; 212:81.
2. Virchow R. Uber den Cretinismus, namentlich in Franken, and uber Patholoische Schadelformen. Verh Phys Med Gesellsch Wurzburg 1851; 2:230.
3. Moss ML. The pathogenesis of premature cranial synostosis in man. Acta Anat 1959; 37:351.

4. Eaton A, Cheverud J, Marsh J. The effect of artifical calvarial modification on endocranial base morphology. Winner, Plastic Surgery Educational Foundation Essay Competition. 1997.
5. Park EA, Powers GF. Acrocephaly and scaphocephaly with symmetrically distributed malformations of the extremities. Am J Dis Child 1920; 20:235.
6. Levine J, Bradley J, Roth D, McCarthy J, Longaker M. Studies in cranial suture biology: regional dura mater determines overlying suture biology. Plast Reconstr Surg 1998; 101(6):1441–1447.
7. Most D, Levine J, Chang J, Sung J, McCarthy J, Schendel S, Longaker M. Studies in cranial suture biology: up-regulation of transforming growth factor-B1 and basic fibroblastic growth factor mRNA correlates with posterior frontal cranial suture fusion in the rat. Plast Reconstr Surg 1998; 101(6):1431–1440.
8. Marsh JL, Koby M, Lee B. 3-D MRI in craniosynostosis: identification of previously unappreciated neural anomalies. Presented 5th Congress International Society Craniofacial Surgery, Oaxaca, Mexico, October 1993.
9. Mulliken JB, Steinberger D, Kunze S, Muller U. Molecular diagnosis of bilateral coronal synostosis. Plast Reconstr Surg 1999; 104(6):1603–1615.
10. Gault D, Renier D, Marchac D, Jones B. Intracranial pressure and intracranial volume in children with craniosynostosis. Plast Reconstr Surg 1992; 90(3):377–381.
11. Cohen S, Pershing J. Intracranial pressure in single-suture craniosynostosis. Cleft Palate Craniofac J 1998; 35(3):194–196.
12. Marsh JL. Personal communication, December 2000.
13. Argenta LC, David LR, Wilson J, Bell WO. An increase in infant cranial deformity with supine sleeping position. J Craniofac Surg 1996; 7:5.
14. http://www.jpanchal.com
15. Mulliken JB, Vander Woude DL, Hansen M, LaBrie RA, Scott MR. Analysis of posterior plagiocephaly: deformational versus synostotic. Plast Reconstr Surg 1999; 103:371.
16. Lun-Jou Lo, Marsh JL, Vannier MW, Patel V. Craniofacial computer-assisted surgical planning and simulation. Clin Plast Surg 1994; 21:501.
17. Baas MB. Human Osteology: A laboratory and field manual of the human skeleton. In: Evans RE, ed. Human Osteology. Special Publications, Missouri Archaeological Society, University of Missouri, Columbia, MO, 1971:54–74.
18. Vu H, Panchal J, Parker E, et al. The timing of physiologic closure of the metopic suture: a review of 159 cases using reconstructed three-dimensional CT scans of the head. J Craniofac Surg 2001; 12(6):527–532.
19. Hansman CF. Growth of interorbital distance and skull thickness as observed in roentgenographic measurements. Radiology 1966; 86(1):87–96.
20. Lo LJ, Marsh JL, Yoon J, Vannier MW. Stability of fronto-orbital advancement in nonsyndromic bilateral coronal synostosis: a quantitative three-dimensional computed tomographic study. Plast Reconstr Surg 1996; 98(3):393–409.
21. Kane AA, Kim YO, Eaton A, Pilgram TK, Marsh JL, Zonneveld F, Larsen P, Kreiborg S. Quantification of osseous facial dysmorphology in untreated unilateral coronal synostosis. Plast Reconstr Surg 2000; 106(2):251–258.
22. Bayley N, Bayley, Nancy. The Bayley Scales of Infant Development, Second Edition. San Antonio, TX: The Psychological Corporation, 1993.
23. Kapp-Simons KA, Figueroa A, Jocher CA, Schafer M. Longitudinal assessment of mental development in infants with nonsyndromic craniosynostosis with and without cranial release and reconstruction. Plast Reconstr Surg 1993; 92:831.
24. Kapp-Simon KA. Mental developmental and learning disorders in children with single suture craniosynostosis. Cleft Palate Craniofac J 1998; 35:197.

25. Speltz ML, Endriga MC, Mouradian WE. Presurgical and postsurgical mental and psychomotor development of infants with sagittal synostosis. Cleft Palate Craniofac J 1997; 34:374.
26. Panchal J, Amirsheyabani H, Gurwitch R. Neurodevelopment in children with single suture craniosynostosis and plagiocephaly without synostosis. Plast Reconstr Surg 2001; 108(6):1492–1498.
27. Sidoti EJ, Marsh JL, Marty-Grames L, Noetzel MJ. Long-term studies of metopic synostosis: frequency of cognitive impairment and behavioral disturbances. Plast Reconstr Surg 1996; 97:276.
28. Rozzelle A, Marty-Grames L, Marsh JL. Speech-language disorders in nonsyndromic sagittal synostosis. Presented at the Annual Meeting American Cleft Palate-Craniofacial Association; April 1995; Tampa, FL.
29. David LR, Genecov DG, Camastra AA, Wilson JA, Watson NE, Argenta LC. Positron emission tomography studies confirm the need for early surgical intervention in patients with single-suture craniosynostosis. J Craniofac Surg 1999; 10:38.
30. Marsh JL, Vannier MW. Cranial base changes following surgical treatment of craniosynostosis. Cleft Palate J 1986; 23 Suppl 1:9–18.
31. Venes JL, Sayers MP. Sagittal synostectomy: technical note. J Neurosurg 1976; 44:390–392.
32. Francel PC. Evolution of the treatment for sagittal synostosis. A personal record, in Craniofacial Anomalies: Growth and Development from a Surgical Perspective. (Goodrich JT, Hall CD eds.) New York: Thieme Medical publishers. New York, 1995.
33. Panchal J, Marsh JL, Kauffman B, Park TS, Pilgram T. Sagittal craniosynostosis: Outcome assessment for two methods and timings of intervention. Plast Reconstr Surg 1999; 103:1574–1584.
34. Jimenez DF, Barone CM. Endoscopic craniectomy for early surgical correction of sagittal craniosynostosis. J Neurosurg 1998; 88(1):77–81.
35. Panchal J, Francel P. Unicoronal Synostosis. Neurosurgical Operative Atlas. In: Setti Rengachary, Robert Wilkins: The American Association of Neurological Surgeons, 1999; Volume 9:103–112.
36. Francel P, Panchal J. Metopic Synostosis. Neurosurgical Operative Atlas. In: Setti Rengachary, Robert Wilkins: The American Association of Neurological Surgeons, 1999; Volume 9:91–111.
37. Panchal J, Marsh J, Hapcic C, Francel P, Levine N. Reossification of the orbital wall following ventral translocation of the fronto-orbital bar and cranial vault remodeling. Plast Reconstr Surg 2001; 108(6):1509–1514.
38. Panchal J, Francel P. The efficacy of use of hydroxyapatite (MIMIX®) in management of osseous defects of the calvarium, calvarial augmentation and malar augmentation. Presented at the American Cleft Palate Craniofacial Society Meeting, Minneapolis, Minnesota: April 2001.
39. Ilizarov GA, Lediaev VI. [Replacement of defects of long tubular bones by means of one of their fragments]. [Russian] Vestnik Khirurgii Imeni Grekova 1969; 102(6):77–84.
40. McCarthy JG, Schreiber J, Karp N, Thorne CH, Grayson BH. Lengthening the human mandible by gradual distraction. Plast Reconstr Surg 1992; 89(1):1–10.
41. Hollier LH, Kim JH, Grayson B, McCarthy JG. Mandibular growth after distraction in patients under 48 months of age. Plast Reconstr Surg 1999; 103(5):1361–1370.
42. Molina F, Monasterio F. Mandibular elongation and remodeling by distraction: A farewell to major osteotomies. Plast Reconstr Surg 1995; 96:825–840.
43. Rowe NM, Mehrara BJ, Dudziak ME, Steinbreck DS, Mackool RJ, Gittes GK, McCarthy JG, Longaker MT. Rat mandibular distraction osteogenesis: Part I. Histologic and radiographic analysis. Plast Reconstr Surg 1998; 102(6):2022–2032.

44. Mehrara BJ, Rowe NM, Steinbrech DS, Dudziak ME, Saadeh PB, McCarthy JG, Gittes GK, Longaker MT. Rat mandibular distraction osteogenesis: II. Molecular analysis of transforming growth factor beta-1 and osteocalcin gene expression. Plast Reconstr Surg 1999; 103(2):536–547.
45. Cohen S, Simms C, Burstein F. Mandibular distraction osteogenesis in the treatment of upper airway obstruction in the children with craniofacial deformities. Plast Reconstr Surg 1998; 101:312–318.
46. Panchal J, Marsh J, Hapcic C. Neonatal mandibular distraction osteogenesis: an alternative to tracheotomy for severe upper airway obstruction due to Robin sequence. Submitted Plast Reconstr Surg
47. Gateno J, Teichgraeber JF, Aguilar E. Computer planning for distraction osteogenesis. Plast Reconstr Surg 2000; 105(3):873–882.
48. Polley JW, Figueroa AA. Rigid external distraction: its application in cleft maxillary deformities. Plast Reconstr Surg 1998; 102(5):1360–1372.
49. Vu Hugh, Panchal J. Combined Simultaneous Distraction Osteogenesis of the Maxilla and Mandible Using a Single Distraction Device in Hemifacial Microsomia: A Case Report. Journal of Craniofacial Surgery (in Press).
50. Sugawara Y, Hirabayashi S, Sakurai A. Gradual cranial vault expansion for the treatment of craniofacial synostosis: A prelimnary report. Annals Plast Surg 1998; 40:554–565.

12
Management of Facial Nerve Paralysis

Joseph G. Feghali
Albert Einstein College of Medicine, New York, New York, U.S.A.

Jose N. Fayad
House Ear Institute, Los Angeles, California, U.S.A.

Mark R. Murphy
New York Presbyterian Hospital, New York, New York, U.S.A.

INTRODUCTION

Over the past few decades, surgeons have come to appreciate the severe social and functional impacts of facial paralysis. As a consequence, various surgical techniques have been devised to preserve or restore facial nerve function whenever possible. In terms of function, facial paralysis interferes with facial movement and eye closure. It also contributes to difficulty with chewing, speech, and swallowing. Facial paralysis can also be psychologically and emotionally devastating. Proper prevention and management of facial paralysis require a thorough understanding of facial nerve anatomy, physiology, as well as available medical and surgical treatment modalities. A full understanding of all considerations relating to the facial nerve is not easy. The long course of facial nerve places it in the surgical fields of surgeons from a variety of disciplines, including: head and neck surgery; neurosurgery; otology and neurotology; skull base surgery; facial cosmetic and reconstructive surgery; craniofacial, maxillofacial, and oral surgery. This chapter reviews, from a surgeon's perspective, the various anatomical, physiological, surgical, and reconstructive considerations pertaining to the facial nerve.

MACROANATOMY

The facial nerve is the seventh cranial nerve. Its intracranial segment originates within the pons and exits between the olive and inferior cerebellar peduncle. It then traverses the cerebellopontine angle medial and anterior to the vestibuloacoustic nerve. The intracranial segment measures 15–17 mm in length and terminates at the porus of the internal auditory canal (IAC) of the temporal bone.

The meatal segment of the facial nerve traverses the IAC where it eventually occupies the anterior–superior quadrant of the canal. At the lateral end of the IAC, the nerve starts its labyrinthine segment after entering the meatal foramen superior to the crista transversalis and anterior to the crista verticalis (*Bill's bar*). The crista transversalis separates the facial and cochlear nerves while the crista verticalis separates the facial and superior vestibular nerves (1–3).

The labyrinthine segment contains the narrowest aspect of the bony course of the facial nerve. This segment runs 2.5–6.0 mm in length. The cochlea lies anteroinferior to the nerve at this point. Of note is that the nerve is most vulnerable to injury in this area. Injury can be secondary to trauma (e.g., fracture, middle fossa surgery) or edema (e.g., viral infections, ischemia). Two factors contribute to the vulnerability of the nerve in this area. The first is that the blood supply of this portion is variable in this watershed area for the carotid and vertebrobasilar arterial systems. The second is that, within the labyrinthine segment, the nerve is closely surrounded by a narrow bony canal. As a consequence, edema of the nerve easily leads to its impingement and strangulation.

After leaving the labyrinthine segment, the nerve starts its tympanic portion. This portion starts at the geniculate ganglion and runs for approximately 11 mm. At the level of the ganglion, the nerve gives off the greater superficial petrosal nerve (GSP) and then makes a 40–80 degree turn (the external or first genu) and courses posteriorly and slightly inferiorly above the cochleariform process and the oval window. This segment has frequent dehiscences that make the nerve susceptible to injury during middle ear surgery (4). The nerve then turns at a severe angle of 110–120 degrees into the second (pyramidal) genu, before it turns inferiorly into the mastoid (vertical) segment. Here the motor stapedius nerve branches off to innervate the stapedius muscle.

The mastoid or vertical segment measures about 13 mm and ends as the nerve exits from the stylomastoid foramen when it becomes the extratemporal segment. Prior to exiting the temporal bone, the facial nerve gives off the chorda tympani branch that travels retrogradely and curves anteriorly into the middle ear.

Some 15–20 mm distal to the stylomastoid foramen, the facial nerve enters the parotid gland. Here it divides at the pes anserinus into its two main temporofacial and cervicofacial divisions. The nerve then divides into its five main branches: temporal, zygomatic, buccal, mandibular, and cervical. The branching pattern of the facial nerve is variable. There is a vast anastomotic network between the branches of the facial nerve. The zygomatic and buccal branches contain the most comprehensive of these systems. The mandibular branch has the least amount of interconnections. This pattern of anastomoses accounts for the rare appearance of a midface deficit after a distal nerve injury (1). The anastomotic network also helps to explain synkinesis. Following injury to the nerve, regenerating nerve fibers have access not only to their originally innervated structures but also to other areas through the anastomotic network. As one would expect, synkinesis is most pronounced in the area where this network is most extensive (1).

Of the five branches, the buccal branch is perhaps the most vital. This branch innervates more emotionally important muscles of facial expression than any other, including the zygomaticus major, zygomaticus minor, risorius, levator anguli oris, and buccinator. As expected, when paralyzed, loss of the buccal branch

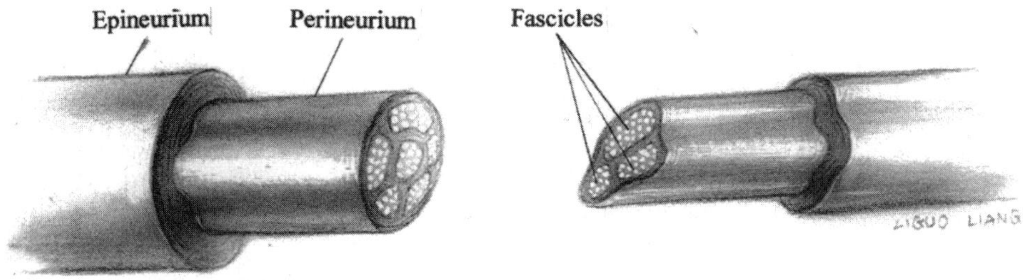

Figure 1 Cross-sectional anatomy of the facial nerve.

produces a profound cosmetic deficit with a loss of the ability to smile and collapse of the oral commissure.

The facial nerve contains 10,000 fibers and 7000 are myelinated motor fibers. Most of the motor fibers travel to the extratemporal portion of the facial nerve and innervate the muscles of facial expression. The remaining 3000 fibers branch off prior to the stylomastoid foramen and provide autonomic and special sensory innervation to the salivary and lacrimal glands and the lingual taste buds (GSP and chorda tympani nerves) (1). They also provide sensory fibers to the posterior aspect of the external auditory canal.

MICROANATOMY

The cross-sectional anatomy of the facial nerve is shown in Figure 1. Facial nerve axons are surrounded by a layer of Schwann's cells forming the myelin sheath. The myelin sheath is in turn surrounded by endoneurium. Multiple axons aggregate into fascicles. Fascicles are also encased within a connective tissue layer, the perineurium, which is a strong, thin layer of neural connective tissue resembling epithelium. The epineurium encases the fascicles to form the definitive nerve sheath. The layout and multiple layers of the nerve sheath are not uniform in the different segments of the nerve. For example, the perineurium in the meatal segment is very thin if even present. This renders this segment of nerve particularly susceptible to iatrogenic injury. The fascicular arrangement of the nerve is also variable. The intracranial segment is monofascicular while the distal mastoid segment is multifascicular. In addition, in the latter segment, the fascicles are arranged in a topographical pattern with each fascicle segregating the motor fibers that are destined for each of the distal branches of the nerve (1).

PATHOPHYSIOLOGY OF INJURY TO THE FACIAL NERVE

Physical injury to the facial nerve can result from a variety of causes: temporal bone and skull fractures and iatrogenic or intentional surgical injury. Acoustic neuroma and parotid surgery often require dissection of the facial nerve and can result in facial nerve paresis or paralysis.

Classification

In 1953 Sunderland created a detailed classification system of the degrees of nerve injuries summarized here (5):

1. First degree (neuropraxia): Electrical conduction is blocked but axoplasmic flow continues bidirectionally. In neuropraxia, the distal aspect of the nerve retains normal electrical stimulability, but voluntary motor function is abnormal. Usually neuropraxia is the result of a compressive lesion or mild trauma to the nerve during surgery. Following neuropraxia, nerve function usually returns to normal after the offending compression or injury subsides.
2. Second-degree (axonotmesis): Axonal continuity is lost and wallerian degeneration sets in distally. In this type of injury, the proximal myelin sheath remains intact and the endoneurial sheaths are preserved. The prognosis following axonotmesis is good because of the preservation of the endoneurium, which helps channel the growing axons to the distal facial muscles.
3. Third degree: The endoneurial tube is disrupted.
4. Fourth degree: The endoneurium and perineurium are disrupted and the fascicles are no longer segregated.
5. Fifth degree: The endoneurium, perineurium, and epineurium are disrupted.

In third-, fourth-, and fifth-degree injury, the endoneurium and axons are disrupted. Neurotmesis is the term used to describe these more severe degrees of injury. Wallerian degeneration and a loss of endoneurial structure characterize these lesions. This form of injury has variable and sometimes unpredictable outcomes. When various elements of the nerve sheath are severed, the regenerating nerve fibers can be rerouted randomly to the distal branches of the facial nerve. This faulty rerouting results in the phenomena known as mass movement and synkinesis.

Electrodiagnosis

Multiple electrodiagnostic tests have been devised to help surgeons decide on the advisablity and timing of surgery for the rehabilitation of facial paralysis. These tests are useful in situations where the outcome of a facial paralysis is not readily predictable. As an example, let us consider the case of patients who undergo surgery for an acoustic neuroma or parotid tumor and in whom the facial nerve is anatomically preserved at surgery. If such patients develop a complete postoperative facial paralysis, the surgeon must try to predict whether the postoperative paralysis is temporary or permanent. In this clinical setting, electrodiagnostic tests may be of help. These tests study the degree of denervation of facial muscles or injury to the facial nerve itself to help prognosticate the final outcome of facial paralysis. Despite their usefulness, these tests are not dependable enough to serve as the sole basis of a treatment plan. Four tests will be considered in this chapter: the minimal nerve excitability test, the maximal nerve excitability test, electromyography, and electroneuronography.

The minimal nerve excitability test is performed by placing an electrode on the angle of the mandible or stylomastoid foramen and another over the face on the skin overlying the various distal branches of the facial nerve. All facial nerve branches are stimulated using this technique. The current subsequently delivered is increased gradually until a visible muscle contraction is noted. The same procedure is then repeated on the normal side and the thresholds that elicit stimulation are compared (6,7).

The maximal nerve excitability test became more popular due to controversy surrounding the validity of the minimal nerve excitability test. The method is similar to that of the minimal excitability test; however, individual branches are stimulated with a stimulus intensity that generates the largest response. The strength of the facial contractions is then compared to the normal opposite side. The results are classified in three categories: minimally diminished (50% normal), markedly diminished (<25% normal), and absent (no response on the paralyzed side) (1). Studies have shown that patients with a markedly diminished or absent response within the first 2 weeks of paralysis had an 86% rate of incomplete recovery. In addition, absent response inside 10 days was correlated with incomplete recovery. In comparison, symmetrical responses within the same time period were associated with excellent recovery in more than 90% of patients (8).

Electromyographic recordings are obtained with needle electrodes placed into the facial muscle. Fibrillation potentials can usually be recorded 10–21 days after severe injury or transection of the nerve (Fig. 2). Fibrillation potentials are due to spontaneous muscle firing after muscle denervation has begun. These potentials will appear only if wallerian degeneration has occurred. Electromyography can also detect evidence of nerve regeneration. Regeneration potentials are polyphasic potentials seen when the muscle has been reinnervated (1,2,9,10).

Electroneuronography uses a supramaximal threshold stimulus to the main trunk of the facial nerve while recording the compound muscle action potential (CMAP) from the distal muscles (e.g., nasalis muscle). This test records the responses obtained from the affected side and compares them to those from the normal side. The response latency is the time difference between the onset of the stimulus and that of the CMAP and is an indicator of residual facial nerve function (11). Electroneuronography is commonly used in the evaluation of Bell's palsy, but could also be utilized in the early stages of posttraumatic facial paralysis (e.g., temporal bone fractures) (12,13).

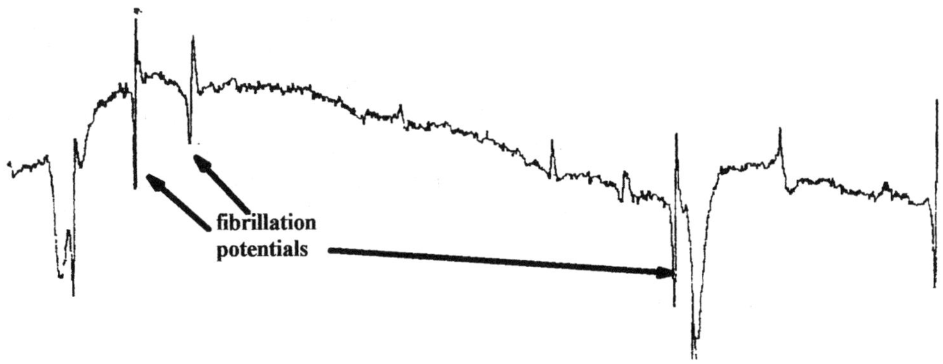

Figure 2 Fibrillation potentials of the facial nerve typical of severe injury.

EXAMINATION OF THE PARALYZED FACE

The assessment of facial function requires experience and an understanding of the natural progression and appearance of the face in patients with facial weakness or paralysis. In the case of immediate postoperative facial paralysis, it is important to be aware that even a complete transection of the facial nerve does not always result in a strikingly asymmetrical face on the same day of injury. The tone of the facial muscles may persist for a few days after the onset of paralysis and can give a symmetrical appearance to the face at rest. Moreover, when the patient blinks, the relaxation of the levator palpebrae muscle (innervated by the oculomotor nerve) may allow the eyelid on the paralyzed side to drift down in synchrony with the eyelid on the normal side. An examination of facial motion therefore requires an examination of the face at rest and during voluntary movement. With the patient at rest, the examiner watches for symmetry of the face including symmetry of the nasolabial fold and forehead lines. The nasolabial fold tends to flatten with facial paralysis, but the onset of this finding may be delayed several days. Observation of the face during blinking is also usually revealing. A lid lag is typically noted and is usually the most sensitive indicator of facial nerve dysfunction and the last finding to normalize in the final stages of recovery (Fig. 3). Lid lag becomes more pronounced a few days after the onset of paralysis when the lower lid starts to lose its natural tone, thus widening the aperture of the eye. The face is then examined during active motion. The patient is asked to move various areas of the face. When the patient is asked to close the eyes, specific instructions should be given to close the eyes tightly since many patients tend to close the eyes without squeezing. As noted above, patients with total paralysis can close the eyelids while the facial motor function is completely paralyzed. If the facial paresis is severe or if there is complete paralysis, it is sometimes difficult to determine whether the weak side is moving actively or whether the movement is secondary to the good side dragging the soft tissues of the weak side across the midline. In this situation, the examiner should apply pressure with the finger at the midline prior to asking the patient to move the face. In typical cases, pressure has to be applied over the forehead, the root of the nose, the midline of the upper lip, and the midline of the lower lip during the examination. In cases of severe paresis, a slight twitch may be the only sign of residual or regained function. In fact, regained function can be as subtle as the regaining of the definition of the nasolabial fold or a stronger facial tone at rest.

All these signs are subtle but consistent. Experience can teach the examiner the nuances of progressive facial weakness or recuperation, but it remains difficult to classify or describe, in a consistent fashion, the appearance of the face whether its function is normal or weakened. Yet, such a classification is important in standardizing the description and reporting facial nerve function and surgical results. The House-Brackmann classification of facial function is the most widely accepted method of describing facial function in its normal and abnormal states. The various grades of this classification are as follows:

1. House-Brackmann grade I
   Normal facial function in all areas.
2. House-Brackmann grade II
   Gross: slight weakness with possible synkinesis

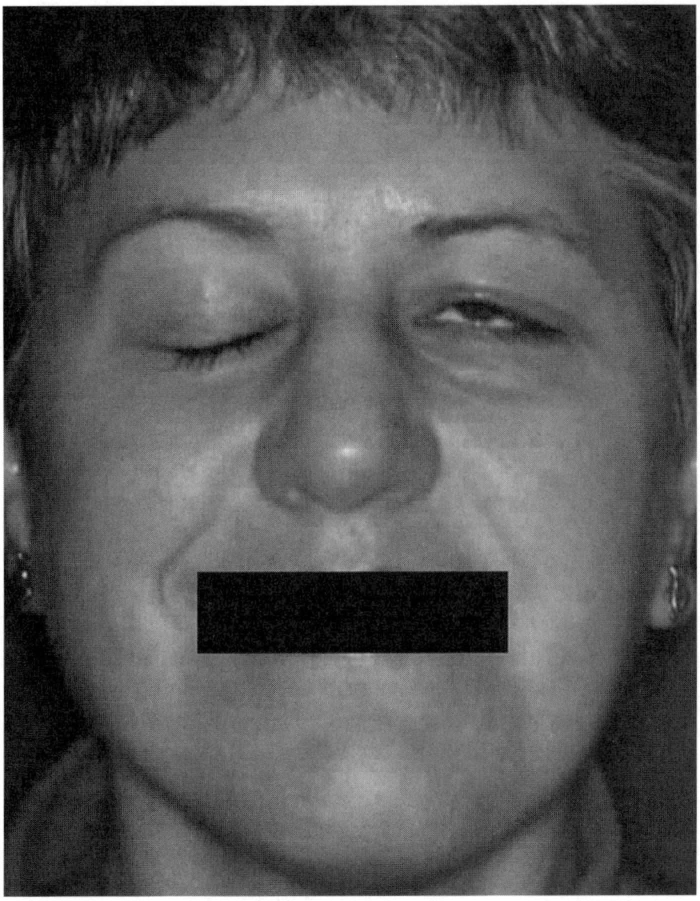

Figure 3 Note lagophthalmos demonstrated as patient attempts to close the eyes: recovering complete facial paralysis on left side.

Rest: normal symmetry and tone
Motion
Forehead: moderate to good function
Eye: complete closure
Mouth: slight asymmetry

3. House-Brackmann grade III
   Gross: obvious difference between sides; Noticeable but not severe synkinesis; contractures with or without hemifacial spasm
   Rest: normal symmetry and tone
   Motion
   Forehead: slight-to-moderate movement
   Eye: complete closure with effort
   Mouth: slightly weak with effort
4. House-Brackmann grade IV
   Gross: obvious weakness with or without disfiguring asymmetry

Rest: normal symmetry and tone
Motion
Forehead: none
Eye: incomplete closure
Mouth: asymmetrical with maximal effort

5. House-Brackmann grade V
Gross: faint motion
Rest: asymmetry
Motion
Forehead: none
Eye: incomplete closure
Mouth: slight movement
6. House-Brackmann grade VI
Complete paralysis (14)

TREATMENT OF FACIAL PARALYSIS

Treatment of facial paralysis must be individualized. Two major considerations have to be addressed in all cases. The first is a functional consideration and relates mostly to the care of the eye on the side of the paralysis. The second consideration is a cosmetic one and relates to the appearance of the face at rest and during motion. Additional considerations relate to speech and swallowing associated with facial paralysis and other associated nerve involvement (e.g., following major head and neck tumor resection).

The care of the eye is of utmost importance in patients with facial paralysis. Corneal exposure and dryness can lead to severe complications including the loss of the eye to enucleation in the most severe conditions. Eye complications are more severe in patients who exhibit a poor Bell's phenomenon resulting in corneal exposure: an upward movement of the eye when the patient closes the eyelids. On the side of the paralysis, this upward movement allows the cornea to be covered and protected by the upper eyelid. Eye complications are also more severe in patients who have an associated fifth nerve compromise with corneal anesthesia. They should be followed more closely and treated more aggressively because they cannot rely on the early symptom of pain or discomfort as an indication of impending corneal damage. In the early stages of facial paralysis, the treatment of the eye is based on generous lubrication with the use of artificial tears and protective ointments. Many physicians suggest the use of eye drops during the day and ointment at night. In some patients with severe exposure of the eye, it is advisable to use lubricating ointment during the day and night, even though the use of ointment blurs the patient's vision. The importance of eye care cannot be overstressed; at the earliest sign of discomfort, hyperemia, or conjunctival injection, an ophthalmological consultation is required. Subsequent care of the eye should be individualized according to the prognosis and expected recovery of the facial paralysis. In patients with severe corneal exposure, temporary procedures that protect the may still be necessary even though the prognosis for recovery of the face may be good. Such temporary procedures include the placement of a gold implant for the upper lid or a tightening suture for the lower lid (Frost stitch; Figs. 4,5). Such procedures can also be used prior to

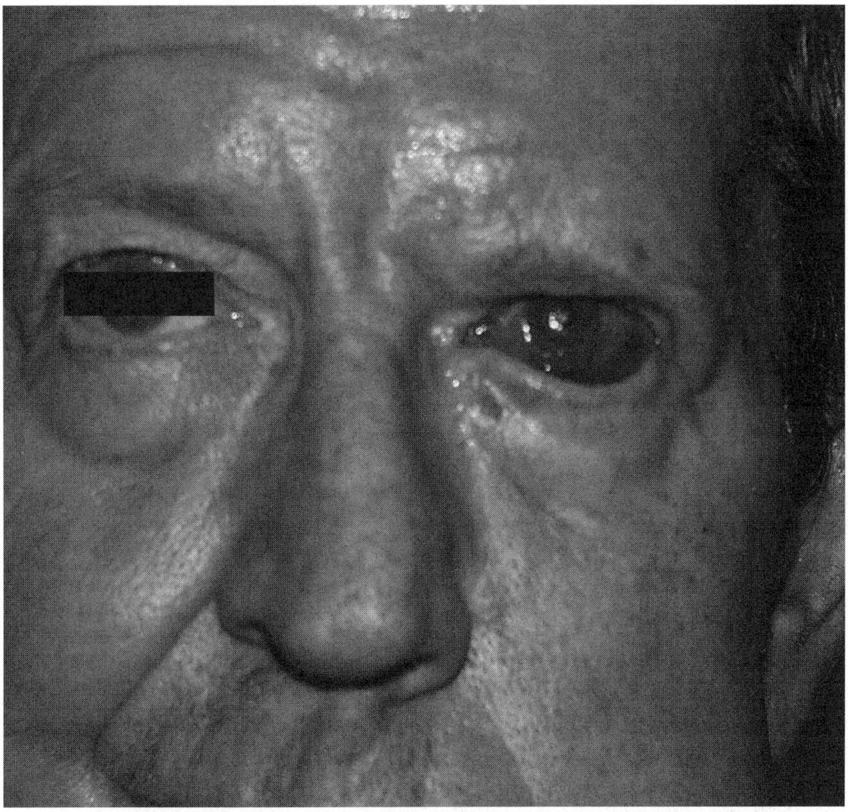

Figure 4 Severe conjunctivitis and corneal exposure in patient's left eye.

definitive eyelid surgery in cases of severe exposure keratopathy and significant paralytic ectropion.

Nonsurgical Treatment

Although early intervention is necessary and advisable in some cases, a more conservative approach is preferred when recovery, albeit incomplete, is expected. Consider the example of a patient who has a total facial paralysis following a superficial parotidectomy. If the facial nerve was anatomically preserved during surgery, management should focus on the care of the eye. The prognosis for recovery is usually excellent, especially if the nerve responded well to low-current stimulation at the end of the surgical procedure. The timing of recovery depends on the mechanism and degree of injury. Nerve stretching can cause degrees of injury varying from neuropraxia to neurotmesis. The prognosis in each case is obviously different. Another factor that should be considered is the timing of the onset of paralysis (i.e., immediate or delayed). Even the faintest active movement of the face after surgery is a good prognostic sign. Therefore, it is extremely important to check facial function immediately after the patient recovers from anesthesia.

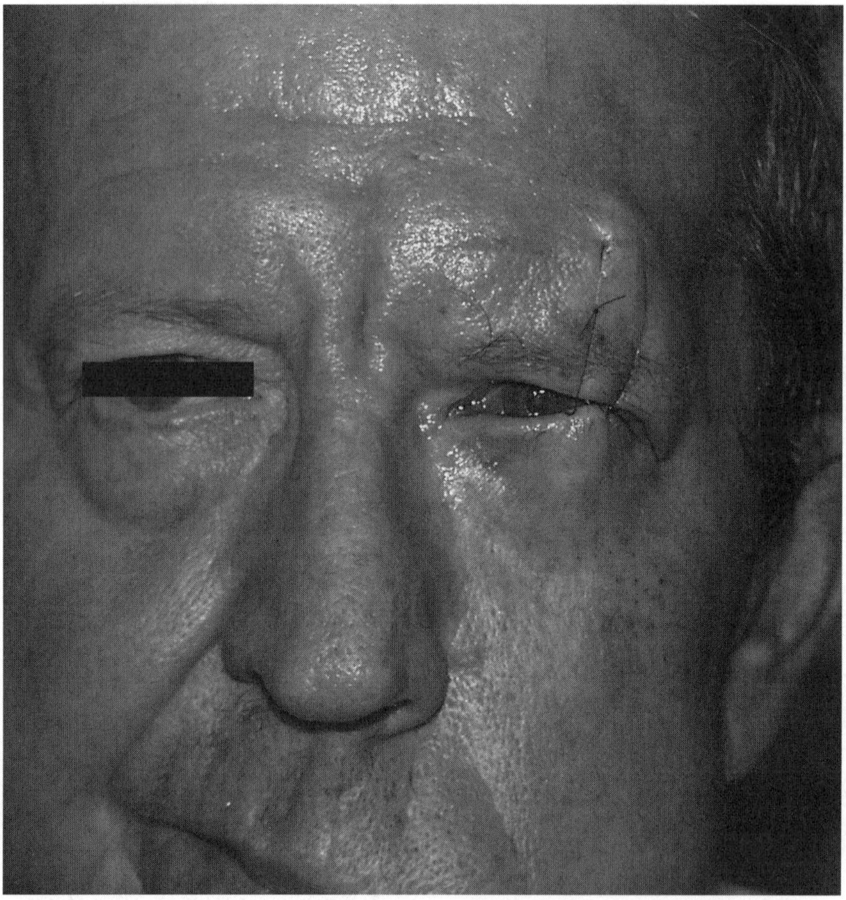

Figure 5 Prior to lower lid tightening procedure, a Frost stitch is placed as an office procedure to protect the eye.

Any residual function postoperatively is typically associated with a good prognosis. However, if the face does not improve over time the surgeon is faced with the possible need for a surgical reanimation procedure.

For patients who require surgery for facial paralysis, several considerations arise: timing of the surgery, interim treatments, and choice of the appropriate surgical procedure best tailored to the individual patient's needs. Timing considerations are crucial but highly variable. For instance, most patients who have a facial paralysis following acoustic neuroma surgery, and in whom the facial nerve was anatomically preserved, should wait for up to 1 year or longer before surgery (except that directed at temporary protection of the eye). Conversely, in patients who had the facial nerve resected as part of the treatment of a cancer do not have to wait as long and may benefit from a procedure performed during or very soon after their initial surgery (e.g., nerve graft). A patient with temporal bone trauma and obvious evidence of bony impingement or transection of the nerve should likewise also have surgery (decompression) as soon as his or her condition allows (15).

In all cases, interim treatments are necessary to ensure that the patient's eye function is preserved. In severe cases, surgery for the sole protection of the eye may be necessary. Other treatments, including speech and swallowing therapy, are helpful to assist the patient in coping with a newly acquired facial dysfunction. They also need increased dental care and hygiene especially on the side of the paralysis where dental and gum diseases are more common. Many patients with facial paralysis ask about the usefulness of facial massages and electric stimulation. The usefulness of these modalities is not established. There is some evidence that supramaximal electrical stimulation of the facial muscles may actually be deleterious.

Surgical Treatment

The choice of a surgical procedure for the rehabilitation or reanimation of the paralyzed face depends on several factors, including the health status and expected survival of the patient (especially in patients with aggressive malignancies). Other factors include the viability of the proximal portion of the paralyzed facial nerve, its distal portion, the status of the paralyzed facial muscles, and the status of other cranial nerves, especially the hypoglossal nerves. The importance of each of these factors depends on the procedure being considered. Most surgeons agree that it is preferable to initiate treatment before 1 year of the onset of paralysis (16). This requirement is somewhat arbitrary because, theoretically, the facial musculature will remain viable and maintain excitability for 18 months or longer postdenervation.

The goals for facial reanimation surgery are achieving movement of all facial muscles, regaining control of specific voluntary and involuntary muscle movements, symmetry in motion and at rest, absence of mass movement and synkinesis, and avoiding the creation of additional sensory or motor deficits. The methods of facial reanimation are broadly classified into four types: neural methods, musculofascial transpositions, facial plastic procedures, and prosthetics. Unfortunately, all goals of facial reanimation are not always achievable with the techniques available. Significant improvement can sometimes be obtained by combining several techniques. Depending on the individual presentation, the surgeon and patient must set realistic goals prior to embarking on any particular course of action.

Surgical Procedures

Neurorrhaphy

A prerequisite for successful neurorrhaphy is the presence of a viable proximal nerve and muscle target. A few days after significant injury to the facial nerve, the distal segment of the nerve cannot be stimulated due to distal axonal degeneration. This axonal degeneration is expected and is not a deterrent to repairing the nerve. However, the inability to stimulate the distal nerve may impede the surgeon's ability to find the distal nerve stump and determine its distribution to the mimetic muscles. The timing of facial nerve repair has been the subject of controversy for many years. Our current philosophy is that the facial nerve should be repaired as soon as feasible. Over time, the facial musculature may atrophy and become less stimulable. However, this time frame is relatively long, in the case of the facial nerve: 18 months–12 years.

Neurorrhaphy is the direct suturing of a severed nerve. It is the most basic form of neural repair (17). When performing a neurorrhaphy, one should be aware of the deleterious effects of physical tension at the suture line. During repair, surgeons often find that the length of the remaining nerve is not adequate, due to injury, tumor resection, or during preparation of the nerve for suturing. Excessive tension at the anastomosis will result in failure due to the growth of scar tissue at the anastomosis site (20). Rerouting the facial nerve can minimize tension. Up to 1 cm of length may be gained by rerouting the nerve in the mastoid–meatal segment. Minimizing tension can also be achieved by interposing a nerve graft.

Unlike many other nerves, the facial nerve presents a specific challenge based on the layout and orientation of the nerve fibers within its trunk. The facial nerve fibers are segregated into fascicles that selectively innervate different groups of facial muscles. This segregation of fibers is referred to as the topographical distribution of the facial nerve fibers (18,19) and can start very proximally in the nerve. Faulty rerouting of the nerve fibers results in synkinesis. In the hope of achieving more precise routing of facial nerve fibers and less synkinesis, some authors have advocated intrafascicular repair of the facial nerve. The results of intrafascicular repair have not proved to be superior to those of traditional epineural neurorrhaphy. One reason may be that, in general, epineural neurorrhaphy causes less trauma to the nerve. It remains our preferred method of neural repair.

Interpositional Grafting

An interposition nerve graft is indicated when the length of the gap between the distal and proximal nerve stumps is greater than the additional length that can be gained by mobilization. It is generally accepted that the use of an autologous graft is superior to end-to-end repair of a nerve under tension (21, 22). The greater auricular nerve is the most commonly used nerve for grafting proximal to the pes anserinus. It is harvested from the ipsilateral side of the injured facial nerve. In cases of suspected malignancy, the contralateral nerve may be utilized. The greater auricular nerve traverses the anterior aspect of the sternocleidomastoid in an anterior–superior fashion towards the auricle and the angle of the mandible. The nerve is easily found by drawing a line between the mastoid tip and the angle of the mandible. The course of the nerve usually bisects this distance and is perpendicular to the line. Between 5 and 10 cm of nerve can be harvested and consists of two or three fascicles (3).

The sural nerve is also commonly used as an interpositional graft for the facial nerve, especially distal to the pes anserinus where the facial nerve branches. The sural nerve provides cutaneous innervation to the side and back of the distal one-third of the leg, ankle, and heel. It lies 1–2 cm lateral to the saphenous vein, medial and posterior to the lateral malleolus of the ankle (3). It is an excellent choice when multiple grafts are needed as well as when long grafts are used such as in cross-facial grafting. More than 35 cm may be harvested with little residual deficit.

Once the donor nerve has been harvested, it must be treated with extreme care. The graft should be longer than the defect: excess length is desirable to minimize tension and allow for a normal amount of contracture. It should be placed in normal saline while awaiting site preparation. The use of a surgical microscope is recommended for accurate placement of the sutures. The least number of sutures that provide adequate alignment is usually employed.

As alternatives to nerve interposition, other interpositional materials have been utilized such as gold foil, collagen tubes, and freeze-thawed muscle (1). More recent reports suggest that the use of neurotrophic factors may become commonplace in the future (23–31). Although these efforts are promising and likely to be included in the surgeon's armamentarium in the future, there are, at present, no established clinical applications for them.

Crossover Techniques

In crossover procedures, the distal branch of the paralyzed facial nerve is anastomosed with a donor nerve other than the ipsilateral facial nerve itself. The most commonly used donor nerve is the ipsilateral hypoglossal nerve. Another nerve that can be used is the ipsilateral spinal accessory nerve. A special mention is given to cross-face grafting in which the source nerves is the distal branches of the contralateral (normal) facial nerve. In this operation, the contralateral distal facial fibers are connected to the corresponding facial fibers on the paralyzed side with the use of an interposition graft, usually the sural nerve.

Nerve crossover operations are usually considered when a simple neurorrhaphy or a neurorrhaphy with an interposition nerve is not feasible. These circumstances typically arise when the proximal portion of the nerve has been damaged or resected (e.g., large acoustic neuroma).

Hypoglossal-Facial Crossover Procedure (XII-VII Crossover)

For this procedure to be successful, it is important to ascertain that the proximal donor nerve (hypoglossal) and the distal facial nerve function properly. It is also essential to establish that the facial musculature is viable and able to accept reinnervation. Electrophysiological testing is helpful in establishing the suitability of these muscles for reinnervation.

The classic procedure is performed through a modified parotid incision extending under the lobule of the ear to approximately 4 cm below the body of the mandible. Flaps are raised and the anterior border of the sternocleidomastoid and posterior belly of the digastric muscles are identified (Fig. 6). The facial nerve is identified by any one of several well-described techniques and dissected into the parotid to the level of the temporofacial and cervicofacial bifurcation. This dissection is continued retrogradely to the stylomastoid foramen and the nerve is cut. The hypoglossal nerve is then dissected under the posterior belly of the digastric muscle. Once found, the nerve is dissected anteriorly and transected as distally as possible. This free end is then folded back over the digastric and anastomosed to the cut end of the facial nerve. The anastomosis is performed in the same manner as a simple neurorrhaphy. The anastomotic site is covered with soft tissue and the wound is closed over a drain (32).

The hypoglossal crossover procedure was first popularized by Baker and Conley and became one of most dependable ways to rehabilitate the paralyzed face. According to Baker and Conley, the procedure has eight distinct advantages: it is uncomplicated requiring only one suture line; it is easier to obtain a good functional result because most facial movements are associated with voluntary and involuntary

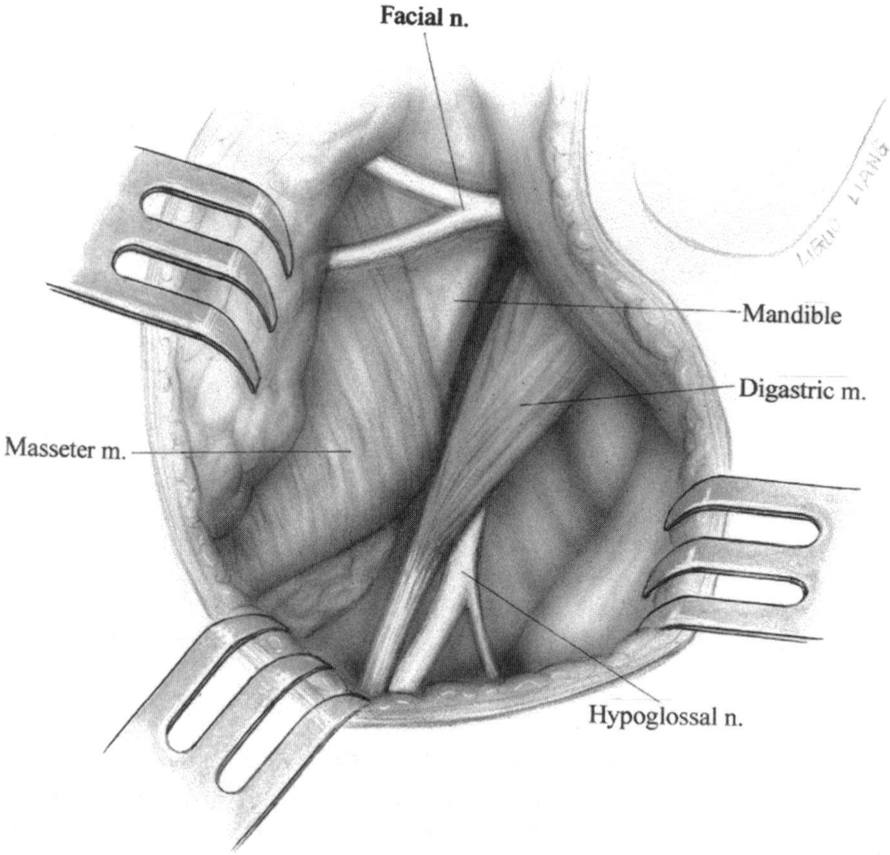

Figure 6 Anatomical relationship of the facial nerve, hypoglossal nerve, and posterior belly of the digastric muscle.

tongue movements; there is better symmetry and more rapid facial movement is gained; there is minimal discomfort from the loss of the ipsilateral twelfth nerve; there is only a mild functional deficit from the loss of the 12th nerve; facial movement is more natural with phonation; an enhanced dynamic functional result is obtained; on a central level, there is a close relationship between the motor region of the cortex of the hypoglossal and facial nerves (33).

At least 90% of patients who are operated within 18 months of the onset of their paralysis have improved facial movement (33–37). The best result is obtained when surgery is performed as close as possible to the time of the insult. The early signs of improvement usually begin within 3–6 months, with continuing improvement in facial tone and movement for the following 18–24 months. Because of the very nature of the XII–VII crossover procedure, a successful result is achieved when the patient develops good facial tone at rest and is able to produce voluntary movement of the face. But even with a so-called successful result, spontaneous and emotive movements are usually not achieved since the face does not move passively or in synchrony with the nonparalyzed side. Patients should

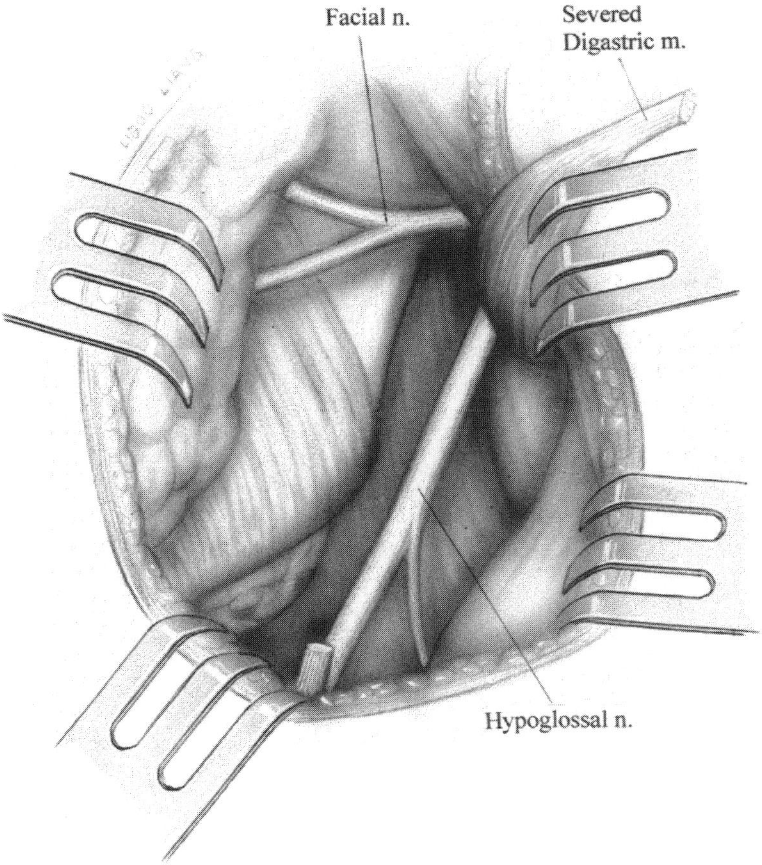

Figure 7 Digastric muscle is divided to facilitate exposure of the proximal hypoglossal nerve.

be counseled preoperatively as to the expectations and chances of success and failure of the procedure. Although 90% of patients have postoperative improvement, it is estimated that only 40% achieve what might be termed an excellent result (1,33,34,36,37).

Recent modifications to the classic XII–VII procedure promise improvement in two common problems or complications of the procedure: tongue atrophy and hypertonia of the face. The modification requires splitting the hypoglossal nerve (thus the term hemihypoglossal) and keeping half of its circumference in continuity. This modification usually allows patients to keep some nerve function to the ipsilateral tongue. The upper half of the nerve is then anastomosed to the trunk of the facial nerve using an interposition graft. The use of the graft is reportedly necessary to avoid tension on the stump of the upper half of the hypoglossal nerve (38,39). In our experience, however, a hemihypoglossal facial crossover is easily achieved without an interposition graft if the hypoglossal nerve is exposed high in the neck and closer to the base of the skull, aided by division of the posterior belly of the digastric muscle (Figs. 7,8). As with any procedure, the use of XII–VII crossover procedures is

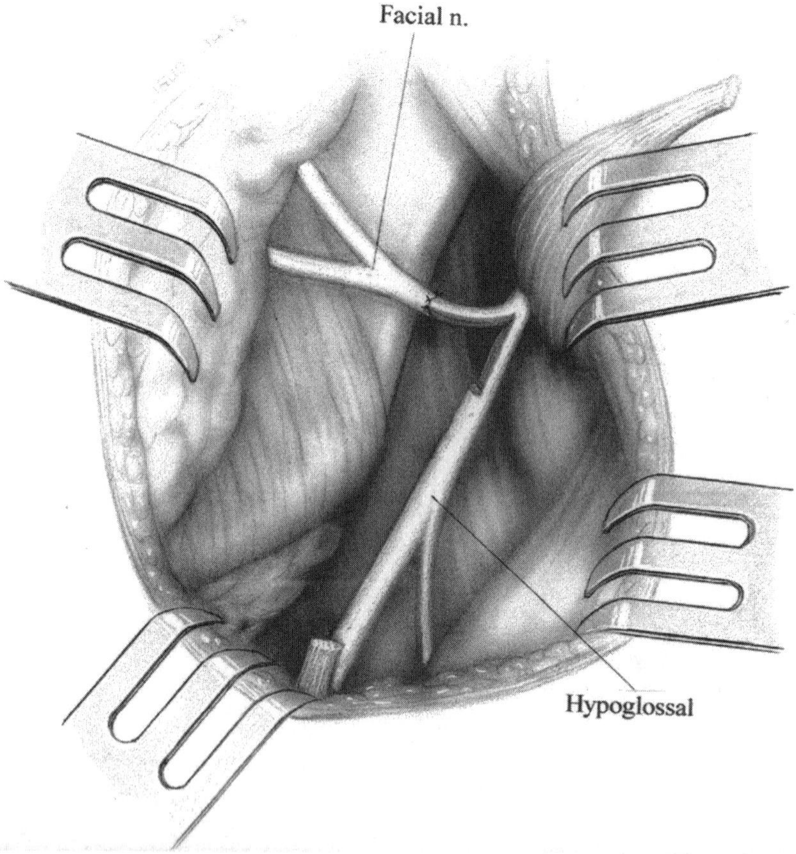

Figure 8 Hemihypoglossal facial crossover.

not highly recommended in patients with multiple cranial nerve deficits on the same or contralateral side of the facial paralysis.

As an alternative to the XII–VII crossover procedure, some surgeons favor the use of the spinal accessory to facial nerve (XI–VII) crossover technique. The theory and technique of this procedure are similar to those of the XII–VII procedure. The disadvantages of the XI–VII crossover technique are similar to those seen after a radical neck dissection: shoulder drop and shoulder pain.

Cross-Facial Grafting

The cross-facial technique uses interposition nerve grafts tunneled across the face to connect facial nerve branches on the nonparalyzed side to the facial nerve branches on the paralyzed side. The rationale for the use of this technique is the theoretical possibility of symmetrical facial movement. Symmetrical and synchronous movement of the face is essential in providing a normal appearance to the face at rest and during nonvoluntary movement. A significant component of one's overall appearance is due to a specific involuntary distribution and intensity of facial muscular tone that reflects one's emotional state. A relaxed appearance and a faint smile are not usually noticed by the subject but are readily apparent to the observer. These emotional and involuntary movements cannot be duplicated by the XII–VII or XI–VII crossover procedures.

The idea that one can coordinate movement with the opposite face is very appealing. In 1970, Scaramella described the use of the contralateral facial nerve branches to reanimate the face (40). Fisch also reported on the use of this procedure and demonstrated that 50% of the very distal facial nerve fibers can be sacrificed with no apparent deficit on the donor (nonparalyzed) side, especially in the distribution of the buccal and zygomatic branches (41). The popularity of this procedure has waned due to concern about damaging a normally functioning facial nerve and, more importantly, because of suboptimal results. The distal branches on the normal side (donor nerves) do not have enough power to move the paralyzed side effectively. In other words, facial movement that results from a cross-facial graft is generally much weaker than the movement generated by a XII–VII crossover operation (42). Although 50% of patients undergoing a cross-facial operation experienced adequate symmetry at rest, only 10% regained satisfactory (strong) voluntary facial movement (43).

There have been recent attempts to combine various procedures to achieve more natural-appearing results. Feghali and Strauch (personal communication) have had a limited but favorable experience with a multiple-stage procedure aimed at combining the advantages of the cross-facial and the XII–VII crossover operations while minimizing the disadvantages inherent in these two operations. The main advantage of the cross-facial operation is that, when the operation is successful, both sides of the face move simultaneously. As discussed, this synchrony is extremely important for the mimetic function of the face. Important aspects of one's appearance are difficult to duplicate unless the movement of the reinnervated face is connected to the innervation of the opposite, nonparalyzed, side. The main disadvantage of the cross-facial procedure has already been mentioned: it does not reinnervate the paralyzed musculature with enough power to exhibit strong voluntary movement of the face. The main advantage of the XII–VII crossover operation is that it provides patients with sufficient power to generate good facial tone and voluntary movement. A disadvantage of this operation is that it seems to provide many patients with too strong a resting tone (tonus phenomenon) and exaggerated voluntary movement. Another is that the resultant movement lacks any synchrony with the opposite nonparalyzed side. Many of the advantages of the two techniques can be retained while avoiding many of the disadvantages by combining the cross-facial with the XII–VII crossover procedure.

In the first stage of the modified hemihypoglossal–facial crossover, a hemihypoglossal facial nerve crossover (without an interposition graft) is performed as described. During the same stage, cross-facial nerve grafts, obtained from the sural nerve, are anastomosed to the donor side and tunneled across the face to the areas of the corresponding branches on the paralyzed side (Fig. 9). During this stage, the cross-facial grafts are tagged but not attached to their recipient facial nerve branches on the paralyzed side. After a wait of about 6 months, the face on the paralyzed side normally gains strength and tone owing to the relatively strong innervation of the donor hemihypoglossal nerve. At this time, the cross-facial grafts are anastomosed to the distal branches on the previously paralyzed side (Fig. 10).

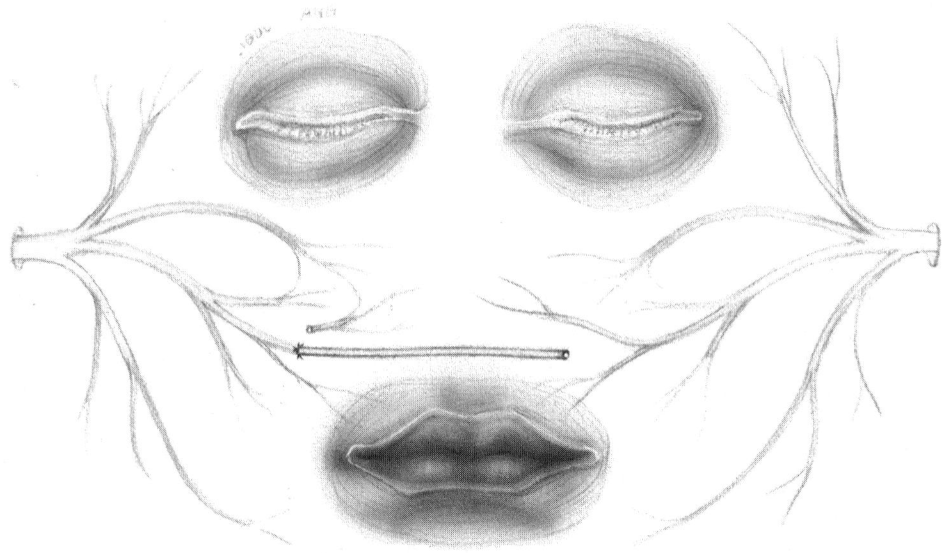

Figure 9 Sural nerve graft tunneled under the upper lip to the opposite paralyzed side.

After another 6 months the outcome is re-evaluated. In three of three patients grade III/VI House-Brackmann results were achieved. All three patients had excellent symmetry at rest. The synchrony and emotional involuntary movement were present in all patients although they were somewhat weak in two. The tongue movement was excellent in all three and there was no tongue atrophy at 1 year postopera-

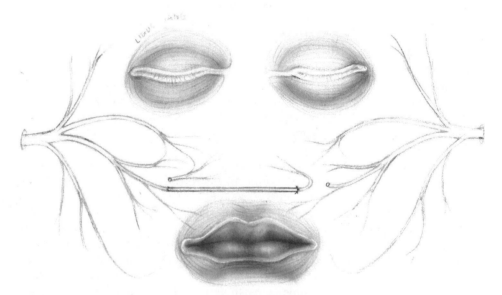

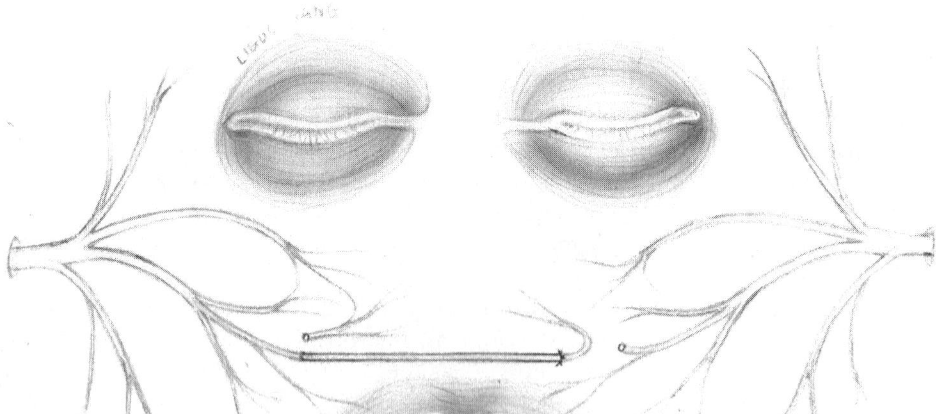

Figure 10 Cross-facial grafts are anastomosed to the distal branches on the previously paralyzed side.

tively. There was a transient partial atrophy of the tongue in one patient that improved over the course of 6 months. One patient had a lid lag that was enhanced with a gold implant and lower lid tightening to achieve a more natural appearance. These three cases illustrate the usefulness of combining procedures to suit a particular patient's needs. They also underscore the need for further developments and refinements to achieve improved results in the future.

Neuromuscular Transfers

Neuromuscular transfer procedures utilize innervated muscles in the head and neck that are rotated and attached to the paralyzed facial muscles, thus achieving dynamic function along with static support of the soft tissues of the paralyzed face. Commonly called dynamic sling procedures, they are typically used when the muscle to be reanimated has atrophied to such an extent that nerve crossover procedures are no longer viable options. Occasionally, neuromuscular transfers are used to augment nerve interposition or crossover procedures that have not attained the desired result. Several muscles have been used in neuromuscular transfers. The temporalis and masseter muscles are the most popular. Less popular are the anterior belly of the digastric, mylohyoid, and sternocleidomastoid muscles.

The temporalis muscle transposition flap is the most versatile and most commonly used muscle for this technique. This fan-shaped muscle is innervated by the trigeminal nerve. For this flap to be successful, the nerve and blood supply and fascia of the muscle must be intact (44). It can used to reanimate the eye but it is more commonly used to reanimate the oral commissure. The procedure begins with a vertical temporal incision from the temporal crest inferiorly to the zygoma. The dissection is continued lateral to the temporalis fascia exposing the central aspect of the muscle. Once an adequate portion of the muscle has been exposed, a vertical incision is made through the muscle to the level of the zygoma and the muscle is elevated with the periosteum intact. The recipient site is then prepared with an incision in the nasolabial fold and the orbicularis oris is exposed. If this muscle is atrophic, the submucosa of the lip is isolated. A tunnel is then created between the temporal fossa and the nasolabial incision coursing just superficial to the body of the zygoma. The distal aspect of the flap is split and folded over the arch of the zygoma through the tunnel to the nasolabial incision. Here it is secured to the muscle or submucosa at the oral commissure. If the muscle does not reach its intended destination it may require extension to attain adequate length. This extension can be achieved by interposing a strip of fascia lata (45). The muscle and its fascial extension will tend to pull the corner of the mouth superiorly and posteriorly. The surgeon should pull on the corner of the mouth in the direction of the muscle and overcorrect the droop at the corner of the mouth during attachment. In fact, the overcorrection can result in a relatively grotesque appearance at the end of the procedure, but with time this overcorrection will give way to a more naturally appearing facial contour. The folding of the muscle results in a bulge in the area of the zygomatic arch and a donor site defect more superiorly. Some surgeons advocate fracture or resection of the zygomatic arch (1,45,46).

May and Drucker reported their results with temporal muscle rotation flaps in 219 patients. They achieved an 80% restoration of a smile and overall improvement in mouth function in 96% of patients. They also noted a 21% complication rate, with the most common being infection in 12%. The same authors suggested several modifications of the technique. They recommended that the procedure be limited to the reanimation of the corner of the mouth and that the central aspect of the muscle alone be sectioned and rotated. They also suggested Gore-Tex as the material to be used for lengthening of the temporal muscle flap instead of fascia lata. If the temporal muscle rotation flap technique is used for reanimation of the corner of the mouth alone, the surgeon can use ancillary procedures to rehabilitate the eye such as a gold implant to the upper eyelid and tightening and elevating the lower eyelid (see below) (47).

The masseter muscle provides the surgeon with an alternative dynamic sling technique when the temporal muscle is not available, such as following temporal bone resection. This flap can be performed intraorally or extraorally. The intraoral application has the distinct advantage of avoiding an external incision, while the extraoral approach provides better exposure and control over the procedure. The incision is typically placed in the submandibular area with exposure of the muscle as it inserts onto the mandible. The fascia overlying the muscle is kept attached. The anterior two-thirds of the muscle is then used as a rotation muscle flap. The neurovascular supply, which enters the muscle from the deep surface at the level of the condylar notch, is kept intact. Another incision is then created at the nasolabial fold and the masseter muscle is attached to the orbicularis oris muscle. The direction of pull of this dynamic sling is superolaterally. An overcorrection of the asymmetry in the face is necessary to compensate for the subsequent relaxation and sagging of the tissues. Some surgeons believe that this technique can allow neurotization of the orbicularis oris by the masseter muscle. To promote neurotization, the undersurface of the masseter fascia must be stripped to allow axons to cross from the masseter muscle to the orbicularis oris muscle. When compared to the temporal muscle dynamic sling, the masseter flap has two main disadvantages. The first is that the masseter muscle is smaller and weaker than the temporalis muscle, providing less support and animation. The second is that the vector of pull of the masseter flap is more horizontal instead of the more favorable superolateral pull of the temporalis.

Static Techniques

Static reanimation procedures should be considered in patients whose condition or preference does not allow them to undergo complex procedures and postoperative rehabilitation. In general, the technique consists of using strips of fascia or synthetic material (e.g., Gore-Tex) to support the corner of the mouth. The strip is tunneled subcutaneously from the temporal fossa and zygomatic arch to the corner of the mouth. It is secured to the oral commissure with nonabsorbing suture through the modiolus. The technique is relatively simple and often combined with rhytidectomies and brow lifts. Recently, because of donor site morbidity, many users of this technique have preferred Gore-Tex to fascia lata as a suspension material (48–50).

Microneurovascular Flaps for Reanimation of the Paralyzed Face

The indications for use of microneurovascular free muscle flaps are similar to those for dynamic muscle slings. In fact, in many centers a free flap has become the treatment of choice in long-standing facial paralysis (51). In 1976, Harii was the first to describe the application of free flaps for the treatment of facial paralysis (52). Free flap reanimation of the face usually requires two stages. In the first stage, a sural nerve graft is used as a cross-facial nerve graft, the distal end lying free within the paralyzed side. In the second stage, 6–9 months later, a free microneurovascular muscle flap is placed in line with the nonviable zygomatic major muscle and its nerve supply is anastomosed to the sural nerve graft. In the usual case, only the corner of the mouth is rehabilitated using this method but it is possible to split the free muscle flap into independently functioning units to reanimate the eye as well. More recently, one-stage procedures have been performed with favorable results (53). Free flaps with nerve pedicles able to reach the opposite face (e.g., latissimus or abductor hallucis muscles) may be transferred to the face in one stage since the cross-facial graft is unneeded. Presently, free flaps are typically used for the reanimation of the lower two-thirds of the face, and are combined with simpler, yet effective, procedures such as upper lid gold implants for rehabilitation of the eye (54).

Aviv et al. described the ideal characteristics of a free muscle that could be used for reanimation of the face: adequate muscle surface area to allow sufficient force of contraction, reliable neurovascular pedicle of adequate length and caliber, segmental innervation so that one nerve supply can innervate muscle segments of varying orientation, low donor site morbidity, and facile harvesting (57). No single muscle is the ideal choice for all patients. Those used include the following: latissimus dorsi, gracilis, pectoralis minor, rectus abdominis, serratus anterior, abductor hallucis longis, extensor digitorum brevis, and rectus femoris (55–60). The most popular of these muscles are the gracilis and latissimus dorsi muscles because they provide enough power and excursion to drive mimetic facial movement with the least amount of bulk (61).

Wei et al. described the one-stage transfer of the latissimus dorsi muscle flap in 86 patients with long-standing facial palsy (Figs. 11,12). A segment of the latissimus dorsi is dissected from the distal part of the muscle so that the flap has an extended neurovascular pedicle. This flap is then split and transferred to the site of implantation. The pedicle is passed through a tunnel in the upper lip to the functioning side of the face. The neurovascular pedicle is anastomosed to branches of the facial nerve, artery, and veins of the functional side of the face. In this series, a satisfactory result was attained in 80 patients, as evaluated at 8 months to 2 years postoperatively. It is interesting that expressive movement is seen not only in the transferred muscle but also in the paralyzed facial muscles covered by the flap. This is postulated to be a result of muscle-to-muscle neurotization (62).

Rehabilitation of the Paralyzed Eye

As described earlier, the care of the eye is essential in patients with facial paralysis. In new-onset facial paralysis, the eye should be cared for with hydration, lubrication, humidity chambers, and other modalities that prevent corneal exposure and drying. If the facial nerve is expected to recuperate quickly, this local care of the eye is usually sufficient. However, if the eye exposure is excessive or if the face is expected to remain paralyzed, more aggressive methods of eye protection may be necessary. Classic tarsorrhaphy or dynamic slings may still have a role in selected patients, but presently the use of various upper and lower eyelid procedures provide patients with functional and more cosmetically pleasing results. Two muscles mediate upper eyelid movement. The levator palpebrae muscle, which

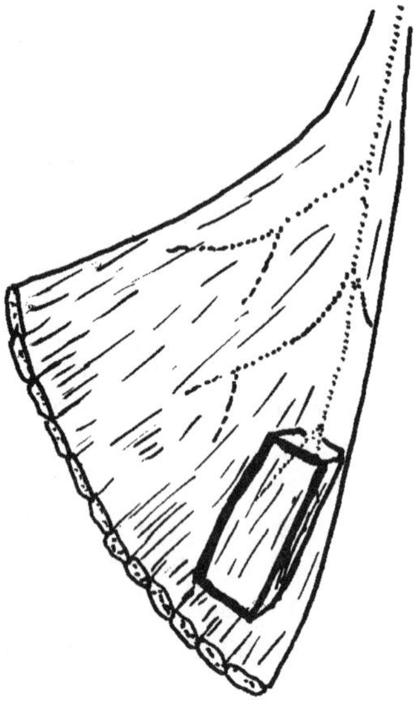

Figure 11 Segmental portion of latissimus dorsi muscle with unique neurovascular pedicle. (From Ref. (62).)

is innervated by the oculomotor nerve, lifts the upper eyelid. The orbicularis oculi muscle, which is innervated by the facial nerve, mediates closure of the upper eyelid. When the facial nerve is paralyzed, the upper eyelid tends to remain open because of the unopposed action of the levator palpebrae muscle. Most procedures are intended to reanimate the upper eyelid in an attempt to compensate for the unopposed action of the levator palpebrae muscle. The spring implant popularized by Levine et al. consists of placing a spring that tends to close the eyelid at rest (63–64). When the levator palpebrae contracts, the upper eyelid opens again. However, this technique is technically difficult and the spring has a high extrusion rate

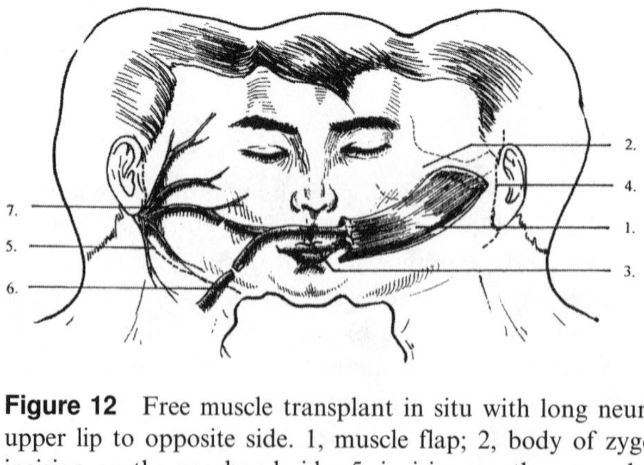

Figure 12 Free muscle transplant in situ with long neurovascular pedicle tunneled under upper lip to opposite side. 1, muscle flap; 2, body of zygoma; 3, neurovascular pedicle; 4, incision on the paralyzed side; 5, incision on the normal side; 6, facial artery and vein; 7, buccal branches. (From Ref. (62).

in the hands of surgeons who are not experienced with its use (65). The use of gold implants is currently the more popular method used to enhance eye closure because of its ease and efficacy. As early as 1974, Jobe reported a greater than 90% success rate by using gold implants modified by manipulating their contour and the addition of holes to secure the implants (66). Several authors have since validated this technique (65,67–69). Gold weights function similarly to the upper eyelid spring, except that it is the weight of the implant (not the action of the spring) that closes the upper eyelid when the levator palpebrae muscle relaxes.

An upper eyelid gold implant can be placed under local or general anesthesia. In a sterile field, an incision is made in the crease of the upper lid. The surgical plane is deep to the orbicularis muscle and superficial to the tarsus. After an adequate pocket has been dissected, a prefabricated 0.6–1.6 g implant is secured to the tarsal plate. The appropriate weight may be selected preoperatively by taping various sizes to the upper lid. Although a heavier weight will result in more effective eye closure, too much weight will cause ptosis by overwhelming the opposing action of the levator muscle. The wound is closed in two layers with fine absorbable suture. If incomplete closure is anticipated, a mullerectomy may be performed. Muller's muscle originating from the levator provides tonic elevation to the lid. This muscle is adherent to the conjunctiva and can be incised through the conjunctiva with a scalpel (65,70). As with all foreign bodies, extrusion of the gold implant is a concern but is rare. Superior migration is more common but does not usually necessitate removal of the implant (65). One important advantage of upper eyelid implants is that they are reversible. Thus many surgeons use them readily for temporary protection of the eye in patients with temporary paralysis, in whom conservative treatment of the eye is not sufficient for protection.

In many patients with facial paralysis, a laxity in the lower eyelid contributes to ectropion and conjunctiva and corneal exposure. Reanimation of the upper eyelid is not sufficient to protect the eye. Therefore, lower lid tightening and elevation are commonly combined with procedures aimed at the upper eyelid such as the gold weight implants. One method of lower eyelid tightening is the lateral tarsal strip procedure (see Blepharoplasty chapter in this volume). In this procedure, a lateral canthotomy is performed and the lateral segment of the lower lid is then separated into musculocutaneous and tarsoconjunctival layers. The tarsoconjunctival layer is abraded to promote adherence and then sutured to the periosteum of the inner orbital rim laterally to shorten and tighten the lower lid. The musculocutaneous layer is then trimmed appropriately and closed with absorbable suture (3,65,71–73). In addition to tightening, many surgeons favor procedures that also provide significant elevation of the lower eyelid. This combination of tightening and elevation of the lower eyelid is more important in patients with severe exposure keratopathy. The lid may be raised by up to 4–5 mm for improved corneal protection with the use of a rigid spacer (e.g., conchal cartilage) placed deep to the inferior tarsus and superficial to the capsulopalpebral fascia (65). Combining upper and lower eyelid procedures has significantly improved the care of the eye in patients with facial paralysis. The success of these procedures has lessened the need for more extensive surgical procedures designed to decrease corneal exposure and has allowed the surgeon to focus more attention on significant functional and aesthetic defects in the cheek and lip.

Ancillary Procedures

The multitude of procedures aimed at reanimating the paralyzed face underscores the fact that no one procedure achieves perfect results in all patients. Many patients who recuperate from facial paralysis are left with various partial deficits. For example, forehead motion rarely recovers in most patients with significant facial paralysis. Patients with very lax or aged skin may still have a significant cosmetic deficit after regaining muscle tone of the face. Conversely, many patients have hypertonia of the facial muscles following XII–VII crossover procedures. For these patients with partially satisfactory results, other ancillary procedures can be considered such as rhytidectomy, blepharoplasty, and brow lifts. Patients with hypertonia may benefit from selective Botulinum toxin injections.

CONCLUSION

This chapter reviewed some aspects of the extensive subject of facial paralysis and reanimation. It is obvious that no combination of procedures has yet been able to restore totally normal facial function for all patients. Yet the concepts and procedures described in this chapter have increased our understanding of facial nerve paralysis and improved our patients' outcome. Further advances are expected in the prevention of facial paralysis, nerve regeneration, and surgical rehabilitation. Such advances will be welcome additions to our imperfect but ever increasing knowledge of this exciting and challenging subject.

REFERENCES

1. Hughes GB, Pensak ML, eds. Clinical Otology. New York: Thieme, 1997.
2. Jackler RK, Brackmann DE, eds. Neurotology, Philadelphia: Mosby, 1994.
3. Bailey B, ed. Head and Neck Surgery Otolaryngology. 2nd ed. New York: Lippincott-Raven, 1998.
4. Schuknecht HF, Gulya AJ. Anatomy of the Temporal Bone with Surgical Implications. Philadelphia: Lea & Febiger, 1986.
5. Sunderland S, Cossar DF. The structure of the facial nerve. Anat Rec 1953; 116:147–162.
6. Gates GA. Nerve excitability testing: technical pitfalls and threshold norms using absolute values. Laryngoscope 1993; 103:379–385.
7. May M. Nerve excitability test in facial palsy: limitations in its use, based on a study of 130 patients. Laryngoscope 1972; 82:2122–2128.
8. May M, Blumenthal F, Klein S. Acute Bell's palsy: prognostic value of evoked electromyography, max stimulation and other electrical tests. Am J Otol 1983; 5:1–7.
9. Sillman JS, Niparko JK, Lee SS, Kileny PR. Prognostic value of evoked and standard electromyography in acute facial paralysis. Otol Head Neck Surg 1992; 107:377–381.
10. Fisch U. Prognostic value of electrical tests in acute facial paralysis. Am J Otol 1984; 5:494–498.
11. Joachims HZ, Bialik V, Eliachar I. Early diagnosis in Bells' Palsy: a nerve conduction study. Laryngoscope 1980; 90(10 part 1):1705–1708.
12. Fisch U. Surgery for Bell's palsy. Arch Otolaryngol 1981; 107:1–11.
13. Fisch U. Maximal nerve excitability testing vs. electroneuronography. Arch Otolaryngol 1980; 106:352–357.

14. House JW, Brackmann DE. Facial nerve grading system. Otolaryngol Head Neck Surg 1985; 93:146–147.
15. Coker NJ. Management of traumatic injuries to the facial nerve. Otolaryngol Clin North Am 1991; 24:215–227.
16. May M. Surgical rehabilitation of facial palsy: total approach. In: May M, ed. The Facial Nerve, 1st ed. New York: Thieme, 1986.
17. Balance C, Duel AB. The operative treatment of facial palsy by the introduction of nerve grafts into the fallopian canal and by other intratemporal methods. Arch Otolaryngol 1932; 15:1–70.
18. Gacek RR, Radpour S. Fiber orientation of the facial nerve: an experimental study in the cat. Laryngoscope 1982; 92:547–556.
19. Kempe LG. Topographic organization of the distal portion of the facial nerve. J Neurosurg 1980; 52:671–673.
20. Millesi H, Berger A, Meissl G. Experimentelle Untersuchungen zur Heiliung durchtrennter peripherer Nerve. Chir Plast 1972; 1:174–206.
21. Samii M, Wallenborn R. Tierexperimentelle Untersuchhungen uber den Einflu*beta* der Spannung auf den Regenerationserfolg nach Nervennaht. Acta Neurochir 1972; 27:87–110.
22. Terris DJ, Fee WE. Current issues in nerve repair. Arch Otolaryngol Head Neck Surg 1993; 119:725–731.
23. Li JM, Brackmann DE, Hitselberger WE, Linthicum FH Jr, Lim DJ. Coexpression of neurotrophic growth factors and their receptors in human facial motor neurons. Ann Otol Rhinol Laryngol 1999; 108(9):903–908.
24. Burazin TC, Gundlach AL. Up-regulation of GDNFR-alpha and c-ret mRNA in facial motor neurons following facial nerve injury in the rat. Brain Res Mol Brain Res 1998; 55(2):331–336.
25. Tong JX, Rich KM. Diphenylpiperazines enhance regeneration after facial nerve injury. J Neurocytol 1997; 26(5):339–347.
26. Kobayashi NR, Bedford AM, Hincke MT, Tetzlaff W. Increased expression of BDNF and trkB in mRNA in rat facial motorneurons after axotomy. Eur J Neurosci 1996; 8(5):1018–1029.
27. Rossiter JP, Rioplelle RJ, Bisby MA. Axotomy-induced apoptotic cell death of neonatal rats facial motorneurons: time course analysis and relation to NADPH-diaphorase activity. Exp Neurol 1996; 138(1):33–44.
28. Oh C, Murray B, Bhattacharya N, Holland D, Tatton WG. (-)– Deprenyl alters the survival of adult murine facial motorneurons after axotomy: increases in vulnerable C57BL strain but decreases in motor neuron degeneration mutants. J Neurosci Res 1994; 38(1):64–74.
29. Ansari KS, Yu PH, Kruck TP, Tatton WG. Rescue of axotomized immature rat facial motorneurons by R(-)-deprenyl: stereospecificity and independence from monoamine oxidase inhibition. J Neurosci 1993; 13(9):4042–4053.
30. Yu WH, Cao CG. Testosterone fails to rescue motorneurons from axotomy-induced death in young rats. Neuroreport 1992; 3(12):1042–1044.
31. Salo PT, Tatton WG–Deprenyl reduces the death of motorneurons caused by axotomy. J Neurosci Res 1992; 31(2):394–400.
32. Bailey B, ed. Atlas of Head and Neck Surgery Otolaryngology, 2nd ed. New York: Lippincott-Raven, 1998.
33. Conley J, Baker DC. Hypoglossal–facial nerve anastomosis for reinnervation of the paralyzed face. Plast Reconstr Surg 1979; 63:63–72.
34. Pitty LF, Tator CH. Hypoglossal–facial nerve anastomosis for facial nerve palsy following surgery for cerebellopontine angle tumors. J Neurosurg 1992; 77:724–731.

35. Sobol SM, May M. Hypoglossal–facial anastomosis: Its role in contemporary facial reanimation. In: Rubin LR, ed. The Paralyzed Face, 1st ed. St. Louis: Mosby Year Book, 1991:137–143.
36. Kunihiro T, Kanzaki J, O-Uchi T. Hypoglossal-facial nerve anastomosis. Acta Otolaryngol (Stockh) 1991; 487:80–84.
37. Pensak ML, Jackson CG, Glasscock ME, Gulya AJ. Facial reanimation with the VII-XII anastomosis: analysis of functional and physiologic results. Otolaryngol Head Neck Surg 1986; 94(3):305–310.
38. May M, Sobol SM, Mester SJ. Hypoglossal–facial nerve interpositional-jump graft for facial reanimation without tongue atrophy. Otolaryngol Head Neck Surg 1991; 104(6):818–825.
39. Hammerschlag PE. Facial reanimation with jump interpositional graft hypoglossal facial anastomoses and hypoglossal facial anastomoses: evolution in management of facial paralysis. Laryngoscope 1999; 109(2 Pt 2 Su 99):1–23.
40. Scaramella LF.Cross-face facial nerve anastomosis: historical notes. Ear Nose Throat J 1996; 75:343, 347–352, 354.
41. Fisch U: Cross-face grafting in facial paralysis. Arch Otolaryngol 1976; 102:453–457, 1976.
42. Cooper TM, McMahon, Lex C, Lenert JJ, Johnson PC. Cross-facial nerve grafting for facial reanimation: effect on normal hemi face motion. J Reconstr Microsurg 1996; 12(2):99–103.
43. Samii M, in discussion, Conley J, De Amicis E, Miehlke A, et al: Rehabilitiation of the face by VII nerve substitution. In Fisch U, ed. *Facial Nerve Surgery*. Birmingham, AL: Aesculapius Publishing Co, 1977.
44. Gomez MM, Pereira H, da Silva AG, Rego JM, Almeida MA. Facial paralysis. Neuromuscular reconstruction techniques. Acta Med Port 1998; 11(3):209–218.
45. May M, Drucker C. Temporaries muscle for facial reanimation. Arch Otolaryngol Head Neck Surg 1993; 119:378–382.
46. Conley J. Discussion: temporalis muscle for facial reanimation. Arch Otolaryngol Head and Neck Surg 1993; 119:383–384.
47. Cheney ML, McKenna MJ, Megerian CA, Ojemann RG. Early temporalis muscle transposition for the management of facial paralysis. Laryngoscope 105(9 Pt 1); 993–1000.
48. Iwahira Y, Maruyama Y. The use of Gore-Tex soft tissue patch to assist temporal muscle transfer in the treatment of facial nerve palsy. Ann Plast Surg 1992; 29(3):274–277.
49. Petroff MA, Goode RL, Levet Y. Gore-Tex implants: applications in facial paralysis rehabilitation and soft-tissue augmentation. Laryngoscope 1992; 102:1185–1189.
50. Konoir RJ. Facial paralysis reconstruction with Gore-Tex soft tissue patch. Arch Otolaryngol Head Neck Surg 1992; 118:1188–1194.
51. Terzis JK, Noah ME. Analysis of 100 cases of free-muscle transplantation for facial paralysis. Plast Reconstr Surg 1997; 99:1905–1921.
52. Harii K, Ohmori K, Torii S. Free gracilis muscle transplantation with microneurovascular anastomoses for the treatment of facial paralysis: a preliminary report. Plast Reconstr Surg 1976; 57:133–143.
53. Jiang H, Guo ET, Ji ZL, Zhang ML, Lu V. One-stage microneurovascular free abductor hallucis muscle transplantation for reanimation of facial paralysis. Plast Reconstr Surg 1995; 96(1):78–75.
54. Aviv JA, Urken ML. Management of the paralyzed face with microneurovascular free muscle transfer. Arch Otolaryngol Head Neck Surg 1992; 118:909–912.
55. Koshima I, Moriguchi, Soeda S, Hamanaka T, Tanaka H, Ohta S. Free rectus femoris muscle transfer for one-stage reconstruction of established facial paralysis. Plast Reconstr Surg 1994; 94:421–430.

56. Harii K. Refined microneurovascular free muscle transplantation for reanimation of the paralyzed face. Microsurgery 1988; 9:169–176.
57. Buncke HJ. Facial Paralysis. In: Buncke HS, ed. Transplantation–Replantation. Philadelphia, PA: Lea & Febiger, 1991:488–506.
58. Mackinnon SE, Dellon AL. Technical considerations of the latissimus dorsi muscle flap: a segmentally innervated muscle for facial reanimation. Microsurgery 1988; 9:36–45.
59. Terzis JK. Pectoralis minor: a unique muscle for correction of facial palsy. Plast Reconstr Surg 1989; 83:767–776.
60. Hata Y, Yano K, Matsuka K, Ito O, Matsuda H, Hosokawa K. Treatment of chronic facial palsy by transplantation of the neurovascularized free rectus abdominis muscle. Plast Reconstr Surg 1990; 86:1178–1187.
61. Bove A, Chiarini S, D'Andrea V, Di Matteo FM, Lanzi G, De Antoni E. Facial nerve palsy: which flap? Microsurgical, anatomical, and functional considerations. Microsurgery 1998; 18:286–289.
62. Wei W, Zuoliang, Xiaoxi L, Jiasheng D, Chuan Y, Hussain K, Hongtai H, Gontur S, Li Z, Tisheng C. Free split and segmental latissimus dorsi muscle transfer in one stage for facial reanimation. Plast Reconstr Surg 1999; 103(2):473–480.
63. Levine RE, House WF, Hitselberger WE. Ocular complications of seventh nerve paralysis and management with the palpebral sling. Am J Opthamol 1972; 73:219–228.
64. May M. Paralyzed eyelids reanimated with the closed eyelid spring. Laryngoscope 1988; 98:382–385.
65. Lauer SA, Feghali JG, Ksiazek S. Facial paralysis: the ophthalmologist's changing role. In: Burde RM, ed. Advances in Clinical Ophthalmology. St. Louis, MO: Mosby, 1994.
66. Jobe RP. A technique for lid loading in the management of lagopthalmos of facial palsy. Plast Reconstr Surg 1974; 53:29–31.
67. May M. Gold weight and wire spring implants as alternatives to tarsorrhaphy. Arch Otolaryngol Head Neck Surg 1987; 113:656–660.
68. Townsend DJ. Eyelid reanimation for the treatment of paralytic lagopthalmos: Historical perspectives and current applications of the gold weight implant. Ophthal Plast Reconstr Surg 1992; 8:196–201.
69. Kartush JM, Lindstrom CJ. Early gold weight eyelid implantation for facial paralysis. Arch Otolaryngol Head Neck Surg 1990; 103:1016–1023.
70. Gilbard SM, Daspit CP. Reanimation of the paretic eyelid using gold weight implantation. A new approach and prospective evaluation. Ophthal Plast Reconstr Surg 1991; 7(2):93–103.
71. Becker FF. Lateral tarsal strip procedure for the correction of paralytic ectropion. Laryngoscope 1982; 92:382.
72. Anderson RL, Gordy DD. The tarsal strip procedure. Arch Ophthalmol 1979; 97:2192–2196.
73. Becker FF. Lateral tarsal strip procedure for the correction of paralytic ectropion. Laryngoscope 1982; 92:382.
74. Naugle TC. Lateral canthoplasty. J Dermatol Surg Oncol 1992; 18(12):1075–1080.

13

Maxillofacial Prosthetics: Intraoral and Extraoral Rehabilitation

Joseph R. Cain and Donald L. Mitchell
University of Oklahoma, Oklahoma City, Oklahoma, U.S.A.

INTRODUCTION

The terminology used in maxillofacial prosthetics has some variation between physicians and dentists. A brief review of the terminology used in this chapter may help eliminate confusion.

Maxilla: Regularly shaped bone that, with its contralateral maxilla, forms the upper jaw (1).
Maxillectomy (maxillary resection): Removal of part or all of a maxilla (1).
  Total maxillectomy: Removal of both maxillae.
  Total palatectomy: Removal all of the hard and soft palate.
Palate: Partition separating the nasal and oral cavities (2).
  Hard palate: Bony portion of the roof of the mouth made from the two palatine bones.
  Soft palate: Movable part of palatal anatomy posterior to the hard palate.
  Palatal vault: Deepest and most superior part of the palate.

Malignant disease of the head and neck often requires aggressive surgical and or radiotherapy treatment to control the disease. These treatment modalities may change the quality of life for the patient requiring rehabilitation. This rehabilitation is often a multistage, time-consuming process. It is of great importance to the patient that he or she understand the consequences of the proposed treatment for his or her malignant disease and the rehabilitation measures that can be undertaken to minimize these consequences before the treatment process begins.

The dental specialty of maxillofacial prosthetics is concerned with the restoration and/or replacement of the stomatognathic and craniofacial structures with prostheses that may or may not be removed on an elective basis. A patient with a diagnosis of a head and neck malignant lesion that is going to undergo a surgical resection, with or without radiation therapy, should be referred to a maxillofacial prosthodontist for a preoperative evaluation. A treatment plan can be created depending upon the location, extension, and histology of the lesion and the proposed surgical resection and/or radiation therapy (3). Preoperative anticipation of anatomical structures to be surgically removed would suggest that rehabilitation be surgical and/or prosthetic. A cooperative effort by the surgeon and the maxillofacial prosthodontist will enable the patient to receive the greatest possible benefit from the rehabilitative effort (4).

The scope of maxillofacial prosthetics includes the fabrication and delivery of surgical, interim, and definitive intraoral as well as extraoral prostheses. The use of maxillofacial prostheses is an option for patient rehabilitation when surgical reconstruction is not possible or when indications for delayed reconstruction exist. Maxillofacial prosthetics is not a replacement for surgical reconstruction, but is indicated when the functional or cosmetic results will be superior.

Surgical resection of the maxilla and associated hard and soft tissues often results in the loss of important anatomical structures, such as bone, teeth, and mucosa. The loss of this tissue can create an oronasal communication resulting in hypernasal speech and loss of fluid or food into the nasal cavity (Fig. 1). A prosthesis fabricated to cover an opening is called an obturator. Patients with surgically acquired maxillary defects can usually receive an obturator to achieve acceptable function and appearance (5). In most instances, maxillary reconstructive surgery is not indicated.

Surgical resection of the mandible presents a greater challenge for patient rehabilitation than the maxilla. A mandibular discontinuity defect leaves the

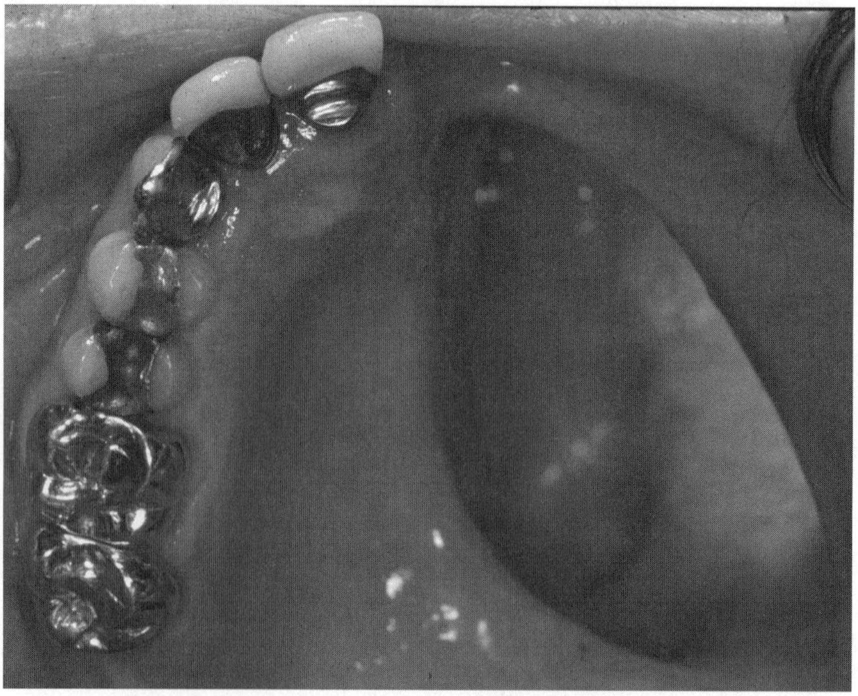

Figure 1 Intraoral palatal defect with oral nasal communication.

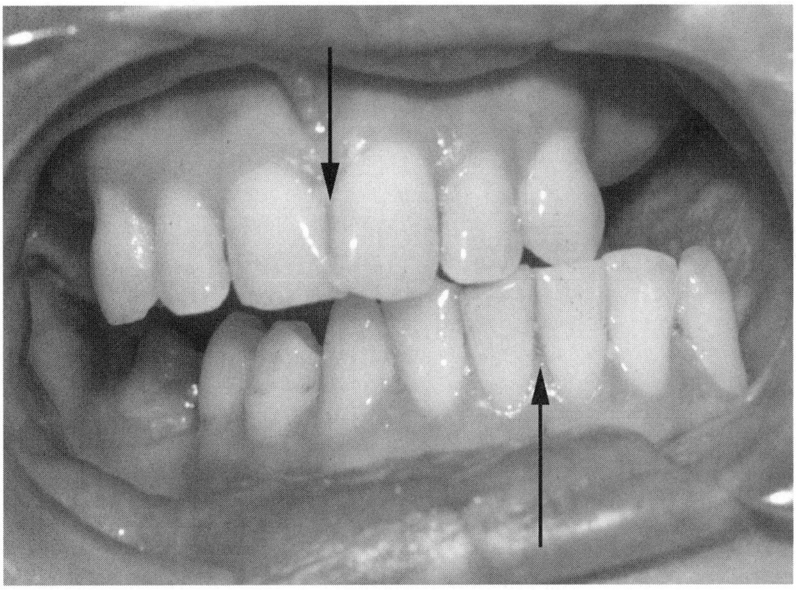

Figure 2 Mandibular discontinuity defect with mandibular deviation. Arrows show midline.

patient with a major functional discrepancy and results in an unstable mandible (Fig. 2). This affects the patient's ability to speak, swallow, and masticate. The availability of microvascular mandibular surgical reconstruction techniques greatly improves the patient's treatment options. However, not all patients are candidates for surgical reconstruction, and those who are not may benefit from a dental prosthesis.

The care of patients with extraoral head and neck malignant disease is not limited to the elimination of disease only. A comprehensive treatment plan for a patient with extraoral disease and requiring extraoral rehabilitation should be drawn up before surgery. Providing a detailed explanation of the treatment phases, side effects expected, and rehabilitation procedures available is the best way to prevent unpleasant surprises for the patient and family.

An extraoral facial prosthesis is a cosmetic bandage utilized to camouflage a surgical defect not amenable to or desirable for surgical reconstruction. An extraoral prosthesis may be considered for the following (6):

1. Large defects not readily closed with available or grafted soft tissue (Fig. 3).
2. Structures not easily reconstructed surgically, (i.e., an eye, nose, or ear) (Fig. 4).
3. Patients not psychologically or physically capable of tolerating a multistage surgical reconstruction.
4. Surgical defects requiring direct visualization to monitor for recurrent disease.
5. Temporary use during multistage surgical reconstruction of a surgical defect.

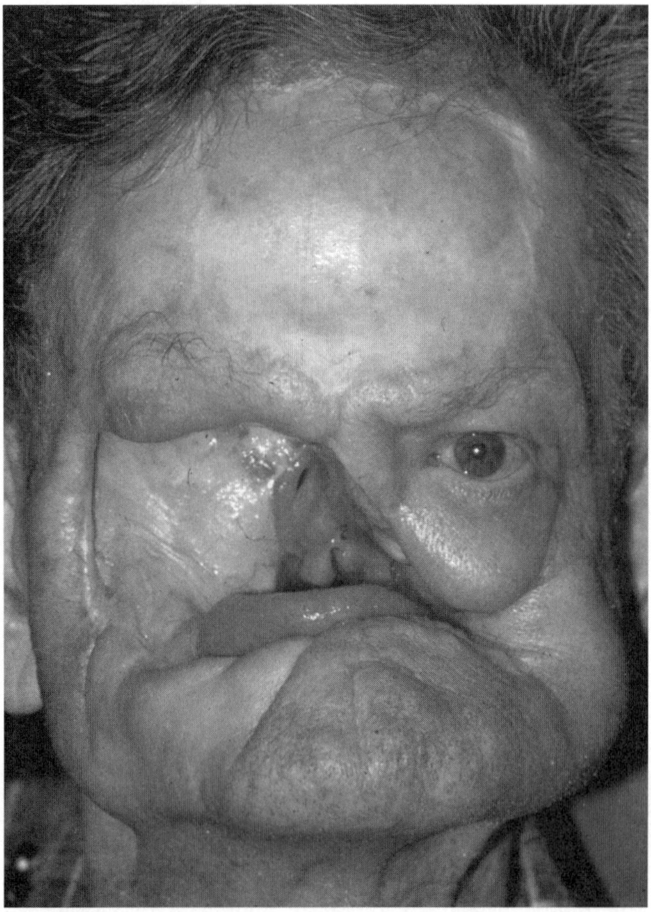

Figure 3 A large facial defect with numerous complex missing anatomical structures.

The use of osseointegrated implants has expanded the prosthetic rehabilitation options for many patients with head and neck cancer. The use of osseointegrated implants has provided patients with prostheses with retentive qualities far greater than could be provided otherwise. Patients with osseointegrated implant-retained prostheses are far more comfortable and confident about resuming their place in society.

Comprehensive management of head and neck malignant disease may include the use of radiation therapy. Salivary glands within the field of radiation will become nonfunctional. The degree of xerostomia experienced by the patient may vary depending the number of major salivary glands irradiated, the type of radiation, and the total dosage. The use of intra- and extraoral shielding can help preserve salivary gland function, reducing postirradiation therapy xerostomia.

In addition to an increased risk of dental caries, xerostomia also reduces a patient's tolerance for an oral prosthesis. Saliva serves as an important lubricant between a prosthesis and the oral tissue and aids in the retention of an oral prosthesis

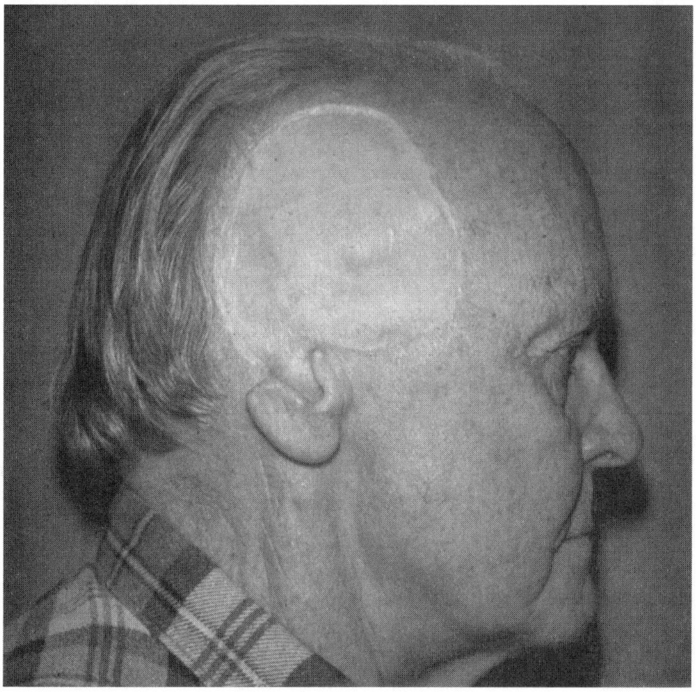

Figure 4 A complex anatomical structure such as an ear is not easily reconstructed surgically.

due to surface tension. Its absence results in increased irritation of oral tissues during prosthesis function because of friction.

PRESURGICAL CONSULTATION

Rehabilitation of a patient with malignant disease of the head and neck is often a multistage, time-consuming process. It is of great importance to patients that they understand the side effects of their proposed treatment and the measures that can be taken to minimize these side effects before initiating the treatment process. Fear of the unknown can be disturbing to many people and the patient's imagination of the unknown can be far more vivid than reality. A detailed explanation of the treatment phases, side effects expected, and rehabilitation procedures is the best way to prevent unpleasant surprises. Pretreatment consultation with a maxillofacial prosthodontist provides an excellent opportunity to explain rehabilitation options to the patient and family. This opportunity includes showing the patient examples of the prosthesis the prosthodontist anticipates fabricating following surgery.

Maxillofacial prosthodontic evaluation of a patient should be a routine part of that patient's general evaluation before undertaking definitive treatment for a benign or malignant head and neck lesion. Prosthodontic evaluation will usually consist of an oral examination, dental impressions for diagnostic casts, and dental radiographs.

The information from this evaluation, along with the preoperative surgical and radiotherapy plan, allows the patient to be initially grouped into one of the following four M.D. Anderson categories of dental condition (7):

1. Edentulous: The patient has no teeth and may or may not be wearing a complete denture. Existing prostheses should be evaluated for use during and after treatment.
2. Poor: The patient's teeth are beyond repair by ordinary dental means, due to significant caries and/or periodontal disease. All remaining teeth are to be extracted and bony prominences recontoured prior to the oncological surgical resection. Elective dental extractions at the time of oncological surgical resection could increase the possibility of seeding the tumor cells during surgical excision. Primary closure of all dental surgical sites is recommended to promote healing. Dental extractions after a surgical resection are more stressful for the patient and may delay rehabilitative efforts.
3. Fair: Teeth can be restored by ordinary dental means. There is minimal periodontal disease. Some selected extractions may be required.
4. Good: Teeth and periodontium are in good condition; oral hygiene is good to excellent.

Patients who have undergone treatment for head and neck malignant disease require periodic maxillofacial prosthetic follow-up care to evaluate the current status of their hard and soft tissues in addition to the serviceability of any prosthesis. Irradiated dentate patients should receive lifelong daily topical fluoride for prevention of dental caries.

A pretreatment consultation is also valuable for the patient with extraoral disease. This affords the maxillofacial prosthodontist an opportunity to educate the patient and family on the advantages and disadvantages of prosthetic rehabilitation.

MAXILLARY SURGICAL DEFECTS

The dental diagnostic casts and radiographs made during the presurgical consultation are reviewed with the referring surgeon to define the proposed surgical outline. A surgical defect of the hard and or soft palate will affect the patient's ability to speak, swallow, and masticate. Patients with a maxillary surgical defect will experience hypernasal speech as well as loss of fluid and food into the nasal cavity. Therefore, surgical, interim, and definitive prostheses are necessary for these patients.

Malignant lesions of the hard palate, nasal and paranasal areas involve common areas of surgical resection. Aramany (8) classified six hard palatal defects based their frequency of occurrence. A seventh maxillary defect listed is a total maxillectomy, which is uncommon but may occur and has been included for completeness (Fig. 5).

Class I: Involves half of the hard palate using the midline suture as the resection guide (Fig. 6).

Class II: Involves a posterior unilateral defect. The anterior teeth on the surgical side are retained (Fig. 7). By retaining anterior teeth and/or alveolar ridges, the obturator's effectiveness is greatly enhanced.

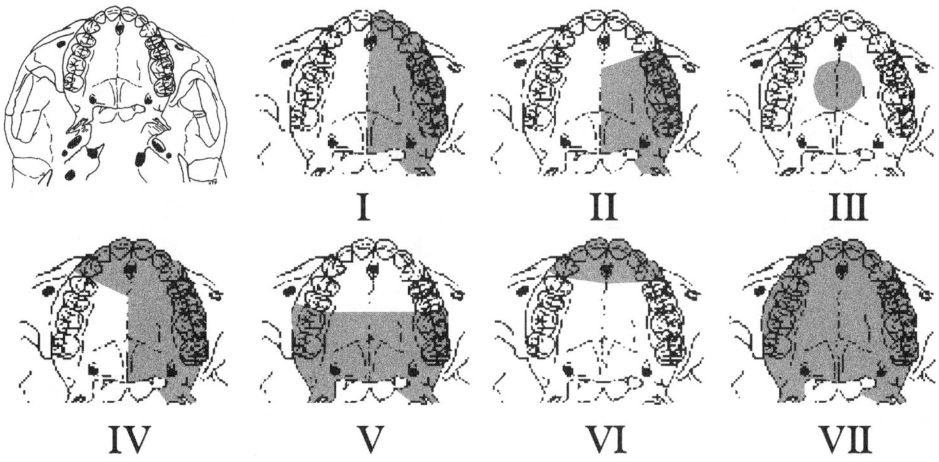

Figure 5 Seven areas of hard palate resection, in order of frequency.

Class III: Involves only the palatal vault. The remaining teeth or alveolar ridges are not involved (Fig. 8).
Class IV: Involves the entire premaxilla and a unilateral maxilla (Fig. 9). This is very difficult to restore with a functional prosthesis.
Class V: Involves the posterior hard palate bilaterally (Fig. 10). Retention of prosthesis depends on the anterior hard palate and soft palate, if intact.

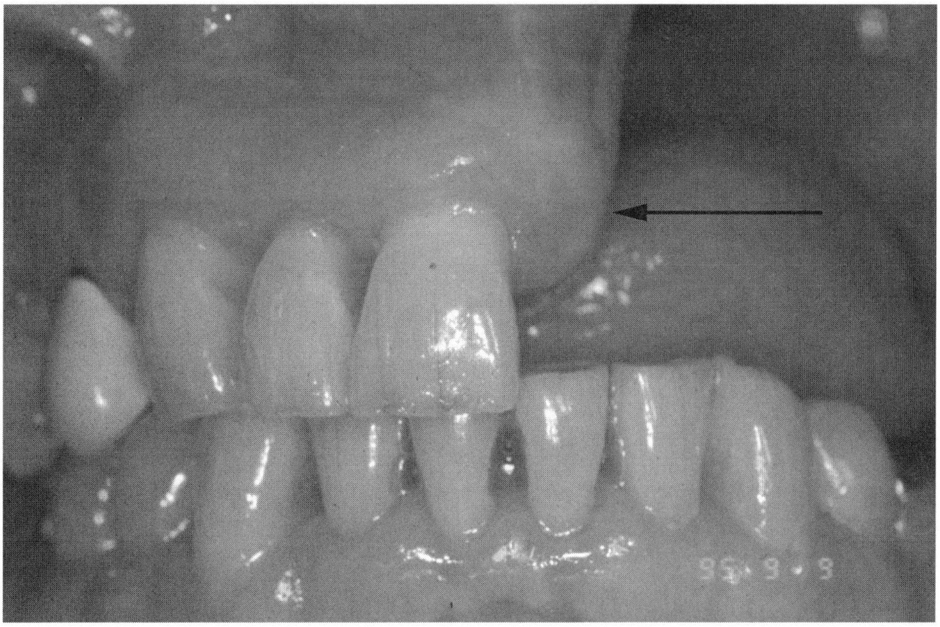

Figure 6 Class I: a midline resection of the hard palate.

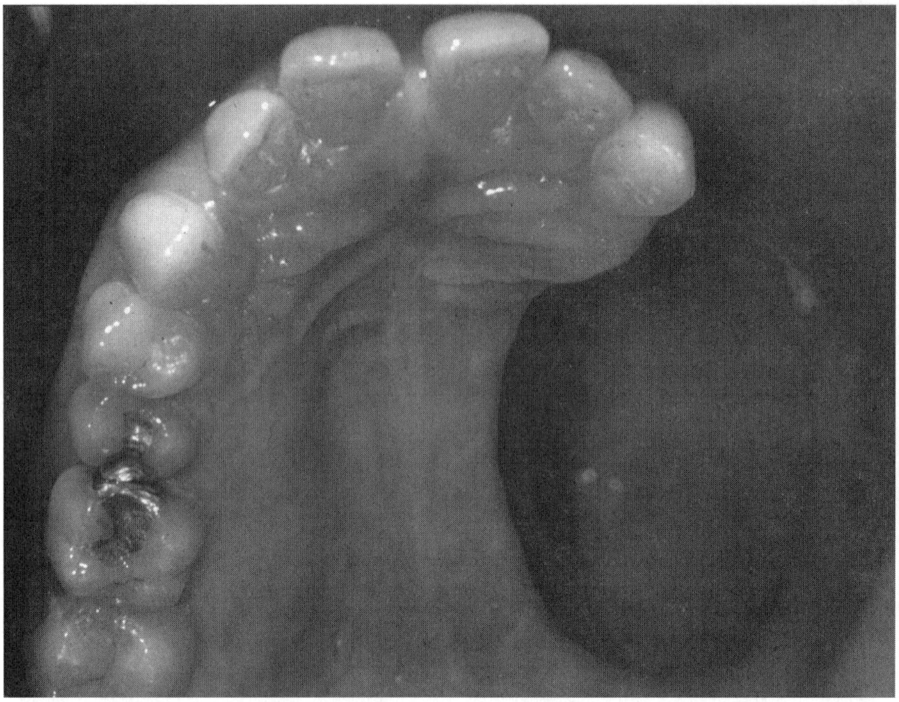

Figure 7 Class II: unilateral posterior defect retaining the premaxilla.

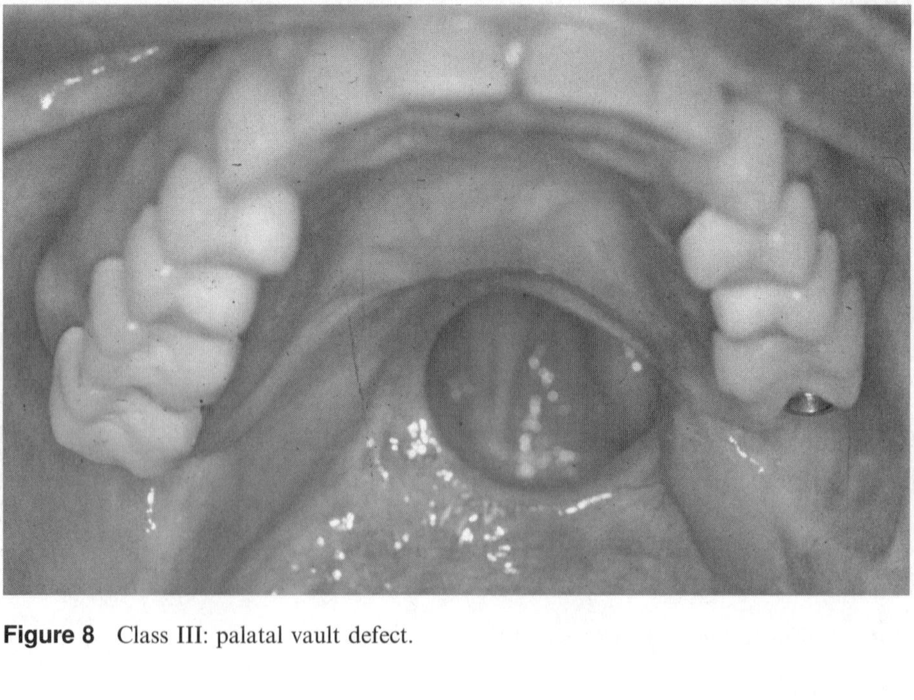

Figure 8 Class III: palatal vault defect.

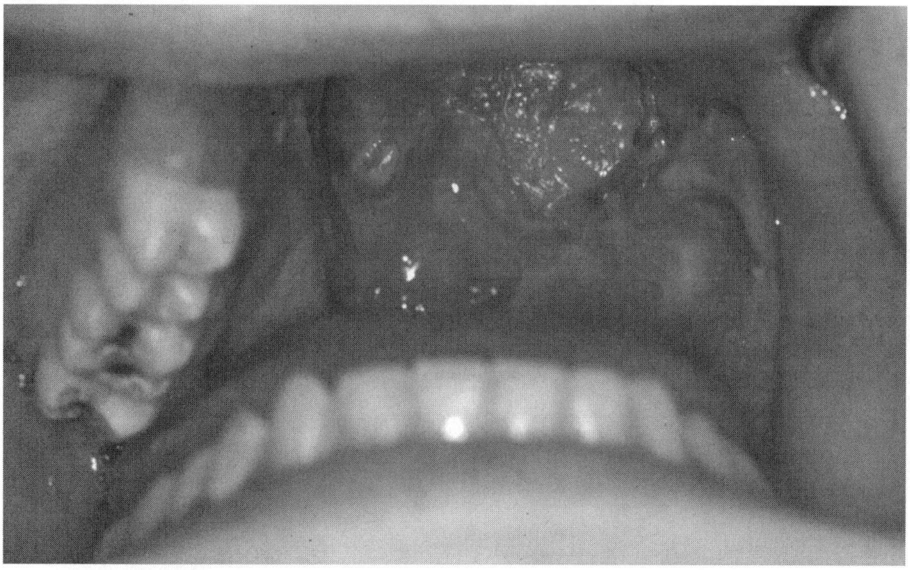

Figure 9 Class IV: resection of premaxilla and half of the hard palate.

Class VI: Involves loss of the premaxilla (Fig. 11). This is rare, but when it occurs, there is a complete collapse of the maxillary lip and the tip of the nose.

Class VII: Involves the total maxilla (Fig. 12). Due to loss of the entire hard palate, retention of an obturator will be significantly diminished (9).

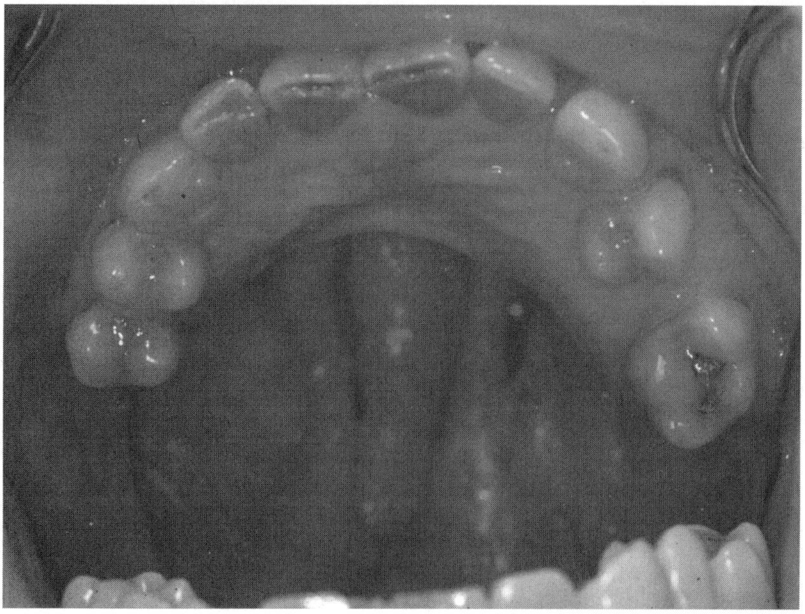

Figure 10 Class V: resection of posterior hard palate bilaterally.

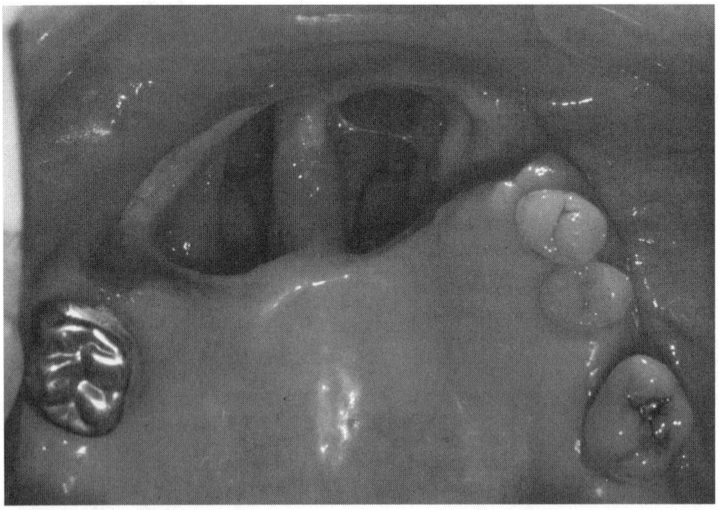

Figure 11 Class VI: resection of the premaxilla only.

From the viewpoint of patient rehabilitation, the more hard palate that is surgically excised, the more difficulty the patient will experience with the prosthesis. A class I palatal defect, the most common, is difficult to restore because one-half of the maxilla is missing. The prosthesis will rotate about the sagittal plane, along the anterior posterior surgical resection. A class II or III palatal defect has a better prognosis

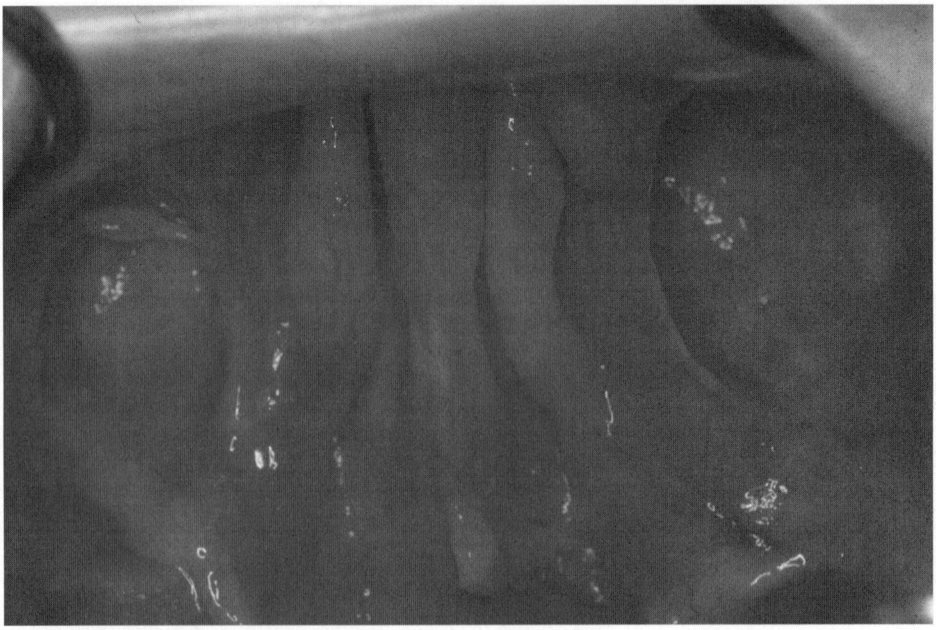

Figure 12 Class VII: total maxillectomy.

because it involves a smaller surgical resection, resulting in minimal alveolar ridge loss, and does not cross the midline. Prostheses for a class II or III surgical defect are generally the easiest for a patient to utilize. A class IV palatal defect is prosthetically challenging because the premaxilla and a unilateral maxilla crossing the midline are missing. A class V or VI palatal defect results in a prosthesis that will have rotation in the transverse axis. Retention and support of an obturator in a class VII palatal defect depend upon anatomical structures within the nasal cavity. These anatomical structures are usually inadequate to provide usable retention and support for an obturator prosthesis. A class VII palatal defect presents the greatest challenge to the patient and the maxillofacial prosthodontist.

MAXILLARY SURGICAL CONSIDERATIONS

Adequate presurgical planning can expedite postsurgical recovery. Rehabilitative success can be enhanced by preparation of a sound prosthodontic foundation. At the time of surgery, dental considerations for the successful use of an obturator prosthesis should include the following:

1. The canine on the surgical side should be retained, if possible. It has a large root that provides good support for a prosthesis (Fig. 13).
2. When teeth are present, the surgical cut through alveolar bone should be through an extracted tooth socket, not between two teeth. A surgical cut

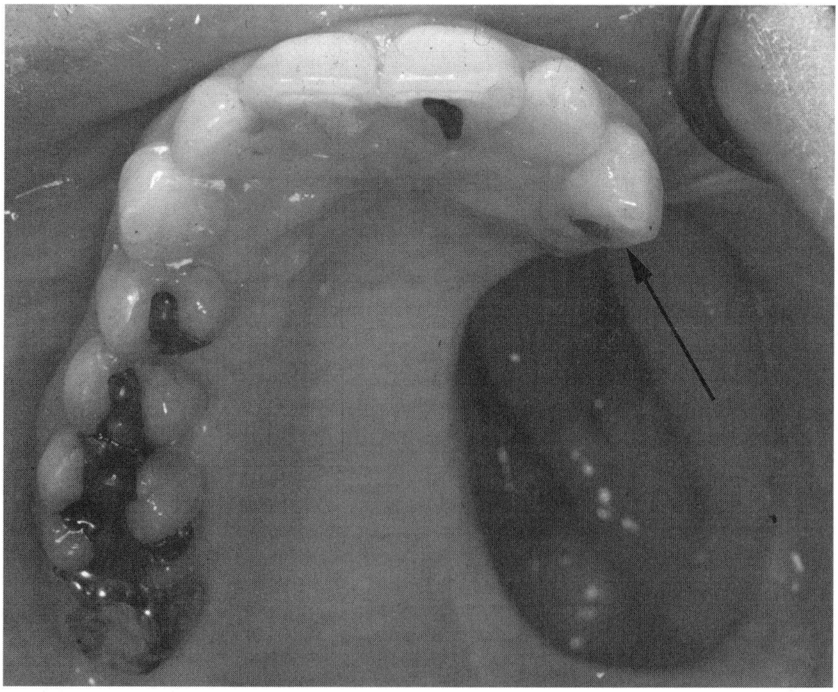

Figure 13 Canine tooth retained as support for a prosthesis.

between two teeth will result in an inadequate amount of bone remaining on the root of the tooth proximal to the cut, causing its eventual loss (Fig. 14).

3. When possible, the cut osseous margins of the alveolus and palate should be covered with palatal mucosa at the time of surgical closure. This can usually be accomplished by making the soft tissue incision lateral to the osseous cut. The palatal mucosa can be sutured over the cut edges of the palatal and alveolar bone. Great care should be taken to ensure that the edges of the osseous cut are smooth. The junction of the hard palate and surgical defect is a region of constant prosthesis contact and can act as a fulcrum. Thick supporting mucosa and round, smooth bone will facilitate the construction of a comfortable prosthesis (Fig. 15).
4. Anatomical structures in the nasal cavity will be exposed after a surgical maxillectomy. Structures such as the inferior and middle turbinates should be electively removed because they will interfere with the insertion and removal of the prosthesis into the palatal defect. In addition, they are covered with respiratory mucosa and will not tolerate any pressure from the prosthesis (Fig. 16).
5. The placement of a split-thickness skin graft on the cheek of a maxillary defect will facilitate healing and patient comfort. A well-defined scar band will form where the graft meets the oral mucosa (Fig. 17) that aids in retention of an obturator prosthesis. A full-thickness tissue graft is usually contraindicated in covering a maxillary defect in case the use of a prosthesis is anticipated because it provides a poor foundation on which to fabricate a dental prosthesis and may contribute to prosthesis movement.
6. At the time of palatal surgery, or before, nonsalvageable teeth and undesirable exostoses, such as palatal tori, should be removed. Perform-

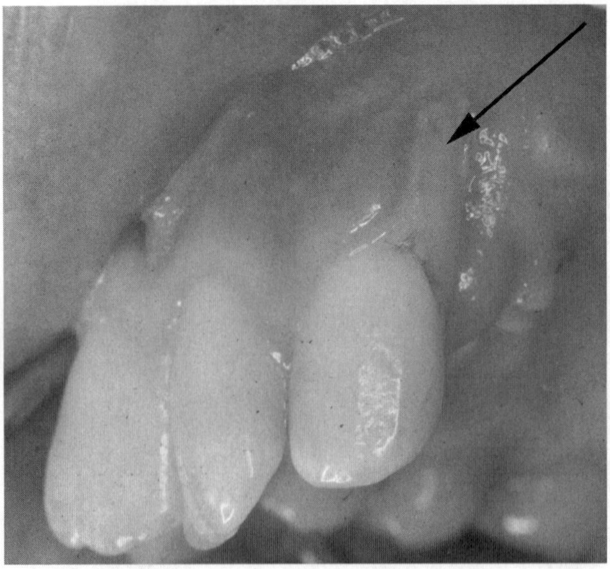

Figure 14 Exposed root resulting from surgical cut between two teeth.

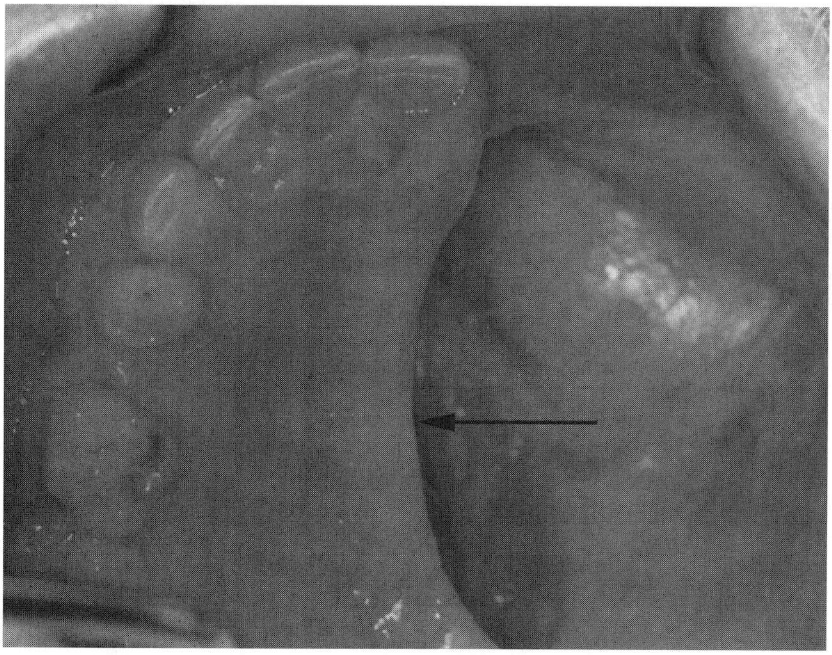

Figure 15 An osseous margin covered with palatal mucosa.

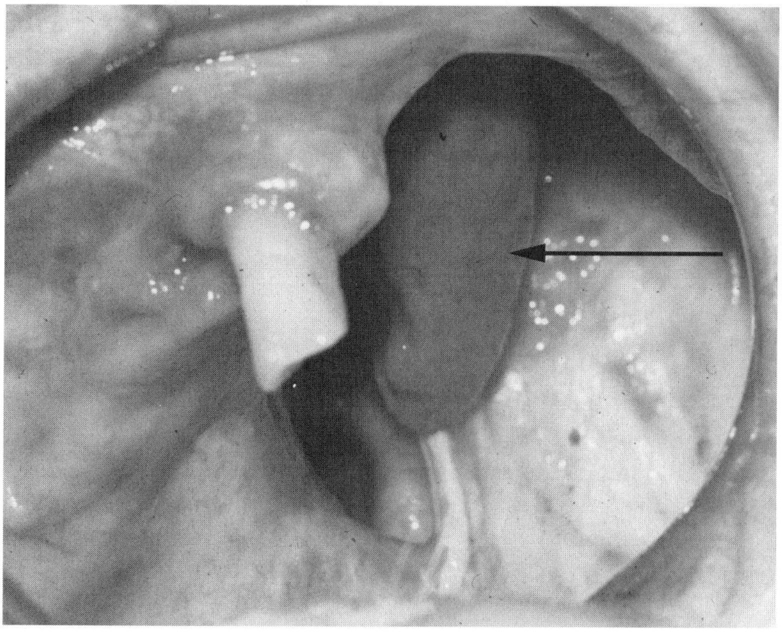

Figure 16 Turbinates covered by respiratory mucosa may interfere with an obturator.

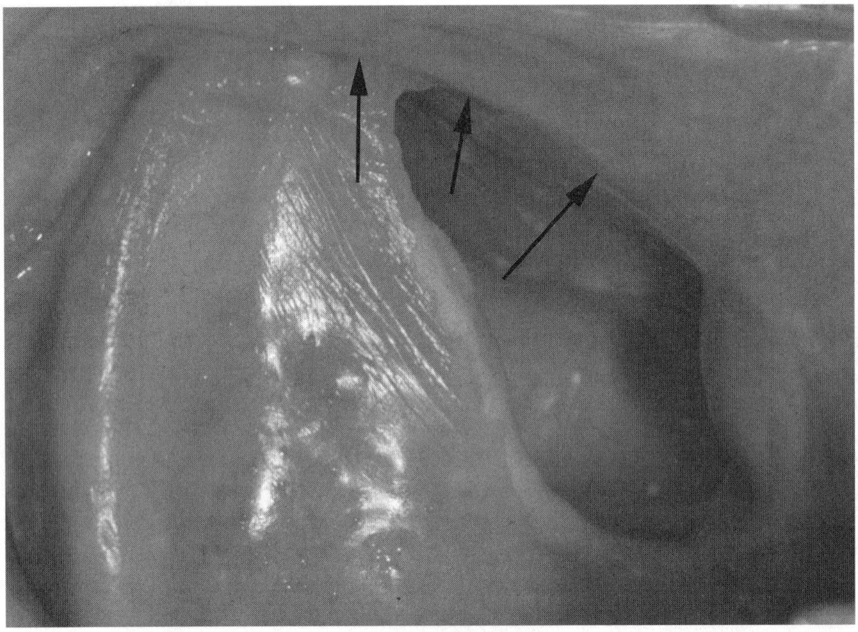

Figure 17 Scar band at the junction of the skin graft and oral mucosa.

ing these procedures after palatal surgery is more stressful for the patient.

7. It is desirable to retain the soft palate at the time of surgery. The natural motion of the soft palate for closure of the oral pharynx is superior to that provided by a prosthesis (10). The prosthesis must obturate the velopharyngeal space vertically as well as laterally, yet leave enough room to breathe and speak. If the soft palate must be resected during surgery, it is important that its natural position be maintained as closely as possible during repair. A posterior band of soft palatal tissue 1 cm wide is usually considered prosthetically advantageous. A band less than 1 cm wide is a prosthetic disadvantage and should be excised. It will interfere with placement of the prosthesis, complicating rehabilitation by compromising speech and deglutition.
8. The anterior mucosal incision of a maxillectomy will produce a fibrous scar band when sutured to the skin graft. The anterior cut edge of the maxilla is an area of intimate contact between the prosthesis and soft tissue. Attention should be directed to not obliterating the buccal vestibule during surgical closure. Surgical obliteration of the anterior buccal vestibule will require excessive prosthesis relief, resulting in reduced stability.
9. When surgical resection involves the pterygoid plates, the surgical defect created will be bounded laterally by the mandibular coronoid process. The latter will interfere with extension of the prosthesis into the surgical defect, decreasing obturation. If the coronoid process is present, movement of the mandible will contribute to prosthesis movement. Consideration should be

given to elective resection of the coronoid process in anticipation of this problem.

TYPES OF OBTURATORS

Fabrication of an intraoral obturator prosthesis usually involves three separate phases:

1. Surgical obturator: placed at the time of surgery and utilized for approximately 1 week while the surgical packing is in place.
2. Interim obturator: used from the second week postsurgery until the patient is well healed. This prosthesis is modified as needed while the surgical defect heals. This may be as long as 6 months, if radiation therapy is a part of the patient treatment plan.
3. Definitive obturator: intended for long-term use with minimal modifications.

Surgical Obturator

A surgical obturator is placed by the surgeon or prosthodontist at the time of the surgical resection. The surgical obturator fulfills many functions (4,5,11):

1. Improves the patient's ability to swallow, decreasing the need for a nasogastric tube.
2. Aids speech by restoring palatal contour and reducing hypernasality.
3. Holds the surgical dressing in place.
4. Helps to keep the surgical area clean, which aids healing.
5. Provides a psychological benefit to the patient by improving speech quality and deglutition, and covering the surgical margins.
6. Reduces the hospital stay by restoring the patient to independent function.

The surgical obturator is fabricated based on a preoperative dental cast (Fig. 18). The cast is modified to simulate a normal palatal contour minus the teeth expected to be lost at the time of surgery (Fig. 19). The prosthesis primarily covers the hard palate. A normal palatal contour is maintained to facilitate deglutition and speech. The prosthesis has minimal extension into the area of the soft palate surgical excision. Potential interference from mandibular movement makes it desirable to underextend a surgical prosthesis in the posterior lateral aspect. An underextended prosthesis can be augmented at a later time, whereas an overextended prosthesis will result in discomfort (Fig. 20).

Artificial teeth are not usually placed on a surgical obturator, because dental occlusion is difficult to re-establish during this phase of treatment. Also, it is desirable to prevent the patient from functioning dentally on the side of the surgical resection and the absence of artificial teeth facilitates this.

Primary retention of a surgical obturator is accomplished with palatal screws, (Fig. 21) circumzygomatic wires, transalveolar pins, or circumdental wires. The use of the palatal screw for retention of a surgical obturator, especially if the patient is edentulous, is preferable. The palatal screw is easier to remove than circumzygomatic wires or transalveolar pins and results in less patient discomfort when the surgical obturator is removed postoperatively.

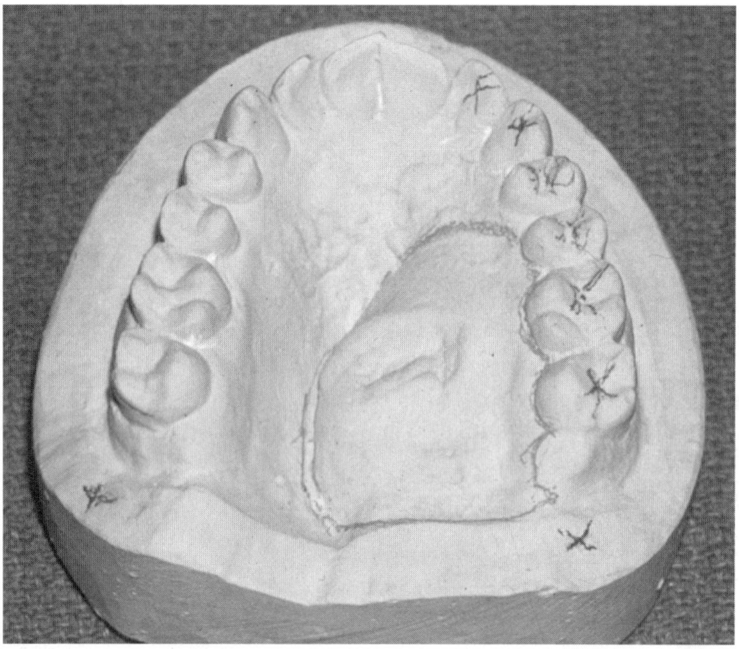

Figure 18 Dental cast shows outline of tumor.

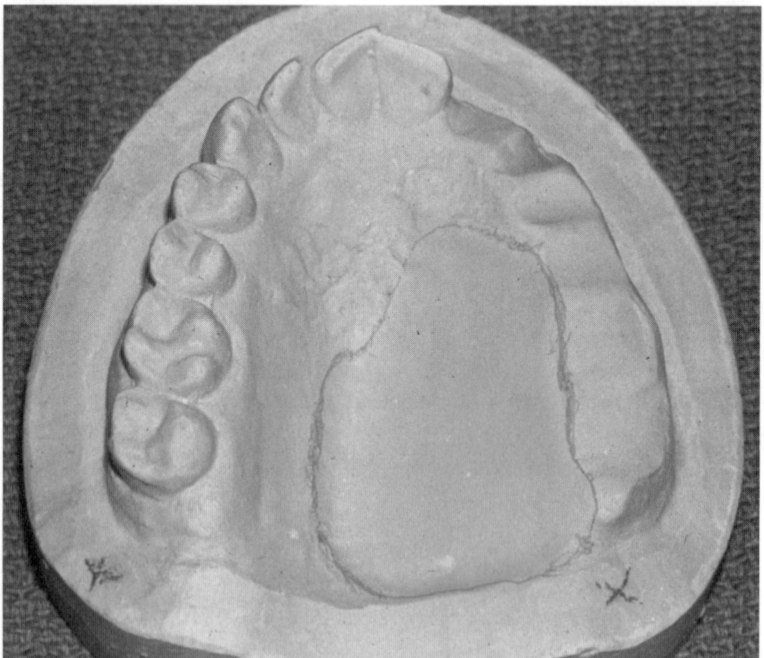

Figure 19 Preoperative dental cast modified to simulate normal palatal contour and removal of teeth included in surgical resection.

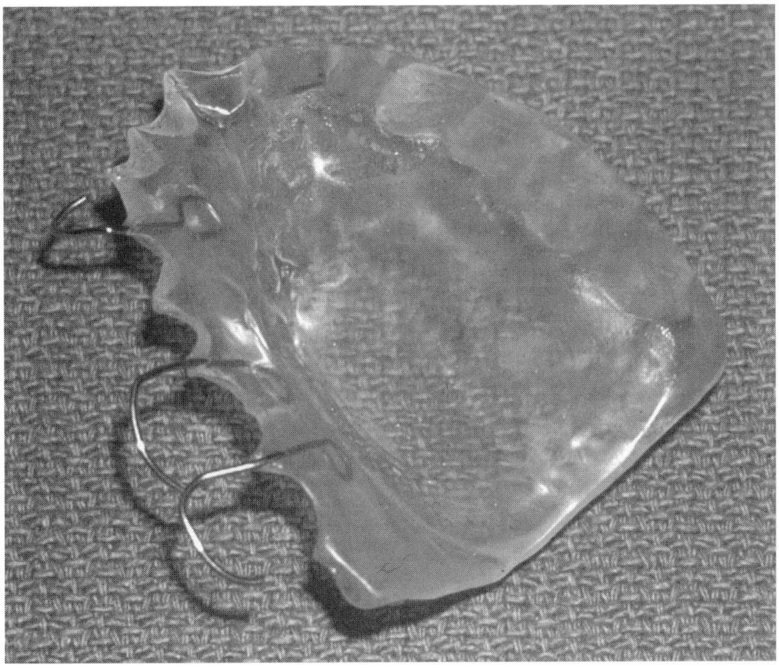

Figure 20 Surgical obturator with wire clasps.

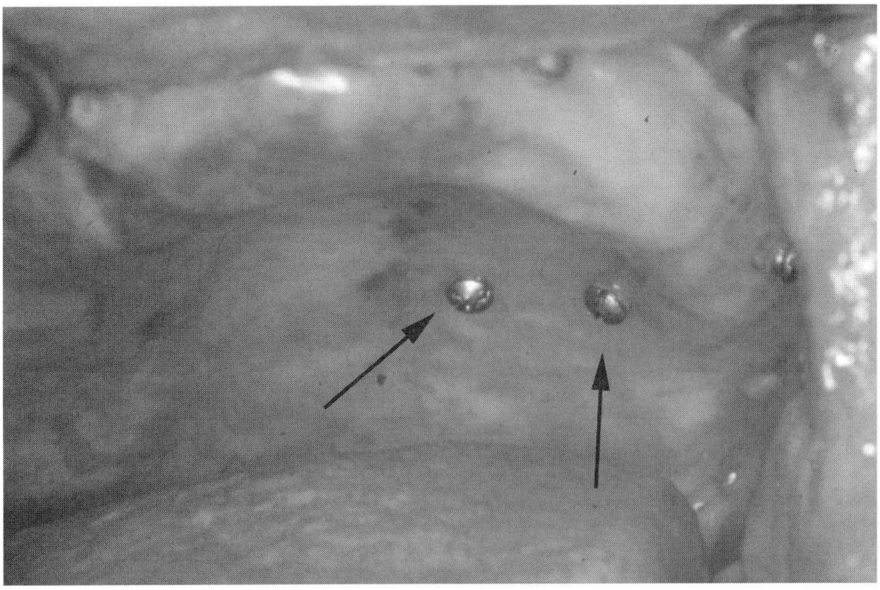

Figure 21 Edentulous surgical obturator retained with palatal screws.

Secondary retention of a surgical obturator is achieved with wire clasps on the teeth remaining after the surgical excision of the tumor. These clasps will become the primary means of retention when the surgical obturator is converted to an interim obturator (Fig. 22). If a patient is completely edentulous, the maxillary complete denture can be used as a surgical obturator if it is in acceptable condition. It should be evaluated for fit and cleanliness prior to use.

Approximately 1 week after surgery, the surgical obturator and surgical packing are removed. The palatal defect is cleaned and examined. Physiotherapy should begin approximately 1 week after the surgical obturator and surgical packing are removed to regain an adequate oral opening. The patient may complain of discomfort and resist oral physiotherapy. It is insufficient for the patient only to open their mouth to a comfortable opening. Maximum opening of the mandible must be done using the patient's fingers, tongue blades, or an acrylic resin corkscrew (Fig. 23). The patient will only regain maximum oral opening by stretching the scar tissue before adhesions occur. Damage to the surgical site will not occur with aggressive physiotherapy. If maximum oral opening is not achieved prior to the initiation of radiation therapy, it is unlikely that the presurgical vertical opening will be regained. Patients who achieve an anterior opening of three fingerwidths will have an opening adequate for eating and postoperative care.

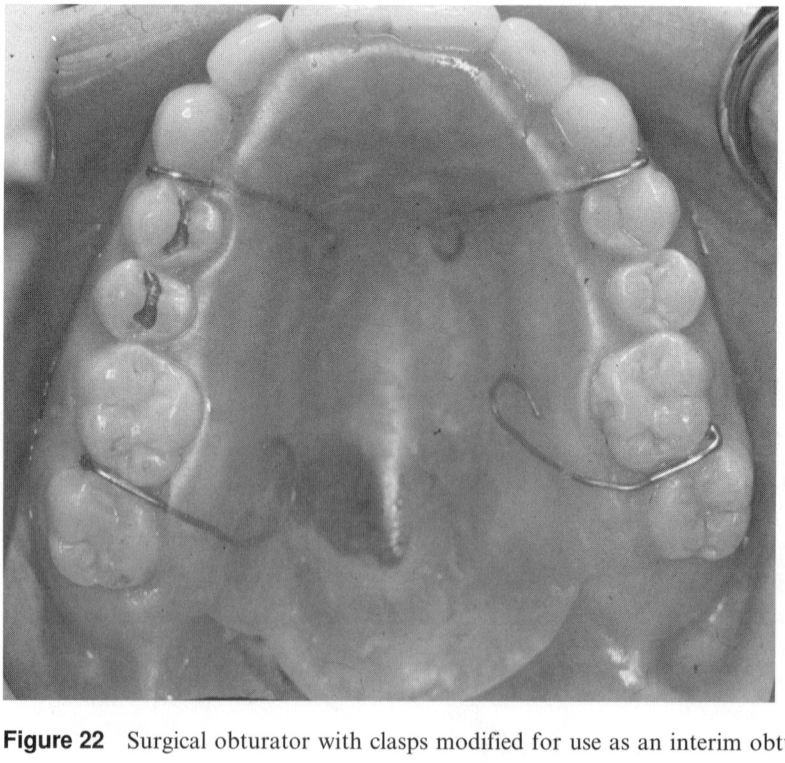

Figure 22 Surgical obturator with clasps modified for use as an interim obturator.

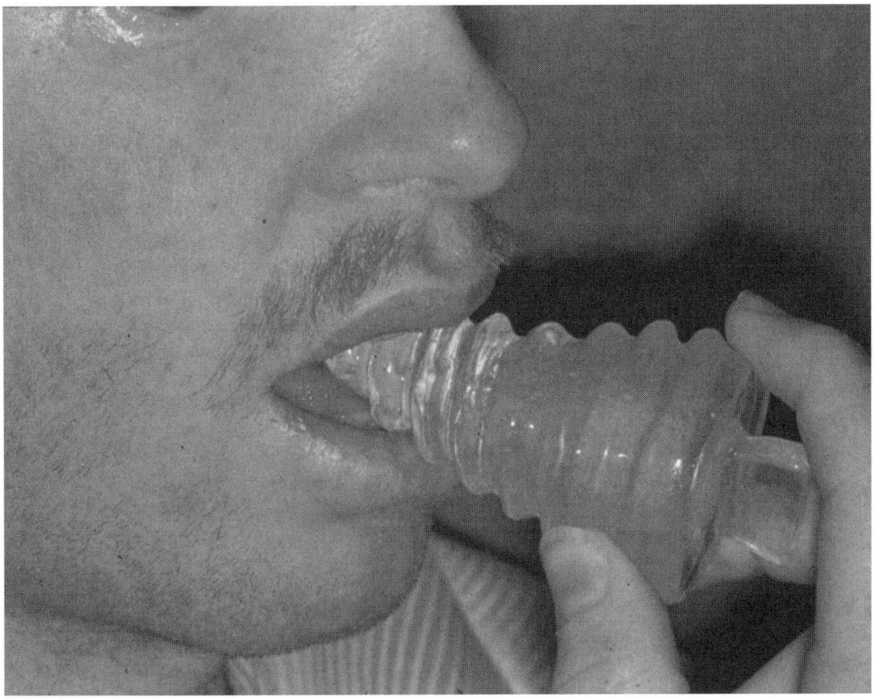

Figure 23 Custom-made acrylic resin cork screw may be utilized for restoring vertical opening.

Interim Obturator

It is preferable to convert the surgical obturator into an interim obturator when the surgical obturator is removed. This can be accomplished with the addition of a soft, autopolymerizing dental material (COE-SOFT, GC America Inc., Chicago, IL) to the surgical obturator (Fig. 24). The dental material is added to the prosthesis to obturate the surgical defect and can be added or subtracted sequentially depending upon the patient's rate of healing and level of comfort. Material can be added to or subtracted from the prosthesis to compensate for voids or pressure spots created due to tissue contraction during healing. After the initial rapid tissue changes have occurred (2–4 weeks), the temporary material can be replaced with a more durable acrylic resin.

If a surgical obturator was not fabricated, or if conversion of the surgical obturator is not possible, an impression of the maxilla must be made and an interim obturator fabricated. Making a maxillary impression shortly after surgery is unpleasant for the patient. The patient is debilitated and unable adequately open the oral cavity to allow fabrication of dental impression. An immediate postsurgical impression should seldom be necessary if proper planning and presurgical consultations have been completed.

The primary reason for fabrication of an interim obturator is to allow the patient to swallow without the loss of significant amounts of fluid into the nasal cavity and to reduce hypernasality of speech. The interim obturator is usually made

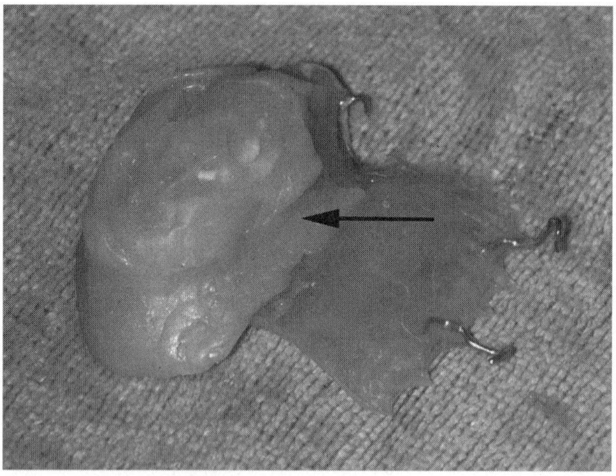

Figure 24 Surgical obturator converted for interim use by addition of COE-SOFT autopolymerizing dental material.

entirely of acrylic resin, allowing for easy modifications. Artificial teeth are usually not placed on an interim obturator because it is undesirable for the patient to function dentally on the side of the surgical defect and the addition of artificial teeth may complicate prosthesis modification during this period of rapid tissue change. If cosmetics are a major concern to the patient, anterior teeth may be added to the interim prosthesis.

During the immediate post surgical phase (8–12 weeks) the patient should only remove the interim obturator to clean the prosthesis and the defect. The interim obturator is not to be removed at night. It will function as a tissue stent during the postsurgical healing period. Removal of the interim obturator during the early stages of healing, even for a few hours, may prevent reinsertion of the prosthesis due to the rapid tissue contraction that can occur in the surgical defect. If the interim obturator cannot be reinserted, it must be modified before it can be reseated and the patient can again function. Continuous use of the interim obturator is also recommended during radiation therapy. Soft tissue and scar contracture can be minimized with the use of an interim obturator acting as a stent.

Definitive Obturator

A definitive obturator is an intraoral prosthesis intended for long-term use with minimal modifications (Fig. 25). Fabricating a definitive obturator is appropriate when the surgical defect and surrounding tissues have stabilized. A 2–3 month postsurgical healing period is usually sufficient before initiating fabrication of a definitive obturator. The utilization of radiation therapy will delay fabrication of a definitive obturator for 3 or more months.

The location and number of a patient's remaining teeth play an important part in the stability and retention of a definitive obturator (12). Bilateral dental support may reduce the need to use the surgical defect to retain the prosthesis. If the tooth

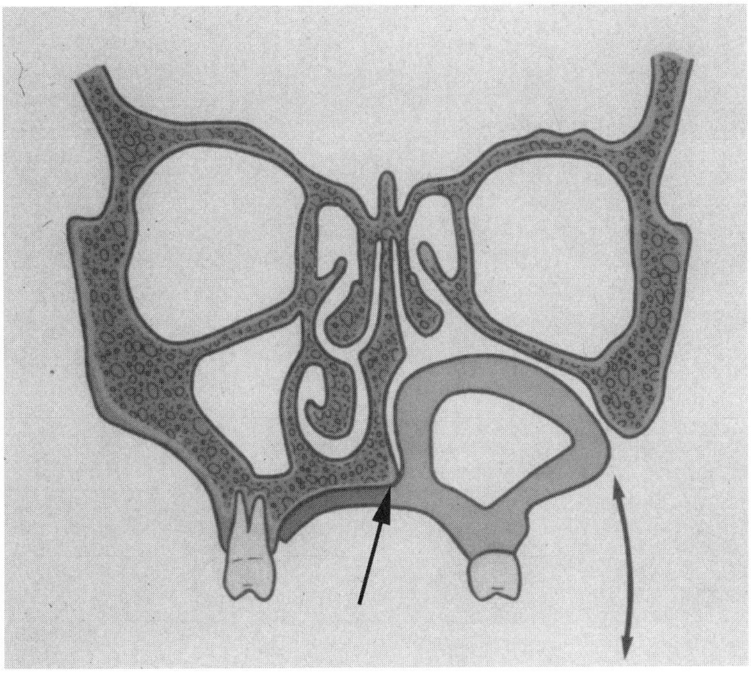

Figure 25 Diagrammatic representation of a prosthesis obturating a class I maxillary defect.

support of a prosthesis is only unilateral or concentrated in one area, the surgical defect will need to be used to aid in the retention of the definitive obturator.

Placement of a split-thickness skin graft on the lateral aspect of a surgical defect facilitates healing and the formation of a scar band (Fig. 17). The skin graft allows vertical extension and intimate contact of the definitive obturator with the cheek (Fig. 26). Prosthesis extension into the surgical defect aids in stability and retention of the definitive obturator (13,14). If the cheek is allowed to heal by granulation without a split-thickness skin graft, it will result in a poor prosthesis-bearing surface. The presence of granulation tissue in the surgical defect will result in excess scar tissue formation and contracture.

The scar band formed at the junction of the split-thickness skin graft and oral mucosa becomes evident about 8 weeks postsurgery. This scar band forms a constriction that plays an important role in the stability and retention of a definitive obturator. By engaging the scar band both superiorly and inferiorly, the obturator is made more stable. The smaller the surgical defect, the less critical the scar band is for prosthesis retention. However, the scar band is still important as a seal to prevent fluids from escaping into the nasal cavity.

The prosthesis will have an axis of rotation about the medial border of the surgical defect. Therefore, the cut edge of the palatal bone should be rounded and covered with palatal mucosa or a split-thickness skin graft. Although minimal prosthesis retention is gained from the medial aspect of the surgical defect, it is important to treat this area with care. Patient comfort and enhanced palatal defect obturation are the goal of restoration.

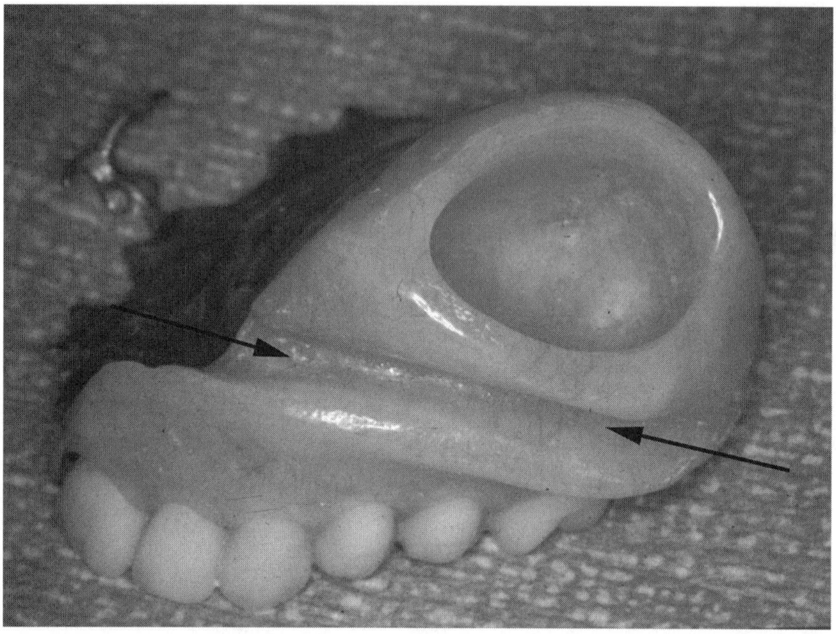

Figure 26 Definitive obturator: arrow identifies concave area for skin graft scar band.

Design considerations of the definitive obturator are complex. The prosthesis has greater functional and dislodging forces placed on it than a conventional removable dental prosthesis. The forces transmitted to the remaining dentition by a definitive obturator are greater because of the increased weight of the bulb in the surgical defect and its resulting lever arm effect. Occlusal forces will displace the prosthesis superiorly. The forces of gravity will displace the prosthesis inferiorly. To compensate for the greater functional and dislodging forces applied by the obturator prosthesis, the maximum area of palatal tissue should be covered. In designing the prosthesis, clasps and rests should be placed on as many teeth as possible to prevent overloading an individual tooth.

Osseointegrated Implants in the Maxilla

An edentulous patient with a complete denture prior to surgery has an advantage over a patient made edentulous just prior to or during surgery. A recently edentulous patient must adjust to the presence of the surgical defect as well as coping with a removable prosthesis. This is very challenging for most patients. A patient with difficulty utilizing a removable prosthesis may benefit from the placement of osseointegrated dental implants. Dental implants have proven to be very reliable and can dramatically improve the support and retention of an oral prosthesis.

MANDIBULAR SURGICAL DEFECTS

Surgical resection of a portion of the mandible will result in a discontinuity defect unless reconstructed (Fig. 2) and presents a greater challenge for rehabilitation than a resected maxilla because it leaves the patient with an unstable mandible and a major functional discrepancy. This affects the patient's ability to speak, swallow, and masticate. The availability of microvascular mandibular surgical reconstruction techniques has greatly improved a patient's treatment options. Patients not candidates for surgical reconstruction may benefit from a dental prosthesis.

In general, the greater the portion of mandible resected, the greater a patient's functional difficulty. The mandibular remnant will deviate toward the side of the surgical resection. The unrestored, resected mandible will also rotate in the sagittal plane because of the pull of the masseter muscle. The resultant mandibular deviation prevents the patient from achieving presurgical alignment of the remaining mandible with the maxilla. If the patient has remaining natural dentition, a malocclusion will occur, which may be as minor as rotation of the occlusal table or as severe as failing to make tooth contact. A patient with a removable dental prosthesis experiences greater difficulties because of the additional challenge of controlling it. Dental implants can be useful in prosthesis stabilizaton and retention (Figs. 27–29).

The patient with a nonsurgically restored, resected mandible cannot produce a protrusive or lateral movement. This patient can only produce an abnormal angular opening and closing motion with their mandible.

Physiotherapy should begin approximately 1 week after surgery. Its purpose is to regain an adequate oral opening and range of motion. The patient may complain of discomfort and resist oral physiotherapy. It is insufficient physiotherapy for the patient to only open their mouth to a comfortable opening, as detailed previously. It is unlikely that the surgical site will be damaged with aggressive physiotherapy. If maximum range of motion is not achieved prior to the initiation of radiation therapy, it is unlikely that the presurgical mandibular range of motion and alignment will be regained.

Having the dentate patient attempt to guide the mandible manually into a normal occlusal relationship will allow evaluation of the progress of the physiotherapy.

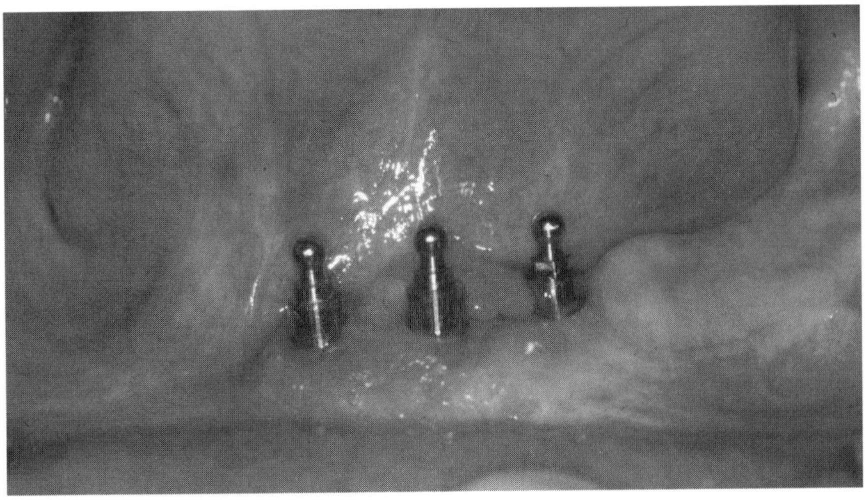

Figure 27 Resected mandible with three dental implants in residual mandible.

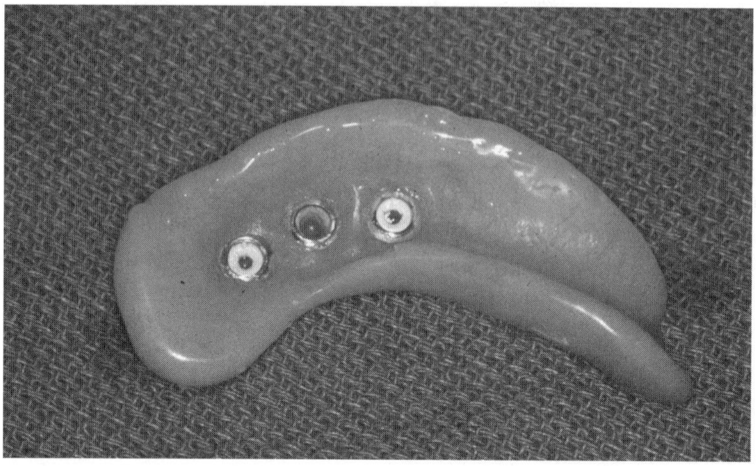

Figure 28 Tissue surface of dental implant supports a mandibular resection prosthesis.

If the dentate patient can only accomplish the presurgical maxillomandiblar relationship with manual assistance then a prosthesis is indicated. Two types of prostheses can be fabricated to provide assistance with acheiving a satisfactory maxillomandibular relationship.

One type is a maxillary prosthesis with an inclined palatal ramp. As the patient's mandibular teeth contact the inclined plane in the palate, the mandible is guided laterally into occlusion. The second type of prosthesis is a buccal guiding flange consisting of two parts: maxillary and mandibular. The mandibular prosthesis has a vertical bar in the buccal vestibule on the nondefect side while the maxillary prosthesis has a horizontal bar in the buccal vestibule on the nondefect side. The mandibular vertical bar rides over the maxillary horizontal bar guiding the mandible into occlusion. Both the palatal ramp and the buccal flange prosthesis require

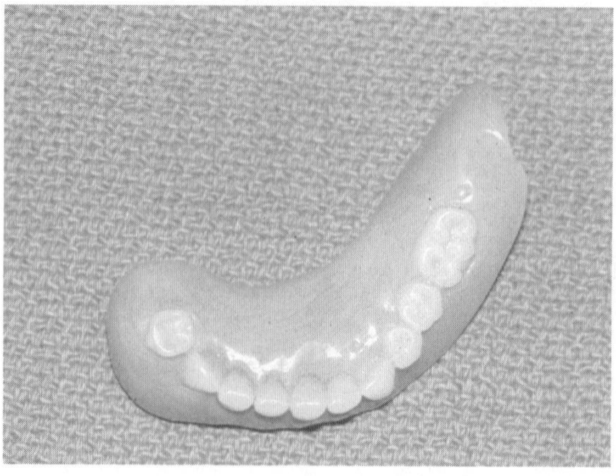

Figure 29 Superior surface of dental implant supports a mandibular resection prosthesis.

natural dentition to work. Therefore, neither of these designs is beneficial for the edentulous patient.

Rehabilitation of a patient that cannot manually move his or her mandible into a presurgical occlusion is more challenging and requires fabrication of a maxillary prosthesis that provides opposing mandibular contact in the area of the palatal vault. This will constrict the palatal vault and can impair the patient's speech.

Rehabilitation of an edentulous patient with a mandibular discontinuity defect is very challenging. Removable dental prostheses require coordinated tongue and mandibular movements to remain stable, as well as adequate alveolar height and vestibular depth. A mandibular removable denture needs cross-arch stability in order to be effective. This involves covering both retromolar pads. All of these requirements are compromised in the patient with a mandibular discontinuity defect. The greater the mandibular segment resected, the smaller the denture foundation, and the less stable and retentive the mandibular prosthesis. Rehabilitation consists of fabricating a maxillary prosthesis that provides opposing mandibular contact in the palatal vault. This type of prosthesis will constrict the palatal vault and can impair the patient's speech.

Most edentulous patients with a resected nonsurgically restored mandible will not be able to use a removable prosthesis for mastication but may find the prosthesis useful as a mandibular vertical stop, something to close against, and for esthetics.

The resected mandible can be surgically restored many ways. Two commonly used techniques are the use of bone plates and bone grafting. The advantage of a surgically reconstructed mandible is that stabilization of the segments results in a more controllable mandible with a more normal range of motion.

Removable dental prostheses should not be fabricated over bone plates covered only by soft tissue. This may result in soft tissue erosion, exposing the bone plate, with subsequent infection and loss of the bone plate.

Removable dental prosthesis fabrication over a bone-grafted mandible benefits from presurgical treatment planning. Bone-grafted mandibles often have insufficient interarch space or alignment to allow dental rehabilitation. Preprosthetic surgery is usually indicated prior to any dental restoration on a bone-grafted mandible, usually involving the release of scar tissue in the buccal and lingual vestibules. It is also necessary to debulk the full-thickness soft tissue grafted with the bone, because this area will be necessary to support the prosthesis. It is important that the prosthesis-bearing area be covered with keratinized, attached, nonmobile soft tissue, which can be accomplished with a split-thickness skin graft on the periosteum.

Palatal Drop Prosthesis

Mandibular surgery often involves the tongue. Surgical resection of a portion of the oral tongue will impair the patient's ability to speak and swallow. The speech impairment occurs because the tongue can no longer make adequate contact in the palatal vault, the swallowing impairment due to decreased tongue mobility (i.e., tethering). Postoperative release of scar tissue and/or grafting can be of great benefit in increasing mobility of the tongue. If the tongue is still unable to make adequate contact with the palatal vault, a palatal drop prosthesis can be fabricated, which recontours the palatal surface, allowing the tongue to make contact (Fig. 30). This prosthesis can be fabricated for either dentulous or edentulous patients.

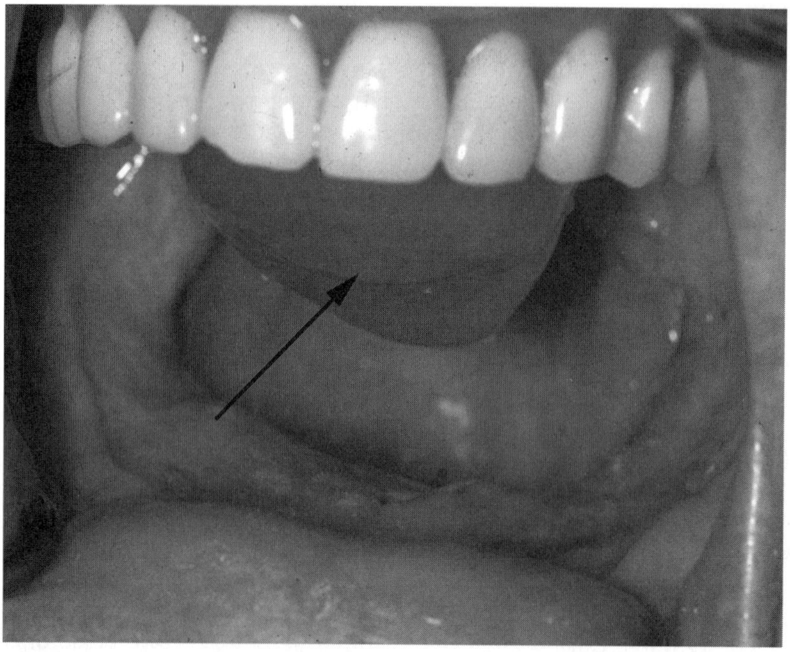

Figure 30 Palatal drop prosthesis.

Osseointegrated Implants in the Mandible

An edentulous patient utilizing a complete denture prior to surgery has an advantage over a patient made edentulous just prior to or during surgery. A recently edentulous patient must adjust to the presence of the surgical defect as well as coping with a removable prosthesis, which is very challenging for most patients. A patient who has difficulty utilizing a removable prosthesis may benefit from the placement of osseointegrated dental implants. Dental implants have proven to be very reliable and can dramatically improve the support and retention of an oral prosthesis (Figs. 27–29). This can be accomplished more predictably if the patient has not received radiation therapy to the oral cavity. As with teeth, the number, size and location of dental implants are important in the retention and stability of mandibular prostheses.

Tongue, Jaw, and Neck Resection

A malignant lesion of the tonsillar pillar often requires surgical resection involving the base of the tongue, tonsillar pillar, posterior lateral aspect of the soft palate, and partial mandibulectomy (Fig. 31). This surgical procedure is often referred to as a tongue, jaw, neck, resection. Velopharyngeal incompetence and difficulty with deglutition are common postoperative complaints. The velopharyngeal incompetence results in hypernasal speech and leakage of fluid and food into the nasal pharynx. Difficulty with deglutition may result in choking and/or aspiration of food or fluid due to impaired mobility of the epiglottis.

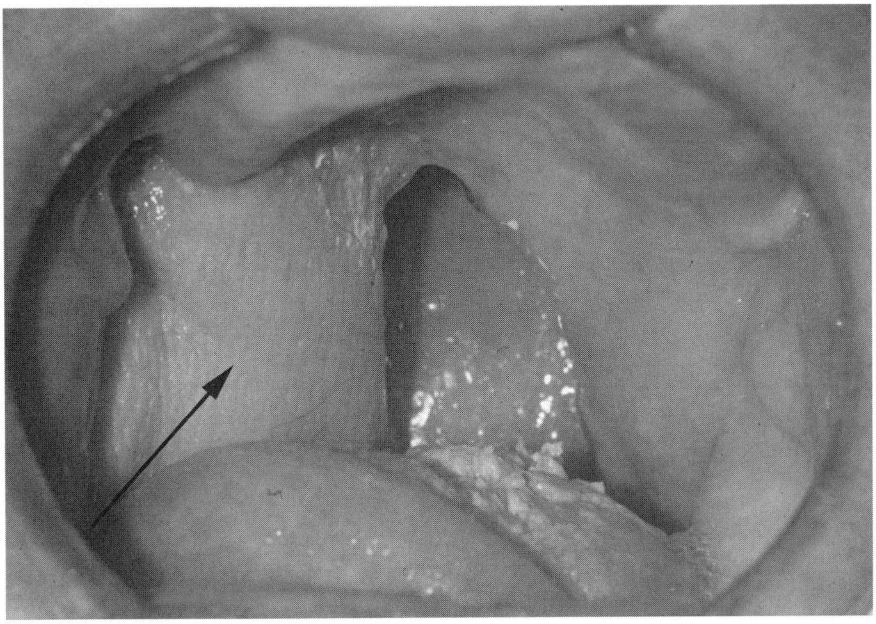

Figure 31 Tongue, jaw, and neck resection with full-thickness tissue graft. Note bulk of full-thickness tissue graft.

Fabrication of a prosthesis to obturate a soft palate defect may decrease the hypernasal speech and reduce leakage of fluids into the nasal cavity. However, the prosthesis will not appreciably affect the patient's ability to swallow. Most problems with deglutition are the result of surgical scar tissue in the oropharynx and not the result of velopharyngeal incompetence. A patient who is to undergo a tongue, jaw, neck resection must be informed about the procedure's expected side effects.

EXTRAORAL PROSTHESES

The care of patients with extraoral head and neck cancer is not limited to the elimination of disease. A comprehensive treatment plan for patient rehabilitation must be considered before surgery. Preoperative anticipation of anatomical structures to be surgically removed would suggest that patient rehabilitation be surgical and/or prosthetic.

An extraoral facial prosthesis is a cosmetic bandage utilized to camouflage a surgical defect that is not amenable to or desirable for surgical reconstruction. An extraoral prosthesis may be considered in the following situations (6):

1. A large defect not readily closed with available or grafted soft tissue (Fig. 3)
2. A structure not easily reconstructed surgically (i.e., an eye, nose, or ear) (Fig. 4)
3. A patient not psychologically or physically capable of tolerating a multistage surgical reconstruction

4. A surgical defect requiring direct visualization to monitor for recurrent disease
5. Temporary use during multistage surgical reconstruction of a surgical defect

Patient Factors

Esthetic and psychological factors are both important when considering rehabilitation with an extraoral facial prosthesis. As MacGregor has said, "the face is the mirror of the soul" (15). The face, always exposed, is the focus of attention and the first thing people see. A change to the face quickly draws unwanted attention. From the patient's esthetic and psychological perspective, how well an extraoral prosthesis camouflages the defect is important.

To be acceptable to the patient, an extraoral prosthesis must blend into the anatomical area. A well-made extraoral prosthesis can be effective in camouflaging an extraoral surgical defect (Figs. 32,33). An ideal extraoral facial prosthesis should have the following features (16):

1. Light weight: the heavier the prosthesis, the more difficult it is to retain.

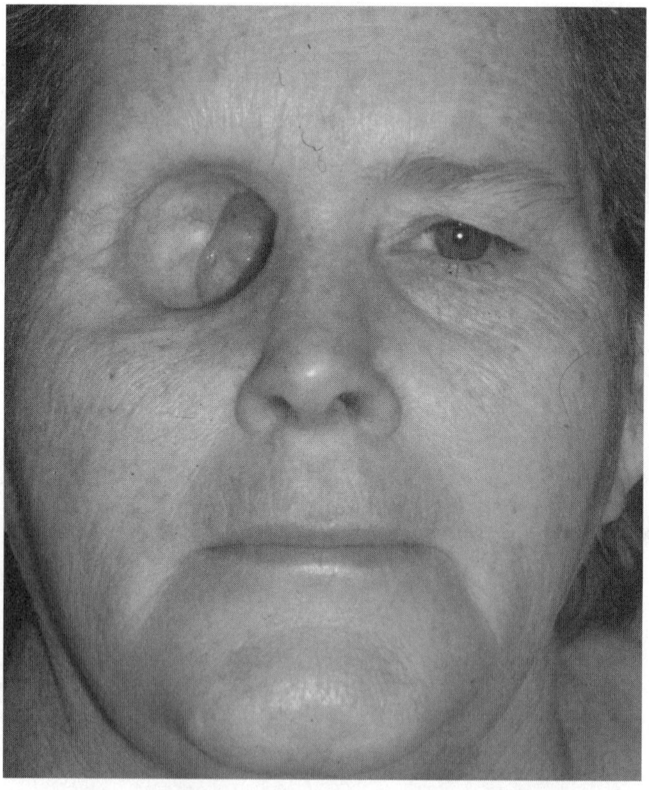

Figure 32 Patient with exenteration of the right eye. Orbital defect has well-formed tissue undercuts.

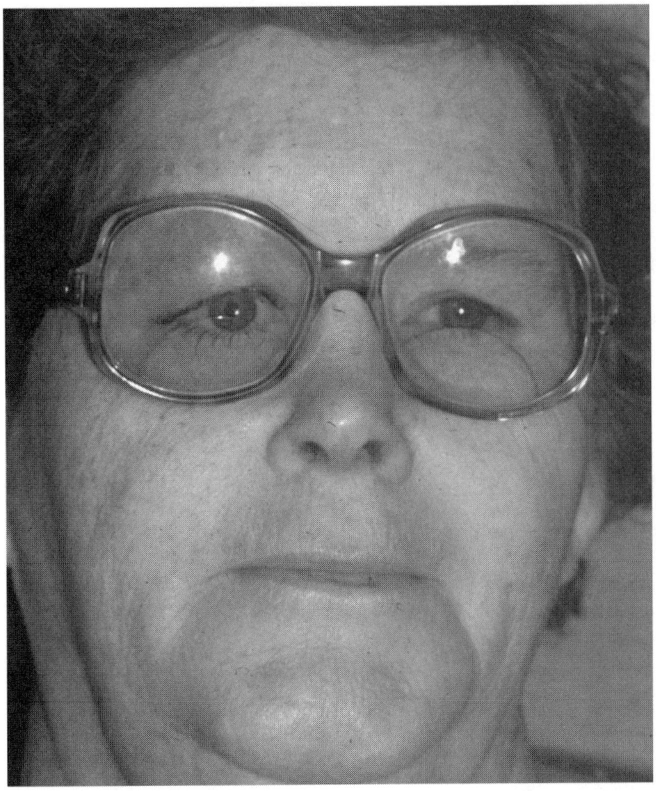

Figure 33 Orbital prosthesis retained by soft tissue undercuts. Tinted glasses help to camouflage margins of the prosthesis.

2. Camouflage the defect: a patient should be able to walk down the street without attracting undue attention.
3. Color-compatible: it should blend in with the patient's natural tissue. A patient's tissue color may change with the seasons, and more than one prosthesis may be necessary for a patient.
4. Retentive: this is important from the psychological perspective of a patient. The patient must feel confident with the retention of the extraoral prosthesis.
5. Durable: because of the cost and the time required to fabricate, the prosthesis should last 6–12 months.

Prosthetic Margins

One of the most common and esthetically superior extraoral prostheses is the ocular prosthesis (Figs. 34,35). An ocular prosthesis only replaces the globe of the eye, which can not be restored surgically (16,17). It is usually esthetic because it resides within the orbit and can be retained by the eyelids, which also camouflage its margins.

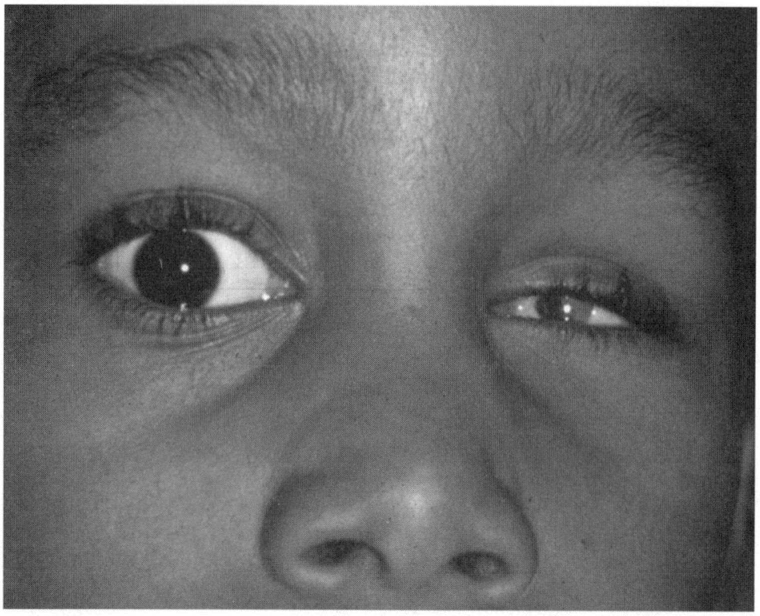

Figure 34 Ocular defect resulting from low-velocity projectile.

As the surgical field expands, more anatomical structures are removed. A larger surgical field dictates a larger prosthesis, with more exposed margins that create cosmetic weak points. The quality of the tissue adjacent to the surgical defect is very important in camouflaging the prosthesis margins. Thin, attached,

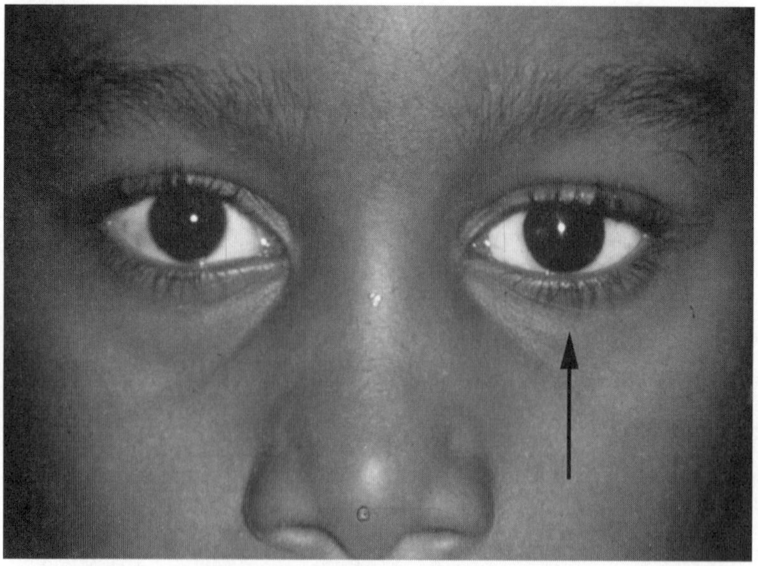

Figure 35 Ocular prosthesis retained by eyelids.

keratinized tissue of natural color provides the ideal surface to terminate the margin of an extraoral prosthesis. Tissue that is thick, nonattached, and mobile will be affected by the movement of adjacent facial musculature. Anatomical areas with mobile soft tissue result in difficulty with prosthetic margins. The prosthesis margins will open. Movement of the orbicularis oris muscle can affect the inferior margin of a nasal prosthesis where it contacts the upper lip. The area inferior to the external auditory meatus, which consists of soft tissue covering the ascending ramus of the mandible, can affect the retention of an auricular prosthesis during mandibular movement.

Surgical Considerations

Surgical considerations that can affect the outcome of an extraoral prosthesis may include the following:

1. The periphery of the surgical defect should be covered with attached, keratinized tissue extending over the margin of the defect. This result can be accomplished through the placement of a split-thickness skin graft (Fig. 36) or by undermining the surgical defect margin to allow the epithelium to wrap over the edge of the defect (Fig. 37).
2. A split-thickness skin graft is preferable to a full-thickness graft because it will attach to the tissue base and offer a more stable surface for prosthetic adhesion.
3. Full-thickness tissue grafts are rarely suitable as a foundation for a facial prosthesis because they do not provide stability.

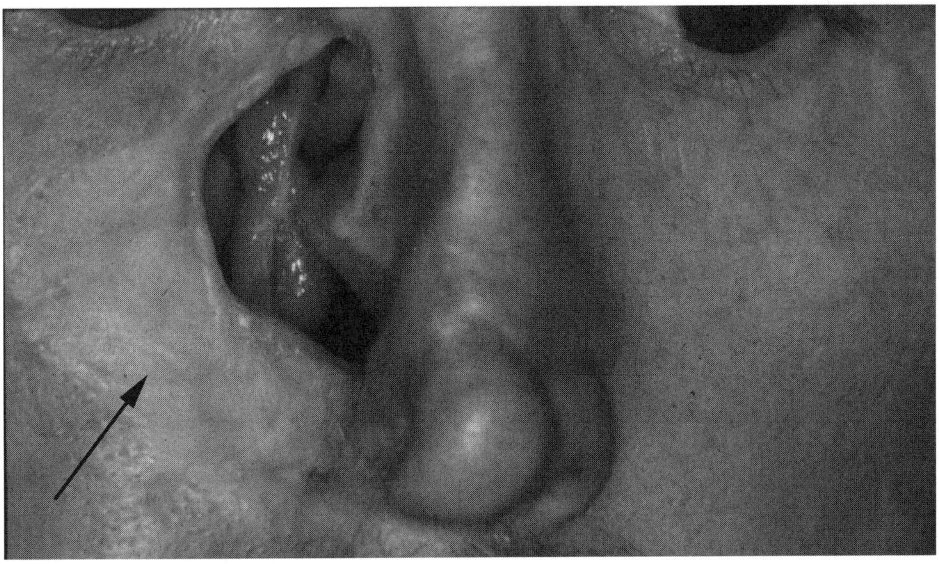

Figure 36 Split-thickness skin graft provides an immovable base and a good surface for adhesive.

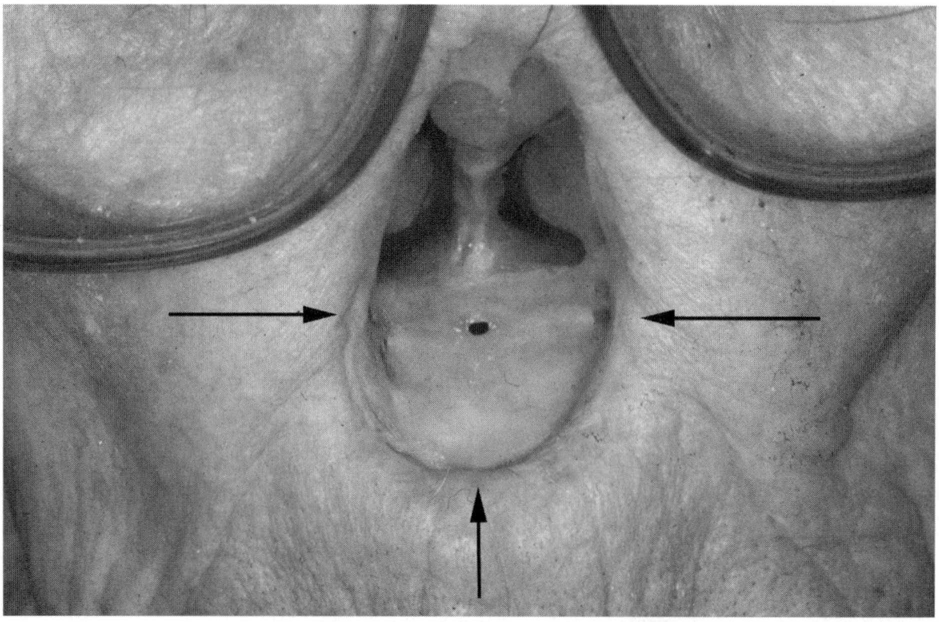

Figure 37 Epithelium covers edges of defect and provides a suitable surface for adhesive.

4. Small remnants of soft tissue should be excised unless there is a strong probability of surgical reconstruction. A rhinectomy, leaving a small portion of the ala, is prosthetically undesirable (Fig. 38). The prosthesis will have to overlay the soft tissue remnant, resulting in a prosthesis that is too large for the patient and unnatural looking. An exception to the removal of small soft tissue tags is the superior half of the ear: the helix. Retaining the helix is desirable because it has a cartilaginous foundation that provides orientation and lends stability to the prosthesis. The tragus can also provide orientation for the construction and placement of an auricular prosthesis (Fig. 39) (6).

The face is a complex area of form, color, and movement. A well-made prosthesis on a well-developed surgical foundation should allow the patient to take his or her place within society with confidence.

Fabrication of an Extraoral Prosthesis

A facial prosthesis is often fabricated from silicone elastomer or acrylic resin (polymethylmethacrylate). The basic technique of fabricating an extraoral prosthesis consists of the following:

1. Making an impression of the surgical defect to fabricate a plaster cast. Dental impression material such as reversible or irreversible hydrocolloid (alginate) is most commonly employed.
2. Sculpting the missing tissue from wax or clay.

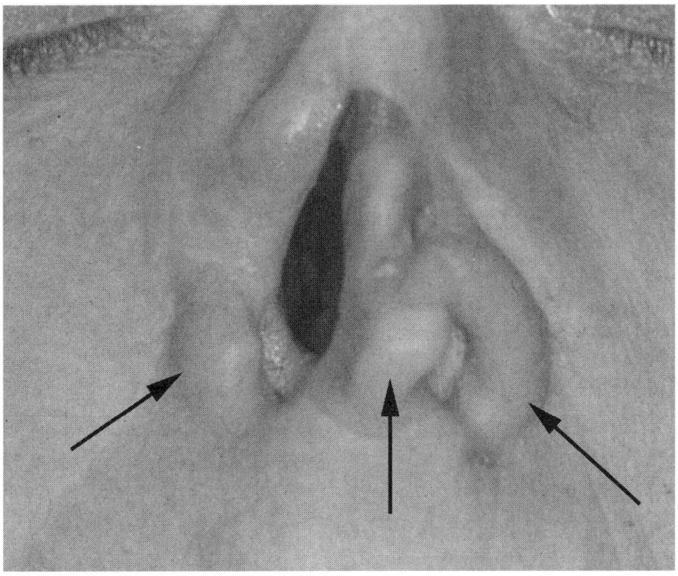

Figure 38 Partial rhinectomy with residual tissue tags.

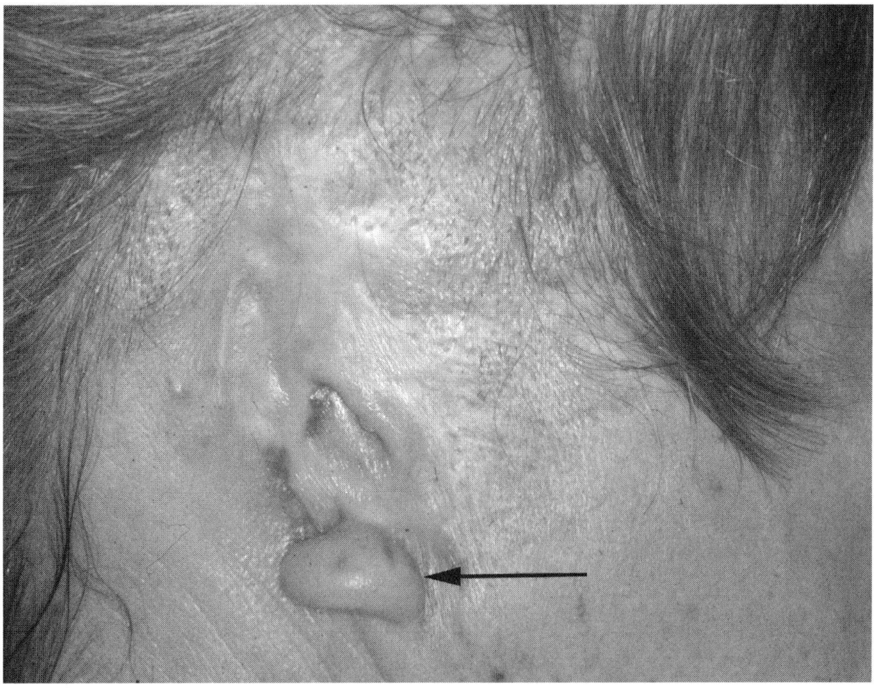

Figure 39 The tragus should be retained, if possible, because it camouflages the anterior margin of the prosthesis.

3. Fabricating the prosthesis mold using the plaster cast as a base.
4. Adding colors to the uncured prosthetic material to simulate the patient's base skin color.
5. Placing the uncured prosthetic material in the mold to cure.
6. Final coloring and delivery of the prosthesis to the patient.
7. Educating the patient about the use and maintenance of the prosthesis.

The extraoral prosthesis should be removed at least once a day for cleaning of the prosthesis, the surgical defect, and surrounding tissue. The extraoral prosthesis should be cleaned with mild soap and water.

Retention of an Extraoral Prosthesis

Retention of an extraoral facial prosthesis is most commonly achieved by engaging soft tissue undercuts, applying surgical adhesives, or the use of extraoral osseointegrated dental implants. The simplest retention of a facial prosthesis is with soft tissue undercuts. An ocular prosthesis, which only replaces the globe of the eye, is retained and its margins camouflaged by the eyelids (Figs. 34, 35). Retention of the ocular muscles at the time of enucleation results in a mobile, soft tissue foundation, imparting life-like motion to an ocular prosthesis.

An orbital prosthesis replaces the globe of an eye, associated musculature, and the eyelids. An orbital defect has naturally occurring, well-formed tissue undercuts (Fig. 32). These undercuts usually retain an orbital prosthesis well. The use of a heavy-rimmed eyeglass frame and tinted lenses can help camouflage the margins of an orbital prosthesis (Fig. 33).

It is not recommend to attach an orbital or any other extraoral prosthesis to an eyeglass frame (Fig. 40). If the facial prosthesis is attached to the eyeglass frame, it is critical that the frame fit precisely and not move. If the eyeglass frame moves, the prosthesis will move and not be well adapted over the surgical defect (Fig. 41). It is advantageous for the patient to be able to remove the eyeglasses independent of an extraoral prosthesis.

Larger surgical defects are usually deficient in the quality and quantity of soft tissue undercuts. The use of a surgical skin adhesive becomes necessary for retention of a larger extraoral prosthesis (i.e., stoma adhesive). Although surgical adhesives can be effective in retaining a facial prosthesis, some undesirable side effects include the following:

1. Efficacy of retention: a mobile tissue foundation may disrupt the adhesive barrier. Adhesive may be less effective in hot, humid weather or on oily skin.
2. Tissue irritation: mechanical irritation of skin during repeated adhesive removal.
3. Hard to clean: difficult to remove adhesive from the prosthesis without damaging thin margins.
4. Messy: difficult to apply adhesive to the small areas of the prosthesis necessary for retention. The adhesive can retain dirt.
5. Difficult to use: patients with poor eyesight or the loss of depth perception will have difficulty managing surgical adhesives for prosthesis retention.

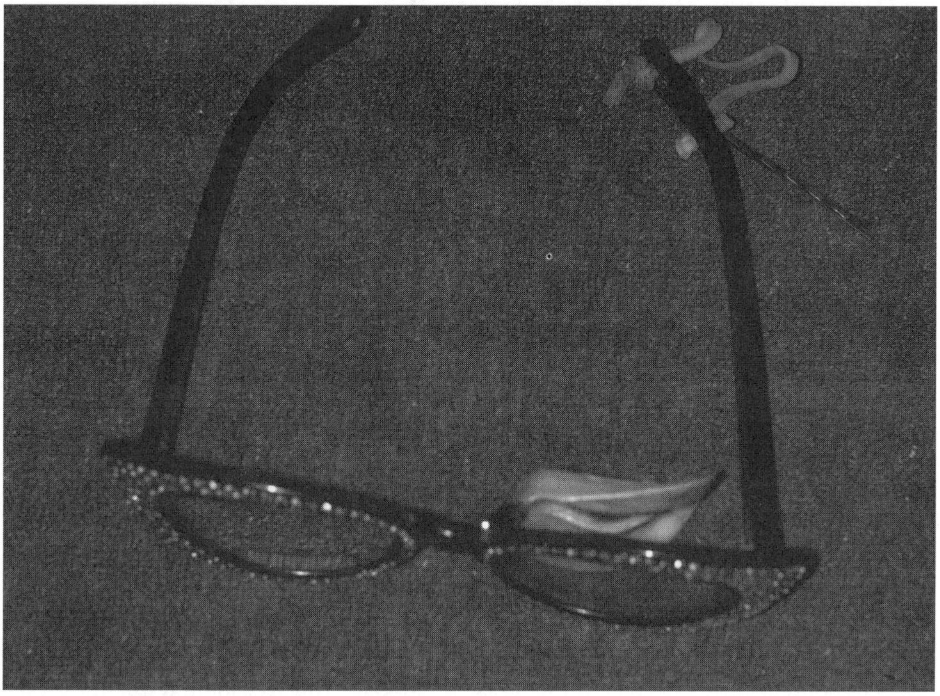

Figure 40 Orbital prosthesis attached to eyeglass frame.

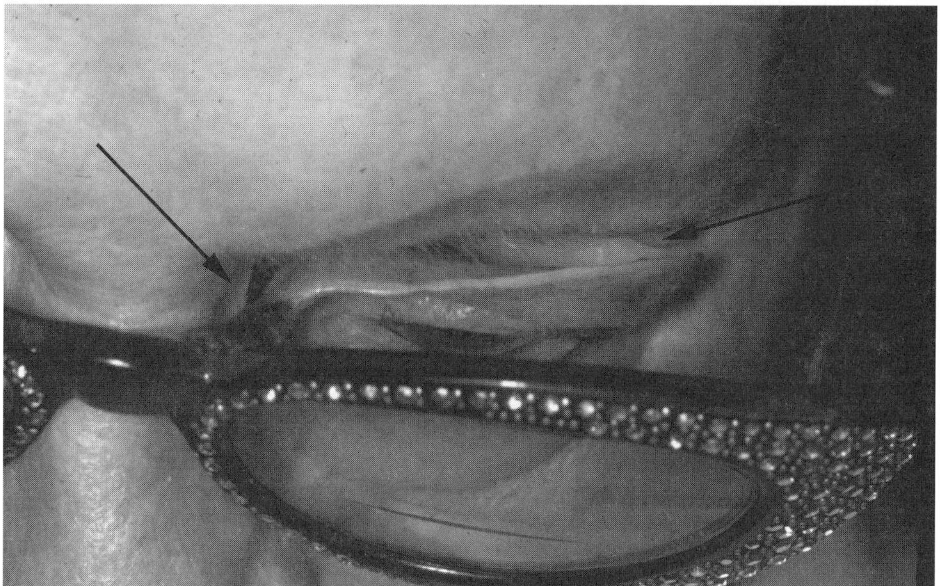

Figure 41 Orbital prosthesis attached to eyeglass frame moves when frame moves.

EXTRAORAL OSSEOINTEGRATED IMPLANTS

A recent advance in the retention of extraoral prostheses involves the extraoral placement of modified osseointegrated dental implants (18–20) that have their anchorage in bone. The use of two to five implants can provide facial prosthesis retention that eliminates the need for surgical adhesive. Osseointegrated implants have proven most beneficial in the auricular area, due to tissue mobility and a lack of prosthesis orientation (Figs. 42, 43).

Rehabilitation of a patient with an extraoral defect can be complex. Although surgical reconstruction of an extraoral defect is ideal, it is not always possible or desirable. The benefits of an extraoral facial prosthesis can be enhanced through presurgical planning and a surgical awareness of facial prosthetic needs. The rehabilitation of a patient with an extraoral surgical defect is most effective when all the members of the team are aware of the others' needs.

OSSEOINTEGRATED IMPLANTS

Dental implants have proven to be very reliable and can dramatically improve the support and retention of a prosthesis. This can be accomplished more predictably if the patient has not received radiation therapy to the area of implant placement. The use of hyperbaric oxygen has proven beneficial in improving the success rate of dental implants placed in irradiated osseous tissue. However, dental implants have

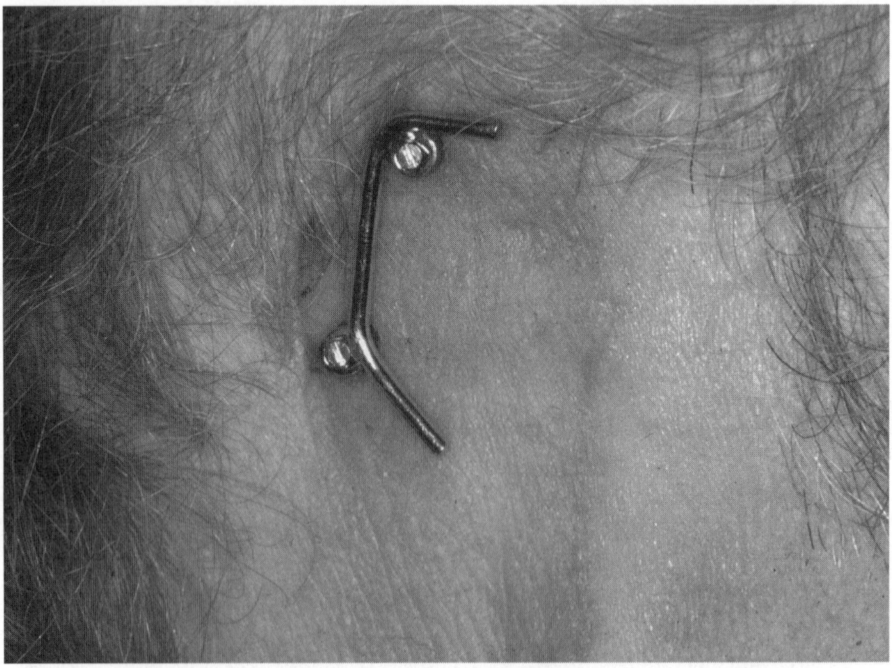

Figure 42 Two osseointegrated implants provide mechanical retention for an auricular prosthesis.

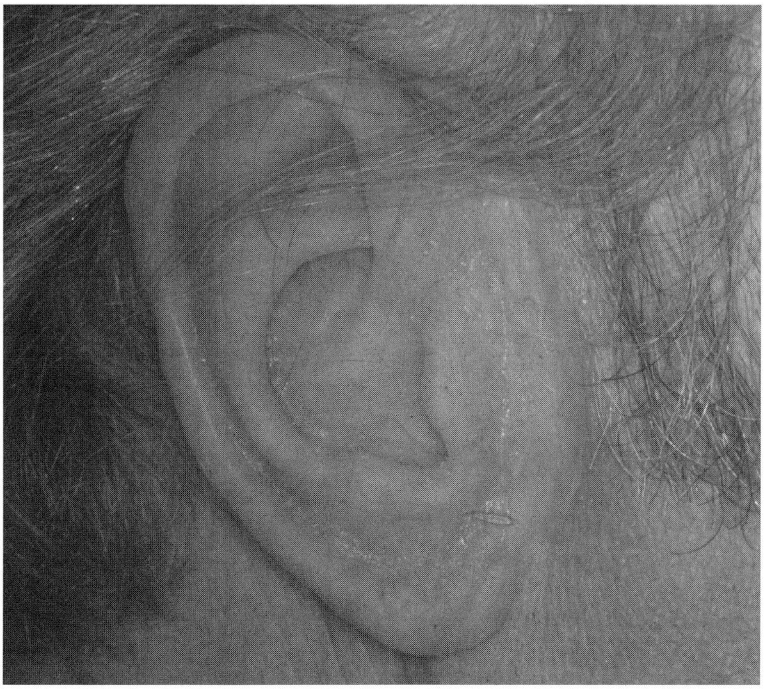

Figure 43 Auricular prosthesis is retained by osseointegrated implants.

been successfully placed in the irradiated mandible both with and without the use of adjunct hyperbaric oxygen (21,22).

Branemark made the serendipitous observation of a bone–metal fusion in 1952 while attempting to remove titanium optical chambers implanted into rabbit femurs. Branemark coined the term osseointegration to describe this metal-bone fusion and performed animal studies that progressed to the clinical placement of implant cylinders into the anterior mandible of edentulous patients in 1965. Between 1965 and 1982, clinical trials progressed the use of dental implants in edentulous mandibles. Branemark presented his research on the clinical use of dental implants to the North America dental community in 1982. His statistical success of osseointegrated dental implants in the anterior nonirradiated edentulous mandible was 95% at 5 years.

Branemark's tenets for the successful osseointegration of an implant include the following:

1. The implant must be sterile, free of contamination, and in a reactive state. The reactive state is a surface layer of titanium oxide.
2. A gentle surgical technique. This includes a minimal elevation of periosteum and not overheating the bone while drilling. This temperature was determined to be less than 47°C for 1 min in animal studies.
3. The implant must be stable when placed in the osteotomy site. This is accomplished by slightly undersizing the surgical receptor site. Intimate contact of the implant and the bone will result in the formation of embryonic bone that will mature into lamellar, load-bearing bone.

4. The implant must be left submerged under soft tissue to heal in an undisturbed state for 3–6 months, depending upon bone quality. Micromovement of an implant during the healing phase disrupts the normal osseous remodeling process leading to fibrous encapsulation rather than osseointegration.

The success of osseointegrated implants is dependent on bone quantity and quality. The open trabecular pattern of cancellous bone provides less surface area for implant contact and initial stabilization. However, very dense cortical bone has a poor blood supply and reduced regenerative capabilities. A desirable osteotomy site will have some cortical bone for implant stabilization and some cancellous bone for vascularity.

The statistical success of osseointegrated implants is very high. A patient in good health is usually a candidate for osseointegrated implants and age is not a contraindication. Medical diseases or conditions can compromise the success rate of osseointegrated implants, including uncontrolled diabetes, blood dyscrasias, or radiation therapy to the implant site. Autoimmune diseases such as Sjögren's syndrome, make it difficult to work in the oral cavity and can be relative contraindications to the placement of osseointegrated implants. Patients who smoke tobacco demonstrate an increased osseointegrated implant failure rate (23).

Osseointegrated implants are placed in individual osteotomy sites. While the statistical success of osseointegrated implants is very high, they can fail to osseointegrate for a variety of reasons: surgical factors such as overheating the bone, failure to stabilize the implant at placement, and/or compromising local vascularity.

An advantage of individual cylindrical implants is that the loss of one implant in a healthy, nonsmoking patient does not necessarily mean the loss of all implants. However, the loss of one implant in a medically compromised patient or one who smokes tobacco often indicates that the remaining implants will eventually fail.

Implants are manufactured in various lengths, diameters, and surface coatings. The philosophy of bank vault construction posits that the longer, the wider, and the increased number of implants placed, the more likely they will withstand the work load imposed by a prosthesis. An intraoral implant 4 mm in diameter by 13 mm in length is a commonly used size. Implants less than 10 mm in length have a significantly reduced success rate intraorally.

Intraoral Maxilla

Patients with a removable maxillary complete denture usually manage well with their prosthesis. A maxillary denture is retained with a denture-style retention (i.e., suction) derived from a border seal. Palatal surgery for malignant disease that disrupts the border seal or perforates the palatal vault will prevent the formation of a border seal and retention of the maxillary denture. Support of a maxillary prosthesis requires the entire intact alveolar–palatal foundation. Loss of any of this foundation will adversely affect the stability of the patient's denture, resulting in significant prosthesis movement.

Dental implants are a proven elective procedure to be considered for a patient desiring improved retention and stability of a dental prosthesis (Figs. 44, 45). This can be accomplished more predictably if the patient has not received radiation

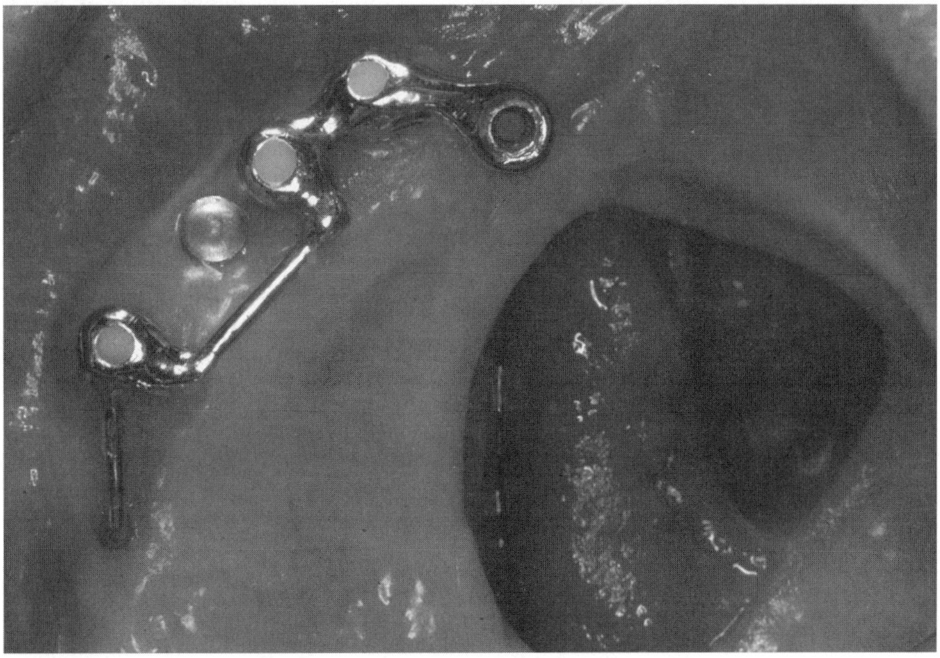

Figure 44 Four dental implants placed to aid retention and stabilization of an obturator.

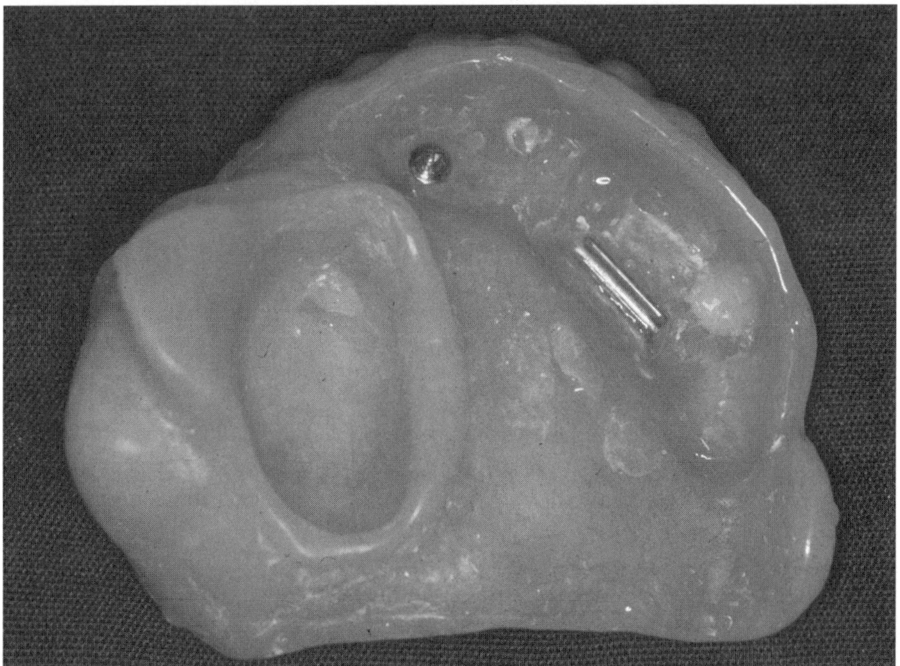

Figure 45 Interior surface of obturator with attachments used for retention of prosthesis.

therapy to the oral cavity. As with teeth, the number, size, and location of dental implants are important. In the ideal situation, dental implants should be dispersed and located where the greatest amount of bone is found. This is usually in the premaxilla and tuberosity.

The success of dental implants in the maxilla is dependent upon the quantity and quality of bone available for osseointegration.The presence of the maxillary sinus complicates the placement of dental implants on the nonsurgical side due to the minimal amount of alveolar bone overlying the sinus. This thin alveolar bone prevents the placement of dental implants of sufficient length. Surgical techniques for bone grafting the maxillary sinus are available, allowing the use of implants of adequate length.

An alternative to bone grafting the maxillary sinus for the placement of a dental implant is a zygomatic implant. A zygomatic dental implant is 40–50 mm long and engages the zygoma by transecting the alveolus, medial to the area of the first molar.

Osseointegrated dental implants must be placed 4–6 months prior to the time of utilization to allow for adequate integration. The placement of dental implants into a surgical defect may be technically possible; however, they are usually difficult to restore and keep clean. Attached keratinized tissue should surround a dental implant where it protrudes through the soft tissue to provide a healthy environment. If these criteria cannot be met, then a dental implant should probably not be placed.

Intraoral Mandible

Edentulous patients, in general, have more difficulty utilizing a removable mandibular prosthesis than a maxillary prosthesis. A mandibular removable complete denture needs cross-arch stability to have a reasonable opportunity of being beneficial. This involves covering both retromolar pads. Mandibular complete denture prostheses require coordinated tongue and mandibular movements to remain stable, as well as adequate alveolar height and vestibular depth. All of these requirements are compromised in the patient with a mandibular discontinuity defect. The greater the mandibular segment resected, the smaller the denture foundation, and the less stable and retentive the mandibular prosthesis. Most edentulous patients with a resected, nonsurgically restored mandible will not be able to use a removable prosthesis for mastication.

Dental implants have proven to be very reliable and can dramatically improve the support and retention of a resected mandibular prosthesis (Figs. 27–29). Dental implants should be dispersed and located where the greatest amount of bone is found, usually the anterior mandible. Implant placement in the posterior mandible must avoid the mandibular nerve and vascular bundle. Osseointegrated dental implants must be placed approximately 4 months prior to the time of utilization to allow for adequate integration. Attached keratinized mucosa should surround a dental implant where it protrudes through the soft tissue to provide a healthy environment.

A mandibular discontinuity defect can be restored with a bone graft or a bone plate. When restored with a bone plate, it can only receive dental implants in the nonresected mandible. When restored with a bone graft, it can have dental implants placed in both the nonresected mandible and the graft. However, bone grafts are not always prosthetically suitable for dental implant placement. Dental implants placed in a bone graft with inadequate interarch space or poor graft orientation cannot be used for prosthodontic rehabilitation.

The surgical repair of a resected mandible with a bone graft requires that the bone graft be covered with a full thickness of soft tissue for vascularity and graft survival. Surgery to release scar tissue in the buccal and lingual vestibules of a bone-grafted mandible is indicated prior to the placement of any dental prosthesis. It is also necessary to debulk the full-thickness soft tissue graft. It is important that the bone-grafted mandible expected to support a prosthesis be covered with keratinized, attached, nonmobile soft tissue. This can be accomplished with a split-thickness skin graft placed on the periosteum.

Extraoral Osseointegrated Implants

The clinical success of osseointegrated dental implants in edentulous and partially edentulous patients has led to the modification of these implants for extraoral use. This modification included the addition of a flange at the top of the implant to prevent overseating during placement. These extraoral implants are 4 mm long and are for use where the bone is thin, such as the mastoid area.

The initial use of extraoral osseointegrated implants was in 1977 for the retention of bone-conductive hearing aids. Osseointegrated implants were first used for the retention of auricular prostheses in 1979 (24).

Implant-Supported Auricular Prothesis

A patient who has lost an auricle has several rehabilitation options: no treatment, surgical reconstruction, or prosthetic reconstruction. The cosmetic results of surgical reconstruction have been less than desirable and in the past prosthetic rehabilitation has been the treatment of choice.

The retention of an auricular prosthesis usually involves a surgical adhesive. The presence of perspiration, skin oils, mandibular movement, hair, and a mobile tissue bed all compromize the retention of the prosthesis. Difficulties with the retention of auricular prostheses led Branemark and co-workers to place the first implant-supported auricular prosthesis in 1979 (Figs. 42, 43) (25).

An auricular prosthesis needs a minimum of two, preferably three, implants in the mastoid area. These are allowed to heal submerged and undisturbed for 4–6 months. The skin that surrounds the transmucosal portion of an extraoral osseointegrated implant must be keratinized, thin, and attached to the periosteum. At the time the implants are uncovered, the elevated flap must be thinned to achieve these desired qualities.

An implant-supported auricular prosthesis requires advanced planning and careful implant placement. A surgical stent facilitates the correct placement of the implants. The use of osseointegrated implants for the retention of an auricular prosthesis significantly increases the patient's confidence in the prosthesis.

Implant-Supported Orbital Prothesis

Orbital exenteration requires rehabilitation due to the high visibility of the surgical defect. Although an orbital exenteration lends itself to an easy closing of the surgical defect with a full-thickness tissue flap, this surgical procedure is contraindicated in any patient desiring prosthetic rehabilitation because the soft tissue fills the orbit. An orbital prosthesis requires substantial anterior–posterior depth to be cosmetically similar to the nonsurgical side. The periphery of an orbital exenteration defect needs to be lined with keratinized tissue. The superior and inferior eyelids are an excellent source of this tissue.

An orbital prosthesis is primarily retained mechanically, achieved with undercuts posterior to the supra- and infraorbital rims. The surgical treatment of the malignant disease may result in the loss of these naturally occurring undercuts. The loss of naturally occurring undercuts requires other methods of prosthesis retention (i.e., surgical adhesive or osseointegrated implants).

Placing osseointegrated implants for the retention of an orbital prosthesis is highly desirable. Unfortunately, the bone surrounding orbital defects is usually thin and of poor quality, which limits the number and location of possible implant placement sites. This results in a lower osseointegration rate for implants placed in the exenterated orbit. The placement of implants in an orbital defect requires preplacement planning to avoid undesirable cosmetic consequences.

Implant-Supported Nasal Protheses

Surgical reconstruction of a total rhinectomy is difficult because of the loss of the cartilaginous skeleton. Prosthetic rehabilitation has produced the most satisfactory cosmetic results. If the patient is to be rehabilitated with a nasal prosthesis, the surgical defect margins should be covered with keratinized skin and the nasal septum removed. The primary retention of a nasal prosthesis has been surgical adhesive. The naturally occurring undercuts in the nasal cavity are unusable for mechanical retention because the nasal mucosa will not tolerate prosthesis contact.

Retention of a nasal prosthesis can be problematic with surgical adhesive because of perspiration, oily skin, exhaled water vapor, and soft tissue mobility (i.e., upper lip). It would seem that a simple solution to retention of a nasal prosthesis would be to attach it to the patient's eyeglasses frame. The disadvantages of this technique include any movement of the eyeglass frame, which opens the prosthesis margins. Removal of the eyeglasses includes removal of the prosthesis. The prosthesis provides no anterior support for the eyeglasses, which are designed to sit on the bridge of the nose.

Osseointegrated implants offer a tremendous benefit for the support of a nasal prosthesis when they integrate. However, the anatomical sites available for implant placement provide bone of poor quality and limited quantity, resulting in a poor rate of success.

Combination Implant-Supported Protheses

A combination prosthesis combines more than one extraoral area and may include an intraoral maxillary defect. The large size and weight of a combination prosthesis result in difficulty with retention. Osseointegrated implants offer a superior method of prosthesis retention. The opportunity for using osseointegrated implants may be greater with the combination prosthesis than with other facial prostheses: the large size of the surgical defect allows use of implant placement sites such as the zygomatic arch and the maxilla.

RADIATION THERAPY

Comprehensive management of head and neck malignant disease may include the use of radiation therapy. Salivary glands within the field of radiation will become nonfunctional. The degree of xerostomia experienced by the patient may vary depending on the number of major salivary glands irradiated, the type of radiation, and the total dosage. The use of intra- and extraoral shielding can help preserve salivary gland function, thus reducing postirradiation therapy xerostomia.

Radiation-induced xerostomia predisposes the patient to dental caries of any remaining teeth (Fig. 46). Additional patient factors, including diet and oral hygiene, will influence the propensity to radiation caries.

Radiation-induced dental caries can be a very aggressive form of dental disease involving smooth surfaces of teeth that are not normally prone to caries. This usually includes the cervical area where the tooth enters the gingiva. Cervical caries are often circumferential and very difficult to restore. Placing a complete artificial crown on a tooth can be a short-term treatment. An artificial crown for a tooth is not a definitive answer because the caries will resume below the margin of the artificial crown.

Radiation-induced dental caries can be dramatically reduced with a daily application of topical fluoride (7,26) daily for the remainder of the patient's life. Xerostomia will continue indefinitely, as will the susceptibility to dental caries. The need for routine dental hygiene and the use of daily topical fluoride will continue indefinitely.

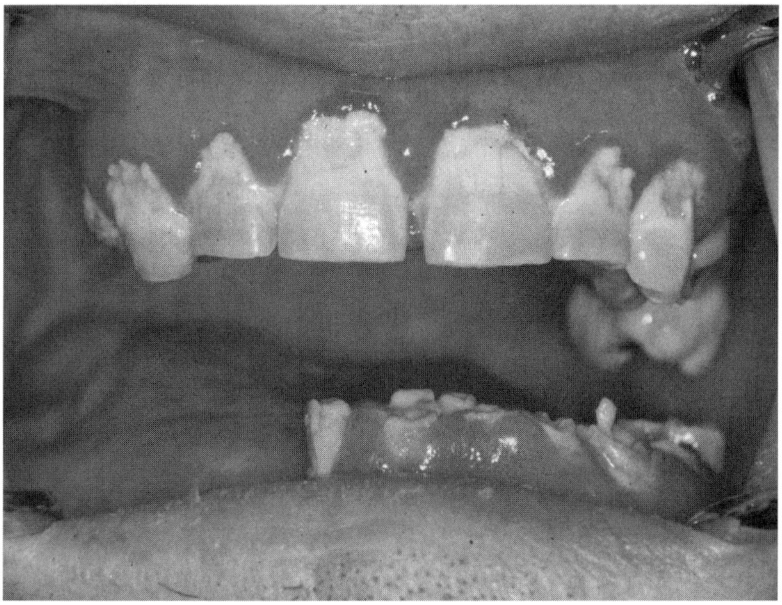

Figure 46 Radiation-induced caries with severe breakdown of teeth.

The fluoride of choice for daily topical application is 0.4% stannous fluoride. The stannous and fluoride ions are both effective in bonding to the dental enamel hydroxylapatite to make the tooth more caries resistant. The stannous ion has a disagreeable taste and flavoring agents must be added.

Some irradiated patients find the taste of the stannous ion or flavoring agents unacceptable. An alternative is 1% sodium fluoride, which is less reactive than 0.4% stannous fluoride. Therefore, it must be in contact with the tooth surface for a greater period of time to provide resistance to caries. Use of a custom-made fluoride carrier is effective to achieve the recommended contact time.

Acidulated phosphate fluoride (APF) is routinely used in the dental office for periodic topical application. This fluoride has a very low pH and, used on a daily basis, will dissolve the enamel and erode natural dentition. It is therefore contraindicated.

In addition to an increased risk of dental caries, xerostomia also reduces a patient's tolerance for an oral prosthesis. Saliva serves as an important lubricant between a prosthesis and the oral tissue. Its absence results in increased irritation of oral tissues during prosthesis function because of friction. Saliva is also an important aid in the retention of an oral prosthesis because of surface tension.

The literature demonstrates that significant soft tissue changes occur within the field of radiation (27), including a reduced blood supply and thinning and atrophy of the oral epithelium. The underlying connective tissue becomes fibrotic and avascular. These changes make the construction and use of an intraoral prosthesis more difficult and increase the risk of osteoradionecrosis.

A preoperative dental evaluation and placement within one of the four M.D. Anderson dental categories is important to minimize the need for postradiation dental complications. Dental extractions in an irradiated patient have an increased risk of healing complications. It is, therefore, important that a patient be dentally stable before undergoing radiation therapy.

REFERENCES

1. The glossary of prosthodontic terms. 7th ed. J Prosthet Dent 1999; 81:48–110.
2. Dorland's Illustrated Medical Dictionary, 25th ed. W. B. Saunders, Philadelphia, 1990.
3. Curtis TA, Beumer J. Restoration of acquired hard palate defects: etiology, disability, and rehabilitation. In: Beumer J, Curtis TA, Firtell DN, eds. Maxillofacial rehabilitation: prosthodontic and surgical considerations. St. Louis: C.V. Mosby, 1979:188–243.
4. Desjardin RP. Early rehabilitative management of the maxillectomy patient. J Prosthet Dent 1977; 38:311–318.
5. Curtis TA, Beumer J. Restoration of acquired hard plate defects. In: Buemer J, Curtis TA, Marunick MT, eds. Maxillofacial rehabilitation: prosthodontic and surgical considerations. St. Louis: Ishiyaku EuroAmerica Inc, 1996:225–284.
6. Beumer J, Ma T, Marunick M, Roumanas E, Nishimura R. Restoration of facial defects: etiology, disability and rehabilitation. In: Buemer J, Curtis TA, Marunick MT, eds. Maxillofacial rehabilitation: prosthodontic and surgical considerations. St. Louis: Ishiyaku EuroAmerica Inc, 1996:377–453.
7. Daly TE. Management of dental problems in irradiated patients. In: The Radiographical Society of America refresher course. Chicago. Nov 2–30, 1971; 2–16.
8. Aramany MA. Basic principles of obturator design for partially edentulous patients. Part I Classification. J Prosthet Dent 1978; 40:554–557.

9. Desjardins RP, Laney WR. Typical clinical problems and approaches to treatment. In: Laney WR, ed. Maxillofacial prosthetic: postgraduate handbook. Littleton Co: PSG Publishing Co., 1979:115–137.
10. Aramany MA, Myers EN. Prosthetic reconstruction following resection of the hard and soft palate. J Prosthet Dent 1978; 40:174–178.
11. Chalian VA, Drane JB, Standish SM. Intraoral prosthetics. In: Chalian VA, Drane JB, Standish SM, eds. Maxillofacial prosthetics: multidisciplinary practice. Baltimore: Williams & Wilkins, 1972:133–142.
12. Desjardins RP. Relating examination findings to treatment procedures (treatment planning). In: Laney WR, ed. Maxillofacial prosthetics: postgraduate handbook. Littleton, Co: PSG Publishing Co., 1979:86–106.
13. Brown KE. Peripheral consideration in improving obturator retention. J Prosthet Dent 1968; 20:176–181.
14. Desjardins RP. Obturator prosthesis design for acquired maxillary defects. J Prosthet Dent 1979; 39:424–435.
15. Macgregor FC. Appearance, interaction and identity. In: Macgregor FC. Transformation and identity: The face and plastic surgery, New York: Quadrangle/The New York Times Book Company, 1974:30–31.
16. Bulbulian AH. Essentials of successful facial prosthetic restoration and prosthesis of the ear part I: Anatomy and part II: types of deformities. In: Bulbuian AH, eds. Facial prosthetics, Springfield, IL: Charles C. Thomas, 1973:40–53 and 278–299.
17. Cain JR. Custom ocular prosthetics. J Prosthet Dent 1982; 48:690–694.
18. Parel SM, Branemark P-I, Tjellstrom A, Gion G. Osseointegration in maxillofacial prosthetics. Part II: extraoral applications. J Prosthet Dent 1986; 55:600–606.
19. Parel SM, Holt GR, Branemark P-I, Tjellstrom A. Osseointegration in facial prosthetics. Int J Oral Maxillofac Implants 1986; 1:27–29.
20. Sugar A, Beumer J. Reconstructive prosthetic methods for facial defects. Oral Maxillofac Surg Clin North Am 1994; 6:755–764.
21. Larsen PE. Placement of dental implants in the irradiated mandible: A protocol involving adjunctive hyperbaric oxygen. J Oral Maxillofac Surg 1997; 55:967–971.
22. Keller EE. Placement of dental implants in the irradiated mandible: a protocol without adjunctive hyperbaric oxygen. J Oral Maxillofac Surg 1997; 55:972–980.
23. Bain CA, Moy PK. The association between the failure of dental implants and cigarette smoking. Int J Oral Maxillofac Implants 1993; 8:609–615.
24. Tjellstrom A. Other applications of osseointegrated implants. In: Branemark PI, Zarb GA, Albrektsson T, eds. Tissue Integrated Prostheses: Osseointegration in Clinical Dentistry, Chicago: Quintessence Publishing Co., 1985:336.
25. Tjellstrom A. Osseointegrated implants for replacement of absent or defective ears. Clin Plast Surg 1990; 22:355–366.
26. Myers RE, Mitchell DL. Fluoride for the head and neck radiation patient. Milit Med 1988; 153:411–413.
27. Beumer J, Curtis TA, Morrish RB. Radiation complications in edentulous patients. J Prosthet Dent 1976; 36:193–203.

14

Surgical Approaches to the Facial Skeleton in Trauma

Robert W. Dolan
Lahey Clinic Medical Center, Burlington, Massachusetts, U.S.A.

INTRODUCTION

Modern techniques of exposing the facial skeleton evolved in the last half of the 20th century from the combined experiences of several surgical disciplines including otolaryngology–head and neck surgery, plastic surgery, maxillofacial surgery, and neurosurgery. Exposure of facial fractures previously consisted of making several small incisions over fracture sites, with little concern for visible scars or sensorimotor deficits. Although limited surgical access is often all that is required for selected simple facial fractures, complex or comminuted fractures demand more extensive exposure for accurate reduction and fixation. The modern approach to complex facial fractures (which represent the majority of facial fractures) is wide surgical exposure that facilitates a three-dimensional assessment of fracture displacement and application of rigid internal fixation appliances and bone grafts (1). These surgical approaches emphasize minimally invasive techniques that spare neurosensory structures while maximizing exposure of the facial skeleton. Craniofacial incisions are hidden in areas such as behind the hairline, within the oral cavity, in the conjunctiva, or under the eyelids. Incisions camouflaged by placement within a border of a topographical subunit or natural skin crease are also acceptable (e.g., subciliary). Examples include

Coronal approach to the upper and midface
Transcutaneous approach to the orbital floor
Transconjunctival approach to the orbital floor
Endoscopic subcondylar approach for the condylar neck
Subcranial approach for the deep upper and midface
Open sky approach for the naso-orbital complex
Extracranial transsphenoethmoidal approach for the optic foramen and canal

CORONAL APPROACH

Description and Indications

The coronal approach provides the greatest potential surface exposure of the craniofacial skeleton including the frontal bone and calvaria, the superior and upper lateral orbital rims, the zygomatic arches, the temporomandibular joints, and the nasal bones. This approach is useful for the open treatment of severely comminuted zygomatic fractures (2). It also provides ample exposure for the zygomaticofacial suture, lateral orbit, malar eminence, and nasoethmoid complex. Most important is that the coronal approach provides wide exposure of the anterior cranial fossa including the frontal sinuses, frontal lobe, cribriform plate, orbital roofs, and orbital apices.

The incision for the coronal approach is usually made behind the hairline from ear to ear. More anteriorly placed incisions (pretrichial, midforehead, and suprabrow) will result in similar exposure but also create noticeable incisions and post-incisional numbness from interruption of the supratrochlear and supraorbital sensory nerves. The pretrichial incision is placed just inside the anterior hairline and may be used for patients with a stable hairline. The midforehead incision is placed within a prominent midforehead rhytid and is used for patients with prominent forehead wrinkles (usually elderly men or women). The suprabrow incision is placed just above the eyebrows, joined by an incision across the nasal root. It has several disadvantages including total forehead and lower anterior scalp hypothesia, limited access laterally, and obvious scarring.

Surgical Anatomy

The coronal incision traverses the skin, subcutaneous tissue, galeal aponeurosis, loose areolar tissue, and pericranium. The aponeurosis merges with its muscular counterparts anteriorly (the frontalis muscle) and posteriorly (the occipitalis muscle). As the scalp flap is dissected anteriorly toward the orbital rims and zygomatic arches, several important neurovascular structures are encountered including the frontal branch of the facial nerve, the supraorbital and supratrochlear arteries and sensory nerves, and the superficial and middle temporal arteries (Fig. 1). In addition, the fascial relationships become more complex as the dissection is continued anterolaterally.

The frontal branch innervates the ipsilateral half of the frontalis muscle laterally and is primarily responsible for elevation of the eyebrow. Frontal nerve injury results in paralysis of the frontalis muscle and a progressive descent of the ipsilateral eyebrow. The approximate course of the nerve follows a line along the inferior part of the tragus and a point 1.5 cm lateral to the lateral extent of the eyebrow (Fig. 2). As it exits the parotid gland, it travels with the superficial temporal artery (its anterior branch) deep to the temporoparietal fascia. The temporoparietal fascia is also known as the superficial temporal fascia and is the superior extension of the superficial musculoaponeurotic fascia (SMAS) and the anterolateral extension of the occipitogaleafrontalis (galeal aponeurosis). Above the level of the zygomatic arch, as the frontalis nerve courses toward the frontalis muscle, the temporoparietal fascia thins leaving a scant amount of tissue between the overlying skin and nerve. Subcutaneous dissection within this area raises the risk of iatrogenic injury to the frontal branch. As the dissection approaches the zygomatic arches, the intricate relationships of the fascias gain importance in avoiding neurovascular injury. First, the temporal line

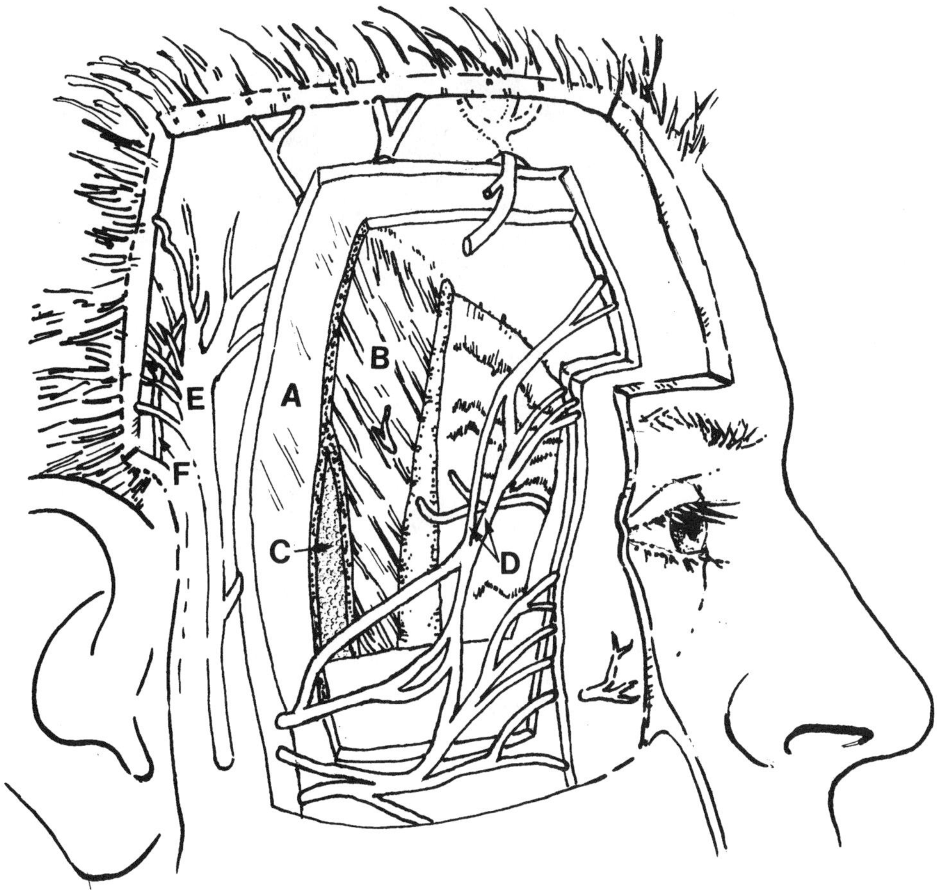

Figure 1 A, deep temporal fascia; B, temporalis muscle; C, deep temporal fat pad; D, frontal nerve; E, superficial temporal artery and vein; F, auriculotemporal nerve.

is encountered where the pericranium and deep temporal fascias meet and adhere to the skull. Beyond this line, the deep temporal fascia continues directly over the temporalis muscle to the temporal line of fusion at the level of the superior orbital rims. Inferior to the temporal line of fusion, the deep temporal fascia splits into superficial and deep layers. The superficial layer continues inferiorly to insert onto the superficial aspect of the zygomatic arch. The deep layer inserts onto the medial aspect of the arch. The deep temporal fat pad occupies the space between the superficial and deep layers of temporal fascia. The buccal fat pad (on the surface of the temporalis muscle) is separated from the deep temporal fat pad by the deep layer of deep temporal fascia. To avoid injury to the frontalis nerve, a safe plane of dissection is below the superficial layer of deep temporal fascia within the deep temporal fat pad.

The auriculotemporal and zygomatic nerves provide sensation to the lateral forehead. The auriculotemporal nerve exits the infratemporal fossa between the mandibular condyle and the ear canal to cross the root of the zygoma in the subcutaneous plane posterior to the parietal (posterior) branch of the superficial temporal

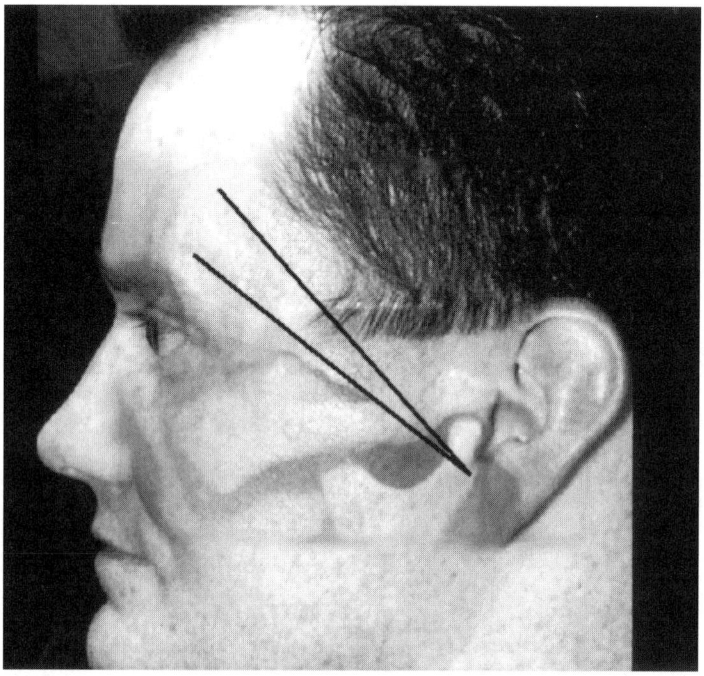

Figure 2 Course of frontal nerve (within the lines).

artery. The zygomatic nerve, a branch from the maxillary division of the trigeminal nerve, enters the orbit through the infraorbital fissure and divides into the zygomaticofacial and zygomaticotemporal nerves. The zygomaticofacial nerve exits the orbit via the zygomaticofacial foramen and supplies the skin over the malar eminence; this nerve is not encountered in the coronal approach. However, the area of distribution of the other division of the zygomatic nerve, the zygomaticotemporal nerve, is encountered using the coronal flap. This nerve exits the orbit via the sphenozygomatic suture and pierces the temporal fascia 2 cm above the level of the zygomatic arch to supply the anterior temporal region. Despite its distribution pattern, the integrity of the nerve is rarely an issue during elevation of a coronal flap. The vessels in proximity to the lateral forehead include the frontal and parietal branches and the middle temporal branch of the superficial temporal artery. The middle temporal artery branches from the superficial temporal artery just above the zygoma and perforates the temporal fascia and muscle to ascend on the squamous portion of the temporal bone. This artery is often sacrificed in exposure of the zygomatic arch via the coronal approach. Approximately 5 cm above the zygoma, the superficial temporal artery divides into frontal (anterior) and parietal (posterior) divisions that travel within the temporoparietal (superficial temporal) fascia. The frontal division courses tortuously upward toward the lateral frontal region, and the parietal division courses upward and backward above the ear.

The supraorbital and supratrochlear neurovascular bundles provide sensation and blood supply to the central forehead. The supraorbital neurovascular bundle exits the orbit through a foramen or notch located in the center of the supraorbital rim, on line with the infraorbital and mental foramina. The bundle ascends approximately 2 cm, just above the periosteum, into the forehead before piercing the frontalis muscle to continue in the subcutaneous plane. The supratrochlear neurovascular bundle is smaller than the supraorbital and exits the upper medial angle of the orbit to supply the skin and subcutaneous tissues of the medial portion of the upper eyelid and medial forehead.

Surgical Technique

The incision for the coronal approach extends between the preauricular creases over the vertex. Inadequate preauricular extension of the incisions hampers release of the flap and exposure of the craniofacial skeleton. The vertex part of the incision should be placed behind the hairline. However, placement of the incision too posteriorly will provide a flap that is excessively long, making its anterior transposition awkward. In male patients, the incision may have to be placed more posteriorly due to a receding hairline. Subcutaneous injection of an epinephrine-containing local anesthetic along the proposed incision line is helpful for hemostasis. A limited head shave extending approximately 1 cm out from the incision is helpful to avoid the annoyance of having to sweep unruly hairs out of the wound. The incision is carried down to, or through, the periosteum depending on the plane of dissection. Hemostasis at the wound edge may be controlled with electrocautery or semicircular hemostatic clips (Raney clips). The coronal flap may be dissected in an avascular plane, above the level of the periosteum, or in a subperiosteal layer. Dissection below the periosteum preserves a potential pericranial–galeal flap on the undersurface of the coronal flap. The pericranial-galeal layer may be dissected off the coronal flap later in the case, if needed. Completion of the preauricular dissections allows flap eversion to facilitate inferior exposure. A few centimeters above the supraorbital rims the periosteum is incised horizontally and further dissection proceeds in a subperiosteal plane. Dissecting under the periosteum protects the supraorbital and supratrochlear neurovascular bundles. If a pericranial flap is planned, the periosteum must be incised to the desired length of the flap. The supraorbital and supratrochlear neurovascular bundles must be released medially by curetting their bony attachments, if necessary, allowing full exposure of the medial orbits and nasal bones. The temporoparietal fascia is preserved laterally within the flap, and, approximately 1 cm above the level of the zygomatic arch, the superficial layer of deep temporal fascia is incised horizontally along the entire length of the arch (at the temporal line of fusion). This exposes the temporal fat pad and represents the new plane of dissection for exposure of the zygomatic arch. Entering the deep temporal fat pad space provides an additional tissue layer between the plane of dissection and the frontal branch of the facial nerve (Fig. 3). Previous surgery or trauma in the area may distort tissue planes and alter the usual course of the nerve. Therefore, entering this deeper plane, below the level of the superficial layer of deep temporal fascia, is essential to protect the nerve. Subperiosteal dissection, anterior and posterior to the arch, provides ample exposure to displaced and comminuted zygomatic arch fractures. Joining this dissection with the medial dissection, along the temporal line, allows full exposure of the lateral orbital rim and zygomaticofacial suture. Wound closure after replacement of the coronal flap consists of either a layered closure or a full-thickness single-layered closure.

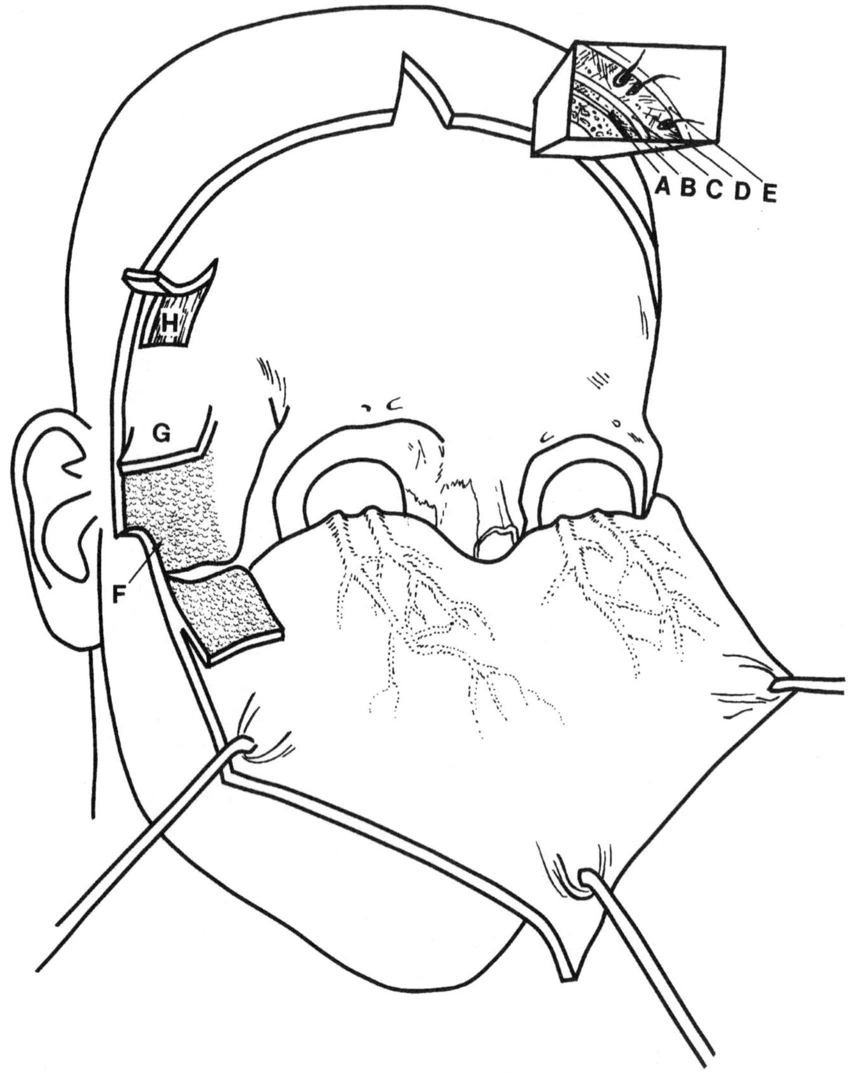

Figure 3 A, periosteum; B, loose areolar tissue; C, galeal aponeurosis; D, connective tissue; E, skin; F, deep temporal fat pad; G, superficial layer of deep temporal fascia; H, temporalis muscle.

Complications

Complications include widened scars, peri-incisional hair loss, sensory deficits, frontalis nerve injury, temporal fossa depression, hematoma formation, infection, and corneal abrasion. Few patients complain of widened scars, but minor depressions in the areas where split calvarial bone grafts are harvested may be of concern to the patient. Hair loss within 1 cm of the incision may be seen, possibly from prolonged use of Raney clips. The hair loss usually resolves over a period of several

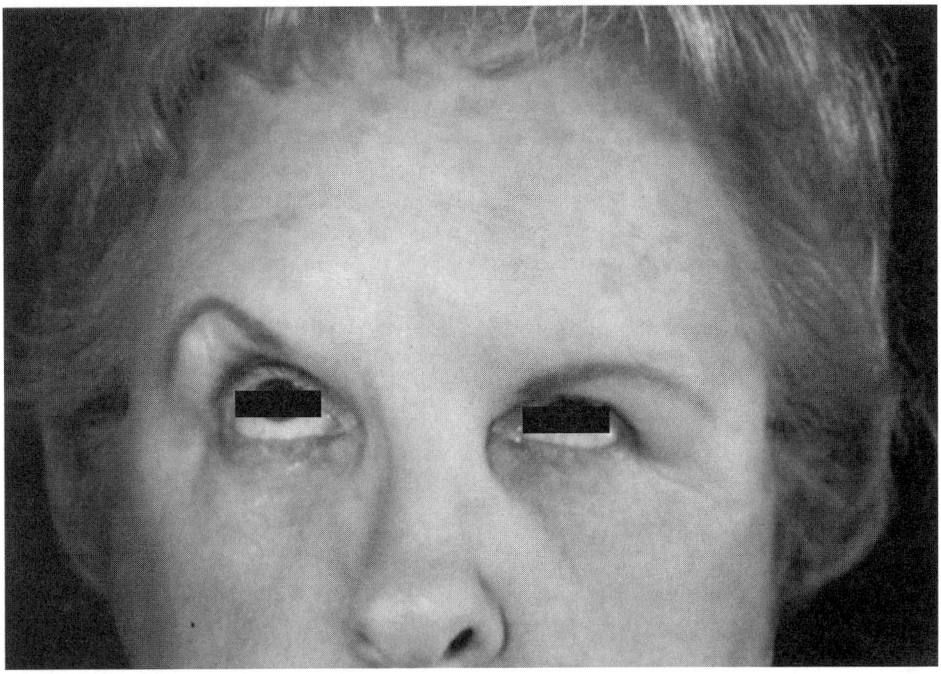

Figure 4 Left frontal nerve paralysis with resulting eyebrow ptosis.

months. Sensory deficits posterior to the incision are common but usually well tolerated. Most patients will experience altered sensation of the vertex that improves dramatically within 1 month. Forehead sensory deficits from injury to the supraorbital or supratrochlear nerves are uncommon. Permanent frontalis nerve deficits are more common in revision cases in which scarring may obscure the division of fascial layers (Fig. 4). Temporal fossa depressions are usually only seen in patients who have experienced severe underlying trauma to the region. Hematomas and infections are rarely seen due to the excellent collateral vascularity of the scalp. Corneal abrasions may be secondary to the pressure exerted on corneal protectors after flap eversion; simple temporary lateral tarsorrhaphy will usually avoid this complication.

TRANSCUTANEOUS AND TRANSCONJUNCTIVAL APPROACHES TO THE ORBIT

Transcutaneous Approaches

Three transcutaneous incisions are described for exposure of the orbital rim and floor: subciliary, lower eyelid, and orbital rim (3). The subciliary incision is placed 2 mm below the lower lid margin extending medially on an imaginary line dropped from the punctum and laterally into a skin crease. The pretarsal orbicularis is preserved by raising a skin-only flap over the lower lid. The orbicularis muscle can be transected horizontally at the inferior border of the tarsus or closer to the orbital rim. Once the muscle is breached, the orbital septum is encountered and the dissection proceeds inferiorly to the rim and arcus marginalis. The periosteum is sharply incised over the orbital rim inferior to the confluence of the orbital floor periosteum, orbital septum, and maxillary periosteum (i.e., arcus marginalis).

The lower eyelid incision is placed through a skin crease midway between the inferior tarsus and the inferior orbital rim. A skin–muscle or skin-only flap is raised and the rim and floor are exposed as in the subciliary approach. The orbital rim incision is placed at the level of the inferior orbital rim and deepened directly to periosteum. Exposure of the orbital floor proceeds as in the subciliary and lower eyelid approaches.

A visible scar results from all of the transcutaneous approaches, but only rarely is the scar prominent or noticeable to the casual observer. Ectropion is the major concern after a transcutaneous approach, and it is most often associated with the subciliary incision. To minimize the incidence of postoperative ectropion, the pretarsal portion of the orbicularis oculi muscle should be preserved to support the lower lid and lessen the effects of scar contracture. The lower eyelid and orbital rim incisions are less likely to cause ectropion despite the creation of more conspicuous scars.

Transconjuctival Approach

The transconjunctival approach was described in the early 1900s and popularized in the 1970s by Converse et al and Tessier (4,5). It was originally viewed as an approach that minimized scarring and morbidity while providing adequate access only for orbital floor fractures. However, when the conjunctival incision is combined with a lateral canthotomy and inferior cantholysis, access to the orbital floor and inferior orbital rim is equivalent to that attained by the transcutaneous routes. As experience with these techniques increased, the transconjunctival approach, with or without lateral canthotomy and cantholysis, was found to be associated only rarely with lower lid malpositions (e.g., ectropion) compared to the transcutaneous approaches. The transconjunctival approach avoids violation of the lower eyelid skin and orbicularis oculi muscle. In addition, the lower eyelid retractors are divided, resulting in a reduced tendency for postoperative lower eyelid retraction, scleral show, and ectropion. A transconjunctival approach may occasionally be impossible due to factors that tend to obliterate the inferior fornix such as persistent chemosis, orbital proptosis, intense lower eyelid edema, or traumatic lower eyelid avulsion or injury. In these cases, a transcutaneous approach is warranted.

The transconjunctival approach is often used in cosmetic surgery for excision of excess orbital fat. There are important differences in the technique for exposure of orbital fat and the more extensive dissection necessary for exposure of the orbital rim and floor without breaching the orbital septum and fat. In addition, superior cantholysis, a technique used for wide exposure of the lateral rim and orbit for tumor surgery, is useful for exposing and plating the zygomaticofacial suture.

Surgical Anatomy

A thorough understanding of the anatomy of the lower eyelid is essential to maximize surgical exposure while minimizing the risk of injury to adjacent structures.

An intimate knowledge of the following spaces and structures is necessary: inferior fornix, inferior tarsus, inferior lid retractor, capsulopalpebral fascia, orbital septum, orbital fat, orbicularis oculi muscle, inferior rectus muscle, and inferior oblique muscle. The inferior fornix is the space between the lower eyelid and the eyeball and is enveloped by conjunctiva. The inferior tarsus is a fibrocartilaginous structure approximately 5 mm high that spans the free edge of the lower eyelid. The capsulopalpebral fascia is the anterior aponeurotic extension of the inferior rectus muscle. On downgaze, the capsulopalpebral fascia probably acts to maintain apposition of the lower lid and globe. The lower lid also passively moves inferiorly a few millimeters assisted by relaxation of the pretarsal orbicularis muscle, gravity, and contact with the cornea. There is no well-developed nonstriated muscle (ostensibly known as Horner's muscle) similar to Mueller's muscle of the upper eyelid present in the lower eyelid complex. The orbital septum is an extension of the orbital periosteum and the periosteum over the face of the maxilla. This trifurcation of fascias along the inferior orbital rim represents the inferior arcus marginalis. The orbital septum encloses the orbital fat and extends anterosuperiorly to within a few millimeters along the inferior border of the tarsus. The inferior oblique muscle lies within the orbital fat near the anterior margin of the orbit. It originates from the orbital floor in the medial one-third, and, coursing in a posterolateral direction below the inferior rectus muscle, inserts into the sclera beneath the lateral rectus muscle. The inferior oblique muscle is often visualized during exploration of the orbital floor or during procedures that violate the orbital fat (e.g., blepharoplasty) and is susceptible to inadvertent injury.

Surgical Technique

The first consideration is protection of the cornea and globe. Corneal protectors (crescent-shaped plastic or metal shields) offer good protection against corneal abrasions and burns but they can migrate over the surface of the globe and expose the cornea to inadvertent injury. A variety of retractors designed to protect the cornea in lieu of, or in addition to, a corneal shield are available, the most popular of which is the Jaëgar retractor (Storz, St. Louis, MO) (Fig. 5). This retractor is contoured to the shape of the globe and extends into the inferior fornix. The operator is usually constantly aware of its position since it requires manipulation during the procedure for optimal visibility in the depths of the wound. The protective function of the Jaëgar retractor can be supplanted later in the procedure by pulling the inferiorly-based conjunctivo-capsulopalpebral flap over the corneal surface using traction sutures.

Loop magnification is helpful to identify accurately the layers of the lower eyelid. There are two basic methods to expose the orbital rim and floor via the transconjunctival approach: the retroseptal approach and the preseptal approach. The retroseptal approach involves creating a horizontal incision between the lower border of the tarsus and fornix through the capsulopalpebral fascia and entering orbital fat. As the fat is retracted posteriorly, the dissection proceeds to the orbital floor where the periosteum is incised widely to expose the rim and the floor of the orbit. Although the retroseptal approach is a popular method for transconjunctival blepharoplasty (this procedure is limited to fat excision without further dissection),

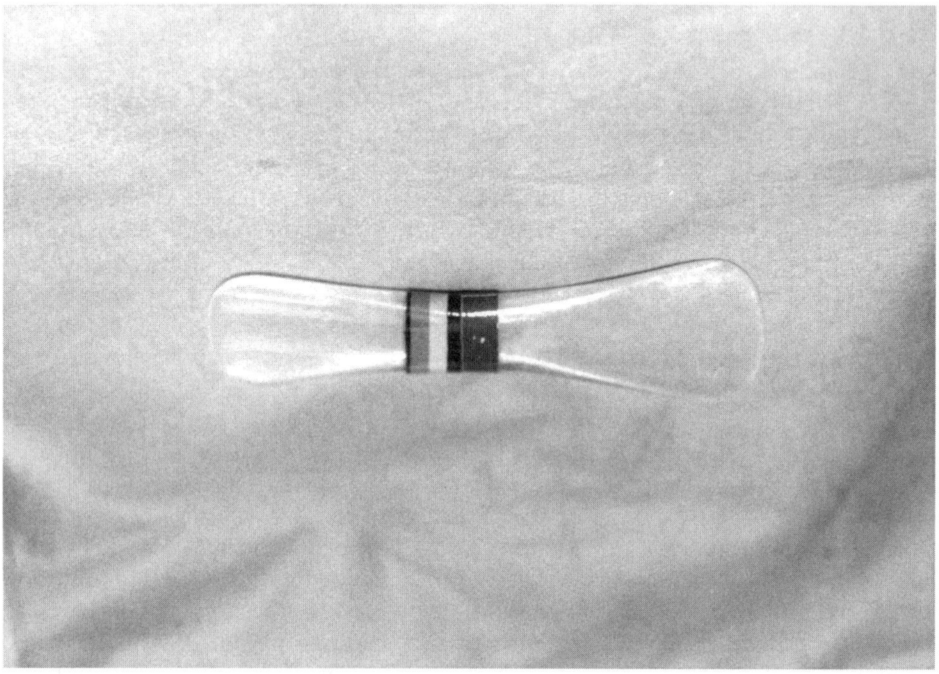

Figure 5 The Jaëgar retractor.

the prolapsing fat can be a nuisance in exposing the orbital rim and floor. Avoidance of orbital fat is helpful to maximize the surgical exposure and prevent inadvertent injury to the inferior oblique muscle that may be obscured by the prolapsing fat. The preseptal approach does not breach the orbital fat and is the preferred method with which to expose the orbital floor (Fig. 6).

In preparation for the preseptal approach to the orbital floor, the surgeon should stand at the head of the operating table and evert the lower eyelid to view the inner aspect of the inferior tarsus. A horizontal incision is made inferior to the tarsus (approximately 6 mm below the lid margin, or 1 mm inferior to the inferior border of the tarsus) extending just lateral to the orifice of the inferior canaliculus. Bleeding is minimized with use of a sharp-tipped electrocautery device for the incision and subsequent dissection. Deepening the incision through the capsulopalpebral fascia above the divergence of the fascial layers that enclose the orbital fat (capsulopalpebral fascia and orbital septum) prevents orbital fat from prolapsing into the wound. The capsulopalpebral flap is pulled over the surface of the globe to protect the cornea (Fig. 7). The orbicularis oculi muscle is visualized and the plane between the muscle and orbital septum anterior to the orbital fat is developed by a combination of blunt and sharp dissection. The orbital rim is encountered and the dissection continues over the rim approximately 1 mm before the periosteum is sharply divided anterior to the inferior arcus marginalis. A subperiosteal plane is entered and widened posteriorly over the bony orbital floor and anteriorly over the inferior orbital rim. This exposure allows evaluation and repair of fractures involving the orbital

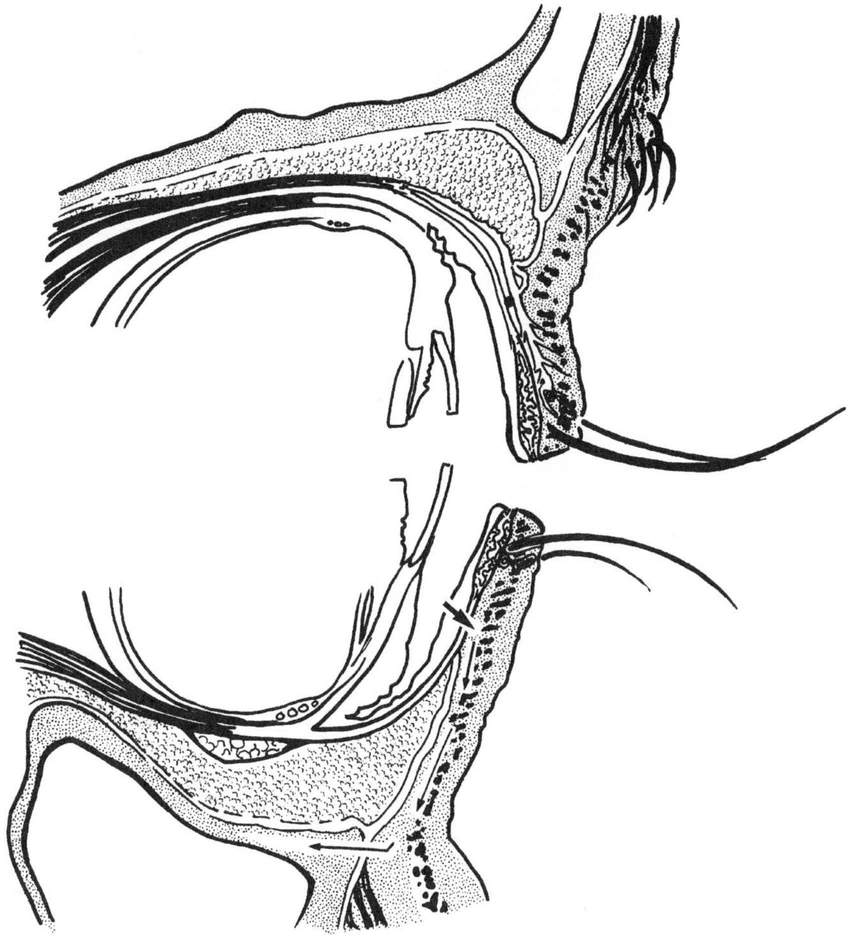

Figure 6 The transconjunctival preseptal approach to the orbital floor and rim.

floor and inferior orbital rim. Closure is accomplished by sutureless repositioning of the wound edges; care should be taken to avoid any overlap that could lead to horizontal shortening of the lower lid and ectropion. Lower eyelid support using Steri-strips or a Frost suture will aid in avoiding conjunctival wound edge overlap.

Although the transconjunctival approach provides ample exposure for the orbital floor, lateral canthotomy and inferior cantholysis improve access to the orbital rim for open fracture reduction and fixation. The addition of these procedures adds little morbidity to the procedure and can be useful adjuncts in selected patients. At the conclusion of the procedure, the inferior canthal tendon should be carefully sutured (nonabsorbable suture) above and slightly behind its original attachment at Whitnall's tubercle. The orientation of the lower eyelid with respect to the upper eyelid in this area should be confirmed visually so that the lower eyelid curves gently superiorly to fall just behind the lateral extent of the upper eyelid. The lateral canthotomy incision is closed in layers.

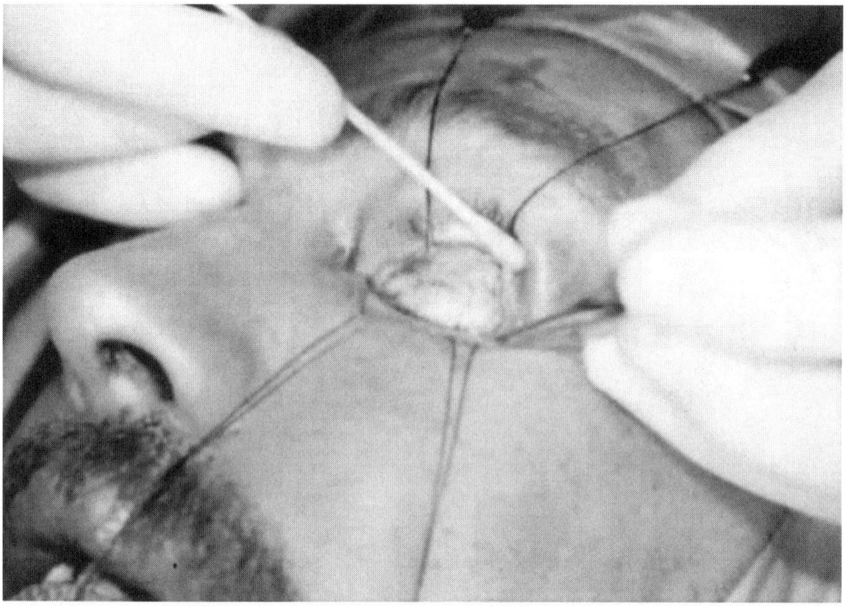

Figure 7 The capsulopalpebral flap is pulled over the surface of globe to protect the cornea.

Although beyond the usual domain of the transconjunctival approach, the lateral orbital rim can be exposed in continuity with the inferior orbital rim, orbital floor, and lateral orbital wall by combining the transconjunctival approach with a lateral canthotomy and superior cantholysis. This combination is useful for exposing important landmarks and fracture sites in zygomatic complex fractures. The technique, after a typical lateral canthotomy is performed, involves grasping the superior lateral lid and locating the tendon by tweaking it while on stretch. Before the tendon is cut, a fine nonabsorbable suture is passed both proximally and distally to the proposed cut mark the exact location of the tendon stumps for reapproximation. After cantholysis, the lid is freed to retract upward and a subperiosteal dissection is developed over the lateral rim including wide exposure of the zygomaticofacial suture. After manipulation and rigid fixation of the lateral rim fracture(s), the ends of the previously placed sutures are tied resulting in precise relocation of the lateral upper lid.

Complications

The reported complication rate using the transconjunctival approach for cosmetic purposes is relatively low (6). Complications using this approach for trauma include transient lower eyelid retraction and scleral show, noticeable lateral canthal scar, and inferior displacement of the lateral canthus. Potential complications including prolonged chemosis, granulation tissue, infection, true ectropion, canthal dehiscence, canalicular injuries, and iatrogenic eye injuries were not observed by Fedok in his review using the transconjunctival approach in cases of trauma (7). However,

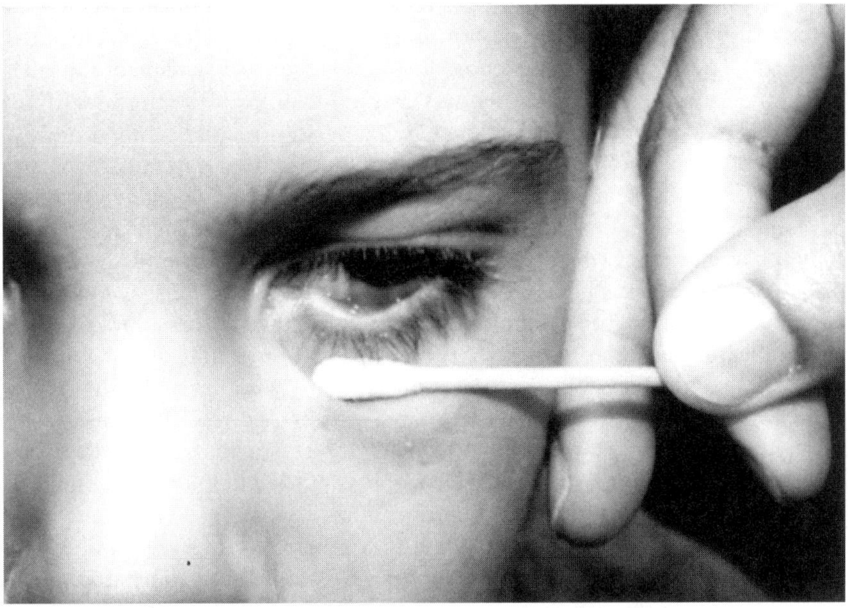

Figure 8 Incisional granuloma occuring after surgery using the transconjunctival approach.

granuloma formation resulting in a pedunculated mucosa-covered mass along the transconjunctival incision may occur more often than reported (Fig. 8). If it is distressing to the patient or obscures the visual axis, it will require secondary excision. Cicatrical ectropion due to excessive overlapping of the free edges of the incision along the horizontal extent of the lower eyelid can result in scleral show requiring scar release later. This can be avoided by carefully pulling the lower eyelid superiorly at the conclusion of the operation to prevent any incisional overlap or by suspending the lower eyelid with a Frost suture or Steri-strips for 24–48 h. Overall, the occurrence of ectropion is much lower using the transconjunctival approach (3%) than the conventional transcutaneous approach (28%).

ENDOSCOPIC SUBCONDYLAR FRACTURE REPAIR

Description and Indications

The endoscopic approach for subcondylar fracture repair provides a magnified view of the lateral mandible and condylar space for percutaneous trocar-assisted fracture manipulation and plating (8). Conventional surgical approaches to the condyle for trauma are via transcutaneous preauricular and submandibular (Risdon) incisions. However, these conventional approaches are associated with a significant risk of stretch-related neuropraxia or transection of the facial nerve and significant facial scarring. The endoscopic approach drastically reduces the risk of transection and stretch-related injuries to the facial nerve and may broaden the indications for the open repair of displaced condylar fractures.

Several preoperative factors must be evaluated before deciding to treat a subcondylar fracture using the endoscopic approach. In adults, the condylar head is rarely (10–20%) displaced out of the glenoid fossa and, even if it is displaced, it does not preclude an endoscopic approach. However, the location of the proximal fracture has a major impact on the difficulty of reducing the fracture endoscopically. The proximal condylar fracture segment is usually displaced laterally over the ascending ramus. This is a favorable position since the proximal segment can be depressed from the lateral direction and pushed back into its normal anatomical position much like a partially displaced puzzle piece. However, if the proximal segment is displaced to the medial side of the ramus, or if there is extensive comminution, endoscopic distraction and reduction are very difficult and this approach may not be successful. Intracapsular fractures or fractures without sufficient intact distal bone to allow two-screw fixation are also not amenable to this approach. Subcondylar fractures in pediatric patients should be treated with closed reduction since open treatment may result in stunted mandibular growth. These fractures are better tolerated in children, and with continued growth of the mandible the posterior mandibular height and condylar malpositions often normalize.

Endoscopic repair of midface and zygomatic complex fractures is described but offers few advantages over conventional techniques. In these cases, the endoscope is primarily used to visualize direct placement of plates over the zygomatic arch (9,10). However, direct plating of the zygomatic arch is rarely necessary. Lee et al. introduced the endoscope through the dehiscent anterior maxillary sinus to repair an orbital floor defect from below. This was accomplished by removing bone fragments from the orbit, reducing orbital structures back into the orbital space, and identifying the stable edges of the floor defect. Titanium mesh was then inserted into the orbital space supported by the remaining stable bony margins of the orbital floor defect. In cases of isolated orbital blowout fractures, the transantral endoscopic approach requires further study. It may be a valuable alternative approach that avoids dissection of the preseptal tissues and eyelids.

Surgical Technique

The patient should be placed in maxillomandibular fixation using rubber bands to allow a minor degree of mandibular adaptation while reducing the subcondylar fracture. A 30 degree endoscope is inserted through an intraoral buccal sulcus incision over the oblique line of the mandible. The endoscope is connected to a video monitor to provide a magnified view. A space for the endoscope is created by elevating the periosteum off the entire lateral ramus of the mandible. A trocar is inserted percutaneously to keep the cavity expanded and for fracture manipulation and screw placement. In the usual case, the proximal fragment of the condyle protrudes over the ramus, allowing fracture reduction by manipulating the trocar over this segment and maneuvering the displaced condylar segment back into alignment. A miniplate is introduced through the buccal incision and screws are placed through the trocar to achieve rigid fixation. At the conclusion of the operation, the maxillomandibular fixation may be removed. Clinical experience with this technique is limited. With existing instrumentation, this approach is difficult and awkward. However, the promise of new instruments designed for the purpose of endoscopic repair of subcondylar fractures should surmount the technical difficulties.

Complications

Compared to the conventional transcutaneous approaches, the endoscopic approach has been associated with few problems. Lee et al., in a series of 20 patients undergoing endoscopic subcondylar fracture repair, found that only one complication occurred: a temporary facial nerve palsy. This occurred in a patient in whom the proximal segment of the fracture was displaced medial to the ramus, resulting in prolonged and aggressive manipulation using the trocar.

SUBCRANIAL APPROACH

Description and Indications

The subcranial approach was popularized by Raveh et al. as an alternative to frontal craniotomy for the open repair of extensive frontonaso-orbital and skull base fractures (11). Since patients with extensive craniofacial trauma often have frontal lobe contusions, treatment is often delayed using the traditional methods of fracture exposure through combined frontal craniotomy and inferior (facial) surgical approaches due to the added risk of frontal lobe retraction. The subcranial approach provides extensive access to the anterior skull base, allowing the open repair of upper facial and intracranial injuries while avoiding craniotomy and frontal lobe retraction. In some cases, a conservatively tailored craniotomy may be added to the subcranial approach, if required. It is possible to repair dural tears along the cribriform plate and orbital roofs, align the entire subcranial undersurface with fascia lata, debride and reduce herniated brain tissue, and reduce intracranial bone fragments. The anatomical structures that can be exposed within the same surgical field include the orbits, nasoethmoid complex, optic canals, lateral orbital rims, frontal sinuses, undersurface and face of the frontal lobe posterior to the frontal sinuses, and cavernous sinuses.

Extensive fractures surrounding the frontal lobes, including those involving the posterior wall of the frontal sinus, and extensive cribriform plate or orbital roof disruptions, have traditionally been approached via frontal craniotomy. The bone flap, consisting of the frontal bone and frontal sinuses, was taken to a back table and the posterior sinus walls removed. The fractures, including those involving the anterior table of the frontal sinus, would then be wired or plated. At the surgical site, fractures and dural tears along the anterior skull base were repaired, necessitating retraction of the frontal lobe. Optic nerve decompression, if necessary, was performed simultaneously. At the completion of the procedure, the bone flap was replaced to allow the frontal lobe to fall forward, resulting in cranialization and obliteration of the frontal sinuses after the frontonasal ducts were plugged.

The subcranial approach often obviates the need for craniotomy, frontal lobe retraction, and manipulation that could lead to iatrogenic frontal lobe and dural injury. In addition, in patients with severe frontal lobe brain injury and optic nerve compression, the subcranial approach can provide access for optic nerve decompression that avoids retraction on the acutely injured frontal lobe. The advantages of the subcranial approach over the intracranial approach include the following:

- No need for frontal lobe retraction
- Preservation of the olfactory nerves

Decreased risk of iatrogenic brain and dural injury
Combined simultaneous access to all the components of a severe frontonaso-orbital and skull base injury
The ability to align the entire subcranial undersurface with fascia lata
More complete optic nerve decompression (vs. via an intracranial route)
Reduction of telecanthus through bilateral open visualization of the medial canthal ligaments and associated dislocated bony fragments
Ease and accuracy of placement of bone grafts
Early definitive management of the skull base and external facial fractures in one stage

Although the subcranial approach is possible in most cases of frontonaso-orbital fractures, bone fragments involving the sagittal sinus may require a craniotomy for proximal and distal vascular control. Orbital pathological conditions may preclude or limit the amount of inferior traction that can be applied during the subcranial approach. Preoperative consultation with a neurosurgeon and ophthalmologist is essential. In cases that require craniotomy to assess and treat associated frontal intracranial injuries not accessible via the subcranial approach, addition of the subcranial approach with the transfrontal approach (craniotomy) is usually unnecessary (12).

Early definitive repair (within 48 h) is desirable for severe upper facial and anterior skull base fractures. Raveh et al. refer to the initial 24–48 h after the injury as the golden period: an ideal time of fracture repair. Repair within this time period avoids several disadvantages associated with delaying fracture repair for a period of several days to weeks: sinus obstruction, lymphatic disruption, edema, infection, granulation tissue and unfavorable scar formation, delay of optic nerve decompression (if needed), and prolonged stays in the intensive care unit. Once this window of opportunity passes, a delay of 10–20 days is appropriate to allow for resolution of soft tissue swelling and ecchymosis.

Early definitive fracture management (within 24–48 h) is one of the foremost advantages of the subcranial approach in patients in whom craniotomy and frontal lobe manipulation are contraindicated because of severe frontal lobe injury. To justify using this approach in this circumstance, the advantages of early single-stage fracture repair must outweigh the risk to the patient of the operation itself. Early definitive fracture repair is advantageous, but the risks of any operation on the well being of the patient must be carefully considered. Any additional risk cannot be justified if definitive fracture repair can be safely performed within 3 weeks. Only in approximately half of the patients was definitive one-stage management possible less than 48 h after the injury in a large series (13).

Surgical Technique

The subcranial approach is performed via a coronal incision with a coronal flap turned down over the superior and lateral orbital rims, providing access to the nasal bridge, ethmoids, orbits, and frontal bone. The anterior skull base is exposed laterally by retracting the orbital contents inferiorly (Fig. 9). Medial exposure is facilitated by complete ethmoidectomy and judicious removal of the fovea ethmoidalis while preserving the olfactory nerves. The face of the frontal lobe is exposed by removing the posterior wall of the frontal sinus. The optic canal is exposed after

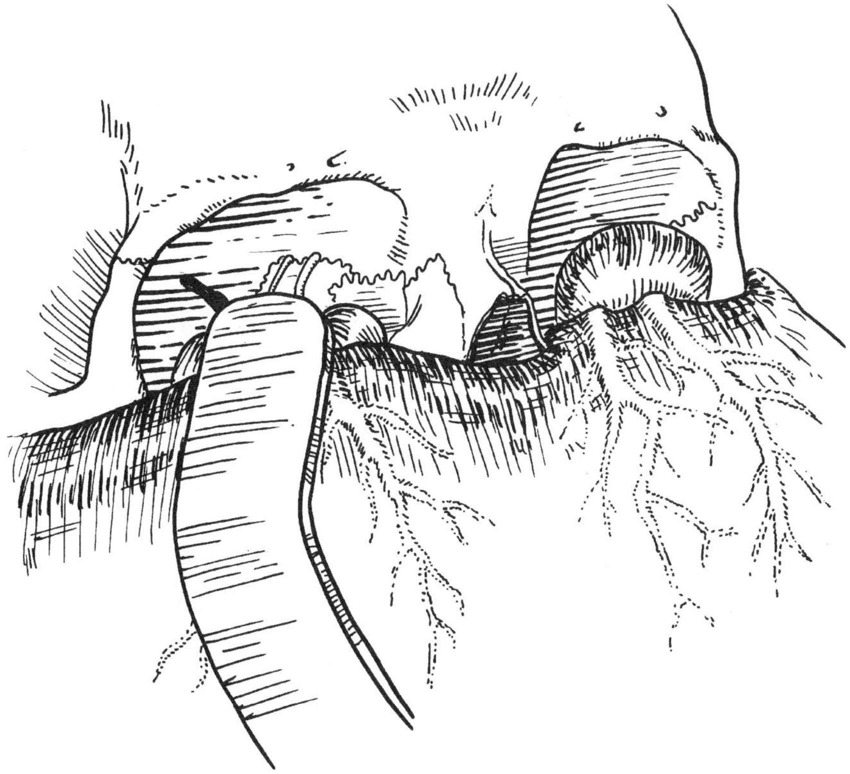

Figure 9 Typical surgical exposure for the subcranial approach.

complete ethmoidectomy and wide sphenoidotomy, allowing the medial optic canal wall to be removed.

Bone fragments are disimpacted and removed from the anterior skull base, and dural lacerations closed or repaired with large continuous sheets of fascia lata. Disimpacted and free bone fragments are replaced or the skull base is reconstructed with split calvarial bone grafts, if necessary. The posterior wall of the frontal sinus is replaced or reconstructed and a large Portex tube is placed within the area of the frontonasal duct and left in situ for several weeks. External facial fractures of the orbital rims, floor, and nose are repaired in the usual manner. Traumatic telecanthus can be repaired accurately because of the wide exposure provided by this approach. The naso-orbital complex and canthal ligaments are precisely positioned and compressed into place by a combination of wire osteosynthesis and plates.

Complications

Blockage or loss of the Portex tube may result in acute frontal sinusitis in the subcranial compartment and vision loss due to pressure at the orbital apex. Revision surgery and replacement or opening the bore of the tube can be therapeutic but vision loss may be permanent despite these maneuvers. The complications associated with the coronal flap are described above.

OPEN SKY TECHNIQUE

Description and Indications

The open sky technique was described by Converse in 1970 as a surgical approach to comminuted naso-orbital fractures (14). The nasal framework is the weakest and most vulnerable portion of the facial skeleton, and severe blunt trauma over the bridge of the nose can result in a telescoping impaction of nasal, orbital, and intracranial structures. Typical findings in a patient with a naso-orbital fracture include a depressed nasal root, prominent epicanthal folds, widened intercanthal distance, and foreshortened palpebral fissures. Naso-orbital fractures are frequently associated with orbital blowout fractures, maxillary Le Fort fractures, zygomatic complex fractures, or intracranial injury. Computed tomographic (CT) scanning is necessary to evaluate for associated regional injuries because they may warrant a different or more extensive surgical approach. The open sky approach allows a complete examination and open repair of the nasofrontal ducts, medial canthal tendons, nasal bones, frontal processes of the maxillae, medial orbital walls, ethmoid labyrinths, orbital apex, lacrimal bone, and lacrimal sacs.

Surgical Technique

Bilateral vertical incisions are placed (Lynch-type) over the lateral wall of the nose midway between the nasal dorsum and medial canthus. The incision extends no more than 1 cm below the medial canthus and may extend into the medial eyebrow. The vertical incisions are joined by a transverse incision across the nasal root and subperiosteal dissection proceeds over the nasal dorsum, lateral nasal walls, and frontal processes of the maxillae (Fig. 10). To improve the cosmetic appearance of the scars and minimize distortion of surrounding structures, the vertical incisions should be in the form of a running W-plasty. The lacrimal sac may be lifted laterally in the subperiosteal plane and further dissection can proceed intraorbitally to expose the ethmoidal arteries, lamina papyracea, and face of the sphenoid. The floor of the frontal sinus can be widely opened and stented, if desired. Wire osteosynthesis and plating can proceed after the bone fragments and medial canthal ligaments are repositioned. Repair of the lacrimal apparatus can be done under direct vision.

Complications

Complications associated with the open sky approach include conspicuous or malpositioned scars and iatrogenic injury to the globes. The corneas should be meticulously protected with corneal shields or by temporarily suturing the eyelids.

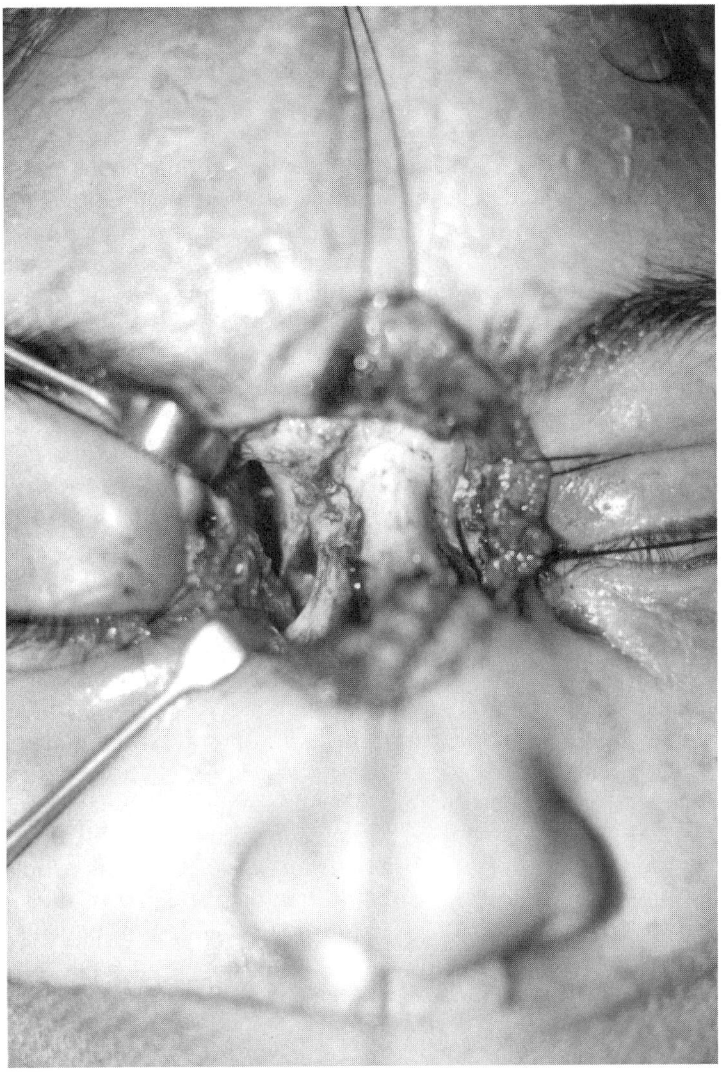

Figure 10 Open sky approach.

EXTRACRANIAL TRANSSPHENOETHMOIDAL APPROACH FOR OPTIC NERVE DECOMPRESSION

Description and Indications

Profound visual loss following maxillofacial injury is uncommon, occurring in approximately 2% of cases (15). The causes of traumatic profound visual loss are myriad and include hyphema, dislocated lens, retinal detachment, vitreous hemorrhage, scleral rupture, retrobulbar hematoma, cortical blindness, and optic neuropathy. Surgical decompression of the optic nerve is indicated only for traumatic optic neuropathy that results from nerve contusion, compression, or impingement, and represents a vast minority of cases. Nevertheless, the seriousness of the injury and the potential gain from surgical decompression have brought the subject of optic nerve decompression to the forefront in the surgical planning of the open reduction of severe facial fractures.

Proposed mechanisms of injury to the intracanalicular portion of the optic nerve include posttraumatic edema and ischemia as the nerve swells within the canal, stretching injury at the anterior foramen as the nerve is tethered in opposition to the firmly fixed nerve within the canal, and direct fracture impingement or impalement of the nerve. A patient can have traumatic optic neuropathy with no fracture of the optic canal. However, a nearly universal finding in patients with traumatic optic neuropathy is impact over the area of the ipsilateral brow. Even a relatively minor degree of pressure on the brow has been shown to result in deformation of the bone of the optic foramen (16).

Vision that progressively deteriorates after impact suggests a reversible process, such as extra-axial hemorrhage or direct nerve compression, which may be successfully treated by optic nerve decompression surgery. However, blindness immediately lost on impact suggests irreversible damage, such as laceration, avulsion, or severe contusion, and surgical decompression will probably not be effective (17). Given the current level of understanding regarding the benefits of optic nerve decompression in the trauma setting, decompression should be reserved only for patients with sight who experience vision deterioration or fail to recover a significant sight deficit (20/200). Although this action is based mainly on inferential evidence from spinal trauma studies, all patients should be given a trial of high-dosage corticosteroid therapy prior to decompression. The corticosteroid regimen and time course leading to surgical decompression vary among institutions. The International Optic Nerve Trauma Study in 1999 prospectively compared the outcome of 133 patients with traumatic optic neuropathy treated with corticosteroids, optic canal decompression surgery, or observed without treatment (18). Based on treatment received within 7 days of the injury, there were 9 untreated patients, 85 corticosteroid-treated patients, and 33 patients who underwent decompression surgery. There were no significant differences in the improvement in visual acuity between any of the groups. Timing of surgery and the timing and dosage of corticosteroid therapy also did not affect the visual outcome. The main conclusions of the study were that no specific therapy should be considered standard of care and that decisions to treat or not to treat should be made on an individual basis (18).

Traumatic optic neuropathy may be present when loss of vision results from facial injury that cannot be explained by pathological conditions in the globe, intracranial portion of the optic nerve, or visual cortex. The first sign of visual loss may be subtle, such as a decrease in color vision (detection of the color red), visual field defects, or acuity. Peripheral retinal fibers travel on the peripheral part of the optic nerve, making them more vulnerable to traumatic injury. Documentation of visual fields is required since constriction of the optic fields due to optic nerve compression may be present with normal central visual acuity. A detailed neuro-ophthalmological examination is essential prior to the diagnosis and treatment of traumatic optic neuropathy.

Visual acuity and field testing may be impossible in intoxicated, sedated, or unconscious patients. Even the assessment of pupil size and reactivity may be impossible due to preseptal swelling and ecchymosis. Although not widely used, visual evoked potential (VEP) recordings can detect the function of optic nerve initially in patients who have abnormal pupillary function, and VEPs are more accurate than pupillary function in assessing the true state of the optic nerve (19). In cases of pupillary dysfunction, VEPs can corroborate the clinical findings. If the pupils cannot be assessed adequately, VEPs may be the only functional testing available on which to base a decision regarding the need for optic nerve decompression.

Recording of flash VEPs is a noninvasive electrophysiological technique that assesses the integrity of the visual pathway. A stroboscopic light stimulus is presented to each eye with the aid of goggles containing a set of light-emitting diodes. Computer-aided signal amplification of the cortical responses results in a typical peak with an approximate latency of 100 ms. The visual stimulus (strobe light) must reach an intact retina, and conditions resulting in diminution of the stimulus such as eyelid closure, edema, or hematoma can result in attenuation of signal amplitude. Although these factors must be considered, even in their presence a sufficient amount of light can usually filter through to stimulate the retina and optic nerve. However, adequate stimulation may not be possible in cases of hyphema, vitreous hemorrhage, and severe retinal detachment. The output is variable and each laboratory must establish its own standard. Only extinct or extremely prolonged VEPs should be considered abnormal. Corneal and retinal abnormalities must be ruled out, as well as intracranial pathology.

Several questions pertinent to optic nerve decompression remain, including the following

1. Which patients benefit from decompression?
2. When should treatment begin?
3. Should steroids be given in conventional or megadoses?
4. How long should the steroids be given?
5. Are corticosteroids always helpful?
6. Are the various extracranial approaches equivalent?
7. To what extent should the optic canal be opened?
8. Should the annulus of Zinn also be opened?

It is difficult to determine which patients will benefit from optic nerve decompression. The literature is replete with reports of patients benefitting from decompression in cases of tumor or Grave's orbitopathies, even after long periods of visual loss (20–22). A recent meta-analysis of several retrospective traumatic optic neuropathy studies revealed several important findings. First, patients with traumatic vision impairment benefitted from either steroids or decompression surgery compared with patients receiving no treatment. Second, recovery of vision was related to the severity of the initial injury. Patients with no light perception did not regain vision regardless of treatment modality. Despite the analysis of a relatively large number of studies, there were no conclusions regarding absolute indications for optic nerve decompression surgery. Management of patients with traumatic optic neuropathy in institutions offering optic nerve decompression surgery includes the following recommendations:

1. Patients with no light perception do not benefit from decompression surgery.
2. All patients should be give a trial of high or megadose intravenous steroids before being considered for decompression.
3. The best candidates for decompression are patients in whom vision was documented to be present or normal, who then experienced visual loss despite administration of steroids.
4. Patients without optic canal fractures demonstrable by CT scanning have a better prognosis after optic nerve decompression.
5. The extracranial approach provides superior access and more complete decompression of the optic nerve than the intracranial approach.

Megadose steroid treatment involves the use of methylprednisolone sodium phosphate in divided dosages of 15–30 mg/kg/day for 3 days followed by an oral tapering dose. Vision is monitored; if it deteriorates during the taper, the dosage is increased and the regimen is repeated. The timing of surgery is dependent upon the results of serial vision evaluations. If vision deteriorates despite administration of megadose steroids, surgical decompression is offered, ideally within the first 48–72 h. Postoperative care consists of three doses of an intravenous antistaphylococcal antibiotic and steroid administration for an additional 24–48 h. An oral antibiotic is given for 10 days.

Optic nerve decompression describes decompression of the optic nerve in its bony canal and can be accomplished by an intracranial route or by various extracranial routes. Extracranial nerve decompression appears to be more effective for patients with traumatic optic neuropathies, providing better access for decompression of the anterior aspect of the optic foramen and the fibrous annulus of Zinn.

Surgical Anatomy

The intracranial portion of the optic nerve is enveloped by arachnoid and dura, and, as the optic nerve exits the canal to enter the orbital cavity, the dura splits into an outer layer and an inner layer. The outer layer is continuous with the orbital periosteum and the inner layer continues as the nerve's dural cover. The intracranial portion is approximately 10 mm in length, the intracanalicular portion is also approximately 10 mm, and the intraorbital portion measures 30 mm from the optic canal to the back of the globe.

The optic canal narrows distally as it approaches the orbit, and the densest and narrowest part is found at the optic ring. The bony partition that separates the ethmoid sinus from the sphenoid sinus forms a significant part of the optic ring medially. The thickness of the medial canal wall averages 0.21 mm while the medial wall of the optic ring averages 0.57 mm (23). The length of the optic canal varies from 5.5 to 11.5 mm. The mean distance from the anterior lacrimal crest to the anterior ethmoidal foramen is 23 mm; to the posterior ethmoidal foramen, 36 mm; and to the optic canal, 41 mm. In more than 3% of cases bone is missing over the optic nerve, posterior to the optic ring, as it traverses the sphenoid sinus. This leaves the nerve and its dural sheath covered only by sphenoid sinus mucosa.

Surgical Technique

A medial approach to the optic nerve is the route of choice in most cases, even if the CT scan demonstrates a fragment of bone impinging on or compressing the optic canal laterally. The medial approach is technically easier than the lateral approach and will allow decompression of the orbital apex and canal without manipulation of surrounding bone fragments. Nevertheless, a lateral facial approach is described to decompress the optic nerve for patients with comminuted lateral orbital fractures (24). The lateral facial approach is a well-described surgical approach to the nasopharynx and infratemporal fossa for tumor excision. Instead of a resection of the zygomatic arch and lateral orbital wall, these structures are simply lifted away as components of the facial fracture. Removal of the greater wing of the sphenoid and retraction of the frontal and temporal lobes is necessary to visualize and decompress the optic canal completely. Although the lateral facial approach may be effective in selected patients, the medial approach is often more direct and technically easier in the majority of patients.

The most common surgical approach for extracranial optic nerve decompression is external transethmoidal (25). Other notable extracranial approaches include

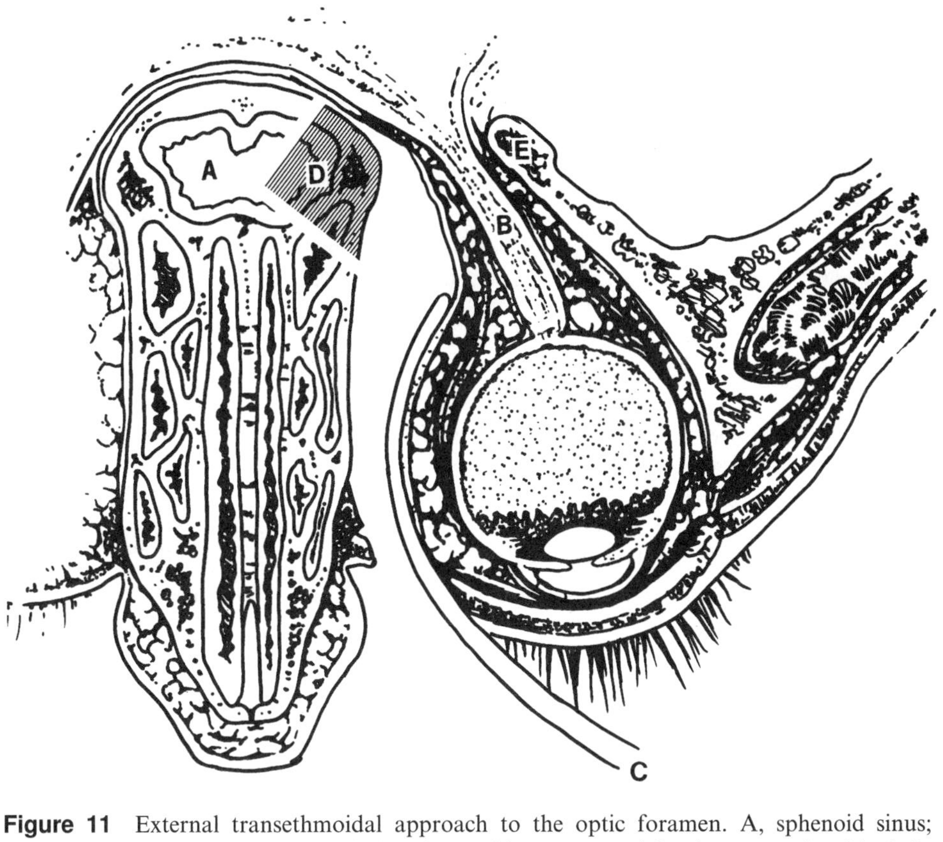

Figure 11 External transethmoidal approach to the optic foramen. A, sphenoid sinus; B, optic nerve; C, retractor; D, medial optic canal bone removed for decompression (shaded); E, lateral optic bony canal.

the endonasal transethmoidal (26), endonasal microscopic transethmoid–sphenoid (27), endoscopic endonasal transethmoid–sphenoid (28), sublabial transnasal (29), and transantral transethmoidal (17).

The incision for the external transethmoidal approach is placed vertically midway between the nasal dorsum and medial canthus, from the frontoethmoidal suture to the inferior margin of the lateral nasal bone. Through a subperiosteal dissection along the medial orbital wall, the lamina papyracea is breached and fractured medially to reach the ethmoidal air cells. A complete ethmoidectomy is performed and the anterior ethmoidal artery is identified. The superior margin of the lamina is followed posteriorly to the optic foramen (Fig. 11). The sphenoidal ostium is enlarged superomedially, and the optic foramen is located at the junction of the ethmoidal roof, the laminal papyracea, and the face of the sphenoid. The optic canal is on the same plane as the ethmoidal arteries. The anatomy of the sphenoid sinus should be evaluated preoperatively by CT scan to define the extent of pneumatization and location of septations. The nerve travels superomedially from the optic foramen toward the roof of the sphenoid sinus. The location of the optic canal is confirmed by observing the thickening of the fibrous tissues representing the fusion of the periorbital and meningeal tissues and the circumferential pattern of the fibers at the annulus of Zinn. The optic tubercle (the thickened anteromedial portion of the optic canal) is removed with a fine burr. The annulus of Zinn is divided, and the optic canal posterior to the optic foramen is very thin and easily removed. The bone posterior to the optic foramen represents the medial wall of the optic canal, while further posteriorly the bone removed represents the inferior wall of the optic canal. Since the narrowest part of the optic canal is anterior, near the optic foramen, it may be sufficient to limit the decompression to the anterior-most optic canal, including the optic foramen and the annulus of Zinn. At the completion of the decompression procedure, other fractures in the vicinity may be treated. If a cerebrospinal fluid (CSF) leak is evident through the sphenoid sinus, the sinus can be filled with abdominal fat.

Complications

The risks of extracranial optic nerve decompression include worsening vision, CSF leak and meningitis, carotid bleeding, and carotid–cavernous fistula. A CSF leak can interfere with healing of surrounding skull base fractures. Carotid artery injury is the most feared complication and can result from iatrogenic injury or an unrecognized traumatic carotid–cavernous fistula.

REFERENCES

1. Jones WD III, Whitaker LA, Murtagh F. Applications of reconstructive craniofacial techniques to acute craniofacial trauma. J Trauma 1977; 17:339–343.
2. Stanley RB Jr. The zygomatic arch as a guide to reconstruction of comminuted malar fractures. Arch Otolaryngol Head Neck Surg 1989; 115:1459–1462.
3. Holtmann B, Wray RC, Little AG. A randomized comparison of four incisions for orbital fractures. Plast Reconstr Surg 1981; 67:731–737.
4. Converse JM, Firmin F, Wood-Smith D, Friedland JA. The conjunctival approach in orbital fractures. Plast Reconstr Surg 1973; 52:656–657.

5. Tessier P. The conjunctival approach to the orbital floor and maxilla in congenital malformation and trauma. J Maxillofac Surg 1973; 1:3–8.
6. Fedok FG, Perkins SW. Transconjunctival blepharoplasty. Facial Plast Surg 1996; 12:185–195.
7. Fedok FG. The transconjunctival approach in the trauma setting: avoidance of complications. Am J Otolaryngol 1996; 17:16–21.
8. Lee C, Mueller RV, Lee K, Mathes SJ. Endoscopic subcondylar fracture repair: functional, aesthetic, and radiographic outcomes. Plast Reconstr Surg 1998; 102:1434–1443.
9. Lee C, Jacobovicz J, Mueller RV. Endoscopic repair of a complex midfacial fracture. J Craniofac Surg 1997; 8:170–175.
10. Lee CH, Lee C, Trabulsy PP. Endoscopic-assisted repair of a malar fracture. Ann Plast Surg 1996; 37:178–183.
11. Raveh J, Laedrach K, Vuillemin T, Zingg M. Management of combined frontonaso-orbital/skull base fractures and telecanthus in 355 cases. Arch Otolaryngol Head Neck Surg 1992; 118:605–614.
12. Wolfgang GL. The management of fractures in the patient with multiple trauma [letter]. J Bone Joint Surg [Am] 1987; 69:152.
13. Raveh J, Laedrach K, Vuillemin T, Zingg M. Management of combined frontonaso-orbital/skull base fractures and telecanthus in 355 cases. Arch Otolaryngol Head Neck Surg 1992; 118:605–614.
14. Converse JM, Hogan VM. Open-sky approach for reduction of naso-orbital fractures. Case report.. Plast Reconstr Surg 1970; 46:396–398.
15. Holt JE, Holt GR. Ocular injuries in craniofacial trauma. Facial Plast Surg 1988; 5: 237–242.
16. Gross CE, DeKock JR, Panje WR, Hershkowitz N, Newman J. Evidence for orbital deformation that may contribute to monocular blindness following minor frontal head trauma. J Neurosurg 1981; 55:963–966.
17. Kennerdell JS, Amsbaugh GA, Myers EN. Transantral–ethmoidal decompression of optic canal fracture. Arch Ophthalmol 1976; 94:1040–1043.
18. Levin LA, Beck RW, Joseph MP, Seiff S, Kraker R. The treatment of traumatic optic neuropathy: the International Optic Nerve Trauma Study. Ophthalmology 1999; 106:1268–1277.
19. Cornelius CP, Altenmuller E, Ehrenfeld M. The use of flash visual evoked potentials in the early diagnosis of suspected optic nerve lesions due to craniofacial trauma. J Craniomaxillofac Surg 1996; 24:1–11.
20. Li KK, Teknos TN, Lauretano A, Joseph MP. Traumatic optic neuropathy complicating facial fracture repair. J. Craniofac Surg 1997; 8:352–355.
21. Kelman SE, Elman MJ. Optic nerve sheath decompression for nonarteritic ischemic optic neuropathy improves multiple visual function measurements. Arch Ophthalmol 1991; 109:667–671.
22. Kelman SE, Heaps R, Wolf A, Elman MJ. Optic nerve decompression surgery improves visual function in patients with pseudotumor cerebri. Neurosurgery 1992; 30:391–395.
23. Maniscalco JE, Habal MB. Microanatomy of the optic canal. J Neurosurg 1978; 48:402–406.
24. Knox BE, Gates GA, Berry SM. Optic nerve decompression via the lateral facial approach. Laryngoscope 1990; 100:458–462.
25. Joseph MP, Lessell S, Rizzo J, Momose KJ. Extracranial optic nerve decompression for traumatic optic neuropathy. Arch Ophthalmol 1990; 108:1091–1093.
26. Fujitani T, Inoue K, Takahashi T, Ikushima K, Asai T. Indirect traumatic optic neuropathy—visual outcome of operative and nonoperative cases. Jpn J Ophthalmol 1986; 30:125–134.

27. Takahashi M, Itoh M, Kaneko M, Ishii J, Yoshida A. Microscopic intranasal decompression of the optic nerve. Arch Otorhinolaryngol 1989; 246:113–116.
28. Kountakis SE, Maillard AA, Urso R, Stiernberg CM. Endoscopic approach to traumatic visual loss. Otolaryngol Head Neck Surg 1997; 116:652–655.
29. Sofferman RA. Sphenoethmoid approach to the optic nerve. Laryngoscope 1981; 91:184–196.

15

Fractures of the Midface, Naso-Orbital-Ethmoid Complex, and Frontal Sinus

Khal Chowdhury
Center for Craniofacial and Skull-Base Surgery, Denver, Colorado, U.S.A.

Brad Andrews
University of Colorado Health Sciences Center, Denver, Colorado, U.S.A.

FRACTURES OF THE MIDFACE

Anatomical Considerations

Midface fractures represent 10–20% of all facial fractures. A detailed understanding of the major support structures and anatomy of the midfacial skeleton is required to appreciate the fracture patterns that occur and were initially described by the pioneering work of Lefort. Only key points in the surgical anatomy are briefly reviewed here, while a more detailed review using a skull model is highly recommended.

The midface is characterized by horizontally and vertically arranged buttresses or pillars that establish a relationship between the palate and alveolar process (occlusal plane) and the (superior) frontal cranium and skull base region. The major vertical buttresses of the midface include the zygomaticomaxillary buttress anterolaterally, the nasomaxillary buttress anteromedially, and the posterior buttress involving the pterygoid plates (Figs. 1,2). Less important are anterior horizontal buttresses formed by the lower alveolar region supporting the maxillary dentition and, superiorly, the infraorbital rim. Between these structurally reinforced buttresses, the bone of the maxilla is quite thin and represents the bone overlying or surrounding the pneumatized maxillary sinus cavity. The thin roof of the maxillary sinus is also the orbital floor: noteworthy because fractures of the upper midface invariably result in orbital fractures. Thus, the midfacial skeleton contributes to form and function by establishing vertical facial height, providing anterior facial projection, and anchoring the maxillary dentition in establishing a functional occlusal relationship.

Fracture Pathophysiology and Classification

Common causes of midface fractures are motor vehicle accidents, assaults, falls, and industrial accidents. Lefort's 1901 classification of midface fractures was based on experimental work using cadaver heads; the recurring fracture patterns he described

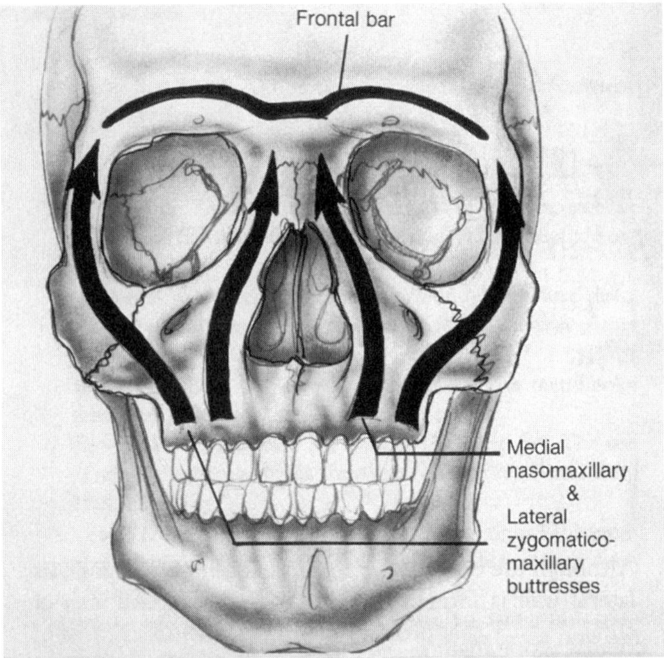

1

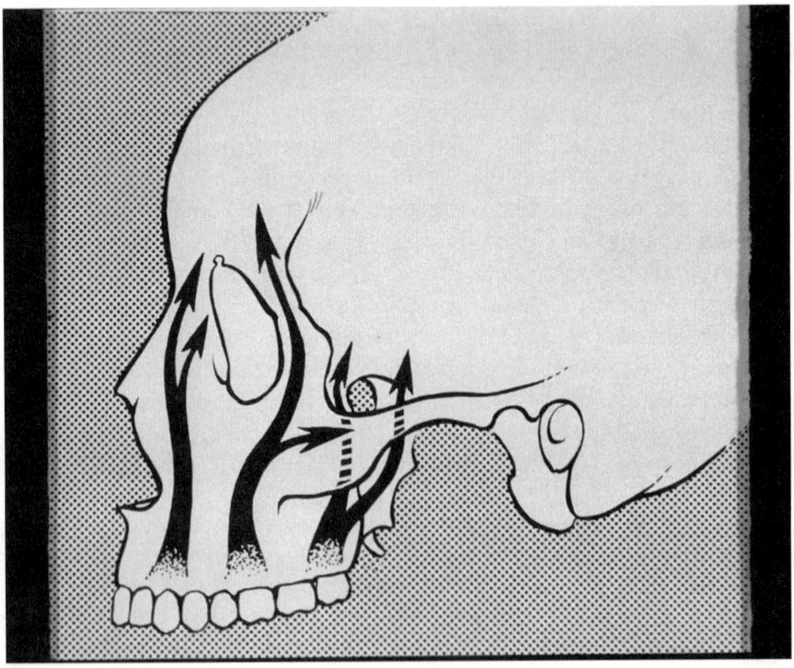

2

Figures 1, 2 Key buttresses of the mid and upper face. Note the medial and lateral buttresses of the midface and the frontal bar.

are still commonly utilized. Lefort's classification defines the fracture pattern based on the most superior fracture involved.

Lefort I Fractures

These are essentially transverse maxillary fractures and represent the lowest level. These are low horizontal fractures that separate the lower alveolar and palatal regions from the upper maxilla.

Lefort II Fractures

These are pyramidal intermediate horizontal fractures that traverse through the orbital floor and nasal bones (Figs. 3,4).

Lefort III Fractures

These represent the most superior fracture pattern and are characterized as complete craniofacial dysjunction (1). Lefort III fractures usually result from high-velocity trauma and the fracture line involves the lateral orbit, midface, and medial orbit including the nasoethmoid complex and anterior skull base. Therefore, Lefort III fractures are often associated with head injuries, dural tears with associated cerebrospinal fluid (CSF) leaks, significant orbital trauma, and other fractures of the craniofacial skeleton.

Fractures of the midface may also occur in a non-Lefort pattern. Segmental alveolar fractures of the tooth-bearing region can occur without a Lefort I. Fractures of the thin maxillary wall without buttress involvement are common. Parasagittal fractures of the palate also occur, often in combination with Lefort midface fractures. Recently, Manson et al. devised a classification system for palatal fractures (2,3):

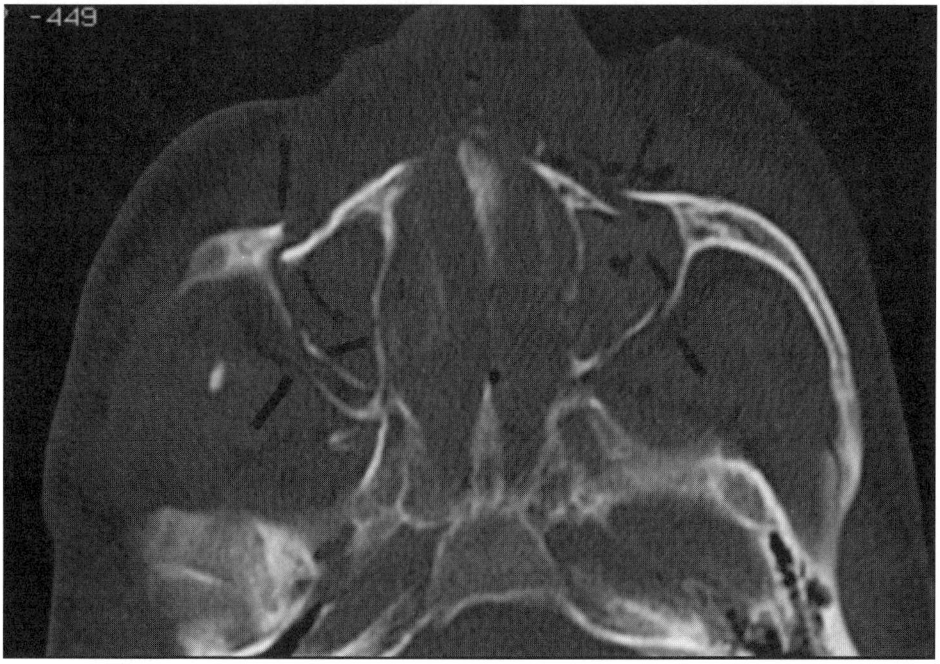

Figure 3 Patient with LeFort II midface fractures as shown on axial computed tomography.

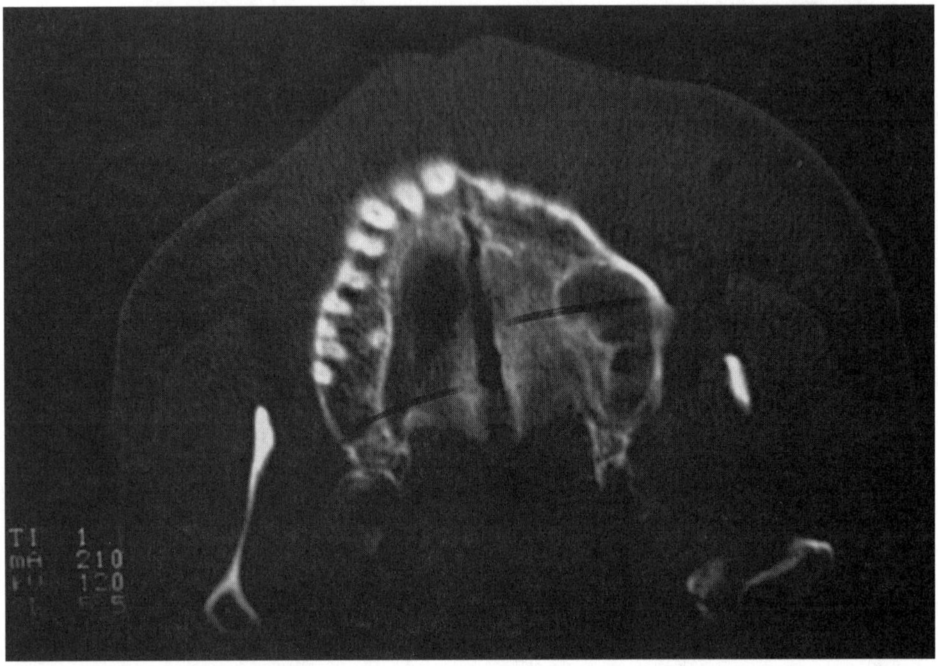

Figure 4 Patient with LeFort II midface fractures as shown on axial computed tomography. Shows the extension of the fracture through the palate.

Type 1: Alveolar fractures—either anterior involving the incisor teeth or posterolateral involving the molar region
Type II: Sagittal fractures—a midline split of the palate
Type III: Parasagittal fractures—the fracture exists between the cuspids anteriorly and posteriorly towards the midline or laterally towards the tuberosity
Type IV: Para-alveolar fractures—fracture is medial to the maxillary alveolus
Type V: Complex fractures—either comminuted fracture pattern or fracture divides the palate transversely and obliquely
Type VI: Transverse palatal fractures—divides the maxilla in a coronal plane

Fractures can be discovered on physical examination and are confirmed with coronal and axial CT scans.

Clinical Evaluation and Diagnosis

After initial stabilization of the trauma patient, evaluation of the facial injuries should commence with reassessment of the patient's airway and neurological status.

Oral bleeding, loose teeth, edema, or associated mandible fractures may lead to airway problems. Head injuries are often associated with midface fractures and CSF leaks should be suspected in patients with Lefort II or III type fractures. The presence and extent of other injuries in patients with multiple trauma may influence the timing of fracture repair and patient outcomes.

A careful and thorough evaluation of the eye and orbit is paramount, and should document visual acuity, extraocular movement, suspected globe injury, eyelid injuries, and suspected orbital fractures. Associated soft tissue injuries of the face need to be cleansed and evaluated regarding the need for early repair. Intraoral assessment of the patient's dentition and occlusion should begin with examination of the palate and maxillary alveolus for loose or missing teeth, lacerations, bleeding, and abnormal mobility. Midfacial fractures will characteristically affect the patient's occlusion. They often give rise to an open bite deformity because of premature contact of the molars posteriorly as the medial pterygoid pulls the posterior maxilla inferiorly (4). The maxilla and palate will often be unstable and mobile on bimanual examination with Lefort fractures and the midface may have a characteristic retrusion with loss of projection. Nasal fractures and associated epistaxis are common in patients with midface fractures.

Radiological assessment with plain films has limited value and should be reserved for situations in which computed tomography (CT) is not readily available. CT scans have dramatically changed the evaluation of midface fractures and all patients with suspected midface fractures should be scanned. Besides axial CT scans, coronal imaging (true coronals when feasible or coronal reformats of axial scans) is frequently useful in better evaluating the extent of orbital fractures. Although the Lefort classification system is still widely employed and useful for describing fracture patterns, CT scans are better able to evaluate and delineate precisely the exact location and extent of fractures. Most fractures in this region are comminuted and usually involve different components of pure Lefort-type fractures. CT scans provide superior guidance for treatment planning.

Management Considerations

Perioperative prophylactic antibiotic coverage should be used in patients with midface fractures. Careful coordination with the anesthesiologist regarding airway management using nasal vs. oral intubation merits consideration. Nasal intubation may interfere with reduction of nasal and midface fractures, while oral intubation may hamper evaluation and restoration of occlusal relationships. Occasionally, a planned change from oral to nasal intubation during the case, although inconvenient, may be helpful in achieving reduction while avoiding a tracheostomy. A planned tracheostomy is usually reserved for patients with multiple trauma, airway problems, or in those requiring mechanical ventilation. Early repair of midface fractures, when the patient's condition is stable, is advantageous, cost-effective, and should result in less morbidity with fewer complications.

Treatment of midface fractures aims to restore preinjury facial appearance and occlusion by restoring anterior facial projection and vertical facial height accurately. Fracture treatment should be customized to the extent and location of the fractures based on clinical evaluation and CT scan findings. Examples would be an edentulous patient or a patient with extensive orbital or mandibular fractures that would influence the treatment approach. Nondisplaced fractures may require minimal treatment. A "cookbook" approach to fracture treatment with inflexible theoretical and pre-conceived notions regarding points of fixation and other variables is highly inadvisable and may result in inappropriate treatment decisions.

Early methods of treatment for Lefort midface fractures involved open reduction of fractures of the inferior orbital rim and closed reduction via mandibular–maxillary fixation (MMF) and wire suspension (5). However, the earlier techniques of closed reduction alone led to frequent complications including lack of midface projection and loss of vertical height (4). As a result, extended open reduction techniques were developed initially using wire and subsequently miniplate fixation of the maxillary buttress system, along with concurrent treatment of associated fractures in order to avoid or minimize such complications.

Open reduction and internal fixation of midfacial fractures are usually accomplished via an intraoral sublabial approach with gingivobuccal incisions placed unilaterally or bilaterally, depending on the extent of fractures requiring subperiosteal exposure and reduction. This approach can be combined with various other methods including a transconjunctival approach to the orbital floor and rim, again depending on fracture extent (6). Lefort III fractures will often require an additional coronal approach for adequate exposure and reduction of the upper midface and orbital regions. Management of palatal fractures consists of a combination of intermaxillary fixation, acrylic splints as supplements, and plate fixation (if required) for stability (3).

The importance of achieving accurate three-dimensional reduction of the fractures along with accurate alignment of the occlusion prior to applying internal fixation cannot be overemphasized. Accurate reduction and titanium miniplate fixation of the fractured nasomaxillary and zygomaticomaxillary buttresses are key elements in stabilizing Lefort I and II fractures (Figs. 5–7). This should be accomplished after associated fractures are addressed, especially in patients with

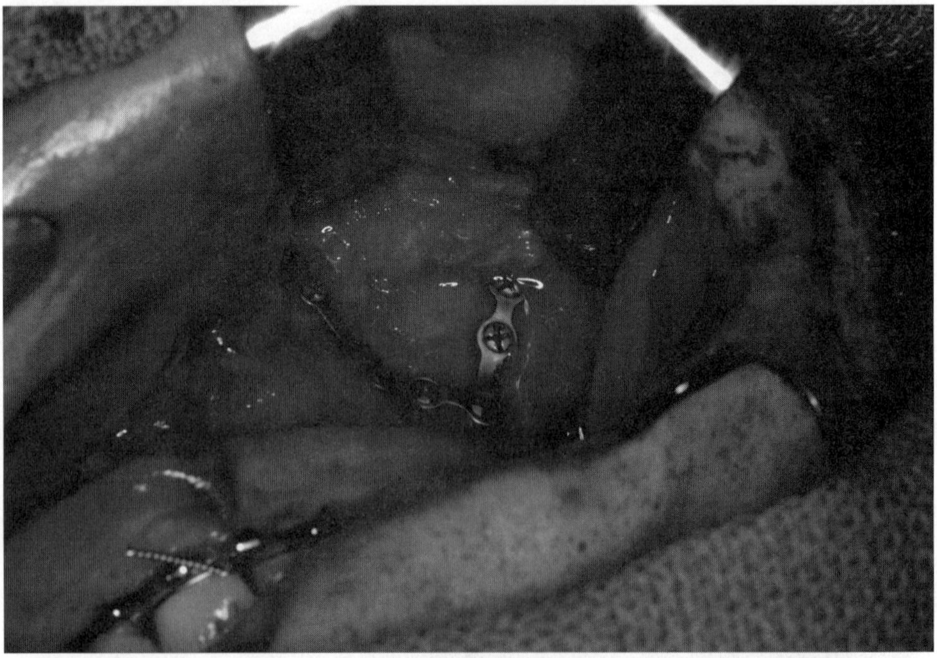

Figure 5 Placement of titanium miniplates on the medial and lateral buttress of the left midface through a midface degloving approach.

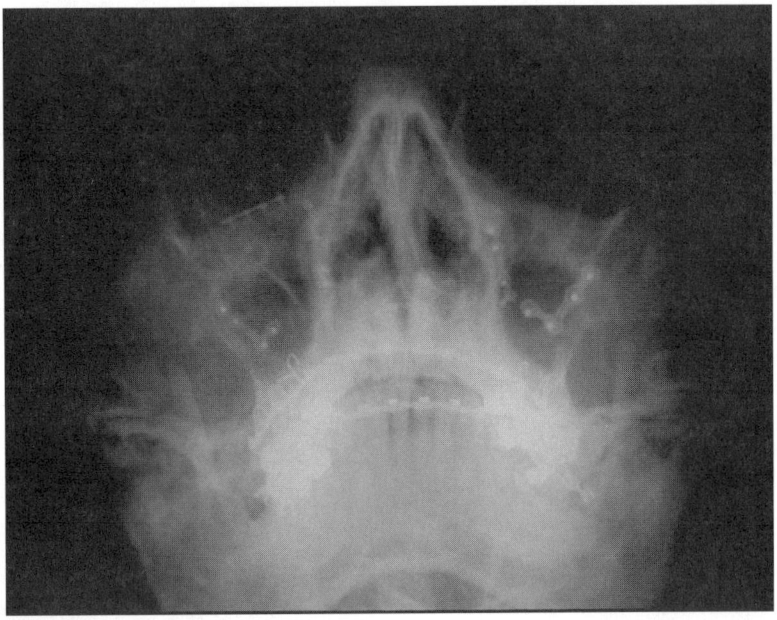

Figure 6 Postoperative radiograph of the patient in Figure 5.

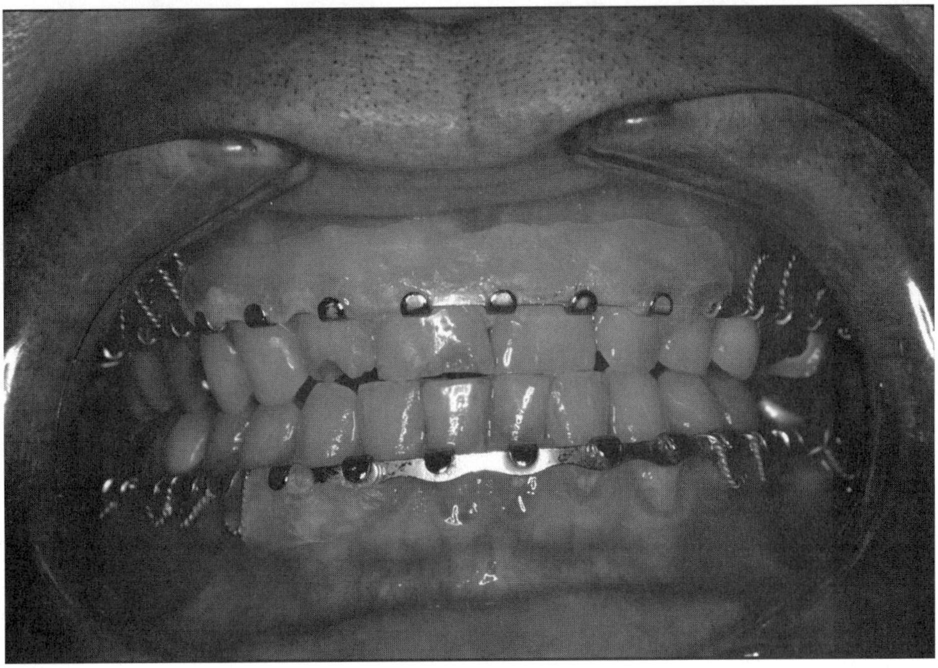

Figure 7 Occlusal view of patient in Figures 5 and 6.

Lefort II and III fractures, and the patient is placed in MMF for occlusal alignment. Temporary MMF during reduction serves to address the posterior height of the facial skeleton by utilizing the height of the ramus of the mandible, since the posterior maxillary buttress is not directly opened (Figs. 8–12). Associated fractures of the mandible, including subcondylar fractures, must also be reduced to establish facial height adequately (4).

Additional use of MMF in the postoperative period for 2–4 weeks may be necessary depending on the fracture pattern and stability achievable in individual situations. Over the last 20 years, the introduction and acceptance of low profile titanium miniplates (1.5–2.0 mm screws) have improved our ability to stabilize the major load-bearing midface buttresses, while diminishing our reliance on prolonged MMF (7). Even smaller microplates (1.0–1.3 mm screws) assist in stabilizing multiple comminuted segments in non-load-bearing regions after fixation of the major buttresses (Fig. 6). The use of plate fixation should be kept to the minimum required to achieve fracture stabilization.

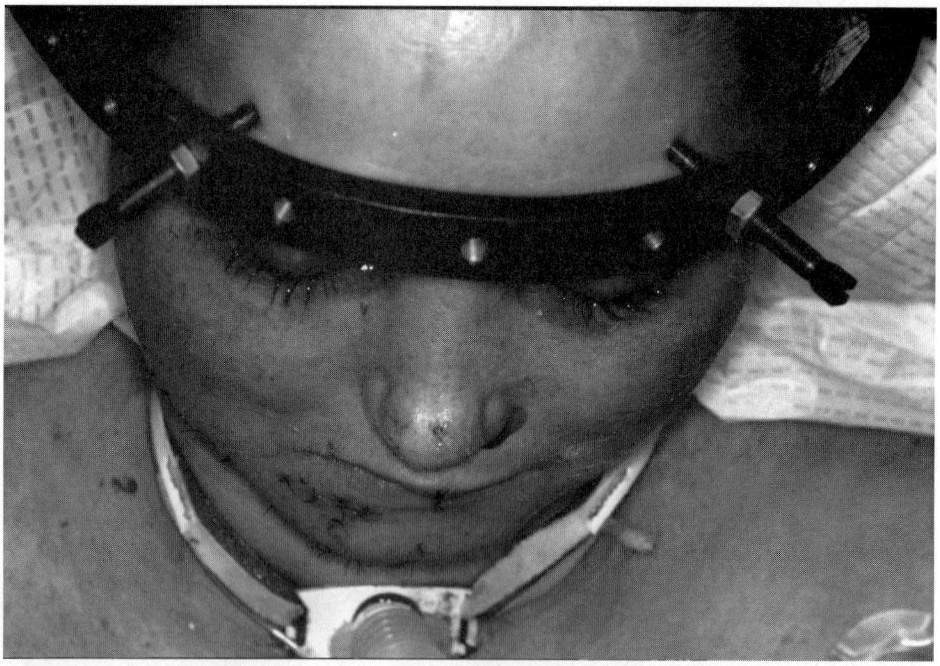

Figure 8 A 34-year-old woman sustained bilateral LeFort III midface fractures with multiple mandible fractures in a motor vehicle accident. She had numerous associated injuries, which included cervical spine fracture with no spinal cord injury. She also had an intimal tear of her carotid artery with a transient cerebrovascular accident. However, she experienced a full neurological recovery. Not shown are temporal bone fractures with facial paresis. The patient was in a cervical halo traction apparatus for stabilization of her cervical spine fractures prior to repair of her facial fractures. This apparatus prevented our use of a coronal incision for access to the Lefort III fractures.

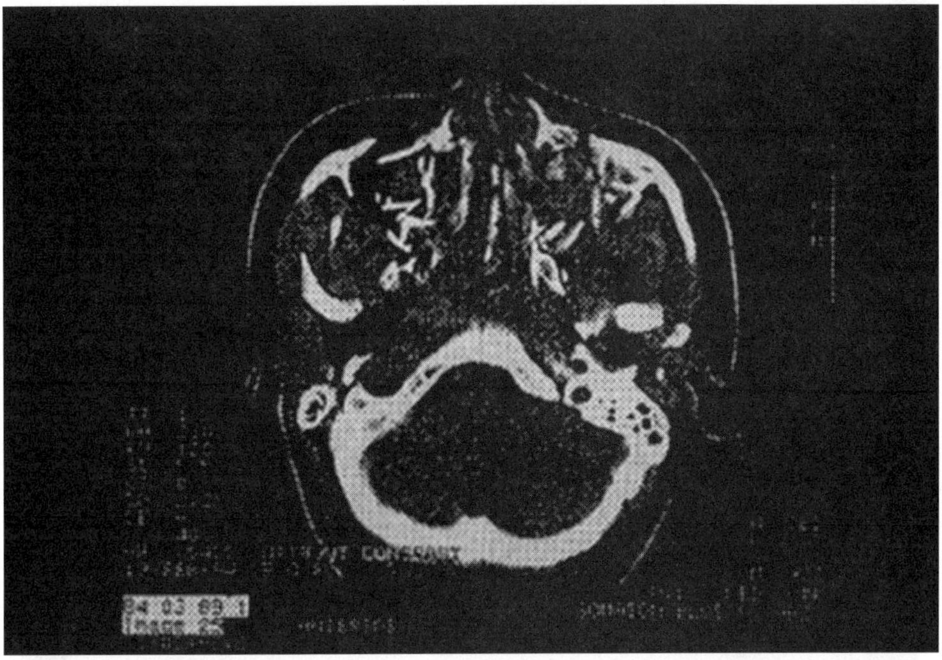

9

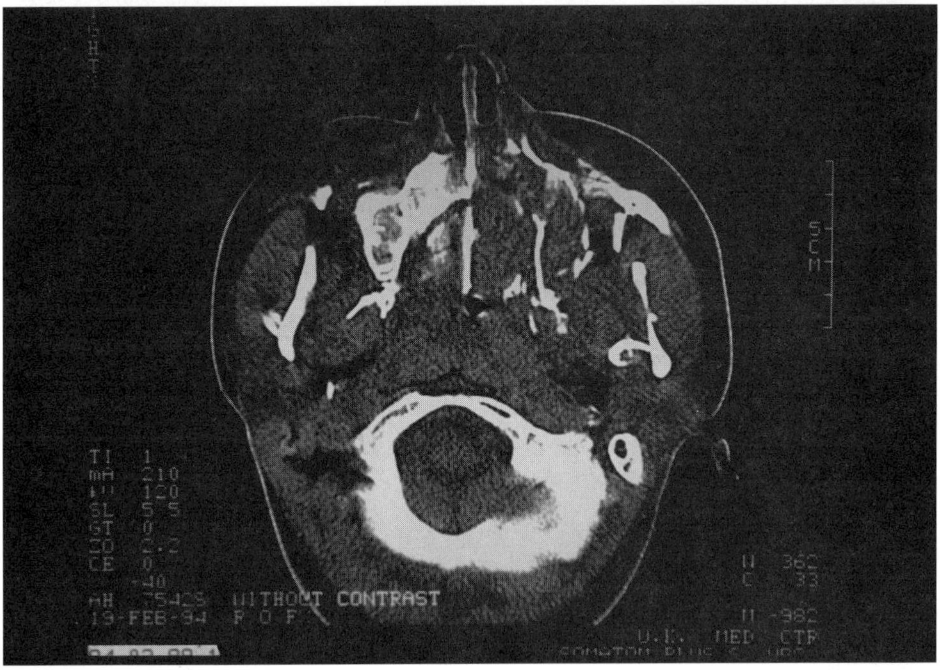

10

Figures 9, 10 Extensive midface disruption.

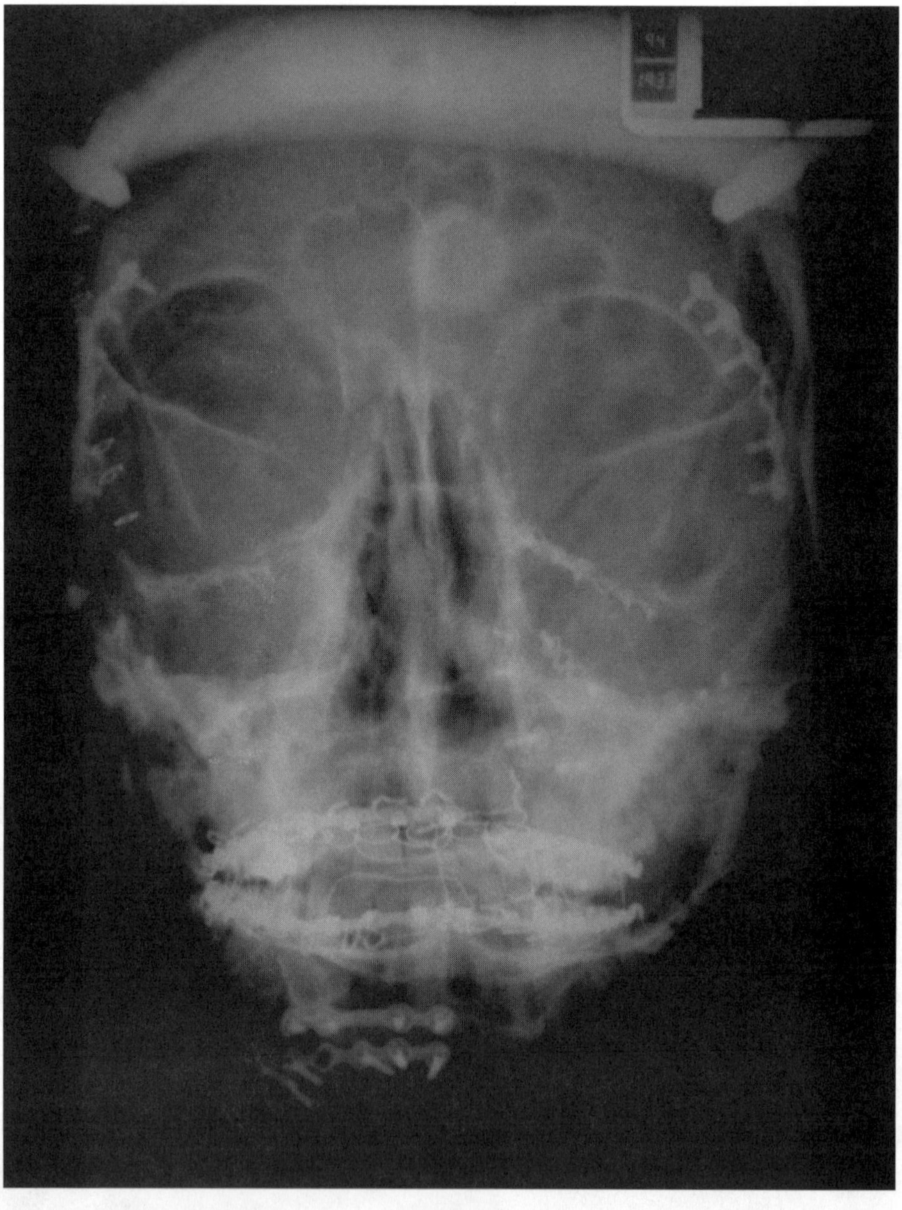

Figure 11 Postoperative radiograph following reduction of fractures.

FRACTURES OF THE FRONTAL SINUS AND NASO–ETHMOID–ORBITAL COMPLEX

Anatomical Considerations

The adult frontal sinus is divided into right and left sections by an intersinus septum. There can be tremendous variation in the size and shape of the frontal sinus both between individuals and occasionally even between the two sides in the same patient.

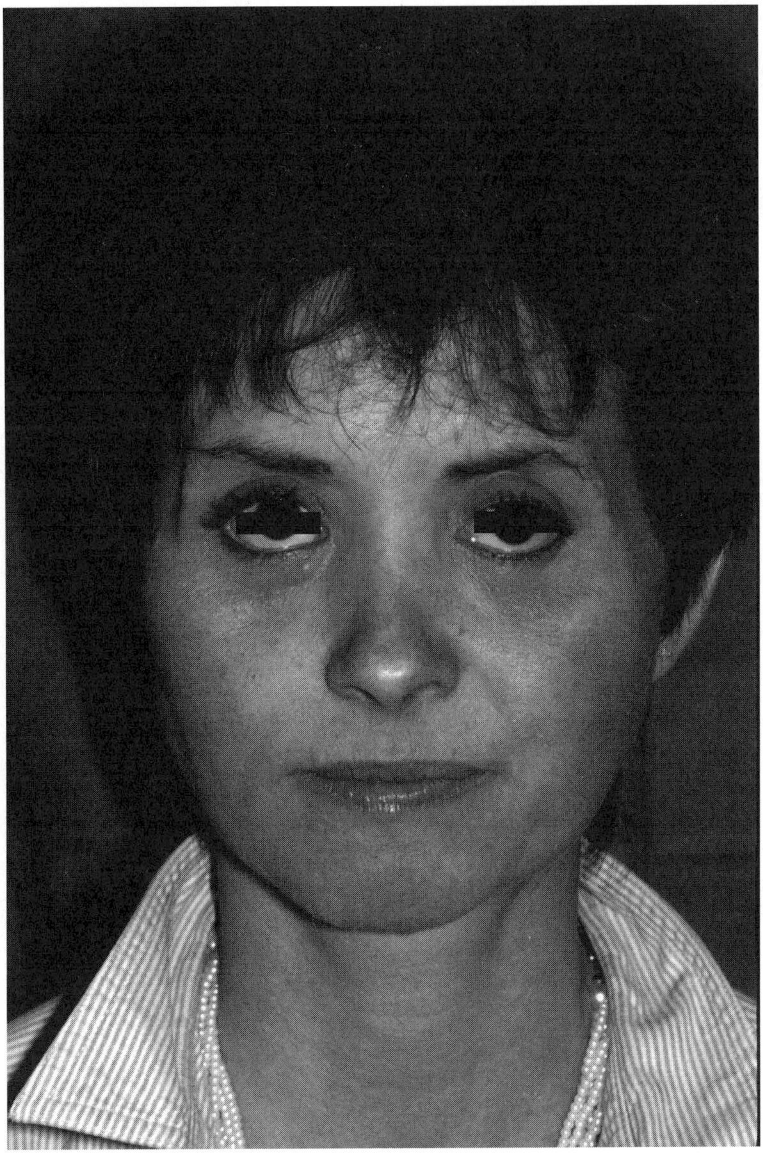

Figure 12 Appearance of the patient 1 year after surgery.

The sinus is composed of a relatively thick anterior table that forms the central and inferior portion of the forehead. A thinner plate of bone forms the posterior table that separates the sinus from the anterior cranial fossa (Figs. 13,14). The floor of the frontal sinus contains even thinner bone and also forms the medial portion of the orbital roof. The floor also contains the drainage or outflow tract (nasofrontal duct) of the frontal sinus. The nasofrontal duct is located in the posterior medial portion of the frontal sinus floor. It is an outflow tract that drains into the facial recess

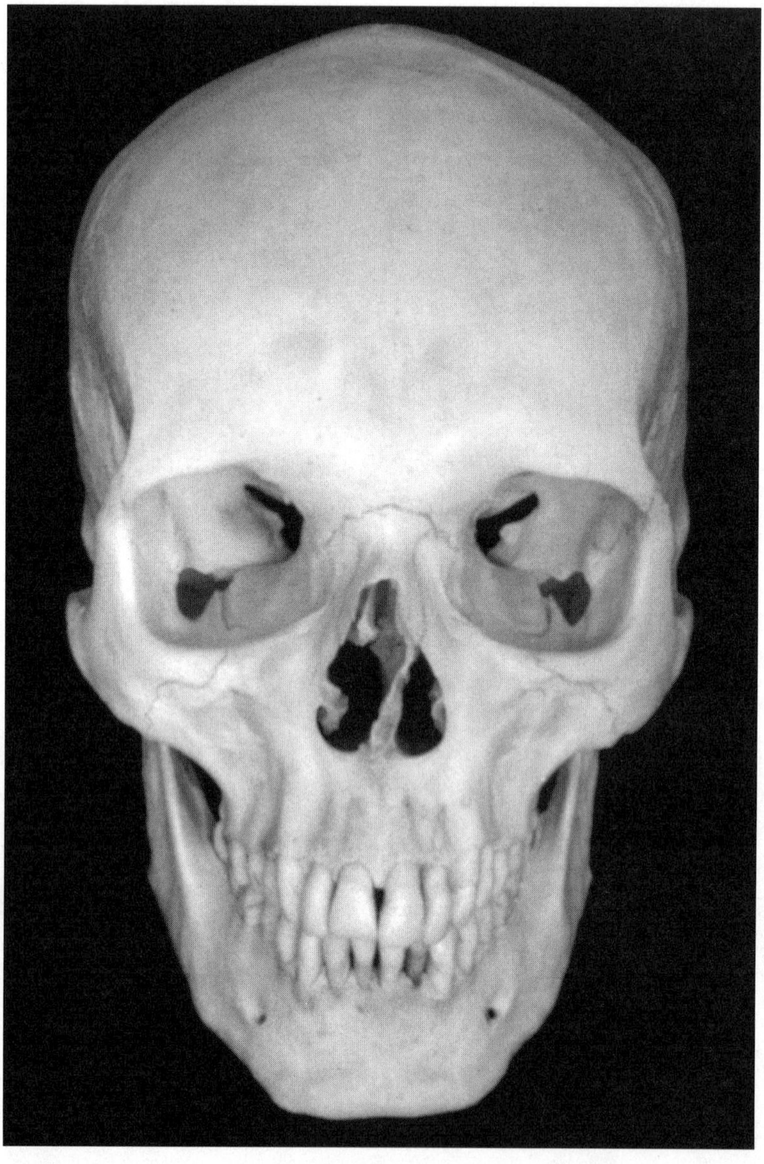

Figure 13 Anatomical view of fronto-orbital area.

located in the anterior portion of the middle meatus between the anterior attachment of the middle turbinate and the lateral nasal wall.

The frontal sinus is normally lined with pseudostratified columnar epithelium that propels mucus at a rate of 1 cm/min medially up the intersinus septum, then laterally over the superior portion to the lateral wall, and finally medially again towards the floor to the nasofrontal duct (8). The integrity of the mucociliary clearance system and the anatomical drainage or outflow provided by the nasofrontal duct is crucial to the evaluation of both frontal sinus and naso–ethmoid–orbital (NOE) fractures.

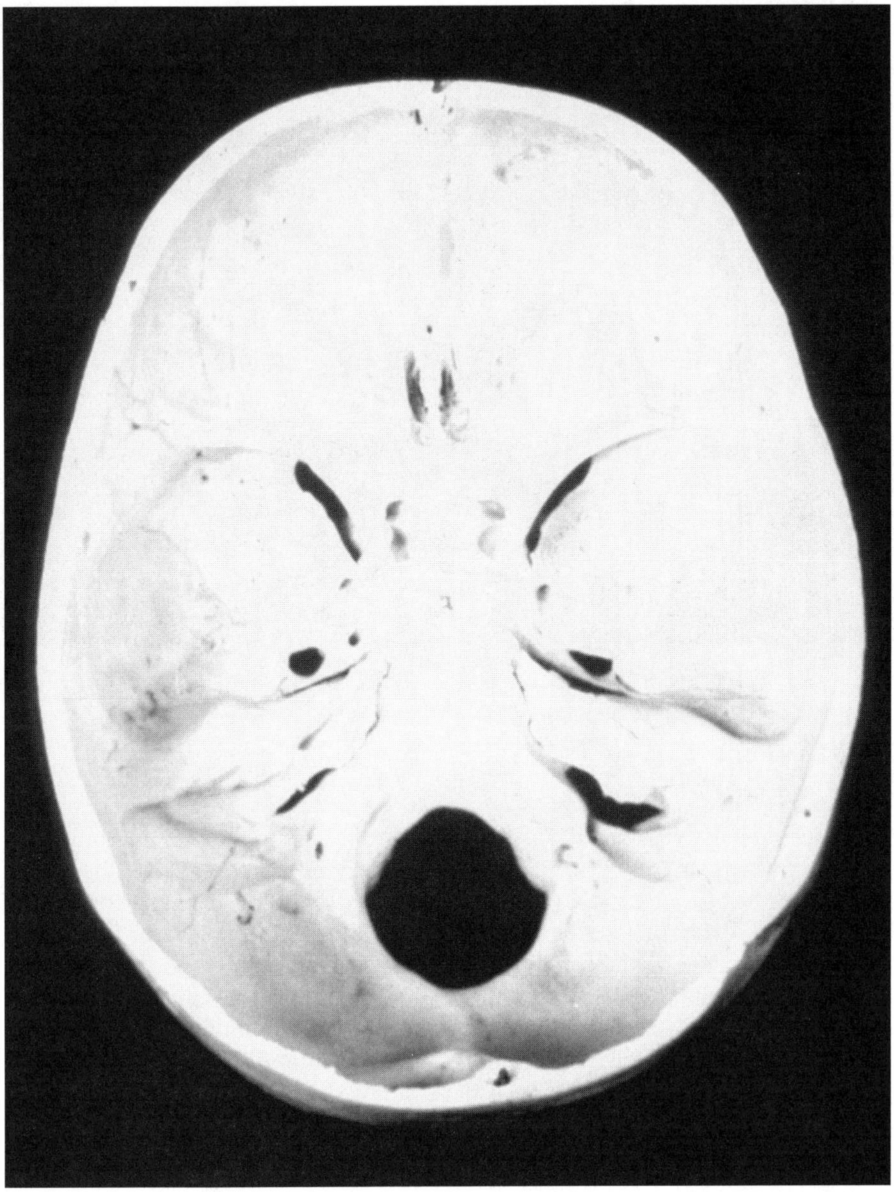

Figure 14 Intracranial view of orbital roof and anterior skull base region. In this anatomical model, the frontal sinus has been cranialized.

The NOE region, as the name implies, involves the nasal bones, the frontal processes of the maxilla, the bones making up the medial orbital walls, and the ethmoid air cells (Fig. 15). The medial orbital walls are made up of the lacrimal bones, the thin lamina papyracea, and posteriorly by the body of the sphenoid bone. The anterior and posterior ethmoid vessels travel in the ethmoidal foramina near the frontoethmoidal suture line; disruption of these vessels with fracture may cause orbital hematoma. Fractures that extend posteriorly through the body of the sphenoid bone may

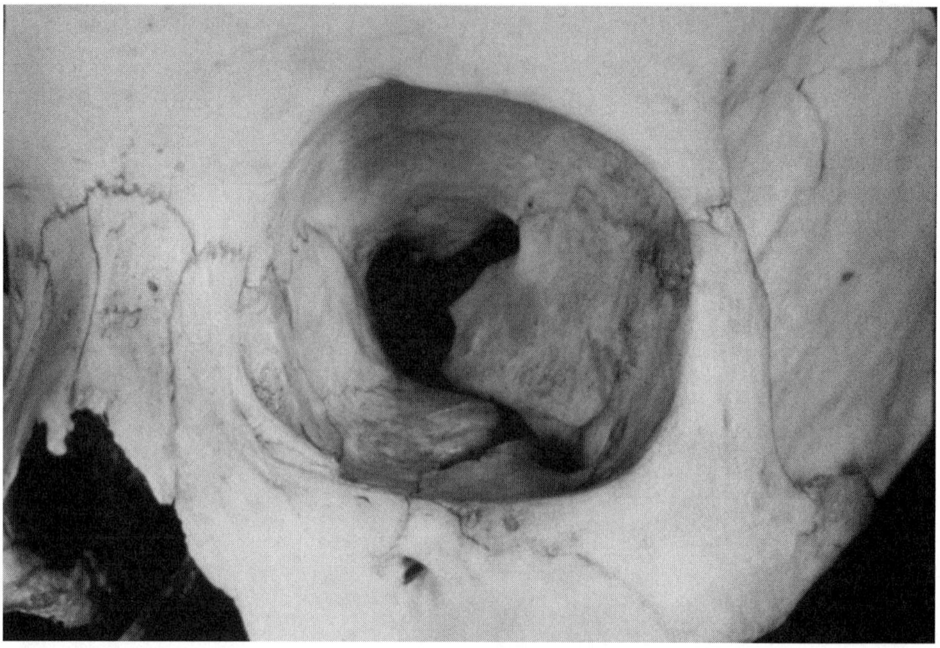

Figure 15 Medial orbital region and naso–ethmoid–orbital complex and its anatomical relationships to the midface and anterior cranial base.

involve the optic nerve canal and the superior orbital fissure. Superior orbital fissure syndrome may be caused by a fracture in this area and is characterized by ophthalmoplegia, ptosis, pupillary dilation, and decreased sensation over the forehead (9). When superior orbital fissure syndrome is associated with damage or injury to the optic nerve, a true orbital apex syndrome exists.

The interorbital area (between the medial orbital walls) is made up of the ethmoid sinuses, cribriform plate, perpendicular plate of the ethmoid, and vomer. All of these thin bones are fragile and subject to comminution. The interorbital area is separated from the intracranial side of the anterior skull base by the cribriform plate that can easily be disrupted. The dura in this area is adherent to the bone and fractures can easily result in dural tears, pneumocranium, and CSF leaks.

The anatomy of the medial canthal tendons and lacrimal system is a critical consideration in NOE fractures. The medial canthal ligament anchors the tarsal plate of the eye to the medial orbital wall and consists of three separate tendons inserting on different areas and giving the system a three-dimensional contour. The three tendons attach to the anterior and posterior lacrimal crests as well as superiorly to the frontal process of the maxilla and frontal bone (10). The anterior attachment to the anterior lacrimal crest is the most firmly adherent. The three separate components surround the lacrimal sac within the lacrimal fossa and serve an important part in the lacrimal pump mechanism, propelling tears into the nasolacrimal duct and eventually into the nasal cavity through the inferior meatus. Disruption of this arrangement results in traumatic telecanthus and possibly epiphora.

Fracture Pathophysiology and Classification

Frontal Sinus Fractures

Fractures of the frontal sinus are relatively uncommon fractures of the maxillofacial skeleton, comprising up to 12% of all facial fractures. They are usually associated with high-impact or velocity trauma; given this high-energy mechanism, significant head injuries are frequently associated with these fractures. It has been stated that forces of 800 to 2200 lbs may be required to cause fracture of the anterior table of the frontal sinus (11). The force required to elicit fracture is two times that for mandible fractures and five times the force needed for maxillary fractures (12).

Considering the amount of force required to cause frontal sinus fractures, associated fractures of the NOE, skull base, and other areas of the maxillofacial skeleton should be suspected. The resilience of the frontal sinus is in large part due to the frontal bar, which is the superior-most horizontal buttress in the facial skeleton. The frontal bar extends between the zygomaticofrontal suture lines and includes the anterior table of the frontal sinus, the superior orbital rims, and the thick glabellar bone of the forehead (13). The relatively thin bone of the maxilla lacks any sagittal buttresses. Therefore, associated fractures of the upper midface, zygoma and NOE (areas largely dependent upon the frontal horizontal buttress for support) are common (14).

Injury to or obstruction of the nasofrontal drainage system creates additional hazards in the treatment of frontal sinus fractures. Treatment of these fractures needs to restore mucociliary clearance and the patency of the nasofrontal outflow tract duct to avoid long-term sequelae or complications. As an alternative, complete ablation of the sinus and all its mucosa may prevent complications resulting from retained or trapped mucosa. These late complications include postoperative infections, meningitis, mucocele formation, and brain abscess.

Frontal sinus fractures should be classified based on the extent of fractures, anterior and/ or posterior table, and whether the fracture involves the nasofrontal duct. Ioannides et al. devised a classification system that encompasses the above characteristics and used it to devise a treatment algorithm (15):

- Type I:Anterior wall fractures
  - Ia: Anterior wall fracture without dislocation, no injury to the duct
  - Ib: High anterior wall fracture with dislocation, no injury to the duct
  - Ic: Anterior wall fracture with loss of tissue or bone, no injury to the duct
  - Id: Low anterior wall fracture with injury to the duct
  - Ie: Whole anterior wall fractured with injury to the duct
- Type II: Posterior wall fractures
  - IIa: Posterior wall fracture without dislocation, no CSF leak
  - IIb: Posterior wall fracture with dislocation and or loss of bone, no CSF leak
  - IIc: Posterior wall fracture with dislocation and presence of CSF leak
  - IId: Extensive comminuted posterior wall fracture and CSF Leak, large sinus
- Type IIIa: Any type I and IIa or IIb
- Type IIIb: Any type I and IIc or IId
- Type IV: Severe comminution of the whole nasofronto-orbital area

NOE Complex Fractures

Successful treatment of NOE complex fractures requires detailed knowledge of the bone and soft tissue anatomy of the region as well as correct evaluation and diagnosis. Suspicion of NOE fractures should arise with localized trauma to the midface severe enough to cause nasal fracture or with generalized high-velocity injury to the mid or upper facial skeleton. Compressive forces of only 30 g. may disrupt the areas of the medial orbital wall, ethmoids, and cribriform plate (16). NOE fractures are produced by force applied to the frontal processes of the maxillae (unilateral or bilateral) and nasal bones and transmitted into the orbit with secondary disruption of the medial orbital wall and ethmoids.

The nasal bones will appear flattened on clinical examination and the medial canthal tendons may be disrupted resulting in telecanthus and epiphora. Furthermore, as mentioned earlier, with high-velocity injury there may be concomitant injury to the frontal sinus, cribriform plate, and anterior skull base. This may result in CSF leakage manifesting as CSF rhinorrhea. Direct compression of the optic nerve by displaced medial orbital bone fragments can cause vision loss or indirect pressure from hematoma or edema may lead to orbital apex syndrome (Fig. 16).

Several different classification systems have been described for NOE injuries. A true NOE fracture requires fracture through five separate bones. However, the degree of displacement of the different fractures is variable. The five bones include nasal, inferior orbital rim, medial orbital wall, piriform aperture, and frontal process of the maxilla (17).

Manson et al. have proposed a classification system based on the degree of disruption of a critical central fragment that includes the bone of the lower portion of the medial orbital wall and the insertion of the medial canthal tendon (18):

Type I: The central fragment is fractured as a single segment and is not com minuted; the degree of displacement is variable.

Type II: The central fragment is comminuted but the communited section does not involve the section of the medial canthal tendon attachment.

Type III: The comminuted section involves the attachment of the medial canthal tendon.

The class of fracture sustained has implications for the degree of exposure required and therefore the surgical approach needed.

Fractures sustained in the central upper midface as a result of high-velocity or high-impact injury will often involve the frontal sinus and skull base in addition to the NOE complex. Furthermore, as discussed above, fracture lines extending along the medial orbital wall can extend back to the sphenoid bone and involve the optic canal. In a series of 475 facial fractures involving combined frontal sinus and skull base injuries reviewed by Raveh et al., 355 involved the NOE complex (19). They proposed a more unified or integrated classification system for these severe injuries that accounts for associated fractures involving adjacent areas:

Type I: Fractures of the NOE complex and anterior wall of the frontal sinus. The posterior table of the frontal sinus is intact, as is the skull base.

Type Ia: Same fracture pattern as in Type I except fracture extends along the medial orbital wall and involves the orbital apex and medial wall of

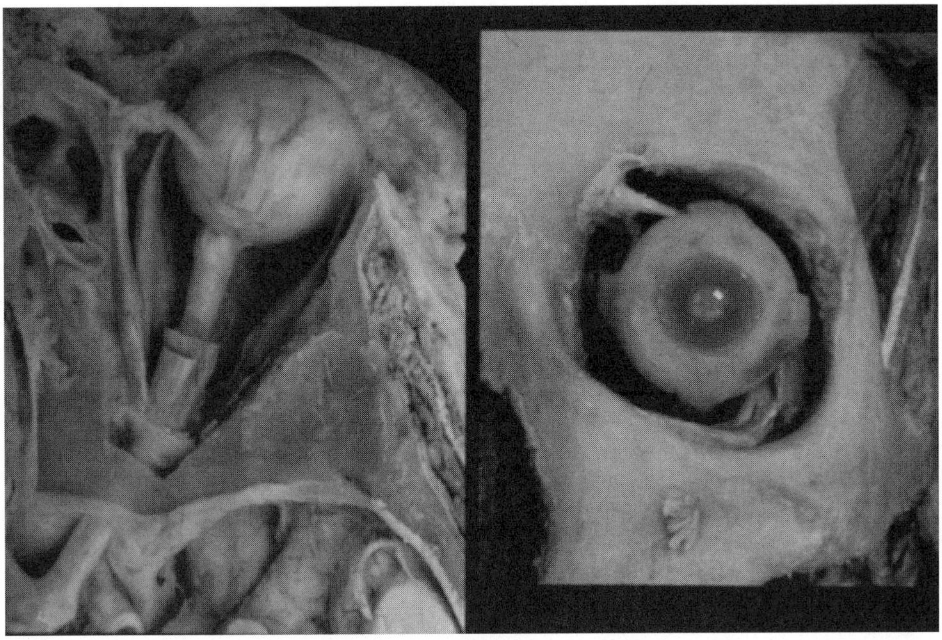

Figure 16 Note relationship of optic nerve at orbital apex to the posterior ethmoid sinuses, cavernous carotid, and sphenoid region. In this cadaveric specimen, the orbital roof has been removed to show the anatomical relationships.

optic canal; may cause orbital nerve compression or orbital apex syndrome.

Type II: Fracture not only includes the NOE and anterior wall of frontal sinus but also involves the posterior table of the frontal sinus or anterior skull base with subsequent dural tears, CSF leaks, pneumocranium, and possible brain herniation into the ethmoids or orbit. Associated injury to the orbital apex is common with this type of more severe injury.

Clinical Evaluation and Diagnosis

Patients with a high-impact injury to the area of the forehead and upper midface must be evaluated for the presence of a frontal sinus fracture. On Clinical examination, there is often profound edema, soft tissue swelling, and ecchymosis that may make initial clinical determination difficult. However, there may be clinical evidence of depression at the area of the frontal sinus and forehead region. Epistaxis, diplopia, visual disturbance, forehead lacerations, and CSF leakage or rhinorrhea may be present. Broad evaluation of the facial skeleton is crucial because fractures of the frontal sinus are often associated with other fractures and complications due to the high-velocity nature of these injuries. It would be safe to assume that most of these patients experience some degree of closed head injury, from very mild to severe frontal lobe contusion or hematoma. Therefore, careful re-evaluation of the neurological status and evaluation of the visual system merit emphasis.

Evaluation of patients with trauma to the central midface should include a search for signs of NOE fractures that may include (see figure 44) flat nasal dorsum, telecanthus, shortened palpebral fissure, enopthalmos and diplopia, subconjunctival hematomas, epistaxis, and CSF rhinorrhea (17). Evaluation of the type or extent of injury may be difficult secondary to edema and soft tissue trauma. NOE fractures frequently accompany frontal sinus fractures, so evaluation should include thorough neurological, orbital and eye examinations. High-impact injuries are often associated with posterior table frontal sinus or cribriform plate fractures, raising the possibility of CSF leak, pneumocephalus, and intracranial injury.

Patients with NOE fractures likewise require careful evaluation of the eye and orbit for signs of entrapment, retrobulbar hematoma, and possible injury to the optic nerve. This evaluation should, at a minimum, include evaluation and recording of visual acuity in each eye separately, presence of an afferent pupillary defect, range of extraocular movements, and the presence of diplopia. Additional forced-duction testing or measurement of intraocular pressure may be necessary and a formal ophthalmology consultation should be considered.

A hallmark finding in NOE fractures is presence of traumatic telecanthus. The average intercanthal distance in white persons is 30–35 mm. Variations occur based on race, ethnic background, gender, and age. Traction on the lower eyelid may reveal laxity or loss of normal tautness in the medial canthal attachment; however, this can be difficult to ascertain when marked edema is present. Normally, the intercanthal distance should be about 50% of the interpupillary distance; when the difference is greater than 50% telecanthus should be suspected. If the intercanthal distance is greater than 35 mm it is suggestive of telecanthus; distances greater than 40 mm are strongly suggestive of telecanthus and NOE fracture (20). Epiphora may also be present with disruption of the lacrimal apparatus; however, it is often difficult to detect in the acute evaluation of the trauma patient.

All patients with significant trauma to the midface, NOE, or frontal sinus area should be evaluated with high-resolution axial CT scans and coronal reformats if available. This will best delineate the fracture extent and severity, permits classification, and facilitates optimal treatment planning. Furthermore, associated intracranial injuries and additional facial fractures can be evaluated simultaneously.

A key point in the radiographic evaluation is to determine the extent or severity of injury to the nasofrontal outflow tract. Although treatment of anterior table fractures that do not involve the nasofrontal duct may be primarily for restoring appearance, fractures involving the nasofrontal duct will require either meticulous restoration of the mucociliary clearance system (while restoring patency of the duct) or obliteration of the sinus. Furthermore, fractures involving the posterior table may require repair of dural defects, obliteration of the sinus, or possibly sinus cranialization.

Management of Frontal Sinus and NOE Fractures

Treatment planning requires meticulous clinical evaluation of the patient's injuries, and detailed analysis of the fracture types, severity, and location from appropriate CT scans. Poor treatment planning resulting from inadequate evaluation or imaging studies will invariably result in less favorable outcomes or complications despite skillful surgery. Treatment of these fractures aims to prevent deformity by restoring preinjury appearance, function, and avoid complications related to the paranasal sinuses and adjacent intracranial areas. Treatment of pediatric patients with NOE or frontal sinus fractures should minimize the use of plate fixation and utilize resorbable plates when possible. This is especially true for patients under the age of 14, in whom restriction of growth resulting from plate fixation may be a concern.

Anterior Table Fractures

Frontal sinus fractures limited to the anterior table only and without involvement of the nasofrontal duct or NOE complex are treated primarily to prevent collapse and depression or deformity of the forehead region. Linear fractures of the anterior table without significant displacement may require no surgical treatment, with outpatient follow-up and observation. Depressed fractures are treated to prevent forehead deformity. The CT scan will show the extent of displacement and comminution of the anterior table while confirming the integrity of the posterior table (Figs. 17–21).

When existing lacerations are present they can sometimes be used with extensions into existing skin creases to provide adequate access for fracture repair. Occasionally, these forehead lacerations can be extended in an intrabrow fashion to provide access (Figs. 22–25). Bilateral brow incisions can provide limited access to the nasofrontal area and are well described, although we would advise against joining the brow incisions over the nasion–glabellar region since this produces more noticeable scars (Figs. 21,26–29). There are also recent reports of the use of endoscopic methods for fracture reduction and fixation that avoid large external incisions when aesthetic concerns are paramount and there are no associated posterior table

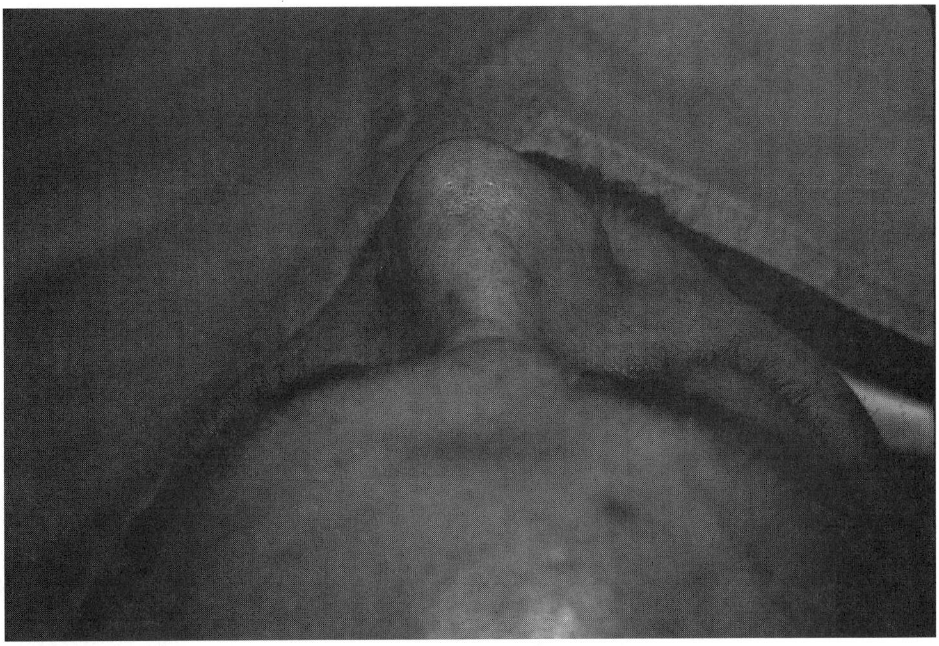

Figure 17 Patient treated at another institution with open reduction of anterior table and frontal sinus fractures through an open sky approach. The patient has poor reduction with residual central forehead deformity.

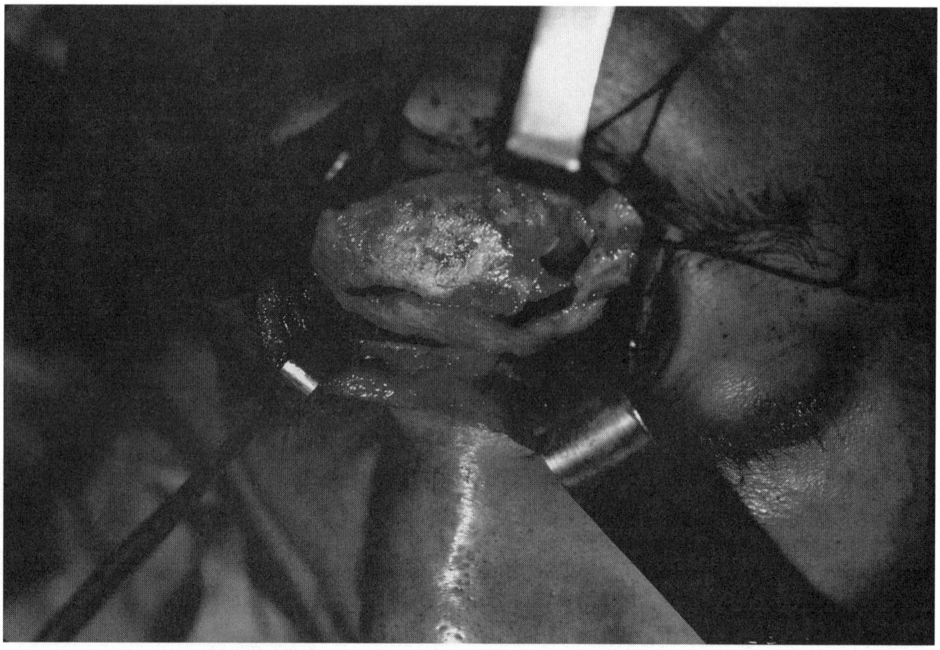

Figure 18 Intraoperative view through the same approach. Note the depressed anterior table fracture.

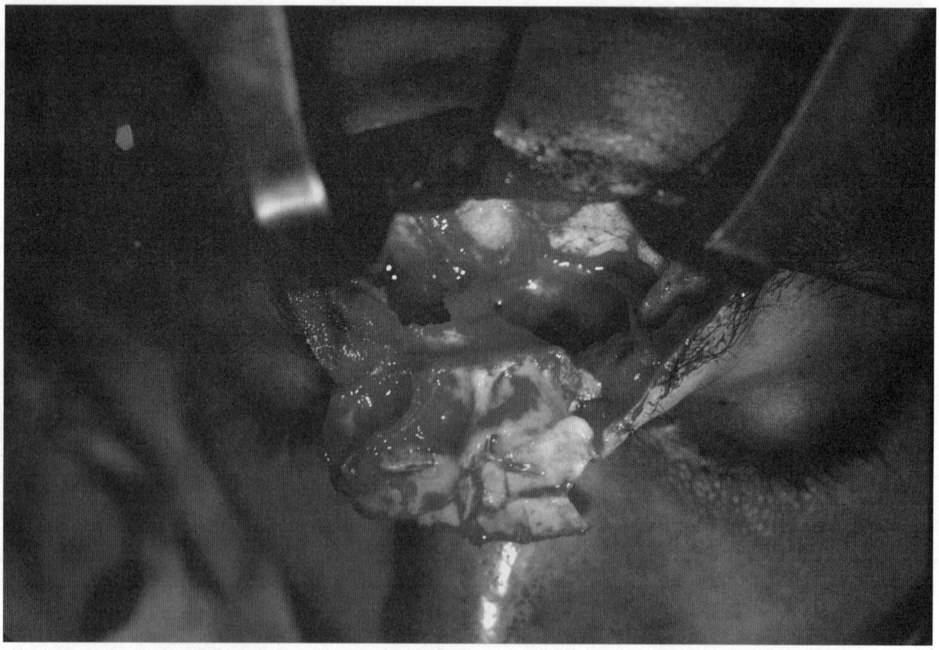

Figure 19 Anterior table of the frontal sinus has been removed. Note the widely patent nasofrontal out flow tracts on either side of the midline.

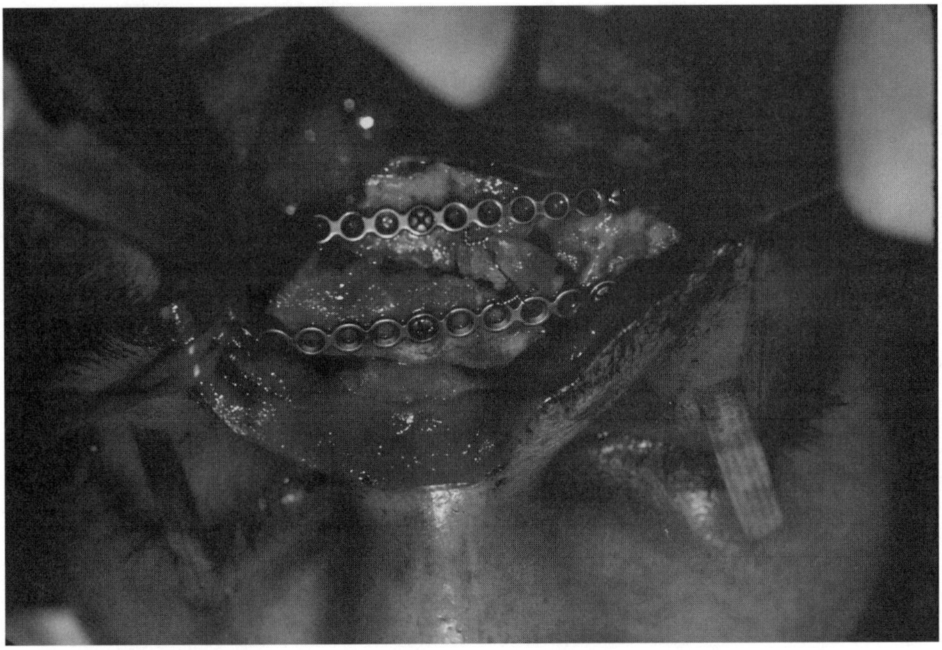

Figure 20 Titanium plate and screw reduction of the anterior table.

or nasofrontal duct injuries (21). However, a coronal incision placed well behind the hairline to camouflage the scar remains a key approach for access to these fractures. The coronal incision has been well described and provides wide and versatile access to the entire NOE and frontal sinus area. In our opinion, there is no justification for shaving or cutting a patient's hair for the purpose of using a coronal incision. The patient's hair can be washed, prepped, parted, and preserved without an increase in infection rates (22,23).

Many different techniques have been used to manage isolated anterior table fractures, depending on the degree of fracture present and the materials available for fixation. Stainless steel wires have been used for fixation; however, over the past 15 years these have been supplanted by titanium plates (miniplates and microplates). Depressed segments of the anterior table should be elevated, reduced, and fixation performed with low-profile titanium microplates (1.0–1.5 mm diameter screws) applied to maintain reduction (Figs. 17–29). Resorbable fixation with polylactide plates and screws should be considered in pediatric and perhaps in selected adult cases (24).

During reduction, the posterior table of the sinus, condition of the sinus mucosa, and the nasofrontal ducts can be inspected. Devitalized sinus mucosa should be removed while untraumatized mucosa may be left intact. Blood clots, debris, or small bone fragments should be removed but meticulously preserved and the sinus cavity copiously irrigated prior to applying fixation. The importance of saving small bone fragments rather than discarding them cannot be overemphasized (Figs. 30–37). These small fragments can then be fitted like the pieces of a jigsaw

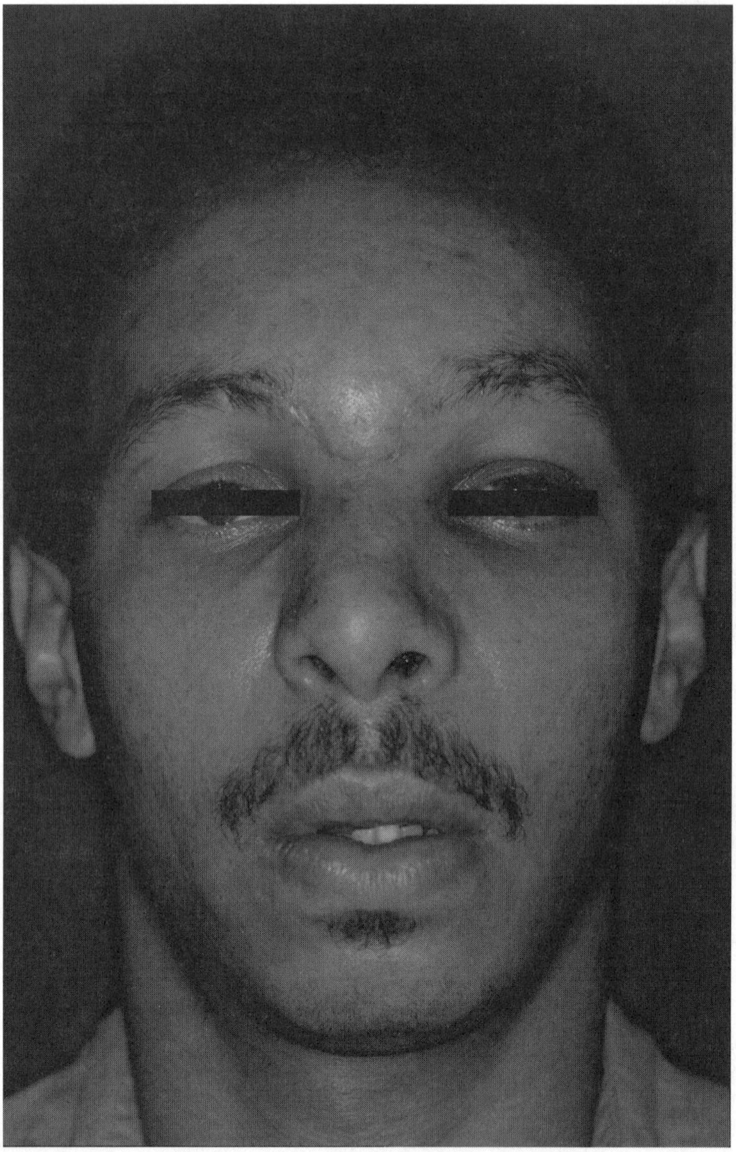

Figure 21 Four-week postoperative view of patient. Note the unsightly central portion of the open sky approach. In our opinion, this part of the incision over the glabella should be avoided unless there are existing lacerations.

puzzle to restore the preinjury configuration, obviating the need for primary bone grafting in most situations (25). Titanium mesh has been utilized and advocated for the repair of severely comminuted anterior table fractures (11). The reduced individual fragments are secured with screws to an overlay of titanium mesh used to maintain contour and stability of the fracture segments. Only in those rare situations in which loss of bone has occurred through open wounds is there a need to resort to primary bone grafting. The coronal approach provides versatile access for harvesting

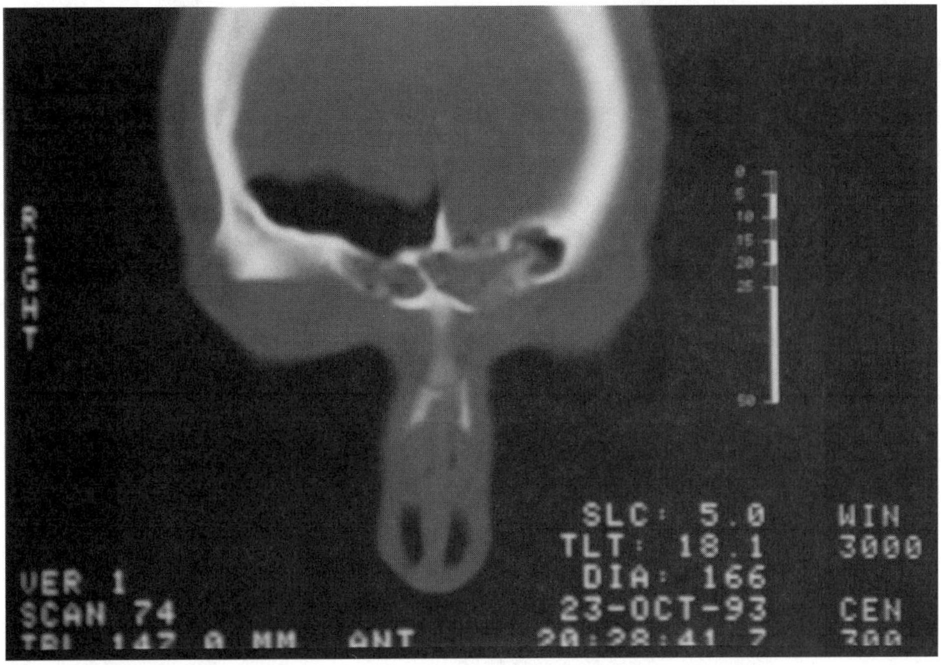

Figure 22 Coronal CT scan shows pneumocephalus resulting from a posterior table fracture involving both tables of the frontal sinus. The patient had been in a motor vehicle accident.

split calvarial bone grafts used in reconstructing the critical supraorbital rim areas first when this is necessary. Besides access and availability, calvarial bone grafts may theoretically suffer less from resorption, although autogenous bone graft stability may be a more important factor than its source (26–28).

Posterior Table Fractures and Associated Nasofrontal Duct Injury

We discussed the high-velocity injury mechanism required to produce posterior table fractures of the frontal sinus. As a result, nasofrontal outflow tract injury, anterior table fractures, additional facial fractures, and head injury are frequently associated with this type of injury. Before the routine use of CT scans, it was often necessary to remove and replace the fractured anterior table segments to examine the posterior table of the frontal sinus and ensure its integrity (25). However, based on CT findings the status of the posterior table can now be predicted preoperatively, making such exploration of the posterior table unnecessary.

Considerable controversy exists regarding the treatment of both posterior table fractures and nasofrontal outflow tract injuries. Management of frontal sinus fractures associated with injuries to the nasofrontal duct are controversial with arguments ranging from obliteration of the sinus to restoration of the integrity of the sinus and subsequent cannulation of the nasofrontal outflow tract to maintain its patency. The obliterative approach aims to exenterate all frontal sinus mucosa in creating a safe reconstruction while the restorative approach aims to restore physiological drainage of the frontal sinus. The aim of both approaches in repairing these fractures is to prevent secondary mucocele formation and delayed infectious

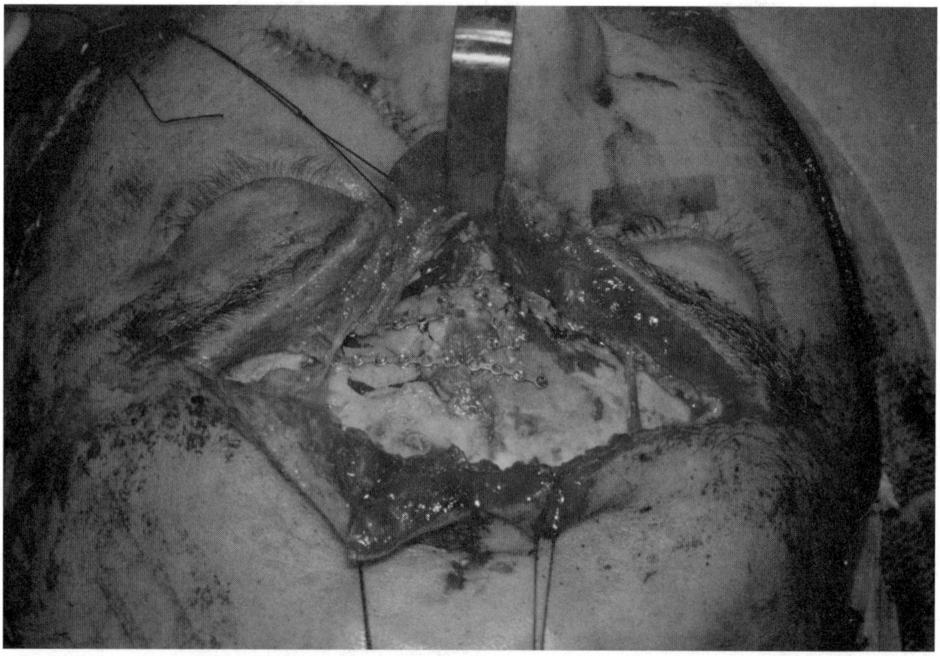

Figure 23 The frontal sinus fractures were accessed through extension of existing lacerations. Note preservation of the supraorbital neurovascular bundle and titanium microplate fixation of the anterior table. The posterior table was preserved, the dura sealed, and a subcranial ethmoidectomy was performed with Silastic tube stenting to maintain frontal sinus drainage.

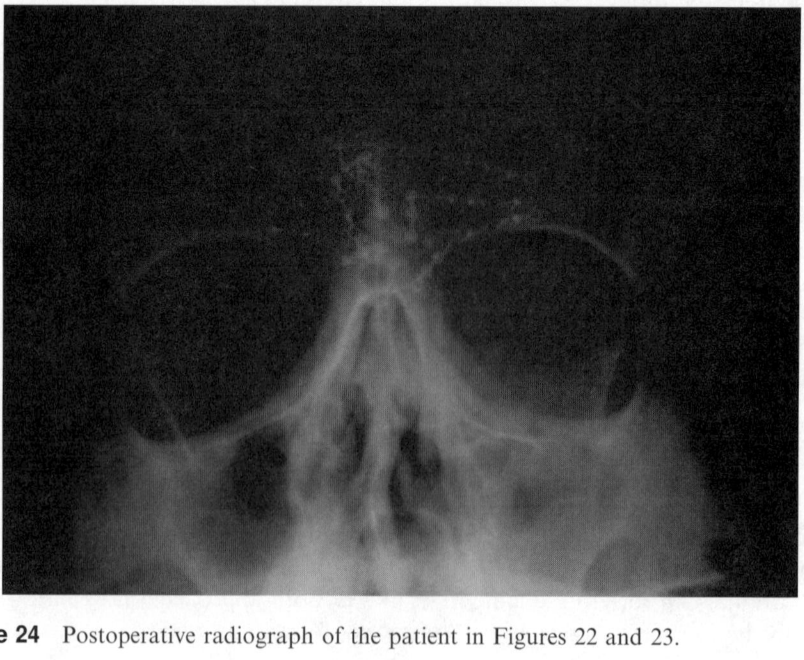

Figure 24 Postoperative radiograph of the patient in Figures 22 and 23.

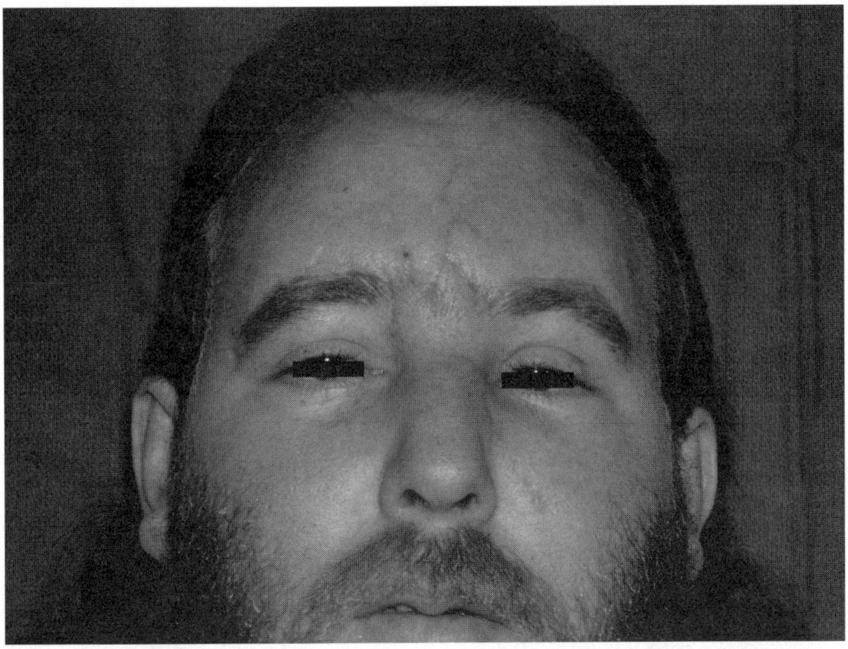

Figure 25 One month postoperative photo of patient in Figures 22–24. There is still some residual swelling in the glabellar area.

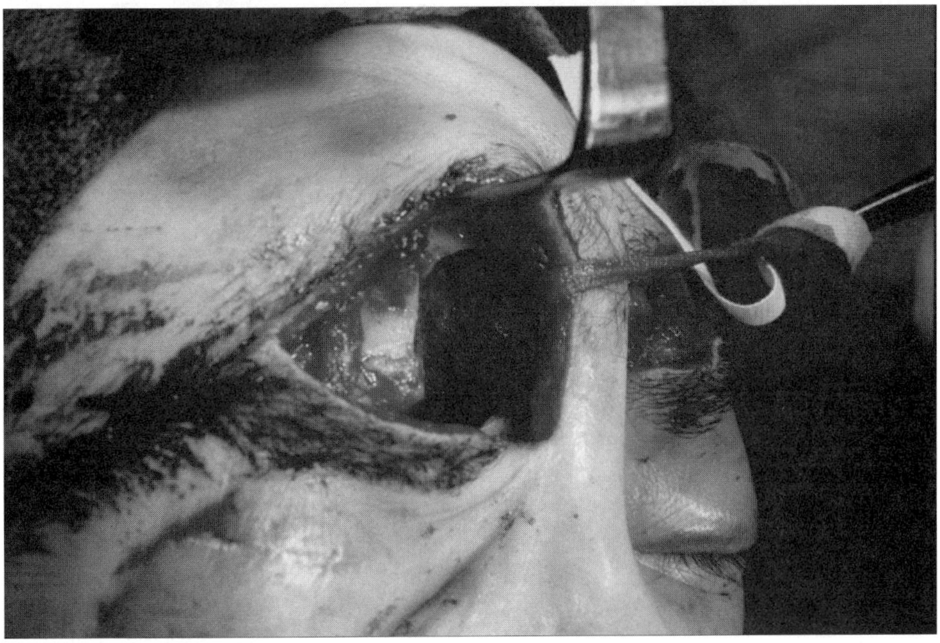

Figure 26 A bilateral brow approach was used in a patient with anterior table frontal sinus fracture, who preferred that we avoid a coronal approach. The incisions are kept primarily within the brow without joining the central portion over the glabella.

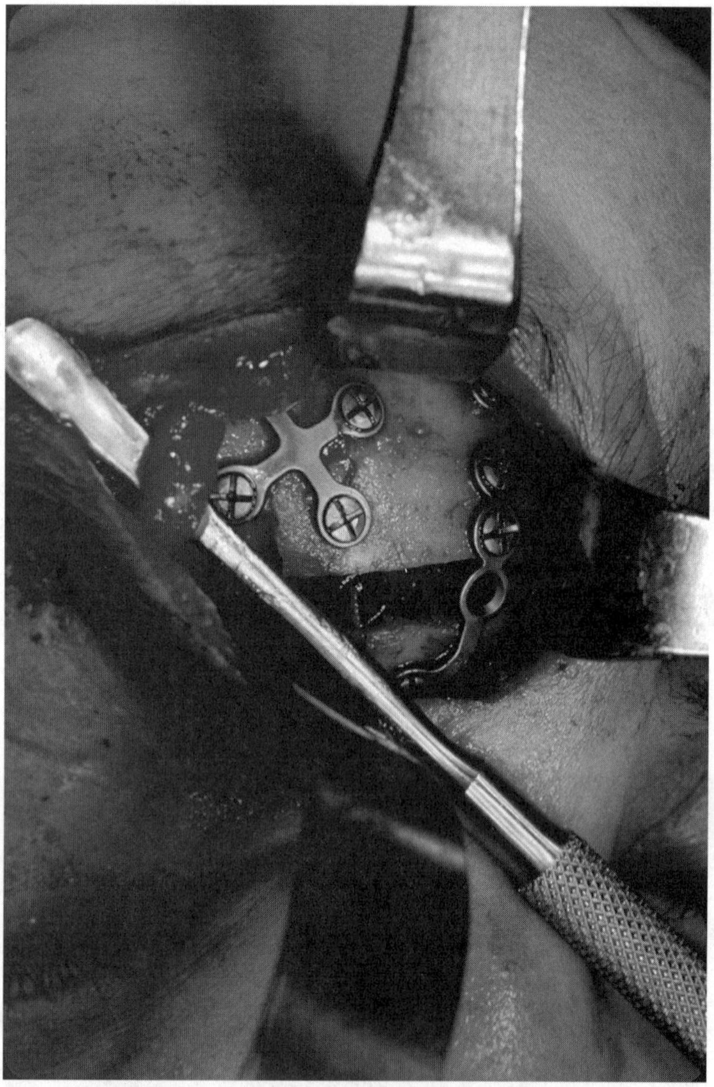

Figure 27 Note preservation of the supraorbital neurovascular bundle.

complications with the potential for intracranial spread (29). Furthermore, the restorative approach has been influenced by advances in endoscopic sinus surgery over the past 20 years that emphasize functional restoration of frontal sinus drainage pathways and the mucociliary clearance system whenever possible.

Proponents of the restorative approach with meticulous reconstruction of the sinus and maintenance of the patency of the nasofrontal duct cite a low incidence of secondary infection and mucocele formation postoperatively. Raveh et al. reported on a series of 355 patients with combined frontal sinus, NOE, and skull base fractures in whom the frontal sinus was reconstructed when feasible and the

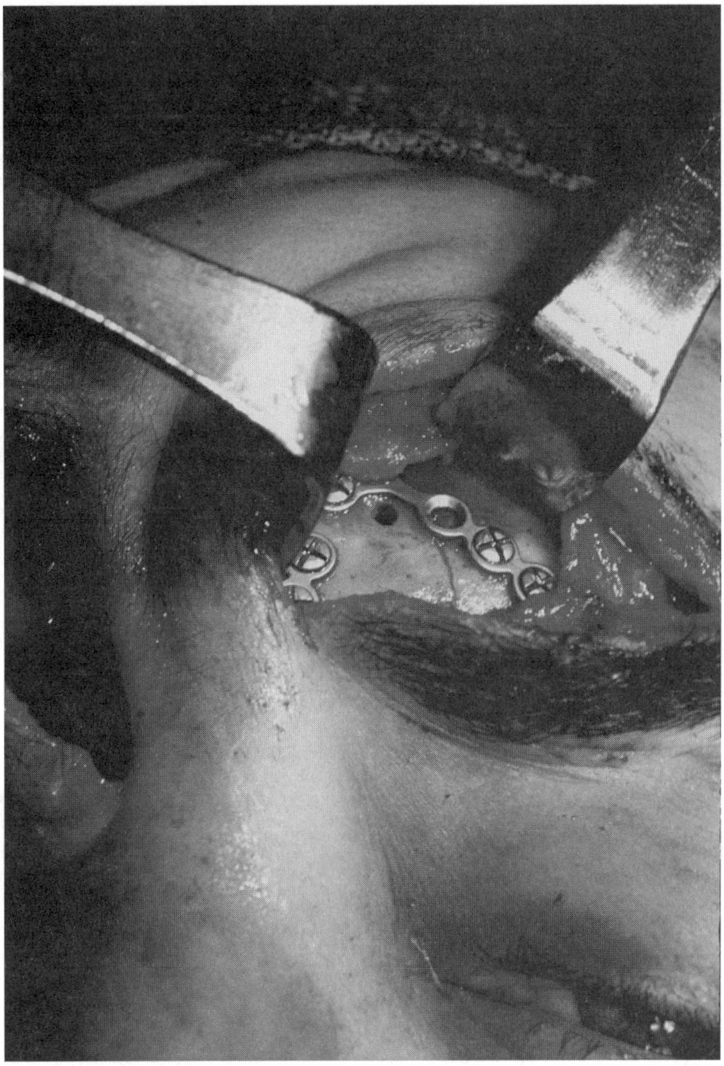

Figure 28 Plate and screw open reduction and internal fixation of the anterior table through the brow approach.

nasofrontal duct was stented with a Silastic pediatric endotracheal tube. With long-term follow up of greater than 1 year the postoperative incidence of infection was 1.7% and the incidence of mucocele formation was 3.0% (19). There is also debate about the ideal material to use for stenting of the duct since Silastic pediatric endotracheal tubes, Silastic sheets, rubber, and gold have all been used. There is also no consensus on the actual need for stenting and about the length of time the stent should be left in place: from 6 weeks to 6 months (15,49).

Obliteration of the frontal sinus in response to significant injury to the frontal sinus mucosa and nasofrontal duct is an option that has been advocated and

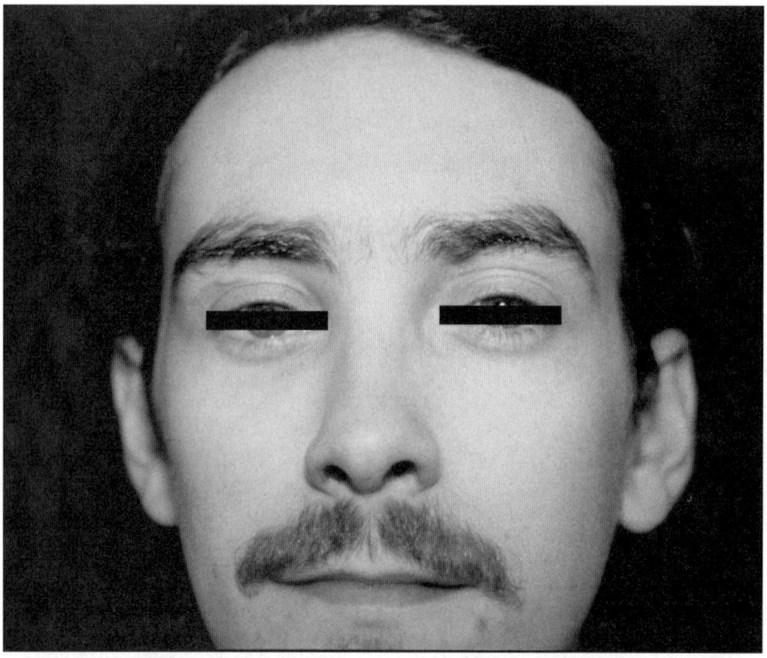

Figure 29 Six-week postoperative view of patient in Figures 26–28.

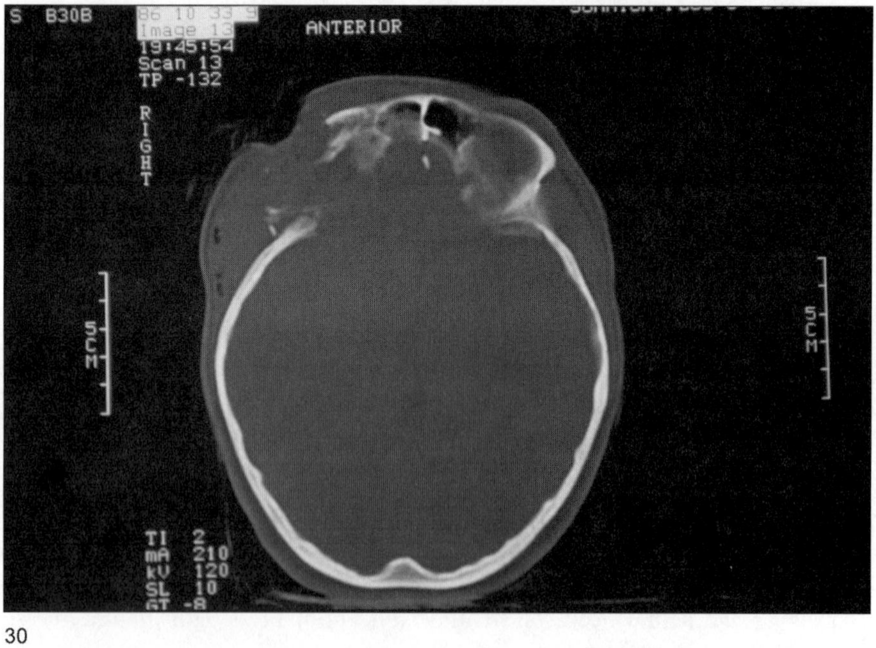

30

Figures 30, 31 Highly comminuted frontal sinus, fronto-orbital, orbital roof, and lateral orbital fracture in a 13-year-old girl who was a passenger ejected from an automobile accident.

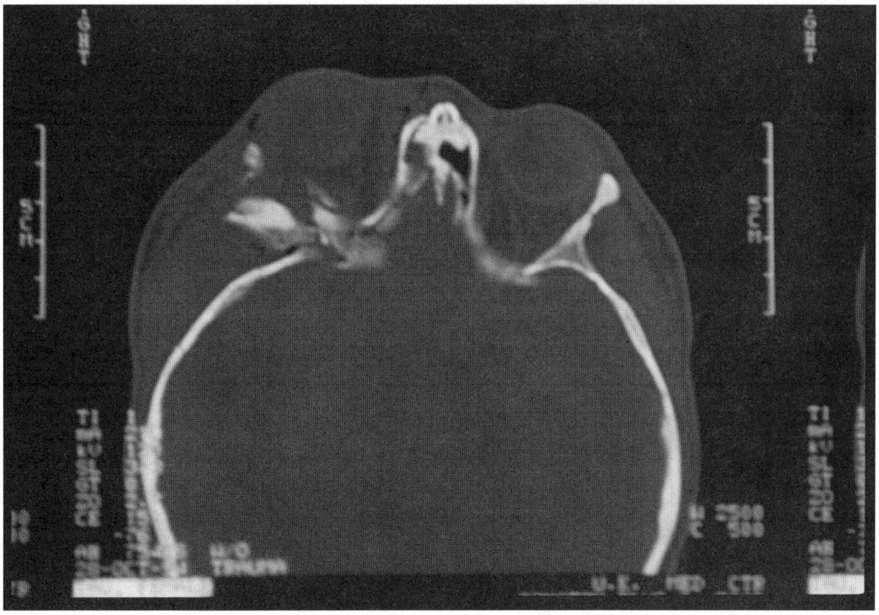

31

Figures 30, 31 (Continued)

utilized to prevent postoperative infection and mucocele formation. Montgomery popularized the use of autogenous fat for obliteration of the human frontal sinus in patients with chronic or refractory frontal sinusitis. A report on their experience and complications with 250 patients undergoing obliteration with fat found an overall perioperative complication rate of 18% (30). However, the length of postoperative follow-up was inadequate to obtain an accurate assessment of mucocele formation and other infectious long-term complications. Weber et al. studied the long-term effectiveness of fat obliteration of the sinus, in which the indications for obliteration included not only frontal sinus fractures but also cases of recurrent or chronic sinusitis in which intranasal drainage could not be restored or in patients with mucoceles. They studied the patients postoperatively with magnetic resonance imaging (MRI) scans and demonstrated mucocele formation in 9.8% of cases and further estimated that the half-life of fat within the sinus to be 15.4 months (31).

Additional autogenous materials, allogenic tissue, and alloplasts have also been explored for obliteration of the frontal sinus (32–36). However, the critical first step in frontal sinus obliteration is meticulous removal of all remnants of the mucosal lining of the sinus, since any residual mucosa can lead to mucocele formation. Donald has described that the mucosa of the frontal sinus is tenacious and can be difficult to remove completely (37). Accordingly, Donald advocated complete ablation of the frontal sinus by cranialization when there is extensive comminution or missing bone in the posterior table. Cranialization involves complete removal of the posterior wall

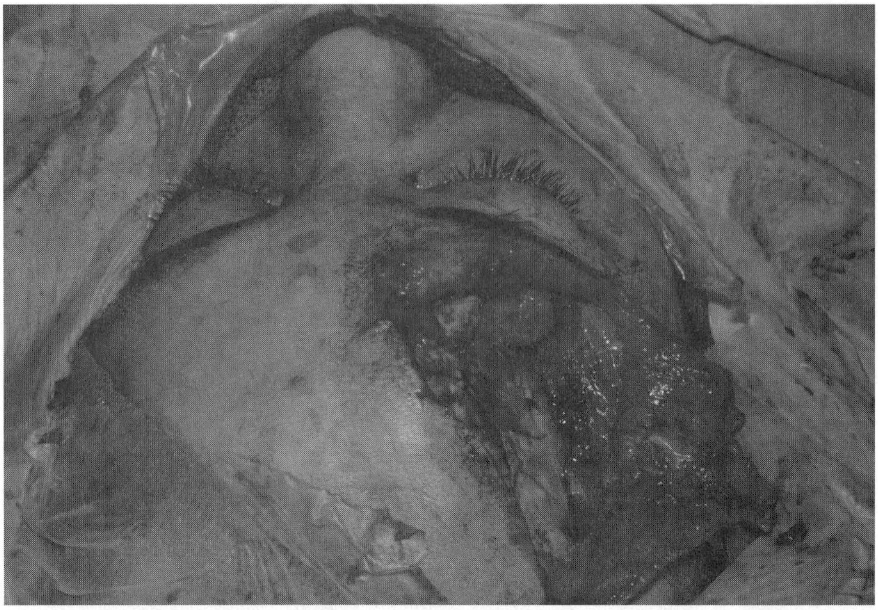

32

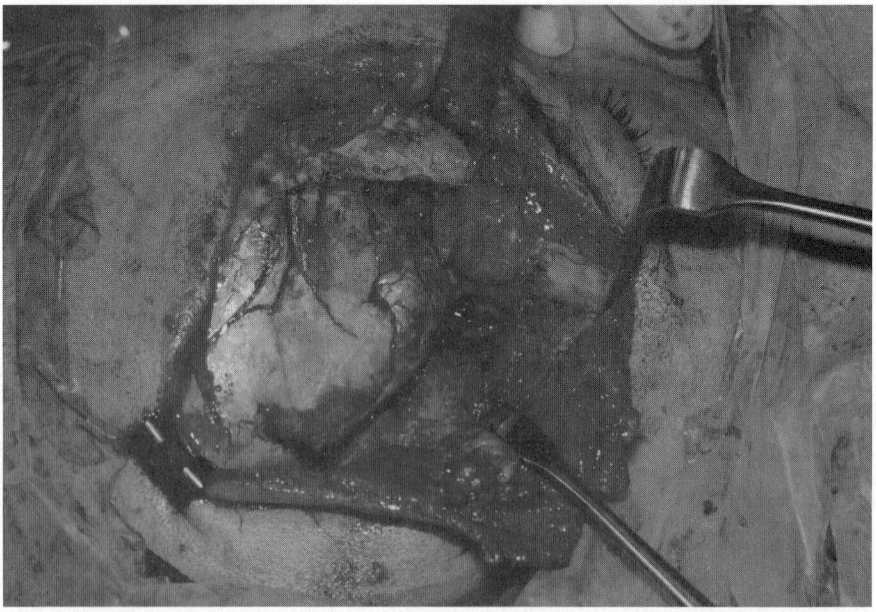

33

Figures 32, 33 Intraoperative view through the patient's existing laceration. Note the extensive orbital roof and skull fractures. Figure 33 shows the exposed brain and dura. Neurosurgical repair of the dura was performed prior to bony repair.

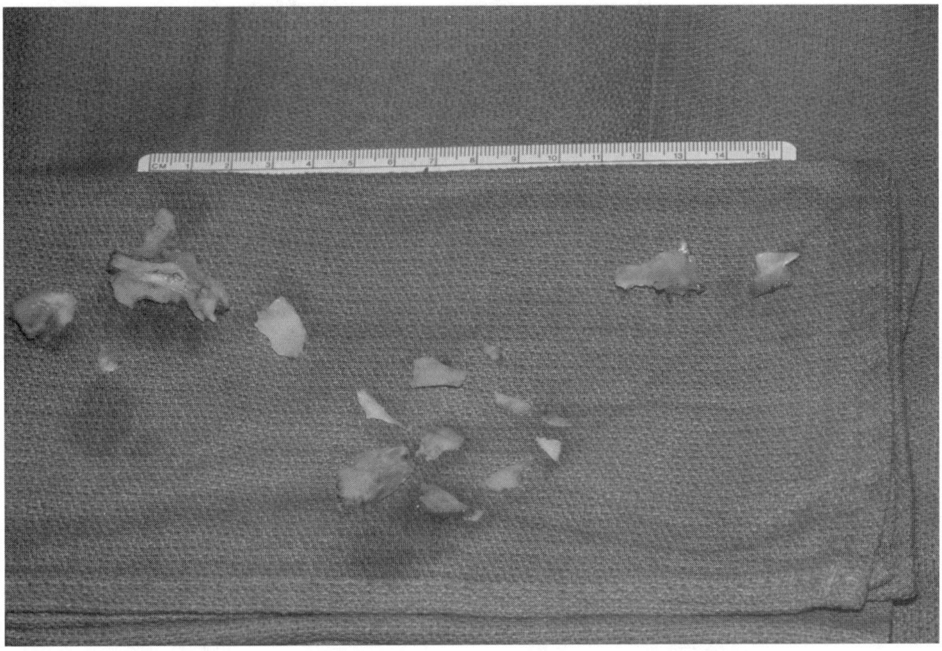

Figure 34 Collected bone fragments from the orbital roof and lateral orbital region in this patient. These pieces were collected, saved, preserved, and replaced in a jigsaw puzzle fashion. This obviated the need for primary autogenous bone grafting.

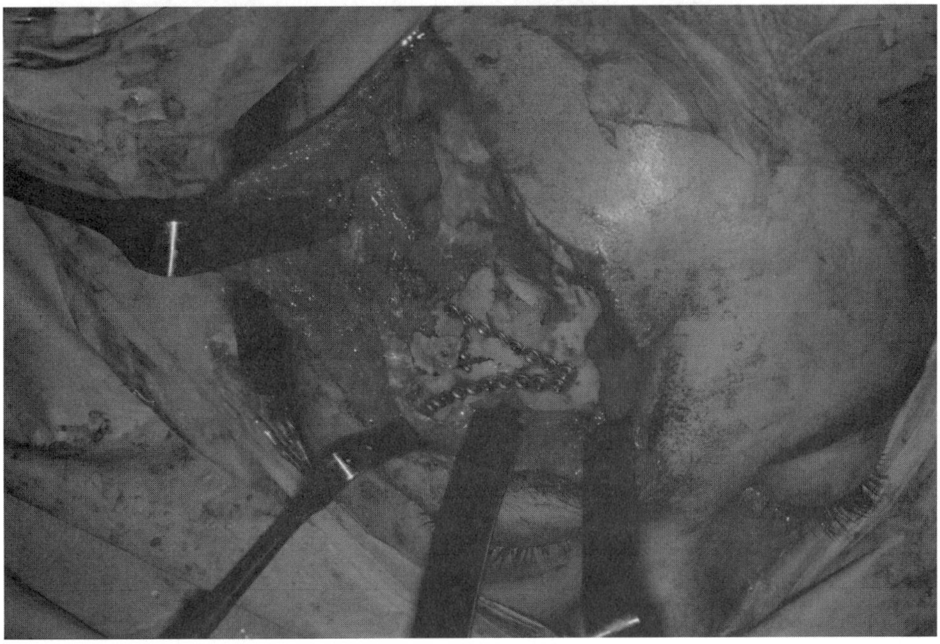

Figure 35 Intraoperative view with replacement of the collected bone fragments in their proper position and the use of titanium plate fixation.

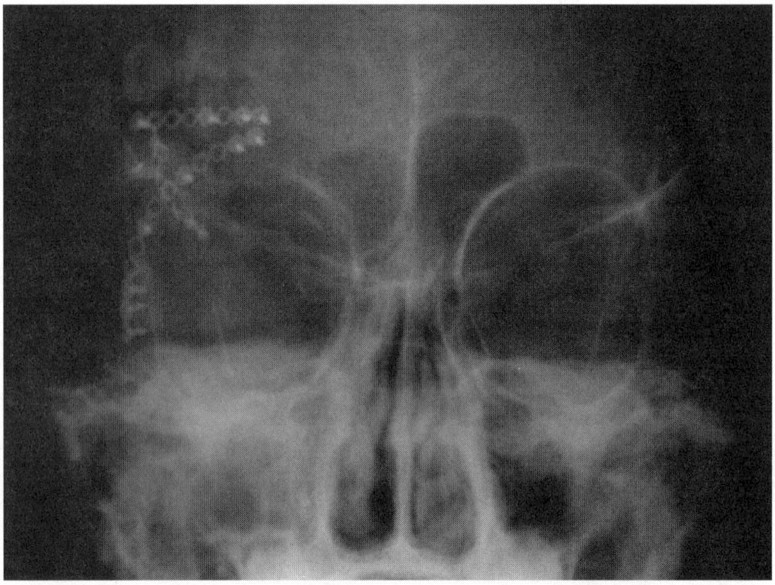

Figure 36 Six-month postoperative radiographic view of patient in Figures 30–35.

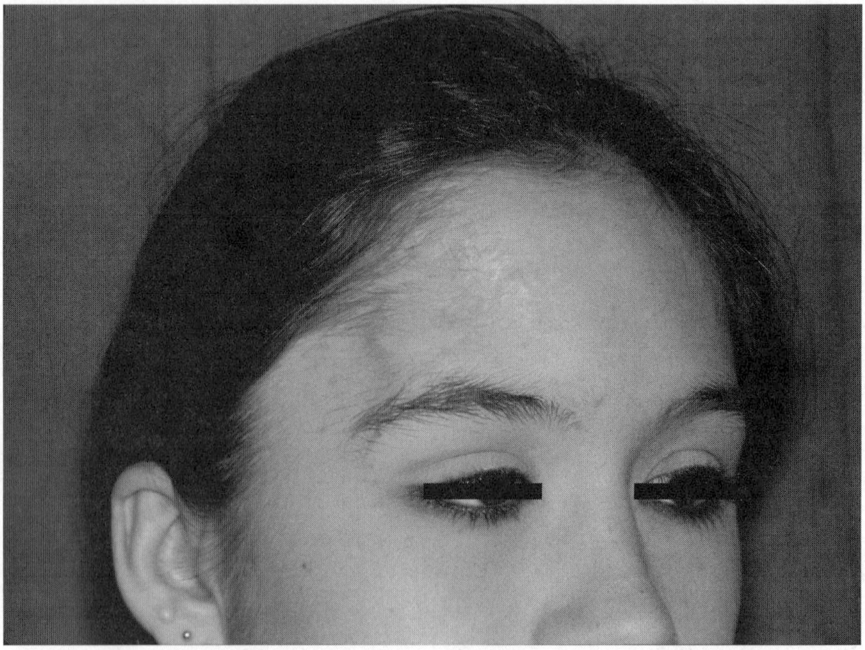

Figure 37 One-year postoperative view of patient in Figures 30–36. She sustained no significant permanent neurological sequelae, despite the significant head injury, and is now attending college.

of the frontal sinus with subsequent forward expansion of the brain into this space (38,39). It is debatable whether complete removal of all frontal sinus mucosa is feasible even with extensive drilling of the sinus walls. Furthermore, since complications such as mucocele formation have been reported as long as 20 years after the original insult, long-term follow-up is necessary to ascertain the efficacy of different techniques, including obliteration with various materials. This length of follow up is seldom attained, with a few exceptions (19), and cranialization of more extensive injuries attempts to create a safe and secure result by ablating the entire frontal sinus.

We advocate a restorative approach with restoration of frontal sinus drainage when nasofrontal outflow tract injury occurs with NOE or anterior table fractures of the frontal sinus. When nasofrontal outflow tract disruption is associated with posterior table fractures, if cranialization of the frontal sinus is not necessary, restoration of drainage in a similar fashion is accomplished as described by Raveh (19). The key steps of this approach are as follows:

1. Determine the need for frontal sinus cranialization when posterior table fractures are present, since this would be a contraindication to restoring drainage. Devitalized mucosa should be removed or stripped from the frontal sinus and supraorbital ethmoid region.
2. A complete subcranial ethmoidectomy is performed on the ipsilateral injury side, essentially removing the entire frontal sinus floor and creating a very wide opening between the frontal sinus and the nasal cavity. This is a critical step for success in restoring drainage and requires ligation or bipolar cautery of the anterior ethmoid vessels.
3. Following reduction of anterior table or NOE fractures, a 2.5–3.5 mm pediatric Silastic endotracheal tube is introduced via the hiatus and placed at the base or the previous floor of the sinus. The superior end of the tube is secured with a 2–0 Vicryl suture to the adjacent frontal sinus anterior table bone. The tube is trimmed intranasally so that its inferior extent is visible emanating from the hiatus. Additional nasal packing is used when indicated but should be removed within a few days postoperatively.
4. Outpatient follow-up 2 weeks postoperatively allows visualization of the tube via anterior rhinoscopy. The patient is started on inhaled nasal aqueous steroids and nasal irrigations if there are no contraindications. The tube is not a drain but a stent that prevents mucosal healing from blocking the frontal sinus outflow tract.
5. Between 3 and 6 months postinjury, the tube is removed under topical intranasal anesthesia with anterior rhinoscopy using a hemostat clamp. Inhaled nasal steroids are continued and subsequent imaging (CT or MRI) can be used to demonstrate an aerated frontal sinus cavity (see Fig. 53).

When posterior table fractures of the frontal sinus are present, neurosurgical consultation should be obtained preoperatively. During surgical repair, the posterior table requires careful inspection and a diligent search for a CSF leak. Comminuted or depressed segments should be carefully dissected free and the dura inspected for tears or leakage sites. With neurosurgical assistance, direct suturing of dural tears or repair with fascial grafts should be completed first. Following dural repair or even when no overt CSF leakage is present, an additional layer of pericranium is placed over the dura with Tisseel fibrin glue (Figs. 38–43). This can be a free graft used in a postage stamp fashion or a pedicled, vascularized pericranial flap similar to those used in skull base reconstruction (33,34).

If there is extensive bone loss or disruption of the posterior table with dural tears, restoration of physiological drainage to the frontal sinus is contraindicated. In these situations, we prefer cranialization to obliteration of the sinus with various materials. Obliteration with autogenous fat is not physiological, is less secure, and is more prone to long-term complications such as mucoceles, meningitis, or other infectious complications due to mucosal remnants. Besides lingering questions about the ability to remove all of the tenacious frontal sinus mucosa without bone removal, cranialization of such severe injuries seems to be a more reasonable approach with greater efficacy and security in preventing potentially serious long-term complications.

During cranialization, complete removal of bone and tissue from the posterior table of the frontal sinus is accomplished with neurosurgical assistance and using a subcranial approach as described below. The nasofrontal duct areas are plugged with

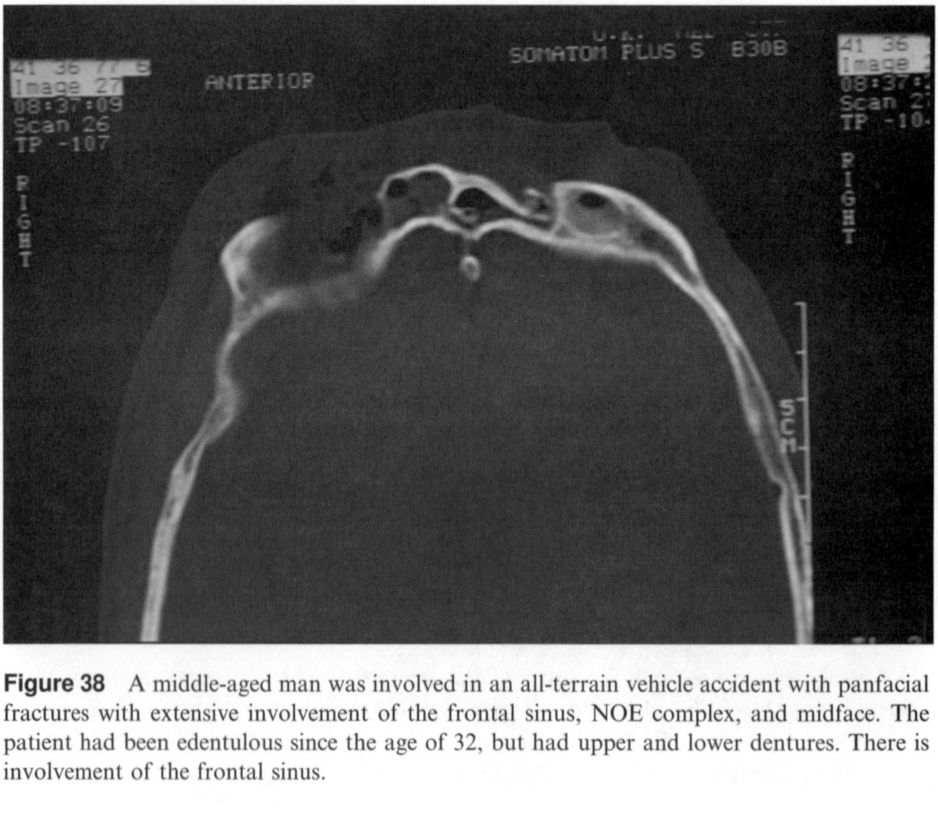

Figure 38 A middle-aged man was involved in an all-terrain vehicle accident with panfacial fractures with extensive involvement of the frontal sinus, NOE complex, and midface. The patient had been edentulous since the age of 32, but had upper and lower dentures. There is involvement of the frontal sinus.

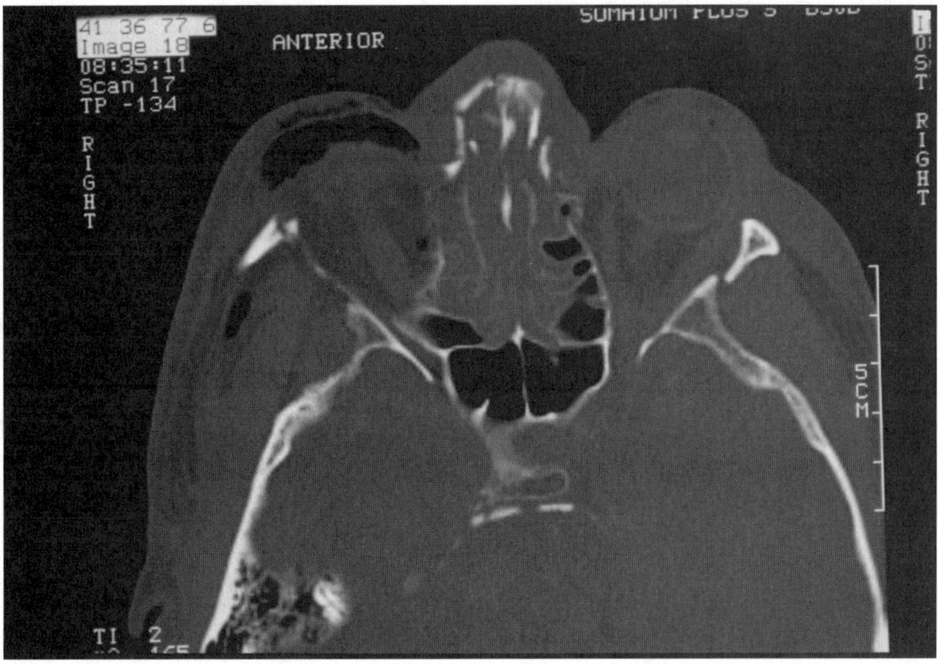

Figure 39 There is involvement of both orbits with nasoethmoid complex and bilateral LeFort III fractures.

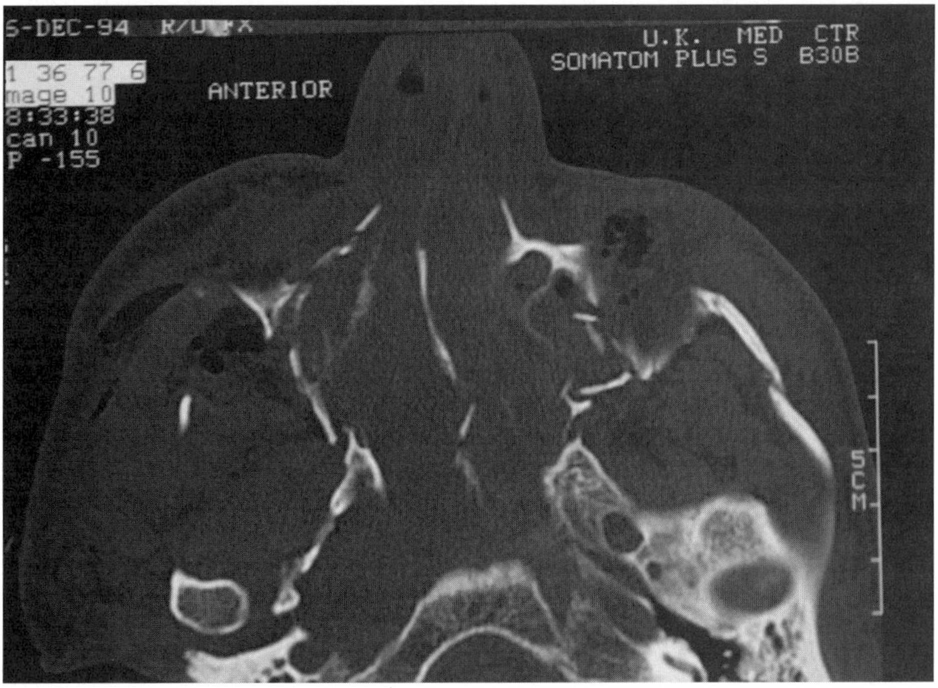

Figure 40 Extensive bilateral comminuted midface fractures are present.

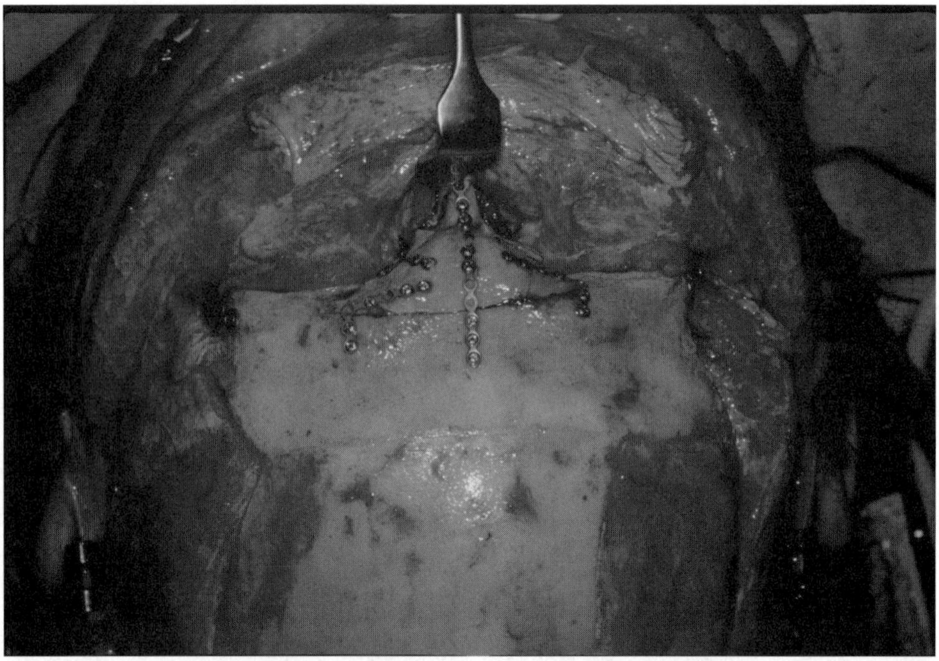

Figure 41 Coronal incision used for exposure of the fractures. Note that the pericranial flap has been raised and the anterior table of the frontal sinus has been replaced with titanium microplates following cranialization of the posterior table. Retractor is on patient's bony nasal dorsum.

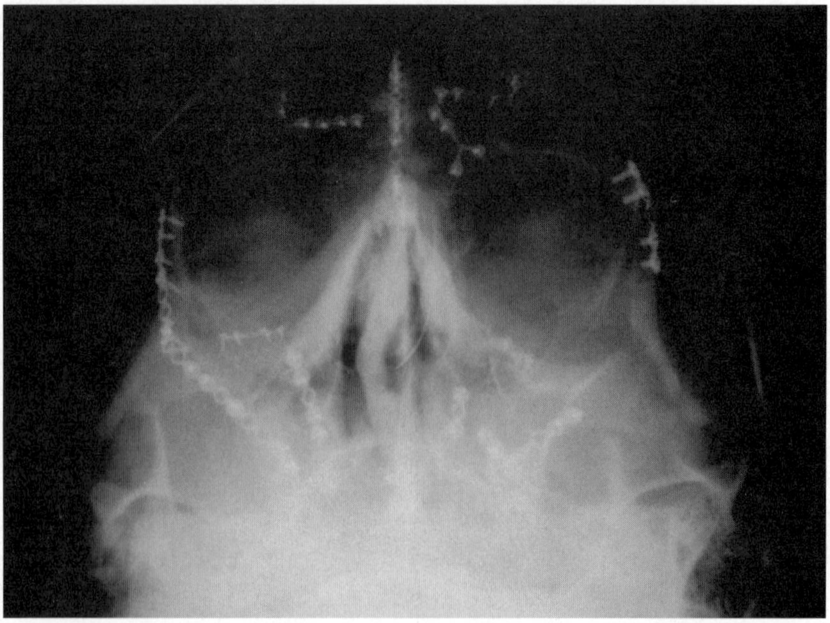

Figure 42 Postoperative Water's radiograph. Note the extensive plates used to restore midface vertical height and anterior facial projection. Patient also had additional mandible fractures treated with internal fixation.

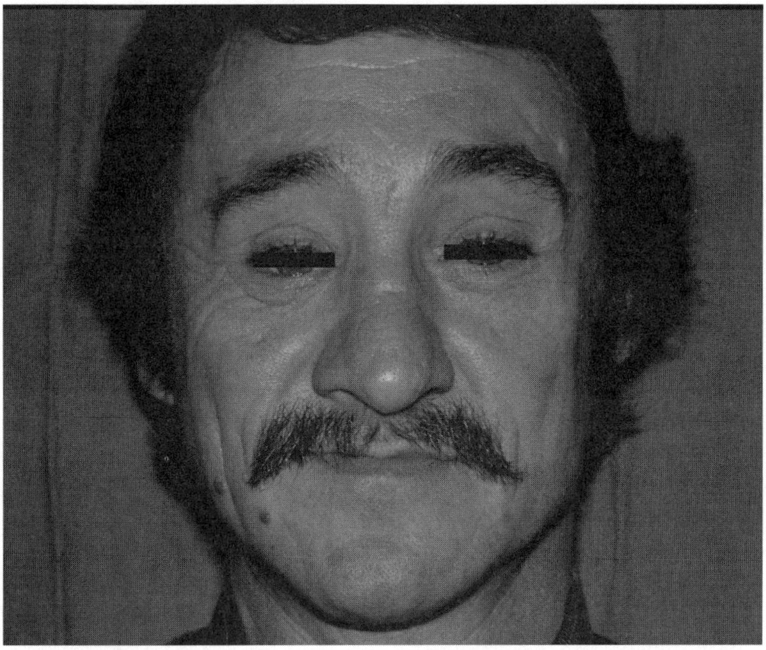

Figure 43 One-year postoperative appearance of the patient in Figures 38–42.

fascia or muscle after inversion of the mucosal lining at the orifice (40). Sharp edges or bony recesses and the back wall of the anterior table are burred carefully with a drill before placement of a vascularized, pedicled pericranial flap against all exposed dural surfaces with Tisseel fibrin glue. This acts as an additional barrier or roof to separate the paranasal sinuses and the intracranial frontal dura. The anterior table bone is then reconstructed as described earlier.

NOE Fractures

Fractures of the NOE complex, by definition, usually result in variable amounts of damage to the nasofrontal outflow tract and are often associated with adjacent fractures of the frontal sinus and midface. Treatment of NOE fractures aims to restore normal dorsal nasal projection and contour, and restore the preinjury intercanthal distance and medial canthal soft tissue relationships. Nondisplaced or minimally displaced type I NOE fractures, based on clinical assessment and CT scan analysis, may require no operative treatment. High-quality CT imaging, preferably in both axial and coronal planes, is invaluable in treatment planning for NOE fractures.

Closed reduction with percutaneous wires and lead plate stabilization are still utilized by some surgeons. These methods seldom result in adequate reduction or correction of telecanthus, and may produce skin necrosis in the medial canthal area. These methods should be relegated to the historical archives; instead, proper reduction and stabilization should be performed through an open approach, when indicated. When concomitant forehead or nasal lacerations are present, these can be utilized with careful extensions into the brows to provide access. As an alternative, a bilateral brow incision can provide limited access when no lacerations are present. However, the coronal incision, as described earlier, provides the best access. Exposure of NOE fractures involves further dissection via the coronal approach over the nasal dorsum, orbital roof, and medial orbital wall and lamina papyracea.

Management of the nasofrontal outflow tract has already been outlined in the previous section. Once this is accomplished, reduction of the fractured and displaced type I NOE fracture is done with microplate fixation of the thin bones. Larger plates are unnecessary and should be avoided since they may be easily palpable under thin skin. The final step involves a medial canthopexy for restoration of the preinjury intercanthal distance and adjacent soft tissue relationships.

Type 2 NOE injuries are considerably more problematic because they involve significant disruption of the anterior skull base with posterior displacement of the nasal buttress underneath the skull base. As a consequence, dural tears with CSF leakage, pneumocranium, and frontal lobe brain contusion occur frequently with this type of injury (Figs. 38–43). These fractures can extend along the cribriform plate into the orbital apex and sellar regions, possibly resulting in contusion or compression of the optic nerve (19). Ophthalmology consultation should be obtained and treatment planning of these fractures requires coordination and cooperation with neurosurgical consultants.

Exposure of type 2 NOE fractures via a coronal incision and a subcranial approach is initially followed by debridement of bone fragments along the ethmoid compartment and orbital apex, and optic nerve decompression when indicated. Next, dural tears are sutured and additional layers of fascia with fibrin glue (Tisseel) are placed along the skull base to ensure watertight separation of the dura from the paranasal spaces. The third step involves meticulous reduction and microplate or wire fixation of fractured bone segments. The final step involves a Raveh-type medial canthopexy that not only reduces the intercanthal distance but also posteriorly reduces the medial canthal tendons into a more accurate position (19). This remains the best method for correcting traumatic telecanthus, providing superior results to other available methods for canthopexy such as transnasal wiring (Figs. 44–55).

The subcranial or subfrontal approach has been recommended for treating posterior table frontal sinus fractures and type 2 NOE fractures and merits further explanation. The subcranial/subfrontal approach was developed by Raveh and others to provide wide access to anterior skull base tumors without excessive frontal lobe retraction and contusion that contribute to postoperative morbidity (19). The numerous advantages of this approach can be applied to craniofacial fractures involving the anterior skull base such as type 2 NOE or posterior table frontal sinus fractures (41). Surgeons involved in the treatment of these fractures should become familiar with the techniques for subcranial/subfrontal access to provide optimal and early treatment of these injuries. Since many of these patients have some degree of frontal lobe contusion due to the nature of the injury, the subcranial approach is especially advantageous in permitting early repair of these fractures without compromising access while avoiding frontal lobe retraction.

Before the availability of CT imaging, treatment of these fractures was commonly deferred or delayed 7–10 days to allow stabilization of the patient's

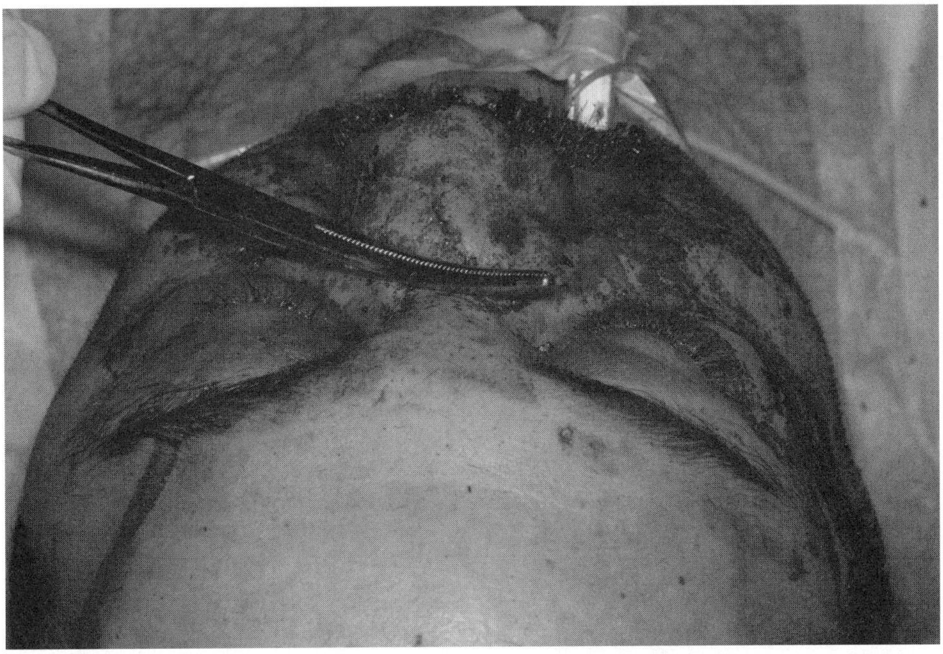

Figure 44 Patient with extensive NOE complex and midface fractures. Note the traumatic telecanthus and telescoping of the nasal buttress underneath the skull base.

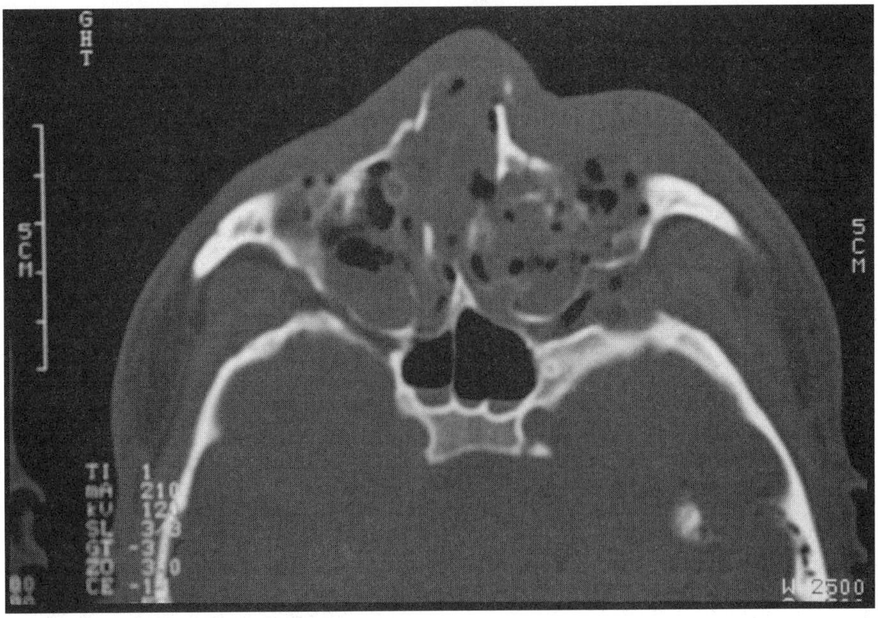

45

Figures 45–47 Axial and coronal CT scans show the nasoethmoid complex, midface, and extensive orbital fractures.

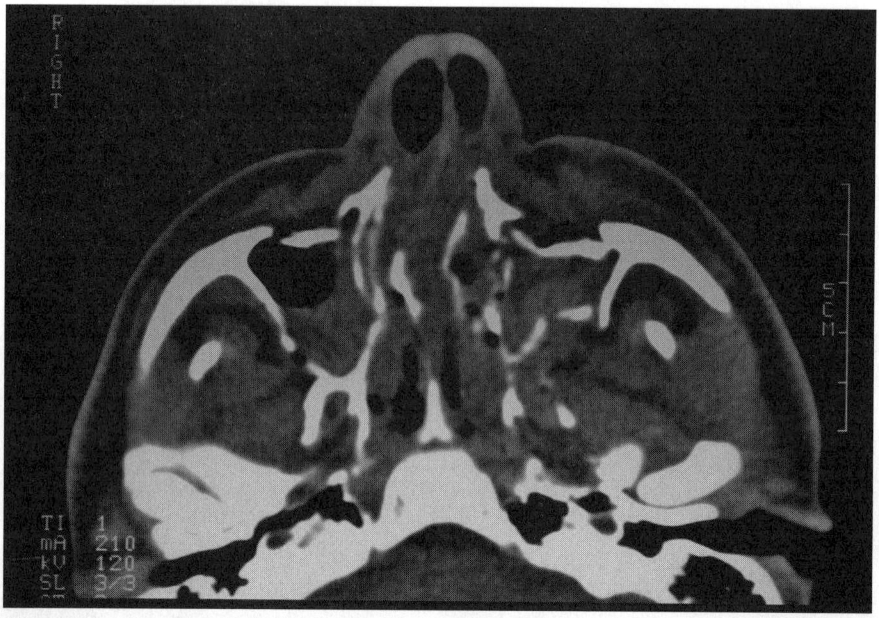

46

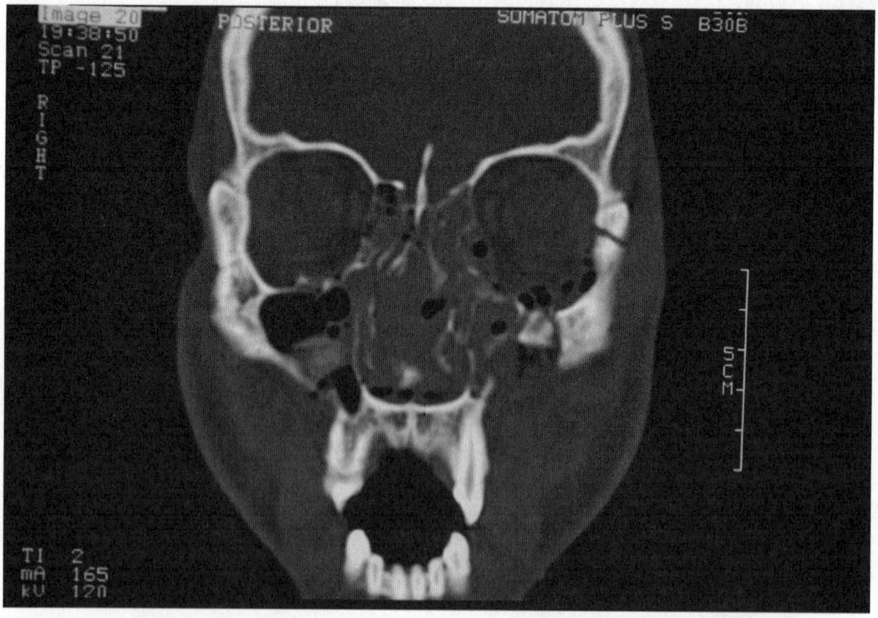

47

Figures 45–47 (Continued)

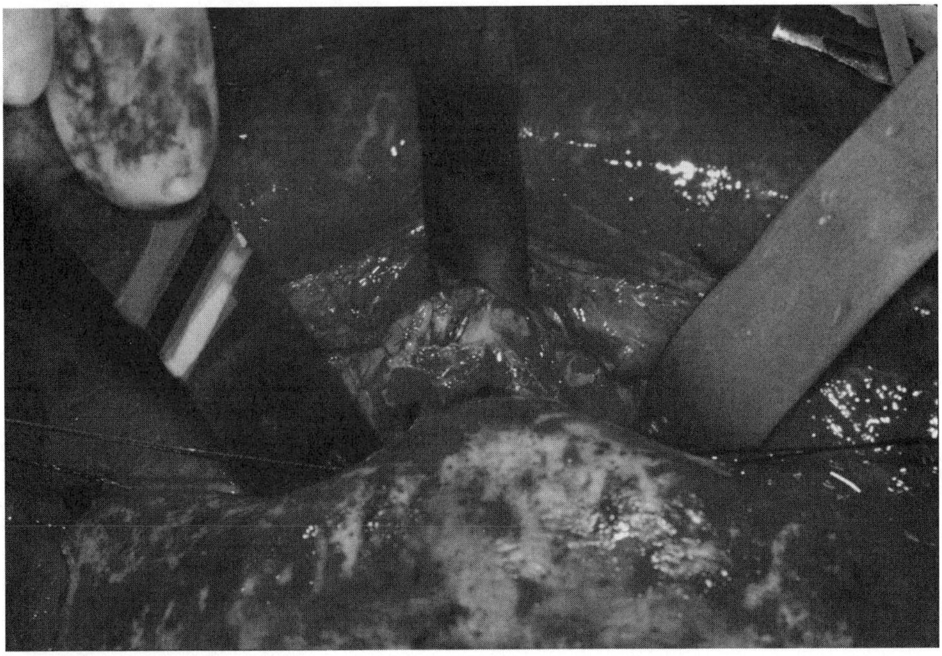

Figure 48 Intraoperative view via a coronal incision. Note retractor on the nasal buttress or dorsum. The sutures show a Raveh crossover medial canthopexy being performed. The sutures on the patient's right represent the left medial canthal tendon with the sutures having been passed underneath the nasal frame to the opposite side.

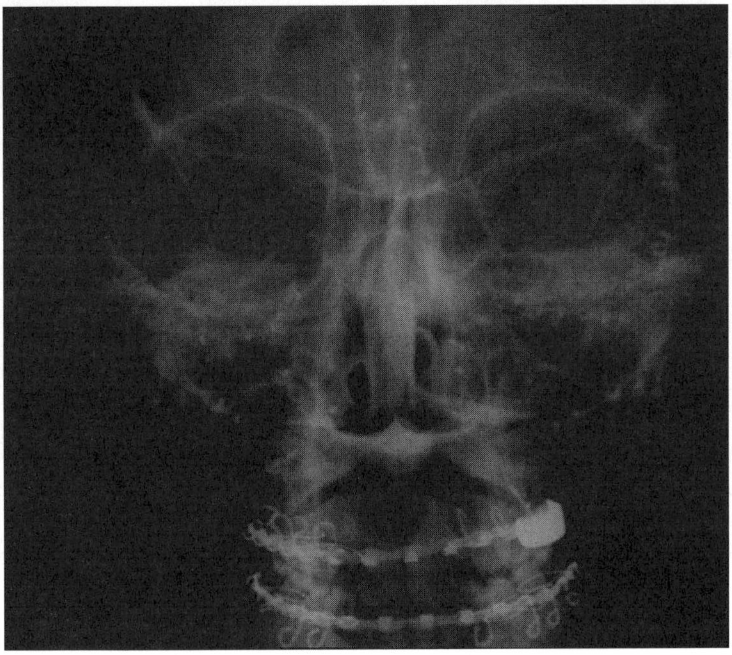

Figure 49 Postoperative radiograph of the patient in Figures 44–48.

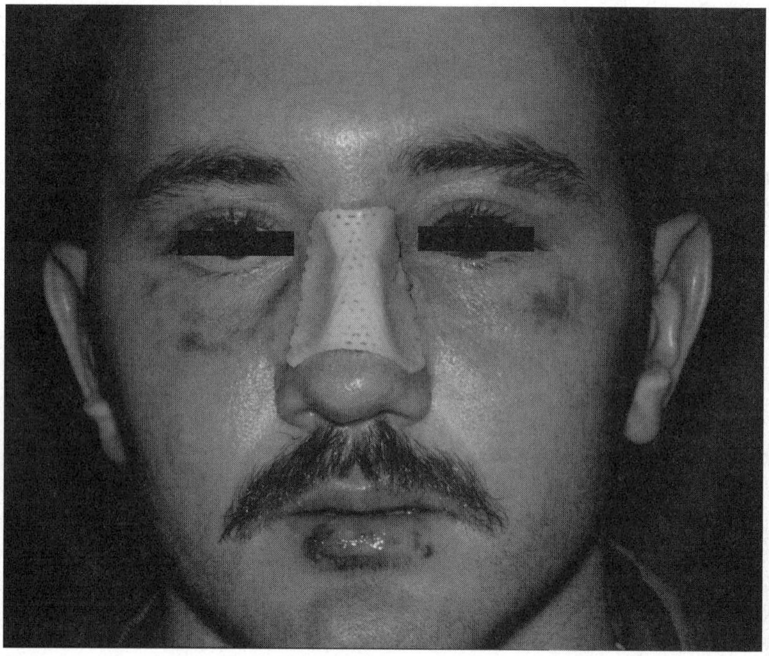

50

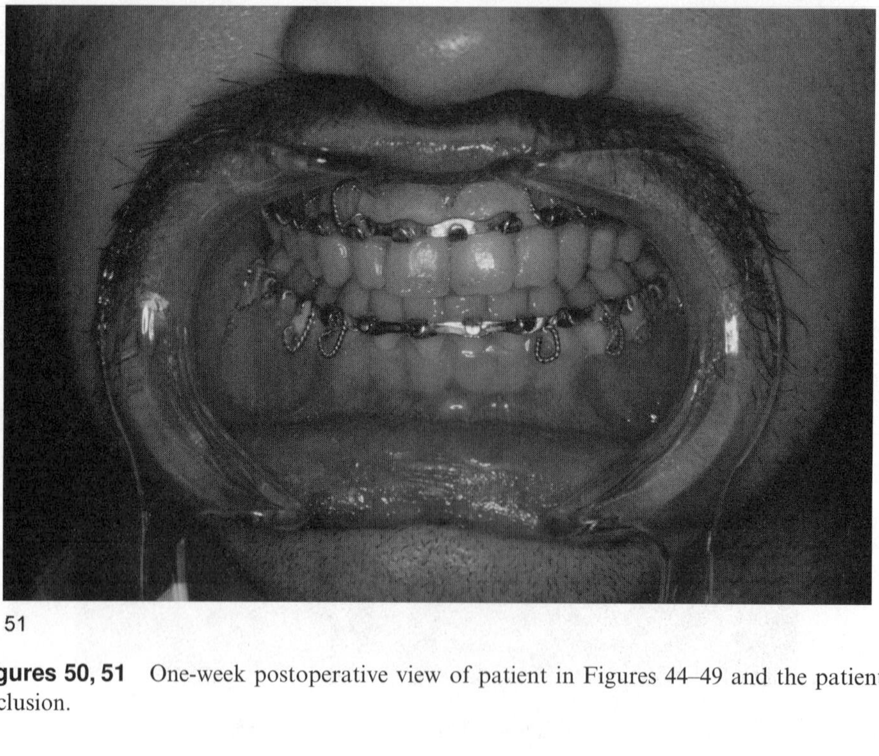

51

Figures 50, 51 One-week postoperative view of patient in Figures 44–49 and the patient's occlusion.

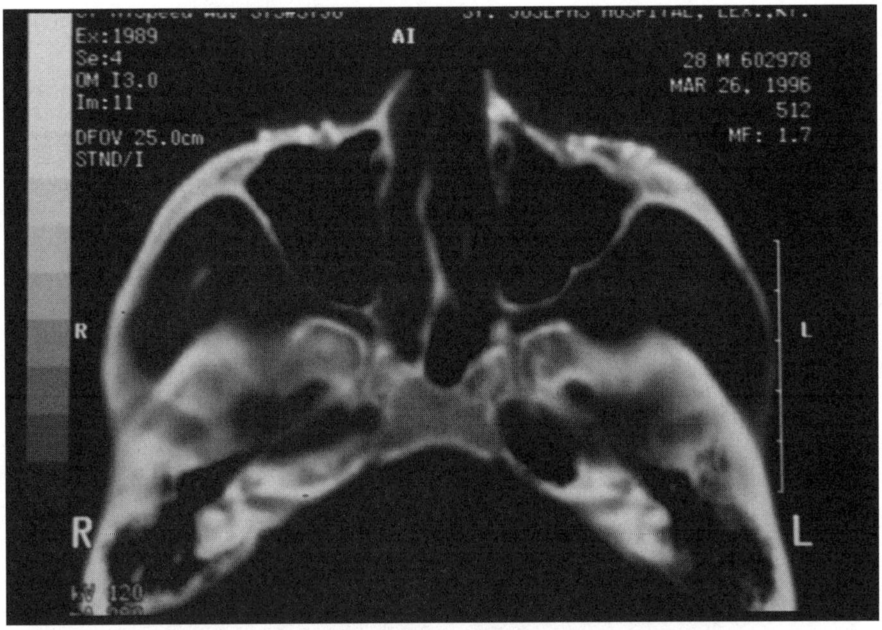

52

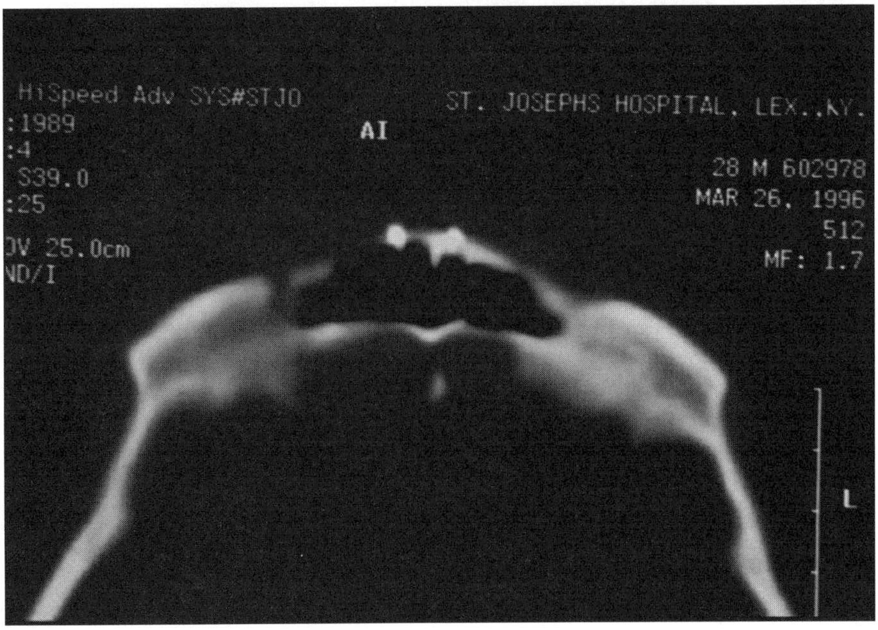

53

Figures 52, 53 Six-month postoperative CT scans of the patient in Figures 44–51. Note the well-aerated frontal sinus in Figure 53.

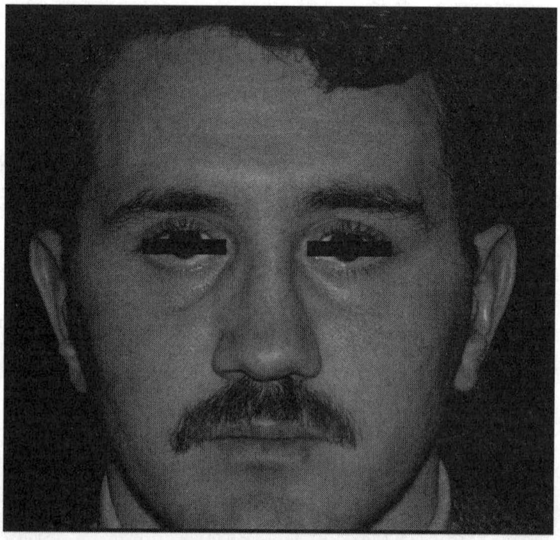

54

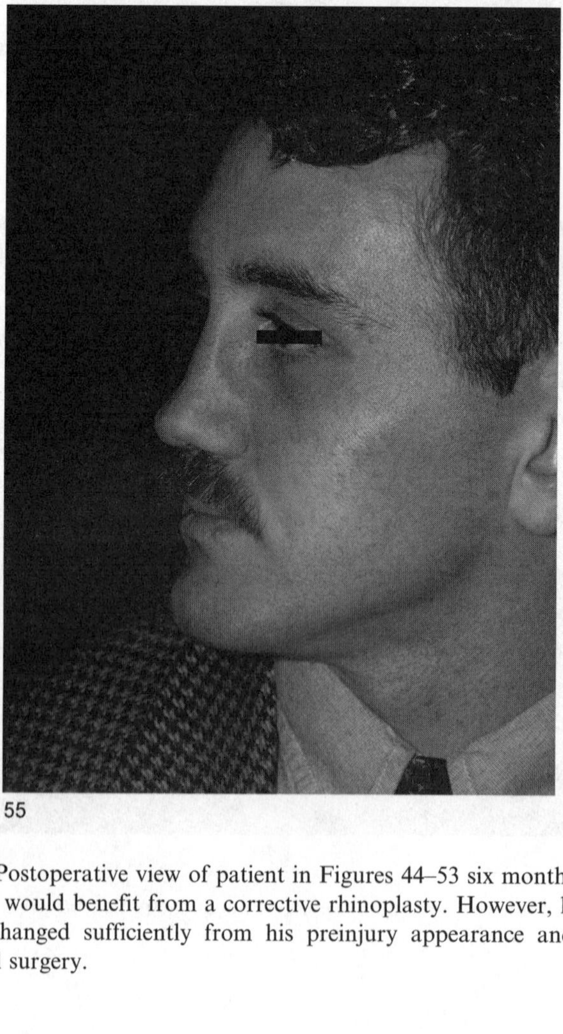

55

Figures 54, 55 Postoperative view of patient in Figures 44–53 six months after injury. We believe the patient would benefit from a corrective rhinoplasty. However, he did not feel his appearance had changed sufficiently from his preinjury appearance and decided not to proceed with nasal surgery.

condition and to allow brain and facial edema to subside. Over the past 25 years, some of the relevant key advances that have occurred are availability of high-quality CT imaging to delineate fractures clearly, improvements in neuroanesthesia, advances in invasive monitoring and critical care, and development of skull base surgical techniques such as the subcranial approach. Despite these numerous advances, many surgeons continue to cling to obsolete concepts from the past, and delay or defer treatment of these fractures without justification. If CT imaging clearly reveals fractures needing repair, then there is no benefit to delaying treatment. Only if the patient's medical condition is unstable due to multiple-trauma or severe head injury, or if there is uncertainty about the need to treat the fractures, should treatment be deferred. Furthermore, if the surgeon is familiar with the subcranial approach then mild head injury or frontal lobe contusion should not be used as excuses for delaying treatment. Earlier treatment of these fractures, preferably within 72 h of injury when possible, will produce better results, reduce patient morbidity and length of hospitalization, and provide more advanced and cost-effective care. The subcranial approach and the timing of surgery are discussed further in Chapter 14.

REFERENCES

1. Stanley RB, Nowak GM. Midfacial fractures: Importance of angle of impact to horizontal craniofacial buttresses. Otolaryngol Head Neck Surg 1985; 93:186–191.
2. Manson, PN, Shack RB, Leonard LG, et al. Sagittal fractures of the maxilla and palate. Plast Reconstr Surg 1983; 72:484.
3. Hendrickson M, Clark N, Manson PN et al. Palatal fractures: classifcation, patterns, and treatment with rigid internal fixation. Plast Reconstr Surg 1998; 101:319.
4. Manson PN, Crawley WA et al. Midface fractures: advantage of immediate extended open reduction and bone grafting. Plast Reconstr Surg 1985; 76:1–9.
5. Adams WM. Internal wiring fixation of facial fractures. Surgery 1942; 523.
6. Shumrick KA, Kersten RC et al. Extended access/ internal approaches for the management of facial trauma. Arch Otolaryngol head Neck Surg 1992; 118:1105–1111.
7. Evans GRD, Clark N, Manson PN. Role of mini and micorplate fixation in fractures of the midface and mandible. Ann Plast Surg 1995; 34:453–456.
8. Messerklinger W. On the drainage of the normal frontal sinus of man. Acta Otolaryngol 1967; 63:176–181.
9. Heine RD. Naso-orbital-ethmoid injury: report of a case and review of the literature. Oral Surg Oral Med Oral Pathol. 1990; 69:542–549.
10. Anderson, RL. The medial canthal tendon branches out. Arch Ophthalmol 1977; 95:2051–2052.
11. Lakhani RS, Shibuya TY, Mathog RH et al. Titanium mesh repair of the severely comminuted frontal sinus fracture. Arch Otolaryngol Head Neck Surg 2001; 127:665–669.
12. Nahum AM. The biomechanics of maxillofacial trauma. Clin Plast Surg 1975; 42:59–64.
13. Cummings CW, Fredrickson JM, Harker LA, Krause CJ, Richardson MA, Schuller DE. Third edition, Otolaryngology Head and Neck Surgery. Vol 1. Mosby, MO: St. Louis, MO, 1998.
14. Manson PN, Clark N, Robertson B et al. Subunit principles in midface fractures: the importance of sagittal buttresses, soft- tissue reductions, and sequencing treatment of segmental fractures. Plast Reconstr Surg 1999; 103:1287–1305.

15. Ioannides C, Freihofer HP. Fractures of the frontal sinus: classification and its implications for surgical treatment. Am Otolaryngol 1999; 20:273–280.
16. Heine RD, Catone GA, Bavitz JB, Grenadier MR. Naso-orbital-ethmoid injury: report of a case and review of the literature. Oral Surg Oral Med Oral Pathol 1990; 69:542–549.
17. Evans GRD, Clark N, Manson PN. Identification and management of minimally displaced nasoethmoidal orbital fractures. Ann Plastic Surg 1995; 35:469–473.
18. Markowitz, BL, Manson PN et al. Management of the medial canthal tendon in nasoethmoid orbital fractures: the importance of the central fragment in classification and treatment. Plast Reconstr Surg 1991; 87:843–853.
19. Raveh J, Laedrach K, Vuillemin T et al. Management of combined frontonaso-orbital/skull base fractures and telecanthus in 355 cases. Arch Otolaryngol Head Neck Surg 1992; 118:605–614.
20. Ellis E. Sequencing treatment for naso-orbito-ethmoid fractures. J Oral Maxillofac Surg 1993; 51:543–558.
21. Lappert PW, Lee JW. Treatment of an isolated outer table frontal sinus fracture using endoscopic reduction and fixation. Plast Reconstr Surg 1998; 102:1642–1645.
22. Amano T, Inamura T, Inoha S, Shono T, Ikezaki K, Matsushima T, Mizoguchi J, Fukui M. (Influence of scalp shaving on prevention of postoperative intracranial infection). No Shinkei Geka 1999; 10:883–888.
23. Sheinberg MA, Ross DA. Cranial procedures without hair removal. Neurosurgery. 1999; 6:1263–1265.
24. Imola MJ, Hamlar DD, Shao W, Chowdhury K, Tatum S. Resorbable plate fixation in pediatric craniofacial surgery: long-term outcome. Arch Facial Plast Surg 2001; 2:79–90.
25. Stassen LFA, McGuinness AJ. A simple method of plate fixation of fractures of the frontal bone. Br J Oral Maxillofac Surg 1999; 37:438–439.
26. Kohan D, Plasse HM, Zide BM. Frontal bone reconstruction with split calvarial and cancellous iliac bone. Ear Nose Throat J 1989; 68:845.
27. Schortingbuis J, Zeebregts CJ, Bos RRM. Frontal bone reconstruction using patellar bone: a case report. J Oral Maxillofac Surg 1999; 57:1132–1133.
28. Powell NB, Riley RW. Cranial bone grafting in facial aesthetic and reconstructive contouring. Arch Otolaryngol Head Neck Surg 1987; 113:713–719.
29. Dolan RW, Chowdhury K. Diagnosis and treatment of intracranial complications of paranasal sinus infections. J Oral Maxillofac Surg 1995; 53:1080–1087.
30. Hardy JM, Montgomery WW. Osteoplastic frontal sinusotomy: an analysis of 250 operations. Ann. Otolaryngol Rhinol Laryngol 1976; 85:523.
31. Weber R, Draf W et al. Osteoplastic frontal sinus surgery with fat obliteration: technique and long term results using magnetic resonance imaging in 82 operations. Laryngoscope. 2000; 110:1037–1044.
32. Mickel TJ, Rohrich RJ, Robinson JD. Frontal sinus obliteration: a comparison of fat, muscle, bone and spontaneous osteoneogenesis in the cat model. Plast Reconstr Surg 1995; 95:586–592.
33. Thaller SR, Donald P. The use of pericranial flaps in frontal sinus fractures. Ann Plast Surg 1994; 32:284–287.
34. Ducic Y, Stone TL. Frontal sinus obliteration using a laterally based pedicled pericranial flap. Laryngoscope 1999; 109:541–545.
35. McNeil RA. Surgical obliteration of the frontal sinus. Laryngoscope 1967; 77:202.
36. Rohrich RJ, Mickel TJ. Frontal sinus obliteration: in search of the ideal autogenous material. Plast Reconstr Surg 1995; 95:580–585.
37. Donald PJ. Recent advances in para-nasal sinus surgery. Head Neck Surg 1981; 4 146–153.

38. Donald PJ. The tenacity of the frontal sinus mucosa. Otolaryngol Head Neck Surg 1979; 87:557.
39. Donald PJ. Frontal sinus ablation by cranialization. Arch Otolaryngol 1982; 108:142.
40. Schenck NL, Rauchbach E, Ogura JH. Frontal sinus disease II. Development of the frontal sinus model. Occlusion of the nasofrontal duct. Laryngoscope 1974; 84:1233.
41. Kellman RM. Use of the subcranial approach in maxillofacial trauma. Facial Plast Surg Clin North Am 1998; 64:501–510.

16

Practical Diagnosis and Management of Mandibular and Dentoalveolar Fractures

Robert E. Lincoln
Boston Medical Center, Boston, Massachusetts, U.S.A.

INTRODUCTION

The clinician who diagnoses and treats facial trauma should be guided by a comprehensive practical clinical and radiographic examination of the patient combined with a thorough knowledge of applicable treatment modalities. The information in this chapter is meant to be practical, not exhaustive. It is the hope that the reader, whether student or experienced practitioner, will develop and implement an approach to treatment of these injuries both to suit his or her skill level and provide predictable and acceptable outcomes for patients.

EPIDEMIOLOGY

Mandibular fractures and dentoalveolar injuries are most commonly the result of motor vehicle accidents, interpersonal violence and assault, sporting accidents, or falls (1). Most fractures occur in the mandibular body, angle, or condyle regions, with lower percentages in the mandibular ramus, coronoid and symphysis regions (2) (Fig. 1). The literature demonstrates that many patients with mandible fractures have more than one fracture location. This may be due to a number of variables such as direction and force of the blow, mechanism of injury, teeth present or not, among others. A number of classification schemes have been presented to describe mandible fractures, the most notable being type of fracture and site of fracture. *Dorland's Medical Dictionary*'s definitions for fractures are sufficient to describe simple, compound, comminuted complex, and pathological mandible fractures (3). However, fractures in children, edentulous atrophic mandible fractures, and complex fractures (i.e., secondary to gun shot wounds, avulsive injuries, or panfacial injuries) deserve special consideration. The muscles of the facial skeleton also influence the classification of mandible fractures depending on their action at the fracture site.

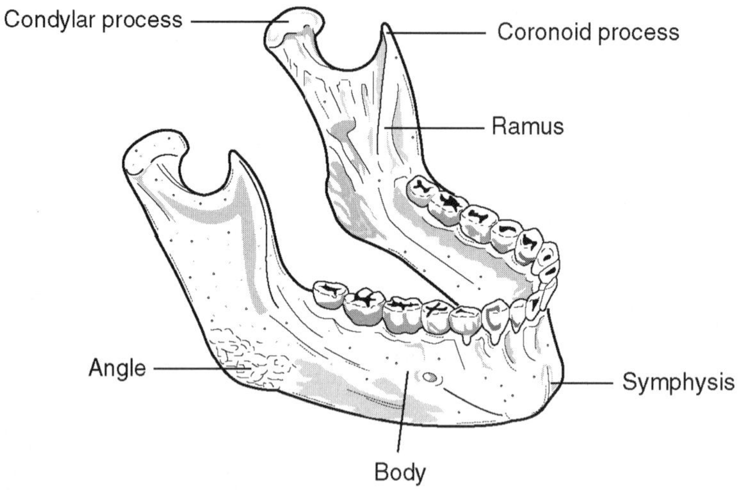

Figure 1 Mandible anatomy.

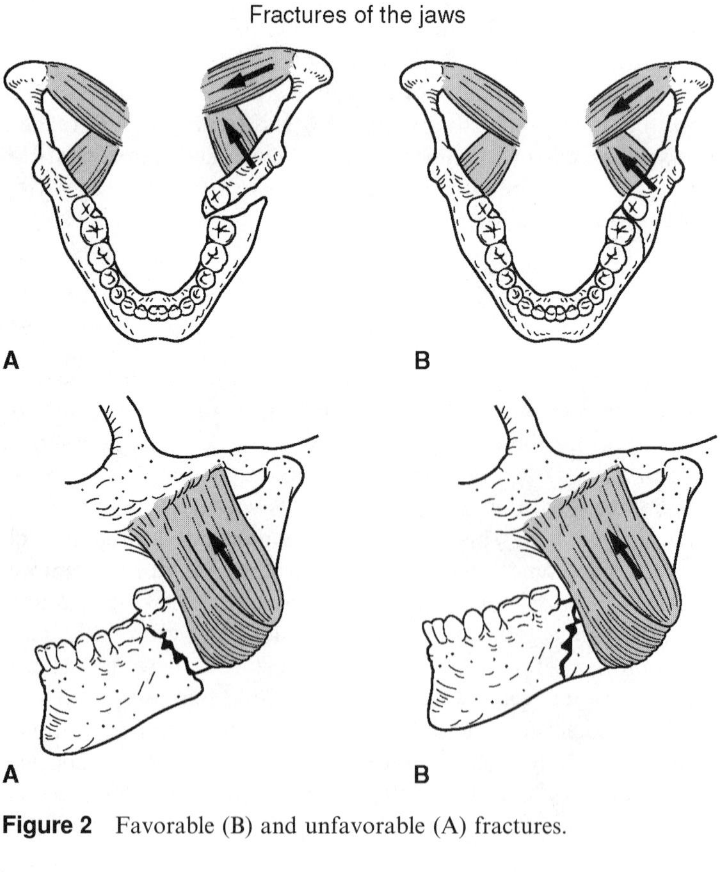

Figure 2 Favorable (B) and unfavorable (A) fractures.

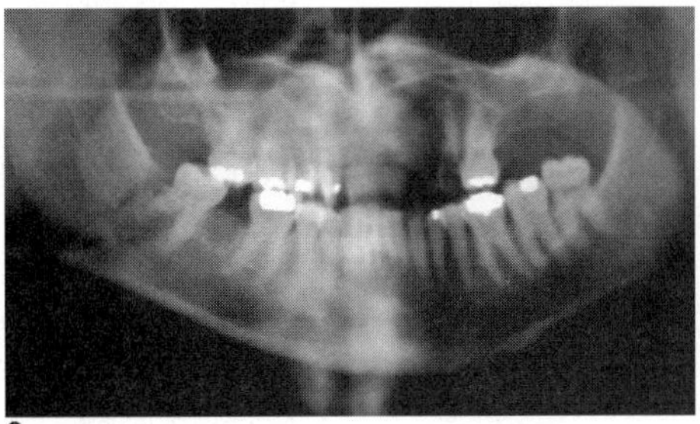

3

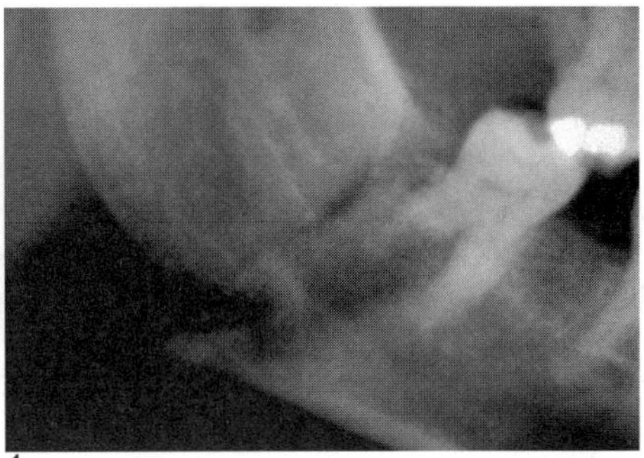

4

Figures 3, 4 Vertically unfavorable fracture of the mandibular angle. Note superior distraction of proximal segment.

Fractures of the mandibular angle may be horizontally favorable (reduced) or unfavorable (displaced) depending on the direction of the fracture and the action of the pterygomasseteric sling. Conversely the same fracture may be vertically favorable or unfavorable depending on the action of the medial and lateral pterygoid muscles on the proximal segment (the angle) Figs. 2–4.

MANDIBLE FRACTURES

Diagnosis

In the treatment of mandible fractures, a successful diagnosis is an absolute necessity as the first step to predictable treatment. An unsuccessful or missed diagnosis will almost certainly jeopardize a favorable outcome. A thorough history of the injury coupled with a comprehensive clinical examination and high-quality radiographic studies serve as the roadmap to treatment. For practitioners training or practicing in a level I trauma center, emergency room, or trauma team, the Advanced Trauma Life Support (ATLS) protocol will dictate the need for emergency evaluation of facial injuries. With mandibular fractures, immediate concerns can range from control of hemorrhage to airway control compromised by aspirated teeth, loss of tongue support, or edema. For example, a maxillofacial surgeon who quickly recognizes a stridorous patient with bilateral mandibular condyle fracture dislocations with a midline symphysis fracture, a hematoma in the floor of the mouth, with avulsed and missing teeth, should direct the trauma team to secure the airway for both immediate and future management of the patient. All practitioners should, regardless of practice setting, be aware of the need to triage facial treatment patients for injuries known to occur in conjunction with mandible fractures such as closed/open open head injuries, cervical spine injuries, injuries of the larynx and hyoid, and vascular injuries (4).

In a stable patient, a thorough history should be obtained. What was the mechanism of injury: fist, shod foot, baseball bat, fall, motor vehicle accident? Was the injury witnessed? Was there any loss of consciousness? Is there a previous history of facial trauma or fractures, either treated or untreated? Were there any pre-existing dental conditions such as deviated or limited opening of the mouth;

a cross-bite, open bite, or other malocclusion; or the use of partial or complete dentures? The patient's medical history, allergies, and medications are important, as well as the patient's social situation and habits. Patients with a history of alcohol or drug abuse have posttreatment compliance issues, which compromise their treatment outcome (5). The age of the fracture upon presentation is important as well. Compound fractures that present 5–10 days after injury may be acutely or chronically infected, and may drastically change the practitioner's approach to management.

The practitioner should make a concerted effort to correlate the findings from the clinical examination with both the history and any available radiographs. A thorough clinical examination should start with an extraoral review of the patient and then move intraorally. Areas of abnormal facial contour or asymmetry should be noted. Preauricular swelling is often indicative of a condyle fracture. Loss of prominence of the mandibular angle may be a sign of an unfavorable fracture in this region. Chin deviation often indicates a condyle fracture with deviation towards the injured side. Diminished chin prominence with lip incompetence and bilateral preauricular swelling may indicate bilateral condyle fractures. The skin of the face and neck should be examined for areas of redness, ecchymosis, lacerations, or hematomas. Skin lacerations should be cleaned and inspected for extension to bone. No wounds should be comprehensively repaired prior to a definitive diagnosis of bony injury. The patient should be asked if he or she is experiencing numbness or paresthesia in the distribution of the inferior alveolar nerve. While not definitively diagnostic, it can be a clue to fractures in the mandibular body, angle, and, occasionally, ramus. This finding is absent in patients with condyle fractures and fractures of the mandibular symphysis anterior to mental foramen. The external auditory meatus should be checked for the presence of blood, which is often seen in conjunction with condyle fractures and blows to the symphysis. Patients may complain of diminished hearing capacity. The patient should also be asked if he or she has difficulty opening their mouth, or if the bite "feels" different than preinjury. This should be correlated

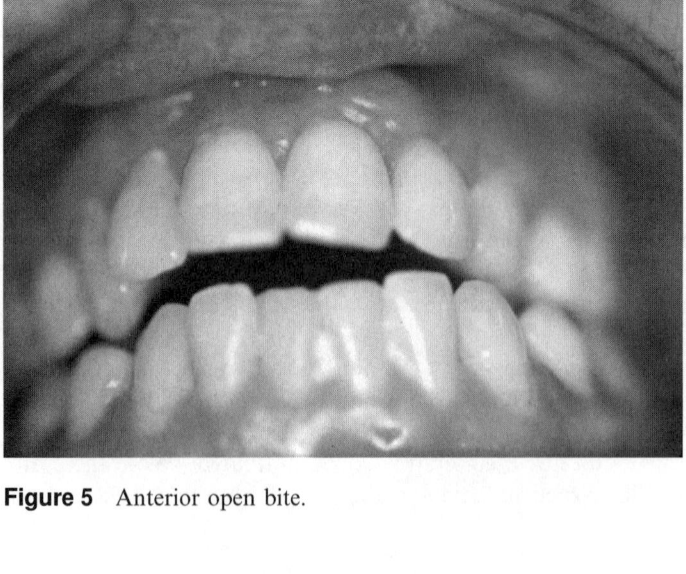

Figure 5 Anterior open bite.

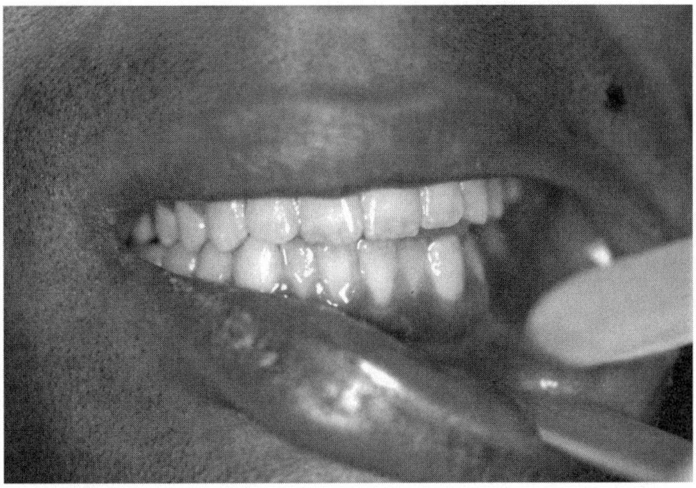

Figure 6 Posterior open bite.

with an assessment of range of mandibular motion, any trismus, deviation, or an inability to close the mouth. A wide range of combinations of mandible fractures can account for a variety of occlusal discrepancies (Figs. 5–7). However, dental injuries, dentoalveolar fractures and temporo mandibular joint (TMJ) arthroses (hemarthrosis, for example) can confound the diagnosis, accounting for occlusal discrepancies despite an otherwise negative clinical and radiographic examination.

The presence of teeth, supported by ligaments within bone, is the unique factor in these particular orthopedic injuries. Knowledge of dental anatomy and occlusion, both normal and abnormal, is critical to the re-establishment of a functional and harmonious bite. Most patients can generally indicate if their bite feels different after

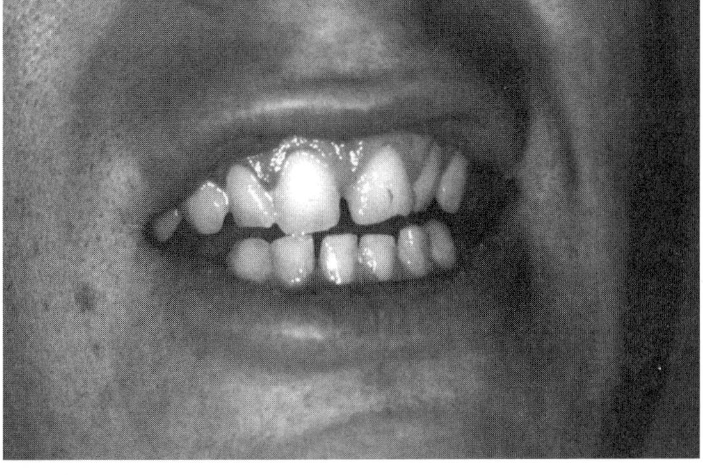

Figure 7 Midline deviation: note separation of central and lateral incisors in line of fracture.

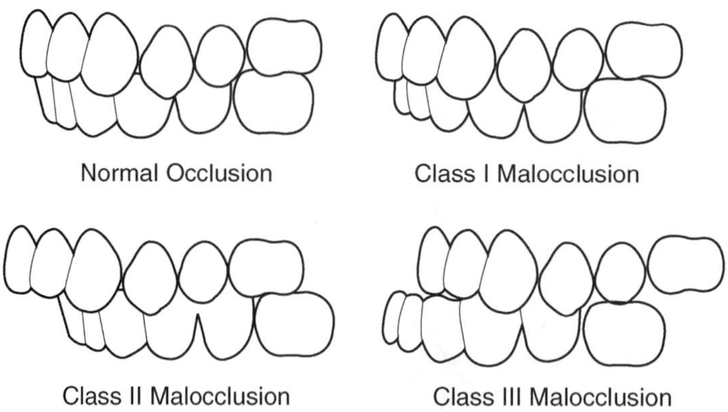

Figure 8 Angle's classification scheme of dental occlusion.

an injury, but they cannot always give practitioners an idea of their preinjury occlusion. Angle has classified dental occlusion into four distinct classes: normal, and malocclusions types I, II, and III (6) (Fig. 8).

Class I: normal molar relationship but incorrect line of occlusion due to dental rotations, or malpositioned teeth
Class II: mandibular molar distally positioned relative to maxillary molar
Class III: mandibular molar mesially positioned relative to maxillary molar

As the examination progresses intraorally, the clinician should examine not only the individual teeth for injuries but also how the mandibular and maxillary arches come together. The practitioner should look for fractured, loose, or avulsed teeth, obvious step-offs between adjacent teeth, and flail segments of alveolus or mandible. The status of the gingiva, including ecchymosis, bleeding, tears, or hematomas (especially sublingual), is strongly suggestive of underlying fractures. If possible, the mandible should be evaluated in a bimanual fashion for segmental mobility and an attempt to delineate fracture patterns. This will generally initiate rebleeding at the fracture sites, so the patient's head should be elevated to 45 degrees if possible with suction and gauze available. Gentle manual reduction will often control persistent bleeding. During the intraoral examination, all dental prostheses (partial dentures, full dentures, retainers, etc.) should be retained (broken or not) for possible future use in treatment of the acute injury.

The final diagnostic consideration is the radiographic examination. Studies should be ordered by the practitioner both to confirm fractures and to rule out suspicious clinical findings. Not all patients require computed tomographic (CT) scans for diagnosing mandibular fractures. However, CT scans can be useful in identifying complex condyle fractures; specifically, those fractured sagitally or dislocated out of the glenoid fossa (Figs. 9,10). CT scans can also be useful in severely injured patients, such as those with a penetrating gun shot wound or a severely comminuted fracture (Fig. 11). The panoramic radiograph is considered by many to be the most versatile study used to image mandible fractures. Its only limitations are its availability within medical center facilities and the ability of the patient to access the machine. Familiarity in interpreting the study is obviously essential. When a Panoramic radio-

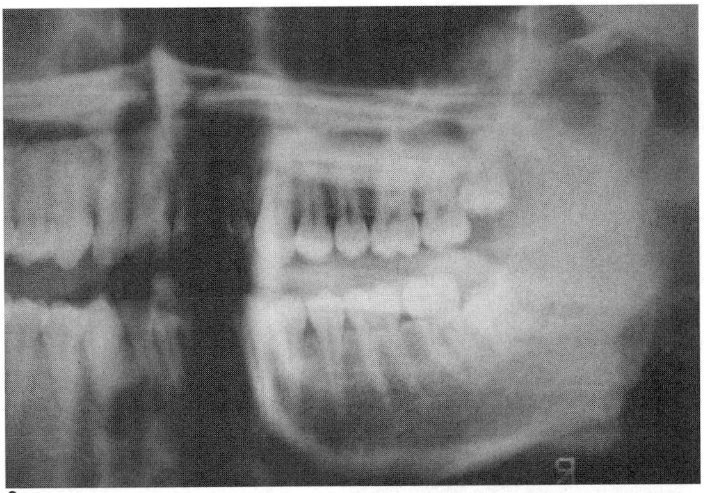

9

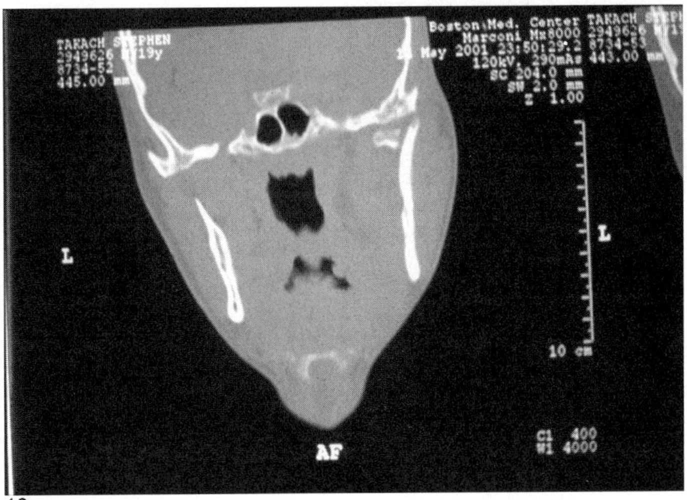

10

Figures 9, 10 Panoramic radiograph demonstrates poorly defined condylar neck fracture. Note degree of displacement and dislocation from glenoid fossa on corresponding CT scan.

graph is unavailable or fails adequately to image the condyles or symphysis, a combination of lateral oblique, posteroanterior, and reverse Towne's views should provide information necessary for diagnosis (Figs. 12–15). An occlusal view taken intraorally is excellent at demarcating minimally displaced or nondisplaced symphysis fractures.

Treatment

Mandibular fractures, once properly diagnosed, should be treated in a timely fashion. Coordination of treatment of the multiply injured patient by all involved

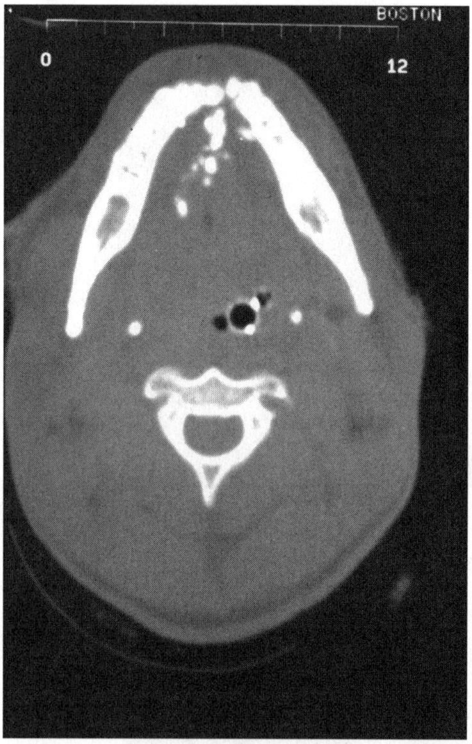

Figure 11 CT scan of mandibular symphysis fracture as a result of gunshot wound. Note degree of edema around endotracheal tube and fragments (bone, teeth) in floor of mouth.

services (general or trauma surgery, oral and maxillofacial surgery, otolaryngology, neurosurgery, etc.) is critical to ensure optimal patient care. For example, a patient with a subdural hematoma and facial injuries should certainly undergo emergent neurosurgical measures immediately, with delayed treatment of facial fractures when the patient is cleared neurologically. Elderly and debilitated patients with significant mandibular fractures may benefit from concomitant tracheostomy or feeding tube placement if a prolonged recovery is expected and intermaxillary fixation is required. Most fractures can and should generally be treated within 48 h of initial presentation. Because many mandible fractures involve gingival tears extending to the teeth and alveolus, they are by definition compound into the oral cavity and prone to invasion by saliva and oral bacteria (7). Early immobilization of segments has been shown to reduce the risk of wound infections (8). Because of the high risk of bacterial contamination in mandible fractures, antibiotic adjunctive treatment is a necessity in all compound mandible fractures both pre- and postoperatively. In a prospective randomized study of dentate mandible fractures, Zallen found that antibiotic coverage greatly diminished the rate of postoperative (9).

Teeth adjacent to fracture sites should be evaluated and assessed for their relative value for retention vs. risk to treatment. Teeth in the line of the fracture that are periodontally compromised, grossly mobile, or fractured beyond restorability should be removed prior to definitive treatment (Figs. 16,17). These pose the risk of

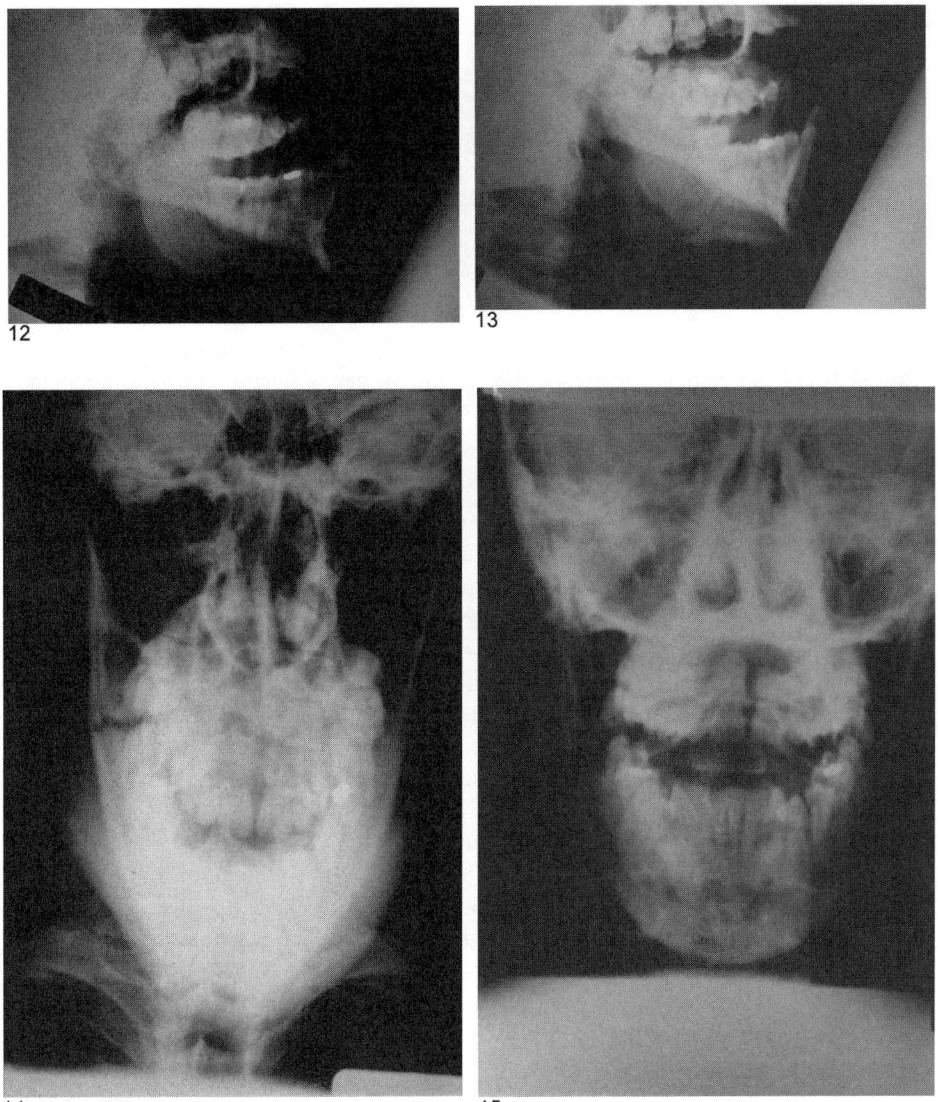

12 13 14 15

Figures 12–15 Bilateral mandibular fractures demonstrated by lateral oblique, Towne's, and posteroanterior views: the classic mandible series of plain radiographs.

infection (and nonunion) as well as recuperative-phase pain to the patient. Partially fractured teeth in a patient with limited dentition may be useful to aid in closed reduction. In this situation, the tooth could be retained until the fracture treatment is complete before a final decision is made to remove or restore the tooth. Wisdom teeth (third molars) in the line of mandibular angle fractures can pose a significant infection risk. The decision to retain or remove these teeth is not simple, and should be made considering such factors as patient compliance and hygiene, interference with proper bony segment reduction, difficulty and risk of removal, relative bone

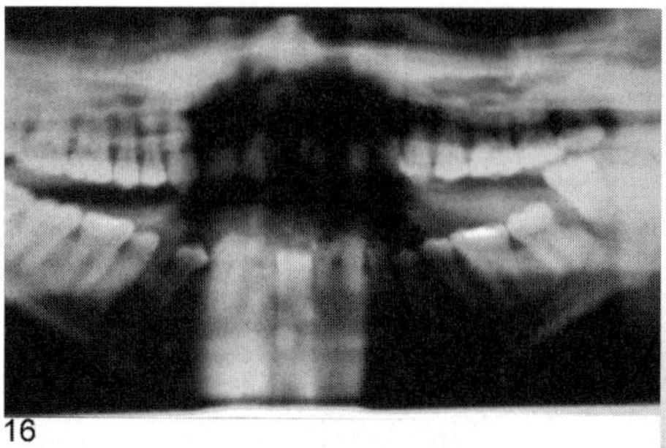

16

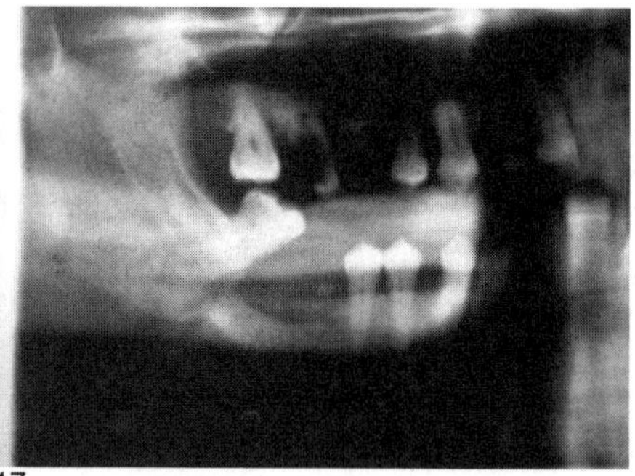

17

Figures 16, 17 In mandible fractures with teeth in the line of fracture, strong consideration should be given to removal of teeth if considerable root exposure is evident.

available at the fracture site, open vs. closed reduction, and favorable vs. unfavorable fracture.

Maintenance of proper oral hygiene, both pre- and postoperatively, is an important treatment adjunct in the management of mandible fractures. Loss of tissue barriers to bacterial invasion due to compound fractures in the line of teeth, gingival tears, hematomas, edema, and interference with natural cleaning mechanisms all increase infection risk. Proper oral hygiene using saline, peroxide, or medicated (chlorhexidine gluconate) rinses should be encouraged. Increased frequency of tooth brushing should be encouraged and the use of pulsatile irrigating devices is helpful in selected patients.

A proper diet and maintenance of nutritional status are additional requirement during postoperative care. Enduring 4–6 weeks of mandibular immobilization with maxillomandibular fixation (MMF) makes nutritional intake more difficult and weight loss is inevitable. However, a large selection of nutritional supplements is available to patients in liquid form that will minimize weight loss and malnutrition (10).

Pre- and postoperative patient positioning and bedside suction devices can simplify the ability of patients to manage oral secretions and bleeding in the immediate postinjury or postsurgery period. Elevating the head of the bed to a 45 degree angle allows patients to clear secretions effectively. Postoperative steroids and the use of ice compresses can be effective at reduction of edema.

Closed Reduction

Accurate reproduction of the pre-existing occlusal state of the patient is the cardinal rule in treatment of mandible fractures. Mandible fractures can be treated with a variety of techniques (open reduction, closed reduction, pin fixation, etc.) and with a wide variety of materials (wires, alloy plates, resorbable plates, lag screws, splints, etc.) However, proper treatment should be guided by using the simplest method to achieve the most predictable favorable result. Mandible fractures amenable to treatment by closed reduction are the following (all in dentate patients with a pre-existing, reproducible occlusion):

1. Minimally to moderately displaced simple or compound fractures (favorable)
2. Most condyle fractures
3. Fractures in children
4. Severely comminuted fractures or fractures in which overlying blood supply has been compromised

Simple, time-tested, and predictable closed reduction techniques for use in the four aforementioned categories are Ivy loops and circumdentally affixed arch bars (Figs. 18–22). Ivy loops, named for their proponent Dr. Robert Ivy, can be a simple and effective means of reducing and immobilizing minimally displaced favorable fractures in compliant patients with a stable occlusion (11). A 24-gauge wire can be used to fabricate a loop on itself, and is affixed to teeth (Fig. 23) utilizing a needle driver, local anesthetic, and a wire cutter. Pigtails can be left on the wire ends to affix elastic or wire traction, elastics being preferred for patient safety. If the patient becomes nauseous or vomits, elastics can be easily cut. Ivy loops can be affixed to each dental quadrant singly or in pairs.

Arch bar fixation is a time-tested and reliable technique that results in more stable fixation than Ivy loops alone (Fig. 24). Arch bars come in a variety of styles, both malleable (Erich type) and semirigid (Winter or Jelenko type). Semi rigid varieties offer improved transarch stability and can be useful in cases in which the maxilla or mandible is missing multiple teeth. The most commonly accepted technique for affixing arch bars to the dentition is via circumdental 24-gauge wires. The two force ends of the wire are tightened in a pigtail fashion over the bar under continuous apical pressure. Arch bar ligatures should typically run from the first or second molars to the canines. Anterior teeth can be utilized, when necessary, but caution should be used because 24-gauge wires have been known to orthodontically move incisors labially or rotationally. A smaller 26-gauge wire is recommended if anterior tooth ligation is needed. Reduction of segments should be with elastic or box wire traction of arch bars into an acceptable occlusion before definitive tightening of circumdental wires, proximal to the fracture site. Arch bars should be affixed tightly without evidence of vertical or horizontal mobility. Tooth-bearing fractures (symphysis, body) should, as a general rule, be reduced prior to non-tooth-bearing fractures (angle, ramus). Arch bars also provide a stable point of fixation for luxated mobile teeth and dentoalveolar segment fractures. Following closed reduction of fractures, it may be determined that a previously nondisplaced fracture, for example, in the angle, is now significantly displaced and nonreducible. In such cases, the practitioner will need to weigh the indications for open reduction and at times change the initial treatment plan. Closed reduction techniques demand patient compliance with maxillomandibular elastic traction (immobilization) for 4–6 weeks prior to release. Thus, patients with behavioral difficulties or those at risk for significant aspiration (alcoholics, patients with Alzheimer's disease) may require more predictable, definitive treatment or overtreatment to effect a more predictable outcome. Mobility at the fracture site has been shown to lead to malunion, nonunion, and osteomyelitis (2). Persistent trismus often results from prolonged maxillomandibular fixation; physical therapy is often useful to obtain a return to normal range of motion.

Two other techniques categorized as closed reduction methods for treating mandible fractures apply to situations in which a dentate mandible opposes an

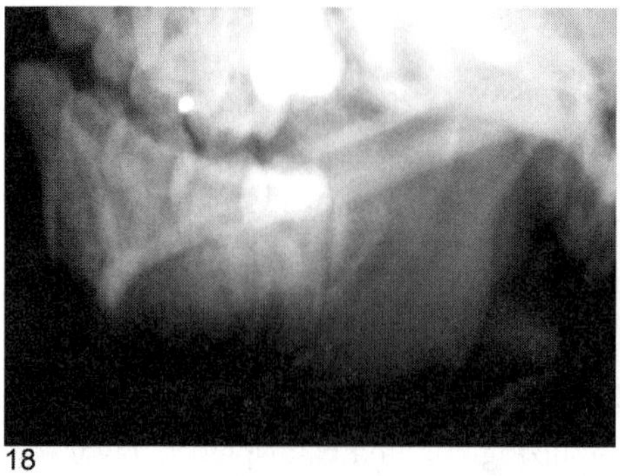

18

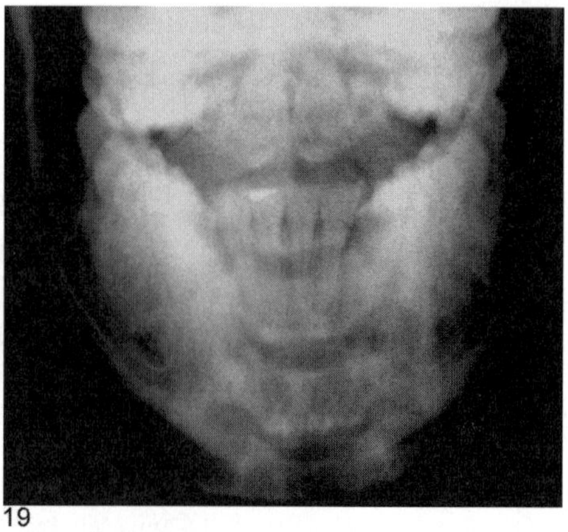

19

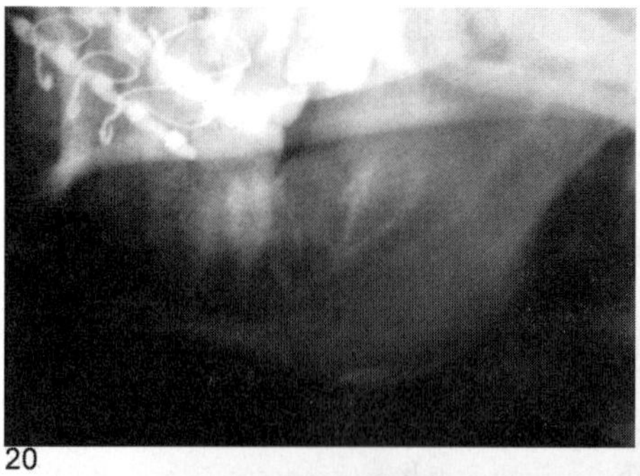

20

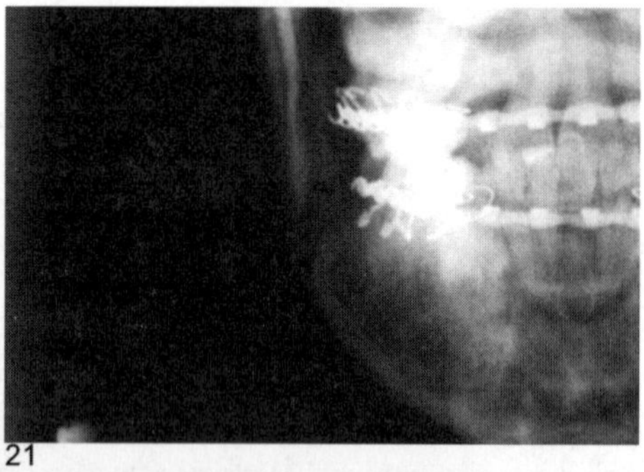

21

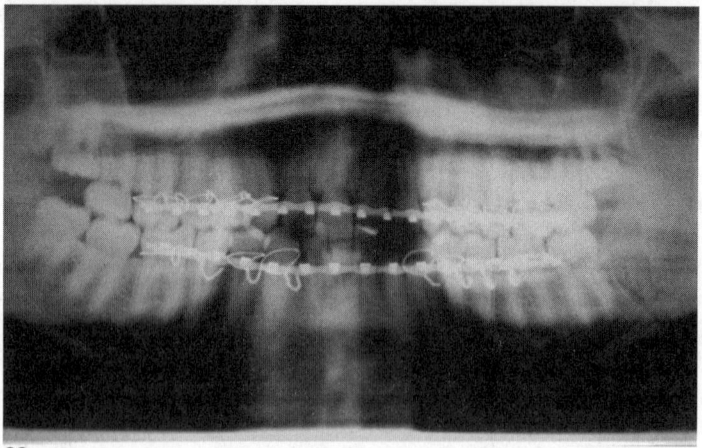

22

Figures 18–22 Management of a nondisplaced mandibular angle fracture through a wisdom tooth. Removal of the wisdom tooth followed by a closed reduction with arch bars resulted in anatomical alignment.

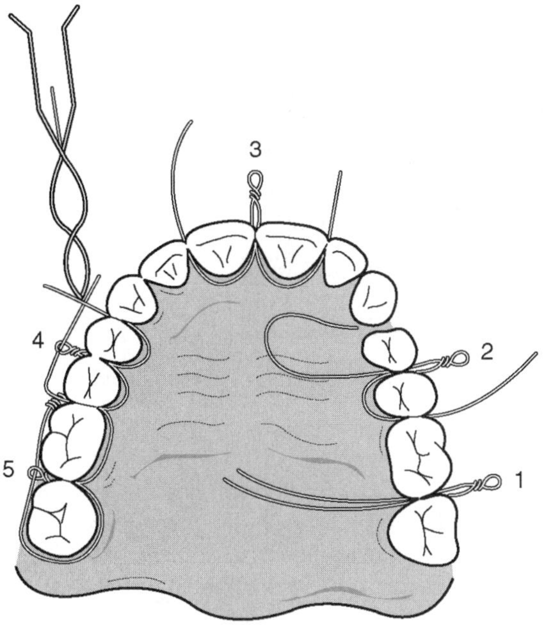

Figure 23 Ivy loop application.

edentulous maxilla, or vice versa. In the first scenario, the patient's pre-existing denture can be modified (Fig. 25) with acrylic to affix an arch bar or a Gunning-type splint can be fabricated from acrylic (12). This is then affixed to the maxilla by screw fixation at the pyriform rims, zygomatic buttresses, or palate. Pyriform rim wires or perialveolar wires can also be used. An arch bar is then

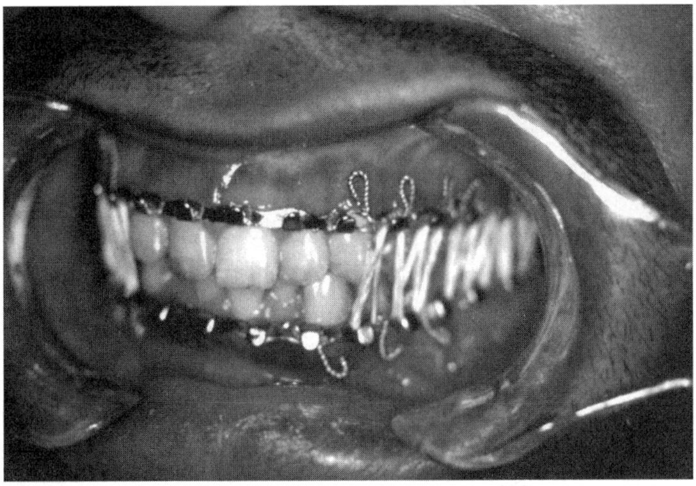

Figure 24 Maxillomandibular fixation with elastics.

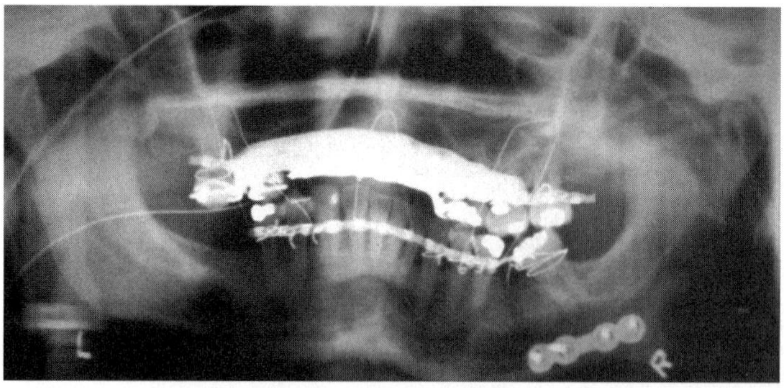

Figure 25 Use of the patient's maxillary dental prosthesis to aid in establishment of proper occlusion in conjunction with open and closed reductions.

affixed to the dentate mandible and a standard closed reduction is then performed using the maxillary denture as the occlusal basis for proper alignment followed by elastic traction fixation (Figs. 26–28). Wires and/or screws are removed at the time treatment is completed. If a dentate maxilla opposes a fractured mandible with a limited number of teeth, a modification of the patient's mandibular partial denture or fabrication of an acceptable splint can be performed in a similar fashion. This can then be affixed to the mandible via circummandibular wires, with care being taken to avoid wire proximity to the fracture site. Care should also be taken to avoid injury to the mental nerve as it exits the mandible and to the submandibular duct and contents of the floor of the mouth. A standard closed reduction can then be created via elastic traction fixation.

Open Reduction

Mandible fractures amenable to treatment by open reduction include the following:

1. Moderate to severely displaced simple or compound fractures
2. Fractures nonreducible by closed means
3. Fractures opposing an edentulous maxilla or nonoccluding maxilla
4. Unfavorable fractures

Excluded from these indications for special consideration are edentulous mandible fractures, mandible fractures in conjunction with panfacial fractures, and avulsive or pathological fractures.

Open reduction techniques for treating mandible fractures are numerous, ranging from both intra- and extraoral approaches, with variations in materials such as wires, wire mesh, plates and screws, lag screws, eccentric dynamic compression plates, resorbable plates, and others. However, the basis for treatment by open reduction or closed reduction should be the same: re-establishment of an acceptable occlusal relationship for the patient in a predictable and safe fashion. In most cases requiring open reduction, a closed reduction is performed initially to approximate an occlusal relationship. A closed reduction serves to guide the practitioner in a functional as well as anatomical alignment of mandibular segments. With the occlusal relationship established, open reduction techniques then provide a means of rigidly or semirigidly immobilizing and maintaining bony segments in an acceptable posi-

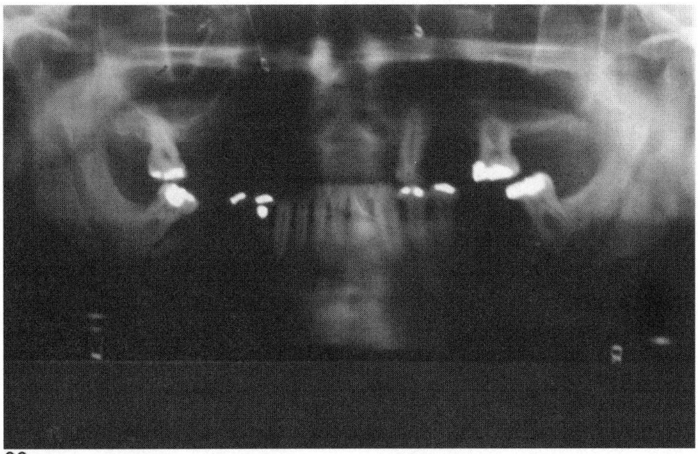

26

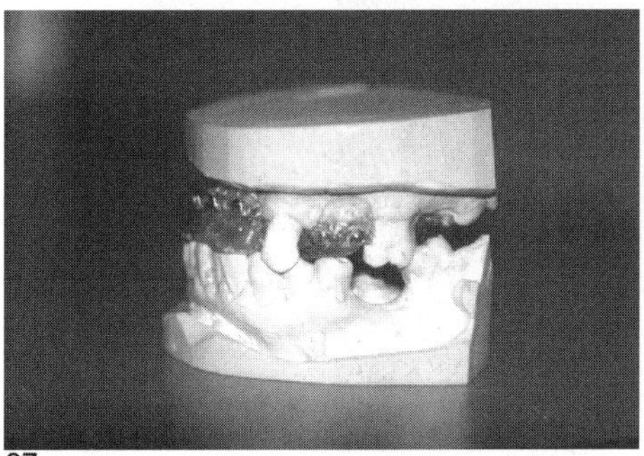

27

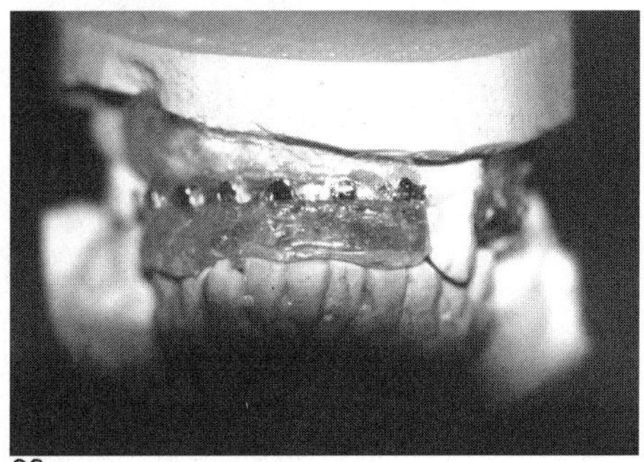

28

Figure 26–28 In the case of a dentate mandibular fracture opposing a limited maxillary dentition, dental models can be utilized to fabricate acrylic splints with arch bars to establish a stable occlusal relationship.

tion with or without compression. Bone edges approximated under compression are thought to undergo more rapid osseous healing (2).

Extraoral approaches to the mandible include the submandibular or Risdon approach, the retromandibular approach, the submental approach, the preauricular approach, and through existing lacerations. Each approach has its particular strengths and weaknesses. Intraoral access can be gained to most anatomical regions of the mandible via a vestibular incision in the mucosa or by a traditional Obwegesser approach to the ramus and low condylar neck/coronoid regions (13). Extraoral approaches lend themselves well to the use of bone screws and rigid plating systems of all types, allowing wide visualization and the ability to place bicortical screws safely. Intraoral approaches are useful to access oblique fractures of the anterior mandible when lag screw fixation is desired and for placement of plates and screws (low condyle fractures) or border wires (Figs. 29–31).

Wire osteosynthesis is a time-honored method for the treatment of mandible fractures. However, with the advent of rigid fixation techniques many practitioners now have limited experience in the use of direct transosseous wiring. Perhaps the

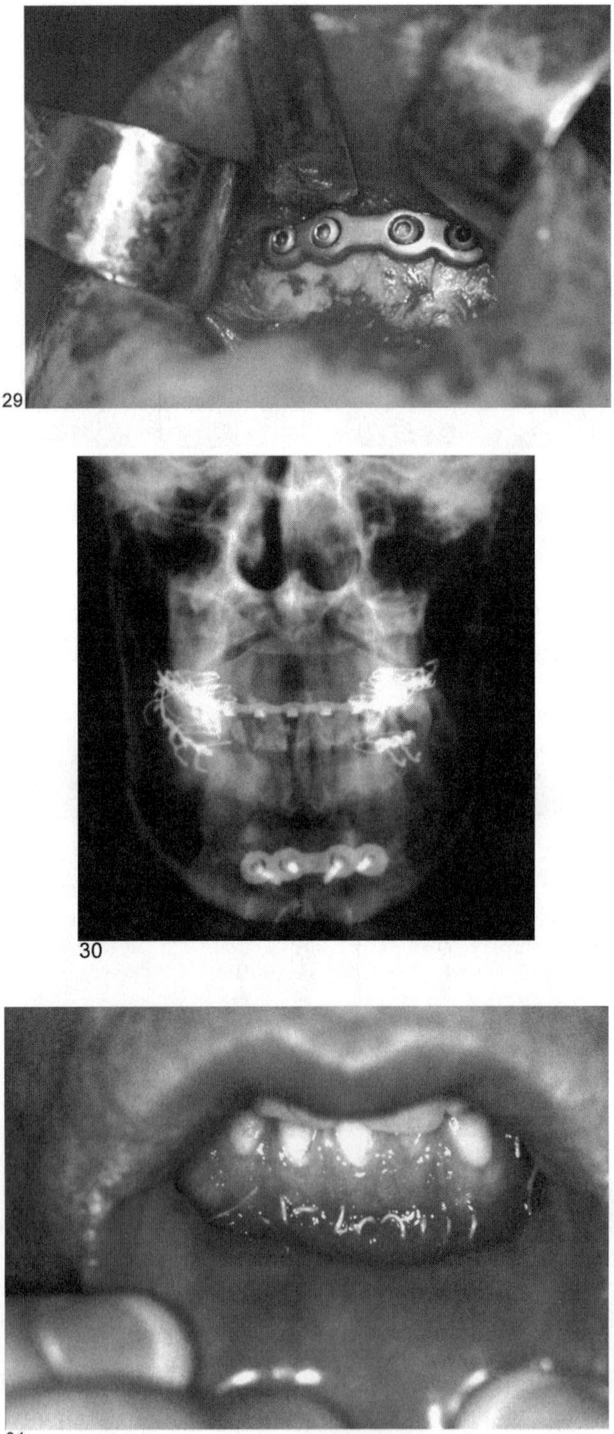

29

30

31

Figure 29–31 Intraoral approach to anterior mandibular symphysis fracture.

most common use currently is the intraoral superior border wire, for the treatment of mandibular angle fractures. Long-term intermaxillary fixation is required when wire osteosynthesis is used as a treatment option due to the wire's inability to limit multidimensional mobility at the fracture site during typical mandibular function. Wires can also be useful adjuncts to manipulate segments in conjunction with extraoral open reduction techniques.

Rigid fixation techniques (or semirigid techniques) differ from wire fixation techniques in several important ways. Rigid fixation techniques maintain stability across a fracture site with an increased surface area (of device) to bone interface compared to wires and these techniques generally do not require prolonged intermaxillary fixation. However, there is a wide variety of alternatives to consider within this particular technique category: plate material and thickness, screw size and thread pitch, mono- or bicortical crews, tension band plates, neutral zone plates, compression plates, lag screws, reconstruction plates, wire meshes, and resorbable plates. Lag screws generate substantial cross-fragment compression and load sharing. The concepts of tension band plates, neutral zone (static plates), and compression plates are well documented in the literature (14). Compression plates (thicker bicortical-affixed plates) compress bony segments when placed across a fracture via eccentrically placed holes (Fig. 32). This compression is believed to promote enhanced bony healing with no intervening callus formation. Tension band plates (smaller monocortical-affixed plates) resist tensile forces along the superior aspect of the mandible. Arch bars have been described as effective tension bands. Neutral or static bone plates (bicortical-affixed) do not offer compression across fracture lines. Wire mesh does offer some three-dimensional stability depending again on size and material. These meshes generally are indicated in avulsed or severely comminuted fractures requiring bone grafting. Resorbable plates and screws, currently under close scrutiny regarding biodegradation issues, still have considerable mechanical limitations over equivalent alloy plates and screws (15).

Fractures of the edentulous mandible are categorized unto themselves. The appropriate management option selected to treat the edentulous mandible fracture should take into consideration the age of the patient, the degree of functional disability postoperatively, the severity and type of fracture, and, most importantly, whether the mandible is edentulous and atrophic (pencil thin). Closed reduction techniques

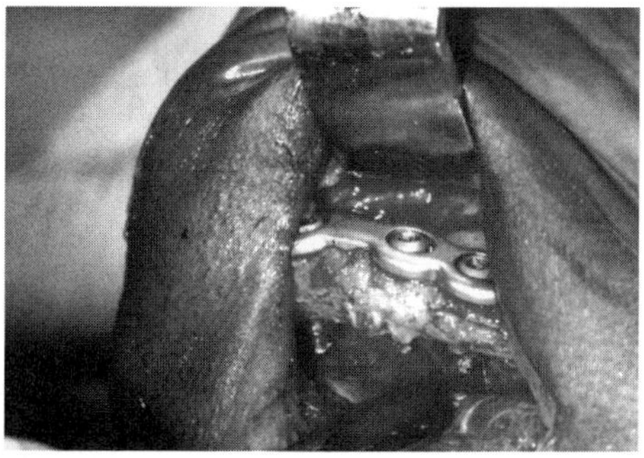

Figure 32 Extraoral approach to mandibular body fracture. Note bicortical penetration of screw.

using the patient's existing dentures (modified) or Gunning-type splints are indicated when MMF with splints will offer adequate segment control and reduction. Circummandibular wires (24-gauge) are used to affix the denture or splint with an arch bar to the maxilla. The dentures or splints should be modified by placement of arch bars (or sections thereof) along the labial flanges and interocclusal keys should be developed occlusally to serve as occlusal stops to prevent sliding displacement (Figs. 33–44). Since the blood supply to the atrophic mandible is nearly entirely supplied by the periosteum, open reduction techniques on these fractures should only done if closed reduction techniques (or biphasic pins) are unsuccessful (16). As stated by Rowe and Williams, "adequate opposition of the fractured bone ends by closed methods is often difficult, and even in comparatively undisplaced fractures, there may be periosteal stripping by the hematoma to a degree which renders the area ischemic. Non union is not at all uncommon in these circumstances" (17). Open reduction with immediate bone grafting is another method advocated for treating severely atrophic mandible fractures.

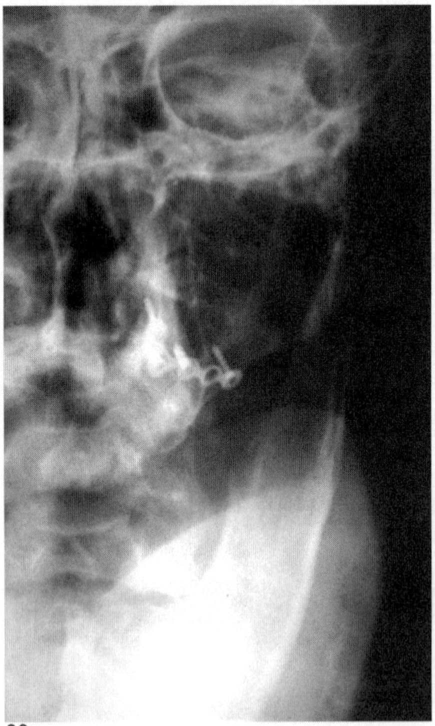

33

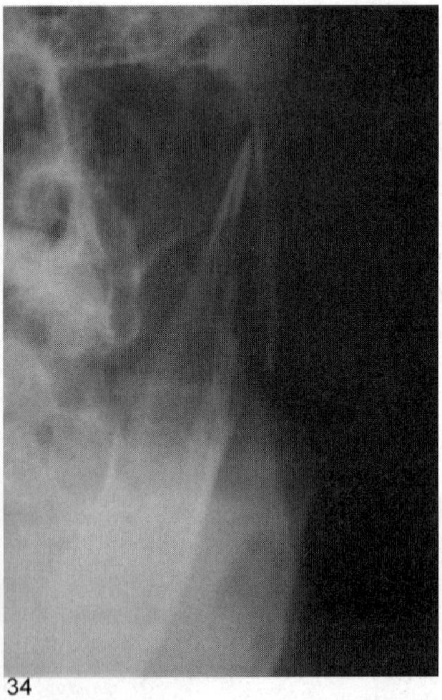

34

Figures 33–44 Management of a bilateral mandible fracture (condyle, ramus) in an edentulous patient. A maxillary splint is fabricated and affixed to the maxilla with transplated screws and piriform rim wires. A mandibular splint is fabricated and affixed to the mandible with circummandibular wires. Maxillomandibular fixation is achieved with elastics. An open reduction is performed after establishment of a proper occlusal relationship.

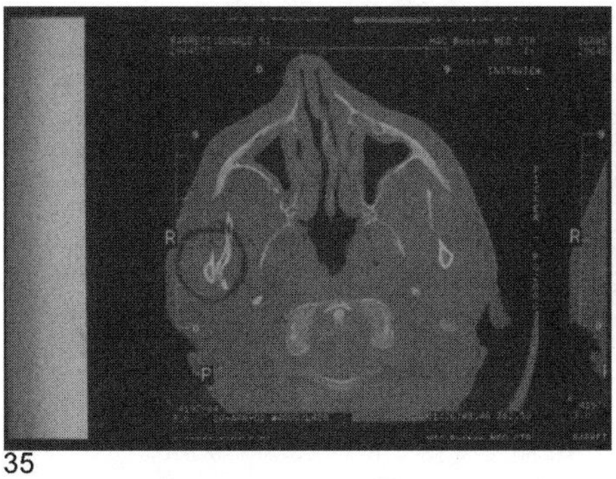
35

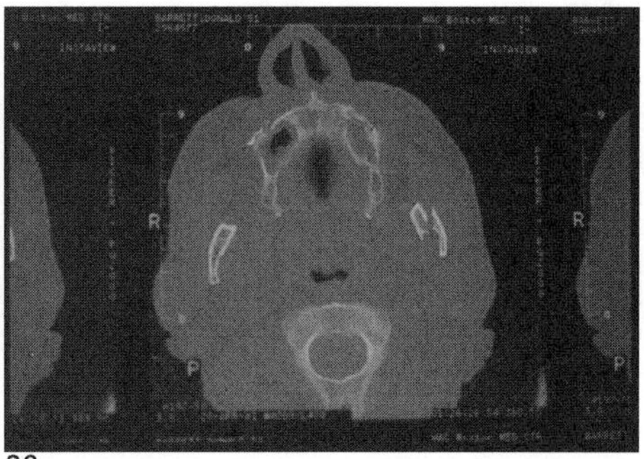
36

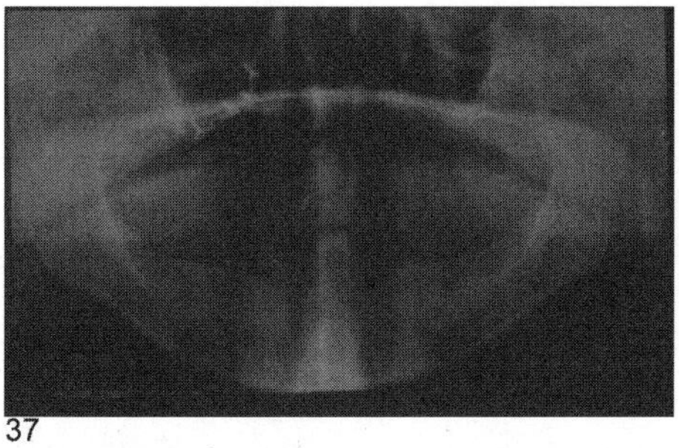
37

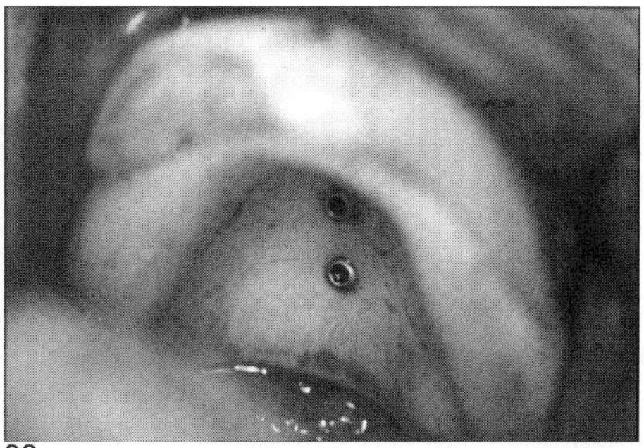
38

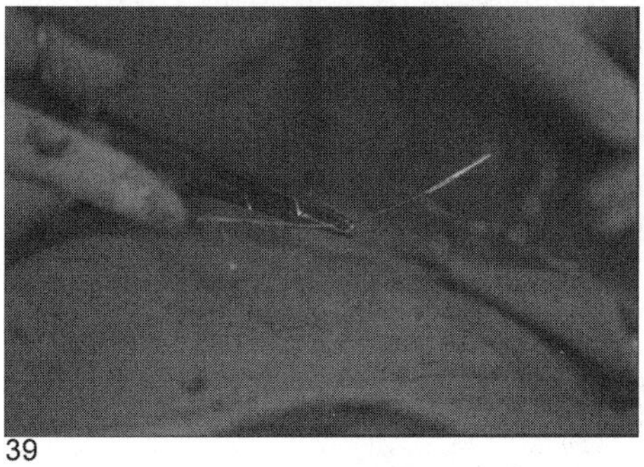
39

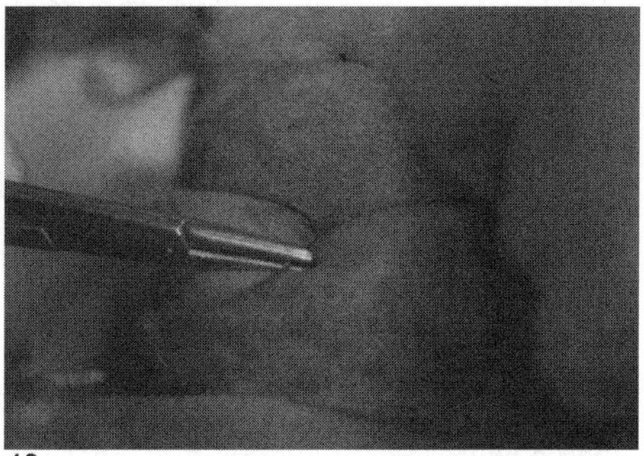
40

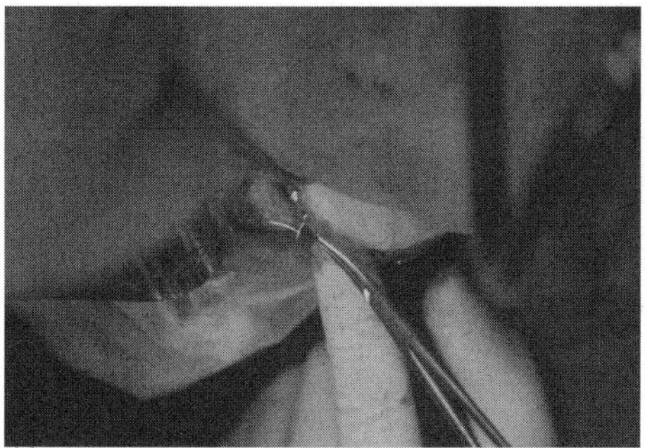
41

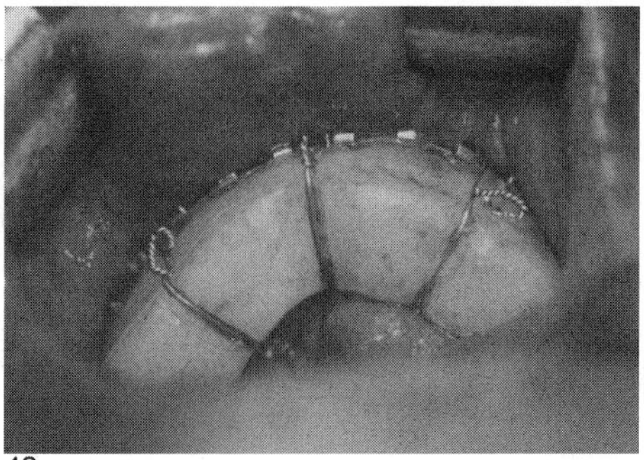
42

Figures 33–44 Continued.

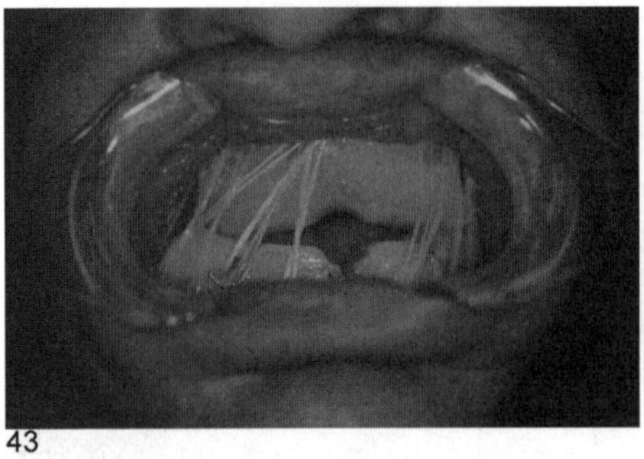

43

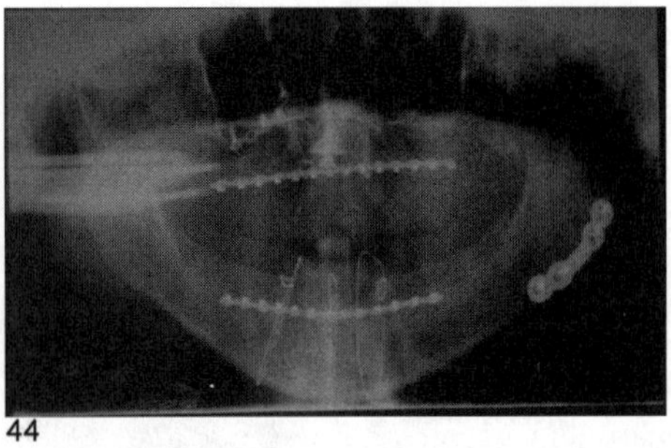

44

Figures 33–44 Continued.

Complications

Avoiding complications is critical to successful management of all injuries. Complications associated with treating mandible fractures have been discussed in previous sections, but a number of observations warrant further mention. Infection is the most common complication seen, ranging from 5 to 10% on average. Most practitioners would agree that closed reduction techniques exhibit the lowest rate of infection. Conversely, the highest infection rates are found in cases managed with open nonrigid techniques, most likely because of the lack of rigidity at the fracture site (2). Several factors are associated with postoperative infections including the presence of mobile, carious, or periodontally involved teeth in the line of the fracture; fracture severity and compromise of overlying soft tissue; pre-existing systemic illnesses that impair wound healing (e.g., diabetes); mobility at the fracture site; and patient noncompliance (alcohol, drug abuse, poor dietary control).

Malocclusion is a significant complication associated with the treatment of mandible fractures. Numerous studies in the literature associate an increased inci-

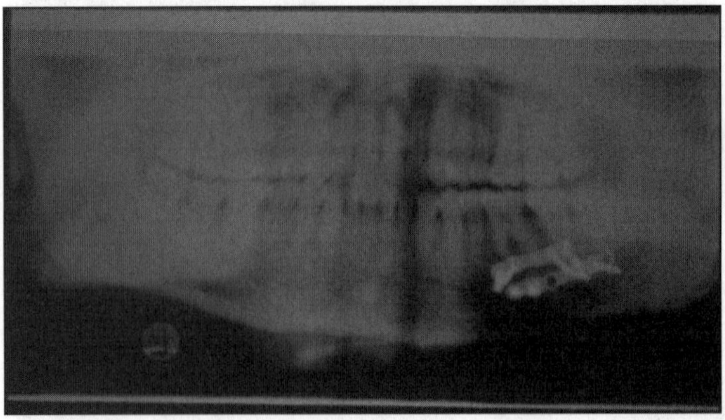

Figure 45 Injudicious screw placement can jeopardize not only tooth roots but also the inferior alveolar nerve.

dence of malocclusion to cases treated with rigid fixation. The practitioner must constantly remind himself that improperly adapted or applied hardware will result in malocclusion. Also, no patient should leave the operating room until the occlusion has been repeatedly verified to be proper and sound. This may require removal and replacement of elastics, splints, or intraoperative radiographs to correlate and confirm the clinical findings. If the mandibular condyle is torqued or displaced out of the glenoid fossa during treatment, a malocclusion will exist. Malocclusions can be treated postoperatively depending upon the severity and time of detection. All but the most minor cases will require operative intervention. Attempts to correct postoperative malocclusions should be made quickly prior to definitive bony healing, or osteotomy may be the only effective therapy.

Nonunion and fibrous union of mandible fractures are uncommon and most often related to mobility at the fracture site, infection, and poor patient compliance (2). The practitioner should always be aware of the risk of iatrogenic injury to cranial nerves 5 (inferior alveolar nerve) and 7 as well as injuries to tooth roots by injudicious screw or wire placement (Fig. 45). Teeth whose roots are injured by a drill or penetrated by hardware will likely devitalize, necessitating removal of not only the teeth but also the hardware.

DENTOALVEOLAR FRACTURES

Examination

A brief mention of dentoalveolar injuries (fractured, subluxed, avulsed teeth, and dentoalveolar segment injuries) is warranted because these wounds often accompany mandible fractures and can even mimic mandible fractures (18). However, they are significant injuries themselves and deserve prompt attention and treatment. These injuries are more likely to be seen in a younger patient population (children and adolescents). A thorough history and examination should account for all teeth in any given individual, especially in patients with mixed (deciduous and permanent) dentition. Teeth that cannot be accounted for by the patient, parents or by examination warrant radiographic studies of the abdomen, chest, neck, and facial soft tissues to rule out their presence in these areas. The right main stem bronchus is the frequent site of aspirated teeth secondary to tracheopulmonary anatomy; these require bronchoscopy for removal.

Diagnosis and Treatment

The teeth should be carefully inspected for fractures of enamel or dentin, especially those that extend to the neurovascular supply (pulp) of the tooth. Mobility of teeth should be evaluated in an attempt to ascertain whole-tooth luxation or avulsion vs. a fracture involving the root of the tooth. Movement of two or more teeth in unison suggests an en-bloc fracture of the alveolus. A distinction should be made between deciduous (baby) teeth and succedaneous (permanent) teeth: significant injury to deciduous teeth (mobility, fractures exposing the pulp, severe intrusions) should generally guide the practitioner toward removal of the injured tooth, whereas the same is not always true of permanent teeth. Of course, many factors including the age of the patient, concomitant injuries, patient cooperation, alveolar injury, and length of time from injury to treatment should all be considered. General anesthesia or sedation may be required for a thorough examination in some patients. Dental periapical radiographs may not be available in a given practice setting to help evaluate such injuries. In such cases, it may be better to defer definitive treatment until the patient can see a dentist or an oral and maxillofacial surgeon for a thorough evaluation. Totally avulsed teeth stand the best chance for successful reimplantation if replaced and stabilized within 30 min. Most reimplantations are not successful if reimplanted after more than 2 h, usually failing due to external root resorption (19). Deciduous teeth are generally not reimplanted. Dentoalveolar segment fractures should be manually reduced into proper occlusion and immobilized using acrylic splints, existing dental orthodontic retainers, acid etch resins, or circumdental wiring to a secured Erich arch bar. A generally accepted time frame for immobilization is 4–6 weeks. Gingival health is critical for the successful outcome of dentoalveolar fractures, any splint should exert minimal pressure on the gingival tissues and underlying alveolus. Pressure in these areas can compromise periosteal blood supply to the underlying bone, leading to mucosal ulceration and breakdown with an increased risk of infection.

CONDYLAR INJURIES

The temporomandibular region is involved in a significant percentage of facial and mandibular injuries. Condylar fractures account for 25–35% of all mandibular fractures (17). Fractures, effusions, hemarthroses, and dislocations are found that can result in significant morbidity if not properly treated, including joint ankylosis, malocclusion, internal meniscal derangement, and growth disruption (20). As with all mandible fractures, the age of the patient, mechanism of injury, and force play major roles in determining the type, location, and severity of the injury. While dislocation at the TMJ can occur in all planes, the most common is anterior dislocation caused by a blow, yawning, vomiting, (some may be self-reducing). Dislocations can occur unilaterally or bilaterally. The two most comprehensive classification systems for condylar injuries are described by Lindahl and MacLennan (21,22). Important differentiating characteristics include the degree of displacement across the fracture, the degree of deviation of the condylar process with respect to the distal fragment, the location of the fracture (condylar head, condylar neck, or subcondylar), and the degree of displacement of the condyle from its fossa.

Diagnosis

A history and clinical examination should be directed toward suggestive signs and symptoms of condylar injuries such as deviation of the mandibular midline, preauricular pain, swelling, tenderness, malocclusion, bleeding from the external auditory canal, and chin contusions or lacerations. Plain radiographs should be obtained initially. Any injured patient for whom a high level of clinical suspicion remains despite negative lateral oblique, Towne's, posteroanterior, or panoramic views should undergo CT scanning to assess for subtle fractures (e.g., sagittal fractures may be missed by plain radiography). The Towne's view is exceptional at displaying the degree of medial displacement; an empty glenoid fossa on CT scan should raise a strong suspicion of a fracture dislocation out of the fossa.

Treatment

Dislocations

Patients can present with TMJ dislocation injuries that are acute or chronic, and unilateral or bilateral. Often precipitated by yawning or vomiting, these injuries should be radiographically documented and diagnosed prior to commencing with attempts at reduction. Because reduction of long-standing dislocations has a relatively low success rate, every attempt should be made to ascertain the duration of the dislocation (hours, days, weeks, or months). Chronic dislocations, refractory to manual reduction, will likely require surgical management. Acute dislocations can generally be managed by manual manipulation and reduction, with or without the aid of local anesthesia or intravenous sedation. Refractory cases may require a general anesthetic in rare cases. Reduction is accomplished by seating the patient in an upright position, in front of the practitioner, and placing the thumbs over the posterior mandibular molars (or mandibular retromolar pads in edentulous patients). With a strong tilting motion, the mandible is pushed in a posteroinferior fashion with steadily increasing force and the patient is instructed to close down at the first sign of posterior movement. Once the baseline occlusion has been re-established, immobilization via intermaxillary fixation, a Barton bandage, or other means is generally indicated because muscle spasms can easily cause repeat dislocation (23). Cases of prolonged dislocation (greater than 1 month's duration), while rare, are unlikely to reduce and may require surgical management via condylotomy, condylectomy, or osteotomy. Cases of persistent, recurrent dislocation can be managed by numerous techniques beyond the scope of this chapter.

Fractures

The treatment of condyle fractures is an area of frequent debate in the oral and maxillofacial literature. These fractures can be managed conservatively by closed reduction and intermaxillary fixation or by open reduction and direct fixation of segments. The goal of both methods is to establish a proper occlusal relationship while mobilizing the TMJ apparatus as soon as is functionally possible. Complications, inherent in any condyle fracture, may be aggravated by attempted open surgical repair including malocclusions, mandibular deviations, facial asymmetry (facial nerve paresis), trismus, internal derangements (meniscal dysfunction), and growth disturbances in growing patients. The literature is replete with evidence suggesting that closed reduction methods (MMF via Ivy loops or arch bars, with training elastics and proper diet) are successful with minimal complications for the vast majority of patients.

Integral to conservative (closed) therapy is determining the appropriate duration of intermaxillary fixation, determination of the need for training elastics, and a properly instituted dietary advancement from full liquids to soft solids to no restrictions. Minimally displaced fractures with minor occlusal disturbances will require less MMF (7–14 days), whereas more significantly displaced fractures or fractures causing significant occlusal disruption (bilateral fractures) will require more time in MMF (4 weeks). This time allows for bony union to occur. During this period, close follow-up is required and elastics can be removed to assess for lingering occlusal disharmony. Following release of MMF, if deviation or prematurity is apparent in the occlusion, training elastics should be utilized to guide the patient in a straight up and down, even midline, motion. Training elastics can be used, generally up to 3 weeks, once the practitioner believes bony union has occurred. The patient is instructed on dietary advancement and physical therapy to enhance joint mobilization. After elastics are no longer needed, the arch bars or Ivy loops can be removed. If slight posttreatment deviation is noted, or occlusal prematurities are evident, occlusal adjustment (selective grinding of teeth) and orthodontic consultation may be of benefit.

In cases of intracapsular fracture or severe comminution of the condylar head and neck, open reduction is contraindicated and fixation is often not an option. Open reduction of condyle fractures, while a viable treatment option, is often reserved for cases clearly demanding of its merits. Inability to establish occlusion, fracture dislocation into the middle cranial fossa, and lateral extracapsular fracture dislocation of the condyle have been noted by Zide and Kent and by Raveh and others as absolute indications for open reduction (24),(25). Relative indications include the patient's inability to comply with closed reduction methods and fractures associated with panfacial trauma. Advantages of open reduction techniques over closed techniques include a shortened interval of MMF and early mobilization of the joint.

The practitioner is wise to perform an initial closed reduction, if possible, on patients undergoing open reduction of condyle fractures to establish the occlusion properly. Proper rigid fixation techniques will then immobilize an anatomical reduction (Fig. 46). Open reduction with wires still requires a period of MMF. The principal surgical approaches to condylar fractures are the preauricular approach (and

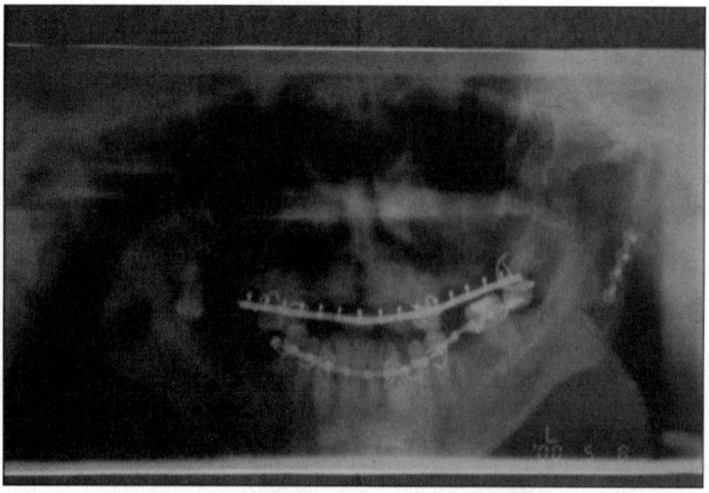

Figure 46 Closed reduction in conjunction with open reduction of a mandibular condyle fracture.

its modified versions), the submandibular (or Risdon approach), and the intraoral approach. An endoscopic approach is also described. Fracture location and displacement may dictate multiple approaches.

It is acceptable to treat condyle fractures (when minimally displaced to nondisplaced with no occlusal deviation, discrepancy, prematurity, or otherwise) in the compliant patient with a liquid diet for 7–14 days to achieve an adequate bony union. However, close follow-up must be maintained in these patients; if a malocclusion should occur, intermaxillary fixation is indicated. Condyle fractures in the edentulous mandible can be managed in a similar fashion if minimally displaced. If there is significant displacement (e.g., bilateral fracture cases), closed and/or open reduction may be indicated but the degree of occlusal disharmony should be the guide in dictating treatment, not necessarily the radiographic findings. Coronoid fractures, as a rule, do not require reduction or fixation. They are generally treated by removal of the segment only if they interfere with reduction of other fractures or pose a risk of bony ankylosis to the zygomatic arch.

MANDIBULAR FRACTURES IN CHILDREN

The treatment of the child with a mandible fracture presents a challenge for the practitioner. Approximately 25% of all facial fractures in children occur in the mandible (26). Rowe has classified children into four groups based on their dental development, which can be used as guides for choice of treatment (27). Patients up to 2 years of age with mandible fractures are best managed by splinting the mandible and its associated erupting deciduous teeth. A single jaw splint, without MMF, should be fabricated to accommodate the maxillary dentition in a noninterfering fashion and secured with circummandibular wires. Two to 3 weeks is sufficient for early union. Open reduction is possible for fractures that are nonreducible by conservative means, with wires or miniplate fixation. Great care should be taken to avoid injury to the tooth buds. Patients aged 2–4 years can be treated in closed fashion with Ivy loops or circumdental wires to effect a closed reduction with elastics, or an open reduction can be utilized as in the earlier age group. Children between the ages of 5 and 8 will display varying degrees of deciduous tooth loss (or loss of root length as they shed) and succedaneous tooth eruption (teeth may be partially submerged and unavailable for wire ligation). In most cases, the deciduous molars act as the anchoring teeth for closed reduction techniques with wires. Ivy loops and circumdental wires with pigtails can be effective for unilateral fractures, but an open reduction or combined open and closed approach may indicated based on the severity of fracture, relative tooth stability, and the number of teeth available. Patients approximately 9 years older and up can be treated like adults, depending on their individual dental development.

In children, a closed reduction (MMF) of 2–4 weeks duration is generally satisfactory to obtain early bony union. The condyle is fractured in 40–60% of all pediatric facial fractures (28). According to the now-accepted functional matrix theory proposed by Moss, the condyle responds to growth in the surrounding soft tissue envelope of the mandible (29). Therefore, in growing children (prior to their teens), the condyle exhibits an amazing capacity to remodel and compensate for traumatic insults (30). Growth disturbances seen in children who have sustained TMJ trauma

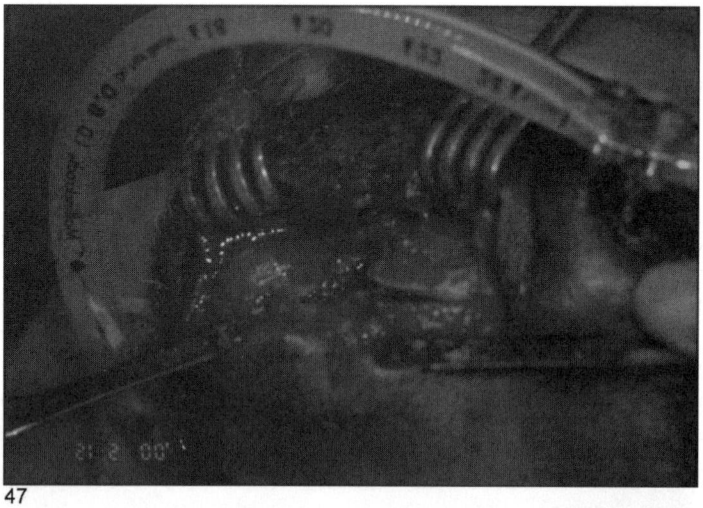

47

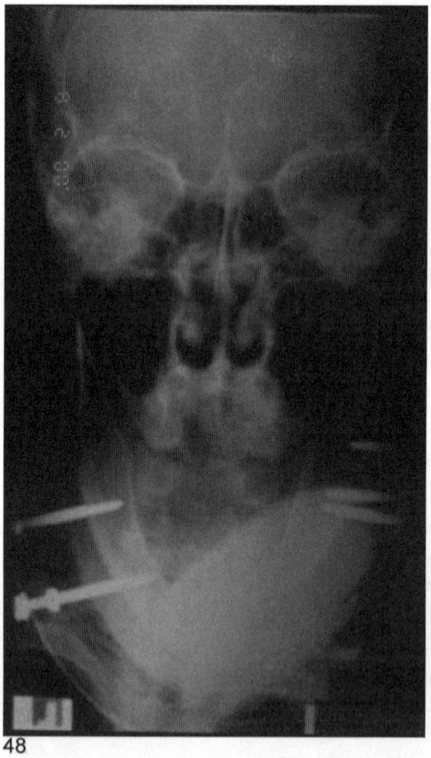

48

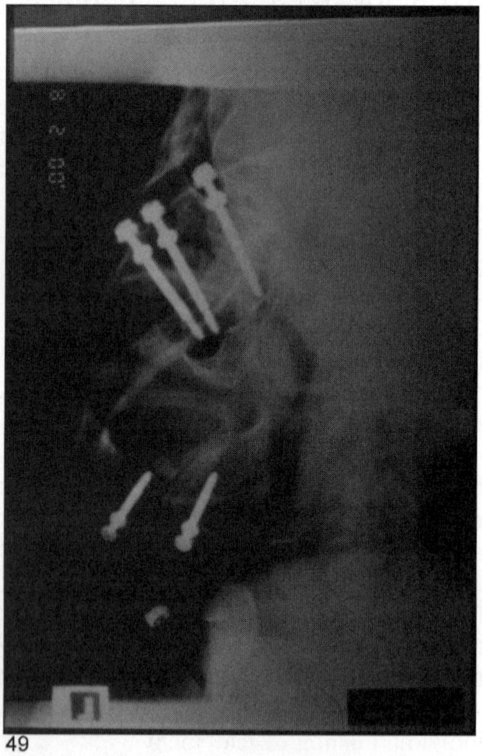

49

Figure 47–49 Debridement of necrotic bone in osteomyelitis superimposed a previously untreated mandible fracture. Note radiographic reduction via biphasic pin fixation and indwelling irrigation catheter.

include ankylosis, deviation, facial asymmetry, diminished ramus height, and internal derangements. Following trauma, especially in untreated fractures, fibrosis and bony ankylosis may have significant detrimental effects on mandibular growth. Hence, early treatment, close follow-up, and appropriately timed periods of MMF (7–14 days) with close monitoring for judicious use of training elastics and physical therapy (exercises to mobilize and properly load the joint) are essential components of treatment to ensure a successful outcome. Given the plasticity of the pediatric mandible, minor aberrations in occlusion and dental alignment are usually of no concern. When these inherent compensations prove inadequate after treatment, orthodontic therapy provides another adjunct to manage the child after a mandible fracture.

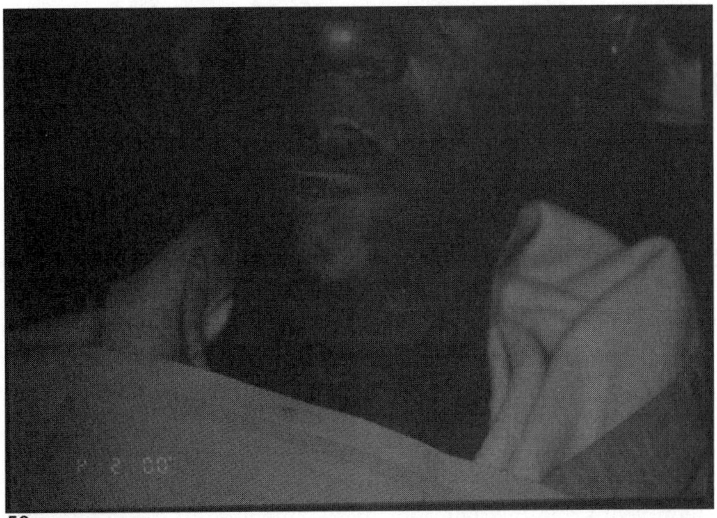

50

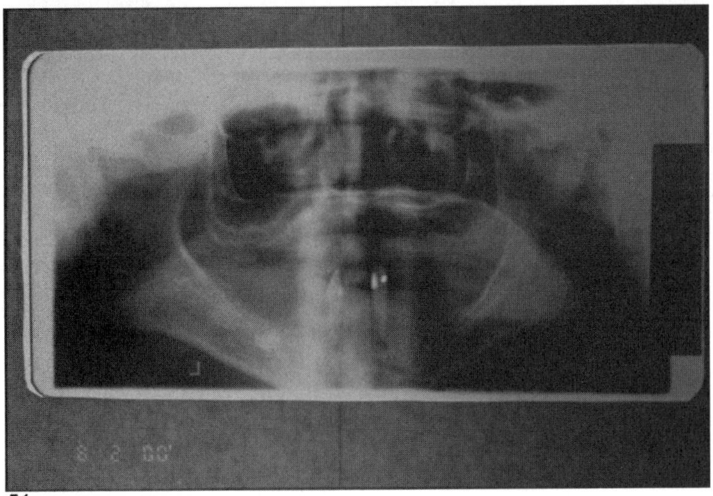

51

Figures 50, 51 An untreated mandible fracture resulting in acute osteomyelitis.

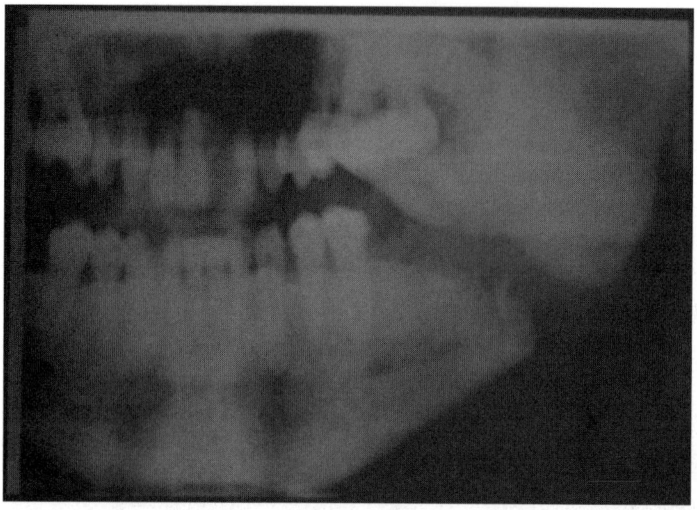

Figure 52 Acute osteomyelitis in a fracture of the mandibular angle. Note bony sequestrum.

AVULSIVE MANDIBULAR INJURIES

Treatment of avulsive mandibular injuries should be viewed from three perspectives: triage, setup surgery, and definitive (reconstructive) treatment. In some cases, these three objectives can be met with one surgery. In other cases, multiple operating room visits may be required. In most circumstances, re-establishment of occlusion is not the only consideration. Restoring facial contour, tissue bulk, deglutition, and speech are also goals. When discussing infected mandible fractures, a diagnostic distinction between osteomyelitis and overlying soft tissue infection or dental infection (pericoronitis) is not always clear. However, because most mandible fractures are compound through the dentition, the risk of bacterial invasion to medullary bone poses a significant risk of osteomyelitis. Risk factors for development of osteomyelitis in fractures of the mandible include old, untreated compound fractures; inadequate immobilization or fixation; a devitalized tooth in the line of fracture; and diminished host defense (usually in diabetics or alcoholics) (1,2).

Treatment of a mandible fracture in the presence of osteomyelitis demands aggressive surgical therapy coupled with targeted antibiotic coverage. Incision and drainage are often required, and debridement of necrotic cortical and medullary bone should be performed until healthy bleeding bone is encountered (Figs. 47–49). Placement of irrigation or drainage mechanisms is often helpful, especially in extensive cases. Immobilization of fracture segments is a critical element to successful treatment and multiple means of fixation (biphasic pins, reconstruction plates, closed reduction) have been advocated. Secondary delayed reconstruction and bone grafting is often required in cases of limited remaining bone volume or in discontinuity defects.

Treatment of avulsive mandibular injuries (e.g., gunshot wounds) and grossly infected mandible fractures is inherently more complex (Figs. 50,51). The biphasic pin fixation system is a simple technique that is often useful under these circum-

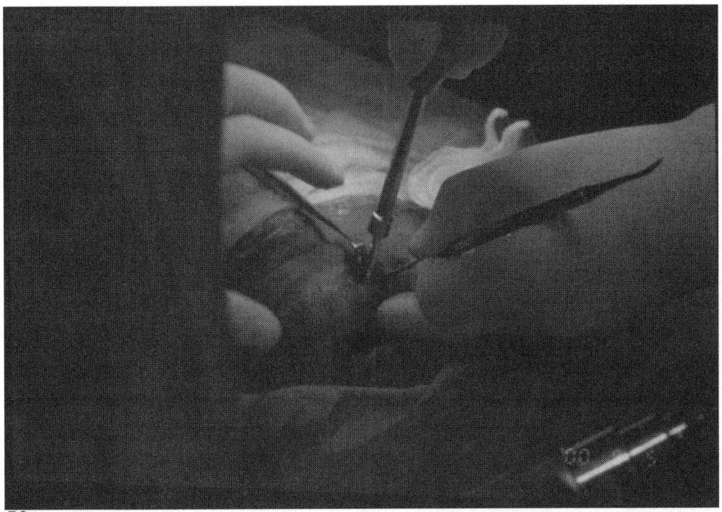

53

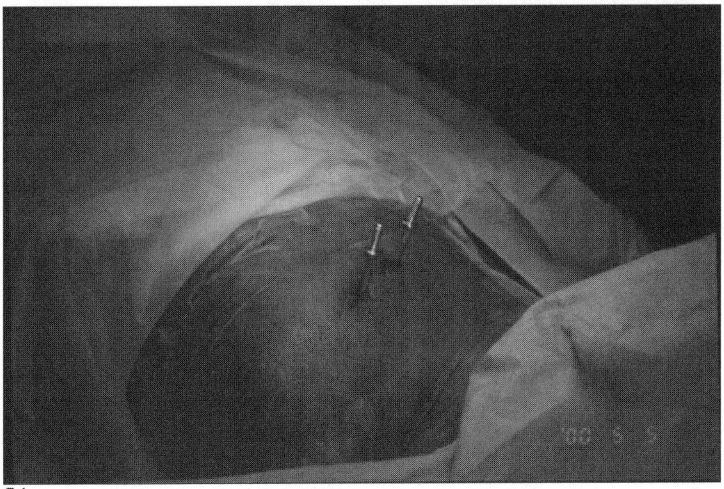

54

Figures 53,54 Placement of percutaneous screws in biphasic pin fixation.

stances (31). This treatment method that can be utilized in a closed or open fashion, alone or in conjunction with other techniques. The biphasic pin method allows mandibular function and movement across broad gaps of tissue loss or infection with limited segmental mobility. This method should be avoided in maximally irradiated patients, osteoporotic mandibles, and in grossly contaminated wounds involving loss of cheek tissue over the mandible (32). The technique is useful in complex fractures of the edentulous mandible. Proficiency is required to master the technique, but its clinical success is well documented. It has two phases of application. The first is initial placement of percutaneous bicortical lag-type screws to the underlying mandible at a distance from the gap or infection (Figs. 52–54) to which attaches an external fixation jig used to reduce the segments (Fig. 55). In the second phase, a

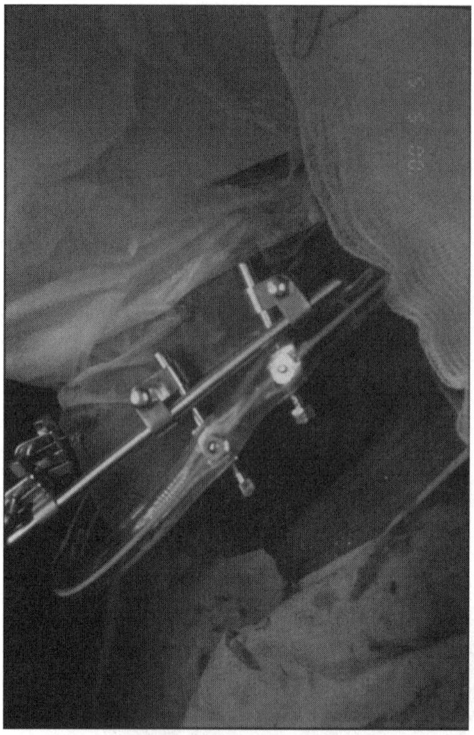

Figure 55 Placement of external fixation jig and template for acrylic bar (a modified endotracheal tube) in biphasic pin fixation.

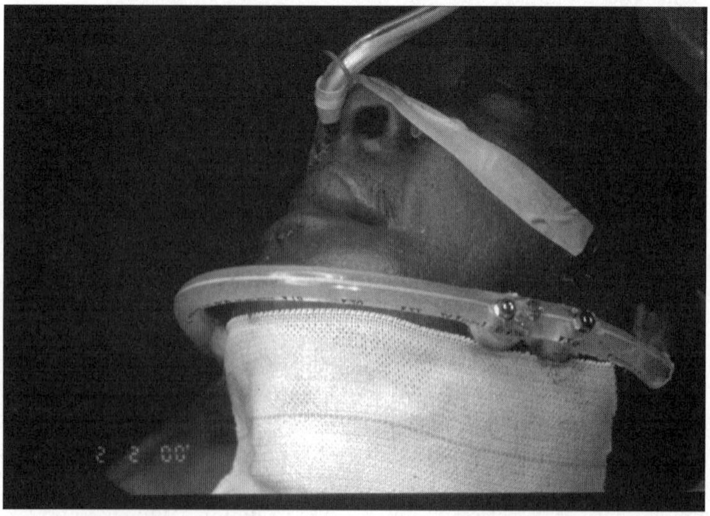

Figure 56 Acrylic bar stabilizing mandible fracture in biphasic pin fixation.

continuous acrylic bar is applied to the screws to maintain alignment and immobilization and to allow removal of the jig (Fig. 56). Great care must be taken to avoid injury to tooth roots and the inferior alveolar nerve when placing biphasic pins. Some facial scarring is expected at the site of screw penetration into the skin. Due to the severity of the injury, prolonged fixation beyond 4–6 weeks is commonly required.

SUMMARY

The proper treatment of mandible fractures and dentoalveolar injuries requires the practitioner to correlate a detailed patient history with results from a comprehensive examination and pertinent good-quality radiographs. Re-establishment of a proper occlusal relationship in a predictable fashion while minimizing foreseeable complications should be the guiding rule for clinicians. This will often necessitate coordination of care with other surgical specialties, as in the multitrauma patient, so that proper sequencing of treatment optimizes surgical outcomes. This is especially true in the patient with panfacial trauma. Numerous treatment schemes have been proposed in the literature to sequence care in the panfacial trauma patient (bottom to top, inside to outside, etc.). Practitioners who treat these patients realize that neurosurgical, ophthalmological, orthopedic, and critical care concerns may dictate restructuring one's traditional approach to such cases. The clinician's judgment (in choosing an appropriate treatment method) is ultimately responsible for the overall successful management of a case. It should be our responsibility as practitioners to evaluate critically our treatment outcomes to ensure that our clinical skills and judgement remain timely and sharp.

REFERENCES

1. Rowe NL, Williams JL. Maxillofacial Injuries. Vol. 1. Edinburgh: Churchill, Livingstone, 1986.
2. Barber HD, Woodbury SC, Silverstein KE, Fonseca RJ. Mandibular fractures. In: Fonseca RJ, Walker RV, eds. Second Edition. Oral and Maxillofacial Trauma, WB Saunders, Philadelphia, PA, Vol. 1. 1997:473–526.
3. Dorlands' Illustrated Medical Dictionary, Philadelphia, PA: WB Saunders, 1988.
4. Ruskin JD, Tu HK. Integrated management of the maxillofacial trauma patient with multiple injuries. Oral Maxillofac Surg Clin North Am 1990; 21:15–27.
5. Passeri LA, Ellis e, Sinn DP. Relationship of substance abuse to complications with mandibular fractures. J Oral Maxillofac Surg 1993; 51:22.
6. Angle EH. Classification of malocclusion. Dent Cosmos 1899; 41:248, 305.
7. Maloney PL et al. A protocol for the management of compound mandibular fractures based on the time from injury to treatment. J Oral Maxillofac Surg 2001; 59:8.
8. Maloney PL et al. Early immobilization of Mandible Fractures. J Oral Maxillofac Surg 1991; 49:698.
9. Zallen RD, Curry JY. A study of antibiotic usage in compound mandibular fractures. J Oral Surg 1975; 33:431.
10. Ziccardi VB, Bergen-Shapiro M. Metabolic and nutritional aspects of facial trauma. Oral Maxillofac Surg Clin North Am 1998; 10(4):507.
11. Ivy RH, Curtis L. Fractures of the Jaws. Philadelphia: Lea & Febiger, 1931.

12. Gunning TB. Treatment of fractures of the lower jaw by interdental splints. Br J Dent Sci 1866; 9:481.
13. Obwegesser H. The surgical correction of mandibular prognathism and retrognathia with consideration of genioplasty. I. Surgical procedures to correct mandibular prognathism and reshaping of the chin. Oral Surg 1957; 10:677.
14. Assael LA. Principles of rigid internal fixation in Oral and Maxillofacial Surgery Knowledge Update. Alpharetta, Georgia: AAOMS Publications. Vol. I, part II, 1995.
15. Bos RM. Discussion. J Oral Maxillofac Surg 2001; 59:25.
16. Bradley JC. A Radiological investigation into the age changes of the inferior dental artery. Br J Oral Surg 1975; 13:82.
17. Bradley P. Injuries of the condylar and coronoid process. In: Rowe NL, Williams JL, eds. Maxillofacial Injuries, Edinburgh: Churchill Livingstone, Vol. 1, 1986:337–362.
18. Abubaker, AO, Giglio JA, Strauss RA. Diagnosis and management of dentoalveolar injuriesOral Maxillofac Surg Knowl Update. Vol. 3, 2001, 29–45.
19. Powers MP, Quereshy FA. Diagnosis and management of dentoalveolar injuries. In: Fonseca R, Walker R, eds. Oral and Maxillofacial Trauma, Philadelphia, PA:WB Saunders, Vol. 1. 1997; 419–472.
20. Rombach DM, Quinn PD. Trauma to the temporomandibular region. In: Fonseca RJ, Walker RV, eds. Second Edition. Oral and Maxillofacial Trauma, WB Saunders, Philadelphia, Vol. 1. 1997:527–570.
21. Lindahl L. Condylar fractures of the mandible I. Classification and relations age, occlusion, and concomitant injuries of the teeth and teeth supporting structures, and fractures of the mandibular body. Int J Oral Surg 1977; 6:12.
22. MacLennan WD. Consideration of 180 cases of typical fractures of the mandibular condyloid process. Br J Plast Surg 1952; 5:123.
23. Barton JR. A systematic bandage for fractures of the lower jaw. Am Med Record 1819; 2:153.
24. Zide MF, Kent JN. Indications for open reduction of mandibular condyle fracture. J Oral Maxillofac Surg 1983; 41:89.
25. Raveh J et al. Open reduction of the dislocated, fractured condylar process: indications and surgical procedures. J oral maxillofacial surg 1989; 47:120.
26. James D. Maxillofacial injuries in children. In: Rowe NL, Williams JL, eds. Maxillofacial Injuries, Edinburgh: Churchill Livingstone, Vol. 1. 1986:538–558.
27. Rowe NL. Fractures of the jaws in children. J Oral Surg 1969; 27:497.
28. Lehman JA, Saddaw ND. Fractures of the mandibile in Children. J Trauma 1976; 16:773.
29. Moss ML. The primary of functional matrices in orofacial growth. Dent. Pract 1968; 19:65.
30. Lindahl L, Hollender L. Condylar fractures of the mandible II. A Radiographic study of remodeling processess in the temporomandibular joint. Int J oral surg 1977; 6:153.
31. Fleming ID, Morris JH. use of acrylic external splint after mandibular resection. Am J Surg 1969; 118:708.
32. Hopkins R. Mandibular fractures; treatment by closed reduction and indirect skeletal fixation. In: Rowe NL, Williams JL, eds. Maxillofacial Injuries, Edinburgh: Churchill, Livingstone, Vol. 1. 1986:232–292.

17
Zygomatic Complex and Internal Orbital Fractures

Robert W. Dolan
Lahey Clinic Medical Center, Burlington, Massachusetts, U.S.A.

ZYGOMATIC COMPLEX FRACTURES

Etiology, Definition, Demographics, Signs, and Symptoms

A zygomatic complex (ZMC) fracture is characterized by traumatic disarticulation of the zygomatic bone from the facial skeleton along four major sutures including the frontozygomatic, sphenozygomatic, zygomaticomaxillary, and zygomaticotemporal. A ZMC fracture is also often incorrectly referred to as a tripod fracture. This fracture is more accurately termed a tetrapod due to its separation from the facial skeleton along four (not three) suture lines. Any classification scheme must differentiate zygoma fractures that are isolated to one segment of the zygoma bone (e.g., zygomatic arch) from those involving disarticulation of the zygoma bone from the facial skeleton (tetrapod).

A ZMC fracture is usually caused by a low-energy blunt blow over the lateral orbital rim and malar eminence during a motor vehicle accident or assault. ZMC fractures are the second most common facial fracture (nasal fractures are most frequent) occurring most often in men 20–40 years of age.

The signs and symptoms of a ZMC fracture include periorbital, buccal, and conjunctival ecchymoses; epistaxis; malar flattening; palpable bony steps over the inferior and lateral orbital rims and the zygomaticomaxillary buttress under the lip; numbness over the cheek (in more than one half of cases); trismus (one-third of cases); enophthalmos (rare); and the Pulfrich phenomenon (very rare) (1) (Fig. 1). The Pulfrich phenomenon describes a disturbance in stereoscopic vision that occurs due to aberrancies in retinal latency (2). It is detectable in fewer than 4% of patients. Central stereoscopic processing is impaired and objects moving in a straight line are perceived as moving along a hyperbolic curve. This is particularly evident when driving a car, since oncoming traffic may appear to be crossing the centerline. Correction requires the use of a tinted lens over the normal eye to increase retinal latency to match the affected eye.

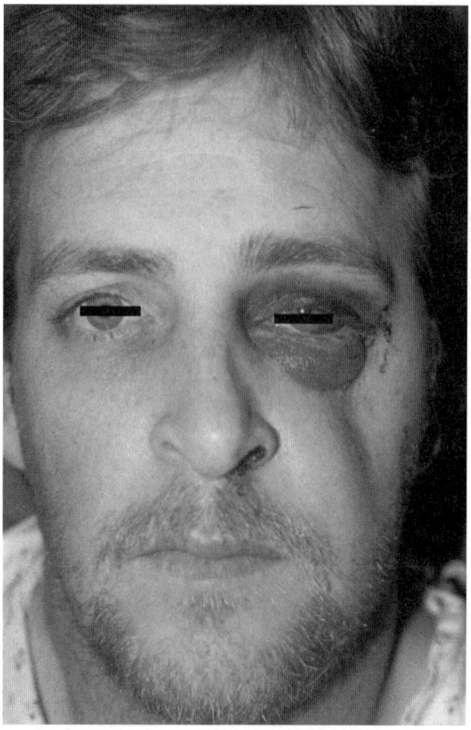

Figure 1 Patient sustained a left ZMC fracture. Note periorbital ecchymosis and obvious malar flattening.

The zygomatic bone tends to displace inferomedially, crushing the anterior wall of the maxillary sinus resulting in a palpable bony step over the area. The step is felt under the lip over the face of the maxilla. Epistaxis results from lacerations in the maxillary sinus mucosa. The infraorbital canal creates an area of weakness along the orbital floor and the fracture line usually follows this structure posteriorly from the zygomaticomaxillary suture line at the orbital rim. As a consequence, contusion and dysfunction of the infraorbital nerve is a common finding. Although trismus is often thought to be due to impaction of the zygomatic process onto the coronoid process of the mandible, it is more likely due to spasm of the temporalis and pterygoid muscles. Enophthalmos in the immediate post-injury period indicates a significant defect in the bony orbital cavity that may require surgical intervention beyond reduction and fixation of the zygomatic bone. Separation of the zygomaticomaxillary and sphenozygomatic suture lines increases orbital volume and allows orbital contents to escape. Muscle impingement, double vision, and globe malposition are possible sequelae. An antimongoloid slant to the palpebral fissure is common due to inferior displacement of Whitnall's tubercle and the lateral palpebral ligament. Globe injury occurs in approximately 5% of cases and ophthalmological consultation is mandatory (3). Common injuries involving the globe itself include vitreous hemorrhage, hyphema, optic nerve contusion, and corneal abrasion.

Pertinent Anatomy

Surface Anatomy

The malar eminence, globe, and lateral canthus are the main surface anatomical structures affected by a ZMC fracture. These structures are difficult to assess acutely in the presence of edema and bruising. Malar (cheek) symmetry is the most useful external indicator of accurate reduction. However, cheek prominence and apparent

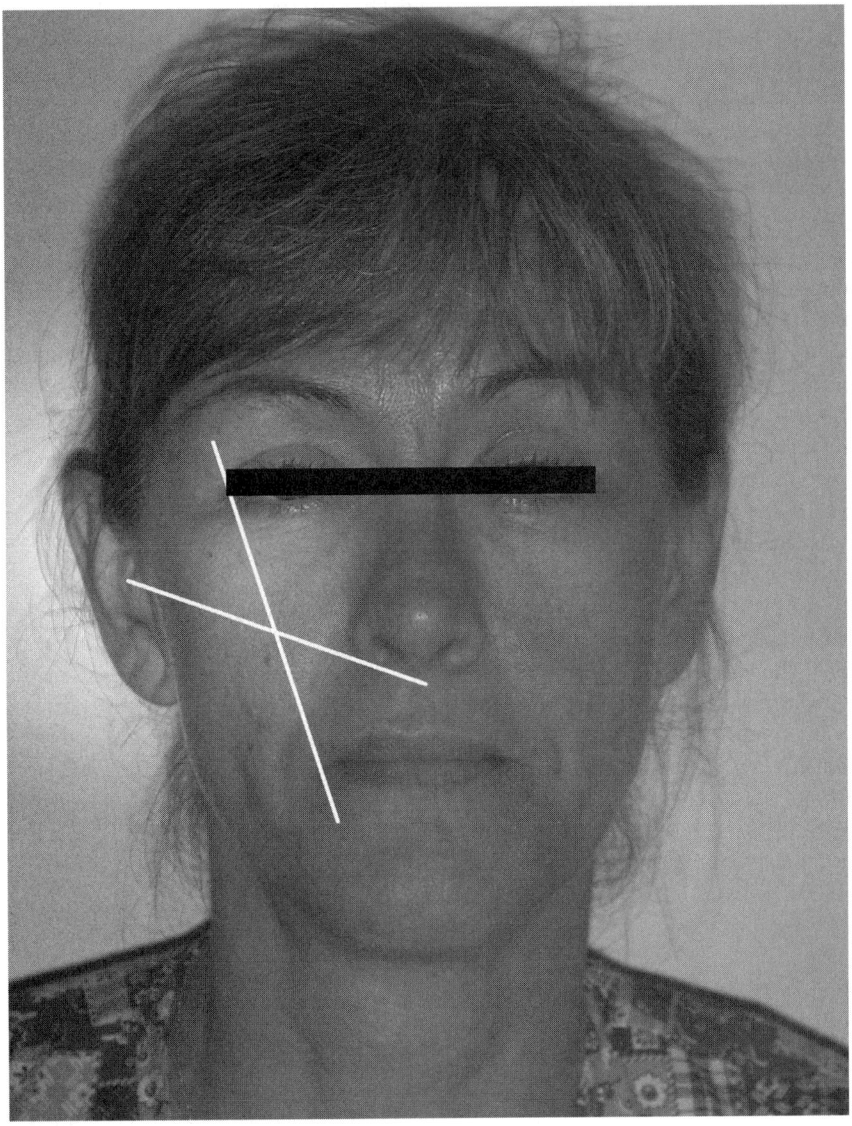

Figure 2 The area posterosuperior to the intersection of lines tangent to the tragus and inferior edge of nasal ala and oral commissure and lateral canthus represents the expected most prominent area of the malar eminence.

symmetry alone are inadequate in all but the most straightforward cases. Nevertheless, it useful to appreciate the aesthetics of the malar eminence and to appreciate where the most prominent area of the eminence is normally located. In the frontal view, a line is drawn from the lateral oral commissure to the ipsilateral lateral canthus. Another line is drawn from the tragus to the inferior edge of the nasal ala. The area posterosuperior to the intersection of these two lines represents the most prominent area of the malar eminence (4) (Fig. 2).

The globe is intimately associated with the zygomatic bone and is invariably affected by ZMC fractures. The zygomatic bone forms a major portion of the floor and lateral wall of the orbit through its frontosphenoidal and orbital processes. Although the bony orbital floor is disrupted, anatomical reduction of a simple ZMC fracture usually results in restoration of normal orbital volume and bony floor support. In addition, Lockwood's ligament provides further support for the globe. However, in cases with extensive disruptions of the orbital floor and medial wall associated with herniation of the periorbita, significant permanent enophthalmos may result. Enophthalmos greater than 2 mm is usually noticeable. Enophthalmos associated with disruption of the orbital walls that is noted preoperatively is an ominous sign and an absolute indication for orbital exploration and reconstruction. Disruption of the orbital floor posterior to the axis of the globe results in enophthalmos and disruption anterior to the axis of the globe results in vertical dystopia.

Inferior displacement of the ZMC (including the frontosphenoidal process) results in inferior displacement of its attached lateral retinaculum and lateral canthus. The palpebral slit slants (antimongoloid) and often becomes foreshortened. An inaccurate reduction may result in retention of these features postoperatively. The lateral palpebral ligament includes superficial and deep limbs that course from the orbital septum and lateral tarsal borders to the lateral orbital rim. The superficial component is thin and ill-defined, inserting into the fascia over the superficial aspect of the lateral orbital rim. The deep limbs are distinct fascial bands that originate at the lateral borders of the superior and inferior tarsal plates and insert onto the medial aspect of the lateral orbital rim at Whitnall's tubercle. The normal position of the lateral canthus is variable depending on the age, gender, and race of the patient. Young women tend to have lateral canthi that are slightly elevated compared to their medial canthi. With age, the lateral canthi tend to descend and lie on the same horizontal plane. Another important feature of the lateral canthus is its relationship to the upper lid fold. The lateral aspect of the lower lid should gently slope upward toward its lateral insertion, and should appear to tuck slightly under the upper lid fold (Fig. 3).

Zygomatic Bone

The zygomatic bone has four processes: the frontosphenoidal, orbital, maxillary, and temporal. These processes articulate with the surrounding facial skeleton at the frontozygomatic, sphenozygomatic, zygomaticomaxillary, and zygomaticotemporal sutures, respectively. The frontosphenoidal and orbital processes form the majority of the lateral and inferolateral bony orbit. In addition, Whitnall's tubercle is an important anatomical landmark located approximately 9 mm inferior to the frontozygomatic suture and 3 mm posterior to the lateral orbital rim (5). Whitnall's

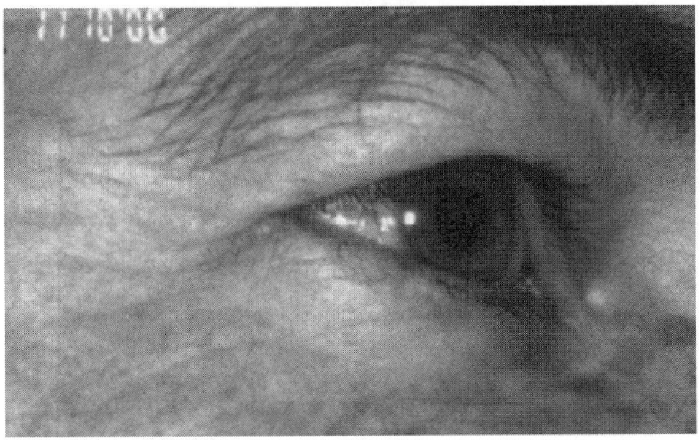

Figure 3 Note subtle tuck of the lateral lower eyelid into the lateral upper eyelid.

tubercle serves to anchor several essential structures including the lateral canthal tendon, check ligament of the lateral rectus muscle, suspensory ligament of Lockwood, and lateral extension of the levator aponeurosis.

The zygomaticofrontal (ZF), zygomaticotemporal, zygomaticomaxillary (ZM), and sphenozygomatic sutures define the articulations of the zygomatic bone with the surrounding facial skeleton (Fig. 4). The thickest bone is found within the frontozygomatic suture and is an excellent site for the application of wires or plates for fixation. The zygomaticotemporal suture delineates the relatively long zygomatic process of the temporal bone from the short temporal process of the zygomatic bone. The zygomatic bone's broadest attachment is with the maxilla both in the orbit and along the zygomaticomaxillary buttress. The sphenozygomatic suture is formed from the union of the upper portion of the orbital process of the zygomatic bone with the greater wing of the sphenoid. This suture line is curvilinear, thus providing a valuable guide to accurate three-dimensional alignment of the ZMC. The lower portion of the orbital process unites with the roof of the maxilla to form the orbital aspect of the zygomaticomaxillary suture. ZMC fractures involve at least four skeletal disruptions: sphenozygomatic suture, inferior orbital rim and floor, ZF suture, and the zygomaticomaxillary suture (hence the term "tetrapod" fracture).

The zygomatic arch is surrounded by muscle and fascia that helps to prevent the displacement of fracture fragments. The temporal muscle passes deep to the arch within the temporal fossa and the temporal fascia attaches along the superior edge. The masseter muscle attaches along its inferior border providing firm inferior pull on fracture fragments against the unyielding temporal fascia. This results in a stabilizing effect that tends to maintain the contour of the arch despite the lack of rigid fixation or wires.

Sensory Nerves

The maxillary division of the trigeminal nerve is at risk of injury (e.g., neurapraxia and neurotmesis) in a ZMC fracture. The main terminal branch of the maxillary nerve is the infraorbital nerve. The infraorbital nerve is at the highest

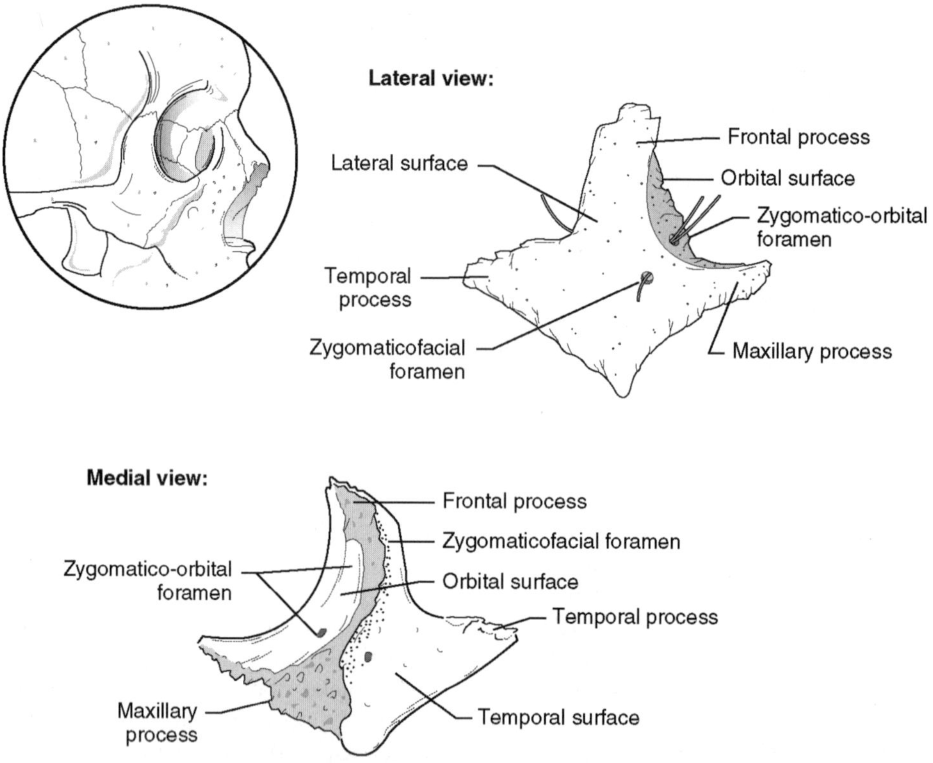

Figure 4 Note the many articulations of the zygomatic bone with the surrounding facial skeleton. These suture lines are the typical areas of separation seen in patients with ZMC fractures.

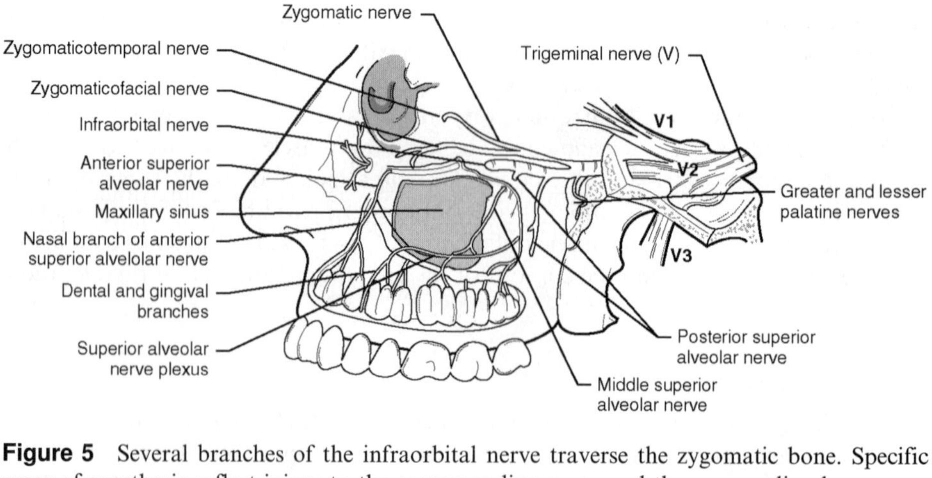

Figure 5 Several branches of the infraorbital nerve traverse the zygomatic bone. Specific areas of anesthesia reflect injury to the corresponding nerve and the surrounding bone.

risk of injury while branches within the orbital cavity are proportionally less at risk as one proceeds posteriorly toward the inferior orbital fissure and pterygopalatine fossa. Proceeding from anterior to posterior from the infraorbital foramen, the branches include anterior superior alveolar, middle superior alveolar, and zygomatic nerves (6) (Fig. 5). The anterior superior alveolar nerve is given off just proximal to the infraorbital foramen and descends in a groove in the anterior wall of the maxillary sinus to supply the ipsilateral incisor and canine teeth. The middle superior alveolar nerve arises from within the posterior part of the infraorbital canal and runs in a groove in the lateral wall of the maxillary sinus to supply the ipsilateral two premolar teeth. The zygomatic nerve branches from the maxillary nerve after it passes through the foramen rotundum within the pterygopalatine fossa. The zygomatic nerve enters the orbit via the inferior orbital fissure and divides into the zygomaticotemporal and zygomaticofacial branches. The temporal division emerges on the face, exiting the orbit via the zygomaticotemporal foramen along the sphenozygomatic suture line. The zygomaticofacial nerve continues anteriorly within the bony orbit to exit through the zygomaticofacial foramen in the body of the zygoma. The zygomaticofacial and zygomaticotemporal nerves are branches of the zygomatic nerve of V2. The zygomaticofacial nerve penetrates the orbicularis oculi muscle over the malar area to supply the skin overlying this area. The zygomaticotemporal nerve passes around the anterior border of the temporalis muscle to penetrate the temporalis fascia 2 cm above the zygomatic arch to supply the temple area. These nerves have substantial crossover supply from neighboring sensory nerves including the auriculotemporal and lacrimal nerves.

The infraorbital nerve divides into three branches including the inferior palpebral, external nasal, and superior labial. Inferior palpebral branches ascend to supply the lower eyelid; the external nasal branches supply the nasal sidewall; and numerous superior labial branches descend to supply the cheek, upper lip, and opposing mucous membrane.

Patients may complain of dysesthesia or anesthesia of the upper teeth following a ZMC fracture. Sensory disturbances of the incisor and canine teeth indicate a nerve injury anteriorly near the infraorbital canal. Sensory disturbance involving the premolar teeth indicates nerve injury in the posterior orbit. Rarely do patients complain of sensory disturbances in the territories of the zygomaticofacial or zygomaticotemporal nerves despite the fact that these nerves are vulnerable to injury as they exit directly through the zygomatic bone. Perhaps, with the significant cross innervation in the areas that these nerves serve, the sensory deprivation is negligible. The incidence of long-term sensory disturbances within the distribution of the infraorbital nerve is reported to be approximately 45% (7,8). Significant permanent nerve injury (Sunderland's third or fourth degree) can be found in more than one-third of patients (9). Third-degree nerve injury (endoneurotmesis) involves disruption of the endoneurium and axons but the perineurium and epineurium remain intact. Wallerian degeneration occurs, but since the perineural and epineural layers remain intact partial reinnervation and incomplete recovery occurs. Fourth-degree nerve injury (perineurotmesis) involves disruption of the perineurium, endoneurium, and axons. Wallerian degeneration occurs with incomplete and misdirected axonal regeneration. Nerve recovery is poor.

Radiological Examinations

Any patient with a complex midface fracture should be evaluated with a computed tomographic (CT) scan (5 mm slices in the axial and coronal planes). Plain radiographs provide limited information and are usually inadequate for preoperative planning. Axial CT scanning is useful in evaluating the involvement and degree of displacement and comminution of the sphenozygomatic suture, zygomatic arch, and malar eminence. Asymmetry in the height of the cornea is also a good indication of the presence of enophthalmos or exophthalmos. The coronal images are most useful in evaluating the degree of injury to the bony orbital walls, herniation of periorbita, and the displacement and comminution of the inferior and lateral orbital rims (Fig. 6). The information gained by careful consideration of the preoperative CT scan is invaluable to planning of the surgery including the various surgical approaches, the type of reduction likely to be successful (closed vs. open), and the type and extent of wire or rigid fixation necessary. Objective criteria for orbital exploration and classification systems based on preoperative CT scanning exist that assist the clinician in obtaining favorable results. The use of intraoperative CT scanning during the repair of ZMC fractures is possible using mobile units. In institutions that have mobile units, rapid post-reduction CT scanning should be considered in patients with complex ZMC and midfacial fractures. Intraoperative CT is especially useful in detecting errors in reduction of the orbital walls, since these are often missed using plain films. The advantages of this approach include potential cost savings in reducing the need for revision surgery and improved outcomes including fewer cases of late enophthalmos and fracture misalignment (10).

Apart from obtaining a CT, a plain radiograph can be obtained immediately after reduction and fixation while the patient is still under general anesthesia. Although the information gained from this type of x-ray is limited, it is valuable for the detection of gross errors. A single Water's view (a posterior–anterior projection with the head positioned at a 27 degree angle to the vertical) is obtained and several parameters are checked, including stray bony fragments, neglected fractures, bony orbital volume asymmetry, inferior or lateral orbital rim misalignments, and malar

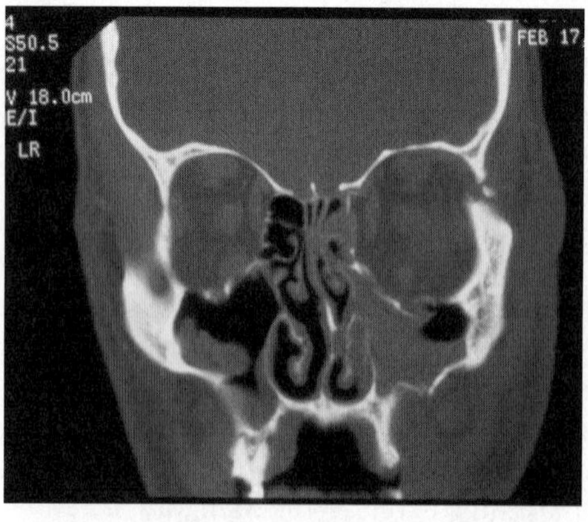

Figure 6 Coronal CT scan shows inferolateral displacement of the ZMC associated with a trapdoor orbital floor defect.

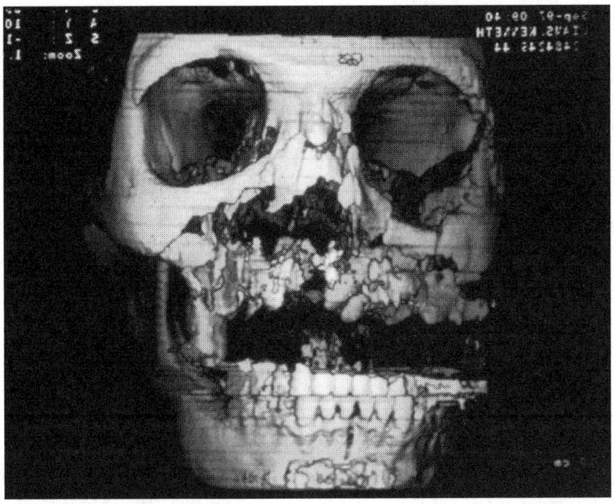

Figure 7 Three-dimensional CT scan shows a complex ZMC fracture secondary to a high-energy injury.

depression. A submentovertex (base) view is useful both preoperatively and intraoperatively for the accurate assessment of the position of the zygomatic arch. Plain films are especially poor at detecting fractures involving the medial orbital wall (11).

Newer three-dimensional CT scan reformations (3D CT) are available that may assist the surgeon in preoperative planning of unusual or complicated cases. In a small study of patients presenting with routine facial fractures ($n = 20$) there was no improvement in the accuracy of interpretations with the addition of 3D CT (12). However, 3D CT is superior to 2D CT and multiplanar reformation scans for localization and anatomical characterization of complex fractures (13) (Fig. 7). Several classification schemes based on radiological criteria attempt to group fractures according to their likely causative, therapeutic and prognostic implications. Zingg et al. present a simple classification of zygomatic fractures based on over 1000 cases (14). It consists of five types of fractures based on a combination of standard radiographs and axial and coronal CT (Fig. 8): A (incomplete), B (complete monofragment), and C (multifragment). The most common type was B (57%) followed by C (35%) and A (8%). The fracture sites are as follows: A1— isolated zygomatic arch; A2—isolated lateral orbital rim; A3—isolated infraorbital rim; B—monofragment (classic) ZMC fracture; and C—multifragmented ZMC fracture (including fracture through the body of the zygoma, typically a high-energy injury). In general, open reduction is required for displaced types A2 and A3 fractures, selected type B fractures, and all type C fractures. Adverse outcomes including late enophthalmos and malalignment are more common with type C fractures.

OPEN SURGICAL APPROACHES

Open reduction of type B and C ZMC fractures may require multiple surgical approaches for access to the inferior orbital rim and orbital floor, sphenozygomatic suture, zygomaticofacial suture, and zygomaticomaxillary suture. Often the incisions

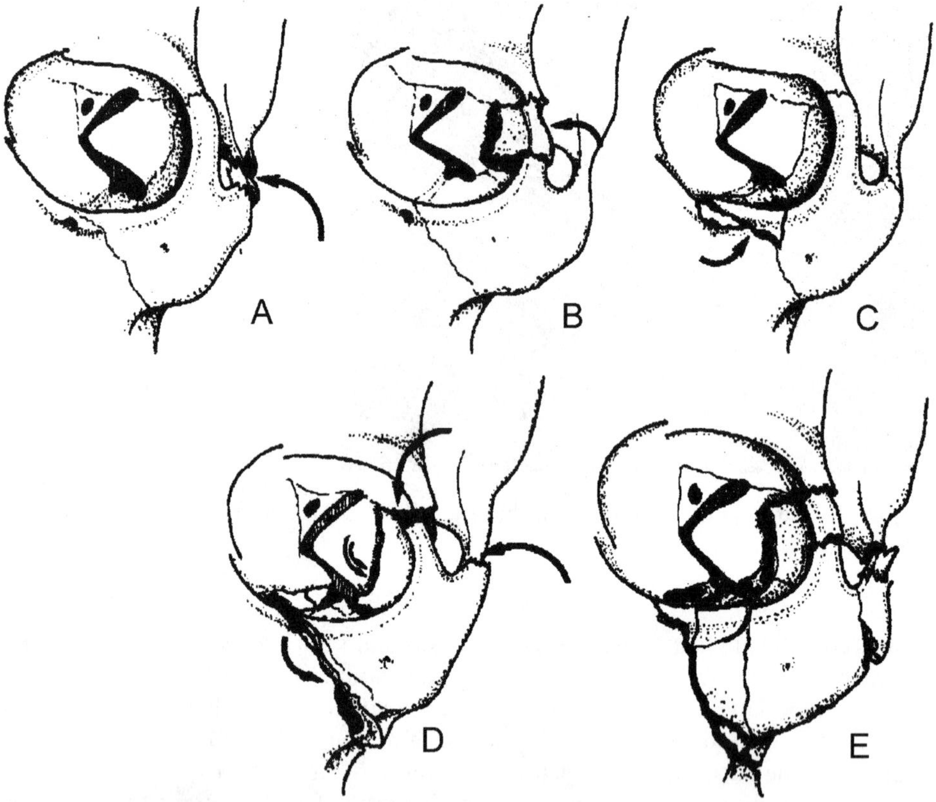

Figure 8 Classification system for ZMC fractures. Isolated fractures includes types A1, A2, and A3. Type A1 (A) are isolated zygomatic arch fractures; type A2 (B) are isolated lateral orbital wall fractures; type A3 (C) are isolated infraorbital rim fractures. Type B (D) fractures are traditional tetrapod fractures and type C (E) fractures are multifragmented ZMC fractures. (From Ref. 14.).

are remote from the fracture to avoid visible scars or sensorimotor deficits. Although limited surgical access is often all that is required for selected simple facial fractures, complex or comminuted fractures demand wider exposure for accurate reduction and fixation. The modern approach to complex facial fractures is wide surgical exposure that facilitates a three-dimensional assessment of fracture displacement and application of rigid internal fixation appliances and bone grafts. These craniofacial surgical approaches emphasize minimally invasive techniques that spare neurosensory structures while maximizing exposure of the facial skeleton. Craniofacial incisions are hidden in areas such as behind the hairline, within the oral cavity, in the conjunctiva, or under the eyelid.

Surgical exposure of the infraorbital rim and orbital floor involves a transconjunctival or transcutaneous route. The transconjunctival approach to the orbital rim and floor has proved to be superior to the transcutaneous approaches (e.g., subciliary) in the avoidance of postoperative lower lid malposition including ectropion (15). However, access to both the inferior and lateral orbital rim is often required in ZMC fractures and can be facilitated by the addition of a lateral canthotomy. A lateral canthotomy may also be added if the exposure to the orbital floor is inadequate. Exposure of the lateral orbital rim via a lateral canthotomy alone is described but it requires extensive tissue retraction and the exposure is often inadequate for hardware placement. The addition of a superior cantholysis greatly facilitates the exposure of the lateral orbital rim and ZF suture (16). Lateral canthotomy and superior cantholysis provide generous exposure of the ZF suture while avoiding a cutaneous scar in the lateral brow. Exposing the ZF suture in this manner frees the tissues of the lateral orbit, enhancing the exposure of the sphenozygomatic suture (aiding reduction). The transconjunctival route to the orbital floor requires a detailed understanding of the anatomy of the lower eyelid and meticulous surgical technique. During the procedure, loop magnification is helpful to identify accurately the layers of the lower eyelid. A preseptal approach is preferred to prevent orbital fat from prolapsing into the wound. The preseptal route will also avoid injury to the inferior oblique and rectus muscles.

Transconjunctival exposure of the orbital rim and floor begins by placement of a corneal shield (crescent-shaped plastic or metal conforming cup). The shield is supplanted later in the operation by pulling the inferiorly based conjunctivocapsulopalpebral flap over the corneal surface using fine silk traction sutures. The surgeon stands at the head of the table and the inner aspect of the lower eyelid is everted to visualize the inferior tarsus. The tarsus is usually approximately 5 mm wide and a horizontal conjunctival incision is made approximately 1 mm inferior to the tarsus (6 mm inferior to the lid margin). This incision extends from the lateral canthus to just lateral to the orifice of the inferior canaliculus. Bleeding and prominent blood vessels are controlled with bipolar electrocautery. The conjunctival incision is deepened through the capsulopalpebral fascia above the divergence of the fascial layers that enclose the orbital fat (capsulopalpebral fascia and orbital septum). If the transcapsulopalpebral incision is placed too low, the orbital fat will be inadvertently entered. The deep surgical plane is the orbicularis oculi muscle whose fibers are visualized through the capsulopalpebral incision. The muscle is not entered and a dissection plane is developed toward the inferior orbital rim between the muscle fibers and the orbital septum. The orbital septum blends with the periosteum over the rim and face of the maxilla. As the rim is encountered, the dissection continues anteriorly about 1 mm and a horizontal incision is made through the periosteum anterior to the arcus marginalis. The arcus marginalis represents the junction of three layers of fascia along the inferior orbital rim including the orbital septum, maxillary periosteum, and periorbita. A subperiosteal plane is developed along the rim and retrodissected under the periorbita exposing the orbital rim and floor. Wider exposure of the orbital floor is possible via a lateral canthotomy and inferior cantholysis.

After reduction, fixation, and placement of the orbital floor implant (if necessary) the inferior canthal tendon is carefully sutured (nonabsorbable suture) above and slightly behind its original attachment at Whitnall's tubercle. The orientation of the lateral lower eyelid with respect to the upper eyelid is visually confirmed so that the lower eyelid curves gently superiorly to fall just behind the lateral extent of the upper eyelid. The lateral canthotomy skin incision is closed in layers. The conjunctival incision requires no suturing. At the conclusion of the operation, the lower lid should be pulled superiorly to eliminate overlap of the capsulopalpebral flap and

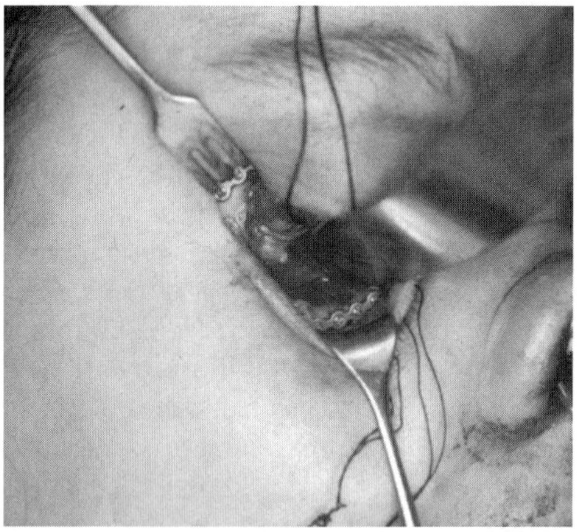

Figure 9 Exposure obtained after a transconjunctival approach combined with superior cantholysis. Note excellent exposure of both the infraorbital rim fracture and the ZF suture simultaneously.

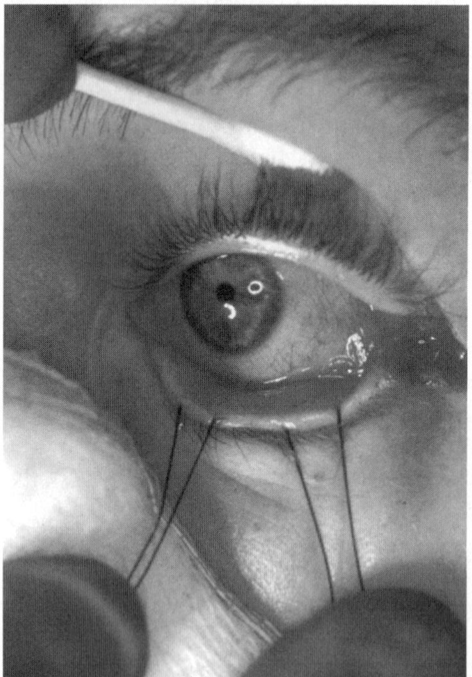

Figure 10 Lateral canthotomy and inferior cantholysis. Note that the through-and-through lateral canthal incision extends through the lateral retinaculum and overlying skin no more than 1 cm lateral to the lateral commissure.

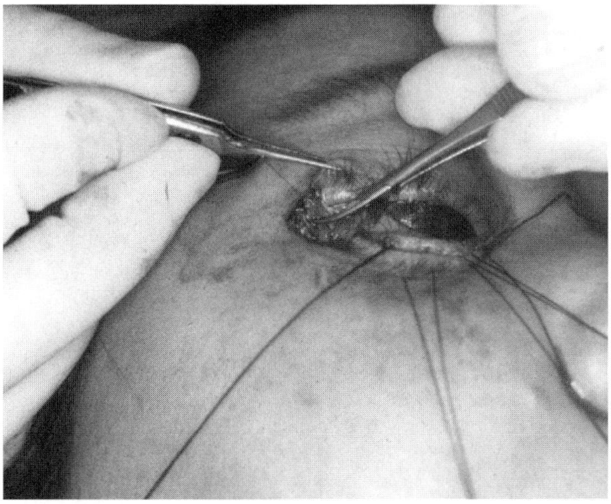

Figure 11 A superior cantholysis is being performed to facilitate exposure of the zygomaticofacial suture. Note that a marking suture is placed through the tendon prior to its transection.

the transconjunctival incision. A Frost suture or inferior lid taping for 48 h is helpful to prevent poor appositional healing and cicatrical ectropion.

Lateral canthotomy and superior cantholysis is performed to expose the ZF suture for miniplate application (Fig. 9). The skin incision for the lateral canthotomy extends to no more than 1 cm beyond the lateral palpebral slit (Fig. 10). The deep limb of the superior canthal tendon is located by pulling the eyelid margin laterally and strumming the tendon with a fine forceps. Distal and proximal to the midportion of the exposed tendon, 4–0 nonabsorbable sutures are passed and held away with hemostats and the tendon is cut between the sutures (Fig. 11). The upper eyelid is lifted away from the lateral orbital rim, exposing the periosteum over the ZF suture. The periosteum of the lateral orbital rim is incised vertically and peeled away from the underlying ZF suture a few millimeters above the insertion of the lateral canthal tendon. The periosteum is stripped to accommodate a miniplate with two proximal and two distal screw holes. The superior canthal tendon must be precisely reapproximated, but this is easily accomplished by simply tying together the stay sutures previously placed distal and proximal to the original cut. The lateral canthotomy is best reapproximated by first passing a deep absorbable suture through the lateral palpebral slit and then closing the skin incision in layers.

Although approaching the ZF suture by superior cantholysis is very useful, it is a recently described technique. The most frequently used method to expose the ZF suture is via a transcutaneous lateral brow incision. Other methods include a coronal flap, lateral extension of an upper lid blepharoplasty incision, and lateral canthotomy alone. The coronal approach provides wide exposure of the ZF suture and the zygomatic arch, but should be reserved for comminuted ZMC fractures associated with midfacial and/or cranial fractures (Fig. 12). Extension of an upper blepharoplasty beyond the lateral canthus tends to cause obvious scarring. The incision may be camouflaged with make-up in woman but is more difficult to conceal in men.

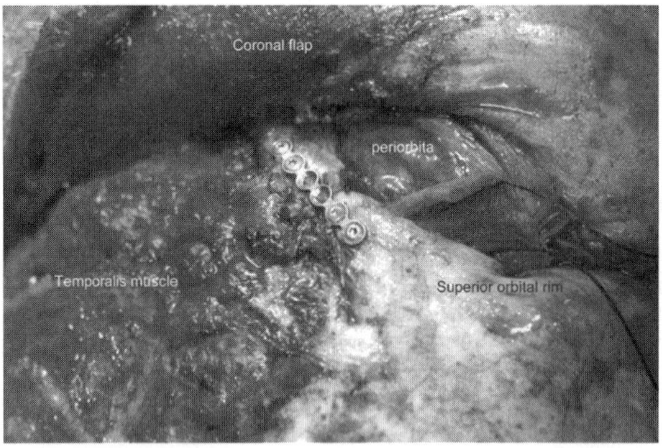

Figure 12 Exposure of the ZF suture via a coronal approach. Note miniplate application across suture line.

To avoid a cutaneous scar, access to the ZF suture is described via a lateral canthotomy alone. This requires forceful retraction and complete mobilization of the lateral canthal ligament (lateral retinaculum), periorbita along the lateral orbital rim, and soft tissues over the lateral orbital rim. The ZF suture is often inadequately exposed for miniplate application and the retraction required results in prolonged edema and subcutaneous fibrosis (17).

The zygomaticomaxillary suture over the face of the maxilla is approached via an intraoral upper buccal sulcus incision immediately posterior to the zygomatic buttress (Fig. 13). Dissection for adequate exposure and application of miniplates proceeds over the suture and malar eminence. Miniplates are placed along the zygomaticomaxillary buttress, avoiding the thin anterior wall of the maxillary sinus. Limited bone loss over the anterior wall of the maxillary sinus is inconsequential and attempts at rigidly fixing this bone in place should be avoided.

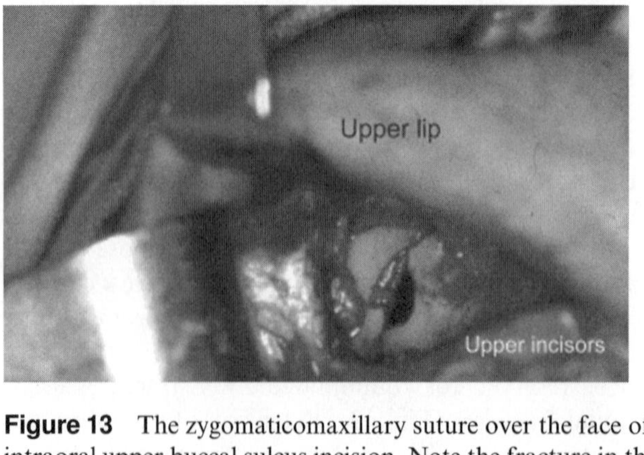

Figure 13 The zygomaticomaxillary suture over the face of the maxilla is approached via an intraoral upper buccal sulcus incision. Note the fracture in the background over the face of the maxilla.

REDUCTION

Reduction of facial bone fractures must be delayed if the patient has other more urgent or life-threatening injuries. Prior to reduction, the globe must be carefully examined since urgent intervention may be needed. If the extent of a patient's injuries is limited, reduction of the ZMC may proceed. To avoid the confounding effects of soft tissue edema, the usual practice is either to repair the ZMC fracture within 6–12 h or delay the repair up to 10–14 days. Although some advocate early repair, delayed signs of occult intracranial or ocular injury may occur. By taking the patient immediately to the operating room for reduction, these signs may be missed. Delaying the repair permits a period of observation and does not significantly compromise the outcome.

Type A1 zygomatic arch fractures are the classic type of ZMC fracture amenable to closed reduction via Gillie's temporal fossa approach (Fig. 14). Gillie's approach involves an incision in the temporal scalp behind the hairline. The incision is deepened to the temporalis muscle deep to the deep temporal fascia. Dissection continues inferiorly under the deep temporal fascia to the zygomatic arch. This plane preserves the zygomaticotemporal branch of the facial nerve. The displaced zygomatic arch fragments are reduced and are splinted by the posterior attachment of the temporal fascia.

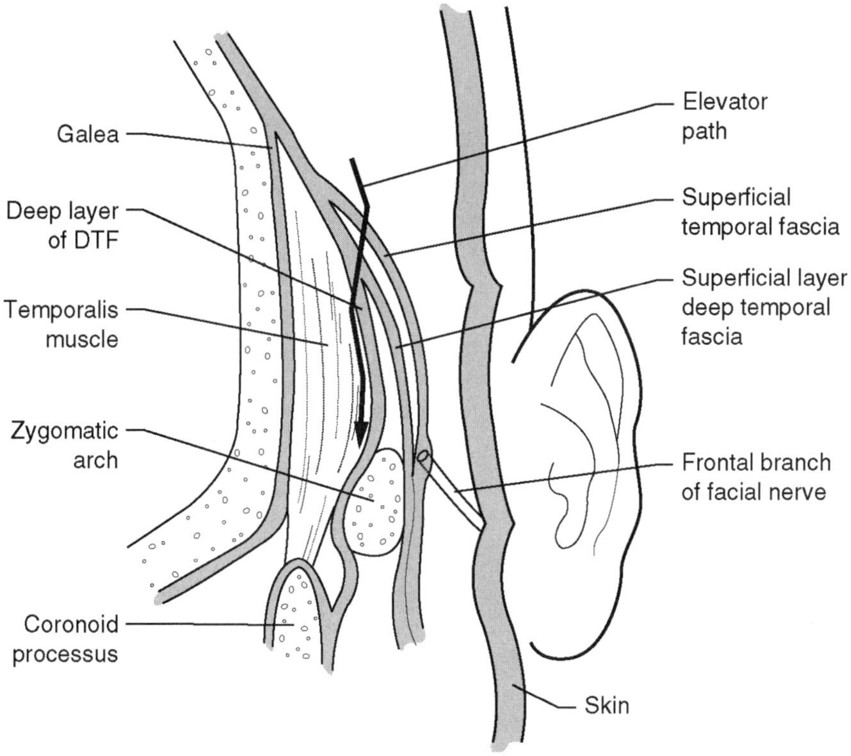

Figure 14 Gillie's approach shows the layers through which the elevator is passed to avoid injury to the frontal branch of the facial nerve.

Rarely is open reduction necessary for isolated zygomatic arch fractures. Open reduction of the arch via a coronal approach is occasionally necessary and the single best criterion for predicting whether open reduction of the arch will be necessary is lateral displacement of the arch (18). Other factors that predict this need include extreme posterior displacement of the malar eminence and a ZMC fracture associated with a facial crush injury (comminuted panfacial fracture) or a Lefort III fracture.

Isolated lateral orbital rim and infraorbital rim fractures usually require open reduction if displaced. Isolated lateral rim fractures are best approached either through a lateral canthotomy and superior cantholysis or via a transcutaneous lateral brow incision. Infraorbital rim fractures are approached through a transconjunctival approach and the fragments pieced together, if necessary. If there are multiple fracture fragments, a microplate is used to support the segments.

Accurate three-dimensional reduction of types B and C ZMC fractures is essential to avoid serious adverse sequelae including enophthalmus, diplopia, malar flattening, and eyelid malposition. Closed reduction is all that is necessary in many cases of type B monofragment fractures. In a large series, 28% of type B fractures underwent closed reduction (14). Closed reduction is often possible in minimally displaced fractures in which at least one articulation is intact (e.g., the ZF suture). Postreduction instability or significant orbital floor disruption necessitates fixation and open reduction. Regardless of the approach used, accurate alignment in three dimensions is critical. To this end, three-point alignment is sufficient; the three points usually used are the zygomaticofrontal suture, inferior orbital rim, and zygomaticomaxillary suture. An important alternative site of alignment that is often intact despite comminution of the zygomatic bone is the sphenozygomatic suture. It is curvilinear and in a much deeper plane than the ZF or orbital rim. Alignment of this suture line has proved to be a very reliable measure of adequate reduction. Type B fractures associated with multiple other complex facial fractures and most type C fractures require additional points of verification. Small fragments of bone should be preserved and replaced along the points of verification to ensure adequate spacing and accurate reduction of the major fragments. The ZF suture, inferior orbital rim, sphenozygomatic suture, and zygomaticomaxillary suture all need to be exposed and assessed to optimize the chances for accurate reduction. In addition, the zygomatic arch may need to be exposed via a coronal flap, especially if there are surrounding facial fractures that make it difficult to assess the proper position of the zygomatic bone in the sagittal plane (projection).

METHODS OF FIXATION

Accurate reduction is the key to a successful outcome regardless of the method of fixation. Methods of reduction and fixation of ZMC fractures differ widely among clinicians. This is not surprising considering that several authors strongly espouse seemingly disparate methods yet report very similar results. However, the common thread in these studies is the absolute requirement that the ZMC be reduced accurately. Maintaining the reduction properly is the greatest source of controversy. Wire osteosynthesis was the mainstay of fracture fixation from the 1940s through the 1970s. The miniplate was introduced in the 1970s and clearly provided more precise control of bone fragments and rigid fixation in three dimensions. Miniplate fixation has become the most common method of fixation of ZMC fractures in the United States (19). The use of miniplates has been associated with improved outcomes including fewer malunions, improved cheek sensation, and fewer cases of enophthalmos and globe dystopias. However, it is likely that the additional exposure necessary to place the miniplates also aids the surgeon in obtaining a more accurate reduction.

It is worthwhile to review several methods of fracture fixation because each has merit and is used by experienced surgeons with good results. Kirschner wires (K-wires), wire osteosynthesis, external pins, miniplates, microplates, and absorbable plates are among the many types of fixation appliances available. Properly used and applied, any of these appliances will be successful.

A K-wire is a rigid stainless steel wire (at least 0.062 inches in diameter) drilled percutaneously through stable bone and through the body of the reduced ZMC. Steinmann pins are often used in similar circumstances; they are similar to K-wires except that they are threaded and usually larger. The leading point of the wire rests within the reduced zygoma body with no penetration of the overlying skin. The proximal wire can be trimmed to the skin surface so that the wire is internal. This method of fixation was introduced for the zygoma in 1950 by Fryer and he subsequently published a 20 year review of his cases (20). The methods of fixation using a K-wire differ mainly in the part of the facial skeleton the proximal pin passes through. A transfacial K-wire passes through the opposite normal zygoma body traversing the lateral nasal walls and septum to reach the reduced zygoma body. A transnasal K-wire passes through the frontal process of the maxilla on the opposite side of the nose and traverses the nasal cavity to enter the reduced zygoma body. The advantages of using K-wires include a minimal equipment requirement; the method takes only a few minutes once the ZMC is reduced; minimal scarring; fixation is in three planes; and infection is rare. The disadvantages of using a K-wire include a tendency for the reduced zygoma to become laterally displaced as the wire enters the deep surface of the zygoma body; the pin must be removed in 4–6 weeks; if the wire is misdirected, direct globe injury could result; and the method is ineffective if the zygoma body is fractured or comminuted. Since the method can be performed with minimal exposure of the ZMC, a surgeon may be mislead into fixing the ZMC that is inaccurately reduced. This is particularly true in cases of significantly displaced or comminuted fractures. K-wires have largely been supplanted by more direct means of fracture fixation including wire osteosynthesis and plating. Even in very experienced hands, K-wire fixation has limited application. Advances in the surgical exposure of the facial skeleton have provided the surgeon with the means to reduce most ZMC fractures accurately. This exposure also provides a direct route for the application of wires and plates obviating the need for remote wire stabilization. A notable exception is an unstable zygomatic arch fracture that requires fixation. Although the arch could be directly fixed via a hemicoronal flap, the use of K-wires is described (21). Two K-wires are used: one inserted percutaneously into the unstable arch fragment and the other inserted percutaneously into the stable zygoma body. The proximal exposed (external) K-wire in the arch fragment is twisted around the backward-bent K-wire from the zygoma body. The wires are removed 2 weeks postoperatively.

External pins and wires suspended by headgear are other forms of fixation that has occasionally been reported (22) (Fig. 15). The external pin method consists of placing rigid threaded rods percutaneously into the fractured zygoma (into the solid

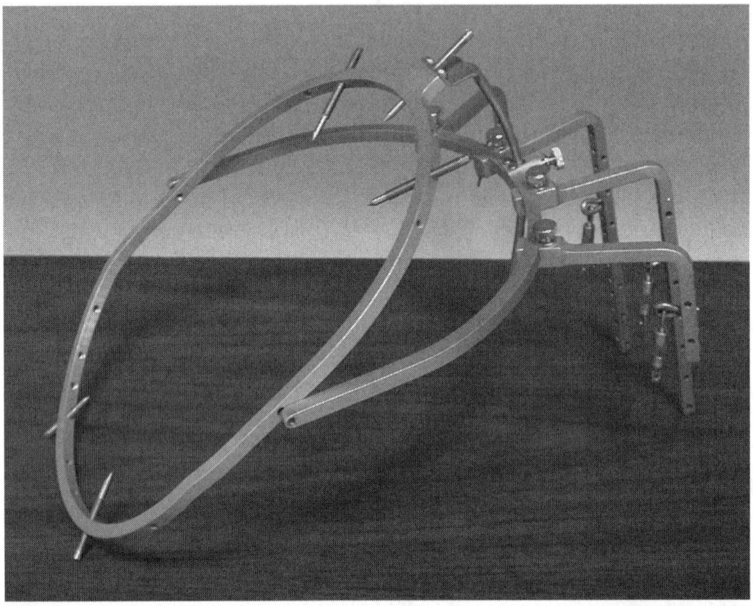

Figure 15 A Georgiade visor halo fixation apparatus for distraction and stabilization of facial fractures including ZMC fractures. This is of historical interest only.

zygoma bone) and into the solid supraorbital rim. The external portions of the pins are joined together with a universal joint locking system or a tube filled with methylmethacrylate. The suspension method utilizes wires connected to a head frame providing outward traction to the ZMC. The pins or wires are removed in 4–6 weeks. The suspension method is inherently unstable because the vector of force is singularly outward. The main disadvantages to the external pin method include cutaneous scarring and the unwieldy external appliance. Internal fixation devices in the form of mini- and microplates have superseded these methods of fixation in the vast majority of cases.

Wire osteosynthesis is a very popular method of fracture fixation and is often used in combination with miniplates. Application of wires requires minimal surgical exposure and the wires are very well tolerated (they are unlikely to extrude or result in erosion of the overlying soft tissue). The thicker bone surrounding the ZF suture and ZM buttress are able to accommodate wire up to 24 gauge and the thinner bone along the infrarbital rim and arch can accommodate a wire up to 26 gauge. Wire along the infraorbital rim is often used in place of miniplates because the latter is associated with a greater incidence of removal due to patient discomfort. The main disadvantages to using wires is that this method of fixation is not rigid in three planes. The distal and proximal fracture segments are prone to rotation resulting in imprecise reduction. In addition, accurate reduction of comminuted fragments is very tedious, often leading to loss of multiple bone fragments.

Monocortical miniplates for the midface are approximately 0.85 mm thick with 2.0 mm or 1.5 mm diameter screws. The diameter of the screw is an indication of the size (not thickness) of the plate. In the late 1980s, microplates were developed with plate thicknesses ≤0.6 mm with ≤1.5 diameter screws (23). Resistance of the screw to dislodge or pull out is inversely proportional to the diameter of the screw. Although dynamic compression miniplates are available, their use in the midface is unnecessary because only adaptation osteosynthesis is required. Dynamic compression is to be avoided because it will result in greater bone loss when adjacent small fracture fragments are being fixed, and it may spoil an otherwise perfect reduction as the screws are tightened. Some authors make a distinction between rigid internal fixation and semirigid internal fixation (24). The term rigid internal fixation is often reserved for compression osteosynthesis. Semirigid internal fixation refers to the type of noncompression fixation provided by miniplates (i.e., adaptive internal fixation without compression). Examples of microplates include 1.0 mm (Leibinger, Freiburg, Germany) and 1.5 mm (Martin, Tuttlingen, Germany) plates. Modern mini- and microplates are manufactured from titanium since this material is considered more biocompatible than its predecessor (stainless steel). Titanium forms an oxide film (titanium dioxide) when exposed to oxygen. This layer is extremely biocompatible with surrounding bone and new bone forms directly over the surface of the implant with no intervening capsule or fibrous tissue (i.e., osseointegration). Allergic reactions to titanium are unknown. An additional benefit to fracture assessment is the fact that titanium produces significantly fewer artifacts on CT scanning.

Plates possess several advantages over wires including three-dimensional stabilization, the ability to secure small fracture fragments in anatomical position, minimal bone loss when compared to wire osteosynthesis, and superior rigid fixation (25). Plates are useful in spanning gaps over comminuted bone while still providing stability across the fracture line. Loose bone fragments can be drawn to the plate with screws (lag screws); despite gaps between the fragments a continuous bony union between the stable fracture ends is achieved with healing. Wiring these bony fragments together results in greater bone loss. Miniplates are sufficiently strong to resist the deformation forces encountered clinically in ZMC fractures. However, microplates are significantly weaker and may deform under the similar biomechanical forces (26). Microplates are inadequate to resist soft tissue deforming forces along the infraorbital rim and the zygomatic arch in high-energy injuries (27). Moreover, microplates should not be used at sites that require substantial rigidity (e.g., ZF suture or ZM buttress). Instead, microplates are best suited for sites that require a very low profile plate yet maintenance of a bony gap is desirable with little expected deforming force (e.g., infraorbital rim or zygomatic arch in cases of mild to moderate comminution and displacement). In a study of complications associated with microplates placed within the maxillofacial skeleton region for fracture fixation (124 microplates in 44 patients), the overall complication rate was 2% (28). Complications included screw breakage, insertion of a screw in a tooth root, screw loosening, and plate removal in three patients who complained of a vague discomfort in the area of the plate. These complications did not affect the clinical outcome and were considered insignificant. Major concerns in children are alterations in growth and deep migration of permanent hardware, including mini- and microplates. This phenomenon has been demonstrated clinically and in animal models. In the animal model, there were demonstrable histological alterations in the underlying brain and meninges as the plates migrated intracranially when originally placed over the cranium (29). Nonabsorbable plates and screws should probably be removed in children once healing has occurred (4–6 weeks). Absorbable plates and screws are available for midface application and should be considered in pediatric ZMC fractures that require fixation.

Biodegradable (absorbable) plates and screws (1.5–2.0 mm screws) are most often used in semirigid fixation after the correction of congenital craniofacial abnormalities. The use of absorbable plating systems began in the 1980s with polyglycolic acid. However, this substance tended to produce a significant amount of inflammation within 4 months after transplantation due to its relatively rapid rate of degradation and release of acids. In addition, the strength of this polymer was not maintained during the healing period of bone (4–6 weeks). Over the last 6 years, poly-L-lactic acid implants have been developed that degrade much more slowly, maintain strength during the healing period of bone, and incite significantly less inflammation. Although biodegradable plates (2.0 mm) provide significantly less holding strength than titanium miniplate systems, they are probably adequate for most monofragmented ZMC fractures (30). Further studies regarding the stability of these resorbable plates in resisting the forces of the masseter muscle are needed. There is concern about the residual materials and degradation products left behind after the plates and screws dissolve. In a study of orthognathic patients using absorbable plating systems (LactoSorb, Walter Lorenz Corp Jacksonville, FL) after maxillary and mandibular osteotomies, the authors found that the plates and screws underwent complete resorption by 18–24 months postoperatively (31). LactoSorb, introduced in 1996, retains 70% of its strength for 6–8 weeks during the period of greatest biological bone healing.

EXTENT OF FIXATION

Reduction should be considered separate from fixation since the best anatomical sites to determine whether a fracture is properly reduced are not necessarily the best sites for the application of hardware or wires. Open reduction does not necessarily mean that hardware was needed or applied. The three best sites to determine whether a ZMC fracture is accurately reduced are the ZM buttress, sphenozygomatic suture, and the infraorbital rim. However, miniplate (semirigid) fixation should be applied to only the load-bearing buttresses including the ZM buttress and ZF suture, since these sites will best withstand the pull of the masseter muscle (primary deforming force in ZMC fractures). The most stable site for a miniplate is the ZF suture followed by the ZM buttress. Application of a miniplate to the infraorbital rim should be avoided because the plate is too thick and can often be readily palpated under the thin skin of the lower eyelid. This creates a dilemma since wire osteosynthesis of the infraorbital rim is problematic, often leading to increased bone resorption (especially with comminuted fragments) and increased long-term dysfunction of the infraorbital nerve. Microplates will provide sufficient stability for bone fragments minimizing bone loss and nerve impingement. They are also significantly thinner and are less likely to be palpable.

Miniplate fixation is superior to wire osteosynthesis in terms of stabilization and clinical outcome including malar symmetry and globe position (32). Although clinical and experimental evidence has supported the contention that miniplates provide superior stabilization, there is little consensus regarding the degree of semirigid fixation that is necessary. In a biophysical study in cadavers, a variety of plate combinations (mini- and microplates) were compared in their ability to maintain the reduced position of a fractured ZMC, while a deforming force of 2–22 kg was applied along a vector defined by the pull of the masseter muscle (33). A miniplate at the ZM buttress and microplates at the ZF suture and infraorbital rim provided the optimal balance of aesthetics and stability. Plate combinations were more stable than any combination of plates and wires. A criticism of this study is that the deforming force (maximum = 22 kg) was too small since normal subjects can generate forces over 130 kg. However, Dal Santo (1992) found that masseteric muscle force decreased significantly after a ZMC fracture, and even at more than 4 weeks postinjury the force was well below normal (34). Few clinical studies help to clarify the degree of rigid fixation that is necessary. Despite the experimental evidence that at least two-point fixation is needed for optimal stabilization, clinical studies report excellent results using a variety of methods including no fixation and ZF suture fixation alone. In a review of surgical practice repairing ZMC fractures, Ellis et al. found that regardless of the number of fixation devices applied there was no difference in post-reduction displacement (35). Treatment consisted of reduction without fixation to four-point fixation. The majority of patients underwent one-point fixation using a miniplate over the zygomaticomaxillary buttress or zygomaticofrontal suture. Clinical determination of post-reduction stability is the key to determining the degree of fixation required. The zygomatic bone is manipulated intraoperatively, with moderate pressure; if it falls out of alignment or seems unstable, fixation devices are applied until the bone is stable. The order in which the sites are treated is not crucial, however, the initial sites are usually the zygomaticomaxillary buttress and the ZF suture. Unfortunately, determining if the bone is stable relies heavily upon the judgment and experience of the surgeon. Many classification systems exist that attempt to assist the clinician in deciding which fractures require more aggressive treatment. The classification scheme promoted by Zingg et al. (previously outlined) is a simple system that broadly categorizes fractures, allowing the clinician some leeway in treatment. This approach more accurately represents clinical experience because more than one treatment strategy can be successful. The main distinction between ZMC fractures is whether the zygoma bone is intact or multifragmented. Monofragment fractures respond to a variety of treatment methods and minimal fixation. However, multifragmented fractures require much more aggressive exposure and fixation. According to the classification scheme, orbital rim fractures often require open reduction and fixation while arch fractures are usually treatable by simple closed reduction alone.

Types A2 and A3 ZMC fractures require open reduction and fixation since they are rarely stable after closed reduction alone. An isolated type A2 fracture (lateral orbital rim) is rarely encountered. Surgical access is attained via a lateral brow percutaneous incision or through release of the lateral retinaculum via a canthotomy and superior cantholysis. In either case, a single bridging miniplate is used and the fragments are lag-screwed into place. A type A3 ZMC fracture is often associated with an orbital floor dehiscence as the fracture tracks posteriorly along the infraorbital canal or along the zygomaticomaxillary suture line. A percutaneous subciliary or transconjunctival route is required to assess and reduce the fracture and apply a small miniplate or wire. If the orbital floor is significantly disrupted, titanium mesh can be placed on the orbital floor and draped over the orbital rim. The portion of the mesh over the rim is fixed with screws for stabilization of the mesh itself and the fracture fragments.

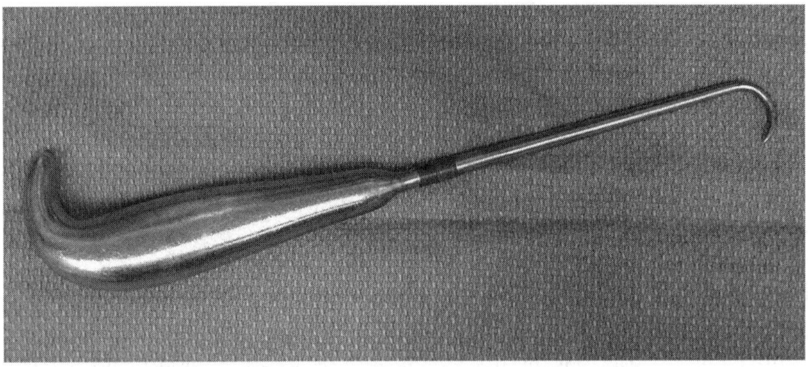

Figure 16 Orthopedic J hook for reduction of a ZMC fracture. The hook is inserted under the body of the zygomatic bone through a small stab incision. Superolateral traction will reseat the bone into a reduced state.

A type B monofragment ZMC fracture may be amenable to closed reduction if the orbital floor is not extensively disrupted and the reduced bone is stable, resisting the inferior-displacing forces of the masseter muscle. Reduction of the ZMC should not be done in the presence of unreduced orbital contents since this could lead to

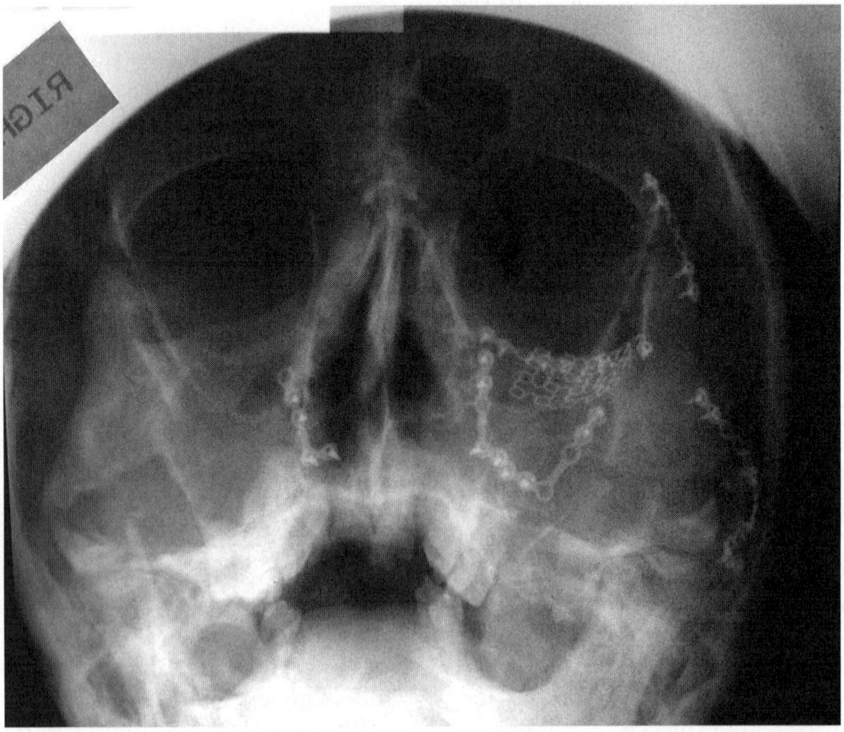

Figure 17 X-ray study shows multiple sites of rigid fixation. Typical use of hardware for a patient with a type C fracture.

muscle and fat entrapment, diplopia, and enophthalmos. The preoperative coronal CT will be the guide as to whether to proceed with attempts at closed reduction without addressing the orbital floor. There are no absolute rules concerning the size of the orbital defect, but with clinical signs of entrapment and obvious herniation of orbital contents into the maxillary sinus by CT, exploration of the orbital floor should precede reduction. In these cases, an open approach to the orbital floor (percutaneous subciliary or transconjunctival) can be combined with ZMC reduction. This allows the orbital contents to be manually reduced before the ZMC is reduced. If the bone is stable and the orbital floor appears closed after reduction, no other surgical approach or fixation need be performed. Closed reduction of the ZMC is done with a J hook inserted through a stab incision parallel to the facial nerve branches just inferior to the body of the zygoma bone. The tip of the hook is engaged under the body of the zygoma and superolateral traction is applied (Fig. 16). The ZMC is reduced when the malar eminence appears similar to the opposite side and no step-offs can be appreciated over the infraorbital rim and zygomaticofrontal and zygomaticomaxillary (intraoral) suture lines. Confirmation in the operating room is obtained using a single Water's view. The stability of the ZMC is tested by placing moderate pressure over the malar eminence. If the bone falls out of alignment, rigid fixation is required. The type of fixation required for a type B fracture is controversial but some type of internal miniplate fixation is standard. A miniplate (e.g., 1.7 mm titanium miniplate) over the ZF suture combined with wire osteosynthesis for the inferior orbital rim is sufficient in the majority of cases. If the ZMC remains unstable, an additional miniplate should be placed over the zygomaticomaxillary buttress.

Type C multifragmented ZMC fractures require multiple surgical approaches and semirigid internal fixation at multiple sites (Fig. 17). Exploration of the orbital floor should be performed early and cotton pledgets should be placed under the reduced periorbita to prevent entrapment during reduction of the ZMC. The ZF suture, sphenozygomatic suture, zygomaticomaxillary buttress and suture, and the infraorbital rim should be exposed in preparation for surgical reduction. Despite fragmentation of the zygoma bone, the malar portion (body) nearly always provides a stable surface for manipulation. A small orthopedic hook is inserted through a stab incision inferolateral to the malar eminence and seated under the bone. Traction is placed on the bone by pulling out on the hook, reducing the ZMC. Confirmation of adequate reduction is obtained by visualizing the alignment and closure of the multiple points of alignment previously mentioned. Especially important is accurate alignment of the sphenozygomatic suture for precise reduction. Final confirmation of the adequacy of reduction is obtained by assessing symmetry with respect to the opposite side and by obtaining Water's radiograph of the facial skeleton after application of the miniplates. At least two-point fixation is required with miniplates along the ZF suture line and zygomaticomaxillary buttress. Wire osteosynthesis is also beneficial for the infraorbital rim. Rarely is a hemicoronal scalp flap justified for rigid fixation of the zygomatic arch unless other complex facial fractures impede accurate alignment using the standard points of alignment. Once the bone is reduced and fixed, the orbital floor is inspected. Often there is a dehiscence along the intraorbital zygomaticomaxillary suture line and infraorbital nerve. If the gap is greater than 1 cm, some form of rigid material should be used. Several materials have been advocated including titanium mesh, septal cartilage, split calvarial bone, anterior maxillary sinus wall bone, Medpor (Porex Surgical Inc., College Park, GA), blocks of hydroxyapatite, among others (36). For very large defects, split calvarial bone grafts are favored but this is rarely necessary in the primary setting. Titanium mesh is a simple and effective alternative for significant orbital floor defects. Soft tissue is incorporated around the mesh, reducing the chances of late extrusion. In addition, further trauma to the area is unlikely to cause posterior displacement of the implant because of its pliability. Smaller orbital floor defects can simply be covered with Gelfilm (Pharmacia and Upjohn Inc., Kalamazoo, Mich).

ORBITAL EXPLORATION

Orbital floor exploration is a controversial subject. The literature is replete with recommendations regarding orbital floor exploration, ranging from exploration in all cases to highly selective exploration based on clinical or radiographic findings. The orbital floor is disrupted in all ZMC complex fractures due to impaction or distraction of the intraorbital sutures associated with the zygomatic bone. In addition, a blowout fracture (impure) may occur that is characterized by comminution and outward displacement of the bony orbital walls. In simple ZMC fractures, lateral displacement of the zygomatic bone results in an increase in the volume of the bony orbit and, left uncorrected, will result in enophthalmos. However, accurate open or closed reduction of a simple ZMC fracture will result in re apposition of the intraorbital zygomaticomaxillary and sphenozygomatic sutures. This re-establishes the integrity and positions of the inferior and lateral bony orbital walls and corrects the volumetric relationships that are crucial in preventing late enophthalmos. In these simple cases, there is no need to explore the orbital floor. Orbital exploration involves a surgical approach to the orbital floor through the lower eyelid (or via an existing laceration) with exposure of the anterior, posterior, and lateral walls of the orbit. Considering that there are significant complications associated with the surgical approach (e.g., ectropion and lid malposition), selective criteria are needed. Orbital floor exploration is generally needed in more severe cases in which the volume of the orbit is not restored despite apparent reduction of the ZMC. This occurs in the presence of significant impure blowout fractures and severely displaced or comminuted fractures of the ZMC. Prior to the advent of CT, it was difficult to determine the true extent of a midface or ZMC fractures. The development of late post-traumatic enophthalmos was difficult to predict based on the limited diagnostic information available.

The basic abnormality that results in enophthalmos is an increase in orbital volume posterior to the axis of the globe. Fat atrophy or loss is not a factor. Volumetric changes anterior to the axis of the globe (just posterior to the infraorbital rim) have little effect on the final position of the globe (37). Operative exploration is needed in cases of significant posterior disruptions of the bony orbit. A difference of 2 mm between the normal globe and the abnormal globe is noticeable and clinically significant. Therefore, posterior volumetric changes that are likely to result in globe displacement greater than 2 mm must be surgically corrected. Impure blowouts involving outward displacement of the medial and inferior walls of the orbit may be responsible. However, inaccurate reduction of the ZMC also results in significant posterior increases in bony orbital volume due to inferolateral displacement of the frontosphenoidal and orbital processes. This is more likely to occur in cases of fragmented (type C) ZMC fractures. Orbital exploration is justified in these cases to ensure adequate apposition of the intraorbital sutures and to repair dehiscences in the inferior and lateral orbital walls. Blowout fractures resulting in loss of bone or outward displacement of the medial or inferior orbital walls posterior to the axis of the globe are often responsible for late enophthalmos. In a clinical study based on CT-based volumetric measurements, an approximate 5% increase in orbital volume (1.25 ml) will result in 1 mm enophthalmos (38). Therefore, a 10% (2.5 ml) increase in volume would be expected to result in clinically significant enophthalmos. This is roughly equivalent to 3 mm of inferior displacement of the posterior orbital floor (39). Medial displacement of the medial orbital wall (medial blowout) associated with inferior displacement of the orbital floor seems to compound the increase in orbital volume. In fact, the majority of patients with late enophthalmos after a ZMC fracture have a medial blowout component. The mean increase in orbital volume (CT-based measurement) in a small series of patients (n=11) with late enophthalmos was 4.4 ml or 17.9% (38).

The majority of patients with ZMC fractures do not require exploration of the orbital rim and floor. Clinical indications for orbital exploration are based on a combination of clinical and radiographic criteria (40). Orbital floor exploration is indicated in the following situations:

Comminution of the inferior orbital rim
Multifragmented ZMC fractures
Rectus muscle entrapment / persistent diplopia
Presurgical enophthalmos
CT evidence of comminution of $>50\%$ of the orbital floor
CT evidence of combined orbital floor and medial wall defects
CT evidence of fracture segments impinging on periorbita or globe

The presence of late enophthalmos correlates with the severity of the initial fracture more than any other variable (e.g., type of fixation). Comminution of the inferior orbital rim or body of zygoma usually indicates that a severe ZMC fracture exists with a significant chance of misalignment and late enophthalmos regardless of treatment. In these cases, orbital exploration not only improves the chances of adequate restoration of the orbital volume but also provides additional landmarks (sphenozygomatic suture) for accurate reduction of the ZMC. Exposure of the orbital rim also allows placement of microplates to stabilize the fractured fragments of bone. Rectus muscle entrapment with a positive forced duction test and evidence of herniation of orbital contents on CT is also a firm indication for orbital exploration.

In 1930 Pichler drew attention to the limitation of passive movement of the traumatized globe when an attempt was made to move the anesthetized eyeball with forceps: the basis of forced duction test. A forced duction test is useful to differentiate mechanical restriction of gaze from muscle weakness or swelling. A positive test indicates that the patient has a mechanical restriction such as entrapment of the (most commonly) inferior rectus muscle. The test is performed by first instilling a local anesthetic solution into the conjunctival fornices. The tendon of the inferior rectus muscle is grasped with a fine forceps through the fornix and an attempt is made to rotate the globe upward. Resistance indicates a mechanical obstruction (positive test). Reasons for a positive forced duction test include herniation of periorbital fat and entrapment of the inferior rectus muscle; impingement of bone fragments directly into the periorbita and muscle; and, in the long term, cicatrix formation with muscular adhesions.

The inferior rectus muscle lies posterior to the axis of the globe, so entrapment of the muscle is a clinical sign of a significant breach within the posterior orbital floor. Clinically significant enophthalmos (>2 mm) that is noted within 2 weeks of the injury is a reliable sign of a pathological increase in orbital volume. Enophthalmos may be difficult to detect in the presence of acute swelling and only the preoperative CT may reveal the presence of this abnormality. Several findings on CT scanning indicate the need to consider orbital exploration. Determination of orbital volume relationships is usually not helpful in the acute fracture setting because a pathological increase in orbital volume is the norm due to the lateral displacement of the zygoma. However, an (impure) blowout fracture is detectable by preoperative CT and may indicate the need for orbital exploration. Comminution of the orbital floor posterior to the axis of the globe associated with herniation of orbital contents indicates that exploration should be considered. Comminution of greater than 50% of the bone in this area is an absolute indication for exploration and possible reconstruction. The combination of orbital floor and medial wall defects is associated with large pathological increases in orbital volume; orbital exploration and reconstruction are indicated. The presence of bony spicules impinging on the periorbita is an indication for exploration and disimpaction of the fractured bony fragments.

Complications

Complications associated with ZMC fractures can be classified into those that are fracture-related, technique-related, or iatrogenic. Fracture-related complications include malar depression and asymmetry, facial widening, maxillary sinus dysfunction, infraorbital nerve dysfunction, and various ophthalmological complications. Technique-related complications include those associated with the various surgical approaches. Serious iatrogenic injuries usually involve the cornea (e.g., abrasions). The incidence of complications is generally related to the severity of the trauma.

Outcome is dependent upon the type of fracture and the accuracy of reduction (both initially and during the healing period). Type A incomplete ZMC fractures are straightforward and require only two-dimensional reduction. Outcome is nearly uniformly good with regard to adequacy of reduction and postoperative symmetry. Adverse sequelae are mainly associated with type B and C fractures, especially severely comminuted type C fractures, including malar asymmetry (type B, 12%; type C, 16%), maxillary sinus dysfunction (type B, 5%; type C, 13%), infraorbital nerve dysfunction (type B, 31%; type C, 23%), and enophthalmus with diplopia (type B, 2%; type C, 9%) (14). Malar asymmetry (malar over or under projection) is better tolerated than lateral displacement of the ZMC both cosmetically and functionally. A minor degree of malar asymmetry is a common finding after a ZMC fracture but is often overlooked by the patient and is not typically associated with a significant increase in orbital volume or enophthalmos. However, even a minor degree of lateral displacement will result in obvious asymmetry and lead to a significant increase in orbital volume as the entire lateral aspect of the orbit is expanded. Secondary correction of the malar eminence is straightforward:it involves the addition or substraction of bone over the eminence via a transbuccal approach.

However, correction of facial widening (lateralized ZMC) will usually require multiple osteotomies through the articulations of the ZMC with the facial skeleton and medial repositioning of the entire bony complex. Maxillary sinus dysfunction (chronic or recurrent sinusitis) is most often found in patients who have sustained a severe ZMC or midface fracture. Overall, the incidence is approximately 8% (14).

Approximately 80% of patients with a ZMC fracture will have some degree of cheek and upper lip numbness due to injury to the infraorbital nerve. Permanent dysfunction occurs in 22–50% of cases (41,42). The dysfunction of the nerve most often involves a third or fourth degree nerve injury (43). The persistence and nature of the dysfunction seem to be most closely related to the type of injury and the method of repair. The highest incidence of long-term dysfunction occurs in fractures with an undistracted ZF suture (43). This finding may indicate that maintenance of this articulation during impact results in greater compression along the infraorbital canal. Long-term sensory disturbances are also associated with patients who have undergone closed reduction without miniplate fixation of the infraorbital rim (44). This finding may be related to the fact that ZMC fractures with undistracted ZF sutures are often amenable to closed reduction. However, several other studies have corroborated that open reduction and fixation are beneficial, and that plate osteosynthesis of the infraorbital rim is superior to wire osteosynthesis with regard to long-term nerve function (45). It is assumed that plate osteosynthesis results in less compression of the bony fragments and infraorbital canal compared to wire osteosynthesis. As mentioned, miniplates along the infraorbital rim are often problematic; microplates may be better tolerated yet provide a similar degree of adaptation and stability of bony fragments.

Severe ocular trauma is uncommon in patients with ZMC fractures; a decrease in visual acuity is the main long-term clinical finding (46). However, severe ocular disorders are common in high-energy injuries (e.g., road traffic accidents), occurring in up to one-third of patients (47). Several eye-related findings are associated with ZMC fractures including enophthalmos, diplopia, hyphema, globe rupture, and blindness. Enophthalmos is essentially caused by either an increase in the volume of the bony orbit or significant herniation of orbital contents through one or more of the orbital walls. A significant increase in the volume of the orbit can occur if the ZMC is not reduced accurately (Fig. 18). In addition, unrepaired dehiscences of the inferior and/or medial orbital walls will result in an increase in the volume of the orbit and herniation of orbital contents. In principle, loss of intra- and extraconal fat located posterior to the axis of the globe will result in posterior displacement of the globe and enophthalmos. Diplopia may indicate clinically the presence of a significant fracture within the posterior orbit with herniation and entrapment of the inferior rectus muscle. This finding must be correlated with forced duction testing and the CT findings. Persistent diplopia is more common in children than adults. Little information is available regarding persistent diplopia in patients with ZMC fractures; however, Cope et al. found that more than half of children with pure blowout fractures experienced persistent diplopia compared to less than one-third of adult patients (48). Timely surgical reconstruction of midfacial fractures with expectant management of the diplopia will minimize persistent cases (49).

An acute finding in some cases of severe ocular trauma is hyphema (blood in the anterior chamber of the eye). Traumatic hyphemas tend to be more common in children and men and are caused by rupture of the vessels in the iris stroma and

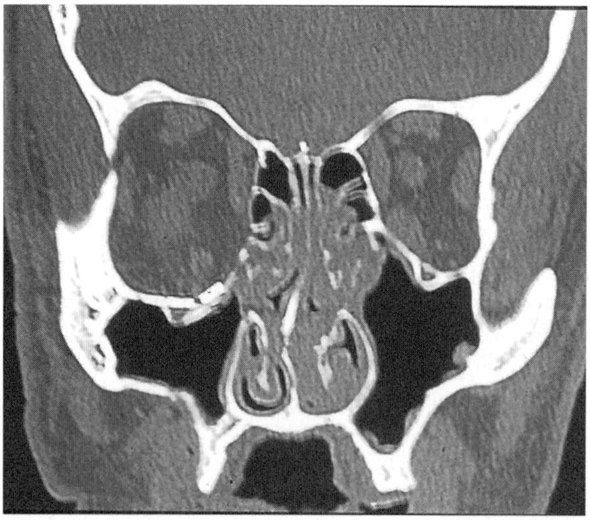

Figure 18 Coronal CT shows inadequately reduced right ZMC fracture with the zygomatic bone displaced inferomedially. Note marked increase in orbital volume associated clinically with significant enophthalmos.

ciliary body (50). A slit lamp examination is useful for diagnosis and the hyphema is graded 1–4 (a grade 4 hyphema indicates that blood completely fills the anterior chamber). Complications associated with hyphemas include blood staining of the cornea and increased intraocular pressure (glaucoma). There is also a significant risk of rebleeding usually within 5 days of the initial bleed. Corneal blood staining and increased intraocular pressure (IOP) can occur with any grade hyphema, but more commonly result from large hyphemas (51). Prolonged increased IOP can result in optic nerve atrophy and blindness. Treatment is usually conservative including eye protection,elevation of the head of the bed, rest, topical beta-blockers, carbonic anhydrase inhibitors, mannitol, and close follow-up. Resistant increased IOP, persistent large hyphema, or corneal blood staining may be indications for surgical intervention by an ophthalmologist.

Acute and subacute blindness result from a ruptured globe, acute retrobulbar hemorrhage, or traumatic optic neuropathy. Most commonly, optic neuropathy results from severe complex facial fractures and frontobasilar fractures, not ZMC or blowout fractures (52). The incidence of blindness after a facial fracture is approximately 3%; the incidence is much less in isolated ZMC fractures (53). Direct globe perforation or orbital compartment syndrome secondary to retrobulbar hemorrhage is responsible for blindness in the vast majority of ZMC fractures. Retrobulbar hemorrhage is characterized by a rapid deterioration of vision after a variable period of orbital swelling and increased IOP. The globe is usually very tense and proptotic. Orbital decompression must commence immediately because the optic nerve and retinal tissues are extremely sensitive to anoxia. Irreversible damage to the optic nerve can occur after only 1–2 h of uncorrected ischemia (54). Orbital decompression consists of medical and surgical therapies including systemic carbonic anhydrase inhibitors, steroids, mannitol, lateral canthotomy and inferior cantholysis, and possible direct evacuation of an orbital hematoma (usually subperiosteal). Close monitoring and ophthalmological consultation are mandatory.

The most common technique-related complications include plate failure and lower eyelid malposition secondary to the surgical approach to the infraorbital rim. Miniplate mechanical failure is rare. Occasionally, patients complain of a vague discomfort or palpable deformity caused by a plate. Removal of the plate is necessary in these cases and the symptoms usually (but not always) resolve. Nonabsorbable plates should be removed after healing in children to avoid complications associated with plate migration during growth. Complications associated with the transconjunctival approach to the inferior orbital rim and floor include transient lower eyelid retraction and scleral show, a noticeable lateral canthal scar, and inferior displacement of the lateral canthus. Potential complications include prolonged chemosis, granulation tissue, infection, true ectropion, canthal dehiscence, canalicular injuries, and iatrogenic eye injuries. However, these were not observed by Fedok in his review using the transconjunctival approach in cases of trauma (55). Cicatrical ectropion due to excessive overlapping of the free edges of the incision along the horizontal extent of the lower eyelid can result in scleral show requiring scar release at a later setting. This can be avoided by carefully pulling the lower eyelid superiorly at the conclusion of the operation to prevent any incisional overlap or by suspending the lower eyelid with a Frost suture or Steri-strips for 24–48 h. The occurrence of ectropion is much lower using the transconjunctival approach (3%) compared to the conventional transcutaneous approaches (28%).

Iatrogenic injury is rare and most commonly involves corneal abrasion. Corneal shields are helpful but they can also cause an abrasive corneal injury. Temporary tarsorrhaphy may be the safest approach in protecting the cornea. A serious iatrogenic injury that may lead to blindness is an undetected retrobulbar hemorrhage; the approximate incidence of this complication is 0.3% (56). During the first 12–24 h postoperatively, the patient's eye and vision should be checked every 2 h. A tense proptotic globe, even in the presence of normal vision, should alert the clinician to the possibility of retrobulbar hemorrhage. Other iatrogenic injuries that have been reported to lead to vision loss include direct injury to the optic nerve by bony fragments or extreme posterior placement of an orbital implant (57,58).

INTERNAL ORBITAL BLOWOUT FRACTURES

Definition, Demographics, and Causes

Smith and Converse in 1957 suggested that the term *blowout* be used when referring to an isolated fracture of the orbital floor. However, this term is also applicable to orbital fractures that are characterized by external displacement of segments of any of the bony orbital walls. The more rare blow-in fracture is characterized by implosion of portions of the bony orbital walls associated with a reduction in the volume of the orbital cavity, proptosis, and impalement of the periorbita. Blowout fractures are further classified into pure fractures (no involvement of the orbital rim) and impure fractures (concomitant orbital rim fracture). Pure blowout fractures may be described as trapdoor or punched-out (59). A trapdoor fracture indicates that a partially attached bone fragment has recoiled against an intact bony edge. This type of fracture is often associated with incarceration of the periorbita. A punched-out fracture indicates that the bone fragment is detached on all sides with no tendency to return to its original position; tissue incarceration is unlikely. Trapdoor fractures are more common in the orbital floor and punched-out fractures are common in the medial wall.

There is a bimodal age distribution for orbital fractures, peaking between ages 21–30 years and 41–50 years (60). Isolated orbital floor fractures make up 4–16% of facial fractures. The majority of internal orbital fractures occur in men and the causes include assaults, falls, motor vehicle accidents, and sports-related traumas. Blowout fractures usually involve the orbital floor but may involve (in descending order) the medial, lateral, and superior orbital walls (61). However, the majority of pure orbital blowouts with a concomitant nasal fracture will involve the medial orbital wall (59). A medial wall blowout will be associated with an orbital floor blowout in at least 20% of cases. In pediatric patients, orbital floor fractures are by far the most common fracture type (71%) (62).

There are three standard theories regarding the pathophysiology of pure orbital blowout fractures: the hydraulic theory, the bone conduction theory, and the direct globe-to-wall theory. The hydraulic theory implied by Pfeiffer in 1943 and later explicitly stated by Smith and Converse in 1957 is the most widely accepted theory regarding the mechanism of a pure orbital blowout fracture. The hydraulic theory states that pressure over the globe causes a generalized increase in intraorbital pressure sufficient to outfracture the weakest walls of the bony orbit. This theory was seriously challenged based on the experimental work of Fujino, who demonstrated that pressure over the orbital rim alone is sufficient to fracture the orbital floor via buckling forces (63). However, Fujino also demonstrated that direct pressure over the globe causes an orbital wall fracture but he considered that the orbital rim was more vulnerable in most cases and probably was the major factor in most orbital blowouts. A direct globe-to-wall mechanism has been proposed but it states that the globe itself is impacted so radically that it actually contacts and ruptures the orbital walls directly (64). It is unlikely that the globe-to-wall mechanism plays a significant role in blowout fractures in which the orbital rim remains intact.

Blow-in fractures are more commonly found in the roof and lateral wall of the orbit. These fractures are often impure, associated with fractures of the orbital rim and adjacent areas of the facial skeleton. In cases of blunt periorbital trauma, buckling forces are primarily responsible for internal displacement of segments of the orbital wall. The orbital process of the frontal bone, greater wing of the sphenoid bone, and zygomatic bones are most often involved (65).

Pertinent Anatomy

Seven bones make up the bony orbit including the ethmoid, frontal, lacrimal, maxillary, palatine, sphenoid, and zygomatic. The orbit is shaped like a pyramid with its base formed by the thick orbital rims and its apex terminating in the inferior and superior orbital fissures and optic canal. The orbital roof is composed mainly of the orbital surface of the frontal bone with a small contribution from the lesser wing of the sphenoid bone. The medial wall is formed by maxillary (frontal process forming the rim), lacrimal, frontal, ethmoidal (lamina papyracea), and sphenoidal bones (lesser wing). The optic canal is formed by the junction of the lesser wing to the body of the sphenoid bone. The orbital floor is composed of the orbital surface of the maxilla, orbital process of the zygomatic bone, and a small posterior contribution from the palatine bone. The lateral wall is composed of the frontal process of the zygomatic bone and greater wing of the sphenoid. The limits of the lateral wall are the superior and inferior orbital fissures.

The structures associated with the orbital roof include the trochlea, superior orbital fissure, the supraorbital notch, anterior and posterior ethmoid canals, and the frontal lobe. Approximately 4 mm posterior to the superomedial orbital rim lies the trochlear fovea. The trochlear fovea is a small depression in the roof of the orbit near its medial margin that serves to anchor the sling for the superior oblique tendon (66). Careful subperiosteal dissection with detachment of the trochlea does not result in extraocular muscle dysfunction or diplopia as long as the orbital soft tissues and periosteum are simply reapproximated (67). Fractures of the orbital roof often occur in the region of the superior orbital fissure because the bone is thinnest in this area. Superior orbital fissure syndrome or orbital apex syndrome can occur (see section on Signs and Symptoms). The supraorbital notch is located at the junction of the medial one-third and lateral two-thirds of the superior orbital rim. It is a true foramen in approximately 25% of individuals. Fractures of the superior orbital rim can affect the integrity of this nerve. The anterior and posterior ethmoidal canals that transmit the ethmoidal vessels are formed by the junction of the frontal bone with the ethmoid.

The medial orbital wall is the most complex and consists of several bones, but the lamina papyracea forms the majority of this wall. The lamina papyracea represents the thinnest wall of the orbit (0.25 mm) and is evidently the area within the orbit most prone to fracture. However, the floor is the most common site of a pure orbital blowout fracture. This may be because the usual location of blunt trauma to the eye is over the inferior orbital rim or that the lamina is actually more resistant to fracture because of the additional support provided by the ethmoid labyrinth.

The floor of the orbit is formed primarily by the orbital processes of the maxilla and zygoma. The orbital process of the maxilla forms the majority of the floor. The floor is divided into lateral and medial parts by the infraorbital groove that defines the passage for the infraorbital vessels and nerve. Pure orbital floor fractures most often involve the medial part of the orbital floor (medial to the infraorbital groove) (59). In fact, pure orbital fractures often involve the lower medial orbital wall in addition. The bone in this area of the orbit is actually inclined at least 30 degrees in an anterior–posterior direction toward the orbital apex. Therefore, fractures not only disrupt the support of the periorbita but also reverse the natural constriction of the orbital contents, increasing the likelihood of enophthalmos. Combined fractures of the floor and medial wall compound this effect. On coronal CT scanning, the so-called bony buttress demarcates the medial orbital wall from the orbital floor (59) (Fig. 19). The buttress is the thick bony extension of the superomedial maxillary sinus to the floor of the orbit. It separates the maxillary sinus from the anterior ethmoids and is partially deficient at the maxillary antrum (midportion). Overlying the buttress anteriorly, opposite the lacrimal groove, is the origin of the inferior oblique muscle. The buttress is thickest anteriorly, underlying the origin of this muscle. Traumatic collapse of the bony buttress usually occurs in the middle and posterior portions. Collapse signifies a more severe displacement of periorbita and orbital volume, making enophthalmos more likely without intervention.

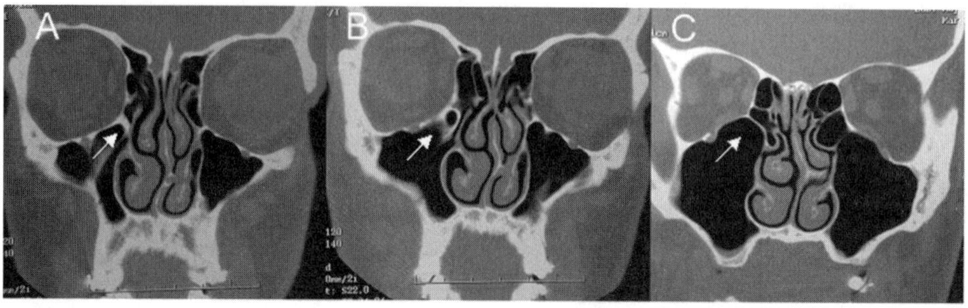

Figure 19 The bony buttress (arrows) separates and helps to support the medial and inferior orbital walls. The buttress is present anteriorly (A) and posteriorly (C) but is dehiscent in the area of the middle meatus (B).

Pure blowout fractures involving the lateral wall are rare. Lateral internal orbital fractures are usually associated with zygomatic complex fractures and are impure. Zygomatic complex fractures are the most common underlying causes for blow-in fractures that are characterized by implosion of bony fragments into the orbital cavity reducing the volume of the orbit. Blow-in fractures may result in impalement injury to the globe or periorbita and proptosis.

Knowledge of the anatomy of the orbital apex is critical in evaluating and treating patients with internal orbital fractures. The location and contents of the annulus of Zinn, superior and inferior orbital fissures, and the optic nerve are particularly relevant. The four recti muscles (inferior, lateral, superior, and medial) arise from a common fibrous ring common called the annulus of Zinn that surrounds the upper, medial, and lower margins of the optic foramen and surrounds the optic nerve (68). The contents of the superior orbital fissure include cranial nerves III, IV, VI, the first division of the trigeminal nerve (V1), sympathetic contributions of the cavernous plexus, and the orbital branch of the middle meningeal artery (68). The contents of the inferior orbital fissure include the maxillary (infraorbital) nerve and its zygomatic branch, the infraorbital vessels, sphenopalatine ganglion branches, and communicating veins (orbital, pterygoid) (68). The optic nerve traverses the bony optic canal and exits into the orbit surrounded by the annulus. The optic nerve is located in the superomedial aspect of the orbital apex and is approximately 42 mm posterior to the anterior lacrimal crest and between 40 and 45 mm posterior to the inferior orbital rim. The distance between the soft tissues of the orbital apex (including the contents of the fissures) and the orbital rim differs depending on the quadrant of the orbit being dissected. Based on dissections of human cadavers, Danko et al. found the mean distances to be 44.5 mm superiorly, 44.1 mm medially, 39.4 mm inferiorly, and 38.3 mm laterally (69). No distance was less than 31.0 mm or greater than 51.0 mm and there was no significant difference noted between the left and right orbits. Subperiosteal dissection along the orbital floor is less likely to impinge on the optic nerve because of the nerve's superomedial location within the orbital apex. However, dissection along the medial orbital wall directly approaches the nerve and dissection posterior to the posterior ethmoid artery risks injury to the optic nerve.

Diplopia and limitation of extraocular movement are important clinical findings that may indicate the need for surgical exploration. A positive forced duction test may be secondary to true incarceration of an extraocular muscle, but this circumstance is uncommon. More commonly, only the periorbital fat is incarcerated and the fine reticular fibrous network within the fat restricts the motion of the extraocular muscle. Koornneef described this fine orbital connective tissue in 1977 (70). Each eye muscle has its own connective tissue system that is part of a generalized and highly organized musculofibrous system within the periorbita.

Symptoms and Signs

The mechanism of injury in a pure fracture vs. an impure fracture is fundamentally different and the symptoms and signs differ. A pure fracture is more likely to be associated with serious ocular injury and, by definition, will have no associated rim fracture. Impure blowout fractures are less likely to be associated with serious ocular injury. Blow-in fractures are often associated with severe ocular injuries that require emergency surgical exploration and decompression. Proptosis, diplopia, globe rupture, superior orbital fissure syndrome, and orbital apex syndrome are associated with blow-in fractures (71).

The cardinal symptoms and signs associated with a pure orbital floor fracture include diplopia, periorbital ecchymosis, orbital dystopia, and cheek dysesthesia. Diplopia is a subjective symptom and is present when a single object is perceived as double. Diplopia is present in most cases but usually resolves. It may be due to a variety of self-limited pathologies including edema, muscle contusion, or neuropraxia; or it may be secondary to actual entrapment of the inferior rectus muscle or surrounding fat. Trap-door fractures of the orbital floor are relatively common, resulting in entrapment of the periorbita. True entrapment of the periorbita associated with limitation of extraocular movement is an indication for surgical exploration. Therefore, it is important to differentiate entrapment from self-limited diplopia. Forced duction testing combined with coronal CT will help to differentiate between these two entities. Orbital dystopia caused by proptosis is the most common finding acutely in the majority of the internal fractures due to soft tissue swelling. However, acute enophthalmos indicates that a significant increase in orbital volume has occurred resulting from a significant defect in an orbital wall. Pseudo ptosis may be present once edema resolves, but is rarely present acutely. Vertical dystopia most often indicates that there has been a significant pathological alteration in the support of the globe anterior to its axis with disruption of the ligamentous sling. This finding is uncommon in pure internal orbital fractures because the majority of the floor defects are posterior to the axis of the globe. Multiple other serious ocular problems are associated with pure orbital blowout fractures including globe rupture, hyphema, optic neuropathy, vitreous hemorrhage, retinal detachment, dislocated lens, and corneal injuries. All patients with internal orbital fractures require evaluation by an ophthalmologist. Patients with cheek numbness often have fractures involving the orbital rim. Although infraorbital nerve dysfunction is associated with pure orbital floor fractures, it is usually mild and most patients experience complete recovery.

Pure medial blowout fractures are usually reported as somewhat less common than pure orbital floor fractures. A medial blowout is associated with periorbital ecchymosis, orbital emphysema, diplopia, and orbital dystopia. Enophthalmos was present in approximately 40% of patients, diplopia in 25%, and mechanical restriction of gaze in 13% in a study by Burm et al. (59). Fracture of the medial orbital wall occurs concomitant with a pure orbital floor fracture in 25–30% of cases (59,60). Combined fractures have a greater tendency to result in clinically significant enophthalmos (>2 mm), especially if there is collapse of the bony buttress (72). In patients with combined fractures, Burm et al. found that enophthalmos was present in 62% of patients, diplopia in 81%, and mechanical restriction of gaze in 48%. Only mechanical restriction of gaze was more common in isolated orbital floor fractures. True entrapment of the medial rectus muscle is rare since these fractures are usually of the punched out variety, with little tendency for the bone fragments to recoil. However, temporary diplopia on medial and lateral gaze secondary to muscle contusion is a common finding.

Blowout fractures of the lateral wall without disruption of the orbital rim are rare. Most fractures involving the lateral wall are associated with ZMC fractures. An important characteristic differentiating pure orbital floor fractures from lateral blowout fractures is that the major portion of a floor fracture is medial to the infraorbital groove and the majority of a lateral fracture is lateral to the infraorbital groove. Impaction of the zygoma bone can result in a blow-in fracture that produces proptosis or even impalement of the globe.

Internal orbital roof fractures are uncommon but have the greatest blow propensity to cause serious intracranial and optic nerve damage. Pure orbital roof fractures are most often of the blow-in variety involving the posterior orbital cavity and the superior orbital fissure. Associated intracranial injuries include contusion and hemorrhage of the frontal lobe, brain herniation into the orbital cavity, dural tears, and cerebrospinal fluid leak. Acute meningitis and pseudomeningoceles are also reported (73). The optic nerve is particularly vulnerable to injury because pressure over the supraorbital rim is indirectly transmitted to the orbital apex. Optic nerve contusion and blindness are associated with blunt injuries to the supraorbital rim even in the absence of a severe orbital roof or rim fracture. Ocular injuries result from implosion and collapse of the orbital roof resulting in globe rupture, proptosis, retrobulbar hematomas, superior orbital fissure syndrome, and orbital apex syndrome. Superior orbital fissure syndrome is a constellation of clinical findings caused by disruption of the cranial nerves that travel through the fissure (cranial nerves III, IV, V, and VI). This results in ophthalmoplegia, ptosis, and a fixed dilated pupil. Orbital apex syndrome is a superior orbital fissure syndrome plus optic nerve dysfunction (74). The majority of patients with supraorbital roof fractures will have an associated skull fracture and a frontal sinus fracture (75). Epidural and subdural hematomas may be associated.

Radiological Examinations

Plain radiography is of limited usefulness in internal orbital fractures, especially for the diagnosis of fractures involving the medial and orbital roof. Water's view is classically described as having a teardrop sign in the presence of an orbital floor blowout. The teardrop presumably results from the herniation of the periorbita into the maxillary sinus. However, this sign can be misleading since a subperiosteal hematoma involving the roof of the sinus will also give the appearance of a teardrop. Bone fragments within the teardrop (look for spotty opacities) are a good indication of the presence of a true blowout. With the advent of CT scanning, detection and characterization of the fracture have become possible. Herniation, muscle entrapment and dislocation, and several fracture-related details are easily identifiable by CT scanning and can be used to direct treatment and predict results. Scanning in the coronal plane provides the most useful information with regard to the degree and composition of herniated soft tissue and the details of the fracture itself (size, location, and type) (Fig. 20). In the presence of diplopia and limitation of extraocular movement, it is important to differentiate simple herniation of the periorbital fat from true entrapment of an extraocular muscle. Although both of these radiographic findings support the need for exploration, true entrapment of an extraocular muscle may result in avascular necrosis and irreversible muscle dysfunction. Other significant soft tissue findings on CT scanning include involvement of the origin of the inferior oblique, which indicates that diplopia may be permanent without surgical intervention (76). Characteristics of the fracture uniquely obtained by CT scanning include an accurate assessment of the size and location of the defect, which may be important in the decision to explore the fracture surgically; in addition, the type of fracture (trap door vs. punched-out) may direct operative treatment.

Criteria for Surgical Exploration

The goals of treatment of internal orbital fractures are prevention and correction of globe malposition, restoration of orthoscopic vision, and maintenance or improvement of visual acuity. Additional considerations when confronted with an impure orbital fracture are restoration of orbital rim and facial skeletal contour and restora-

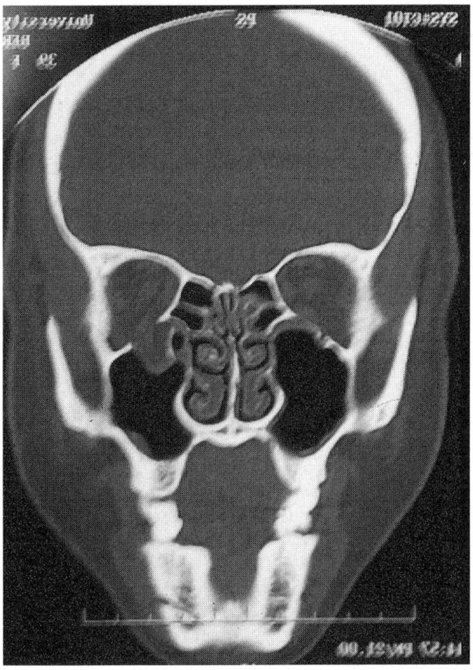

Figure 20 Coronal CT shows a typical internal blowout fracture of the orbital floor.

tion of cheek sensation. Early repair within 3 weeks is associated with an improved outcome compared to late repair or significant delay (77). Delayed correction of enophthalmos is difficult or impossible because of scarring and irreversible muscle injury. However, significant delays in surgical exploration may be warranted if there is coexisting serious globe trauma or other life-threatening injuries or if the involved eye is the only-seeing eye (78). Enophthalmos and diplopia are the most common debilitating late sequelae of pure medial wall and orbital floor blowout fractures. The decision to explore the fracture surgically is based on the likelihood that the injury will result in long-term problems with enophthalmos and diplopia. Before the availability of CT scanning, the decision to explore was sometimes arbitrary. In the 1960s, these fractures were considered emergencies and most were explored immediately. Reduction of periorbita and reconstruction of the orbital floor were performed to reduce the risk of late enophthalmos and diplopia. As a direct challenge to this approach, Putterman and colleagues reported on 57 patients with pure orbital floor challenges who were simply followed without surgical intervention regardless of the severity of their fractures and symptoms. No patient experienced late cosmetically unacceptable enophthalmos or debilitating diplopia. However, approximately 20% of the patients experienced enophthalmos of up to 3 mm and 20% had diplopia in upgaze. This study demonstrated for the first time that the majority of patients with pure orbital blowout fractures do not require surgical intervention.

Enophthalmos of less than 2 mm is usually not obvious and no treatment is necessary. Enophthalmos is most commonly measured with a Hertel exophthalmometer, which is the most popular instrument to measure globe position. It uses either mirrors or prisms to determine the position of the globe. Two footplates fit over the temporal margin of the lateral orbital rims, allowing measurement of both globes for increased accuracy and reproducibility. The key measurement for each orbit is the distance between the lateral orbital rim and the corneal apex. The examination is performed with the patient seated looking straight ahead. The lateral orbital rim is palpated to determine the deepest angle; this will serve as the first reference point. The Hertel exophthalmometer is positioned over the lateral orbital rims and adjusted so that the mirrors view the corneal profiles and millimeter scale. The position of the corneal profile in millimeters is noted for each globe. The results can be reported as millimeters over the base value (i.e., distance between the lateral orbital rims) or simply in terms of the actual distance in millimeters between the orbital rim and corneal apex for both globes. Average readings in adults are between 15 and 17 mm, but vary according to race and gender. A difference of greater than 2 mm between sides is significant. The main source of error using this method is positioning the footplates over the lateral orbital rims.

The presence of the following signs and symptoms indicates the need for open treatment to prevent clinically significant (>2 mm) late enophthalmos:

1. Acute enophthalmos despite significant periorbital edema
2. Combined medial and inferior orbital wall fractures
3. Isolated medial wall fracture with medial displacement >3–5 mm
4. Isolated orbital floor fracture with inferior displacement ≥ 3 mm

Although the volume of the orbital cavity is consistently increased in cases of posttraumatic enophthalmos, it is an oversimplification to attribute enophthalmos to this solely. To avoid postoperative enophthalmos, several factors must be considered before surgical exploration, including the extent of orbital wall displacement and collapse and herniation of the retrobulbar soft tissues. Various criteria have related the extent of the floor fracture, amount of soft tissue herniation, location of the fracture, and the shape of the retrobulbar fat. Isolated medial wall fractures are less likely to produce enophthalmos because the medial wall is lacking the striking retrobulbar convexity present in the orbital floor. This retrobulbar convexity is important in maintaining the shape of the retrobulbar fat and forward position of the globe (Fig. 21). In addition, displacement of the medial orbital wall is associated with smaller increases in orbital volume than to similar displacements of the orbital floor. Approximately 1 mm medial displacement of the medial wall results in a 0.4 ml increase in orbital volume, whereas 1 mm inferior displacement of the floor results in a 0.8 ml increase in orbital volume (79). An increase in orbital volume of approximately 1.25 ml will result in 1 mm enophthalmos (38). Therefore, a 10% (2.5 ml) increase in volume would be expected to result in clinically significant enophthalmos. This is roughly equivalent to 3 mm inferior displacement of the orbital floor (39). It is interesting to note that medial orbital wall fractures often accompany orbital floor fractures in many cases of late posttraumatic enophthalmos. It appears that the combination of a medial and inferior orbital wall fracture, especially when accompanied by collapse of the bony buttress, is likely to cause posttraumatic enophthalmos (38).

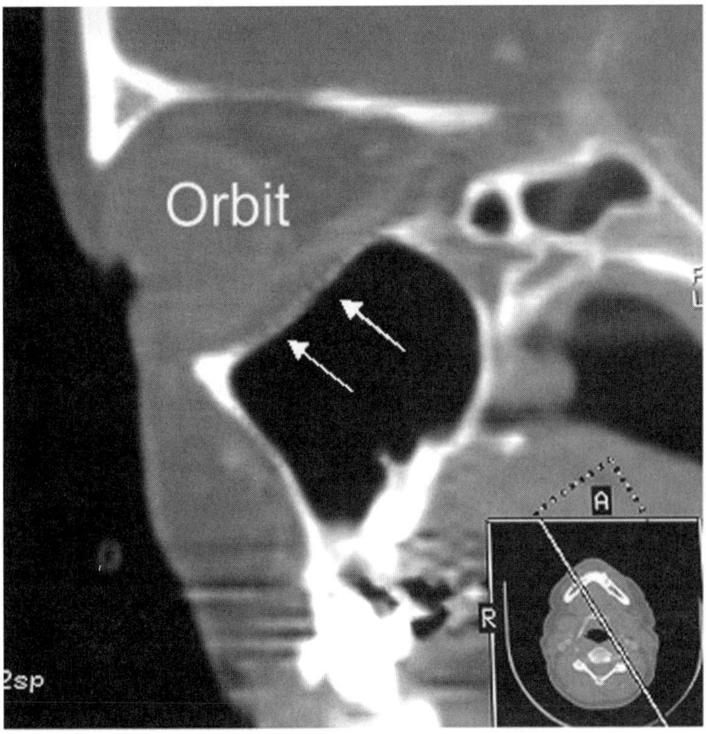

Figure 21 Sagittal CT scan shows natural convexity (arrows) in the posterior orbit that is important in maintaining the forward position of the globe.

The presence of the following signs and symptoms indicate the need for open treatment to prevent clinically significant late diplopia:

1. Diplopia and positive forced duction testing
2. Diplopia and depression or significant displacement of the origin of the inferior oblique muscle
3. Acute entrapment of an extraocular muscle

Although diplopia is a very common symptom associated with a blowout fracture, the majority of patients experiencing diplopia (>95%) will be symptom free in 6 months. Therefore, surgery for diplopia must be reasonably selective. Even in those at risk for permanent diplopia, if the problem occurs only in upgaze it is usually well tolerated. Diplopia in primary or down-gaze will interfere with everyday activities including reading and will be disabling. True mechanical restriction of gaze is the most common significant risk factor resulting in persistent disabling diplopia. Force duction testing is crucial in differentiating true entrapment from diplopia secondary to contusion, neuropraxia, or edema. Usually only the periorbita is entrapped and the muscle is restricted by virtue of its fibrous attachments to the entrapped tissue. In rare cases, the muscle itself becomes entrapped (identified by CT scanning). The fracture should be explored as soon as possible because the entrapped muscle may undergo avascular necrosis. In rare cases, diplopia may be permanent in the absence of positive forced duction testing. This is evident in cases of depression or significant displacement of the origin of the inferior oblique muscle seen on CT scanning (76).

Blow-in (impacted) fractures more commonly involve the roof and lateral orbital walls and may be associated with decreased visual acuity and restriction of gaze. The vast majority of patients so injured should undergo early surgical exploration to remove the impacted segments of bone from the periorbita. Restoration of the volume of the orbital cavity is a secondary gain and support of bony fragments with plates and screws is often necessary (80).

Surgical Approaches

Numerous surgical approaches to the bony orbit are useful in trauma. The orbital floor can be approached via an intraorbital route or through the maxillary sinus. The various intraorbital routes include transcutaneous approaches (e.g., subciliary) and transconjunctival approaches, which are reviewed elsewhere. Approaches through the maxillary sinus involve an initial incision under the lip between the maxillary buttress and canine. The sinus is entered through its thin anteroinferior wall and the floor of the orbit is visualized directly or with an endoscope. Although clinical experience using the endoscope for fracture reduction is limited, certain benefits seem clear. Determinations of the actual size of the floor fracture and the possibility of ruling out an orbital fracture clinically without the need for orbital exploration through the eyelid are potential benefits (81). Reduction of orbital contents and repair of the orbital floor are feasible using the endoscope: however, there is a risk of injury to the periorbita by misdirected fragments of bone.

The medial orbital wall is approached via a transcutaneous incision between the medial canthus and nasal dorsum or through the nose using an endoscope. The transcutaneous route is direct, simple, and allows complete mobilization of the periorbita and placement of implants as necessary. The incision is staggered and placed well away from the medial canthus to prevent web formation (82,83). A subperiosteal dissection proceeds posterior to the posterior lacrimal crest on to the lamina papyracea. The anterior ethmoid artery is clipped and divided to improve exposure and hemostasis. The posterior limit of the dissection is the posterior ethmoid artery, which can be left intact or also clipped and divided for hemostasis. Although endoscopic repair of a medial blowout fracture is described, there are several limitations to this approach (84). Moderate to severe fractures may distort important intranasal landmarks that are used by the surgeon to avoid critical areas including the cribiform plate, sphenoid recess and sinus, and posterior orbit. Most orbital implants cannot be placed intranasally and require an external approach. Like the transmaxillary sinus approach to the orbital floor, impalement of bone fragments into the periorbita is possible.

The orbital roof can be approached directly through a laceration over the superior orbital rim, transcranially, or subcranially. The orbital roof is approachable via a limited or frontal craniotomy. All aspects of the fracture can be addressed including reconstruction. However, this approach requires manipulation and retraction of the frontal lobe; such extensive exposure of the anterior cranial fossa may not be required in all cases. Raveh et al. developed the subcranial approach as an alternative to frontal craniotomy for the open repair of extensive frontonasoorbital and skull base fractures (85). Via a coronal incision, the subcranial approach allows complete access to the superior aspect of the orbit and inferior aspect of the anterior cranial fossa and frontal sinuses. Manipulation and reduction of bone fragments, repair of dural defects, split calvarial bone grafting, and repair of frontal sinus fractures are all possible without the need for craniotomy or retraction of the frontal lobe.

Treatment Overview

Routine surgical treatment of pure internal orbital fractures consists of disimpaction of bone fragments, exploration and replacement of herniated periorbita, and freeing of entrapped extraocular muscles. Of course, treatment of ocular, intracranial, and optic nerve injuries must take precedence. Management of trauma to the globe should be done in conjunction with an ophthalmologist and treatment of intracranial and optic nerve injuries (most commonly found in association with orbital roof fractures) should be individualized. Blindness is rarely associated with internal orbital fractures. However, with the assistance of an ophthalmologist the signs of ongoing or impending optic nerve dysfunction should be sought. The first sign of visual loss may be as subtle as a decrease in the detection of the color red, a visual field defect, or decreased visual acuity. Peripheral retinal fibers travel on the peripheral part of the optic nerve, making them more vulnerable to injury. Constriction of the visual field may be present due to optic nerve compression; central visual acuity may be normal despite the constricted field.

Surgery should be delayed in cases of optic nerve injury that is improving. Avoidance of further surgical trauma (e.g., implant insertion) is important to maximize recovery and minimize the chances of postoperative blindness (86). Surgical decompression of the optic nerve may be considered in selected cases of stagnant or worsening visual acuity. Impacted bone fragments associated with blow-in fractures often require urgent reduction or removal, especially if there is impalement of intraorbital structures. This can be found in high-energy ZMC fractures resulting in proptosis and increased intraorbital pressure. In these rare cases, reduction and disimpaction of the zygomatic bone must be done as soon as possible. Herniated periorbita and entrapped muscles must be replaced in the orbital cavity and the dislocated orbital wall fragments replaced.

Treatment of orbital roof fractures usually consists of repositioning bony fragments, stabilization with miniplates, and reconstruction using autologous calvarial bone grafts (87). Associated intracranial injuries are repaired in conjunction with a neurosurgeon via either a subcranial or a transcranial approach. Treatment of isolated pure orbital floor and medial wall fractures consists of reducing displaced and entrapped periorbita and extraocular muscles. These walls must be reconstructed to support the reduced periorbita and recreate the natural convexity of the postbulbar bony orbital cavity. The choice of material used for orbital implantation depends on many factors and is a source of controversy (see section on Orbital Implant Materials below). Once the graft is in place, intraoperative forced duction is performed to ensure that there is no residual entrapment. When repairing the orbital floor, the graft should be placed behind the orbital rim and supported by a posterior lip of stable bone. The natural convexity present in the medial aspect of the floor posterior to the globe should be recreated with the graft to restore the shape and position of the intraconal fat.

Orbital Implant Materials

Many autologous, alloplastic, and allogenic materials are available for reconstruction and augmentation of the orbital floor. The choice of material often depends as much on surgeon preference as the characteristics of the defect and implant. The ideal implant should be sufficiently firm to support the periorbita yet be unlikely to result in significant posterior displacement in case of repeated trauma. It must also be of sufficient size, readily available, and compatible with the surrounding bone and soft tissue so that the likelihood of infection or extrusion is negligible. Typical autologous materials include ear or septal cartilage, iliac crest, anterior maxillary sinus wall, and split calvarial bone. Alloplastic materials include titanium mesh, Marlex mesh (Phillips Chemical Co, Houston, TX), Medpor (Porex Surgical Inc, College Park, GA), Gelfilm (Pharmacia and Upjohn Inc, Kalamazoo, MI), and hydroxyapatite blocks or cement. Allogenic materials include lyophilized dura or cartilage and banked cadaveric bone.

A bone graft is the time-honored implant material for orbital floor reconstruction and augmentation. Both endochondral (iliac crest) and mesenchymal (split calvarial) grafts are commonly used for large defects of the orbital floor (larger than $2\,cm^2$). Bone grafts provide sufficient firmness and bulk to reconstruct subtotal or total defects of the orbital floor, roof, or walls. Large orbital floor defects may lack a sufficient rim of uninjured bone to support a bone graft and a titanium mesh implant may be needed to act as a scaffold. It is a popular misconception that the titanium mesh enhances resorption of the bone (88). The disadvantages of using autogenous bone, especially when correcting moderate to severe enophthalmos, include gradual resorption of the implant, increased operative time, and potential donor site morbidity. Sullivan et al. found that approximately one-third of the thickness of an intraorbital iliac bone graft is resorbed over a 28 week period (88). The embryonic origin of the bone graft (mesenchymal vs. endochondral) may be important with regard to the rate of resorption and final volume of the graft. It is commonly believed that bone grafts of mesenchymal origin (e.g., split calvarium) tend to resorb at a much slower rate and maintain greater volume than bone grafts of endochondral origin (e.g., iliac crest). Ozaki et al. challenged this perception by comparing mesenchymal cortical grafts to endochondral cortical and cancellous grafts in rabbits (89). The cortical bone grafts maintained their volumes significantly better than the cancellous bone grafts independent of embryonic origin. Bone grafts are nevertheless considered the gold standard for implant materials within the orbit but their drawbacks (resorption, operative time, and donor site morbidity) are significant enough to warrant the use of alternative methods under most circumstances. Bone grafts are generally reserved for patients undergoing revision surgery for correction of moderate to severe enophthalmos or globe malposition. However, split calvarial bone grafts are sometimes used in the primary setting in cases of significant bone loss, most often for floor defects over $2.5\,cm^2$, especially if a coronal flap is already in use. Routine use of the thin bone overlying the anterior wall of the maxillary sinus is advocated by some for repair of moderate-sized orbital wall and floor defects (90,91). Lee et al. found that this method was highly reliable, with little or no tendency for the bone to resorb (91).

Cartilage grafts (conchal and septal) are readily available in most cases and can be used to span large defects of the orbital floor, walls, and roof. Despite its accessibility, only a few cases of cartilage grafts for orbital reconstruction are reported. The grafts seem to be well tolerated with very low infection and extrusion rates. In a study by Wiseman et al., the volume of cartilage grafts actually increase because of fibrous tissue formation when transplanted from ear to ear in rabbits (92). There are also reports of diced conchal cartilage for augmentation of the medial orbital wall for correction of enophthalmos (93).

A variety of synthetic biomaterials are available for repair of orbital wall defects. Some biomaterials have clearly been proved inferior with relatively high infection and extrusion rates (e.g., Silastic) (94). Extrusions or compulsory removal of the implant may occur from months to years after insertion. Implant failure has been linked to dental surgery, upper respiratory tract infection, cutaneous fistula formation, cocaine use, postoperative infection, and implant migration (95). Commonly used materials today include methylmethacrylate, Medpor (Porex Surgical Inc., College Park, GA), Marlex mesh (C.R. Bard, Inc., Murray Hill, NJ), Gelfilm (Pharmacia and Upjohn Inc., Kalamazoo, MI), and titanium mesh. Methylmethacrylate is exothermic while curing and implants should be prefabricated ex vivo before placing in the orbital cavity near the periorbita. A soft tissue capsule eventually envelops the methylmethacrylate implant, making it easier to remove if required. However, it is prone to extrusion upon minor repeated trauma or infection. Medpor (porous polyethylene) allows both bone and soft tissue ingrowth, creating a stable implant that is unlikely to extrude. The implant also provides a significant amount of bulk to the orbital cavity and is especially useful for the secondary correction of enophthalmos (96). Although this alloplastic implant appears to hold promise, there are no long-term clinical studies regarding infection and extrusion rates. There is also a concern that tissue ingrowth may lead to tethering and limitation of extraocular movement (97). Marlex mesh provides insufficient support for prolapsing periorbita and is rarely used (98). Gelfilm is thin (0.075 mm) and is manufactured from denatured collagen. It is useful for small defects with very limited herniation of periorbita. Gelfilm is eventually resorbed and replaced by fibrous tissue (99). Although titanium mesh is

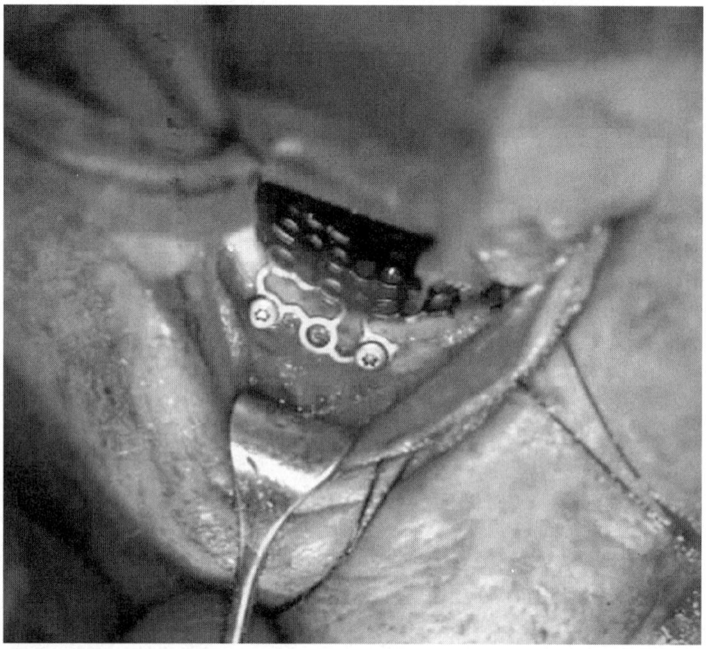

Figure 22 Titanium mesh implant used for repair of a large floor defect in the right orbit. The inferior lid is retracted inferiorly while the periorbita is supported superiorly using a wide ribbon retractor. Note that the implant is bent over the inferior orbital rim and two microscrews are used to hold the implant in place. Posteriorly, the impant should rest on a stable bony shelf.

of proven benefit in supporting large bone grafts, it is also useful alone for repair of orbital floor and medial orbital wall defects up to 2.5 cm^2 (Fig. 22). Of course, the mesh will not provide much bulk but it is useful to restore intraorbital contour and prevent herniation of the periorbita.

Late Diplopia and Enophthalmos

Despite proper initial surgical and medical treatment of internal orbital fractures, long-term disabling diplopia and enophthalmos may still occur. The occurrence of long-term diplopia and enophthalmos correlates most closely with the severity of the fracture regardless of treatment. Diplopia is especially disabling if it occurs in primary or downgaze. Diplopia in upgaze or in the extremes of gaze is not significant and requires no treatment. The foundation of correcting diplopia is extraocular muscle surgery. Selection of the appropriate procedure is based on the degree and nature of the ocular muscle dysfunction (101). Diplopia may also be correctable by altering the abnormal position of the globe (correcting enophthalmos or vertical globe malposition). In some cases, globe malposition may sufficiently displace the extraocular muscles, or alter the visual axis, to result in diplopia despite the absence of significant extraocular muscle injury. Restoring the globe to a more normal position will improve the diplopia and obviate the need for extraocular muscle surgery (102).

Complete correction of late enophthalmos is often difficult or impossible. The effects of scarring within the periorbita are pervasive and extremely difficult to overcome. Greater success is possible in effecting a change in the vertical position of the globe, but significant changes in the anteroposterior plane are difficult to attain. The volume of the globe and periorbita remain nearly normal in most cases of post-traumatic enophthalmos. Increase in volume of the posterior bony orbit associated with a change in the shape of the retrobulbar fat (from a convex to a more spherical configuration) correlates most closely with the occurrence of clinically significant enophthalmos (103). Therefore, attempts to move the globe forward should focus on augmenting the posterior orbit and recreating the retrobulbar convexity that is present in the orbital floor. These maneuvers will decrease orbital volume and restore the shape of the retrobulbar fat. A common error is to place grafts too anteriorly (anterior to the axis of the globe) thereby changing only the vertical position of the globe with no effect on its anteroposterior position. The most common grafts for the correction of enophthalmos are split calvarial bone grafts but Medpor implants are also frequently used. Medpor implants are easily shaped, allow tissue ingrowth for stability, avoid the potential morbidity of a donor site, and do not resorb. Since long-term experience using Medpor is limited, split calvarial bone grafting remains the gold standard. When using bone grafts, a certain degree of resorption should be anticipated (up to 30%) and overcorrection is advocated. However, in actual practice, movement of the globe is limited and even normalization of globe position is often impossible. The limit of graft material that the posterior orbit will accommodate without undue pressure over the globe and periorbita is usually reached well before the enophthalmos is fully corrected.

REFERENCES

1. Pulfrich C. Die Stereoskopie im Dienste der isochromen und heterochromen Photometrie. Die Naturwissenschaften 1922.
2. Larkin EB, Dutton GN, Heron G. Impaired perception of moving objects after minor injuries to the eye and midface: the Pulfrich phenomenon. Br J Oral Maxillofac Surg 1994; 32:360–362.
3. Livingston RJ, White NS, Catone GA, Thomas RF. Treatment of orbital fractures by an infraorbital–transantral approach. J Oral Surg 1975; 33:586–590.
4. Hinderer UT. Malar implants for improvement of the facial appearance. Plast Reconstr Surg 1975; 56:157–165.
5. Anastassov GE, van Damme PA. Evaluation of the anatomical position of the lateral canthal ligament: clinical implications and guidelines. J Craniofac Surg 1996; 7:429–436.
6. Gray H. Anatomy of the Human Body. Philadelphia: Lea & Febiger, 1918.
7. Nordgaard JO. Persistent sensory disturbances and diplopia following fractures of the zygoma. Arch Otolaryngol 1976; 102:80–82.
8. Jungell P, Lindqvist C. Paraesthesia of the infraorbital nerve following fracture of the zygomatic complex. Int J Oral Maxillofac Surg 1987; 16:363–367.
9. Vriens JP, Moos KF. Morbidity of the infraorbital nerve following orbitozygomatic complex fractures. J Craniomaxillofac Surg 1995; 23:363–368.
10. Stanley RB. Use of intraoperative computed tomography during repair of orbitozygomatic fractures. Arch Facial Plast Surg 1999; 1:19–24.
11. Iinuma T, Hirota Y, Ishio K. Orbital wall fractures. Conventional views and CT. Rhinology 1994; 32:81–83.

12. Broumand SR, Labs JD, Novelline RA, Markowitz BL, Yaremchuk MJ. The role of three-dimensional computed tomography in the evaluation of acute craniofacial trauma. Ann Plast Surg 1993; 31:488–494.
13. Fox LA, Vannier MW, West OC, Wilson AJ, Baran GA, Pilgram TK. Diagnostic performance of CT, MPR and 3D CT imaging in maxillofacial trauma. Comput Med Imaging Graph 1995; 19:385–395.
14. Zingg M, Laedrach K, Chen J, Chowdhury K, Vuillemin T, Sutter F et al. Classification and treatment of zygomatic fractures: a review of 1,025 cases. J Oral Maxillofac Surg 1992; 50:778–790.
15. Converse JM, Firmin F, Wood-Smith D, Friedland JA. The conjunctival approach in orbital fractures. Plast Reconstr Surg 1973; 52:656–657.
16. Dolan RW, Smith DK. Superior cantholysis for zygomatic fracture repair. Arch Facial Plast Surg 2000; 2:181–186.
17. Manson PN, Ruas E, Iliff N, Yaremchuk M. Single eyelid incision for exposure of the zygomatic bone and orbital reconstruction. Plast Reconstr Surg 1987; 79:120–126.
18. Manson PN, Markowitz B, Mirvis S, Dunham M, Yaremchuk M. Toward CT-based facial fracture treatment. Plast Reconstr Surg 1990; 85:202–212.
19. Michelet FX, Deymes J, Dessus B. Osteosynthesis with miniaturized screwed plates in maxillo-facial surgery. J Maxillofac Surg 1973; 1:79–84.
20. Fryer MP, Brown JB, Davis G. Internal wire-pin fixation for fracture-dislocation of the zygoma. Twenty-year review. Plast Reconstr Surg 1969; 44:576–581.
21. Lew DH, Park BY, Lee HB, Lew JD. Simple fixation method for unstable zygomatic arch fracture using double Kirschner's wires. Plast Reconstr Surg 1998; 101:1351–1354.
22. Duckert LG, Boies LR. Stabilization of comminuted zygomatic fractures with external suspension apparatus. Arch Otolaryngol 1977; 103:381–382.
23. Schortinghuis J, Bos RR, Vissink A. Complications of internal fixation of maxillofacial fractures with microplates. J Oral Maxillofac Surg 1999; 57:130–134.
24. Zachariades N, Mezitis M, Anagnostopoulos D. Changing trends in the treatment of zygomaticomaxillary complex fractures: a 12-year evaluation of methods used. J Oral Maxillofac Surg 1998; 56:1152–1156.
25. LaTrenta GS, McCarthy JG, Breitbart AS, May M, Sissons HA. The role of rigid skeletal fixation in bone-graft augmentation of the craniofacial skeleton. Plast Reconstr Surg 1989; 84:578–588.
26. Hegtvedt AK, Michaels GC, Beals DW. Comparison of the resistance of miniplates and microplates to various in vitro forces. J Oral Maxillofac Surg 1994; 52:251–257.
27. Yaremchuk MJ, Del Vecchio DA, Fiala TG, Lee WP. Microfixation of acute orbital fractures. Ann Plast Surg 1993; 30:385–397.
28. Schortinghuis J, Bos RR, Vissink A. Complications of internal fixation of maxillofacial fractures with microplates. J Oral Maxillofac Surg 1999; 57:130–134.
29. Yu JC, Bartlett SP, Goldberg DS, Gannon F, Hunter J, Habecker P. An experimental study of the effects of craniofacial growth on the long-term positional stability of microfixation. J Craniofac Surg 1996; 7:64–68.
30. Kasrai L, Hearn T, Gur E, Forrest CR. A biomechanical analysis of the orbitozygomatic complex in human cadavers: examination of load sharing and failure patterns following fixation with titanium and bioresorbable plating systems. J Craniofac Surg 1999; 10:237–243.
31. Edwards RC, Kiely KD, Eppley BL. The fate of resorbable poly-L-lactic/polyglycolic acid (LactoSorb) bone fixation devices in orthognathic surgery. J Oral Maxillofac Surg 2001; 59:19–25.
32. Rohrich RJ, Watumull D. Comparison of rigid plate versus wire fixation in the management of zygoma fractures: a long-term follow-up clinical study. Plast Reconstr Surg 1995; 96:570–575.

33. O'Hara DE, DelVecchio DA, Bartlett SP, Whitaker LA. The role of microfixation in malar fractures: a quantitative biophysical study. Plast Reconstr Surg 1996; 97: 345–350.
34. Dal Santo F, Ellis E, Throckmorton GS. The effects of zygomatic complex fracture on masseteric muscle force. J Oral Maxillofac Surg 1992; 50:791–799.
35. Ellis E, Kittidumkerng W. Analysis of treatment for isolated zygomaticomaxillary complex fractures. J Oral Maxillofac Surg 1996; 54:386–400.
36. Chowdhury K, Krause GE. Selection of materials for orbital floor reconstruction. Arch Otolaryngol Head Neck Surg 1998; 124:1398–1401.
37. Pearl RM. Surgical management of volumetric changes in the bony orbit. Ann Plast Surg 1987; 19:349–358.
38. Schuknecht B, Carls F, Valavanis A, Sailer HF. CT assessment of orbital volume in late post-traumatic enophthalmos. Neuroradiology 1996; 38:470–475.
39. Parsons GS, Mathog RH. Orbital wall and volume relationships. Arch Otolaryngol Head Neck Surg 1988; 114:743–747.
40. Shumrick KA, Kersten RC, Kulwin DR, Smith CP. Criteria for selective management of the orbital rim and floor in zygomatic complex and midface fractures. Arch Otolaryngol Head Neck Surg 1997; 123:378–384.
41. Afzelius LE, Rosen C. Facial fractures. A review of 368 cases. Int J Oral Surg 1980; 9:25–32.
42. Westermark A, Jensen J, Sindet-Pedersen S. Zygomatic fractures and infraorbital nerve disturbances. Miniplate osteosynthesis vs. other treatment modalities. Oral Surg Oral Diagn 1992; 3:27–30.
43. Vriens JP, Moos KF. Morbidity of the infraorbital nerve following orbitozygomatic complex fractures. J Craniomaxillofac Surg 1995; 23:363–368.
44. Vriens JP, van der Glas HW, Moos KF, Koole R. Infraorbital nerve function following treatment of orbitozygomatic complex fractures. A multitest approach. Int J Oral Maxillofac Surg 1998; 27:27–32.
45. Taicher S, Ardekian L, Samet N, Shoshani Y, Kaffe I. Recovery of the infraorbital nerve after zygomatic complex fractures: a preliminary study of different treatment methods. Int J Oral Maxillofac Surg 1993; 22:339–341.
46. Jayamanne DG, Gillie RF. Do patients with facial trauma to the orbito-zygomatic region also sustain significant ocular injuries? J.R Coll Surg Edinb 1996; 41:200–203.
47. al Qurainy IA, Stassen LF, Dutton GN, Moos KF, el Attar A. The characteristics of midfacial fractures and the association with ocular injury: a prospective study. Br J Oral Maxillofac Surg 1991; 29:291–301.
48. Cope MR, Moos KF, Speculand B. Does diplopia persist after blow-out fractures of the orbital floor in children?. Br J Oral Maxillofac Surg 1999; 37:46–51.
49. al Qurainy IA, Stassen LF, Dutton GN, Moos KF, el Attar A. Diplopia following midfacial fractures. Br J Oral Maxillofac Surg 1991; 29:302–307.
50. Bloom JN. Traumatic hyphema in children. Pediatr.Ann 1990; 19:368–371, 375.
51. Wilson FM. Traumatic hyphema. Pathogenesis and management. Ophthalmology 1980; 87:910–919.
52. Amrith S, Saw SM, Lim TC, Lee TK. Ophthalmic involvement in cranio-facial trauma. J Craniomaxillofac Surg 2000; 28:140–147.
53. Li KK, Caradonna D, Lauretano AM, Iwamoto MA. Delayed blindness after facial fracture repair. Otolaryngol Head Neck Surg 1997; 116:251–253.
54. Tarn DM, Marmor MF. Modulation and mechanisms of electroretinogram recovery after short- term retinal ischemic injury. Doc Ophthalmol 1995; 91:109–116.
55. Fedok FG. The transconjunctival approach in the trauma setting: avoidance of complications. Am J Otolaryngol 1996; 17:16–21.

56. Ord RA. Post-operative retrobulbar haemorrhage and blindness complicating trauma surgery. Br J Oral Surg 1981; 19:202–207.
57. Gonzalez MG, Santos-Oller JM, Vicente Rodriguez JC, Lopez-Arranz JS. Optic nerve blindness following a malar fracture. J Craniomaxillofac Surg 1990; 18:319–21.
58. Nicholson DH, Guzak SW. Visual loss complicating repair of orbital floor fractures. Arch Ophthalmol 1971; 86:369–375.
59. Burm JS, Chung CH, Oh SJ. Pure orbital blowout fracture: new concepts and importance of medial orbital blowout fracture. Plast Reconstr Surg 1999; 103:1839–1849.
60. Brown MS, Ky W, Lisman RD. Concomitant ocular injuries with orbital fractures. J Craniomaxillofac Trauma 1999; 5:41–46.
61. Mathog RH. Management of orbital blow-out fractures. Otolaryngol Clin North Am 1991; 24:79–91.
62. Bansagi ZC, Meyer DR. Internal orbital fractures in the pediatric age group: characterization and management. Ophthalmology 2000; 107:829–836.
63. Fujino T. Experimental "blowout" fracture of the orbit. Plast Reconstr Surg 1974; 54:81–82.
64. Erling BF, Iliff N, Robertson B, Manson PN. Footprints of the globe: a practical look at the mechanism of orbital blowout fractures, with a revisit to the work of Raymond Pfeiffer. Plast Reconstr Surg 1999; 103:1313–1316.
65. Yoshioka N, Tominaga Y, Motomura H, Muraoka M. Surgical treatment for greater sphenoid wing fracture (orbital blow-in fracture). Ann Plast Surg 1999; 42:87–91.
66. Sacks JG. The shape of the trochlea. Arch Ophthalmol 1984; 102:932–933.
67. Haug RH. Management of the trochlea of the superior oblique muscle in the repair of orbital roof trauma. J Oral Maxillofac Surg 2000; 58:602–606.
68. Gray H. 20Anatomy of the Human Body. Philadelphia: Lea & Febiger, 2000, 1918.
69. Danko I, Haug RH. An experimental investigation of the safe distance for internal orbital dissection. J Oral Maxillofac Surg 1998; 56:749–752.
70. Koornneef L. The architecture of the musculo-fibrous apparatus in the human orbit. Acta Morphol Neerl Scand 1977; 15:35–64.
71. Antonyshyn O, Gruss JS, Kassel EE. Blow-in fractures of the orbit. Plast Reconstr Surg 1989; 84:10–20.
72. Raskin EM, Millman AL, Lubkin V, della Rocca RC, Lisman RD, Maher EA. Prediction of late enophthalmos by volumetric analysis of orbital fractures. Ophthal Plast Reconstr Surg 1998; 14:19–26.
73. Smith DK, El Sayed I, Pafundi E, Dolan RW. Presentation and treatment of a posttraumatic pseudomeningocele of the superior orbit. Am J Otolaryngol 2000; 21:219–221.
74. Zachariades N, Vairaktaris E, Papavassiliou D, Papademetriou I, Mezitis M, Triantafyllou D. The superior orbital fissure syndrome. J Maxillofac Surg 1985; 13:125–128.
75. Martello JY, Vasconez HC. Supraorbital roof fractures: a formidable entity with which to contend. Ann Plast Surg 1997; 38:223–227.
76. Cahan MA, Fischer B, Iliff NT, Clark NL, Manson PN. Less common orbital fracture patterns: the role of computed tomography in the management of depression of the inferior oblique origin and lateral rectus involvement in blow-in fractures. J Craniofac Surg 1996; 7:449–459.
77. Bansagi ZC, Meyer DR. Internal orbital fractures in the pediatric age group: characterization and management. Ophthalmology 2000; 107:829–836.
78. Mathog RH. Management of orbital blow-out fractures. Otolaryngol Clin North Am 1991; 24:79–91.

79. Parsons GS, Mathog RH. Orbital wall and volume relationships. Arch Otolaryngol Head Neck Surg 1988; 114:743–747.
80. Stanley RB, Jr., Sires BS, Funk GF, Nerad JA. Management of displaced lateral orbital wall fractures associated with visual and ocular motility disturbances. Plast Reconstr Surg 1998; 102:972–979.
81. Saunders CJ, Whetzel TP, Stokes RB, Wong GB, Stevenson TR. Transantral endoscopic orbital floor exploration: a cadaver and clinical study. Plast Reconstr Surg 1997; 100:575–581.
82. Arthurs B, Silverstone P, della Rocca RC. Medial wall fractures. Adv Ophthal Plast Reconstr Surg 1987; 6:393–401.
83. Burm JS, Oh SJ. Direct local approach through a W-shaped incision in moderate or severe blowout fractures of the medial orbital wall. Plast Reconstr Surg 2001; 107:920–928.
84. Jin HR, Shin SO, Choo MJ, Choi YS. Endonasal endoscopic reduction of blowout fractures of the medial orbital wall. J Oral Maxillofac Surg 2000; 58:847–851.
85. Raveh J, Laedrach K, Vuillemin T, Zingg M. Management of combined frontonaso-orbital/skull base fractures and telecanthus in 355 cases. Arch Otolaryngol Head Neck Surg 1992; 118:605–614.
86. Cullen GC, Luce CM, Shannon GM. Blindness following blowout orbital fractures. Ophthal Surg 1977; 8:60–62.
87. Piotrowski WP, Beck-Mannagetta J. Surgical techniques in orbital roof fractures: early treatment and results. J Craniomaxillofac Surg 1995; 23:6–11.
88. Sullivan PK, Rosenstein DA, Holmes RE, Craig D, Manson PN. Bone-graft reconstruction of the monkey orbital floor with iliac grafts and titanium mesh plates: a histometric study. Plast Reconstr Surg 1993; 91:769–775.
89. Ozaki W, Buchman SR. Volume maintenance of onlay bone grafts in the craniofacial skeleton: micro-architecture versus embryologic origin. Plast Reconstr Surg 1998; 102:291–299.
90. Mandel MA. Orbital floor "blowout" fractures. Reconstruction using autogenous maxillary wall bone grafts. Am J Surg 1975; 130:590–595.
91. Lee HH, Alcaraz N, Reino A, Lawson W. Reconstruction of orbital floor fractures with maxillary bone. Arch Otolaryngol Head Neck Surg 1998; 124:56–59.
92. Wiseman JB, Holt GR, Keefe MA, Holck DE, Canaan RL, Clark WD. The fate of fresh, layered, nonsutured and sutured, autogenous cartilage in the rabbit model. Arch Facial Plast Surg 2000; 2:256–259.
93. Lee J. Preplanned correction of enophthalmos using diced cartilage grafts. Br J Plast Surg 2000; 53:17–23.
94. Morrison AD, Sanderson RC, Moos KF. The use of silastic as an orbital implant for reconstruction of orbital wall defects: review of 311 cases treated over 20 years. J Oral Maxillofac Surg 1995; 53:412–417.
95. Mauriello JA, Jr., Hargrave S, Yee S, Mostafavi R, Kapila R. Infection after insertion of alloplastic orbital floor implants. Am J Ophthalmol 1994; 117:246–252.
96. Purdy EP. Oculoplastic and orbital applications of porous high-density polyethylene implants. Curr Opin Ophthalmol 1997; 8:57–63.
97. Choi JC, Bstandig S, Iwamoto MA, Rubin PA, Shore JW. Porous polyethylene sheet implant with a barrier surface: a rabbit study. Ophthal Plast Reconstr Surg 1998; 14:32–36.
98. Haug RH, Nuveen E, Bredbenner T. An evaluation of the support provided by common internal orbital reconstruction materials. J Oral Maxillofac Surg 1999; 57:564–570.
99. Raz S. Gelfilm and blowout fractures. J Laryngol Otol 1976; 90:699–702.
100. Sugar AW, Kuriakose M, Walshaw ND. Titanium mesh in orbital wall reconstruction. Int J Oral Maxillofac Surg 1992; 21:140–144.

101. Van Eeckhoutte L, De Clippeleir L, Apers R, Van Lammeren M, Janssens H, Baekeland L. A protocol for extraocular muscle surgery after orbital floor fracture ("blow-out"). Binocul Vis Strabismus Q 1998; 13:29–36.
102. Rubin PA, Rumelt S. Functional indications for enophthalmos repair. Ophthal Plast Reconstr Surg 1999; 15:284–292.
103. Manson PN, Grivas A, Rosenbaum A, Vannier M, Zinreich J, Iliff N. Studies on enophthalmos: II. The measurement of orbital injuries and their treatment by quantitative computed tomography. Plast Reconstr Surg 1986; 77:203–214.

18

Management of Massive Traumatic Tissue Loss

Robert W. Dolan
Lahey Clinic Medical Center, Burlington, Massachusetts, U.S.A.

EPIDEMIOLOGY

Although in the first 45 years of life personal assault is the most common cause of craniofacial injury, massive tissue loss is most often associated with motor vehicle accidents and gun shot wounds (GSWs). Injury and death rates are decreasing from motor vehicles and increasing from firearms. In the United States, the majority of firearm injuries are caused by handguns.

Motor vehicle accidents (MVAs) generally cause blunt trauma that only occasionally is avulsive in nature. However, crashes involving alcohol or drugs are particularly likely to cause moderate to severe facial trauma. This may be due to the effect that these substances have on the normal and protective reflexes at the time of an accident (1). Drivers and front seat passengers are significantly more likely to be injured than occupants seated in the rear (2). The most common vehicle contact point resulting in facial injury (all severities) in unbelted passengers is the windshield or seats. When seat belts are worn, the most common contact point and source of injury is the steering wheel (3). Seat belts significantly reduce the incidence of facial laceration and the number of facial fractures but may not prevent mandibular fractures, further supporting a need for improved safety belt design (4). Air bags reduce the risk of brain damage, facial laceration, cervical spine injury, and death in severe car crashes (5).

GSWs are more often responsible for massive tissue loss. The differing nature of bone loss between MVAs and GSWs is significant since penetrating injuries, especially from high-velocity missiles, often result in explosive, destructive, and indiscriminate tissue injury. The missile tends to traverse bony structures, leaving them shattered and resulting in a loss of viable bone. In contrast, MVAs generally cause blunt injury, resulting in fractures along the weakest planes of the facial skeleton:

instead of shattering bone, it leaves intact bone segments that can be reduced without a net loss of viable bone.

Injuries due to firearms are approximately equally divided between suicides and homicides. Patients who attempt suicide by placing the muzzle of the gun under the chin will often reflexively extend their head when firing the weapon. This results in a facial high-energy avulsive wound as the cranial cavity is jerked out of the path of the missile.

HISTORICAL PERSPECTIVE

Before the 20th century, experiences gained from treating war casualties led to the only significant advances in reconstructive surgery. The nature of war injuries dramatically changed after gunpowder was introduced in Europe in the 14th century. Gunpowder is believed to have originated in 9th century China where it was used for making fireworks. It is a mixture of saltpeter (75%), sulfur (10%), and charcoal (15%). Saltpeter is a chemical compound (KNO_3) that releases oxygen when heated. Gunpowder was largely outmoded by nitroglycerin for use in the manufacture of smokeless powder and dynamite. Nitroglycerin was first produced commercially by Alfred Nobel. Concerned about the potential uses of nitroglycerin, he established a fund to provide annual awards in the sciences, literature, and the promotion of international peace.

The small arm (firearm) was initially a crude handheld cannon fired by igniting the gunpowder at the touchhole. Later, the matchlock handgun provided a trigger to move the flame to the touchhole, its successors being the wheel lock and flintlock (spark generating). The musket and the pistol were shoulder-braced and handheld variations of this technology. In the 15th century, it was discovered that by creating spiral grooves in the barrel (rifling) it would impart a spinning motion to the bullet greatly improving its accuracy. Rifled muskets first came into prominent use in the American Civil War. All long-barreled guns subsequently became rifled with the exception of shotguns that fire either a single slug or, more commonly, several pellets. By the 19th century, breechloaders (rear loading), magazine loading, smokeless powder, and bolt action firearms came into common use. The modern handgun with a revolving cylinder for semiautomatic firing was introduced by Samuel Colt in 1835. Most of the subsequent developments in small weaponry involved rapid-firing machine guns (e.g., the Thompson submachine gun or so-called Tommy gun in the 1920s) and semi-automatic lightweight rifles (e.g., the American M-16 and the Russian AK-47).

GSWs during the 15th and 16th centuries were created by low-velocity missiles ($< 600\,m/s$) that caused tissue injury limited to the path of penetration. The foremost danger in patients who survived the initial injury was infection. The bullet was dirty and harbored several pathogens that, when propelled into soft tissue, could lead to fatal infection within a few days. In addition, laceration of the bowel was also a major cause of sepsis. During this period, wound management after GSWs mainly consisted of removal of all bullet fragments, even by the use of additional incisions, to reduce the incidence of infection. Physicians instilled a variety of caustic concoctions into the wound including hot oil to neutralize the poisons associated with the bullet fragments. With the introduction of the rifle and higher-velocity weapons, direct tissue injury became a much more prominent cause of postinjury morbidity and mortality.

Improvements in the immediate treatment of wounds and rapid transport to hospitals resulted in a dramatic decrease in mortality associated with battle wounds in World War I. Further improvements in morbidity and mortality resulted with the widespread use of sulfonamides in the World War I. The benefits of instituting treatment early and the routine use of antibiotics have led to more conservative management of GSWs, especially those involving the maxillofacial region.

BALLISTICS

Classifying firearms is helpful in predicting their wounding capabilities. The first consideration is the weapon's caliber (diameter of its muzzle bore) and the projectile's velocity. The wounding potential and lethality of handguns are proportional to the caliber of the weapon. Handguns range in caliber from 0.22 to 0.45 (hundredths of an inch). If the caliber of a bullet is essentially its mass (m), then the kinetic energy (KE) with respect to caliber and velocity (v) is expressed:

$$KE = \frac{mv^2}{2}$$

The most important variable in energy transfer is the velocity of the missile. The relevant value of velocity is at the entrance to the body (impact velocity), not within the muzzle. If the bullet exits the body, not all of the KE is dissipated, and the amount of KE actually spent to wounding tissue is expressed:

$$KE = \frac{m(v_1 - v_2)}{2}$$

Handguns are considered low-velocity weapons with muzzle velocities ranging from 200 to 450 m/s. High-velocity weapons have muzzle velocities over 1000 m/s. Magnum handguns increase the powder charge to propel the bullet at a higher velocity, but are still classified as low-velocity weapons. High-velocity weapons, such as the typical rifle with calibers ranging from 0.17 to 0.460, have muzzle velocities over 1000 m/s and are able to propel a bullet accurately at high velocity over long distances.

Other factors that influence the degree of tissue injury secondary to gunshots include the composition and flight characteristics of the bullet. The modern bullet usually has a lead core encased in a copper jacket. A fully copper-encased bullet travels more true through the air, with improved accuracy and velocity retention. The copper casing also minimizes bullet deformation both in flight and after tissue penetration. Bullet deformation increases the effective diameter of the wound, resulting in a significant increase in tissue damage. Although not approved by the Hague Convention (1908) for military use, some bullets are designed to deform on impact (e.g., dum-dum, hollow-point, or soft-nose). These expanding bullets tend not to exit the tissues but expend all their potential KE within the tissue.

The flight characteristics of a bullet influence the interactions of the bullet with the penetrated tissue. A high-velocity bullet demonstrates several types of movement, both because of the velocity and the spin imparted on it by the rifled bore. The types of movement are yaw: oscillation around the long axis of the bullet; precession: oscillation in a spiral form; and nutation: rotational movement in small circles forming a rosette pattern on forward flight (6). When the bullet hits tissue, these movements increase the drag and release of KE, resulting in greater tissue damage. A bullet that is steady in flight with minimal yaw will tend to undergo less destabilization on impact and will be more likely to pass through tissue without significant loss of KE.

Shotguns are unique in their dramatically different wounding capabilities, depending on the distance from the victim. Other factors include the gauge of the shotgun, cartridge size, pellet load, power charge, and the angle of the shot. Although a shotgun has a muzzle velocity of 370 m/s, (higher than most handguns), the projectile's velocity decreases rapidly after departing the muzzle. At approximately 30 yards, its impact velocity and wounding capability are dramatically reduced. Most penetrating shotgun injuries in humans occur at less than 10 yards (7). Shotgun injuries within 3 feet of the muzzle are characterized by massive soft and hard tissue destruction, often with large chunks of tissue blown out of the wound.

TISSUE INJURY

As the impact velocity of a typical bullet exceeds 600 m/s, shock waves and temporary cavitation phenomena occur within the penetrated tissues. Cavitation is caused by the tendency of the tissue surrounding the path of the bullet to flow forward briefly, creating a wavelike sucking and vapor-filled cavity lasting several milliseconds. The degree of tissue necrosis, up to 30–40 times the diameter of the bullet, depends upon the elasticity and density of the tissues along the bullet's path. Solid, less elastic tissues tend to suffer the greatest injury while air-filled spaces (e.g., lung or bowel) tend to suffer the least damage. With regard to maxillofacial injuries, high-velocity bullets tend to cause the most damage to bony tissues, while bullets that traverse the air-filled spaces of the oropharynx, nasopharynx, and sinuses tend to cause the least amount of damage. The mandible is affected in approximately 25%, the maxilla in 25%, and combined mandible, maxilla, and orbit in 50% of cases involving avulsive high-energy ballistic wounds (8).

The pathological changes to blood vessels surrounding the path of the bullet are of concern when considering free tissue transplants. The temporary cavity produces a blunt crushing injury to blood vessels in proximity to the path of the projectile. The pathological changes include microthrombus formation, endothelial loss, breaks in the internal elastic layer, and necrosis. In a study of dogs receiving high-velocity bullet wounds (a 1 g steel ball traveling 1300–1500 m/s) to the head, microangiopathic injury occurred within 3 cm of the path of the bullet. Mild pathological changes occurred between 2–3 cm, and these tended to recover 7 days after injury. Prior to 3 days after the injury, small vessel anastomoses tend to fail within this zone of injury. Therefore, if free tissue transplantation is planned, it should be done after 3 days following the injury, and the donor vessels should originate at least 3 cm away from the path of the bullet (9).

The principal mechanism of injury from low-velocity bullets is laceration and crushing of tissues along the path of the bullet. Single or multiple bone fractures are present in the majority of low-velocity missile wounds in the head and neck. Most common are comminuted fractures of the mandible, followed by fractures involving the maxilla and midface. In low-velocity injuries, damage is limited to tissues immediately proximate to the path of the bullet; however, a bullet is often deflected multiple times and its path may not be predictable. Simply tracing a line between the entrance and exit wounds is not an adequate indicator of the path the bullet; looking for a trail of lead fragments on CT scanning may be more predictive. The entrance wound in handgun injuries is characteristically small and well formed. Often, there is no exit wound due to the lower energy of the bullet and its frequent contact with bone.

WOUND CLASSIFICATION

GSWs can be classified according to the terminal location of the missile and its wounding effect as penetrating, perforating, or avulsive. The bullet is retained within the tissue in penetrating wounds (either superficial or deep). The bullet traverses the tissue (there is an exit wound) in perforating wounds. In avulsive wounds, tissue damage is massive and large chunks of tissue may explode from the wound. Penetrating injuries are usually caused by low-velocity bullets typically from handguns. The perforating wound is usually caused by higher-velocity bullets from high-powered handguns or rifles, creating a small entrance wound and a relatively larger or gaping exit wound. High-velocity bullets, heavy arms, or close-range shotgun blasts cause avulsive injuries. The entrance wound may be small if caused by a conventional rifle, and gaping if caused by heavy arms or shotgun. Although this classification is useful for a basic description of the type of wound and its potential for tissue injury, it lacks any specific reference to the extent of tissue injury.

No uniform classification of handgun injuries exists. However, in an analysis of 40 cases of low-velocity handgun injuries, Cohen et al. devised a simple classification scheme based on the severity of soft and hard tissue injuries (10):

Type I: Soft tissue injury alone
Type II: Single fracture without comminution
Type III: Single fracture with localized comminution of the fracture site
Type IV: Severe comminution of a large area of bone
Suffix "s": associated significant soft tissue injury

A classification of ballistic and avulsive facial injuries should be based on the causes and anatomical tissue loss (gunshot, shotgun, or high-energy avulsive). Any extensively avulsed facial injury can produce an evolving pattern of tissue loss; however, high-energy ballistic and close-range shotgun injuries are the usual causes.

EMERGENCY TREATMENT

The initial emergency room encounter with a patient who has sustained a massive traumatic facial tissue loss consists of

1. Rapid assessment of all entrance and exit wounds

2. Assessment of the ABCs for immediate resuscitation (airway, breathing, circulation)
3. Establishing an airway, usually by endotracheal intubation, before blood or edema impede access to the airway
4. Performing a tracheotomy or cricothyroidotomy, if necessary
5. Control of hemorrhage by pressure and selective hemostasis
6. Protection of the cervical spine via immobilization or cervical collar

Delay non-life-threatening maxillofacial injury assessment until the patient is stabilized. Two major problems in the initial management of patients with facial trauma are bleeding and difficulty in obtaining an airway. In all cases of severe maxillofacial injuries, an airway should be established as soon as possible. Foreign bodies such as teeth or debris are commonly found in the upper airway after massive facial trauma and should be sought in the initial encounter. If attempts at endotracheal intubation (either directly or with a fiberoptic laryngoscope) are unsuccessful, or if there is laryngotracheal separation or overwhelming bleeding, an airway should be established in the neck. This can be accomplished by routine tracheotomy, cricothyroidotomy, or direct tracheal intubation in the case of a gaping neck wound. An endotracheal tube or tracheostomy tube directly sutured to the trachea or surrounding skin should be used. Difficult-to-control oral bleeding can be controlled with pharyngeal packing after the airway is secured. The approach to nasal bleeding should be more judicious since the haphazard placement of packing can exacerbate or create a cranial base injury. In cases of nasal hemorrhage, a Foley catheter can be placed through the nose with the distal balloon in the nasopharynx. The balloon should be carefully filled with water, followed by the placement of standard anterior nasal packing.

Specific assessment of the cervical spine is essential in any patient with a severe facial injury. Midface injures are most often associated with cervical spine injuries at the level of C5–7. Injuries to the lower third of the face tend to be associated with injuries of the upper cervical spine. The incidence of cervical spine injury associated with injuries of the maxillofacial region varies between 0.3 and 19.3% (11).

DIAGNOSTIC TESTING AND INJURY CLASSIFICATION

Subsequent acute care management will depend on whether the patient can safely undergo various radiographic studies including computed tomography (CT) or magnetic resonance imaging (MRI) and angiography. Angiography is the standard method for detecting clinically occult vascular injury. Magnetic resonance angiography may be appropriate for selected patients, but it does not render adequate definition to rule out subtle vascular injuries that may require operative intervention. Uncontrollable hemorrhage, expanding hematoma, or intra-abdominal injuries are the usual reasons for emergency transfer to the operating room without first having the patient undergo radiographic assessment of the wound and surrounding vital structures.

Radiographic assessment prior to fracture reduction and soft and hard tissue reconstruction consists primarily of CT scanning. The entire facial skeleton can be assessed with fine cut (2 mm) CT scanning in the coronal and axial planes. With this degree of detail, a very accurate three-dimensional CT can be obtained that can assist the surgeon in visualizing the extent of injury (Fig. 1). Based on these types of scans, stereolithographic models can also be constructed that allow the surgeon to view and manipulate the pertinent anatomy prior to surgery (12).

Separating the head and neck into zones of injury can be useful. Zone I lies between the clavicle and the cricoid cartilage; zone II lies between the cricoid cartilage and the mandibular angle; zone III lies between the mandibular angle and the base of the skull. These divisions become obscured and arbitrary in massive avulsive and high-energy facial injuries. Even in wounds caused by low-velocity bullets, secondary bullet fragments or propelled tissue fragments can cause injury to an adjacent zone despite clearly defined entrance and exit wounds that seemingly are confined to a single zone. Vascular injuries in zone I and zone III are more likely to be clinically silent and are more difficult and treacherous to approach surgically. Angiography, both diagnostic and therapeutic, should be performed in cases of suspected injury involving zones I and III. Zone II is easier to access surgically, and proximal and distal control of vascular hemorrhage is straightforward. Therefore, injuries limited to zone II may be surgically explored to rule out significant vascular injury. Patients with massive tissue loss due to high-energy GSWs will have injuries that involve at least zone III, and in most cases should undergo cervical angiography as soon as possible upon presentation. Significant findings include arterial thrombosis, arteriovenous fistula, bullet embolus, pseudoaneurysm, and intimal disruption or tear.

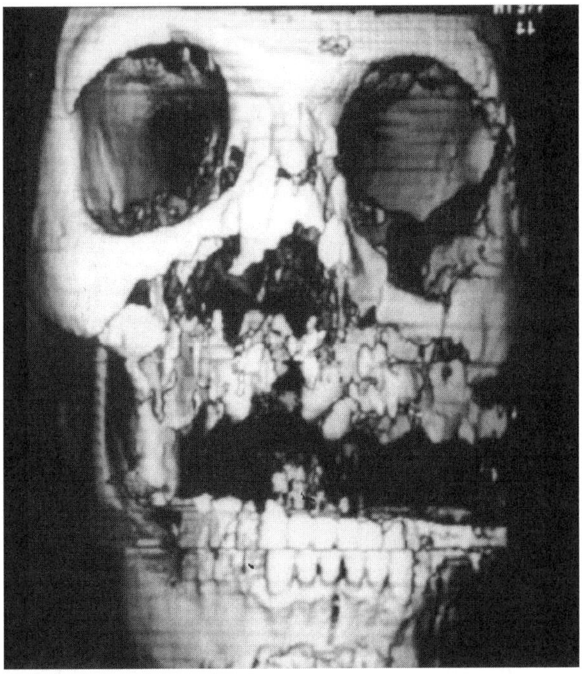

Figure 1 Three-dimensional CT scan is useful for operative planning and assessing the extent of injury.

EARLY WOUND MANAGEMENT

Tetanus prophylaxis and broad-spectrum antibiotics are indicated in all cases. The degree of tissue injury from GSWs is often difficult to assess accurately during the first several hours of injury. This is due to several problems associated with the acute GSW:

1. Evolving tissue necrosis surrounding the bullet, especially relevant to high-velocity bullet injuries
2. Secondary bullet and tissue fragments that act like small missiles to cause injuries apparently well away from the presumed path of the bullet
3. Unpredictable injuries due to bullet deflection within the tissues
4. Imminent tissue changes including edema that may affect surrounding vital structures such as the cranial nerves or airway
5. The often moribund condition of the patient, making examination of vital functions such as vision difficult

Ballistic wound management was originally described as a guide to managing ballistic injuries in the 18th century. The method was designed to minimize tissue necrosis and infection and involved wound packing and serial debridement followed by delayed reconstruction. The basic tenets of this method include frequent open wound assessments to accomplish the following:

1. Evacuate hematomas
2. Debride nonviable and infection-prone tissue
3. Eliminate dead space
4. Immediate stabilization and anatomical reduction of existing bone
5. Check for viable tissue alignment

Any wound with an extensive soft and hard tissue or avulsive injury may behave like a high-energy ballistic wound, and a ballistic wound protocol is effective in reducing the degree of ultimate tissue loss.

The patient with a GSW must be carefully monitored and repeatedly examined over the first 48–72 h after the initial injury. This is despite the variety of initial studies such as CT scanning, MRI, and angiography that may show negative results. Tissue injury, especially ophthalmic and avascular tissue necrosis, may be evolving or unrecognized during the initial encounter and radiological assessments. Ophthalmological consultation should be sought for deeply penetrating injuries involving the upper third of the facial skeleton. Continuing loss of vital tissues is common, especially in high-energy and avulsive wounds. Early debridement and antibiotics significantly decrease the eventual amount of tissue loss in GSWs. Debridement of obviously necrotic tissue under general anesthesia (assessment of tissue necrosis includes color and capillary bleeding) within 6 h is required to minimize the ultimate amount of tissue devitalization. However, intravenous penicillin has been shown to increase this window of opportunity effectively to 12 h (13). Repeated debridements every 12–24 h are usually necessary, but early intervention lessens the need for subsequent debridements. Wound debridement may need to be delayed if the patient is unstable or if a developing problem such as vision deterioration is detected.

During the initial evaluation and exploration of massive tissue injuries, a variety of problems may be encountered including of bullet fragments, severed facial nerve branches, a severed parotid duct, an injured globe, and exposed auricular cartilage. In most circumstances, removing bullet fragments is unnecessary. However, fragments may migrate and occasionally extrude either through the skin or into the airway several months to years after the injury. This is particularly true when the fragments are within a mobile area such as the neck or posterior pharynx. If a large fragment is near a major vessel within the neck, it can erode the vessel and lead to hemorrhage in the future. Factors such as the size of the fragment necessary to cause erosion are unknown. However, an easily accessible bullet fragment should be removed if it is resting near a major neck vessel.

Severed nerve branches may be tagged or repaired during the initial surgical exploration depending on the need for continuing debridement within the area. The distal segments of the facial nerve may be stimulated (using a facial nerve electric stimulator) within 72 h of the injury. This is valuable to locate the distal cut segments. The nerve ends may be reanastomosed primarily with three to four nonabsorbable fine sutures through the epineurium. If the nerve ends are separated and primary anastomosis is not possible, a nerve graft should be exploited using either the greater auricular nerve or sural nerve.

Injury to the parotid duct can be detected by cannulating the duct papule with an 18–22 gauge catheter and injecting diluted methylene blue. Extravasated dye represents either a complete duct transection or a laceration. The potential sequelae of this injury are parotid duct stenosis, salivary fistula, and sialocele formation. To minimize the occurrence of these problems, primary duct repair should be performed (under loop magnification) using fine nonabsorbable sutures. Salivary fistulas and sialoceles will usually resolve spontaneously, even without salivary duct repair. Parotid stenosis is usually more difficult to manage and may require repeated dilation (14,15).

Globe injury may lead to delayed blindness in the opposite eye due to sympathetic ophthalmia. Sympathetic ophthalmia is a rare granulomatous uveitis associated with either a perforating globe injury in the region of the ciliary body or a retained foreign body in the eye. The injured eye becomes inflamed first and the other eye follows (sympathetically), usually at least 10 days after the initial injury. The cause is unknown, but it may be a T-cell-mediated autoimmunity to uveal and retinal antigens. Systemic steroids may help suppress the autoimmune response and delay the onset of blindness (16,17). Symptoms include photophobia, redness, blurred vision, and occasionally pain. The most effective prevention is enucleation of the injured eye within 10 days following the injury. If the injured eye is not enucleated, the patient must be vigilant and seek medical attention immediately at the first sign of blurred vision, redness, or photophobia. Sympathetic visual loss can occur even years following the injury.

It is common to find exposed ear cartilage associated with these types of injuries. If primary skin closure over the area of exposed cartilage is not possible, the cartilage should be carefully preserved and buried in postauricular skin. This prevents chondritis and further tissue loss and leaves the cartilage in the area for subsequent reconstruction. If the perichondrium is intact, split-thickness skin grafting will also be effective in covering the cartilage in wounds that are not grossly contaminated.

TRAUMATIC AMPUTATIONS OF FACIAL STRUCTURES

Replantation of traumatically amputated facial parts without re-establishment of the blood supply is usually unsuccessful unless the part is very small. A nonvascularized replanted part may survive if it is precisely amputated with minimal crushing injury and if there is no more than 1 cm between all areas of the part and the vascularized bed. Larger amputated facial parts must be replanted with reconstitution of their blood supply. This is often very difficult due to the small size of the arteries and frequent lack of veins suitable for anastomosis. A variety of tissue parts can be considered for reimplantation including the scalp, nasal tip, ear, lip, and eyebrow.

The scalp is particularly suitable for replantation because the entire unit can survive on a single superficial temporal artery and vein, and, in avulsive injuries, these vessels are usually well preserved. Techniques for improving the venous outflow in revascularized flaps include leeching, creation of arteriovenous fistulas, and repeated pin pricking. Repeated pricking is rarely successful. Creation of an arteriovenous fistula involves anastomosing one of the arteries from the amputated part to a vein in the recipient bed. This method is probably most successful when a suitable donor vein is unavailable. Leeching can be successful in many cases; however, blood loss can be significant and there is an increased risk of bacterial infection. The leech can ingest up to 8–10 ml blood, and the wound can continue to ooze another 50 ml blood from the bite site (18). Wound infection is most commonly caused by *Aeromonas hydrophila*, a facultative gram-negative rod that is part of the normal flora in the leech gut flora. Prophylactic antibiotics should be administered to counteract this organism, commonly third-generation cephalosporins (ceftriaxone), ciprofloxacin, aminoglycosides, sulfa drugs, or tetracycline (19). The overall success rate for reimplantation of amputated facial parts is approximately 50%. However, an aggressive attempt at microsurgical reimplantation will result in more tissue survival and a better cosmetic outcome than any other reconstructive procedure (20).

DELAYED PRIMARY RECONSTRUCTION

Delayed primary reconstruction describes initiating the reconstruction process during the same hospitalization after a period of delay to allow for wound stabilization (usually within 7 days of the injury). Reconstruction in the past was delayed for several months to allow for wound and scar maturation and healing of oral cavity wounds to minimize salivary contamination of secondarily placed grafts, flaps, and implants. Nonvascularized bone grafts will not survive in the presence of inadequate soft tissue coverage, salivary contamination, or infection. The patient was usually reconstructed in several stages by first providing adequate soft tissue to seal the oral cavity and a well-vascularized bed for future placement of bone grafts. However, secondarily placed bone grafts often cannot fully restore the contour of the overlying soft tissues due to dense scarring. Multiple smaller revision procedures were required to shape the soft tissue flaps and to revise scars.

In the late 20th century, remarkable technological improvements in flap selection and design have made primary reconstructive efforts much more effective. Primary reconstruction has become more reliable due to the availability of composite tissues including vascularized composite tissue grafts and a greater understanding of wound care in high-energy avulsive injuries. These tissues can be placed without compromise in fields grossly contaminated with saliva and can actually fight infection and improve vascularity. Early definitive reconstruction requires fewer procedures and fewer hospitalizations during the course of treatment (21).

The greatest achievements in reconstructive surgery involve the ability to replace missing bone and restore the facial skeletal framework. Advancements in antibiotics, craniofacial surgical techniques, accurate preoperative planning using CT scanning, techniques of open reduction, and the sophisticated use of regional and free tissue transfers have made the near-perfect restoration of the facial skeleton a reasonable goal. However, there are substantial deficiencies in the ability to restore muscular function and soft tissues. To achieve an optimal cosmetic result, the skeletal framework must be accurately reconstructed allowing the much more difficult task of soft tissue replacement to proceed unhampered by gross contour deformities and cicatrical collapse. The most important considerations during the initial phases of reconstruction of massive tissue deficits include the following:

1. Open reduction and fixation of facial fractures
2. Replacement of missing bone
3. Replacement of missing soft tissue
4. Intraoral and pharyngeal reconstruction to maximize speech and swallowing
5. Careful planning of future stages so as not to disrupt adjacent tissue transfer or proceeding with ill-conceived and unrealistic attempts at primary reconstruction.

Fractures should be reduced and fixed with miniplates, wire osteosynthesis, and external fixation devices as needed. Augmentation of lost bone in the midface and orbit can be done with free bone grafts, preferably split-thickness bone grafts from the calvarium. Preoperative planning together with an anaplastologist and a maxillofacial prosthodontist is essential. Definitive reconstruction in areas of bone loss using microvascular bone grafts should proceed despite a possible lack of overlying skin. If the overlying skin is intact and the bone is destroyed, especially in the areas of the premaxilla and mandible, primary bone reconstruction is crucial to prevent cicatricial contraction of the skin envelope. This is particularly relevant to low-velocity missile injuries since the underlying bone injuries are usually much more substantial than the soft tissue injuries.

A massive wound resulting from a low-velocity missile typically will have extensive underlying bone injury, including multiple displaced and devitalized fragments associated with minimal soft tissue cover and skin injury. This type of wound is similar to those caused by severe blunt injuries and is characterized by complex facial fractures with minimal skin loss. However, the fractures resulting from GSWs do not follow the typical fracture patterns seen in blunt facial trauma. They follow the path of the bullet and usually do not occur along areas of weakness in the facial skeleton such as typical Lefort or zygomatic complex fractures. Nevertheless, these wounds can be treated similar to complex facial fractures using all the typical craniofacial approaches and rigid internal fixation. However, the need for bone replacement using microvascular bone grafts is higher in wounds created by GSWs because the underlying bone may be destroyed.

During the initial reconstruction, several key areas of the skeleton must be corrected with respect to symmetry, contour, support, and function including the orbit, maxilla, and mandible.

PRIMARY ORBITAL RECONSTRUCTION

The orbital rims should be verified to be symmetrical and in good position to minimize eyelid malposition and contour abnormalities. Proper eyelid and canthal position is obtained by confirming that the distance between the medial canthi (between the eyes) is equal to width of the palpebral fissures (from lateral canthus to medial canthus). Measurements are referenced to a horizontal line across the nasion. The distances between this line and the lateral canthus, medial canthus, and pupil (in primary gaze) on the uninvolved side can be used as a guide for accurate globe and canthal repositioning for the abnormal side (Fig. 2).

Globe projection can be assessed with a Hertel prism exophthalmometer by measuring the height of the dome of the cornea based on the plane of the lateral orbital rim (normal values = 12–20 mm). A 2 mm difference between the projection of the globes is usually obvious. Excessive orbital volume is a common finding in patients with severe penetrating and blunt facial trauma. The orbital volume must be restored by sufficient reduction and reconstruction of the walls of the orbit, especially medially and inferiorly. Failure to restore orbital volume will result in an inferiorly displaced globe that is enophthalmic and rigidly enveloped in scar. The main cause of enophthalmos is an increase in the volume of the posterior orbital cavity due to bone

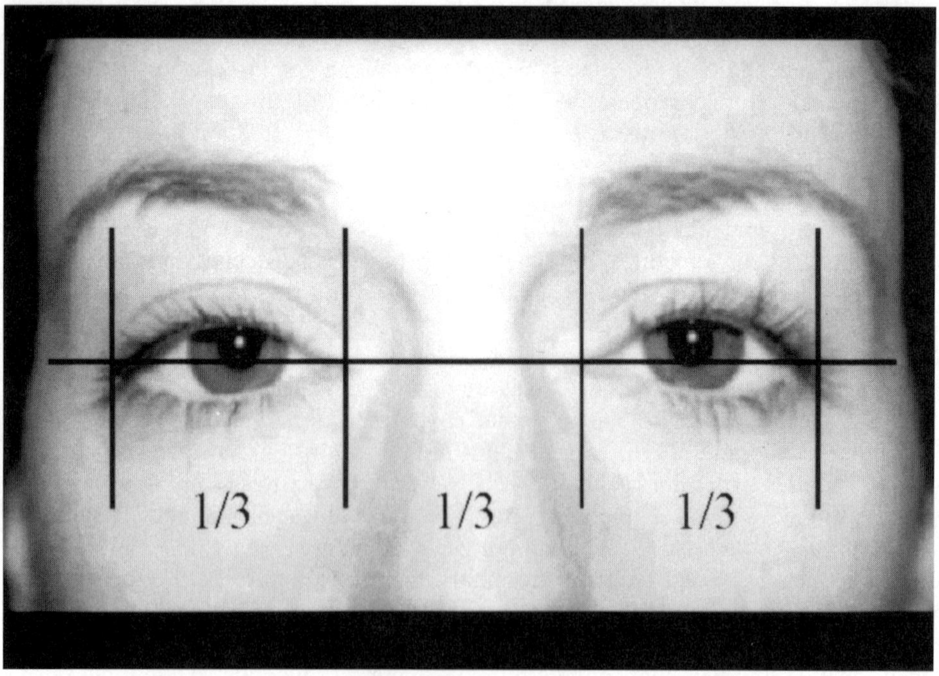

Figure 2 Relationships of the lateral and medial palpebral commissures.

loss and malposition. The anterior–posterior projection of the globe is primarily dependent upon volumetric and support mechanisms posterior to the equator of the globe. Failure to correct deficiencies of bone mass and support in the posterolateral, posteromedial, or posterior orbital floor will result in enophthalmos. Even if a defect in the bone is not evident, bone grafts should be placed in the posterior orbit to restore its conal shape and correct volume deficits. Deficiencies of bone and support in the anterior orbit (anterior to the equator of the globe) tend to affect the vertical position of the globe. The final position of the globe is determined by the orbital volume, inferior support of the periorbital contents, and size and location of bone grafts. The anteroposterior(AP) axis (projection) can be measure with a Hertel exophthalmometer and is the distance from the corneal apex to the lateral orbital rim.

Approximately 13% of patients with severe, complex facial fractures will require autogenous bone or cartilage grafting in the primary setting (22). Intraorbital and periorbital reconstruction can generally be achieved using split calvarial onlay bone grafting to repair gaps and restore orbital volume. The superior orbital rim is the most common area of injury requiring immediate bone grafting. Block grafts from the iliac crest (endochondral bone) tend to undergo more resorption (75%) than split calvarial bone grafts (membranous bone) that only lose 10–20% of their volume. The cancellous portion of the bone should be in contact with the recipient bone and preservation of the periosteum may help to minimize absorption. Once skeletal fixation is completed with rigid miniplates, areas of bone loss over the orbital rims or internal orbit become apparent. Bone grafts are used to span the bony gaps over the orbital rims and are fixated to the previously placed rigid miniplates. Defects within the bony orbit are repaired with an onlay technique with or without

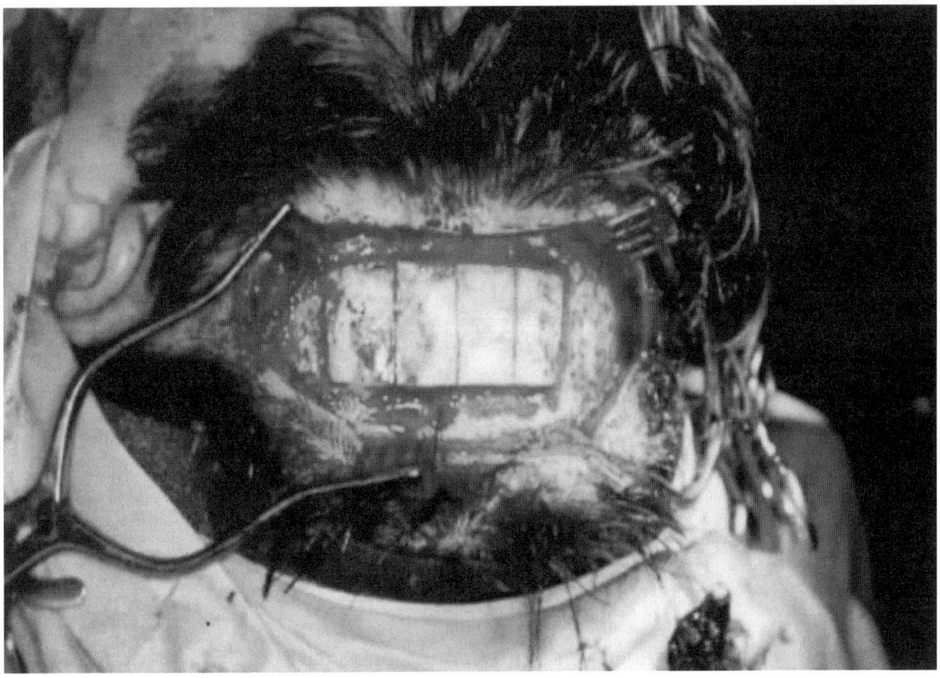

Figure 3 Split calvarial bone grafts harvested through a separate scalp incision.

fixation of the bone grafts. Primary bone grafting is successful in most cases of cranial and midface reconstruction, and split calvarial bone grafts will survive despite having one side facing an open cavity (8). Multiple calvarial bone grafts can be harvested through a hemicoronal scalp incision Fig. 3). In cases of massive tissue loss over the orbital rims, the primary placement of free bone grafts is more difficult and may lack an adequately vascularized tissue bed to support the bone. In these cases, a rotational flap or free vascularized tissue must be used for coverage. An osteocutaneous free flap should be considered if there is orbital rim bone loss and severe bony maxillary deficiencies, especially associated with large cheek defects.

RECONSTRUCTION OF THE MAXILLA

The vital areas of the maxilla where tissue loss must be addressed include the frontal process of the maxilla, the zygomaticomaxillary (ZM) buttress, hard palate, and the pyriform apertures. Isolated anterior or medial wall (lateral nasal wall) losses are of no consequence. Frontal process and ZM buttress loss results in destabilization of the midface and some minor contour deficiencies. Lacrimal sac and duct injuries are often associated. Instillation of dye (fluorescein) into the upper and lower canaliculi can uncover canalicular, lacrimal sac, or duct injuries. The canaliculi can be stented with fine polyethylene tubing (Jones' tubes) if injury is found isolated to these structures. Lacrimal sac tears should be sutured with fine nonabsorbable sutures. Injured lacrimal ducts can be bypassed by primary or secondary dacryocystorhinost-

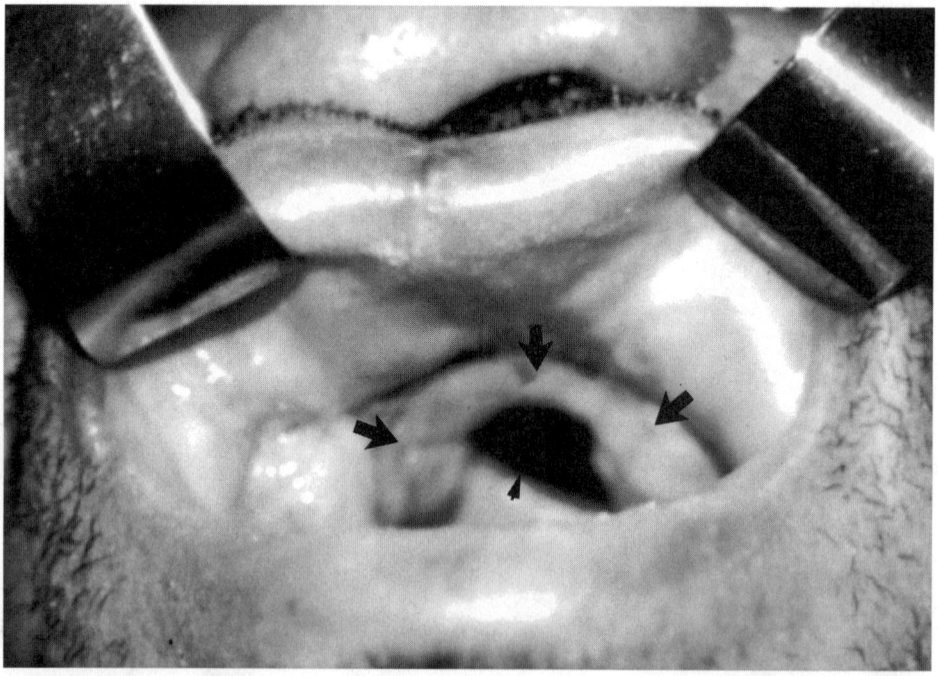

Figure 4 Palatal defect: fibular bone transferred to reconstruct entire hard palate that disintegrated after a GSW to the face. Large arrows, fibular bone; small arrow, oronasal fistula.

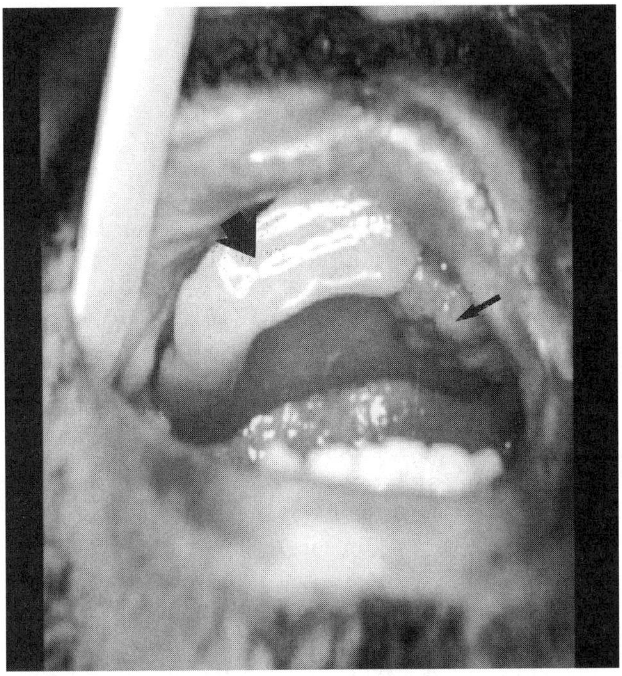

Figure 5 Larger arrow points to palatal prosthesis anchored to underlying fibular bone. Smaller arrow indicates surface of fibula.

omy. The frontal process contributes to the medial orbital rim, and bony deficiencies in this area must be corrected to prevent eyelid malposition. Bone remnants or split calvarial bone grafts may be placed primarily if there is adequate soft tissue coverage. In avulsive facial injuries, a soft tissue flap may be necessary to cover the free bone grafts.

Hemipalatal defects are relatively common in handgun injuries and can be obturated easily using a custom prosthesis. Smaller palatal defects (those that do not extend past the midline) may be effectively closed using the temporalis muscle flap or the buccinator musculomucosal flap (23). However, total palatal loss or significant coronal anterior palatal losses will result in collapse of the midface and leave little support for prostheses. An osseous free flap is required to provide an anchor for a palatal prosthesis to close the oronasal fistula and to prevent velopharyngeal incompetence in the case of associated soft palate injury. The cutaneous portion of the osseus free flap may be used to close the oronasal defect that can potentially avoid the need for prostheses. A palatal prosthesis is the best method available for the prevention of velopharyngeal incompetence (VPI) in patients with significant defects of the soft palate (Figs. 4,5).

Osseointegrated fixtures implanted into the adjacent intact alveolus or the newly placed reconstructed bone are an excellent method to retain maxillary prostheses. Secondary placement of these fixtures is more accurate than primary placement at the time of the initial reconstruction in terms of their three-dimensional alignment. Primary placement is hampered by the fact that the configuration and dimensions of the maxilla will change with healing and many of the osseointegrated implants primarily placed will become malpositioned. After 4 months, the wound will have matured sufficiently for reliable placement.

RECONSTRUCTION OF THE MANDIBLE

The first attempts at bone replacement surgery date back to World War I using bone–periosteal grafts from the mandible to span gaps and fill defects in other areas of the mandible. This experience formed the basis of several subsequent developments in mandibular reconstruction, including the use of bone from distant sites, most often the ilium, and the use of rigid metal trays and cancellous bone packing (24). After World War II, the technique of mandibular reconstruction using cancellous bone and absorbable trays was refined and is still widely used today (25). The major drawback to this method is that there is a very high failure rate if the recipient bed is ischemic or subject to salivary contamination. Therefore, nonvascularized bone grafts must often be placed secondarily after one or more preliminary surgeries for soft tissue coverage to seal the recipient site from saliva and provide a vascularized bed for the bone graft. Placing the bone graft in this setting requires extensive lysis of adhesions, scar release, and expansion of the soft tissue envelope. Scar release is often inadequate, leaving a tight and distorted compartment for the bone graft. Additional soft tissue may be required to cover and expand the recipient site adequately to accommodate the bone graft, often leaving additional scars and contour deformities. This was the prevailing method of reconstruction for patients undergoing segmental mandibular resections prior to the advent of microvascular bone grafts. Microvascular bone grafts are successful and survive completely without bone loss in more than 95% of cases despite ischemic tissue beds and gross salivary contamination (Fig. 6). No preliminary surgery is necessary to prepare the recipient site and, since the flap can be placed primarily, the problems of scarring and soft tissue collapse are avoided. Primary replacement of segmental defects of the mandible should be undertaken, especially in patients with intact overlying skin. Vascularized bone restores a functional mandible, minimizes the chances of hardware exposure, maintains the mandibular profile, and prevents soft tissue collapse. Secondary reconstruction should be considered a compromise and reserved for patients who cannot undergo or refuse primary surgical repair.

SECONDARY RECONSTRUCTION

The orbit and midface are the most difficult areas to reconstruct in the secondary setting, primarily due to the effects of scarring. In contrast, the nose and auricle are best left for secondary correction because of the difficulty in obtaining acceptable results in the primary setting. Flaps and grafts must also be adapted for use in the secondary setting. Minor contour deformities of the skull can be corrected with onlay grafts, preferably from the calvaria. Newly available calcium phosphate cement that sets to solid microporous hydroxyapatite may be very valuable in correcting contour deficiencies of the face and skull. The material is applied directly to bone and molded in its paste form (Figs. 7–9). It solidifies within minutes and over a period of several months is progressively replaced by bone that is indistinguishable from the surrounding bone. Experimental evidence to date suggests that

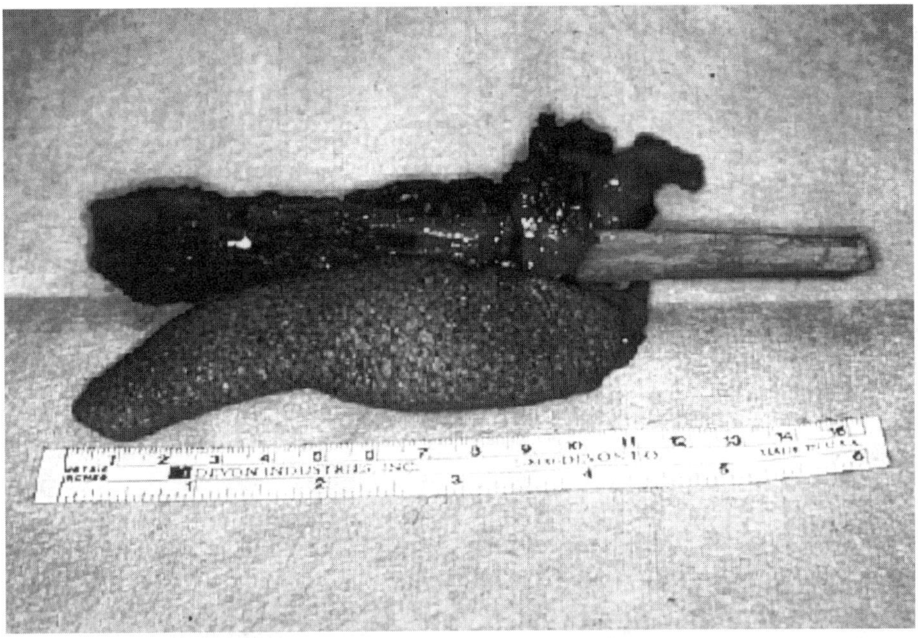

Figure 6 Example of the most commonly used microvascular bone graft: the fibular free flap.

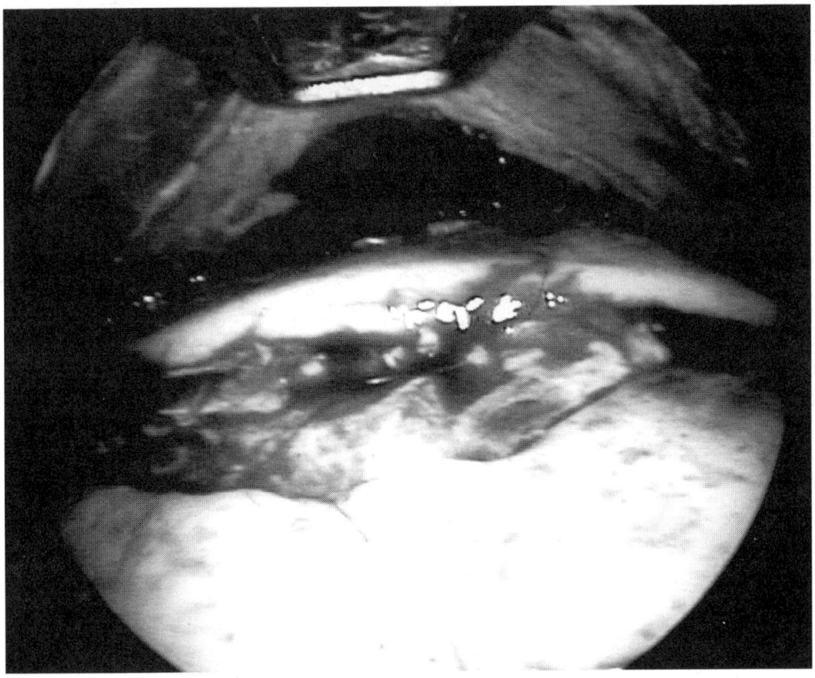

Figure 7 Endoscopic view of frontal bone defect after craniotomy; above the retractor is the scalp. The arrow marks the defect with exposed dura.

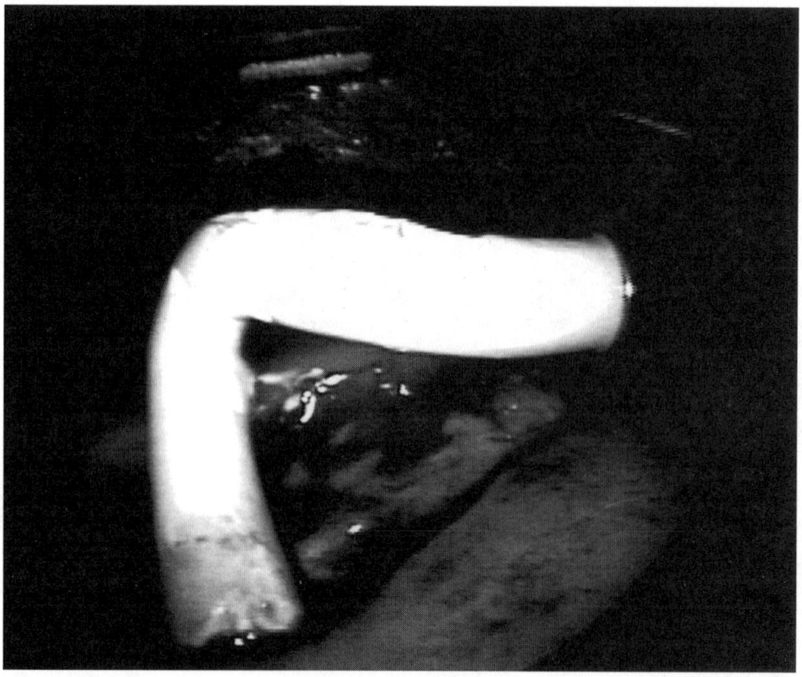

Figure 8 Hydroxyapatite cement as it is applied endoscopically over the defect shown in Figure 7.

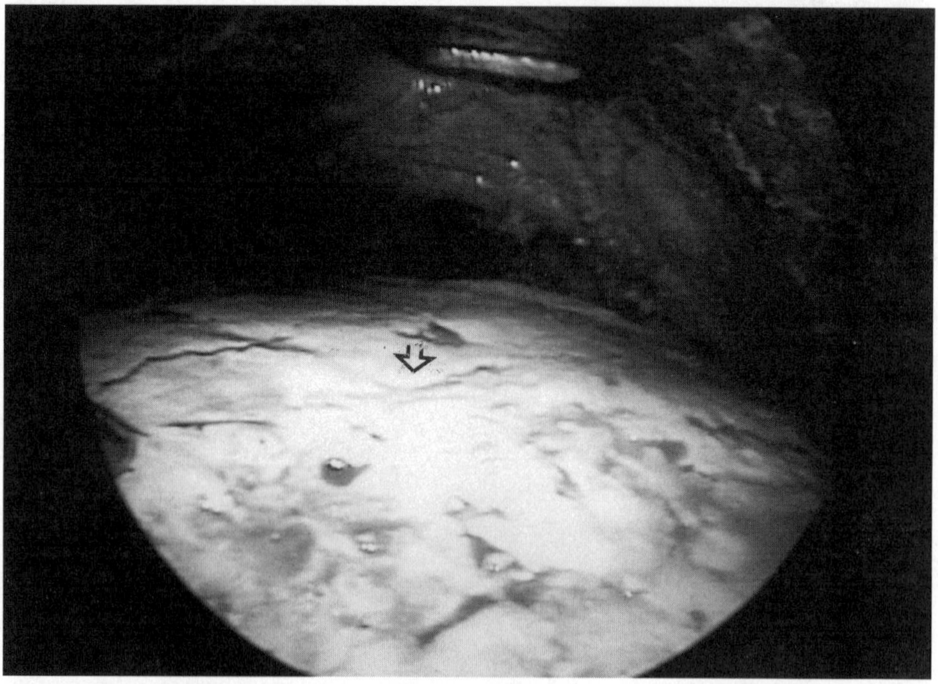

Figure 9 Repaired defect shows smooth contour with bone paste in place (arrow).

the implant maintains its shape and does not undergo any resorption or loss of volume (26).

SECONDARY ORBITAL RECONSTRUCTION

Secondary correction of post-traumatic enophthalmos and dystopia is difficult. Several factors are often cited as responsible for globe malposition, including displaced or missing periorbital bone, loss of orbital fat, and scar contracture. However, the major factor responsible for post-traumatic enophthalmos and dystopia is a pathological increase in dimensions of the bony orbit, most often because of a dislocated zygomatic bone. A displaced and rotated zygomatic bone separates from its natural articulations with the greater wing of the sphenoid and maxilla. This results in gaping fissures along the floor and lateral wall of the orbit, and a substantial increase in the volume of the orbital cavity. In addition, severe nasoethmoid complex injuries often result in significant canthal distortion and malposition. Telecanthus and canthal height distortions are equally difficult to correct, especially if significant amounts of bone and soft tissue are missing.

Dystopia (excess or deficiency in the horizontal position of the globe) is easier to correct than enophthalmos. Horizontal dystopia (inferior displacement) is correctable by subperiosteal augmentation of the anterior orbital floor, anterior to the axis of the globe. This is a very effective method to produce superior movement of the eyeball but does little to correct enophthalmos despite an overall decrease in orbital volume.

To correct enophthalmos, the volume of the orbital cavity must be reduced posterior to the axis of the globe. Refracturing and rearticulating the skeletal framework, including the zygomatic bone, is effective in restoring the three-dimensional anatomical features of both the external and internal structure of the bony orbit. Complete exposure of the zygomatic bone is required using craniofacial techniques to cut and free the bone and to re-establish the correct alignment. Through a coronal flap, the zygomaticofrontal suture and zygomatic arch are fully exposed and the fascial and muscular connections are released, including the masseter muscle. Through a lower eyelid incision, the inferior orbital rim and orbital floor is exposed: through an upper lip gingivobuccal incision, the zygomaticomaxillary articulation is uncovered. Using a reciprocating saw, bony cuts are created that mimic those found in a typical zygomatic complex fracture (i.e., zygomaticofrontal, zygomatic arch, orbital rim, and zygomaticomaxillary). The zygomatic bone is freed and replaced into its new position and rigidly fixated. Bone grafting then proceeds to close the gaps and augment orbital volume, as needed. If autologous bone is used to augment orbital volume, the globe should be made slightly exophthalmic (1–2 mm) in anticipation of some absorption of the bone grafts over the ensuing several months; however, this is often difficult to achieve because of the extensive scarring present. The grafts should be placed external to the intramuscular cone. Inadvertent placement of grafts or postoperative displacement of grafts into the intramuscular cone can result in severe dysfunction of the extraocular muscles or injury to the optic nerve (27). To avoid this complication, careful dissection of the periorbita off the underlying bone is necessary, creating safe pockets for the grafts. If the periorbita is disrupted from previous trauma, the extraocular muscles may be visualized and the grafts placed external to them.

Inherent risks to secondary correction of enophthalmos include worsening vision, diplopia, dystopia, and enophthalmos. Dramatic changes in vision may occur, especially if the grafts are misplaced or there is retrobulbar hematoma. However, more subtle changes in Snellen acuity may occur from the pressure exerted by the grafts on the posterior aspect of the globe, resulting in retinal folds and ischemia (28). Diplopia may improve, but only to a limited degree because the majority of patients have permanent cicatrical reductions in ocular motility. Enophthalmos and dystopia can worsen postoperatively due to scarring or implant displacement and absorption. However, the vast majority of patients experience at least a moderate improvement in globe position that is long-lasting (27).

Lateral displacement of the medial canthus (telecanthus) can be corrected using similar principles of skeletal rearrangement using a medial orbital osteotomy (29). Creating bone cuts along the lines of fracture that are typical in nasoethmoid complex fractures frees a segment of bone that includes the insertion point of the tendon. Medial relocation of the bone into its normal anatomical position draws the tendon and overlying soft tissue medially correcting the telecanthus. The bone is then rigidly fixed to surrounding stable bone over the inferomedial forehead and maxilla, and missing bone segments are replaced with autologous bone grafts.

SECONDARY USE OF FLAPS AND GRAFTS

The principles of secondary reconstruction of post-traumatic deformities using flaps and grafts include the following:

1. Reconstruction of cutaneous defects should follow standard aesthetic principles and defectsshould be altered in size, shape, and outline to conform to the topographical unit principle.
2. Multiple revisions are usually necessary to achieve the optimal aesthetic result.
3. Adjacent aesthetic units should be reconstructed with separate flaps, or the flap should be tailored to conform to the unit principle.
4. The use of local tissues should be maximized, including through the use of tissue expansion.

Although massive tissue losses often require the use of large composite flaps for coverage, the topographical unit principle should still apply whenever possible. Replacing soft tissue defects of the face with identically sized flaps or grafts often produces an obviously patched area. There are definite regions in which skin differs in color, texture, mobility, and thickness. The boundaries of these regions represent the natural transition zones where incisions and flap or graft borders can escape notice. Gonzalez-Ulloa et al. outlined the patterns of the shape of seven facial regions on cadavers as templates for flaps and grafts (30) (Fig. 10).

Reconstructing an entire aesthetic unit allows the placement of incisions at the unit borders so that scars, contractures, and depressions become less noticeable. Even trapdoor scarring and bunching of the flap are less noticeable and may result in a net aesthetic improvement in areas that are naturally bulbous (e.g., the nasal ala or chin). The principle of removing the remaining portion of a topographical unit if a large part of a unit is missing (e.g., $> 50\%$) is as applicable in post-traumatic cases as in patients who have undergone resection for treatment of cancer, provided the area

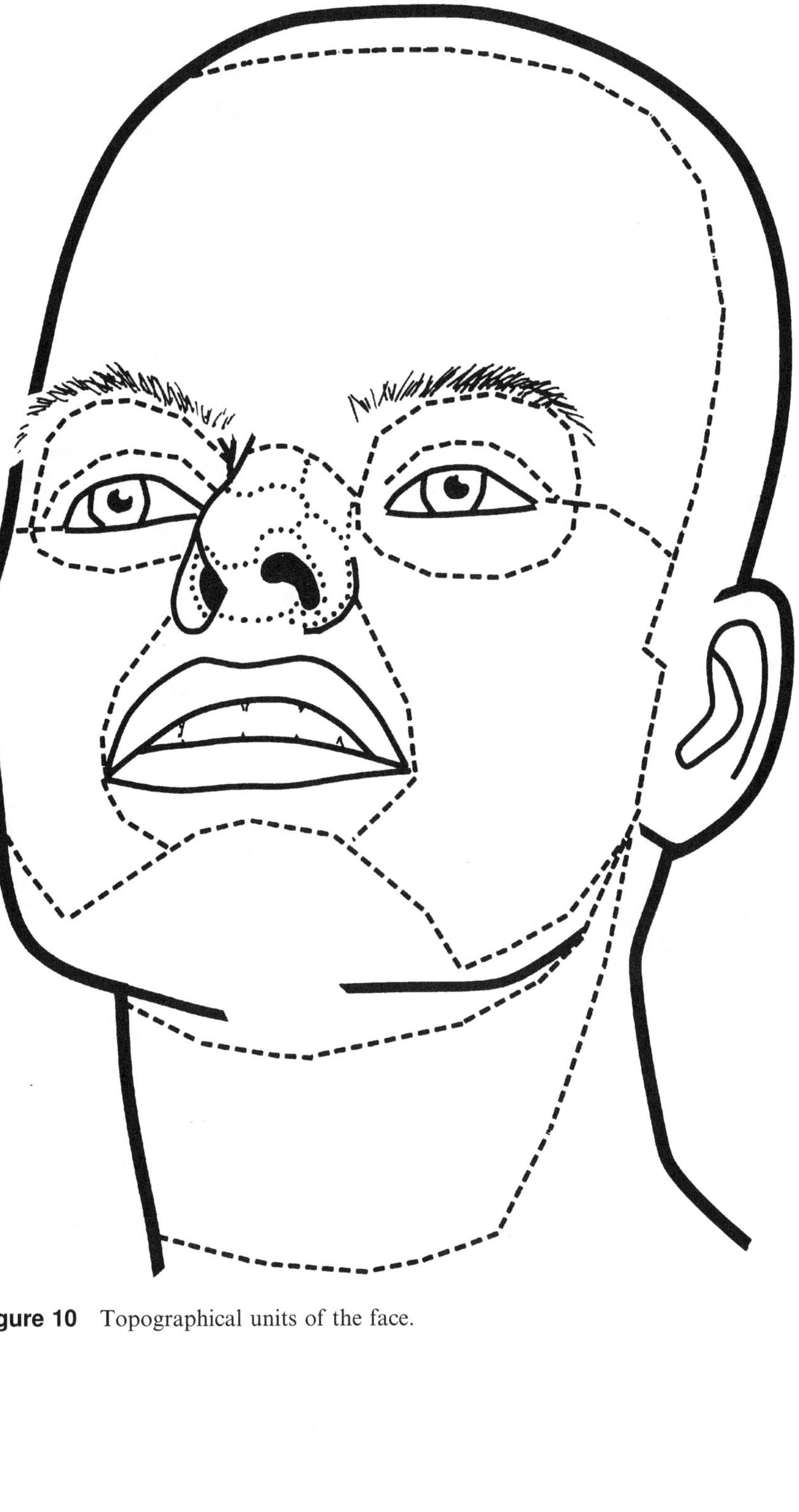

Figure 10 Topographical units of the face.

surrounding the unit is relatively normal and unaffected. The nose was considered a single topographical (aesthetic) unit by Gonzalez-Ulloa et al.; however, it is useful to subclassify the nose further into aesthetic subunits with borders that fall into natural visual rifts created by subtle shadows, concavities, and convexities (31). The facial regions (topographical units) and subunits do not necessarily correspond to the resting skin tension lines (RSTLs). If incisions are within a topographical unit, attention to the RSTLs is important to maximize camouflage and to attain the thinnest scar possible by following the natural skin tension lines. However, in most cases, the unit principle will take precedence.

The reconstructive surgeon should also be familiar with the technique and application of basic scar revision and lengthening procedures (e.g., Z-plasty, W-plasty); the basic local flaps (e.g., rotation, rhombic); perinasal local flaps (e.g., mid-forehead, cheek advancement); and the variety of flaps for local eyelid and lip reconstruction (e.g., Karapandzic, Bernard-Burow). Regional (off the face) flaps may also be considered for facial reconstruction, but they are often aesthetically unacceptable. The shortcomings of regional flaps include less flap selection, bulkiness, poor reliability of composite tissues, persistent problems with marginal necrosis, secondary contour irregularities from the pedicle, and sagging. However, the galeal frontalis and temporoparietal fascia flaps are commonly used for post-traumatic facial defects. These flaps can be useful for reconstruction of anterior skull base injuries and traumatic ear defects, respectively (Figs. 11,12).

Although local tissues are preferred, distant tissue may be required because of lack of adequate tissue bulk or quality available for transfer. Distant tissue (micro-

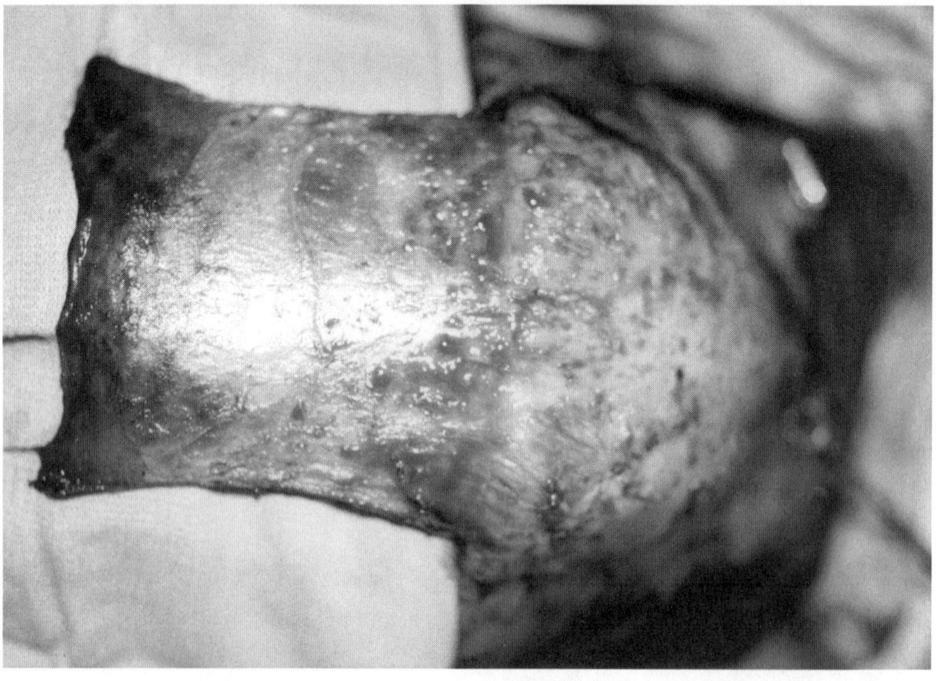

Figure 11 Pericranial–galeal flap harvested from turned down coronal flap.

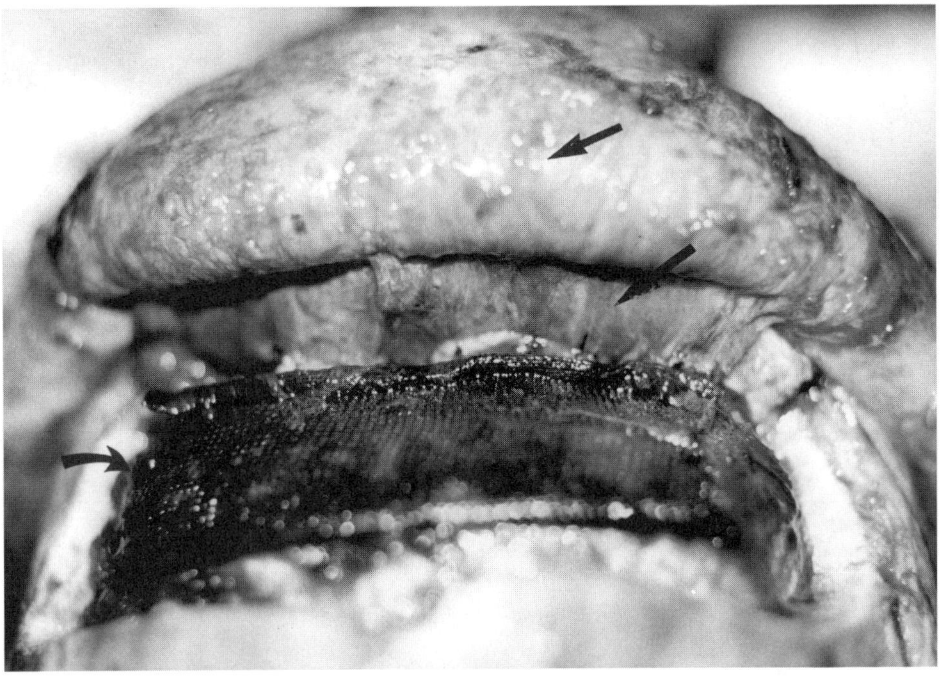

Figure 12 Pericranial–galeal flap inset under frontal lobe. Large arrow, flap; small arrow, coronal flap; curved arrow, hemostatic dressing placed over frontal lobe dura.

vascular autografts) is available to fulfill the needs of a variety of complicated cervicofacial defects, yet they often cannot provide aesthetically acceptable skin and soft tissue bulk. The most common microvascular flaps for posttraumatic cervicofacial reconstruction include the radial forearm, fibular osteocutaneous, scapular osteocutaneous, and rectus abdominus.

Prolonged tissue expansion is a useful method for scalp reconstruction and is the method of choice for this purpose in most circumstances. It can also be useful to camouflage the cutaneous component of composite tissue flaps. Skin from composite tissue flaps is often a poor match to facial or neck skin in texture and color. Tissue expansion allows adjacent cervicofacial skin to be advanced over a composite flap after its skin is removed (de-epithelialized). In addition, cutaneous scarring from the original insetting of the composite flap can be eliminated by advancing adjacent expanded skin. The disadvantages to prolonged tissue expansion include the requirement for at least two separate procedures; expansion takes several weeks; and the expander balloon creates a significant temporary cosmetic deformity. When expanding the forehead skin, the expander is placed submuscularly (subgaleally) and is expanded over an 8–10 week period. Expander placement is usually in the subcutaneous plane in the face, under the platysma for neck expansion (avoiding placement over vital vascular structures), and under the galea for scalp expansion. Contraindications to prolonged tissue expansion include prior irradiation, patients with major psychiatric illness, and patients who may be poorly compliant. Prior irradiation increases the risk of expander exposure, but it is not an absolute contraindication if the expander is used with caution (32). Within the head and neck, the scalp is asso-

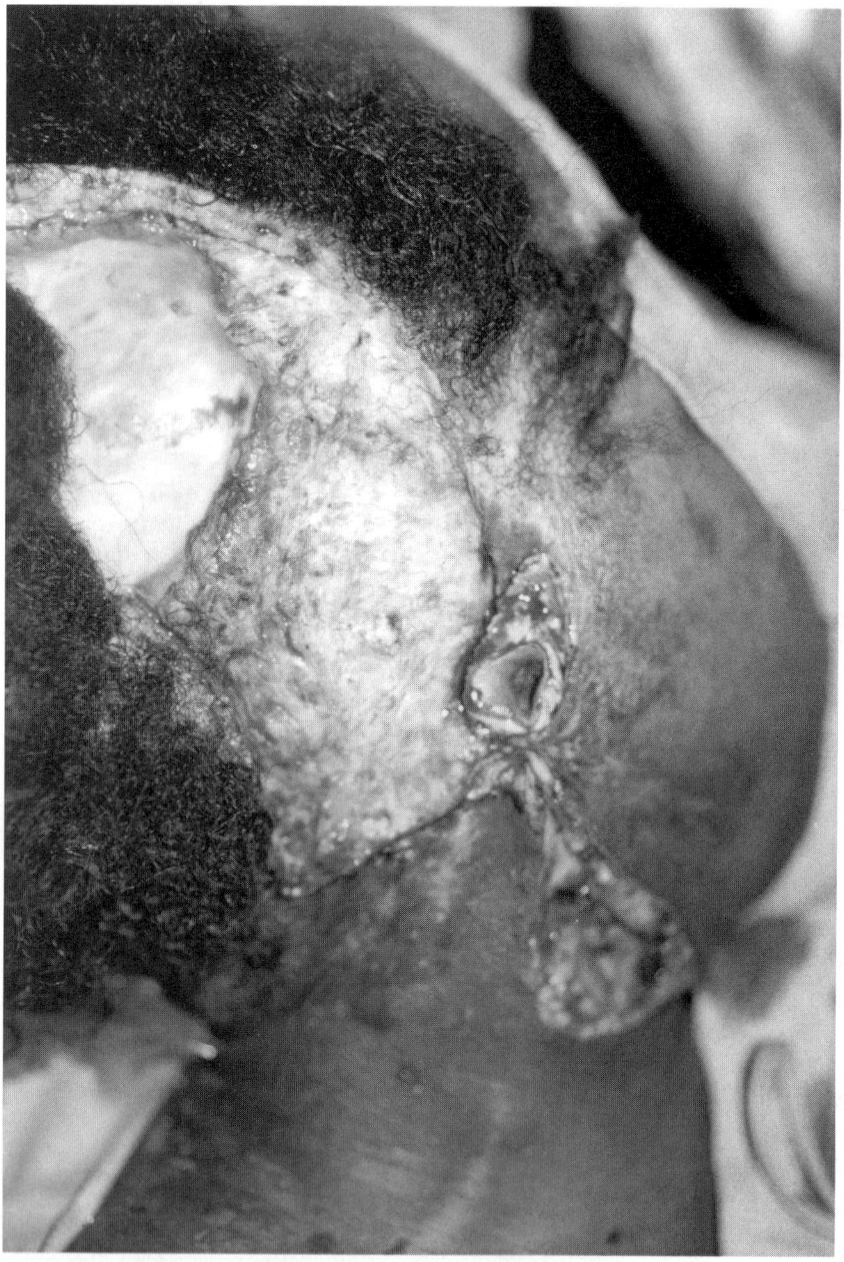

Figure 13 Traumatic hemicoronal scalp and total auricular defect.

ciated with the lowest complication rate. Complications, most commonly implant exposure, occur in fewer than 10–30% of patients (33). The most common complications are implant or filling port exposure, implant infection, overlying skin ischemia, hematoma, and bone absorption under the expander balloon. Bone absorption in patients undergoing scalp expansion is rare. A patient recently undergoing tissue

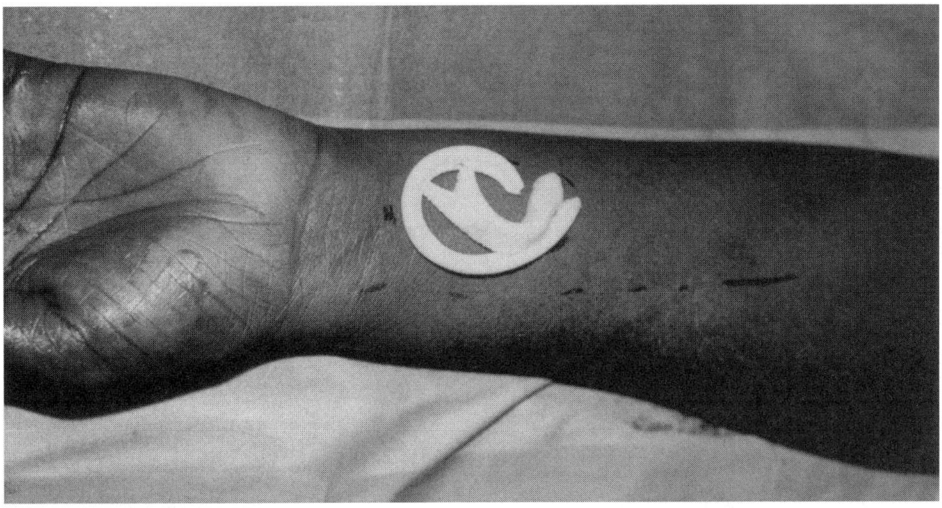

Figure 14 Medpor (Porex Surgical Inc. College Park, GA) ear form about to be subcutaneously transplanted into area encompassed by radial forearm flap.

expansion for a large scalp defect found that she was pregnant just prior to the planned expander removal and scalp rotation. The expander was left in place for an additional 10 months with no evidence of underlying bone erosion documented by routine skull films and on inspection at reoperation.

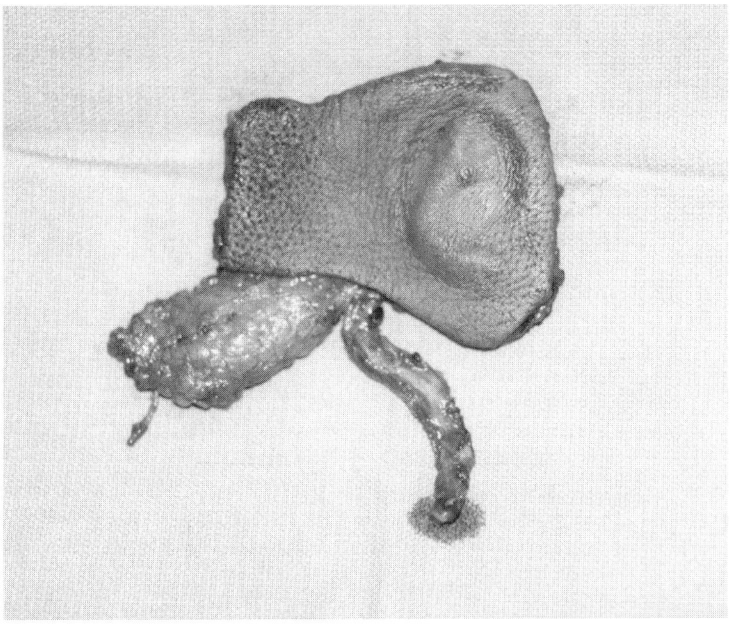

Figure 15 Several months after ear form implantation, radial forearm flap is transferred to the scalp; vascular pedicle is seen draped inferiorly. Note harvest of additional tissue skin tissue posterior to ear form to fill in postauricular hairless area.

RECONSTRUCTION OF THE AURICLE AND NOSE

It is particularly difficult to achieve acceptable results in primary reconstruction of total or subtotal auricular and nasal defects. Attempts to address these areas during the initial phases of reconstruction often result in poor results and wasted effort. Primary reconstruction should focus on providing a platform for osseointegrated prostheses or autogenous composite tissues. The patient is often not satisfied with the retention and feel of a nasal or pinna prosthesis. However, the use of a temporary prosthesis should be encouraged initially to allow time for planning definitive reconstruction.

Aesthetic restoration of the nose after total rhinectomy is described using the radial forearm free flap. The skin of the flap is interiorized and the raw surface skin grafted. At a second stage, the skin graft is removed and supporting framework is placed under a midline forehead flap. Several minor revisions are usually necessary, and the free tissue only acts as an inner lining. Aggressive thinning of the free flap is necessary to maintain the nasal airway.

Off-the-face flap prefabrication using autogenous or synthetic forms for structural support is a useful and appealing alternative for many patients. Subcutaneous implantation of bone, cartilage, or synthetic materials into the tissues encompassed by a microvascular free flap allows the prefabrication of a nose or ear in a less conspicuous area than the face. The area encompassed by the radial forearm free flap site is ideal because it offers a thin, pliable, tissue base that can be easily molded by structural elements implanted subcutaneously. Several stages may be necessary to achieve an acceptable form, but the site can be hidden under a shirtsleeve and each stage can be done under local anesthesia comfortably. Once the composite tissues appear to match the requirements for the recipient site, the flap is transferred using standard microvascular techniques (Figs. 13–15).

REFERENCES

1. Nakhgevany KB, LiBassi M, Esposito B. Facial trauma in motor vehicle accidents: etiological factors. Am J Emerg Med 1994; 12:160–163.
2. Bradbury A, Robertson C. Prospective audit of the pattern, severity and circumstances of injury sustained by vehicle occupants as a result of road traffic accidents. Arch Emerg Med 1993; 10:15–23.
3. Worrall SF. Mechanisms, pattern and treatment costs of maxillofacial injuries. Injury 1991; 22:25–28.
4. Reath DB, Kirby J, Lynch M, Maull KI. Patterns of maxillofacial injuries in restrained and unrestrained motor vehicle crash victims. J Trauma 1989; 29:806–809.
5. Jordan KS. Air bags: a major advance in injury control. Orthop Nurs 1999; 18:37–41.
6. Peters CE, Sebourn CL, Crowder HL. Wound ballistics of unstable projectiles. Part I: projectile yaw growth and retardation. J Trauma 1996; 40:S10–S15.
7. Zide MF, Epker BN. Short-range shotgun wounds to the face. J Oral Surg 1979; 37: 319–330.
8. Clark N, Birely B, Manson PN, et al. High-energy ballistic and avulsive facial injuries: classification, patterns, and an algorithm for primary reconstruction. Plast Reconstr Surg 1996; 98:583–601.
9. Zhou S, Lei D, Liu Y, Tan Y, Gu X. Experimental study on firearm wound in maxillofacial region. Chin Med J (Engl.) 1998; 111:114–117.

10. Cohen MA, Shakenovsky BN, Smith I. Low velocity hand-gun injuries of the maxillofacial region. J Maxillofac Surg 1986; 14:26–33.
11. Lalani Z, Bonanthaya KM. Cervical spine injury in maxillofacial trauma. Br J Oral Maxillofac Surg 1997; 35:243–245.
12. Stoker NG, Mankovich NJ, Valentino D. Stereolithographic models for surgical planning: preliminary report. J Oral Maxillofac Surg. 1992; 50:466–471.
13. Dahlgren B, Berlin R, Janzon B, et al. The extent of muscle tissue damage following missile trauma one, six and twelve hours after the infliction of trauma, studied by the current method of debridement. Acta Chir Scand Suppl 1979; 489:137–144.
14. Hallock GG. Microsurgical repair of the parotid duct. Microsurgery 1992; 13:243–246.
15. Lewis G, Knottenbelt JD. Parotid duct injury: is immediate surgical repair necessary? Injury 1991; 22:407–409.
16. Rao NA, Wong VG. Aetiology of sympathetic ophthalmitis. Trans Ophthalmol. oc U.K. 1981; 101 (Pt 3):357–360.
17. Hebestreit H, Huppertz HI, Sold JE, Dammrich J. Steroid-pulse therapy may suppress inflammation in severe sympathetic ophthalmia. J Pediatr Ophthalmol Strabismus 1997; 34:124–126.
18. de Chalain TM. Exploring the use of the medicinal leech: a clinical risk-benefit analysis. J Reconstr Microsurg 1996; 12:165–171.
19. Utley DS, Koch RJ, Goode RL. The failing flap in facial plastic and reconstructive surgery: role of the medicinal leech. Laryngoscope 1998; 108:1129–1135.
20. Baker SP, O'Neill B, Haddon W, Jr., Long WB. The injury severity score: a method for describing patients with multiple injuries and evaluating emergency care. J Trauma 1974; 14:187–196.
21. Vasconez HC, Shockley ME, Luce EA. High-energy gunshot wounds to the face. Ann Plast Surg 1996; 36:18–25.
22. Antonyshyn O, Gruss JS. Complex orbital trauma: the role of rigid fixation and primary bone grafting. Adv Ophthalmic Plast Reconstr Surg. 1987; 7:61–92.
23. Licameli GR, Dolan R. Buccinator musculomucosal flap: applications in intraoral reconstruction. Arch Otolaryngol Head Neck Surg 1998; 124:69–72.
24. Donelan MB. Reconstruction of electrical burns of the oral commissure with a ventral tongue flap. Plast Reconstr Surg 1995; 95:1155–1164.
25. Jacob OJ. Reconstruction of total loss of upper lip with hair-bearing flaps. Aust NZ J Surg 1995; 65:251–253.
26. Shindo ML, Costantino PD, Friedman CD, Chow LC. Facial skeletal augmentation using hydroxyapatite cement. Arch Otolaryngol Head Neck Surg 1993; 119:185–190.
27. Marin PC, Love T, Carpenter R, Iliff NT, Manson PN. Complications of orbital reconstruction: misplacement of bone grafts within the intramuscular cone. Plast Reconstr Surg 1998; 101:1323–1327.
28. Iliff N, Manson PN, Katz J, Rever L, Yaremchuk M. Mechanisms of extraocular muscle injury in orbital fractures. Plast Reconstr Surg 1999; 103:787–799.
29. Cohen SR, Kawamoto HK Jr. Analysis and results of treatment of established posttraumatic facial deformities. Plast Reconstr Surg 1992; 90:574–584.
30. Gonzales-Ulloa M. Preliminary study of the total restoration of the facial skin. Plast Reconstr Surg 1954; 13:151.
31. Burget GC, Menick FJ. The subunit principle in nasal reconstruction. Plast Reconstr Surg 1985; 76:239–247.
32. Swenson RW. Tissue Expansion. In: Papel ID, Nachlas NE, eds. Facial Plastic and Reconstructive Surger. St. Louis: Mosby, 1992:56–67.
33. Antonyshyn O, Gruss JS, Zuker R, Mackinnon SE. Tissue expansion in head and neck reconstruction. Plast Reconstr Surg 1988; 82:58–68.

19
Laceration and Scar Revision

Christine M. Puig
Ear, Nose, and Throat Plastic Surgery Associates, Auburn, Washington, U.S.A.

Keith A. LaFerriere
University of Missouri, Columbia, Missouri, U.S.A.

Revision of facial scars presents a significant diagnostic and technical challenge to the facial plastic and reconstructive surgeon. Being more difficult to conceal, facial scars are often more stress-provoking than scars on other areas of the body. Appropriate planning and technical skills are essential to achieving a result that is both functionally and cosmetically advantageous for the patient. Following injury and primary repair, the wound healing process leads to scar formation that is influenced by many variables. The nature and extent of the initial injury are of paramount importance in determining the ultimate need for scar revision. Scar revision should not be considered until the patient has recovered from the emotional trauma and anger associated with the facial injury, and until the injury has matured past the stage of acute inflammation. This period of time must be tailored to the individual patient, and is generally in the range of 6 weeks to 6 months. A thorough understanding of the factors that influence undesirable scars is necessary for a successful outcome.

EVALUATION

The human eye regards features on the face by scanning the components and noticing anything that appears outside the norm of expected facial anatomy. Creases and lines are normal on the face as long as they conform to what the viewer's eye perceives as compatible with past experience of observing facial features. The fact that a scar exists is not an indication for revision. Only when a scar deviates from what one expects to see on a face does it become noticeable, and thus a candidate for improvement. Any of the techniques used for scar revision are not designed to eliminate or erase the scar, but to make it more compatible with what appears to the viewer's eye as a normal feature. If the surgeon keeps this in mind when designing the most appropriate approach, and communicates this effectively to the patient, everyone involved in the process will be more satisfied with the final result.

With careful planning, scar tissue produced by scar revision surgery can be minimized. The surgeon's judgement and attention to detail are critical in scar revision. There is no incision that will not produce a scar, therefore, it is important that the surgeon be thoroughly familiar with the factors that lead to favorable scars. A thorough understanding of the significance of relaxed skin tension lines and aesthetic units and subunits of the face is essential in evaluating scars for revision.

Relaxed Skin Tension Lines and Facial Subunits

Relaxed skin tension lines (RSTL) of the face are shown in Figure 1. Lacerations and elective incisions placed precisely within or close to the RSTL have minimal tension, and will heal in a fine line with less visibility when closed appropriately. The exact location of the RSTL varies between individuals. In older patients these lines parallel the natural creases and wrinkles of the face. The general rule is that the RSTL lie perpendicular to the underlying facial musculature, and in the neck they are found perpendicular to areas of flexion. The RSTL run horizontally across the forehead, where the frontalis muscle is directed vertically. They are directed in a curved fashion over the cheeks, and radiate outward from the oral cavity over the lips due to the

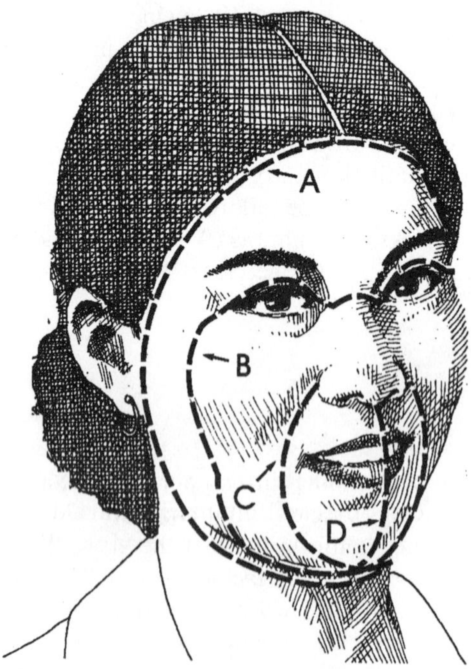

Figure 1 Relaxed skin tension lines of the face. A. Marginal. B. Palpebral. C. Nasolabial. D. Median.

circular orbicularis oris muscle. An exception to this rule is the central eyelids, where the RSTL run horizontal, and are nearly parallel to the underlying muscle fibers of the orbicularis oculi. By asking the patient to go through a series of facial expressions (smile, frown, laugh, squint), while in the upright and sitting position, prior to the injection of local anesthesia, one can usually identify the RSTL. The RSTL are often identifiable in children with enough patience and close examination. Scars that do not follow the RSTL closely are antitension line (ATL) scars (1).

Aesthetic Units and Subunits

Facial aesthetic units are comprised of the forehead, eyes, nose, lips, and chin. These esthetic units can be further classified into subunits based on skin thickness, color, elasticity, and underlying structural support. Incisions are best placed at the junctions of these units, subunits, or in the midline of the face for least perceptible scars (2).

Unsightly or functionally significant facial scars can be evaluated for revision by the following six parameters: length, width, elevation or depression in relation to the surrounding skin, color, direction, and distortion of facial landmarks. These characteristics of scars are very interdependent and must be considered collectively before a decision regarding scar improvement can be made.

SCAR CHARACTERISTICS

Any scar longer than 2.0 cm has the potential to be unsightly. A long, relatively straight scar is conspicuous because, as the eye perceives a part of this line, it naturally follows it throughout its length. In the absence of other characteristics of unfavorable scars such as ATL scars, those less than 2 cm will generally not benefit significantly from revision. Even longer but thin scars, if they parallel the RSTL, may not need revision because they may appear as normal facial creases. Scars wider than 1–2 mm resulting from inadequate closure or from ATL scars are frequently candidates for improvement.

Elevation or depression of the scar in relation to the surrounding skin is often seen in scars that were not repaired primarily, in stellate scars, or when the edges of a laceration were inadequately approximated. Abrasion scars frequently result in significant unevenness of the skin surface.

Color is an important consideration. Scars may be red when they are immature, whiter than the surrounding skin when fully mature, or tattooed from debris at the time of the original injury. Erythematous scars in the early stages of maturation are not usually good candidates for revision unless the redness is narrowly confined to the scar. In the absence of other factors that will ultimately demand scar revision, allowing the red scar to mature may lessen the need for revision. White scars are often perplexing because that may be the only disturbing characteristic of the scar; it is highly likely that any revision will ultimately produce a similar white scar. Tattooing of these scars to approximate the normal surrounding skin color may be the best solution. Tattooed scars from the original injury are best treated at the time of original repair. When significant discoloration from debris is present in the mature scar, it is always unsightly and usually a candidate for revision.

Scars may significantly distort facial landmarks. If structures such as the eyelid, eyebrow, lip, or nose are distorted from the scar, it is likely that revision will be needed since these changes are often the most disfiguring injuries on the face.

LINEAR SCAR REVISION TECHNIQUES

When considering options for scar revision, it is important to examine the area closely for skin thickness, elasticity, texture, hair growth, and RSTL. A fine-tip surgical marking pen is invaluable in the initial planning stages. Ideas should be drawn, measured, and remeasured before the skin is incised. If it is then decided that there is a better option, the marks can be easily erased and the patient has suffered no harm.

Tension at the wound edges is an important variable in wound healing. Excessive tension can cause tissue slough due to compromised blood flow to the margins of the flap, it can distort surrounding local and regional landmarks, and may result in hypertrophic and widened scars.

The tensile strength of a mature scar is 80% of normal skin. A long-lasting absorbable or permanent subcutaneous suture closure is imperative to relieve tension over time and prevent scar widening during healing (2).

The workhorse techniques for linear scar revision are the fusiform, Z-plasty, W-plasty, and geometric broken line (GBL). These can be used alone or in any combination to achieve a more cosmetic or functional scar. The choice of revision depends on evaluation of the scar using the six scar characteristics discussed previously.

Fusiform Scar Revision

The simplest technique used for scar revision is the fusiform scar revision (FSR). The scar is excised within a fusiform shape that is widest at its center and tapered at each end to 30 degree angles or less. A 3:1 length/width ratio in a fusiform shape will best produce a closure without leaving a standing cone deformity, often called a dog ear, at either end. (Fig. 2a,b). The scar is excised and closed in a line parallel to the RSTL, a skin crease, or a natural anatomical boundary line. This technique is useful for small, round, stellate or elliptic scars that are widened and when the closure comfortably lies in a facial crease or RSTL. The de-epithialized scar bed is often left intact to lessen postoperative depression of the revised scar. FSR is the technique of choice whenever the final scar will lie in the RSTL.

A fusiform incision can be shortened at its ends using an M-plasty, which preserves skin at the tapered end of the fusiform by creating two smaller angles of closure. The M-plasty design shortens the scar length along its central axis. It is most useful when the end of a fusiform incision encroaches on a landmark structure such as the lateral canthus, or when the fusiform design results in an excessively long linear scar (Fig. 2c,d).

Z-plasty Scar Revision

The Z-plasty technique consists of two triangle flaps designed in the shape of a Z, or a reversed Z, that are undermined, raised, and transposed into each other's bed.

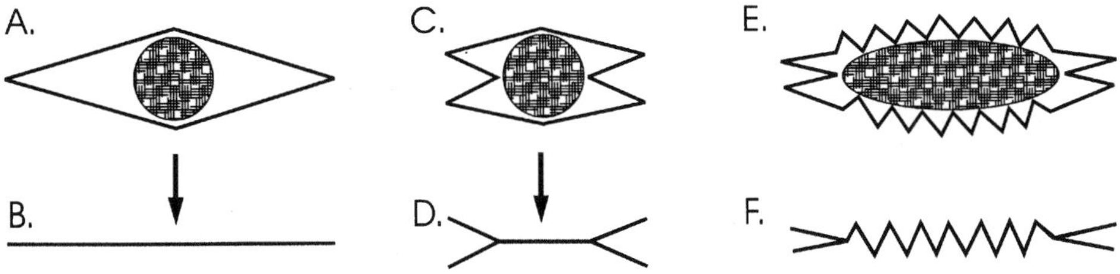

Figure 2 A. Fusiform excision of a circular lesion. B. Closure of the fusiform defect in Figure 2A. C. Excision of a cirular lesion utilizing bilateral M-plasty excisions. D. Closure of the excision in Figure 2C. E. W-plasty excision of an elongated oval lesion, also utilizing bilateral M-plasty excisions. F. Closure of excision in Figure 2E. Note that none of the lines should lie perpendicular to the RSTL.

In the head and neck, Z-plasties are typically used to lengthen a contracted or webbed scar, level a severely depressed scar, realign distorted anatomical landmarks, or break up a scar into multiple shorter segments.

The Z-plasty has three arms of equal length (unlike an actual letter Z, which has a long diagonal and two shorter limbs) and two equal angles. The scar being revised is usually the diagonal and is often excised in a fusiform fashion. The peripheral arms are parallel when the angles of divergence from the diagonal are equal. The peripheral limbs should lie as close as possible to the RSTL: this will facilitate the most tension-free closure and least perceptible scar. The Z-plasty is incised along the three arms and then undermined in all directions to allow easy transposition and a tension-free closure. When these flaps are undermined and transposed, there is an increase in length in the direction of the original central arm. The ideal angle of divergence from the diagonal is 60 degrees: this will give the best balance between gain in length along the direction of the central arm without causing distortion, or a standing cone deformity, at the ends. The 60 degree Z-plasty rotates the central arm 90 degrees and is the only design that results in right-angle rotation (Fig. 3). The angle of divergence from the diagonal can vary from 30 to 75 degrees, with the gain in length along the direction of the central limb proportional to the increase in degrees. Less than 30 degrees can risk flap viability and greater than 75 degrees leads to standing cone deformities. A 30 degree Z-plasty will increase the scar length 25%, a 45 degree angle 50%, and a 60 degree angle 75% (Fig. 4). Gain in length, however, is dependent on the amount of tissue available laterally, and whether it has normal elasticity or is also involved with scar.

In the Z-plasty revision of a scar that is ATL, the orientation of the peripheral limbs is of utmost importance. There are two choices in any Z-plasty, and they are mirror images of each other. The correct design is the one in which the peripheral arms of the Z-plasty are as close to parallel to the RSTL as possible. With scars nearly parallel to the ATL, it is often not possible to align the limbs parallel to the RSTL, but they should come as close as possible with the limbs in the range of 60 degrees from the scar. The ideal length of the limbs for a Z-plasty in the head and neck area is 1.5 cm, but they can be slightly smaller or considerably larger depending on the circumstances.

One of the most frequent indications for the Z-plasty scar revision is a webbed scar spanning a concave area such as the neck (Fig. 5). A long scar can

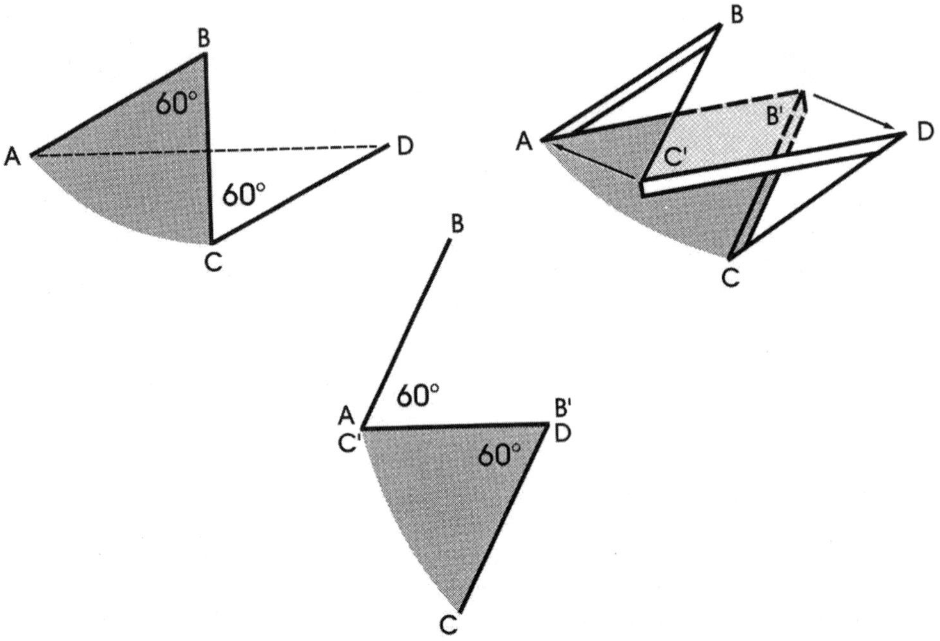

Figure 3 A 60 degree angle Z-plasty.

be divided into a number of segments, and within each segment a Z is designed (Fig. 6). Multiple Z-plasties are frequently used to diffuse the tension on the closure, cause less lateral distortion, and result in a less conspicuous scar due to the smaller limbs used. The leveling effect of multiple scars with tension directed

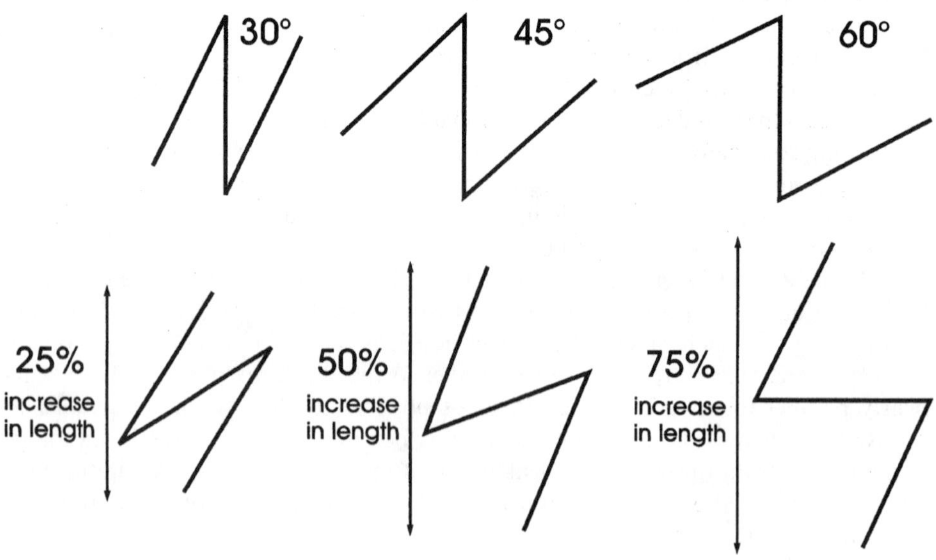

Figure 4 The larger the Z-plasty angle, the greater the increase in scar length.

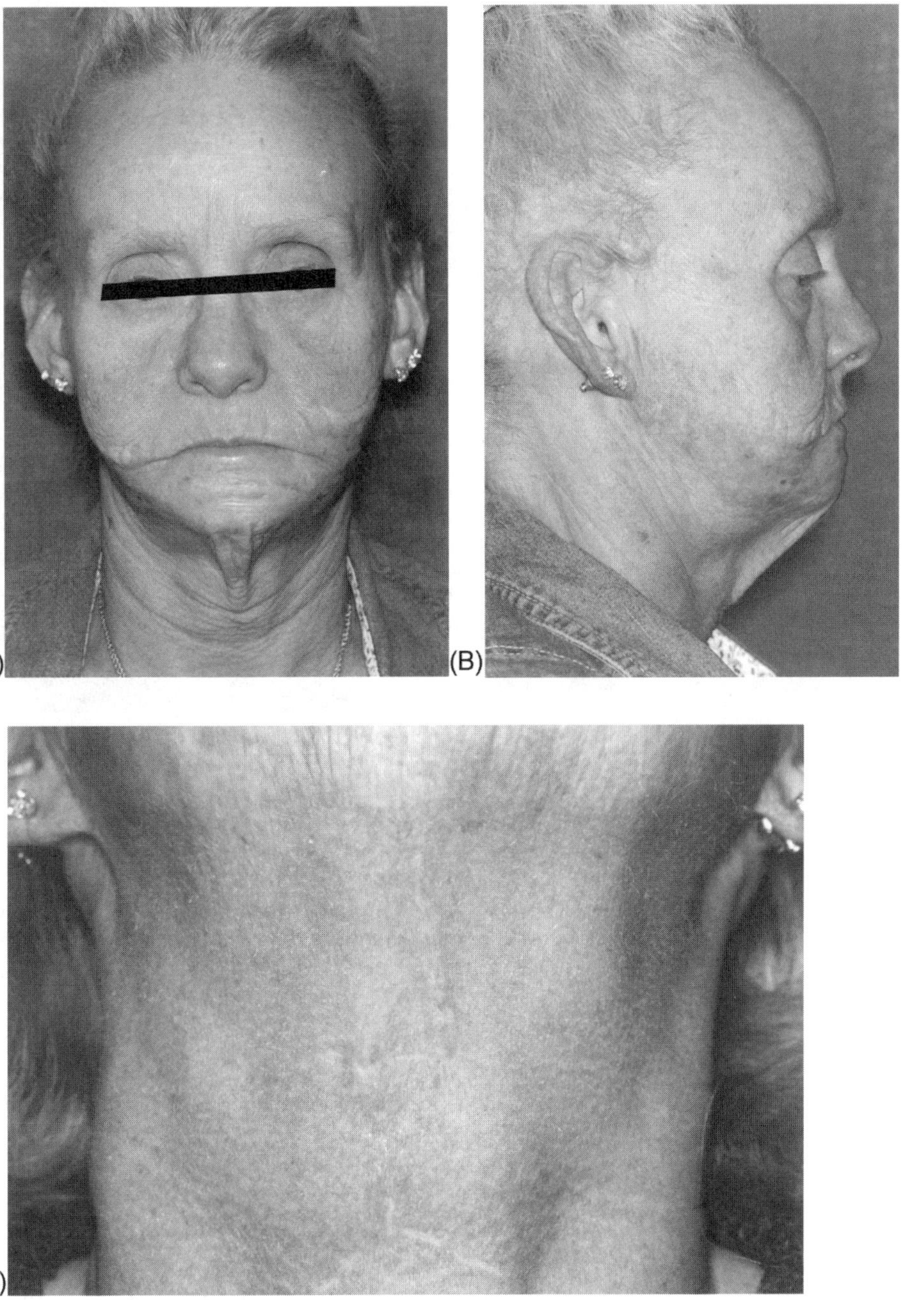

Figure 5 A, B. Preoperative burn scar contractures and redundant skin of the neck with webbing. C. Superior and inferior horizontal fusiform excisions, central vertical fusiform excision of redundant skin, and Z-plasty in the midportion of the vertical segment to break up and lengthen the scar. D, E. Result 9 months after surgery. Lengthening of the scar resulting from the Z-plasty prevented recurrence of the webbing.

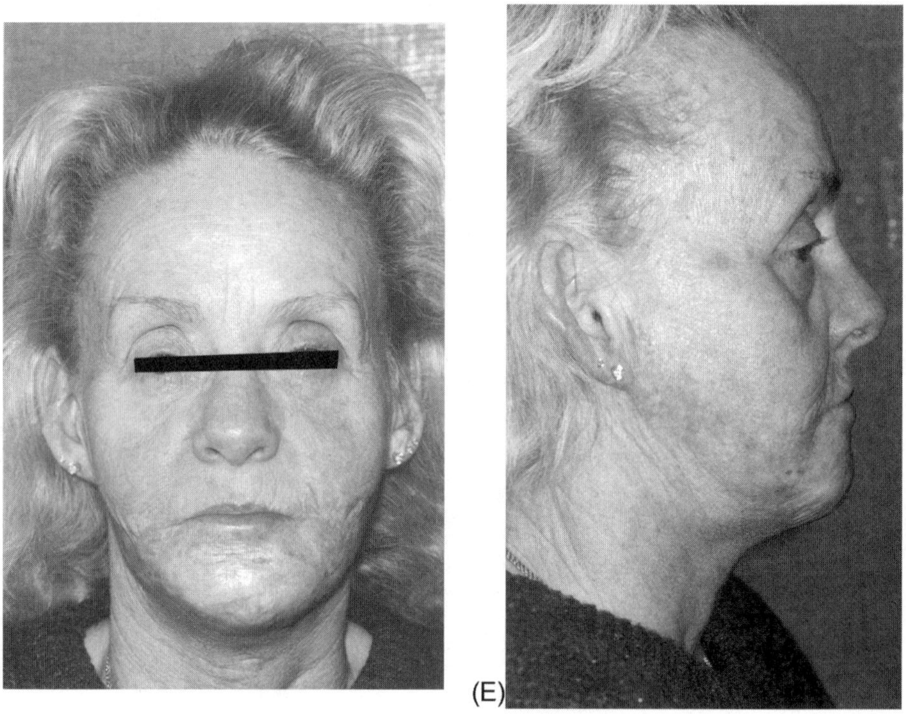
(D) (E)

Figure 5 (Continued)

in multiple vectors also makes the Z-plasty especially useful for severely depressed ATL scars (Fig. 7).

The Z-plasty technique is uniquely suited for the realignment of distorted anatomical areas, such as scars crossing the melolabial fold (Fig. 8), the corner of the mouth, the lip or the eyelids. It is necessary to orient the limbs of the Z-plasty so that the maximal gain in length is in the appropriate direction.

Variations of the classic Z-plasty include curvilinear rather than straight arms. This changes the Z to an S. Transposition and advancement occur in both. The S-plasty modification has been found advantageous for larger flaps over loose subcutaneous tissues, such as the anterior neck (3).

W- plasty Scar Revision

The W-plasty is a zigzag excision of scars closed by advancement without rotation of tissue to produce a less apparent scar. First described by Borges in 1959 (4) for the correction of straight or curved ATL scars, the running W-plasty consists of a series of side-by-side triangular flaps cut along each side of the scar in such a way that the tips on one side are aligned with the recipient defect on the other side (Fig. 2e,f). The resultant zigzag scar breaks up the linear appearance of the scar into small segments that are more closely aligned to the RSTL with a blending effect in relation to the surrounding tissue. When used on the face, the limbs of the triangles should be 6 mm or less; the angles of the limbs to the scar edge ideally

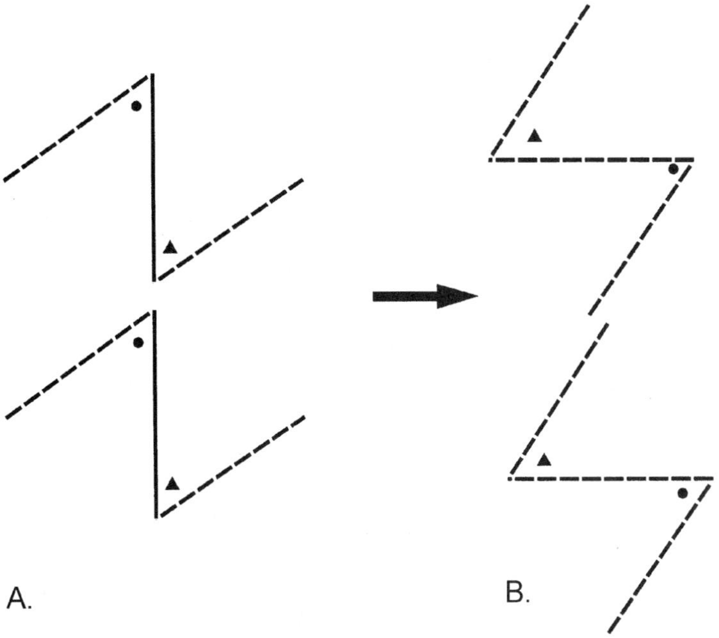

Figure 6 Multiple Z-plasty. A. A long scar is divided into segments. The peripheral arms of the Z-plasty lie parallel to the RSTL of the region. B. Z-plasty flaps are transposed for an overall lengthening and release of scar contracture.

should be in the range of 50–60 degrees and oriented as close as possible to the RSTL. Wide angles tend to lessen the accordion effect, resulting in reduced elasticity; narrow angles make the revision more technically difficult and have the potential to compromise the blood supply to the tips of the flaps. To avoid a regular or repeating pattern, it is desirable to vary the width, angles, and length of the triangles when possible. In spite of the inevitable regularity that comes with the running W-plasty scar revision, it is an excellent technique for camouflaging linear ATL scars on the forehead, cheek, and chin areas, and is frequently used in conjunction with fusiform or Z-plasty techniques (Fig. 9). The amount of scar tissue excised in a W-plastic scar revision is roughly comparable to that of a fusiform excision.

Attention to technical details is essential in achieving a good result with W-plasty scar revisions. Each incision should be marked as close to the scar being excised as possible to minimize the amount of normal tissue excised. It is easiest to begin centrally, marking each incision first on one side of the scar and its counterpart on the other side of the scar, so that the correct number and size of the triangles are created. The size of the individual triangles can vary in size and should diminish slightly toward the ends. Each end is completed with a small triangle to eliminate a standing cone deformity. Incisions are best made with a no. 11 blade sequentially from side to side to ensure matching triangles and to stabilize the tissues. It is desirable to leave the scar bed in place to efface the wound when closed and to undermine the edges sufficiently to allow as tension-free closure as possible. Closure is facilitated by placing a sub-dermal monofilament suture from

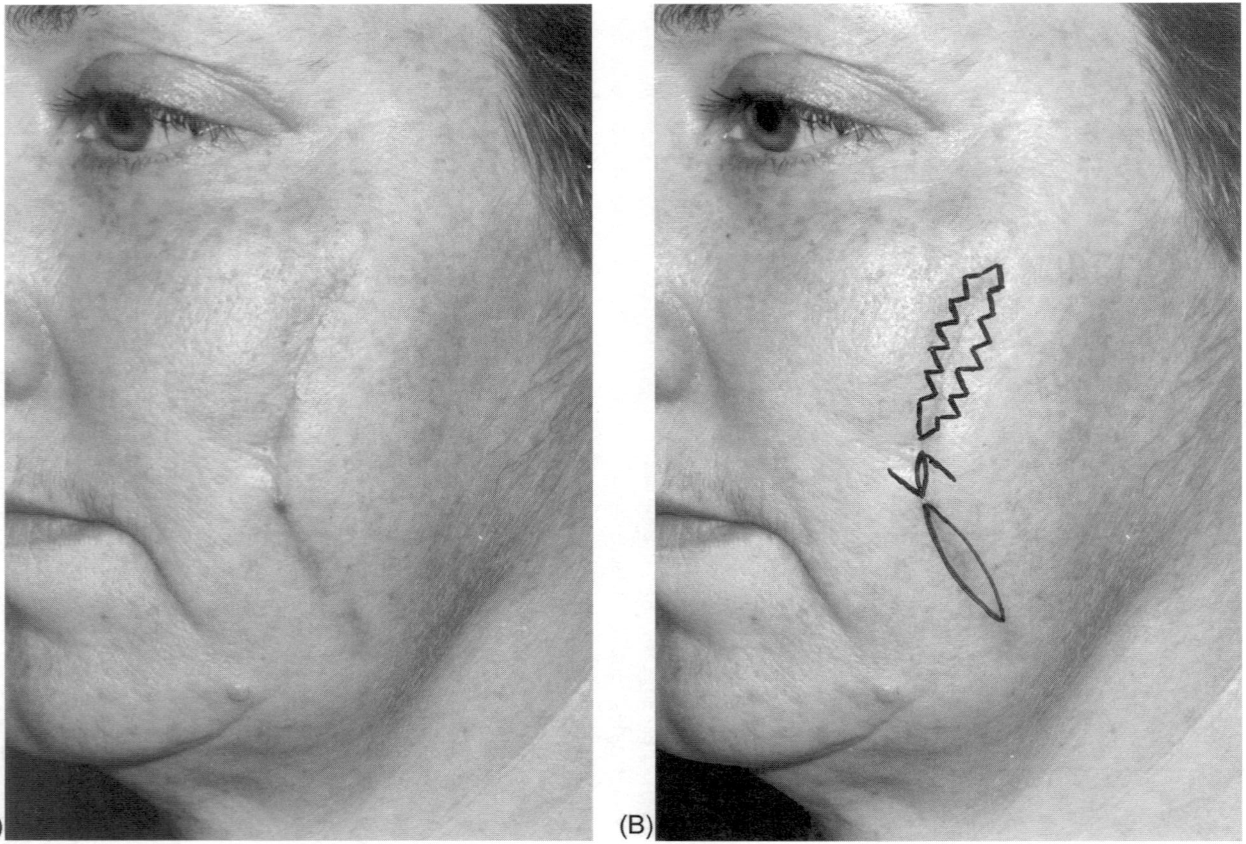
(A) (B)

Figure 7 Cheek scar. A. Appearance 3 months after emergency room repair of initial cheek laceration. The superior aspect of the scar is 80–90 degrees ATL, with the midportions depressed and dimpled. The inferior aspect of the scar closely follows the RSTL. B. Outline of scar revision utilizing a W-plasty for the 80–90 degree ATL portion, a Z-plasty at the most depressed areas of transition, and a fusiform revision for the segment less than 30 degrees ATL. C. Appearance 1 year after scar revision.

(C) 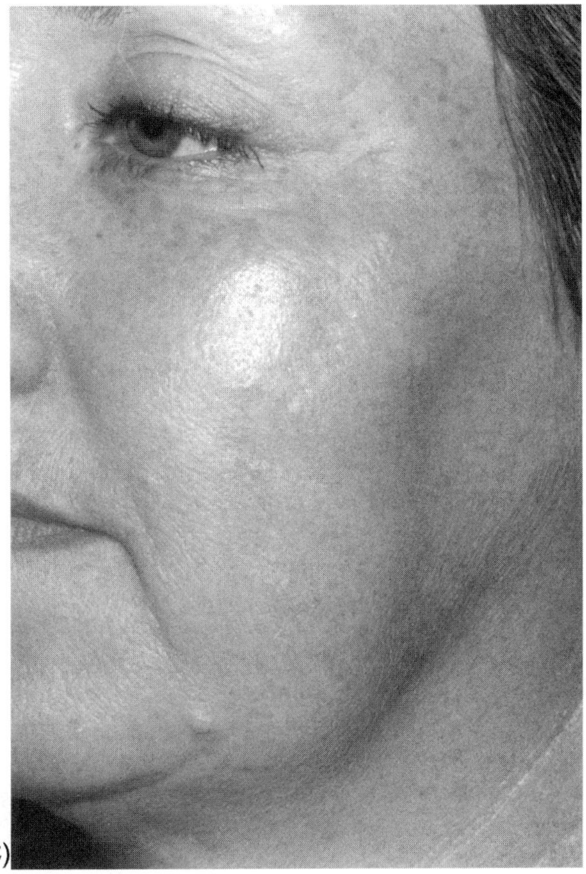

Figure 7 (Continued)

end to end through the midportion to each triangle for stabilization and approximation of the skin edges.

W-plasty scar revision is a powerful technique with many variations and nuances (1). It is indicated for scars that are 30–90 degree ATL and is especially helpful on the forehead, chin, and cheek areas. The W-plasty technique is contraindicated in scars less than 30 degrees ATL. These are more appropriately improved with a Z-plasty or fusiform scar revision.

Geometric Broken Line Closure

Combinations of triangular, square, crescentic, and rectangular interposed skin flaps on the edges of the advancement flaps have been termed geometric broken line closure. The GBL is more time-consuming in both planning and performing the scar revision than with the Z-plasty or the running W-plasty. Its proponents claim that the deliberate random shapes makes the line less easily perceived than the more predictable running W-plasty. In general, the rectangular and square segments produce a superior cosmetic result when kept small and as parallel to the RSTL as possible

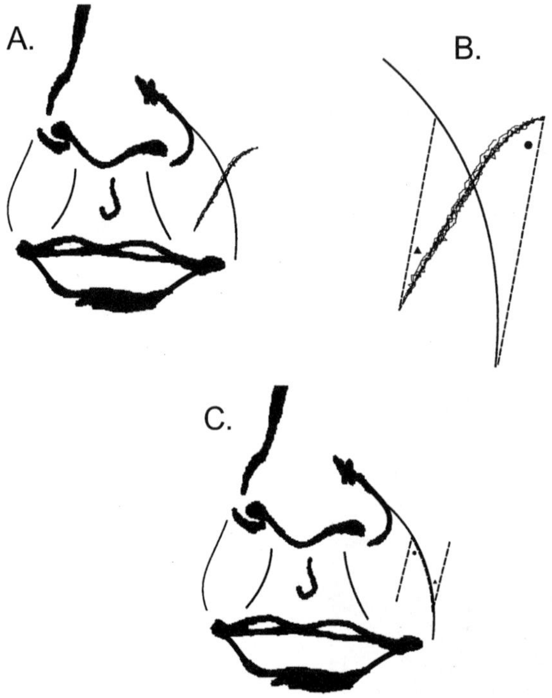

Figure 8 A. Facial scar lying oblique to the nasolabial line. B. Peripheral arms of the Z are drawn. The central arm of the Z is the scar to be excised. Angles of the Z-plasty are marked with a triangle and a circle to assist in identifying the transposition of the triangular Z-plasty flaps to their final placement seen in Figure 4C. C. The Z-plasty flaps are elevated and undermined for ease of rotation and transposition. The central arm of the Z now lies parallel to the nasolabial line.

(Fig. 10). The crescent-shaped components can result in small trap door scars and should be kept to a minimum in the design of the GBL closure. For facial scar revisions, no segment should be longer than 6 mm (5). As with the running W-plasty, to be aesthetically superior the resultant scar must be narrow, flush with the surrounding surfaces in movement and at rest, and should have components running in directions favorable to the RSTL when possible. Like the W-plasty technique, the GBL is contraindicated is scars less than 30 degrees ATL. These are best treated with fusiform or Z-plasty revisions.

Summary of linear scar revision techniques

When evaluating a linear scar for improvement, knowing when to use the various techniques is crucial in achieving the best result possible. In general, with scars less than 30 degrees ATL, a fusiform excision will produce the best result because the scar can be converted to lie in the RSTL. The limiting factor is the ultimate length of the final scar. If a fusiform revision of a less than 30 degree ATL scar will result in an excessively long scar that will be readily visible, breaking it up in one or more areas with a small Z-plasty will improve its appearance. Scars 70–90 degrees ATL

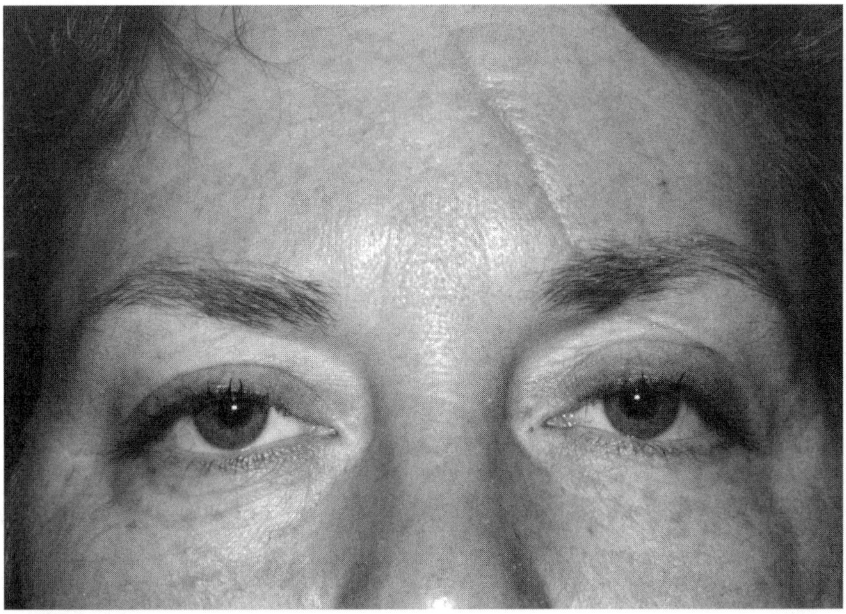
(A)

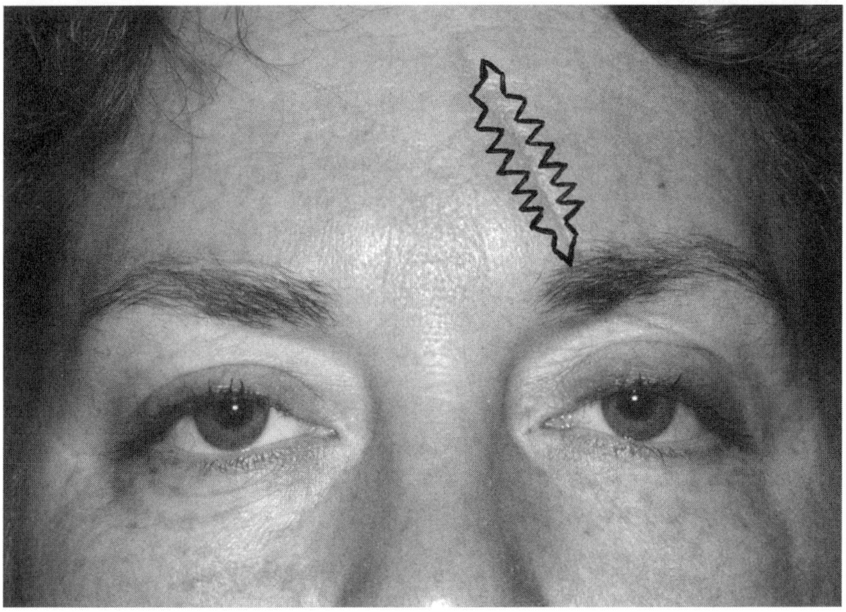
(B)

Figure 9 Forehead. A. Appearance 3 months after emergency room repair of forehead laceration. The resultant scar is approximately 60 degrees ATL. B. Outline of scar revision with a W-plasty technique. C. Nine years after scar revision.

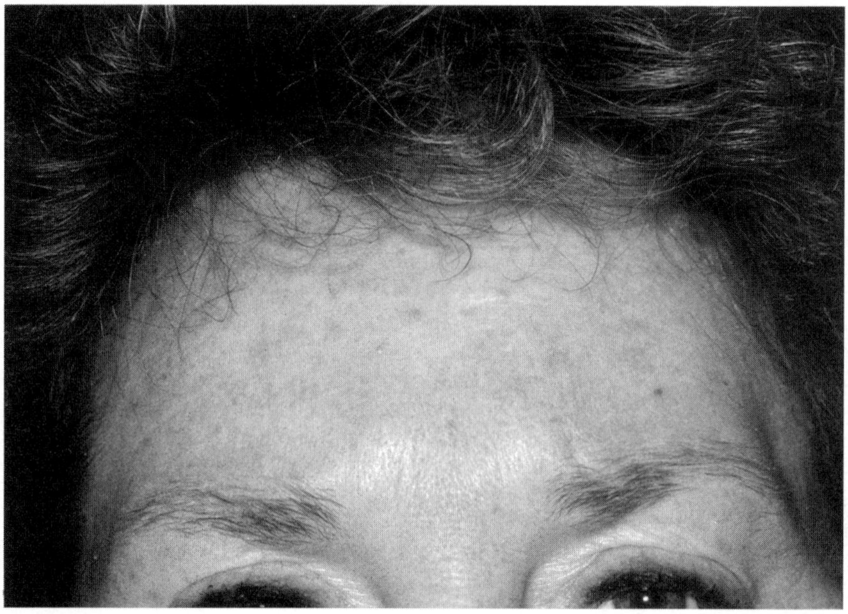
(C)

Figure 9 (Continued)

are most frequently amenable to running W-plasty or GBL revisions, especially on the forehead and cheek. Scars that lie 30–70 degrees ATL will benefit from Z-plasty, running W-plasty, or GBL revision. A combination of two or three of these techniques is often used on different aspects of the same scar, depending on the relation of the various segments to the RSTL (Fig. 10). Breaking scars into components relative to the RSTL is the most useful approach to evaluating linear scars.

SERIAL SCAR EXCISION

Serial scar excision (SSE) may be used to remove full- or partial-thickness skin grafts, burns, congenital lesions (Fig. 11), and very wide scars. The undesirable scar or lesion can be gradually excised and the final scar line placed in a RSTL, or at a junction between facial aesthetic subunits. The success of SSE is achieved by placing a continuous stretch on the tissues. This is supplied by each successive excision creating, in effect, a tissue expansion of the surrounding normal skin. Caution is advised when excising previously grafted skin: underlying structures such as the facial nerve, parotid duct, and significant blood vessels may be located more superficially because the normal surrounding subcutaneous tissues may be missing.

SSE should begin by determining where the final scar is to lie in relation to the RSTL. Whenever possible, each stage of the excision should lie within the confines of the scar, with the last excision or two encompassing the normal edges and any extra tissue necessary to allow the scar to follow the RSTL. Depending on the size of the scar, three, four, or more sessions may be needed to excise the scar completely and orient the final scar in the RSTL. It is important to undermine the tissue sufficiently

(A)

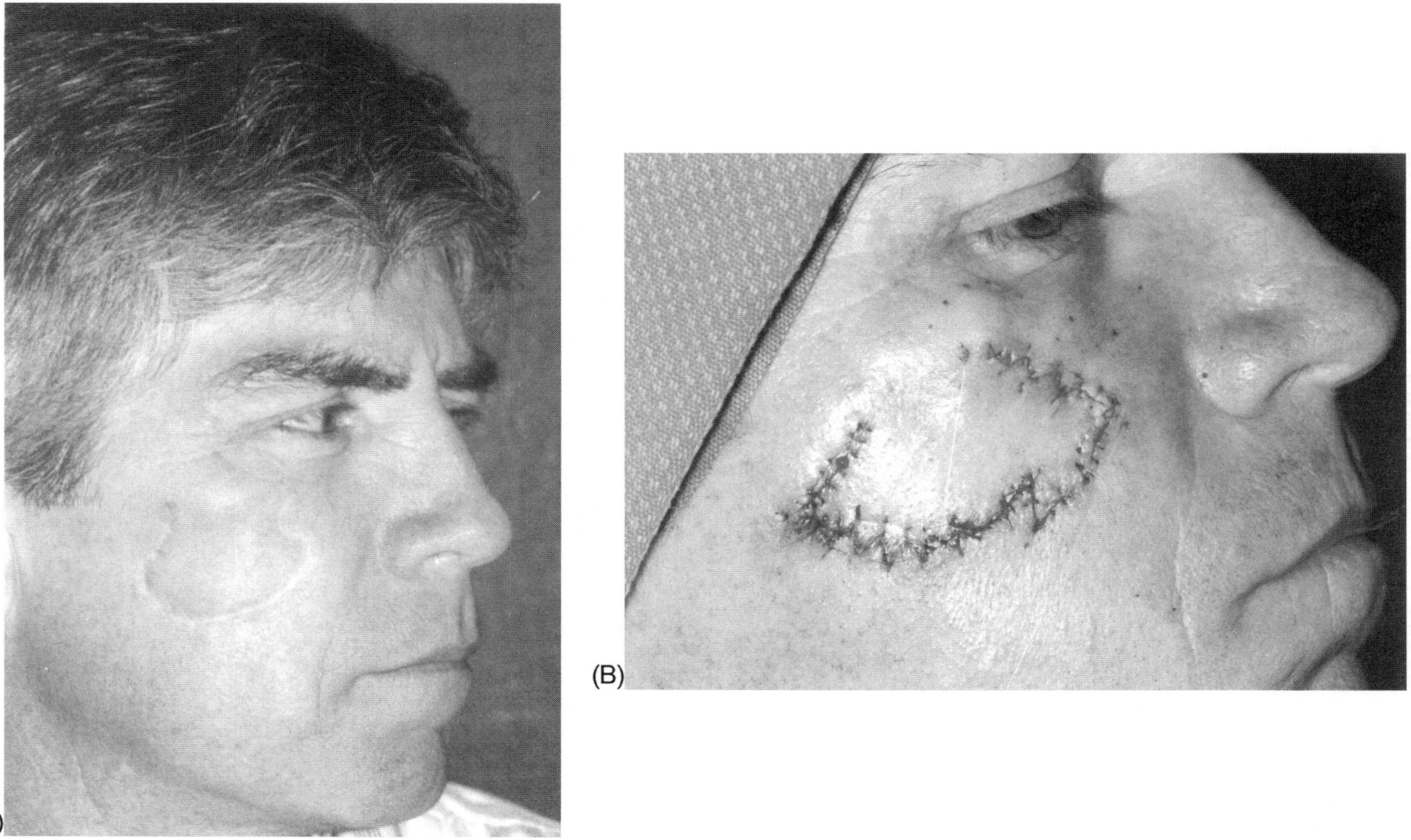

(B)

Figure 10 Cheek. A. Tangential cheek laceration with resultant trap-door deformity. B. Immediate postoperative scar revision using two W-plasties for the 90 degree ATL segments, two fusiform revisions for the RSTL scars, and a Z-plasty for the 45 degree ATL portion of the scar. C. Nine months after scar revision: result shows significant leveling of the trap-door deformity.

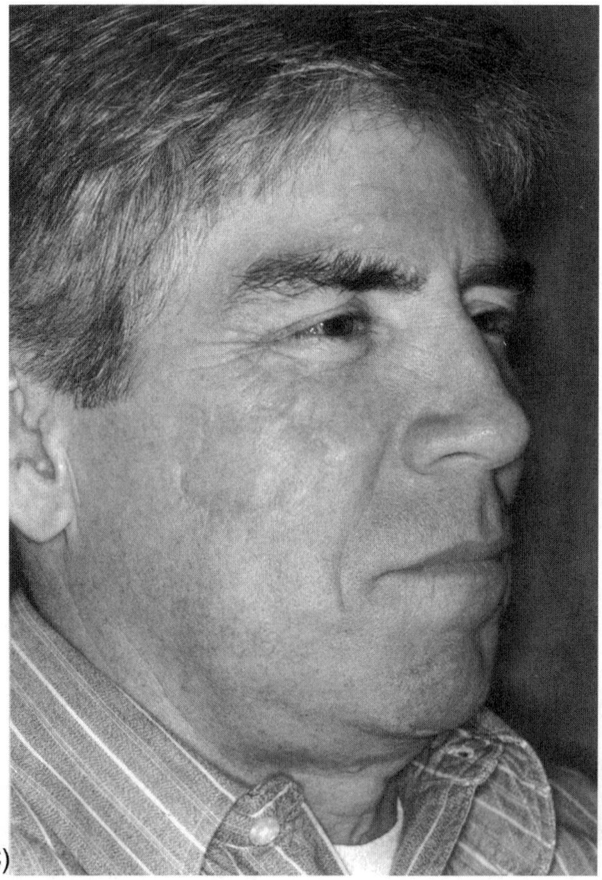

(C)

Figure 10 (Continued)

in all directions to allow a closure as free of tension as possible. Widening of the scar between sessions is often encountered, but if the final stages are designed and executed with as tension-free closure as possible, the ultimate scar can be relatively inconspicuous. Appropriate time between sessions can vary, but 3 months is probably the minimum. With extremely large scars or grafts, some distortion of the surrounding landmarks may occur with a complete SSE, but this will gradually improve over time and rarely will require compensatory procedures.

TISSUE EXPANDERS

Tissue expansion is indicated for revision or excision of a scar that cannot be readily reconstructed by a local or regional flap, or can only be done at the cost of significant donor or recipient site deformity. Most commonly, tissue expansion is utilized in the scalp and forehead for scar revision, but large area scars in any location may benefit. The scalp is especially inelastic and does not readily allow for primary or

(A) (B)

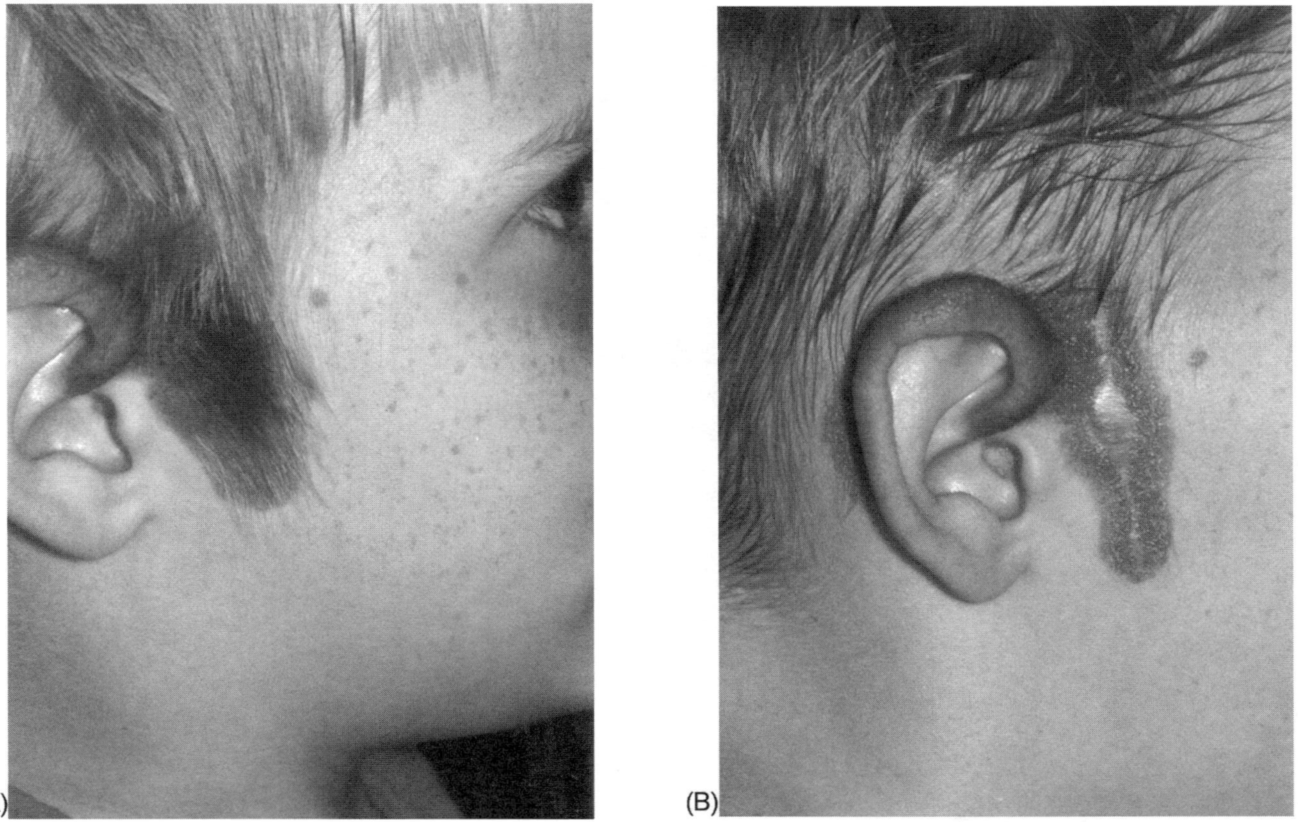

Figure 11 Giant hairy nevus. A. Preoperative appearance. The axis of the nevus is approximately 20 degrees ATL. This will be adjusted at the final stage to lie along the RSTL, at the expense of increasing the final length of the scar. B. Results after two serial scar excisions. Note the location of the scar within the confines of the lesion. C. Result after the fourth serial excision. The preauricular portion of the lesion is entirely excised. Another stage will be necessary to obtain maximal cosmetic improvement after complete maturation of the existing scar.

(C)
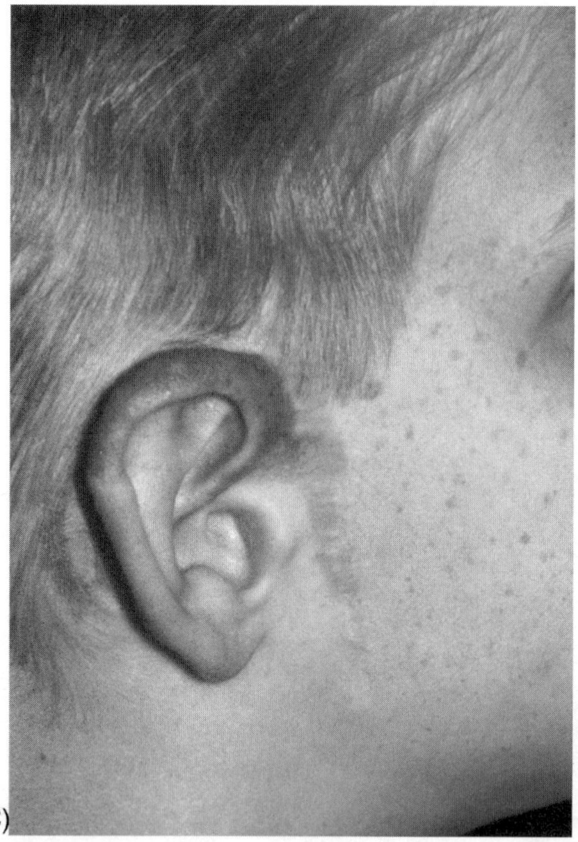

Figure 11 (Continued)

local flap closure of large defects, making tissue expansion ideally suited for scalp defects (Fig. 12). Tissue expansion allows for replacement of scar tissue with tissue from neighboring areas that is of similar color, texture, adnexal structures, and innervation.

Tissue expanders are Silastic balloons with self-sealing valves or reservoirs that are completely implanted beneath the skin. They come in different shapes and sizes, and can be custom-made to fit the very irregular defect. Regardless of the type of expander selected, it must be of sufficient size to provide the required expansive forces necessary to gain tissue needed for reconstruction. With rectangular or crescentic expanders, the surface area of the expander needs to be 2.5 times that of the scar to be replaced. With circular expanders, the diameter of the base needs to be 2.5 times that of the scar (6). Expanders should be located in positions that take advantage of simple advancement, rotation, or transposition flaps. The placement of the expander in relation to the scar is crucial: expansion on the adjacent normal tissue is the goal, not expansion of the scar. Areas of scarring, atrophy, or prior radiation therapy should be avoided due to increased rate of surface necrosis and tissue breakdown leading to exposure of the expander (7). The expander must be of sufficient volume that the apical circumference of the dome of the skin overlying the fully

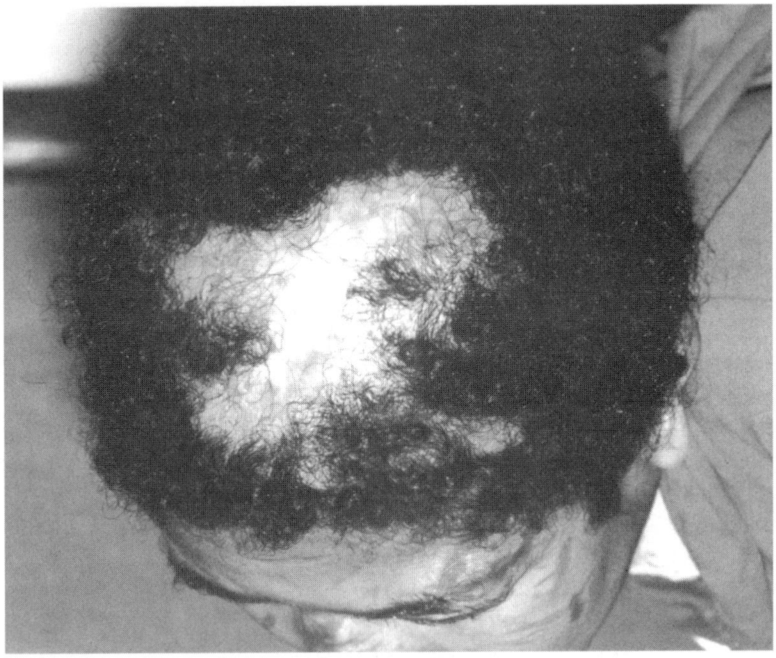

(A)

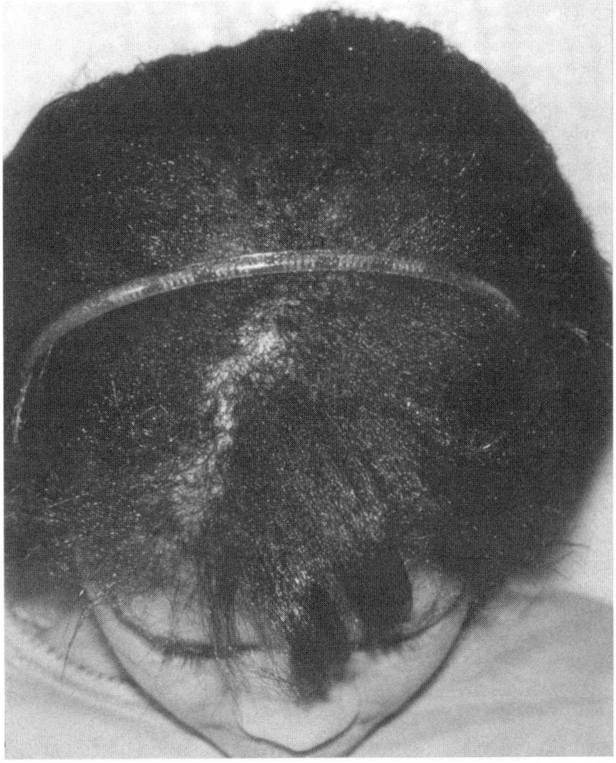

(B)

Figure 12 Scalp expansion. A. Traumatic alopecia secondary to scalding. B. Result following placement of a rectangular tissue expander posterior to the defect and subsequent closure with an advancement flap of expanded scalp.

inflated expander is two to three times the width of the defect. This will allow coverage by the expanded skin of both the defect and the donor site (8). This generally takes 6–8 weeks for the skin of the forehead and neck, and sometimes up to 12 weeks for the scalp.

Biomechanical properties of controlled expansion of the skin result in the creation of additional new epidermal skin, with thinning of the dermis and subcutaneous tissues. Hair follicle morphology and number remain the same, which is important for use of expanders in scalp expansion (9). Tissue expansion stimulates proliferation of blood vessels; it has been demonstrated that flaps raised in expanded tissue have a 117% increase in survival length over acutely raised random-pattern flaps (10). The gradual stretching of skin over an expanding subcutaneous mass is known as biological creep. Placing a Silastic balloon and going through a series of inflations and deflations to stretch the skin and soft tissues can be performed as acute intraoperative tissue expansion. This can be very useful when less tension on the wound edges during closure is needed. This ability of the skin to stretch beyond its inherent extensibility is called mechanical creep. The effects of mechanical creep are due to the relative dehydration of tissue by displacement of fluids, parallel alignment of the random positions of collagen fibers, microfragmentation of elastic fibers, and the migration of tissue into the field by stretching force (11).

The major advantages of tissue expansion for large area scar revisions over distant or free flaps are that the local increase of tissue includes the preservation of sensation, vascularity, and adnexal structures. These features are especially important in the head and neck for both functional and cosmetic reasons. Disadvantages include the necessity of two operative procedures and the need for frequent inflations of the expander. A temporary visible deformity occurs as the expander reaches its fully inflated state, which may be objectionable to a patient who must continue to work in a job that requires interacting with the public.

Complications of tissue expanders include but are not limited to infection, implant exposure, implant failure, pain, bony erosion beneath the implant, and psychological stress for the patient as expansion progresses.

ADJUNCTIVE TECHNIQUES

Shave excision (Dermaplaning)

Dermaplaning is used to shave down any portions of a mature scar that continue to be elevated from the surrounding tissue. This will flatten the irregular scar and make it level with the remaining scar. Dermaplaning can be performed with a scalpel or a single hand-held razor blade; alone or as a valuable adjunct to dermabrasion or laser resurfacing preparatory to removal of the high spots before a more generalized resurfacing is undertaken.

Resurfacing Techniques

Dermabrasion and laser resurfacing are the most commonly used techniques for smoothing irregular scar surfaces. Resurfacing procedures can be used to level high areas within the scar or to blend depressed scars with the surrounding normal tissues. Dermabrasion is the time-honored technique that mechanically removes the epidermis and a portion of the superficial dermis with a wire brush or a diamond fraize (11). More recently, CO_2 laser resurfacing has frequently been employed to accomplish the same end by vaporizing the epidermis and upper dermis and creating thermal injury (12). Both techniques result in a smoother scar that blends into the surrounding normal tissue, making the scar less conspicuous. Scars with large, irregular surface area, as seen with abrasion injuries and those with tattoos from debris left in the wound from the primary repair, are treated with resurfacing techniques. If the area to be treated is large, it is desirable to resurface at least the entire facial esthetic unit and often the entire face to blend the final color and texture. Both of these techniques have the potential to cause permanent hypopigmentation if the deeper layers of the dermis are reached. Postinflammatory hyperpigmentation occurs in about 15% (personal communication, LaFerriere, 1999) to 37% of the time and is responsive to topical treatment with bleaching agents such as hydroquinones and kojic acid (17). Dermabrasion and CO_2 laser resurfacing should not be utilized in the lower two-thirds of the neck because fewer adnexal structures are present and scarring is likely. Caution should also be exercised over the jaw line and upper neck.

Augmentation of Depressed Scars

Depressed scars are often amenable to improvement with subcutaneous or intradermal materials. Injectable medical-grade silicone was once used for the permanent augmentation of depressed scars, but the U.S. Food and Drug Administration withdrew its approval for its clinical use because of intracutaneous granuloma formation; its use is currently illegal in the United States. Bovine collagen (Zyderm, Zyplast, Collagen Biomedical, Palo Alto, CA), autologous dermal collagen (Autologen, Collagenesis Corporation, Beverley, MA), and various other injectable substances have been developed for the augmentation of depressed scars but have the disadvantage of being temporary. Fat transplant efficacy for the treatment of facial contour defects remains uncertain (13,14). Autogenous dermal–fat grafts and acellular dermal grafts (AlloDerm, LifeCell Corporation, The Woodlands, TX) may result in a long-lasting improvement in the depressed scar, require implantation rather than injection, and are more technically difficult to use. Expanded polytetrafluorethylene (e-PTFE) (Gore-Tex, W.L. Gore & Associates, Flagstaff, AZ) is a permanent augmentation material with use in improving subcutaneous deficits of varying size (15). Gore-Tex subcutaneous augmentation material (SAM) is frequently used for facial augmentation purposes, but is of little value in depressed cutaneous scars.

HYPERTROPHIC AND KELOID SCARS

Hypertrophy of surgical and posttraumatic scars occurs most frequently when the wounds were closed under tension or are ATL scars that, by nature of their direction, are subject to increased tension on the wound edges. Hypertrophied scars are characterized by erythema, tenderness, pruritis, elevation, and thickening. A hypertrophic scar that persists for more than 12 months and the margins of which extend beyond the original wound into neighboring tissues is a keloid scar. Hypertrophic scars generally regress with time but frequently leave the area widened and depressed, whereas keloids rarely diminish in size without treatment. Both hypertrophic and keloid scars are more common in younger, darker-skinned patients, and when the wound is closed under tension (16). Areas under constant movement, such as the upper lip and neck region, may produce more wound tension and induce hypertrophy. A common area to find a hypertrophic or keloid scar is the ear (Fig. 13). Histological differentiation between hyertrophic and keloid scars is extremely difficult in the early phases of scar formation and is not clinically necessary in the mature scar (17–20).

Any consideration of the treatment of hypertrophic and keloid scars should start with a discussion of prevention. Gentle soft tissue handling at the initial wound closure, planning incisions to lie as close as possible to the RSTL, adequate undermining to lessen tension on the wound, and closing in layers to avoid dead space are technical details that help prevent hypertrophic scar formation. Postoperative splinting of the wound with tape or other topical dressing is helpful in reducing the motion and tension on the healing wound, and should be continued after suture removal for

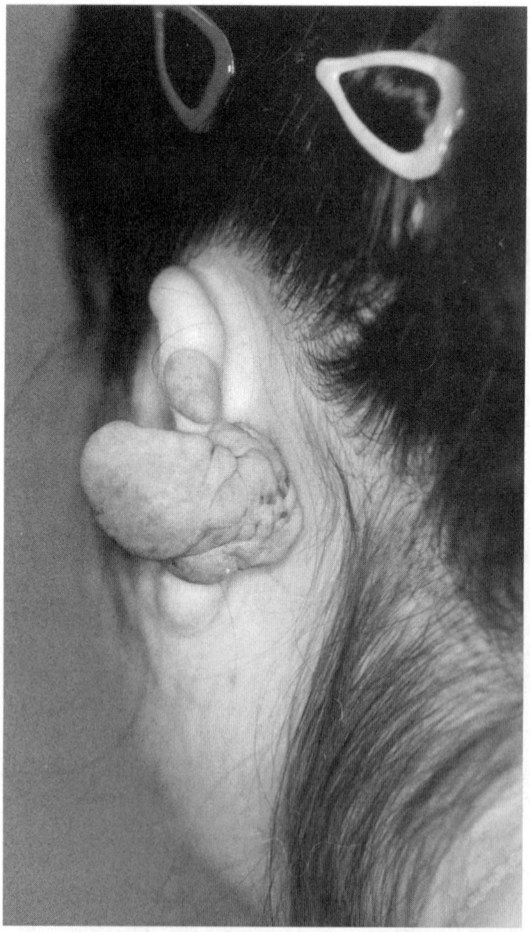

Figure 13 Pedunculated keloid scar of the auricle secondary to ear piercing.

up to 1 month in areas susceptible to excessive movement or tension. When revising scars, proper tissue management is essential to avoid the occurrence or reoccurrence of hypertrophied or keloid scars.

Hypertrophic scars respond to intralesional steroid injections. Triamcinolone acetonide, 10 mg/ml, is most commonly used, injected with a 30 gauge needle at intervals of 4 weeks until there is a significant clinical change in symptoms or regression of the scar. Most scars begin to show signs of improvement, such as softening, flattening, and decreased itching, by the third injection, and often do not require further intralesional steroid. The amount injected is dependent on the size of the scar but rarely approaches the maximum dosage of triamcinolone per month: 120 mg in adults, 80 mg in children 6–10 years, and 40 mg in children 1–5 years of age. It is thought that steroids work by increasing the rate of collagen degradation, and by decreasing collagen synthesis, the inflammatory process, and fibroblast proliferation (21). Care must be taken to avoid injection of the steroid into normal skin and subcutaneous fat because atrophy of these tissues is likely. In addition to tissue atrophy, complications include telangectasia formation and hypopigmentation.

Keloid scars are much more difficult to treat. Repeated steroid injections are helpful in softening and reducing the bulk of the scar, and surgical excision is frequently required. To improve the results of surgery, steroid injections in the wound margins, application of external pressure dressings, cryosurgery, and radiation at the time of surgery have been used. Even with aggressive perioperative and postoperative care, keloid recurrence rates can approach 41% after combination steroid and surgical therapy (22). Keloids that are too large to be excised and closed primarily with a tension-free closure may best be treated with excision followed by a thin (8–10/1000 in) split-thickness skin graft, or be left to heal by secondary intention (26). The CO_2, argon, and neodymium–yttrium–aluminum–garnet (Nd:YAG) lasers have been used to treat keloid scars with variable results (24–32).

Pressure-treated keloid scars have been demonstrated to have decreased intercollagen cohesiveness and fibroblast content, possibly due to local hypoxia caused by external mechanical occlusion (33). Pressure dressings should be used when possible for 4–6 months to decrease the risk of scar contracture or scar hypertrophy after removal of the splint. These pressure dressings may range from an elasticized garment, paper tape casting, to Silastic sheeting. These are all self-administered, painless, and may provide the patient with scar improvement and symptomatic relief.

The existence of multiple treatments for keloid scars reflects the inadequacy of any one method, and at this time no definitive procedure is available to the surgeon faced with these lesions.

REFERENCES

1. Borges AF. Scar Revision. 1st ed. Boston: Little Brown and Company, 1973, 20–24.
2. Larrabee WF, Sherris DA. Principles of Facial Reconstruction. Philadelphia, PA: Lippincott-Raven, 1995,
3. Davis JS. The relaxation of scar contractures by means of the Z or reversed Z-type incision. Ann Surg 1931; 94:871–884.
4. Borges, AF. Improvement of antitension-lines scar by the W-plastic operation, Br. J Plast Surg 1959; 12:29.

5. Webster RC, Davidson TM, Smith RC. Broken line scar revision. Clin Plast Surg 1977; 42:263–274.
6. Van Rappard JHA, Molenaar J, Van Doorn K, Sonneveld GJ, Borghouts JMHM. Surface are increase in tissue expansion. Plast Reconstr Surg 1988; 82:833–837.
7. Kane WJ, McCaffrey TV, Wang TD, Koval TM. The effects of tissue expasion of previously irradiated skin. Arch Otolaryngol Head Neck Surg 1992; 118:419–426.
8. Roenigk RK, Wheeland RG. Tissue expansion in cicatricial alopecia. Arch Dermatol 1987; 123:641–646.
9. Kabaker SS, Kridel RWH, Krugman ME. Tissue expansions in the treatment of alopecia. Arch Otolaryngol 1986; 112:720.
10. Cherry GW, Austed ED, Pawyk KA. Increased survival and vascularity of random pattern skin flaps elevated in controlled expanded skin. Plast Reconstr Surg 1983; 72:680.
11. Gibson T. The physical properties of skin. In: Converse JM, ed. Reconstructive Plastic Surgery, I., Philadelphia, PA: WB Saunders, 11977:70–77.
12. Kurtin A. Corrective surgical planing of skin. Arch Dermatol Syphilol 1953; 681:389.
13. Nehal KD, Levine VJ, Ross B, Ashinoff R. Comparison of high-energey pulsed carbon dioxide laser resurfacing and dermabrasion in the revision of surgical scars. Dermatol Surg 1998; 246:647–650.
14. Nanni CA, Alster TS. Complications of CO_2 laser resurfacing. An evaluation of 500 patients. Dermatol.-Surg 1998; 24(3):315–320.
15. Briscoll M. Autologous fat tissue augmentation. Am J Cosmet Surg 1987; 4:141.
16. Ersek RA. Transplantation of purified autogenous fat: a 3 year follow-up is disappointing. Plast Reconstr Surg 1991; 87:219.
17. Schoenrock LD, Reppucci AD. Gore-Tex in facial plastic surgery. Int J Aesth Reconstr Surg 1993; 1:63–69.
18. Farrior RT, Stambaugh KI. Keloids and hyperplastic scars. In: Thomas JR, Holt GR, eds. Facial Scars, Revisions, and Camouflage., St Louis: CV Mosby, 1989:83–97.
19. Blackburn WR, Cosman B. Histologic basis of keloid and hypertophic scar differentiation. Arch Pathol 1966; 82:65–71.
20. Sherris DA, Larrabee WF, Murakami CS. Management of scar contractures, hypertrophic scars, and keloids. Otolaryngol Clin North Am 1995; 28:5.
21. Curtis ASG, Seehar GM. The control of cell division by tension or diffusion. Nature 1978; 274:52–53.
22. Murray JC, Pinnell SR. Keloids and excessive dermal scarring. In: Cohen IK, Diegelman RF, Lindblod WS, eds. Wound Healing: Biochemical & Clinical Aspects., Philadelphia: WB Saunders, 1992:500–509.
23. Ketchum LD, Robinson DW, Master FW. The degradation of mature collagen: a laboratory study. Plast Reconstr Surg 1967; 40:89–91.
24. Cosman B, Wolff M. Bilateral earlobe keloids. Plast Reconstr Surg 1974; 53:540–543.
25. Bailin P. Use of the CO_2 laser for non-PWS cutaneous lesions. In: Arndt KA, Noe JM, Rosen S, eds. Cutaneous Laser Therapy: Principles and Methods., New York: John Wiley & Sons, 1983:187–200.
26. Ben-Bassat M, Ben-Bassat M, Kaplan I. A study of the ultrastructural features of the cut margin of skin and mucous membrane specimens excised by carbon dioxide laser. J Surg Res 1976; 21:77–84.
27. Henderson DL, Cromwell TA, Mes LG. Argon and carbon dioxide laser treatment of hypertrophic and keloid scars. Lasers Surg Med 1984; 3:271–277.
28. Apfelberg DB, Maser MR, Lash H, White D, Weston J. Preliminary results of argon and carbon dioxide laser treatment of keloid scars. Lasers Surg Med 1984; 4:283–290.
29. Castro DJ, Abergel RP, Johnston KJ, Adomian GE, Dwyer RM, Uitto J, Lesavoy MA. Wound healing: biological effects of Nd:YAG laser on collagen metabolism in pig skin in comparison to thermal burn. Ann Plast Surg 1983; 11:131–140.

30. Abergel RP, Meeker CA, Lam TS. Control of connective tissue metabolism by lasers: recent developments and future prospects. J Am Acad Dermatol 1984; 11:1142–1150.
31. Diegelmann RF, Cohen IK, McCoy B. Growth kinetics and collagen synthesis of normal skin, normal scar, and keloid fibroblast in vitro. J Cell Physiol 1979; 98:341–346.
32. Abergel RP, Dwyer RM, Meeker CA, Lask G, Kelly AP, Uitto J. Laser treatment of keloids: a clinical trial and an in vitro study with Nd:YAG laser. Lasers Surg Med 1984; 4:291–295.
33. Kischer CW, Shetlar MR. Collagen and mucopolysaccharides in the hypertrophic scar. Connect Tissue Res 1974; 2:205–213.

20
Basic Rhinoplasty

Robert W. Dolan
Lahey Clinic Medical Center, Burlington, Massachusetts, U.S.A.

INTRODUCTION

The first known description of nasal surgery is found in a 3000-year-old Egyptian papyrus containing a detailed account of the diagnosis and treatment of a nasal fracture. Until the mid-19th century, nasal surgery was reserved for the correction of severe acquired and congenital malformations. Modern rhinoplasty began with the advent of cocaine and the pioneering efforts of Dieffenbach, Roe, and Joseph. Dieffenbach and others during the late 19th century corrected nasal deformities through external incisions along the side or dorsum of the nose. John Orlando Roe, an otolaryngologist from Rochester, New York, performed the first aesthetic intranasal rhinoplasty in 1887. Jacques Joseph, an orthopedic surgeon from Berlin, Germany, subsequently did seminal work on aesthetic rhinoplasty and is considered by most to be the father of modern rhinoplasty and facial plastic surgery. The technique that Dr. Joseph used for intranasal rhinoplasty was the standard for the majority of rhinoplasty procedures performed through the 1960s. His technique included intercartilaginous and full transfixion incisions, hump removal with an osteotome, medial osteotomy with a chisel, lateral osteotomy with a saw, and tip cartilage reduction. His technique came to be known as reduction rhinoplasty in contrast to the more modern technique of augmentation rhinoplasty. Grafts (e.g., autografts, allografts, and synthetics) were not commonly used in routine rhinoplasty, although they were often used for the correction of nasal deformities such as a saddle nose. As the aesthetic norms shifted away from the operated look of a patient who had undergone a typical reduction rhinoplasty, the techniques of augmentation rhinoplasty took hold. Aside from the cosmetic concerns over reduction rhinoplasty, several functional problems emerged as these patients were followed over the long term. Cartilage excision produced noses that lacked support in the lower and middle thirds resulting in collapse of the nasal valve and nasal obstruction. As cosmetic and functional concerns mounted in the late 1960s, surgeons and patients began to embrace a different philosophy. Techniques were adapted that would result in a natural-appearing and well-supported functional nose. Cartilage reshaping and augmentation, often through open techniques (i.e., external rhinoplasty), enhanced the short- and long-term results of aesthetic rhinoplasty. Subsequent developments up to the present have continued to improve on this modern philosophical and technological paradigm.

ANATOMY

The nose is the most prominent feature on the face and figures highly in facial balance and beauty. Many men have either been belittled, as the Dauphin of France, or extolled, as Caesar, for the size and shape of the their noses. It is the rhinoplastic surgeon's role to ensure that the nose fits harmoniously with the rest of the face. Ethnicity, patient desire, and overall facial balance must be considered. As it does with an architect, the adage "form will follow function" plays an essential role in the procedures performed. Hence, the surgeon must have a keen sense of the anatomy of the nose and how it relates to function. Anatomy and function are intertwined and the surgeon must be cognizant of both to achieve the desired aesthetic result.

Topography

The nose is a pyramid of bone, cartilage, and soft tissue (Fig. 1). It is divided into thirds corresponding to the bony nasal vault (upper third), middle vault (middle third), and lower vault (lower third). Important anatomical landmarks in the upper two-thirds are useful in delineating and describing pathology of the external nose.

The nasion is the junction of the frontonasal suture with the midsagittal plane.

The radix nasi is the soft tissue correlate of the nasion and refers to the point of origin of the nasal root.

The rhinion is the landmark corresponding to the tip of the nasal bones in the midsagittal plane. It is located at the junction of the nasal bones and cartilaginous septum.

The landmarks in the lower third of the nose include the lobule, nasal tip, domes, columella, and nasal alae. The lobule is the area of the nose bounded by the upper free edge of the nostrils and the supratip breakpoint. It is subdivided into the tip (most projecting portion of the lobule), supratip, and infratip lobules. The (clinical) domes represent the junctions of the medial and lateral crura of the lower lateral cartilages. The dip just superior to the highest part of the domes corresponds to the supratip depression (break). This depression is not so much a true anatomical landmark as an aesthetic landmark.

Skin and Muscles

The skin is thickest at the nasofrontal groove (1.25 mm) and thinnest over the rhinion (0.6 mm) (1). Subcutaneous fat is nearly absent at the rhinion and most abundant in the supratip. Muscle mass is most prominent at the nasofrontal groove, consisting of the procerus and corrugator supercilii.

The quality of the skin has important implications in rhinoplasty, especially with respect to the nasal tip. Very thick skin can mask improvements made to the underlying cartilages and, despite a favorable cartilage framework, tip refinement

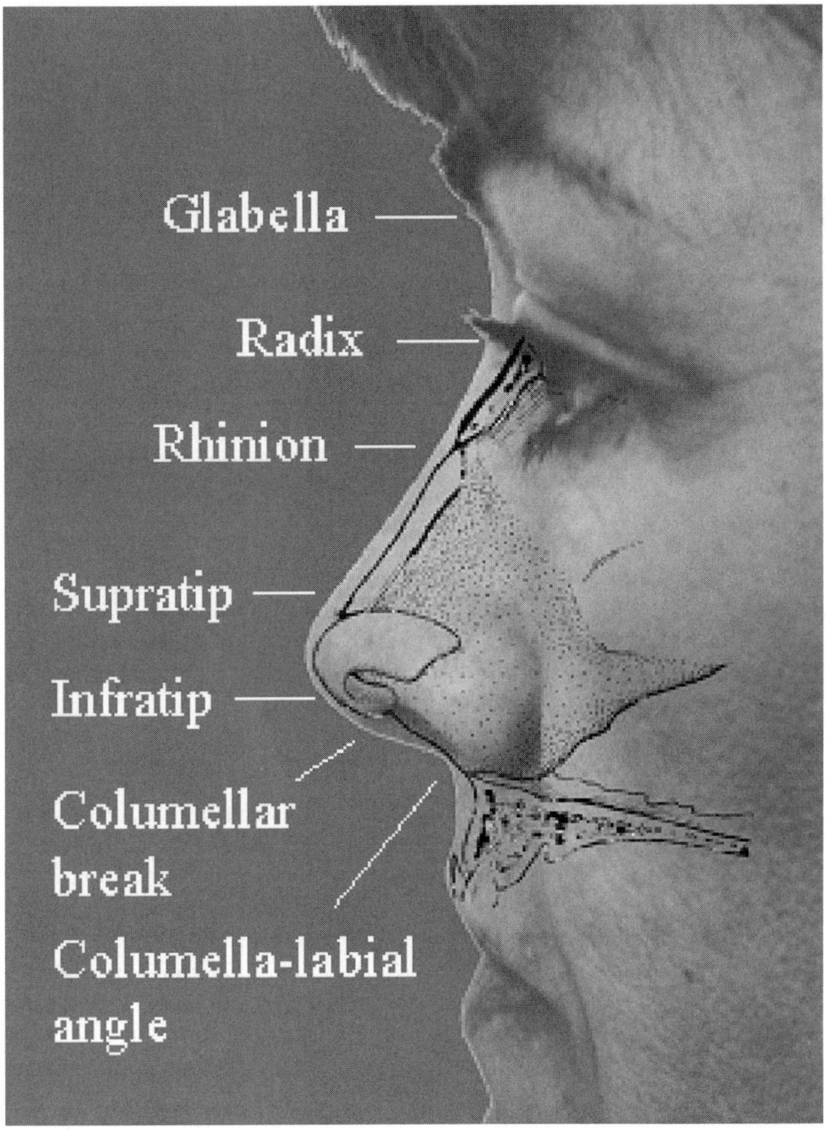

Figure 1 Topographical landmarks of the external nose.

and definition may remain poor. However, thin skin with sparse subcutaneous tissue can also be problematic. The cartilage framework is easily seen and even minor contour problems will be obvious. For example, a bifid nasal tip appears to have widely separated domes, yet this may result from a combination of thin skin and a lack of intervening soft tissue rather than an abnormality of lower lateral cartilage formation.

The muscles of the nose include the procerus, pars transversa (compressor naris) of the nasalis muscle, and depressor septi (2) (Fig. 2). The procerus muscle is a single pyramidal slip of muscle arising from the nasal bones and upper lateral

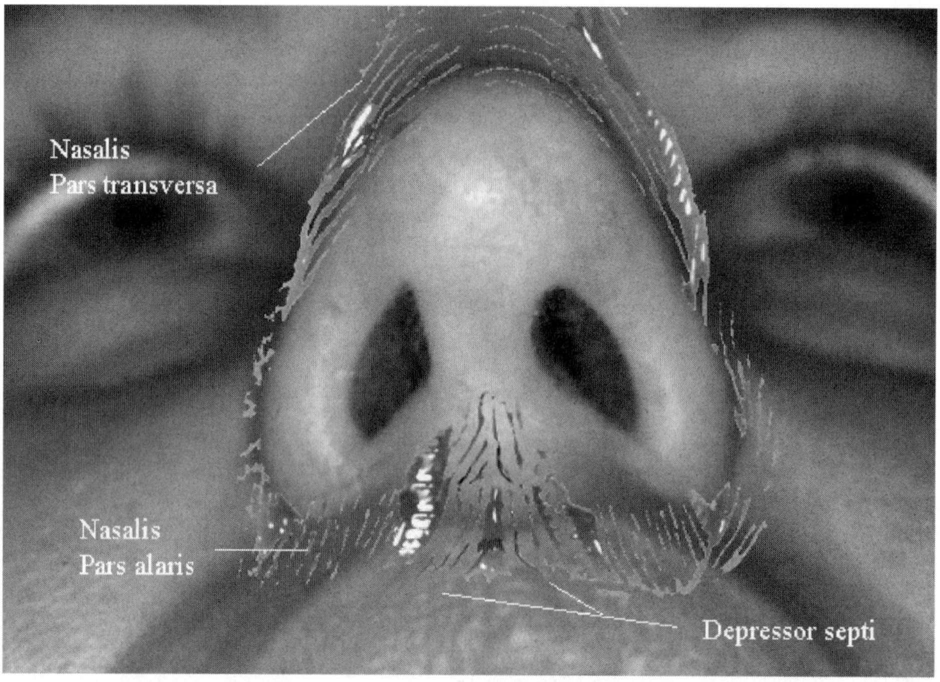

Figure 2 Muscles of the nose.

cartilages. It inserts into the frontalis muscle and skin between the eyebrows. The pars transversa is a paired muscle that takes origin from the canine eminence of the maxilla and inserts into a fibrous aponeurosis shared with the opposite muscle along the cartilaginous nasal dorsum. The pars alaris (paired) takes origin above the labial incisor tooth and inserts into lower and lateral margin of the nasal ala. The depressor septi is perhaps the most important muscle in rhinoplasty since it can cause a functional tip ptosis. The muscle is paired, takes origin from the premaxilla, and inserts into the base of the columella and medial crural footplates. It plays an important role in nasal ventilation in deep inspiration by tensing the columella and membranous septum.

All of the muscles appear to function to dilate the nasal aperture and improve airflow by flattening and widening the nasal dorsum (pars transversa), flaring the nostrils (pars alaris), and elongating the columella (depressor septi). The muscles are supplied entirely by the buccal branch of the facial nerve.

Arteries and Nerves

The arteries of the nose include the lateral nasal branch of the facial artery, nasal branch of the infraorbital artery, dorsal nasal branch of the ophthalmic artery, and external nasal branch of the ethmoidal artery (2). The lateral nasal branch of the facial artery supplies the ala and a portion of the dorsum. The infraorbital artery branches under the levator labii superioris to supply the nasal base and ala via its branches. The dorsal nasal artery is a terminal branch of the ophthalmic artery that emanates from the medial orbit superior to the medial palpebral ligament to supply the nasal dorsum. An external nasal branch from the ethmoidal artery (from the ophthalmic) reaches the nasal dorsum between the nasal bone and upper lateral cartilages to supply the nasal dorsum. The venous system follows the arterial system closely.

The sensory nerves of the nose include the external nasal branches of the infraorbital nerve, infratrochlear nerve, and external nasal branch of the anterior ethmoidal nerve (2). The infraorbital nerve divides under the levator labii superioris muscle and gives rise to external nasal branches that supply the base of the nose and ala. The nasociliary nerve divides into the infratrochlear nerve and the anterior ethmoidal nerve at the anterior ethmoidal foramen. The infratrochlear nerve travels lateral to the lamina papyracea and leaves the orbit between the superior oblique muscle and the medial palpebral ligament to supply the superomedial and upper dorsal aspects of the nose. The anterior ethmoidal nerve enters the nose within the ethmoidal air cells and continues medially entering the anterior cranial fossa just superior to the cribriform plate. The nerve travels anteriorly and re-enters the nasal cavity through the ethmoidal fissure at the side of the crista galli. Besides supplying the neighboring mucosal structures, an external nasal branch emerges on the nasal dorsum between the nasal bone and upper lateral cartilages to supply the nasal dorsum from the rhinion to the tip.

Nasal Fascia

The nose is covered with a superficial muscular aponeurotic system (SMAS) that surrounds the nasal musculature and intimately attaches to the overlying dermis (3). The main arteries and nerves and perichondrium are deep to the SMAS. The perichondrium thickens between the medial crura and domes and forms the transverse and intradomal ligaments, respectively. In most cases, the transverse ligament between the medial crura is continuous with the intradomal ligament.

Nasal Bones

The upper nose approximates the shape of a pyramid and its structure results from the shape and articulation of the paired nasal bones, frontal processes of the maxillae, nasal processes of the frontal bones, and perpendicular plate of the ethmoid. The nasal bones average 25.1 mm in length from the frontonasal suture. The frontonasal suture is 10.7 mm above the intercanthal line (1). The midline nasal suture is a solid syndesmosis and is often replaced completely by bone after nasal growth is complete, resulting in a synostosis. The fused caudal nasal bones overlap several millimeters of the cephalic upper lateral cartilages. The nasal bones, upper lateral cartilages, quadrilateral cartilage, and perpendicular plate of the ethmoid form a confluent solid mass called the keystone area (4). The nasal bones are thin inferiorly but gradually thicken to approximately 6 mm at the nasal root. At the intercanthal line, the nasal bones are sufficiently thick to resist osteotomy, and most osteotomies approaching this area are deflected medially. An osteotomy should not be forcibly carried to the frontal bone since narrowing of the nasal root above the intercanthal line is rarely indicated.

The perpendicular plate of the ethmoid articulates with the nasal bones along their inner dorsal surfaces at the keystone area. Marked deviation of the nasal septum in this area may affect the position of the nasal bones after infracture. If this is the case, a septoplasty involving the high bony septum must performed first to ensure that the proper position of the nasal bones after osteotomy and medialization is attained.

Nasal Cartilages

The nasal cartilages consist of the quadrilateral septal cartilage, paired upper lateral cartilages, paired lower lateral cartilages, sesamoid cartilages, and accessory cartilages. The cartilaginous vault lies anterior to the pyriform aperture and constitutes the largest part of the nasal anatomy.

Upper Lateral Cartilages

The upper lateral cartilages are triangular and are bounded superiorly by the nasal bones, inferiorly by the lower lateral cartilages, laterally by the face of the maxillae, and pyriform sinuses, and medially by the septum. They are connected to the upper two-thirds of the dorsal septum by a firm fibrous aponeurosis. The upper lateral cartilages form a 10–15 degree angle with the dorsal septum. The nasal valves are formed at the distal aspect of the upper lateral cartilages because of this slight separation. The medial upper lateral cartilages are continuous with the dorsal cartilaginous septum forming a T configuration, except near the septal angle where the cartilages tend to separate with intervening connective tissue. Near the rhinion, this trifurcation tends to thicken and often contributes significantly to the nasal hump deformity. The T configuration causes the upper lateral cartilages to splay, which contributes in part to a slight normal widening of the middle and lower nasal vaults. The caudal end of the upper lateral cartilages most often ends in a scroll configuration interwoven with an opposing scroll from the lower lateral cartilage (lower lateral cartilage). The scroll is most prominent medially and, if excessive, contributes to widening of the lower middle vault and supratip lobule. Loss or removal of the scroll area can result in narrowing of the nasal valve. Excessive scroll may also contribute to obstruction.

Patency of the nasal valve is crucial to the function of the nose and is an important consideration in any aesthetic nasal surgery. The structures that bound the upper lateral cartilages also act to maintain the valve's patency. The upper lateral cartilages form an unyielding attachment to the caudal aspect of the nasal bones. Medial movement of the nasal bones (e.g., after lateral osteotomy) will result in medialward rotation of the upper lateral cartilages and narrowing of the nasal valve. The integrity of the mucosal cover is important to maintain laminar flow through the nasal valve. Disruption of this mucosa after rhinoplasty may result in scarring and obstruction.

Lower Lateral Cartilages

The lower lateral cartilages (Fig. 3) are complex three-dimensional structures vital to nasal tip support and shape. They are C-shaped and, although the cartilage is one

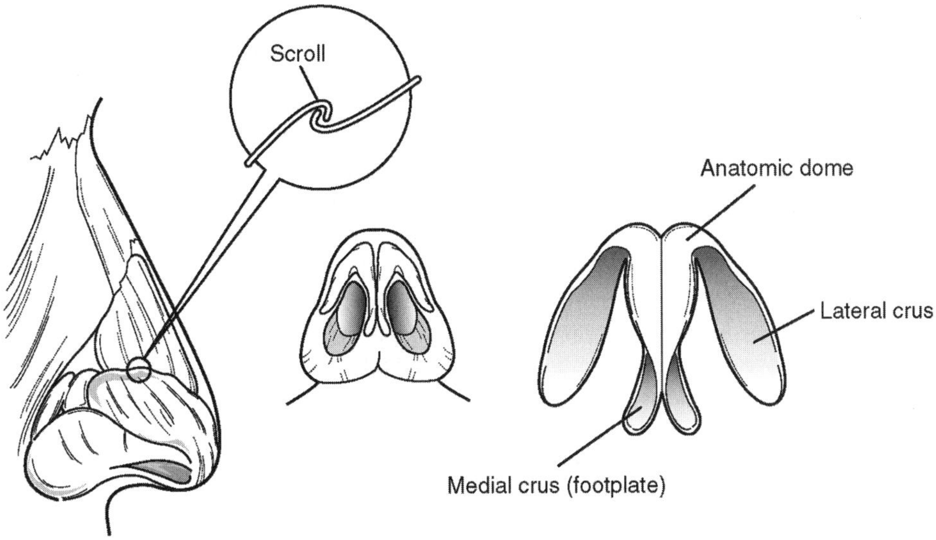

Figure 3 Upper and lower lateral cartilages. Note that the lateral crus courses superolaterally away from the nostril rim. The scroll area is defined by the relationship and articulation of the caudal margin of the upper lateral cartilage and the cephalic margin lower lateral cartilage.

piece, it is divided into three anatomically unique segments: the medial crus, the middle or intermediate crus, and the lateral crus (5). The medial crus is a thin, delicate extension of cartilage within the soft tissues of the columella. It includes the footplate and columellar segments. The length of a footplate is between 4 and 7.5 mm and the thickness ranges from 0.80 to 1.5 mm (6). The footplates tend to separate as they course inferiorly and will wrap around the caudal septum. The range of separation of the footplates is between 7.5 and 15 mm. The width of the base of the columella is determined primarily by the degree of flaring of the medial crural feet. The columellar segments of the medial crura are separated by a variable amount of connective tissue that also contributes to the width of the columella.

The middle (intermediate) crus is subdivided into lobular and domal segments. The lobular segment begins after an acute cephalic bend in the medial crus at the columella–lobule angle (columellar break). It is vertically oriented, blending into the domal segment as the cartilage folds posteriorly and becomes convex along its cephalic border. The caudal border of the domal segment is deficient at the domal notch, giving rise to the soft tissue facet or soft triangle near the apex of the nostril. The domal segment ends as it blends into the lateral crus at the domal junction. The tip defining points fall on the domal junction line near its caudal margin (7). The configuration of the dome is extremely variable, ranging from gently curved to sharply angulated with multiple projecting points. In aesthetic terms, the dome is defined in four ways: anatomical, clinical, vestibular, and surgical. The anatomical dome is located at the junction of the middle and lateral crura. The clinical dome is the part of the tip cartilage identified externally. In thinned-skin individuals, the anatomical dome may closely match the appearance of the clinical dome. The most projected point of the clinical dome is the tip-defining point. The vestibular dome is the counterpart to the clinical dome internally and is at the apex of the concavity formed between the medial and lateral crura. The surgical dome is the dome established at surgery (8).

The lateral crus may be concave, convex, or straight with a scroll evident superomedially that articulates with a reverse scroll at the caudal edge of the upper lateral cartilages. The shape of the lateral crus has been classified by Lessard et al. as type 1: smooth, convex (10%); type 2: convex, concave (30%); type 3: concave, convex (25%); type 4: concave, convex, concave (25%); type 5: concave (5%); and type 6: complete convex (5%) (1). The most aesthetically pleasing configuration of the domal junction is formed by a convex domal segment merging with a concave lateral crus at the domal junction. A common misconception is that the caudal border of the lateral crus closely parallels the nostril rim. In fact, the lateral crus diverges widely from the rim, curving superomedially at a 30–40 degree angle. There may be an exaggerated cephalic rotation of the lateral crura, in some cases actually running parallel to the dorsal septum, adding to lobular and supralobular (supratip) fullness. This condition has been described by Sheen as cephalic malposition or "parentheses tip" (9) (Fig. 4). The free lateral edge of the lateral crus does not reach the pyriform aperture. It is indirectly attached through connective tissue and a series of variable true accessory cartilages distributed along a curvilinear line from the lateral tip to the nasal sill (10). The accessory cartilages must be differentiated from the inconsistent sesamoid cartilages found scattered between the caudal upper lateral cartilages and the cephalic lower lateral cartilages.

Septum

Approximately 1 cm of the dorsal and caudal quadrilateral cartilage (i.e., dorsocaudal strut) must be preserved to maintain nasal support and projection. The bony portions of the septum, including the vomer and perpendicular plate of the ethmoid bone, are not directly responsible for nasal support. Of course, deviations in these bones will cause nasal obstruction, and irregularities of the perpendicular plate between the nasal bones may cause bony dorsal asymmetry after osteotomy and infracture.

Important landmarks involving the quadrilateral cartilage include the rhinion, anterior septal angle, inferior septal angle, and nasal valve (Fig. 5). The anterior septal angle is the angle formed at the junction of the dorsal septum with the caudal septum. This portion of the nasal septum does not usually project beyond the domes of the lower lateral cartilages and it is at or slightly caudal to the supratip depression. The inferior septal angle is formed as the caudal septum makes a distinct bend toward the anterior nasal spine in its lower half. The caudal aspect of the quadrilateral cartilage is an essential component of the nasal valve, forming its medial border. Even minor deviations of the cartilage in this area will cause nasal valve narrowing and the perception of nasal obstruction.

The membranous septum is a distinct anatomical structure that connects the caudal septum to the columella. It is covered by vestibular mucosa and composed of connective tissue surrounding the medial crura. The upper half of the columella is separated from the caudal septum by the membranous septum. The lower half of the columella travels much closer to the caudal septum and the feet of the medial crura overlap the septum to a variable extent. Due to the elasticity of the

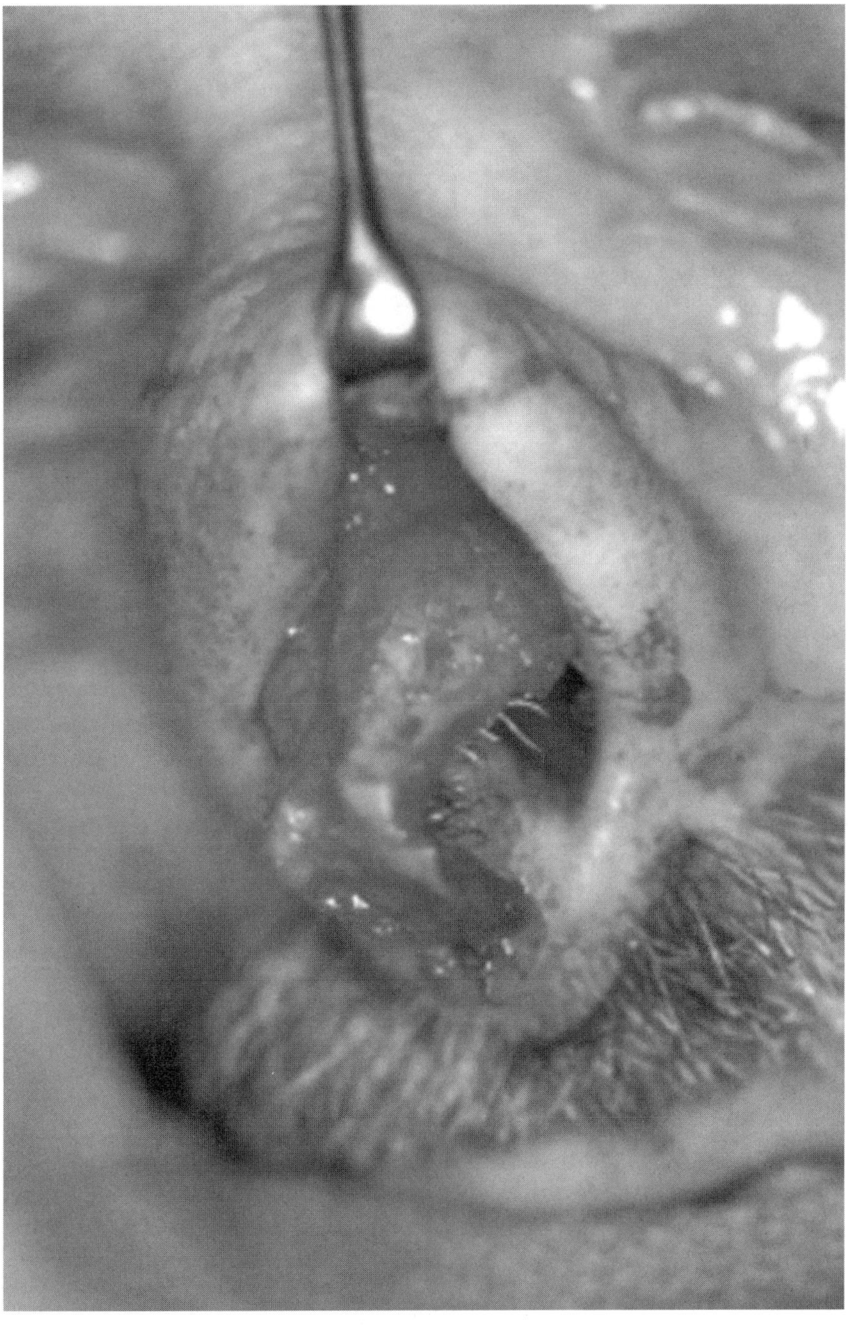

Figure 4 Cephalically malpositioned lateral crura seen through an open approach. Note how the lateral crus nearly parallels the dorsal nasal septum.

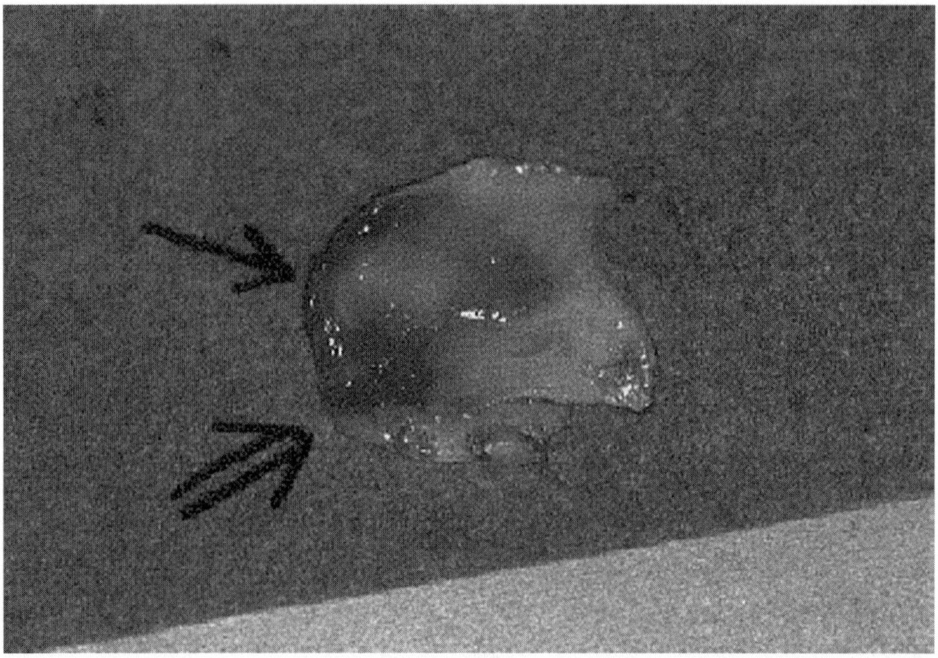

Figure 5 Quadrilateral cartilage ex vivo shows the anterior (single arrow) and inferior (double arrow) septal angles. The anterior septal angle is found between the domes and the inferior septal angle is seated over the maxillary spine.

membranous septum and mucoperichondrium over the caudal septum, the columella and medial crura are easily retracted away from the caudal septal edge.

Tip Support

Nasal tip resiliency and projection are maintained by major and minor structural supports. The major tip support mechanisms are the size, shape, and strength of the lower lateral cartilages; the medial crura and footplates and their attachment to the caudal septum; and the attachments of the lower lateral cartilages with the upper lateral cartilages (scroll area). The minor tip support mechanisms include the soft tissues of the membranous septum and interdomal area, the cartilaginous dorsum (the upper lateral cartilages and the dorsal septum), and the fibrous attachments of the lower lateral cartilages with the overlying skin. Uncorrected disruption of the major support mechanisms will result in tip depression and/or caudal rotation (ptosis). The minor tip support mechanisms may assume greater significance if they are overdeveloped or if the major supports are significantly weakened.

Tripod Concept

Understanding what is termed the tripod concept is fundamental in predicting nasal tip projection and rotation changes resulting from a variety of surgical interventions.

The theory states that three legs representing the lateral crura and conjoined medial crura support the nasal tip. The axis of rotation for the tripod is located at the base of the columella and the tripod itself is sloped caudally because the medial crura are shorter than the lateral crura. Since the axis of rotation is at the base of the columella and nasolabial angle, augmenting or reducing the legs of the tripod will have unequal effects on projection and rotation of the nasal tip. For example, augmenting the conjoined medial crura will increase nasal projection more than a similar degree of augmentation of the lateral crura. Conversely, augmentation of lateral crura will result primarily in caudal rotation of the nasal tip. Maximum projection without cephalic rotation is achieved by augmenting both the medial crura and lateral crural elements of the tripod.

Nasal Valve

Mink in 1940 originally described the nasal valve as the narrowest portion of the nasal cavity and as "the passage between the lower margin of the upper lateral cartilage and the septum and the most important regulator of airway resistance" (11). The nasal valve is the two-dimensional slit-like opening between the caudal edge of the upper lateral cartilages and the septum (Fig. 6). The angle formed by the junction of the upper lateral cartilages with the septum is normally 15–20 degrees. Since most of the inspired air must pass through the nasal valve, even small changes in its cross-sectional area will result in significant changes in nasal resistance. The nasal

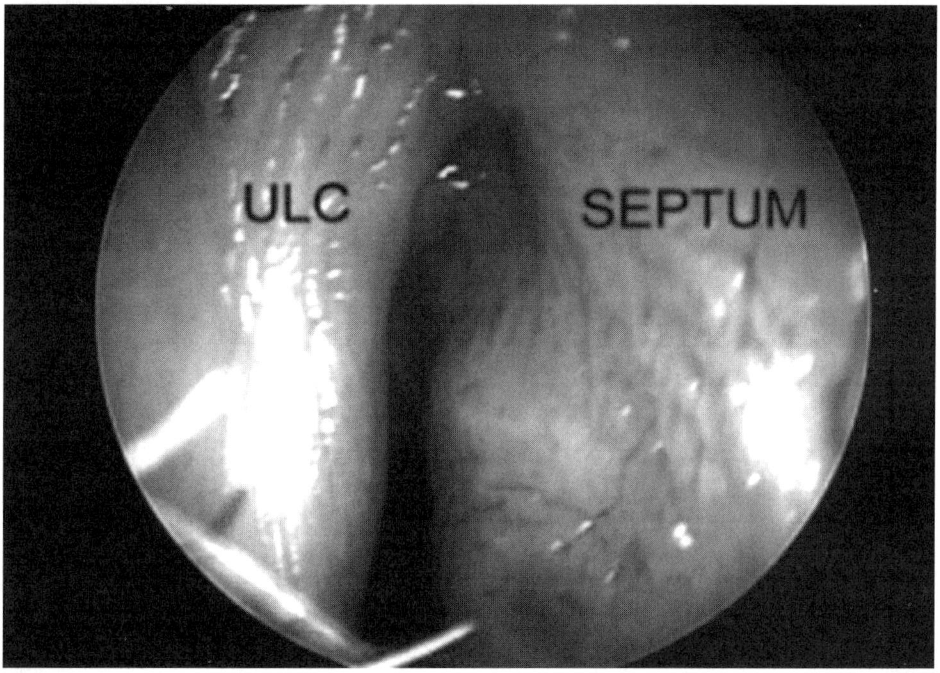

Figure 6 The nasal valve. Note the boundaries of the nasal valve: the caudal upper lateral cartilage (ULC) and nasal septum.

valve narrows in response to pressure changes generated within the nasal cavity by the act of inspiration. A dysfunctional nasal valve is a significant cause of nasal obstruction, especially in the patient who has undergone rhinoplasty.

The nasal valve has been called the internal nasal valve to differentiate it from the external nasal valve (the nasal ala). Since the nasal alae possess a valvular function only in pathological conditions, the term nasal valve should be reserved for the internal valve. The term external nasal valve should be discarded and nasal ala used instead. The nasal valve is a component of the nasal valve area and represents the narrowest part of the nasal cavity. The nasal valve area is a pyramidal space within the anterior nasal cavity bounded at its apex by the nasal valve, inferolaterally by the head of the inferior turbinate, and inferiorly by the rim of the pyriform aperture. The lateral boundaries include the lateral crus and fibrous-attached accessory cartilages (the so-called hinge area) and the soft tissue corresponding to the medial aspect of the supra-alar melolabial fold (external lateral triangle). Airflow during inspiration is deflected superiorly towards the nasal valve by the pyriform aperture. Obstructions within the nasal valve area will produce greater increases in nasal resistance than partial obstructions in areas outside of the nasal valve area. However, obstruction at the nasal valve itself will produce the greatest increase in nasal resistance because the predominant airstream is directed through this site.

The physiological benefit of the nasal valve is not known. It may serve to slow the airstream to allow for humidification, olfaction, filtration, or temperature regulation. Over-resection or weakening of the upper lateral cartilages will indirectly cause valvular narrowing by allowing the soft tissue in the lateral nasal wall to contract, drawing the upper lateral cartilages medially. This is commonly seen as a pinched nose in patients who have undergone traditional reduction rhinoplasty (Fig. 7). However, even in standard or augmentation rhinoplasty, the upper lateral cartilages are often cut free from the septum and the support and spring from the T configuration are lost. The upper lateral cartilages will then fall onto the septum, effacing the nasal valve. In addition, soft tissue and the upper lateral cartilages are moved medially after lateral osteotomies because of the firm attachment that the upper lateral cartilages share with the nasal bones. This causes the valves to narrow and become less flexible and, hence, less functional.

Nasal Alae

The nasal alae are the soft tissue portions of the nostrils that have scant skeletal support. They consist primarily of skin, subcutaneous tissue, vestibular mucosa, and muscle. The dilator naris muscle is a major component, opening the nostril through its attachment to the lateral crus. It does not affect nasal airflow in non-pathological conditions. However, collapse or obstruction of one or both nasal alae can abruptly stop nasal airflow. Nasal alar narrowing can also cause secondary collapse of the nasal valve.

The lower lateral cartilages also contribute to the stability of the nasal alae because the lateral crura course within the cephalic aspect of the nasal alae to a variable extent. Disruption or weakening of the lower lateral cartilage may cause alar flaccidity and collapse. Facial nerve paresis or paralysis can also result in functional nasal alar collapse due to motor loss and lack of tonicity in the dilator naris muscle.

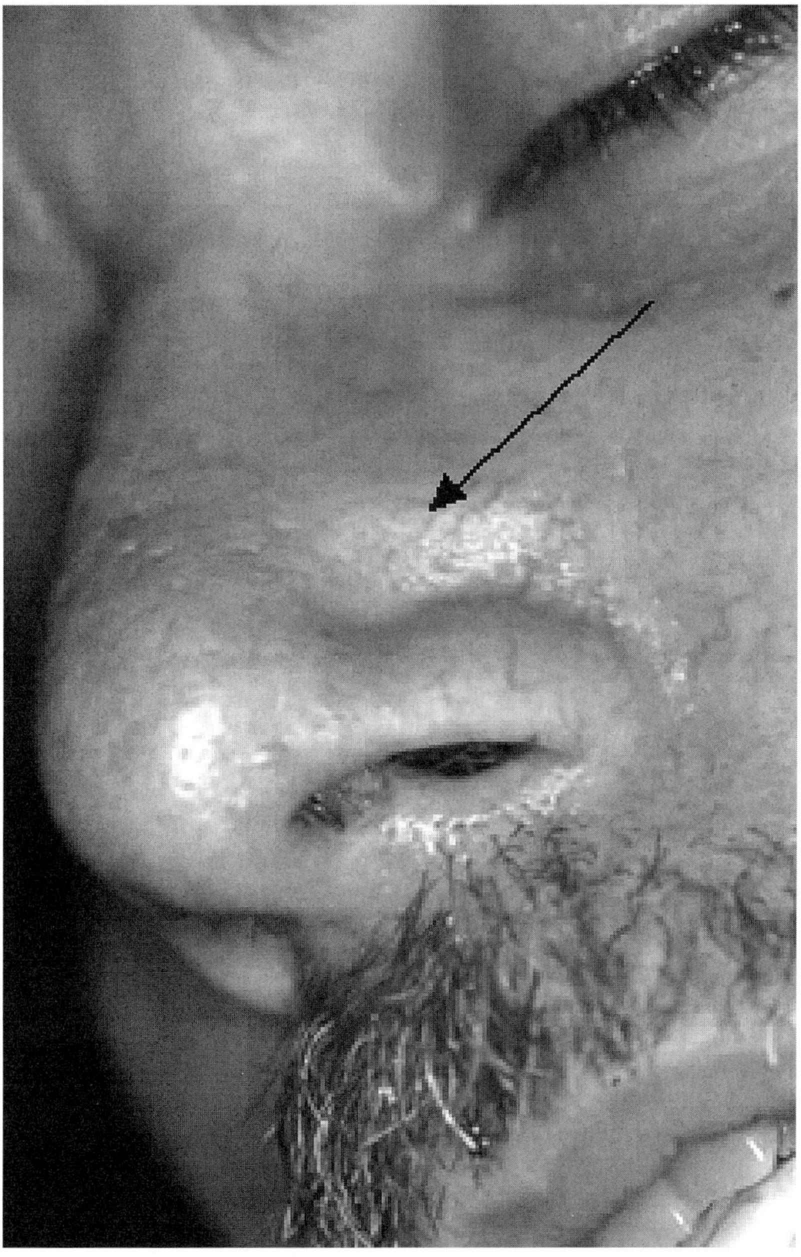

Figure 7 Example of a pinched nose deformity (arrow, supra-alar depression) due to over-resection of the lateral crus.

PREOPERATIVE EVALUATION

In addition to the intrinsic properties of the nose, age, gender, race, and stature are factors to be considered in the preoperative evaluation (12). The anatomy of the nose changes significantly as a person matures through childhood and adulthood. Two peaks of nasal growth occur in childhood: prior to the age of 8 years, and during puberty. A baby's or toddler's nose differs most dramatically from that of an adult in its upper third. There is often an open roof with widely separated nasal bones in children through the age of 5 years. The nasal bones gradually close and nasal growth goes into dormancy until puberty when there is a rapid increase in the rate of growth and bony and cartilage size. Nasal growth plateaus at the conclusion of puberty and young adulthood as the bony and cartilaginous framework become increasingly defined. With advancing age, the soft tissue cover and underlying musculature become increasingly lax, eventually resulting in nasal tip elongation and ptosis. Besides the nasal tip, aesthetic aberrations common in the aging patient also include elongation of the nose and an acute nasolabial angle. This change in anatomy also leads to nasal obstruction from the collapse of the nasal valve area and nostrils. Rhinoplasty in the aging patient must be directed at reversing these age-related functional and aesthetic problems.

Racial differences profoundly affect planning and the final result in rhinoplasty. For example, the African-American nose typically has relatively weak skeletal support, with flaring nostrils and inadequate tip projection. The nasal base is often excessively wide and the lobule is ill-defined with excessively thick skin. The typical rhinoplasty in the African-American patient entails increasing tip support and projection, narrowing the nasal base, and defatting the lobule. Although the tip cartilages may be of similar size to white patients, they are usually weaker and less resilient. Autogenous cartilage grafts are often required to increase tip support and projection.

Another important consideration is the patient's stature, especially with regard to the perception of tip rotation and nasal length. Taller patients who have undergone rhinoplasty often appear to have nasal tips that are over-rotated despite a nasolabial angle that falls within the aesthetic standard. The over-rotated appearance then leads to the perception of an overly shortened nose. Nostril show, cephalic tip rotation, and opening of the nasolabial angle should be minimized and nasal length should be maintained in taller patients.

During the initial consultation, a series of photographs should be taken including full frontal views, basal views, and left and right lateral and angled views. If digital photography is used, photos can be viewed immediately by surgeon and patient. This can be valuable since the patient can see views of the nose not possible using a standard mirror. Balance with other facial structures can easily be pointed out to the patient. Thoughtful nasal analysis cannot be done immediately with the patient waiting or present. However, with the patient's desires in mind, an analysis can be done prior to the procedure and reviewed with the patient preoperatively. Some patients may want to see potential changes demonstrated on the computer. This may be best left to a second visit after a definitive analysis has been done. Although this portends a strong rapport between surgeon and patient, it does not come without risks. Patients must be warned that the outcomes created on the computer might not be identical to real results due to problems that occur with healing such as shifting of structures, scarring, and the like. Patients should be warned that the results seen are not guaranteed but can give them a good idea of the possible outcome.

Nasal Analysis

Although many factors play a role in the overall appearance of the nose, including race, age, and ethnicity, several basic landmarks and relationships are common to any analysis of the nose prior to cosmetic rhinoplasty. Nasal analysis includes assessment of skin quality and texture, support (tip recoil), surface landmarks and features, and facial balance.

Skin thickness and pathology such as rhinophyma or scarring are noted. The quality of the skin has important implications especially relating to the nasal tip. For example, patients with thick skin and bulbous tip structures are well suited for extensive tip refinement. The thick skin tends to efface the sharp angles and slight irregularities within the underlying cartilaginous framework created by such extensive work. The opposite holds true in thin-skinned individuals, so cartilaginous work on the tip is usually more conservative.

Tip recoil is fundamental to any examination of the nasal tip. By gently depressing the nasal tip, the examiner can estimate resiliency and tip support. Poor recoil is present when the spring in the nasal tip is greatly diminished, indicating attenuated underlying cartilaginous support. In these cases, the need for additional cartilaginous support in the form of grafts or sutures should be anticipated.

Other conditions that may cause tip projection abnormalities include a hypoplastic premaxilla resulting in retropositioning of the entire nasal base. The nasolabial angle is also usually less than 90 degrees and there is some degree of tip ptosis. This condition is most commonly found in patients with a history of cleft palate and those with Binder's syndrome (maxillonasal dysplasia) (13).

Important surface landmarks in basic nasal analysis include the supraorbital ridges; clinical domes; nasal lobule; alar margins, grooves, and creases; medial canthi; radix nasi; rhinion; nasal tip; subnasale (Sn); columellar break; upper vermilion (Vu); pogonion; glabella; alar fold; columella base; and medial crural footplates. These landmarks are used to define structures and aesthetic relationships that are important in nasal analysis. The nose is initially assessed from three perspectives: anteroposteriorly (portrait view), laterally (profile view), and inferiorly (basal view) (Table 1). The portrait view includes assessment of the nasociliary lines, alar–lobule contour, nasal width, nasal width-to-length ratio, and overall symmetry (Fig. 8). The profile view includes assessment of the contour of the dorsum and supratip, columella–lobule–tip configuration, radix height, nasofrontal angle, nasolabial angle, nasal tip projection, chin projection, columellar position, and alar fold position (Fig. 1). The basal view includes assessment of footplate flaring, caudal septal deviation, nostril shape, lobule width-to-base ratio, and lobule height-to-columellar height ratio (Fig. 9).

Portrait View

Nasociliary Lines. Each nasociliary line outlines the ipsilateral silhouette created by the contour of the supraorbital rim, nasal dorsal ridge, and tip-defining

Table 1 Preoperative Rhinoplasty Evaluation Report

Landmarks	Aesthetic relationships (normative values)	Findings
Portrait View		
Supraorbital ridges; domes	Nasociliary lines	
Alae and lobule margins	Ala–lobule line	
Alar margins; medial canthi	Nasal width	
Alar margins; radix; nasal tip	Width/length (0.70)	
Radix; rhinion	Symmetry	
Profile View		
Upper 1/3; mid 1/3	Dorsum contour	
Nasal tip	Supratip contour	
Sn; columellar break	Columellar-lobule-tip config.	
Nasal root	Radix height (supratarsal crease)	
Dorsum; glabella	Nasofrontal angle (120–135 degrees)	
Columella; upper lip	Nasolabial angle (90–110 degrees)	
Vu; Sn; nasal tip	Nasal tip projection lip height/columella-tip (1:1)	
Alar crease; nasal tip; radix	Projection/length (0.55–0.60)	
Pogonion; glabella	Nasomental angle (130 degrees)	
Pogonion; glabella; dorsum	Nasofacial angle (36 degrees)	
Alar crease; ant. nostril margin	Ala–cheek junction	
Nostril rim; columella	Columellar position	
Nostril rim; columella; alar fold	Alar position	
Basal View		
Columellar base; footplates	Footplate flare	
Columella; septum	Caudal septum deviation	
Alar grooves; alar creases	Lobule width/base (< 0.75)	
Nostril rim; canthi; nasal base	Nostril flare	
Nasal tip; Sn; columellar break	Lobule height/columella (1:2)	
General		
Skin	Tip Recoil	Premaxillary support
Nasal valve	Septum	Turbs

Preoperative Pathology Initial • Revision	Operative Plan Open • Closed
	Implants:
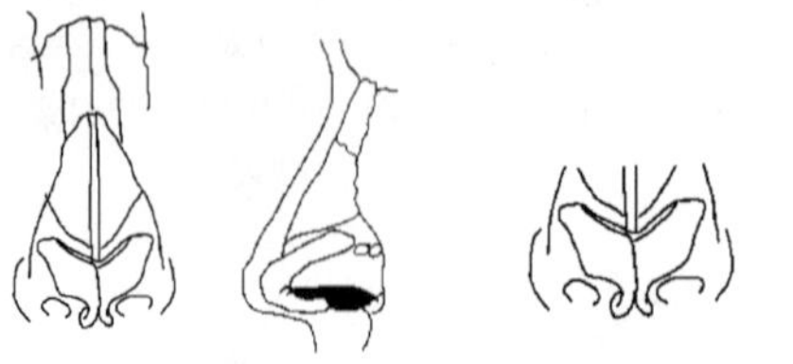	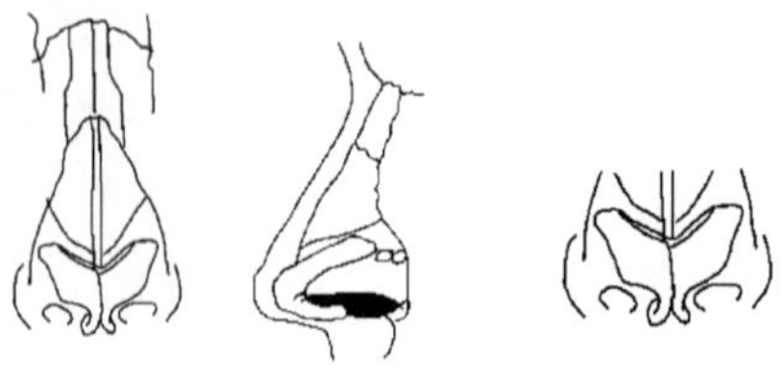

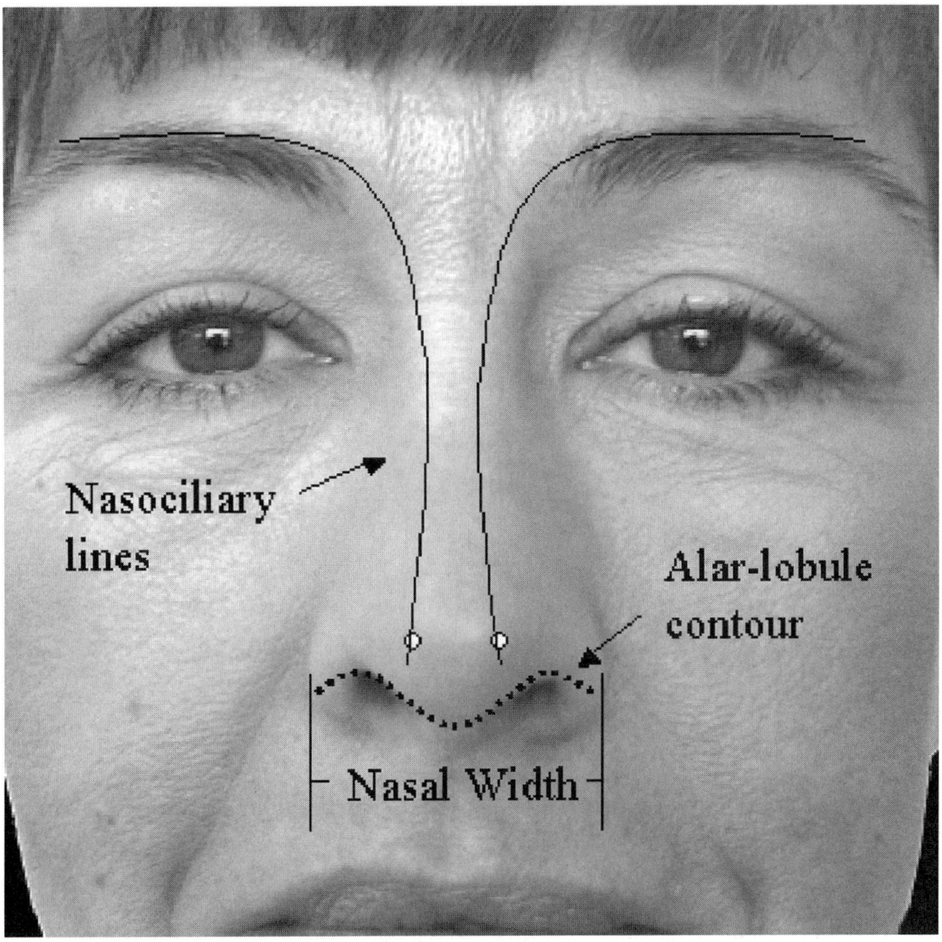

Figure 8 Important landmarks on portrait view (see text).

point. The nasociliary lines should course gracefully as mirror images from the supraorbital ridges onto well-defined dorsal ridges ending at distinct tip-defining points. If there is excessive widening, narrowing, or asymmetry of the nasal dorsum, the nasociliary lines will be uneven. The usual anatomical abnormality detected is excessive widening of the upper third (nasal bones). Widening of the middle third may be due to excessive size or splay of the upper lateral cartilages or an exaggerated scroll. Flat, disparate, or irregular domes are typical abnormalities found in the lower third of the nose. The nasociliary lines are useful guides to determine if narrowing or widening the nose is necessary through osteotomy (upper third) or cartilage grafting (middle third).

Ala–lobule Contour. The ala–lobule contour follows the free inferior edge of the alae and columella–lobule angle and is most aesthetic when it forms a graceful gull-wing-like silhouette. The lobule itself should be symmetrical and highlighted by clear domal tip-defining points and a well-defined columella–lobule angle. Alar rim abnormalities such as notching, asymmetry, or irregular inclinations are readily

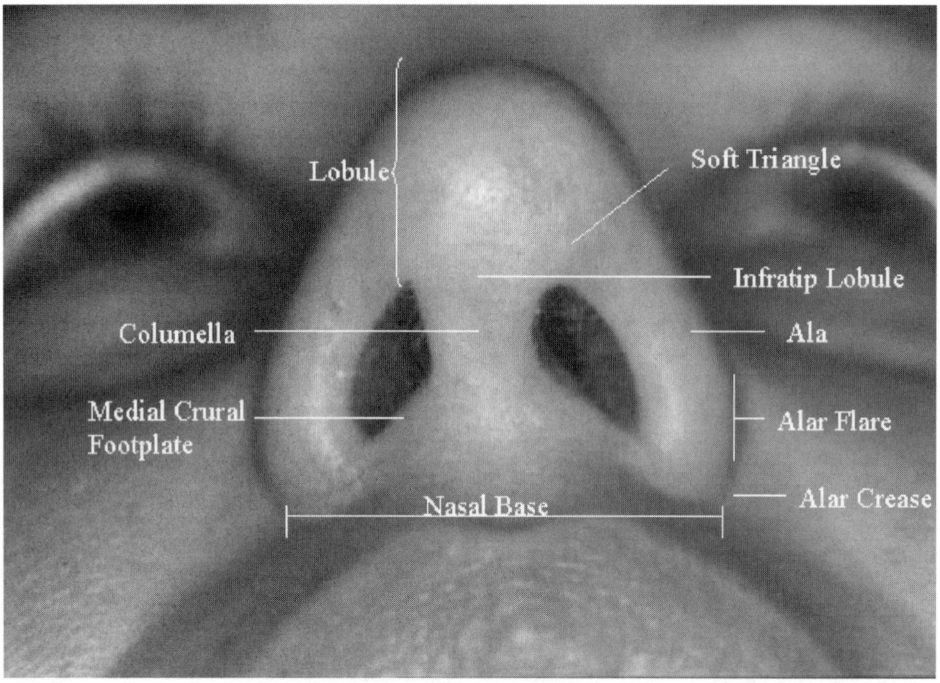

Figure 9 Important landmarks on basal view (see text).

noted by carefully noting the ala–lobule contour. The tip-defining points and clinical domes should correlate. Elements of the lobule that should be noted include bifidity, bulbosity, horns, and asymmetry. Widely separated domes and a flat or depressed nasal tip characterize a bifid tip. A bifid tip appears trapezoidal and surgical techniques should be employed to efface this geometric configuration to a more rounded one. A bulbous tip appears fat and ball-like. This can be due to excess or wide lower lateral cartilages, skin, subcutaneous tissue, or a combination of all three.

Nasal Width. The nasal width in the anteroposterior view is the distance between the flared aspects of the alae and is evaluated in relation to the eyes. The alae are most aesthetically aligned with lines dropped from the medial canthi. Hence, nasal width should approximately equal the width of an eye from canthus to canthus. If the alae flare outside the intercanthal lines, then alar-narrowing procedures may be indicated.

Overall Symmetry. Ideal nasal length is proportional to the total facial height. It can be assessed using Leonardo da Vinci's facial thirds: forehead height (trichion–glabella) = nose length (nasion–subnasale) = lower face height (subnasale–gnathion). These thirds should be equal.

The Profile View

Contour of the Dorsum and Supratip. The contours of the dorsum and supratip are important aesthetic parameters in rhinoplasty. The contour is described as convex, concave, straight, or irregular. Typically, a nasal hump is a

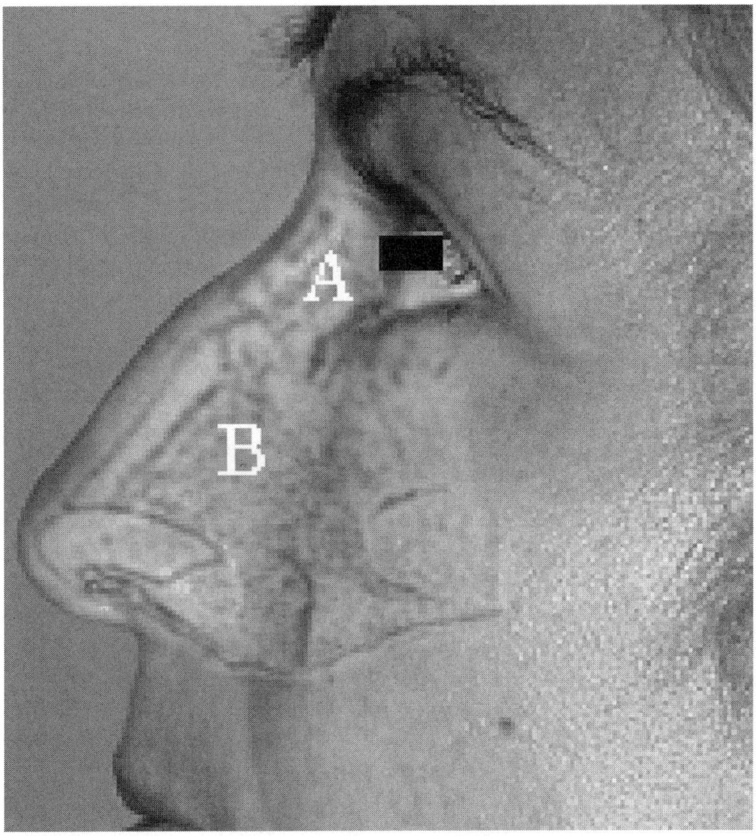

Figure 10 Typical nasal hump consisting of a combination of bone and cartilage. The underlying nasal bone (A) and cartilage (septum and upper lateral cartilages; B) have been introduced into the profile to demonstrate the complex nature of the usual nasal hump.

convexity at the rhinion and is composed of a complex of bone and cartilage (Fig. 10). It is usually secondary to overdevelopment of the cephalic upper lateral cartilage–quadrilateral cartilage–caudal nasal bone complex (the keystone area). Removal of the nasal hump as performed in a typical reduction rhinoplasty will result in the separation of the upper lateral cartilages from the septum, disruption of the keystone area, and creation of an open roof deformity exposing the upper nasal vault and perpendicular plate of the ethmoid. The ideal contour of the supratip differs between men and women, at least in white patients. The supratip break is an aesthetic feature more common to the female profile. Excessive break in the male nose is to be avoided. The break is a slight concavity in the supratip lobule formed by the projection of the nasal tip, dome position, and the height of the dorsal septum.

Columella–lobule Tip Configuration. The columella–lobule tip configuration is essentially an evaluation of the existence and quality of a columellar double break. The double break is more an aesthetic landmark than a true anatomical landmark. On profile view, it is seen as an acute columella–lobule angle creating a distinct soft tissue platform over the lobular segment of the middle crus (Fig. 11). The

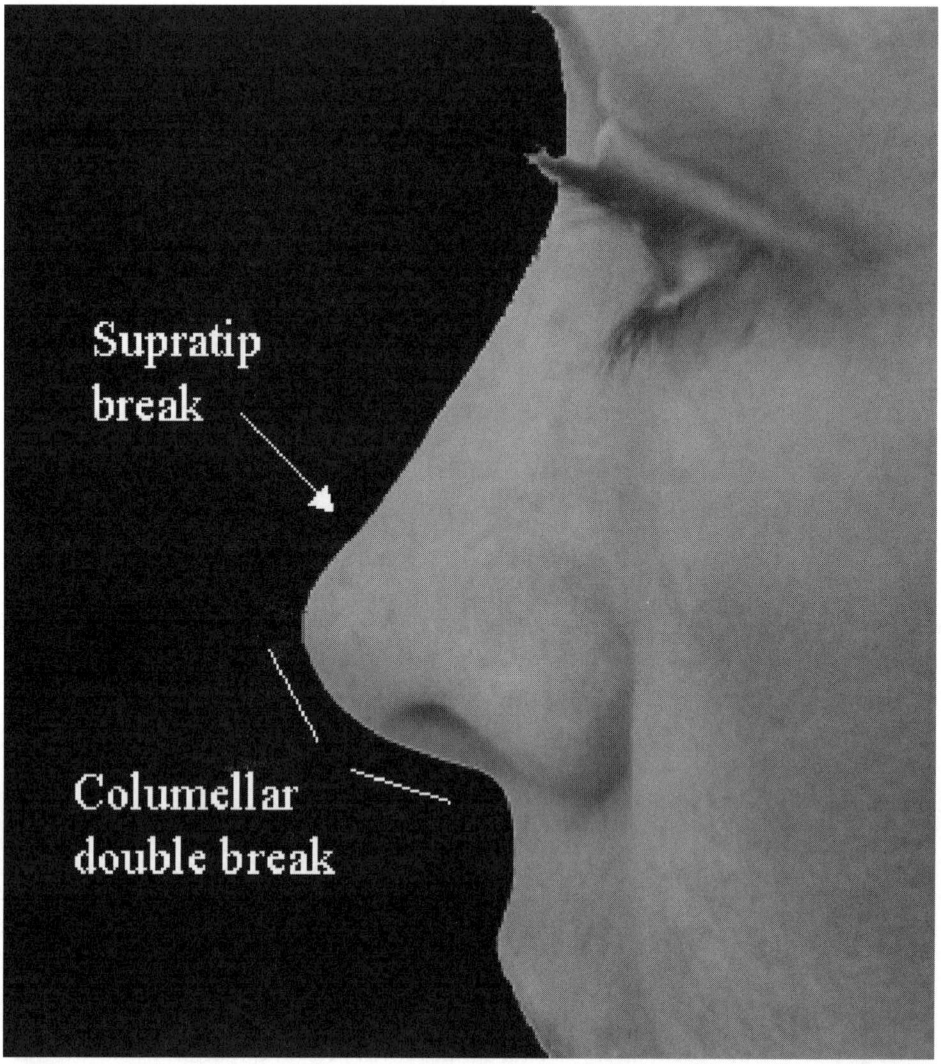

Figure 11 The columella–lobule double break. This is an aesthetic aspect of the nasal tip on profile that is sought after in white patients undergoing rhinoplasty.

columella–lobule angle is ideally approximately 37 degrees. The platform extends to the anterior-most point on the lobule (nasal tip).

Radix Depth and Position. The radix nasi is the root of the nose and is located at the depths of the nasofrontal angle formed at the intersection of vertical lines parallel to the glabella and nasal dorsum. The nasofrontal angle normally measures between 120 and 135 degrees and the radix is most aesthetically at the level of the supratarsal fold (or approximately 1 cm above the canthi) (14,15). A high radix is associated with an obtuse nasofrontal angle and an overly long nose (e.g., Grecian profile). A low radix often gives the illusion of a foreshortened nasal dorsum and short nose. An obtuse nasofrontal angle (shallow radix) is associated with a Grecian profile, although this profile was appealing in ancient Greek culture, it is not considered attractive by today's standards. A useful index that reflects modern aesthetic standards regarding the depth of the radix is the ratio of the radix-to-corneal surface distance (r–c) to the corneal surface-to-lateral (external) canthus distance (c–ex). The index (r–c / c–ex) should be slight less than or equal to 1 (16) (Fig. 12). Overdevelopment of the proximal nasal bones results in a prominent (projecting) nasofrontal angle whose most posterior extent (radix) is above the level of the supratarsal fold. The caudal portions of the nasal bones are

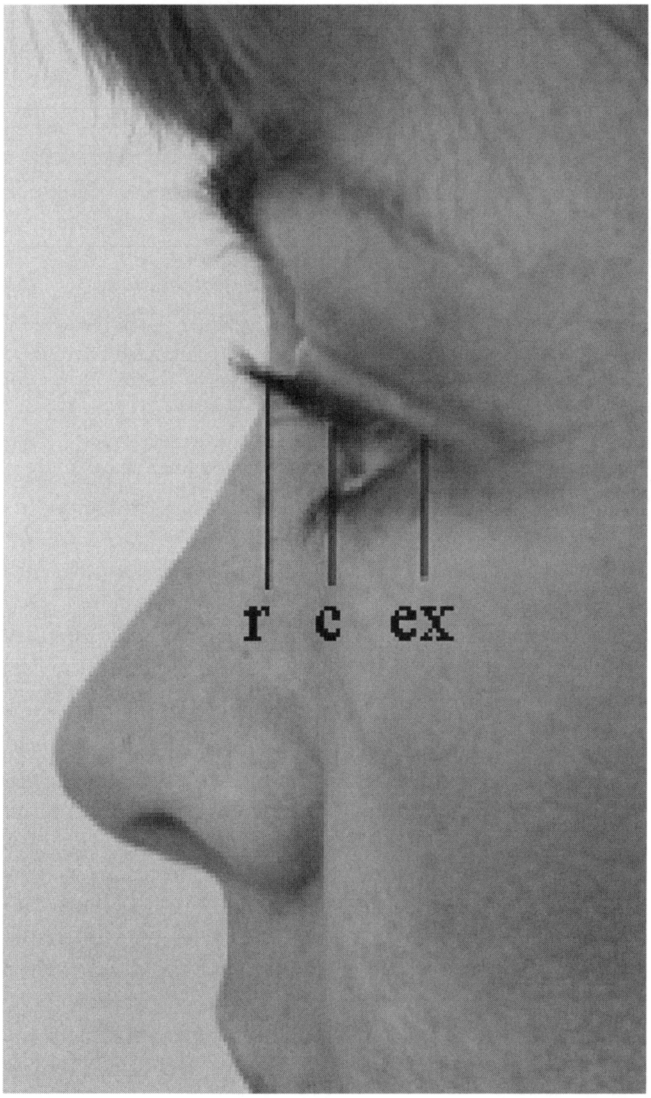

Figure 12 The ratio of the radix-to-corneal surface distance (r–c) to the corneal surface-to-lateral (external) canthus distance (c-ex) is a useful measure of radix depth. The index (r–c / c–ex) should be slight less than or equal to 1.

usually also overdeveloped, resulting in a slight hump. The nose appears larger and longer, often diminishing the appearance of the nasal tip. Conversely, underdevelopment of the proximal portion of the nasal bones results in a depressed (deep and inferior) nasofrontal angle and radix (17). This abnormality is also associated with mild-to-moderate overdevelopment of the caudal nasal bones, resulting in an exaggerated hump. The nose appears smaller and a normally projecting tip may appear overly projected and out of proportion with the foreshortened nasal dorsum. It is essential to consider the level of the nasofrontal angle and radix in surgical planning before modifications to the nasal dorsum are undertaken. If the unwary surgeon removes a hump in a patient with a depressed nasofrontal angle, the nose will appear small and out of balance with the face and nasal tip. The nasal dorsum will be foreshortened and the nasal tip will appear overprojected. A high radix would be an indication for glabellar rasping and a low radix would indicate a need for grafting. In routine rhinoplasty, the nasofrontal angle is generally not displaced and the surgeon need only address the nasal hump.

Nasolabial Angle. The nasolabial angle is the angle formed by the columella and upper lip in the midsagittal plane and is a useful measure of nasal tip rotation. Premaxillary deficiency and columellar malposition may significantly influence the appearance of this angle. A more precise method when the columellar position is not ideal is to assess nasal rotation by measuring the angle formed by the long axis of the nostril with the vertical facial plane. The aesthetic standard for this angle is 90–95 degrees in males and 95–100 degrees in females. An overly rotated tip will usually accompany a truly short nose and the nasolabial angle will invariably exceed the accepted aesthetic standard. Conversely, a so-called closed nose is characterized by an underrotation of the tip with a lack of projection, acute nasolabial angle, and nasal dorsum convexity. Similar findings may become evident in some patients during smiling and activation of their depressor septi muscles. The cause is unclear but muscular slips have been found that extend between the medial crura to insert into the tip lobule. If this condition is present, preoperative planning should include division of these fibers near the base of the columella. This will reduce tip hypermobility and enhance the effect of techniques designed to strengthen and project the medial crural component.

Nasal Tip Projection. Nasal tip projection is assessed by measuring the distance between the alar crease and the nasal tip. This measurement must be in balance with the rest of the nose. There are two common methods employed to determine if nasal projection is in balance with the face and nose. The first is Goode's method in which nasal length (radix to nasal tip) is used for comparison. According to Goode's method, the ideal nasal projection/nasal length ratio is 0.55–0.60 (Fig. 13). The main problem using this method is that the reference value (nasal length) may be abnormal, thus confounding the formula. For example, projection may be underestimated in a patient with an excessively long nose.

To avoid this pitfall, Crumley's method uses a straight reference line from the radix to the upper lip vermilion–cutaneous border. The length of the reference line (i.e., reference value) represents a measure of facial height independent of nasal length. Nasal projection is measured from the nasal tip along a line perpendicular and anterior to the reference line. According to Crumley's method, the ideal ratio of nasal projection to the reference value equals 0.2833 (18). Goode's method of

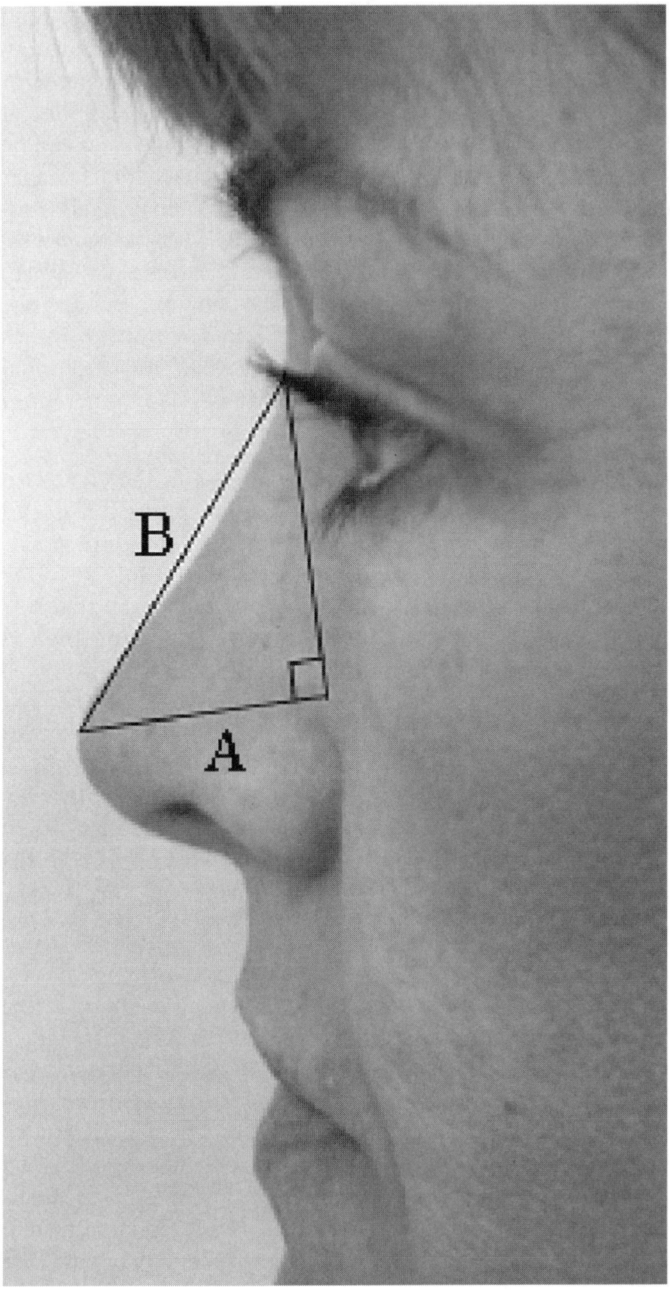

Figure 13 A useful measure of nasal projection is Goode's formula. The ideal nasal projection (A) nasal length (B) ratio is between 0.55 and 0.60.

objectively gauging nasal tip projection in a patient with an excessively long nose will erroneously indicate inadequate projection due to its reliance on nasal length in the equation. Crumley's method obviates the need to rely on nasal length or other intrinsic nasal features and can be more predictive of true abnormalities of nasal tip projection. Despite objective measurements, the illusion of inadequate nasal tip projection is created in patients with a long nose or a large dorsal hump. The nasal tip must be in balance with the rest of the nose and appropriately projected from the face. The most basic of rhinoplastic procedures with the most predictable results come from surgeries in which no tip work has been performed. Once the tip structure and support mechanisms have been violated by surgery, healing will guide the final outcome. This is the most demanding portion of rhinoplasty and is sometimes fraught with the most uncertainty. Evaluation is essential to know what structures need altering and what aesthetic traits already inherent in the tip should be preserved.

Chin Projection. The visual relationship between the nose and the chin is so intimate that to change the size and shape of one influences the apparent size and shape of the other. Chin projection is most directly evaluated by determining its relationship to a line dropped perpendicular to Frankfort's line from the radix. The pogonion is most aesthetically tangent to or slightly posterior to this line (Fig. 14). In nasal analysis, it is also helpful to evaluate the position of the chin in relation to nasal and facial projection using the so-called aesthetic triangle of Powell and Humphries (14). The base of the triangle is along a line connecting the radix and pogonion and its apex is at the nasal tip. Angles formed by the triangle that reflect the dynamic relationship between the nose and the chin include the nasomental angle and the nasofacial angle. The nasomental angle is formed at the junction of the tip–pogonion line with the tip–radix line; ideally, it is between 130 and 140. The nasofacial angle is formed at the junction of the nasal dorsum with the base (radix–pogonion line) and is ideally between 35 and 40 degrees. Abnormalities of chin projection, frontal bosselation, or saddle nose will affect the depth of the angle and give an indication of the correction needed.

Columellar and Alar Fold Position. On lateral view, columellar show is the amount of columella visible below the nostril margin. The ideal profile displays 2–3 mm of columella show (5). A more refined way of evaluating columellar show is to assess critically the positions of both the alar rim and the inferior edge of the columella. This is accomplished by using a reference line through the long axis of the nostril. The distance between this reference line and the alar rim and/or columella should be 1–2 mm. If the distance between the reference line and the columella is greater than 2 mm it is considered hanging, usually due to excessively large medial crura, excess membranous or caudal septum, or an enlarged nasal spine. A retracted columella is one less than 1 mm from the reference line. If the distance between the reference line and the alar rim is more that 2 mm, the ala is considered retracted. An alar rim that dips to within less than 1 mm of the reference line is characterized as hanging. A retracted or hanging ala should be differentiated from an ala that inserts too high or too low into the cheek (ala–cheek junction). If the insertion is abnormal, the long axis of the nostril may be altered and the reference line used to judge the position of the columella and ala will be fallacious. The ala–cheek junction should be at a level superior to the caudal posterior columella, resulting in some columellar

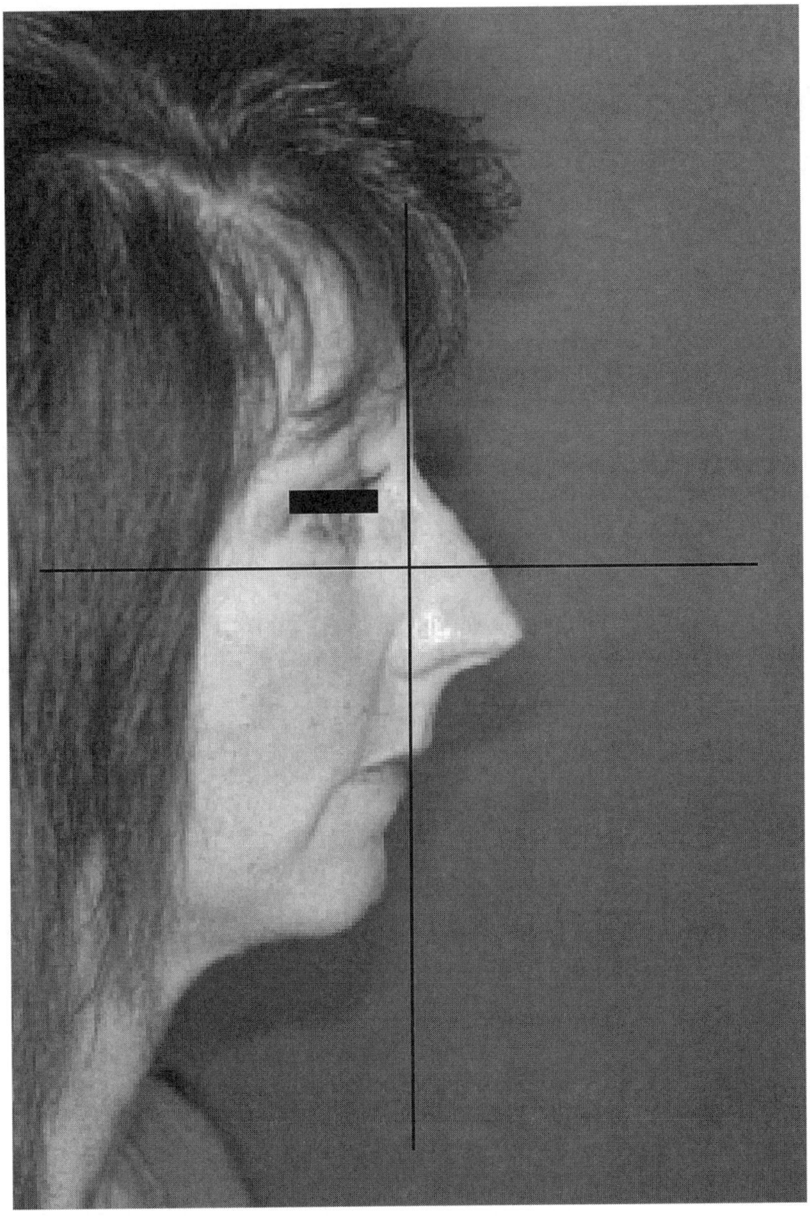

Figure 14 Example of a patient with chin retrusion based on a line dropped from Frankfurt's horizontal. The pogonion is most aesthetic tangent to or slightly posterior to this line.

show. An inferiorly or superiorly attached ala often appears excessively straight and long. By evaluating individually the positions of the nostril margin, columella, and ala–cheek junction, misdiagnoses can be avoided. Repositioning the columella requires augmentation (e.g., cartilage grafting) in cases of retraction and cartilage and/ or membranous septum reduction in cases in which the columella is hanging.

Correction of a retracted alar rim may require cartilage grafting or alteration of the level at which the ala joins the cheek in cases of a high ala–cheek junction.

Basal View

Aesthetic tip architecture is a rounded, thin appearance that looks like an equilateral triangle on basal view. Important elements in the basal view include footplate flare, caudal septum deviation, nostril flare and shape, and lobule width and height. Problems with the configuration of the nasal base and nostrils may only become evident after the nasal tip has been modified. Nostril flaring and nasal base widening are commonly encountered after an overly projecting tip is reduced.

Footplate Flare and Caudal Septal Deviation. The medial crural footplates play a significant role in the shape of the lower half of the columella and inferomedial nostril. Excessive flaring of the footplates produces characteristic symmetrical widening in the lower half of the columella. The combination of excessive flaring and inadequate nasal projection is common. In these cases, approximating the footplates with suture will improve projection and reduce the flaring deformity.

Deviation of the caudal septum will also affect the shape appearance of the columellar nasal base (Fig. 15). Septoplasty in this area often requires separation of the footplates from the septum, replacement of the deflected caudal strut centrally, and re-establishment of the connection between the footplates and the septum.

Nostril Flare. Nostril flare is the outward curvature of the ala. Excessive flare can cause an apparent increase in the width of the nose in its lower third. A certain amount of flaring is desirable and must be in balance with the face and nasal base. Flaring and facial balance can be assessed by examining vertical lines dropped from the medial canthi on frontal view. The external surfaces of the nostrils should ideally fall tangent to these lines. Ideally, the nasal creases also fall on the intercanthal lines. Therefore, nostril flaring can be considered excessive if the external aspects of the nasal lobules extend beyond the intercanthal lines and alar creases. The level of excess flare is important since flaring at the midlobule level is treated differently than a widened nasal base or flaring at or below the nasal sill. The overall shape and thickness of the alar lobules should also be noted. The ideal nose in a white patient has nostrils that are pear-shaped and the thickness of an alar lobule should be less than one-fifth of the total width of the nasal base. Typical surgical alar modifications involve reducing flaring, narrowing the nasal base, and (less commonly) defatting excessively thick alar lobules. These modifications are needed only occasionally in white patients but are routinely needed in non-white patients undergoing rhinoplasties. Surgical planning must include the anticipated changes in flaring and shape of the alar lobules that occur following surgical adjustments in nasal projection.

Lobule Width/Base Ratio. The tip lobule is the portion of the tip that lies above the apex of the nostrils on basal view and consists of the domes and soft tissue covering. The descriptions of the boundaries of the lobule are inconsistent. The nasal lobule is frequently defined as including the nasal tip, alae, and columella: essentially the lower third of the nose between the alar creases. For the purpose of nasal analysis, the nasal lobule is defined more specifically as including, in the horizontal plane, the area encompassed by the lower lateral cartilages. The lateral borders of the lobule correspond to the alar grooves, which are usually easily discernible on

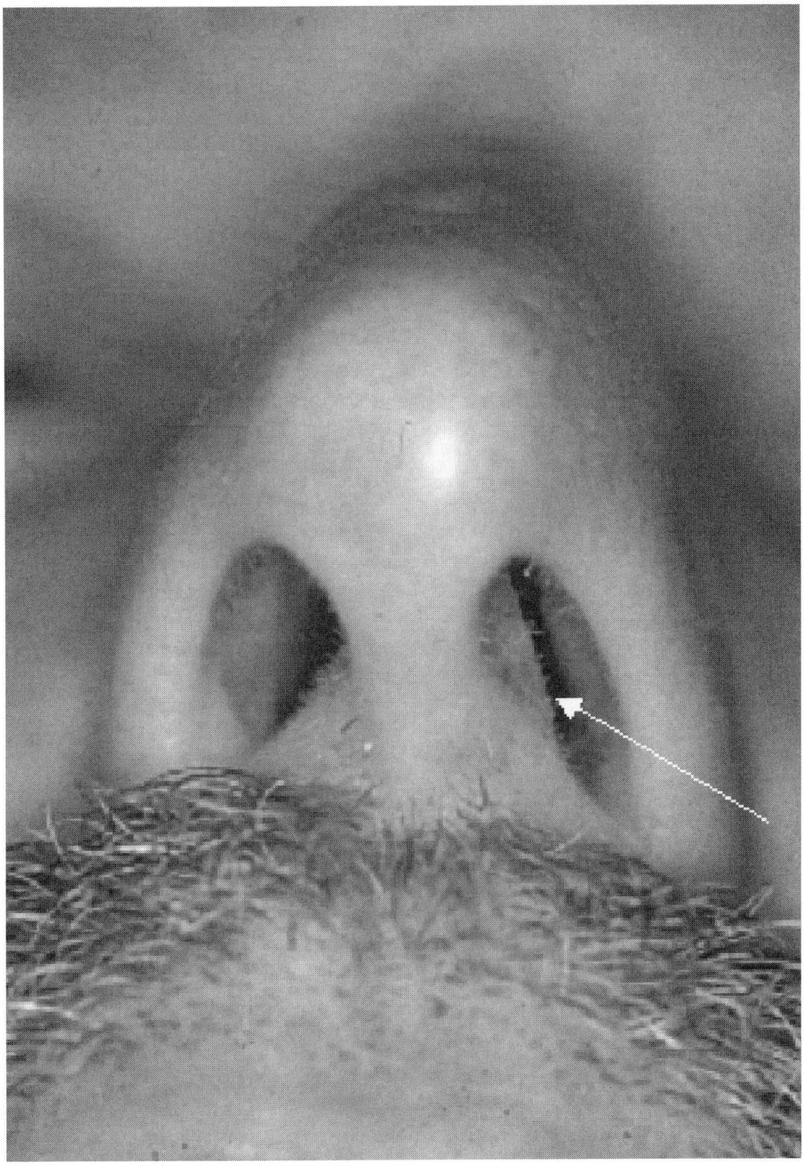

Figure 15 Caudal septal deviation on basal view (arrow).

the basal view. More specifically, the horizontal extent of the nasal lobule is defined as the demarcation between the soft tissue of the alae and the outer edges of the lower lateral cartilages accentuated by the cephalic sweep of the lateral crura. In basic nasal analysis, it is helpful to compare the width of the lobule to the width of the nasal base because these structures must be in balance. The ideal lobule width-to-nasal base width ratio is less than 0.75. Tip bifidity or bulbosity are common abnormalities leading to excessive lobular width.

Lobule Height/Columella. The height of the lobule on basal view is determined by measuring the distance between the nostril apex (columellar–lobular angle on profile) and the nasal tip. The columella is defined by the nostril apex (columellar–lobule angle on profile) and the nostril sill (nasolabial angle on profile). The ideal columella/lobule height ratio should be 2:1 and the length of the columella should equal the height of the philtrum. An overly projected nasal tip will commonly contain an overly tall lobule, bringing the proportion closer to 1:1.

Nasal Valves. The nasal valve (internal) is examined with the patient's head tilted backward and the examiner looking directly into the nostrils. Behind the apex of the nostril lies the nasal valve formed by the junction of the caudal upper lateral cartilage and the dorsal nasal septum. The normal angle formed by these structures is 10–15 degrees. The valve is considered dysfunctional if it is collapsed (static dysfunction) or collapses with mild inspiration (dynamic dysfunction). Static dysfunction is most common and is characterized by a valve permanently obstructed due to collapse or scarring. Dynamic dysfunction is characterized by premature closure as the airstream velocity increases. A variably dysfunctional valve is open and functional under some conditions but becomes statically or dynamically dysfunctional under other conditions, such as allergic rhinitis or turbinate hypertrophy associated with the nasal cycle. To determine if the patient will experience significant relief by the valve being opened, the valve can be manually opened by lateralization the upper lateral cartilage. Either the Cottle maneuver (lateral traction on the cheek) or direct lateralization by pushing the caudal end of the upper lateral cartilage with a cotton-tipped applicator may be used. Nevertheless, it is commonly used as a gross indication of valve function and the need for spreader grafts in complicated cases. The function and patency of the nasal valve are better assessed by direct visualization. By gently retracting the nasal ala and probing the upper lateral cartilages using the back end of a cotton-tipped applicator, static patency and pathology can be assessed.

Nasal valve dysfunction is commonly found in rhinoplasty patients who have undergone some degree of cephalic trimming of their lower lateral cartilages or removal of a dorsal hump. Removal of a dorsal hump or the act of separating the upper lateral cartilages from the septum disrupts the T configuration that the upper lateral cartilages share with the dorsal septum. The upper lateral cartilages tend to fall against the septum, closing the nasal valve. Externally, this is often associated with an overly narrowed middle vault and an inverted "V" deformity as the caudal edge of the nasal bones are brought into relief against a collapsed middle vault. Nasal valve obstruction may also occur in some patients with naturally narrow noses or deviated nasal bones or in rhinoplasty patients who have undergone lateral osteotomies and infracture of their nasal bones. A medialized nasal bone may cause secondary collapse of the nasal valve due to the rigid connection that the cephalic upper lateral cartilages share with the caudal nasal bone. A closed or narrow valve (static dysfunction) is the usual cause of nasal valve dysfunction and can be due to septal deviation, medial displacement of the caudal upper lateral cartilages, or scarring. Medialization of the upper lateral cartilages and scarring across the nasal valve are common findings, especially in post-rhinoplasty patients.

Nasal alar obstruction is diagnosed when there is obstruction of airflow along the nostril rim due to static abnormalities (deficient soft tissue, masses, or scarring)

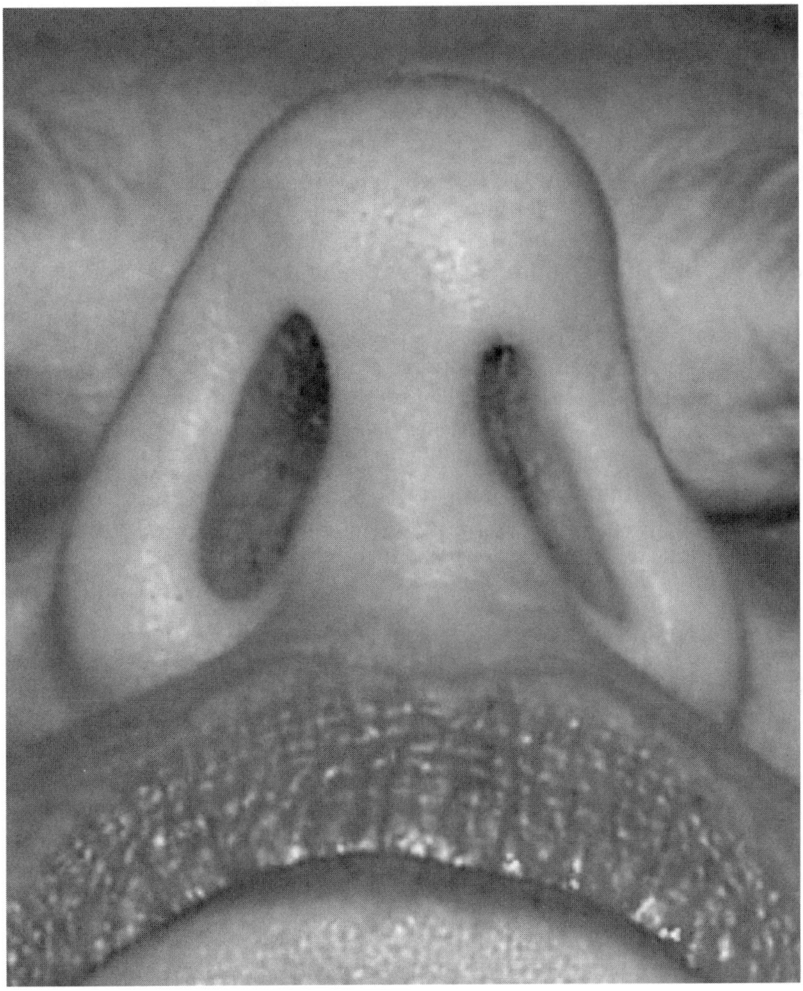

Figure 16 Dynamic alar collapse (left) due to brisk inhalation. This patient had lack of cartilaginous support due to cephalic malposition of the alar cartilage.

or dynamic alar collapse. Nasal alar dysfunction in patients undergoing primary or revision rhinoplasty is often due to dynamic alar collapse upon moderate to brisk inspiration (Fig. 16). This may occur in patients with thin alar sidewalls, overly projecting nasal tips, or slit-like nostrils.

ESSENTIALS OF RHINOPLASTY

Modern primary rhinoplasty is more complicated than the standard reduction rhinoplasties of the past. Each case is tailored to achieve the goals of rhinoplasty that reflect current trends including a natural, nonoperated look, a well-balanced nose and face, a stable and permanent result, and a functional nose. The same surgical maneuvers may result in different results in different noses. Facial analysis and an awareness of a variety of surgical techniques and their potential outcomes are critical to success. This individualized approach to modern rhinoplasty calls for a variety of specialized techniques. Nevertheless, certain techniques are used commonly for typical problems in patients seeking primary rhinoplasty. Most patients desire reduction of a nasal hump and tip refinement. Minor changes in tip rotation and projection may also be needed. Despite these seemingly simple goals, the preoperative analysis may uncover subtle problems that require techniques often considered to be advanced, such as grafting or suture modification of the lower lateral cartilages.

Surgical access is also an important consideration. Although a typical primary rhinoplasty can be done through a closed approach, many surgeons prefer an open approach for wide access and teaching. Therefore, familiarity with a variety of approaches and access incisions is required in basic rhinoplasty. After exposure of the dorsum and tip is accomplished, the first decision with regard to surgical corrections is whether to begin with the dorsum or the nasal tip. Traditional reduction rhinoplasty involved correcting the dorsum first with subsequent matching of the nasal tip. This done routinely will result in an overly reduced nasal tip in many patients. In general, it is better to begin with the more complex nasal tip and project it appropriately before altering the nasal dorsum.

Surgical correction of the nasal tip (tip-plasty) calls for a variety of techniques that are generally cartilage-sparing. Interrupted cartilage techniques, including dome division, are usually avoided. Although increasing nasal projection may be a part of the preoperative plan, it is accomplished by redistribution of cartilage within the nasal framework, not by the use of cartilage grafts or radical cartilage techniques. Nevertheless, some cartilage grafting may be used to improve tip definition (shield grafts), improve tip stability and projection (columellar strut grafts), and to counteract the effects of nasal osteotomy and cartilage excision on the nasal valves (spreader grafts).

Prior to working on the nasal dorsum, the projection of the nasal tip and position of the radix must be established. If the radix and nasal tip are appropriately projected and positioned preoperatively, and only tip refinement is planned, it makes no difference whether the dorsum is treated (e.g., removal of the nasal hump) before or after the nasal tip. Cosmetic improvement of the nasal dorsum generally entails reducing the width of the upper and middle cartilaginous vaults and correcting contour irregularities of the dorsum (e.g., eliminating a nasal hump). Altering the projection and vertical position of the nasofrontal angle is also considered. Reducing the widths of the upper and middle nasal vaults is accomplished by osteotomies within the upper third of the nose (bony vault). The firm attachments of the cephalic upper lateral cartilages to the caudal nasal bones ensure that medial movement of the nasal bones will also result in medial movement (narrowing) of the upper lateral cartilages and middle nasal vault. Multiple osteotomies may be required to accomplish the desired effect. The most common osteotomies that simply narrow the nasal bones include the medial osteotomy and the lateral osteotomy. If a dorsal hump has been removed, a so-called open roof deformity is created and medial osteotomies are not required because the medial aspects of the nasal bones are already released. Hence, in the typical primary rhinoplasty only lateral osteotomies are required.

After tip-plasty, nasal dorsum work, and establishment of the radix, the nasal valves are carefully examined. The nasal valves are often narrowed excessively due to medialization of the upper lateral cartilages. Insertion of spreader grafts can reverse this phenomenon by splinting open the nasal valves. A secondary effect of spreader grafting is slight widening of the middle third of the nose (middle vault). This can bring the middle and upper thirds of the nose into better balance while preventing the operated look of an inverted V deformity.

Anesthesia

Rhinoplasty can be done under local anesthesia with sedation without difficulty. Benzodiazepines (e.g., Diazepam 10–20 mg) are given 1–2 h prior to surgery. Intraoperative sedative anesthesia (Propofol or Fentanyl) is administered in the presence of a trained anesthesiologist. Locally injected anesthesia effectively desensitizes the nose in preparation for rhinoplasty. Initially, cotton pledgets immersed in 2–4% cocaine (or 1:10,000 epinephrine or an over-the-counter nasal decongestant) are inserted into the nasal cavities. This causes intense vasoconstriction that improves access and makes it less likely that the injectable anesthetic will be accidentally infused intravascularly. The typical injectable anesthetic solution contains 1 or 2% lidocaine with 1:100,000 or 1:200,000 epinephrine. Specific nerve blocks may be performed but the usual method is simply to inject the entire nasal dorsum and tip in the subcutaneous and submucosal planes. This results in complete anesthesia of the external nasal branches of the infraorbital nerve, the infratrochlear nerves, and the external nasal branches of the anterior ethmoidal nerves. The amount of anesthetic solution should be limited so that minimal soft tissue distortion occurs; the entire nose can usually be anesthetized with less than 2 ml. Additional anesthetic may be needed for the septum and turbinates. Ten to 15 min should elapse prior to the first incision to allow the epinephrine to cause maximal vasoconstriction.

Access Incisions

Several unique incisions are useful to expose and alter important structural elements in rhinoplasty (Fig. 17). It is essential to understand the nomenclature, the secondary effects of the incision on the major and minor tip support mechanisms, and the role the incision has with regard to the overall surgical approach and exposure.

Intercartilaginous

An intercartilaginous incision is placed between the cephalic border of the lateral crus and the caudal border of the upper lateral cartilage. It disrupts the major tip-supporting attachments of the lower lateral cartilage with the upper lateral cartilage (scroll area). However, without resection of the cephalic border of the lower lateral cartilage, there is no tissue void left after the incision and postoperative healing rarely results in long-term loss of tip support. The intercartilaginous incision provides access to the entire middle and upper nasal vaults and, through retrograde vestibular mucosal dissection, the cephalic aspect of the lateral crus.

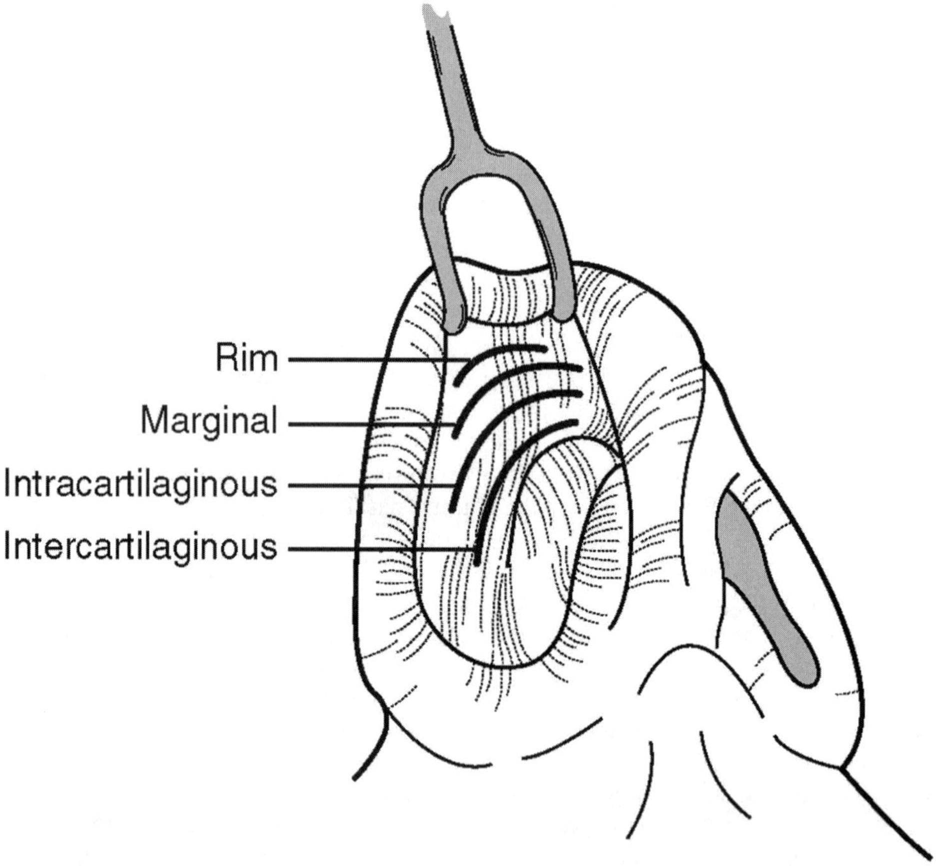

Figure 17 Various nasal access incisions including rim, marginal, intracartilaginous, and intercartilaginous. The latter three incisions must follow the superolateral curvature of the nasal ala and will deviate significantly from the nostril rim as one proceeds from medial to lateral.

Intracartilaginous (cartilage-splitting)

An intracartilaginous incision is made caudal to the cephalic border of the lateral crus resulting in transection of the cartilage. This incision allows direct excision of the desired amount of cartilage (cephalic border of the lateral crus) with minimal manipulation of the surrounding tissue. The typical intracartilaginous incision will result in a complete strip. This incision also disrupts the major tip-supporting attachments of the lower lateral cartilages with the upper lateral cartilages (scroll area). The impact of this incision on tip support and cephalic rotation is proportional to the width of the cartilage excised and volume loss between the lateral crus and caudal border of the upper lateral cartilages. Like the intercartilaginous incision, this incision provides access to the middle and upper nasal vaults. Drawbacks to this incision include limited visualization of the lower lateral cartilage. Manipulation and shaping of the cartilage are impeded and symmetry is difficult to assess. Correction of boxy or bulky nasal tips is best performed through incisions designed to deliver or fully expose the cartilages. Although an intercartilaginous incision is typically used to deliver the lower lateral cartilage, an intracartilaginous incision can also be used.

Marginal

A full marginal incision is made along the entire caudal border of the lower lateral cartilage. Additional incisions must be made to expose the cartilage since a marginal incision alone will not be sufficient to expose any more than the caudal border of the medial and lateral crura. A full marginal incision is combined with a transcolumellar incision in the open rhinoplasty approach. A partial marginal incision encompassing the lateral and middle crura is combined with an intercartilaginous incision in the delivery approach for exposure of the medial and lateral crura. The caudal border of the lateral crus does not follow the nostril rim but extends cephalically and is most closely related to the cephalic border of the nasal vibrissae. When making a marginal incision, whether for an open approach or to deliver the lower lateral cartilage, the most critical area is at the soft triangle. If the marginal incision is brought too close the nostril rim in this area, scar tissue may form and obliterate the concavity that defines the soft triangle. The incision must follow the caudal aspect of the lower lateral cartilage closely to avoid this complication. The marginal incision does not disrupt any of the tip-support mechanisms.

Transcolumellar

A transcolumellar incision may be oriented vertically or horizontally. A vertical incision in the midcolumella is useful for the direct placement of columellar strut grafts. It heals very well and leaves an insignificant scar. Several types of horizontally oriented transcolumellar incisions can be used to approach the nasal septum and nasal cartilages. The most common indication for a transcolumellar incision is for external rhinoplasty, and it is usually in the form of a W or inverted V placed just superior to the feet of the medial crura (midcolumellar). The incision is brought around the medial crura to merge with the intranasal marginal incisions along the caudal borders of the lower lateral cartilages. Combining the transcolumellar incision with the marginal incisions provides access to all of the structural elements (hence the designation open structure rhinoplasty or simply open rhinoplasty).

Transfixion

A nasal transfixion incision is performed by passing a knife through-and-through the membranous septum anterior to the septal angles. It is usually joined with an intercartilaginous incision. If the transfixion is brought down to the medial crural feet it is referred to as partial transfixion; if it is carried through the junction of the footplates with the caudal septum (i.e., the medial crural feet are separated from the caudal septum) it is referred to as a full transfixion. A partial transfixion incision provides enhanced exposure to the septal angle and dorsal septum while preserving the attachment of the medial crural footplates to the caudal septum. A full (complete) transfixion incision provides maximal exposure to the caudal septum but interrupts the major tip-support mechanism provided by the connection of the footplates to the caudal septum. A full transfixion incision may be combined with procedures designed to attenuate the lateral crura to bring about retrodisplacement of the nasal tip. A full transfixion incision (without fixation of the footplates to the caudal septum) will result in tip ptosis in some patients with otherwise normally projecting nasal tips.

Modified Transfixion

A modified transfixion incision is used in rare cases or revisions when work is only needed near the septal angle. It is commonly used as a surgical approach to either reshape the angle due to pollybeak or place a graft for definition or projection. This incision only extends 2–3 mm inferior to the anterior septal angle.

Hemitransfixion

A hemitransfixion incision courses through the ipsilateral membranous septum only without disrupting the medial crus. It is most often used to approach the septum during routine septoplasty. A Killian incision is similar to a hemitransfixion incision except it is made on the quadrilateral cartilage approximately 1 cm behind its caudal edge.

Alar Base (Nasal sill)

Sometimes it is necessary to narrow the nasal base, alae, or floor of the nasal vestibule (nasal sill). The incision bridges the vestibular mucosa of the nasal sill and the skin overlying the attachment of the ala to the base of the nose. A section of skin and soft tissue of the medial ala is removed at the base and the ala is then sutured medially. A classic Weir incision involves removal of a crescent-shaped piece of ala in its midportion by incisions created in the ala itself.

Closed vs. Open Approach

There are several methods to expose the nasal cartilages in rhinoplasty. Modern rhinoplastic surgery is performed through either a closed or an open approach. Closed approaches utilize only transmucosal intranasal incisions while an open approach uses a combination of transmucosal incisions and a transcutaneous (transcolumellar) incision. Conventional practice is first to consider closed approaches because they avoid cutaneous scarring, tend to be less time-consuming, and often require less tissue undermining. Nevertheless, closed approaches tend to disrupt the major tip-support mechanisms.

Closed approaches may involve manipulation of the cartilages in situ (i.e., nondelivery) or exteriorization of the lower lateral cartilages (i.e., delivery). A nondelivery approach is least invasive and involves altering the upper lateral cartilage in situ via an intercartilaginous or intracartilaginous incision. A complete strip procedure is possible either through retrograde dissection of the vestibular mucosa from the lateral crus or by directly incising the cephalic edge of the lateral crus through the vestibular lining. Retrograde dissection is performed through an intercartilaginous incision; direct cartilage excision is performed via the intracartilaginous incision. Either method disrupts the upper lateral cartilage–lower lateral cartilage attachment and results in tip rotation and a minor degree of loss of tip support. A nondelivery approach is useful in patients who require only minimal tip rotation and some volume reduction. Delivery of the lateral crus requires marginal and intercartilaginous incisions. Dissection proceeds between the perichondrium and skin over the dome and lateral aspect of the lateral crus. A cotton-tipped applicator or retractor is inserted into the pocket to evert the lateral crus and bring it into the nasal cavity. Delivery of the lateral crus allows direct observation of the anatomical variations that may be present. Cartilage delivery is indicated when the anatomy is unknown or irregular, or if full access to the cartilage is necessary for the accurate placement of sutures, struts, or contouring grafts. Correction of asymmetrical cartilages often requires a delivery or external rhinoplasty approach. Techniques that often require cartilage delivery or full visualization include interrupted cartilage techniques or placement of transdomal and interdomal sutures. This approach is ideal for patients with slightly asymmetrical nasal tips and irregular lateral crura that require refinement and rotation of the tip. Tip defatting and scar excision are also possible with this approach.

Padovan introduced the open (external) rhinoplasty approach to North America in 1973 from France (19). After the transcolumellar and marginal incisions are made, subcutaneous dissection proceeds raising the skin and SMAS off the perichondrium of the lower and middle thirds of the nose. The dissection plane over the nasal tip and middle vault should remain submuscular (i.e., under the SMAS) to preserve the blood supply to the skin and prevent skin necrosis over the nasal tip. As the caudal aspect of the nasal bones is approached, the plane of dissection shifts to a subperiosteal level. The entire nasal dorsum is exposed allowing direct visualization and manipulation of the nasal cartilages, septum, and nasal bones (Fig. 18). The septum may be exposed via a caudal or dorsal approach. The caudal approach involves separation of the medial crura and dissection through the membranous septum to reach the caudal aspect of the nasal septum (Fig. 19). The dorsal approach involves careful separation of the upper lateral cartilages usually starting at the septal angle and proceeding in a cephalic direction (Fig. 20). The medial aspects of the upper lateral cartilages must be sharply separated from the dorsal septum with care taken not to disrupt the underlying mucosa surrounding the nasal valves. Mucoperiosteal flaps may then be widely dissected to allow modification or removal of the entire septum.

At the completion of the procedure, the medial crura may be sutured to the caudal septum to re-establish this major tip support mechanism. In addition, a single buried 4-0 chromic suture is used to approximate the transcolumellar incision in the midline. Additional cutaneous sutures are placed along the lateral aspects of the transcolumellar incision and along the marginal incisions within the nasal vestibule. Carefully reapproximating the mucosal incision avoids healing irregularities and covers grafts and cartilage sutures. Small intercartilaginous stab incisions can be safely made to promote drainage, if necessary.

The primary indication for the external rhinoplasty approach is for improved exposure of the nasal tip. It is useful in revisions when the operative anatomy of the nasal tip is irregular or unknown; in cases of moderate to severe nasal bone or cartilage asymmetry (twisted nose); congenital malformations including cleft lip; and for primary rhinoplasty that requires extensive tip alterations and grafts. Advantages of the open approach include direct and accurate assessment and treatment of cartilage and bone abnormalities, ease and accuracy of suture placement, direct access to the nasal cartilaginous dorsum (including the quadrilateral septal cartilage), and teaching. Direct visualization of the complex anatomy facilitates learning and mastery of rhinoplasty. The disadvantages to the open approach include that it is more time-consuming, cutaneous scarring, operative edema, subcutaneous scarring, and nasal

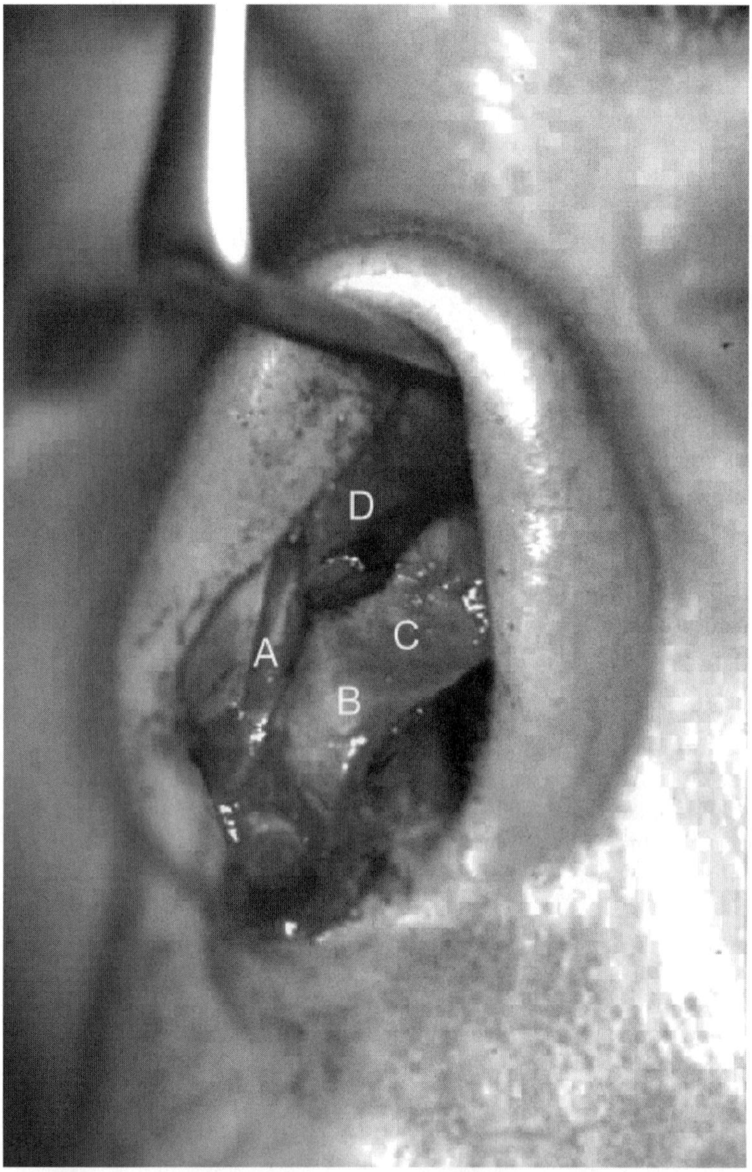

Figure 18 Exposure obtained through the open approach. Note the septal angle (A), anatomical dome (B), alar cartilage (C), and upper lateral cartilage (D).

tip anesthesia (temporary). The cutaneous (transcolumellar) scarring is of minimal concern and, if properly performed, is rarely problematic.

THE NASAL TIP

In the typical rhinoplasty, trimming and suture modification of the lower lateral cartilages to improve the nasal tip are all that is needed. Overuse of grafts, interrupted

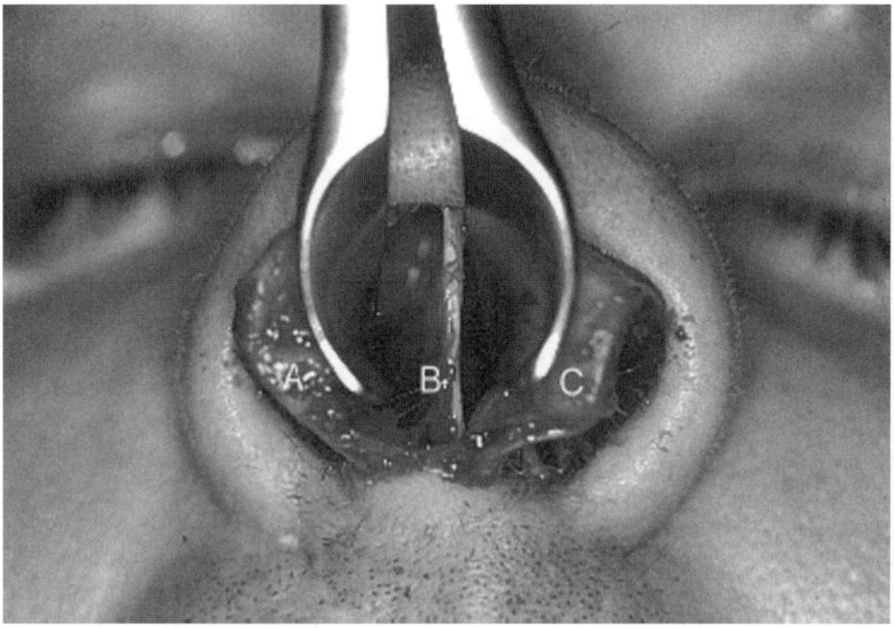

Figure 19 Caudal approach to the nasal septum in an open rhinoplasty. Note the right lower lateral cartilage (LLC) (A), caudal septum (B), and left LLC (B).

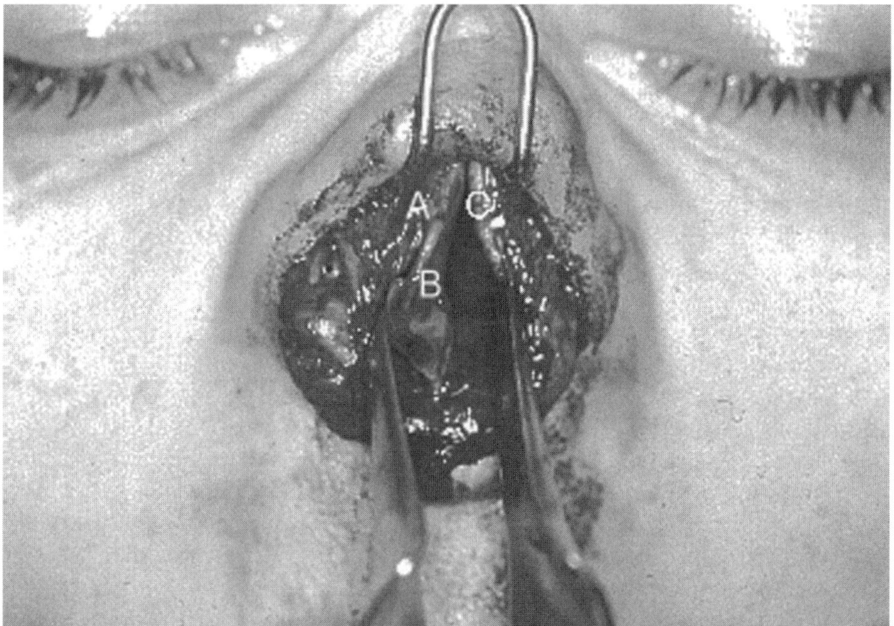

Figure 20 Dorsal approach to the nasal septum in an open rhinoplasty. Note the right ULC (A), anterior septal angle (B), and left upper lateral cartilage (ULC) (B).

strip procedures, and radical excisional techniques are to be avoided. Structural grafts (e.g., columellar strut or lateral crural strut grafts) are being used more liberally in primary rhinoplasty because minor postoperative warping and resorption problems are less noticeable compared to surface grafts (e.g., tip onlay or shield grafts), but are not the standard in uncomplicated cases (Fig. 21). Volume reduction, cephalic rotation, and increase in definition are the most common objectives in nasal tip surgery. These can be achieved using conservative complete strip procedures, limited morselization, and approximating suture techniques (Table 2).

The Lower Lateral Cartilages

Complete Strip

The lateral crura are often modified during nasal tip surgery to correct deformities or increase tip definition (Fig. 22). The complete strip technique removes a portion of the cephalic edge of the lower lateral cartilage (intermediate and lateral portions) leaving a *complete* intact strip of cartilage laterally (Fig. 23). The strip, in all of these procedures, refers to portion of cartilage that remains. This is the most common form of volume reduction performed. It acts to reduce supratip fullness by removing the scroll area of the lower lateral cartilage, narrow the tip at the dome, and create tip rotation (albeit minimal). To preserve nasal support and minimize cephalic tip rotation, the remaining cartilage strip should be at least 5 mm in width (usually 8–10 mm). Preserving an adequate strip is essential to prevent postoperative complications including asymmetrical healing, alar notching, and unpredictable cephalic rotation. Loss of projection is usually not associated with this technique.

A complete strip procedure is possible through a retrograde (intracartilaginous), delivery, or open approach. Retrograde dissection is performed through an intercartilaginous incision and the delivery approach is performed via intercartilaginous and marginal incisions. The intracartilaginous approach is used in cases where the domes are not thought to be bifid and do not need modification, or when the tip may be bulbous or just in need of thinning. Delivery is used when the anatomy is unknown, irregular, or if full access to the cartilage is necessary for the accurate placement of sutures, struts, and contouring grafts. Of course, an external rhinoplasty approach may also be used and will provide a direct in-situ view of the entire nasal skeleton including the lower lateral cartilages. The open approach is superior in terms of diagnosis, ease of graft placement, and cartilage modification.

The retrograde approach should begin with the surgeon measuring the diameter of the lower lateral cartilages on the vestibular side of the nostril. A decision is made as to where the incision should be placed: remember to preserve at least 4–5 mm cartilage. The incision is made through the vestibular skin and cartilage paralleling the direction of the cartilage up to the dome internally. Converse scissors can be used to dissect the cartilage away from its surrounding soft tissue through the incision as an assistant puts gentle traction on the incised edge of vestibular mucosa. The cleaned cartilage to be removed is then dissected from the vestibular mucosa with care taken not to damage the lining. Once the cartilage is removed, the mucosa is replaced and sutured back with 4–0 chromic gut sutures.

Marginal incisions are made at the edge of the lower lateral cartilages along the vestibular lining paralleling the edge from lateral to medial, through the domal area.

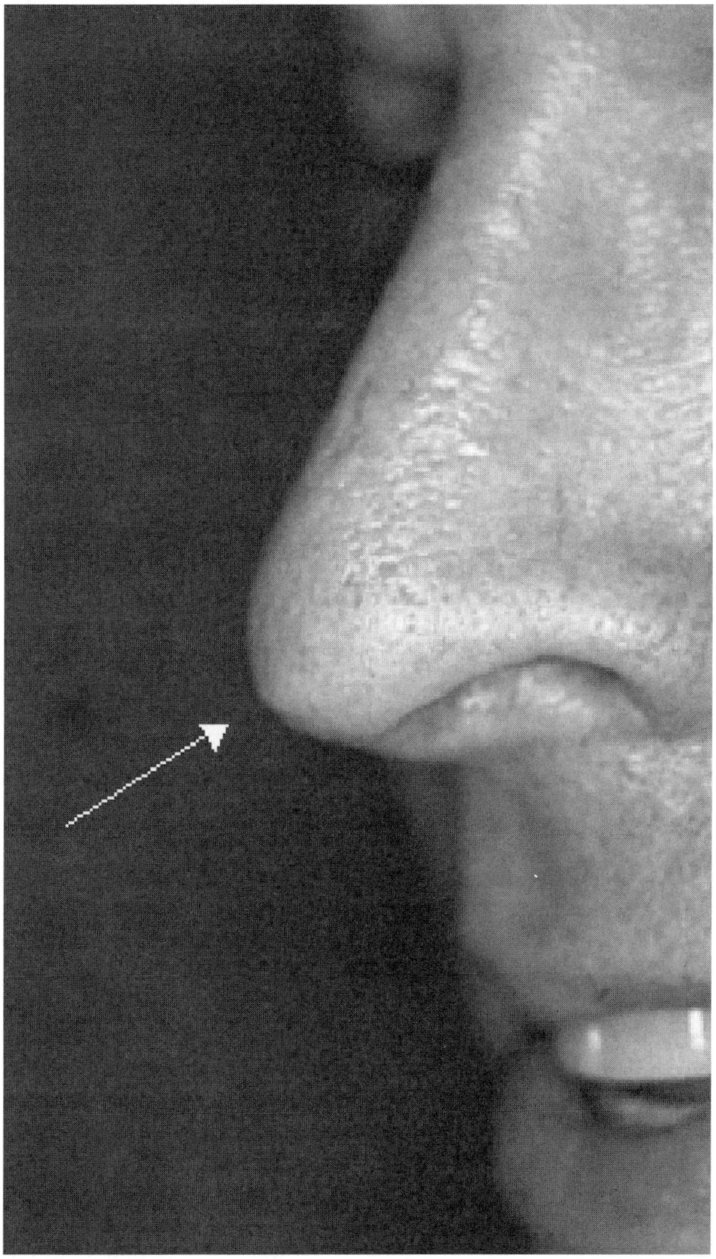

Figure 21 Example of a noticeable shield graft placed during primary rhinoplasty that was later removed. Note the unwanted acute convexity under the arrow indicating the cephalic aspect of the graft.

Table 2 Surgical Modifications of the Lower Lateral Cartilage and Their Effects on Tip Projection, Rotation, and Nasal Length

		Projection	Cephalic rotation	Nasal length
Lateral Crura and domes	Complete strip	−	+	−
	Lateral crural flap	−	++	−−
	Rim strip	−	++	−−
	Morselization of dome	+/−	+/−	~
	Lateral crus division	−	+++	−−
	Dome division	−−	++++	−−−
	Goldman's vertical dome division and advancement	+++	+++	−−−
	Shield grafting	++	~	++
	Onlay grafting	+++	~	+
	Marginal grafting	~	~	+
	Cephalic interposition grafting	+	−−	++
Medial crura	Columellar strut graft	+++	+	−
	Plumping graft	+	+	−
	Lateral crural steal	+++	++	−−
	Septocolumellar sutures	+	+	~
	Suture approximation	+	+	~
	Full transfixion incision	−−	−	~
	Medial crural segmental resection	−−−	−	~

A cotton-tipped applicator or Goldman groove director is inserted into the pocket to evert the lateral crus and bring it into the nasal cavity. Delivery of the lateral crus allows direct observation of the anatomical variations that may be present. At this point a complete or rim strip procedure can be performed with removal of the superior aspect of the lower lateral cartilage with precision. Correction of asymmetrical cartilages often requires a delivery technique or external rhinoplasty approach. This approach is ideal for patients with slightly asymmetrical nasal tips and irregular lateral crura that require refinement and rotation of the tip. Tip defatting and scar excision are also possible.

Rim Strip

The cartilage incision that produces a rim strip extends from near the dome through the lateral crus, posteriorly transecting its caudal margin (20). This procedure leads to more pronounced changes in tip rotation and volume reduction. The incision parallels the nostril margin, leaving a large island of lateral crus superolaterally to be resected. This results in a large structural void between the rim strip and caudal upper lateral cartilage. It is usually performed through a delivery approach. Removing more cartilage near the dome produces greater cephalic rotation while removing more cartilage posteriorly produces greater tip retrodisplacement. However, the amount of tip retrodisplacement and cephalic rotation is often unpredictable and

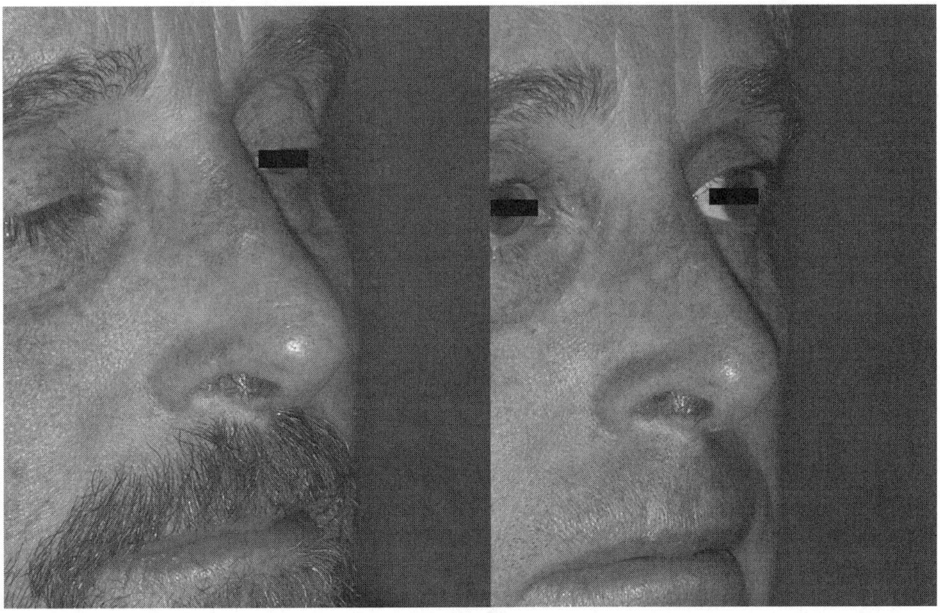

Figure 22 Preoperative and postoperative views of a patient undergoing complete strip to better define the nasal tip. The patient had a bulbous nasal tip with fullness apparent in the supratip lobule (left photo). After conservative trimming of the cephalic upper lateral cartilages, the bulbosity and fullness are significantly improved (right photo).

problems with alar rim notching and irregularities are common. A rim strip is rarely used except in cases requiring scar debulking to correct a severe pollybeak deformity or in patients with thick skin that require marked cephalic rotation. It may be helpful in cases when vertical dome division is not needed but rotation is desired.

Interrupted Strip

Goldman described vertical dome division over 40 years ago (21). He emphasized the use of the medial crura in augmenting tip projection and narrowing the nasal tip by recruiting cartilage from the lateral crura. The technique involves complete transection of the lateral crura just lateral to the dome including the underlying vestibular mucosal, removal of the intervening connective tissue between the medial crura, and suturing the medial crura and associated lateral crura remnants together in the midline to form a projecting strut of cartilage beneath the tip lobule (Fig. 24). This procedure can be safely used in patients with relatively thick skin in which the cut edges of the cartilage will be adequately camouflaged. The lateral crus should be divided no more than 3 mm lateral to the anatomical dome. This maneuver will result in significant cephalic tip rotation while avoiding asymmetrical healing and scar contracture over the more vulnerable medial areas. Problems include borrowing too much of the lateral crura, which will create a pinched appearance to the nasal tip; unpredictable healing, often leading to an asymmetrical tip, cartilage bosses; alar notching; and undesirable pronounced cephalic rotation of the tip. Routine use of this procedure to increase projection and narrow the nasal tip has been abandoned.

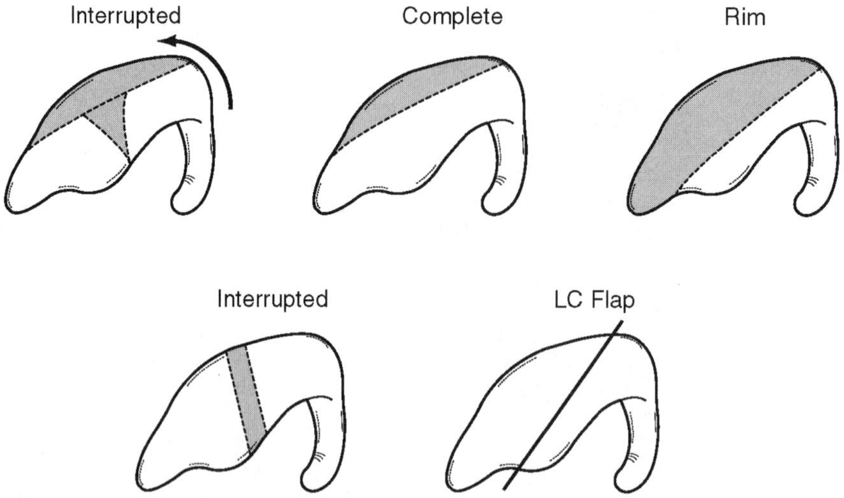

Figure 23 A variety of common incisional and excisional techniques are useful in shaping and rotating the nasal tip. A complete strip leaves the majority of the alar cartilage intact, trimming away an appropriate portion to improve tip definition and reduce fullness in the supratip lobule. A rim strip only leaves a remnant (rim) of alar cartilage, resulting in significant cephalic rotation of the nasal tip and reduced fullness in the supratip lobule and lateral aspect of the nose. An interrupted strip entails an incision or excision of cartilage along the alar cartilage or lobule. Depending on where the interrupted strip is placed along the cartilage, there can be minor cephalic rotation (lateral cut) or major cephalic rotation and dome sharpening (medial cut). An interrupted strip is sometimes combined with a complete strip to weaken the cartilage further. This is useful in cases of extremely boxy and bulbous tips with resilient cartilages. A lateral cural flap is useful to achieve a measure degree of cephalic rotation with more predictable postoperative healing.

The procedure is nevertheless used in selected cases of boxy tips, ptotic tips, so-called closed noses in which the columella–labia angle is acute, foreshortened columella, and in patients with thick skin (ethnic rhinoplasty). There is still controversy between proponents of Goldman's tip division technique and the more modern techniques that involve suture modification and cartilage grafting.

Morselization

Morselizing the lower lateral cartilages, although not commonplace, is a good method for refining misshapen cartilages. Morselization can aid in smoothing out lateral crura bosses as well as domal irregularities prior to suturing. The technique involves using a guarded morselizer. The guard should be placed on the mucosal side of the cartilage to prevent destruction of the underlying soft tissue. If the cartilage has been dissected away from its mucosal attachments, as in the lateral crural flap or steal procedures, then the morselizer need not be guarded.

Suture Modifications

Although sutures may be required to stabilize altered cartilages or to secure grafts, they are also capable of bringing about significant structural changes, especially in

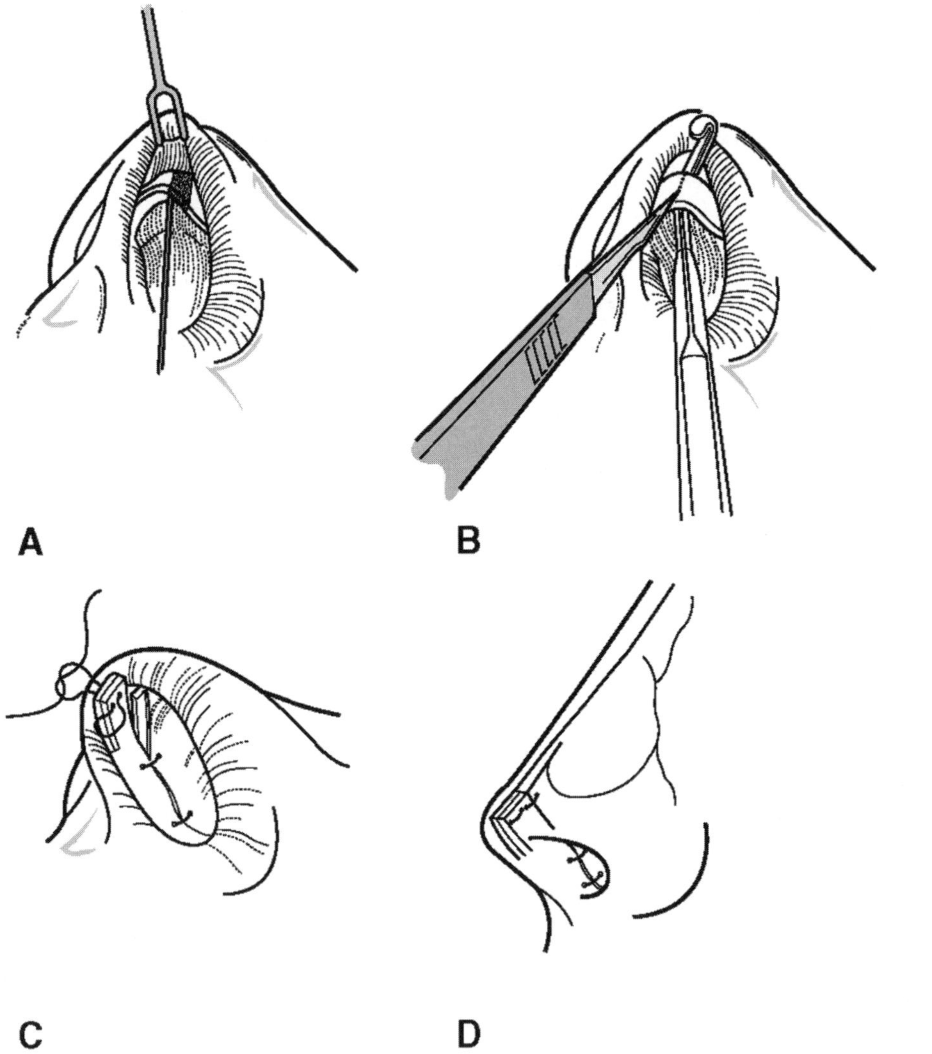

Figure 24 Goldman's vertical dome division. Note that the medial aspects of the lateral crura are recruited to enhance nasal projection.

the lower lateral cartilages and nasal tip. Most commonly, sutures are useful to change a trapezoidal tip into a more rounded configuration by bringing the domes into apposition, effacing bosselation and boxiness, and refining the overlying soft tissue.

Single Dome-Binding Suture (transdomal)

A single dome-binding stitch entails placing a stitch of 4–0 chromic PDS (Ethicon, NJ) in a mattress pattern through the domes to bring them together (23). The knot should be buried between the domes so that they will be encased in the soft tissue scar postoperatively. This stitch is used most commonly in cases of boxy or amorphous tips and rounded tip and dome cartilages. The dome angle is left intact but the lobule is narrowed and refined. It is preferable to maintain the integrity of the lateral crura by limiting cartilage work to a complete strip, thus enhancing support of the nasal tip.

Double Dome-Binding Suture (Transdomal and Interdomal)

The double dome-binding suture involves three separate stitches used to create a dome on each lower lateral cartilage and a third stitch to bind them in the midline (24). The dome stitches act to make a distinctive knuckle of cartilage to act as a new dome. This technique is useful in cases of bifid and boxy tips, asymmetrical tips, long intermediate crura with lack of dome definition, and tips with poor structural support.

Double-dome sutures can be used in intact or interrupted units. The intact method involves simply placing the stitches without cartilage incision or division. The interrupted method involves dividing the newly formed dome through the cartilage but not through the underlying vestibular mucosa. This creates greater narrowing of the domal segment and refinement of the lobule. The height of the lobule can be reduced by systematic incision of the cartilages and trimming of the cut edges. Overall, the technique produces predictable rotation and projection changes, enhanced stability of the tripod, and, with the use of columella or tip grafts, more exact refinement of the lobule complex.

Basic Grafting

Spreader Grafts

Spreader grafts are effective in widening the nasal valve and improving nasal airflow (5). The grafts are harvested from the conchal bowl or septum and typically measure 2.5 cm in length, 3 mm in height, and 2 mm in thickness. An endonasal or open rhinoplasty approach can be used for graft placement. The endonasal approach requires a separate submucoperichondrial pocket along the nasal dorsum through an access incision on the anterior caudal septum, anterior to the nasal valve. The graft is inserted into the pocket and the incision is closed with a single stitch of absorbable suture. The open rhinoplasty approach involves creating a dorsal incision between the upper lateral cartilages along the dorsal septum beginning near the anterior septal angle. Submucoperichondrial dissection proceeds to separate the upper lateral cartilages from the septum creating a crib for the graft. Usually, one graft is placed on either side of the septum and secured with 5–0 PDS horizontal mattress sutures that pass through the upper lateral cartilages, grafts, and septum.

Placement through a dorsal approach is usually indicated in patients already undergoing open rhinoplasty. Separation and dorsal trimming of the upper lateral cartilages and septum are usually already done, revealing the space into which the spreader graft will be placed. It is essential that the underlying mucosa be preserved as much as possible to prevent scarring in the area of the valve. The graft is inset into the space between the upper lateral cartilages and septum and is sutured into position. Aside from opening the nasal valves, spreader grafts can be used to lengthen a short nose, camouflage or redirect a twisted nose, and widen a narrow nose. Slight widening of the dorsal middle vault is to be expected when spreader grafts are used, and the patient should be informed of this preoperatively.

Columellar Strut Graft

A columellar strut is a straight rectangular graft that usually measures 5 mm wide, 20 mm long, and 2 mm thick. It functions as a rigid support within the columella and provides superb, precise tip projection and partial rotation. The best source is the septum along the maxillary crest or perpendicular plate of the ethmoid. It is inserted between the medial crura and domes from a surgically created cradle anterosuperior to the anterior nasal spine. The graft is positioned between the medial crura inferior to the domes of the lower lateral cartilages. The strut can be placed through several types of incisions including marginal, vertical columellar, intraoral, and (most precisely) through the open rhinoplasty approach. It is fixed to the medial crura with two or three buried 5–0 PDS sutures to project the tip to the desired position.

A columellar strut graft can stabilize a poorly supported tip and is a useful adjunct in combination with other grafting procedures to provide a stable cartilaginous framework that will resist the forces of scar contracture. Strut grafts provide for a variable degree of cephalic rotation depending on the extent of surgical attenuation or suspension of the lateral crural component of the tripod. To maximize the effect of the columellar strut graft for tip projection, the depressor septi should be divided near the base of the columella. Problems associated with the graft include reduced mobility of the nasal tip in the early postoperative period, improper positioning causing an obtuse nasolabial angle, buckling of the medial crura due to too large a pocket being created, and unfavorable appearance of the columella.

Shield Graft

A shield graft is a triangular flat or slightly convex piece of cartilage originally designed to recreate the domal tip-defining points in revision rhinoplasty. The graft is designed with two points representing the new domes tapering inferiorly toward the midcolumella. The inferior aspect of the graft enhances the columella–lobule angle and provides the appearance of an aesthetic double break. Shield grafts are mainly used to rebuild deficient or extremely irregular domes in secondary rhinoplasty and should only rarely be used in primary rhinoplasty cases unless the domes are extremely attenuated. They can be used to assist in lengthening a short nose, with little or no effect on cephalic rotation. A shield graft, like any other surface or onlay graft, should be used with caution in patients with thin skin. The edges of these grafts should always be tapered and sutured into position with buried mattress 5–0 PDS sutures. Placing the graft via an open rhinoplasty approach ensures accurate placement and ease of suturing.

Stacking tapered rectangular-shaped onlay grafts directly over the domes can create a more dramatic increase in nasal projection. The horizontal extent of an onlay graft should be sufficient to cover the domes and the interdomal areas. The width of the grafts should approximate the width of the intermediate and lateral crura. Conchal cartilage is ideal because of its inherent gentle curvature. The concave side is placed down and its edges are tapered. The grafts may be placed via a rim incision into a pocket or directly sutured into place via an open rhinoplasty approach.

Changing Nasal Rotation

Other than correcting anatomical abnormalities of the tip cartilages, the one major objective of tip-plasty is correcting abnormalities of projection and rotation. Nasal tip projection and rotation are intimately related to one another and are a function of the placement and structure of the lower lateral cartilages. The degree of projection and rotation is predictable based on the type and extent of surgical modification to the lateral crura and domes (Table 2). Conservative tip techniques (complete strip, single dome binding suture) will lead to predictable results with few adverse sequelae. The complete strip procedure is the workhorse of tradition tip-plasty and more radical procedures should be considered only in the hands of experienced surgeons.

Often only the illusion of projection or rotation is actually achieved. Although the tip-plasty techniques described will create some degree of actual projection and rotation, several adjunctive techniques will give the illusion of nasal tip rotation. For example, nasolabial cartilage plumping grafts will appear to increase tip rotation while dorsal and tip grafts will appear to decrease tip rotation. The grafts may be cartilage or synthetic material. Synthetics such as Gore-Tex (Gore and Associates, Flagstaff, AZ) are used as a plumping graft because of their deep location and thick soft tissue cover.

Appreciating the intimate relationship between rotation and projection is vital to a successful outcome. The relationship can be explained by the tripod concept (Fig. 25). If all three legs are shortened then tip retrodisplacement occurs. Shortening or weakening the lateral crural legs and augmenting the medial crural component will cause the nasal tip to project and rotate upwards while opening the nasolabial angle. To attain an actual decrease in tip rotation it will be necessary to augment the lateral crural legs with interposition grafts (cartilage-only or composite grafts). If the medial crural leg is also shortened, the tip will fall forward and lose projection without much rotational change.

Several advanced procedures designed to increase tip projection will also result in some degree of cephalic rotation. For example, columellar struts, plumping grafts, and the lateral crural steal technique will result in mild to moderate degrees of cephalic rotation secondary to lengthening the medial crural component of the tripod. However, several basic techniques that improve tip definition (refinement and narrowing) will also result in cephalic rotation including the complete strip, rim strip, and dome division techniques. Procedures designed specifically to address the problem of tip ptosis include the use of the lateral crural flap, lateral crural steal, and several techniques that involve division of the lateral crura.

Changing Nasal Projection

Several techniques are available to increase nasal projection. Simple techniques described above can be employed that will increase tip projection without the use of grafting materials. Vertical dome division and single- or double-dome binding stitches are most commonly used for this purpose (Fig. 26).

Augmenting the medial crura is the primary method by which an increase in nasal projection is attained. Modification of the existing cartilaginous framework involves special suturing techniques alone or in combination with surgical

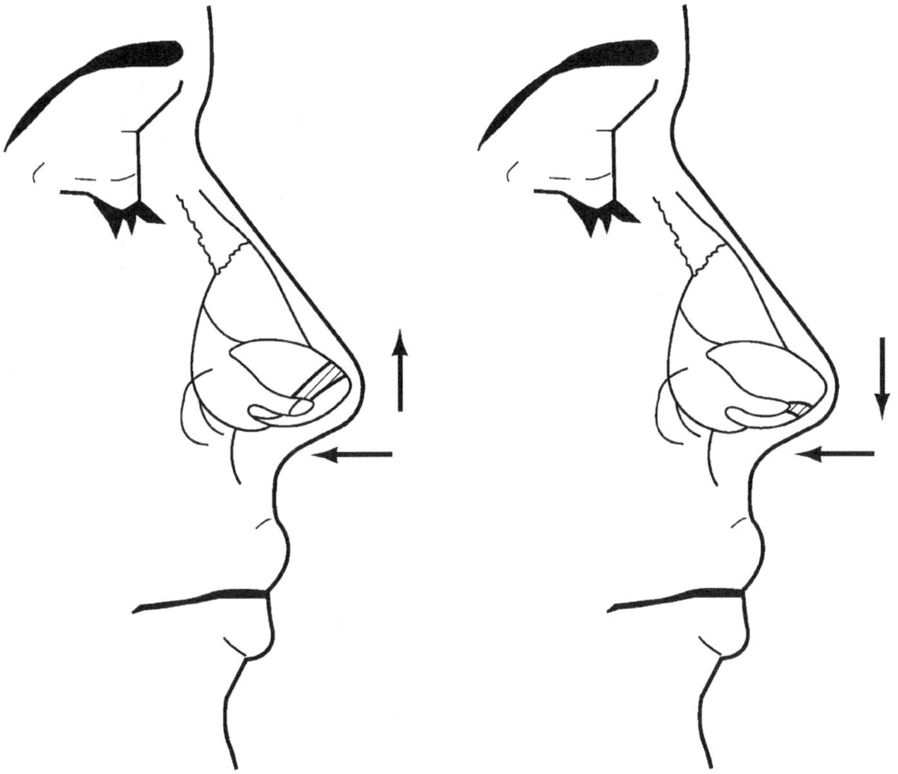

Figure 25 The nasal tip can be likened to a camera tripod, with the three legs represented by the lateral crura and conjoined medial crura. Shortening or lengthening the legs will rotate or project the tip in a predictable fashion based on the tripod concept.

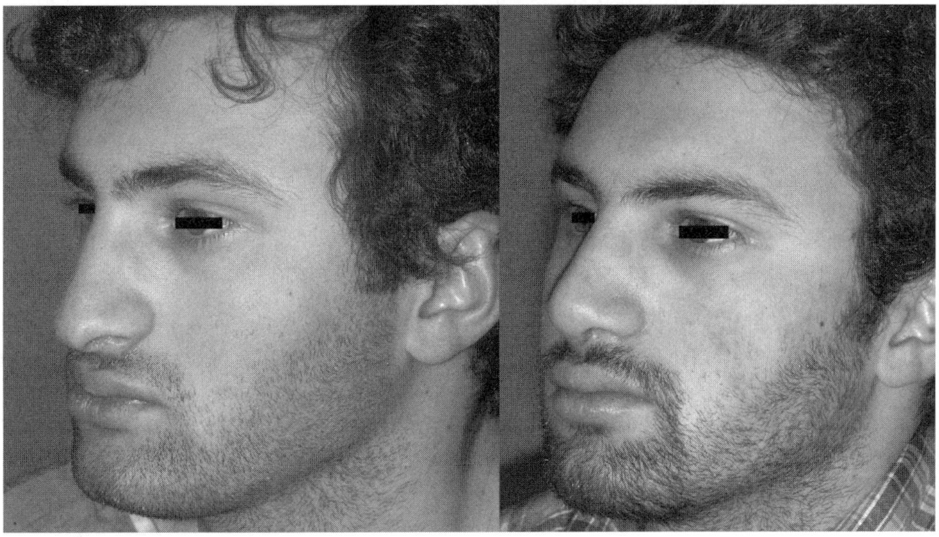

Figure 26 Preoperative (left photo) and postoperative (right photo) three-quarter views of a patient who underwent vertical dome division to increase nasal tip rotation.

modification of the lower lateral cartilages and grafts. Suturing alone can result in modest increases in tip projection such as suture approximation of the medial crura, septocolumellar sutures, or transdomal sutures. Suture approximation of divergent medial crural footplates will result in modest lengthening and an increase in projection. The technique involves first removing the intervening soft tissue and placing one or two buried 5–0 PDS mattress sutures to cinch the footplates together. Septocolumellar sutures are placed between the caudal nasal septum and the medial crura at slightly divergent levels to lift the tip. Transdomal and interdomal sutures are useful to increase tip definition and projection. Transdomal sutures placed through the domes enhance the tip-defining points of each dome. The interdomal suture is placed below the transdomal sutures in a buried mattress fashion through-and-through the domes. This results in narrowing the tip and a minor increase in projection.

A variety of grafting techniques will also increase nasal projection. The majority are cartilage grafts obtained from the septum or conchal bowl. Plumping grafts are used for premaxillary augmentation and are inserted directly behind the nasolabial angle. The main effect of a plumping graft is to open the nasolabial angle. The secondary effects are creating the illusion of cephalic rotation and a modest increase in nasal projection.

A shield graft will moderately enhance nasal projection while providing for new tip-defining points. It will not result in cephalic tip rotation. A columellar strut graft will increase nasal projection and provide increased stability to the nasal tip to resist scar contracture during healing. A strut graft will result in cephalic rotation of the nasal tip especially if the lateral crura are attenuated.

Decreasing tip projection is easier than increasing it. The nose can actually be shortened or the illusion of shortening can be obtained. Rim strip and complete strip procedures are the most useful and easiest ways to cause tip retrodisplacement, but the degree of cephalic rotation associated with these procedures may be undesirable. Removal of the dorsal hump will also give the illusion of tip retrodisplacement, although measurements have shown that the tip does not actually shorten. Actual shortening can be accomplished by directly excising a segment of medial crura. Along with attenuation of the lateral crural components, significant tip retrodisplacement will occur (Fig. 27). Vertical dome division can also be used for deprojection. Rather that stealing from the lateral crura and creating a new dome with lateral crura cartilage to enhance projection, this portion of crura can be resected and a new dome created at the level of the intermediate crura.

The Nasal Dorsum

Taking the Hump

A nasal hump is usually the result of a prominent convexity involving both the lower bony and upper cartilaginous vaults (Fig. 28). A mild convexity to these structures is necessary to achieve a straight nasal profile because the skin over the rhinion is thin relative to the skin over the root of the nose and the nasal tip. Surgical creation of a perfectly straight cartilaginous and bony platform would result in a scooped out appearance (concavity) along the nasal dorsum after the skin envelope is replaced (Fig. 29). The classic method of hump removal involves excision of the cartilaginous and bony components en bloc up to the intercanthal line. Heavy scissors are used to plane off the anterior cartilaginous dorsum up to the nasal bones. A straight

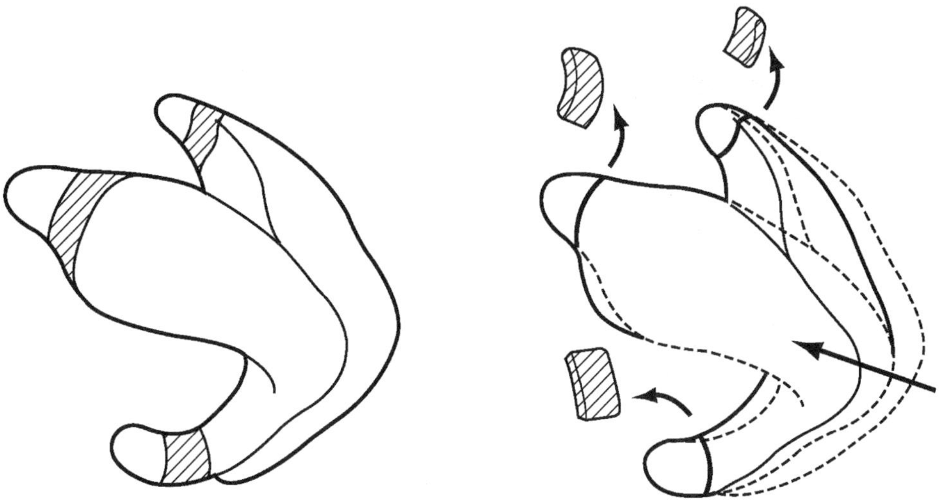

Figure 27 Decreasing nasal tip projection through segmental resection of tip cartilages. By shortening all three legs of the tripod, there will be an incremental decrease in nasal tip projection. Rotation will also occur but will be less pronounced.

osteotome is then inserted against the caudal nasal bones along the line of cartilage excision. The osteotome is advanced through both nasal bones and is deflected anteriorly by the gradual thickening of the nasal bones, usually disengaging about the level of the intercanthal line. The hump is thus removed as an intact unit consisting of the anterior caudal nasal bones and upper dorsal quadrilateral cartilage. After the hump is removed, the nose is unroofed to reveal the free edges of the nasal bones, perpendicular ethmoid plate, upper lateral cartilages, and quadrilateral cartilage.

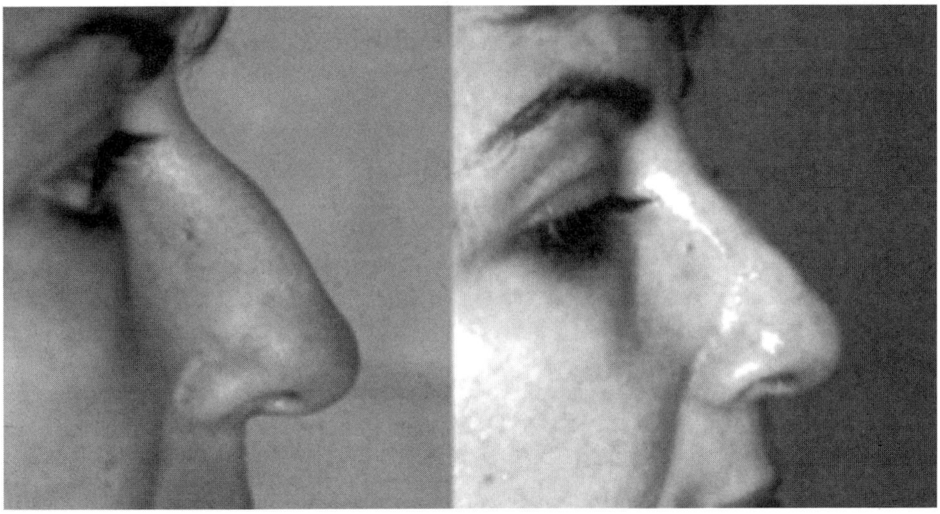

Figure 28 Preoperative and postoperative views of a patient with resection of a prominent nasal hump.

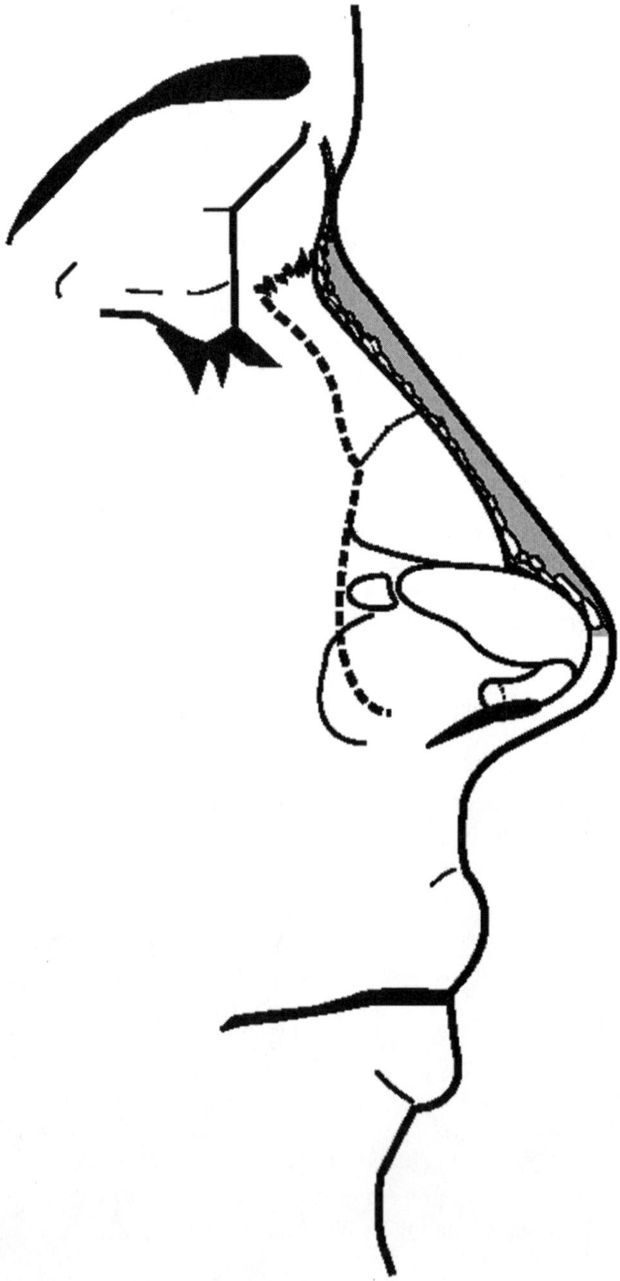

Figure 29 Maintenance of a convex osseocartilaginous dorsum is required to achieve the appearance of a straight dorsum due to the differing skin thicknesses along the nasal dorsum. Note that the skin over the mid-dorsum is quite thin. To achieve an apparently straight dorsum, the underlying bone must kept slightly convex after removal of a nasal hump.

The underlying mucosa is also disrupted so that the nasal contents are visible. Closure of the open roof requires lateral osteotomies that allow the nasal bones and upper lateral cartilages to fall toward the midline. If the ethmoidal perpendicular plate is deviated it must be partially removed or straightened to allow the nasal bones to close the midline gap fully. Medialization of the upper lateral cartilages occurs because they are firmly attached to the nasal bones.

Refinements to the classic method of hump removal have been reported since Joseph's original description in 1931. An extramucosal hump removal is commonly used today to preserve the integrity of the mucosa in the upper nasal vault. The technique involves sharp dorsal division of the upper lateral cartilages from the dorsal septum and careful dissection of the underlying mucosa away from the proposed area of cartilage excision. The dorsal quadrilateral cartilage is excised as needed followed by appropriate reduction of the bony pyramid using a rasp or osteotome. Despite the popularity of this method, significant problems may be encountered when the hump is excised. The exposed sharp edges of the nasal bones, perpendicular ethmoid plate, and septum may cause contour irregularities over the nasal dorsum that are difficult to camouflage, especially in patients with thin skin. Disruption of the T configuration and excessive medialization of the upper lateral cartilages may result in excessive narrowing of the middle vault, an inverted V deformity, and nasal valve obstruction. Several alternative methods of hump removal have been proposed. Most notably, Cottle in 1954 described a mucosal-sparing technique of "pushing down" the hump after intermediate and lateral osteotomies and excision of a cephalodorsal strip of septum. Skoog in 1966 described a technique to restore the nasal roof and eliminate the sharp edges of the osteotomized nasal bones by replacing the intact osseocartilaginous components of the hump. The hump, once removed, is trimmed, straightened, and replaced as a free graft. This is a useful concept because it may occasionally be necessary to replace a portion of an excised hump following an overly aggressive application of the classic method.

The Skoog technique (removal and replacement of the hump) is rarely used today. Most rhinoplastic surgeons are not adept at removing the cartilage and bony hump en bloc. Most prefer an alteration of the method called the double hump deformity. The incisions are the same. Intercartilaginous incisions and transfixion incisions are made to deglove the nose. The upper lateral cartilages are separated from the septum sharply, sparing mucosa if possible. The cartilaginous hump is removed to the surgeon's satisfaction. This creates the double hump deformity in which the first hump is actually the tip and the second is the remaining bony hump. It looks somewhat like a camel back. At this point, the bony hump can be removed by a number of methods. Rasping is an easy but time-consuming method, but it produces definable results and is safe in the hands of inexperienced surgeons. Prior to rasping, the periosteum should be elevated and rasping should be performed subperiosteally if possible. While rasping, it is important to use the rasp intermittently with the teeth pointing towards the skin to sweep away residual bone fragments gently. Remaining bone fragments can create a foreign body reaction or act as a nidus for neo-osteogenesis, creating a new bony hump or bony nubbins postoperatively. Coarse rasps (no. 6 or 8) are used first to remove a large portion of bone, followed by finer rasps in the final stages. The other popular technique is to use a straight guarded or unguarded osteotome. Large humps, especially those that extend into the nasofrontal area, can be removed en bloc. Precise placement and guidance of the osteotome are essential to avoid removing too much tissue. A fine rasp is used to smooth the free edges of the nasal bones after hump removal using an osteotome. Excessive removal of tissue will leave the patient with a low-set nasofrontal angle and foreshortening of the nose. If too much bone is removed, do not attempt to correct it by resecting more dorsal septum or tip to match the over-resected dorsum. Immediate grafting is indicated usually with a portion of the removed piece.

At the conclusion of hump removal, the finger test should be performed. This involves placing an index finger at the base of the columella and pressing inferiorly towards the nasal spine. If the septal angle becomes visible upon pressing, there is a possibility of a pollybeak postoperatively. Further resection of the septal angle, septal dorsum, or both should be considered. Finally, the overprojecting dorsal edges of the upper lateral cartilages should be trimmed to lie in line with the nasal dorsum. Medialization of the upper and middle nasal vaults is necessary to close the open roof. This is accomplished using standard osteotomies.

Osteotomies and Narrowing the Nasal Dorsum

An osteotomy (Fig. 30) may be accomplished with a variety of osteotomes, saws, or powered instrumentation. The curved or straight, guarded or unguarded, osteotomes are most frequently used. Once the hump is removed some surgeons choose to perform tip-plasty, while others choose to finish the nasal pyramid work by performing

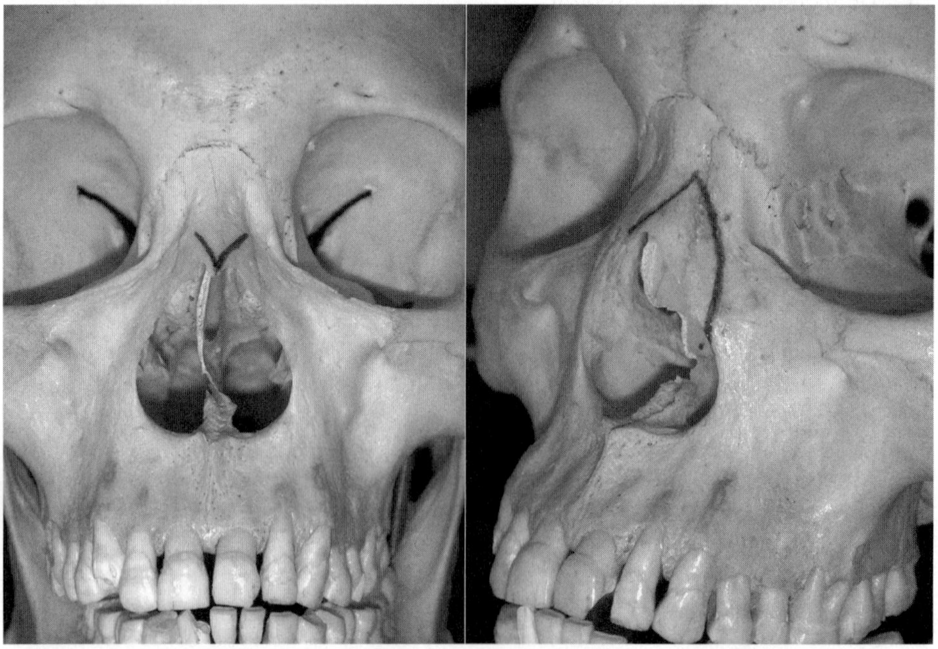

Figure 30 Medial and lateral osteotomies demonstrated on a skull. Note that medial osteotomies begin at the midline of the nasal bones and proceed in a superolateral direction at a 40 degree angle (left photo). Lateral and medial osteotomies are demonstrated in the photo on the right. Note how the lateral osteotomy begins high along the pyriform aperture and travels primarily through the ascending process of the maxilla.

osteotomies to close the open roof (the gap between the nasal bones created by removing the hump).

Lateral Osteotomy. Reducing the width of the bony nasal dorsum is a component of most cosmetic rhinoplasties (Fig. 31). Infracture of the nasal bones becomes a necessity when removal of the bony component of a nasal hump leaves the dorsal aspect of the nasal bones separated (i.e., an open roof deformity). Low lateral osteotomies allow the nasal bones and a portion of the frontal processes of the maxillae to move toward each other, closing the open roof and narrowing the nasal dorsum. A low lateral osteotomy lies within the nasofacial groove in the substance of the frontal process of the maxilla. The osteotomy is gently curved and designed to preserve the piriform aperture (i.e., "high–low–high" osteotomy). Superiorly, the osteotomy curves medially across the nasomaxillary suture as it begins to meet resistance at the intercanthal line where the nasal bones thicken. The superomedial nasal bone is not usually osteotomized but is fractured secondarily with light pressure. It is important that the initial greenstick fracture created by finger pressure at the nasion be complete, otherwise the bones can float and lateralize during healing and create an open roof deformity. Other problems include a shelf effect laterally if the osteotome is placed too high along the nasal bones, and rocker deformity. Rocker deformity is present if the osteotomy was incomplete and the nasal bone teeters as pressure is applied to its inferior or superior edge. Repeat intermediate and low lateral osteotomies with or without overlay camouflage grafts may be required for correction.

A lateral osteotomy may be done via either an intranasal or a transcutaneous approach. Despite improved exposure in an external rhinoplasty approach, lateral

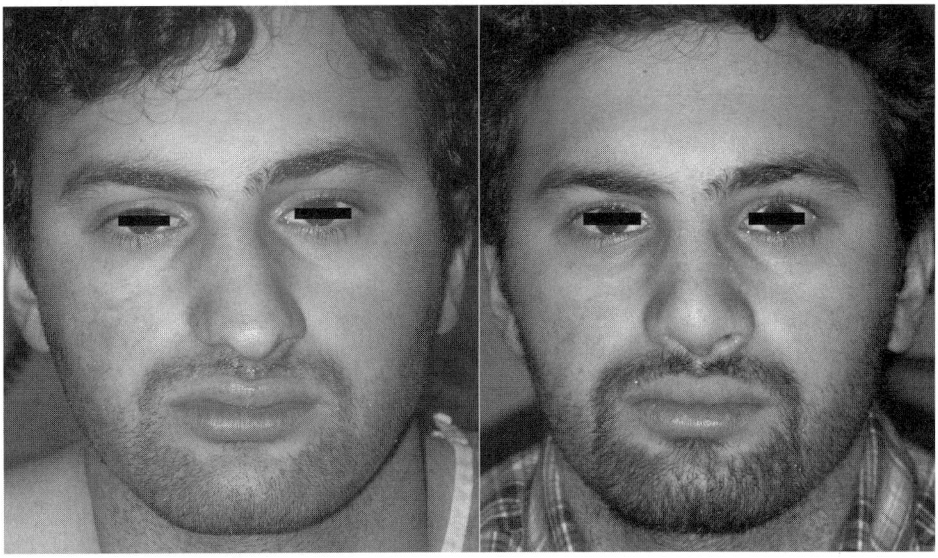

Figure 31 Narrowing the nasal dorsum and restoring aesthetic nasociliary lines. Note that the patient presented with a severely deviated and widened nasal dorsum. Symmetrical nasociliary lines were restored by correcting the deviation and narrowing the bridge of the nose.

osteotomies are still performed the traditional way (i.e., intranasal or transcutaneous). An intranasal approach is more popular and consists of making a stab incision at the pyriform aperture within the nasal vestibule to allow insertion and advancement of a guarded 2–4 mm osteotome. The osteotomy is continuous, cutting through bone and periosteum. Despite the guard being turned intranasally, mucosal injury and tearing are seen in most cases (25). The transcutaneous technique involves creating a stab incision along the nasofacial groove at the level of the infraorbital rim. A 2 mm unguarded osteotome is inserted and the bone and periosteum are perforated at closely spaced noncontiguous points along the nasofacial groove. The transcutaneous approach possesses several advantages over the intranasal approach including that the intranasal mucosa is rarely injured, the fracture segments are more stable since the periosteum is not completely disrupted, less ecchymosis and edema, more accuracy, and greater ability to create a controlled osteotomy along the nasal root. The major drawback to the transcutaneous approach is obvious cutaneous scarring but this is uncommon.

Medial Osteotomy. Medial osteotomies are bone cuts along each side of the perpendicular plate of the ethmoid about two-thirds the length of the nasal bones. If medial osteotomies are planned, they are always completed prior to other planned osteotomies. A 5 mm straight osteotome is introduced between the cephalic medial border of the ipsilateral upper lateral cartilage and dorsal septum and advanced through the ipsilateral nasal bone. At the level of the canthus the osteotome is directed laterally to meet up with the previous (or to-be created) lateral osteotomy. This lateral extension of the medial osteotomy has been termed an oblique osteotomy but it is just the superior extension of a medial osteotomy as previously stated. The opposite side is done in an identical manner leaving a 2 mm wide midline longitudinal portion of nasal bone supported by the underlying perpendicular plate of the ethmoid. Medial osteotomies are typically useful in three situations: to create a midline release of the nasal bones to allow fracture after lateral osteotomies in the absence of an open roof, to allow a more controlled removal of the dorsal bony hump in open rhinoplasty, and to complete the release of the nasal bones cephalically to allow infracture in the presence of an open roof and lateral osteotomies. It is also used in cases where bony hump removal was not done by a sharp osteotome but by rasping. Rasping will smooth the dorsum and remove the hump but usually does not completely create an open roof. The medial osteotomy is used to complete the procedure and create the open roof needed so that infracture of the nasal bones can be accomplished after lateral osteotomies. If the procedure is performed improperly, the perpendicular plate of the ethmoid may be fractured and dislocated, which may result in an immediate saddle deformity. This should be corrected immediately with grafting or splinting.

Intermediate Osteotomy. An intermediate osteotomy is performed similarly to a lateral osteotomy. It is used when there is a previous nasal fracture and portions of the fractured nasal bone are abnormally positioned, when a rocker deformity has occurred during lateral osteotomy, or in the presence of nasal horns that are protuberances of nasal bone in the midportion of the bone. If rasping does not efface the horn, an intermediate osteotomy is useful. This osteotomy is used in conjunction with the other two and should not be used as the sole means to infracture the nose.

Establishing the Radix

Movement of the radix is performed to change the depth or angle of the nasofrontal angle. This correction is usually a byproduct of hump removal. However, in some cases movement of the radix is necessary either to lengthen or shorten the nasal dorsum. It is rarely necessary in primary rhinoplasty in white patients but may play a prominent role in cases of revision rhinoplasty and in patients of other races. A prominent radix will usually be displaced superiorly along the nasal dorsum of the nose and a deep-set radix is often displaced inferiorly. Rasping or removal of bone is usually required to deepen and lower the radix and grafting is required to efface and raise the radix. Movement of the radix in a purely posterior direction (retrodisplacement) requires removal of bone and soft tissue from both the nasal and frontal components of the nasofrontal angle. Anterosuperior displacement of the radix opens the nasofrontal angle, lengthens the nose, and gives the illusion of decreased projection of the nasal tip. Posteroinferior displacement of the radix makes the nasofrontal angle more acute, shortens the nasal dorsum, and gives the illusion of increased projection of the nasal tip.

FUNCTIONAL SURGERY

The Nasal Valve

Nasal obstruction due to narrowing at the nasal valve area is a commonly overlooked problem before and after rhinoplasty. Typical abnormalities leading to nasal obstruction that involve the nasal valve area include collapse of the upper lateral cartilages, nasal bone deviation, septal deviation or thickening near the nasal valve, turbinate hypertrophy, scarring, and iatrogenic medialization or attenuation of the lateral crura.

Collapse of the Upper Lateral Cartilages and Nasal Bone Deviation

Static nasal valve dysfunction due to collapse of the upper lateral cartilages and medialization is most commonly corrected by the use of cartilage grafts. Deviated nasal bones may also cause medialization of the upper lateral cartilage and nasal valve narrowing. In some cases, repositioning the nasal bones by osteotomy may result in lateralization of the upper lateral cartilage and opening of the nasal valve. If osteotomies are planned, they should be performed prior to the more direct remedial techniques such as cartilage grafting or suture suspension.

The spreader graft is a very effective method to widen the nasal valve and improve airflow (Fig. 32). Usually two grafts are placed: one on each side of the septum. The grafts are held in place using 5–0 PDS horizontal mattress sutures that pass through the upper lateral cartilages, grafts, and the septum. In addition, flaring sutures can be placed to stent the nasal valve open. A flaring suture is placed in a horizontal fashion into the caudal lateral portion of each upper lateral cartilage and tied across the midline. Slight nasal widening along the dorsal middle vault is to be expected when spreader grafts are used and the patient should be informed of this preoperatively.

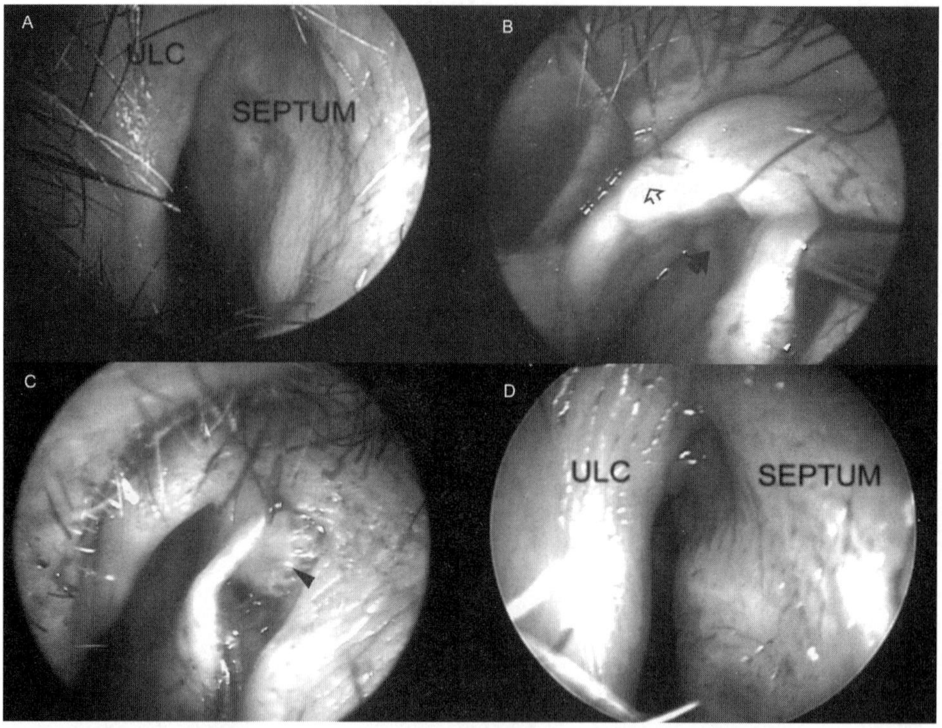

Figure 32 Correction of nasal valve narrowing using a spreader graft via an endonasal approach. A cartilage strip measuring approximately 2 cm long by 4 mm wide is placed within a submucoperiosteal pocket along the dorsal septum to lateralize the upper lateral cartilage and stent the nasal valve open. A. The septum is lying directly against the ULC, indicating a static nasal valve narrowing. B. A freer elevator is inserted into a submucoperiosteal pocket along the dorsal septum (solid arrow), thereby lateralizing the upper lateral cartilage (hollow arrow). C. A cartilage strip is inserted into the pocket (arrow). D. Final result indicating an open nasal valve.

A splay graft spans the nasal dorsum under the upper lateral cartilages to reinforce the cartilage, stent open the nasal valves, and widen the middle nasal vault (26). The graft is harvested from the conchal bowl to take advantage of the natural curvature and inherent spring in the cartilage. A splay graft can be more effective than a spreader graft when the upper lateral cartilages are greatly attenuated. However, splay grafts cause more dramatic widening of the middle nasal vault. The technique involves placing the graft over the septum (convex side up) and under each upper lateral cartilage, which is best done via an open rhinoplasty approach. The mucoperichondrium must be dissected carefully away from the septum and the undersurface of the upper lateral cartilages. The dissection is tedious and small perforations are common but will not affect the viability of the graft. After the dissection is completed, a pocket is created that will accept the graft. The septum will be the fulcrum point of the graft and should be lowered in selected cases. The cartilage graft will extend to the lateral border of the upper lateral cartilages or to the pyriform apertures, depending on the desired affect.

Nasal valve suspension involves suture-suspending the lateral nasal wall and lateral crus to the maxilla (27). A nonabsorbable suture is passed through a subciliary or transconjunctival incision just above the maxillary periosteum through the lateral crus and into the nose. The suture is again passed from the nose approximately 5 mm separated from the original pass through the lateral crus toward the inferior orbital rim. As the suture is pulled taught, the lateral nasal wall is lateralized and opens the nasal valve. The suture may be secured to the periosteum under the inferior orbital rim by passing it through the periosteum, around a screw, or through a drill hole. This method has only recently been described and the permanence of the procedure is unknown. There may be significant widening of the lateral nasal subunit; this method will not work well in the presence of lateral nasal scarring or soft tissue deficiency.

Conservative resection of the caudal upper lateral cartilage is effective for excessive scrolling, deviations, or thickening that result in narrowing of the nasal valve (28). It avoids widening the middle nasal vault. The procedure is performed through an intercartilaginous incision, exposing the caudal surface of the upper lateral cartilage. The mucosa from the undersurface of the upper lateral cartilage must be dissected away. This is the most tedious portion of the procedure. After the caudal 3–4 mm of the upper lateral cartilage is exposed, a triangular portion is excised. The base of the triangle corresponds to the lateral aspect of the upper lateral cartilage preserving the articulation of the upper lateral cartilage with the dorsal septum. The removed cartilage represents the abnormally thickened or deviated portion of the upper lateral cartilage causing the obstruction at the nasal valve. The full thickness of the mucosa is reapproximated using interrupted absorbable suture. This reestablishes the connection between the caudal upper lateral cartilage and the cephalic border of the lower lateral cartilage, pulling the upper lateral cartilage laterally and opening the valve.

Septal Deviation/Thickening

Minor septal deviations or pathological septal thickening in the area of the nasal valve can be corrected by selective thinning (shaving) with a scalpel or by lateralization of the upper lateral cartilage. Scoring the cartilage may be effective in some cases but this technique tends to weaken the cartilage and may not adequately correct the problem.

Moderate and severe septal deviations may also cause deviation of the nasal dorsum below the level of the rhinion. Straightening the dorsocaudal strut may be all that is necessary to correct the external nasal deformity and open the nasal valve. However, correcting a substantial septal deviation in this area is very difficult using standard septoplasty techniques. An open rhinoplasty approach is best in these situations and will allow selective resection of the upper lateral cartilages and septum, and cartilage grafting. Total removal of the dorsocaudal strut and correction on a back table using cartilage grafts may be necessary. After the dorsocaudal strut is reformed and strengthened, it is replaced and suture-fixated to the upper and lower lateral cartilages.

Turbinate Hypertrophy

The anterior one-third (head) of the inferior turbinate is an important component of the nasal valve area that must be considered in the diagnosis and treatment of nasal obstruction. Turbinate reduction may be achieved through medical or various forms of surgical management. Medical management should be attempted prior to any form of surgical management. Long-term pharmacological modalities include inhaled steroids, injected steroids, anticholinergics, and cromolyn sodium. The relative benefits of these treatments are unclear, but for patients with allergy and non-allergy-related turbinate hypertrophy, inhaled steroids can be effective. Turbinate steroid injection is also effective but may last only a few months. Patients whose condition does not respond to these medical therapies are candidates for surgical intervention including various mechanical (turbinate outfracture), submucosal destructive (electrocautery, cryosurgery, or radiofrequency), or turbinate resection (submucosal, partial, or total) procedures. Complications associated with surgical management include hemorrhage, prolonged nasal crusting, and atrophic rhinitis. The less aggressive surgical modalities, including the mechanical and submucosal destructive procedures, are less prone to complications but may not result in permanent turbinate regression. Submucous resection is often considered aggressive but offers the best chance of long-term turbinate reduction while minimizing the occurrence of hemorrhage, nasal crusting, and atrophic rhinitis. The method involves creating an incision along the inferior margin of the turbinate and removing the majority of the turbinate bone and glands while preserving the mucosal cover. Only the anterior half to one-third of the turbinate needs to be treated because only this portion falls within the nasal valve area.

Scarring

Scarring in the nasal valve will obliterate the space despite adequate separation of the caudal upper lateral cartilage and the septum. Attempts to place flaps or mucosal grafts into the area will usually fail. Simple scar lysis and silastic stenting will be successful in the majority of cases. The stent should be left in place for 3–5 weeks.

Medialization of the Lateral Crura

Excessive medial displacement of the lateral crura may occur after suture correction of a boxy tip deformity or other maneuvers that tend to constrict the nasal tip. A common cause of problematic medial displacement is sometimes found after suture correction of a boxy nasal tip when an interdomal suture pulls the lateral crura medially. Correction of this deformity is best performed during the primary rhinoplasty using a lateral crural strut graft.

Supra-alar Pinching

Alar batten grafts are useful in correcting pinching in the supra-alar region, stabilizing the lateral nasal wall, and maintaining the patency of the nasal valve and nasal ala. Batten grafts can also be used to correct dynamic nasal alar dysfunction by placing the graft in a more caudal position.

The typical batten graft is harvested from either curved septal cartilage or concha and is approximately 6 mm in width by 10–15 mm in length. The graft may be placed via an endonasal or open rhinoplasty approach. When an endonasal approach is used, the access incision is placed at the site of maximal collapse. A subcutaneous pocket is created so that the graft will fit securely, spanning the pyriform aperture. The curvature of the graft should follow the contour of the alar rim and should not extend cephalic to the supra-alar crease. When the graft is placed using an open rhinoplasty approach, the subcutaneous pocket is created caudal to the caudal border of the lower lateral cartilage extending over the pyriform aperture. The graft should not extend pass the central point of the lateral crus and should be sutured in place. The graft will stabilize the lateral nasal wall to prevent dynamic nasal valve collapse and correct the cosmetic deformity of supra-alar pinching. There may be an increase in the thickness of the lateral nasal wall because of graft placement. Batten grafts are ineffective in the presence of scar.

The Nasal Ala

The nasal ala also may be the cause of increased airway resistance because of permanent narrowing (static nasal alar dysfunction) or inspiratory collapse (dynamic nasal alar dysfunction) (Table 3). Aside from soft tissue deficiencies and scarring, static nasal alar dysfunction is most commonly encountered in patients with overprojected nasal tips associated with tense, slit-like nostrils. Tip deprojection is usually all that is required to correct this problem. Dynamic nasal alar dysfunction may be due to a weakened lateral crus, especially in the female patient with a small nose. In addition, patients with excessive cephalic rotation of the lateral crus may have a weakened alar sidewall due to the loss of cartilage support. The lateral crus and alar sidewall must be strengthened to correct the problem. Batten and lateral crural strut grafts are effective. A batten graft is placed caudal to the caudal border of the lower lateral cartilage, inferior to the position that would be used for the correction of dynamic nasal valve dysfunction.

Patients with cephalically malpositioned lateral crura may have dynamic nasal alar collapse due to loss of skeletal support at and inferior to the supra-alar crease. This deformity is best treated by an open rhinoplasty approach with inferior reposi-

Table 3 Causes and Treatment of Nasal Alar Valvular Dysfunction

Classification	Cause	Treatment
Static	Alar rim collapse	Lateral crural strut Rim graft
	Soft-tissue deficiency/scarring	Lysis and stenting Local flap Nasolabial w/rim graft Forehead w/rim graft Composite cartilage graft
Dynamic	Nasal alar and lower lateral cartilage flaccidity	Batten graft Lateral crural strut Suspension suture
	Malpositioned lateral crura (cephalic rotation)	Open rhinoplasty w/upper lateral cartilage repositioning Lateral crural strut Batten graft

tioning of the lateral crura and placement of lateral crural struts along their caudal edge. Additional batten grafts can be used if a lateral crural strut does not provide sufficient rigidity.

Prevention of Nasal Valve Dysfunction

Prevention of nasal valve dysfunction should be considered fundamental to any rhinoplasty procedure. Pre-existing abnormalities involving the nasal valve area tend to worsen after rhinoplasty unless these areas are specifically addressed during the primary procedure. Identification of preoperative nasal valve dysfunction and anticipation of the secondary effects of various treatment options should be incorporated into the operative plan. In addition, some nasal valve abnormalities are preventable while others are inevitable and should be corrected during the primary procedure.

Common preventable post-rhinoplasty problems that lead to obstruction of the nasal valve include synechiae and scarring in the nasal valve and weakened or overresected lower or upper lateral cartilages. Separation of the upper lateral cartilages from the septum and dissection of the underlying mucosa away from the planned cartilage excision or hump removal are necessary to preserve the mucosal lining of the nasal valve. Without these pre-emptive maneuvers, the mucosa at the apex of the nasal valve can be injured, causing scarring, synechiae, and obstruction. Weakening or overresection of the nasal cartilages should be avoided. Primary application of the various upper lateral cartilage lateralization procedures, lateral crural grafts, or batten grafts is useful for patients with excessively pliable cartilages or those that require significant cartilage resection or repositioning for aesthetic reasons.

Common procedures that will cause nasal valve narrowing or obstruction include hump removal and interdomal suture to correct a boxy tip. Hump removal disrupts the articulation of the upper lateral cartilages with the dorsal septum. The T configuration is lost and the upper lateral cartilages fall toward the septum, obliterating the nasal valves. Spreader grafts placed at the time of hump removal will restore the position of the upper lateral cartilages and keep the nasal valves open. As part of the preoperative plan, the spreader grafts may also be used to help straighten a crooked nose or lengthen a congenitally short nose. Primary placement of a lateral crural graft may be necessary when an interdomal suture is used to medialize the lower lateral cartilages. The graft prevents medial encroachment of the lateral crus into the nasal valve area.

Nasal bone osteotomies and intercartilaginous incisions may produce nasal valve obstruction. The integrity of the firm osseocartilaginous connection between the upper lateral cartilages and nasal bones must not be violated. Injury or avulsion of the upper lateral cartilage from the nasal bone destabilizes the upper lateral cartilage and leads to collapse of the lateral nasal wall and nasal valve. An intercartilaginous incision, if not carefully performed, may injure the scroll of the caudal upper lateral cartilage, weakening the cartilage that forms the lateral wall of the nasal valve. Combining a transfixion incision with the intercartilaginous incision increases the likelihood of scarring in the nasal valve. The mucosal incisions should be carefully reapproximated to minimize the risk of scarring and synechiae formation.

Septoplasty

Septal deviations involving the dorsocaudal strut can be difficult to correct because surgical modifications may result in loss of nasal support, unintentional cephalic tip rotation, or a saddle nose deformity (Fig. 33). Minor septal deviations or cartilage

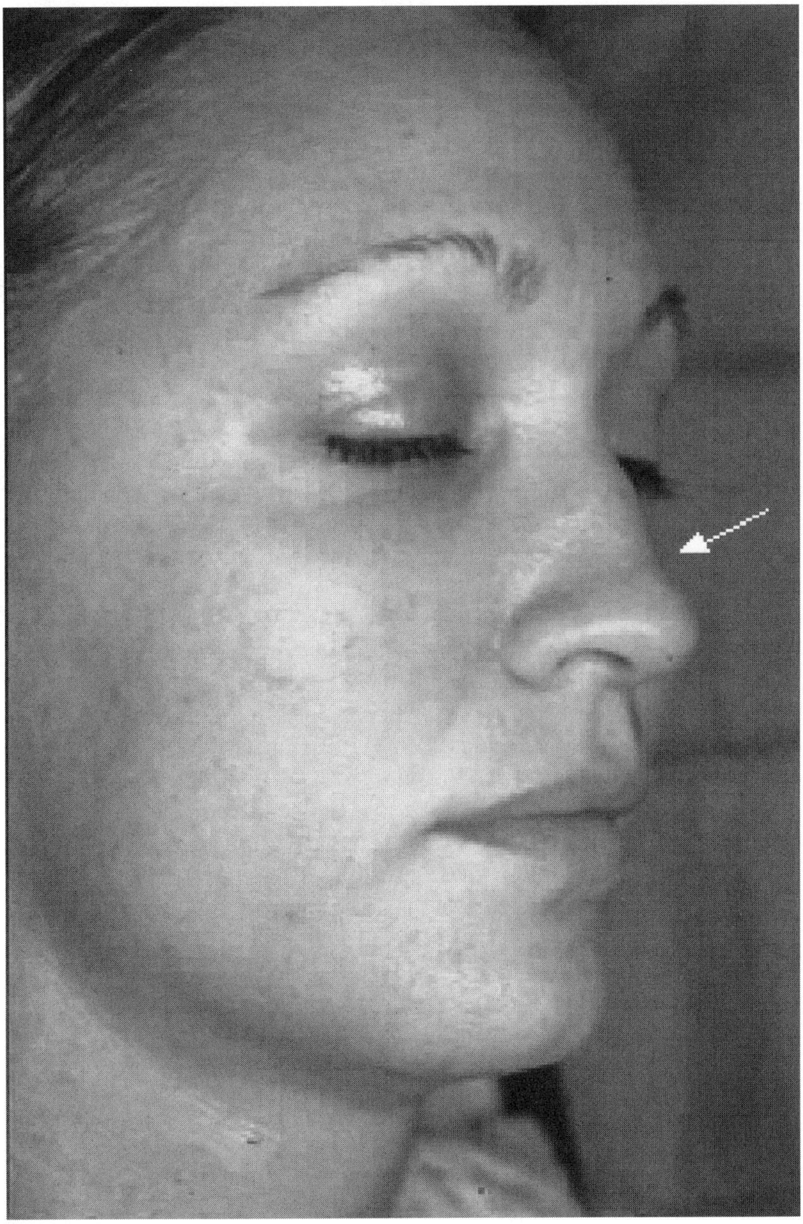

Figure 33 Saddle nose deformity after septoplasty. The scooped-out appearance in the supratip area (arrow) is secondary to overzealous resection and weakening of the dorsocaudal septal cartilage.

thickening at the nasal valve can lead to significant increases in nasal resistance and nasal obstruction. This is correctable during rhinoplasty by shave excisions or upper lateral cartilage lateralization. Rarely do minor septal deviations cause rotation or distortion of the external nose.

Occasionally, moderate-to-severe deviations involving the dorsal strut are associated with deviation of the nasal dorsum (i.e., twisted nose deformity). Although the septal deviation is usually not the sole cause of the external nasal deformity, straightening the nasal dorsum will require correction of the septal deviation in addition to modifications of the other nasal cartilages. Dorsal strut curvature can be corrected using either an open or closed approach. In-situ modifications include extensive cross-hatching, selective removal of cartilage, and suture fixation. In selected cases, the quadrilateral cartilage is removed completely and modified ex-vivo. Modifications may entail extensive cross-hatching, suturing, and application of thin cartilage strips to add strength to the weakened modified cartilage. The strut is then replaced and suture-fixated to the feet of the medial crura and upper lateral cartilages.

Caudal septal deflections require a special note. These deflections can alter tip architecture, mid vault shape, and columellar symmetry. These are typically repaired through full transfixion incisions. If the problem appears to be displacement off the maxillary crest anteriorly, then creating a trap door incision and swinging the remaining portion of the septum into the midline will suffice. This is accomplished by removing a small horizontal piece of septum at the base of the cartilage near the maxillary crest. A tunnel is then made with a Freer elevator raising the septal mucosa off the contralateral maxillary crest and inferior septal cartilage. The cartilage is then swung onto the maxillary crest and sutured in place either to the crest itself or to the periosteum behind the nasal sill. If the caudal end is too twisted to perform such a maneuver, then the end can be removed, reshaped, and then sutured back in place in the midline. This technique may cause a saddle nose that will need to be supported because the tip and dorsal support mechanisms of the septum are interrupted.

Septoplasty in children deserves special consideration because the septum may play a significant role as a growth center in the midface. The anterior free end and the suprapremaxillary areas have the greatest growth activity, especially during early childhood and puberty (29). Resection of septal cartilage from these areas should be avoided in the growing child. Simply raising mucoperiosteal flaps or resecting cartilage from the posterior aspect of the septum has not been associated with long-term growth problems.

Appendix Terminology

Term	Definition
Accessory cartilages	String of cartilages distributed along a curvilinear line from the lateral tip of the lateral crus to the nasal sill (pyriform aperture)
Alae	The lateral nostril walls extending from the nasal tip to the cheek and base of columella; resembling wings
Alar crease	Trough/demarcation formed by the junction of the ala with the cheek

(Continued)

Appendix (continued)

Term	Definition
Alar groove	The external skin crease overlying the caudal margin of the lateral crus; separates the lobule from the ala
Anatomical dome	The junction of the middle and lateral crura
Angle of the lower lateral cartilages	Area where the medial and lateral crura merge
Angle of divergence	The degree of separation between the two middle crura
Angle of rotation	See columella–lobule angle
Anterior septal angle	Angle formed by the junction of the dorsal and caudal septum
Binder's syndrome	Midfacial hypoplasia and an absent anterior nasal spine; not usually considered a true genetic syndrome: a nonspecific abnormality of the nasomaxillary complex (30)
Boss	A knoblike protuberance of the nasal tip
Cephalic malposition	Excessive superomedial rotation of the lateral crus; results in lobular and supralobular fullness; also known as parentheses tip
Clinical dome	Part of the lower lateral cartilage that is identified externally; corresponds to the ipsilateral tip-defining point
Columella	Column of skin, connective tissue, and underlying cartilage separating the nostrils at the base of the nose
Columellar base	Deepest aspect of the nasolabial angle; the transition point of the columella with the upper lip; corresponds to level of inferior nostril sills
Columella breakpoint	Columella–lobule angle; transition between the columella and infratip lobule
Columella–lobule angle	Angle formed by the junction of the columella with the infratip lobule; it is most aesthetically approximately 37 degrees; forms the basis of the columellar double break
Columellar show	Amount of columella visible below the nostril margin on profile
Complete strip	Removal of the cephalic edge of the lower lateral cartilage (intermediate and lateral portions) leaving a *complete* intact strip of cartilage laterally; the strip refers to the portion of cartilage that remains, not taken away
Delivery	Exteriorizing the middle and lateral crura via marginal and intercartilaginous incisions
Depressor septi	Paired muscle originating from the premaxilla and inserting into the base of the columella and medial footplates; most important muscle in rhinoplasty since it can cause a functional tip ptosis
Domal junction line	Junction of the middle and lateral crura
Domal notch	Indentation in the caudal border of the domal segment of the middle crus; responsible for the overlying soft tissue soft triangle and facet
Dome	Highest part of the nasal vestibule corresponding to the highest projecting point of the lateral crus; see also anatomical dome, clinical dome, vestibular dome, and surgical dome
Dorsocaudal strut	Approximately 1 cm of the caudalmost and dorsalmost areas of the quadrilateral cartilage; important in maintenance of support of the tip and dorsum; excessive resection of loss of cartilage may result in a characteristic saddle nose deformity

(Continued)

Appendix (continued)

Term	Definition
Double break	Aesthetic interruption of the columella near the superior nostril margin by an acute bend in the lower lateral cartilage between the medial and middle crura; the bend forms a distinct platform over the lobular segment of the middle crus extending form the columella–lobule angle to the nasal tip
External nares	The alar margin
External nasal valve	Putative airflow regulator only in pathological states corresponding to collapse of the fibrofatty nasal ala; it is bounded medially by the caudal cartilaginous and membranous septum, laterally by the nasal ala and caudal edge of the lower lateral cartilage, and inferiorly by the soft tissues anterior to the inferior rim of the pyriform aperture
Frankfurt line	Imaginary line extending through the facial profile passing through the superior tragal margin and inferior orbital rim
Glabella	The most prominent portion of the forehead in the lateral plane; area just above the nasofrontal angle and radix nasi
Hemitransfixion incision	Incision through one side of the membranous septum exposing the caudal septum and medial crura
Hinge area	Lateral boundary of the nasal valve area consisting of the lateral crus, fibrous-attached accessory cartilages, and surrounding soft tissue
Inferior septal angle	Angle formed at the junction of the caudal septum with the maxillary crest
Infratip lobule	Portion of the lobule between the tip defining points and the columella–lobule angle
Intermediate crus	See middle crus
Internal nares	Area of the nose that corresponds to the caudal margin of the lateral crus of the lower lateral cartilage
Internal nasal valve	Also referred to as simply nasal valve (see nasal valve definition)
Interrupted strip	Vertically sectioned lower lateral cartilage
Keystone area	Area of the dorsum at the rhinion representing the confluence of the fused nasal bones, perpendicular ethmoid plate, quadrilateral cartilage, and upper lateral cartilages
Lateral crus	Portion of the lower lateral cartilage; begins at the lateral border of the middle crus; extends superomedially mostly above the alar groove
Lateral crural steal	Technique to increase nasal tip projection through recruitment of the lateral crura to lengthen the medial crural component of the tripod; accomplished without division of the lateral crura
Limen vestibuli	Junction of the vestibular skin with the nasal mucosa corresponding to the junction of the cephalic margin of the lateral crus with the caudal margin of the upper lateral cartilage
Lobule	Lower mobile part of the nose bounded by the supratip depression superiorly, the upper nostril margins inferiorly, and the alar grooves laterally
Marginal incision	Incision that follows the caudal border of the medial and lateral crura

(Continued)

Appendix (continued)

Term	Definition
Medial crus	Thin, delicate extension of lower lateral cartilage within the soft tissues of the columella; includes the footplate and columellar segments
Membranous septum	Mobile subcutaneous tissue between the caudal septum and columella; the medial crura are contained within its most anterior portion
Middle crus	Middle portion of the lower lateral cartilage, subdivided into lobular and domal segments
Nasal base	Lower nasal platform extending from alar crease to alar crease
Nasal dorsum	Upper two-thirds of the nose
Nasal height	Distance between the radix and subnasale
Nasal pyramid	Upper one-third of the nose corresponding to the nasal bones and frontal processes of the maxillae
Nasal sill	Part of the alar margin adjacent to the base of the columella
Nasal tip	Apex of the lobule; the most projecting point of the nasal tip on profile
Nasal valve	Two-dimensional slitlike opening between the caudal end of the upper lateral cartilages and the septum; the narrowest part of the nasal cavity; acts as a dynamic airflow regulator during inspiration
Nasal valve area	Three-dimensional correlate of the nasal valve; bounded by the apex of the nasal valve, head of the inferior turbinate, inferior rim of the pyriform aperture, and soft tissues overlying these areas
Nasion	Midpoint of the frontonasal suture in the sagittal plane under the soft tissue nasofrontal angle
Nasofrontal angle	Angle formed by the junction of the nasal dorsum with the glabella
Nasofrontal groove	Angle formed by the soft tissue covering the frontonasal suture; corresponds to the starting point of the nasal dorsum
Nasolabial angle	Angle formed by the junction of columella with the upper lip; indirect measure of nasal tip rotation; abnormal position of columella is a source of error
Non-delivery	Method of altering the lower lateral cartilage (e.g., complete strip) in situ without exteriorizing (delivering) the cartilage
Pars alaris	Paired muscle originating above the labial incisor tooth and inserting into the lower margin of the nasal ala
Pars transversa	Paired muscle originating from the canine eminence and inserting into a fibrous aponeurosis along the cartilaginous nasal dorsum
Pogonion	Most anterior point of soft tissue chin
Pollybeak deformity	Unaesthetic fullness in the supratip
Procerus muscle	Single pyramidal slip of muscle arising from the nasal bones and upper lateral cartilages; insertion is into the frontalis muscle and skin between the eyebrows
Radix nasi	Soft-tissue correlate of the nasion; refers to the root of the nose; most aesthetic at level of the supratarsal fold in primary gaze
Retrograde approach	A method of exposing the lateral and middle crura through an intercartilaginous incision and retrograde dissection of vesibular mucosal from the undersurface of the cartilage
Rhinion	Anterior bony–cartilaginous junction often corresponding to the typical location of a nasal hump
Rim incision	Incision that follows the nostril rim along the inner vestibular surface

(Continued)

Appendix (continued)

Term	Definition
Rim Strip	Removal of most of the cephalic edge of the lower lateral cartilage (intermediate and lateral portions) leaving a few millimeters of an intact *rim* strip of cartilage; strip refers to the portion of cartilage that remains, not taken away
Rocker deformity	Results from an incomplete osteotomy: the osteotomized segment rocks back and forth with digital pressure
Saddle nose deformity	Concavity or depression of the nasal dorsum that results in a saddlelike appearance on profile; also known as pug nose or boxer's nose
Scroll	Redundant cephalic margin of the lower lateral cartilage; this area articulates with an opposite scroll from the ipsilateral upper lateral cartilage
Sellion	Deepest point in the hollow beneath the glabella in the sagital plane
Septal angle	Angle formed by the caudal and dorsal aspects of the septal quadrilateral cartilage
Sesamoid cartilages	Inconsistent islands of cartilage scattered between the caudal upper lateral cartilage and cephalic lateral crus
Soft Triangle	Soft tissue of the lobule opposite the domal notch; depression here is referred to as a facet
Subnasale (Sn)	Bony landmark under the soft tissue nasolabial angle; junction of the columella with the upper cutaneous lip
Supratip area	Transition between the nasal dorsum and supratip lobule; formed by a slight inferior descent of the dorsal septum and the cephalic convex lateral crura; a supratip depression is an aesthetic landmark denoting a slight concavity
Supratip lobule	Portion of the nasal lobule between the supratip break and the tip-defining points
Surgical dome	Dome established at surgery
Tip-defining points	Soft tissue landmarks representing the most projecting areas on each side of the nasal tip; overlies the domal junction line near their caudal margins
Transfixion incision	Incision through and through the membranous septum exposing the caudal septum and medial crura; a full transfixion incision separates totally the medial crural feet from the caudal septum; a partial transfixion incision stops proximal to the feet
Tripod concept	Simplified model of the nasal tip stipulating that three legs representing the lateral crura and conjoined medial crura support the nasal tip
True horizontal	An imaginary horizontal line extending through the profile as the patient stares straight ahead; also known as the natural horizontal facial plane
Upper vermilion (Vu)	Upper vermilion lip–skin border
Vertical facial plane	Perpendicular plane to the true horizontal
Vestibular dome	Counterpart to the clinical dome internally; located at the apex of the concavity formed between the medial and lateral crura
Vestibule	Space inside the nostril bounded medially by the membranous septum and columella, laterally by the ala, superiorly by lower border of the lateral crus and bony pyriform aperture, and inferiorly by the nasal sill and mucocutaneous junction of the nostril rim

REFERENCES

1. Lessard ML, Daniel RK. Surgical anatomy of septorhinoplasty. Arch Otolaryngol 1985; 111:25–29.
2. Woodburne RT. The head and neck. 7th ed. New York: Oxford University Press, 1983, 198–243.
3. Letourneau A, Daniel RK. The superficial musculoaponeurotic system of the nose. Plast Reconstr Surg 1988; 82:48–57.
4. Natvig P, Sether LA, Gingrass RP, Gardner WD. Anatomical details of the osseous–cartilaginous framework of the nose. Plast Reconstr Surg 1971; 48:528–32.
5. Sheen JH. Aesthetic Rhinoplasty. St. Louis: C.V. Mosby Co., 1978.
6. Guyuron B. Footplates of the medial crura. Plast Reconstr Surg 1998; 101:1359–63.
7. Hoasjoe DK, Stucker FJ, Aarstad RF. Aesthetic and anatomic considerations for nasal reconstruction. Facial Plast Surg 1994; 10:317–321.
8. Perkins SW. Anatomy and Physiology. In: Pastorek N, Mangat DS, eds. 1. Aesthetic Facial Surgery, Philadelphia: J.B. Lippincott Co., 1991:5–31.
9. Sheen JH. Aesthetic Rhinoplasty. 2nd ed. St. Louis: C.V. Mosby Co., 1987.
10. Daniel RK, Letourneau A. Rhinoplasty: nasal anatomy. Ann Plast Surg 1988; 20:5–13.
11. Mink PJ. Le nez comme voie respiratorie. Presse Otolaryngol (Belg) 1903; 481:.
12. Schoenrock LD. Nasal Analysis. In: Pastorek N, Mangat DS, eds. Aesthetic Facial Surgery, 1st ed. Philadelphia: J.B. Lippincott Co., 1991:45–63.
13. Rune B, Aberg M. Bone grafts to the nose in Binder's syndrome (maxillonasal dysplasia): a follow-up of eleven patients with the use of profile roentgenograms. Plast Reconstr Surg 1998; 101:297–304.
14. Powell N, Humphries B. Proportions of the Aesthetic Face. New York: Thieme-Stratton, 1984.
15. Salyer K, Joganic E. Analysis of facial proportions. Procedures in plastic and reconstructive surgery—how they do it. Boston: Little, Brown and Co., 1991, 6.
16. Mommaerts MY, Van Butsele BL, Abeloos JS, De Clercq CA, Neyt LF. Rhinoplasty with nasal bone disarticulation to deepen the nasofrontal groove. Experimental and clinical results. . J Craniomaxillofac Surg 1995; 23:109–114.
17. Molenaar A. The depressed nasofrontal angle in aesthetic rhinoplasty. Plast Reconstr Surg 1988; 82:698–706.
18. Crumley RL, Lanser M. Quantitative analysis of nasal tip projection. Laryngoscope 1988; 98:202–208.
19. Goodman WS, Gilbert RW. The anatomy of external rhinoplasty. Otolaryngol Clin North Am 1987; 20:641–652.
20. Webster RC. Advances in surgery of the tip: intact rim cartilage techniques and the tip–columella–lip esthetic complex. Otolaryngol Clin North Am 1975; 8:615–644.
21. Goldman IB. The importance of the mesial crura in nasal-tip reconstruction. Arch Otolaryngol 1957; 65:143–147.
22. Micheli-Pellegrini V, Ponti L, Ponti G, Guidarelli P. Interrupted and continuous strip technique for tip surgery during traditional rhinoplasty. Facial Plast Surg 1996; 12: 347–355.
23. Tardy ME, Jr., Patt BS, Walter MA. Transdomal suture refinement of the nasal tip: long-term outcomes. Facial Plast Surg 1993; 9:275–84.
24. Petroff MA, McCollough EG, Hom D, Anderson JR. Nasal tip projection. Quantitative changes following rhinoplasty. Arch Otolaryngol Head Neck Surg 1991; 117:783–788.
25. Rohrich RJ, Minoli JJ, Adams WP, Hollier LH. The lateral nasal osteotomy in rhinoplasty: an anatomic endoscopic comparison of the external versus the internal approach. Plast Reconstr Surg 1997; 99:1309–1312.
26. Guyuron B, Michelow BJ, Englebardt C. Upper lateral splay graft. Plast Reconstr Surg 1998; 102:2169–2177.

27. Paniello RC. Nasal valve suspension. An effective treatment for nasal valve collapse. Arch Otolaryngol Head Neck Surg 1996; 122:1342–1346.
28. Kern EB. Surgical approaches to abnormalities of the nasal valve. Rhinology 1978; 16:165–189.
29. Vetter U, Pirsig W, Heinze E. Growth activity in human septal cartilage: age-dependent incorporation of labeled sulfate in different anatomic locations. Plast Reconstr Surg 1983; 71:167–171.
30. Quarrell OW, Koch M, Hughes HE. Maxillonasal dysplasia (Binder's syndrome). J Med Genet 1990; 27:384–387.

21

Traditional, Revision, and Augmentation Rhinoplasty

Robert W. Dolan
Lahey Clinic Medical Center, Burlington, Mansachusetts, U.S.A.

Laurence Milgrim
Trumbull, Connecticut, U.S.A.

Advanced rhinoplasty encompasses a wide range of rhinoplasty techniques and challenges. However, much of what is considered within the scope of advanced rhinoplasty relates to the diagnostic and therapeutic methods used in revision rhinoplasty. Advanced rhinoplasty has been considered synonymous with revision rhinoplasty, but this notion has changed over the last 20 years. Revision techniques are now being applied routinely to primary cases under the guise of 'augmentation rhinoplasty.' Revision rhinoplasty usually involves reconstitution of lost cartilage and bone and reconstruction of the nasal framework. This approach, when applied to patients undergoing primary rhinoplasty, is termed augmentation rhinoplasty. Augmentation of the nasal framework in primary rhinoplasty has come to be favored over radical cartilage excision and destruction because the former achieves a more stable and natural-appearing long-term result. What is included under the general heading of "advanced" is sometimes arbitrary. Nevertheless, this chapter will include a review of revision rhinoplasty, augmentation rhinoplasty including grafts and implants, the open rhinoplasty technique, and challenging special conditions including lengthening a short nose, straightening a crooked nose, cleft rhinoplasty, rhinoplasty in the aging patient, rhinoplasty in nonwhite patients, and repair of nasal fractures.

TRADITIONAL RHINOPLASTY

Traditional rhinoplasty incorporates a variety of reduction and cartilage division techniques including those used in the classic Joseph reduction rhinoplasty and techniques described specifically for improving tip projection and rotation without grafts or implants. Although the universal application of reduction techniques leads to many of the typical adverse sequelae associated with reduction rhinoplasty, many of the traditional reduction and cartilage modification techniques are safe and useful when used in selected patients. The application of these traditional techniques is indicated in patients with anatomical characteristics that can tolerate relatively radical (by today's standards) cartilage reduction and division. These characteristics include a substantial cartilaginous framework, good pre-existing nasal support and projection, and relatively thick skin to help camouflage the ends of the cut and altered cartilage.

Certain objectives can only be accomplished through the application of a reduction or cartilage division technique. For example, correction of true excessive projection of the nasal tip requires the unfettered application of reduction rhinoplasty principles. Pure retrodisplacement of the tip with no caudal rotation will require a concomitant shortening of all legs of the tripod (see Fig. 27 in Chapter 20 on Basic Rhinoplasty). Cephalic trimming of the upper lateral cartilage associated with an unsecured full transfixion incision will result in retrodisplacement of the nasal tip. However, for patients with medial crura that extend the entire length of the columella, a full transfixion incision will have little effect on nasal support or projection. In these cases, the medial crural component of the tripod must be reduced in some other way (e.g., segmental resection). A significant reduction in nasal tip projection is achieved by trimming the dorsal septum (including the septal angle) combined with segmental resection of the medial crura. The lateral crura may also require weakening to avoid caudal rotation of the nasal tip and the creation of a pollybeak. This can be achieved through a combination of cephalic trimming and wedge resection. To maintain nasal tip support and avoid notching or surface contour irregularities, the free ends of the medial crura must be carefully reapproximated.

Nasal Tip Rotation and Projection Techniques

Cephalic rotation of a dependent nasal tip is an objective most effectively achieved using traditional reduction techniques. Of course, nasal tip projection and rotation are intimately related. Cephalic rotation of a ptotic nasal tip may result in some coincident gain or loss of projection depending on the technique chosen. Cephalic tip rotation may be achieved by interruption of the dorsal tip-supporting elements, especially the lateral crura, consistent with the tripod concept. The degree of cephalic rotation is predictable based on the type and extent of surgical modification to the lateral crura and domes. Several commonly used techniques are designed to improve tip definition (refinement and narrowing) and also result in some cephalic rotation including the complete strip, rim strip, and dome division. The lateral crura are often modified during nasal tip surgery to correct deformities or increase tip definition. Trimming a longitudinal strip of cartilage along the cephalic border of the lateral crura will enhance tip definition and may result in cephalic rotation of the nasal tip. A residual so-called complete strip of cartilage (at least 5 mm) must remain to maintain the strength of the lower lateral cartilage and nasal tip support.

Lateral Crural Flap

A rim strip will result in significant cephalic rotation of a dependent nasal tip. However, if what is termed a 'lateral crural flap' is left in place after a typical rim strip procedure, healing and the degree of cephalic rotation are more predictable (1). This technique is similar to the rim strip operation except the superolateral portion of the lateral crus that is excised in a rim strip is left in situ. This island of cartilage is left attached to the stable nasal framework superiorly, including the upper lateral cartilage, sesamoid cartilages, and the pyriform aperture. The lateral crural flap fills the void between the narrow rim strip and the upper lateral cartilage and pyriform aperture. In a typical rim strip operation, this void is obliterated with scar tissue, leading to unpredictable superior traction on the remaining lower lateral cartilage. The degree of tip retrodisplacement and cephalic rotation is variable and problems with alar rim notching and irregularities are common. Like the rim strip, tip retrodisplacement and cephalic rotation are the main indications for the use of the lateral crural flap technique. However, as mentioned, these changes are more predictable using the lateral crural flap, the postoperative problems of asymmetry and alar notching secondary to uncontrolled scar contracture are lessened.

The lateral crural flap technique involves delivering the cartilage followed by a complete or rim strip procedure (Webster). The remaining strip is transected through the intermediate and caudal lateral crus area. This incision parallels the alar rim, leaving a large portion of the superolateral crus intact as this portion of the lateral crus curves cephalically. The anterior portion of the cartilage is then undermined to the dome, sparing the underlying mucosa. This strip is then rotated posteriorly, resulting in overlapping of the free ends of the rim strip and posterior crural flap remnant. Some surgeons prefer not to undermine and leave the mucosal–cartilage flap intact. The overlapping portion of the lateral crural flap is excised, and buried sutures are used to approximate and stabilize the cartilage segments. The amount of cartilage excised is calibrated according to the desired degree of cephalic rotation and tip retrodisplacement (Fig. 1). Despite the advantages of leaving the lateral crural flap in situ after a rim strip procedure, there are persistent problems inherent in any technique that involves a rim strip and division of the lateral crus. A severely weakened dome may result in ptosis of the nasal tip because it cannot resist the natural forces of even minimal scar contracture of the soft tissue envelope. This may result in an undesirable supratip fullness (pollybeak deformity) as the tip migrates inferiorly, bringing into relief the superior septal angle and the scrolls of the upper and lower lateral cartilages. In addition, the cut edges of the lateral crura tend to medialize into the vestibule despite suture fixation, causing nasal obstruction by narrowing the nasal valve area. The rim strip and lateral crural strip techniques should only be used in patients with relatively thick skin and dependent, overprojected nasal tips.

Goldman's Vertical Dome Division and Lateral Crural Steal

It is possible to increase nasal tip projection significantly using cartilage division techniques. However, these techniques may be considered in selected patients only since augmentation techniques (grafts) generally provide a safer and more predictable result. A significant degree of cephalic rotation is a common side effect of techniques designed to increase nasal projection. Nevertheless, direct surgical modification of the lower lateral cartilages can result in significant gains in nasal projection in patients with a suitably resilient and an abundant cartilage framework. Modification of the existing cartilages to increase tip projection is usually

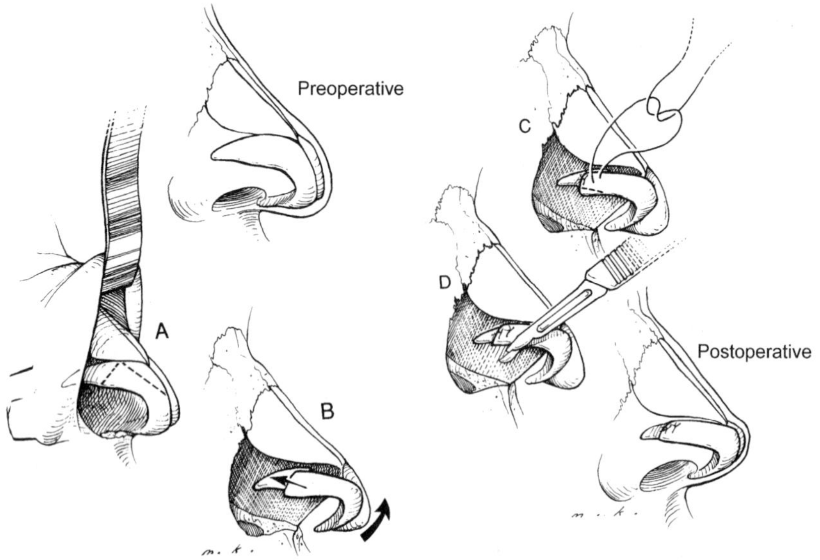

Figure 1 Lateral crural flap technique as performed through an open rhinoplasty approach. A. After a conservative complete strip is performed, the lateral crus is divided. B. The crus is moved posteriorly, resulting in tip rotation. C. The desired configuration is stabilized using 5-0 PDS suture. D. The inferior edge of the cartilage is trimmed to remove irregularities created as the crural segments were overlapped. (From Kridel RW, Konior RJ. Controlled nasal tip rotation via the lateral crural overlay technique. Arch Otolaryngol Head Neck Surg 1991; 117(4):411–5.)

not possible in revision or secondary rhinoplasty cases. The basic idea is to recruit the lateral crura to lengthen the medial crural component of the tripod. This results in tip narrowing, increased definition, cephalic rotation, and significant increases in tip projection. Two commonly used procedures that recruit the lateral and intermediate crura are the Goldman vertical dome division and (2) the lateral crural steal. Dr. Goldman described vertical dome division over 40 years ago (2). He emphasized the use of the medial crura in augmenting tip projection and narrowing the nasal tip by recruiting cartilage from the lateral crura. The technique involves complete transection of the lateral crura just lateral to the dome, including the underlying vestibular mucosa, removal of the intervening connective tissue between the medial crura, and suturing the medial crura and associated lateral crura remnants together in the midline to form a projecting strut of cartilage beneath the tip lobule (see Fig. 24 in Chapter 20 on Basic Rhinoplasty). This procedure can be safely used in patients with relatively thick skin in which the cut edges of the cartilage will be adequately camouflaged. The lateral crus should be divided no more than 3 mm lateral to the anatomical dome. Division of the lateral crura well lateral to the dome within the thicker supra-alar skin is preferable when the domes do not require much modification. This maneuver will result in significant increases in projection while avoiding asymmetrical healing and scar contracture over the more vulnerable medial areas. Risks include creation of a pinched appearance to the nasal tip, an asymmetrical nasal tip due to unpredictable healing, cartilage bossing, alar notching, and undesirable pronounced cephalic rotation. These complications are seen with some frequency and the routine use of the Goldman tipplasty has been abandoned. Nevertheless, the procedure is used in selected cases of boxy tips, ptotic tips, so-called closed noses in which the columella–labial angle is acute, foreshortened columella, and in patients with thick skin (ethnic rhinoplasty). Modifications of the Goldman tipplasty have been devised to reduce the postoperative sequelae of bosselation, pinching, and the typical 'operated look' that results from this procedure. Dr. Ponti of Rome, Italy, who trained under Goldman, altered the procedure by preserving the vestibular lining (3). He also cut the cartilage more lateral to the dome than Goldman and resected additional lateral crura to achieve more volume reduction. This was known as the 'butterfly' technique because, on basal view, the cut edges of the dome and lateral crural segments resembled butterfly wings. However, this modification can lead to lateral pinching of the nose and a clown effect, with a rounded ball-like tip juxtaposed against thinned lateral walls.

The lateral crural steal technique also recruits the lateral crura to lengthen the medial crural component of the tripod but does so without division of the lateral crura (4). This technique also results in tip narrowing, increased definition, cephalic rotation, and significant increases in tip projection. The procedure requires an external rhinoplasty approach to allow full visualization of the lower lateral cartilages. The vestibular lining is separated from the undersurface of the intermediate and lateral segments of the lower lateral cartilage. Both lateral crura are released from their fibrous attachments to mobilize the cartilage. Conservative cephalic trimming (i.e., conservative complete rim strip) may be done at this point if necessary. Transdomal sutures are placed to move the intermediate and lateral crura medially, thus increasing the height of the medial crural component of the tripod and projecting the tip. Since the lateral crura are shortened, the increase in nasal projection is accompanied by a proportional increase in cephalic tip rotation and nasal shortening. The lateral crural steal procedure preserves the integrity of the lateral crura, minimizing the potential problems associated with division of the lateral crus and dome. These include alar notching, unpredictable healing and tip asymmetry, and obvious dome irregularities.

The techniques of traditional and reduction rhinoplasty rely heavily on the intrinsic nasal cartilage framework to achieve various aesthetic objectives including improved tip definition, rotation of the nasal tip, and changes in tip projection. Although it is clear that reduction techniques are needed for patients with dependent and overprojected nasal tips, the majority of patients benefit from a combination of conservative reduction (e.g., complete strip) and augmentation (sutures and grafting). The key in determining the appropriate technique is the preoperative nasal analysis and diagnostic acumen of the clinician. In a sense, rhinoplasty has become a much more complicated endeavor because of this highly individualized approach. No longer is a rhinoplasty performed in a standard way. For example, in the past, inadequate tip projection was often compensated for by reducing the height of the nasal dorsum. The ratio of nasal tip projection to nasal length normalized and the nose became intrinsically balanced. As was typical of reduction rhinoplasty, the nose was small and out of proportion with the rest of the face. Pollybeak deformity occurred due to overreduction of the nasal dorsum. The excess dead space and cartilage division or reduction resulted in scar contracture and excessive cephalic rotation of the nasal tip. Modern rhinoplasty is based in large part on the shared experiences of clinicians treating patients seeking revision rhinoplasty who had undergone standard reduction rhinoplasty several years earlier. It is useful to review this common experience of revision rhinoplasty and the adverse consequences of reduction rhinoplasty.

REVISION RHINOPLASTY

Revision rhinoplasty is most often done to correct the adverse sequelae of undercorrection or overresection of the cartilaginous structures of the nose. Overresection of cartilage (reduction rhinoplasty) is the most common reason for revision. In the lower third of the nose there is collapse and buckling of the lower lateral cartilages producing tip ptosis, asymmetry, pollybeak deformity, and nostril flaring. In the middle third, medial collapse of the upper lateral cartilages may produce 'pinched nose' and inverted 'V' deformities associated with narrowing of the nasal valves and nasal obstruction. In the upper nasal third, the nasal dorsum may be overreduced or irregular. Correction of abnormalities in the upper third is usually more straightforward than in other parts of the nose. The typical specific adverse functional and aesthetic effects of reduction rhinoplasty are reviewed below.

Nasal Tip

Reduction rhinoplasty techniques have the greatest deleterious effect on the nasal tip. Attenuation of the cartilages in the nasal tip and disruption of the major and minor tip supporting mechanisms result in many of the typical adverse sequelae associated with reduction rhinoplasty: nasal alar collapse, supra-alar pinching, nostril flaring, loss of tip support, pathological cephalic rotation, asymmetry, pollybeak deformity, and tip deprojection. Although weakening of the cartilage framework is a significant underlying factor, the creation of tissue voids due to the loss of cartilage is the predominant factor leading to many of these abnormalities. A bed of scarring is created in areas of cartilage loss that leads to soft tissue contraction. The existing weakened cartilage framework is unable to prevent the scar contraction and the cartilages may buckle, leading to surface abnormalities and asymmetry. Weakening or division of the alar cartilages may result in dynamic collapse of the nasal alae, causing nasal obstruction and significant cephalic rotation of the nasal tip proportional to the degree of cartilage attenuation and loss. The loss of tip support relates to weakening and detachment of the medial crura and alar cartilages commonly resulting from full transfixion incisions and rim strips, respectively. Overresection in the area of the anterior septal angle will result in a tissue void over the supratip. This void fills with scar tissue and will eventually lead to the formation of an unattractive fullness in the supratip and pollybeak deformity (Fig. 2).

Aggressive division of the lower lateral cartilages along the alae or through the domes increases the likelihood that abnormalities within the nasal tip will develop during healing including knuckle (bossae) formation, lateral wall instability, and asymmetry. Unequal reduction of tip volume, uneven scar formation, or misplacement of dome-binding stitches can also result in asymmetry. Scar-related abnormalities can occur secondary to any procedure on the nasal tip but, as a rule, the more aggressive the primary resection and reshaping, the greater the likelihood of scar

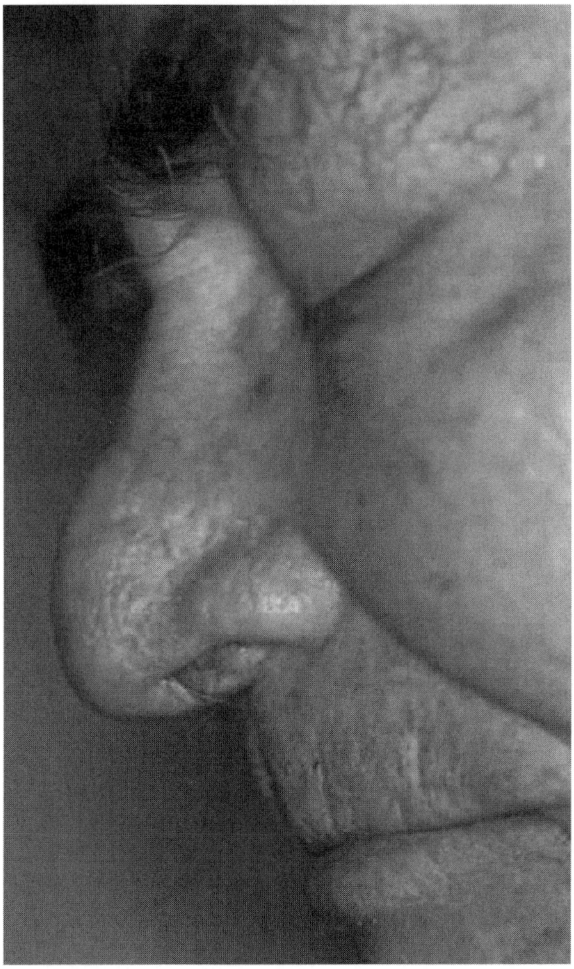

Figure 2 Pollybeak deformity. Note the fullness and rounding effect in the supratip. This patient is a relatively extreme example of pollybeak due to placement of a forehead flap in the area. The supratip was subsequently defatted.

contracture abnormalities. A variety of augmentation rhinoplasty techniques (reviewed below) are needed to correct these deformities.

Nasal Dorsum

The nasal dorsum is often overreduced to match an attenuated and retrused nasal tip. In doing so significant tissue voids are created that have the potential to lead to either a saddle nose deformity or pollybeak deformity. Saddle nose deformity is usually due to overzealous removal of a nasal hump by an inexperienced surgeon. Correction is relatively straightforward and involves onlay grafts obtained from the septum, conchal bowl, or the resected portions of the tip cartilages. Sequelae that are more difficult to correct include abnormal fractures and bone spurs. Abnormal fractures such as rocker deformity occur from misalignment of the osteotome and aberrant fractures. A shelf effect can occur if the osteotome and fracture are placed too high along the ascending process. A 'rocker' deformity occurs if the osteotomy was incomplete (see definition in Chapter 20 on Basic Rhinoplasty). Correction of a rocker deformity requires repeat intermediate and low lateral osteotomies with or without onlay camouflage grafts. Bone spurs occur when the lateral osteotomy is placed too high. The inferior edge of the face of the maxilla often protrudes and creates a noticeable ledge between the infractured superior portion and the remnant attached to the face of the maxilla. Perforating osteotomies or a repeat low lateral osteotomy is needed to efface the ledge.

Nasal Valve

Excision of a nasal hump disrupts the T configuration that the upper lateral cartilages share with the dorsal septum. Once the splaying effect of this articulation is lost, the upper lateral cartilages tend to fall toward the septum, narrowing the internal nasal valves. Further medialization is seen after lateral osteotomy and medialization of the nasal bones because of the rigid connection between the cephalic upper lateral cartilages and the caudal nasal bones. In addition to this functional problem, some patients experience adverse aesthetic effects including a pinched middle nasal vault and inverted V deformity.

Narrowing within the nasal valve area also contributes to nasal obstruction although it is not as dramatic as narrowing within the internal nasal valve itself. Medialization of the lateral crura narrows the nasal valve area along the nasal sidewall (the so-called hinge area). This finding is associated with previous rhinoplasty when the domes or lateral crura have been sutured in the midline, pulling the lateral crura medially.

Scarring across the nasal valve is a common finding after a poorly performed rhinoplasty. This is usually secondary to disruption of the mucosal lining at the apex of the nasal valve during excision of the dorsal septum near the anterior septal angle. If the dorsal cartilaginous septum requires significant reduction during primary rhinoplasty, it should first be separated from the surrounding mucosa in the area of the nasal valve. This preserves the mucosal lining and prevents scarring and nasal valve obstruction. As previously mentioned, dynamic nasal valve dysfunction (collapse during inspiration) is often due to overresection of the lateral crura and weakening of the nasal sidewall in the hinge area. This abnormality is most commonly encountered in patients who have undergone a traditional reduction rhinoplasty. The typical external nasal deformity that accompanies this functional abnormality is pinching in the supra-alar region.

Patient Selection

If the techniques of reduction rhinoplasty are universally applied, many patients will display the problems described above. However, these maneuvers will be quite successful in achieving an aesthetic and long-lasting result in a subset of patients. Determining which patients require cartilage division and relatively radical cartilage attenuation is sometimes difficult. Whenever cartilage is divided or significantly weakened, there is a chance of an adverse result due to the unpredictable way in which such injuries heal. For this reason, radical cartilage manipulation (e.g., division or rim strip) should be reserved for patients with thick skin and ample preoperative nasal support in whom a relatively radical change is desired. For example, a patient with a boxy, overprojecting, and drooping nasal tip with widely divergent domes is a candidate for cartilage division and attenuation. Conversely, certain unique anatomical traits predispose patients undergoing rhinoplasty to a poor outcome. If these traits are identified during the preoperative nasal analysis, the operative plan can be altered accordingly. In the majority of cases this means that cartilage grafting or suture techniques will be needed instead of cartilage excision or other typical 'reduction' techniques. An example of an anatomical trait that is useful in predicting the need for augmentation instead of reduction is poor nasal tip recoil. Poor recoil is present when the spring in the nasal tip is greatly diminished, indicating pre-existing attenuated underlying cartilaginous support. In patients with this finding, the need for additional cartilaginous support in the form of grafts or sutures should be anticipated. Anatomical traits present preoperatively that were found frequently by Constantian in those seeking revision rhinoplasty included low radix, narrow middle vault, cephalic malposition of the alar cartilages, and inadequate tip projection. An interesting finding was that these traits are also common sequelae of reduction rhinoplasty. Furthermore, both groups of patients share the need for augmentation techniques to correct these abnormalities adequately and safely. This is an illustrative example of how what was once solely in the realm of revision rhinoplasty is now expanded to include patients undergoing primary rhinoplasty. The approach to both revision and primary rhinoplasty has melded, resulting in a highly individualized approach based on the principles of augmentation rhinoplasty, which is a unified approach of cautious reduction and selective augmentation.

AUGMENTATION RHINOPLASTY

Augmentation of the nasal framework is the hallmark of revision rhinoplasty but the same techniques are now used routinely in primary rhinoplasty to strengthen and supplement the existing cartilage structure. In fact, the surgical planning and methods of revision and primary rhinoplasty are similar and the modern rhinoplasty surgeon should consider each case individually and apply the appropriate techniques when indicated.

Augmentation rhinoplasty describes a philosophical approach to rhinoplasty involving the use of a variety of techniques and grafts that tend to preserve and augment the structural integrity and shape of the nose. This approach to modern rhinoplasty was cultivated in the 1970s when multiple revisions were being performed on patients who had undergone standard reduction techniques. Reduction rhinoplasty, as the method has come to be known, was a rote approach to primary rhinoplasty that consisted of often radical (by today's standards) excision and division of tip cartilage, dorsal hump removal, and nasal bone infracture. The structural and functional integrity of the nose was largely ignored. The loss of cartilaginous support and mucosal lining eventually resulted in scar contracture with surface irregularities, collapse or severe retraction of the nasal tip, collapse of the middle vault (inverted V deformity), and nasal valve obstruction. As mentioned, revision rhinoplasty is most often done to correct adverse sequelae of overresection of cartilage. Revision cases inevitably required scar lysis and surgical techniques using a variety of grafts to restore the structural and functional integrity of the nose. Revision surgery using grafts and conservative reconstructive techniques led to predictable long-term results with a nose that was functionally and structurally sound and in balance with the rest of the face. Taking lessons from these revision cases, the approach to primary rhinoplasty changed dramatically. Cartilage excision and violation of the mucosal linings were minimized. Cartilage grafts were more likely to be used instead of cartilage excision or division to create a change in the balance or shape of the nose. Thus, the era of primary augmentation rhinoplasty was inaugurated. Subsequent developments have included the increasing popularity of the open structure rhinoplasty to facilitate the accurate manipulation and placement of cartilage grafts and sutures. There is also an increasing appreciation of the aesthetic balance between the shape and size of the nose and the rest of the face. This is especially relevant to the position of the radix, projection of the premaxilla, and projection of the chin. A variety of difficult rhinoplasty problems also exists that require a specialized approach that includes correcting a high or low radix, lengthening a short nose, straightening a crooked nose, and performing cleft rhinoplasty. In addition, the approach to rhinoplasty in the aging patient and in the non-white patient requires special consideration. The need for augmentation in those presenting for primary rhinoplasty is predictable based on the preoperative nasal analysis. Universal application of reduction techniques, as was the practice in the era of 'reduction rhinoplasty,' results in a poor aesthetic and functional result in many but not all patients. A subset of patients who undergo traditional reduction rhinoplasty do well but the majority of patients will experience aesthetic or functional problems. Several factors account for these findings, including the type and extent of primary cartilage modification and the preoperative anatomical configuration of the nose.

Although augmentation rhinoplasty techniques are an integral part of many primary rhinoplasties, a variety of traditional reduction techniques are still required in the majority of patients seeking primary rhinoplasty. Often the nose is first reduced and reassessed on the operating table. This rapid intraoperative assessment may reveal several adverse sequelae typical of reduction rhinoplasty. At this point, application of the principles and techniques of augmentation rhinoplasty serve to reconstruct and stabilize the nose in its new favorable aesthetic and structural configuration.

Trimming, morselization, and suture modification of the lower lateral cartilage to improve the nasal tip are all that is needed in uncomplicated primary rhinoplasty cases. Overuse of grafts, interrupted strip, and radical excisional techniques are to be avoided. The use of structural grafts (e.g., columellar strut or lateral crural strut grafts) rather than surface grafts (e.g., tip onlay or shield grafts) may be more liberal in primary rhinoplasty because minor postoperative warping and resorption problems are less noticeable. Volume reduction, slight cephalic rotation, and an increase in definition are the most common objectives in nasal tip surgery. These can be achieved using conservative complete strip, limited morselization, and approximating suture techniques.

A typical primary augmentation rhinoplasty would consist of the following steps:

1. Establish goals with the preoperative nasal analysis.
2. Perform open rhinoplasty to facilitate graft placement.

3. Assess anatomy and symmetry of the lower lateral cartilages.
4. Set tip projection using cartilage modification, suture, and grafting techniques.
5. Correct asymmetries of the nasal bones and set the radix using osteotomies, rasping, and onlay grafts.
6. Reconstitute the middle third and nasal valves using spreader grafts and sutures.
7. Set dorsal projection in the middle and upper thirds using grafts and selective sculpting.
8. Reassess tip and establish tip-defining points, if necessary, using shield grafts and suture techniques.
9. Redrape skin envelope and carefully remove subcutaneous scar tissue as necessary to increase tip definition and eliminate soft tissue pollybeak.

Familiarity with anatomy and nasal analysis (see Chapter 20 on Basic Rhinoplasty), grafts and implants, the open approach, and a variety of procedures directed at correcting common specific aesthetic and functional nasal abnormalities is essential.

The Open Approach

Padovan introduced open or external rhinoplasty to North America in 1973 from France (6). This approach provides improved exposure of the nasal tip and dorsum for diagnosis, cartilage manipulation, and graft placement. It affords superior visualization of the lower lateral cartilages, upper lateral cartilages, internal nasal valve, dorsal septum, and dome areas.

The most dramatic difference between the open rhinoplasty approach and the closed approaches is the far superior visualization of the nasal tip cartilages provided by the former. Therefore, the main indication for using the open approach is to facilitate work on the nasal tip. Typical indications include tip asymmetry, unknown anatomy (e.g., revision cases), and a need for grafting. The procedure is outlined in Chapter 20 on Basic Rhinoplasty. A transcolumellar incision is created that is an extension of the marginal incision used in delivering the lower lateral cartilages. The shape of the incision varies from surgeon to surgeon, but most use either a 'W' or upside-down 'V'-shaped incision approximately two-thirds down along the columella from the tip.

The procedure begins with the creation of both marginal and transcolumellar incisions that are eventually connected over the soft triangle. The soft tissue columella is raised over the medial and middle crura and the columellar and marginal incisions are joined as the dissection continues over the domes and the lateral crura. A combination of sharp and blunt dissection proceeds over the upper lateral cartilages and dorsum in a supraperichondrial plane. An intercartilaginous incision is only made if needed. The dissection should remain submuscular (i.e., under the superficial musculoaponeurotic system [SMAS]) to preserve the blood supply to the skin and prevent skin necrosis over the nasal tip. As the caudal aspect of the nasal bones is approached, the plane of dissection shifts to a subperiosteal level in the midline. The entire nasal dorsum is exposed, allowing direct visualization and manipulation of the nasal cartilages, septum, and nasal bones. The septum may be exposed via a caudal or dorsal approach. The caudal approach involves separation of the medial crura and dissection through the membranous septum to reach the caudal aspect of the nasal septum. The dorsal approach involves careful separation of the upper lateral cartilages, usually starting at the septal angle and proceeding in a cephalic direction. The medial aspect of the upper lateral cartilages must be sharply separated from the dorsal septum, with care taken not to disrupt the underlying mucosa surrounding the nasal valves. Mucoperiosteal flaps may then be widely dissected, allowing modification or removal of the entire septum. At the completion of the procedure, the medial crura should be secured to the caudal septum to re-establish this major support mechanism, if necessary. In addition, a single buried 4–0 chromic suture is used to approximate the transcolumellar incision in the midline. Additional cutaneous sutures are placed along the lateral aspects of the transcolumellar incision and along the marginal incisions within the vestibule. Carefully reapproximating the mucosal incisions prevents healing irregularities and covers grafts and cartilage sutures. Small intercartilaginous stab incisions can be safely made to promote drainage, if necessary.

The advantages of the open approach include direct and accurate assessment and treatment of cartilage and bone abnormalities, ease and accuracy of suture placement, direct access to the nasal cartilaginous dorsum (including the quadrilateral septal cartilage), and teaching opportunities. Direct visualization of the complex anatomy facilitates learning and mastery of rhinoplasty. Disadvantages of the open approach include additional operative time, cutaneous scarring, operative edema, subcutaneous scarring, and nasal tip anesthesia. The cutaneous (transcolumellar) scarring is of minimal concern and, if the procedure is properly performed, rarely is problematic. Permanent anesthesia of the nasal tip is rare. The connection between the medial crura and caudal septum is disrupted in the caudal approach to the nasal septum. Since this is a significant tip-supporting element, the medial crural attachment should be reestablished with suture to avoid postoperative loss of nasal support.

Grafts and Implants

The use of a variety of grafts in primary and revision rhinoplasty has become commonplace. Cartilage grafts have traditionally been reserved for use in revision cases for the correction of a retused tip, saddle nose deformity, or lateral nasal wall or nasal valve collapse. However, modern augmentation rhinoplasty frequently calls for the use of grafts including tip shield grafts, columellar struts, and plumping grafts.

The most common grafting material for the nasal tip is either septal or conchal cartilage. A variety of allografts and alloplasts are available to shape, augment, and support the nasal tip, but the long-term retention and stability of these materials are poor. Two popular alternatives to autogenous grafts are porous high-density polyethylene (alloplast: Medpor, Porex Surgical Inc, Atlanta, GA) and homologous dermis (allograft: Alloderm dermal graft, LifeCell Corporation, Woodlands, TX). The nasal tip is the most mobile portion of the nose and excess graft movement is often responsible for graft extrusion or absorption. Medpor is especially prone to exposure in the nasal tip area and, because of the disastrous consequences of this complication, it is rarely used. Alloderm has proved to be a useful alternative in selected cases. However, its performance as a volume expander (e.g., correction of a saddle nose deformity) is poor due to absorption that occurs over a period of several months after placement. Alloderm is better used to camouflage slight surface irregularities and to augment thin overlying skin. Irradiated homologous cartilage grafts have been used with success and little risk of extrusion. Despite graft resorption rates in excess of 75%, there may be little loss of volume because the graft is replaced with fibrous tissue (7). However, autogenous cartilage grafts are undoubtedly the graft material of choice considering the material's long-term stability and extremely low extrusion rates.

Septal cartilage provides relatively stiff and straight pieces of cartilage ideal for columellar struts and spreader grafts. The thickest cartilage is found along the maxillary crest and ethmoid plate. Conchal cartilage is softer than septal cartilage and possesses a natural curvature. It is ideal for grafts that must span the nasal dorsum, such as a splay graft. Conchal cartilage is harvested through a curvilinear incision through the anterolateral aspect of the conchal bowl. Preservation of the perichondrial layer may improve graft volume retention through the growth of new cartilage (8). Using a subperichondrial dissection on the anterior surface and a supraperichondrial dissection on the posterior surface preserves the posterior perichondrial layer. Preserving the posterior perichondrium is straightforward because it is tightly adhered to the cartilage.

Spreader Graft

Spreader grafts (Fig. 3) are very effective in widening the nasal valve and improving nasal airflow (9). They are harvested from the ear or septum, typically measuring 2.5 cm in length, 3 mm in height, and 2 mm in thickness. An endonasal or open rhinoplasty approach can be used for graft placement. The endonasal approach

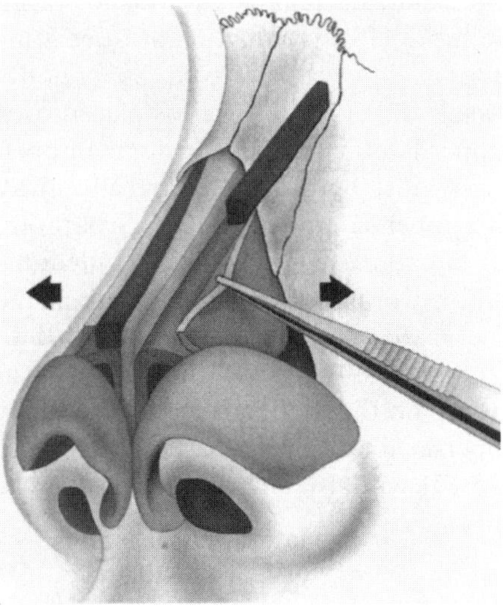

Figure 3 Spreader graft placed during an open rhinoplasty. Note that the upper lateral cartilage is separated sharply from the dorsal septum and the graft is placed between it and the septum; the underlying mucosa remains intact. (From Dolan RW. Nasal ala and internal valve insufficiency. In: Holt R, ed. Facial Plastics Clinics. Philadelphia: W.B. Saunders, 2000: 8(4); 447–464.)

requires a separate sub-mucoperichondrial pocket along the nasal dorsum through an access incision on the anterior caudal septum, anterior to the nasal valve. The graft is inserted into the pocket and the incision is closed with a single absorbable suture (see Fig. 32 in Chapter 20 on Basic Rhinoplasty). The open rhinoplasty approach requires that a dorsal incision be made between the upper lateral cartilages along the septum beginning near the anterior septal angle. Submucoperichondrial dissection proceeds to separate the upper lateral cartilage from the septum to create a crib for the graft. Usually, one graft is placed on either side of the septum and secured with 5-0 PDS (Ethicon, NJ) horizontal mattress sutures that pass through the upper lateral cartilages, grafts, and septum.

Placement of the spreader graft through a dorsal approach is usually indicated in patients undergoing open rhinoplasty. Separation and dorsal trimming of the dorsal upper lateral cartilage and septum have usually already been done, revealing the space into which the spreader graft will be placed. It is essential that the underlying mucosa be preserved as much as possible to prevent scarring in the area of the valve. Dissecting the mucosa away from the undersurface of the upper lateral cartilages is difficult and meticulous sharp technique is needed. The graft is inset into the space between the upper lateral cartilages and septum and sutured into position. Aside from opening the nasal valves, spreader grafts can be used to lengthen a short nose, help camouflage or redirect a twisted nose, and widen a narrow nose. Slight widening of the dorsal middle vault is to be expected when spreader grafts are used and the patient should be informed of this preoperatively.

Splay Graft

An upper lateral splay graft (Fig. 4) spans the nasal dorsum under the upper lateral cartilages to reinforce the cartilage and open the nasal valves (10). The graft is harvested from the conchal bowl to take advantage of the natural curvature and spring inherent in the cartilage. A splay graft can be more effective than a spreader graft when the upper lateral cartilages are greatly attenuated or overresected. Splay grafts also result in greater widening of the middle nasal vault. A splay graft is placed over the septum (convex side up) and under each upper lateral cartilage through an open rhinoplasty approach. The mucoperichondrium must be dissected carefully away from the septum and the undersurface of the upper lateral cartilages. Separating the mucosa from the undersurface of the upper lateral cartilages is extremely tedious and small perforations are common; however, this will not affect the viability of the graft. The septum acts as the fulcrum for the graft and may require lowering in selected cases. The cartilage graft will extend to the lateral border of the upper lateral cartilages or to the pyriform apertures, depending on the desired affect. A butterfly graft is similar to a splay graft but is placed superficial to the upper lateral cartilages and deep to the lower lateral cartilages (Fig. 5). It will also significantly widen the middle nasal vault.

Onlay Graft

A splay graft is a type of onlay graft. Onlay grafts lie along the surface of the septum, upper lateral cartilages, or both and consist of cartilage, cartilage and bone, or alloplastic material. They are used to efface saddle nose deformities or to correct deficiencies of the lateral nasal wall. In overrotated tips, they are used to bring the tip back into alignment or to act as camouflage. In open rhinoplasty, these grafts can

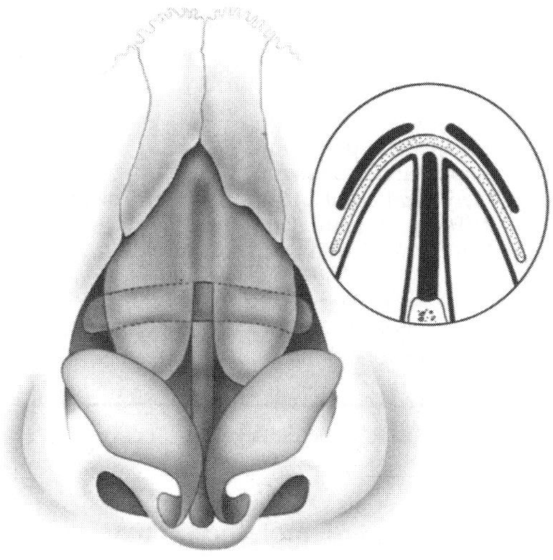

Figure 4 Upper lateral splay graft placed to open the nasal valves. Note that the graft spans the dorsal septum and is secured under the upper lateral cartilages, thereby splaying open the nasal valves. Although this is effective in opening the nasal valves it will usually result in marked widening in the middorsum. (From Dolan RW. Nasal ala and internal valve insufficiency. In: Holt R, ed. Facial Plastics Clinics. Philadelphia: W.B. Saunders, 2000: 8(4); 447–464.)

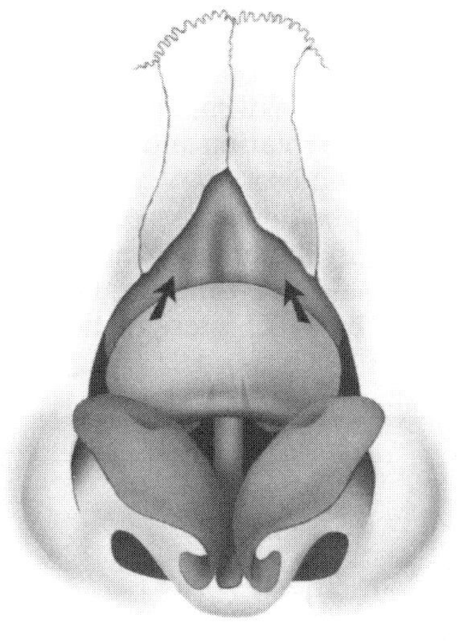

Figure 5 Butterfly graft placed to open the nasal valves. This graft is similar to the splay graft but is placed and secured over the upper lateral cartilages. This graft will also markedly widen the middorsum. (From Dolan RW. Nasal ala and internal valve insufficiency. In: Holt R, ed. Facial Plastics Clinics. Philadelphia: W.B. Saunders, 2000: 8(4); 447–464.)

be directly sutured to the underlying cartilage framework for long-term stability. In the closed approach, a pocket is created, if not already formed from nasal degloving, and the graft is inserted. It can be temporarily secured to the skin of the dorsum by a chromic stitch placed through-and-through.

Lateral Crural Strut Graft

A lateral crural strut graft (Fig. 6) directly addresses the problem of a weakened and medialized lateral crus (1). The graft should measure approximately 4 mm in width and 20 mm in length and be slightly curved. It is placed convex side out under the lateral aspect of the lateral crus (between the cartilage and vestibular mucosa) via an open rhinoplasty approach. The graft should extend from the midlateral crus to over the pyriform aperture and be secured to the lateral crus with two interrupted 5-0 PDS sutures. The graft corrects medialization of the lateral crus and supports a weakened and collapsing nasal ala. The position of the alar rim can be lowered if the lateral crus–lateral crural strut complex is secured in a more caudal position. The lateral crural strut will not function well in the presence of scar or soft tissue deficiency.

Batten Graft

A batten graft (Fig. 7) is the generic term for a thin and narrow piece of cartilage used to strengthen and augment the underlying cartilaginous structure of the nose. These grafts are most commonly placed along the caudal septum and over the lateral aspect of the lateral crura. An alar batten graft is a slightly curved rectangular piece of septal or conchal cartilage measuring approximately 6 mm in width by 10–15 mm in length. It is placed in a precise subcutaneous pocket either via an endonasal or open rhinoplasty approach. Alar batten grafts are mainly used to correct functional

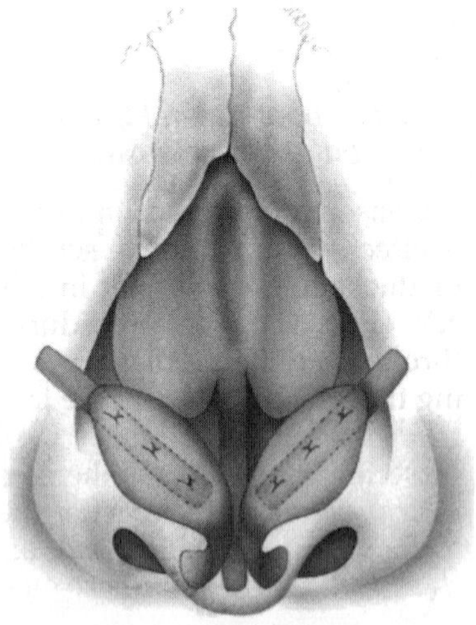

Figure 6 Lateral crural strut graft placed to open the nasal valve area and to reverse pinched nose deformity. The graft is placed under the lateral crus and over the pyriform rim. Although effective in some patients, there is a tendency for counterproductive excessive thickening within the lateral nostril due to the graft itself. (From Dolan RW. Nasal ala and internal valve insufficiency. In: Holt R, ed. Facial Plastics Clinics. Philadelphia: W.B. Saunders, 2000: 8(4); 447–464.)

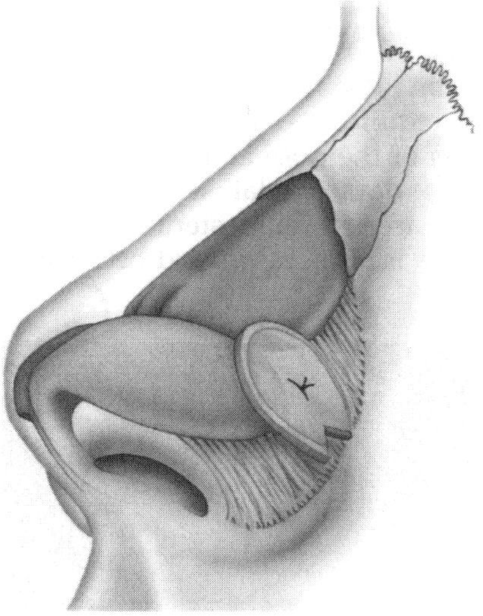

Figure 7 Batten graft placed for reversal of pinched nose deformity and stabilization of the lateral wall of the nose. This graft will assist in correcting static and dynamic narrowing within the nasal valve area. (From Dolan RW. Nasal ala and internal valve insufficiency. In: Holt R, ed. Facial Plastics Clinics. Philadelphia: W.B. Saunders, 2000: 8(4); 447–464.)

breathing problems commonly found in patients seeking revision surgery. Overresection of the cephalic border of the lateral crus (e.g., aggressive complete strip) will result in the loss of support of the lateral nasal wall, supra-alar pinching, and dynamic or static airway obstruction at the nasal valve. Replacing the lost cartilage in the area in the form of a batten graft will restore support and volume in the area. A batten graft is effective in strengthening a floppy nasal ala due to inherent problems with support, such as cephalically malpositioned lateral crura or surgically weakened lateral crura. It is ineffective in cases of scar or soft tissue deficiency.

In cases of nasal valve collapse, the batten graft is placed mostly cephalic to the lateral crus, corresponding to the area of previous cartilage removal. To correct a collapsing nasal ala, the graft is placed mostly caudal to the lateral crus and allowed to span the pyriform aperture. In either position, there will be widening of the side of the nose, although this will diminish with time as the wound contracts.

Columellar Strut Graft

A columellar strut (Fig. 8) is a straight rectangular graft that is typically 5 mm wide, 20 mm long, and 2 mm thick. It functions as a rigid support within the columella and provides superb, precise tip projection and partial rotation. The best source is the septum along the maxillary crest or perpendicular plate of the ethmoid. It is inserted between the medial crura and domes from a surgically created cradle anterosuperior to the anterior nasal spine. The graft is positioned between the medial crura inferior to the domes of the lower lateral cartilages. The strut can be placed through a variety of incisions including marginal, vertical columellar, and intraoral. However, it is most precisely placed through the open rhinoplasty approach. The graft is fixed to the medial crura with two or three buried 5–0 PDS sutures to project the tip to the desired location.

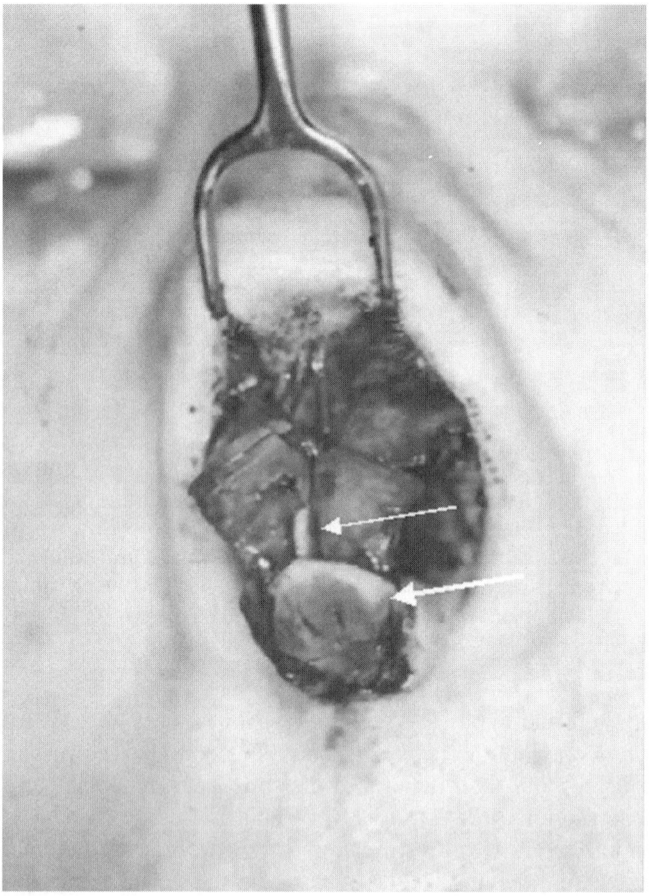

Figure 8 Columellar strut graft placed to stabilize and support the nasal tip. Note the strut (thin arrow) placed in a pocket between the medial crura. The graft extends from the anterior maxillary spine to just below the level of the anatomical dome and secured with buried 5-0 PDS suture. Note also a shield graft (thick arrow) to define better the nasal tip and domes and lend additional projection to the tip.

A columellar strut graft can stabilize a poorly supported tip and is a useful adjunct to other grafts to provide a stable cartilaginous framework that will resist the forces of scar contracture. Strut grafts can also be used to project the nasal tip and provide for a variable degree of cephalic rotation, depending on the extent of surgical attenuation or suspension of the lateral crural component of the tripod. The depressor septi muscles should be divided near the base of the columella to maximize the effect of the columellar strut graft for tip projection. Problems associated with the graft include reduced mobility of the nasal tip in the early postoperative course, improper positioning causing an obtuse nasolabial angle, buckling of the medial crura due to too large a pocket being created, and columellar distortion.

Shield Graft

A shield graft (Fig. 9) is a triangular flat or slightly convex piece of cartilage originally designed to recreate the domal tip-defining points in revision rhinoplasty. The graft is designed with two points representing the new domes tapering inferiorly toward the midcolumella. The inferior aspect of the graft enhances the columella–lobule angle and provides for the appearance of an aesthetic double break. Shield grafts are mainly used to rebuild deficient or extremely irregular domes in secondary rhinoplasty and should only rarely be used in primary rhinoplasty cases unless the domes are extremely attenuated. They can be used to assist in lengthening a short nose with little or no effect on cephalic rotation. A shield graft, like any other surface or onlay graft, should be used with caution in patients with thin skin. The edges of these grafts should always be tapered and sutured into position with buried mattress 5-0 PDS. Placing the graft via an open rhinoplasty approach ensures accurate placement and ease of suturing.

Stacking tapered rectangular onlay grafts directly over the domes can create a more dramatic increase in nasal projection. The horizontal extent of an onlay graft should be sufficient to cover the domes and the interdomal areas. The width of the grafts should approximate the width of the intermediate and lateral crura. Conchal

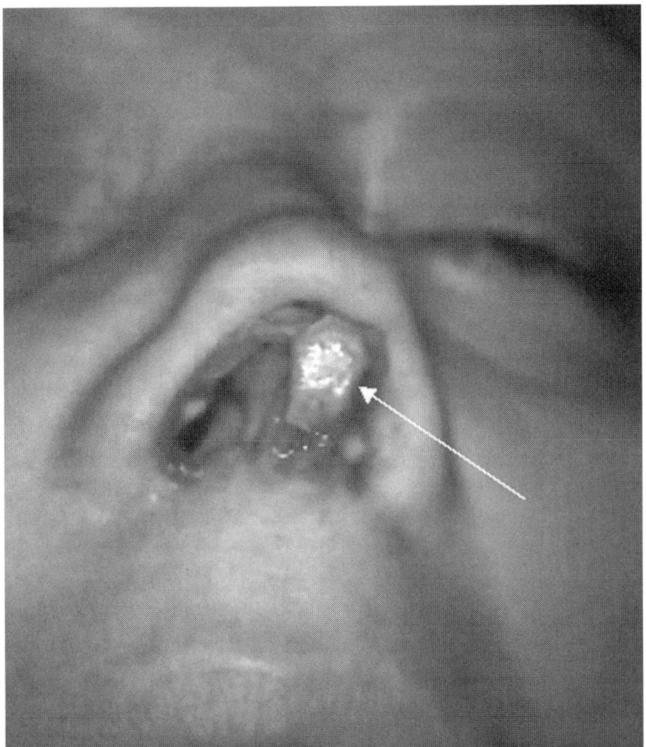

Figure 9 Shield graft placed during open rhinoplasty to create well-defined domes and the appearance of a double break.

cartilage is ideal because of its inherent gentle curvature. The concave side is placed down and its edges are tapered.

Premaxillary Graft

Premaxillary grafts fulfill several functions, including supplementing nasal tip support and bringing nasofacial aesthetic relationships into balance. The choice of graft material placed is wider because the deep location of these grafts makes extrusion unlikely. Plumping grafts are placed in the soft tissue in front of or directly under the nasal spine. The graft is usually stacked cartilage or bone. Folded Goretex (Gore and Associates, Flagstaff, AZ) is another viable option. It is introduced through an incision made below the feet of the medial crura and placed into a premaxillary pocket. If placed in front of the spine, it can be seated and sutured to this structure to prevent it from extruding or moving. If placed below the spine, the graft can be secured with a stitch through the skin similar to an onlay graft. It is used in cases of columellar retraction when tip projection and rotation have been optimized but the nasolabial angle is still blunted or acute. Grafts can be placed posterior to the feet of the medial crura for correction of short or weak medial crura contributing to inadequate projection of the nasal tip.

Advanced Nasal Tip Techniques

Many challenging conditions affecting the nasal tip require specialized techniques both in primary and revision rhinoplasty including: cephalic malposition of the alar cartilages, pollybeak deformity, inadequate tip projection, and underrotation of the nasal tip.

Cephalic Malposition

Cephalic malposition of the alar cartilages is a commonly overlooked cause of supratip fullness (pollybeak deformity) and dynamic or static alar collapse. The alar cartilages normally lie at a 30–40 degree angle from the alar rim. Cephalic malposition describes a condition in which the alar cartilages more closely follow the dorsal septum, resulting in an abnormal fullness over the anterior septal angle. This condition also leaves the alar lobules without cartilaginous support, often resulting in flaccidity and alar collapse during inspiration. The clinician must be aware of this condition since lack of preoperative diagnosis could lead to inappropriate and excessive cartilage excision in an attempt to resolve the supralobular fullness and bulbosity of the nasal tip. Accurate preoperative diagnosis is necessary since treatment requires unique surgical modifications to the nasal tip and alar cartilages that entail only limited cartilage excision.

Correction of this deformity requires only cartilage repositioning. Through an open rhinoplasty approach, the alar cartilages are completely freed from the vestibular mucosa. This results in alar cartilages attached to the nose only via the intermediate crura. Further inferior soft tissue dissection beyond the alar crease on each side is performed to create a pocket to accept the caudalmost aspect of the lateral alar cartilage. The alar cartilages are then repositioned to a more inferior location aligned approximately 30 degrees with the alar rims (Fig. 10). Buried 5-0 PDS sutures are used to secure the cartilages into place. A conservative complete strip is performed to enhance tip definition further over the anterior septal angle.

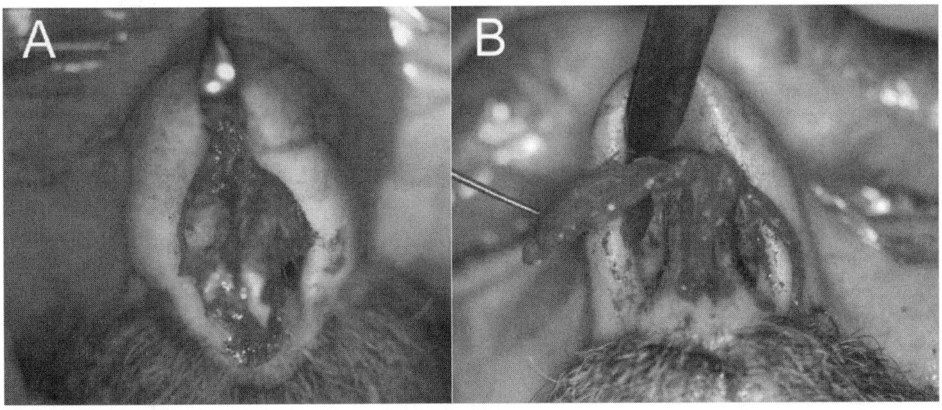

Figure 10 Method of lateral crura repositioning to correct cephalic malposition and the so-called parenthesis tip. Note how the lateral crura parallel the nasal dorsum (A). To reposition the lateral crura, they are completely freed from the beds by meticulous dissection of the overlying SMAS and underlying vestibular mucosa. Once the lateral crus is freed (B), it is displaced and secured in a more inferolateral position.

The skin is replaced and complete reversal of the 'parenthesis tip' should be noted (Fig. 11). Once this anatomical abnormality is corrected, the rest of the rhinoplasty can proceed as usual.

Pollybeak Deformity

Pollybeak deformity is an unaesthetic fullness in the supratip due either to excess cartilage or soft tissue. Approximately 10% of patients presenting for primary

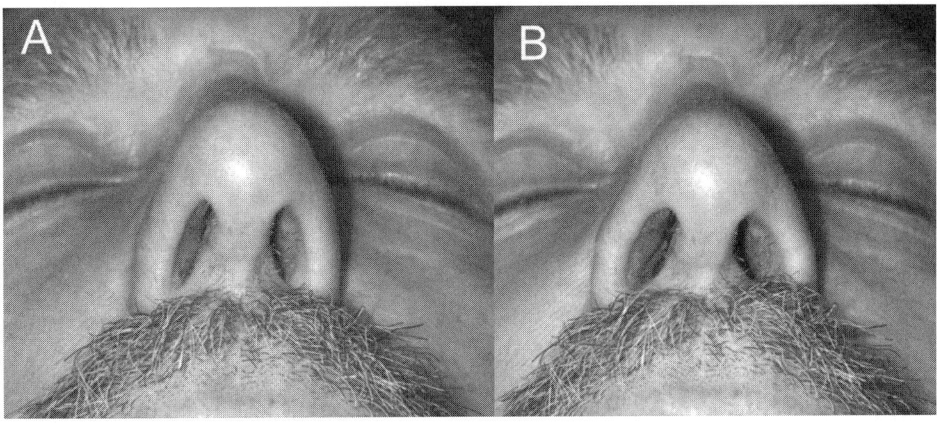

Figure 11 Reversal of parenthesis tip and static and dynamic nostril narrowing in a patient with cephalic malpositioning of his alar cartilages (same patient as in Fig. 10). Preoperatively (A) the patient experienced collapse of his alae upon deep inspiration. Once the lateral crura were placed in a more inferolateral position the nostrils widened (B) and were structurally stiffer thereby preventing inward collapse of the alae during inspiration.

rhinoplasty may exhibit this deformity. Patients seeking primary rhinoplasty will usually have excess septal caudodorsal projection and inadequate tip projection, bringing the septal angle and soft tissue into prominence over the supratip. Cephalic malposition of the alar cartilages is another common finding in those initially presenting with pollybeak deformity. In revision cases, the most common cause is exuberant subcutaneous scarring. The deformity is present predominantly in those seeking revision rhinoplasty. Pollybeak deformity is commonly believed to be secondary to overresection of the nasal dorsum with subsequent scarring and swelling in the supratip area (11). This contention has been borne out in experience but other causes must also be considered.

Patients presenting for revision rhinoplasty will have postoperative sequelae that result in this deformity. As mentioned, the most common cause is overresection of the caudal dorsum. This creates dead space that is prone to fill in with scar tissue that creates a convexity in the supratip. Other causes include underresection of the caudal septum, especially in the presence of inadequate tip projection similar to that found in patients presenting for primary rhinoplasty. In the usual case, supratip fullness and pollybeak are not obvious in the immediate postoperative period. As scar formation builds and the fullness in the supratip increases, pollybeak deformity is noted, usually within 1–2 months postoperatively. Treatment should initially consist of subdermal steroid injections of 0.1–0.2 ml triamcinolone acetate (40 mg/ml). This is repeated every 2 weeks if necessary. If this treatment is ineffective, then surgical correction is necessary consisting of scar excision and graft placement. Surgical repair is performed through an open approach and the supratip is completely exposed. Scar is excised and a cartilage graft is sutured into place over the anterior septal angle to fill the dead space, and another suture is passed from the subcutaneous tissue under the supratip and into the graft. This latter supratip suture fixates the overlying skin to the graft minimizing postoperative fluid collection and scarring.

Inadequate Nasal Tip Projection

Several techniques that involve minimal manipulation of the existing cartilage structure are available to increase projection of the nasal tip. First, an illusion of increased nasal projection can be created by removing a prominent nasal hump or by decreasing nasal length (e.g., lowering the radix). Second, modest increases in nasal projection are possible using sutures. Suturing alone can result in modest increases in tip projection such as suture approximation of divergent medial crura, septocolumellar sutures, or transdomal sutures. Suture approximation of divergent medial crural footplates will result in modest columellar lengthening and an increase in projection. The technique involves first removing the intervening soft tissue between the footplates and placing one or two buried 5–0 PDS mattress sutures to cinch the footplates together. Septocolumellar sutures are placed between the caudal nasal septum and the medial crura at slightly divergent levels to lift the tip. Transdomal and interdomal sutures are useful to increase tip definition and projection. Transdomal sutures enhance the tip-defining points of each dome. The interdomal suture is placed below the transdomal sutures in a buried mattress fashion through-and-through the domes, resulting in narrowing of the tip and a minor increase in projection.

Augmentation along the medial crura is the primary method by which a significant increase in nasal projection is accomplished. A variety of grafting techniques will increase nasal projection. Plumping grafts are used for premaxillary augmentation and are inserted directly behind the nasolabial angle. The main effect of a plumping graft is to open the nasolabial angle. Secondary gains include creating the illusion of cephalic rotation and a modest increase in nasal projection. A columellar strut graft will result in a considerable increase in nasal projection while providing increased stability to the nasal tip to resist scar contracture during healing. To increase projection further and resist cephalic rotation due to the columellar strut, the lateral crura and dorsum should be augmented. This can be achieved with spreader grafts that extend beyond the dorsal septum, with the free ends projecting against a shield graft. As an alternative, the cephalic aspect of the alar cartilages can be augmented with interpositional cartilage grafts to push the nasal tip inferiorly.

Underrotation of the Nasal Tip/Dependent Tip

The choice of technique to achieve cephalic rotation of the nasal tip depends largely on the additional need for an increase in nasal projection. The illusion of a minor degree of cephalic tip rotation can be achieved by blunting the nasolabial angle with cartilage-plumping grafts or synthetic grafting material. In some cases, nasal tip projection may be adequate or excessive. Standard reduction techniques including alar cartilage reduction with or without suture fixation are appropriate to achieve cephalic rotation with a variable degree of deprojection. In addition, caudal resection of the nasal septum may be needed. To achieve significant cephalic rotation and an increase in nasal projection, the Goldman tipplasty or lateral crural steal may be used (see above). As mentioned, these techniques require significant dissection and alteration of the tip cartilages. Scarring, contour irregularities and asymmetry are common side effects. In contrast, augmentation rhinoplasty techniques use cartilage grafts that are inset into the nasal tip and require little manipulation of the existing cartilaginous framework. Cephalic rotation is primarily achieved by augmenting the strength and length of the medial crural component of the tripod using columellar struts. An increase in projection of the nasal tip is a byproduct. Combined with interdomal sutures and modest complete strips, this technique will result in a well-projected and rotated tip with good definition. Healing is predictable with minimal scarring and the cartilage grafts lend support to the tip to resist contracture during normal healing.

Advanced Nasal Dorsum Techniques

Low Radix

The position of the radix is an important consideration in rhinoplasty. On profile, a low radix can make an appropriately projected nasal tip appear overprojected. In contrast, a high radix essentially lengthens the nasal dorsum, making an otherwise normal nasal tip appear inadequately projected. By positioning the radix at the appropriate height and normalizing the relationship between dorsal length and nasal tip projection, the surgeon can achieve apparent cosmetic benefits in nasal tip projection without ever touching the nasal tip. For example, an apparent decrease in tip projection and restoration of nasal balance may be achieved by placing a radix graft.

A prominent radix will usually also be displaced superiorly and a deep-set radix is often displaced inferiorly. Anterosuperior movement of a low radix will require augmentation over the upper nasal dorsum. Posteroinferior movement requires removal of nasal bone and soft tissue above the desired level of the radix. Movement of the radix in a purely posterior direction (retrodisplacement) requires removal of bone and soft tissue from both the nasal and frontal components of the nasofrontal angle (12).

Anterosuperior displacement of the radix opens the nasofrontal angle, lengthens the nose, and gives the illusion of decreased nasal tip projection. Posteroinferior displacement of the radix makes the nasofrontal angle more acute, shortens the nasal dorsum, and gives the illusion of increased projection of the nasal tip.

To move a prominent radix posteriorly, a combination of bone and soft tissue (subcutaneous tissues including procerus muscle) must be removed. To deepen the radix, the portion of the nasal bones cephalic to the intercanthal line must be planed down. The nasal bones above the intercanthal line are quite thick, approaching 6 mm, and resist osteotomy. A typical lateral osteotomy rarely extends above the intercanthal line because of the thickening nasal bones in this area. Removal of the anterior projection of nasal bone between the intercanthal line and the nasofrontal suture (approximately 10.7 mm in length) is difficult and routine osteotomy is inadequate. Although removal of bone above the nasofrontal suture (glabella) can be performed conservatively it carries the risk of entering the frontal sinus. Removal of the cephalic-most nasal bone and soft tissue over the inferior glabella should provide sufficient retrodisplacement of the radix in most cases. A few millimeters of cephalic nasal bone can be effectively planed using a curved osteotome placed in the midline through a transnasal approach. However, there is only a 25% soft tissue response to bone reduction in this area (13). Therefore, removal of 4 mm of bone at the nasion results in 1 mm of soft tissue retrodisplacement at the radix. Deeper gouging requires additional osteotomies oriented in an anteroposterior direction to release the osteotomized bony segment. The anteroposterior osteotomies must be performed percutaneously (12,13). Alternative methods of removing bone and reducing the anterior projection of the nasal bones include using a powered guarded burr and using a straight osteotome up to the nasofrontal suture. One disarticulates the nasal bone from the frontal bone and removes the segment (13,14). Bony refinement is accomplished with a rasp subsequent to en-bloc removal of nasal bone.

Anterosuperior displacement of a deep radix requires augmentation of both the nasal and forehead components of the nasofrontal suture. Superior vertical movement of the radix is possible with midline augmentation of the cephalic-most nasal bones up to the frontonasal suture. Often a small nasal hump must be removed and this can be done prior to placement of the radix graft. The graft may be obtained from the septum, conchal bowl, or remnants of lower lateral cartilage after a complete rim strip. The cartilage can be morselized to follow the contour of the nasal root and stacked as needed. A cartilage graft placed over the upper nasal dorsum can be introduced into the nose using a suture. The suture is introduced percutaneously at the desired location of the cephalic edge of the graft and pulled through under the skin, feeding it out through the intercartilaginous incision or the opened nose in the case of open rhinoplasty. The suture is then passed through the cephalic aspect of the graft and again through its caudal aspect. The needle is then reintroduced into the nose and passed through the skin at the desired caudal aspect of the graft. When the surgeon pulls on both the superior and inferior sutures, the graft is pulled into the nose over the dorsum. The free ends of the suture are tied holding the underlying graft in place. The suture may be safely removed in 1 week.

Narrow Middle Vault and Nasal Valve Dysfunction

The association of narrow middle vault and obstruction of the nasal valves is common. A variety of grafting techniques are available to widen the nasal valves. Most commonly, spreader grafts are used because they cause relatively minor degrees of nasal widening. Spreader grafts are placed between the upper lateral cartilage and the septum. In addition, flaring sutures (secured to the upper lateral cartilages in a horizontal mattress fashion and tied across the midline), splay grafts, butterfly grafts, and nasal valve suspension sutures are useful in selected patients.

Spreader grafts will slightly widen the cartilaginous dorsum and prevent an overly narrowed appearance (i.e., the inverted V deformity) after reduction rhinoplasty. The spreader graft is harvested from the cartilaginous septum or ear as previously noted. The endonasal (closed) approach is a convenient and quick way to place the graft. A splay graft is placed via an open rhinoplasty approach. The graft takes advantage of the dorsal septum, using it as a fulcrum to suspend the upper lateral cartilages. It must be placed under the upper lateral cartilages. These grafts tend to stent the nasal valves open and widen the nasal dorsum to a greater extent than spreader grafts. Since the external appearance of the nose is subject to overwidening, the application of the graft is limited. The upper lateral cartilage can also be pulled laterally, opening the nasal valve through traction on the lateral nasal wall and lateral crura. The technique of nasal valve suspension takes advantage of this mechanism by suspending the lateral nasal wall to the orbital rim periosteum using a buried nonabsorbable suture (15). This is a novel technique with little long-term follow-up. As the suture is pulled taught, there can be significant widening of the lateral nasal subunit.

The nasal valve area can also be narrowed most commonly by iatrogenic medialization of lateral crura. This occurs after suture medialization of the domes that results in medial movement of the alar cartilages. It should be corrected during the primary procedure either by altering the tip sutures or by placing lateral crural strut grafts to support the medialized edges.

Scarring across the nasal valve most commonly occurs after rhinoplasty. Local flap rotation and free mucosal grafts are rarely successful in correcting this problem because of excessive bulk or scar reformation. Appropriate treatment consists of scar lysis and placement of a small Silastic stent that should remain for 3–5 weeks.

SPECIAL CONDITIONS

Lengthening a Short Nose

The three principles of repairing a short nose are wide undermining, restoration and augmentation of structure and function, and release of internal lining. The open approach is preferred to allow complete visualization and access to the lower two-thirds of the nose. Complete separation of the cartilages and wide undermining of the skin envelope and inner lining proceed. Once the nose is completely degloved and disassembled, the nasal tip is pulled inferiorly to simulate lengthening the nose.

This will cause separation of the upper and lower lateral cartilages that should be maximized by dissecting the upper and lower lateral cartilages apart at the scroll areas. At this point, the inner lining will restrict further caudal displacement of the tip despite previous wide separation of the lining over the quadrilateral cartilage. Nonopposing releasing incisions are created through the mucoperiosteum perpendicular to the dorsal edge of the quadrilateral cartilage about 1–2 cm in length (16). The nasal tip moves caudally as these releasing incisions expand. In moderate-to-severe cases, three areas of soft tissue and structural (cartilaginous) voids are created. First, with inferior traction on the nasal tip, the vertical staggered incision through the mucoperiosteum along the dorsal septum leaves wide (about 1 cm) areas of exposed cartilage. Since there is rigid framework (i.e., the quadrilateral cartilage), there is little tendency for retraction during healing and the raw areas readily heal. Second, release of the upper lateral cartilage from the lower lateral cartilage creates a void between these structures. The lack of cartilage in the scroll area will result in significant cephalic pull on the nasal tip during healing. Therefore, this defect must be filled in with a rigid graft. In the absence of an underlying vestibular mucosal incision and defect, a simple cartilaginous interposition graft sutured into place is sufficient. The graft is usually triangular and placed with its base secured along the septum. In cases of moderate-to-severe retraction, a vestibular-releasing incision is often required along the cephalic border of the lateral and intermediate crura. With further inferior traction on the nasal tip, the vestibular incision gapes, resulting in a composite defect that must be filled in with a composite graft. A conchal chondrocutaneous composite graft is ideal. The graft is taken from the anterior conchal bowl because the skin is tightly adherent and over the concave (inner) side of the graft (Fig. 12). The composite graft may be triangular or designed as a gull-wing to achieve more inferior displacement of the medial aspect (including the medial crus) of the lower lateral cartilage (17). The void along each lateral crus should be adequately filled to prevent inordinate superior traction on the ala. Lengthening the dorsum without expansion of the nasal sidewalls will result in distortion of the alar–columellar relationship and alar notching. The third void created is along the caudal aspect of the septum and septal angle. Substantial structural support, especially caudal to the septal angle, is necessary. Support and grafting in this area are most often combined with dorsal augmentation (from radix to nasal tip) and augmentation of the medial leg of the tripod (i.e., the columella). Grafts placed along the nasal dorsum are perhaps the most important component of the repair because they serve to secure the nasal tip in its new position. Without adequate dorsal structural support, the strong vertical contractile forces during healing would overwhelm the interpositional grafts and the deformity would recur.

The most significant variations in the technique to lengthen a short nose involve structural correction along the caudal septum and nasal dorsum. The more severe the short nose deformity, the more substantial and rigid the repair must be. Grafts for augmentation and structural rigidity range from a simple caudal septum batten graft to a full dorsal onlay graft from radix to nasal tip, consisting most commonly of an osseocartilaginous rib graft or interlocking split calvarial bone grafts. In the simplest case with a mild-to-moderate deformity, a batten graft is secured along the caudal septum caudal to the septal angle (approximately 2.5×1 cm). The graft serves effectively to extend the caudal septum and anterior septal angle less than 1 cm and provides support and projection to the tip in the form of a columellar strut.

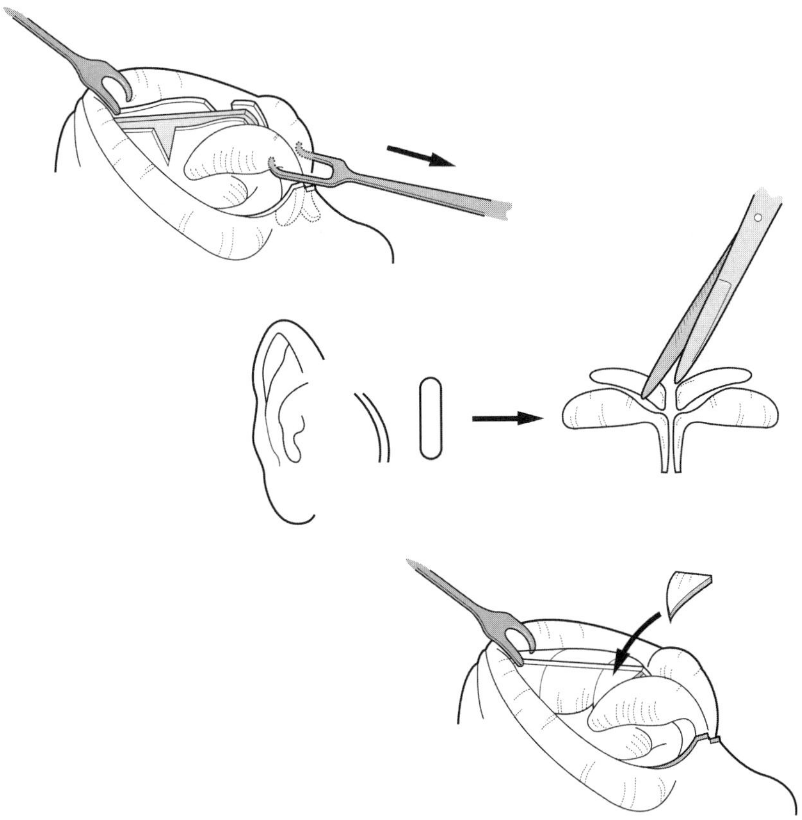

Figure 12 Vertical septal releasing incisions and composite grafts to lengthen a short nose. Note the offset vertical incisions placed through the mucoperiosteum to allow advancement of the nasal tip. These incisions open as the nasal tip is brought forward. A composite conchal graft is taken to act as a spacer between the caudal aspects of the upper lateral cartilages and alar cartilages. The dehiscent inner lining is resurfaced with the skin of the conchal bowl.

This technique will be inadequate to resist the contractile during healing in most cases. Additional stability is provided if extended spreader grafts are placed as well. These grafts are fashioned so that their caudal ends extend beyond the caudal septum to the desired position of the nasal tip. The caudal ends are secured to the batten graft that lies between the medial crura and domes (flying buttress technique) (18). This technique is useful if the deformity is mild-to-moderate in degree and nasal dorsal augmentation is not needed. The spreader grafts will also improve pre-existing nasal valve obstruction in the absence of scarring. Unfortunately, spreader grafts are best obtained from the septum but adequate septal cartilage is often unavailable in these cases.

A rib graft along the dorsum is most commonly used. This provides substantial rigid support while serving to augment a deficient dorsum (saddle nose deformity). The rib graft is harvested from the costochondral junction of the seventh through the tenth ribs via an inframammary incision. The graft is harvested as an 'L' shape to include a columellar strut placed in the usual position between the medial crura and domes. The bony portion of the graft is secured to the nasal bones either end-to-end for minimal dorsal augmentation or to the nasion to augment the profile in this area. The graft may be secured to the nasal bones using micromini plate fixation, wire osseointegration, or temporary Kirschner wire fixation (14 days) (17). The main disadvantage of this method is that the rib graft has a tendency to warp over time. In an attempt to prevent this significant problem, Gunter et al. have placed a buried Kirschner wire through the graft's longitudinal axis (19). An alternative method that provides similar rigid fixation with a much-reduced risk of warping is split calvarial grafting. Split calvarial grafts are harvested through an incision in the parietal scalp. The grafts are thinned to approximately 1 mm and measure 1×5 cm (20). A single graft is placed flat over the nasal dorsum and secured to the nasal bones as an overlay or end-to-end depending on the need for dorsal augmentation. The distal (caudal) end can be grooved to accept a split calvarial columella strut in a tongue-in-groove fashion (21). The two segments are secured with a single screw and the distal conjoined end is burred to eliminate sharp edges. The major drawback to this method is the excessive rigidity created in the nasal tip. This effect can be minimized with adequate tip grafting and suture modification of the domes.

The final steps in correcting the short nose involve techniques to improve the nasal valve and to provide strategically placed grafts that enhance nasal length visually. A sculpted radix graft is needed in patients with a low radix that remains uncorrected after dorsal grafting. This will enhance the effect of nasal lengthening and adds to the overall result. Single or stacked nasal tip grafts (e.g., shield grafts) will serve two purposes. First, the graft(s) will camouflage the sharp caudal end of a rigid dorsal overlay graft and create aesthetic dome-defining points. Second, stacked grafts will aid in nasal lengthening. Once all the grafts are secured, the nasal access incisions are closed in the standard fashion. Prior to closure, further undermining over the pyriform apertures and ascending processes of the maxilla and glabella may be necessary to provide adequate soft tissue release to allow a tension-free closure.

Crooked Nose

A true crooked nose deformity is characterized by deviation of the nasal dorsum or tip from the midsagittal plane. The illusion of a crooked nose (pseudo-crooked nose deformity) is created when the dorsum and tip are aligned in the midsagittal plane but there is a relative deficiency of tissue along the nasal sidewall. True crooked nose deformities are classified into nasion-related, rhinion-related, or mixed. Nasion-related deformities are characterized by departure of the nose from the midsagittal plane beginning at the nasion with good intrinsic alignment of the dorsum and nasal tip. Rhinion-related deformities are characterized by a nose that deviates at the rhinion with an upper nasal dorsum that is aligned with the midsagittal plane. A mixed deformity is characterized by deviation at both the nasion and rhinion, usually in opposite directions, giving rise to the classic 'C'-shaped (rightward deviation at the nasion) or a reverse 'C'-shaped (leftward deviation at the nasion) appearance to the nasal dorsum (Fig. 13). This classification is useful not only for descriptive purposes but also for determining the appropriate surgical approach. Pure nasion-related deviations may only require osteotomies via a closed approach for repair

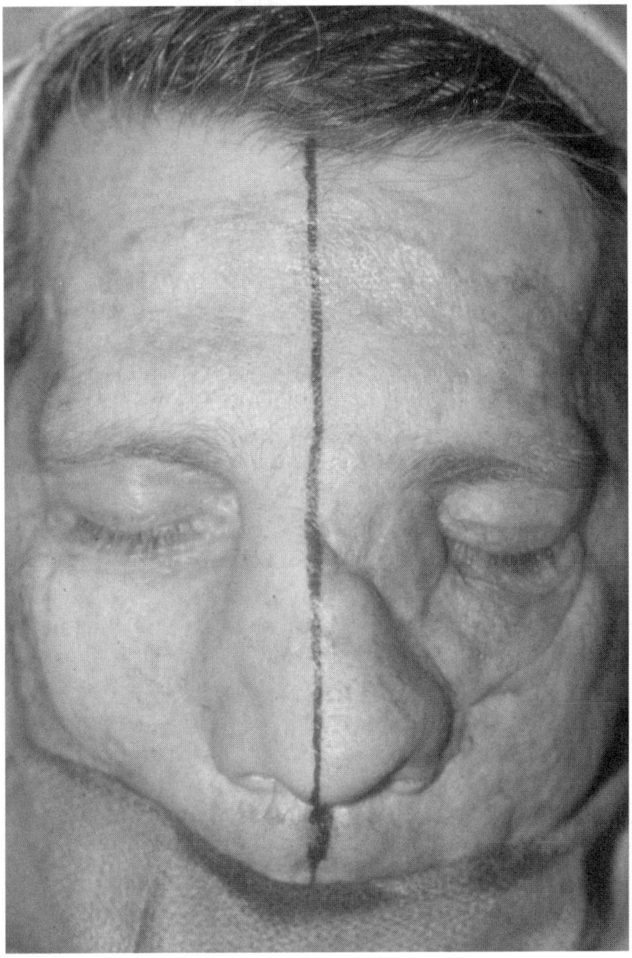

Figure 13 Typical C-shaped twisted nose deformity. Note how the nasal dorsum deviates from the midline, first to the right at the nasion and then to the left at the rhinion.

while most rhinion and mixed deformities are more difficult to repair and require an open approach and extensive bony and cartilaginous work.

Additional deformities often associated with a twisted nose include severe caudal septal deflections, asymmetrical nostrils, nasal valve obstruction, and deviation of the nasal septum. The correction of these deformities is usually incorporated into the overall plan for reconstruction.

The majority of crooked noses arise as a result of prior trauma, especially in childhood. Traumatic deformities in childhood may worsen as the nose matures, principally during puberty which is typically a period of rapid nasal growth. Prior nasal surgery may lead to a twisted nose deformity from flawed osteotomies, disarticulated upper lateral cartilages, unrecognized septal deformities, malpositioned sutures, or errant scarring causing misalignment of the upper or lower lateral cartilages.

The problems encountered when treating the twisted nose are multiple and deceivingly complex. In the usual case, all parts of the nose are involved including the upper third, middle third, lower third, and nasal septum. The rigid and supportive keystone area and the intricate interface between the middle third and the nasal tip are the most problematic areas to correct. Special areas of concern intranasally that are difficult to correct include deviations of the nasal septum that involve the dorsocaudal strut and internal nasal valve. The nasal bones (upper third) require osteotomy or camouflage grafts for correction and, although the problem of memory is of least concern in this area, the surrounding structures often impede accurate and stable repair. Deviations of the perpendicular plate of the ethmoid under the nasal bones may impede movement of the nasal bones after osteotomy. The rigid and three-dimensional connection of the caudal nasal bones, upper lateral cartilages, and upper cartilaginous septum at the keystone area will also greatly impede movement of the nasal bones after osteotomy. Disassembly and reconstruction of the keystone area will be required. In long-standing deviations involving the middle and lower thirds of the nose, discrepancies in the lengths and heights of the upper lateral cartilages are often present. Intractable deviation of the dorsal septum and nasal valve obstruction will accompany this deformity in all cases. Deviation and moderate-to-severe twisting of the nasal tip may be secondary to a vast array of problems. The support and structure of the nasal tip are entirely cartilaginous and the major and minor tip support mechanisms are intricately related. For example, long-standing deviation of the nasal tip may be associated with buckled or foreshortened middle and lower medial crura on the side of the deviation. Deviation of the caudal septum may also be associated with irregular or deficient medial crura and nasal valve obstruction or alar collapse. Despite correction of the nasal septum, the nasal tip deformity persists because of these secondary deformities. Structural grafts and redirecting sutures are commonly needed to correct even minor twisting of the nasal tip, which are best placed through an external rhinoplasty approach.

Three basic surgical methods are used to correct the twisted nose depending on existing pathology. The first is osteotomy alone through a closed approach with minimal degloving of the surrounding soft tissue envelope. This approach is used to correct deviations of the nasal dorsum emanating from misdirected nasal bones (nasion-related). Once the upper third of the nose is realigned with the midsagittal plane, the middle and lower nasal thirds should follow suit because the nose itself is intrinsically straight. The second method involves cartilaginous reconstruction alone through a closed or open approach without osteotomy. This approach is reserved for cases of mild deviation limited to the dorsum at or below the rhinion (rhinion-related). The focus of this operation is correction of deviation of the dorsocaudal strut portion of the quadrilateral cartilage and asymmetries of the upper lateral cartilages. More severe deviations may require osteotomies to redirect the upper portions of the upper lateral cartilages at their rigid connection with the caudal aspect of the nasal bones. The third method involves osseous and cartilaginous reconstruction through an open rhinoplasty approach. This is useful for correction of moderate-to-severe rhinion-related and mixed deviations of the nose. Although this approach is seemingly more ‘radical’, it is the most common approach used because of the difficulty in achieving a favorable and long-lasting result in the majority of patients with a twisted nose deformity. In cases of a moderate-to-severe deviation of the nasal tip, an open rhinoplasty approach is preferred. This facilitates accurate assessment of the problem, placement of grafts and sutures, and access to the dorsal septum and anterior septal angle. In general, the endonasal approach has more limited application in the treatment of the twisted nose. The endonasal approach is used if the dorsocaudal strut is minimally involved and there exists only mild deviation of the middle third of the nose at or below the rhinion.

Patients with pseudodeviation may be lacking soft tissue or bone, giving the appearance of a twisted nose. However, realignment is unnecessary because the nasal dorsum does not deviate from the midsagittal plane. If the only goal is to make the nose appear straight, correction most often will be limited to the use of onlay grafts placed through a closed approach within the areas of tissue deficiency.

Camouflage techniques using grafts are often useful in cases of true twisted nose deformities and to even out irregular areas or to make a mildly deviated dorsum appear straight. Nasal septal quadrilateral cartilage is the graft of choice and is harvested by a traditional submucous resection of the septum. There is little long-term resorption and a variety of struts, splay, and onlay grafts can be fashioned from a single piece. In revision cases, the nasal septum may be missing so alternative sources of cartilage must be sought. Most commonly, the cartilage from the conchal bowl is harvested. It is curved and is less ideal for many applications but may be used effectively for camouflage. Onlay camouflage grafts should be trimmed and tapered to eliminate sharp edges. To make the grafts maximally conformable, they may be morselized. Morselization will increase absorption of the graft, so slight overcorrection will be necessary. Acellular dermis (AlloDerm, LifeCell Corporation, Branchburg, NJ) is a useful product consisting of sheets of skin that allow fibrous ingrowth and collagen deposition. Maintenance of volume is poor over the long term but this product can be used to smooth surface irregularities.

Surgical correction of deviated nasal bones must address the nasal bones themselves, ascending processes of the maxilla, perpendicular plate of the ethmoid, and the complex keystone area. Camouflage grafts may be used efface minor irregularities but multiple osteotomies are usually required. The types of osteotomies differ from those typically used in primary or even revision rhinoplasty. Unilateral osteotomy or a combination of medial, transverse, intermediate, and lateral osteotomies may be required. A basic fact that must be remembered when considering the types of osteotomies required is that an osteotomy will result in medial collapse of the osteotomized segment. This is particularly relevant to the lateral osteotomy where there is no medial bony support. Attempts to lateralize a concave nasal bone-ascending process complex through a combination of medial and lateral osteotomies will fail despite internal splinting and packing. Instead, medialization of the opposite nasal bone or ipsilateral onlay grafting should be considered. Correction of a deviated nasal bone complex is most commonly accomplished through a series of osteotomies referred to as 'the open-book method.' Particularly relevant using this method is the conspicuous absence of the lateral osteotomy on the concave side for reasons mentioned previously. The open-book method consists of sequential osteotomies that result in movement of the nasal bones that is likened to turning the pages of a book from the concave to the convex side (22) (Fig. 14). In the typical case, the nasal bones are deviated from the nasion towards the right side, resulting in a relative medial position of the left aspect of the nasal pyramid and a relative rightward shift of the right nasal pyramid. Since lateralization of the left nasal pyramid is not feasible or desirable

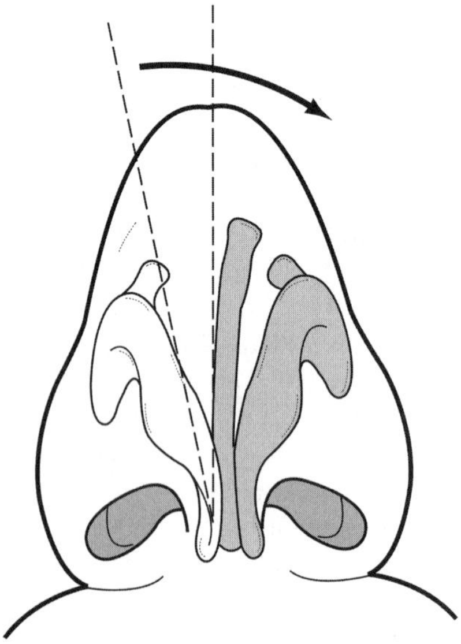

Figure 14 Open book method of osteotomy to correct a twisted nasal dorsum. For a nasal pyramid that is deviated to the right, the sequence of osteotomies is as follows: (1) left medial osteotomy, (2) left transverse osteotomy, (3) right medial osteotomy, (4) transverse root osteotomy, (5) right transverse oblique osteotomy, and (6) right low lateral osteotomy. The initial osteotomies (1 and 2) will allow the left nasal bone and underlying septum to be fractured toward the left side, creating an open nasal dorsum as demonstrated. An additional intermediate osteotomy may be required to accomplish this step. The right nasal bone then is collapsed medially after the subsequent right-sided osteotomies are completed.

in most cases, the right aspect of the nasal pyramid is medialized using this method.

The sequence of osteotomies is as follows: left medial osteotomy, left transverse osteotomy, right medial osteotomy, transverse root osteotomy, right transverse oblique osteotomy, and right low lateral osteotomy. The medial osteotomies also serve to disarticulate the cephalic upper lateral cartilages from the septum in the midsagittal plane at the keystone area. Following the left medial and transverse osteotomies, the left nasal bone is rotated to the left, leaving an open dorsum to the left of the nasal septum. An intermediate osteotomy may be required prior to rotation if the nasal bone is fixed. Following the right medial and transverse root osteotomies, the nasal septum (perpendicular plate) is rotated to the left, closing the open roof on the left but creating an open roof on the right. The perpendicular plate is fractured during this maneuver. If the perpendicular plate is deviated, then limited resection may be necessary. The right transverse oblique and low lateral osteotomies allow medial collapse of the right aspect of the nasal pyramid that finally closes the open roof. Separation of the skin from the nasal bones (undermining) should be limited so that the skin envelope will help to stabilize the multiply osteotomized bony segments. For this reason, performing the lateral osteotomy with a 2 mm osteotome percutaneously through a small stab incision between the ipsilateral dorsum and medial canthus is useful. The scar is not visible in the vast majority of cases.

A benefit of the percutaneous osteotomy is that the periosteum is merely perforated and not stripped from the underling nasal bones, lending stability and limiting medial collapse. If the concave side remains too depressed, then a graft should be placed to efface and fill the defect.

Deviations at the rhinion involve the keystone area and nasal tip, which are two of the most complex areas of the nose. The typical twisted nose will have a rightward deviation beginning at the nasion and a leftward deviation starting at the rhinion ('C'-shaped). These mixed deformities require a host of specialized rhinoplasty techniques including open rhinoplasty, nasal disassembly, sequential osteotomies, specific reshaping of the upper and lower lateral cartilages, unique suture placement, the use of specialized grafts, and extensive septal reconstruction. In some cases, the deviation only involves the middle third of the nose (rhinion-related) and repair may only entail cartilage reconstruction. Yet even in these cases, extensive nasal disassembly and reconstruction may be necessary.

Deviated nasal bones are corrected first through sequential osteotomies since the nasal bones will alter the nature of the deviation at the rhinion owing to their firm attachment to the cephalic upper lateral cartilages and nasal septum. The dorsocaudal strut is always deviated and it is sometimes tempting to blame most of the external nasal deviation on the septum. However, straightening the septum will not significantly affect the appearance of the nose because the vast majority of external deviations are multifactorial. Among the multiple anatomical reasons for a twisted nose, the one often most responsible is malpositioned and asymmetrical upper lateral cartilages. Through the open rhinoplasty approach, the nasal cartilages are exposed and the upper and lower lateral cartilages are separated from the septum in a process of progressive nasal disassembly. First, near the anterior septal angle the nasal septum is exposed sharply with care taken not to disrupt the mucosa surrounding the nasal valves. This is the easiest area in which to expose the nasal septum since the caudal lower lateral cartilages slightly diverge in this area. The nasal septum is relatively thin and delicate at the angle so dissection must proceed with care. With the underlying mucosa preserved, the septum is exposed and submucoperiosteal flaps are dissected widely including along the dorsal septum to the junction of the nasal bones. A knife is passed on each side of the dorsal septum and swept anteriorly to separate the upper lateral cartilages from the septum. Full access to the nasal septum is now possible and the dorsocaudal strut is examined. Severe deviations, including those involving a significant caudal deflection, may be difficult to realign despite scoring and suturing. In these cases, it may be best to remove the quadrilateral cartilage entirely and fashion a reinforced dorsocaudal strut on the back table (Fig. 15). Although the whole cartilage may be curved, it is often possible to suture together two pieces of cartilage with opposite bends that will result in a straight and reinforced segment. With the whole quadrilateral cartilage accessible, there should be ample cartilage available to fashion a straight reinforced dorsocaudal strut. Additional cartilage projecting slightly beyond the native anterior septal angle is desirable for added tip support. As an alternative, spreader grafts harvested from the posteroinferior quadrilateral cartilage can be placed along the dorsal septum. The spreader grafts help to stabilize and strengthen the dorsal strut while maintaining it in the corrected position. The spreader grafts should extend beyond the anterior septal angle to lend additional support and stability to the nasal tip. This technique is most useful when there is an easily correctable or insignificant deviation

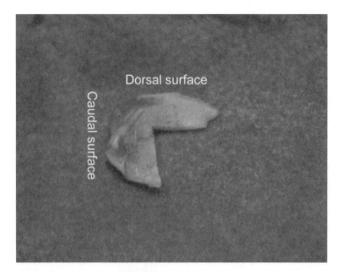

Figure 15 The dorsocaudal strut of quadrilateral cartilage after straightening. The entire quadrilateral cartilage was removed during an external septorhinoplasty and straightened ex vivo. The strut will be replaced in the nose and secured.

along the caudal septum. Once the dorsocaudal strut and nasal bones are in their corrected position, the nose is again examined. It will be evident that the deviation is persistent because of the uncorrected upper lateral cartilages. Manually moving the tip to midline will expose the anatomical reasons for the persistent deviation. In the usual case, the dorsal aspect of the upper lateral cartilage on the side opposite the deviation will project above the level of the dorsal septum after manual correction. This cartilage will also appear too long and resist correction. Dorsal and caudal trimming of the upper lateral cartilage followed by suture fixation of the trimmed caudal end to the ipsilateral lower lateral cartilage at the scroll area will help to maintain the nose in the reduced position. Spacer grafts between the upper lateral cartilage on the deviated side and the ipsilateral lateral crus may also assist in correcting the deviation.

Cleft Rhinoplasty

A cleft lip nasal deformity refers to the pathological anatomy found in association with a congenital cleft lip deformity. The anatomical features and severity of the nasal deformity vary but all cleft lips are associated with a cleft lip nasal deformity regardless of the degree of clefting in the palate. The original unilateral unrepaired cleft is associated with several unique nasal deformities (Table 1). The bilateral cleft lip nasal deformity is similar except that the anatomical abnormalities are bilateral and symmetrical and the columella is uniformly shortened.

Primary cleft repair usually commences in infancy and includes preoperative palatal orthopedics followed by some variation of the Millard cheiloplasty (23) (see Chapter 10 on 'Cleft Lip and Palate'). The modern approach to primary cleft repair includes several techniques aimed at improving nasal tip aesthetics. Primary rhinoplasty during the original cleft repair can achieve good symmetry and aesthetics

Table 1 Unrepaired Unilateral Cleft Lip Nasal Deformity

Retrodisplaced and hypoplastic lower lateral cartilage
Depressed dome
Concave lateral crus
Shortened columella on cleft side
Caudal septal deviation or dislocation toward noncleft side
Absent nasal sill
Hypoplastic maxilla
Flattened or concave ala
Horizontally oriented nostril
Effaced alar facial groove
Alar hooding (flattened nostril apex)
Slanted columella with base toward noncleft side
Alar base substantially inferiorly and laterally displaced

of the nasal base and alae using relatively conservative techniques including cartilage release and temporary suture fixation and bolsters. Secondary correction of the same abnormalities requires more aggressive techniques. Early dissection of the nasal tip and alar base during the initial repair was once avoided because of the presumed adverse effects on nasal growth. This perception was based on the finding that septoplasty involving extensive submucoperiosteal resection is linked to nasal growth retardation in humans and animals. However, no reliable evidence exists to indicate that wide dissection and cartilage repositioning lead to growth disturbances (24–26). In fact, early so-called 'definitive' repair of the cleft lip nasal deformity may lead to a more normal growth pattern while avoiding the social problems that patients with significant orofacial deformities experience (27). Most contemporary surgeons treat the lip and the nose to achieve a complete repair. The main goal during primary repair relating to the nasal tip is symmetry of the nasal base and alae by reshaping and repositioning the affected ala, lower lateral cartilages, and columella. Nevertheless, even aggressive early repair often proves inadequate in the long term because, despite achieving a nearly normal appearance in childhood, the nose will again appear abnormal after the pubertal growth spurt. Some degree of secondary correction will be necessary regardless of surgical therapies before adolescence and must be performed after midface growth is complete (between 16 and 18 years of age in girls and 17 to 20 years in boys).

The appearance and function of the nose vary greatly in adulthood depending on the severity of the original cleft deformity and prior surgical treatments. A thorough preoperative examination including a detailed nasal analysis is necessary prior to secondary rhinoplasty. Typical findings from the preoperative analysis are listed in Table 2. Severe maxillary hypoplasia or crossbite deformities may be an indication for maxillary advancement and Lefort osteotomies. Consultation with an oral surgeon before embarking on secondary rhinoplasty is required in this circumstance. Secondary rhinoplasty can often be limited to work on the middle and lower thirds of the nose and septum, since the upper third of the nose including the nasal bones is generally spared in this deformity. The procedure includes all the typical techniques of open augmentation rhinoplasty including extensive cartilage grafting, open septoplasty, and nasal tip repositioning and reshaping. The main difference between

Table 2 Secondary Unilateral Cleft Lip Nasal Deformity

Hypoplastic maxilla
Acute nasolabial angle
Slightly shortened upper lip
Asymmetrically depressed nasal tip
Flattened ipsilateral dome and nostril
Irregular thin concave alar cartilage
Shortened columella on the cleft side
Alar–columellar (nostril apex) webbing
Caudal septal deviation into the normal side

augmentation rhinoplasty in the patient with a cleft deformity and the patient without a cleft deformity is the need to reposition the underlying alar cartilage, nostril, and ala to achieve symmetry within the nasal tip and base, and to restore vestibular lining. Repositioning the alar cartilage achieves several secondary goals including dome symmetry, a more vertically oriented and symmetrical nostril, and ipsilateral columellar lengthening. Surgical maneuvers unique to the repair of the cleft lip nasal deformity are listed in Table 3. Alar repositioning has been performed using a variety of techniques but most involve some degree of composite repositioning of the lower lateral cartilage with secondary beneficial effects as mentioned. The ipsilateral dome is elevated by recruitment of cartilage and skin either medially or laterally. For example, superolateral rotation of a composite flap that includes vestibular lining, medial crus, and lip scar brings additional lining and cartilage to the dome and lengthens the columella (Fig. 16). Various techniques that have been reported include superolateral sliding rotation flaps using midcolumellar and nasal tip transcutaneous incisions, a marginal incision using a medial crural composite flap advanced toward the ipsilateral depressed dome, and an incision carried into the lip scar that advances the scar superiorly to lengthen the columella (28–30). A chondrocutaneous flap advanced from lateral-to-medial has also been used with success (31). Aside from alar repositioning, premaxillary and pyriform grafting are needed to achieve complete symmetry of the nasal base and correct the often severely closed nasolabial angle. The grafts are placed via a nasal sill, alar groove, or sublabial incision. Subperiosteal pockets are created over the face of the maxilla beneath the nasolabial angle and alar groove. The grafts lie deep within the tissue so rejection is rarely a problem. A variety of grafting materials is well tolerated in this area and, although cartilage can be used, Gore-Tex is an acceptable and widely used alternative.

When significant alar repositioning and columellar lengthening are not needed, a standard open rhinoplasty may be performed (32). The lower lateral cartilage is completely released and separated from the overlying skin and

Table 3 Unique Surgical Techniques for the Unilateral Cleft Lip Nasal Deformity

Composite repositioning of the lower lateral cartilage
Superior advancement of the ipsilateral columella
Pyriform aperture and premaxillary grafting
Placement of draw and trans-alar temporary stay sutures
Repair of the webbed nostril apex

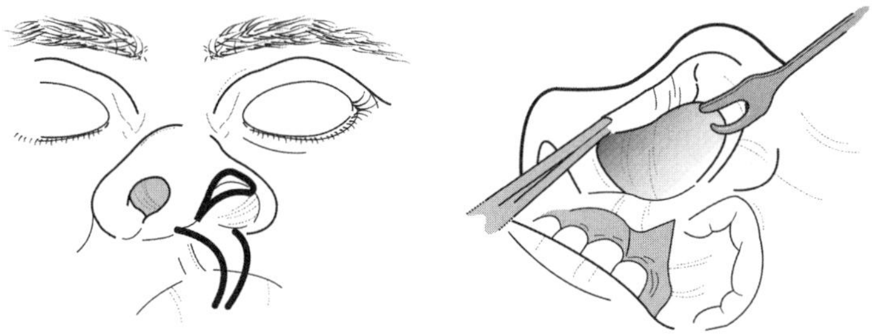

Figure 16 Superolateral rotation of the ala to correct a flat and deficient nostril associated with a cleft lip. Note the proximally based sliding lip flap transposed into the nostril along the lateral crus.

vestibular lining. This allows the cartilage to be repositioned independent from the abnormally positioned linings. The lower lateral cartilage is pulled medially to recruit cartilage and create a new anatomical dome that is elevated and symmetrical with respect to the normal side. The lateral crus is also repositioned to a more normal cephalic position and suture-suspended to the contralateral upper lateral cartilage (33). Batten grafts and a columellar strut are sutured into position and interdomal sutures are used to secure the new dome into place. A dorsal cartilaginous onlay graft may also be necessary. The linings are redraped, supported by the new underlying cartilaginous structural configuration. The lateral alar attachment is thinned and repositioned as needed and plumping grafts are placed along the pyriform rim and maxilla.

A common residual deformity, despite adequate alar repositioning and symmetry, is webbing at the nostril apex. This problem has been corrected using various transcutaneous techniques, the simplest of which involve excision of skin above the nostril rim to efface the web. Contemporary treatment of this deformity involves a simple skin incision along the desired location of the nostril margin. Thus creates a newly positioned nostril rim. The excess skin can be turned in to create additional lining in the area of the dome.

Correction of the bilateral cleft lip nasal deformity requires many of the techniques used in the unilateral cases. However, collapse of the nasal tip and shortening of the columella can be severe in the bilateral cases and requires special techniques for repair. The dorsal middle third of the nose must also be further augmented to match the corrected nasal tip. The main problem is lengthening the columella and, although cartilage grafts are helpful, recruitment of skin and lining from the upper lip and nasal floor is usually required. New concepts and surgical techniques applied during the initial repair, especially using premaxillary orthopedics and primary alar correction, have minimized the problem of a short columella (34). Sufficient tissue exists that a columella of sufficient length can be constructed primarily, thereby avoiding the problem of a foreshortened columella in adolescence and adulthood. Nevertheless, if a shortened columella is present, then a columellar lengthening procedure will be necessary. Two popular columellar lengthening procedures are Cronin's advancement flaps and (2) Millard's forked flap. Cronin advanced tissue into the base of the columella using bilateral V-Y nasal floor advancement flaps (35). Millard's forked flap involves raising two peninsulas of skin, one on either side of the prolabium (along the philtral columns), and advancing each flap in a V-Y fashion to the base of the columella. Millard's forked flap may also be raised during the initial repair and stored within the nasal sills to be used later for columellar lengthening when the child is 2–4 years of age (34,36).

Rhinoplasty in the Aging Patient

The aesthetic goals for the aging patient are subtly different from those of their younger counterparts. Most of their desires lie in the correction of deformities acquired from the aging process, which causes specific changes to nasal architecture and function. The more mobile parts of the nose, including the skin envelope and cartilages, become lax and sag. The lower lateral cartilages thin and undergo partial ossification. There is a loss of support in the nasal tip due to the lack of resiliency of the overlying skin and underlying nasal cartilages and the progressive loosening of the fibrous infrastructure of the nose. The tensile strength of the cartilages and fibrous attachments at the nasal valve also weaken, causing nasal obstruction.

Correction of the multiple deformities associated with aging primarily involves strengthening and restoring the youthful position of the nasal cartilages. Sutures and grafts placed within the nasal tip and middle third of the nose are required. An open approach is needed because the majority of the work is within the nasal tip, with extensive grafting and suture placement. Using the open approach, mucosa can be spared, grafts can be applied, and tip techniques can be used without disrupting the delicate internal architecture of the nose. Typical augmentation techniques may be used to derotate and strengthen the nasal tip. Columellar struts and interdomal suturing are usually needed. Surface grafts (i.e., shield graft) should be used sparingly because of the thin overlying skin. Sutures between the upper and lower lateral cartilages at the scrolls are useful to help shore up the weakened fibrous connections in these areas and derotate the nasal tip. Septoplasty should be conservative to preserve dorsal support.

The major difference between rhinoplasty in the older and the younger patient is the use of external incisions. The overlying skin has lengthened due to the aging process and specifically designed external incisions can aid in creating support and assist in keeping the nose rotated upward during healing. The two most commonly used incisions are the glabellar and supratip. The glabellar incision is a horizontal incision across the nose at the nasion to remove 1–2 cm lax skin. The incision can extend from inner canthus to inner canthus and usually can be placed within a rhytid. Direct excision of skin in the supratip area is done vertically starting at the supratip just superior to the lobule, extending approximately 1–1.5 cm in length. These incisions are very useful because aging skin does not drape well postoperatively and may not shrink in to the newly created nasal architecture due to lack of elasticity. These incisions usually heal well without noticeable scars because of the lack of skin elasticity.

Rhinoplasty in Nonwhite Patients

There are fundamental anatomical and aesthetic differences between the nonwhite (Asian and black) and white nose. Although these differences are recognized anthropologically, the standard of beauty often remains a Western, white look. However, the practice of applying these standards wholeheartedly to nonwhite noses results in unrealistic goals and noses that appear odd and out of balance with the rest of the face. Of course, the true standard of beauty in the world is culturally dependent. Nevertheless, the usual nonwhite patient seeking cosmetic rhinoplasty in the United States is looking for one or more aspects of their nose to take on a more western look. It is sometimes difficult for the typical rhinoplasty surgeon to discern beauty across cultures and the typical nonwhite patient often seeks to keep some racial traits while shedding others. Therefore, it is imperative that the surgeon carefully question the patient with regard to his or her desires and limit the rhinoplasty to those specific goals. Unrealistic expectations or additional information or possibilities should be carefully explored. Rhinoplasty in this group of patients is a balance between achieving a selectively more Western look while preserving most of the unique racial features of the patient's nose and face.

Only certain traits can be changed and some can only be modified. Three aspects of the nonwhite nose that can be changed are a deficient nasal dorsum, an inadequately projected nasal tip, and flaring nostrils. In terms of the actual procedures, most rhinoplasty in nonwhite patients centers on modification of the broad short dorsum with its lack of support and short septum, frail alar cartilages, widened nasal base, and underprojected nasal tip. Maneuvers to counteract each of these problems will be needed.

The typical white nose is characterized by a high dorsum, thin alar wings, a thin well-defined nasal tip, and a supratip break that lies approximately three-fourths the way down the nasal dorsum. This being the standard and the result that should be achieved, the nose is commonly placed into one of three general categories:

Leptorrhine: Typical white nose.

Mesorrhine: Found among Asians and characterized by a short nose, underprojected and slightly overrotated tip with short dorsal height, short septum, and widened nasal bridge. The nasal base is not appreciably wide. The supratip break lies approximately two-thirds of the way down the nasal dorsum.

Platyrrhine: Found among African-Americans. It is characterized by a flat broad dorsum with widely flared nostrils, widened nasal sills and nasal base, overrotated tip, short columella, and paucity of nasal septum. The supratip break lies one-half the way down the nasal dorsum.

These cases strictly call for augmentation rhinoplasty techniques. Most mesorrhine and all platyrrhine noses need both dorsal as well as columellar augmentation. The premaxilla particularly requires augmentation since most nonwhite noses display a relatively retruded premaxilla and short or absent (platyrrhines) nasal spine.

For the dorsal problem, autogenous or alloplastic onlay grafts are useful. Many surgeons in Asia have had success with combined dorsal and columella molded silicone implants. However, others have reported a high incidence (up to 10%) of late complications leading to removal of the implant and implant extrusion (37). The first choice of grafting material should be autologous (e.g., rib, septum, or ear). The most reliable alloplast to date is Medpor and may be suitable for selected individuals. The surgeon may have to stack the grafts to achieve the desired height. With regard to narrowing the upper third of the nose, most patients with mesorrhine noses do not need osteotomies. The broad platyrrhine nose often calls for medial and low lateral osteotomies. Given that the problem is dorsal height vs. width, osteotomies might be counterproductive by excessively narrowing the nose in the presence of a widened lobule and alar complex, leaving a pear-shaped deformity. If osteotomies are performed, it is essential that the nasal bones be made completely mobile. Incomplete osteotomies will result in widening of the nasal bridge postoperatively, accentuating the deformity rather than effacing it.

Tip-plasty has become a point of contention among many surgeons who perform this type of rhinoplasty. Some prefer vertical dome division while others prefer a dome-binding approach with onlay tip grafts. The author prefers the application of a medial crural strut that extends from just below the domes to the nasal spine. Dome-binding sutures are utilized to decrease the bulbosity of the nasal tip along with selective defatting. To define and augment the nasal tip further, a shield graft may be used. Vertical dome division is reserved for patients with relatively hardy alar cartilages and thick overlying skin, especially with platyrrhine noses. Medial crural-binding stitches are used liberally to add firmness and form to the columella. Dorsal septal grafts and premaxillary plumping grafts are often needed to enhance nasal support and efface the nasolabial angle.

A wide alar base and excessive nostril flare are typical findings in a black nose. Correction of excessive flare should be done after the nasal tip is projected adequately since changes in projection have a significant affect on alar flaring. The Western aesthetic standard for the dimensions of the alar base includes the rule that the width of the alar base (between the alar creases) should equal the intercanthal distance. The rule for alar flare states that the external aspects of the nostrils should not protrude beyond the alar–cheek attachments on base view (Fig. 17). Although not usually addressed during nonwhite rhinoplasty, other aesthetic aspects of the nasal base should also be assessed including the vertical position of the alar insertion and the recurvature of the ala into the base of the columella. On profile view, the plane of insertion of the ala into the cheek should be within 2–3 mm above the columellar–labial junction (38). For example, insertion at or below the columellar–labial junction results in an unaesthetic appearance of the ala (alar hooding). Recurvature of the ala is an important aesthetic parameter since lack of appropriate recurvature can be a direct result of surgery performed for correction of a wide nasal base or excessive alar flare. Although the appearance on base view of a nasal ala directly inserting into the cheek, without the typical gentle curve toward the base of the columella, can be found in nonoperated patients, this finding is a common adverse consequence of nasal base surgery. For this reason, any nasal base surgery should be done incrementally since the result will be a delicate balance between an abnormal lack of recurvature and the desired result.

Reduction of alar flare is a realistic goal and achievable in an incremental fashion by variable wedge excision of the nostril floor mucosa, nasal sill, and alar sidewall. As mentioned, direct reduction of alar flare should only be considered after the desired tip elevation and projection procedures are completed, since they will significantly reduce alar flare in and of themselves (Fig. 18). Reduction of nostril flaring will usually result in the appearance of a reduction in nasal base width as well. Any actual reduction in the width of the nasal base requires so-called nasal bunching sutures since excision of skin and associated soft tissues across the nasal base itself (i.e., between the alar creases) will leave obvious scars. A nasal bunching suture is

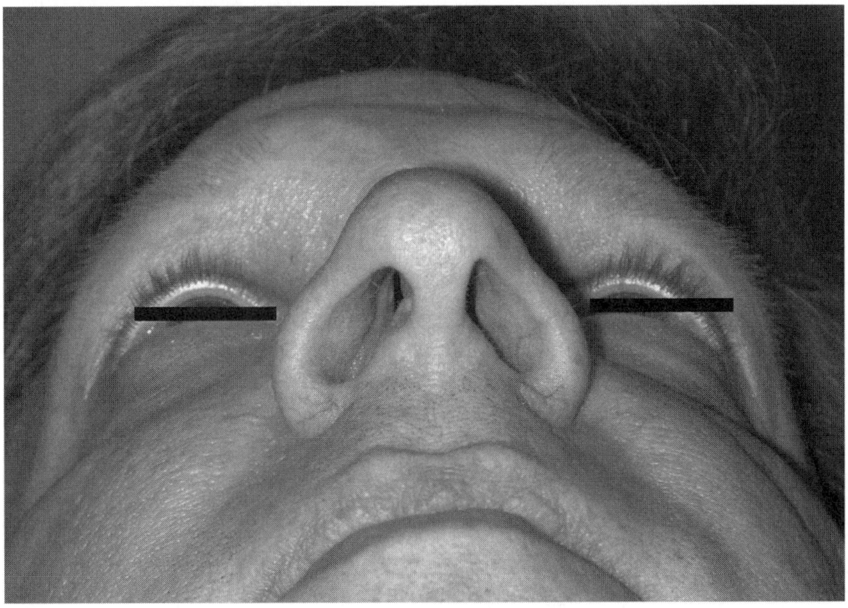

Figure 17 Excessive alar flare. Note that the lateral aspects of the nostrils extend well beyond their attachments to the cheek.

placed through incisions in the mucosa behind the nasal sills bilaterally. A 'U' stitch is placed by passing the suture through the ipsilateral incision and exiting through the opposite incision. The suture is then passed again through the opposite side and brought out the ipsilateral side. As the suture is cinched, the soft tissues within the nasal base are pulled together to bring the alar attachments medially thus narrowing the nasal base.

Alar flaring is reduced by pulling the external aspect of the ala medially. This is accomplished most conservatively by excising a diamond-shaped wedge of tissue within the nasal mucosa behind the sill. A further reduction in flaring is achieved by extending the wedge excision through the nasal sill. This will also narrow the nostril and change its shape, depending on the amount of soft tissue removed. Maximal reduction in flaring and nostril shape and size is done through a combined wedge excision of the nasal mucosa, sill, and alar sidewall (Fig. 19). The width (corresponding to the degree of soft tissue removal) of each component of the wedge will determine the final shape and recurvature of the nostril. Too aggressive an approach will lead to the appearance of a straight ala inserting directly into the cheek, which is a highly undesirable look. When the wedge extends into the alar sidewall, it is important to place it 1–2 mm above the alar crease. This avoids having to suture across a sharp concavity (i.e., the alar crease), thus facilitating good apposition of the cut skin edges.

Nasal Fracture and Posttraumatic Rhinoplasty

The nasal bones are the most commonly injured bones in the facial skeleton. Fractures usually result from lateral blunt trauma sufficient to displace and fracture the

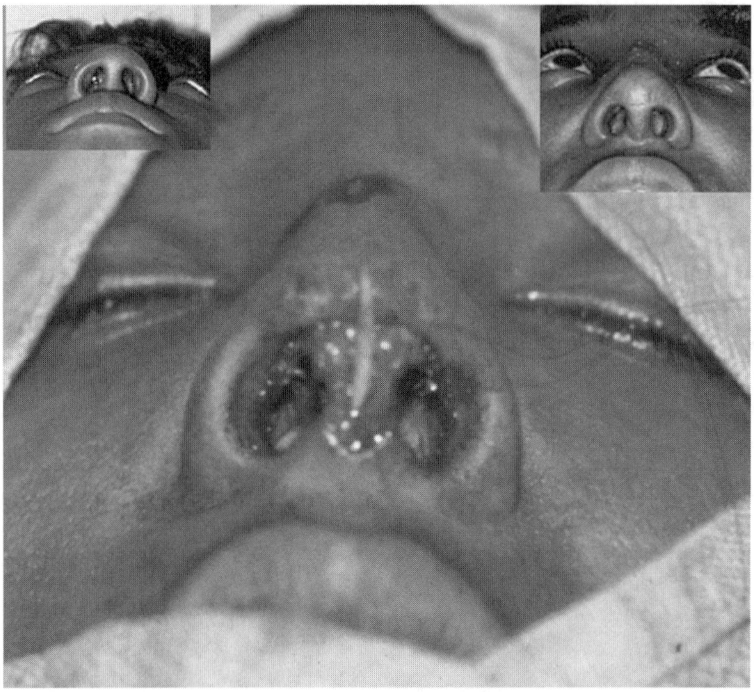

Figure 18 Reducing alar flare by projecting the nasal tip. In many cases of excessive alar flaring (inset, left), simply projecting the nasal tip (in this case, using a columellar strut, center) will significantly reduce the unaesthetic flaring (inset, right).

small paired nasal bones and the ascending processes of the maxillae. This fracture is deceivingly difficult to manage because of the complex nature of the underlying anatomy. Early (within 2 weeks) closed reduction is often successful in restoring the position of the displaced nasal bones, but the underlying septum often remains

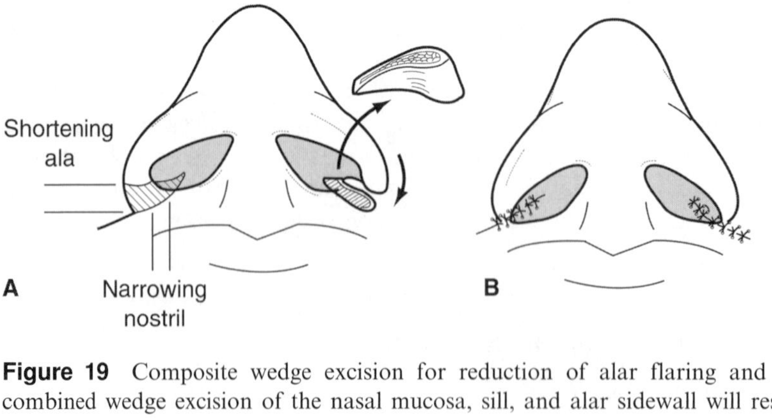

Figure 19 Composite wedge excision for reduction of alar flaring and nostril size. A combined wedge excision of the nasal mucosa, sill, and alar sidewall will result in maximal reduction in flaring and nostril size.

out of place. Undetected and untreated septal deviations may lead to subtle problems with nasal bone alignment and an ultimately undesirable result.

Nasal fractures are more correctly referred to as nasoseptal fractures because of the intimate connection the nasal bones share with the dorsal nasal septum, especially at the rhinion where the septum, upper lateral cartilages, and nasal bones are confluent. Although lateral blows are the usual cause of nasoseptal fractures, the degree of septal displacement is often greater in frontal blows because the quadrilateral cartilage is contacted first. In addition, septal buckling, displacement off the maxillary crest, and septal hematoma are more common in this type of injury. In frontal or lateral impacts, the nasal bones are most often displaced posterolaterally. Severe impacts may result in avulsions of both soft tissue and cartilage, resulting in an unstable open fracture prone to scarring and contracture. Diagnosis is based on clinical examination alone with little role for routine radiography. Plain nasal films are notoriously unreliable and should not be used for diagnosis or management of these fractures (39). If extensive facial fractures are suspected, then computerized tomography should be arranged.

In the typical isolated nasoseptal fracture, there is a window of approximately 2 weeks after the injury in which the nasal bones can be replaced. After 2 weeks sufficient healing has occurred and reduction is more difficult. Initial management should include closure of lacerations both externally and internally if possible, accurate reduction of the bony fractures, and replacement of avulsed or displaced cartilage including the nasal cartilages and septum. Accurate reduction of the septum is important to ensure a long-lasting and functional result. Unfortunately, the septum is the most difficult part of the fracture to reduce and is often inadequately treated. A common management approach to nasoseptal fractures is to allow the edema to resolve and, after 7–10 days, the nasal bones are closed reduced with a Boise elevator or the handle of a Bard Parker surgical scalpel. The septum is grossly evaluated for septal hematoma but little or no effort is expended in reducing it. This approach is justified because the septum often contains overlapping segments that are impossible to realign via a closed approach. The quadrilateral cartilage is elastic and resists replacement in a reduced position once fractured. This approach (simple reduction), however, leads to high rates of failure that require secondary septorhinoplasty. Nevertheless, closed reduction alone is likely to be successful in the case of a simple unilateral or bilateral nasal bone fracture. Comminuted fractures, complex nasal fractures with significant septal disruption, and naso-orbitoethmoid (NOE) fractures usually require open reduction methods.

Regardless of fracture type, a thorough examination of the septum is needed, preferably endoscopically. If there is a significant septal disruption then the septum will require open reduction. This tends to be the case if the nasal bones are deviated more than half the width of the nasal bridge (40). Closed reduction of the nasal septum is usually not successful for reasons already mentioned, so open reduction under a local or general anesthetic is necessary. Open reduction may require a limited inferior resection of the quadrilateral cartilage and reconstruction using sutures and typical conservative septoplasty techniques. A common mistake in initially performing nasal and septal reduction is failure to complete greenstick fractures. The nasal bones should be manipulated so that they are completely mobilized and ready to be placed in proper position, with little likelihood of them springing out of position. An exception to this rule is if the nasal bone is found to snap back into a good reduced position and seems to remain stable despite further gentler manipulation. The septum is quite prone to greensticking and often the only hope of achieving a midline reduction is to fracture the partially tethered remaining septum with a back and forth movement. This may result in fracture of the maxillary crest, but this is acceptable if nasal support is preserved. If a septal hematoma is encountered initially, it is drained via a unilateral Killian incision (over the cartilage). The opposite side drains through the fractured septum or through a surgically created tunnel. A small rubber band drain may be placed within the septum and the nasal cavities gently packed with gauze bilaterally for 2–3 days with antibiotic coverage.

Long-term posttraumatic nasal deformities most often involve the septum, upper lateral cartilages, and nasal bones. A combination of functional and aesthetic problems must be addressed. Nasal obstruction involving the nasal valve may result from scarring across the valve between the septum and caudal end of the upper lateral cartilage or simply from a deviated septum. Disrupted or avulsed upper lateral cartilages may collapse against the septum, resulting in nasal obstruction at the valve and an external nasal deformity manifesting most often as a twisted nose deformity. Injury in the area of the upper lateral cartilage creates a void that is replaced with scar that contracts. With contraction, the nasal tip and dorsum (below the rhinion) are pulled toward the side of the injury. The magnitude of the twist can be dramatic and any attempt at repairing it (i.e., septorhinoplasty) should be delayed until this process has stabilized (at least 6 months).

REFERENCES

1. Gunter JP, Friedman RM. Lateral crural strut graft: technique and clinical applications in rhinoplasty. Plast Reconstr Surg 1997; 99:943–952.
2. Goldman IB. The importance of the mesial crura in nasal-tip reconstruction. Arch Otolaryngol 1957; 65:143–147.
3. Micheli-Pellegrini V, Ponti L, Ponti G, Guidarelli P. Interrupted and continuous strip technique for tip surgery during traditional rhinoplasty. Facial Plast Surg 1996; 12:347–355.
4. Kridel RW, Konior RJ, Shumrick KA, Wright WK. Advances in nasal tip surgery. The lateral crural steal. Arch Otolaryngol Head Neck Surg 1989; 115:1206–1212.
5. Constantian MB. Four common anatomic variants that predispose to unfavorable rhinoplasty results: a study based on 150 consecutive secondary rhinoplasties. Plast Reconstr Surg 2000; 105:316–131.
6. Goodman WS, Gilbert RW. The anatomy of external rhinoplasty. Otolaryngol Clin North Am 1987; 20:641–652.
7. Welling DB, Maves MD, Schuller DE, Bardach J. Irradiated homologous cartilage grafts. Long-term results. Arch Otolaryngol Head Neck Surg 1988; 114:291–295.
8. Breadon GE, Kern EB, Neel HB III. Autografts of uncrushed and crushed bone and cartilage. Experimental observations and clinical implications. Arch Otolaryngol 1979; 105:75–80.
9. Sheen JH. Aesthetic Rhinoplasty. St. Louis: C.V. Mosby Co., 1978.
10. Guyuron B, Michelow BJ, Englebardt C. Upper lateral splay graft. Plast Reconstr Surg 1998; 102:2169–2177.
11. Sheen JH. A new look at supratip deformity. Ann Plast Surg 1979; 3:498–504.

12. Webster RC, Davidson TM, Smith RC. Nasofrontal angle changes in rhinoplasty. Otolaryngol Head Neck Surg 1979; 87:95–108.
13. Guyuron B. Guarded burr for deepening of nasofrontal junction. Plast Reconstr Surg 1989; 84:513–516.
14. Mommaerts MY, Van Butsele BL, Abeloos JS, De Clercq CA, Neyt LF. Rhinoplasty with nasal bone disarticulation to deepen the nasofrontal groove. Experimental and clinical results. J Craniomaxillofac Surg 1995; 23:109–114.
15. Paniello RC. Nasal valve suspension. An effective treatment for nasal valve collapse. Arch Otolaryngol Head Neck Surg 1996; 122:1342–1346.
16. Kamer FM. Lengthening the short nose. Ann Plast Surg 1980; 4:281–285.
17. Lee Y, Kim J, Lee E. Lengthening of the postoperative short nose: combined use of a gull-wing concha composite graft and a rib costochondral dorsal onlay graft. Plast Reconstr Surg 2000; 105:2190–2199.
18. Naficy S, Baker SR. Lengthening the short nose. Arch Otolaryngol Head Neck Surg 1998; 124:809–813.
19. Gunter JP, Clark CP, Friedman RM. Internal stabilization of autogenous rib cartilage grafts in rhinoplasty: a barrier to cartilage warping. Plast Reconstr Surg 1997; 100: 161–169.
20. Romo T III, Jablonski RD. Nasal reconstruction using split calvarial grafts. Otolaryngol Head Neck Surg. 1992; 107:622–630.
21. Leach J. Interlocking calvarial bone grafts: a solution for the short, depressed nose. Laryngoscope 2000; 110:955–960.
22. Larrabee WF Jr., Murakami C. Osteotomy techniques to correct posttraumatic deviation of the nasal pyramid: a technical note. J Craniomaxillofac Trauma 2000; 6:43–7.
23. Millard DR Jr. Cleft Craft. Vol. 1. Boston, Little: Brown, & Company, 1976.
24. Rock WP, Brain DJ. The effects of nasal trauma during childhood upon growth of the nose and midface. Br J Orthod 1983; 10:38–41.
25. Goumas P, Strambis G, Antonakopoulos C, Helidonis E. Long-term results of nasal surgery in children. Ear Nose Throat J 1988; 67:294–296.
26. Verwoerd CD, Urbanus NA, Nijdam DC. The effects of septal surgery on the growth of nose and maxilla. Rhinology 1979; 17:53–63.
27. Salyer KE. Primary correction of the unilateral cleft lip nose: a 15-year experience. Plast Reconstr Surg 1986; 77:558–568.
28. Vissarionov VA. Correction of the nasal tip deformity following repair of unilateral clefts of the upper lip. Plast Reconstr Surg 1989; 83:341–347.
29. Blair VP. Nasal deformities associated with congenital cleft of the lip. JAMA 1925; 84:185–187.
30. Converse JM. Reconstructive Plastic Surgery. Philadelphia: W.B. Saunders, 1964.
31. Potter J. Some nasal tip deformities due to alar cartilage abnormalities. Plast Reconstr Surg 1954; 13:358–366.
32. Farrior RT. The cleft lip nose: an update. Facial Plast Surg 1993; 9:241–268.
33. Rifley W, Thaller SR. The residual cleft lip nasal deformity. An anatomic approach. Clin Plast Surg 1996; 23:81–92.
34. Mulliken JB. Correction of the bilateral cleft lip nasal deformity: evolution of a surgical concept. [Review] [20 refs]. Cleft Palate-Craniofac J 1992; 29:540–545.
35. Cronin T. Lengthening columella by use of skin from the nasal floor and alae. Plast Reconstr Surg 1958; 21:417.
36. Millard DR Jr. Columellar lengthening by a forked flap. Plast Reconstr Surg 1955; 22:254.
37. Pak MW, Chan ES, van Hasselt CA. Late complications of nasal augmentation using silicone implants. J Laryngol Otol 1998; 112:1074–1077.

38. Crumley RL. Aesthetics and surgery of the nasal base. Facial Plast Surg 1988; 5:135–142.
39. Sharp JF, Denholm S. Routine x-rays in nasal trauma: the influence of audit on clinical practice. J R Soc Med 1994; 87:153–154.
40. Murray JA, Maran AG, Mackenzie IJ, Raab G. Open v closed reduction of the fractured nose. Arch Otolaryngol 1984; 110:797–802.

22
Functional and Aesthetic Blepharoplasty

Robert W. Dolan
Lahey Clinic Medical Center, Burlington, Massachusetts, U.S.A.

INTRODUCTION

Blepharoplasty describes any operation designed to correct congenital or acquired eyelid defects. Indications for functional upper lid blepharoplasty include senile blepharoptosis, levator aponeurosis dehiscence, entropion, paralytic lagophthalmos, and prolapsing orbital fat causing an upper visual field deficit. The usual indications for functional lower lid blepharoplasty include entropion, ectropion, scleral show, epiphora, senile lid laxity, and lateral canthal dystopia. The most common cosmetic blepharoplasty procedures include excision of redundant eyelid skin and prolapsing orbital fat, creation of a superior eyelid crease, revision of epicanthal folds, and excision of malar folds and festoons.

Patient selection and a complete anatomically based evaluation of the eyelids are important preoperative considerations. A thorough understanding of the terminology (see Appendix), anatomy, pathophysiology, and potential benefits of each blepharoplasty technique is essential for a successful outcome. Preoperative education with regard to the potential benefits and risks of surgery and alternative nonsurgical treatments should be thoroughly discussed with the patient and documented. The patient should understand that blepharoplasty cannot correct fine wrinkling or dark discoloration often present in eyelid skin. Finally, every patient undergoing aesthetic blepharoplasty should undergo a complete ophthalmological examination preoperatively.

PREOPERATIVE EVALUATION

A complete ocular examination is routinely performed prior to blepharoplasty. The examination may uncover occult ocular abnormalities that represent relative or absolute contraindications to elective surgery. In a medicolegal sense, the examination provides an objective benchmark against which claims of postoperative ocular complications may be measured. The typical examination includes fundoscopy and an evaluation of tear production, measurement of intraocular pressure, visual fields, visual acuity, and a slitlamp examination of the cornea and conjunctiva.

Detecting patients who may be prone to dry eyes is of utmost importance in operative planning. Even conservative upper lid blepharoplasty in patients at risk will exacerbate the symptoms of dry eyes and lead to an unhappy patient despite an acceptable cosmetic outcome (1). Patients at risk include those with paradoxical excessive tearing (intermittent, resulting from irritation), burning, crusting, or the presence of collagen vascular disease (e.g., lupus, scleroderma). Schirmer's test is a useful objective measure of tear production. It is performed by placing a special type of filter paper (Whatman #41 filter paper, 5 mm wide and 35 mm long) in the lateral corner of the eye, with or without anesthetic, avoiding contact with the cornea. After 5 min the paper is removed and the length of moisture that migrated onto the strip is measured. The normal range is 10–15 mm. Schirmer's test is specific but lacks sensitivity. The history may be more helpful in predicting the likelihood of dry-eye syndrome (DES) even in the presence of normal findings on Schirmer's test (2). Deficient tearing can lead to corneal erosions, scarring, or infection. A careful slit-lamp examination of the cornea can sometimes detect subclinical evidence of corneal drying. Patients with a history or physical examination (including an abnormal Schirmer's test) indicative of DES should not undergo cosmetic blepharoplasty of the upper lid. However, these patients may still be candidates for a conservative lower lid blepharoplasty performed with minimal or no resection of eyelid skin.

Any patient who cannot tolerate a general anesthetic for medical reasons should not be considered a candidate for cosmetic blepharoplasty. Drugs or dietary supplements that increase the bleeding time including nonsteroidal anti-inflammatories, cortisone preparations, and vitamin E should be discontinued at least 2 weeks preoperatively. A history of easy bruising or prolonged bleeding time should prompt a more formal hematological work-up. Patients should also be free of underlying diseases that may impede healing (acquired or congenital immunodeficiency or collagen vascular disease) or cause persistent periorbital edema (thyroid dysfunction or renal disease). Although testing every patient for thyroid dysfunction is unnecessary, further testing may be warranted in the presence of signs or symptoms suggestive of hypothyroidism, hyperthyroidism, or Graves' disease. Some patients experience periorbital manifestations of thyroid disease that may be mistaken for signs of aging. In a review of patients seeking aesthetic blepharoplasty, the periorbital findings were attributed to hypothyroidism in 2.6% of cases and hyperthyroidism in 0.3% of cases (3). When these patients received treatment for their thyroid condition, the periorbital signs frequently improved. Patients with hypothyroidism often have nonspecific systemic symptoms consistent with a hypometabolic state. The connective tissue changes consist of myxedema (subcutaneous edema), clammy yellowish skin, brittle hair and nails, and hair loss in the lateral eyebrows. The periocular findings consist of nonpitting periorbital edema, malar erythema, malar bags, and festoons (3). Patients with lower lid or periorbital edema should be screened for thyroid dysfunction (e.g., measurement of thyroid-stimulating hormone [TSH] level). The clinical hallmarks of Graves' disease and thyroid orbitopathy are vertical eyelid retraction, proptosis, lagophthalmos, restrictive extraocular myopathy, chemosis, dilated conjunctival blood vessels, elevation of intraocular pressure, eyelid edema, and optic neuropathy. A typical patient may complain of increased or decreased tearing, blurring and difficulty focusing, pressure sensation, and diplopia. Lacrimal gland dysfunction may lead to either increased or decreased production of tears. Diplopia and difficulty focusing are usually secondary to inflamed extraocular muscles. A Computed tomographic (CT) scan may confirm the diagnosis by demonstrating enlarged extraocular muscles. Chemical evidence of thyroid dysfunction is an unreliable sign of thyroid orbitopathy and may only be present in the minority of cases. However, if a complete set of thyroid laboratory tests is obtained, including measurement of thyroid function and antibody studies, the majority of patients with thyroid-associated opthalmopathy will show an abnormality.

A complete ophthalmological examination is useful for the detection of corneal ulcerations using the slitlamp, optic disk edema and venous dilation by fundoscopy, proptosis by exophthalmometry, and optic neuropathy by visual acuity, field-testing, and color desaturation. A sensitive indicator of optic neuropathy is rapid degradation of hue when the patient is asked to look at a bright red object (red desaturation). Patients with thyroid orbitopathy and vertical eyelid retraction should undergo, at most, only conservative blepharoplasty, and any skin or muscle resection should be kept to a minimum.

The most common postoperative complication in lower eyelid blepharoplasty is lower lid malposition including scleral show and ectropion. Detecting patients who are prone to postoperative eyelid malposition is also an important component of the preoperative examination. Patients particularly prone to this complication include those with pre-existing anatomical lower lid malposition or lower lid laxity. Pre-existing eyelid malpositions are common in patients with proptosis, large globes, thyroid opthalmopathy, and deficient malar support. Patients with prominent globes or deficient underlying bony support often show a reversal in the vector of projection of the globe in relation to the lower eyelid margin. The apex of the cornea projects beyond the lower eyelid margin in these patients. Patients predisposed to lower eyelid malposition should undergo lateral canthoplasty and conservative resection of skin and muscle.

After a complete history and physical examination, the patient desiring a cosmetic improvement of the eyelids should be allowed to point out, with the aid of a mirror and cotton-tipped applicator, specific areas of concern. Standard photographic views are then taken (see Chap. 1), and a complete physical examination of the eyelids is done with documentation of the following pathologic conditions (Table 1): eyebrow ptosis, dermatochalasis, prolapsing orbital fat, orbicularis oculus muscle hypertrophy, lacrimal gland ptosis, lagophthalmos, lid lag and vertical eyelid retraction, blepharoptosis, low or absent upper eyelid crease, epicanthal folds, lower eyelid and canthal malposition, tear trough deformity, and malar folds and festoons.

Eyebrow Ptosis

If the eyebrow is ptotic (Fig. 1) the thicker skin subjacent to the eyebrow tends to fall into the area normally occupied by the thin skin of the eyelid. Performing aggressive skin resection in the upper eyelid to compensate for the ptotic eyebrow leads to further decent of the brow, inadequate definition of the lateral orbit–eyebrow complex, and obvious scarring within the thicker infrabrow skin. Elevating the ptotic brow prior to upper lid blepharoplasty results in significant secondary gains in the aesthetics of the upper eyelid and lateral orbit–eyebrow complex (4). As the brow is elevated, the upper eyelid is relieved of the burden of the thick skin in the infrabrow area and resection of eyelid skin may be more conservative. Upper lid

Table 1 Anatomically Based Evaluation of the Eyelids With Normal Ranges and Pathological Diagnoses

	Pathological diagnoses	Clinical Findings: Females	Clinical Findings: Males
Upper eyelid	Eyebrow ptosis	Eyebrow at or below orbital rim	Eyebrow below orbital rim
	Eyelid fullness	Bulging and sagging due to fat and orbicularis oculus muscle	
	Dermatochalasis	Fine wrinkling of eyelid skin	
	Entropion	Lid margin inversion	
	Ectropion	Lid margin–globe passive separation or eversion	
	Lacrimal gland ptosis	Lateral upper eyelid bulging due to a ptotic lacrimal gland	
	Lagophthalmos	Incomplete eye closure	
	Lid lag	Lagging descent of upper lid margin with downgaze	
	Blepharoptosis	Eyelid fissure <9-mm	Eyelid fissure <8-mm
		Upper lid margin >25 percent overlap of corneal limbus	
	Vertical eyelid retraction	Eyelid fissure >13-mm	Eyelid fissure >10-mm
		Upper lid margin touching or above corneal limbus	
	Epicanthal fold	Medial canthal hooding	
	Low/absent lid crease	Lid crease <10 mm above lid margin	Lid crease <8 mm above lid margin
	Levator muscle dysfunction	Excursion 0–4 mm = poor levator function 5–7 mm fair 8–12 mm good >12 mm = excellent	
Lower eyelid	Lid laxity	Fails "snap back" test	
	Round eye	Slight inferior displacement of the eyelid margin	
	Canthal dystopia	Malposition of the eyelid commissure	
	Scleral show	Lower lid margin below corneal limbus	
	Malar fold	Gross prominences over the malar eminence	
	Festoon	Severe malar fold with a drape-like or swag appearance	

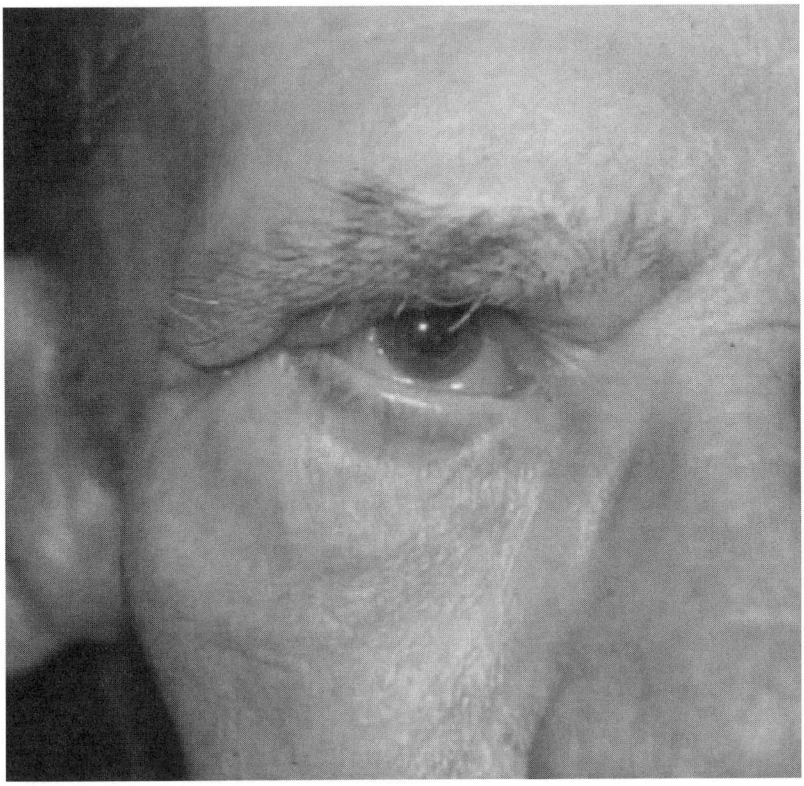

Figure 1 Patient with eyebrow ptosis: a heavy look and redundant upper eyelid skin.

blepharoplasty may be performed during the same operative session or delayed indefinitely to allow a more complete evaluation of the effects of the browplasty on the upper lid–brow complex.

Dermatochalasis

Dermatochalasis (Fig. 2) refers only to the condition of sagging skin although it is often associated with other signs of the aging eyelid including pseudoherniation of orbital fat. Dermatochalasis is usually an acquired condition (aging, environmental, genetic) that is manifested as either fine wrinkling or redundant skin.

Prolapsing Orbital Fat: Upper Eyelid

Medial and central bulges of the upper eyelid are most often caused by pseudoherniation of preseptal orbital fat. Laxity of the orbital septum or changes in the distribution of orbital fat within the confines of the bony orbit due to age-related ligamentous weakness are responsible. A lateral bulge usually represents a ptotic lacrimal gland and is easily differentiated from the adjacent central fat pad (Fig. 3). The medial fat pad is more difficult to locate, more prone to bleeding, and is often responsible for residual bulging after an apparently successful upper eyelid cosmetic blepharoplasty. The medial fat pad is paler and more prone to bleeding due to its greater fibrous content and vascularity.

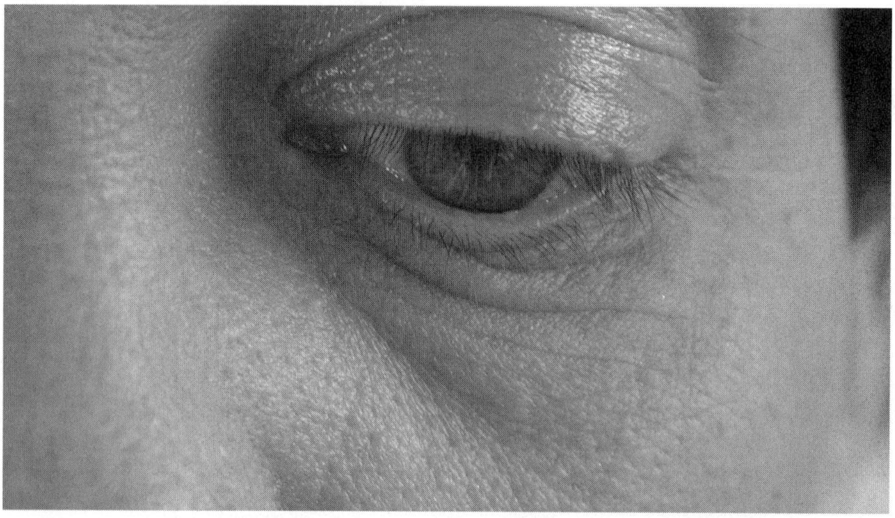

Figure 2 Note skin laxity over eyelids consistent with dermatochalasis or fine wrinkling over lower eyelid.

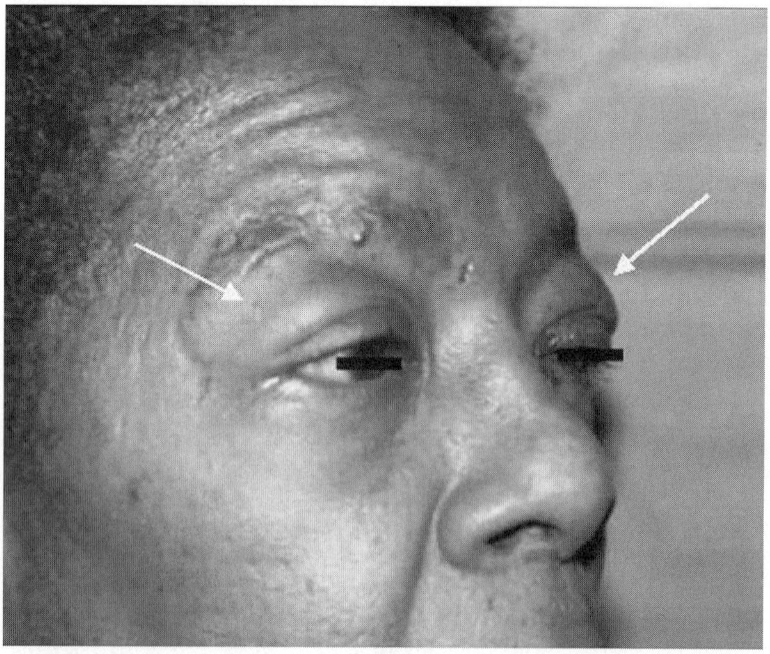

Figure 3 Prolapsing lacrimal glands (arrows), which must be differentiated from prolapsing central fat pads. Treatment consists of resuspension of the glands through an upper blepharoplasty incision. The glands should never be resected.

Prolapsing Orbital Fat: Lower Lid

Bulging of the preseptal eyelid skin in the lower eyelid may be secondary to prolapsing orbital fat, subcutaneous edema, or hypertrophied orbicularis muscle. Orbital fat will be more pronounced when the patient looks up, as the orbicularis muscle relaxes and the orbital fat is brought forward. Squinting will accentuate the folds of hypertrophied orbicularis oculus muscle while minimizing the amount of prolapsing fat. These maneuvers will assist the clinician in differentiating among the various causes of lower eyelid bulging.

A prominent inferior orbital rim or tear trough deformity should be documented as part of the preoperative examination. Orbital fat excision can accentuate these abnormalities and repositioning the orbital fat may be more appropriate in patients with this condition.

Orbicularis Oculus Muscle Hypertrophy

The orbicularis oculus muscle may become hypertrophic in its pretarsal and upper preseptal divisions causing convex contour deformities (i.e., bulging) in these areas. The patient may appear to have double bulges within the lower eyelid representing hypertrophic muscle above and prolapsing orbital fat below. A prominent pretarsal orbicularis muscle is a feature of some younger lower lids and may not be of cosmetic concern. However, in some (especially older) patients, reduction of the bulging in these areas improves the aesthetics after excision of orbital fat by creating a smoother surface from the eyelid margin to the orbital rim.

Lagophthalmos, Lid Lag, and Vertical Eyelid Retraction

Lagophthalmos (Fig. 4) is the amount of separation (in millimeters) between the eyelid margins as the eyes are gently closed. Lid lag describes a phenomenon in which there is a slight delay in complete eyelid closure due to a lag in the movement of the upper eyelid. Vertical eyelid retraction is excessive upper eyelid retraction in primary gaze characterized by a vertical eyelid fissure of greater than 10 mm in men and greater than 13 mm in women. This condition may be due to scarring or, more commonly, secondary to Grave's ophthalmopathy. If lagophthalmos, lid lag, or vertical eyelid retraction is detected on the preoperative examination then traditional cosmetic upper eyelid blepharoplasty may result in dry eye syndrome or exposure keratopathy.

Blepharoptosis

Ptosis is classified as mild, moderate, or severe (5). Mild ptosis is characterized by an eyelid margin 2–3 mm below the limbus in primary gaze; moderate ptosis, 3–4 mm; and severe ptosis, greater than 4 mm. Ptosis may also be quantified by measuring the distance in millimeters between the upper lid margin and corneal light reflex (i.e., the marginal reflex distance [MRD]). The MRD reflects the severity of ptosis more accurately than measurements of the distance of the lid margin overlapping the limbus, since the lid itself obscures the latter structure. The MRD is measured with the patient in primary gaze and the frontalis muscle completely relaxed. A normal

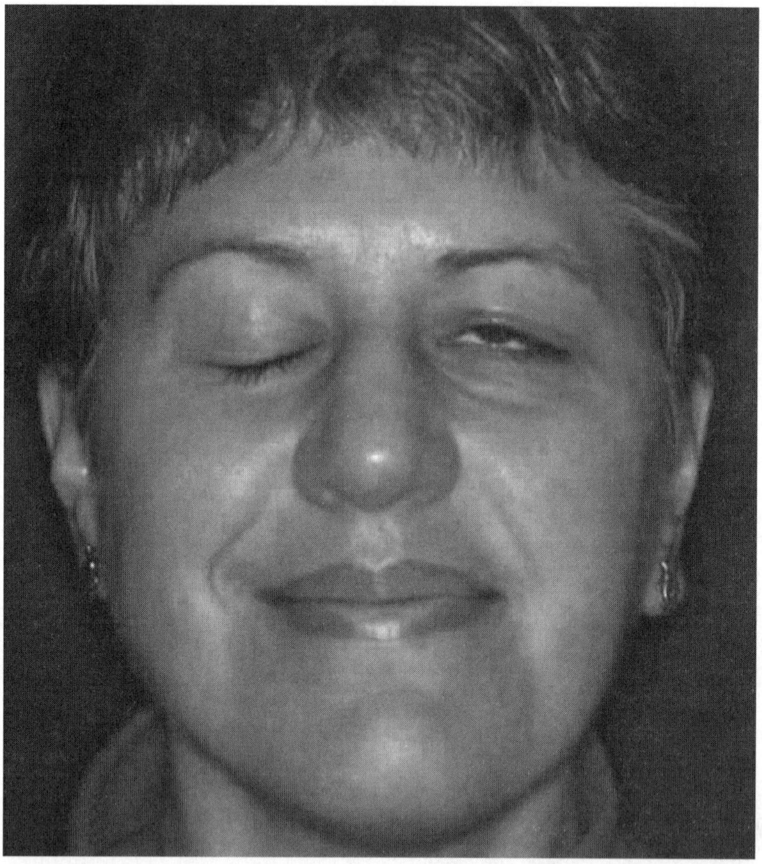

Figure 4 Patient exhibits lid lag from a resolving left facial nerve paralysis. Complete voluntary eye closure is usually the last physical finding to resolve in a patient recovering from a facial nerve injury.

MRD is +4–+5 or 4–5 mm between the lid margin and the light reflex (Fig. 5). This corresponds to an upper lid margin resting 1–2 mm below the corneal limbus. A visual field examination should also document the severity of the superior field deficit.

Blepharoptosis may be congenital or acquired (6). Congenital blepharoptosis is usually sporadic (nonhereditary), unilateral in 70% of cases, and involves dysfunction of the levator muscle. A weak levator muscle with poor excursion characterizes simple congenital ptosis. The levator muscle may also be malformed, resulting in ptosis and lagophthalmos. An interesting phenomenon associated with congenital blepharoptosis is the Marcus-Gunn jaw-wink. It is present in approximately 5% of patients with congenital ptosis and is a trigemino-oculomotor synkinesis. Patients exhibit eyelid retraction with stimulation of the ipsilateral pterygoid muscles (e.g., mouth opening, chewing) (7).

The most common form of acquired ptosis results from dehiscence of the levator aponeurosis from the tarsus often associated with degeneration and stretching of the aponeurotic expansion in the aging eyelid. The disinserted complex elevates the

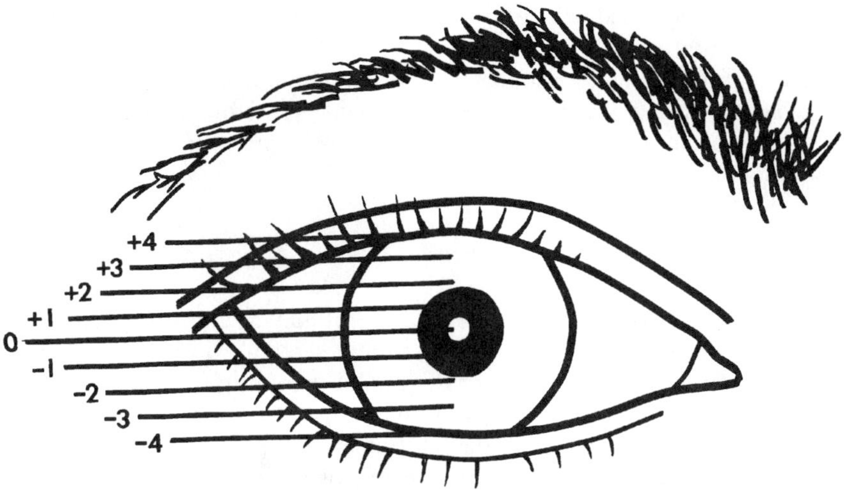

Figure 5 A grading system for the severity of ptosis referred to as the marginal reflex distance (MRD).

orbital (preaponeurotic) fat into the area under the superior orbital rim, resulting in a hollowed superior sulcus, high or absent lid crease, and ptosis. The levator muscle itself is normal, both functionally and anatomically. Other causes of acquired ptosis include traumatic disruption of the aponeurotic sheet or disruption of Whitnall's ligament. Whitnall's ligament suspends the levator muscle under the superior orbital rim; injury to the sling during dissection in the superior orbit can result in ptosis. Acquired myogenic ptosis may be secondary to generalized neuromuscular diseases such as myasthenia gravis. Neurogenic ptosis is secondary to interruption of the nerve supply to the levator muscle (cranial nerve III) or Müller's muscle (sympathetics, Horner's syndrome). Ptosis secondary to Müller's muscle dysfunction is mild because the muscle only provides approximately 2 mm of lift in the upper eyelid. Mechanical ptosis is due to weighting down of the eyelid margin from excessive skin, scarring between the upper and lower eyelid margins, or neoplasm (Fig. 1). Pseudoptosis is the appearance of ptosis secondary to pathological conditions separate from the eyelid such as enophthalmos, vertical dystopia, or phthisis bulbi.

Dehiscence and weakening of the levator aponeurosis is the cause of ptosis in the vast majority of patients who present for cosmetic blepharoplasty. Determination of levator function is required before a surgical plan can be formulated. Levator function is determined by measuring upper lid excursion, which is the distance in millimeters the central lid margin travels vertically from full downgaze to full upgaze. Normal lid excursion is > 8 mm; fair is 5–7 mm; and poor is < 4 mm. If levator function is not normal, an ophthalmologist should be consulted since surgical correction will require techniques beyond those typically used during routine blepharoplasty.

Epicanthal Fold

A medial epicanthal fold is a normal finding in patients of Asian descent. It is formed by an apparent excess of skin that drapes over the medial canthus. The fold gives the appearance of a foreshortened palpebral fissure and a widened intercanthal distance; elimination of the fold is often one of the major goals in blepharoplasty in Asian patients. An epicanthal fold may also form as a result of injudicious medial extension of an upper blepharoplasty incision in a white patient. Therefore, avoidance of the formation of an epicanthal fold is an important consideration in performing cosmetic blepharoplasty in white patients.

Entropion

Entropion is an infolding of the margin of the eyelid. It may result from scarring and contracture of the capsulopalpebral fascia or orbital septum, causing pathological shortening of the posterior lamella that draws the lid margin toward the globe surface. The basic problem stems from irritation of the corneal surface by keratinized skin and eyelashes along the margin of the lid. Entropion may also be due to a lack of rigidity along the lid margin due to weakening of the tarsal plate (e.g., senile entropion) or inadequate reconstruction of the lid margin (i.e., lack of an adequate tarsal replacement after resection).

Ectropion

Ectropion is a rolling outward of the lid margin away from the surface of the globe. It is classified most commonly as cicatricial (Fig. 6), senile (Fig. 7), or paralytic. Ectropion is considered mild if there is only slight separation of the lower eyelid margin from the globe; moderate if there is slight eversion of the eyelid margin

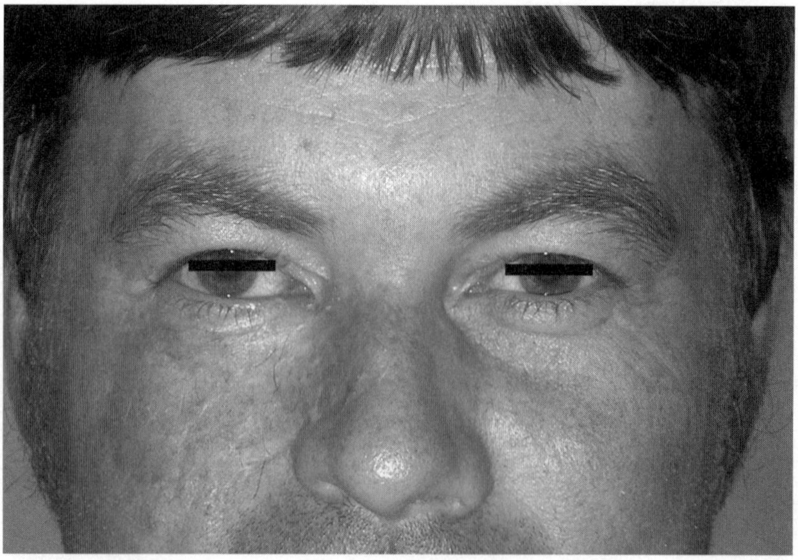

Figure 6 Cicatricial ectropion; appearance following skin graft to the anterior lamella and cheek under the right eye. This was corrected with a full-thickness skin graft placed over the anterior lamella of the lower eyelid.

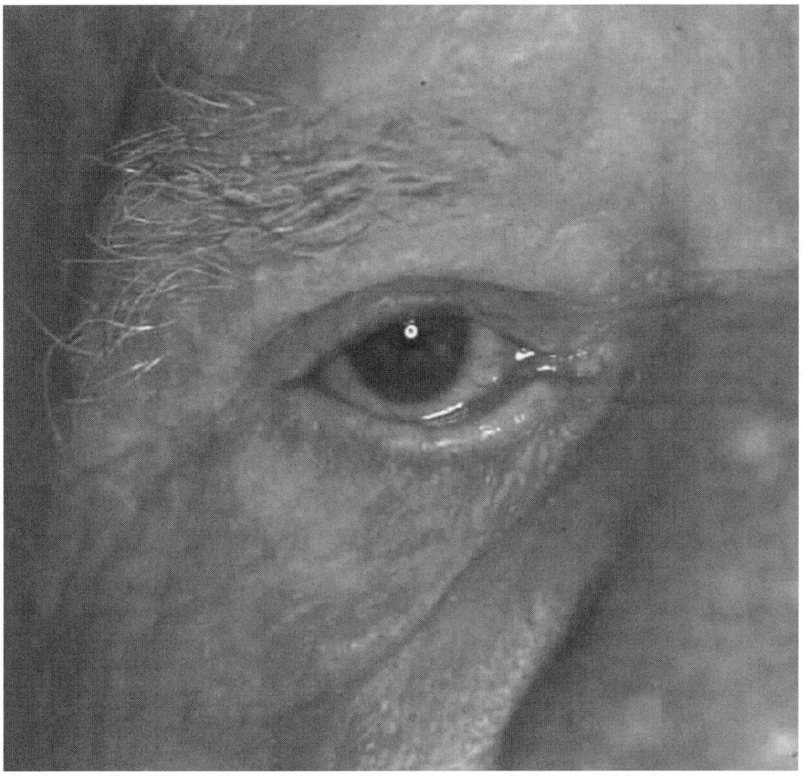

Figure 7 Senile ectropion: note eversion of lower eyelid due to loss of tone and elasticity in the lower eyelid. This is similar to what is found in a patient with paralytic ectropion.

and inferior displacement; and severe if there is obvious eversion and inferior displacement (8).

Lid Laxity

Subclinical lower eyelid laxity is detected with a snap back test and a distraction (pinch) test. The snap back test is performed by pulling the lid away from the surface of the globe and observing its ability to snap back to the globe surface. A distraction test is performed by grasping the inferior eyelid and measuring the distance that the lid margin can be pulled away from the surface of the globe. A distance of greater than 6 mm is abnormal. Patients with an abnormal snap back or pinch test are prone to postoperative eyelid malposition and should undergo canthopexy or canthoplasty in addition to the primary procedure.

Lower Eyelid Retraction

Inferior displacement or fixation of the lower eyelid margin may be congenital or acquired (Fig. 8). The diagnosis is confirmed by grasping the inferior eyelid and noting resistance to superior traction along the entire aspect of the lid. Normally, the

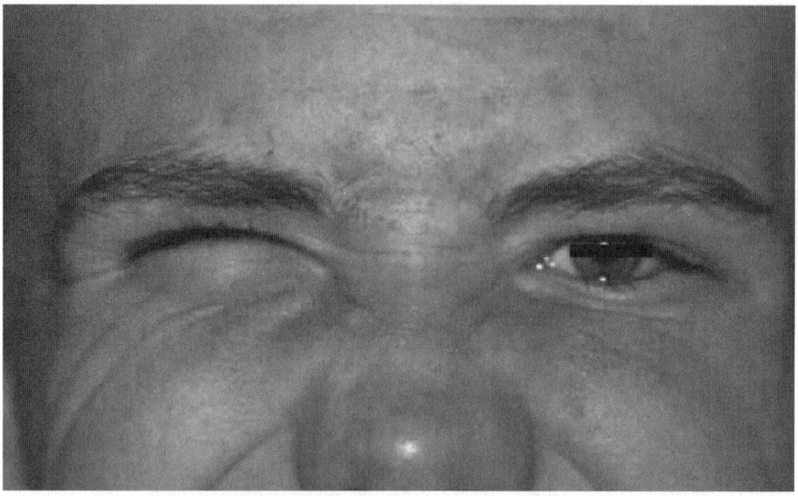

Figure 8 Lower eyelid retraction characterized by an inability to close the left eye completely; the patient was also noted to have resistance to superior traction along the entire aspect of the lower lid.

inferior eyelid margin can be pulled over the midpupillary axis in primary gaze. The pathological change may be isolated to the posterior or anterior lamella and may or may not reflect an underlying soft tissue deficiency. It may result from excessive overlap of the conjunctival–capsulopalpebral flap edges after transconjunctival surgery.

Tear Trough Deformity

A tear trough deformity is characterized by an apparent depression between the inferior orbital rim and the cheek. It can follow the orbital rim but it is usually more prominent medially, presenting as a nasojugal depression. It demarcates the orbital area (corresponding to the preseptal orbicularis oculus muscle) and the cheek (inferior to the orbital rim). The tear trough deformity may be congenital or age-related. Age-related changes that accentuate the tear trough include progressive protrusion of orbital fat, gradual descent of the malar fat pad (especially if a pre-existing bony malar deficiency exists), and loss of subcutaneous fat over the rim and nasojugal areas (9).

Malar Folds and Festoons

Malar folds (Fig. 9) consist of baglike projections of soft tissue below the bony orbital rim and inferior eyelid skin. This may be caused by edema, excess fat in the subcutaneous or suborbicularis spaces, or herniation of suborbicularis fat through an attenuated orbicularis oculus muscle (10,11). Malar bags and festoons are always accompanied by some degree of excess skin and often attenuated (not hypertrophic) orbicularis oculus muscle. The causative factors may be differentiated clinically by observing the malar bag while the patient leans his or her head forward. This man-

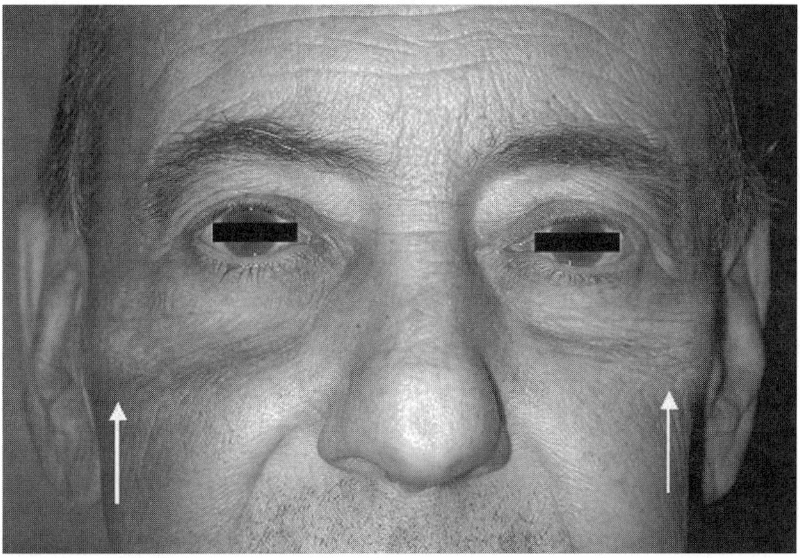

Figure 9 Malar folds (arrows) characterized by baglike projections of soft tissue below the bony orbital rim and inferior eyelid skin.

euver will have little effect if edema is the primary factor but will worsen the condition if fat herniation through the orbicularis muscle is present. The fold should be palpated to determine the relative contribution of edema and underlying fat. If the fold is primarily due to attenuation of the orbicularis oculus muscle, the malar bag should efface when the patient squints (the squinch test). Significant excess in skin can result in a festoon (a severe form of a malar fold that takes on a drapelike or swag appearance).

PREOPERATIVE PREPARATION AND ANESTHESIA

Most patients can tolerate blepharoplasty while lightly sedated with topical (4% tetracaine) and subcutaneous (1% lidocaine w/1/200,000 epinephrine) anesthetic. General anesthesia may be contraindicated if a dynamic upper eyelid shortening or lengthening procedure is done because the patient will be unable to cooperate in the functional assessment of eyelid position during the procedure. The lidocaine solution is injected subcutaneously within the proposed area of skin excision. A small bleb is raised and digitally spread by gentle massage. Hyaluronidase (Wydase) added to the solution assists in spreading the anesthetic through the tissues. The anesthetic should be injected after all the skin markings are made, and only a small amount (1–2 ml) is needed. Additional injections of the individual fat pads will also be necessary. A period of 15 min should elapse between the subcutaneous injection of the epinephrine-containing lidocaine solution to allow for adequate vasoconstriction.

Intravenous sedation is a useful adjunct to the local anesthetics. The patient may benefit from taking diazepam (Valium, 5–10 mg) 20 min prior to the procedure.

A variety of sedative and hypnotic agents can be used during the procedure including midazolam (Versed, 0.015–0.05 mg/kg) and propofol (Diprivan, 0.5–2.5 mg/kg). Versed is useful as a solo agent and can be given in repeated doses of 1 mg in the typical adult woman. Patients' blood pressure, electrocardiogram, and blood oxygen levels (pulse oximetry) should be monitored.

The periorbital area is prepped with diluted (0.25%) povidone–iodine paint solution (diluted with normal saline). No detergent solutions should be used. The povidone–iodine should be flushed from the eyes with a balanced salt solution prior to the procedure.

UPPER EYELID BLEPHAROPLASTY

Surgical Anatomy

Important anatomical structures (Fig. 10) in upper eyelid blepharoplasty include the levator palpebral superioris muscle, levator aponeurosis, the eyelid crease, Whitnall's ligament, Müller's muscle, orbital septum, orbital fat, and the retro-orbicularis oculus fat pad (ROOF).

Levator Palpebrae Superioris

The levator muscle is striated and under voluntary control. The closely associated Müller's muscle is smooth (sympathetic) and involuntary. The levator palpebrae superioris takes origin from the upper orbital apex and fans out anteriorly over

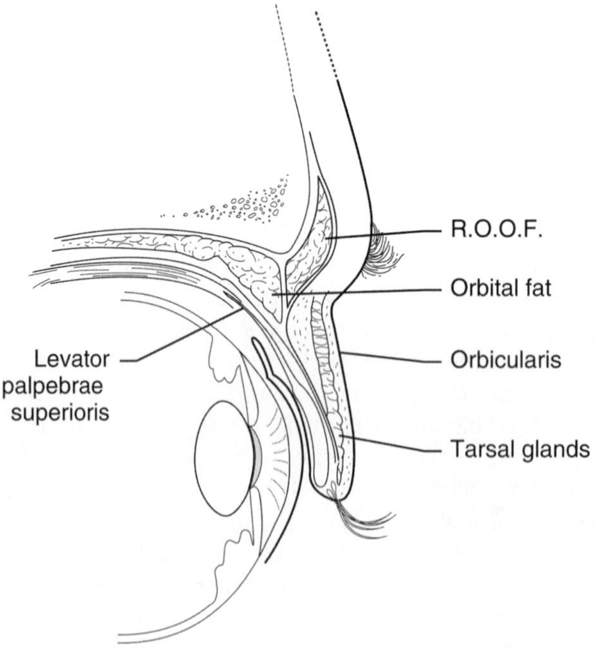

Figure 10 Relevant surgical anatomy for upper eyelid blepharoplasty includes the levator palpebrae superioris, levator aponeurosis, orbital septum, orbital fat, and ROOF.

the superior rectus muscle. It becomes aponeurotic 5–10 mm beyond Whitnall's ligament.

Levator Aponeurosis

The levator aponeurosis inserts anterior to the tarsal plate into a confluence of fascias consisting of the orbicularis oculus fascia and orbital septum. This pretarsal or conjoined fascia spans the length of the tarsus and is tightly adherent to the overlying orbicularis oculus muscle and underlying tarsus. The pretarsal fascia provides an anchor for the levator aponeurosis to pull the lid margin superiorly.

Eyelid Crease

The eyelid crease forms as the eyelid is elevated and the adherent layers overlying the tarsus (pretarsal skin and conjoined fascia) are drawn under the loose skin and muscle superiorly. In addition (consistent with the traditional teaching) direct dermal insertions of slips of aponeurotic fascia may also contribute to the formation of the eyelid crease. The pretarsal platform is the fixed skin under the crease overlying the conjoined fascia and tarsus (Fig. 11). The level of fusion of the fascias that form the conjoined fascia (i.e., the level of the crease) is located approximately at the superior tarsus to 3 mm above in white women's eyelids. The conjoined fascia may degenerate and separate with age resulting in an inferiorly displaced crease and inferior migration of the preaponeurotic orbital fat, giving the upper eyelid a puffy appearance. A high crease corresponds to a premature confluence of the fascias and is often associated with a hollowed-out appearance under the orbital rim because the orbital fat extends only to the confluence of fascias. A low or absent crease (e.g., the Asian eye) corresponds to an acquired or congenitally low confluence of fascias. This type of crease is often associated with an apparent abundance of orbital fat descending over the tarsus because the orbital fat is allowed to extend more inferiorly due to the lower insertion of the levator aponeurosis. In Asian eyes,

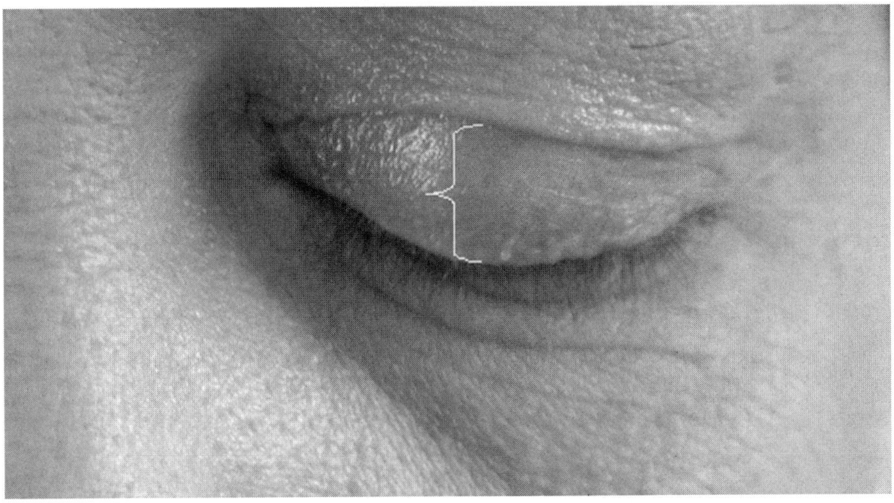

Figure 11 The pretarsal platform (marked): important cosmetic feature of the upper eyelid. A tightened pretarsal platform facilitates placement of makeup.

the fuller eyelid appearance is also due to a greater amount of fat in all of the fascial layers.

Whitnall's Ligament

Some 15–20 mm above the superior tarsal border, the levator sheath thickens to form Whitnall's ligament that extends from the trochlea medially to the lacrimal gland fascia laterally. The levator muscle is suspended in the superior orbit near the superior orbital rim by Whitnall's ligament. The aponeurotic portion of the levator muscle begins approximately 10 mm above the upper border of the tarsus (12).

Müller's Muscle

Müller's muscle takes origin along the transition zone between the levator muscle and aponeurosis and inserts into the upper free border of the tarsal plate. Müller's muscle provides only approximately 2 mm of lift for the upper lid (13).

Orbital Septum

The orbital septum begins at the superior arcus marginalis along the superior orbital rim and descends as a two-layered structure to merge with the levator aponeurosis. The inner layer turns superiorly at the junction of the levator aponeurosis to encapsulate the orbital fat. It continues superiorly to merge with the sheath of the levator muscle and superior transverse ligament of Whitnall (12). The outer layer extends to the pretarsal fascia (conjoined fascia).

Orbital Fat

The orbital fat is deep to the orbital septum and rests on the levator aponeurosis (i.e., preaponeurotic fat). It is cradled inferiorly along the superior border of the conjoined fascia where the outer layer of the orbital septum merges with the levator aponeurosis. Although the orbital fat is traditionally considered to be compartmentalized, many authors believe that the fat is continuous (14). On clinical appearance the fat appears to be partitioned into compartments by fragile septa. In classic cases, only two fat pads are described in the upper eyelid: medial and central (Fig. 12). However, a third fat (lateral) pad may be present located just medial to the lacrimal gland in up to 44% of patients (15). The medial fat pad is paler (due to its higher fibrous content) and more vascular than the other fat pads. Orbital fat volume is unrelated to body habitus and does not regenerate after excision.

Roof

The ROOF pad is located between the orbicularis oculus muscle and lateral orbital rim between the supraorbital nerve and upper lateral orbit. Prominence of this fat pad causes fullness over the lateral orbital rim that is correctable by partial resection and contouring of the fat in this area.

Cosmetic Upper Eyelid Blepharoplasty

A typical upper lid blepharoplasty for cosmetic purposes involves excision of redundant eyelid skin and pseudoherniated orbital fat. Establishing the height and form of the eyelid crease and tightening the levator aponeurosis are also objectives in most cosmetic blepharoplasties.

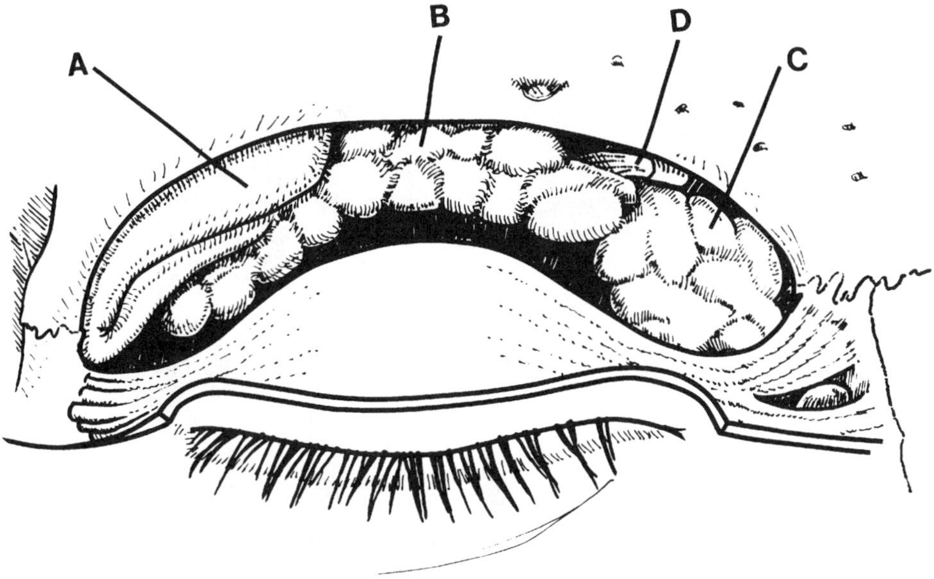

Figure 12 Lacrimal gland and fat pads in the upper eyelid (right eye). A. Lacrimal gland. B. Central fat pad. C. Medial fat pad. D. Trochlea.

Skin Excision

The desired location of the lid crease should be marked first. The height of the crease is gender- and race-dependent. In white women, the crease should be marked approximately 10–12 mm above the eyelid margin at the mid-pupillary axis (Fig. 13). In men, the crease should be at 8–10 mm, and in Asians the crease should be considerably lower at 4–6 mm (16). The incision extends medially and laterally in an arc following the curve of the tarsus. As the incision approaches the superior punctum and lateral canthal angle, it should be no closer than 5 mm from the lash line. The incision should not extend beyond the superior punctum medially and laterally it should not extend beyond the lateral canthal angle. If there is a significant degree of redundant lateral eyelid skin in a woman, the incision can be carried out beyond the lateral canthal angle in a true horizontal plane or gently curved upwards (1). Although the portion of the incision beyond the lateral canthal angle is often noticeable, women are better able and willing to camouflage it with makeup than are men.

The upper incision determines the ultimate extent of eyelid skin resected and the amount of pretarsal exposure on primary gaze. The extent of pretarsal exposure is 1–2 mm less than the distance between the lower incision (i.e., lid crease) and the lash line because the upper eyelid skin will slightly overlap the upper incision. This is beneficial because the incision will be hidden under this fold.

The extent of skin to be excised can be determined by pinching the proposed upper and lower incisions together and observing what effect this maneuver has on lid margin elevation and lid separation. A slight degree of eyelid separation (1 mm lagophthalmos) is acceptable. Most patients can tolerate significant skin

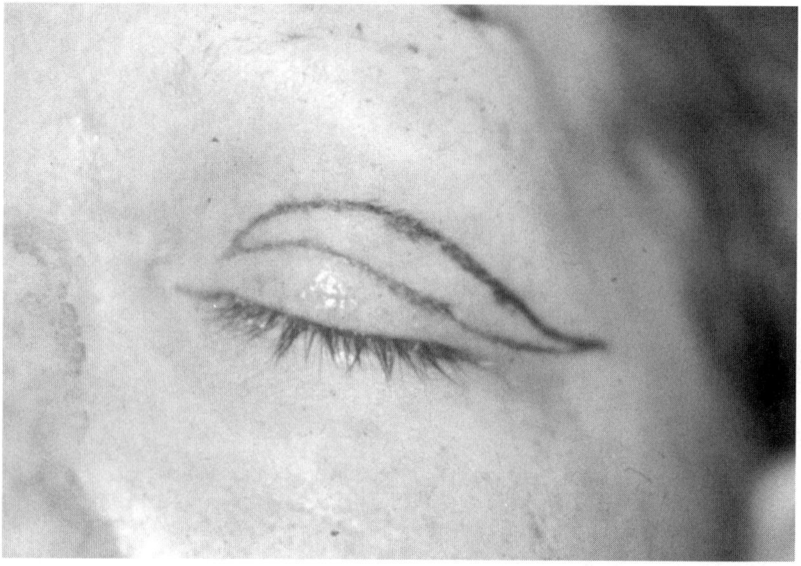

Figure 13 Incision marked for upper lid blepharoplasty in a white woman. Note that the lower limb follows the eyelid crease. The excision of skin can extend well beyond the lateral canthus since scarring in this area is easily camouflaged with makeup.

excision; however, the upper incision should not extend into the thicker infrabrow skin because this area is more prone to prominent scarring (16). The location of the upper incision should be approximately 2 mm below the transition zone between the fine crepe-like skin of the eyelid and the thicker skin of the infrabrow region. Flowers states that at least 20 mm of skin should be preserved between the inferior brow and lash line (9). The upper incision joins the lower incision medially at a 60 degree angle and laterally at a slightly more acute angle.

The skin with a narrow strip of underlying orbicularis oculus muscle is removed from lateral to medial exposing the orbital septum. The septum is opened along the full extent of the incision with a fine scissors over the bulging fat (Fig. 14). The orbital septum over the medial aspect of the incision tends to be thicker and more closely applied to the underlying levator aponeurosis. Careful dissection of the orbital septum in this area is required to avoid injury to the aponeurosis.

After judicious excision of orbital fat, the skin is closed with a running fine nonabsorbable suture (Fig. 15). The lateral aspect of the incision is often closed under minor tension and interrupted sutures may be of benefit. Great care should be taken in accurately approximating the skin edges because skin–edge overlap will lead to more obvious scarring. The sutures are removed in 3–5 days.

Orbital Fat Excision

The areas corresponding to apparent orbital fat pseudoherniations are marked preoperatively. This is an important step because not all bulging in the superior periorbital area is due to prolapsing orbital fat. Correction may require repositioning of the lacrimal gland, resection of retro-orbicularis oculus fat, or subcutaneous fat debulking (17). Partial resection and contouring of the ROOF can correct fullness

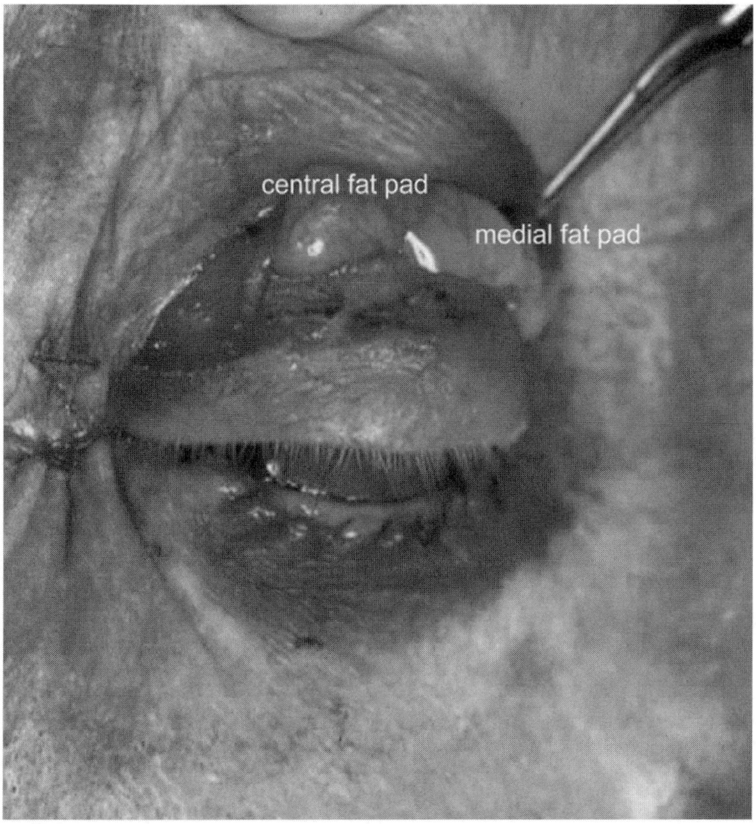

Figure 14 Bulging fat of the upper eyelid after the orbital septum is opened. Note central and medial fat pads.

in the lateral lid area (Fig. 16). This fat pad must be differentiated from a ptotic lacrimal gland; the former is located between the orbicularis oculus muscle and orbital rim, and the latter is found inferior and deep to the orbital rim. Resection of the ROOF is often associated with numbness in the lateral orbital area and carries the risk of partial denervation of the orbicularis oculus and corrugator muscles (18).

A ptotic lacrimal gland is usually responsible for lateral bulging in the upper eyelid. Surgical correction involves resuspension of the gland into the lacrimal fossa under the bony orbital rim. Both arms of a double-armed nonabsorbable suture are placed, slightly separated, under the orbital rim and passed inferiorly through the capsule of lacrimal gland. As the two ends of the suture are cinched down and tied, the lacrimal gland is pulled under the rim and permanently repositioned (Fig. 17). Removal of any portion of the lacrimal gland, except for biopsy purposes, is contraindicated.

If the patient is undergoing blepharoplasty using local anesthesia, the fat pockets are injected with local anesthetic and gently teased into the wound prior to partial excision. The medial fat pocket is sometimes difficult to expose adequately but can be recognized by its relatively pale appearance. Protruding fat from the

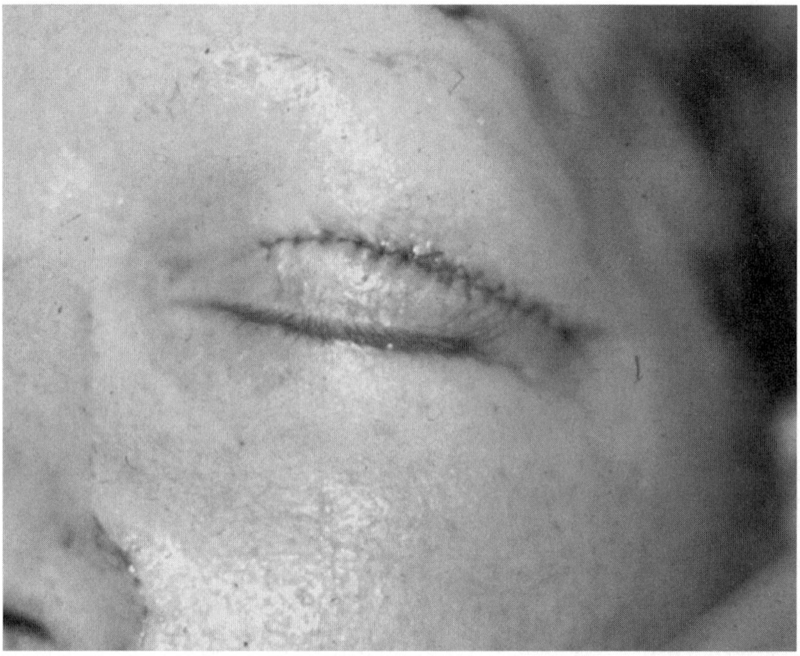

Figure 15 Final appearance immediately after closing the upper blepharoplasty incision in a woman (same patient as in Fig. 13).

central and medial fat compartments is cauterized with a bipolar cautery and excised. Teasing the fat should be conservative since excision of excess fat can lead to a hollowed-out appearance in the infrabrow area.

Technique Synopsis

The typical surgical steps involved in an upper eyelid blepharoplasty include marking incisions, applying tetracaine drops over the sclera and injecting local anesthetic solution into the area of proposed skin excision, preparing and draping the area, placing the scleral shield, and making inferior and superior skin incisions outlining an ellipse of skin that is to be excised. The lid crease incision should be made on the opposite eye immediately after it is placed on the operated eye to ensure symmetry.

The next steps involve removing skin with fine-tipped scissors exposing orbicularis muscle starting at the temporal end, excising a narrow strip of orbicularis muscle to expose the orbital septum, incising the orbital septum along the entire extent of skin and muscle excision exposing preaponeurotic orbital fat and levator aponeurosis. The incision through the orbital septum should be over the bulging orbital fat to avoid injury to the aponeurosis. Next, apply gentle pressure to the globe to facilitate exposure of the fat pads, inject the fat pads with the local anesthetic solution, selectively remove excess orbital fat being careful to cauterize the fat at the base of the excision, suspend the lacrimal gland if necessary, and excise a small strip of orbicularis oculus muscle to the level of the crease. Interrupted fine nonabsorbable sutures (four to six) can be used to secure the levator aponeurosis to the dermis to define the lid crease better and tighten the pretarsal platform. This maneuver is particularly useful in white women. The skin edges are sutured using either an interrupted

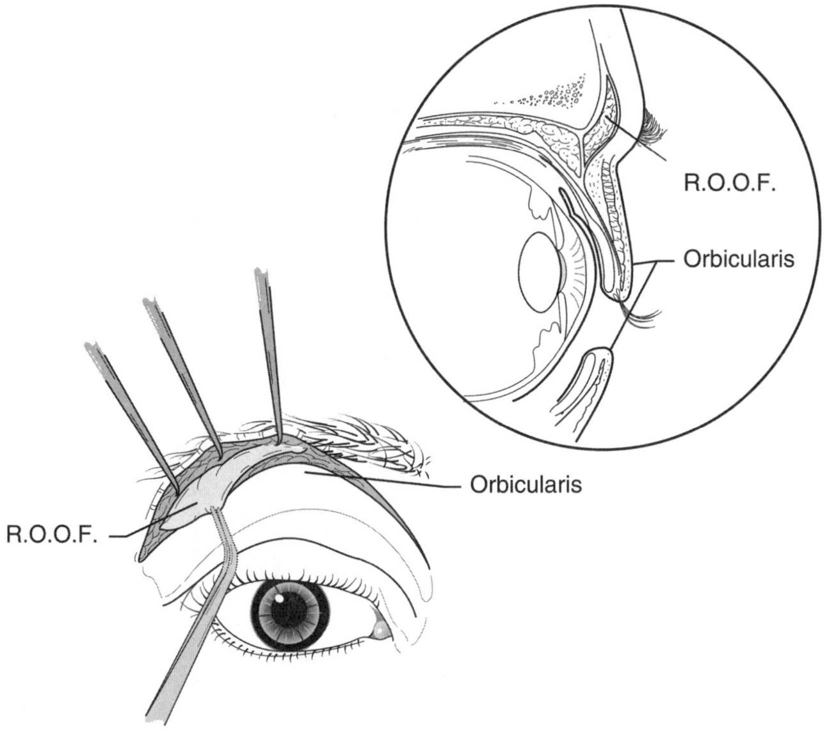

Figure 16 Location of the ROOF pad found between the orbicularis oculus muscle and orbital rim.

or a continuous suturing technique with a nonabsorbable suture, an antibiotic ointment (ophthalmic Bacitracin) is placed over the incision, the scleral shield is removed and an ice pack placed over the area. The sutures are removed 5 days postoperatively.

Correction of Blepharoptosis

Some type of levator aponeurosis advancement or sling (with or without fascial grafts) is required for the surgical correction of blepharoptosis. The appropriate procedure will depend primarily on the function of the levator muscle (excursion) and secondarily on the severity of the ptosis. Congenital ptosis that is mild-to-moderate (1–4 mm of ptosis with > 5 mm of lid excursion) is correctable by advancement and fixation of the levator aponeurosis. Severe cases can be repaired by frontalis suspension. The frontalis suspension procedure involves placing a graft (e.g., fascia lata) between the tarsus below and the frontalis muscle above to provide translational movement from the forehead to the upper eyelid (7). An oculoplastic surgeon should evaluate patients with moderate-to-severe congenital blepharoptosis.

Most adult patients with blepharoptosis have no intrinsic abnormalities of levator muscular function. Eyelid excursion will be good and there will be a mild-to-moderate degree of ptosis. These patients are candidates for aponeurotic resection and repair. This technique involves tightening the aponeurosis and elevating the lid using several interrupted nonabsorbable sutures. The excess aponeurotic sheath is

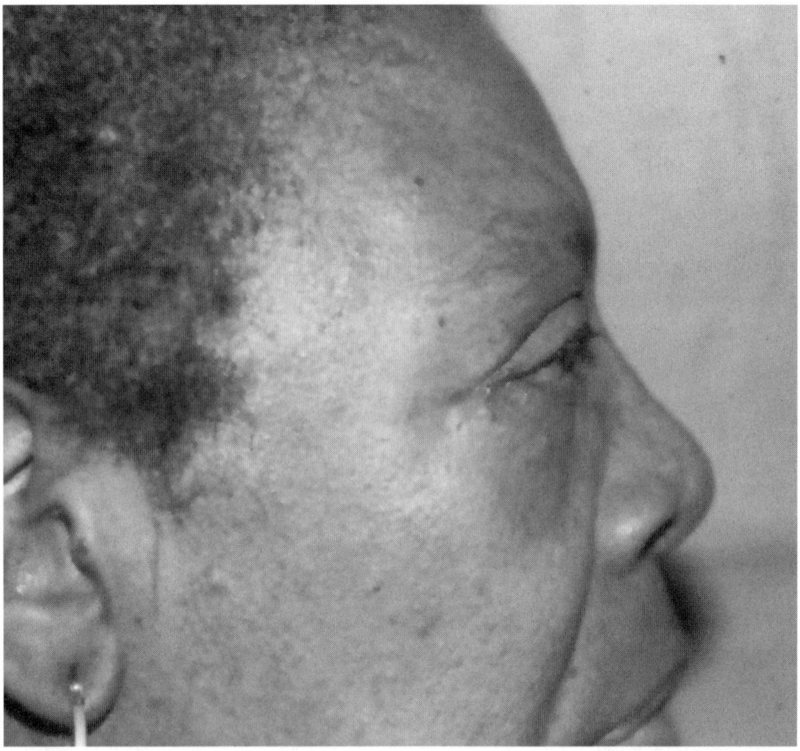

Figure 17 Same patient as in figure 3: postoperative photo shows results of lacrimal gland repositioning.

trimmed and discarded. The patient should undergo the procedure while awake to allow voluntary levator function to assess the final position of the upper eyelid after repair. Despite the apparent symmetry obtained intraoperatively, there can be significant variation in the permanent position of the operated eye due to resolving edema, healing, and muscular action. Because of Hering's law of equal innervation, the opposite eye may fall, resulting in asymmetry between the operated eyelid and the normal eyelid. This phenomenon may occur in up to one-third of patients (19). Revision within 1 week (usually the first postoperative visit) in the office is often possible by limited reopening of the incision line and judicious replacement of the fixation sutures.

The typical surgical steps involved in the correction of blepharoptosis include marking the lid crease and injecting a limited volume (1 ml) of 1% lidocaine with 1:100,000 epinephrine without hyaluronidase to avoid paralysis of the levator muscle; creating the lid crease skin incision to the orbicularis oculus muscle; incising the orbicularis oculus muscle at or slightly superior to the eyelid crease incision to expose the orbital septum; incising the orbital septum along the full extent of the incision to expose the orbital fat; retracting the orbital fat superiorly to expose the thinned or dehisced levator aponeurosis; the central and inferior edge of the aponeurosis is then exposed at the midtarsal level; the aponeurosis is mobilized superiorly revealing the underlying peripheral vascular arcade and Müller's muscle;

and, finally, the aponeurosis is advanced over the tarsus and sutured centrally using a horizontal mattress technique with fine nonabsorbable sutures approximately 3 mm below the superior tarsal border. After the first central suture is placed, the level of the eyelid should be checked for symmetry and function by having the patient open and close the eye both in the upright and supine positions: adjustments are made to achieve an optimal result. Approximately four sutures are then placed centrally between the advanced aponeurosis and tarsus: the aponeurosis should be sutured to the anterior surface of the tarsus to avoid tilting the tarsal plate inward (entropion) or outward (ectropion). A slight overcorrection (1 mm) is beneficial to anticipate the antagonistic action of the orbicularis oculus muscle postoperatively. Excess aponeurosis inferior to the sutures is trimmed (usually 5–10 mm) and the skin crease is reformed by placing buried interrupted dermal fixation sutures through the orbicularis muscle and levator aponeurosis.

Creation of the Upper Eyelid Crease

Creation of a well-defined lid crease should be considered in all women undergoing cosmetic blepharoplasty, particularly in cases that involve partial aponeurotic dehiscence. An essential feature of a partially dehisced levator is a misplaced and ill-defined lid crease. However, even patients with a lid crease at the proper height preoperatively may benefit from a fixation procedure to tighten the pretarsal platform and improve ptotic eyelashes. A tight pretarsal platform also provides a good surface to accept makeup. The fixation procedure first involves trimming the orbital septum and orbicularis oculus muscle to the inferior skin edge. Five to seven buried interrupted fine sutures spaced out along the length of the tarsus bind the underlying aponeurosis to the muscle and dermis. The sutures should not enter the tarsus because this would create a permanent crease that may be evident on eye closure. Any asymmetry between the lid creases is often obvious, so the fixation sutures must be placed in exactly the same locations in the opposite eyelid.

The level at which the orbicularis oculus fascia, orbital septum, and levator aponeurosis fuse to form the conjoined fascia determines the level of the skin crease. Merging of these fascias occurs high in patients with high lid creases and normal levator anatomy and function. Since the orbital fat is above the conjoined fascia, patients with high lid creases (15–20 mm) tend to have a hollow-appearing superior orbital area. Separation of the fascial layers and inferior migration of orbital fat are probably responsible for the puffiness and low lid creases in some older patients (13).

Understanding the fascial components of the Occidental eyelid that produce the lid crease and compartmentalization of the orbital fat is helpful in appreciating the anatomical basis for the configuration of the Asian eyelid (13). The upper lid crease in most Asian subjects is usually low or not visible and the pretarsal lid has a puffy appearance. Formation of the conjoined fascia occurs at a lower level (corresponding to the level of the crease), allowing the orbital fat to migrate inferiorly over the tarsus (Fig. 18). In addition, abundant fat may be present in the subcutaneous and suborbicularis planes.

Many of the basic surgical principles in reconstituting an eyelid fold in the senile eyelid in non-Asian patients apply to creating a lid crease in the Asian patient's eyelid. However, some important differences do exist. The subcutaneous and

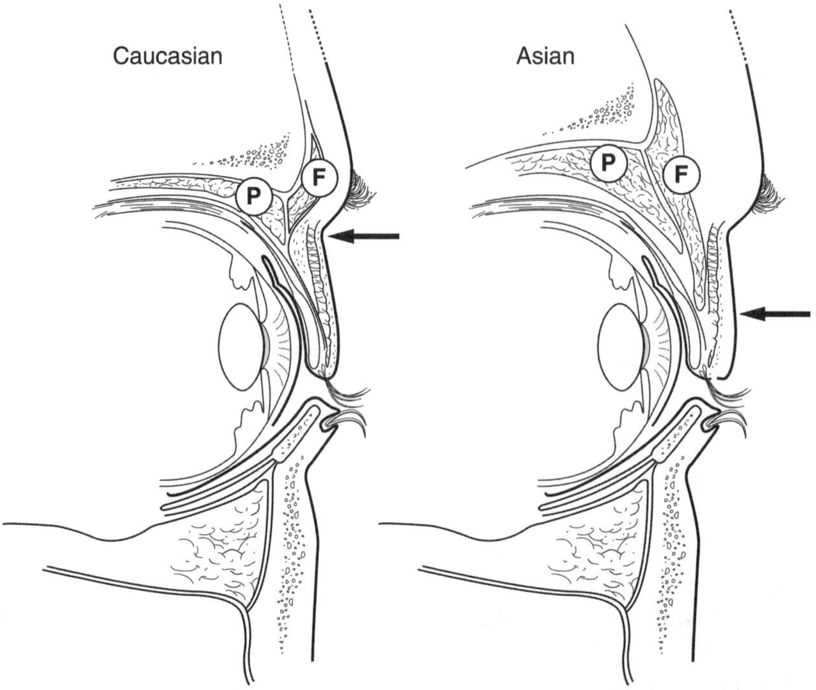

Figure 18 Upper eyelid (right) in an Asian patient displays typical inferior location of orbital fat due to formation of the conjoined fascia at a lower level compared to the typical Occidental eyelid (left). P=orbital fat; F=ROOF.

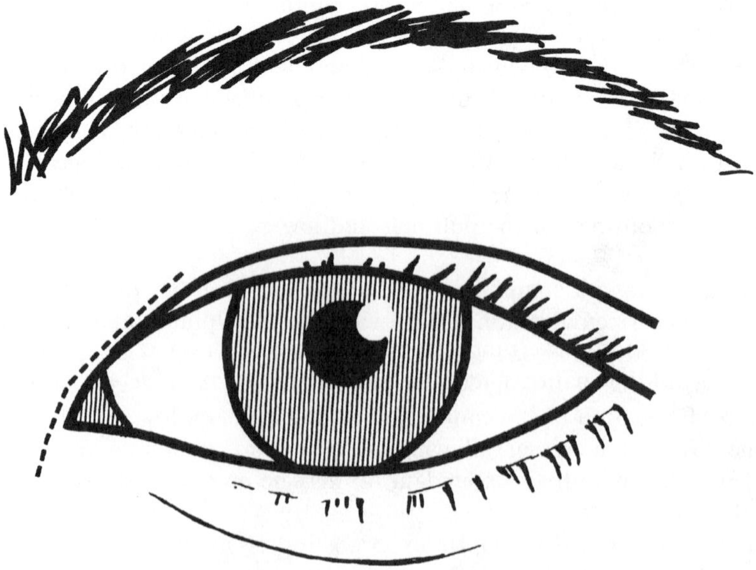

Figure 19 Epicanthoplasty, step 1: initial incision along the free edge of fold.

suborbicularis fat is more abundant, fibrotic, and less amenable to easy removal and sculpting. The dimensions of the Asian eye are smaller, including smaller and thinner tarsal plates. Finally, epicanthal folds are a unique characteristic of the Asian eyelid and are challenging to modify surgically.

The usual goals in Asian blepharoplasty are creating or elevating a lid crease, diminishing the epicanthal fold, and selective orbital fat removal for eyelid debulking. Although there may be a desire to create a more western-appearing eyelid, placing the crease too high tends to produce an unnatural appearance. The eyelid crease in the Asian eyelid should be placed no more than 7 mm above the lid margin.

The fundamental surgical principle in creating a lid crease in the Asian eyelid is to increase the height of the conjoined fascia and lift the orbital fat away from the pretarsal platform. In addition, excision and sculpting of the orbital and subcutaneous fat are usually required to reduce the bulkiness of the skin superior to the crease. The upper eyelid skin (eyelid fold) will overlap the upper incision to a greater degree in an Asian patient's eyelid than in a white patient's eyelid. Therefore, the amount of pretarsal exposure on primary gaze will be proportionally less. To maintain the unique ethnic characteristics of the Asian eye, pretarsal exposure should be no more than 3 mm, and, as previously mentioned, the upper eyelid incision should be placed no more than 7 mm from the ciliary margin (20). The most commonly used method to create a lid crease in an Asian eyelid (i.e., double fold operation) is to suture the levator aponeurosis to the dermis at the new level of the crease (21).

The typical surgical steps involved in creation of a lid crease in the Asian eyelid include making a lid crease incision from 5 to 7 mm above the lid margin and incising the orbicularis oculus muscle at or slightly superior to the eyelid crease incision exposing orbital septum. The orbital septum is incised along the full extent of the incision to expose the orbital fat, which is conservatively removed to reduce the puffiness of the eyelid and expose the levator aponeurosis. Subcutaneous fat is removed from the superior aspect of the wound to improve the contour of the future eyelid fold and from the inferior aspect of the wound to reduce and tighten the pretarsal platform. Conservative removal of skin from the inferior wound edge is sometimes warranted to tighten the pretarsal platform further (overresection will produce ectropion). Five to seven permanent buried or temporary sutures are placed along the desired crease, joining the pretarsal fascia with the superior and inferior skin edges. The temporary sutures are allowed to remain for 10 days to foster fibrous fixation between the newly created crease and underlying tarsus.

Epicanthoplasty

Many procedures are described for the correction of an epicanthal fold including direct excision, V-Y advancement, transposition flap, and Z-plasty (22). Incisions over the nasal skin in Asian patients tend to become hypertrophic scars. All the common corrective procedures are associated with a significant risk of scarring, under- or overcorrection, and recurrence. Fuente del Campo describes a simple and effective epicanthoplasty involving the creation of a medially based transposition flap (23).

The surgical steps involved in epicanthoplasty include incising the free edge of the fold (Fig. 19), pulling the dorsal nasal skin medially to open the incision and expose the medial aspect of the fold. A curved incision is placed in a supero-

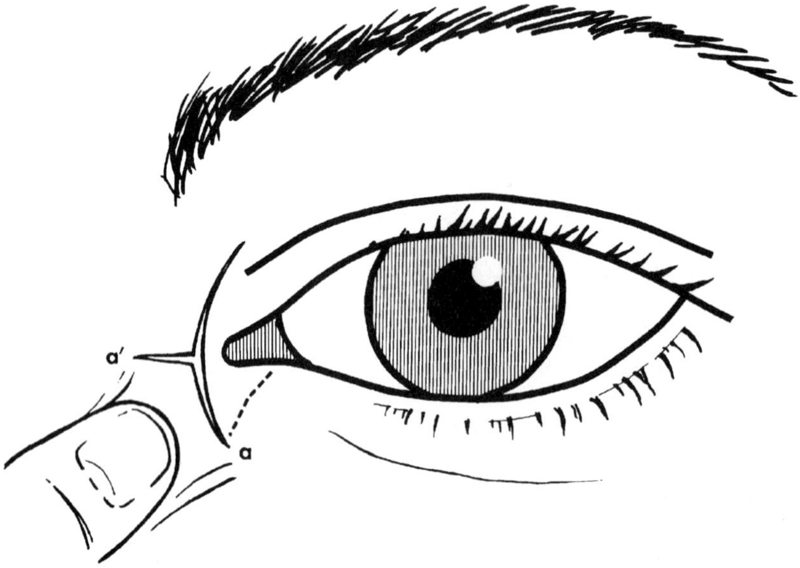

Figure 20 Epicanthoplasty, step 2: vertical and horizontal incisions within the medial canthus to create a laterally based transposition flap.

lateral direction from the inferior end of the fold to 2 mm below the medial punctum, creating a laterally based transposition flap. Another incision is extended from the mid fold medially to accept the transposition flap (Fig. 20). The flaps are elevated, exposing the medial canthal tendon and a medial canthopexy may be performed if necessary. The transposition flap is placed into the medial incision and secured with a 4–0 Vicryl dermal–periosteal stitch (Fig. 21). The wounds are closed with fine nonabsorbable sutures that are removed in 1 week (Fig. 22).

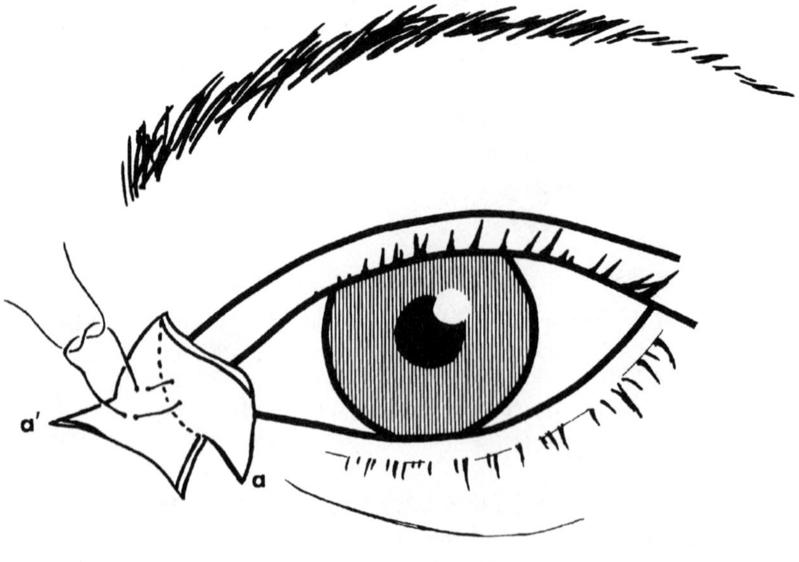

Figure 21 Epicanthoplasty, step 3: the transposition flap is placed into the medial horizontal incision and secured with a 4–0 Vicryl dermal–periosteal stitch.

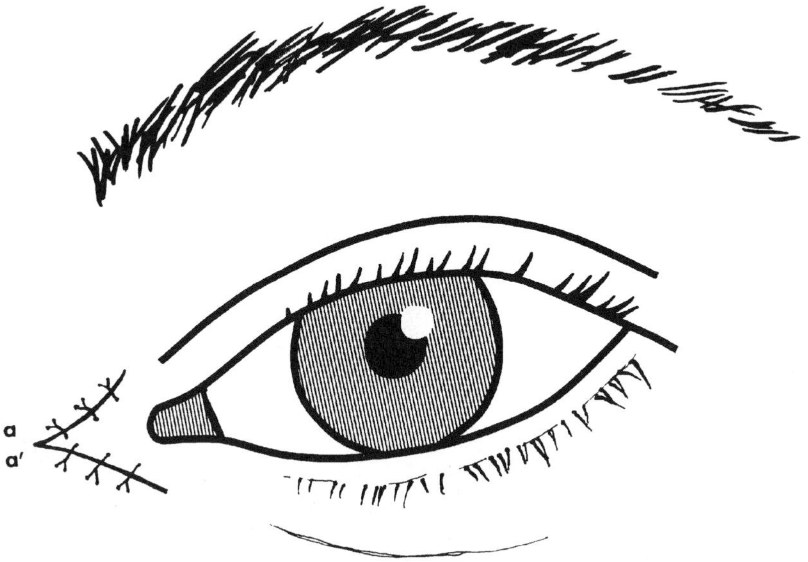

Figure 22 Epicanthoplasty, step 4: final skin closure and effacement of the epicanthal fold.

LOWER EYELID BLEPHAROPLASTY

Surgical Anatomy

The eyelids are divided into anterior and posterior lamellae separated by the orbital septum (often referred to as the middle lamella). The anterior lamella consists of skin and orbicularis oculus muscle. The posterior lamella consists of capsulopalpebral fascia, tarsus, and conjunctiva. The fibrous tarsus is approximately 5 mm in height in the midline and spans the free edge of the lower eyelid (see Chapter 7, Eyelid Anatomy).

Important anatomical structures in lower eyelid blepharoplasty include the capsulopalpebral fascia, orbital septum, orbital fat, suborbicularis oculus fat pads, orbicularis oculus muscle, inferior rectus muscle, inferior oblique muscle, Lockwood's ligament, and canthi (Fig. 23).

Capsulopalpebral Fascia

The capsulopalpebral fascia is the anterior aponeurotic extension of the inferior rectus muscle. Although the dynamic function of this complex is unknown, it probably assists in keeping the lower eyelid apposed to the globe on downgaze. The lower eyelid also moves inferiorly on downgaze, but this is most likely a passive action facilitated by relaxation of the pretarsal orbicularis muscle, gravity, and translational contact with the cornea. There is no well-developed involuntary muscle (ostensibly known as Horner's muscle) within the lower eyelid complex similar to Müller's muscle of the upper eyelid.

Orbital Septum

The orbital septum is an extension of the orbital periosteum and the periosteum over the face of the maxilla. The trifurcation of fascias along the inferior orbital rim represents the inferior arcus marginalis. The orbital septum (anteriorly) and the capsulo-

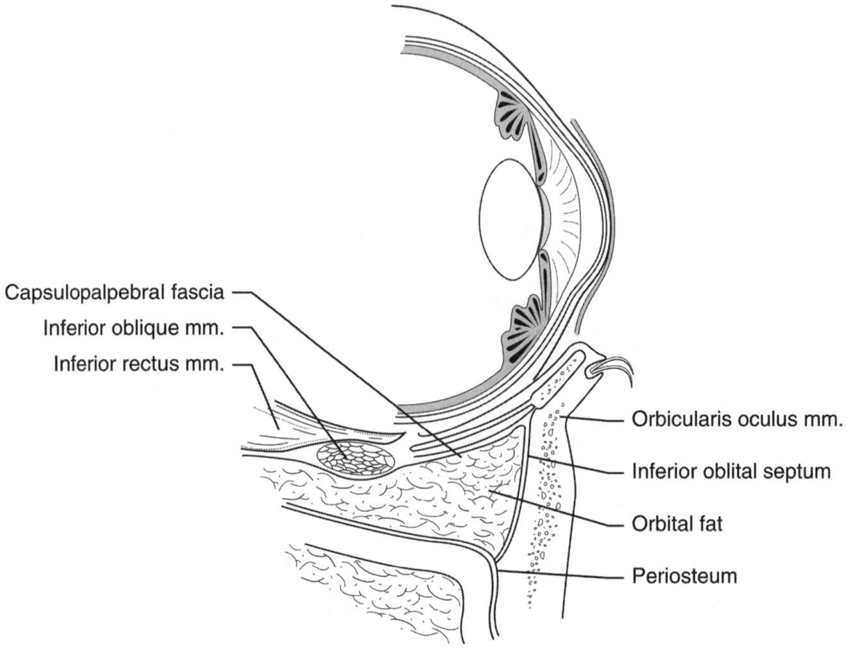

Figure 23 Surgically important landmarks in lower eyelid blepharoplasty.

palpebral fascia (posteriorly) enclose the orbital fat behind the inferior eyelid. The orbital septum extends superiorly to merge with the capsulopalpebral fascia a few millimeters below the inferior border of the tarsus.

Orbital Fat

The orbital fat (Fig. 24) is surrounded by fine connective tissue septa. An anterior fascial extension from the inferior oblique muscle (the arcuate expansion) separates the medial fat pad from the central fat pad. Another anterior fascial extension near the origin of the inferior rectus muscle separates the central fat pad from the lateral

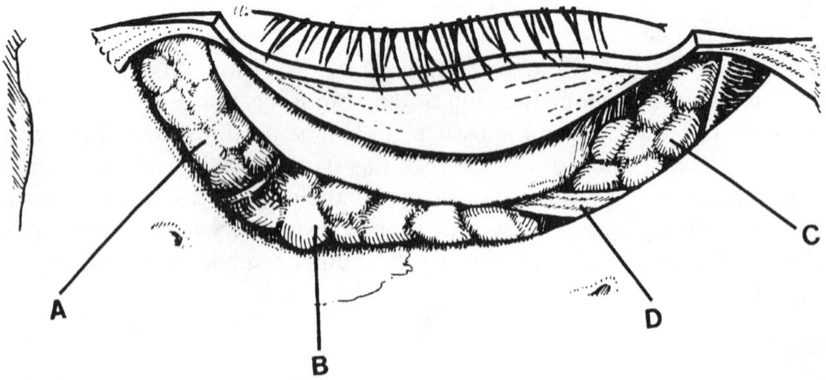

Figure 24 Orbital fat of the inferior eyelid (right eye). A. Lateral fat pad. B. Central fat pad. C. Medial fat pad. D. Inferior oblique muscle origin.

fat pad. The medial fat pad is paler in appearance due to its greater fibrous tissue content and it is more prone to bleeding. Although the majority of the orbital fat is contained behind the orbital septum, a small dehiscence in the orbital septum just below the lateral canthal tendon allows a small bulge of orbital fat to emerge (16).

Suborbicularis Oculi Fat Pads

The suborbicularis oculus fat (SOOF)(Fig. 25) pad is made up of deep fat situated inferior to the inferior orbital rim, below the orbicularis oculus muscle and above the periosteum (24).

Orbicularis Oculus Muscle

The muscular fibers of the orbicularis oculus muscle encircle the orbit including the eyelids and beyond the orbital rims. There are three components, depending on the underlying structure that the muscle is covering: pretarsal, preseptal, and orbital (outside the orbital rims) (25). The muscle is intimately associated with the overlying skin with little intervening subcutaneous tissue and fat.

Inferior Rectus and Inferior Oblique Muscles

The inferior rectus muscle takes origin in the posterior orbit and inserts into the inferior aspect of the globe 6.5 mm inferior to the corneal limbus (26). The inferior oblique muscle takes origin from the bone in the anteromedial orbit (the only extra-

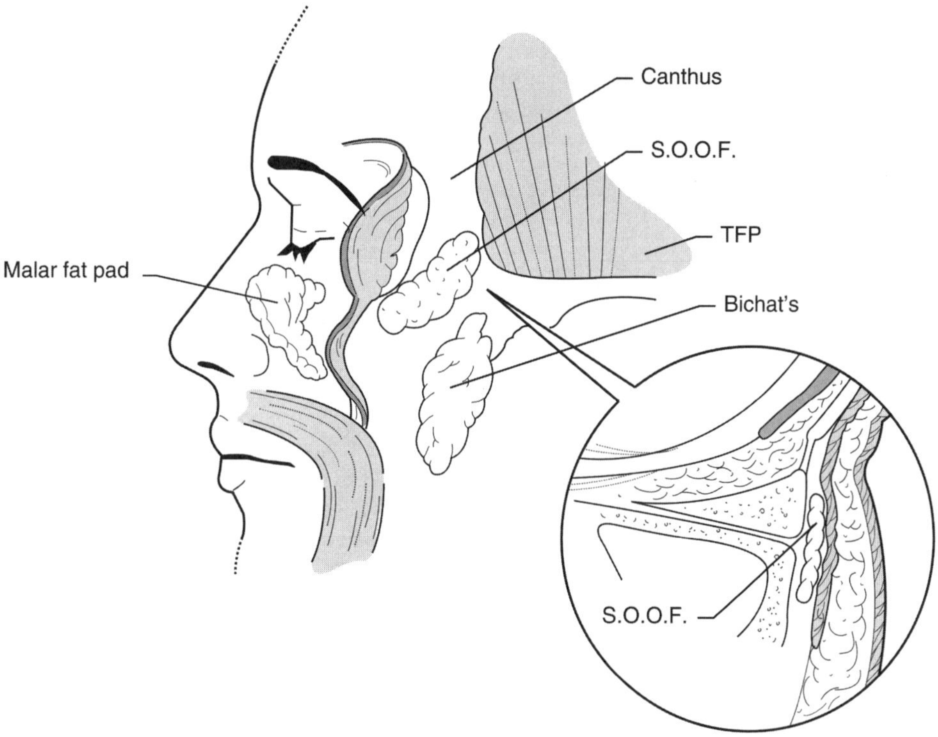

Figure 25 SOOF: this fat pad is situated deep and inferior to the inferior orbital rim, below the orbicularis oculus muscle and above the periosteum.

ocular muscle to take origin from the anterior orbit) and courses within orbital fat posterolaterally to insert onto the globe. The inferior oblique muscle passes under (inferior to) the inferior rectus muscle 9 mm posterior to the inferior rectus insertion (15.5 mm posterior to the inferior limbus) (26). The origin of the inferior oblique muscle and the insertion of the inferior rectus muscle are often visualized during routine cosmetic blepharoplasty.

Lockwood's Ligament

Lockwood's ligament is an inferior transverse suspensory ligament formed by a condensation of capsulopalpebral fascia at the axis of the globe. It acts as a supportive sling for the globe preventing downward displacement (vertical movement), even in the absence of the bony orbital floor (e.g., maxillectomy defects).

Canthi

The lateral canthus consists of a complex fusion of several structures including fibrous extensions of the upper and lower tarsal plates, the lateral extension of the levator aponeurosis, Lockwood's ligament, and the check ligament of the lateral rectus muscle (5). This complex is termed the lateral retinaculum and serves to attach the tarsal plates to the lateral orbital rim. It has superficial and deep limbs that insert into the periosteum over the lateral orbital rim and into Whitnall's tubercle, respectively. The superficial limb is thin and insubstantial. Whitnall's tubercle is approximately 4 mm deep to the lateral orbital rim and 9 mm below the zygomaticofacial suture (27).

The vertical position of the lateral palpebral commissure changes with age. Younger individuals tend to have their lateral commissures 1–2 mm above the medial commissure, giving the palpebral fissure a superolateral slant. The lateral commissure descends with age, resulting in an equal or a slightly inferior relationship to the medial commissure (9,27).

Cosmetic Lower Eyelid Blepharoplasty

The most common reason for performing a cosmetic lower eyelid blepharoplasty is for the correction of orbital fat pseudoherniation (steatoblepharon) and the most common functional indication is for acquired lower eyelid laxity (e.g., senile ectropion). Other indications include reconstruction of postsurgical defects, ectropion, entropion, dermatochalasis, malar folds, and festoons.

There are two basic techniques for surgical access to the orbital fat: transcutaneous and transconjunctival. Many surgeons use one or the other approach exclusively; however, each approach has merit depending on the pathology and goals of the operation. The best approach depends on three factors: pre-existing lower lid laxity, degree of skin redundancy, and presence of orbicularis oculus hypertrophy. Pre-existing lower lid laxity and the need for some type of lid tightening procedure may require a transcutaneous approach to provide for sufficient elevation and resection of the lateral tarsus. Mild lid laxity may be amenable to lesser procedures designed to suspend the inferior tarsus through a transconjunctival or upper blepharoplasty incision. In cosmetic cases, the amount of skin redundancy is the major factor in determining the need for a transcutaneous approach. If only fine wrinkling is evident over the lower eyelid, a transconjunctival approach is appropriate combined with a procedure that will address the fine wrinkling such as laser resurfacing (CO_2 or erbium), chemical peel, or dermabrasion. Excising a small strip of subciliary skin is also commonly done by the pinch technique to address this problem. However, if there is moderate-to-severe skin redundancy with or without orbicularis muscle hypertrophy, a transcutaneous approach is indicated. Orbicularis oculus muscle hypertrophy involves, most prominently, the pretarsal portion of the muscle. It is accessed through a standard subciliary incision during a routine transcutaneous (skin-only flap) blepharoplasty. The hypertrophied muscle is carefully planed down by excising the raised surface along the direction of the muscle fibers (28). The muscle is never divided.

Transcutaneous Approach

The subciliary incision is placed 2 mm below the lower lid margin, extending from the level of the punctum medially to approximately 1 cm lateral to the lateral commissure. A skin-only or a skin–muscle flap is created and dissected inferiorly to the level of the orbital fat. In either case, the pretarsal orbicularis oculus muscle is preserved to lend support to the eyelid margin. The skin is intimately related to the underlying orbicularis muscle and dissection between these layers is difficult. Injury to the skin and ecchymoses are common. The skin-only technique is useful for correction of extensive dermatochalasis or for resection of an excessive amount of lax skin. Once the dissection reaches the level of the orbital fat, the muscle and orbital septum are penetrated and the fat is resected as needed.

A skin–muscle flap is much more common and the dissection is relatively easy (16). After the subciliary incision, a limited skin-only dissection proceeds to just inferior to the pretarsal portion of the orbicularis oculus muscle. At this point, the muscle is penetrated and the new plane of dissection is between the orbital septum and muscle. This is a bloodless plane and the septum and muscle are easily separated.

A visible scar results from all of the transcutaneous approaches but only rarely is the scar prominent or noticeable to the casual observer. Ectropion is the major concern after a transcutaneous approach and is most often associated with the subciliary incision. To minimize the incidence of postoperative ectropion, the pretarsal portion of the orbicularis oculus muscle should be preserved to support the lower lid and lessen the effects of scar contracture.

Technique

The typical surgical steps involved in a transcutaneous lower eyelid blepharoplasty include creation of a subciliary incision 2 mm below the free lid margin from just below the lower punctum to 1 cm lateral to the lateral commissure. A submuscular dissection plane is then established below the pretarsal orbicularis oculus and at the level of the bulging orbital fat along the entire horizontal extent of the orbital septum. The central fat pad is usually the most prominent and is treated first by grasping the portion overlapping the orbital rim, cauterizing the base, and excising it. The medial and lateral fat pads are resected in a similar manner; the medial fat pad is particularly prone to bleeding and should be well cauterized. The medial fat pad, lying slightly deeper, is close to the inferior oblique muscle and the area around the proposed fat excision should be gently explored to identify the muscle. The amount of fat to be resected is determined by repeatedly checking the contour of the eyelid after replacing the flap, aided by light pressure on the globe. The skin–muscle flap is redraped and a triangle-shaped portion of excess flap tissue is excised laterally. The flap edge should rest without tension against the subciliary incision line. A fine absorbable suture (5-0 PDS) is placed through the lateral orbicularis oculus muscle and the periosteum overlying the lateral orbital rim to suspend the lower lid and minimize the risk of ectropion and lid malposition. The skin is closed with either a running or a continuous suture in a single layer.

Transconjunctival Approach

The transconjunctival approach was originally described in the early 20th century and popularized by Converse and Tessier for access to the orbital floor fractures (29,30). Today, it is a popular method of approaching the orbital fat in cosmetic blepharoplasty of the lower lid. The dissection is from the inner surface of the eyelid and the globe must be protected. A variety of surgical instruments are specifically designed to protect the globe during lower lid blepharoplasty, including corneal shields and specialized retractors. The Jaëgar retractor is contoured to the shape of the globe and assists in retracting the globe posteriorly after it is placed deep into the inferior fornix. With the Jaëgar and Desmarres (lid retractor) retractors in place, the capsulopalpebral fascia is fully exposed. The Jaëgar retractor may be replaced later in the procedure by the inferiorly based capsulopalpebral flap as it is pulled over the surface of the cornea using fine traction sutures. Corneal shields can be useful but can involve some stretching of the eyelids and patient discomfort for placement. They can slide freely over the surface of the globe, exposing the cornea to inadvertent injury.

Loop magnification is helpful for the novice surgeon to identify accurately the layers of the lower eyelid. There are two methods to expose the orbital fat via the transconjunctival approach: the retroseptal approach and the preseptal approach (Fig. 26). The retroseptal approach involves creating a horizontal incision between the lower border of the tarsus and fornix through the capsulopalpebral fascia directly entering orbital fat. The preseptal approach involves entering the potential space between the orbicularis oculus muscle and orbital septum through an infratarsal incision. The orbital fat is visualized through the thin orbital septum similarly to the transcutaneous approach. Orbital fat excision in cosmetic blepharoplasty is performed via the retroseptal approach by most surgeons.

Retroseptal Approach

The typical surgical steps involved in a retroseptal lower eyelid blepharoplasty begin by placing medial and lateral silk retaining sutures through the gray line to aid in lid eversion. As the lid is everted, a Jaëger retractor is placed against the globe to expose the proposed incision fully. The globe is slightly depressed to highlight the areas of fat protrusion through the capsulopalpebral fascia. The conjunctiva–capsulopalpebral fascia is opened fully from the level of the medial punctum to the lateral canthus, exposing the medial, central, and lateral fat pads. The fat pads are identified and trimmed after cauterization along the base of the incision. The effects of trimming the orbital fat are evaluated by observing the external lower eyelid both at rest and with gentle pressure over the globe. A mild-to-moderate degree of excess skin can be trimmed using the pinch technique. At the completion of the procedure, the edges of the incised conjunctiva–capsulopalpebral fascia are apposed

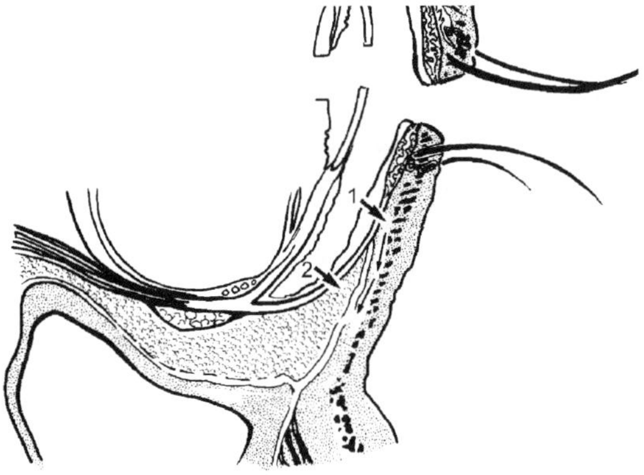

Figure 26 Sagittal view of the lower eyelid shows the retroseptal (2) and preseptal (1) approaches to the orbital fat during transconjunctival blepharoplasty.

by lifting the lid superiorly (no suturing is needed). A Frost suture can be placed to ensure no overlapping of the conjunctival incision if desired (Fig. 27).

The retroseptal approach to the orbital fat is a more direct method of excising protuberant orbital fat compared to the preseptal approach, which probably accounts for its popularity. However, if the retroseptal incision is placed too posteriorly, injury to the extraocular muscles is more likely. The preseptal approach requires more skill and is slightly more time-consuming but has significant advantages. The orbital fat is exposed via the orbital septum similarly to the transcutaneous approach, allowing dissection and excision of prolapsing orbital fat in a more anteriorly oriented approach away from the extraocular muscles (Fig. 28). The fat pads are easier to identify, especially the lateral orbital fat pad (Fig. 29). In addition, a capsulopalpebral flap is developed prior to fat excision that can be pulled over the corneal surface to prevent corneal injury (Fig. 30). The incision through the orbital septum may result in further tightening of this structure, enhancing the aesthetic outcome. Although not yet proven, the preseptal approach to the orbital fat may be associated with less serious complications, such as extraocular muscle injury, than the retroseptal approach.

Tranconjunctival Orbital Fat Repositioning

A recent concept in the treatment of the aging face is preservation and repositioning (vs. excision) of fat. Repositioning prolapsing orbital fat may be beneficial in treating fat-deficient areas over the orbital rim that are created with the age-related descent of the midfacial structures including skin, subcutaneous fat, and malar fat pad. Fat repositioning is especially helpful in camouflaging the tear trough deformity present in many patients due to soft tissue ptosis. The orbital fat in the medial and central compartments is amenable to repositioning to soften the area over the orbital rim and upper medial cheek.

The technique of orbital fat repositioning involves the following surgical steps. Preoperative marking of fat-deficient areas is required with respect to the tear trough deformity while the patient is upright. A retroseptal or preseptal transconjunctival approach is used to expose the orbital fat. Inferior dissection exposes the full extent

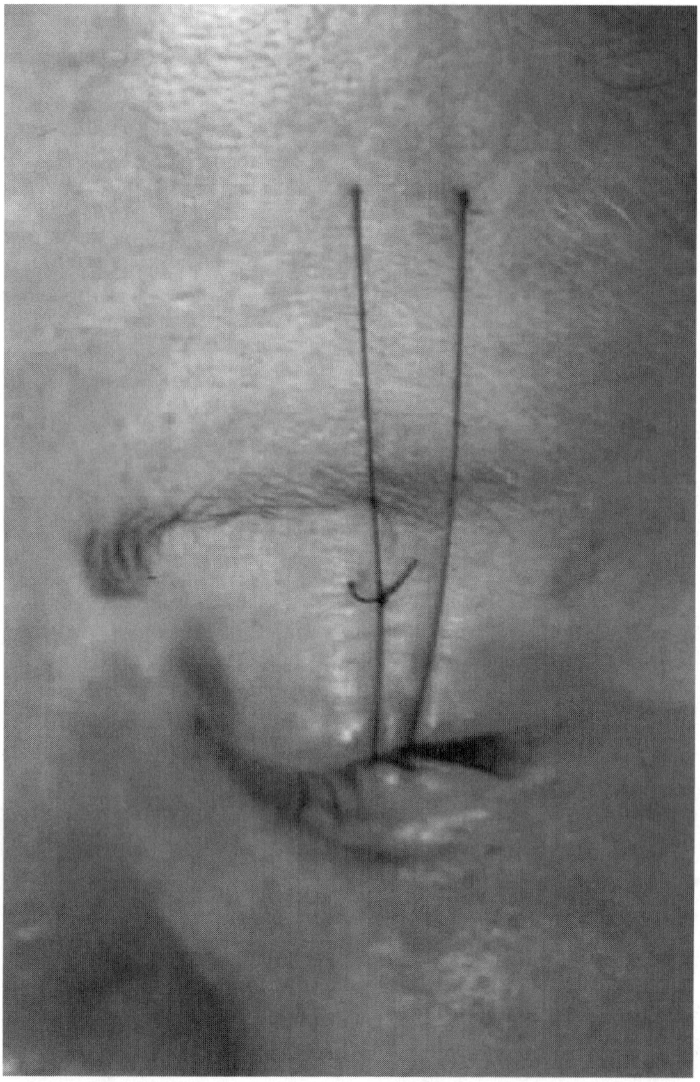

Figure 27 Frost suture in place to lift lower eyelid. This is useful in promoting healing and avoiding eyelid malposition problems.

of the arcus marginalis. The arcus is incised and a subperiosteal dissection proceeds, creating a pocket according to the preoperative markings. The pedicled orbital fat is carried over the orbital rim and placed into the subperiosteal pocket, trimming as necessary. The distal portion of the pedicled fat is secured to the SOOF or overlying periosteum with fine buried absorbable sutures.

Transconjunctival (preseptal) SOOF Lift

The SOOF lift is a method of midface rejuvenation to correct ptosis of the skin, subcutaneous fat, and the malar fat pad. The SOOF itself is closely attached to the maxillary periosteum and probably does not descend markedly with age. However,

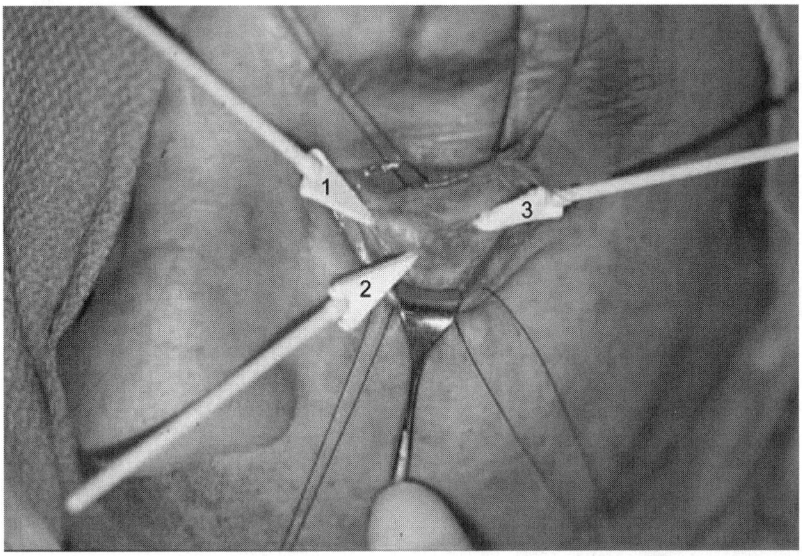

Figure 28 Orbital fat pads as seen via the preseptal approach; note the medial (1), central (2), and lateral (3) collections.

SOOF suspension will camouflage contour deficiencies in the upper cheek and orbital rim areas (but does not address the tear trough deformity). Overlying skin and subcutaneous fat are also lifted, resulting in an actual increase in skin and muscle available in the lower eyelid. A transconjunctival SOOF lift is useful to bring needed tissue into the lower eyelid to correct a deficient anterior lamella (eyelid skin and muscle) associated with vertical eyelid retraction (31). A transcutaneous midface lift by SOOF suspension is a reasonable alternative when there is no pre-existing vertical eyelid retraction (32).

The technique of the SOOF lift involves the following surgical steps. A lateral canthotomy and inferior cantholysis are performed to free the lower eyelid. A full horizontal incision is created inferior to the inferior tarsal border to enter the preseptal space. The space between the orbicularis oculus muscle and orbital septum is dissected to the arcus marginalis. The periosteum is incised horizontally across the inferior orbital rim and below the canthotomy incision. The periosteum over the face of the maxilla and malar eminence is undermined. Approximately 15 mm below the inferior orbital rim, the periosteum is incised and released to allow superior transposition of the SOOF and attached structures. The superior aspect of the SOOF and its attached periosteum are anchored to the orbital rim periosteum with horizontal mattress 4–0 Prolene sutures. The lateral canthal tendon is reattached using typical canthoplasty procedures.

Correction of Lower Lid Laxity and Malposition

Patients undergoing cosmetic blepharoplasty may benefit from prophylactic canthoplasty to prevent postoperative lid malpositions (Table 2). Pre-existing clinical conditions that warrant prophylactic canthoplasty include proptosis, lid margin posterior

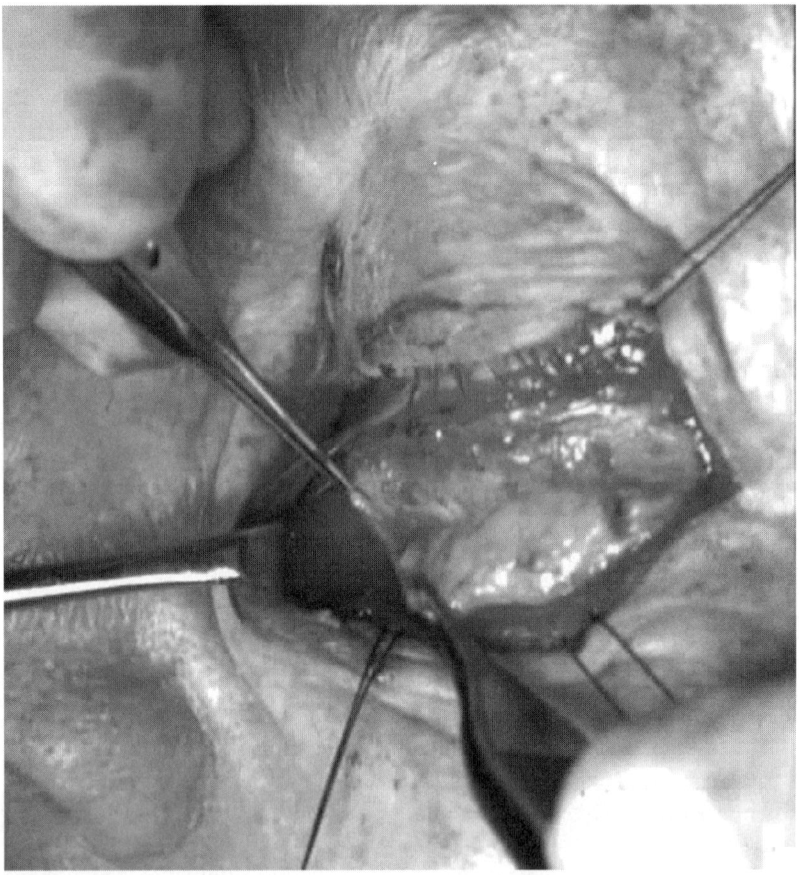

Figure 29 Preseptal exposure of orbital fat; the forceps is grasping the central fat pad.

to corneal apex (negative vector deformity), malar deficiency, and mild lid laxity (not associated with malposition). All transcutaneous subciliary blepharoplasties should include prophylactic canthoplasty. Patients with predisposing conditions who are undergoing cosmetic blepharoplasty are candidates for inferior retinacular suspension (33). The inferior retinacular lateral canthoplasty results in tightening of the lower lid margin via the lateral extension of the upper blepharoplasty incision. It is easily combined with a transconjunctival lower lid blepharoplasty. In cases that require only minimal lower lid tightening, a canthopexy (without cantholysis) may be performed. Inferior retinacular lateral canthoplasty involves the following surgical steps: elevate a skin-muscle flap over the lateral orbital rim from the lateral extension of the upper blepharoplasty incision; cut and mobilize the lower lid component of the lateral retinaculum (inferior cantholysis) (Figs. 31,32); pass a horizontal mattress suture of 4–0 Prolene between the lower lateral canthal tendon and the lateral rim periosteum at the level of the pupil (in primary gaze) (Fig. 33); tighten and tie the suture to secure the lateral canthal tendon in its elevated position; and confirm that the lower eyelid margin slightly overlaps the inferior limbus

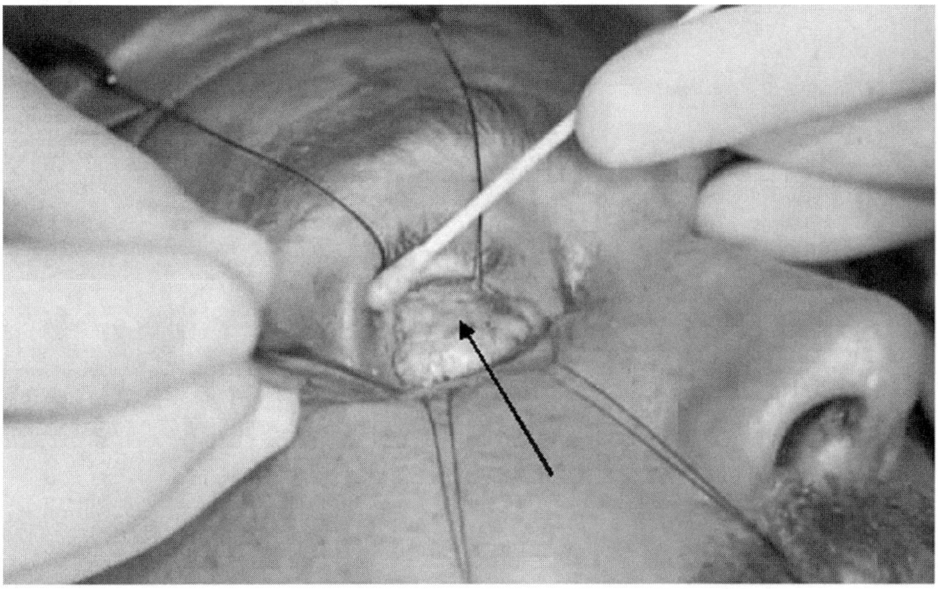

Figure 30 A capsulopalpebral flap (arrow) elevated and pulled over the corneal surface protects the globe from inadvertent injury.

Table 2 Lateral Canthoplasty Techniques and Indications

Procedure	Indications	Comments
Pentagonal wedge resection	Excess horizontal lid length with lid laxity	Rarely used; associated with lid margin notching; lateral canthal procedures often required anyway
Tarsal strip	Senile ectropion Paralytic ectropion Substantial lid laxity	Disrupts commissure; leads to some rounding of the canthal angle and shortening of the palpebral slit; reliably corrects lower lid laxity, ectropion, and canthal dystopia
Dermal pennant stitch	Lid laxity associated with minor lid malpositions and canthal dystopia	Preserves integrity of the commissure; postoperative edema and dog ears are common; should be used with caution in patients undergoing cosmetic blepharoplasty; best in patients with >1 cm between the commissure and lateral orbital rim
Inferior retinacular suspension	Negative vector relationship Minor lid laxity	Good choice for cosmetic blepharoplasty patients to prevent postoperative lid malposition; no need for lower eyelid incision; ideal for use in combination with the transconjunctival approach

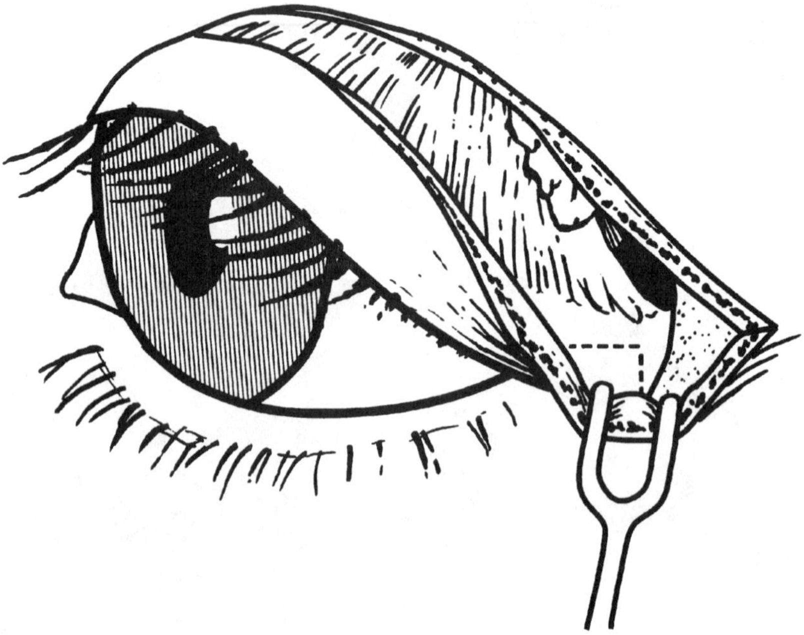

Figure 31 Inferior retinacular canthoplasty, step 1: the lower lid component of the lateral retinaculum is cut via the lateral extension of the upper blepharoplasty incision.

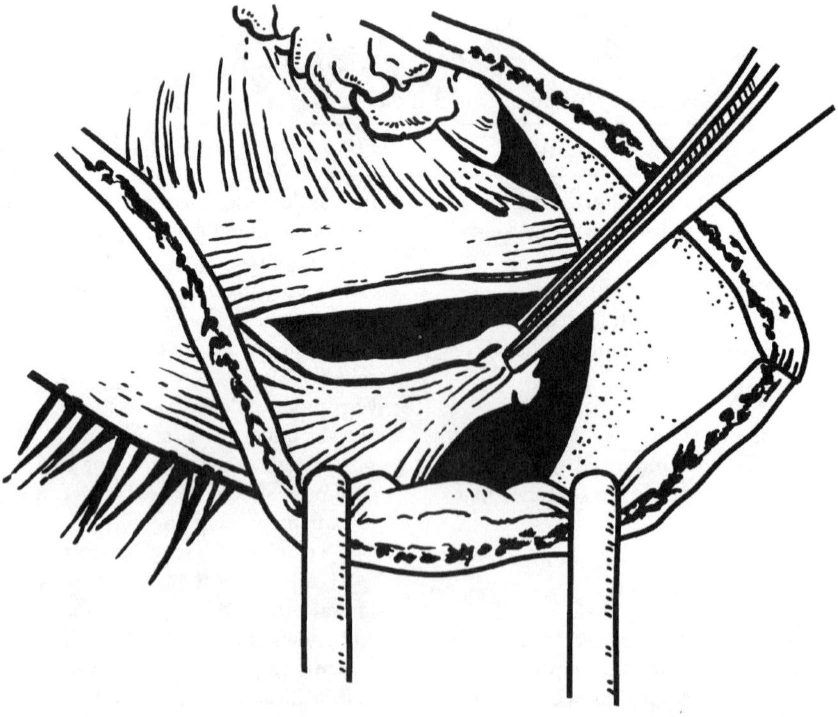

Figure 32 Inferior retinacular canthoplasty, step 2: the lower lid component of the lateral retinaculum is mobilized.

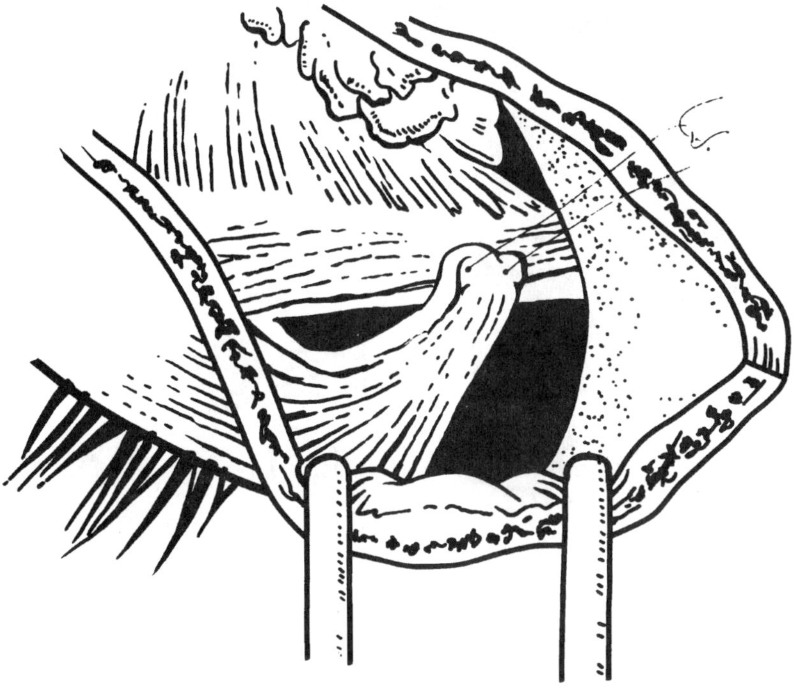

Figure 33 Inferior retinacular canthoplasty, step 3: a suture is passed through the mobilized component of the inferior retinaculum, through the lateral orbital rim periosteum, and tied.

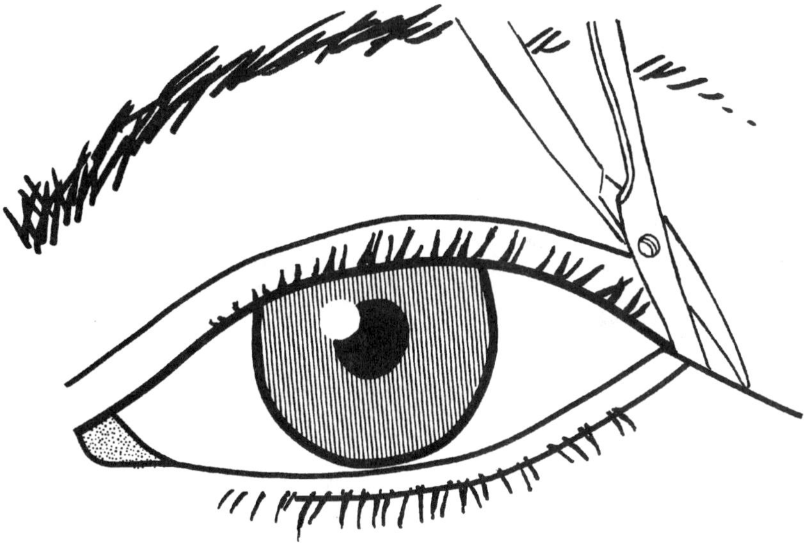

Figure 34 Lateral tarsal strip, step 1: depicted is a lateral canthotomy; an inferior cantholysis is performed to complete this step of the operation.

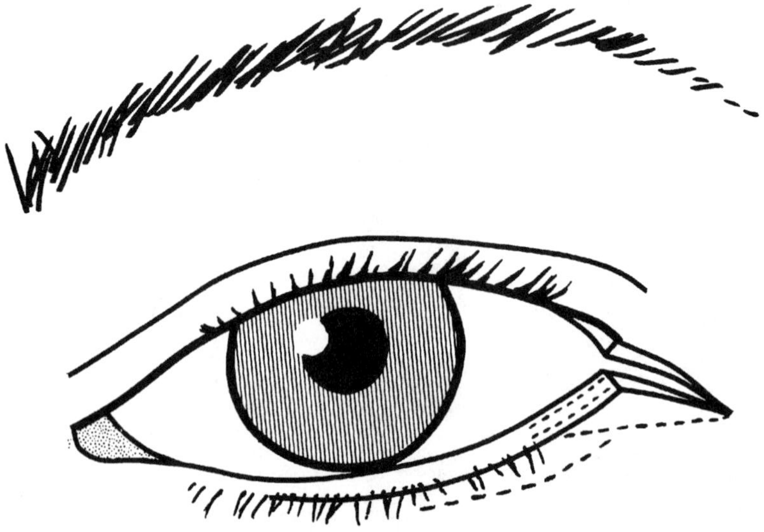

Figure 35 Lateral tarsal strip, step 2: an inferior cantholysis is performed with scissors as the lower eyelid is retracted away from the globe.

approximately 2 mm (slightly overcorrected). The upper eyelid blepharoplasty incision is closed as usual.

Correction of Ectropion

Senile ectropion, paralytic ectropion, and lids with substantial laxity require techniques that involve lid margin shortening and resuspension. The most common and successful technique for moderate-to-severe ectropion is the tarsal strip procedure (34), which involves a lateral canthotomy with inferior cantholysis. The incision can be carried into the lateral extension of the lower blepharoplasty incision when using the subciliary transcutaneous approach (Figs. 34, 35). A tarsal strip is

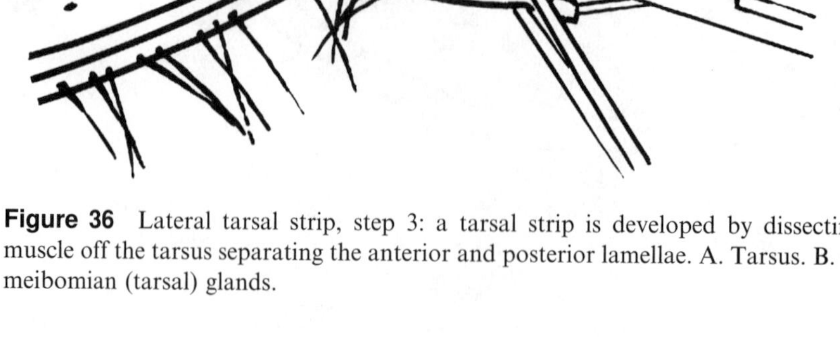

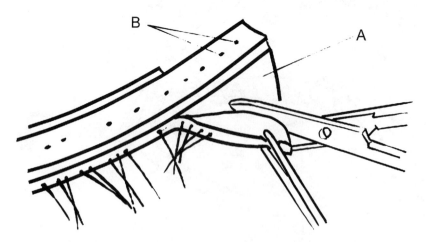

Figure 36 Lateral tarsal strip, step 3: a tarsal strip is developed by dissecting skin and muscle off the tarsus separating the anterior and posterior lamellae. A. Tarsus. B. Openings of meibomian (tarsal) glands.

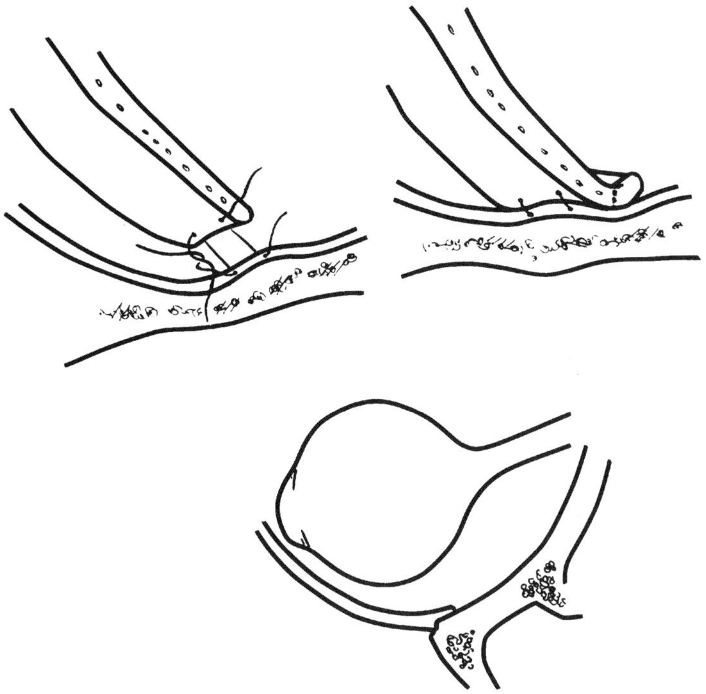

Figure 37 Lateral tarsal strip, step 4: the lateral tarsus is secured with a mattress suture (5-0 Prolene) to the lateral orbital rim.

developed by dissecting skin and muscle off the anterolateral aspect of the tarsus and mucosa and conjunctiva from its posterolateral aspect (Fig. 36). The tarsal strip is pulled laterally to tighten the eyelid margin, with excess tarsus trimmed as needed. The tarsus is secured with a mattress suture (5-0 Prolene) to the lateral orbital rim slightly superior to its original attachment at Whitnall's tubercle (Fig. 37). A buried suture is placed to appose the upper and lower gray lines laterally to re-create the lateral commissure accurately (Fig. 38). The cutaneous incision is closed with a running 5–0 prolene suture.

The tarsal strip is indicated for moderate-to-severe cases of ectropion not associated with cicatrix or tissue deficiencies in the posterior or anterior lamellae (see section on *Inferior Lid Retraction*). The procedure results in actual horizontal shortening of the eyelid margin and a slight superior repositioning of the lateral canthus. The disadvantages of this procedure include slight rounding of the lateral commissure and a slightly narrower palpebral slit. In less serious cases of simple ectropion or scleral show, inferior retinacular suspension or orbicularis oculus suspension is performed.

Correction of Entropion

Surgical correction of entropion must be designed to rotate the lid margin away from the surface of the cornea. This usually requires the use of cartilage grafts (senile entropion) or cartilage–mucosa grafts (cicatricial entropion). However, senile

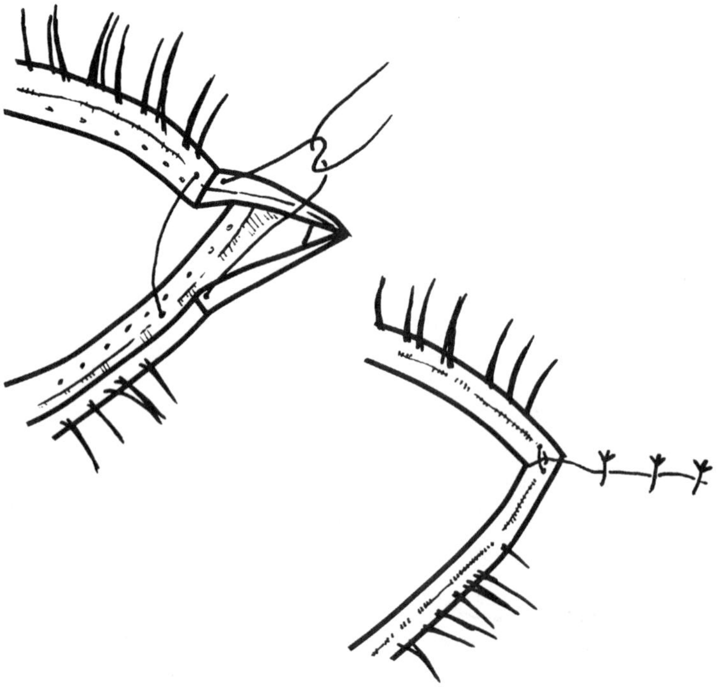

Figure 38 Lateral tarsal strip, step 5: a suture is placed to appose the upper and lower gray lines laterally to re-create the lateral commissure.

entropion is often effectively managed by the lateral tarsal strip procedure alone. If the entropion is limited to less than 25% of the lid margin, it may be corrected by full-thickness excision and primary closure.

Correction of Lower Eyelid Retraction

Correction of lower eyelid retraction must be based on the underlying pathological condition. Deficiency of skin or muscle in the anterior lamella or deficiency of the soft tissues within the posterior lamella will often require the use of grafts for adequate correction. After horizontal division of the structures that are vertically deficient (e.g., capsulopalpebral fascia, orbital septum, orbicularis muscle, or skin), a combination of cartilage grafts and skin may be required. If the lid retraction is due to scarring without loss of soft tissue, then simple scar lysis and temporary lid support may be adequate (e.g., Frost suture). This may be feasible after transconjunctival blepharoplasty when the edges of the conjunctiva–capsulopalpebral flaps heal in an overlapping position, resulting in eyelid retraction and scleral show.

Moderate-to-severe cases of vertical eyelid retraction may also be corrected through recruitment of skin and orbicularis muscle from the cheek. Recruitment may be accomplished by pulling the eyelid margin superiorly using a fascial graft (e.g., palmaris longus tendon). The tendon is routed through a suborbicularis pocket and fixed medially and laterally along the orbital rim. This procedure is usually used in cases of severe paralytic or involutional ectropion. Significant recruitment of cheek tissue can also be accomplished by SOOF suspension. Subperiosteal dissection inferior to the arcus marginalis mobilizes cheek tissue and the SOOF. Superolateral suspension of this complex moves both the posterior and anterior lamellae superiorly, thereby correcting lid retraction. Severe cases that are not amenable to repair by these procedures will require grafting in addition to suspension.

Correction of the Tear Trough Deformity

A tear trough deformity may be effectively corrected by repositioning the orbital fat over the inferior orbital rim. However, the deformity may also be masked by simply excising protruding orbital fat, as in routine blepharoplasty, and may need no further treatment. Although fat and fascial grafts have been used, they often resorb (9).

The medial and central fat pads can be repositioned to efface a tear trough during routine lower eyelid blepharoplasty (35). The tear trough is marked preoperatively while the patient is in an upright position. The orbital fat is draped over or under the periosteum. A subperiosteal pocket is generally preferred because it is bloodless and there is less risk of entering the angular vessels. The orbital fat is then brought over the orbital rim still pedicled to its vascular supply and placed into the subperiosteal pocket. The leading edge of the transposed fat is fixated using absorbable suture to the depths of the subperiosteal pocket. Even distribution of the fat within the pocket results in effacement of the tear trough and significant improvement in the appearance of the nasojugal area.

Correction of Malar Folds and Festoons

Surgical treatment of malar folds has traditionally been accomplished by direct excision but they can also be treated through a standard transcutaneous blepharoplasty incision (10). An ordinary subciliary skin–muscle flap is developed with a lateral canthal extension of no more than 1.5 cm. Excision or redraping of the orbital fat proceeds as usual followed by further inferior submuscular dissection to the superior margin of the fold. The plane of dissection then shifts to the supramuscular (subcutaneous) layer under the thicker malar skin (Fig. 39). The dissection proceeds to the inferior extent of the fold and the protruding tissues are removed, including slips of orbicularis oculus muscle and fat, as needed. Subcutaneous suspension sutures are placed at the inferior aspect of the wound and secured to the lateral aspect of the bony orbital rim and arcus marginalis to counteract the downward pull of this large infraorbital flap. The remaining surgical steps including redundant skin–muscle resection at the superior edge of the wound proceed as in standard blepharoplasty. Although festoons may also be treated via standard blepharoplasty approaches, large deformities may still require direct excision.

COMPLICATIONS

A thorough preoperative evaluation (history, physical, eye examination) is essential to detect patients at increased risk for complications. Complications associated with blepharoplasty are outlined in Table 3.

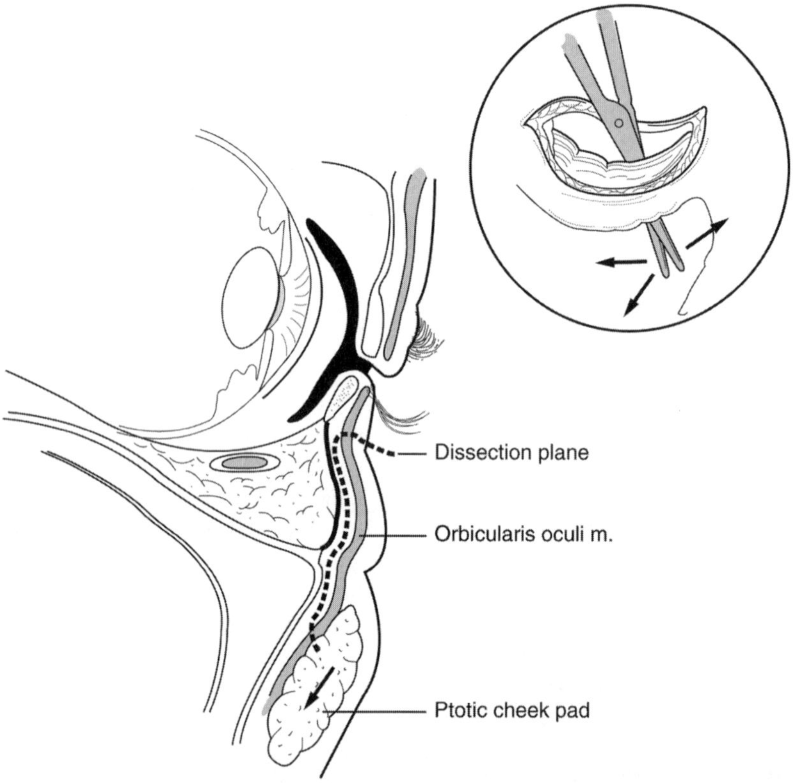

Figure 39 Dissection plane to reach the malar fold for correction of a malar fold deformity.

Eyelid Malposition

Scleral show, eyelid eversion (ectropion), and vertical eyelid retraction are most often associated with blepharoplasty of the lower lid. Failure to tighten a lax lower lid is the

Table 3 Complications of Blepharoplasty

Eyelid malposition
Superficial hematoma
Conjunctival granuloma
Infection
Chemosis
Canthal webbing
Dry eye syndrome
Overresection of fat
Underresection of fat
Underresection of skin
Upper lid crease asymmetry
Ptosis
Diplopia
Visual loss

most common cause of postoperative lower lid malposition. Excision of excess skin or muscle is the second most common cause of postoperative lid malposition, resulting in vertical eyelid retraction and scleral show (lower lid) or lagophthalmos (upper lid). If postoperative ectropion or lagophthalmos is moderate-to-severe and due to excess skin excision, the patient's excised skin can be replaced as a free graft. This can be done immediately if the problem is noticed in the operating room. The original excised skin should be saved in a saline-soaked surgical sponge and refrigerated. This banked skin can be used as a free graft up to 48 h postoperatively. As an alternative, a full-thickness skin graft from the postauricular area or clavicle may be required.

Lower lid malposition and scleral show noted in the early postoperative period should be treated conservatively by massage and suspending the eyelid with tape (Fig. 40). The eyelid should return to a normal position within 3 weeks. After an upper lid blepharoplasty it is common to note a slight separation of the upper lid from the lower lid (approximately 1 mm of lagophthalmos). This amount of lagophthalmos will spontaneously resolve after the edema and function of the orbicularis oculus improve.

The transconjunctival approach to the lower eyelid fat and inferior orbit is associated with less risk of postoperative scleral show and ectropion than the transcutaneous approaches. This may be the case because, in transconjunctival

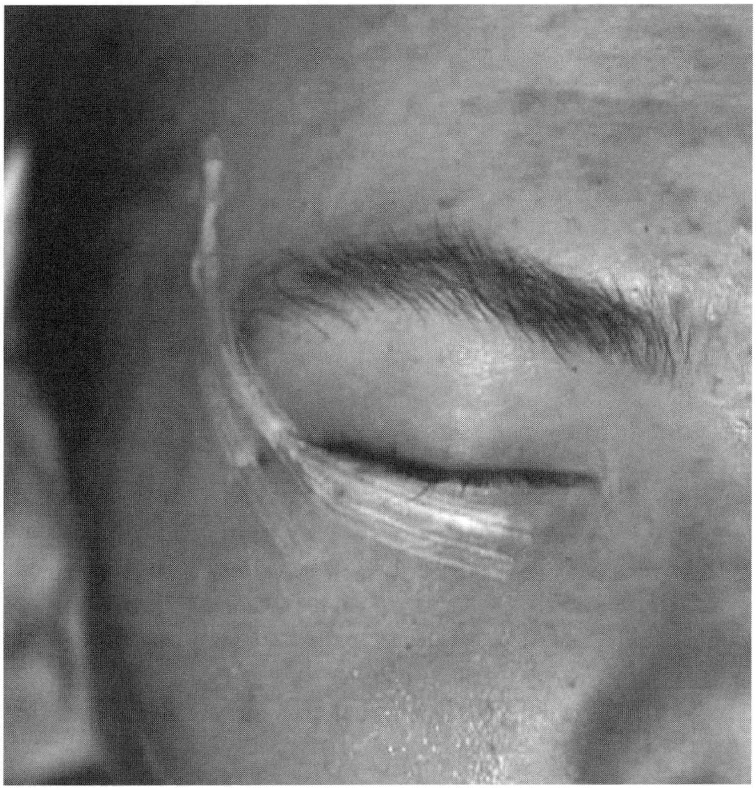

Figure 40 Temporary suspension of the lower eyelid after blepharoplasty using Steri-strips is useful in preventing postoperative eyelid malposition.

blepharoplasty, the anterior lamella (skin and orbicularis oculus muscle) is not violated and the capsulopalpebral fascia is divided, resulting in less downward pull on the lower eyelid margin. However, cicatricial ectropion may result after transconjunctival blepharoplasty due to excessive overlapping of the free edges of the conjunctival incision along the horizontal extent of the lower eyelid. This can be avoided by carefully pulling the lower eyelid superiorly at the conclusion of the operation to prevent any incisional overlap or by suspending the lower eyelid with a Frost suture or tape for 24–48 h. Nevertheless, the occurrence of ectropion is much lower using the transconjunctival approach ($< 5\%$) than the conventional transcutaneous approaches ($> 25\%$).

Superficial Hematoma

Hematomas involving the subcutaneous tissues are best treated by aspiration to minimize fibrosis and scarring. If one assumes that the patient was screened for clotting abnormalities, it is difficult to predict which patients will experience prolonged ecchymoses or hematomas.

Granuloma

Granuloma formation along the conjunctival incision occurs unpredictably. The granuloma presents as a pedunculated mucosa-covered mass along the transconjunctival incision. If it is distressing to the patient or obscures the visual axis, it will require simple secondary excision.

Infection

Although infection after blepharoplasty is rare, once the septum is surgically breached serious deep orbital infection is a risk. At the first signs of orbital infection, such as pain, redness, or purulent discharge, the patient should be given antibiotics. If an orbital abscess is suspected a CT scan should be obtained. An abscess can usually be drained via the original incisions.

Chemosis

Chemosis (conjunctival edema) occurs unpredictably, usually following lower lid blepharoplasty. However, it can occur after transconjunctival or transcutaneous surgery. Supportive care is all that is needed, including eye lubricants. It will resolve spontaneously within 3–4 months (16).

Canthal Webbing

Epicanthal webs may result if the upper blepharoplasty incision is carried beyond the level of the medial punctum. It usually must be corrected by direct excision with W-plasty scar revision. Minor webbing in the early postoperative period may be managed with subcutaneous steroid injections.

Dry Eye Syndrome

Even minor dysfunction of upper eyelid closure can result in corneal drying, especially in patients at risk. Any complaints of dry eye symptoms (stinging, irritation, lack of tears/lubrication) preoperatively may worsen, even after a conservative upper eyelid blepharoplasty. Damage or inadvertent resection of the lacrimal gland will result in an irreversible condition of dry eyes and corneal injury. The lacrimal gland must be carefully differentiated from the upper central fat pad. The gland may be prolapsed and the inexperienced surgeon could misidentify it as orbital fat. However, the gland is usually easily differentiated from adjacent orbital fat. The gland will have a thicker capsule and will be firmer with light gray coloring. The prolapsed lacrimal gland can be safely resuspended under the upper lateral orbital rim using interrupted 5–0 Prolene sutures.

Overresection of Fat

Excessive removal of fat can lead to a hollowed appearance to the lid or restrictions in lid movement. Deep orbital fat resection can lead to inadvertent injury to extraocular muscles, especially the inferior oblique and inferior rectus muscles. Treatment of this condition is rarely satisfying and consists of free fat transplants or fat injection. In cases of vertical dystopia resulting from excess fat excision anterior to the axis of the globe, the condition may be improved by augmenting the orbital floor with grafts including bone. However, even with aggressive fat removal, vertical dystopia is rarely observed because of globe support from Lockwood's ligamentous sling.

Underresection of Fat

Underresection of orbital fat is most commonly encountered after transconjunctival lower eyelid blepharoplasty, especially involving the lateral orbital fat pad. This is often noticed after the edema has resolved. Revision blepharoplasty will be required to correct the problem.

Underresection of orbital fat in the upper eyelid most often involves the medial fat pad. One method to treat this problem without reopening the skin over the area is to approach the fat pad under the eyelid through the conjunctiva (i.e., transconjunctival upper blepharoplasty) (17). The medial fat pad lies medial to the levator aponeurosis and is the only fat pad in the upper eyelid to do so. Therefore, only the medial fat pad is accessible by this approach.

Underresection of Skin

Underresection of skin is most commonly encountered in the upper eyelid. Before revision, the level of the eyebrow must be re-evaluated. Lateral hooding involving an apparent excess of skin in the lateral orbit may be due to a ptotic brow. Removal of skin in the area will result in further decent of the eyebrow and incisions within the thicker infrabrow skin could lead to obvious scarring. A brow lift may be all that is necessary to correct the problem.

Upper Lid Crease Asymmetry

Lid crease asymmetry may be secondary to actual differences in the height of the crease or secondary effects from an asymmetrical lid fold. An asymmetrical lid fold may be caused by differences in the amount of skin or orbital fat resected. This abnormality should be observed to await complete resolution of edema and the effects of scar contracture. Altering the height of one of the creases, if necessary, can then done secondarily.

Ptosis

Mild blepharoptosis is common after upper lid blepharoplasty and is secondary to temporary dysfunction of the levator and Müller's muscles. As the edema subsides and muscular function returns to normal (usually within a few days), the ptosis will resolve. Persistent blepharoptosis may be secondary to injury to the levator muscle or inadvertent separation of the levator aponeurosis from the conjoined fascia. This usually occurs along the inferior aspect of the incision where the aponeurosis is closely apposed to the overlying orbicularis oculus muscle. Aponeurotic injury can also occur if the orbital septum is opened inferior to the orbital fat. The orbital fat serves as a protective layer and the orbital septum should only be opened over the bulging fat, not inferior to it.

Subclinical ptosis may be unmasked in the postoperative period after ptosis repair in the opposite eye. This phenomenon is an example of the effect of Hering's law of equal innervation. Subclinical ptosis can be detected in the preoperative evaluation by manually elevating the obviously ptotic lid. If Hering's law is a factor, the opposite lid will become ptotic. The operative plan should include correction of ptosis for both lids.

Diplopia

Temporary diplopia lasting several hours after an uneventful blepharoplasty may be due to dysfunction of the extraocular muscles from the local anesthetic. Mild diplopia may be present for several days (or weeks) due to hematoma and edema. Permanent diplopia typically results from direct injury to the extraocular muscles.

The most common extraocular muscle to be injured during transcutaneous blepharoplasty is the inferior oblique muscle. However, the inferior rectus muscle is injured at least as often as the inferior oblique muscle with use of the retroseptal transconjunctival approach (26). During routine transcutaneous or preseptal transconjunctival blepharoplasty, the origin of the inferior oblique muscle is often exposed and may be injured. Many surgeons prefer to identify the belly of the muscle prior to fat excision to avoid inadvertent injury. Since the origin of the muscle is somewhat variable, and possibly more anteriorly positioned in some patients, identifying the muscle is warranted in most cases.

Placing the transconjunctival retroseptal incision too posteriorly (deep in the fornix) may result in direct injury to the inferior rectus or oblique muscles. Dissection and excision of the orbital fat through a posterior incision may also result in adjacent muscle injury or scarring that could lead to muscle dysfunction and strabismus. Injury to the inferior oblique muscle results in problems with extorsion and inferior rectus injury results in limitations in inferior rotation.

Visual Loss

Blindness after blepharoplasty is the most dreaded complication and occurs in about 1:40,000 cases. The usual mechanism involves retrobulbar hemorrhage that increases extra- and intraocular pressure beyond the perfusion pressure of the retinal artery (ischemic optic neuropathy) (25). Factors associated with hematoma include use of anticoagulants, hypertension, advanced age, and metabolic disease (1). The cause of the retrobulbar hemorrhage is unknown but shearing of the fine blood vessels that supply the deep orbital fat may be a contributing factor. Therefore, gentle handling of the fat is essential to prevent postoperative hemorrhage. Patients should be counseled regarding postoperative care including participating in only light activities, avoidance of straining, and avoiding medications that interfere with clotting for 7 days postoperatively. No occlusive or pressure dressings should be applied to the eye after blepharoplasty.

Signs of retrobulbar hemorrhage include proptosis, pain, and vision changes including field and color changes, and diffuse ecchymosis. Retrobulbar hemorrhage and blindness are most often associated with excision of fat from the lower lid medial fat pocket. Hemorrhage and visual loss are seldom associated with upper eyelid blepharoplasty. Prompt evaluation and treatment are required to prevent blindness in patients with a retrobulbar hematoma. Therapeutic steps include: opening the wound at the bedside, lateral canthotomy and inferior cantholysis, and administration of mannitol and steroids. An ophthalmological surgeon should be consulted promptly. If vision remains impaired despite these measures, consideration of bony orbital decompression is next. Decompression proceeds by removal of the inferomedial orbital floor, and, if necessary, removal of the medial wall (via a Lynch incision), and, finally, removal of the lateral wall.

Other causes of postoperative blindness have been reported including embolic retinal artery occlusion or migration of substances within the subarachnoid space to the contralateral eye (causing temporary vision loss in the opposite eye). The risk of amblyopia is high in children under the age of 8 years when visual stimulation is interrupted for even a few days. Prolonged use of occlusive dressings or blurring eye ointments should be avoided (7).

SPECIAL TOPICS

Medicare Rules for Blepharoplasty as a Covered Benefit

Blepharoplasty is a Medicare-covered benefit if it is performed for functional reasons (usually to improve vision) according to the Medicare Part B regulations published in 1996. Blepharoplasty is considered functional when excision of excessive skin, fat, or muscle results in correction of the upper lid to allow for proper positioning of eyeglasses; blepharoptosis repair improves vision impaired by paresis of the levator muscles; and excision of excess skin improves chronic, symptomatic dermatitis of the pretarsal platform. To establish medical necessity as a covered service under Medicare Part B regulations, one or more of the following criteria must be met: malpositioning of spectacles due to excessive lower lid tissue, with photographic documentation; upper eyelid margin is within 2.5 mm of corneal light reflex on primary gaze; excessive eyelid tissue rests on the eyelashes; and/ or visual fields demonstrate a minimum of 8 degrees or 20% loss of upper field vision, correctable by taping. The rules regarding blepharoplasty as a covered benefit may vary according to unique state regulations, year, and insurance carrier. Other functional problems that are covered by most third-party payers include correcting prosthesis problems and chronic blepharitis.

Laser Blepharoplasty

After the skin markings are completed, a CO_2 laser (5–10 W, continuous mode) can be used to complete the operation including skin, muscle, and fat excision. The advantages of the laser include improved precision, minimal manipulation of the tissues, improved hemostasis, and decreased operative time. In addition, with the beam slightly out of focus, the orbital fat can be more precisely sculpted. The disadvantages include laser eye injury, fire hazard, and the lack of feel or tactile feedback when cutting through the tissues. Typical laser precautions and a metal laser-proof corneal shield should used. The handpiece is held away from the operative field and a collimated laser beam is projected over the planned incision. The surgeon does not actually touch the tissues with the cutting instrument and lacks tactile feedback typically present with use of the knife or scissors. The surgeon must have a thorough knowledge of the anatomical landmarks and a period of acclimatization to ensure a favorable outcome.

REFERENCES

1. Pastorek NS. Upper-lid blepharoplasty. Facial Plast Surg 1996; 12:157–169.
2. Rees TD, La Trenta GS. The role of the Schirmer's test and orbital morphology in predicting dry-eye syndrome after blepharoplasty. Plast Reconstr Surg 1988; 82:619–625.
3. Klatsky SA, Manson PN. Thyroid disorders masquerading as aging changes. Ann Plast Surg 1992; 28:420–426.
4. Sykes JM. Surgical rejuvenation of the brow and forehead. Facial Plast Surg 1999; 15:183–191.
5. Spinelli HM, Forman DL. Current treatment of post-traumatic deformities. Residual orbital, adnexal, and soft-tissue abnormalities. Clin Plast Surg 1997; 24:519–530.
6. Gausas R. Technique for combined blepharoplasty and ptosis correction. Facial Plast Surg 1999; 15:193–201.
7. Brady KM, Patrinely JR, Soparkar CN. Surgery of the eyelids. Clin Plast Surg 2000; 25:579–586.
8. Pospisil OA, Fernando TD. Review of the lower blepharoplasty incision as a surgical approach to zygomatic–orbital fractures. Br J Oral Maxillofac Surg 1984; 22:261–268.
9. Flowers RS. Tear trough implants for correction of tear trough deformity. Clin Plast Surg 1993; 20:403–415.
10. Farrior RT, Kassir RR. Management of malar folds in blepharoplasty. Laryngoscope 1998; 108:1659–1663.
11. Furnas DW. Festoons, mounds, and bags of the eyelids and cheek. Clin Plast Surg 1993; 20:367–385.
12. Hwang K, Kim DJ, Chung RS, Lee SI, Hiraga Y. An anatomical study of the junction of the orbital septum and the levator aponeurosis in Orientals. Br J Plast Surg 1998; 51: 594–598.
13. Siegel RJ. Essential anatomy for contemporary upper lid blepharoplasty. Clin Plast Surg 1993; 20:209–212.
14. Hugo NE, Stone E. Anatomy for a blepharoplasty. Plast Reconstr Surg 1974; 53:381–383.
15. Niechajev IA, Ljungqvist A. Central (third) fat pad of the upper eyelid. Aesth Plast Surg 1991; 15:223–228.
16. Wolfley D. Blepharoplasty. In: Krause CJ, Mangat DS, Pastorek N, eds. Aesthetic Facial Surgery, Philadelphia: J.B.Lippincott, 1991:571–599.

17. Januszkiewicz JS, Nahai F. Transconjunctival upper blepharoplasty. Plast Reconstr Surg 1999; 103:1015–1018.
18. May JW Jr., Fearon J, Zingarelli P. Retro-orbicularis oculus fat (ROOF) resection in aesthetic blepharoplasty: a 6-year study in 63 patients. Plast Reconstr Surg 1990; 86:682–689.
19. Tucker SM, Verhulst SJ. Stabilization of eyelid height after aponeurotic ptosis repair. Ophthalmology 1999; 106:517–522.
20. Yoon KC, Park S. Systematic approach and selective tissue removal in blepharoplasty for young Asians. Plast Reconstr Surg 1998; 102:502–508.
21. Boo-Chai K. Some aspects of plastic (cosmetic) surgery in orientals. Br J Plast Surg 1969; 22(1):60–69.
22. Kao YS, Lin CH, Fang RH. Epicanthoplasty with modified Y–V advancement procedure. Plast Reconstr Surg 1998; 102:1835–1841.
23. Fuente dC. A simple procedure for aesthetic correction of the medial epicanthal fold. Aesth Plast Surg 1997; 21:381–384.
24. Aiache AE, Ramirez OH. The suborbicularis oculi fat pads: an anatomic and clinical study. Plast Reconstr Surg 1995; 95:37–42.
25. Furnas DW. The orbicularis oculi muscle. Management in blepharoplasty. Clin Plast Surg 1981; 8(4):687–715.
26. Ghabrial R, Lisman RD, Kane MA, Milite J, Richards R. Diplopia following transconjunctival blepharoplasty. Plast Reconstr Surg 1998; 102:1219–1225.
27. Anastassov GE, van Damme PA. Evaluation of the anatomical position of the lateral canthal ligament: clinical implications and guidelines. J Craniofac Surg 1996; 7:429–436.
28. Bernardi C, Dura S, Amata PL. Treatment of orbicularis oculi muscle hypertrophy in lower lid blepharoplasty. Aesth Plast Surg 1998; 22:349–351.
29. Converse JM, Firmin F, Wood-Smith D, Friedland JA. The conjunctival approach in orbital fractures. Plast Reconstr Surg 1973; 52:656–657.
30. Tessier P. The conjunctival approach to the orbital floor and maxilla in congenital malformation and trauma. J Maxillofac Surg 1973; 1:3–8.
31. Aldave AJ, Maus M, Rubin P. Advances in the management of lower eyelid retraction. Facial Plast Surg 1999; 15:213–224.
32. Patel BC. Midface rejuvenation. Facial Plast Surg 1999; 15:231–242.
33. Jelks GW, Glat PM, Jelks EB, Longaker MT. The inferior retinacular lateral canthoplasty: a new technique. Plast Reconstr Surg 1997; 100:1262–1270.
34. Anderson RL, Gordy DD. The tarsal strip procedure. Arch Ophthalmol 1979; 97:2192–2196.
35. Goldberg RA, Edelstein C, Balch K, Shorr N. Fat repositioning in lower eyelid blepharoplasty. Semin Ophthalmol 1998; 13:103–106.

Appendix Terminology of Blepharoplasty

Amblyopia	Decreased vision in one eye; most often describing unilateral vision loss in childhood due to lack of visual stimulation
Asthenopia	Subjective feeling of ocular fatigue and strain
Bichat's fat pad	See "buccal fat pad"
Blepharitis	Inflammation of the eyelids
Blepharochalasis	An idiopathic syndromic disorder seen in young and middle-aged women characterized by recurrent unilateral or bilateral upper eyelid edema giving rise to thin excess eyelid skin, blepharoptosis, and weakening or dehiscence of the lateral canthal tendon
Blepharedema	Edema of the eyelids
Blepharophimosis	A narrowed or stenotic palpebral fissure
Blepharoptosis	Drooping or ptosis of the upper eyelid; vertical eyelid fissure <8 mm in men, or <9 mm in women
Blepharophimosis syndrome	A dominant hereditary condition characterized by synkinetic ptosis: an involuntary motion of the eyelid
Buccal fat pad	Encapsulated fat in the cheek resting on the external surface of the buccinator muscle
Canthal dystopia	Malposition of the lateral or medial eyelid commissure
Capsulopalpebral fascia	Anterior aponeurotic extension of the inferior rectus muscle spanning the full extent of the lower eyelid
Cicatricial ectropion	Ectropion caused by a deficiency of eyelid skin or skin and muscle (anterior lamella) secondary to congenital, traumatic, irradiation, burns, or inflammatory causes
Ciliary part of the eyelid	Lash-bearing part extending from the lateral canthus to the lacrimal punctum (at which point the lacrimal portion begins)
Dermatochalasis	An acquired condition (due to aging, environmental, or genetic causes) of excess skin and abnormal laxity leading to cutaneous rhytidosis; often associated with prolapsing orbital fat
Dry eye syndrome	A collection of symptoms typical of patients with deficient tear production including paradoxical excess tearing, burning, stinging, pain, sensitivity to windy conditions, and corneal inflammation
Ectropion	Separation or a rolling over of the eyelid margin away from the surface of the globe
Entropion	Inversion of the eyelid margin
Epiphora	Excess accumulation of tears
Excursion, upper eyelid	Distance in millimeters that the upper eyelid margin travels vertically from a position of full downgaze to full upgaze in the midpupillary axis
Festoon	Severe malar folds taking on a drapelike or swag appearance

Gray line	A well-known surface anatomical landmark along the upper and lower eyelid margins useful in the repair of lid margin lacerations; corresponds histologically to the most superficial portion of the orbicularis muscle, known as the muscle of Riolan. The superior tarsus border is posterior to the gray line with its meibomian gland orifices
Hering's law of equal innervation	Equivalent innervation of matched muscles may cause nonphysiological overactivity of the normal side while compensating for weak side; pertains to increased height of the eyelid on the normal side in response to blepharoptosis on the abnormal side
Horner's muscle	Lacrimal portion of the orbicularis oculi muscle; arises from the lacrimal bone and fans out to insert along the medial edge of the tarsus, within the subcutaneous tissues along the eyelid margin, and the lateral commissure; primarily responsible for directing the flow of tears toward and through the lacrimal apparatus
Hypotropia	One globe is positioned lower than the other globe
Inferior fornix	The space between the lower eyelid and the eyeball; enveloped by conjunctiva
Lacrimal part of the eyelid	Eyelid margin is divided into a ciliary portion and a lacrimal portion. The lacrimal portion extends from the punctum to the medial canthal angle
Lagophthalmos	Separation (in millimeters) between the eyelid margins as the eyes are gently closed
Lateral hooding	The appearance of excess skin along the lateral upper lid effacing the superior eyelid crease and prolapsing over the pretarsal skin and eyelashes; may be secondary to prolapsing orbital fat, lacrimal gland ptosis, eyebrow ptosis, or a prominent or malpositioned lateral orbital rim
Levator aponeurosis disinsertion	Dehiscence of the levator–orbital septum conjoined fascias from the surface of the superior tarsus. This results in a high or absent lid crease and retraction of orbital fat into the superior sulcus and under the superior bony orbital rim.
Levator palpebrae superioris muscle	Major elevator of the upper eyelid; takes origin from the orbital roof anterior to the optic canal; becomes aponeurotic (i.e., levator aponeurosis) several mm above the upper tarsus and inserts into full length of the upper tarsal border; the upper lid crease, most prominent in white patients' lids, is formed from the insertion of slips of the aponeurosis into the orbicularis muscle and skin; the motor nerve supply is from the oculomotor division of the trigeminus nerve
Lid lag	Upper eyelid lags behind the descent of the globe during the act of downgaze
Lower eyelid retraction	Congenital or acquired soft tissue deficiency in the anterior or posterior lamella resulting in inferior migration of the lower eyelid margin and inability to elevate the lid margin above the pupillary axis
Malar folds	Gross prominences over the malar eminence, below the bony orbital rim, consisting of excess skin, subcutaneous fat, orbicularis oculus muscle, and suborbicularis fat; edema may also be present
Marginal reflex distance	Distance in millimeters between the corneal light reflex and the upper eyelid margin; useful in judging the degree of blepharoptosis

(Continued)

Appendix (Continued)

Mechanical ptosis	Blepharoptosis caused by external forces such as excess skin with no intrinsic abnormalities in the levator or Müller's muscles
Meibomian (tarsal) glands	Approximately 30 sebaceous meibomian glands are embedded in the tarsi that open into the lid margin; they secrete a lipid barrier along the lid margin that helps prevent spillage of tears from the conjunctival sac
Müller's muscle	Involuntary (smooth) muscle in the upper eyelid responsible for approximately 2 mm lid elevation
Ocular limbus	Junction of the sclera with the free edge of the cornea
Paralytic ectropion	Lower eyelid ectropion due to paresis or paralysis of the orbicularis oculus muscle
Phthisis bulbi	Shrinkage of the globe usually after an inflammatory condition; may lead to pseudoptosis
Pseudoptosis	Appearance of ptosis in the absence of eyelid pathology
ROOF	Lateral fibrofatty pad under the orbicularis oculus muscle along the upper lateral orbital rim sometimes responsible for fullness in the lateral eyelid area
Muscle of Riolan	Within the ciliary part of the eyelid; occupies nearly the entire thickness of the lid margin traversed by lash follicles, glands of Moll, and the ducts of the Meibomian glands; corresponds exactly to the gray line
Scleral show	Lower eyelid malposition resulting in a show of sclera below the level of the inferior corneal limbus in primary gaze
Secondary blepharoptosis	Excess skin overhangs a normally positioned eyelid margin, resulting in pseudoptosis
Senile ectropion	Lower eyelid ectropion caused by laxity of the lid retractors, tarsus, and canthal ligamentous structures
Snap back test	A test to detect excessive lower lid flaccidity; performed by manually pulling the eyelid margin away from the surface of the globe and observing its ability to snap back
Steatoblepharon	True or pseudoherniation of orbital fat causing discrete or diffuse distensions in the eyelid
SOOF	Relatively fixed area of fat below the orbital rim, above the periosteum and deep to the orbicularis oculus muscle
Superior palpebral lid crease	Formed by the insertion of levator aponeurotic slips into the pretarsal and preseptal orbicularis muscle and skin; the height of the crease is determined by measuring the distance from the lash line to the crease, at the pupil, as the patient slowly retracts the upper eyelid from the relaxed closed position
Tarsus	Elongated fibrous (not cartilaginous) strip responsible for the structural support of the free edge of upper and lower eyelid; the upper eyelid tarsus measures approximately 10 mm in height at the pupil; the lower eyelid tarsus is approximately 5 mm in height at the pupil
Vertical eyelid fissure	The distance between the upper and lower eyelids in primary gaze
Vertical eyelid retraction	Excessive upper eyelid retraction in primary gaze; vertical eyelid fissure >10 mm in men, >13 mm in women
Whitnall's tubercle	Orbital tubercle (prominence) of the zygomatic bone, serving as the insertion point of the deep component of the lateral retinaculum (lateral canthal tendon)

23
Otoplasty

Raffi Der Sarkissian
Boston University School of Medicine, Boston, Massachusetts, U.S.A.

Cosmetic and reconstructive correction of auricular deformities and construction of the auricular framework are among the most challenging procedures for the plastic surgeon. The task begins with a thorough knowledge of the intricate embryology and anatomy of this complex structure. The proportional, positional, and angular relationship of the ear to adjacent structures must also be respected. Sound surgical technique is required as the surgeon seeks to create a natural and aesthetically appealing replica of this complex form.

EMBRYOLOGY

The auricle develops from six mesenchymal proliferations known as hillocks that arise from the dorsal ends of the first (mandibular) and second (hyoid) branchial arches on either side of the first branchial cleft during the sixth week of gestation (1) (Fig. 1). Initially described by His, the origin of these six hillocks has been debated (2). The original description accounted for formation of the tragus, root of the helix, and superior helix from three hillocks arising from the first branchial arch and the antihelix, antitragus, and lobule from three hillocks arising from the second branchial arch. Subsequent embryological data, as presented by Wen, Wood-Jones, and Streeter, suggest that the entire ear, with the exception of the tragus, is of second branchial cleft origin (2,3). The first and sixth hillocks are thought to maintain a fairly constant position at the site of the tragus and antitragus, respectively, with the fourth and fifth hillocks expanding and rotating across the dorsal end of the cleft to give rise to the anterior helix, crus helicis, and body of the auricle (Fig. 2). The mandibular arch is suppressed and gives rise only to the tragus (2). The fusion of the hillocks is completed by 12 weeks of gestation and the ear begins to take on the adult form by 20 weeks. The auricles are initially positioned in the lower neck. With development of the mandible in a caudal dimension, they ascend to the side of the head (1). This embryologic developmental relationship helps to explain the association of malpositioned or malformed ears with mandibular hypoplasia or deformity. The ear continues to grow after birth, reaching approximately 85% of adult size by age 3, 90–95% by age 6, and nearly full adult size by age 9.

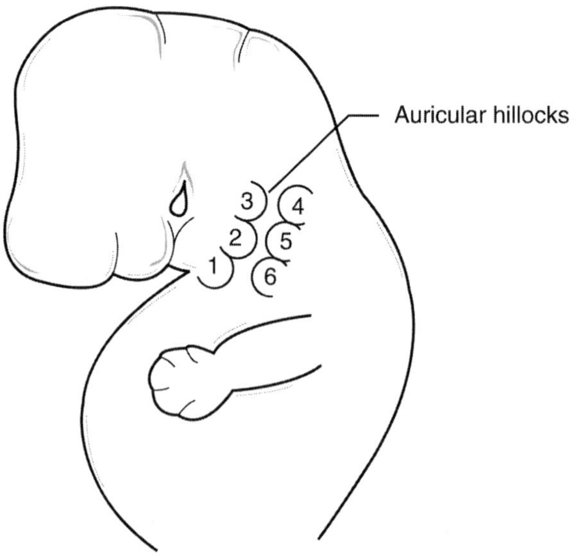

Figure 1 Six mesenchymal hillocks derived from the first and second branchial arches arise on either side of the first branchial cleft.

ANATOMY

The complex concavities and convexities of the elastic cartilage auricular framework are covered by thin skin that is more closely adherent laterally than medially (4). The helical border terminates anteriorly above the external auditory meatus. The antihelix diverges superiorly into the superior and anterior crura, creating the fossa triangularis. Between the helix and antihelix is the scaphoid fossa. The concha is separated into a concha cymba and concha cavum by the crus helicis. The tragus is at the anterior edge of the concha cavum and the antitragus lies along the posterior edge. The auricular cartilage framework ends inferiorly at the cauda helicis, with the fibrofatty lobule being devoid of cartilage. The cartilage framework is continuous with the cartilaginous external auditory canal (Fig. 3).

Three ligaments secure the auricle to the bony skull. The anterior ligament attaches the helix and tragus; the superior ligament attaches the spine of the helix to the superior margin of the bony canal; and the posterior ligament attaches the medial surface of the concha to the mastoid process (5). Six rudimentary muscles of the ear are described. The three extrinsic muscles (anterior, superior, and posterior auricular) are better developed than the intrinsic muscles. These muscles serve little function in humans, however, in lower animals, they help to orient the auricle toward sound sources.

The blood supply to the auricle is extremely rich, arising from the posterior auricular artery and auricular rami of the superficial temporal artery. Despite this rich blood supply, the absence of protective overlying soft tissue allows this vascular plexus to be easily compressed by tight dressings or vasoconstrict in response to severe cold temperatures. The venous drainage from the auricle is via the superficial temporal vein that further drains into the retromandibular vein and the posterior

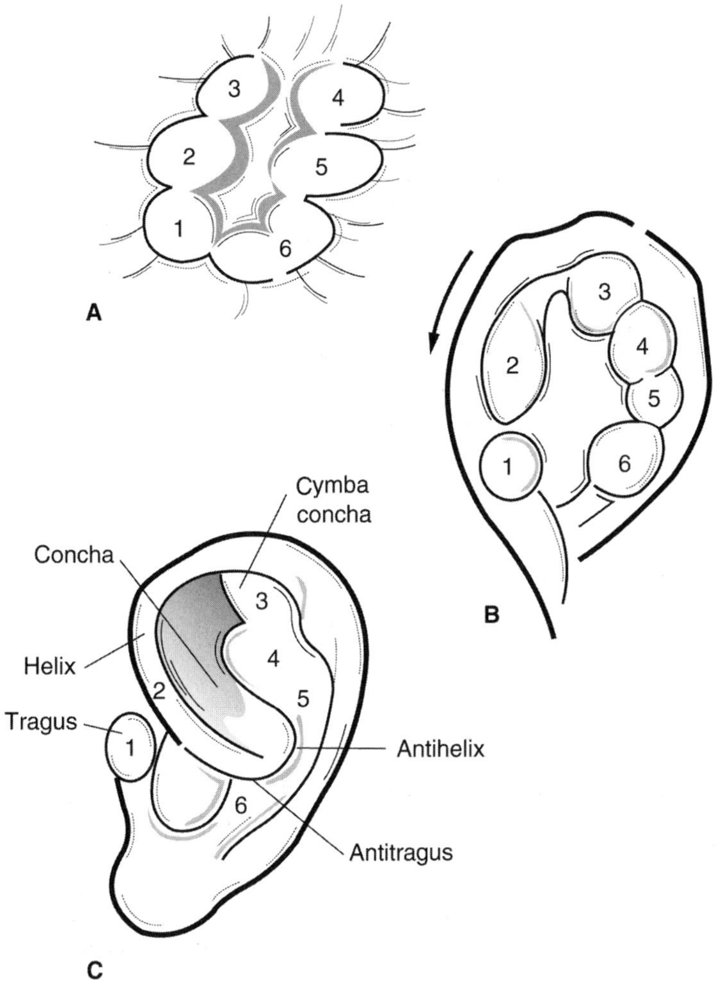

Figure 2 The first and sixth hillocks remain in relatively constant position while the remaining hillocks rotate around the cleft to their new positions, giving rise to different parts of the auricular anatomy.

auricular veins, which drain into the external jugular and, occasionally, into the sigmoid sinus via emissary veins (5). The lymphatics of the ear drain into the parotid (preauricular) lymph node chain, the superficial cervical nodes along the external jugular vein (infraauricular), and the mastoid (postauricular/retroauricular) lymph nodes.

The nerve supply to the ear is relatively complex, with varying contributions from several sensory nerves. The auriculotemporal branch of the mandibular division of the trigeminal nerve supplies the anterior portion of the helix and the tragus. The greater auricular nerve originating from cervical roots C2 and C3 supplies the majority of the posterior surface of the auricle. The skin overlying the mastoid is supplied by the lesser occipital, also originating from C2 and C3. Both the greater auricular and lesser occipital nerves supply the upper medial portion of the auricle. The concavity of the concha is supplied by fibers of the ninth and tenth cranial

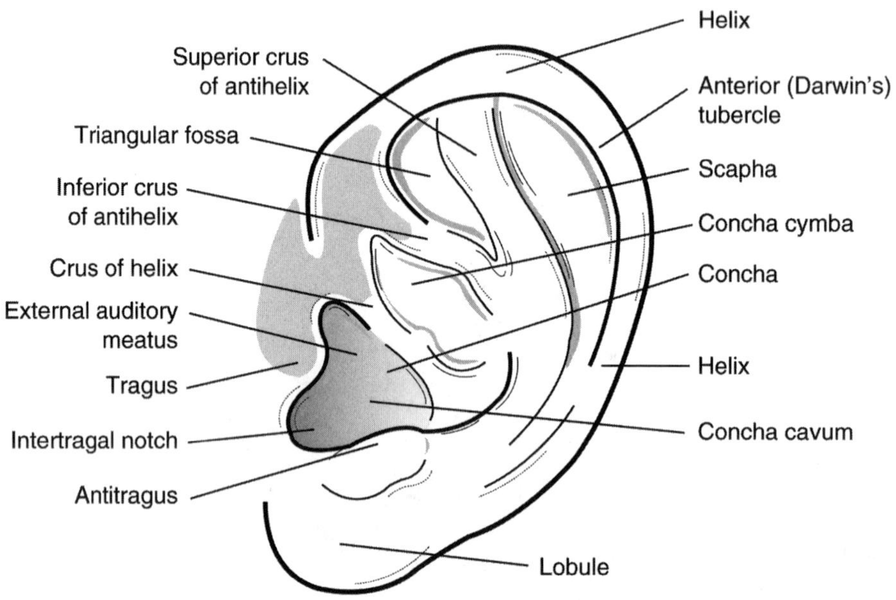

Figure 3 Numerous named concavities and convexities of the ear contribute to its complex morphology.

nerves with a contribution from sensory branches of cranial nerve seven (5). This complex innervation requires consideration when performing an anesthetic block of the ear for procedures to be performed under local anesthesia.

The adult auricle, on average, measures 6.5 cm in vertical height and approximately 3.5 cm in width (Fig. 4). The width is 55–60% of the height. The superior aspect is at the level of the lateral brow and the inferior aspect at the level of the nasal ala. The angle created with the mastoid is 20–30 degrees and corresponds to a distance between the superior helix and squamous portion of the temporal bone of 15–25 mm. The normal cephaloconchal angle is approximately 90 degrees. The normal scaphoconchal angle measures between 90 and 120 degrees. The long axis

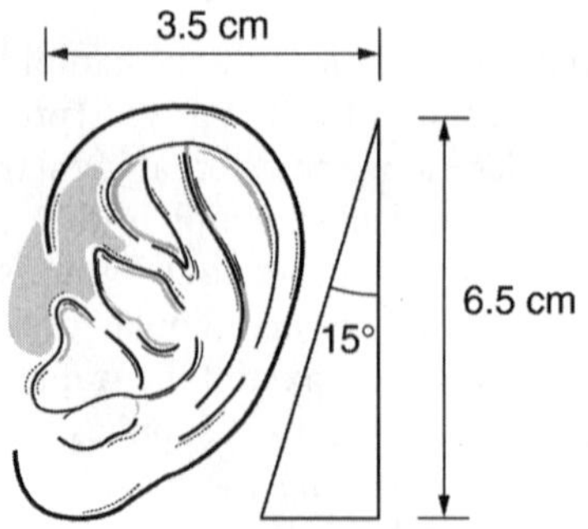

Figure 4 On average, the adult auricle measures 6.5 cm in vertical height and 3.5 cm in width. The posterior margin is angled anteriorly approximately 15 degrees from vertical.

of the auricle is angled posteriorly approximately 15 degrees from vertical, with the posterior edge of the auricle roughly parallel to the slope of the dorsum of the nose.

NOMENCLATURE

There are over 40 terms in the literature, including cup ear, lop ear, snail shell ear, and bat ear, describing abnormalities of the auricle relating to size, shape, or position. To avoid confusion, the term "prominauris" can be applied to any ear that is prominent or outstanding. The most common causes of abnormal positioning of the auricle are absence of the antihelical fold, prominence of the conchal cartilage, or anterior angulation of the lobule. The term "macrotia" can be applied to larger than average-sized ears related to excess height or width of the cartilage framework or excess length or size of the lobule. "Microtia" can be used to describe any ear smaller than average size. Thought to be related to factors interfering with normal development of the first and second branchial arches, microtia occurs in 1:7000 live births. High maternal fevers and exposure to ototoxic medications, radiation, rubella, thalidomide, vitamin B deficiency, and retinoic acid in the first trimester have all been implicated as possible causes (6).

PROMINENT AURICLE

Surgical treatment of prominent auricles begins with a meticulous evaluation of the angular or structural anomolies producing the deformity. A cephaloconchal angle greater than 90 degrees or an auriculomastoid angle greater than 40 degrees suggests conchal excess. A scaphoconchal angle greater than 120 degrees suggests absence of an antihelical fold. A distance of greater than 20 mm between the helical rim and the skull can result from either conchal excess or absent antihelical fold (Fig. 5). Lobular position and angulation should also be assessed in presurgical evaluation of the prominent ear. After meticulous evaluation of the abnormal auricle, the surgeon should plan to re-establish more normal angular and dimensional relationships.

Surgical techniques have run the gamut from skin excision only to cartilage scoring, cross hatching and shaving, to cartilage excision, conchal setback techniques, and mattress suture techniques. A synthesis of several of these techniques is often required to achieve excellent results in treatment of the prominent ear. In the majority of cases, some combination of a mattress suture reconstitution of the antihelical fold, varying amounts of conchal cartilage disc excision, and a concha-to-mastoid setback technique is performed.

Operative Markings

Preoperative planning consists of applying downward and posterior pressure on the superior helical rim to establish where the new antihelical fold will be created. A 25 gauge needle is dipped in methylene blue and used to pierce the anterior skin,

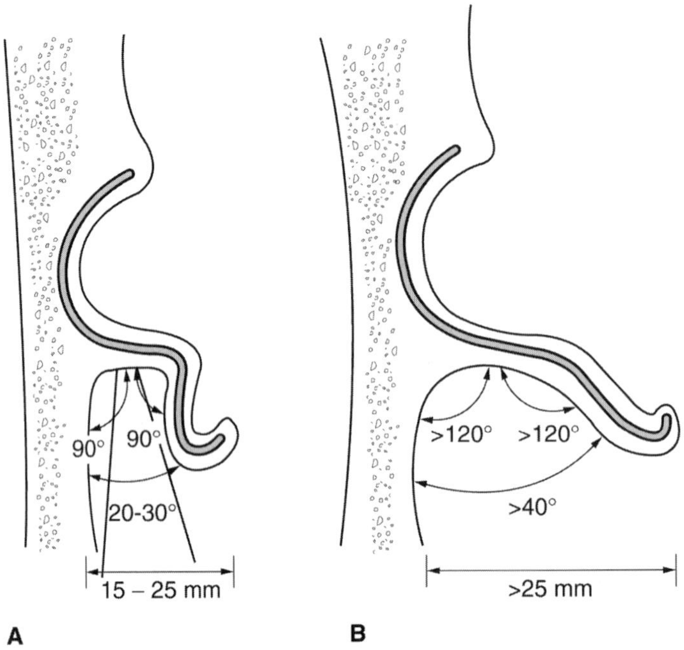

Figure 5 A. Normal cephaloconchal angle of 90 degrees. Normal scaphoconchal angle of approximately 90 degrees. Normal auriculomastoid angle of 20–30 degrees that corresponds to a distance of 15–25 mm between the helix and skull mastoid. B. Obtuse cephaloconchal and scaphoconchal angles greater than 120 degrees each. Abnormal auriculomastoid angle greater than 40 degrees with a distance greater than 25 mm between helix and skull.

cartilage, and posterior skin to mark the cartilage along the proposed new fold. Some surgeons prefer to place the needles approximately 8 mm from either side of the proposed fold to leave approximately 16 mm between needle marks and allow for creation of a natural antihelical fold. Next, a postauricular incision is marked approximately 1 cm onto the posterior cartilage, parallel to the post auricular sulcus. This incision should lie posterior to the needle insertion marks. If necessary, the incision can be converted to an elliptical excision of skin to address postauricular skin excess. A small volume of 1% lidocaine with 1:100,000 epinephrine is infiltrated in a submucoperichondrial plane to help hydrodissect the skin and perichondrium off the cartilage. The postauricular skin and perichondrium are dissected anteriorly to the free edge of the helical rim, with dissection carried approximately 5 mm onto the anterior surface of the auricular cartilage as well. This allows creation of the new fold without binding of the skin at the helical margin.

Mustardé Suture Placement

After adequate exposure, three to five Mustardé sutures of 4-0 Mersilene are placed. The sutures are placed in a horizontal mattress fashion, passing through the cartilage and anterior perichondrium but not through the anterior skin. This placement is crucial: including the anterior perichondrium helps to prevent the sutures from pulling through the cartilage and keeping the suture material beneath the anterior skin helps to prevent exposure of suture material and potential ulceration and extrusion. All sutures are placed and held, then sequentially tied as the sharpness of the new antihelical fold is assessed. Placement of sutures too close to the helical rim should be avoided to minimize unnatural folding of the rim posteriorly (Fig. 6).

Upon accurate placement of the Mustardé sutures, the ear should be returned to anatomical position and evaluated for the degree of conchal setback required to create a natural auriculomastoid angle and appropriate helical-rim-to-mastoid distance. In some situations, very little needs to be done to achieve a natural contour of the ear, and the mattress suture technique is adequate. In patients requiring moderate conchal setback, the technique, as described by Furnas, is used to place anchoring sutures of 4-0 Mersilene from the conchal cartilage back to the mastoid periosteum (9). Care must be exercised in placing the mastoid sutures sufficiently posterior to prevent anterior displacement of the conchal cartilage that can result in cartilaginous canal stenosis (Fig. 7).

In cases of significant conchal cartilage memory that interferes with adequate retrodisplacement of the auricle, partial-thickness discs of cartilage can be removed to weaken the cartilage memory. In ears with a very significant excess of conchal cartilage, resection of strips of cartilage, parallel to the postauricular sulcus, may be required prior to placement of conchal/mastoid sutures. If a strip excision technique is used, care must be taken to avoid creating a sharp edge of cartilage anteriorly.

After creation of the antihelical fold and conchal setback, the angular relationships of the ear are again evaluated. Necessary changes are made prior to turning attention to the contralateral ear. After all cartilaginous modifications are completed on both sides, the amount of excess postauricular skin is evaluated and an appropriate amount of skin is excised in fusiform fashion. This excision should be done conservatively to avoid obliterating the postauricular sulcus or creating unnecessary tension on the skin closure. Skin is closed in a single layer using 5-0 nylon (Fig. 8).

Special Problems

An often overlooked element of otoplasty is treatment of the abnormally proportioned, or angled, lobule. Lobular excess or anterior displacement of the lobule should be addressed by judicious excision of skin from the posterior aspect of the lobule. Debulking of the fibrofatty tissue of the lobule is performed, as required, to address excess size or thickness. Modification of the lobular size or position often helps to create a more harmonious balance between the upper and lower auricular anatomy.

In some patients, an excessively large auricle can be present, compounding the angular abnormalities leading to prominauris. Treatment of the noncartilaginous lobule has been described. When the cartilaginous framework is abnormally large, wedge or stellate resections of skin and cartilage may be required to decrease the vertical or anteroposterior proportion of the ear to within normal limits (Fig. 9). The technique used is similar to wedge resections for cutaneous neoplasms of the auricle. Prior to skin closure, it is important to reapproximate the cartilage carefully using a clear nonabsorbable suture (e.g., 5-0 clear Prolene) to prevent widening of the scar or notching at the helical rim. This size reduction can be performed simultaneously with antihelical fold creation and conchal setback techniques.

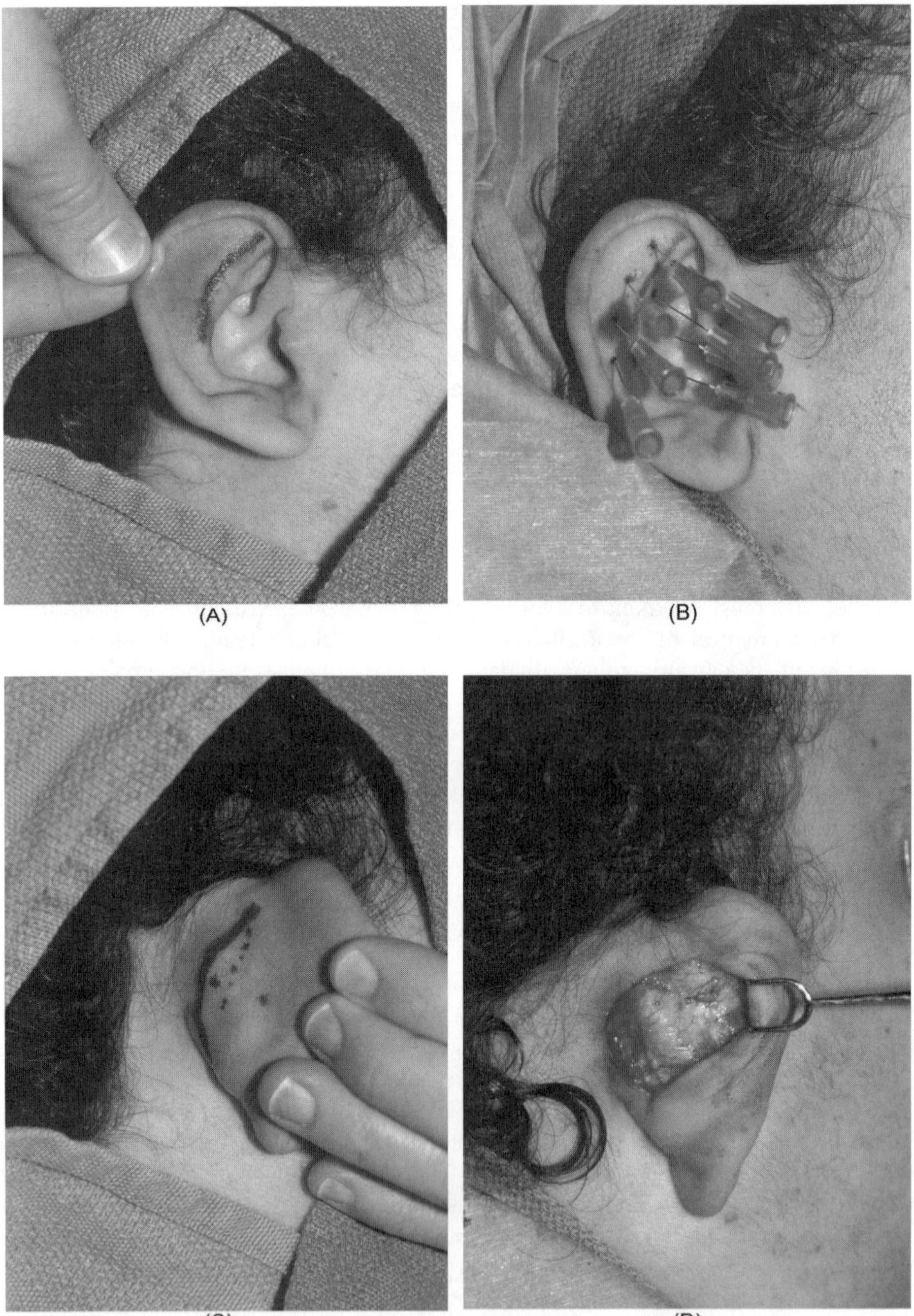

(A) (B) (C) (D)

Figure 6 A. Creation of the proposed antihelical fold with forward pulsion of the auricular helix. B. Placement of needles dipped in methylene blue approximately 8 mm anterior and posterior to proposed new antihelical fold. C. Creation of incision on posterior auricular surface approximately 1 cm posterior to sulcus. D. Elevation of skin over posterior aspect of ear extends to helical rim and approximately 5 mm on anterior aspect or ear.

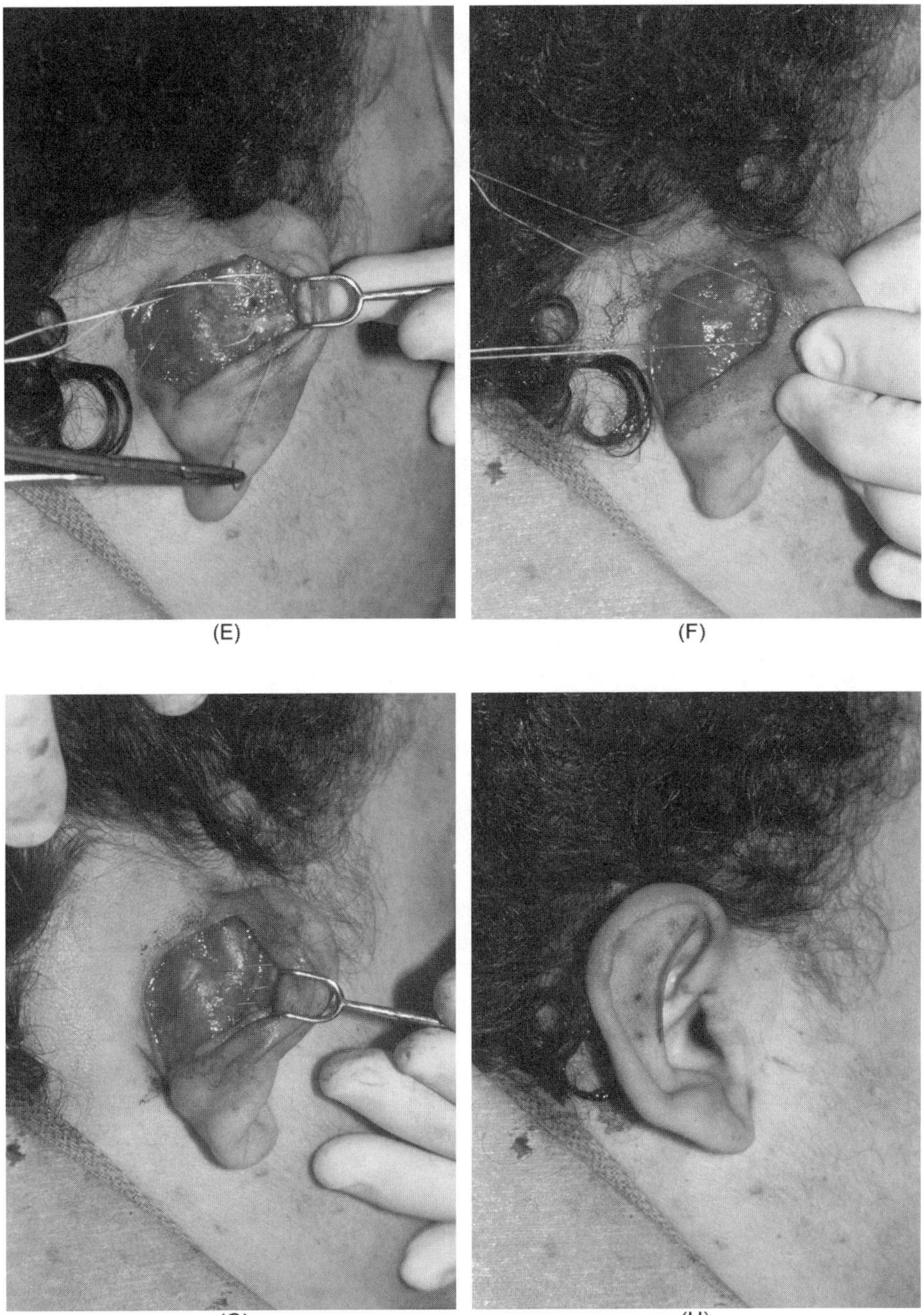

(E) (F) (G) (H)

Figure 6 (Continued). E. Placement of Mustardé mattress sutures in horizontal fashion leaving approximately 2 mm between sutures. F. Placement and tagging of sutures to facilitate exposure for each sequential suture. G. Sutures tied down to create new antihelical fold. H. Antihelical fold created along proposed site.

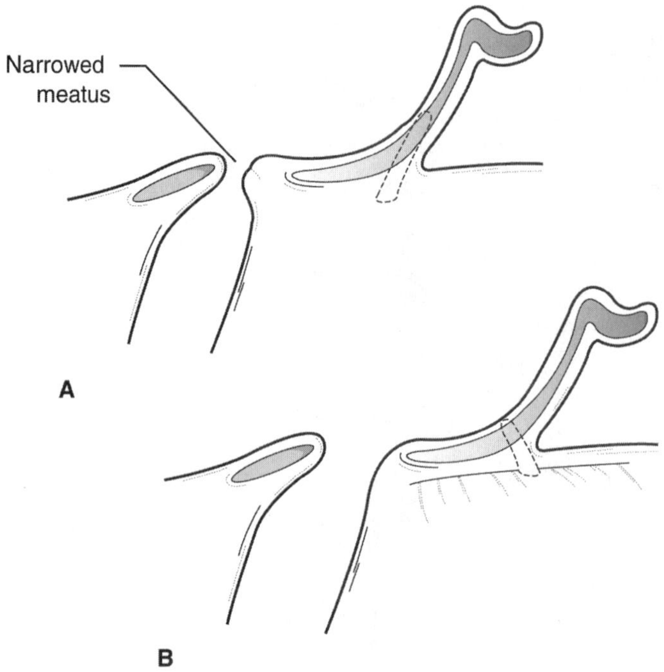

Figure 7 A. Conchomastoid suture secured too far anteriorly to mastoid periosteum will advance anterior conchal margin forward, compromising meatal opening. B. Properly placed conchomastoid suture will maintain meatal patency.

Postoperative Care

Postoperative dressing is extremely important in otoplasty procedures. Strips of iodinated petrolatum gauze are carefully insinuated into all recesses of the ear anteriorly followed by placement of petrolatum-impregnated cotton over the strips and in the postauricular sulcus. A mastoid-type dressing is applied with extreme caution to prevent folding of any part of the helix or lobule while just enough pressure is applied to prevent hematoma formation without ischemia. The dressing is taken down on the first postoperative day and a less compressive dressing is applied until postoperative day 5, when the dressing and sutures are removed.

Complications

Complications in otoplasty are numerous and can range from very simple to very severe. The most common complication is the presence of asymmetry after correction of the prominent ears. In the majority of cases, the asymmetry is minimal. Most patients, noting a dramatic improvement in the appearance of their previously prominent auricles, are not disturbed by the difference from side to side. If the asymmetry is significant, correction of the undercorrected or overcorrected side is an option.

Undercorrection is seen especially after otoplasty in adults who have less pliable cartilage and in those with very thick cartilage or significant conchal excess. Relaxation or pulling through of Mustardé sutures can result in loss of the antihelical fold

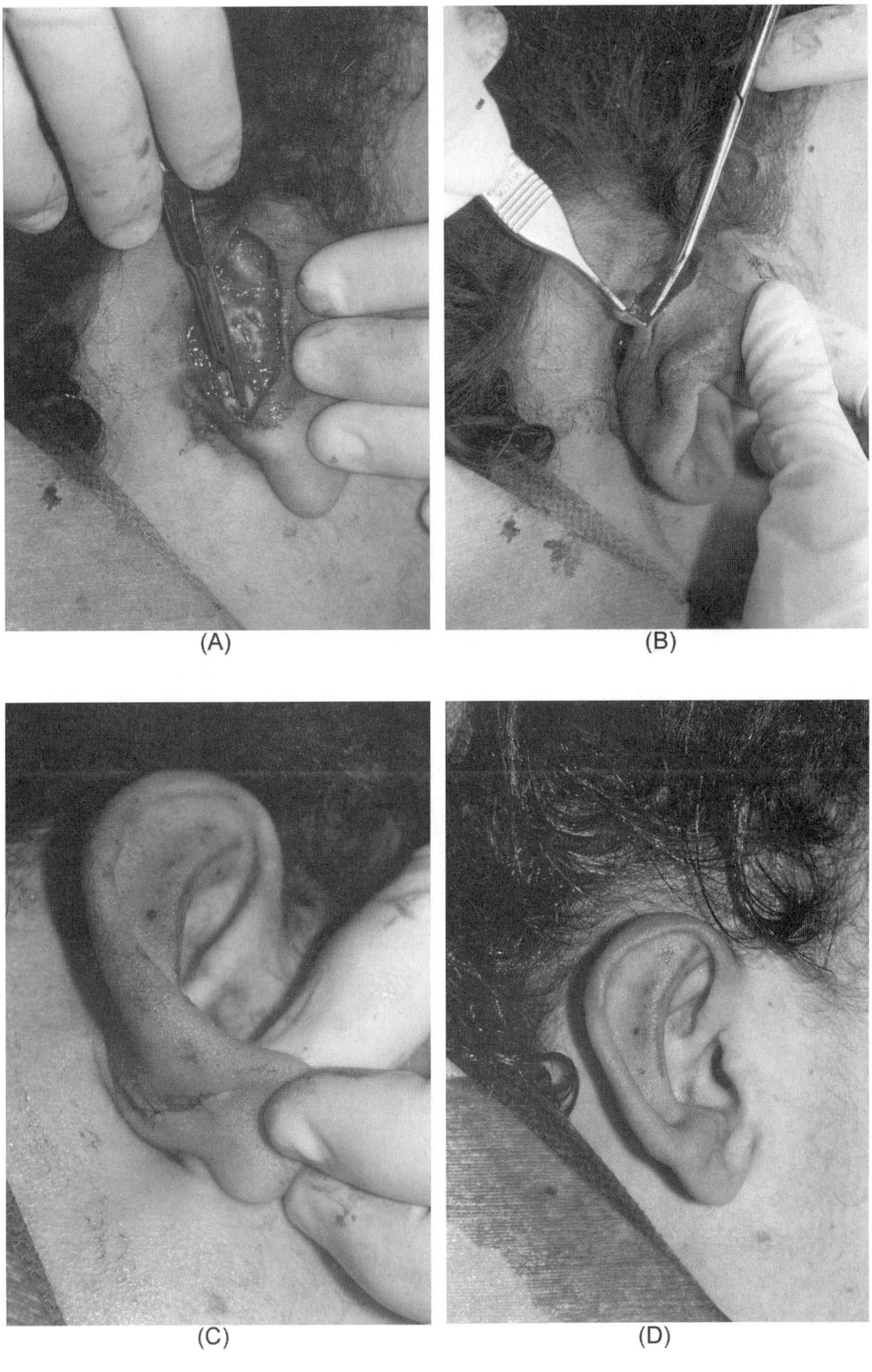

Figure 8 A. Removal of disks to weaken cartilage and allow for conchal setback with less tendency toward loss of correction. B. Appropriate amount of excess skin removed in fusiform fashion. C. Anteriorly displaced lobule addressed by horizontal skin excision posteriorly. D. Completed creation of antihelical fold, conchal setback, and lobule repositioning.

sharpness. Weakening or release of conchal setback sutures can result in prominence of the affected side.

Overcorrection can result from mattress sutures being placed too tightly, or overaggressive conchal setback from excess cartilage or skin excision, or inappropriate placement of conchal setback sutures (Fig. 10). Overcorrection often requires release of the offending sutures and may require tissue replacement in the form of postauricular flap advancement or skin grafting techniques.

Other complications include suture granulomas, bowstringing of sutures from mattress placement, or extrusion of sutures through cartilage. Keloids can be seen in darkly pigmented persons, and preoperative inquiry regarding abnormal wound healing is important. Auricular hematoma can occur if meticulous hemostasis is not achieved at the time of surgery or if an inadequate postoperative compressive dressing is used. Conversely, ischemia of the ear can occur from an inappropriately tight occlusive dressing. Chondritis can be seen in the wake of a hematoma or as a delayed complication of otoplasty.

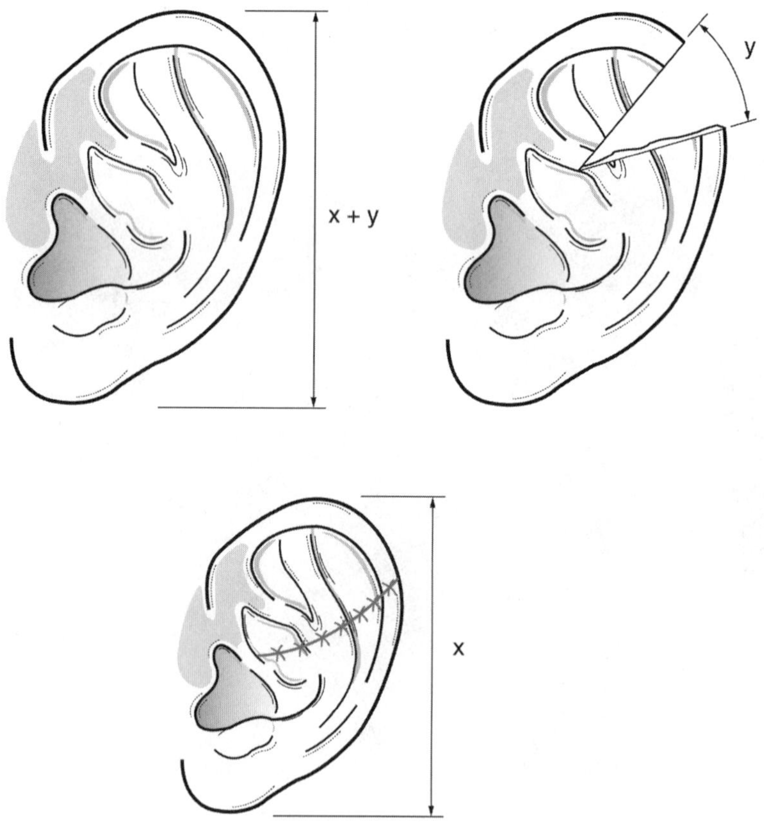

A

Figure 9 A. A simple wedge excision with linear closure in layers can correct a minor macrotia. B. More significant macrotia may require a stellate excision to avoid cupping of the ear upon closure.

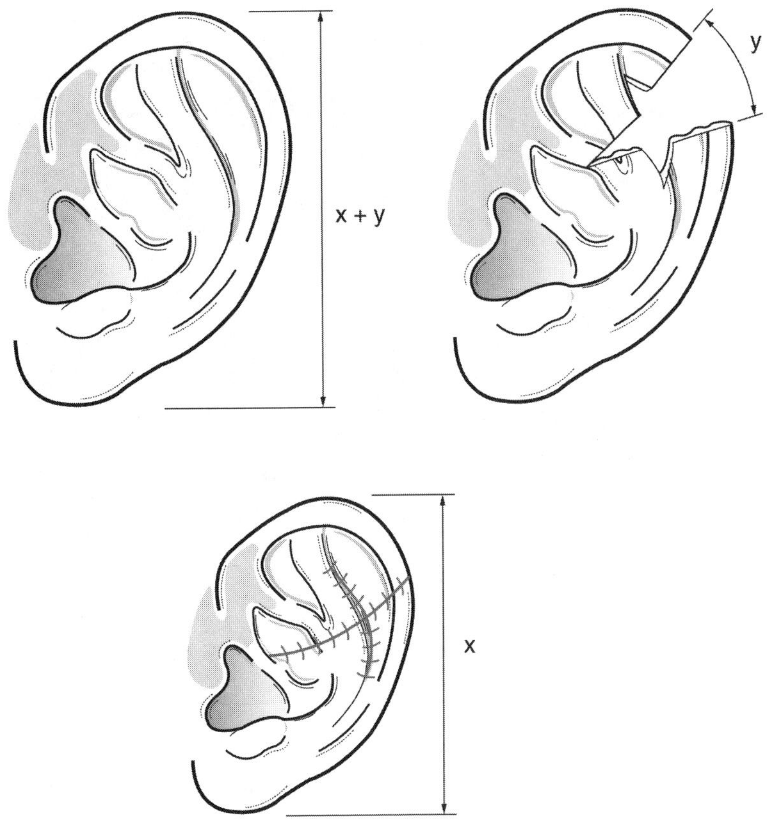

B

Figure 9 Continued

Successful otoplasty relies on careful preoperative evaluation and planning and appropriate treatment of each of the abnormal angles or dimensions of the prominent ear. Long-term follow-up is required, as there may be loss of the correction over time (Fig. 11).

MICROTIA

Microtia can be a devastating anomaly for both parent and child. The deformity can range from a well-formed ear that is simply too small to a grouping of cartilaginous remnants and skin tags that are unrecognizable as an auricle. Even in the most severe cases, a remnant of fibrofatty tissue will be present at the inferior pole of the ear remnant. The condition is most often unilateral but can be bilateral in as many as 27% of patients (6). Abnormal development of the auricle is associated with other first and second arch developmental abnormalities such as hemifacial microsomia, mandibular hypoplasia, and underdevelopment of the ear canal and middle ear structures in greater than 50% of cases (6).

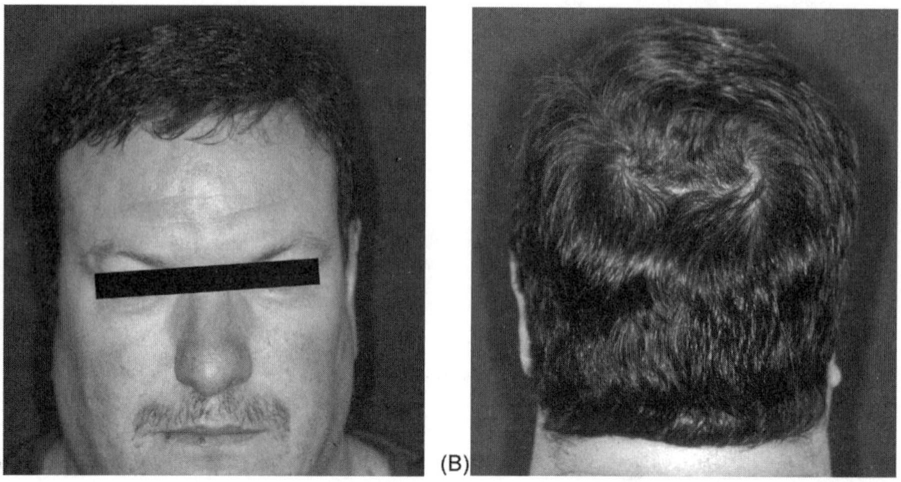

(A) (B)

Figure 10 A. Anterior view of overcorrection from excess conchal setback. B. Posterior view.

Classification

Several classifications of microtia have been popularized. They range from the very simple wide categories as proposed by Rogers, to the more complex classifications that describe the different types of deformity within each subset as proposed by Tanzer (4) and Weerda (7). Among the most useful is the Marx classification that describes three grades of deformity (8). In grade I, the auricle is small, but the different structures of the ear are clearly recognizable. In grade II, the ear is smaller than normal and the auricular remnant retains some structural resemblance to the helix, although less well defined. In grade III, the auricular configuration is absent (Fig. 12). This latter classification seems to be most applicable to microtic deformities by categorizing an abnormal auricle with a grading system and adding verbal descriptions of the specific subunit anomolies to help guide the proposed reconstruction.

Timing of Surgical Repair

The timing of surgical correction of microtia is determined by several factors. By age 4–5, children begin to develop body image and by age 5 or 6, with increasing social interaction in school, the abnormal ear draws greater attention and the child is subject to ridicule. It is well described that the majority of auricular growth occurs by age 5; however, the auricle does not reach full adult size until age 8 or 9 (6). It is also important to consider the development of the ribs to allow for harvest of adequate donor cartilage to construct the new auricular framework. Age 6 tends to be the earliest at which costal cartilage and ear size are adequate. Construction at this age also spares the child undue ridicule by his or her peers. If desired, it is easier to delay auricular construction in girls because they can cover the deformity with

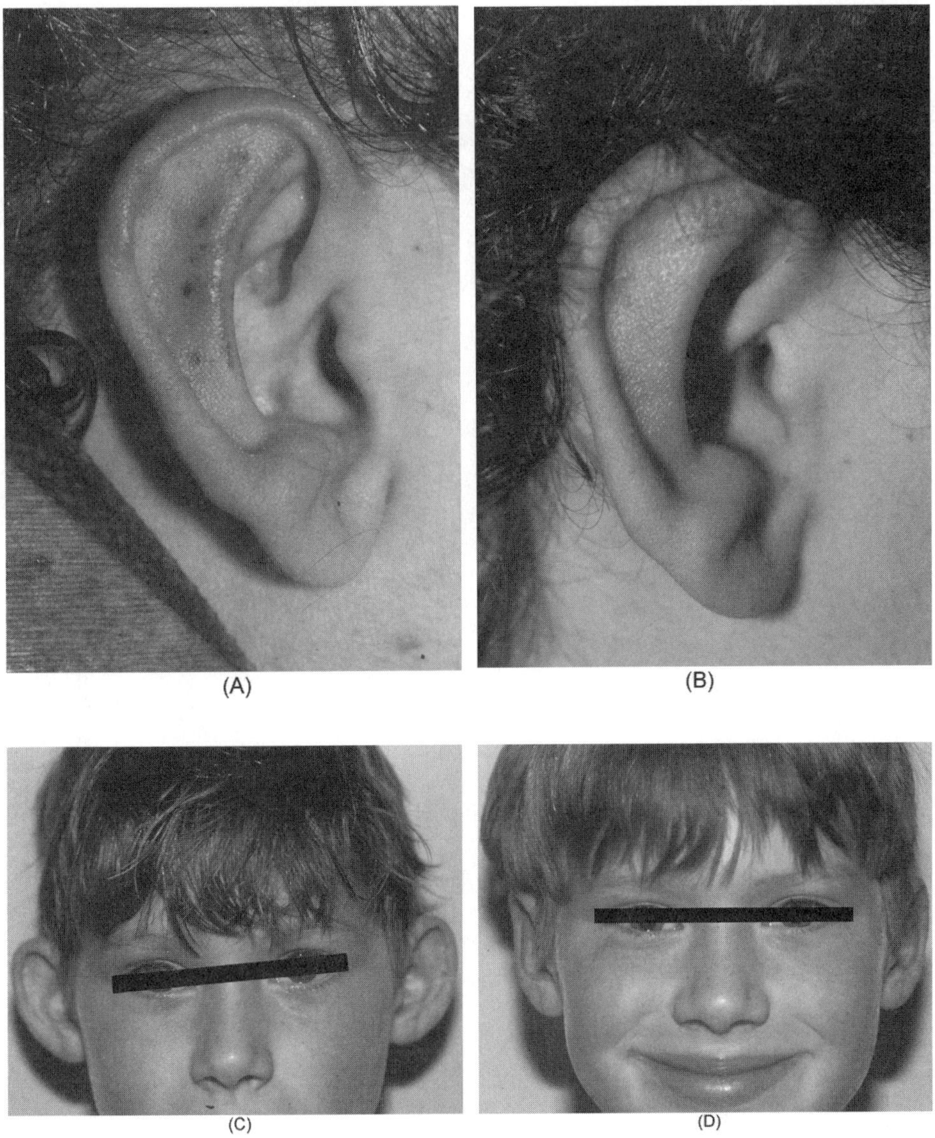

Figure 11 A. Correction of patient in Figure 8 at completion of case. B. Maintenance of correction 18 months postoperatively. C. Preoperative view of child with prominauris at age 6. D. Maintenance of correction 20 months postoperatively.

longer hair. Some parents will encourage their sons with microtia to wear long hair to hide the abnormality and allow for construction at a later age.

Once the decision is made to begin auricular construction, careful planning of the numerous steps is necessary. An otologist with expertise in aural atresia repair is consulted to determine the feasibility and timing of otological intervention. A computed tomographic (CT) scan is obtained in axial and coronal planes to determine the location and degree of aeration of the middle ear, the condition of the

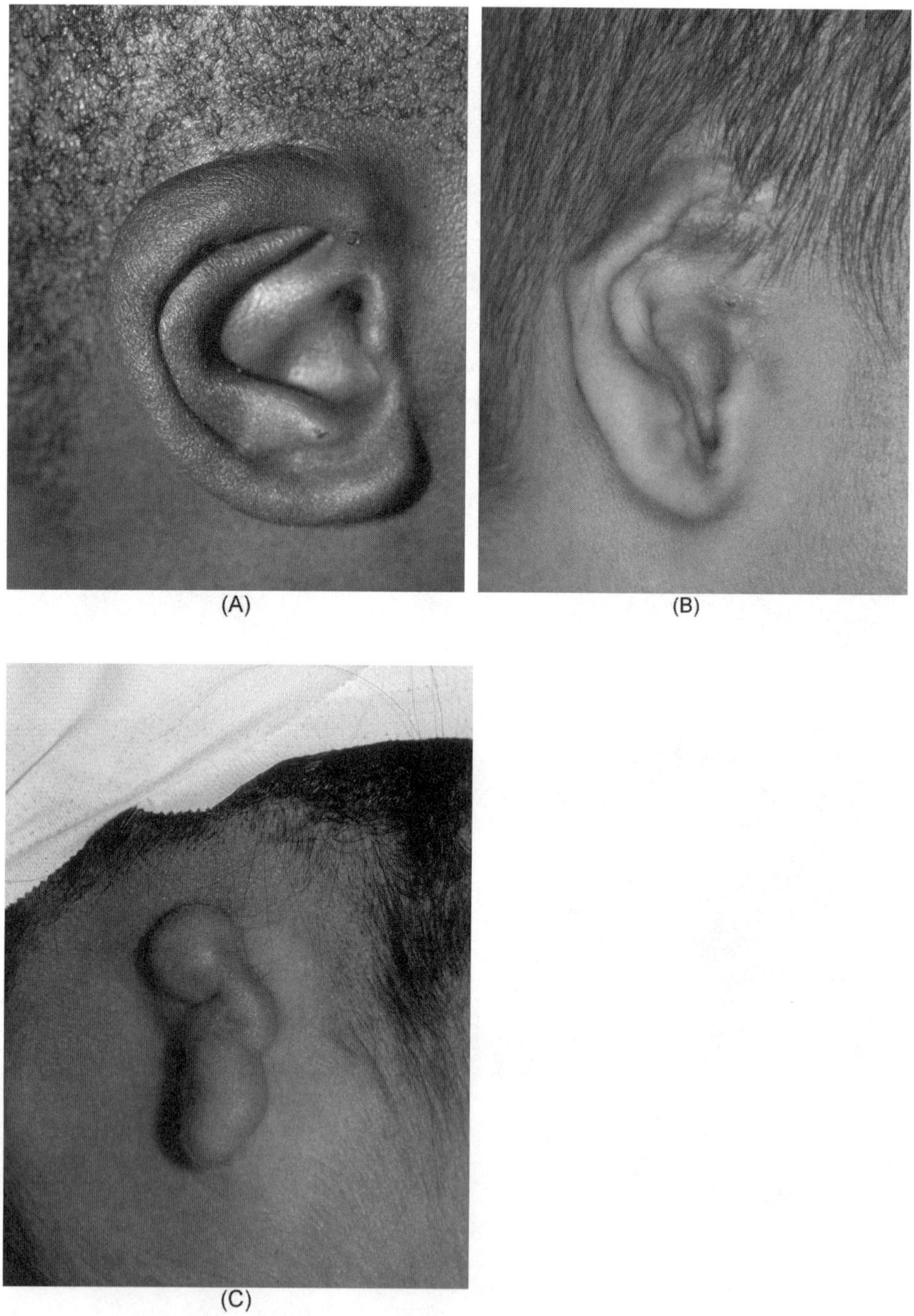

Figure 12 A. Grade I microtia: a smaller than average auricle with clearly recognizable features. B. Grade II microtia: smaller than average with less well-defined features. C. Grade III microtia: absence of auricular configuration.

ossicles (if present), and the position of the facial nerve and tegmen. Should the child or adult be deemed a candidate for reconstruction of the canal and middle ear, the position of the meatus must be carefully agreed upon.

Auricular construction generally follows the sequence of framework fabrication, lobule transposition, creation of the canal and middle ear reconstruction (if indicated), conchal excavation and tragus creation, and elevation of the framework with creation of the postauricular sulcus.

Framework Fabrication

Framework fabrication has been attempted with allograft rib and preformed Silastic. With the former, resorption and loss of architecture were common and with the latter, immediate or delayed infection or extrusion commonly occurred. Recent use of porous polyethelyne has been reported. However, the long-term results are not known and the risk of infection or soft tissue breakdown will likely be similar to other synthetic materials. Autologous costal cartilage remains the best-tolerated material yielding the most reproducible and lasting results. The first use of costal

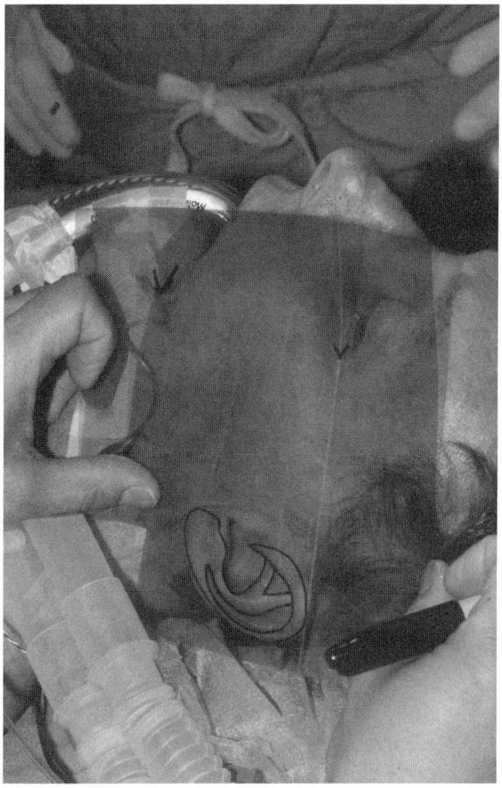

Figure 13 Size and position of normal ear are traced on film along with necessary landmarks (oral commissure, lateral canthus, lateral brow).

cartilage was described by Gillies and has been popularized and used extensively by Tanzer (10–12), Brent (13–16), and Ruder (6).

A thorough preoperative examination should include assessing the skin overlying the proposed construction site; identifying the location and nature of auricular vestiges that are present and the contralateral normal ear, if present; and evaluating the chest anatomy and rib size. Meticulous measurements of height and width of the normal ear and its position and angle relative to the eyebrow, nose, and mouth are taken. These relations are easily traced onto unexposed x-ray film with an indelible marker (Fig. 13). In the case of bilateral microtia, the standard dimensions, angles, and relations are used to construct the first ear, after which the second ear is size- and position-matched to the first. A second tracing of the contours of the normal auricle is used to guide the carving of the microtic ear framework. This tracing should be slightly smaller than the normal ear cartilage framework to account for the overlying soft tissue envelope (Fig. 14). The tracings are scored onto the x-ray film with an 18 gauge needle or #11 blade and placed in povidone–iodine solution for use intraoperatively.

Cartilage is harvested from the contralateral chest with the synchondrotic ribs 6 and 7 most commonly used for the main framework. Adequate exposure of the ribs can be achieved through a 5–8 cm incision created parallel and approximately 2 cm cephalad to the free border of rib 9. After exposure of the appropriate segments of costal cartilage, the x-ray film template is positioned with the ribs in situ to

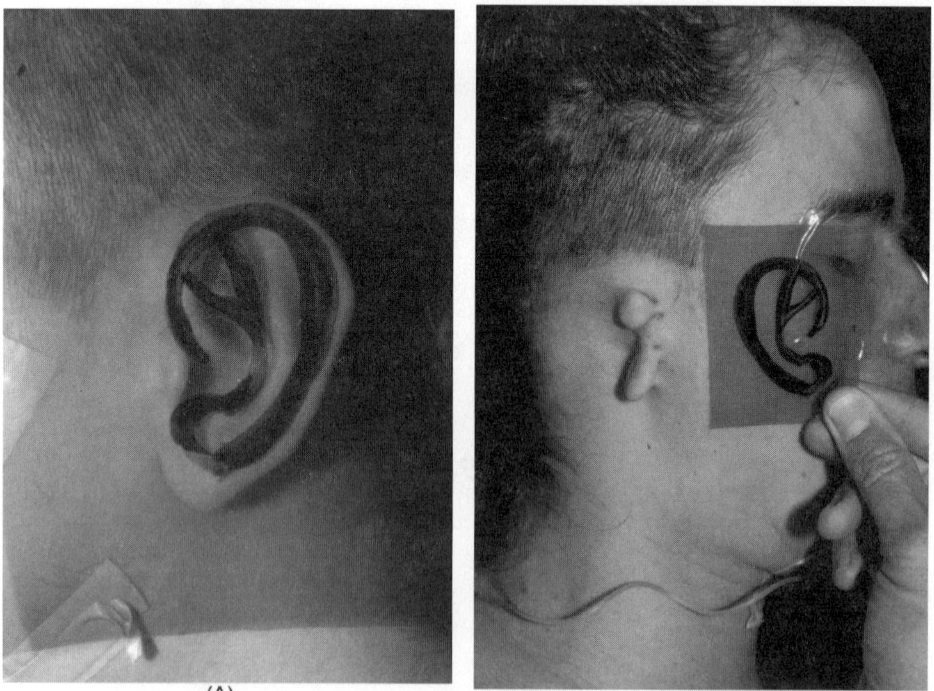

(A) (B)

Figure 14 A. Template of the normal ear traced on unexposed x-ray film. B. Traced image reversed to be used for carving cartilage framework.

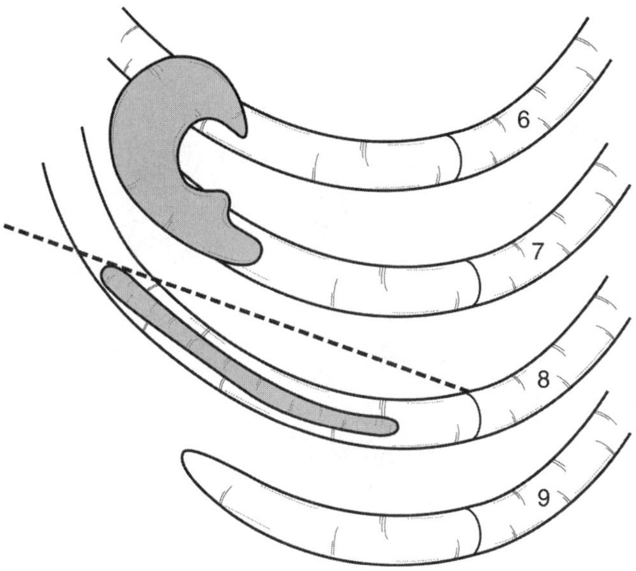

Figure 15 Costal cartilage is harvested for the main framework from the synchondrosis of ribs 6–7. Template is positioned in situ to determine ideal segment of rib(s) to harvest. Cartilage to be fashioned into the helical rim is harvested from the eighth rib.

determine how much rib will need to be taken for the main framework. Rib 8 or 9 is used for harvest of an additional section of cartilage that will be fashioned into the helical rim and sutured to the main framework (Fig. 15). Given the thickness of the soft tissue envelop that will cover the framework, compared to the thin skin that covers the normal auricle, the newly sculpted framework requires exaggerated contours to better resemble the normal ear architecture. As much perichondrium as possible is left on the carved rib cartilage. This helps to anchor the new framework to surrounding soft tissues, encourage neovascularization, and decrease resorption. The x-ray film template is used to guide the carving using a combination of #15, #10, and #20 blades and various U and V gouges (Fig. 16). The gouges can be found at art supply stores and are generally used for carving wood or linoleum.

After the main framework has been carved, the free segment of rib is thinned adequately so that it can be bent to create the helix. Sufficient thickness of this roll should be maintained as this attached segment will give the new auricle much of its anterior projection. The free piece is sutured to the edge of the main framework using 5-0 clear Prolene (Fig. 17). At this point, the framework is set aside and the soft tissue pocket is planned and created.

Framework Placement

An incision is made anterior to the microtic ear. Any remnants of cartilage are carefully removed with extra consideration given to not violating the skin flap. The recipient pocket is then created with meticulous undermining in a subdermal plane, keeping the flap as thin as possible while still maintaining the subdermal plexus. The pocket should be developed approximately 2 cm larger circumferentially than

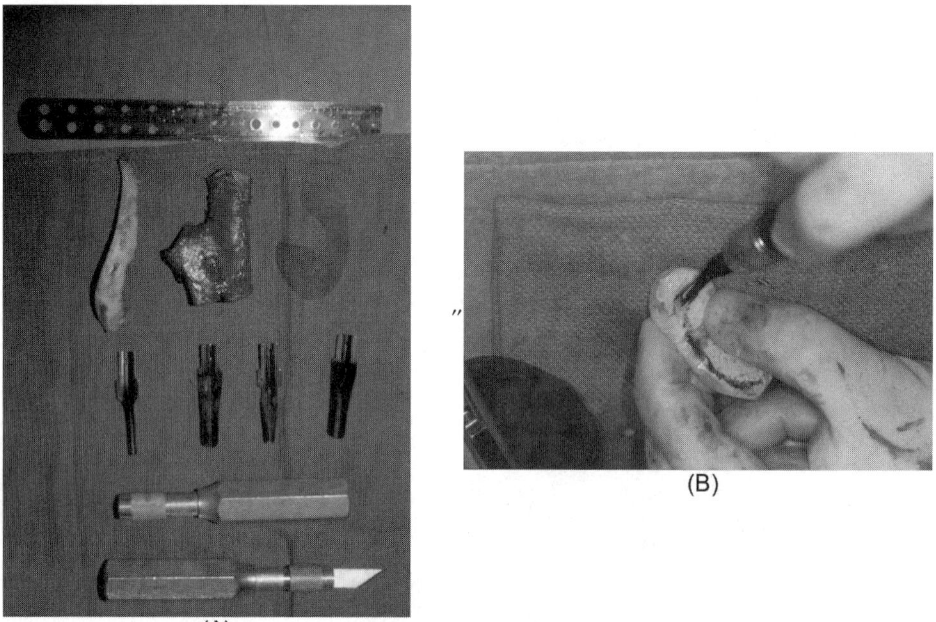

(A) (B)

Figure 16 A. A selection of blades and U- and V-shaped gouges is necessary to carve the cartilage framework accurately. B. Gouges are particularly helpful in excavating the scapha and triangular fossa.

the actual framework size to allow for easy placement of the cartilage and to minimize excess compression of the framework.

Placement of the framework is attempted with modification of the pocket as required. The inferior end of the cartilage is inserted and the framework is rotated into the pocket. When the pocket is deemed adequate, the framework is removed,

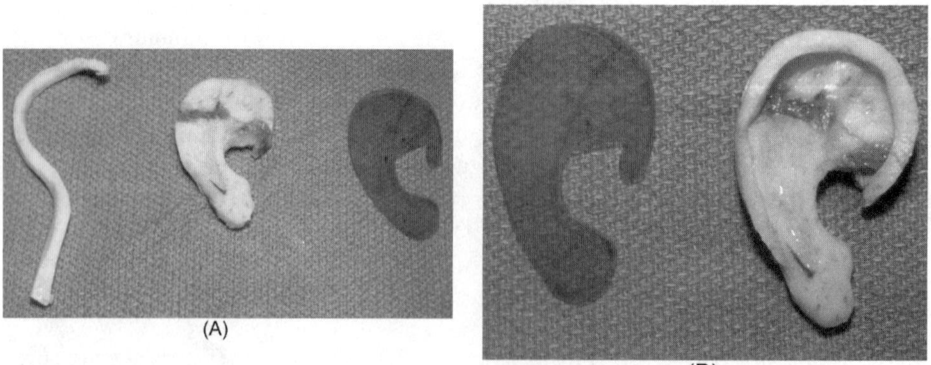

(A) (B)

Figure 17 A. The helix is created by suturing the free carved segment from rib 8 to the main framework. Adequate height of the newly created helical rim is imperative. B. The completed framework ready for implantation.

inspected for integrity, and two narrow round suction drains are placed anterior and posterior to the proposed framework position.

The cartilage is reintroduced and the incision is coapted while suction is applied (Fig. 18). If adequate suction is generated, the contours of the cartilage will be clearly visible. The pocket is flushed with saline to ensure patency of the drains. The absence of adequate suction or the presence of seroma or hematoma can result in acute chondritis and loss of framework integrity. The skin incision is closed with 5-0 nylon, and the sulci are packed with petrolatum-impregnated gauze strips followed by petrolatum-impregnated cotton. A mildly compressive mastoid-type dressing is placed and the drains are kept on 60 mmHg continuous suction for 48 h. The mastoid dressing is removed on the first postoperative day to allow one to check for hematoma formation or drain failure. The dressing is reapplied until postoperative day 2 when the drains are removed. Upon discharge, a removable protective dressing is placed over the operated ear. Sutures are removed in 5 days. The patient is instructed to keep the dressing on at all times for 7 days and thereafter only while asleep for an additional 3 weeks.

Lobule Repair

The next stage, lobule transposition, is performed approximately 3 months after framework construction. Generally, even in the more severe grade III microtia cases, a fibrofatty lobular remnant persists. The remnant generally lies anterosuperior to its proper anatomical location and, therefore, needs to be transposed inferiorly and superiorly to be attached to the inferior aspect of the newly constructed framework. Where an inadequate lobular remnant is present, the cartilage framework should be carved in such a way to provide extra length inferiorly to help create the new lobule. The inferior aspect of the framework is de-epithelialized, and a Z-plasty technique is used to transpose the remnant into correct anatomical position. The remnant is split into anterior and posterior leaflets to facilitate creating a hanging lobule and to allow for insetting and suturing the lobular flap anteriorly and posteriorly (Fig. 19).

Atresia Repair

At this stage, after consultation with the neuro-otologist, a decision is made regarding atresia repair. Some otologists prefer to perform atresia repair at this stage, prior to framework elevation, particularly if a postauricular approach will be used. Others would consider performing atresia repair at the same time as framework elevation. Yet others prefer to delay otological intervention until after all stages of the microtia repair are completed. These different approaches to possible atresia repair underscore the need for close cooperation between otologist and facial plastic surgeon during the microtia/atresia reconstruction.

Framework Elevation

The next stage in auricle construction is framework elevation with postauricular skin grafting. This procedure creates a postauricular sulcus, but will not significantly project the framework anteriorly. For this reason, projection is best achieved by implanting a deeply carved framework at the initial stage of construction. An

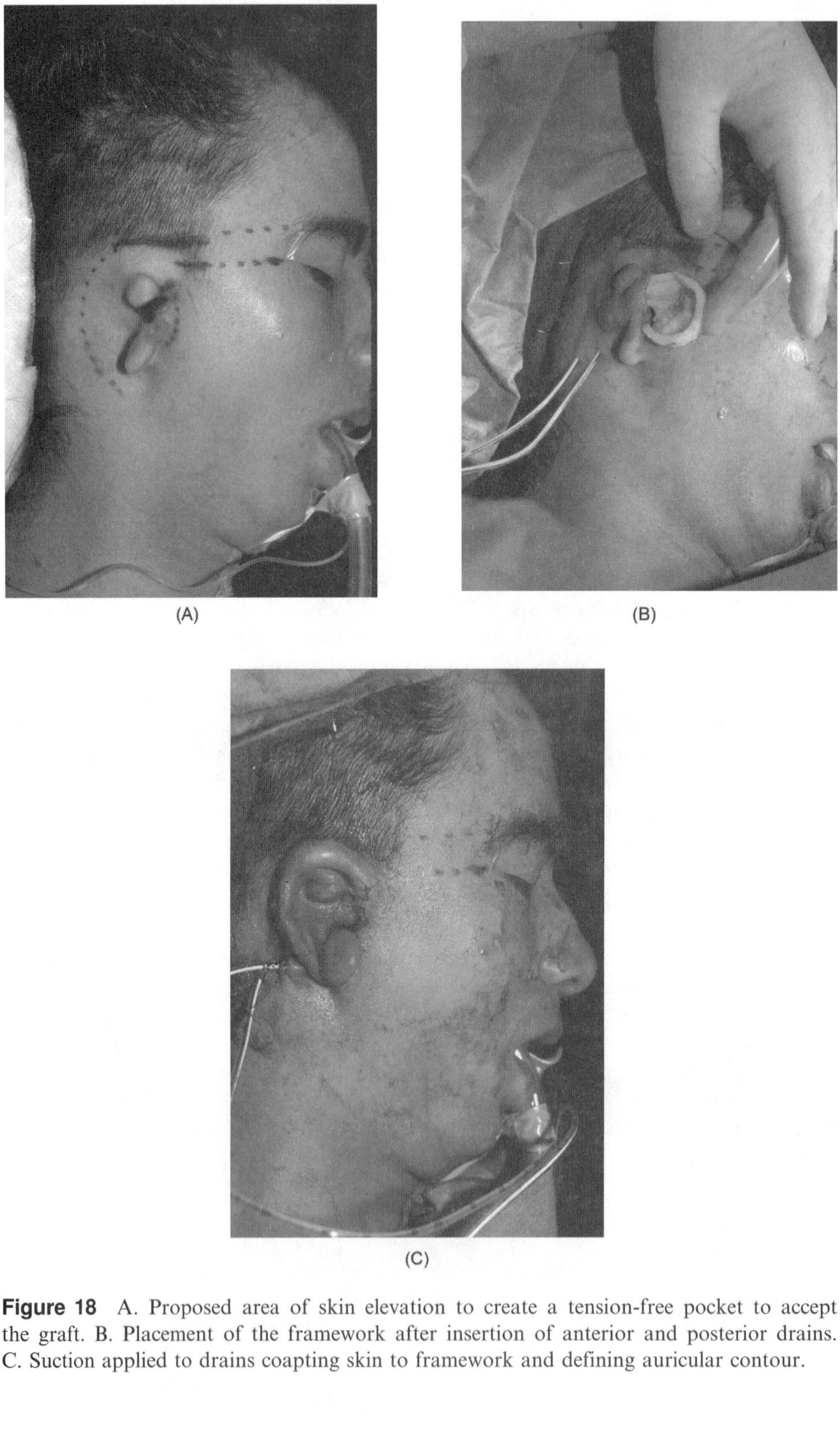

(A) (B) (C)

Figure 18 A. Proposed area of skin elevation to create a tension-free pocket to accept the graft. B. Placement of the framework after insertion of anterior and posterior drains. C. Suction applied to drains coapting skin to framework and defining auricular contour.

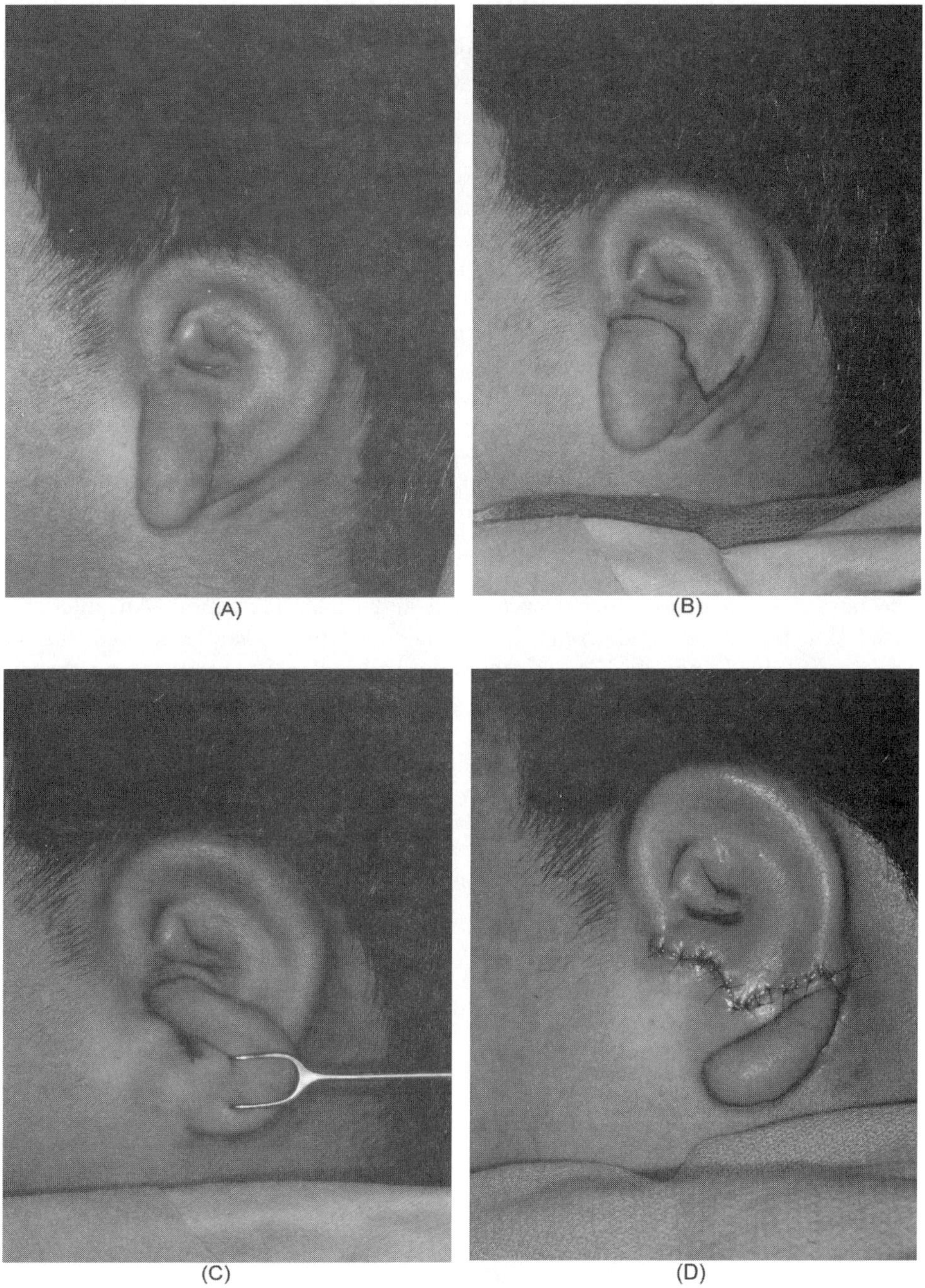

Figure 19 A. Lobular remnant anterior and superior to normal anatomical position. B. Proposed incision to transpose lobule posteriorly and inferiorly. C. Proposed movement of posteriorly pedicled lobule. D. Transposed remnant sutured in place.

incision over the helical rim is created carefully without exposing the cartilage framework. The framework is dissected away from the scalp, maintaining as much attached soft tissue as possible. The scalp is undermined and advanced into the postauricular sulcus and secured down to periosteum using 3-0 or 4-0 PDS. The posterior surface of the framework is covered with a thick, split-thickness skin graft harvested from the buttock or lateral thigh or a thin, full-thickness graft harvested from the abdomen or scapular region (16). Although full-thickness grafts carry a certain risk of incomplete take, the decreased contraction of these grafts helps to maintain an open sulcus and are preferred over split-thickness grafts. We have also noted less donor site morbidity in harvesting full-thickness grafts as described. After application of the graft, it is perforated to allow for drainage. The sutures used to secure the edges of the skin graft are tied over a rolled Xeroform bolster that is left in place for 7 days (Fig. 20). To create enough bolster compression, 3-0 silk is used to provide adequate suture strength and friction during knot tying. If adequate scalp advancement is not possible, the postauricular scalp can be skin grafted as well. Should there be a poor color or texture match, the grafted skin can be serially excised at a later stage.

Conchal Excavation and Tragus Formation

The next stage involves conchal excavation and tragus formation. An anteriorly based skin flap is elevated from the conchal bowl of the newly created auricle. The flap is folded upon itself anteriorly and a cartilage graft, harvested posteriorly

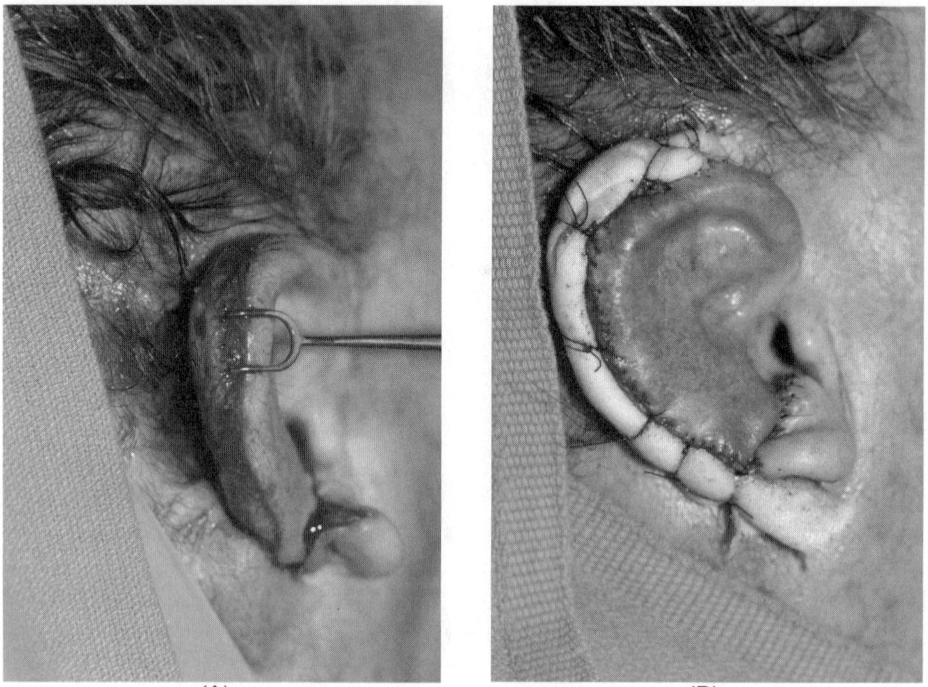

(A) (B)

Figure 20 A. Elevation of framework maintaining perichondrium on cartilage. B. Bolster technique used after placement of skin graft along posterior aspect of framework.

from the contralateral ear, is implanted in this fold of skin to create the tragus. The conchal bowl is excavated by removing soft tissue to approximate the depth and shadow of the normal side. The area is skin-grafted with a full-thickness graft harvested from the contralateral ear (Fig. 21). This harvest technique also allows the surgeon to position the normal ear posteriorly to approximate better the projection of the newly formed ear.

Microtia Repair

Bilateral microtia poses a functional concern regarding the adequacy of hearing and reconstructive concerns because there is no template to fashion the microtic ear to match the normal contralateral side. After CT scanning and auditory brainstem testing of the child with bilateral microtia, bone-conducting hearing aids are applied within the first 3–4 weeks of life (18). Similar planning is involved in the microtia repair as in unilateral cases with the exception of dimensions, contour, and positioning of the auricle being based on cephalometric norms. In addition, even closer cooperation is required with the otologist because early attempts at restoration of hearing are more of a concern in bilateral microtia/atresia cases. Microtia repair is staged starting with the ear more likely to benefit from atresia repair. Some surgeons choose to perform framework creation bilaterally at

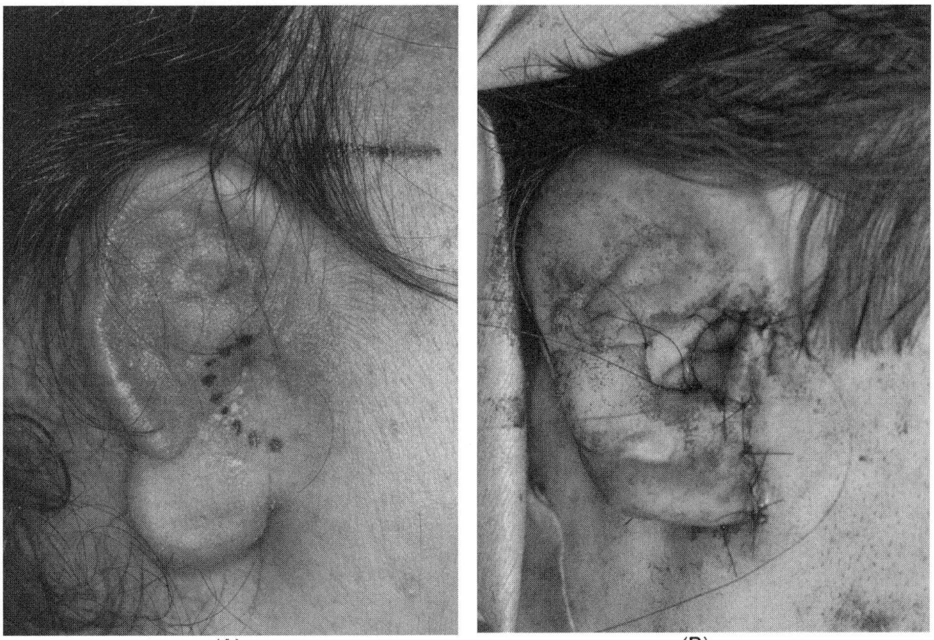

(A) (B)

Figure 21 A. Incision to be created along posterior aspect of conchal bowl. B. Different patient after conchal flap has been advanced anteriorly, folded upon itself, and sutured over a cartilage graft to create the tragus. The conchal flap donor site is grafted with full-thickness skin harvested from the posterior aspect of the contralateral ear.

the first stage; however, the risk of trauma to an operated side is greater using this protocol.

Complications

Myriad complications can occur during each of the stages of auricular construction. Immediate complications during stage I include the risk of pneumothorax, infection at the harvest site, skin ischemia or loss over the implanted cartilage framework, hematoma formation, and infection/chondritis of the framework. With meticulous costal cartilage harvesting, skin flap elevation, and the use of perioperative antibiotics and a two-suction drain system, the incidence of these complications is rare. Delayed loss of cartilage contour has been seen; however, avoidance of heat-generating burrs to contour the cartilage and ensuring adequate flap elevation to avoid significant soft tissue compression of the framework can help to minimize these risks. Malposition and poor projection of the new auricle are far more common complications. Meticulous measurement, pocket creation, and placement of the framework will prevent malposition, and exaggerated depth in the initial framework carving is imperative to ensure adequate projection. Cartilage exposure can occur during any of the stages of reconstruction. Meticulous wound care and prompt local flap coverage for nonhealing areas will help to salvage the remaining framework.

Secondary reconstruction of a failed microtia repair is generally limited by the integrity of the skin overlying the previous reconstruction. In some cases, the skin is sufficiently viable to reimplant a newly fashioned framework after removal of an infected or poorly positioned synthetic framework or a resorbed or poorly fashioned cartilage framework. In the presence of infection, the framework should be removed to allow for complete resolution of infection prior to any attempt at placement of a new framework. Most often, after failed initial repair, the vascularity of the skin in the area is poor, and dense scarring does not allow for use of this skin for further reconstruction. In these situations, the scarred tissue is excised and a new cartilage framework is placed and covered by a vascularized temporoparietal fascia flap and split-thickness skin graft (9,19,20).

SUMMARY

Correction of auricular deformities, ranging from minor angular abnormalities or malposition to near total absence of one or both ears, is a challenging undertaking for the facial plastic surgeon. A thorough understanding of the anatomy of the auricle and cephalometric relationships to other facial structures, and use of sound plastic surgical techniques and judgement are imperative for success in this challenging endeavor.

REFERENCES

1. Sadler TW: *Langman's Medical Embryology*. 5th Ed. Williams & Wilkins, Baltimore, 1985.
2. Wood-Jones F, Wen IC. The development of the external ear. J Anat 1934; 68:525.
3. Streeter GL. Development of the auricle in the human embryo. Contrib Embryol Carnegie Inst 1922; 14:111.

4. Tanzer R. Congenital deformities. In: Converse JM, 2nd ed., Reconstructive Plastic Surgery, WB Saunders: Philadelphia, Vol. 3, 1977.
5. Hollinshead WH. Anatomy for Surgeons: The Head and Neck 3rd Ed. Vol. 1. Philadelphia: JB Lippincott Company, 1982.
6. Ruder R. Microtia reconstruction. In: Papel ID, Nachlas NE, eds. Facial Plastic and Reconstructive Surgery, St Louis: Mosby-Year Book, Inc., 1992.
7. Weerda H. Classification of congenital deformities of the auricle. Facial Plast Surg 1988; 5(5):385.
8. Marx H. Die missbildungen des ohres. In: Denker-Kahler (ed). HandBuch der Hals-Nasen-Ohrenheikunde, Berlin: Bd VI, Springer-Verlag, 1926.
9. Furnas D. Correction of prominent ears by concha mastoid sutures. Plast Reconst Surg 1968; 42:189.
10. Tanzer RC. Microtia—a long-term follow-up of forty-four reconstructed auricles. Plast Reconstr Surg 1978; 61:161.
11. Tanzer RC. Total reconstruction of the auricle: the evolution of a plan of treatment. Plast Reconstr Surg 1971; 47:523.
12. Tanzer RC. Total reconstruction of the external auricle. Plast Reconstr Surg 1959; 23:1.
13. Brent B. A personal approach to total auricular construction. Clin Plast Surg 1981; 8:211.
14. Brent B. Auricular repair with autogenous rib cartilage grafts: two decades of experience with 600 cases. Plast Reconstr Surg 1992; 90:355–374.
15. Brent B. The correction of microtia with autogenous cartilage grafts I. The classic deformity. Plast Reconstr Surg 1980; 66:1–12.
16. Brent B. The correction of microtia with autogenous cartilage grafts II. Atypical and complex deformities. Plast Reconstr Surg 1980; 66:13–22.
17. Eavey RD. Microtia repair: creation of a functional postauricular sulcus. Otolaryngol Head Neck Surg 1999; 120:789–793.
18. Megerian C. Congenital aural atresia and microtia. Facial Plast Surg Clin North Am 1997; 5(4).
19. Nagata S. Secondary reconstruction for unfavorable microtia results utilizing temporoparietal and innominate fascia flaps. Plast Reconstr Surg 1994; 94:254–267.
20. Tegtmeier RE, Gooding RA. The use of a fascial flap in ear reconstruction. Plast Reconstr Surg 1977; 60:406–411.

24

Genioplasty and Malar Augmentation

Steven M. Sullivan and J. Andrew Colgan
University of Oklahoma, Oklahoma City, Oklahoma, U.S.A.

GENIOPLASTY

Introduction

Pleasing aesthetic characteristics vary widely among cultures. They have changed somewhat through history; however, general characteristics associated with the esthetic face as described by Leonardo Da Vinci in the 15th century have changed very little overall. Stereotyping of personality characteristics is often formed based upon the initial evaluation of facial features. Society tends to utilize terms such as "strong" chin or "weak" chin, implying characteristics associated with a personality trait. As one of the more prominent facial features, the chin has been used to characterize masculinity when prominent, and a weak or submissive personality when recessive.

With more focus by society on facial esthetics, genioplasty has been utilized more often to achieve balance of the lower third of the face, often as an adjunctive procedure with orthognathic surgery, rhinoplasty, and rhytidectomy. Computer-aided imaging has assisted the clinician in patient education regarding surgical possibilities. Improvements in surgical technique, instrumentation, and fixation have allowed genioplasty procedures to evolve into outpatient or in-office procedures, utilizing general anesthesia or intravenous (IV) sedation and local anesthesia.

History

The horizontal sliding osteotomy was first described by Hofer for augmentation of the mandibular symphysis in 1942 (1). Access was via an extraoral incision through which a horizontal osteotomy of the anterior one-half of the inferior border was completed. Hofer used transosseous sutures for stabilization of the mobilized fragment, following its advancement. Converse, in 1950, discussed the feasibility of bone grafts introduced through intraoral approaches (2). Trauner and Obwegeser, in 1957, utilized the horizontal osteotomy through an intraoral incision with degloving of the anterior mandible (3). Converse and Woods described various applications for, as well as the versatility of, the horizontal osteotomy (4). Utilizing osteotomies for augmentation of the chin appears to be the primary emphasis of most early surgical approaches. It was not until 1965 that Reichenbach and colleagues proposed wedge osteotomy and vertical shortening of the chin (5). The authors found versatility in this procedure, as the segment could also be advanced or moved posteriorly, in addition to effecting vertical change. Hinds and Kent, in 1969, discussed the importance of maintaining the soft tissue attachments along the inferior segment and the role of these attachments in achieving maximal soft tissue change (6).

Preoperative Evaluation

Chin deformities can manifest in all three planes of space: transverse, vertical, and anteroposterior, with the vast majority being in the anteroposterior plane. Clinical and radiographic analysis should involve careful scrutiny of the osseous, dental, and soft tissue structures. Vertical facial balance can be evaluated by comparing the relative size and proportions of the various structures. Facial balance occurs when the upper, middle, and lower thirds are of approximate equal size and the structures within each segment are proportional. The eyes and nose should be proportional with other structures in the midfacial region. The lips and chin should be in harmonious proportions to the nose and eyes (7) (Fig. 1).

Evaluation of the chin must consider all structures that may be affected by surgery: the depth and shape of the labiomental fold, lower lip position, and the soft

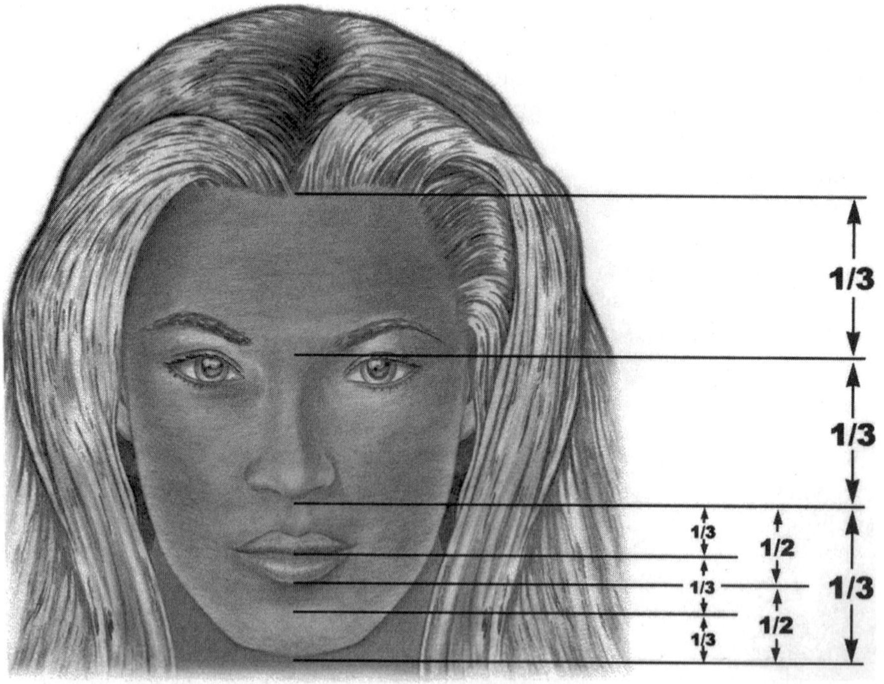

Figure 1 Vertical balance of the face uses proportions rather than absolute dimensions in judging harmony. The face is generally divided into thirds, with upper, middle, and lower thirds being proportionally similar and structures within those divisions also having harmonious proportions.

tissues of the mandibular symphysis. Lower lip position can be affected by the position of the maxilla and tooth-bearing segments, the size of the anterior mandible and position of the lower incisors in the sagittal plane, and the vertical height of the symphysis. Mentalis muscle hyperactivity must be closely evaluated and properly diagnosed. When the chin is viewed in the anteroposterior plane, the osseous contour and overlying soft tissue thickness will influence the soft tissue contour. The labiomental fold is influenced by the relative position of the maxilla and related skeletal malocclusions. The fold may be increased in the presence of a deep bite or skeletal class II malocclusions, or flattened in most class III malocclusions (8,9). All of these components must be evaluated in the frontal plane for optimal treatment planning and decision making as they relate to the surgical treatment plan.

Treatment planning for genioplasty requires a detailed three-dimensional analysis that will integrate the aforementioned components of soft tissue, dental, and skeletal aspects into a final treatment plan individualized to treat the deformity. The clinician must realize that genial deformities are rarely a result of an isolated component and the surgical treatment may require correction in more than one plane.

Cephalometric Evaluation

A variety of methods have been proposed for the evaluation of a patient's profile cephalometrically. Popular analysis include a combination of Down's, Steiner's, and Tweed's analyses to assess the relative relationships of the maxilla and mandible, in addition to the relationships of the maxillary and mandibular teeth (Fig. 2). This ensures that any skeletal and occlusal disparities will be identified and can be corrected prior to, or with, the genioplasty procedure. The bony chin position can be evaluated in the anteroposterior plane by utilizing SN–pogonion (range, 72–88

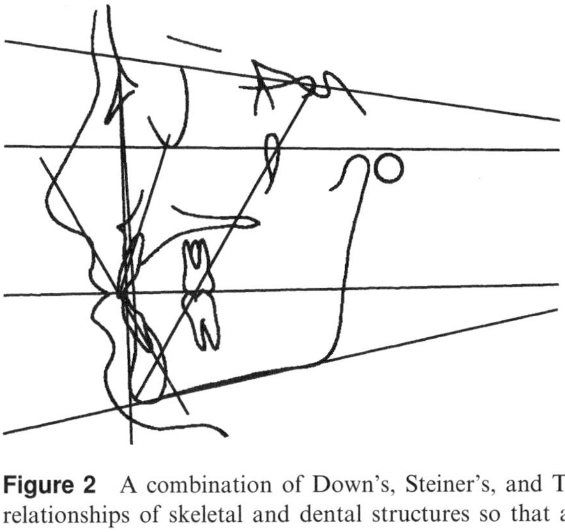

Figure 2 A combination of Down's, Steiner's, and Tweed's analyses is used to assess the relationships of skeletal and dental structures so that an accurate diagnosis of skeletal and dental anomalies can be made. The information obtained from this analysis is considered when performing sagittal or vertical changes in chin position.

degrees, mean 80), SN–B point (72–87 degrees, mean 79 degrees). Other cephalometric evaluations also exist, including the Y growth axis (range, 53–66 degrees, mean 59 degrees) (see Chapter 1) (10).

Soft Tissue Evaluation

Soft tissue profile evaluation can be made utilizing several methods (Fig. 3). Merrifield's Z-angle is formed by a line from the soft tissue chin (pogonion) tangent to the

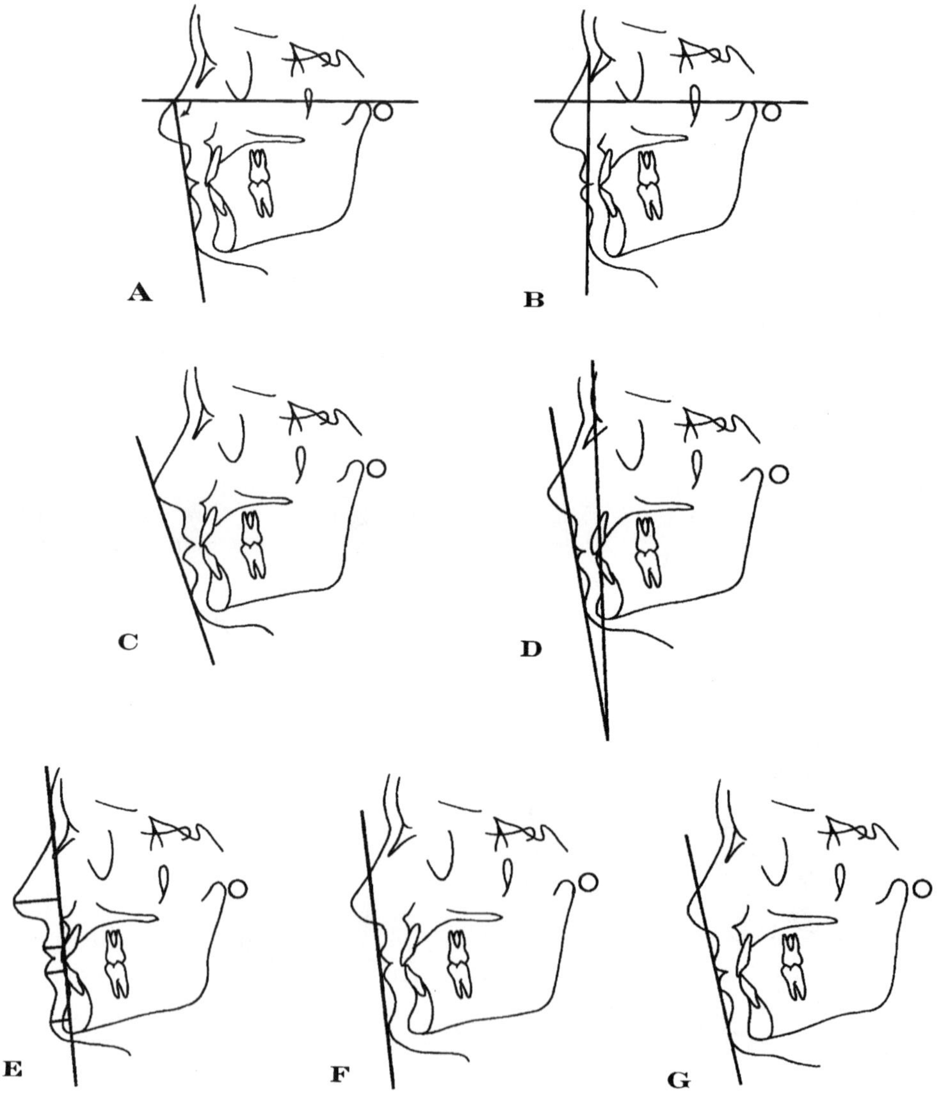

Figure 3 Popular soft tissue evaluations (see text). A. Merrifield's Z-angle. B. Gonzales-Ulloa and Steven's zero meridian for aesthetic soft tissue chin position. C. Rickett's law of lip relationships. D. Holdaway's H-line and H-angle. E. Zimmer's aesthetic plane. F. Riedel's plane, in which the lips and chin fall in a straight line. G. Steiner's aesthetic plane.

most procumbent lip, which forms an angle with the Frankfurt horizontal. The upper lip should fall on the profile line, with the lower lip tangent to or slightly behind the profile line (11). The Z-angle should be 80 ± 5 degrees. A simple method was described by Gonzales-Ulloa and Stevens in which a line perpendicular to Frankfurt horizontal passing through soft tissue nasion is constructed. The soft tissue chin should be tangent to this line (12). The esthetic plane was described by Ricketts (10) as a line from the tip of the nose to the chin. He found that in esthetically pleasing profiles the upper lip was 4 mm and the lower lip was 2 mm behind the esthetic plane, respectively. Holdeway suggested a line tangent to the chin and upper lip that forms an angle with a line between the nasion and basion of 7–9 degrees (13). Zimmer proposed a line from the anterior nasal spine to Down's "B" point and demonstrated that the nose and lips, as well as chin, were almost identical in thickness to this plane and that the nose had an approximate ratio of 5:1 to any of the other soft tissue structures (14). Reidel found that in individuals with pleasing esthetics, the lips and chin generally fell on a straight line (15). Steiner also used soft tissue landmarks to define pleasing profiles. He constructed a plane from the middle of the columella, midway between the curves of the upper lip and nasal tip. The lips should fall on this line (13). All cephalometric assessments should be critically combined with clinical judgment and the individual needs of the patient. The esthetic desires of the patient should be a priority.

Horizontal Osteotomy with Advancement

Osseous genioplasties can be performed under intubated general anesthesia or with intravenous sedation and local anesthetic. When selecting the anesthetic technique, one must consider that in the sedated patient anterior movement of the osteotomized segment can be difficult. Other factors for consideration include the possibility of hemorrhage and airway control. The surgical approach to the anterior mandible consists of an intraoral bidirectional incision. The mucosal incision should be initiated approximately halfway between the depth of the vestibule and the wet–dry line. It should be marked at its midpoint and extend to approximately the canine region bilaterally. The mucosal incision is undermined and the mentalis muscle is divided, beveling towards bone. Sharp incision and reflection of periosteum from the anterior mandible can then be accomplished. Periosteum on the inferior border should not be reflected, maintaining a minimum of 5–10 mm attached periosteum on the anterior mandible at the midpoint. Maintaining the periosteal attachments will ensure soft tissue advancement following repositioning of the osteotomized inferior segment. The mental nerves are identified and the foramina are noted for symmetry. Midline and paramedian orientation lines should be inscribed with a small burr to facilitate orientation and to ensure symmetrical movements with anterior, posterior, or vertical changes.

The proposed line of the osteotomy is inscribed at a level approximately 5 mm below the canine tooth root and 10–15 mm above the inferior border. The osteotomy should extend 3–4 mm below the lowest mental foramen. The angle of the osteotomy as it proceeds proximally can influence both vertical and horizontal changes. The more parallel with the occlusal and mandibular plane, the purer the anteroposterior movement. Care should be taken to mark and reproduce the vertical height if vertical changes are undesirable. To effect vertical shortening, the angle of the osteotomy is

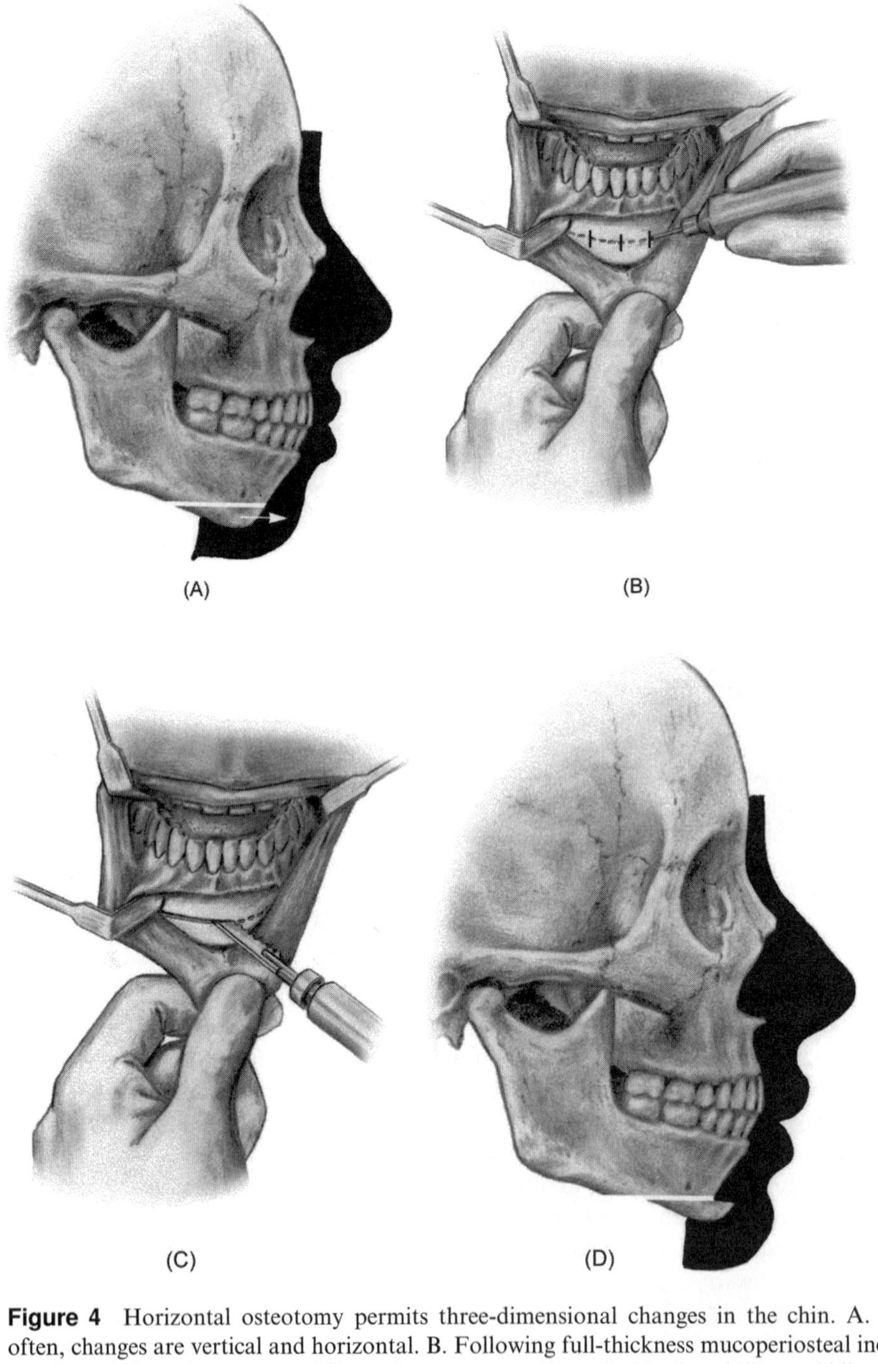

Figure 4 Horizontal osteotomy permits three-dimensional changes in the chin. A. Most often, changes are vertical and horizontal. B. Following full-thickness mucoperiosteal incision and limited dissection, proposed lines of osteotomy are inscribed in the midline and bilaterally, beneath the mental foramina, to ensure accurate symmetrical repositioning. C. A reciprocating saw blade is used to complete a full-thickness osteotomy, ensuring bicortical cuts at the inferior border. D. The inferior segment can then be advanced, shortened, or lengthened and secured with rigid or nonrigid fixation. E-I. Preoperative and postoperative results following genioplasty combined with maxillary and mandibular osteotomies.

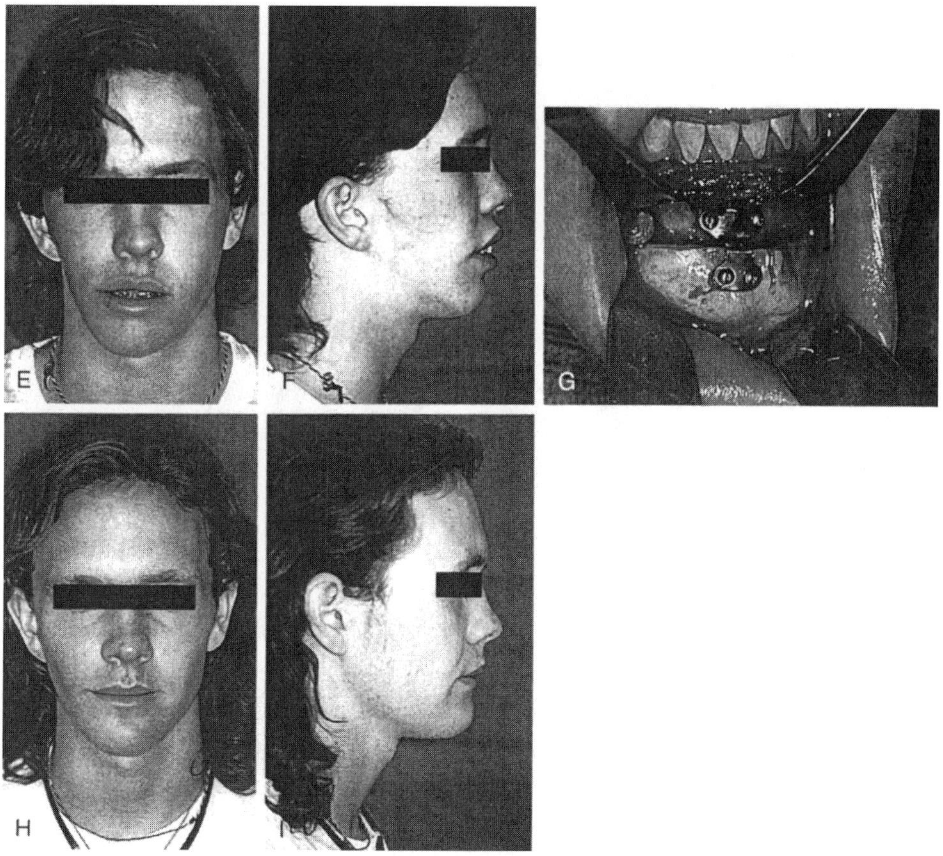

Figure 4 Continued

made less acute with the mandibular plane. The osteotomy can be completed with a reciprocating or ossillating saw. Saw orientation must remain constant to ensure a symmetrical cut through the buccal and lingual cortices. The buccal and lingual cortical cuts must be complete where they join proximally. Failure to complete the lingual cortical cut in this area could result in mandibular fracture necessitating repair, compromise of the inferior alveolar nerve, or unfavorable esthetic results. After completion of the ostetomy, the inferior segment can be repositioned and stabilized utilizing a variety of techniques including unicortical or bicortical wires, adaptation plates, prebent chin plates, or lag screws. Bone deposition and osseous remodeling of the mobilized segments have been demonstrated to be consistent, with bone deposition occurring on the superior edge of the inferior segment and the labial surface of the superior segment (16). Therefore, fixation devices should be placed in areas of bone deposition, if possible. When utilizing transosseous wires for fixation, the degree of advancement must be limited to the overall symphyseal thickness. This must be determined prior to deciding to utilize this stabilization method (Fig. 4).

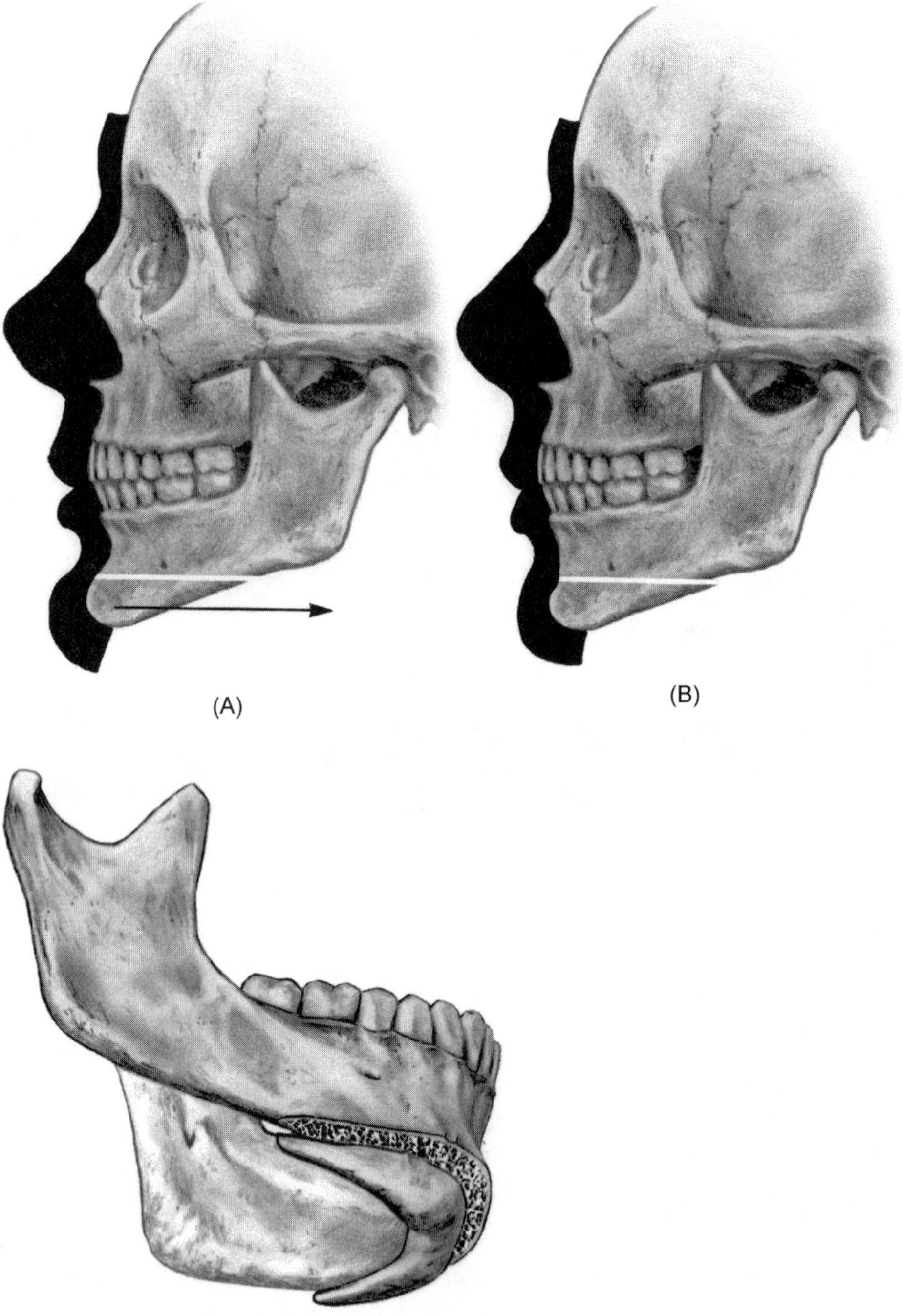

(A) (B)

(C)

Figure 5 Horizontal osteotomy with setback (A) requires special attention laterally at the inferior border (B, C) to ensure a smooth transition between the mobilized segment and mandible.

Horizontal Osteotomy with Anteroposterior Reduction

The surgical approach and osteotomy are completed as described with advancement. It is necessary to reduce the proximal tips from the mobilized segment to avoid palpable steps and to ensure a smooth transition along the inferior border. The surgeon must also be cognizant of potential changes in the anterior vertical height of the mandible and thus take this into consideration when planning the orientation of the osteotomy (Fig. 5).

Tenon Technique

The tenon technique was originally described by Michelet and associates in 1974 (17) and offers several advantages. Symmetry is ensured by the tenon and visual inspection of the proximal extensions. Often only a single lag screw is required for stabilization. Limitations to the amount of advancement also exist relating to the overall thickness of the anterior mandible. Prior to using this technique, the surgeon must ascertain this dimension. The surgical approach is via the previously described degloving technique. A U-shaped monocortical osteotomy is created centrally on the symphysis. Lateral extensions are developed below the mental nerves and connected to the superior aspects of the tenon corticotomy. Full-thickness osteotomies are completed on the lateral extensions and only through the lingual cortex on the superior aspect of the tenon. The resultant full thickness of bone behind the tenon facilitates the mortising of the tenon and lag screw fixation (Fig. 6). When posterior movement is desired, the "U" is inverted and the osteotomies completed as described, with mortising of the tenon on the inferior segment into the superior segment of the mandible.

Double Sliding Horizontal Osteotomy

Occasionally, the chin is so deficient that a double sliding horizontal osteotomy must be utilized (18). The surgical technique involves the creation of a stepped

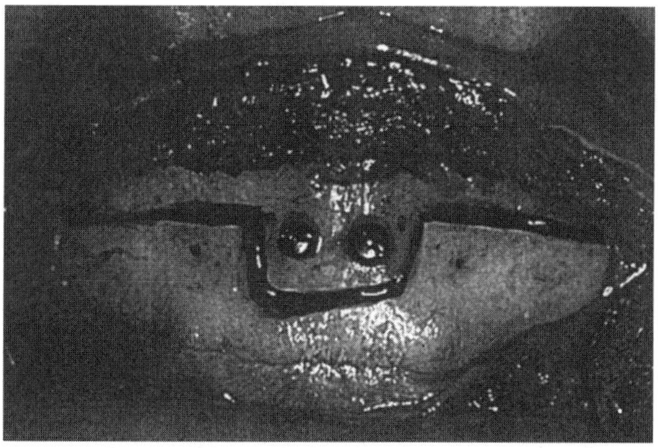

Figure 6 The tenon technique allows for mortising of the tenon into the mobilized fragment when the chin is advanced. In the setback procedure, the tenon is reversed and the mobilized fragment is mortised into the mandible. Lag-screw fixation is usually the only fixation required.

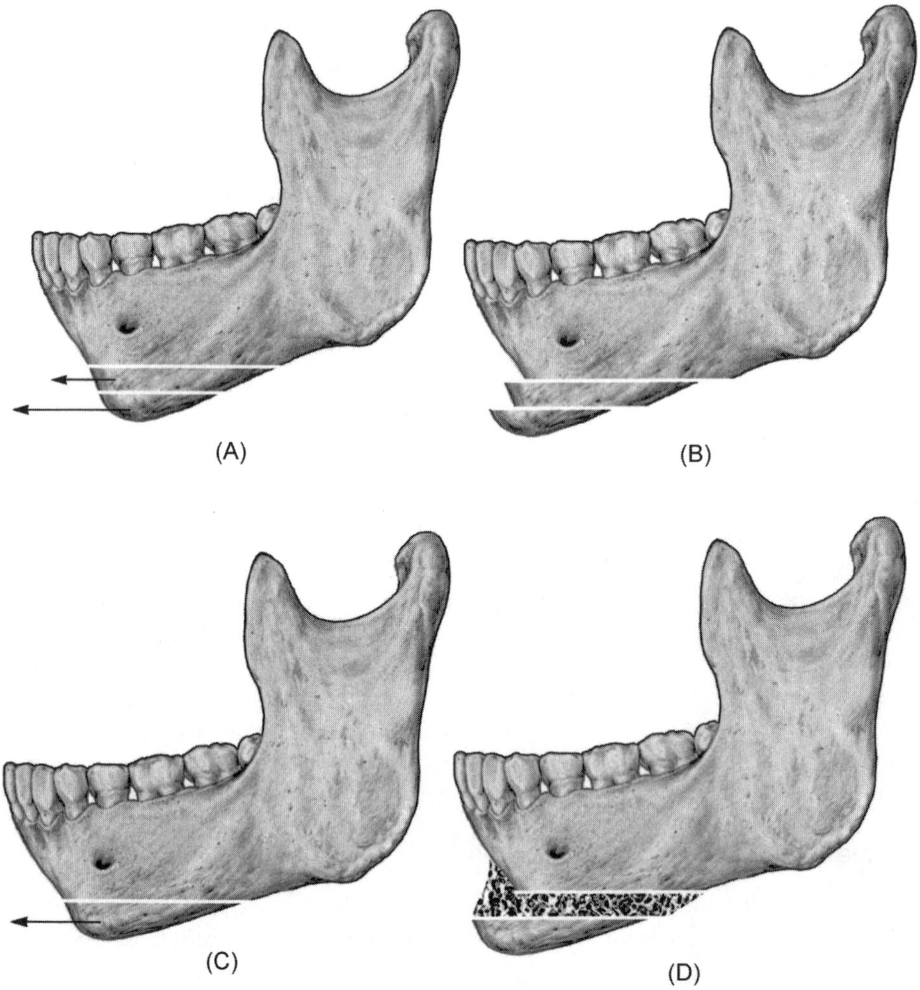

Figure 7 In cases of severe deficiency (A) double sliding genioplasty can be used. B, Often it is necessary to provide bone grafts over the step defects to ensure a predictable contour.

intermediate wafer of bone between the inferior fragment and mandible, which is also advanced to provide bony contact between the upper and lower segments (Fig. 7A,B).

Vertical Augmentation

Vertical augmentation is indicated when the treatment plan calls for an increase in lower facial height, especially when the deficit is in the mandibular alveolus and symphysis. Vertical augmentation is accomplished by interpositional grafting or alloplastic implant placement into the inferiorly repositioned chin segments following horizontal osteotomy of the mandible. Autogenous bone and hydroxyapatite are the most commonly used interpositional materials. It is also possible to make anteroposterior changes if desired (Fig. 7C,D; Fig. 8).

Vertical Reduction Genioplasty

A variety of genioplasty techniques exist to accomplish vertical changes in chin height, which can be effected during advancement or setback by altering the angle of the osteotomy as previously described. The magnitude of the angle is proportional to the amount and direction of horizontal movement. In most instances, only 3–5 mm of vertical reduction can be obtained. If the surgical goal is for a greater decrease in vertical chin height with or without anteroposterior change, a wedge reduction is indicated. This can be accomplished using the tenon technique as well as a horizontal osteotomy. The surgical protocol is as previously described; however, an appropriately sized wedge ostectomy is performed. From a technical standpoint it is easier to remove the wedge from the middle segment. Diligent intraoperative planning is essential to avoid tooth roots and to maintain an adequate inferior segment (Fig. 9).

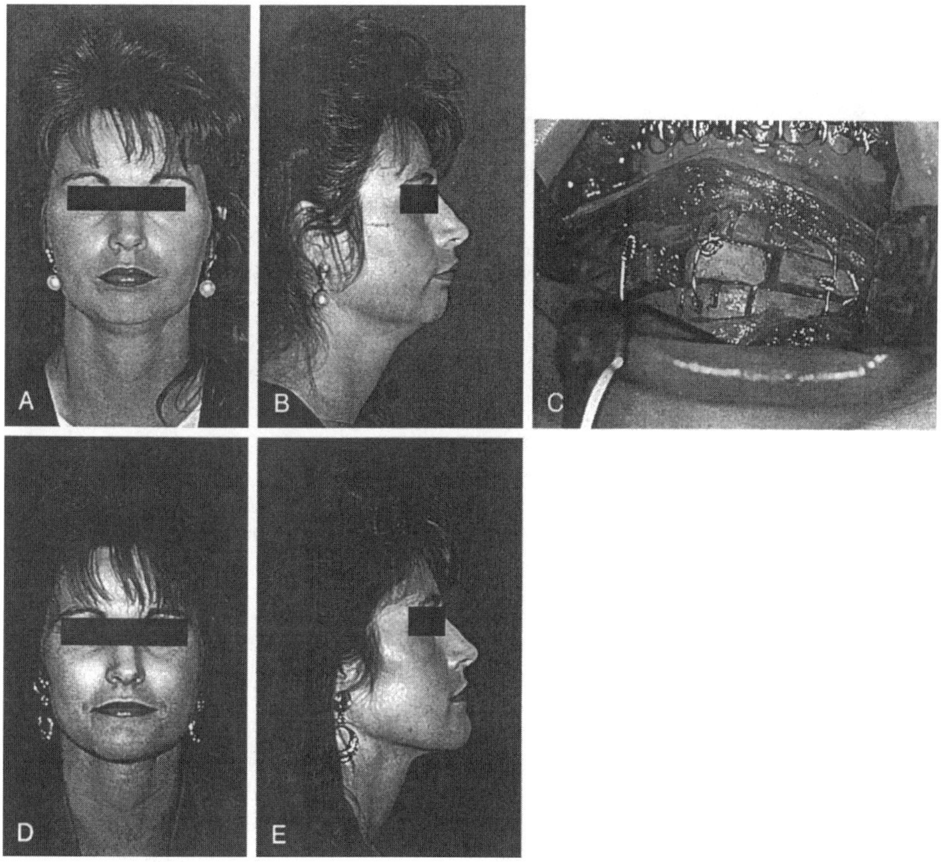

Figure 8 Interpositional grafts of hydroxyapatite or autogenous bone not only facilitate anteroposterior movements but also allow vertical lengthening. Preoperative (A, B), intraoperative (C), and postoperative (D, E) photographs demonstrate the effects of vertical lengthening and advancement of the chin.

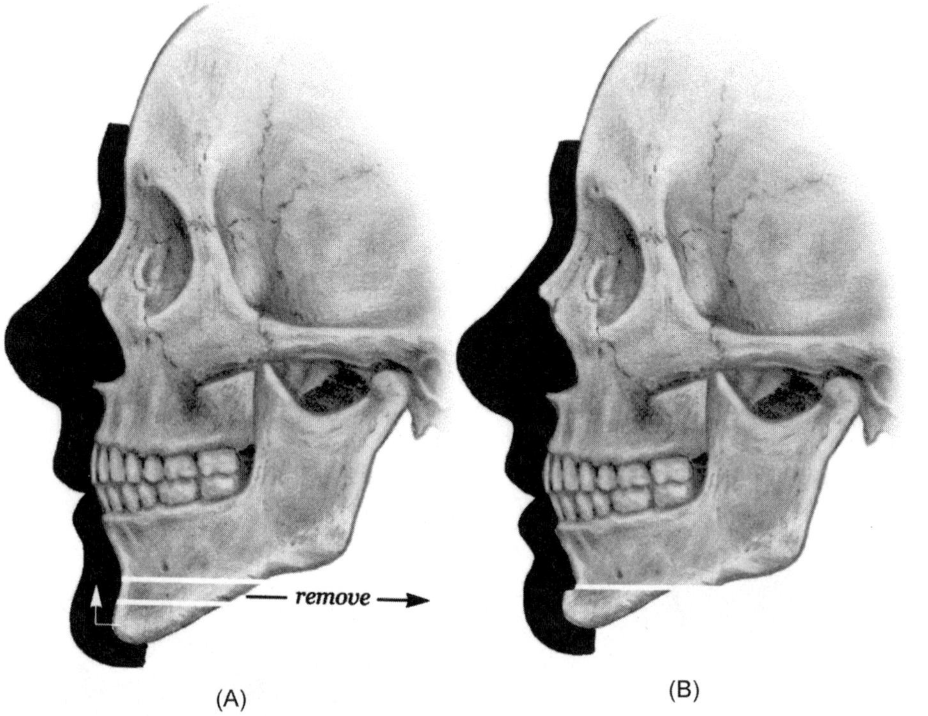

Figure 9 A. Wedge vertical reduction osteotomy allows for anteroposterior repositioning in addition to (B) vertical shortening.

Alloplastic Augmentation Technique

Alloplastic chin implants afford the clinician the ability to augment not only the anteroposterior dimension but also vertical and, more importantly, lateral augmentation. Alloplastic implants with extensions are designed to eliminate some of the disadvantages of osseous genioplasty including the possibility of asymmetrical advancement, inadvertent vertical changes, and surreptitious narrowing of the anterior mandible with large advancements. However, alloplasts have been associated with underlying bony resorption, postoperative infection, and noninfectious inflammatory responses (19). The use of an alloplast, as with osseous genioplasty, should be based upon the individual patient's needs.

A variety of surgical techniques can be used for insertion of an alloplast. Extraoral access via a submental fold incision can be combined with lipectomy or liposuction. Intraoral surgical approaches include a vestibular incision as previously described, or a midline vertical incision with a tunneling technique. Great care must be taken when using limited access incisions to ensure symmetrical placement of the implant, in addition to positioning it appropriately in a vertical plane. Implants can be used to increase anterior height by extending them below the anterior mandibular border and to augment the parasymphyseal regions more so than single piece osseous genioplasty (Fig. 10). Implants should be stabilized

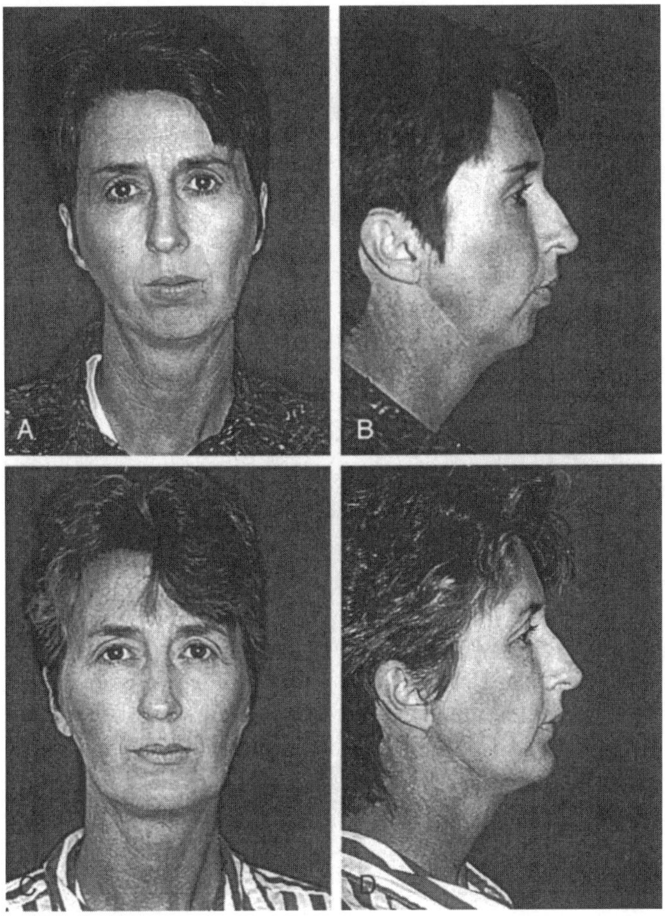

Figure 10 Alloplastic augmentation allows for more parasymphyseal augmentation than does osseous genioplasty. A, B. Preoperative views. C, D. Postoperative views.

with transosseous wires or screws to ensure immobility. Bony resorption under alloplasts has been seen in patients with hyperactive mentalis muscles and lip incompetence (20).

Soft Tissue Closure

Accurate reapproximation of the mentalis muscle is crucial in preventing lower lip malpositions and chin ptosis (witch's chin). Attention is directed first to closing the periosteal–mentalis muscle layer. A single 3-0 resorbable suture is placed in the midline followed by a running 3-0 resorbable suture. Attention is then directed to the mucosal layer where a single 4-0 resorbable suture is placed at the midline followed by a running 4-0 resorbable suture. A pressure dressing is placed to minimize the formation of a hematoma and to facilitate reattachment of degloved soft tissues.

Soft Tissue Changes

Soft tissue changes associated with genioplasty are highly variable. Reports in the literature regarding translation of osseous to soft tissue change range 1:0.6 to 1:1. Reduction genioplasty apppears to have the most variability in osseous to soft tissue change. Several surgical considerations will ensure the greater magnitude of bone to soft tissue change. The most important surgical tenets appear to be limited periosteal stripping and meticulous layered soft tissue closure, including reapproximation of the mentalis muscle (21,22).

Complications

Complications of genioplasty include prolonged neurosensory disturbance (23), avascular necrosis of mobilized segments (24), hemorrhage causing lingual hematoma and possible airway compromise, unesthetic soft tissue changes such as chin ptosis (25) and excessive lower tooth display, bony resorption under alloplasts (20), devitalization of teeth, mandible fracture (26), creation of mucogingival problems, and asymmetry.

Prolonged neurosensory changes are attributable to direct nerve injury or traction neuropraxia. Cumulative injury can occur when other osteotomies, such as sagittal split osteotomy, are simultaneously undertaken (23). In general, minor neurosensory deficits are expected and resolve over time. Direct nerve injury, such as transsection, requires immediate microneural repair for optimal neurosensory recovery. Excessive resorption or avascular necrosis of the mobilized segment can be avoided by maintaining a broad vascularized soft tissue pedicle (22). This is accomplished by minimal stripping of the soft tissues overlying the symphysis and maintaining as much of the lingual muscle attachments as possible.

Hemorrhage and airway compromise are rarely seen. It is vitally important that intraoperative bleeding be controlled promptly and effectively using hemostatic agents or electrocautery. Most causes of lingual hematoma with extension are the result of medullary bone or muscle bleeding once the patient becomes normotensive following anesthesia. Postoperative pressure dressings may aid in controlling minor

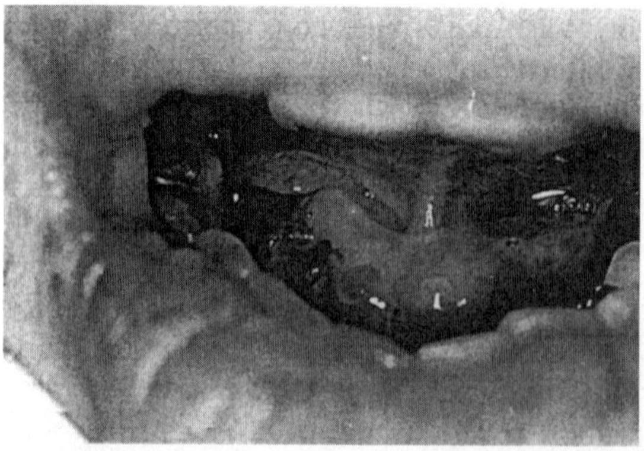

Figure 11 Sublingual hematoma may form as a result of medullary and muscular bleeding following horizontal osteotomy. In this case, treatment required evacuation of the hematoma and placement of an intraoral drain.

soft tissue bleeding and hematoma formation, but there is no substitute for good intraoperative hemostasis (Fig. 11).

Chin ptosis results from inferior redistribution of the soft tissues of the chin. Signs can include redundancy of submental skin or flattening of the labiomental fold, excessive lower tooth display, and, in severe cases, lip incompetence. The usual cause is excessive reflection of the periosteum from the inferior border of the mandible. Other causes include inadequate approximation and suspension of reflected muscle and periosteum. Limited soft tissue reflection and meticulous layered closure will minimize the possibility of ptosis. If ptosis is anticipated, the clinician can support the soft tissues with suspension sutures through the outer cortex of the osteotomy or from microscrews superiorly (25) (Fig. 12).

Bone resorption under alloplastic chin implants has been reported. In one report, mean resorption was 1.3 mm (27). In most cases, this is not clinically significant. Severe resorption has been reported and implant removal and secondary reconstruction have been necessary using traditional osteotomy techniques. The presence of hyperactive mentalis muscles has been identified as a predictor for excessive resorption under alloplasts (Fig. 13).

Devitalization of teeth may result from compromise of pulpal blood flow. It is recommended that osteotomies be carried out a minimum of 5 mm below the longest tooth root. On average, the mandibular canine is 20 mm long. Strict attention to tooth root location is of paramount importance. Long-term loss of vitality with periapical changes may necessitate endodontic intervention.

Mandibular fracture is a very rare occurrence (26). The most common cause is failure to complete the osteotomy proximally through both the buccal and lingual cortices. When the inferior segment is mobilized, an inferior border fracture takes place with extension through the body, angle, or ramus. If this should occur,

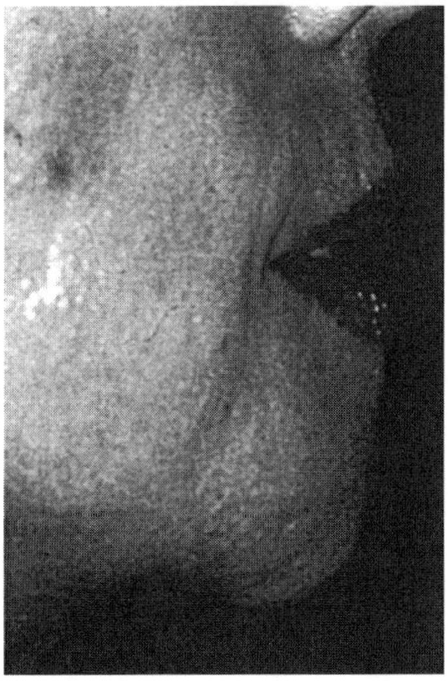

Figure 12 Inadequate mentalis muscle reconstruction and soft tissue closure, in addition to excessive soft tissue stripping of the inferior border, can result in ptosis of the chin and flattening of the labiomental fold.

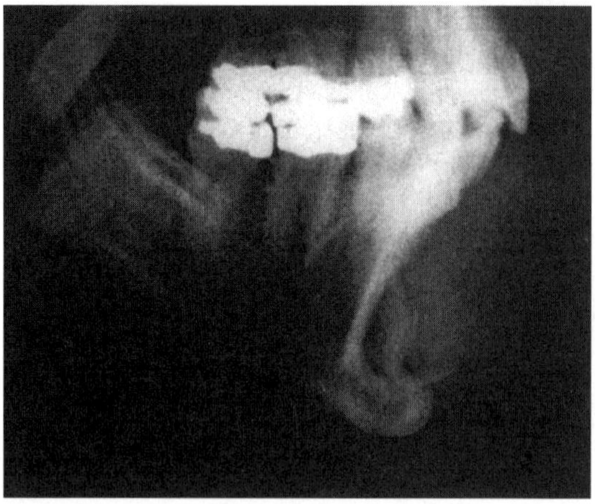

Figure 13 The presence of hyperactive mentalis muscles, in addition to an oversized implant, resulted in bony resorption of approximately 3 mm.

completion of the osteotomy, followed by open or closed reduction of the fracture should take place.

Problematic mucogingival stripping can occur as a result of inappropriate incision placement. Tension on mucogingival tissues may cause inadvertent stripping of gingiva. Placement of the incision between the sulcus and wet–dry line, meticulous layered closure, and identification of underlying mucogingival pathology will minimize this potential complication (Fig. 14).

Asymmetry may occur if the mobilized segment is free-handed into its new position. Orientation marks and visual inspection following stabilization is necessary to avoid this problem. A pre-existing or undiagnosed asymmetry may be more apparent following chin repositioning. Immediate visual inspection and modification will minimize this problem.

Genial procedures afford the surgeon the ability to make small but necessary changes, or dramatic alterations in the overall form of the lower third of the face.

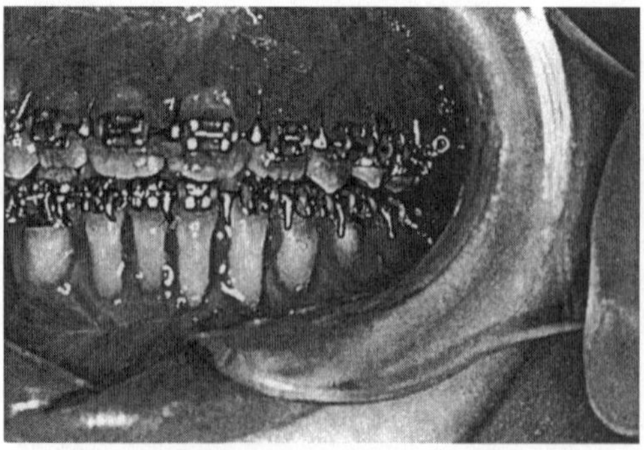

Figure 14 Pre-existing mucogingival problems can be exacerbated by advancement genioplasty. Note loss of mucogingival attachment following advancement genioplasty.

The predictability of a successful outcome is excellent with detailed preoperative planning and conscientious application of good surgical technique.

MALAR AUGMENTATION

Introduction

If the eyes are the window to the soul, then the orbital structures and the malar complex are the window frame and dressing. In American culture the malar complex is the corner stone for an esthetic face. Strong cheek bones also seem to give a more youthful appearance. The malar region is important in determining the oval shape of the face and the character of the face on oblique profile. It has been shown that the oblique profile is most commonly seen in conversation and thus is a very important aspect of confluent facial aesthetics (28). The malar region is unique due to its projection and placement in all three planes of space. However, visualization in all three planes of space makes it difficult to formulate an ideal esthetic value for the malar region.

The appearance of the malar eminence is determined not only by the prominence of the bone but also by the reflection of light and the coinciding shadows. The malar region comprises both soft and hard tissue. The malar eminence, frontal process, and arch provide superior and lateral definition to the contour. The soft tissues help to round out the inferior and medial aspects. Excessive soft tissue may round out the superior and lateral projections and reduce the amount of definition of the complex. The attractive malar prominence should appear round and full but not too angular. It should be proportionate to the rest of the face. A proper malar complex will finish out the oval form of the face, which is the most aesthetic facial form. A flat hypoplastic zygoma makes the face seem dull and aged, also increasing the prominence of the nose and chin.

Evaluation

Several methods have been described for evaluation of the malar complex. Hinderer described a technique of two crossed lines, one extending from the lateral canthus to the commissure and the other extending from the ala to the superior tragus (28) (Fig. 15A). The eminence (and implant) is ideally located in the superolateral aspect of the cheek between the lines just above the cross. Wilkinson locates the eminence just lateral to the lateral canthus at a point one-third the distance from the lateral canthus to the inferior border of the mandible (29) (Fig. 15B). Silver states that the malar prominence is located more anteriorly and described a coordinate system for locating the prominence (30) (Fig. 15C). A vertical line is drawn from the lateral limbus. A horizontal line is drawn from the midpoint of the vermilion border of the upper lip and the nasolabial angle. A line is then drawn from that point to the medial canthus. The angle formed is then transposed to the intersection with the Frankfort horizontal plane, locating the malar eminence. Powell made a practical division of the malar anatomy by organizing the prominence into anteromedial and posterolateral segments (31) (Fig. 15D). Dropping a vertical line from the lateral canthus makes this division. This analysis helps to identify the type of malar deficiency.

The deficiency may be anteromedial, posterolateral, or both. Prendergast and Schoenrock defined the malar eminence as the point below the lateral canthus that gives the impression of being the most prominent point of the malar mound in any view (32). Looking at the face obliquely, they drew a line from the lateral canthus to the commissure. A line drawn 90 degrees off this line at two-thirds the distance from the commissure to the canthus passes through the most prominent point of the malar complex (Fig. 15E). Terino made a similar division of the midface region into anatomical zones (33) (Fig. 16). Zone 1 comprises the major portion of the malar bone and the zygomatic arch. Augmentation of this area will maximize the projection of the malar prominence. Zone 2 is the middle third of the zygomatic arch. Augmentation of this area will increase facial width. Zone 3 is the paranasal area and is composed of the region medial to the infraorbital foramen and lateral to the nasal bones. Augmentation in this area will increase fullness in the infraorbital area. Zone 4 is the posterior third of the zygomatic arch. Augmentation in this zone is rarely indicated. In addition, branches of the facial nerve course through this area and are vulnerable to injury. Zone 5, or the submalar zone, contains the overlying facial musculature, fat, and subcutaneous tissue of the midface region. It is bordered by the inferior

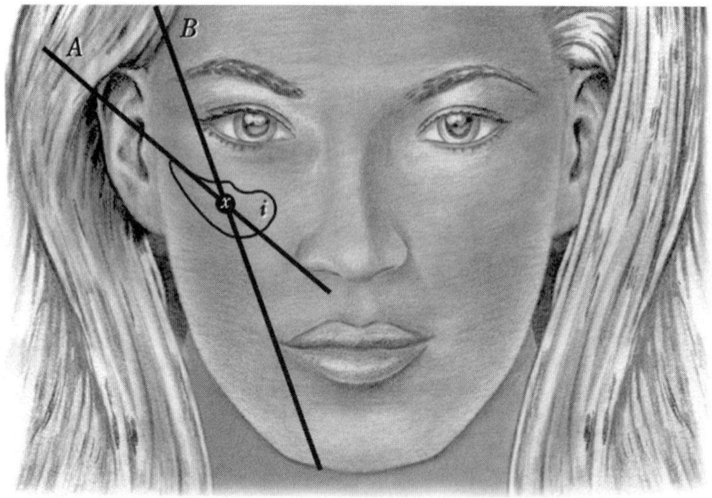

(A)

Figure 15 Hinderer's crossed lines: A. one (A) from the ala to the tragus and the other (B) from the lateral canthus to the commissure. B. Wilkinson's method placed the malar prominence at or just lateral to the outer canthus on a point (A) approximately one-third the distance from the lateral canthus to the inferior border of the mandible. C. Silver's malar prominence triangle. Silver dropped a vertical line (A) from the limbus as the patient looks forward. The horizontal line B is at the midpoint between the vermilion border of the upper lip and the nasolabial angle. A meets B at point X. A line is drawn from X to medial canthus (N). Angle AXN is reflected laterally to form AXP. Where the Frankfort horizontal line C crosses at point P is the malar prominence. D. Powell's method of dividing malar anatomy into anteromedial and posterolateral segments. E. Pendergast and Schoenrock drew a line from commissure to lateral canthus. One-third of the distance down this line is the most prominent point of the malar complex.

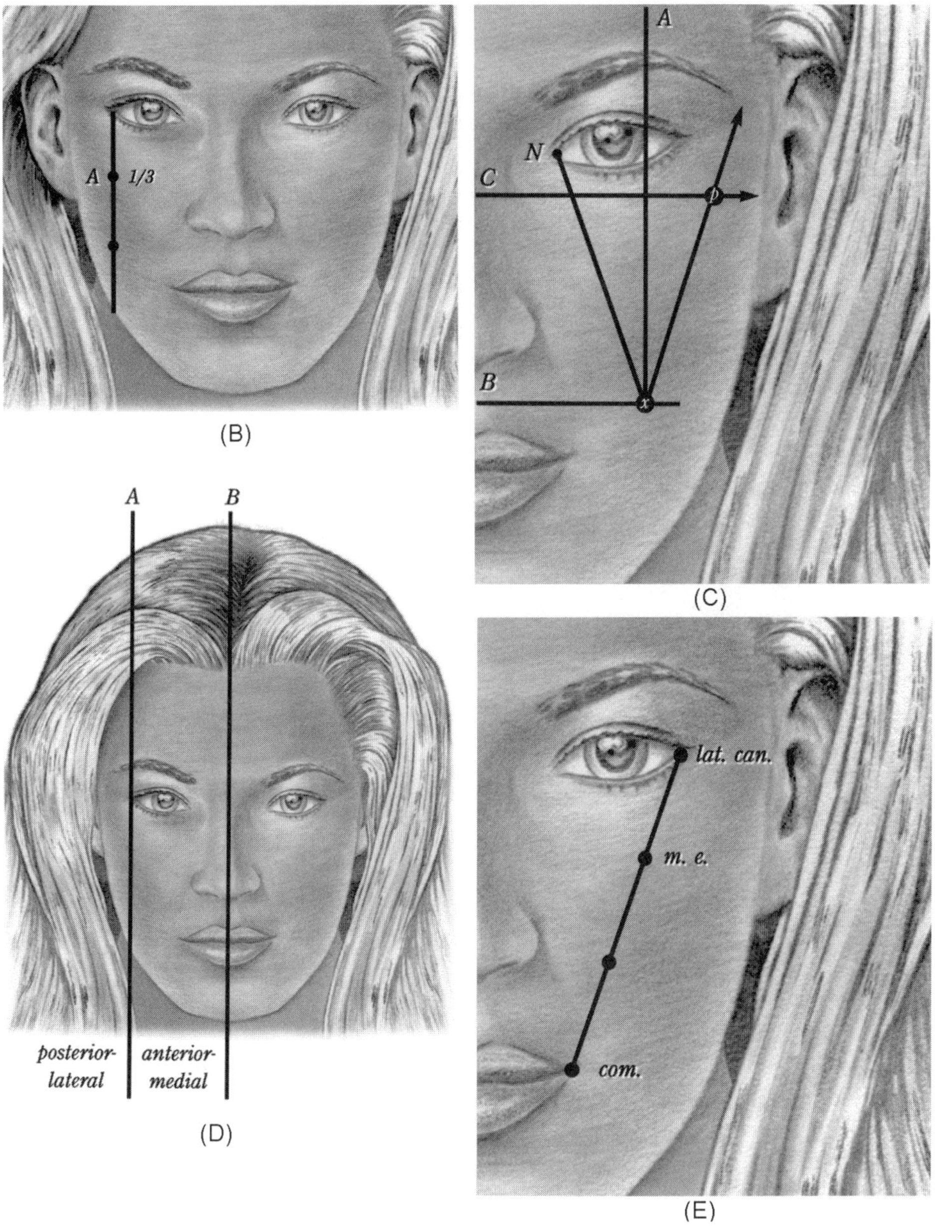

(B) (C) (D) (E)

Figure 15 Continued

bony margin of the malar eminence, the lateral border of the nasolabial fold, and the masseter muscle. Binder (34) and Terino (33) advocate augmentation of the zone by itself, or in conjunction with a rhytidectomy. Other authors have modified or devised alternative methods of evaluation. Regardless of the method of evaluation, accurate and definitive communication with the patient is imperative. The surgeon must duplicate the patient's expectations.

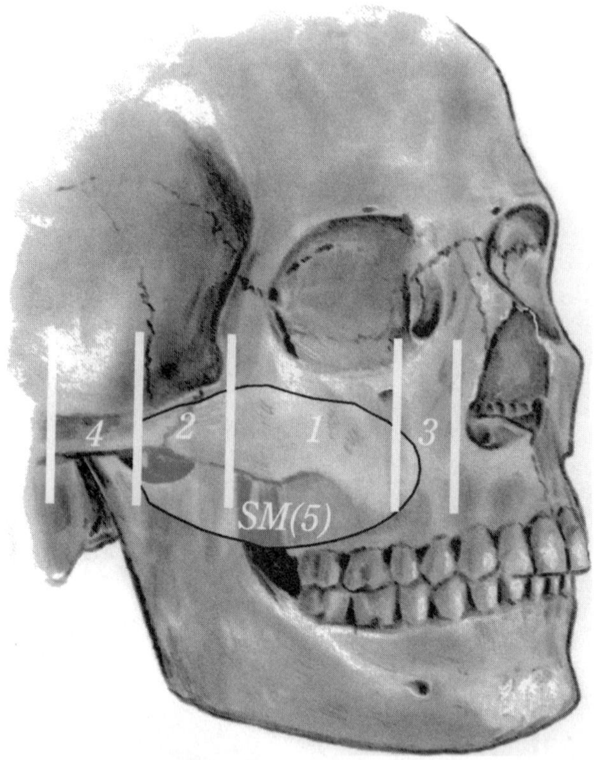

Figure 16 Terino's division of the midface region into anatomical zones.

Patients may present to the surgeon with multiple complaints regarding facial aesthetics; however, it is rare for the patient to complain specifically about the appearance of their malar complex. The surgeon must be able to recognize the type of malar deformity that would benefit from augmentation (35), including the following:

1. Congenital deformities
2. Posttraumatic deformities
3. Flat, concave facial profile
4. Long narrow face
5. Aged face with sag or atrophy of soft tissues
6. Round, full face
7. Asymmetry

Patients who present in the first two categories usually have no trouble understanding the need for malar augmentation. Congenital concave facial profiles may be subtle or so severe that orthognathic or craniofacial surgery is required for correction. If an occlusal discrepancy is present, osteotomies with occlusal correction may result in an improvement in facial appearance. However, some deformities may require both osteotomies and malar implants.

Patients with a long narrow face often receive a more attractive oval shape to the face by placement of the implant to include zone 2, thereby increasing the bizygomatic width.

In the older patient with sag or atrophy of the soft tissues, the potential of malar augmentation should not be overlooked. A face lift with superficial musculoaponeurotic system (SMAS) repair lifts the sagging subcutaneous tissues and imparts fullness to the lateral posterior cheek; anterior malar improvement is often temporary or less than ideal. Malar implants can improve the face lift results and give a long-lasting correction to the malar eminence. Binder (36) advocates a submalar (zone 5) implant alone or in conjunction with rhytidectomy.

A round, full face looks more attractive with a well-defined malar eminence. Placement of the implants is usually more anterior (zone 1), thus avoiding increased lateral width.

Malar Implants

Selection of the proper size and shape of implant is crucial to improving facial aesthetics. The implant itself should be easily modified and inserted, biologically inert, as well as imperceptible to the patient. In addition, the implant should have the ability to be easily exchanged when necessary or desirable with minimal to no removal of adjacent tissues. Unfortunately, no single implant universally satisfies all these qualities. Solid silicone should be considered one of the safest implantable materials currently available in the United States (37). The silicon–oxygen bonds in Silastic are particularly strong, making this material resistant to degradation in the body (38). Silastic implants can be steam autoclaved and sterilized with raditation or ethylene oxide gas (39). Because of capsule formation that occurs around a Silastic implant, removal of the implant, if necessary, becomes easier than with porous implant materials. Whitaker (39) recommended a 6 mm thick implant if the bony hypoplasia is mild or moderate and the soft tissue is normal. If there is exaggerated bony hypoplasia or soft tissue thickness, 8 mm implants should be used. In patients with thin soft tissue cover, a 6 mm implant may need to be reduced by 1 to 2 mm and tapered at both ends, or a 4 mm implant may be used. It is important that the surgeon evaluate the patient for midfacial asymmetry and consider the use of different-sized implants for correction.

Surgical Technique

Some surgeons advocate marking the proposed location for the malar prominence on the skin with the patient in the sitting position. This can be accomplished with an extra implant or an implant sizer. Anesthesia may be local with IV sedation or general endotracheal. Regardless of the anesthesia modality used, local anesthetic with a vasoconstrictor is injected directly against the malar bone as well as the incision and overlying soft tissues.

A variety of surgical approaches may be used to insert the malar implants, including coronal, blepharoplasty, and rhytidectomy. The most common surgical approach is the intraoral maxillary vestibular incision. The incision should be in the buccal vestibule about 1.5 cm in length above the mucogingival junction (Fig. 17). If the implants will be fixated to bone without reliance upon the soft tissue

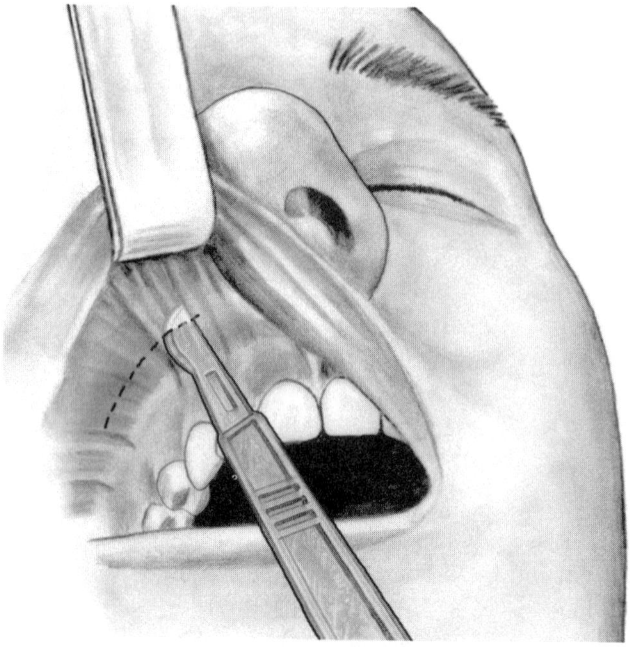

Figure 17 The maxillary vestibular incision is made so that the cut parallels the anterior surface of the maxilla above the mucogingival junction.

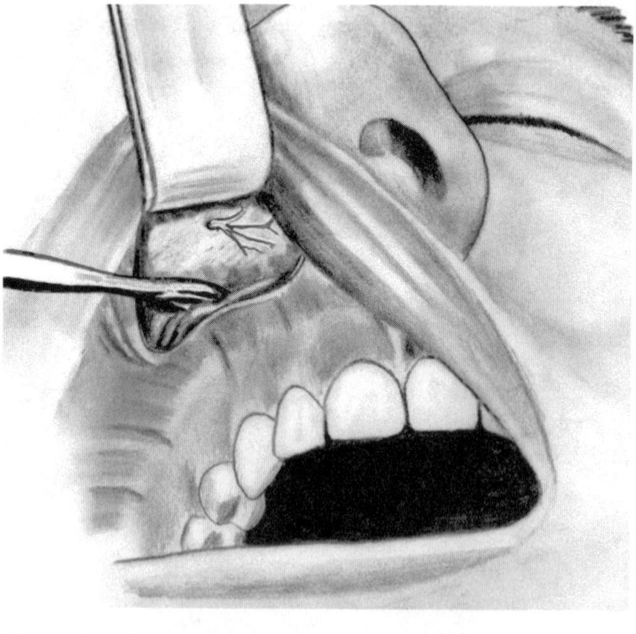

Figure 18 Periosteal elevator is inserted to bone immediately beneath the infraorbital nerve and swept downward, creating a cuff of soft tissue inferiorly which forms a ledge for the implant to sit against. The dissection follows bone laterally onto the zygomatic arch, superficial to the masseter muscle.

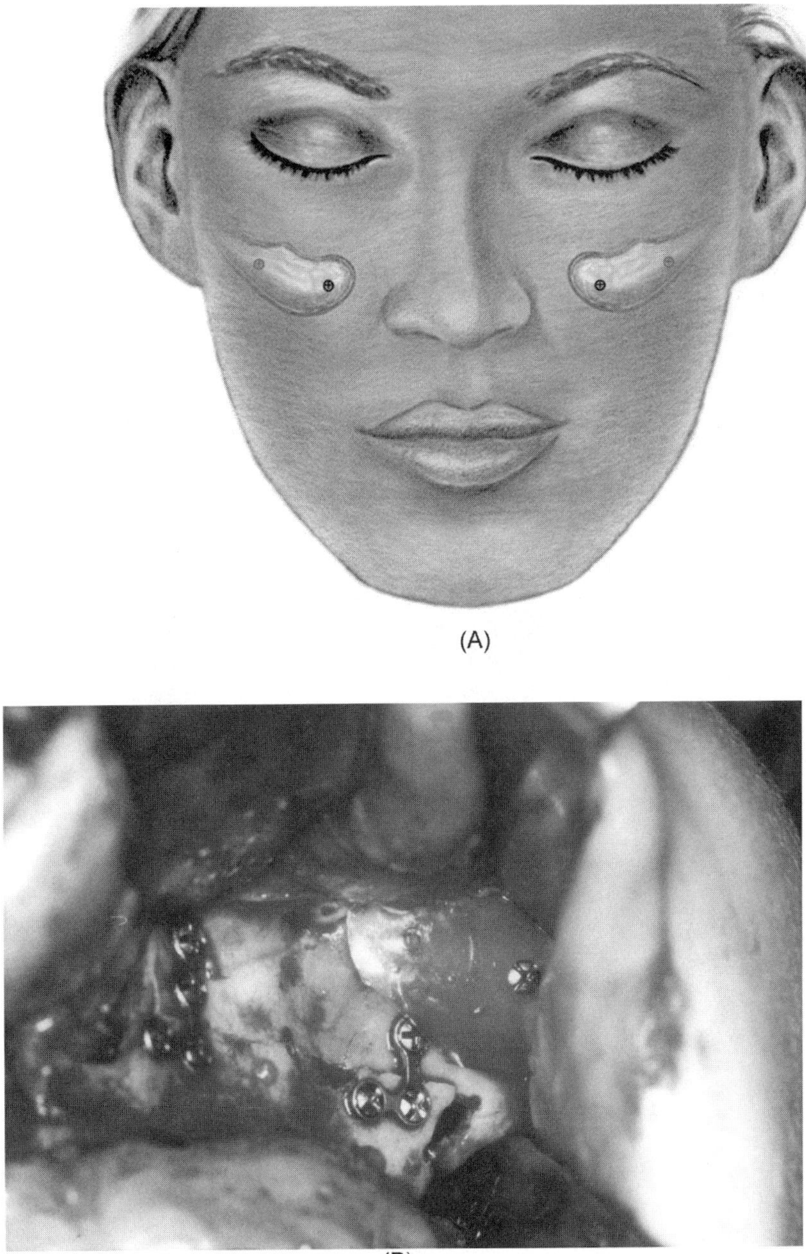

(A)

(B)

Figure 19 Rigid screw fixation provides implant stabilization.

pocket for retention, then the incision can be extended to a LeFort I type incision. A periosteal elevator is used to sweep the soft tissue downward off the bone from just below the infraorbital nerve toward the buccal sulcus, creating a soft tissue ledge for the implant to rest against. The dissection follows bone out onto the zygomatic arch,

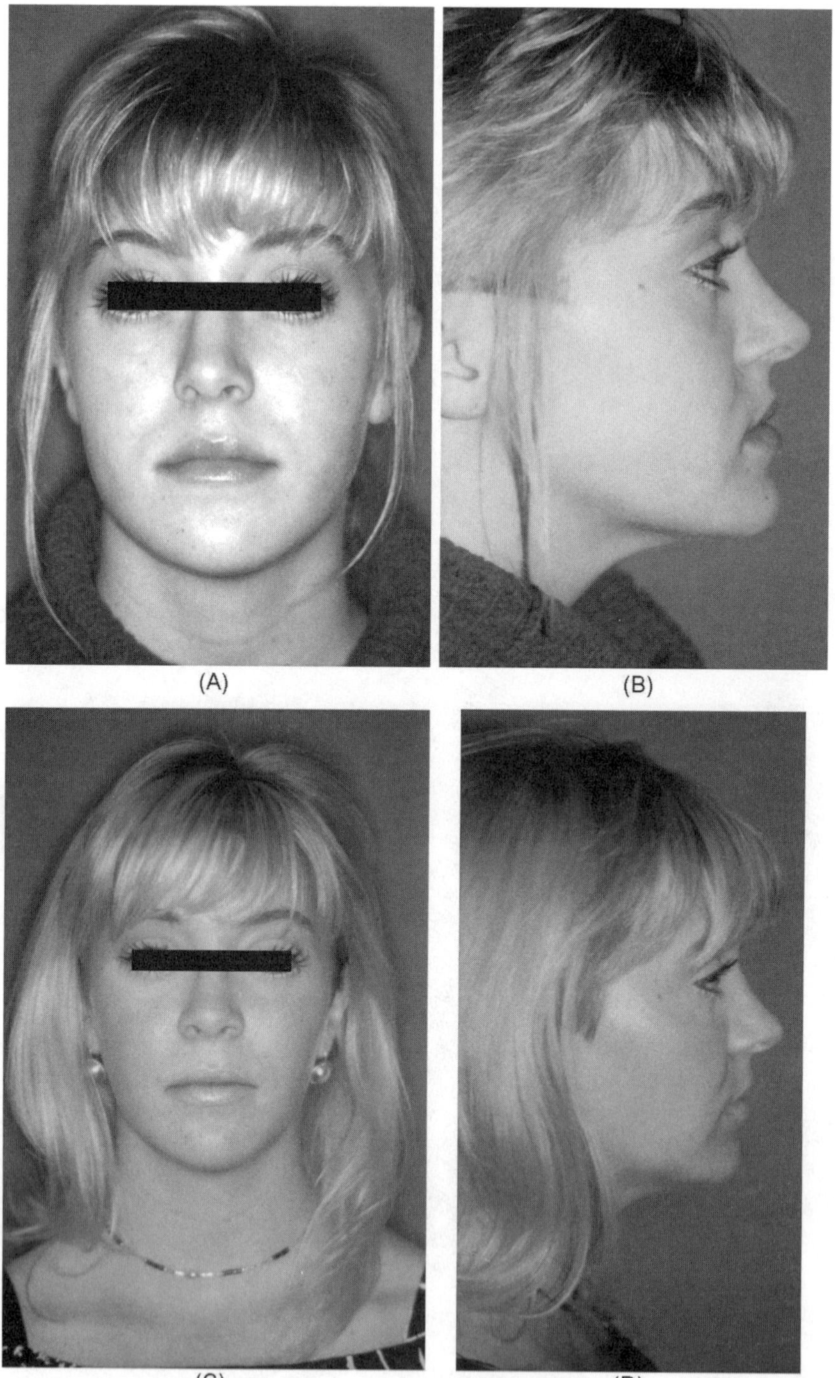

Figure 20 A,B Preoperative frontal and lateral views demonstrate maxillary anteroposterior hypoplasia and malar deficiency. C-E Postoperative frontal, lateral, and oblique views after Lefort I maxillary advancement and malar implant placement.

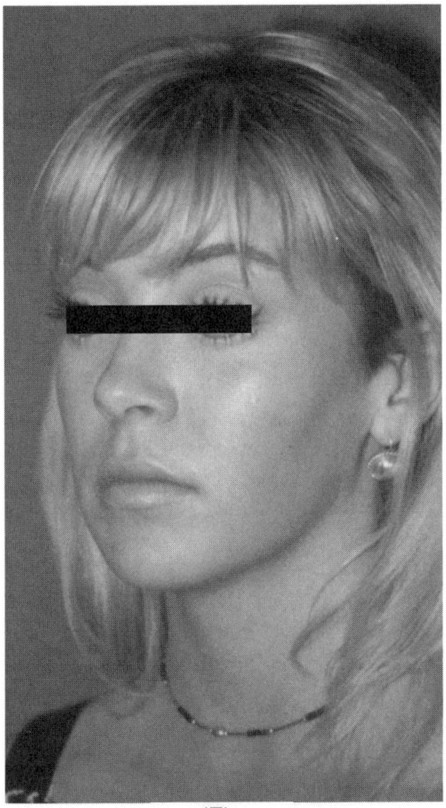

(E)

Figure 20 Continued

providing the tunnel for implant positioning and fixation. Dissection proceeds superficial to the masseter muscle in this region (Fig. 18). The implant is placed and should lie passively within the pocket created. If the pocket is too small, the implant may fold upon itself or it may tend to extrude. If the pocket is too large, the implant will not be stable and may become malpositioned (38). Fixation screws are placed, stabilizing the implant in position (Fig. 19). The incision is closed in a single layer using absorbable sutures. The patient is prescribed postoperative oral antibiotics for 1 week and given appropriate analgesic pain medications.

Complications

Complications from the intraoral approach include dysethesias from damage to the infraorbital nerve or motor dysfunction of the orbicularis oris (41). Nerve symptoms may be attributed to transection of small branches in the lip during incision, damage to the nerve bundle during dissection, or pressure impingement on the nerve from the implant. These complications are rare and minimized if meticulous surgical technique is observed.

Summary

Alloplastic malar augmentation affords the facial surgeon the ability the enhance the natural skeletal framework of the midface region. When performed on the appropriate patient after thorough evaluation, improvement in facial harmony can be expected with minimal morbidity (Fig. 20).

REFERENCES

1. Hofer O. Operation der prognathic and mikerogenie. Dtsch Zahn Mund 1942; 9: 121–132.
2. Converse JM. Restoration of facial contour by bone grafts introduced through the oral cavity. Plast Reconstr Surg 1950; 6:295–300.
3. Trauner R, Obwegeser H. Surgical correction of mandibular prognathism and retrognathia with consideration of genioplasty. Oral Surg 1957; 10:677–689.
4. Converse JM, Wood-Smith D. Horizontal osteotomy of the mandible. Plast Reconstr Surg 1964; 34:464–471.
5. Reichenback E, Kole H, Bruckl H. Chirurgische kieferorthopadie. Johann Amrosious Barth Verlag 1965; East Germany.
6. Hinds EC, Kent JN. Genioplasty: The versatility of the horizontal osteotomy. J Oral Surg 1969; 27:690–700.
7. Bell, Profitt, White. Surgical Correction of Dentofacial Deformities. Vol. 2. Philadelphia: W.B Saunders, 1980: 1212–1213.
8. Burstone CJ. Integumental contour and extension patterns. Am J Orthod 1959; 29: 93–104.
9. Burstone CJ. Lip posture and its significance to treatment planning. Am J Orthod 1967; 53:262–284.
10. Ricketts RH. Planning treatment on the basis of the facial pattern and an estimate of its growth. Angle Orthod 1957; 27:14–37.
11. Merrifield LL. The profile line as an aid in critically evaluating facial esthetics. Am J Orthod 1966; 52:804–826.
12. Gonzales-Ulloa M, Stearns E. Role of chin correction in profileplasty. Plast Reconstr Surg 1974; 41:477–486.
13. Hambleton RS. Soft tissue covering of the skeletal face as related to orthodontic problems. Am J Orthod 1964; 50:405–420.
14. Zimmer GH. Another look at the soft tissue profile. Unpublished manuscript, 1970.
15. Reidel RA. An analysis of dentofacial relationships. Am J Orthod 1957; 43:103–119.
16. Precious DS, Armstrong JE, Morais D. Anatomic placement of fixation devices in genioplasty. Oral Surg Oral Med Oral Pathol 1992; 73:2–8.
17. Michelet FX, Goin JL, Pinsolle J. L'Utilisation le la symphyse mentonniére. Ann Chir Plast 1974; 19:69.
18. Nevner O. Correction of mandibular deformities. Oral Surg 1973; 36:779–789.
19. Cohen SR, Mardach OL, Kawawata HK. Chin disfigurement following removal of alloplastic chin implants. Plast Reconstr Surg 1991; 88:62–67.
20. Matarasso A, Elias AC, Elias R. Labial incompetence: a marker for progressive bone resorption in silastic chin augmentation. Plast Reconstr Surg 1996; 98:1007–1014.
21. Park HS, Ellis E, Fonseca RS. A retrospective study of advancement genioplasty. Oral Surg Oral Med Oral Pathol 1989; 67:481–489.
22. Bell WH, Gallagher DM. The versatility of genioplasty using a broad pedicle. J Oral Maxillofac Surg 1983; 41:763–769.
23. Lindquist CC, Obeid G. Complications of genioplasty done alone or in combination with sagittal split ramus osteotomy. Oral Surg Oral Med Oral Pathol 1988; 66:13–16.

24. Mercuri L, Laskin DM. Avascular necrosis after anterior horizontal augmentation genioplasty. J Oral Surg 1977; 35:296–298.
25. Zide BM, McCarthy J. The mentalis muscle: an essential component of chin and lower lip position. Plast Reconstr Surg 1989; 83:413.
26. Goracy ES. Fracture of the mandible body and ramus during horizontal osteotomy for augmentation genioplasty. J Oral Surg 1978; 36:893–894.
27. Guyuron B, Raszewski RL. A critical comparison of osteoplastic and alloplastic augmentation genioplasty. Aesthetic Plast Surg 1990; 14:199–206.
28. Hinderer U. Malar implants for improvement of the facial appearance. Plast Reconstr Surg 1975; 56:157–165.
29. Wilkinson T. Complications in aesthetic malar augmentation. Plast Reconstr Surg 1983; 71:643–649.
30. Silver WE. The use of alloplast material in contouring the face. Facial Plast Surg 1986; 3:81.
31. Powell NB, Riley RW, Lamb DR. A new approach to evaluation and surgery of the malar complex. Ann Plast Surg 1988; 20:206–214.
32. Prendergast M, Schoenrock LD. Malar augmentation. Arch Otolaryngol Head Neck Surg 1989; 115:964.
33. Terino EO. Alloplastic facial contouring: surgery of the fourth plane. Aesthetic Plast Surg 1992; 16:195–212.
34. Binder WJ. Submalar augmentation: an alternative to face-life surgery. Arch Otolaryngol Head Neck Surg 1989; 115:797–801.
35. Mladick RA. Alloplastic cheek augmentation. Clin Plast Surg 1991; 18:29–38.
36. Binder WJ. Submalar augmentation: a procedure to enhance rhytidectomy. Ann Plast Surg 1990; 24:200–212.
37. Mass CS, Merwin GE, Wilson J, Frey MD, Maves MD. Comparison of biomaterials for facial bone augmentation. Arch Otolaryngol Head Neck Surg 1990; 116:551–556.
38. Constantino P. Synthetic biomaterials for soft-tissue augmentation and replacement in the head and neck. Otolaryngol Clin North Am 1994; 27:223–230.
39. Whitaker LA. Aesthetic augmentation of the malar–midface structures. Plast Reconstr Surg 1987; 80:337–346.
40. Ivy EJ, Lorenc ZP, Aston SJ. Malar augmentation with silicone implants. Plast Reconstr Surg 1995; 96:65.
41. Wilkinson TS. Complications in aesthetic malar augmentation. Plast Reconstr Surg 1983; 71:643–649.

25

Facial Resurfacing: Dermabrasion, Chemical Peel, and Laser Ablation

Darlene Skow Johnson
Lahey Clinic Medical Center, Burlington, Massachusetts, U.S.A.

Valentina R. Bradley
Affiliated Dermatology, Dublin, Ohio, U.S.A.

HISTORY

The concept of applying chemicals to the skin to improve its appearance is not new. The ancient Egyptians applied sour milk to the skin as a way to regain its youthful appearance. Unbeknownst to them, lactic acid, an alpha-hydroxy acid (AHA), was the active ingredient (1). During the French Revolution, women of royalty applied aged wine to their skin not knowing that tartaric acid, also an AHA, was the chemical ingredient improving the appearance of the skin (2). In the late 1800s, Dr. P.G. Unna, a German dermatologist, noted improvement of the skin with the application of acids such as salicylic acid, phenol, resorcinol, and trichloroacetic acid (1). During World War I, a French physician, la Gasse, used phenol covered with tape to heal gunpowder burns. His daughter, Antoinette, later brought the technique to Los Angeles in the 1930s and 1940s to treat scars and wrinkles (1). In the 1950s, a number of dermatologists were actively studying chemical peeling. Dr. Max Jessner at New York University reported the application of a combination of 14% salicylic acid, lactic acid, and resorcinol, known today as Jessner's solution (3). Sir Harold Gillies, a British otolaryngologist, successfully used phenol and tape for peeling of the skin (4). The toxicity associated with using phenol was known and efforts were made to formulate a buffered solution. In 1961, Baker and Gordon developed a saponated formula of 55% phenol mixed with water, hexachlorophene, and croton oil that make up the phenol formulation still used today (1). In the 1980s, animal and human models were used to study the histological depth of penetration of different chemical peels (1). This work resulted in the three-tiered classification of superficial, medium, and deep depth peeling. Today, alpha-hydroxy acids and beta-hydroxy acids are popular for chemical peeling.

Dermabrasion, an in-office procedure for resurfacing of the skin, was introduced in 1953 by Dr. Abner Kurtin who presented 200 cases of "corrective surgical planing of skin" at Mt. Sinai Hospital. A wheel covered with numerous, small, angulated wires were applied via a motor-driven rotating cable to abrade frozen skin rapidly and deeply (5). Small hand-held units powered by electrical engines or manual abrasion with sandpaper are used for dermabrading today.

In 1917, Albert Einstein published a theory describing stimulated emission of radiation by a photon from molecules in an excited state (6). In 1960, Maiman designed light amplification by stimulated emission of radiation (laser) using a ruby crystal and a flashlamp (6). Lasers were popularized in the 1960s and 1970s: ruby lasers for treatment of epidermal lesions, argon lasers for vascular lesions, and the carbon dioxide laser for excision and vaporization (6). In 1983, Anderson and Parrish reported the theory of selective thermolysis, which describes selective tissue injury by laser light that reduces the scarring of surrounding tissue (7). This theory led to the development not only of the flashlamp pulsed dye laser specific for vascular lesions, but also of a number of lasers that selectively target and treat a wide range of lesions. The medical use of a specific laser is directed by its wavelength, depth of penetration, and pulse duration.

INDICATIONS

Photoaging is the most common reason for patients to seek facial rejuvenation via resurfacing procedures. Photoaging occurs as a result of exposure to ultraviolet radiation (UV). UVB (290–320 nm) and UVA (320–400 nm), with its deeper penetrating wavelengths into the dermis, are responsible for photodamage (8). Elastic fiber degeneration occurs coupled with increased collagenase activation resulting breakdown of type I collagen. The subsequent resorption of elastin and collagen leads to a relatively prominent epidermis resting on a relatively diminished dermis, resulting in the formation of a wrinkle (9). The Glogau classification has been used to classify photodamage (Table 1) (10). In addition to rhytides, pigmentary dyschromias are another aspect of photoaging for which patients may seek resurfacing. These include melasma, lentiginies, and ephelides.

Another indication for facial resurfacing is the treatment of scars, resulting from severe acne, prior varicella infection, surgery, or trauma. In addition, actinic keratoses, a type of precancerous lesion that, if left untreated, could result in squamous cell carcinoma, may be successfully treated with resurfacing procedures.

Table 1 Glogau Classification of Photodamage

Type I	Mild No keratoses Little wrinkling
Type II	Moderate Early actinic keratoses Early wrinkling
Type III	Advanced Actinic keratoses Wrinkling at rest
Type IV	Severe Actinic keratoses, skin cancer Wrinkling: actinic, dynamic

Source: From Ref. 10.

Table 2 Fitzpatrick's Classification of Skin Types

Skin Phototype	Sun Exposure History
I	Burns; never tans
II	Burns; minimally tans
III	Burns moderately; moderately tans
IV	Burns minimally; moderately tans
V	Burns rarely; profusely tans
VI	Burns never; profusely tans

Source: From Ref. 11.

Fitzpatrick's classification of skin types I–VI is important in selecting the appropriate mode of treatment for each individual (Table 2) (11). In skin types I–III, pigmentary changes of hypopigmentation or hyperpigmentation usually do not occur, making all types of chemical peels safe. Skin types I–II are the best candidates for treatment with lasers. In skin types IV–VI the risk of postinflammatory hypopigmentation or hyperpigmentation is greater; a test spot at the hairline should be performed before proceeding further. Selection of a procedure is dependent not only on the desired depth of penetration but also on the duration of healing time and patient's ability to tolerate the procedure.

PATIENT EVALUATION

An appropriate amount of time should be spent with the patient so that he or she will not have unrealistic expectations about the outcome of a procedure. Letting the patient point out the area of concern and discuss in his or her own words the desired result may provide more insight. Discussing your perception of the patient's expectations along with realistic goals and outcomes is a cornerstone of any cosmetic procedure. For example, multiple superficial peels or multiple laser treatments may be required to reach the patient's desired outcome.

Photodocumentation before the procedure is important for both the physician and patient to assess results. The office staff should have a predetermined set of photos taken for all patients to ensure reproducible views and distances for comparison: anterior, left lateral, and right lateral views.

A full medical history should be taken and a full skin examination be performed. It is not advisable to treat patients with autoimmune diseases such as lupus, scleroderma, or vitiligo. Patients with lupus have an increased tendency to show Koebner reactions after cosmetic procedures (12). Patients receiving chemotherapy or who have human immunodeficiency virus (HIV) disease are at greater risk for postprocedure infections (13). Patients with a tendency toward hypertrophic scarring or keloid formation should be treated with caution and should have a test site performed prior to the procedure. The knowledge of prior exposure to x-ray treatment for the face is important to note; the potential lack of adnexal structures could impair proper re-epithelialization of the epidermis, which originates from these structures (14). If prior surgical procedures have been performed on the face, an interval of up to 6 months is necessary before treatment to ensure that collagen remodeling has been completed (14). Previous treatment of lesions and the resulting fibrosis may also affect the depth of penetration of the chemical peel or laser.

If the patient has a history of recurrent herpes simplex virus (HSV) infection, prophylactic antiviral treatment should be initiated with suppressive dosages of acyclovir, Valtrex, or Famvir as the trauma of treatment may induce reactivation. This is especially important for treatment with carbon dioxide laser in which the entire epidermis is removed and reactivation of HSV could result in scarring. For instance, treatment with acyclovir 400 mg twice daily perioperatively 5–10 days after peeling is recommended to prevent activation of HSV (15). A patient with a history of HSV infection who is undergoing carbon dioxide laser resurfacing should be prescribed a full 10 day course of antiviral medication (16). All procedures should be avoided in the setting of an active HSV infection.

The physician should review the patient's current and recent oral and topical medications. The prior use of isotretinoin or Accutane, which is utilized for the treatment of severe acne vulgaris, is important to note because it can increase the risk of postprocedure scarring. Isotretinoin suppresses collagenase and decreases the amount of pilosebaceous units in the skin. Collagenase is responsible for collagen remodeling and the pilosebaceous units are necessary contributors to the process of re-epithelialization. The lack of these two vital components in wound healing may result in abnormal hypertrophic or keloid scarring after resurfacing procedures. It is generally recommended that chemical peeling, dermabrasion, or laser treatment not be performed within 1–2 years of its use (17). Use of blood-thinning medications such as aspirin, a nonsteroidal anti-inflammatory, and vitamin E should be noted in the initial consultation and stopped, if approved by the primary care physician, 1 week prior to dermabrasion and laser treatment to prevent petechiae, purpura, or excessive bleeding. It should be noted whether the patient has been pretreating the skin with tretinoin. Tretinoin benefits photodamaged skin by increasing type I collagen formation and decreasing collagen breakdown by inhibiting collagenase (18). Tretinoin has been shown to potentiate the effects of superficial chemical peels and hydroquinone in the treatment of melasma (19). Pretreatment with tretinoin has also been shown to reduce healing time following dermabrasion (20). Daily application of 0.1% tretinoin cream for 2 weeks prior to 35% trichloroacetic acid peeling enhanced the healing time of facial, forearm, and hand skin (21).

PATIENT PREPARATION

Chemical peeling, dermabrasion, and laser treatment are in-office procedures performed by a trained physician. Aestheticians who perform chemical peels in a cosmetology setting are performing peels of lower concentration that are left on the skin for a shorter period of time. A nurse can perform the microdermabrasion procedure (see later). The patient, to ensure that he or she understands the possible risks of the procedure, should sign a consent form. This should be done prior to any anesthesia/analgesia. The patient should be advised to wear comfortable clothing on the day of the procedure. In general, the patient should first remove makeup, then wash the skin with an antibacterial skin cleanser such as Hibiclens. Preprocedure photos should be taken. Once the patient is reclined in the examination chair, a head cover should be placed to cover the hair. Drapes may be placed to protect clothing.

If lasers are being used, standard safety measures should be taken. The appropriate wavelength eye shields should be provided to all persons in the room. "Laser-in-use" warning signs as well as room access restrictions should be in place. Fire prevention steps and equipment should be established. All personnel should be well educated with laser use protocol.

CHEMICAL PEELING

In chemical peeling, moist gauze can be applied to the eyes to prevent the chemical from entering the eye and to encourage the patient to keep the eyes closed. First the skin is prepared by cleansing. Scrubbing the skin to remove the stratum corneum, cutaneous oils, and other debris prior to administration of the peel increases the depth of penetration. Scrubbing the face with acetone for 2–3 min is ideal as it dissolves sebum. Caution should be used, however, because acetone is flammable. Rubbing alcohol is occasionally used. An ointment such as petrolatum or Aquaphor Healing Ointment may be applied with a cotton-tipped applicator to deeper creases such as the alar grooves, oral commisures, and deep periorbital rhytides to prevent collection of the chemical agent in these areas. A fan blowing on the patient greatly decreases patient discomfort through cooling and also removes vapors associated with peel application.

The chemical to be used for the peel is poured into a cup for use to prevent contamination. Application of chemicals can be performed with one or two cotton-tipped applicators, large cervical swabs, a gauze sponge, or a fan-shaped sable brush. A rapid, uniform application is the goal, with the peeling agent fully applied to all parts of the face in approximately 60 s. In this way, the variation of the duration of chemical contact with the skin among the cosmetic units is minimal. Whether the peel is limited by time or patient tolerance, a resulting uniform peel is desired. The chemical peel is generally applied to the following cosmetic units: forehead, glabella, nose, cheeks, temples, upper lip, chin, and mandible. Application can occur superiorly to inferiorly and medially to laterally. This minimizes the risk of any agent being splashed or dripped into the eyes. The peel should be feathered into the hairline and jawline to prevent a noticeable demarcation line. Many peel chemicals pool in hair-bearing areas, resulting in crusting. This should be kept in mind when treating near eyebrows and hairlines.

In application, varying amounts of pressure may change the depth of penetration. Increasing the number of coats applied may also increase the depth of penetration. Adequate time between coats should be allowed to ensure the completion of active chemical penetration prior to applying the next coat. In this way, a deeper than expected peel and scarring may be avoided. Frosting of the skin may occur with application of the peel and is evidence of epidermal protein agglutination. Frosting can be an indication of evenness of peel application but is not a reliable indication of depth of penetration. If prior treatment with tretinoin or an alpha-hydroxy acid has occurred, then frosting occurs more rapidly. Severely photodamaged skin and highly sebaceous skin can slow the appearance of frost.

Superficial

Superficial chemical peels encompass the depth of the epidermis with some penetration to the level of the superficial papillary dermis. Superficial peels are indicated for treatment of fine rhytides, melasma, lentigines, ephelides, acne, superficial acne scarring, and actinic keratoses. Superficial peeling agents include alpha-hydroxy acids such as glycolic acid, trichloroacetic acid 10–35% beta-hydroxy acids such as salicylic acid, Jessner's solution, modified Unna's resorcinol paste, and solid carbon dioxide. Superficial peels are thought to be safe for all Fitzpatrick skin types I–VI and to have a low risk for the complication of postinflammatory hyperpigmentation or scarring. Superficial peeling requires multiple applications approximately once a month for a total of six applications to be effective. However, multiple applications are not equivalent to even one peel of medium depth. It is important that the patient recognize this.

Alpha-Hydroxy Acids

Use of AHAs has gained increasing popularity since the 1990s. Glycolic (2-hydroxyethanoic) acid and lactic (2-hydroxypropanoic) acid are the most commonly used AHAs. AHAs occur naturally, with glycolic acid found in sugar cane, lactic acid in sour milk, malic acid in apples, citric acid in fruits, and tartaric acid in grapes. The mechanism of action of the AHAs is epidermolysis with dyscohesion of the keratinocytes of the stratum corneum. AHAs have been shown histologically to thicken the epidermis and increase glycosaminoglycan deposition in the dermis (22). Glycolic acid has been shown to potentiate the effects of topical treatment of melasma with tretinoin and depigmenting agents such as hydroquinone or Kojic acid (23). The depth of penetration of these bleaching agents is increased when the epidermis is intermittently treated with glycolic acid. Greater epidermal necrosis and peeling have been shown with increased concentration of AHAs and with a more acidic pH (24). The lower the pH used in the chemical peel solution, the greater the amount of free acid available (i.e., the lower the pKa). Strength and depth are also dependent on the amount of buffering or neutralization of the AHA (24). Both are used to decrease irritation of the acid. Therefore, a chemical peel solution of 35% glycolic acid in a buffered solution may actually be equivalent to a 20% glycolic acid peel in a more acidic pH preparation. The physician must take great care to understand the active agents and preparations used. Strength is not a simple comparison of the percentage of acid content of a solution; strength also varies greatly among manufacturers.

Prior to application of glycolic acid, the skin is scrubbed with acetone or alcohol. Initial peeling should commence with 20–30% glycolic acid (a low concentration), to determine the patient's tolerance and cutaneous reaction. Application is with a dry cotton-tipped applicator, gauze, or sable brush. One hand is used to stretch out any skin creases as the agent is applied. Firm pressure with application to deeper folds of skin will increase the peel effectiveness in these areas. Application is continuous and repetitive, limited by time and not number of applications. Duration of chemical contact is determined by a combination of patient tolerance, indication for the peel, desired depth of peel, and/or a predetermined timed endpoint such as 5–10 min. Some patients, even at low doses of agent, may only tolerate 30 s of application. Others may be comfortable with little erythema at 5 min. Uniform erythema is desired. If frosting occurs, immediate neutralization of the glycolic acid should take place. Neutralization occurs with the application of bicarbonate solution resulting in a foaming reaction. A water rinse is applied next and may relieve the initial burning sensation experienced. Weekly or monthly treatments may be performed. Peel duration or the concentration of the acid solution may be increased with each subsequent peel. It is preferred, however, that only one variable change at a time.

Trichloroacetic Acid

Trichloroacetic acid (TCA) is indicated for rhytides, actinic keratoses, postinflammatory hyperpigmentation, melasma, and superficial acne scarring (15). TCA 15–25% acts superficially and has been shown to be effective for localized hyperpigmentation such as lentigines (23). TCA, with its pKa of 0.52, is a stronger acid than glycolic acid, which has a pKa of 3.86 (15). The mechanism of action of TCA is coagulation necrosis of epidermal and dermal proteins. The actual depth of penetration varies with the concentration of TCA used. Mixing TCA crystals with 100 ml distilled water makes the desired TCA concentration. For example, mixing 35 g of TCA crystals with 100 ml water makes a 35% TCA solution. The solution should be kept in a dark glass bottle and refrigerated. It should be poured into a separate container for use and the primary bottle restored to prevent weakening of the acid concentration through exposure to light and air. Mixed TCA solution can be stored for up to 6 months.

Application is with cotton-tipped applicators or a damp gauze sponge. A white frost occurs that is indicative of protein coagulation. Neutralization is accomplished with water through a mist spray or cool wet gauze. Reapplication of TCA to areas of greater photodamage or thicker skin may be made, with 3–5 min elapsing between coats. For subsequent peels, increases in peel duration or acid concentration may be desired based on the prior outcome and reported patient tolerance. For example, after peeling with a 10% concentration for 2 min, future peeling can be performed with a 5% increase in concentration up to 35%. One can then begin again at a 1 min timed application. Frequency of peeling can be weekly or monthly depending on the concentration, duration, and patient tolerance.

Jessner's Solution

Also known as Combes' formula, Jessner's solution consists of 14 g resorcinol, 14 g lactic acid, and 14 g salicylic acid in 95% ethanol to a quantity sufficient to make a total of 100 ml. This combination is important to decrease the total amount of any individual agent used, to decrease the toxicity of all individual components, and to increase the overall keratolytic effect of the peel. Although not as useful as TCA for the treatment of photoaging, Jessner's solution is useful for treating dyspigmentations of the face, neck, and chest (25). Pigment treated may appear darker for 2–3 days after peeling and flaking may be evident for as long as 7 days after treatment. The solution is best applied with a 1 inch sable brush. A gauze or sponge may be used if lighter application is desired. Jessner's solution is neutralized via its chemical reaction with epidermal proteins. Water application will dilute but not neutralize it. If multiple coats are to be applied, 5–15 min should elapse between applications to ensure completion of activity and proper depth of peel. Rapid succession of multiple coats will undoubtedly result in an undesired depth of peeling and possibly scarring. The fact that water dilutes Jessner's solution and does not neutralize it becomes particularly important if multiple peels are combined (for example, Jessner's solution and TCA [see below]). The number of coats of Jessner's solution can be increased with each session up to three coats.

Salicylic Acid

Salicylic acid (ortho-hydroxybenzoic acid) is a beta-hydroxy acid chemically unrelated to AHAs. Although AHAs are hydrophilic, salicylic acid is hydrophobic and lipophilic and is therefore active in sebaceous units. This makes it especially useful as a comedolytic in acne (26). The mechanism of action is a reduction in keratinocyte adhesion. Neutralization occurs with a cold water rinse. Salicylic acid has been reported as superior to glycolic acid for the treatment of acne vulgaris in patients with darker skin types (27). A 20% solution is applied for 3 min for the first application and 5 min in the second application (no sooner than 2 weeks later). Three more peels can be performed using 30% salicylic acid for 5 min application 2 weeks apart. Patients report less stinging and burning with beta-hydroxy acid peels than with glycolic acid peels.

Resorcinol

Resorcinol (m-dihydroxybenzene) is another superficial peel that disrupts the hydrogen bonds of keratin. Although the original paste contained resorcinol, zinc oxide, kaolin, olive oil, wool fat, and petrolatum, modified versions now exist. To detect contact allergy sensitivity, a test site application should be performed in the post-auricular region for 15 min and evaluated 4 days later. At the time of the peel, the paste is warmed for a few minutes in a plastic container surrounded by hot water in order to facilitate application. The paste is then applied for 25 min. The patient will experience a burning sensation. The paste is wiped away with dry gauze and the patient is left with a gray so-called resorcin membrane. Water and moisturizer applied to the face should be avoided for 4–7 days after peeling. The peel may be applied weekly for a month and should not conflict with a patient's immediate return to work.

Carbon Dioxide

Carbon dioxide (CO_2), at −78.5°C, can act as a superficial peeling agent. Solid blocks of carbon dioxide are wrapped in a towel dipped in a 3:1 acetone/alcohol mix that turns the composition into slush. Application is performed in strokes applying pressure for up to 15 s in any one area of treatment. Mild application is 3–5 s, moderate 5–8 s, and hard application 8–15 s. Increasing the pressure of application increases the depth of penetration. Solid CO_2 is an effective comedolytic and is useful for acne and acne excoriée, with freezing of comedones occurring with 5–8 s of application (28).

Medium

Medium depth peeling penetrates to the level of the lower papillary dermis and upper reticular dermis and is useful for the treatment of moderate photodamage. Peeling treats actinic keratoses, softens fine rhytides, decreases pigment, and improves depressed scars. Recovery time for medium depth peels is 7–10 days. Agents for medium depth peeling include combination peels such as 70% glycolic acid followed by 35 percent TCA (29), Jessner's solution followed by 35% TCA (30), solid CO_2 followed by 35% TCA (31), 50% TCA (32), pyruvic acid (33), and the combination of Jessner's and glycolic acid peel (34). On histological examination, 90 days after a medium depth peel, a Grenz zone is evident in the mid-to-upper dermis consisting of a thick band of elastotic fibers. Also seen is an increase of glycosaminoglycans, which, as a component of the ground substance of the dermal matrix, binds water and provides hydration to thicken the dermis and counteract wrinkling (35). Dermal collagen reorganization is complete in 60–90 days and is required before repeat peeling so that scarring does not occur. In other words, no repeat chemical peels should be performed on a patient sooner than 3 months after a medium depth chemical peel. Medium depth peels are often useful in combination with laser skin resurfacing, where the carbon dioxide laser is used over localized areas with greater photodamage while a medium depth peel is applied to the remainder of the face. This decreases healing time and minimizes the scarring risk associated with full-face skin resurfacing (34).

70 Percent Glycolic Acid and 35% TCA

This combination allows the glycolic acid to debride the stratum corneum facilitating dermal penetration of TCA. Glycolic acid is applied to the face with a cotton swab for 2 min and then neutralized with water. Next, 35% TCA is applied with a cotton applicator or gauze and subsequently neutralized with water. Cool saline compresses can be applied to the face to provide symptom relief.

Solid CO_2 and 35% TCA

The technique of solid CO_2 and 35% TCA combination peeling involves application of CO_2 as previously described with a block of CO_2 dipped in alcohol/acetone solution with varying amounts of pressure applied for epidermal destruction. After CO_2 is applied, the skin is wiped with a dry gauze and then 35% TCA is applied as previously described for dermal penetration. Although this peel is beneficial in that it allows for focal control of peel depth and is unique for treating contours of scars, it has the greatest risk of scarring because it can penetrate deeply.

Jessner's Solution and 35% TCA

The Jessner's solution and 35% TCA combination peel is effective for the treatment of actinic keratoses, rhytides, and pigmentary dyschromias. Initial application of Septisol or povidone–iodine solution should occur followed by an acetone scrub to remove the residue of the first cleansing agent. This is necessary not only to thoroughly cleanse the skin but also to remove superficial keratin debris of dry stratum corneum for even peel penetration. Jessner's solution is applied with a cotton applicator, gauze, or a sable brush. Frosting occurs after one coat. After 15 min, 35% TCA is applied followed by water neutralization. Water application dilutes Jessner's Solution and should not be done until after application of TCA. A second or third application of TCA will further increase the depth of penetration but should be avoided except in areas of greater photodamage or thicker skin. The stinging and burning that occur with this peel may be lessened with the use of a short-acting sedative (diazepam 5–10 mg) with analgesia such as meperidine 25–50 mg orally and hydroxyzine hydrochloride 25 mg intramuscularly (34). Postoperative care includes 0.25% acetic acid soaks four times a day followed by emollient application for the first 24 h. After this period, gentle cleansing of the face should be performed. Erythema and desquamation caused by this peel usually last for 1–2 weeks.

Electron microscopy of the skin 90 days following this combination peel reveals activated fibroblasts and collagen remodeling with organized, parallel arrays of collagen (36). Jessner's solution with 35% TCA has been shown in a single treatment to be as efficacious in treating actinic keratoses as treatment with topical 5-fluorouracil twice daily for 3 weeks. There was also a significant decrease in morbidity; post-peel healing time was 10 days compared to 6 weeks healing time with 5-fluorouracil (37). A single-application chemical peel may therefore be useful in poorly compliant patients with actinic keratoses. On histological examination, both Jessner's solution with 35% TCA and 70% glycolic acid with 35% TCA produce a thinner Grenz zone of remodeled collagen and elastotic fibers than does CO_2 with 35% TCA (15).

Pyruvic Acid

Pyruvic acid is an alpha-keto acid that converts physiologically to lactic acid, which is an AHA. Epidermolysis occurs in 30–60 s with dermal penetration in 1–2 min. Full-strength (95–99%) pyruvic acid is not used because of its scarring potential. Griffin reported the successful use of 60% pyruvic acid in ethanol for the treatment of actinic keratoses (33). Increased dermal penetration occurs if 5 ml pyruvic acid is combined with 8 drops Brij 35 (emulsifying agent polyethylene laurel ether) and one drop of croton oil (38). Croton oil comes from the seed of the *Croton tiglium* tree and is an epidermolytic agent. After the skin has been mildly scrubbed the acid is applied with a cotton applicator over 2–5 min. Water can be applied to the face for comfort but neutralization is not necessary. Erythema occurs 1 h after peeling and edema occurs within 48 h. Crusting occurs and resolves in approximately 10 days. Following peeling, skin care should be done with Povidone–iodine, water, hydrogen peroxide, or 0.25% acetic acid soaks with Bacitracin, Polysporin, petrolatum, or Aquaphor Healing Ointment.

50% TCA

This medium depth peel is no longer popular not only because of its unpredictability and increased risk of scarring but also because the combination peels have been shown to be as effective (15). Besides scarring, it is also known to produce hypopigmentation, hyperpigmentation, and prolonged erythema (39).

Deep

Deep peeling with phenol (carbolic acid), also known as Baker's phenol, penetrates to the midreticular dermis. In 1961, Baker and Gordon used 3 ml of 88% phenol, 2 ml of tap or distilled water, 8 drops Septisol liquid soap, and 3 drops croton oil (40). This combination dilutes the phenol to 50–55%. Caution should be used in application of the phenol peel because it can cause cardiac arrhythmias. Phenol peeling is absolutely contraindicated in patients with pre-existing cardiac arrhythmias. Because it is metabolized in the liver and excreted in the kidney, it is absolutely contraindicated in patients with hepatorenal insufficiency (41). A relative contraindication for phenol peeling is concomitant use of coumadin. A preoperative electrocardiogram, complete blood count, and electrolyte levels should be performed and cardiac monitoring is required during the procedure. Lactated Ringer's Solution (500 cc) should be given before, 1000 cc during, and 1000 cc after the procedure. Diazepam 2–5 mg and intramuscular or intravenous meperidine 50–100 mg have been widely used for sedation and analgesia (42). A regional nerve block could also be used, with long-acting bupivicaine infiltrating the supraorbital, infraorbital, mental, superior alveolar, and preauricular nerves. Risks include scarring, hypopigmentation, and a lack of depth control (43). Prior to peeling, a 3 min acetone scrub followed by alcohol application is performed. Using a moist cotton applicator, application occurs in six cosmetic units: forehead, left cheek, right cheek, perioral region, nose, and periorbital region. Peeling of the neck is avoided because scarring is likely. The peel is applied until a gray frost occurs. For a deeper penetrating peel, occlusion with tape is added (44). Waterproof zinc oxide nonporous tape can be applied as a mask to each area of the face. Small strips are applied in an overlapping manner avoiding the eyebrows, eyelids, and earlobes. To decrease toxicity, 10–15 min should elapse between treatments of cosmetic units, with the entire procedure taking 60–90 min. An immediate burning sensation occurs with application and pain can last up to 10 h. Severe edema also occurs that requires analgesia. Ice packs may be applied over the mask. The patient should sleep the first night in a sitting or semireclining position to minimize edema and facial friction with pillows. The mask is removed at 48 h and any exudate is wiped with sterile saline or hydrogen peroxide. To encourage re-epithelialization, the patient should perform wet to dry soaks or washes with povidone–iodine, followed by application of Bacitracin or Polysporin ointment. A side-by-side study comparing the treatment of upper lip wrinkles with application of three passes, 950 s dwell time carbon dioxide laser and unoccluded phenol peel showed a greater improvement on the phenol-treated side when examined at 6 months (45). Phenol peels were shown histologically to result in a thicker zone of newly remodeled collagen than pulsed CO_2 laser (46). The sun should be absolutely avoided during the 14 days of healing time from phenol peeling. Repeat peeling can be peformed in 1 year.

Postprocedure Care

After peeling, a moisturizer such as Cetaphil lotion should be massaged into the skin twice a day to decrease the risk of scarring. The patient should also be advised not to pick off any crusted areas or rupture any blisters that may form. If crusting occurs, a topical antibiotic such as Bacitracin or Polysporin should be applied twice a day to affected areas. However, immediate use of topical antibiotic ointments may increase the likelihood of an allergic or irritant reaction. If a moderate amount of erythema is noted following peeling, a low-potency topical corticosteroid may be applied. Post-peel pain should be treated with acetaminophen. Aspirin or nonsteroidal anti-inflammatory agents should be avoided during the recovery from dermabrasion and carbon dioxide laser resurfacing. One week after peeling, treatment with tretinoin can be restarted.

Sun avoidance and sun protection with sunscreen that has both UVB and UVA protection are important measures to prevent postprocedure pigment irregularities and to minimize further photoaging. The sun should be avoided for the first month after resurfacing. After re-epithelialization, a sunscreen with at least SPF 15 with UVA protection is recommended for daily use. If prolonged exposure to the sun is expected, at least an SPF 30 with UVA protection is required. Wide brimmed hats are a good adjunct to any photoprotective regimen.

Complications

Potential complications of all methods of resurfacing overlap because they all involve a degree of epidermal and dermal injury. Hyperpigmentation can last several weeks. Treatment with topical tretinoin and/or bleaching agents may minimize or reverse this side effect with time. Hyperpigmentation will be exaggerated if the patient has direct sun exposure during the re-epithelialization phase. Patients with skin types IV–VI are at an increased risk for postinflammatory hyperpigmentation. Hypopigmentation is largely an unpredictable outcome of any resurfacing procedure deeper than a superficial peel. This side effect is often not reversible.

Postpeeling infections may occur with aerobic or anaerobic bacteria, fungi, yeast, or viruses. The physician should see the patient soon after a resurfacing procedure to monitor for this. In addition, the patient should be instructed to call the office if any variation in the healing process is noticed or he or she experiences a fever, increased pain, or discharge. If infection is suspected, culture and sensitivities should be done and appropriate therapy begun. Infections can lead to significant scarring and early intervention is key to a good outcome. Patients with a history of HSV may experience reactivation of lesions with these procedures and should receive prophylactic-treatment (see above).

Prolonged erythema and pruritus may last up to 4 weeks. Topical low-potency corticosteroids such as 2.5% hydrocortisone may help to speed recovery and tolerance following the procedure. Ocular irritation may occur with peeling; therefore, caution should be taken to cover the eyes before beginning treatment. If irritation occurs and is significant, evaluation by an ophthalmologist should be done. Milia, or small inclusion cysts, may occur in the postoperative period following any resurfacing procedure as healing takes place. Milia may be treated with extraction using a no. 11 blade. Topical tretinoin used 2 weeks prior to dermabrasion and resumed 1 week after has been shown to reduce the incidence of milia formation (20). Usually this is delayed until full re-epithelialization is complete to minimize irritation. In addition, extensive use of a thick, occlusive moisturizer such as petrolatum may exacerbate this form of epidermal retention. Again, scarring may occur with any of these procedures and is usually related to the depth of treatment. Patients with a history of hypertrophic scar or keloid formation should be treated with caution only after a test site is treated.

DERMABRASION

Dermabrasion, or skin planing, is a procedure in which skin, particularly the epidermis and superficial dermis, is removed in variable amounts. It may be performed manually with sterile sandpaper or with a mechanical hand engine powering either revolving diamond fraises or a wire brush. Dermabrasion is a medium to deep resurfacing procedure (47). In comparing dermabrasion with superpulsed carbon dioxide laser, there was no difference in rhytid scores at 4 months. Less postoperative crusting and more rapid re-epithelialization were noted with the dermabrasion-treated skin (48). Dermabrasion may be performed for treatment of a variety of dermal and epidermal irregularities (Table 3) (47). Dermabrasion for improvement of a scar, traumatic or surgical, is best performed within 4–8 weeks of scar formation (Fig. 1)

Table 3 Indications for Dermabrasion

Acne rosacea
Actinic keratoses
Angiofibromas of tuberous sclerosis
Basal cell nevus syndrome
Chickenpox scars
Chronic radiation dermatitis
Congenital pigmented nevi
Colloid milium
Darier's disease
Decorative tattoo
Dermatitis papillaris capillitii
Elevated recipient sites of hair transplantation
Favre-Rachouchot syndrome
Fox-Fordyce disease
Hailey-Hailey disease
Hidradenitis supporativa
Hypertrophic scars
Keloids
Leg ulcer
Lentigines
Lichen amyloidosis
Lichenified dermatoses
Linear epithelial nevus
Melasma
Molluscum contagiosum
Multiple pigmented nevi (LEOPARD syndrome)
Neurofibromatosis
Neurotic excoriations
Porokeratosis
Postacne scarring
Postoperative scarring
Pseudofolliculitis barbae
Resistant or chronic acne
Rhinophyma
Scars from discoid lupus erythematosus (if disease is inactive)
Scleromyxedema
Seborrheic keratoses
Smallpox scars
Solar elastosis
Striae distensae
Syringoma, multiple
Telangiectasia
Traumatic scarring
Traumatic tattoo
Trichoepithelioma, multiple
Verrucous nevus
Xanthelasma
Xeroderma pigmentosum

Source: From Ref. 47.

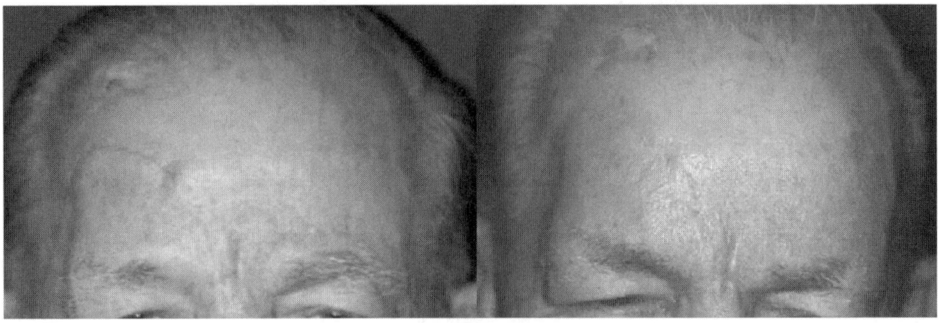

Figure 1 This patient underwent an A-T closure after a Mohs' microsurgical cancer excision over the right temple and forehead. The anterior forehead scar is obvious (left) and was dermabraded to the deep papillary/superficial reticular layer. After 8 weeks the scar is hardly noticeable (right).

(49). Scar improvements have been attributed to an increase in collagen bundle density and size with reorientation of collagen fibers parallel to the epidermis. Also seen is an upregulation of tenascin expression throughout the papillary dermis and an increase of the a6b4-integrin subunits on the keratinocytes of the stratum spinosum (50).

Patient Selection

The cornerstones of good surgical decision-making also apply to this procedure: proper patient selection, thorough medical history, review of systems, and focused physical examination. The need to acquire patient past medical history, medication history, and scarring history has been previously discussed in this chapter. In particular for dermabrasion, a history of bleeding dyscrasias and/or medications that affect blood clotting or bleeding time should be reviewed. Some contraindications for dermabrasion should be kept in mind (Table 4) (51). Adequate preoperative consultation time should be spent to discuss the procedure, its risks, benefits, possible complications, as well as alternative treatments. The patient should be evaluated for the possibility of combining dermabrasion with other surgical techniques for the best cosmetic outcome. For example, removal of ice-pick scars with punch biopsies or subcision of broad tethered scars is performed prior to dermabrasion (52).

Table 4 Contraindications to Dermabrasion

History of abnormal wound healing
History of hypertrophic scars
Recent isotretinoin treatment
Deep thermal burns
Congenital ectodermal defects
Chronic radiation dermatitis
Active infection (herpes simplex, human papilloma virus)
Psychosis

Source: From Ref. 51.

Informed consent should be obtained the day of the procedure before any sedative medication is given to the patient; this also allows time to discuss any last-minute questions. Many surgeons perform a dermabrasion test spot near the planned location of treatment. This may help assess healing and serves to expose the patient to the procedure and the necessary postprocedure care required. Nevertheless, the test site may not be indicative of the final outcome.

Equipment

Equipment varies according to the surgeon's preference. If using manual abrasion with sandpaper, medium-grade sandpaper can be obtained from a hardware store, cut into appropriately sized rectangles (1×2 inches for example), and sterilized. Many hand engines have been developed over the years that provide various rotational speeds (400–33,000 rpm) and torque choices. Most are electrically powered; however, some are driven by nitrogen gas and can be cumbersome because of the need to replenish and store nitrogen gas cylinders. Diamond fraise tips or wire brush heads secure into the hand engine, often with a choice of direction of rotation. The choice of tip is operator- and treatment-site dependent. Fraises and wheels vary in length, diameter, and texture coarseness. Diamond fraises are stainless steel wheels with industrial-grade diamonds bonded to them (53). In general, the coarser the tip, the faster it planes and the deeper the penetration. It is imperative to triple check the insertion and ensure the firm stabilization of the chosen tip in the handle. The hand piece should be easily maneuverable and the speed of the rotating tip easily controllable. All equipment should be easily accessible during the procedure and should be cleaned and sterilized using surgical center protocol. Regular maintenance of the equipment is vital.

Technique

Preoperative photos are essential for the ultimate evaluation of results as well as for documentation. The staff should establish a standardized backdrop and series of facial profiles. The treatment sites should be marked with a skin-marking pen: rhytides and demarcations of cosmetic units will be distorted with injection of local anesthesia.

The type and extent of anesthetic used depend on the location and extent of dermabrasion to be performed. If focal dermabrasion is planned, local anesthesia for infiltration and/or nerve blocks may be sufficient. If a larger area, such as full-face dermabrasion, is to be performed, conscious sedation may be needed. Patient monitoring appropriate for the degree of sedation is critical. Local anesthesia provides many benefits in dermabrading. It tumesces the tissue to provide a firm surface on which to abrade while epinephrine provides mild, local hemostasis throughout the procedure. Tumescent anesthesia, as used for liposuction, can also be readily applied to dermabrasion. This infiltration of saline with dilute lidocaine, epinephrine, and bicarbonate provides excellent tissue turgidity with an extremely low risk for lidocaine toxicity while providing excellent hemostasis via compression and the vasoconstrictive effects of epinephrine. Placing 4×4 gauze pads soaked with 2% lidocaine with epinephrine 1:100,000 with mild pressure onto the skin can augment hemostasis on treated sites. Some surgeons obtain a firm tissue surface by using a cryogenic spray to the skin just prior to dermabrasion. Frigiderm cools the skin to approximately −40°C in 25 s. Care should be taken not to refreeze adjacent areas, since this will increase the depth of tissue damage (53).

The patient should be comfortably positioned and lighting should be adjustable. A surgical tray should be easily accessible containing analgesic/anesthetic, dry gauze 4×4 pads, a basin of 2% lidocaine with epinephrine on 4×4 gauze pads, and cotton-tipped swab applicators. The hand engine, additional tips, and bandaging supplies should also be easily accessible. The patient should be draped to expose only the treatment site, all hair should be secured and covered, and all jewelry removed. The patient's eyes should be covered with gauze or goggles. The skin is prepped in a sterile manner. Due to the use of a rapidly spinning tip, dermabrasion often splatters blood (Fig. 2). The physician and staff should have protective covering according to universal precautions. The staff should wear face shields, gowns, and gloves. Before the procedure begins, the order of treatment sites should be planned according to cosmetic units. The assistant should use firm tension to keep the treatment site stable and taut. The surgeon should be extremely careful not to catch gauze in the rotating tip. The direction of tip rotation should always be away

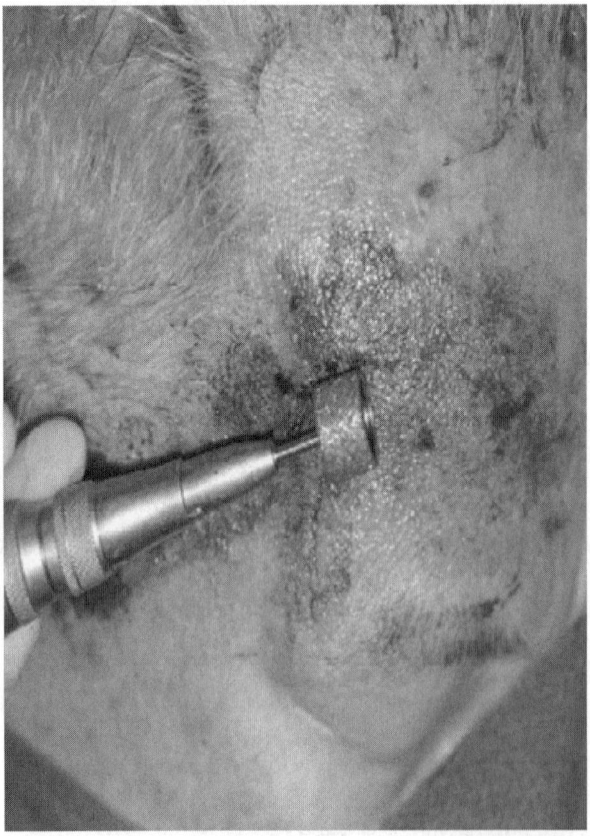

Figure 2 The same patient as in figure 1 as the dermabrasion proceeds with a hand engine diamond fraise.

from vital structures. The desired depth of treatment is no deeper than the midreticular dermis: scarring is significantly more common with treatments deeper than this. This correlates clinically with a change in color and texture of the dermal collagen seen while dermabrading. A surgeon should perform dermabrasion under supervision until this level of depth is firmly established and comfortably recognized. Hemostasis is achieved through firm pressure with gauze pads soaked with 2% lidocaine with epinephrine 1:100,000.

Postoperative Care

After reasonable hemostasis is achieved, postoperative photos are taken and the initial bandage is applied. This again is dependent on the surgeon, but usually consists of a topical antibiotic, a nonadherent dressing, an absorbent layer such as gauze pads, and a stabilizing outer layer for compression. Skin care while at home should be reviewed with the patient and also provided in written form. It is often helpful to have the person who accompanied the patient to the procedure present for these instructions as well. Appropriate pain medication should be made available to the patient. The patient should advised to avoid aspirin, products containing acetylsalicylate, and nonsteroidal anti-inflammatory medications. Applying icepacks and recommending that the patient sleep with the head elevated will help to minimize swelling, throbbing, and pain during the immediate postoperative period. The patient should perform once or twice daily soaks to the treated site always followed by a topical antibiotic or other lubricant to keep the area sealed from the drying air. The patient should be reminded not to leave the treated area open to air. If a crust does form, the patient should be advised not to pick at it. Keeping the treated skin moist and free of crust as wound healing occurs is important to ensure proper re-epithelialization (54). The patient should be scheduled to return to the office within the first week for evaluation since most patients heal in 7–10 days (47). Further follow-up and return to regular activities may be determined after evaluation of the treatment site and assessment of patient healing. Sunscreen use should resume as soon as re-epithelialization is complete; the skin is more sensitive to the sun for 1–2 months following dermabrasion. It is very important that the patient consider that the physician and office staff are always available for questions or problems. It is always better to address questions, concerns, and/or complications earlier rather than later.

Complications

Postoperative edema varies in terms of resolution rates but is often fully resolved 4–6 weeks posttreatment. Occlusive side effects such as milia, rebound oil production, and acneiform eruptions are often transient and usually respond well to skin care alterations as previously discussed. Complications such as infections (viral, bacterial, fungal), hyperpigmentation/hypopigmentation, and persistent erythema are possible with all resurfacing procedures. Scarring, although also possible with other treatment modalities, is a particularly significant risk after dermabrasion. Because the technique is so operator- and experience-dependent with the use of a powered instrument, one can quickly penetrate too deeply in treatment areas, resulting in scarring. Scarring, if it occurs, can be treated with silicon patches, intralesional steroids, or pulsed dye laser. It is of paramount importance to prescreen patients and eliminate those with a history of isotretinoin use in the past year or a history of any irregular scarring. However, the most difficult complication to overcome is unrealistic patient expectations. This again emphasizes the importance of the initial patient consultation as well as documentation with photographs.

MICRODERMABRASION

Microdermabrasion uses the concept of dermabrasion friction for removal of the epidermis using small granules circulated over the skin. This tends to be a more superficial treatment that extends, at maximum, into the papillary dermis. The granules vary depending on the machine and company, but are often aluminum oxide crystals. The speed of circulation over the skin and strength of suction on the skin control the depth of the procedure.

The concepts of appropriate patient selection, medical history, and evaluation apply. The patient is prepped and the skin cleansed before treatment as for chemical peeling. A test site is performed with a mild setting and adjusted according to patient tolerance. No anesthesia is required for this superficial treatment. As in other resurfacing modalities, the face is treated in zones, always moving away from vital structures. As with dermabrasion, it helps to stabilize the skin with firm pressure. Due to the superficial nature of this treatment, the patient may cleanse the skin, apply makeup, and resume regular activities immediately following treatment.

The long-term benefits from this treatment have not been firmly established histologically. Short-term benefits are an immediate soft texture of the skin due to removal of the rough stratum corneum. However, this texture change reverts within a month secondary to maturation of keratinocytes. Improvement of fine rhytides may occur both from the removal of the superficial keratinocytes and as a result of edema produced by the procedure. Some patients feel that improvement is a transient phenomenon. Most patients enjoy the slight erythema produced, which provides a more youthful skin tone than the yellowish hue that occurs with aging. This change also resolves over the subsequent few weeks. Repeated monthly treatments may also result in lightening of hyperpigmented macules such as ephelides and lentigines (55,56).

LASER ABLATION

Laser Physics

A laser emits electromagnetic radiation that consists of a stream of photons that travel in a wave moving at the speed of light. Electromagnetic radiation is ubiquitous and is the type of energy found in radiowaves, microwaves, infrared, ultraviolet and visible light, x-rays, and gamma rays (Fig. 3). The only difference between these types of electromagnetic radiation is the quantity of energy within the photons. Highly energetic photons have very short wavelengths at very high frequencies (e.g., gamma rays). Relatively low energy photons have long wavelengths (e.g., long-wave radio at 1000 m—taller than many buildings) at low frequency. Clinical lasers emit electromagnetic radiation in the infrared, visible, and ultraviolet spectrums

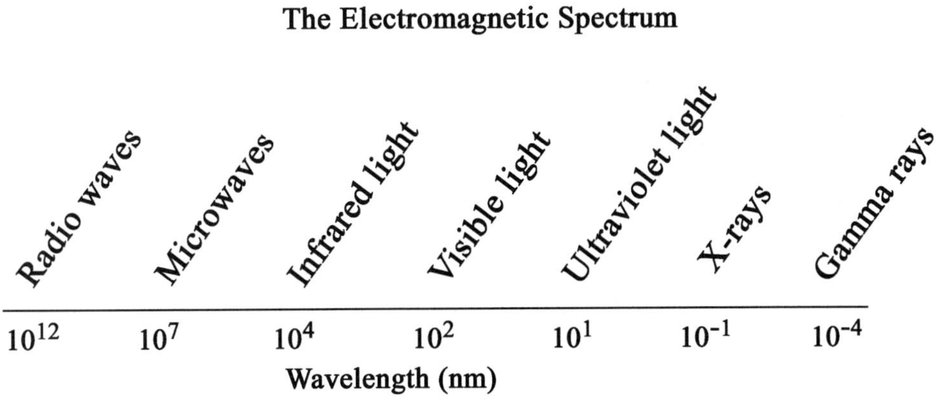

Figure 3 The electromagnetic spectrum.

(Table 5). The lasing material is unique for each type of laser and may be a crystal, dye, gas, or other. There must be an energy source that stimulates the lasing material such as a flash lamp, radiation, or electrical current. As the energy source stimulates the lasing material, the electrons are excited to a higher energy level in a process is known as population inversion. When the electrons return to their steady-state orbits they release quantums of energy in the form of photons that travel in phase at a certain wavelength. They stimulate other electrons to return to their steady state and release photons (stimulated transition). The photons along the optical axis are reflected back and forth, causing a cascading effect of energy and photon release. The light is amplified and a laser beam is produced. Certain lasing materials are capable of producing more than one wavelength of light.

Table 5 Lasers and Their Common Clinical Applications

Laser	Wavelength (nm)	Indications
Pulsed/scanning CO_2	10,600	Resurfacing; atrophic scars
Er:YAG	2940	Resurfacing; atrophic scars
Long pulsed ruby	694	Hair removal
Long pulsed alexandrite	755	Hair removal
Long pulsed diode	800	Hair removal
Long pulsed Nd:YAG	1064	Hair removal
QS ruby	694	Pigmented lesions; tattoo removal
QS alexandrite	755	Pigmented lesions; tattoo removal
Pulsed dye	510	Pigmented lesions; tattoo removal
QS Nd:YAG (freq doubled)/KTP	532	Pigmented lesions; tattoo removal
QS Nd:YAG	1064	Pigmented lesions; tattoo removal
Argon-pumped tunable dye	577, 585	Vascular lesions
Flashlamp-pumped dye	585	Vascular lesions; hypertrophic scars
Pulsed Nd:YAG (freq doubled)/KTP	532	Vascular lesions

Hundreds of lasers are available throughout the electromagnetic spectrum. Depending mainly on their wavelength, each laser releases its energy into the tissues in a unique way. Lasers within the visible spectrum (e.g., argon, KTP) and infrared (e.g., Erbium:YAG, CO_2) cause primarily photothermal injury. Depending upon the wavelength, the target tissues also absorb the energy in unique ways. The primary tissue constituent that absorbs the laser energy is termed the chromophore. The principal chromophores in tissue are water (CO_2), melanin (argon, KTP), and hemoglobin. The color of the target may be the primary attractor of the laser energy. This characteristic is especially useful in tattoo removal. The process of obliterating unique targets (chromophores) within the tissue using a laser is called selective photothermolysis (7). The absorption length of a laser is another critical factor in its effect upon the target tissue. This relates to the depth of the thermal injury that is caused by the laser pulse.

The most basic characteristic of any particular laser (its energy output into the target tissue) is influenced by the power of the laser, the spot (treatment) size, and duration of treatment (dwell time). Laser power is equivalent to laser watts (joules (J)/s). Power density incorporates laser power and spot size and is expressed as follows:

$$\frac{watts}{cm^2} \quad \text{or} \quad \frac{J/\mathrm{s}}{cm^2}$$

Fluence, a critical measure of laser energy, incorporates dwell time into the equation:

$$\frac{watts \times \mathrm{s}(dwell)}{cm^2} \equiv \text{Fluence} \equiv \frac{J}{cm^2}$$

Fluence (J/cm^2) measures the total amount of energy delivered to the target tissue on a pass or pulse of a laser beam. Although, for a given spot size, equivalent laser energy can be delivered by varying the power (watts) and dwell time, the dwell time is the critical factor in the clinical usefulness of the laser for safe and effective resurfacing. If the dwell time is prolonged, there will be significant charring and thermal damage to the tissue leading to deep injuries and scarring.

All laser energy, once absorbed, is converted into heat. This heat is what injures the tissue through a process called photothermolysis. The heat spreads within the tissues under the laser spot in proportion to the total energy delivered, absorption length, and, perhaps most importantly, dwell time. The tissues surrounding the area of primary photothermolysis (target tissue) will cool sufficiently to prevent the conduction of heat if the duration of the laser pulse is sufficiently short and the time between pulses is sufficiently long. The heat diffuses away by a process called thermal relaxation (time for tissue to lose 50% of its heat). If the laser pulse or dwell time is of short duration (less than the thermal relaxation time [TRT]), heat conduction and surrounding tissue injury will be minimized. A target chromophore with a long TRT allows the energy or fluence to be delivered over a longer pulse duration for target destruction while minimizing the thermal bleed into the surrounding nontarget tissue. Delivering laser energy to a target chromophore using a pulse duration or dwell time exceeding the TRT of the target produces thermal bleed (heat dissipation) that results in less peak energy available for target destruction and unwanted damage to the surrounding nontarget tissue. To ablate the target tissue it must be heated and vaporized. This requires a critical energy delivery and power density (critical power density). If an attempt is made to ablate tissue at less than the critical power density, a paradoxical increase in tissue damage may result due to excessive heating (energy usually released with vaporization).

To limit the injury to the target tissue, the thermal effects of the laser must be minimized. Tissue vaporization with minimal thermal spread of energy is ideal and can only be accomplished by severely limiting the dwell time. To achieve this, a high-energy–short-duration laser pulse or beam must be generated. For example, a fluence of at least $5\,J/cm^2$ must be achieved to vaporize a layer of skin during facial resurfacing (57). This energy must be delivered in less than 1 ms to prevent spread of thermal injury to nontarget surrounding tissue. This requires a high-energy laser specifically designed for resurfacing. For example, a laser that delivers a 50 mJ pulse under 1 ms with a spot size of 1 mm will have a fluence of $5\,J/cm^2$. Usually, the spot sizes are much larger (on the order of at least $3\,mm^2$) requiring a pulse energy of at least 400 mJ. There are several types of lasers for clinical use with a seemingly endless number of configurations. Pulsed and scanning type lasers are most useful for facial resurfacing. The key characteristic of most of the clinical lasers is the ability to deliver a very short pulse of a high-energy beam. This is accomplished in several ways including using a laser with a high energy burst capability and quality (Q)-switching mode. Q-switching is used to produce very short (nanoseconds) bursts of energy from a laser. A device within the optical chamber of the laser diffracts light and allows the stimulated emissions to reach very high levels of energy. The energy is then released in short repetitive bursts (laser pulse).

To choose the correct laser, several factors must be considered. These include the laser's primary chromophore, absorption length, and power density. For facial laser resurfacing, the desirable chromophore is water and the most common lasers used are the CO_2 and Erbium:YAG. The absorption length of the CO_2 laser is significantly greater than the Er:YAG and its depth of penetration and thermal effects are significantly enhanced. Both deliver sufficient power but their thermolysis capabilities differ. The CO_2 has a much greater potential for photothermolysis. A CO_2 laser can be operated in a superpulsed mode to minimize its thermal destructive effects. This mode delivers such high energy in such a short time that it vaporizes tissue into a plume by more of a photomechanical effect than a purely photothermolysis effect. Nevertheless, some thermal effect to the nontarget (deeper) tissue is desirable to achieve hemostasis and collagen tightening.

The CO_2 laser beam is collimated and the energy is dispersed over the skin surface in a gaussian distribution. The center of the beam (spot) contains the highest energy, with a fall off of energy toward the periphery. For this reason, there should be a slight overlap of the beam when treating adjacent areas (approximately 10%) to attain a more uniform treatment pattern. Some pulsed CO_2 lasers (e.g., Novapulse) create a beam that has a uniform fluence across the width of the beam. No overlap is necessary with these types of lasers. In addition, no overlapping is necessary with the scanning lasers.

Facial Resurfacing

Two wavelengths and types of lasers are in common use for facial resurfacing: erbium doped yttrium aluminum garnet (Er:YAG, 2940 nm) and the pulsed carbon dioxide (CO_2, 10,600 nm). The chromophore for these lasers and for any laser used for facial resurfacing is water. Most commonly, either laser is used alone to resurface the face and neck; however, each has beneficial effects and using both lasers in a single session is becoming more common. The Er:YAG is generally considered the more gentle of the two and is associated with a shorter time to re-epithelialization and less pain. However, it is less effective in most surgeons' hands in smoothing and tightening the skin than the CO_2 laser.

The depth of injury achieved with a laser is less than that achieved with a deep chemical peel. The depth of laser injury is comparable to a medium-depth trichloroacetic acid chemical peel (57). Nevertheless, the clinical improvement noted with the laser is comparable to a deep chemical peel. The laser is able to achieve these results due to the controlled conduction of heat beyond the zone of tissue injury and vaporization resulting in significant collagen shrinkage, remodeling, and skin tightening. Despite achieving similar results, the laser is associated with fewer adverse events than deep chemical peeling, including scarring and permanent hypopigmentation. The depth of injury per pass at the threshold fluence to ablate tissue using an Er:YAG laser is considerably less than a CO_2 laser. A CO_2 laser vaporizes approximately 50 μm tissue with a residual depth of thermal injury of approximately 100 μm. The Er:YAG resurfacing laser vaporizes 5 μm tissue with a residual depth of thermal injury of less than 20 μm.

Fitzpatrick et al. described three distinct zones of injury within the skin after laser resurfacing (58). The first is the zone of direct interaction in which there is tissue vaporization. The second is the zone of irreversible thermal damage in which there is tissue necrosis. The third is the zone of reversible thermal damage in which there is collagen shrinkage and remodeling. The third zone is probably responsible for the long-lasting skin-tightening effect noted after CO_2 facial resurfacing. The first two zones are responsible for skin smoothing and elimination of epidermal and dermal lesions and pigment irregularities.

Facial resurfacing is safe because re-epithelialization occurs with a low incidence of scarring. Re-epithelialization occurs by virtue of the skin appendages and is more reliable and rapid in areas with a greater concentration of skin appendages. Therefore, facial resurfacing is relatively safe compared to resurfacing other parts of the body, including the neck, that possess fewer appendages. Conventional laser resurfacing should be limited to the face. Regions of the face that tolerate deeper resurfacing include the cheeks, chin, forehead, and perioral areas. So-called light resurfacing, especially with one or two passes of an Er:YAG laser, is safe for the neck. When treating the face, a sharp demarcation is undesirable; therefore, light feathering of the laser over the mandible and into the neck can safely be done. Resurfacing skin in areas with fewer appendages should be performed using significantly less laser energy.

Preoperatively, a thorough medical and surgical history is obtained including a history of prior facial surgery and medications. Prior resurfacing procedures including laser, chemical peeling, or dermabrasion may predispose the patient to delayed wound healing and scarring. Prior blepharoplasty will predispose the patient to lower eyelid malposition after laser resurfacing. Use of isotretinoin (Accutane) within the last year has been associated with an increased incidence of hypertrophic scarring after resurfacing. Accutane use within the last 6 months is an absolute contraindication to resurfacing. A history of facial herpetic infection is noteworthy but is not an absolute contraindication. Smoking is discouraged and may be associated with delayed healing. Prior therapeutic radiation or collagen skin diseases usually preclude resurfacing.

Indications

Skin resurfacing with a pulsed or scanned CO_2 laser is used mostly for improvement of fine or moderate rhytides and dyschromias (Fig. 4). Although deeper rhytides also may be improved, other procedures such as autologous fat transplantation, Gore-Tex/other implantation, or surgical lifting can be used to provide additional benefit. Dyschromias, including solar lentigines, often are improved with laser resurfacing, although they generally are not regarded as a primary indication for treatment. Improvement of melasma has been reported although the recurrence rate after laser resurfacing is high.

Laser resurfacing may greatly improve atrophic scars caused by acne, trauma, or surgery (Fig. 5). Deeper pitted acne scars often require ancillary procedures for

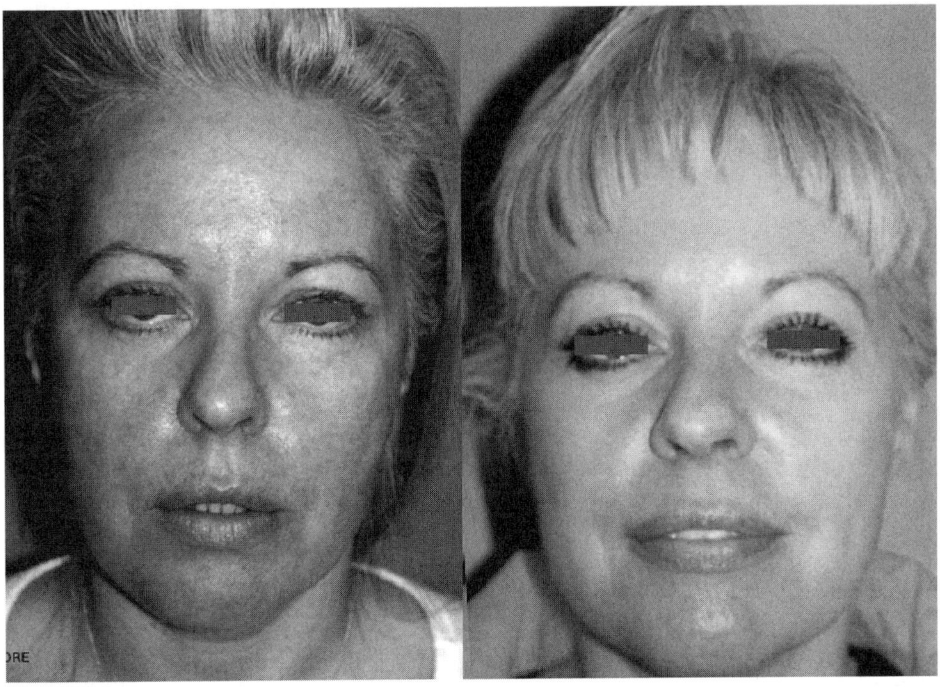

Figure 4 This patient's primary presenting complaints were uneven pigmentary changes (dyschromia) and mild rhytidosis (left). These are ideal indications for laser resurfacing and she underwent CO_2 laser full face resurfacing. Approximately 3 months later (right) her skin is smooth and of uniform color.

optimal results such as excision or punch grafting. These procedures can be performed either prior to or concomitant with CO_2 laser resurfacing.

Other conditions that have been shown to respond favorably to laser resurfacing include rhinophyma, severe cutaneous photodamage (seen in Favre-Racoucho syndrome), sebaceous hyperplasia, xanthelasma, syringomas, actinic cheilitis, and diffuse actinic keratoses. The CO_2 laser was used more often in the past for tattoo removal (in conjunction with dermabrasion); however, its use for this purpose has been largely abandoned due to the availability and efficacy of pigment lasers.

Preoperative Preparation

Preferences for skin preparation for laser resurfacing vary among surgeons. Often no specific preparation is done except perhaps an antibacterial facial wash the night prior to surgery. Pretreatment with tretinoin (Retin-A) has been shown to improve wound healing in animals and to lessen the depth of injury after laser treatment (59). Tretinoin cream (0.025%) applied nightly for at least 14 days prior to the procedure improves healing and postoperative recovery (58). Pretreatment with hydroquinone solution (4%) may be beneficial in patients with darker skin to prevent postoperative hyperpigmentation. However, a study by West et al. refutes the effectiveness of hydroquinone in preventing postoperative hyperpigmentation (60). Perioperative antibiotics and antiviral medication (famciclovir) are administered. Famciclovir is best administered 125 mg twice daily in patients with no history of HSV infection

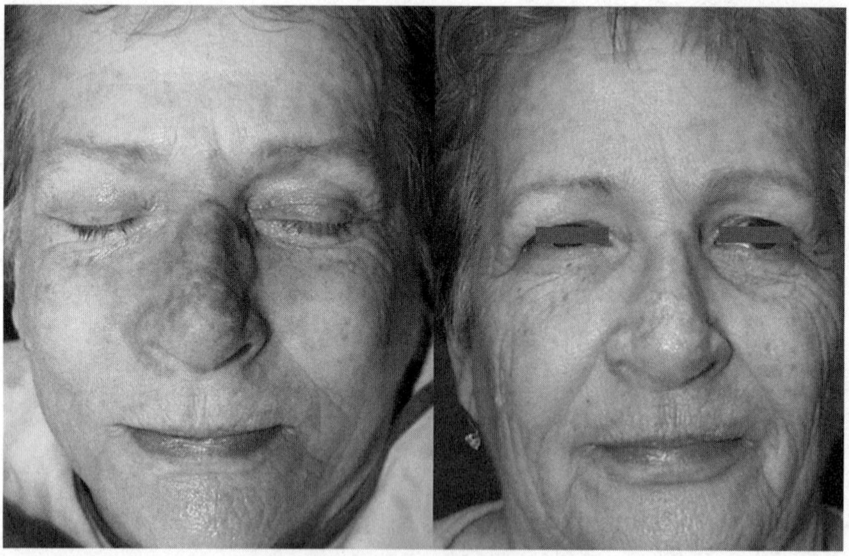

Figure 5 A full-thickness skin graft was placed over a Mohs' microsurgical defect on the upper lateral nasal dorsum. The grafted area was obvious and distressed the patient. The appearance of the graft 8 weeks after placement is shown (left). An Er:YAG resurfacing laser was used to ablate the skin over the graft and onto the surrounding skin of the nose and medial cheek. The skin was ablated to the deep papillary/superficial reticular layer. Six weeks after treatment the scar is not noticeable (right).

and 250 mg twice daily in those with a history of HSV infection (61). On the day of surgery, the face is prepped with dilute povidone–iodine and rinsed with normal saline. The procedure may be done under a general anesthetic or with local sedation and nerve blocks (mental, infraorbital, supraorbital). Resurfacing with a CO_2 laser can be painful and sedation is best administered by an anesthesiologist.

CO_2 Laser Resurfacing

David et al. first reported use of the CO_2 laser for cosmetic facial resurfacing in 1989. They used a conventional laser in a defocused mode to ablate the superficial layers of skin. The precise amount of thermal energy delivered in this manner was unknown but the technique produced results similar to a deep chemical peel. This system was difficult to control and a uniform distribution of thermal energy across the skin surface was difficult to achieve. In addition, prolonged dwell times with this free hand approach were common, leading to deep thermal damage and scarring. In the 1990s, Coherent Medical, Inc. (Palo Alto, CA) and Sharplan Laser, Inc. (Allendale, NJ) produced resurfacing lasers with high-energy output and very brief dwell times. The Coherent Ultrapulse laser produces short pulses of high energy sufficient to vaporize tissue ($> 5\,J/cm^2$) with a dwell time of less than 1 ms. The Sharplan Silktouch (scanning) laser produces a continuous wave laser beam that sweeps across the tissue to keep the dwell time under 1 ms.

A variety of CO_2 skin resurfacing lasers are marketed that either produce short intense pulses of light or are designed to emit a continuous laser beam that is rapidly scanned over the target tissue. The dwell time for each of these types of lasers is < 1 ms while the fluence achieved with each pulse is close to $5\,J/cm^2$. These lasers have microprocessors that configure the manual settings of watts, repetition rate, and spot size so that the dwell time and fluence are maintained at the appropriate levels. The user need only follow the manufacturer's directions to remain within the parameters for effective and safe resurfacing. Although the settings on different lasers may be adjusted to achieve apparently equivalent energy outputs, the ultimate tissue effects may be different. It is best that the surgeon become familiar with a particular machine so that consistent results are achieved. To aid the surgeon in consistent technique a computerized pattern generator (CPG) is available. The CPG creates a patterned treatment area with a predetermined overlap so that freehand manipulation of the laser beam is minimized. The surgeon need only move the CPG-controlled unit to adjacent areas and deliver the pulses. No synchronous movement on the surgeon's part is necessary.

The tissue effects of a laser and clinical outcome are somewhat variable depending upon the preoperative preparation of the face, the laser used, whether it is pulsed or scanning, the unique delivery method of the surgeon, the parameters initially set on the machine (watts, spot size, etc.), whether debris is removed between passes, the number of passes with the laser, and postoperative care. Observation and experience are important factors in achieving consistent results. With the available aids to uniform delivery (CPG) and a relatively wide margin of safety compared to deep chemical peels, laser resurfacing is a relatively safe and effective tool in most hands. The average tissue ablation during the first pass of a CO_2 lasers approximates 20–60 μm. After two or three passes the residual thermal damage (depth) is approximately 100 μm. The appearance of a yellowish color indicates entrance into the upper reticular dermis, which signifies the endpoint of treatment.

The largest difference with respect to energy delivery between the clinically available lasers for resurfacing is whether they are pulsed or scanning. Weisberg et al. studied pulsed and scanning lasers and their histological effects on in vitro human an in vivo porcine skin samples (62). They performed up to five passes with a scanning or short-pulsed CO_2 resurfacing laser. Tissue shrinkage (tightening), depth of thermal injury, the critical fluence needed for clinical effect, and the effects of tissue debridements between passes were studied. Maximal tissue shrinkage per pass was seen with the scanning laser (Sharplan Silktouch) at a fluence of $5.9\,J/cm^2$ and with the pulsed laser (Coherent Ultrapulse) at a fluence of $2.5\,J/cm^2$. The depth of thermal injury was maximal at 77 μm with the scanning laser at a fluence of $9\,J/cm^2$ and 25 μm with the pulsed laser at a fluence of $3.5\,J/cm^2$. Tissue debridement between passes resulted in increased shrinkage and decreased fluence required for the threshold tissue effect. Lowering the amount of energy delivered to the tissue minimizes the morbidity of CO_2 laser resurfacing, just so that it remains above the threshold fluence for tissue ablation. This study supports the contention that the pulsed laser causes less thermal injury than the scanning laser to achieve maximal tissue shrinkage.

Er:YAG Laser Resurfacing

The pulsed Er:YAG laser was introduced into the United States in 1996. This laser emits an infrared light with a wavelength of 2940 nm: near the peak absorption of water. The laser light is absorbed so efficiently that the depth of penetration into the tissue is only approximately 5 μm compared to 25 μm for the CO_2 laser. More importantly, the zone of thermal injury beyond the area of vaporization is much narrower: between 20 and 50 μm (63). Compared to a CO_2 laser, which is the only other type of laser that is commonly used for facial resurfacing, the Er:YAG laser produces much less tissue injury with each pass, especially with respect to the thermal spread of energy. In fact, there is so little thermal injury that collagen shrinkage and hemostasis are negligible. Without significant collagen shrinkage and hemostatic effect, the Er:YAG laser, while being an excellent photomechanical resurfacer, is less effective in initial ease of use (excesssive bleeding) and long-term elimination of rhytides and skin laxity. However, because of the negligible thermal effects, healing time (time to reepithelialization) and pain are significantly less than the CO_2 laser.

Er:YAG laser resurfacing is useful for a variety of epidermal and superficial dermal benign lesions as well as for many patients with photoaging including mild to moderate rhytidosis. Moderate-to-severe photodamage and deeper benign dermal lesions are best treated with the CO_2 laser. For routine laser resurfacing in the appropriate patient, the Er:YAG laser is effective and can be done with relatively little patient discomfort under local anesthesia with sedation. Healing is rapid and prolonged erythema is rare. Nevertheless, most patients will achieve a superior cosmetic result after CO_2 laser resurfacing, albeit with a slightly higher risk of complications and a relatively extended period of re-epithelialization. On average, a single pass of an Er:YAG laser results in a depth of tissue ablation of 10–20 μm. Approximately three passes are necessary to ablate the entire epidermal layer (100 μm). Fluence correlates with the depth of tissue ablation more precisely with the Er:YAG laser than with the CO_2 laser. In addition, since the energy from the Er:YAG is much more efficiently absorbed in the target chromophore (water) and the zone of thermal spread of energy is so small, the mechanism of tissue ablation is more photomechanical than photothermal. In fact, during resurfacing, the debris is thrown off the skin surface so quickly that the particulates actually reach supersonic speeds, creating a distinct popping sound with each laser pulse. The endpoint of resurfacing with an erbium laser is generally signaled by the appearance of punctate bleeding indicating entrance into the papillary dermis. Deeper resurfacing is possible but is impeded by the blood.

Combining the advantages of Er:YAG laser resurfacing (precise ablation, little thermal damage, rapid re-epithelialization) and CO_2 laser resurfacing (deep ablation with fewer passes, hemostatic effect) is a recent advance. Blended CO2/Er:YAG lasers (Derma-K or ESC Sharplan) are available for this purpose. The Er:YAG is often a typical short pulsed laser and the CO_2 is either a typical short-pulsed laser or a continuous-wave laser that is relatively long-pulsed and subablative. The usual reason to combine these resurfacing modalities is to speed the rate of re-epithelialization by minimizing the thermal injury caused by the CO_2 laser. This is achieved by removing or minimizing the zone of thermal damage caused by traditional CO_2 laser resurfacing. CO_2 laser resurfacing followed by Er:YAG resurfacing is reported to reduce discomfort and speed re-epithelialization because the Er:YAG removes the majority of the zone of thermal damage left behind by the CO_2 laser (64). Er:YAG resurfacing followed by a single pass of a CO_2 laser is also reported to decrease patient discomfort and time to re-epithelialization (compared to CO_2 resurfacing alone) while achieving adequate thermal injury to efface rhytides and tighten the skin. Histological examination of the treated skin reveals that thermal injury is less compared to the use of the CO_2 laser alone to achieve similar depths of ablation (65). Another significant advantage to combined-modality resurfacing is the ability of the treating surgeon to tailor easily the amount of thermal energy delivered to different areas of the face, depending on the lesions present and skin thickness.

Further advances in the field of laser resurfacing include the utilization of longer-pulsed Er:YAG lasers and nonablative laser resurfacing. The long-pulsed Er:YAG laser produces a beam with a dwell time longer than the TRT of the target chromophore (water). As a result, there is purported to be a greater zone of thermal damage, better hemostasis, collagen shrinkage, and skin tightening. The long-pulsed (10 ms) Er:YAG laser has been shown to produce greater thermal damage in the dermis than the traditional short-pulsed (350 μs) version (66). The variable-pulsed Er:YAG laser is reported to achieve similar clinical results to the short-pulsed CO2 laser with a risk profile similar to the short-pulsed Er:YAG (67). Nevertheless, the clinical evidence to support the contention that long-pulsed Er:YAG lasers can achieve similar results to the short-pulsed CO_2 with fewer adverse events is still lacking. It is likely that the risk profile is similar when the zone of thermal damage is equivalent.

Nonablative resurfacing is an option for patients with no need for removal of epidermal and dermal lesions but who desire an improvement in mild-to-moderate rhytidosis. Collagen breakdown and remodeling—the processes associated with skin smoothing, tightening, and wrinkle effacement—are possible without ablating the epidermis. The target chromophore in most nonablative resurfacing is oxyhemoglobin, primarily within the dermis. Histological changes within the dermis after nonablative resurfacing are similar to traditional ablative resurfacing. The mechanism by which this occurs is unknown but may be related to the release of cytokines and inflammation leading to collagen breakdown and reorganization. The epidermis is protected by surface cooling and targeting the deeper dermal microvasculature. Laser wavelengths useful for nonablative resurfacing include lasers within the visible light spectrum: 532 nm (green), 585 nm (yellow), and lasers within the infrared spectrum: 1320 nm (infrared) and 1450 nm (infrared). The target chromophore for the visible light lasers is oxyhemoglobin and the target for the infrared lasers is water. Although superficial lesion ablation is not done, certain pigmented and vascular lesions are improved with nonablative resurfacing including facial telangiectasias. Reports using the 532 nm (2 ms pulse duration) Nd:YAG laser indicate a significant improvement in mild-to-moderate rhytidosis and acne scarring with a high safety profile (68).

Postoperative Care

Immediately after ablative resurfacing, cool gauze saturated with topical lidocaine is helpful to relieve the stinging. The famciclovir is continued for 7–10 days until re-epithelialization is complete. Continuation of oral antibiotics is not necessary and may lead to the development of resistant pathological bacteria. Wound care consists of either an open technique or a closed technique. An open technique of wound care allows wound seepage and mild debridement while maintaining a moist environment suitable for re-epithelialization. The patient is instructed to debride accumulated crusts gently using a very dilute vinegar solution or a gentle water wash (shower) followed by copious application of petrolatum jelly until re-epithelialization is complete. Frequent wound checks and debridement are done in the office until the wound is healed. Numerous occlusive creams are available (e.g., Aquaphor, topical vitamin E, aloe vera) but petrolatum jelly is nonreactive and contact dermatitis is not seen.

A closed technique of wound care entails placing an occlusive dressing over the resurfaced skin for at least 24 h postoperatively. Closed dressings may be used up to 3 days postoperatively. Numerous methods are described but, in general, once the occlusive dressing is removed an open technique is used until re-epithelialization is complete. Purported advantages of the closed technique include less postoperative pain and shortened time to re-epithelialization. Batra et al. used a silicone occlusive dressing and found that it significantly reduced erythema, swelling, and crusting compared to the open technique. The eventual outcome remained unchanged (69). Newman et al. found that with a closed dressing technique there was a reduction in crusts, itching, erythema, and pain. No difference was found between the open and closed techniques with regard to the rate of re-epithelialization (54). Regardless of technique, after re-epithelialization is complete, a moisturizing cream is prescribed (e.g., Eucerin, Biersdorf, Norwalk, CT.) along with sunscreen.

Complications

Complications are rare after laser resurfacing and include laser fire, inadvertent organ injury, infection, scarring, prolonged erythema, hypopigmentation, and hyperpigmentation. Laser precautions are of paramount importance to prevent laser fires and inadvertent injury. Laser-safe goggles worn by the treating staff and patient are essential. Appropriate preparations such as signage and securing the operating suite should be undertaken by the ancillary staff. Laser-safe metallic corneal protectors are useful when treating the periocular areas. Minor infections include acne exacerbation and milia. These conditions are best treated with topical retinoic or glycolic acid or mild mechanical debridement. Fungal, bacterial, and herpetic infections are more serious but can be controlled with appropriate treatment. These infections occur during the process of re-epithelialization. Antiviral medications (famciclovir) should be continued until re-epithelialization is complete (at least 5 days postoperatively). Without antiviral prophylaxis, herpetic infections (HSV types I and II) occur in up to 9% of cases (61). If an HSV infection occurs despite prophylaxis, the antiviral medication should be continued for at least 14 days at an increased dosage.

Fungal and bacterial infections are more common in those treated with the closed dressing technique and those undergoing full face resurfacing. *Pseudomonas aeruginosa* is the most commonly found agent, followed by *Staphylococcus aureus, S. epidermidis*, and *Candida* species (70). Candida fungal infections are more common in those with chronic or recurrent vaginal yeast infections. Yeast infections are best treated with topical antifungals (e.g., clotrimazole) in conjunction with oral fluconazole.

Contact dermatitis is most often due to an applied wound emollient including an antibiotic ointment (Bacitracin or Neomycin), sunscreens, or steroid creams. Patients are especially vulnerable during the re-epithelialization phase. Erythema is expected and will resolve in the majority of patients within 6 months: a shorter period of resolution is expected after Er:YAG laser resurfacing. Topical hydrocortisone cream applied twice daily is useful to hasten resolution.

Hypertrophic scarring is fortunately rare, occurring in less than 1% of cases. It is most often seen in the neck, perioral, and mandibular line areas. The depth of the laser injury in these areas is most closely associated with scarring. Treatment includes topical and injectable steroids. Treatment with a vascular 585 pulsed dye laser, silicone gel, or silicone sheets can also be helpful.

Hyperpigmentation is seen with increasing frequency in darker-skinned individuals, usually occurring within 4–6 weeks postoperatively. This condition often resolves spontaneously but topical application of retinoic or glycolic acid is helpful to hasten resolution. Topical application of hydroquinone (5%) is effective for recalcitrant cases and its routine use should be considered in darker-skinned individuals. Hypopigmentation is rare and often not apparent for several months postoperatively. This condition is probably related to damage to melanocytes and may be permanent.

Hair Removal

The laser has made hair removal a more tolerable procedure than traditional methods such as electrosurgical epilation and waxing (71). It is also more effective than the traditional methods even though it rarely achieves complete and permanent hair ablation. The only nonlaser method that compares favorably is intense pulsed-light. This method utilizes a xenon flashlamp with optical filters to produce a multiwavelength light (550–1200 nm).

The chromophore for laser hair removal is melanin and the ideal wavelength for achieving destruction of the hair follicle, considering the need for an adequate depth of penetration of the laser energy, is 700 nm (72,73). Pulse duration is also an important determinant of efficacy. Photomechanical destruction of the hair follicle has been attempted using very short (ns) pulses of laser light. Although a portion of the hair follicle is disrupted, few permanent or long-lasting effects are demonstrated. However, Q-switched lasers have been demonstrated to cause hairs in the anagen phase to switch to telogen and shed. Therefore, using lasers in this mode, hair loss is proportional to the quantity of hairs in anagen (74). Although the TRT of melanin is short (< 1 ms), pulse durations considerably longer must be used. This is apparently because the true TRT of the hair follicle is longer and the thermal energy must be transferred from the melanin to the hair stem cells. The concept of thermal damage time was proposed to explain this phenomenon. It is the time required for the laser energy to diffuse from the treated hair to the hair stem cells. Destroying stem cells is the key to ensuring permanent hair removal. This time requirement ranges from 170 to 1000 ms (super-long pulses). However, it was found that higher fluences with pulse durations near 1000 ms cause greater pain and complications (75). Most hair removal lasers are used with pulse durations in the 2–50 ms range. The shorter pulse durations are better tolerated and few complications are reported using these parameters. The tradeoff may be, however, that laser hair removal is temporary and often incomplete. Although it is generally believed that hair clearance is more effective if the hairs are treated during their anagen phase, it may make little difference using the long pulse systems.

Several lasers designed for hair removal are in common use including the ruby laser (694 nm), alexandrite laser (755 nm), diode laser (800 nm), and Nd:YAG laser (1064 nm). Multiple treatments are usually necessary to achieve near-complete hair removal. Approximately 50% hair clearance is achieved at long-term follow-up (6 months). Ideal candidates are those with light skin (Fitzpatrick I–III) and dark or black hair. Some areas of the body are particularly resistant to treatment including the male face (beard) and pubic area.

The technique of laser hair removal is simple and can be performed by ancillary personnel. Laser safety protocols should be strictly adhered to. If the patient is tanned in the area to be depilated, the treatment is delayed to allow for lightening. If the patient has a history of herpes infections, then prophylaxis is given. The area is shaved or the hairs are trimmed to 1–2 mm the day before. Topical 5% lidocaine or EMLA cream is useful over the treatment area. All laser hair removal systems have an accommodation that allows cooling of the epidermis, often as an integral part of the laser wand (cooling tip). Overlapping treatment areas is avoided. Although a larger spot size is more convenient for the operator, larger spot sizes tend to be more painful (76). Multiple sessions are required to achieve apparent near-complete hair clearance. No commonly used hair removal laser is significantly different from another, except that the Nd:YAG laser, although less effective, is considered safer in dark-skinned patients.

Long-pulsed Ruby (694 nm)

The ruby laser is one of the most commonly used lasers for hair removal. It works by inducing telogen in the treated hair follicles followed by shedding and miniaturization (77). The recommended pulse duration is approximately 3 ms. Epidermal skin reactions tend to be more severe with shorter pulse durations. Increasing the pulse duration up to 20 ms was found to be safe and effective even for dark-skinned patients (78).

In a consecutive series of 346 patients, Chana et al found in using a ruby laser with a mean power setting between 8.6 and 15.7 J that there were few complications, mostly in patients with Fitzpatrick skin types V and VI (79). Pigmentary changes and blistering (mostly temporary) were seen. At 1 year follow-up, a 55% reduction in hair density was found with a median hair-free interval of 8 weeks (median number of treatments = 4).

Long-pulsed Alexandrite (755 nm)

The alexandrite laser is also a commonly used hair removal laser, most often used with a 3 ms pulse duration with fluences ranging from 20 to 50 J/cm^2 depending on skin type. The degree of hair clearance is proportional to fluence. Patients with lighter skin types are able to tolerate higher fluences and greater hair clearance. In a study by Eremia et al. there were no long-term complications in 89 patients (492 treatments) (80).

Long-pulsed Diode (800 nm)

The diode laser (12.5–25 ms pulse duration, 25–40 J/cm^2) was found to be equivalent to the alexandrite laser (2 ms pulse duration, 25–40 J/cm^2) in treating the axillary areas with minimal complications (81). Rogachefsky et al. used a modified diode laser (810 nm, 200–1000 ms super long pulse duration) to study the theory of thermal damage time. This laser was effective in safely removing hair even in dark-skinned patients (75). Lasers with super long pulse durations are rarely used but probably deserve further consideration, especially for patients with dark skin.

Long-pulsed Nd:YAG laser (1064)

The Nd:YAG laser (1064 nm) is more deeply penetrating and possesses a wavelength outside the peak absorption of melanin compared to the usual hair removal lasers. Nevertheless, this laser is useful in hair follicle destruction and is associated with fewer side effects because laser energy absorption by epidermal melanin is negligible. When used in its short-pulsed mode (Q-switched mode), an exogenous chromophore is applied to the hair follicles to encourage targeted thermal destruction. A carbon suspended in paste is applied to the skin and allowed to penetrate the hair follicle prior to treatment. When the laser is used in a long pulsed mode (50 ms) a carbon paste is not used. Alster et al. treated a series of dark-skinned patients with a long pulsed Nd:YAG laser (50 ms pulse duration, three treatments). At 12 months they observed a 70–90% clearance of hair. Adverse effects included mild-to-moderate pain during treatment and temporary pigmentary changes. Their conclusion was in agreement with other authors: the Nd:YAG laser is safe and effective for patients with dark skin (82).

Complications

Complications associated with laser hair removal are usually mild and temporary. Patients with light skin and dark hair are least likely to experience adverse effects. Complications include prolonged erythema, epidermal vesicle formation and crusting, and hypo- or hyperpigmentation. Scarring and pigmentary changes are most concerning. Fortunately, scarring is very rare but may result with high fluences in dark-skinned patients. Hypopigmentation is most often temporary due to the suppression of melanogenesis.

Pigmented Lesions

The chromophores for pigment-treating lasers are melanin and exogenous pigment (tattoo ink). As noted, melanin (within the hair follicle) is also the target chromophore for lasers that specialize in removing hair. The ruby, alexandrite, and Nd:YAG lasers, commonly used for hair removal, are also used as pigment lasers. The fundamental difference between a pigment laser and a hair removal laser is pulse width. Highly energetic short pulse widths (ns) are useful in photoacoustically disrupting melanin, melanosomes, and exogenous pigment. Longer pulse widths (>10 ms) are useful in the photothermal disruption of the hair follicle. Pigment lasers utilize short pulse widths that are less than the TRT of melanin. Hair removal lasers utilize pulse widths greater than the TRT of melanin and less than or equal to the TRT of the melanin–hair follicle framework. The short (several nanosecond) pulses of pigment lasers are produced mainly through Q-switching.

Typical pigment lasers include the red light lasers (QS ruby 694 nm and QS alexandrite 755 nm), green light lasers (pulsed dye laser 510 nm and QS Nd:YAG 532 nm), and near infrared lasers (Nd:YAG 1064 nm). Typically, multiple treatments are needed to clear pigmented lesions. The red light lasers are moderately deeply penetrating and are useful for lesions that involve the deep dermis including various nevi (e.g., blue), solar lentigines, and the nevus of ota (oculodermal melanocytosis). Nevus of Ota is a bluish lesion that is often widespread over the face. Most often found in Asian patients, the birthmark is due to overproduction of melanocytes within the dermis. Although rare, malignant melanoma may arise within nevus of Ota. More commonly, nevus of Ota is associated with melanoma arising in the eye and central nervous system (83). There are so few cases of melanoma arising within nevus of Ota that the effect of laser ablation on risk is unknown.

The green light lasers are less penetrating and are most effective in treating superficial lesions, mainly within the epidermis. Lesions treated effectively including seborrheic keratoses and freckles. Lasers with wavelengths in the near-infrared spectrum are more deeply penetrating but relatively poorly absorbed by melanin. Near-infrared lasers, like their hair-removing cousins, may be safer in clearing pigment in darker-skinned patients. Due to its long wavelength, an infrared pigment laser can more deeply penetrate the skin. It is effective in clearing nevus of Ota and is sometimes used in combination with a red light laser, although such a combination has been associated with an increased incidence of hypopigmentation (84).

Removal of Professional and Amateur Tattoos

Tattoo removal, including tattooing for radiation therapy planning, is an increasingly popular request. Traditional methods of removal, including excision and mechanical abrasion, have been largely supplanted by laser ablation. Tattoo ink is not easily removed because it resides deep within the dermis. The ink particles are predominantely found within perivascular dermal fibroblasts (85). Attempts to remove the ink mechanically will result in scarring. Laser light is meant to disrupt the pigment granules so that inflammatory cells including macrophages subsequently clear them.

Laser ablation requires several treatments and often results in incomplete tattoo removal. Professional tattoos are more difficult to remove due to the types of dyes used and their depth and density (most important) within the dermis. The density of the pigment granules is probably the main reason. A laser beam of a particular wavelength targets specific pigments within a tattoo causing their fragmentation. The TRT of pigment is quite short. Therefore, to confine the laser energy to the target pigment, very short (ns) high-energy pulses are required. Q-switched lasers are used for this purpose. Successful clearing of a particular color is wavelength dependent. Fluence should be sufficient to fragment the pigment. Sufficient fluence is present clinically if there is immediate pallor or whitening without blister formation. Spot size is proportional to beam penetration.

The target chromophore is the pigment within the tattoo. The absorption of energy by the pigment is dependent upon its color. For example, black ink absorbs laser energy in wavelengths that encompass the entire visual spectrum. Therefore, a laser with a wavelength within the visual spectrum (400–800 nm) will be effective in targeting this color. Fortunately, black ink is the most common color found in tattoos. Other colors within the visual spectrum demonstrate bracketed peak absorptions of energy that is wavelength dependent. The range of peak absorption (wavelengths) for various tattoo colors is demonstrated in Figure 6 (86). In general, a color most efficiently absorbs light from the opposing end of the visible spectrum. Black absorbs wavelengths across the visible spectrum well but its peak absorption falls between 600 and 800 nm. Based on these observations, the four lasers commonly used to eliminate tattoos (ruby, alexandrite, Nd:YAG, and pulse dye) should have predictable efficacy against the various colors within a tattoo. It should also be apparent that multiple lasers are often needed to remove a typical multicolored tattoo (87). Tan or flesh-colored pigment is particularly difficult to remove using a laser. These colors are more common in cosmetic tattooing. In fact, there are several reports of immediate darkening of flesh-colored and yellow pigments (88). This effect may be due to a chemical reduction of Fe_2O_3 within the pigment to FeO (black) upon laser contact (89).

The QS ruby laser (694 nm), according to the peak absorption spectrum, should be most effective in treating blue, green, and black pigments. This is found clinically, except that green tends to more resistant despite the expected peak absorption values (90). The QS alexandrite laser (755 nm) should be most effective in clearing blue, green, and black pigments, similar to the ruby laser. Like the ruby laser, clearance of red ink is poor. The QS Nd:YAG (532 nm, 1064 nm) laser operates at a dual wavelength. The 1064 nm Nd:YAG is essentially effective in clearing only dark or black pigment. The primary advantage of this laser is that it is more deeply penetrating due to its longer wavelength and is useful for lightening tattoos in dark-skinned individuals (sparing epidermal melanin more effectively than the shorter-wavelength lasers). The frequency-doubled 532 nm Nd:YAG laser treats red ink well (Q-switched mode) as expected from the peak absorption spectrum. Yellow and orange pigments are resistant to treatment despite the fact that this wavelength falls near the absorption peaks of these colors (91). The flashlamp-pulsed dye laser (510 nm) clears red pigment well. It is more effective against yellow pigment since this lower wavelength is within the upper limit of the peak absorption spectrum for yellow. Because of its shorter wavelength, clearing of pigment within the epidermis is more pronounced (92,93).

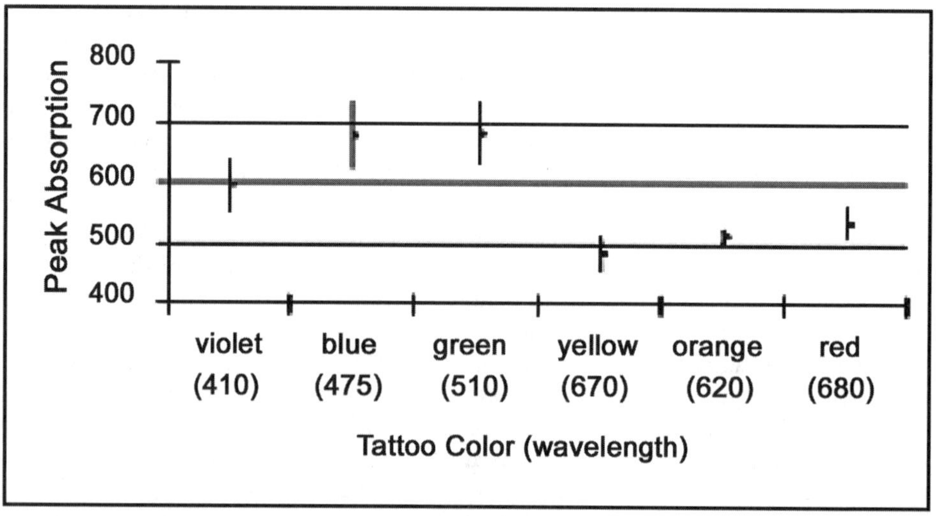

Figure 6 Peak absorption (nm wavelength) and tattoo color (nm wavelength). The vertical bars represent the range of peak absorption for each color.

Vascular Lesions

Many disfiguring congenital and acquired vascular lesions are treatable with a laser. Vascular lesions with large vessels or that are situated deep within the dermis are resistant to treatment. Vascular lesions commonly treated with a laser include spider leg veins, facial telangiectasias, and port-wine stains. Some scars respond well to laser therapy. Lasers have a limited role in the management of childhood hemangiomas.

Telangiectasias (including spider leg veins) are a result of abnormal dilation of existing vessels. The causes are varied and may be related to sun exposure, alcohol use, genetics, hormones (pregnancy), or steroid use (topical or injected). Facial telangiectasias are easier to eradicate by laser ablation than those in the lower extremity. Lower extremity telangiectasias are more deeply situated and are often associated with large feeding vessels. Sclerotherapy remains the treatment of choice for the larger vessels. Nevertheless, more superficial and isolated lesions are amenable to laser treatment, especially using lasers that are more deeply penetrating in the near-infrared spectrum (with an associated epidermal cooling device) (94).

Port-wine stains (PWS) are pink to bluish skin vascular malformations characterized histologically as hyperplastic and ectatic capillaries with the dermis. They tend to grow with the child and in early adulthood may hypertrophy and ulcerate. Port-wine stains are most often found within the V2 dermatome. Those within the V3 dermatome and neck tend to have more superficially situated vessels and are easier to eradicate with laser therapy (95). As with many vascular lesions, port-wine stains require several treatments and often never fade completely.

Laser scar revision is useful but the treatment varies depending on the type of scar. Keloids and hypertrophic scars can be improved using vascular lasers, while atrophic scars are best treated by laser resurfacing (ablation) methods. Atrophic scar revision can be done equally well with dermabrasion or laser resurfacing. Ablation methods should be avoided in treating keloids and hypertrophic scarring. This type of scarring responds best to nonablative methods meant to slow or reverse scar progression, soften the scar, and decrease erythema. Vascular lasers are assumed to work by the selective destruction of capillaries with the dermis. The resulting hypoxia may decrease collagen synthesis (96). The ideal time to treat a scar—whether atrophic or hypertrophic—is unknown but commonly 6 weeks after healing is chosen because of the peak in collagen synthesis at that time. The pulsed dye laser is commonly used for this purpose.

Hemangiomas, most often involving the head and neck, will grow rapidly within the first year of life and then regress slowly. Some hemangiomas should be treated, especially if they interfere with normal birth and development (e.g., obscuring vision). Although a variety of treatments are available (surgery, steroids, cryosurgery), laser therapy has proved successful for selected cases. Despite its efficacy in selected cases, the routine use of laser therapy for uncomplicated hemangiomas is not warranted. Patients treated with a pulsed dye vascular laser were found to be more likely to have skin atrophy and hypopigmentation than those whose hemangiomas were simply observed to resolution (97).

The chromophore for vascular lasers is oxyhemoglobin. The absorption peaks for hemoglobin are at 418 nm, 542 nm, and 577 nm (98). Lasers with wavelengths near these absorption peaks would be expected to be most effective in eliminating vascular lesions. The TRT of oxyhemoglobin is short (nanoseconds) but disruption of endothelial cells requires pulse durations in the microsecond or millisecond range (99). The main competing chromophore to oxyhemoglobin is melanin. To minimize thermal damage to the epidermis due to absorption of laser energy by melanin, a dynamic epidermal cooling device is often used (94). This is especially useful in dark-skinned patients. Common vascular lasers include the argon-pumped tunable dye laser (577 nm, 585 nm), flashlamp-pumped pulsed dye laser (585 nm), and the KTP (532 nm).

The argon laser was one of the original vascular lasers used to selectively target the microvasculature. This early vascular continuous-wave blue–green laser (488 nm and 514 nm) targeted oxyhemoglobin and melanin. The relatively nonselective wavelengths and long dwell times resulted in significant nontarget thermal damage. Subsequent work in developing laser systems with more selective wavelengths and shorter dwell times resulted in the advent of the argon-pumped tunable dye laser (577 nm, 585 nm) and the flashlamp-pumped dye laser (585 nm) (100,101). The shorter dwell times and more selective wavelengths resulted in better ablation of the vascular lesion while minimizing thermal damage and epidermal injury.

Argon-pumped Tunable Dye Laser (577 nm, 585 nm)

The argon-pumped tunable dye laser (577 nm) with a computerized scanning device is useful for treatment of many superficial vascular lesions including telangiectasias and port-wine stains. Increasing the wavelength to 585 nm results in deeper tissue penetration that is beneficial in treating lesions with deeper dermal components, such as most port-wine stains. Although significant success was attained using this laser, the flashlamp-pumped dye laser (577 nm, 585 nm) was found superior with improved lightening of port-wine stains (102).

Flashlamp-pumped Dye Laser (585 nm)

The pumped dye laser (PDL) was introduced in the 1980s for the treatment of vascular lesions but was significantly improved shortly after its introduction by intensifying its selectivity for blood vessels by increasing the wavelength from 577 nm to 585 nm and increasing the pulse duration from 360 to 450 ms (103). The PDL supplanted the argon-pumped dye laser not only because it was more effective but also because it caused significantly less thermal damage and scarring (104). The major problem with the PDL is the significant purpura that results after treatment. This will resolve within 3 weeks but is distressing for the patient. Recently, the pulse duration of the PDL has been increased to over 1.5 ms for deeper tissue penetration and improved hemostasis (103). In addition, the extended pulse duration more closely matches the true TRT of blood vessels (105). The PDL is the laser of choice for most port-wine stains and a variety of common vascular lesions including telangiectasias and superficial hemangiomas. Few side effects are associated with treatment. In a study of over 500 patients using the PDL, there were no cases of hypertrophic scarring ($<0.1\%$ of atrophic scarring) and only 1% of patients showed hyperpigmentation. Transient hypopigmentation occurred in 2.6% after multiple treatments of port-wine stains (106).

Pulsed KTP (532 nm)

Potassium titanyl phosphate (KTP) is the most commonly used crystal for frequency-doubling of Nd:YAG lasers. Because of the shorter wavelength, the depth of penetration of this laser would be expected to be less than the PDL. Although its use in the treatment of port-wine stains has been reported, the KTP laser would be anticipated to be less effective than the PDL in treating the larger deeper vessels within these lesions (further study is needed) (107). The pulse durations used with the KTP laser are on the order of 10 ms, which is significantly longer than typical pumped-dye lasers. Therefore, purpura seen with a traditional PDL is largely avoided. The KTP laser is commonly used for treatment of spider veins of the lower extremities that measure less than 0.75 mm in diameter in patients with light skin types (108). It has also been found effective in softening and lightening hypertrophic pigmented scars and ablating facial telangiectasias without purpura (109,110).

REFERENCES

1. Brody HJ, Monheit GD, Resnik SS, Alt TH. A history of chemical peeling. Dermatol Surg 2000; 265:405–409.
2. Moy LS, Eakin DR. When and how to choose chemical peels. Skin Aging October 2000; 59–69.
3. Brody HJ. Chemical Peeling and Resurfacing. 2nd ed. St. Louis: Mosby-Year Book, Inc., 1997, 82.
4. Brody HJ. Chemical Peeling and Resurfacing. 2nd ed. St. Louis: Mosby-Year Book, Inc., 1997, 2.
5. Kurtin A. Surgical planing of the skin. Arch Dermatol Syphilol 1953; 68:359.
6. Stratigos AJ, Dover JS. Overview of lasers and their properties. Dermatol Ther 2000; 13:2–16.
7. Anderson RR, Parrish JA. Selective photothermolysis: precise microsurgery by selective absorption of pulsed radiation. Science 1983; 220:524–527.

8. Yaar M, Gilchrest BA. Cellular and molecular mechanisms of cutaneous aging. J Dermatol Surg Oncol 1990; 16:915–922.
9. Brody HJ. Chemical Peeling and Resurfacing. 2nd ed. St. Louis: Mosby-Year Book, Inc., 1997, 9.
10. Glogau RG. Physiologic and structural changes associated with aging skin. Dermatol Clin 1997; 154:555–559.
11. Pathak MA, Ngheim P, Fitzpatrick TB. Acute and chronic effects of the sun. In: Freedberg IM, Eisen AZ, Wolff K, Austen KF, Goldsmith LA, Katz SI, Fitzpatrick TB, eds. Fitzpatrick's Dermatology in General Medicine. 5th ed. New York: McGraw-Hill, 1999:1606.
12. Baker B. Cosmetic procedures are not advisable in lupus patients. Skin Allergy News 1999; 3011:22.
13. Brody HJ. Chemical Peeling and Resurfacing. 2nd ed. St. Louis: Mosby-Year Book, Inc., 1997, 50.
14. Brody HJ. Chemical Peeling and Resurfacing. 2nd ed. St. Louis: Mosby-Year Book, Inc., 1997, 49.
15. Nguyen TH, Rooney JA. Trichloroacetic acid peels. Dermatol Ther 2000; 13(2):173–182.
16. Alster TS. Cutaneous Laser Techniques. Philadelphia: Lippincott-Raven, 1997, 14.
17. Rubenstein R, Roenigk HH Jr., Stegman SL, Hanke CW. Atypical keloids after dermabrasion of patients taking isotretinoin. J Am Acad Dermatol 1986; 15(2 Pt 1): 280–285.
18. Brody HJ. Chemical Peeling and Resurfacing. 2nd ed. St. Louis: Mosby-Year Book, Inc., 1997, 12.
19. Brody HJ. Chemical Peeling and Resurfacing. 2nd ed. St. Louis: Mosby-Year Book, Inc., 1997, 101.
20. Mandy SH. Tretinoin in the preoperative and postoperative management of dermabrasion. J Am Acad Dermatol 1986; 15(4 Pt 2):878.
21. Hevia O, Nemeth AJ, Taylor JR. Tretinoin accelerates healing after trichloroacetic acid chemical peel. Arch Dermatol 1991; 127(5):678–682.
22. Ridge JM, Siegle RJ, Zuckerman J. Use of alpha hydroxy acids in the therapy for "photoaged" skin. J Am Acad Dermatol 1990; 23:932.
23. Cotellessa C, Peris K, Onarati MT. The use of chemical peelings in the treatment of different cutaneous hyperpigmentations. Dermatol Surg 1999; 256:450–454.
24. Maddin S. Current review of the alpha-hydroxy acids. Skin Ther Lett 1998; 3(5).
25. Brody HJ. Chemical Peeling and Resurfacing. 2nd ed. St. Louis: Mosby-Year Book, Inc., 1997, 84.
26. Mills OH, Kligman AM. Assay of comedolytic activity in acne patients. Acta Dermato Venereol 1993; 631:68–71.
27. Guttman C. Chemical peel beneficial to dark skin. Dermatol Times 1999; S20.
28. Brody HJ. Chemical Peeling and Resurfacing. 2nd ed. St. Louis: Mosby-Year Book, Inc., 1997, 90.
29. Coleman WP, Futrell JM. The glycolic acid trichloroacetic acid peel. J Dermatol Surg Oncol 1994; 20(1):76–80.
30. Monheit GD. The Jessner's + TCA peel: a medium-depth chemical peel. Dermatol Surg Oncol 1989; 15(9):945–950.
31. Brody HJ. Variations and comparisons in medium-depth chemical peeling. Dermatol Surg Oncol 1989; 15(9):953–963.
32. Brody HJ. Chemical Peeling and Resurfacing. 2nd ed. St. Louis: Mosby-Year Book, Inc., 1997, 128.
33. Griffin TD, Van Scott EJ. Use of pyruvic acid in the treatment of actinic keratoses: a chemical and histopathologic study. Cutis 1991; 47(5):325–329.
34. Monheit GD. Medium-depth combination peels. Dermatol Ther 2000; 13(2):183–191.

35. Van Scott EJ, Yu RJ. Effects of alpha-hydroxy-acids on photoaged skin: a pilot clinical, histologic, and ultrastructural study. J Am Acad Dermatol 1996; 34(2):187–195.
36. Brody HJ. Chemical Peeling and Resurfacing. 2nd ed. St. Louis: Mosby-Year Book, Inc., 1997, 18.
37. Lawrence N, Cox SE, Cockerell CJ. A comparison of the efficacy and safety of Jessner's solution and 35 percent trichloracetic acid vs 5 percent fluorouracil in the treatment of widespread facial actinic keratoses. Arch Dermatol 1995; 131(2):176–181.
38. Brody HJ. Chemical Peeling and Resurfacing. 2nd ed. St. Louis: Mosby-Year Book, Inc., 1997, 130.
39. Brody HJ. Chemical Peeling and Resurfacing. 2nd ed. St. Louis: Mosby-Year Book, Inc., 1997, 128.
40. Brody HJ. Chemical Peeling and Resurfacing. 2nd ed. St. Louis: Mosby-Year Book, Inc., 1997, 138.
41. Asken S. Unoccluded Baker-Gordon phenol peels—review and update. Dermatol Surg Oncol 1989; 15:998–1008.
42. Brody HJ. Chemical Peeling and Resurfacing. 2nd ed. St. Louis: Mosby-Year Book, Inc., 1997, 140.
43. Roenigk RK, Broadland DG. A primer of facial chemical peel. Dermatol Clin 1993; 11(2):349–359.
44. Alt TH. Occluded Baker-Gordon chemical peel: review and update. J Dermatol Surg Oncol 1989; 15(9):980–993.
45. Chew J, Gin I, Rau KA. Treatment of upper lip wrinkles: a comparison of 950 microsecond dwell time carbon dioxide laser with unoccluded Baker's phenol chemical peel. Dermatol Surg 1999; 25(4):262–266.
46. Moy LS, Kotler R, Lesser T. The histologic evaluation of pulsed carbon dioxide laser resurfacing versus phenol chemical peels in vivo. Dermatol Surg 1999; 258: 597–600.
47. Lawrence N, Mandy S, Yarborough JM Jr., Alt T. History of dermabrasion. Dermatol Surg 2000; 262:95–101.
48. Holmkivst KA, Rogers GS. Treatment of perioral rhytides. Arch Dermatol 2000; 136:725–731.
49. Yarborough JM Jr. Ablation of facial scars by programmed dermabrasion. J Dermatol Surg Oncol 1988; 14:292–294.
50. Harmon CB, Zelickson BD, Roenigk RK, et al. Dermabrasive scar revision. Immunohistochemical and ultrastructural evaluation. Dermatol Surg 1995; 21:503–508.
51. Matarasso SL, Hanke CW, Alster TS. Cutaneous resurfacing. Dermatol Clin 1997; 14(4):569–582.
52. Orentreich N, Orentreich DS. Dermabrasion. Dermatol Clin 1995; 132:313–327.
53. Padilla RS, Yarborough JM Jr. Dermabrasion. In: Ratz JL, ed. Textbook of Dermatologic Surgery, Philadelphia: Lippincott-Raven, 1998:473–484.
54. Newman JP, Koch RJ, Goode RL. Closed dressings after laser skin resurfacing. Arch Otolaryngol 1998; 124(7):751–757.
55. Shim EK, Barnette D, Hughes K, Greenway HT. Microdermabrasion: a clinical and histopathologic study. Dermatol Surg 2001; 276:524–530.
56. Tsai R, Wang C, Chan H. Aluminum oxide crystal microdermabrasion: a new technique for treating facial scarring. Dermatol Surg 1995; 21:539–542.
57. Hruza GJ, Dover JS. Laser skin resurfacing. Arch Dermatol 1996; 132:451–455.
58. Fitzpatrick RE, Goldman MP, Satur NM, Tope WD. Pulsed carbon dioxide laser resurfacing of photo-aged facial skin. Arch Dermatol 1996; 132:395–402.
59. McDonald WS, Beasley D, Jones C. Retinoic acid and CO_2 laser resurfacing. Plast Reconstr Surg 1999; 104:2229–2235.

60. West TB, Alster TS. Effect of pretreatment on the incidence of hyperpigmentation following cutaneous CO_2 laser resurfacing. Dermatol Surg. 1999; 25:15–17.
61. Wall SH, Ramey SJ, Wall F. Famciclovir as antiviral prophylaxis in laser resurfacing procedures. Plast Reconstr Surg 1999; 104:1103–1108.
62. Weisberg NK, Kuo T, Torkian B, Reinisch L, Ellis DL. Optimizing fluence and debridement effects on cutaneous resurfacing carbon dioxide laser surgery. Arch.-Dermatol 1998; 134:1223–1228.
63. Walsh JT Jr., Flotte TJ, Deutsch TF. Er:YAG laser ablation of tissue: effect of pulse duration and tissue type on thermal damage. Lasers Surg Med 1989; 9:314–326.
64. McDaniel DH, Lord J, Ash K, Newman J. Combined CO_2/erbium:YAG laser resurfacing of peri-oral rhytides and side-by-side comparison with carbon dioxide laser alone. Dermatol Surg 1999; 25:285–293.
65. Millman AL, Mannor GE. Histologic and clinical evaluation of combined eyelid erbium: YAG and CO_2 laser resurfacing. Am J Ophthalmol 1999; 127:614–616.
66. Adrian RM. Pulsed carbon dioxide and long pulse 10-ms erbium-YAG laser resurfacing: a comparative clinical and histologic study. J Cutan Laser Ther 1999; 1:197–202.
67. Rostan EF, Fitzpatrick RE, Goldman MP. Laser resurfacing with a long pulse erbium:YAG laser compared to the 950 ms pulsed CO(2) laser. Lasers Surg Med 2001; 29:136–141.
68. Bernstein EF, Ferreira M, Anderson D. A pilot investigation to subjectively measure treatment effect and side-effect profile of non-ablative skin remodeling using a 532 nm, 2 ms pulse-duration laser. J Cosmet Laser Ther 2001; 3:137–141.
69. Batra RS, Ort RJ, Jacob C, Hobbs L, Arndt KA, Dover JS. Evaluation of a silicone occlusive dressing after laser skin resurfacing. Arch.Dermatol 2001; 137:1317–1321.
70. Sriprachya-Anunt S, Fitzpatrick RE, Goldman MP, Smith SR. Infections complicating pulsed carbon dioxide laser resurfacing for photoaged facial skin. Dermatol Surg 1997; 23:527–535.
71. Polderman MC, Pavel S, le Cessie S, Grevelink JM, van Leeuwen RL. Efficacy, tolerability, and safety of a long-pulsed ruby laser system in the removal of unwanted hair. Dermatol Surg 2000; 26:240–243.
72. Liew SH. Laser hair removal: guidelines for management. Am J Clin Dermatol 2002; 3:107–115.
73. Grossman MC, Dierickx C, Farinelli W, Flotte T, Anderson RR. Damage to hair follicles by normal-mode ruby laser pulses. J Am Acad Dermatol 1996; 35:889–894.
74. Kolinko VG, Littler CM, Cole A.. Influence of the anagen:telogen ratio on Q-switched Nd:YAG laser hair removal efficacy. Lasers Surg Med 2000; 26:33–40.
75. Rogachefsky AS, Silapunt S, Goldberg DJ. Evaluation of a new super-long-pulsed 810 nm diode laser for the removal of unwanted hair: the concept of thermal damage time. Dermatol Surg 2002; 28:410–414.
76. Eremia S, Newman N. Topical anesthesia for laser hair removal: comparison of spot sizes and 755 nm versus 800 nm wavelengths. Dermatol Surg 2000; 26:667–669.
77. McCoy S, Evans A, James C. Long-pulsed ruby laser for permanent hair reduction: histological analysis after 3, 4 1/2, and 6 months. Lasers Surg Med 2002; 30:401–405.
78. Elman M, Klein A, Slatkine M. Dark skin tissue reaction in laser assisted hair removal with a long-pulse ruby laser. J Cutan Laser Ther 2000; 2:17–20.
79. Chana JS, Grobbelaar AO. The long-term results of ruby laser depilation in a consecutive series of 346 patients. Plast Reconstr Surg 2002; 110:254–260.
80. Eremia S, Li CY, Umar SH, Newman N. Laser hair removal: long-term results with a 755 nm alexandrite laser. Dermatol Surg 2001; 27:920–924.
81. Handrick C, Alster TS. Comparison of long-pulsed diode and long-pulsed alexandrite lasers for hair removal: a long-term clinical and histologic study. Dermatol Surg 2001; 27:622–626.

82. Alster TS, Bryan H, Williams CM. Long-pulsed Nd:YAG laser-assisted hair removal in pigmented skin: a clinical and histological evaluation. Arch Dermatol 2001; 137:885–889.
83. Patel BC, Egan CA, Lucius RW, Gerwels JW, Mamalis N, Anderson RL. Cutaneous malignant melanoma and oculodermal melanocytosis (nevus of Ota): report of a case and review of the literature. J Am Acad Dermatol 1998; 38:862–865.
84. Chan HH, Leung RS, Ying SY, Lai CF, Kono T, Chua JK. A retrospective analysis of complications in the treatment of nevus of Ota with the Q-switched alexandrite and Q-switched Nd:YAG lasers. Dermatol Surg. 2000; 26:1000–1006.
85. Fujita H, Nishii Y, Yamashita K, Kawamata S, Yoshikawa K. The uptake and long-term storage of India ink particles and latex beads by fibroblasts in the dermis and subcutis of mice, with special regard to the non-inflammatory defense reaction by fibroblasts. Arch Histol Cytol 1988; 51:285–294.
86. Hodersdal M, Bech-Thomsen N, Wulf HC. Skin reflectance-guided laser selections for treatment of decorative tattoos. Arch Dermatol 1996; 132:403–407.
87. Jimenez G, Weiss E, Spencer JM. Multiple color changes following laser therapy of cosmetic tattoos. Dermatol Surg 2002; 28:177–179.
88. Chang SE, Kim KJ, Choi JH, Sung KJ, Moon KC, Koh JK. Areolar cosmetic tattoo ink darkening: a complication of Q-switched alexandrite laser treatment. Dermatol Surg 2002; 28:95–96.
89. Fitzpatrick RE, Goldman MP, Dierickx C. Laser ablation of facial cosmetic tattoos. Aesthet Plast Surg 1994; 18:91–98.
90. Leuenberger ML, Mulas MW, Hata TR, Goldman MP, Fitzpatrick RE, Grevelink JM. Comparison of the Q-switched alexandrite, Nd:YAG, and ruby lasers in treating blue-black tattoos. Dermatol Surg 1999; 25:10–14.
91. Ferguson JE, August PJ. Evaluation of the Nd/YAG laser for treatment of amateur and professional tattoos. Br J Dermatol 1996; 135:586–591.
92. Stafford TJ, Tan OT. 510-nm pulsed dye laser and alexandrite crystal laser for the treatment of pigmented lesions and tattoos. Clin Dermatol 1995; 13:69–73.
93. Alster TS. Q-switched alexandrite laser treatment (755 nm) of professional and amateur tattoos. J Am.Acad.Dermatol 1995; 33:69–73.
94. Kauvar AN. The role of lasers in the treatment of leg veins. Semin Cutan Med Surg 2000; 19:245–252.
95. Eubanks LE, McBurney EI. Videomicroscopy of port-wine stains: correlation of location and depth of lesion. J Am Acad Dermatol 2001; 44:948–951.
96. Dierickx C, Goldman MP, Fitzpatrick RE. Laser treatment of erythematous/hypertrophic and pigmented scars in 26 patients. Plast Reconstr Surg 1995; 95:84–90.
97. Batta K, Goodyear HM, Moss C, Williams HC, Hiller L, Waters R.. Randomised controlled study of early pulsed dye laser treatment of uncomplicated childhood haemangiomas: results of a 1-year analysis. Lancet 2002; 360:521–527.
98. Massey RA, Marrero G, Goel-Bansal M, Gmyrek R, Katz BE. Lasers in dermatology: a review. Cutis 2001; 67:477–484.
99. Jori G, Spikes JD. Photothermal sensitizers: possible use in tumor therapy. J Photochem Photobiol B 1990; 6:93–101.
100. Tan OT, Carney JM, Margolis R, Seki Y, Boll J, Anderson RR. Histologic responses of port-wine stains treated by argon, carbon dioxide, and tunable dye lasers. A preliminary report. Arch Dermatol 1986; 122:1016–1022.
101. Greenwald J, Rosen S, Anderson RR, Harrist T, MacFarland F, Noe J. Comparative histological studies of the tunable dye (at 577 nm) laser and argon laser: the specific vascular effects of the dye laser. J Invest Dermatol 1981; 77:305–310.
102. Glassberg E, Lask GP, Tan EM, Uitto J. The flashlamp-pumped 577-nm pulsed tunable dye laser: clinical efficacy and in vitro studies. J Dermatol Surg Oncol 1988; 14:1200–1208.

103. Garden JM, Bakus AD. Clinical efficacy of the pulsed dye laser in the treatment of vascular lesions. J Dermatol Surg Oncol 1993; 19:321–326.
104. Edstrom DW, Hedblad MA, Ros AM. Flashlamp pulsed dye laser and argon-pumped dye laser in the treatment of port-wine stains: a clinical and histological comparison. Br J Dermatol 2002; 146:285–289.
105. Dover JS. New approaches to the laser treatment of vascular lesions. Australas J Dermatol 2000; 41:14–18.
106. Levine VJ, Geronemus RG. Adverse effects associated with the 577- and 585-nanometer pulsed dye laser in the treatment of cutaneous vascular lesions: a study of 500 patients. J Am Acad Dermatol 1995; 32:613–617.
107. van Gemert MJ, Welch AJ, Pickering JW, Tan OT, Gijsbers GH. Wavelengths for laser treatment of port wine stains and telangiectasia. Lasers Surg Med 1995; 16:147–155.
108. Bernstein EF, Kornbluth S, Brown DB, Black J. Treatment of spider veins using a 10 millisecond pulse-duration frequency-doubled neodymium YAG laser. Dermatol Surg 1999; 25:316–320.
109. Bowes LE, Nouri K, Berman B, Jimenez G, Pardo R, Rodriguez L. Treatment of pigmented hypertrophic scars with the 585 nm pulsed dye laser and the 532 nm frequency-doubled Nd:YAG laser in the Q-switched and variable pulse modes: a comparative study. Dermatol Surg 2002; 28:714–719.
110. Cassuto DA, Ancona DM, Emanuelli G.. Treatment of facial telangiectasias with a diode-pumped Nd:YAG laser at 532 nm. J Cutan Laser Ther 2000; 2:141–146.

26

Management of Alopecia

Brian P. Maloney
Maloney Center, Atlanta, Georgia, U.S.A.

The exact function of hair in humans is uncertain. For animals, it provides warmth and protection. In humans it seems to have lost any functional purpose. However, it has retained many mystical qualities. Over the centuries, hair has been associated with the connotations of youth, health, and strength. There is no better example than Samson to demonstrate the sudden effect that loss of hair can have on one's physical well being. In fact, the ancient Everest papyrus (1500 BC) details an Egyptian prescription for hair loss consisting of honey, red lead, powdered alabaster, and garlic (1). For most men and women, loss of hair is associated with significant psychological distress.

ANATOMY OF THE SCALP AND HAIR

The scalp consists of five separate layers, which can easily be remembered by the acronym SCALP: skin, cutaneous tissues, aponeurosis galea, loose areolar, and periosteum. The scalp is innervated anteriorly by the fifth cranial nerve. The posterior one-third of the scalp is innervated by the cervical plexus and the dorsal rami of the second and third cervical nerves. Motor innervation of the scalp is provided by the seventh cranial nerve.

Hair follicles first appear 8 weeks after conception along the embryo's eyebrows, upper lip, and chin areas. As the fetus grows, more follicles appear but none will form after birth. This is very important because, as the child grows and the surface area of the skin increases, the distance between the follicles increases (2).

Three different types of adult hair exist. Negroid follicles have a curly or heliotrichous hair. Caucasoid follicles have wavy or cynotrichous hair. Mongoloid follicles have straight or leiotrichous hair. The shape of the follicle determines the hair form. The negroid follicle is helical, the mongoloid completely straight, and the caucasoid is somewhere in between (3).

On the human body there are three types of human hair that occur at different ages. Lanugo hair is fetal hair and is shed before full-term growth. It is usually unpigmented, lacks a central core, and is very fine and soft. Vellus hair replaces lanugal hair after birth and is spread more or less uniformly over the entire body. This hair similarly is fine, soft, and without pigment. Terminal hair is longer than vellus hair, coarser, and usually pigmented.

The hair follicles transcend the three layers of the skin: epidermis, dermis, and subcutaneous tissue. The hair follicle is an infolding of the epidermis that encloses a small dermal papilla at its base. The follicle is surrounded by a very rich blood supply that provides oxygen and nutrients needed for growth. Within the follicle, the hair shaft is contained in a sheath consisting of several layers. One of these layers, called Huxley's layer, is composed of elongated keratin fibers that contain the coloring of the hair in the form of melanin granules (see Chapter 1, Fig. 14). The hair grows by the formation and dividing of keratin fibers. As the cells divide and grow upward, a dense matrix forms between the keratin filaments (3).

Human scalp hair usually grows for approximately 3 years up to a length of 42 inches if uncut. The hair on the scalp undergoes a cycle of growth consisting of three distinct but overlapping stages: a growth phase, anagen; the phase of regression, catagen; and the resting phase, telogen. There are no specific demarcations between the phases of anagen and catagen. The phase of anagen is the active growth phase and, as the follicle reaches the end of anagen, it reduces and ceases its production of melanin. The base of the hairshaft becomes large with keratin to form a bulb. At this point, it is clearly in catagen, which is the phase in which the dermal papilla is loosened from the epidermis. Approximately 90% of the human terminal hairs are in the growing phase, 1% are in catagen, and the remaining hairs are in the telogen resting stage. The anagen phase is approximately 2–5 years, catagen generally lasts 2–3 weeks, and telogen lasts a few months (4). This cycle is responsible for the loss of approximately 100 hairs per day. Each follicle is independent of its neighbor yet has the same growth control characteristics. This independent pattern is known as a mosaic. Plucking of hairs from resting follicles will cause the cycle to advance to the next stage of activity.

FACTORS AFFECTING HAIR GROWTH

There are many myths about hair growth; for example, many think that cutting hair will make it grow faster. Hair is a dead structure and studies have shown that the frequency of cutting has no effect on hair growth. Hair form and its subsequent growth appear to be controlled by several different genes. The follicular cycle is also influenced directly by hormones (5). The same hormones that promote sexual hair growth after puberty also cause androgenic alopecia of the scalp. Hormones implicated in hair growth include testosterone, adrenal steroids, and thyroid hormones. Up to 10% of patients who complain of hair loss may be suffering from hypothyroidism. There appears to be a decrease in mean hair diameter as well as an increase in the numbers of hairs in telogen in patients with hypothyroidism. During pregnancy, hair growth is increased as estrogen appears to prolong the anagen phase. Postpartum hair loss also appears to be hormonally mediated as a greater percentage of hairs enter the telogen phase, resulting in a transient alopecia about 4–6 months after delivery. Postpartum hair loss is most likely related to a decrease in estrogen and/or progesterone levels (6). Testosterone and/or its metabolites have been known to have a direct effect on follicular activity: castration halts baldness in men.

Hair growth also may show some seasonal changes, being the greatest in spring and early summer. The lowest levels of follicles in the telogen stage are present in December. Mental and physical stresses as well as fever can result in alopecia. This particular type of hair loss is referred to as telogen effluvium and is considered to be a nonspecific response to a wide variety of acute physical or mental stresses. It generally lasts for only a few months before returning to normal. Some systemic disorders that produce telogen effluvium are Hodgkin's disease, leukemia, cirrhosis, renal failure, and severe infections. Alopecia is commonly associated with uncontrolled diabetes. This may be due to poor circulation to the scalp or to insulin regulation of androgen metabolism (insulin is found in the hair follicle). Genetic studies have failed to reveal any correlation between the two conditions (7).

Nutritional alopecia can result from poor nutrition over long periods of time. This type of alopecia occurs not only in underdeveloped regions but also in more well-developed countries where fad diets may result in inadequate nutrition.

Anagen effluvium describes hair loss following chemotherapy or exposure to ionizing radiation (8). A loss of anagen hairs occurs within several days of a metabolic insult. Medications including anticoagulants, antibiotics, and anticancer drugs have also been associated with development of alopecia (9).

Alopecia can be a marker for some medical conditions. Vertex alopecia, especially in men with hypercholesterolemia and hypertension, is linked to an increased risk for coronary heart disease (10). Male pattern baldness also seems to be a risk factor for prostate cancer (11).

THEORIES OF BALDING

Both men and women experience a natural shedding of hair over time. This natural decrease in hair density is due to two factors. The first is a decrease in the diameter of the individual hairs, called miniaturization; the second is a natural decrease in the density of the hairs. A threshold diameter of 60 μm is a sensitive index to evaluate the progression of male pattern baldness (12).

Alopecia can either be hereditary or acquired. Hereditary alopecia can be congenital as a result of dermal and syndromal abnormalities. Hereditary alopecia can also present as male pattern baldness in postpubescent males. This type of hereditary alopecia is very poorly understood; it does not follow traditional genetic patterns and is most likely polygenic. Female pattern hair loss is a more diffuse thinning of the entire scalp hair. However, some women will experience a more classic male pattern baldness.

The most common form of alopecia results from genetic predisposition and androgen dependence. Testosterone is converted to dihydrotestosterone (DHT) by the 5 alpha reductase enzyme (13). This enzyme is found in two forms. Type one is found in the skin and scalp and type two is found in the scalp and prostate. In patients with male pattern baldness the cause is most likely increased 5 alpha reductase activity leading to increased levels of DHT. Especially in female pattern baldness, there are multiple hormonal influences involved with hair loss (14). Androgenic alopecia affects 50–80% of white men. Some 30% of men in their 30s have alopecia, and 40% of men in their 40s. The high incidence may be due to the Western diet high in saturated fat. There is a strong link between cholesterol concentrations and androgen production.

Trichotillomania is a psychological compulsion to pull out the hair commonly seen in children and teenagers. Treatment for this generally involves psychiatric evaluation.

Traction alopecia is a result of aggressive hair styling and may result in early loss of the hair. Discontinuation of the behavior usually results in regrowth of the hair.

CLASSIFICATION OF HAIR LOSS

Baldness as a result of old age or premature androgenic baldness should be thought of as exhibiting patterns. The most popular type of classification system that provides a basis for projection of future baldness is called the Norwood Hamilton Classification. Originally described by Hamilton (15) and later expanded by Norwood (16) it provides the surgeon with a universal method of classifying alopecia. Familiarity with one of the classification systems is important: it will allow the surgeon to project a final hair pattern and therefore recommend an appropriate plan for the patient. The Norwood classification is summarized as follows:

Type 1: Hair pattern with little to no frontal recession.
Type 2: Symmetrical bitemporal recession extending no further posteriorly than 2 cm anterior to a coronal plane connecting the external auditory meatus. No vertex thinning.
Type 3: Symmetrical bitemporal recession extending further posteriorly than 2 cm anterior to a coronal plane but not reaching the plane connecting the external auditory meatus.
Type 3 Vertex: Vertex thinning with or without symmetrical bitemporal recession extending no further posteriorly than a coronal plane connecting the external auditory meatus.
Type 4: Frontal recession extends to the coronal plane with a distinct bridge of dense hair separating the vertex and frontal areas.
Type 5: Types 5–7 all have a horseshoe-shaped pattern. Type 5 has a sparse band of hair separating the frontal and occipital areas.
Type 6: Frontal and vertex may be separated by no bridge of hair. Generally there is a wide fringe along the sides and back.
Type 7: Extensive balding with only a thin fringe along the sides and occiput.

Ludwig described a classification for women consisting of three grades (17):

Grade 1: Normal frontal hair line with only thinning of the crown.
Grade 2: More pronounced thinning of the crown than in grade 1.
Grade 3: Complete absence of hair in the crown.

Many female patients will have a more male pattern type of baldness and the Norwood classification may be more appropriate to classify such patients.

ALOPECIA CONSULTATION

A complete medical history should include the time the patient first noticed thinning hair, the rate of hair loss, and the areas. Patient evaluation needs to include a detailed personal medical history regarding the patient's general health; medications, both prescription and over-the-counter; and any known allergies. An extensive drug history that takes into account patients' nonprescription medications and health supplements is important. With the popularity of natural products as a replacement for pharmaceuticals and also as cosmetic supplements, a detailed accounting is essential because some could have an impact on hair growth. An example of this is soy estrogens used in reducing symptoms of menopause, which may play a role in hair growth. The patient should also be queried as to any skin disorders as well as systemic disorders such as diabetes, bleeding disorders, and a history of drug or alcohol abuse.

Patient expectations and motivations can be better appreciated by seeking answers to the following questions. Why is the patient seeking hair replacement surgery? How long has the patient been thinking about this? Has the patient used any other methods such as Rogaine or Propecia for the treatment of their thinning hair? How long has the patient been thinking about having surgery? What does the patient think the procedure will do for him or her? Does the patient understand that the procedure may not achieve his or her goals? Does the patient understand that multiple procedures may be necessary? Does the patient understand the possibilities of graft failure, infection, and scarring (7). It is very important for the patient to understand the goals of improvement and not perfection. Caution should be exercised with the patient who desires perfection.

Age

Young patients (generally less than 20 years old) presenting with early thinning along the frontal hairline should be encouraged to investigate possible medical treatments as their future pattern may not be fully defined. These patients can be monitored every 6–12 months to note the progression of the thinning. When a hair loss pattern becomes better defined, then the patient can consider hair restoration. This is important, especially if there is a family history of male pattern baldness. Therefore, it is important to ask the patient regarding possible members of the family who have exhibited hair loss. Because the genetics of androgenic alopecia are poorly understood, the clinician should ask about baldness on both the maternal and paternal sides of the family.

Physical Examination

The examination should focus first on the patient's overall facial appearance. Any sign of any facial asymmetries or distortions may suggest an underlying syndrome or medical condition such as Graves' disease or malnourishment.

Hair Color and Texture

Patients with light-colored hair have much less contrast between the hair and the scalp and therefore may present after more advanced thinning is present. The best colors, in order of desirability, for hair transplantation are white, gray, salt and pepper, blonde, red, brown, and black. Because of this color difference, patients with thin, dark hair may benefit from lightening their hair in order to decrease the contrast with the scalp.

Hair texture is important because coarser hairs have a larger diameter and will therefore increase the total bulk of the hair much more rapidly than fine hair.

Hair density is important in hair transplantation. With the advent of follicular grafting, low hair density is not an absolute contraindication; the patient with a low hair density and minimal frontal recession is still a candidate if his or her goals are limited.

Examination of the scalp should include any scaling or scalp disorders. The elasticity of the scalp can be easily assessed by placing thumb and forefinger on each side of the balding area of the vertex of the scalp and pushing towards the central area. This also gives the surgeon an assessment of scalp thickness. The thickness and elasticity of the scalp are importaint in guiding the surgeon to possible flap transplantation or scalp reduction. Female patients should be examined for any excess of facial hair to determine the possibility of excess testosterone.

To evaluate the amount of hair fall out, gently pull about one cm^2 of hair between the thumb and forefinger. Normally one to five telogen hairs may come out. In a patient with active telogen effluvium, one may pull out 30 or more hairs.

MEDICAL TREATMENT FOR ANDROGENIC ALOPECIA

Androgenic alopecia, the most common form of postpubescent balding, can be treated with a variety of medications. Minoxidil is currently available in two over-the-counter nonprescription strengths. Potential side effects are negligible. The age of the patient and type of baldness rather than its duration seem to affect the final success of the use of topical Minoxidil (18). Topical minoxidil is most effective on the vertex scalp, with approximately one-third of male patients noticing an increase in terminal hair growth, another one-third may notice a stabilization of the balding, and the remaining one-third will generally not notice any change. The use of minoxidil is required daily and its cessation will result in relatively quick shedding of any hair the medication had been able to maintain. It will not accelerate the balding process. The mechanism of action of minoxidil is uncertain. Combining it with tretinoin appears to facilitate penetration through the skin layers.

As mentioned, dihydrotestosterone has been implicated as the main androgenic hormone responsible for androgenic alopecia. Finasteride is a synthetic 4-azasteroid that is a specific competitive inhibitor of this enzyme (19). It is interesting to note that the 5 alpha reductase enzyme is only found in the scalp and the prostate in humans. Finasteride was originally developed as a treatment for benign prostate hypertrophy and was found to increase hair growth in many of the patients taking the medication. Potential drug interactions appear to be minimal. Patients taking this medication to treat balding need to inform their urologists that they are taking Finasteride as their prostate screening antigen test (PSA) numbers need to be doubled to give a more accurate reading. It is also recommended that patients 40 or older have a screening PSA prior to treatment with Finasteride. The incidence of side effects is very low, the most common being impotence, decreased libido, and decreased volume of ejaculate. Pregnant women are advised not to handle the tablets because if they are carrying a male fetus there is a possibility of birth defects. Finasteride has not been found in the semen. With cessation of Finasteride treatment, there is a more gradual return to pretreatment levels and not an immediate shedding as noted with minoxidil withdrawal.

For women with alopecia and hirsutism associated with obesity and menstrual abnormalities, the source of the androgen excess is frequently ovarian (20). If the hirsutism is associated with average weight and normal menses, the source is most often adrenal. Nolactone (aldactone) is the most popular antiandrogen therapy for hirsutism in the United States and it is commonly prescribed with oral contraceptives to improve its effectiveness and prevent potential fetal abnormalities. Female patients with normal androgen levels may have increased end-organ sensitivity to androgens. Oral contraceptives may be helpful.

NONSURGICAL MANAGEMENT OF ALOPECIA

The use of hairpieces or additions can be very effective in restoring facial balance due to hair loss. These tools frequently require monthly cleaning and servicing to achieve their optimal appearance and can be effective for many patients, especially those with extensive thinning.

To reduce the contrast between the hair and the scalp, scalp polishes can be used to darken the scalp and thus give the appearance of more hair. Occasionally, permanent cosmetics can be applied to the scalp to provide a more permanent type of scalp darkening. However, care should be advised because the pigment may change color over time (e.g., black to blue).

SURGICAL MANAGEMENT OF ALOPECIA

Designing a Frontal Hairline

This is one of the most important components of the surgical restoration process. Designing a frontal hairline must take into account not only the patient's current degree of balding but also, to some degree, anticipate what pattern the patient is most likely to develop. An improperly placed hairline could be a telltale sign of hair transplantation. Hairlines that are too low or too high or that round off into the temporal hairs are undesirable. Many patients will have fine hairs along the frontal area that may guide the surgeon as to the appropriate placement of the hairline. Caution should be exercised to take into account the age of the patient in these cases. In a young patient, follicular transfer should be performed at a higher level to allow the patient to have a more mature hairline as he or she ages. A hairline that is too low or appropriate for a 21-year old may not be appropriate when the same patient is in his or her 50s.

For the patient with well-defined frontal loss, placement of the hairline in the absence of significant frontal hair can be determined anteriorly by placing two fingerbreadths above the highest forehead crease. This point should serve as the most anterior point of the hair line. The lateral-most points of the hairline should lie at or just medial to a vertical line from each lateral canthus. An arch can then be created between these three points, keeping the arch horizontal. The angle between the frontal hairline and the temporal hairline should be approximately 90 degrees or less. Rounding of this angle generally results in a very unnatural hairline. The surgeon needs to evaluate the hairline from the front and sides and confirm its placement with the patient prior to the procedure.

Surgical hair restoration is best divided into procedures for the frontal area and procedures for the vertex. Surgical techniques to reconstruct the frontal area include follicular transfer and other grafting techniques, short and long flaps, and scalp reduction. Surgical techniques to reconstruct the vertex area include scalp reduction as well as grafting techniques.

Follicular Transfer, Micro-Minigrafts

Description

The history of autotransplantation for the reconstruction of bare areas dates to the early 1800s. However, it was not until Dr. Orentreich popularized the procedure in his article in the 1950s that grafting truly came of age (21). Since that time, the technique of transplanting large round grafts often compared to doll's hair has been refined to the point that surgeons will transplant one- to three-hair groupings, called follicular units. The donor area is chosen based upon the best color and texture match of the hair along either the temple or occipital region. Procedures can generally be performed under oral sedation or twilight anesthesia. The area is supplemented with local anesthetic, generally 1% lidocaine with 1:100,000 epinephrine. After allowing for appropriate hemostatic effect and prepping and draping the patient, the donor area is infiltrated with injectable normal saline to help make the area tense and more rigid. Using a multibladed knife, a strip is then incised across the donor area, being careful to bevel the incision so that the hair follicles are preserved, stopping frequently to check that the follicles are not injured (Fig. 1). Scissors are used to separate

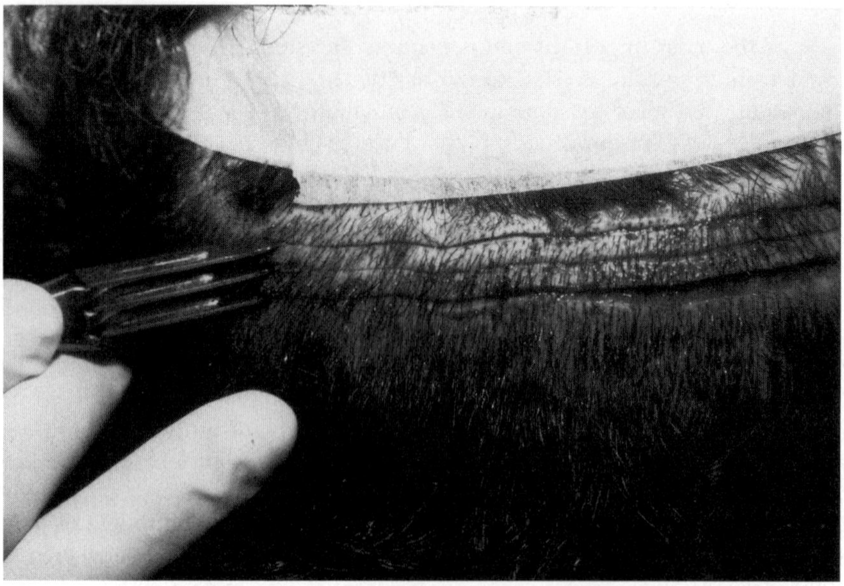

Figure 1 Multibladed knife used to harvest donor hair from the occipital region. Note the bevel of the blades corresponding to the direction of the hair folicle.

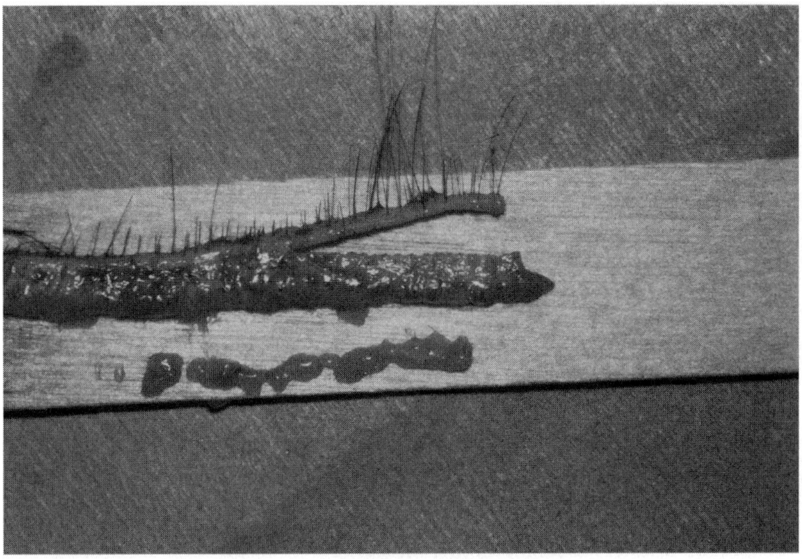

Figure 2 A strip of donor scalp is de-epithelialized superiorly. The excess fat is trimmed, leaving a thin layer of fat attached to the follicle.

the strip from the underlying soft tissues. Care is taken to avoid injuring any of the follicles, which can be easily seen projecting into the subcutaneous fat. Once the strip is removed, hemostasis can be obtained with bipolar cautery and by closing the incision with a running, locking 0-Prolene suture. At this point, the strip is then prepared under magnification, dissecting out the individual follicular units, being careful not to injure the follicle as this may decrease the survivability of the graft. A small amount of fat on the bulb of the follicle is ideal (Figs. 2,3). With this technique, even curly hair such as in African Americans can be more easily prepared for transplantation with much better survival of the thick grafts. The graft should be kept on ice to decrease metabolic activity prior to use. Care should be taken to prevent them from drying out. A moist bandage in a covered petri dish will help to accomplish this.

The recipient site is infiltrated with the local anesthetic prior to making the recipient holes. Using a knife breaker and a double-edged razor blade, appropriate-sized blades can be fashioned to create recipient holes in the donor site. Once a blade is fashioned, one or two holes are made and the size of the grafts is assessed to make sure that the holes will accommodate the grafts. A carbon dioxide laser may also be used to create recipient holes. Some surgeons like this technique because the laser cauterizes resulting in less bleeding. This technology may be helpful on the first session when there is minimal hair in the area. On subsequent sessions, the hair in the recipient area may be singed by the laser. Holes are generally spaced 2–3 mm apart. In a patient who has microvascular disease, a greater distance may be appropriate to ensure appropriate blood supply to the grafts. The recipient holes are made in an irregular fashion along the hairline, generally with a zone of individual hairs along the frontal area. This is feathered more posteriorly into larger follicular units to ensure a gentle transition (Fig. 4). The follicular units are then placed along the frontal area with a slight forward inclination. At the

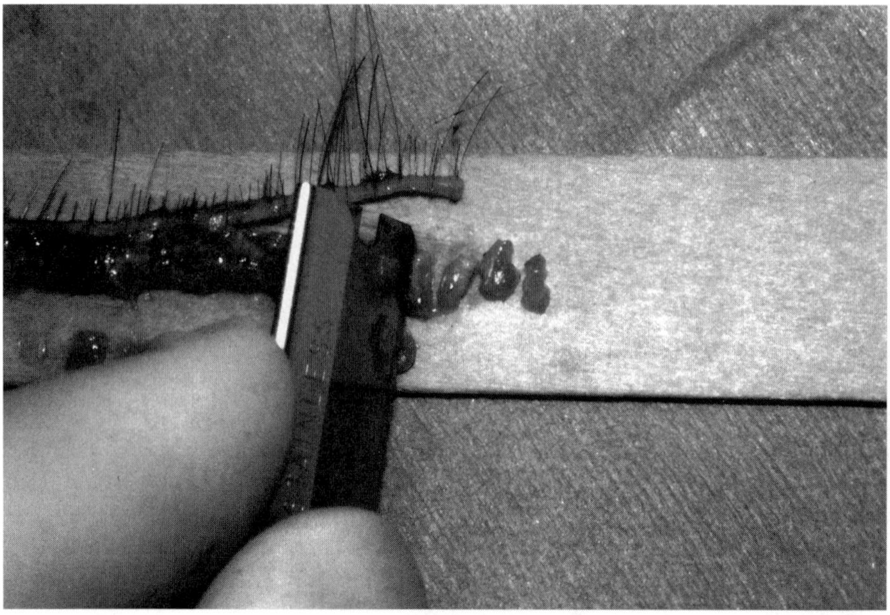

Figure 3 The final stage of graft preparation. The follicles are cut into the desired sizes.

conclusion of the procedure, the placement of the grafts should be checked and the hair can be blown dry to secure the grafts in their new position. No dressing is necessary at this point unless the patient has had significant oozing. If there is oozing, Surgilube may be applied with a layer of absorbent bandage followed by application of a gentle compression dressing (Fig. 5).

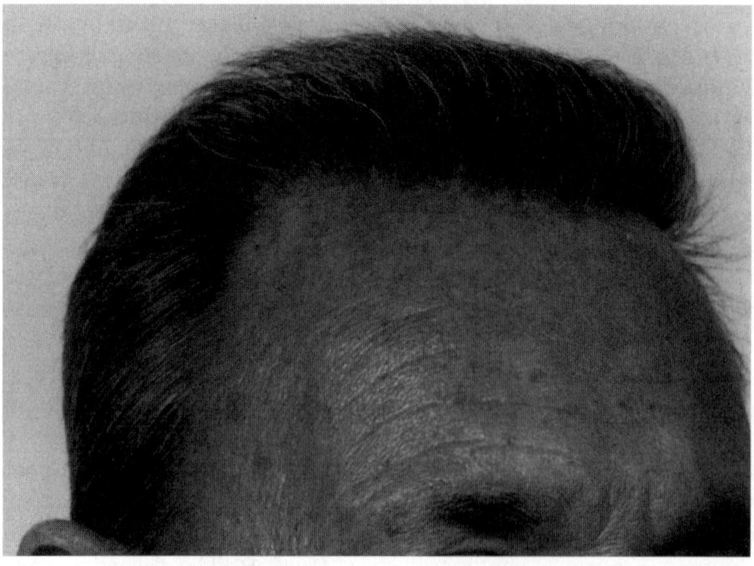

Figure 4 Irregular nature of the transplanted hairline achieves a natural look.

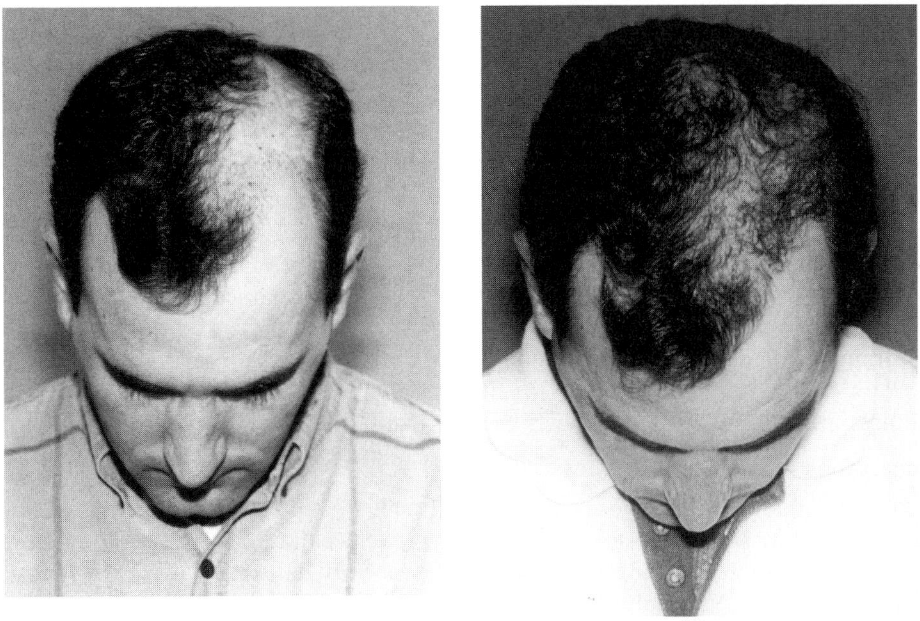

(A) (B)

Figure 5 A. Preoperative photograph shows a patient who underwent radiation to the scalp for intracranial malignancy with subsequent alopecia. B. Postoperative photographic after one session of grafting.

Indications

Both frontal and vertex thinning can be treated with this method. This technique can also be used to reconstruct specialized areas including eyebrows, mustache, and others.

Advantages

The newer techniques generally lead to a very natural look. Due to the smaller graft sizes the hair may not fall out and go through telogen during the postoperative period.

Disadvantages

Patients experience crusting, swelling and generally require multiple treatments. The transplanted hair in the grafts will commonly fall out and begin growing about 3 months after the procedure. It will reach a substantial length approximately 6 months after the procedure.

Flap Reconstruction for Frontal Alopecia

Description

An alternative method of reconstruction of the frontal hairline is a technique first popularized by Juri and then Mayer and Flemming (22,23). This method involves harvesting a long temporal parietal flap based on a posterior branch of the superficial temporal artery. The procedure is generally carried out in three stages. The first stage consists of identifying the posterior branch of the artery using Doppler ultrasound and outlining a flap that is appropriate to cover the width of the forehead. The flap margins are simply incised posteriorly and delayed. One week later, the sutures are removed and distal half of the flap is elevated and replaced on its bed. In the third week, the entire flap is elevated and rotated into its new position. The hairline is determined as previously described and the flap secured into its new position with two-layered closure. If the donor site is not able to be closed primarily, a portion of the skin that was excised from the forehead can be placed in this donor area and then subsequently excised as the scalp relaxes. Proponents of the flap believe that the direction of the hair growth is not a significant problem for the patient and generally does not pose any restrictions on styling. Additional follicular grafting may be necessary anterior to the flap incision to help soften this incision, as well as small procedures to revise the dog-ear at the donor site. Within a week, the sutures are removed from the newly created frontal hairline.

Indications

This technique is ideal for patients who only demonstrate recession of the frontal area with no loss of the posterior hair. If a patient has an exceedingly wide forehead or a very tight forehead, a smaller flap, approximately half this size, can be rotated from each of the temporal regions across the midline. Additional follicular grafting sessions can be performed at approximately 3 months.

Advantages

This technique can offer the patient denser hair than is possible with follicular grafting in a much shorter period of time.

Disadvantages

This is a larger procedure with potential risk of flap necrosis and the need for additional procedures. If a patient has had a previous transplant session, he or she is generally not a candidate for a long flap procedure because the donor incision may have disrupted the blood supply to the flap. The patient could have a short flap from each side that meets in the middle. The donor site may be difficult to close primarily and may require insertion of a portion of the removed frontal scalp temporarily. A dog ear may occur at the point of flap rotation. This generally flattens but may require a revision procedure.

Surgical Reconstruction of the Vertex

The vertex area can be reconstructed using either the grafting technique or scalp reduction. The grafting technique as described earlier can be used to increase the density of hair in the vertex area. The incisions are placed in a ripple or swirling fashion from the center of the vertex with graft orientation radiating outward.

Scalp Reduction or Hair Line Advancement

Description

One of the most popular methods of reducing the balding vertex scalp is scalp reduction or hairline advancement. This has been performed over the years using a variety of techniques, the most common being excising an ellipse of scalp skin down to the galea. The lateral aspects of the dissection are carried down to the ear and to the inferior aspect of the postauricular hairline allowing the free edges of the ellipse to be approximated. Closure is usually performed in the galeal layer with an absorbable suture followed by stainless steel staples for wound edge approximation. After allowing 3–6 months for the scalp to relax, a second scalp reduction can be performed in a similar fashion.

Introduction of the Frechet extender has allowed this process to be accelerated. At the conclusion of the first scalp reduction, prior to closure, an extender (a device with a row of stainless steel hooks) is inserted just beneath the hair fringe on one side. The extender is pulled across the top of the head to 1–2 cm inside the fringe on the other side. The tension on the rows of hooks will pull the fringes closer together over a 3–4 week period. The extender can be left in place up to 6 weeks. With the use of the extender, there is a potential space between the scalp and periosteum where fluid can collect. Either a drain or a dressing may be helpful to reduce this potential complication. A second scalp reduction is then performed at 3–6 weeks following the initial insertion. Patients will generally recognize that the tight feeling of the scalp has dissipated and this is a good indicator for removal. The key to success in using the extender is adequate dissection under the temporal hair—the area that is being stretched to cover the vertex. Care must also be taken to select appropriate candidates for scalp reduction to prevent additional thinning of the side areas. The extender has, in large part, replaced the expander for accelerated management of vertex thinning because it causes no cosmetic deformity and does not require weekly adjustments.

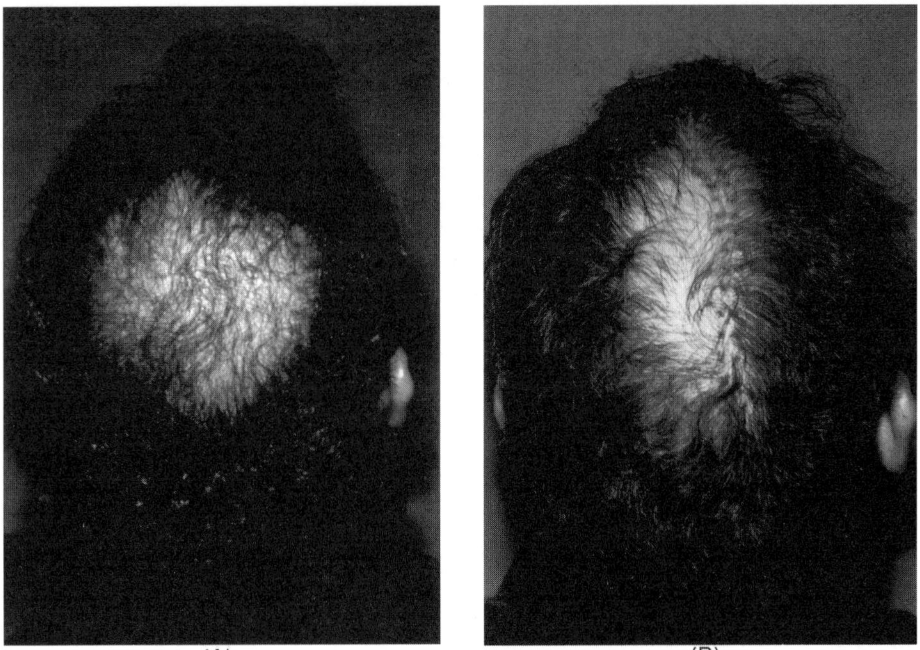

(A) (B)

Figure 6 A. Preoperative photograph. B. Postoperative photograph 6 weeks after initial scalp reduction and subsequent removal of extender and second scalp reduction. Note the degree of bald vertex removed in such a short time.

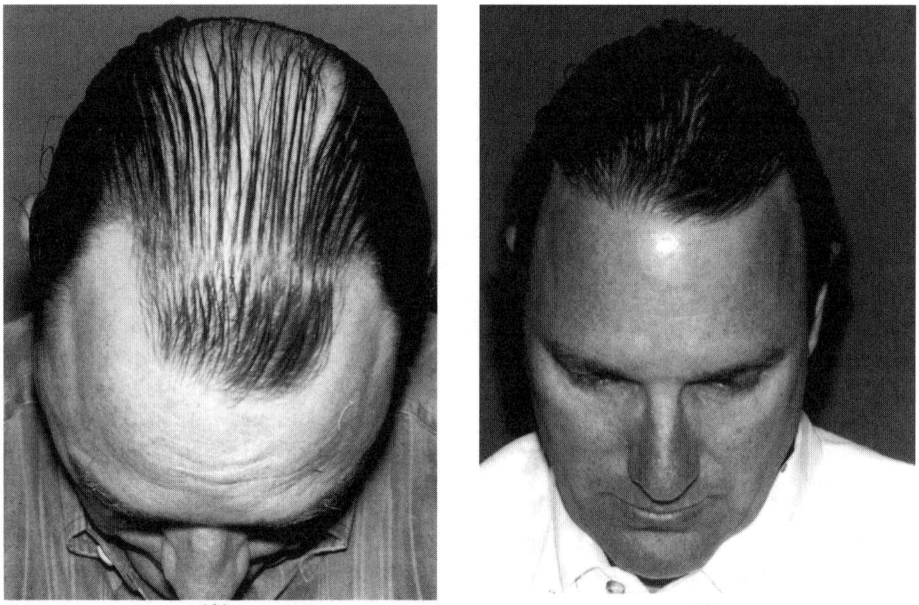

(A) (B)

Figure 7 A. Preoperative appearance of a patient with class 4–5 alopecia. B. Patient after follicular transfer to the bitemporal recessions and scalp reduction with extender to the vertex area.

Sometimes the goal of scalp reduction is not complete obliteration of the vertex balding but just a reduction in size to allow a hairpiece to fit better (Figs. 6,7).

Indications

Patients with vertex alopecia and adequate density of the hair along the sides are ideal candidates. In patients with extensive alopecia, a scalp reduction can be used to reduce the vertex area, allowing a hair piece to fit better.

Advantages

The scalp reduction can generally remove a significant amount of balding scalp very quickly. It can raise the temporal fringe to allow better reconstruction of the frontal hair line.

Disadvantages

A scar that may widen is created on the vertex. Numbness of the scalp may occur and, rarely, be permanent. The procedure may result in thinning of the temporal hair.

A LOOK TO THE FUTURE

Cloning of hair, although a popular media topic, appears to be far in the future. The proper terminology is not cloning but cell therapy, by which a single hair is removed and hundreds are reproduced. This technology has not been perfected and is under study. Because of the large number of patients with male pattern baldness, topical medications are destined to be discovered that will ameliorate the loss of hair. Last year over 40 patents were issued in the United States and several hundred around the world for new hair loss treatments. No universal treatment is successful; individual treatment under a physician's care is generally the best course.

REFERENCES

1. Coiffman F. Square scalp grafts. Clin Plast Surg 1982; 9, 2:221–228.
2. Ferriman D. Human Hair growth and disease, Springfield IL: Charles C Thomas, 1971.
3. Dawber R, Van Neste D. Hair and scalp disorders. Philadelphia: JB Lippincott Co, 1995.
4. Orentreich D, Orentreich N. Androgenic alopecia and its treatment. In: Unger WP, ed. Hair Transplatation Ed II. New York: Marcel Decker, 1988.
5. Schmidt JB. Hormonal basis of male and female androgenic alopecia: clinical relevance. Skin Pharmacol 1994; 7(1–2):61–66.
6. Wallace ML, Smoller BR. Estrogen and progesterone receptors in androgenic alopecia versus alopecia areata. Am J Dermatopathol 1998; 202:160–163.
7. Ellis JA, Stebbing M, Harrap SB. Insulin polymorphism and premature male pattern baldness in the general population. Clin Sci 1999; 966:659–662.
8. Mitchell AJ, Balle MR. Alopecia areata. Dermatol Clin 1987; 53:553–564.
9. Brodin MB. Drug related alopecia. Dermatol Clin 1987; 53:571–579.
10. Lotufo PA, Chae CU, Ajani UA, Hennekens CH, Manson JE. Male pattern baldness and coronary heart disease: the Physician Health Study. Arch Intern Med 2000; 1602:165–171.
11. Hawk E, Breslow RA, Graubard BI. Male pattern baldness and clinical prostate cancer in the epidemiologic follow up of the first National Health and Nutrition Examination Survey. Cancer Epidemiol Biomakers Prev 2000; 95:523–527.
12. Ishino A, Uzuka M, Tsuji, Nakanishi J, Hanzawa N, Imamura S. Progressive decrease in hair diameter in Japanese with male pattern baldness. J Dermatol 1997; 2412:758–764.
13. Ellis JA, Stebbing M, Harrap SB. Genetic analysis of male pattern baldness and the 5 alpha-reductase genes. J Invest Dermatol 1998; 1106:849–853.
14. Legro RS, Carmina E, Stanczyk FZ, Gentzschein E, Lobo RA. Alterations in androgen conjugate levels in women and men with alopecia. Fertil Steril 1994; 624:744–750.
15. Hamilton JB. Patterned hair loss in man: types and incidence. Ann NY Acad Sci 1951; 53:708.
16. Norwood OT. Hair Transplant Surgery. Springfield, Illinois, Charles C. Thomas, 1973.
17. Ludwig E. Classification of the types of androgenic alopecia (common baldness) occurring in the female sex. Br J Dermatol 1977; 973:247–254.
18. Karam P. Topical minoxidil therapy for androgenic alpopecia in the Middle East, The Middle Eastern Topical Minoxidil Study Group. Intl J Dermatol ; 3210:763–766.
19. Sudduth SL, Koronkowski MJ. Finasteide the first 5 alpha reductase inhibitor. Pharmacotherapy 1993; 134:309–325.
20. Redmond GP. Androgens and women's health. Int J Fertil Womens Med 1998; 432: 91–97.
21. Orentreich N. Autografts in alopecias and other selected dermatological conditions. Ann NY Acad Sci 1959; 83:463–479.
22. Juri J. Use of parietal-occipital flaps in the surgical treatment of baldness. Plast Reconstr Surg 1975; 456.
23. Mayer T, Flemming, RW. Aesthetic and Reconstructive Surgery of the Scalp. St Louis, MO: Mosby Year Book, 1992.

27
Face Lifting and Cervicofacial Liposuction

Juan Carlos Giachino Jr.
Plastic Surgery Associates, Stuart, Florida, U.S.A.

Jeffrey H. Spiegel
Boston University, Boston, Massachusetts, U.S.A.

INTRODUCTION

Beauty is defined by Webster as "the quality or aggregate of qualities in a person or thing that gives pleasure to the senses or pleasurably exalts the mind or spirit." For centuries, people have attempted to accentuate or recapture their beauty by various means. It was not until recently, with advances in modern medicine, that safe and effective surgical options have become available. Medical understanding of facial anatomy and the physiology of aging have provided the foundation for current surgical interventions. These interventions have evolved, especially in the last 40 years, to enhance and restore a more youthful and healthy appearance. Most notably, rhytidectomy has proven most effective in achieving these goals. This chapter will provide an analysis of facial aging and various surgical therapies aimed at reversing this process including rhytidectomy, brow elevation, and cervicofacial liposuction.

PATHOPHYSIOLOGY OF AGING SKIN

Several factors are responsible for facial aging. Natural changes occur in the skin, on a microscopic level, as a person grows older. These, along with the constant effect of gravity, contribute to changes in facial architecture associated with an aged appearance. Features noted in elderly individuals include brow ptosis, malar ptosis, deepening of nasolabial folds, development of jowling, submental skin and fat excess, fine skin wrinkles, and pigmentary changes. The various histological changes in the skin that are associated with aging include (1–3)

1. Flattening of the dermoepidermal junction with loss of papillae
2. Decrease in the number of melanocytes
3. Decrease in glycosaminoglycans, proteoglycans, and ground substance
4. Decrease in elastic fibers
5. Decrease in total collagen, especially type III

Sun exposure is the main causative factor in premature aging. Prolonged exposure to the sun (ultraviolet A [UVA] and ultraviolet B [UVB]) causes actinic skin damage including epidermal dysplasia and dermal elastosis (4).

PREOPERATIVE EVALUATION

A thorough history and physical examination are necessary before proceeding with any aesthetic procedure. The patient's medical conditions, current medicines, prior surgical history, and allergies are all routine parts of a preoperative evaluation. Specific factors that increase the risk for postoperative complications should receive special attention. Hypertension and aspirin may cause postoperative hematomas, therefore, patients should continue antihypertensive medicines and maintain a reasonable blood pressure. Aspirin use should be discontinued at least 2 weeks prior to surgery. Another factor that may result in significant postoperative morbidity is smoking. Continuation of smoking can result in microcirculatory changes that may contribute to skin flap necrosis. Cessation of smoking should begin 2–3 weeks before surgery.

Skin Disorders

Ehlers Danlos/Cutis Hyperelastica

Ehlers Danlos/ cutis hyperelastica is a genetically inherited syndrome characterized by hypermobile joints, fragile hyperextensible skin, predisposition to subcutaneous hemorrhages, and dark skin pigmentation. These clinical attributes are due to an abnormality in collagen maturation that retards normal collagen synthesis leading to poor wound healing, postoperative hemorrhage, and dark scar pigmentation. Elective surgery is best avoided (5).

Cutis Laxa

Cutis laxa is also a genetically inherited condition in which there is a decrease in the size and number of elastic fibers in the dermis causing significant skin laxity. Since there is not a derangement in the synthesis of collagen, no wound healing difficulties arise. Therefore, patients with this condition are good candidates for surgery and benefit from rhytidectomy (6).

Peudoxanthoma Elasticum

Pseudoxanthoma elasticum demonstrates both dominant and recessive inheritance patterns. Patients are noted to have degeneration of elastic fibers in the skin causing premature skin laxity. They also show no wound healing abnormalities since collagen synthesis proceeds normally. Rhytidectomy would be a safe and effective treatment in patients with this condition (7).

Werner's Syndrome/Adult Progeria

Werner's Syndrome/ adult progeria is an autosomal recessive condition that presents with systemic manifestations including scleroderma-like skin changes, growth retardation and short stature, premature facial aging, high-pitched voice, muscle atrophy, osteoporosis, premature arteriosclerosis, and various neoplasms. These patients are not candidates for elective cosmetic surgery (8).

Progeria/Hutchinson-Gilford Syndrome

Progeria/ Hutchinson-Gilford Syndrome is also acquired through an autosomal recessive mode of inheritance. Features include growth retardation, craniofacial abnormalities, premature baldness, pinched nose, enlarged ears, micrognathia, and cardiovascular disease secondary to arteriosclerosis and calcification. Life expectancy for these patients is short and they are not candidates for elective surgical procedures.

Physical Examination

The next step in the preoperative evaluation for aesthetic surgery of the face is a thorough physical examination. This should be carried out in a well-lit room. An orderly approach should be taken to evaluate each anatomical subunit of the face as well as the condition of the skin. Notable skin changes include the amount of actinic damage, degree of skin laxity, and extent of skin wrinkling. The facial soft tissues, underlying musculature, and bony anatomy should also be assessed. The facial subunits should be studied beginning with the forehead. Notable features include transverse wrinkling, glabellar wrinkles from overactive procerus and corrugator muscle activity, and eyebrow/upper eyelid ptosis.

Midface assessment includes evaluation of the position and quality of the malar eminences and nasolabial folds. Lower facial evaluation should focus on the mandibular border and the presence of jowling. The neck should be examined for submental or submandibular lipodystrophy. Platysmal banding, laxity in the neck skin, and an obtuse cervicomental angle are also of importance. Included in the initial evaluation should be a detailed examination of facial nerve function for comparison postoperatively.

The preoperative work-up should also include:

1. Preoperative photographs in three views (anteroposterior, lateral, and oblique).
2. Age-appropriate laboratory tests per hospital guidelines.
3. Patient preparation including avoidance of sun exposure, alcohol, and tobacco for two weeks prior to surgery. Use of acetylsalicyclic acid, nonsteroidal anti-inflammatory drugs, estrogen, and anticoagulants should also be stopped 2 weeks before surgery. Patients should remove all makeup the night before with mild soap and water and wash their hair with PhisoHex. An anxiolytic, such as lorazepam, taken the night before may be helpful.

FACELIFT ANATOMY

An intimate knowledge of facial anatomy is paramount when performing a rhytidectomy. Most importantly, knowledge of the anatomy of the facial nerve and the superficial musculoaponeurotic system (SMAS) are crucial to safe, consistent, and pleasing aesthetic results. Throughout the face, the superficial anatomy is composed of five layers that include the skin, subcutaneous fat, superficial musculoaponeurotic system, fascia, and facial nerve. The most important layer in rhytidectomy surgery is the SMAS. First described by Mitz and Peyronie in 1976, it is a fascial layer in continuity with the muscles of facial expression including the frontalis, orbicularis oculus, zygomaticus major and minor, and platysma (9). In the temporal region, the SMAS continues as the temporoparietal fascia (10). The facial nerve (CN VII) travels deep to the SMAS layer to innervate the muscles of facial expression. Exceptions to this rule include the buccinator, mentalis, and levator anguli oris muscles. These muscles receive their innervation from the facial nerve on their superficial surfaces (Fig. 1).

The facial nerve exits the cranial vault via the stylomastoid foramen. The main trunk then proceeds to pass between the superficial and deep lobes of the parotid

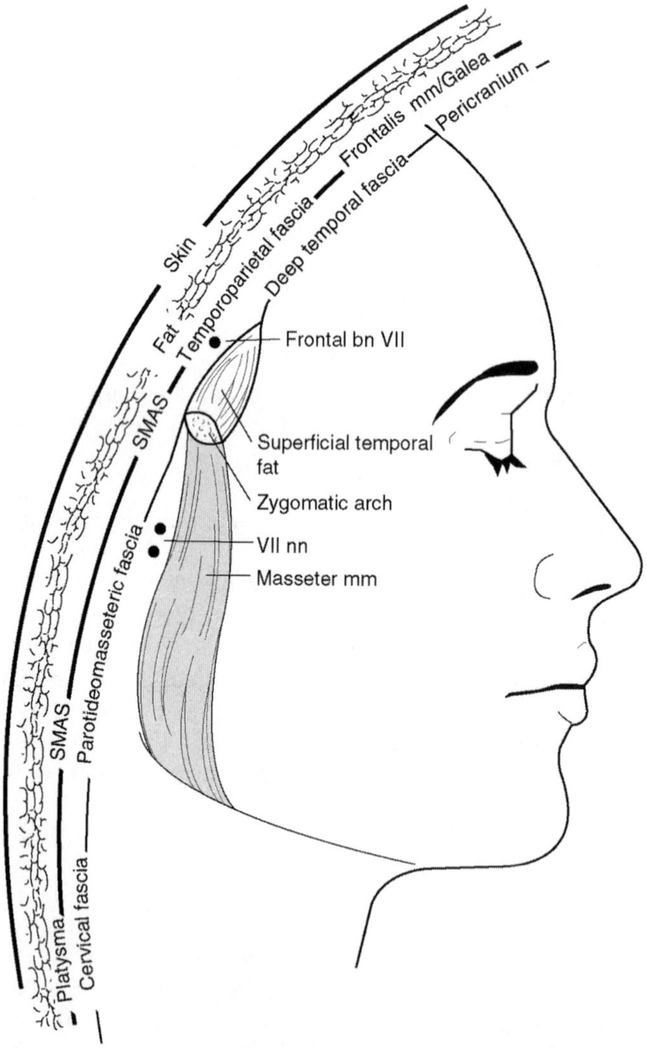

Figure 1 Despite the complexity of anatomical layers of the face, the facial nerve remains deep to the SMAS and innervates the musculature from their deep surfaces.

gland. It is at this point (pes) that the nerve divides into five distinct branches: frontotemporal, zygomatic, buccal, marginal mandibular, and cervical. Studies by Baker and Conley on over 2000 parotid dissections demonstrated communications between the zygomatic and buccal branches in 70% of cases (11). The frontal and marginal mandibular branches communicated with other branches in only 15% of patients. They have also presented data more recently indicating that the marginal mandibular nerve is always found below the inferior border of the mandible. This contradicts prior beliefs espoused by Dingman and Grabb that the marginal mandibular nerve lies above the border of the mandible in 81% of cases (12).

Other significant anatomical structures influencing currently used facelifting procedures include the nasolabial fold, retaining ligaments, and platysma muscle. Prominent nasolabial folds and jowling develop in part due to laxity of the retaining ligaments of the cheek. These include the zygomatic ligaments (McGregor's patch) and the mandibular ligaments (13). In these areas, the overlying skin is anchored to the bone below. By resisting gravitational forces and allowing the intervening cheek skin to descend, the nasolabial folds deepen and jowls develop. In addition, the platysma muscle, in most instances, will decussate at the level of the hyoid cartilage. In the remainder of cases, the medial borders of the muscle run parallel to each other. These findings, along with the effects of aging and gravity, lead to the development of submental banding and the so-called turkey gobbler deformity.

RHYTIDECTOMY

Modern facelift surgery has undergone great advancements over the last 100 years. Facelifting procedures were first described in the early 1900s and consisted of simple skin excision and direct closure. As techniques improved, the concept of raising skin flaps in the subcutaneous plane was proposed with improved aesthetic results. It was not until Skoog in the 1970s that the concept of deep layer suspension came into favor (14). This was the basis for studies by Mitz and Peyronie that defined the SMAS and its role in modern facelift surgery. Since then, several modifications have been proposed including deep plane SMAS advancement and subperiosteal facelifting procedures.

The technique of rhytidectomy varies from surgeon to surgeon depending on their experience and preference. Since the advent of SMAS–suspension rhytidectomy in the 1970s, several technical modifications to this basic rhytidectomy technique have been advocated. Surgeons seeking an improvement in the midface and nasolabial fold (typical problem areas that are undertreated with classic rhytidectomy) have inspired development of these new-generation rhytidectomy techniques. Further medial dissection over or under the SMAS is the essential element in nearly all of the permutations of the classic rhytidectomy. Despite the vast number of rhytidectomy variations espoused by numerous surgeons, they can generally be classified into categories including lateral rhytidectomy, conventional rhytidectomy, extended rhytidectomy, deep plane rhytidectomy, and composite rhytidectomy.

Lateral

Lateral rhytidectomy is perhaps the simplest SMAS–suspension rhytidectomy technique (15). A traditional subcutaneous flap is dissected that extends medially to the malar eminence and beyond the jowls along and below the mandibular line. A narrow strip of SMAS is resected over the parotid along a line 2–3 cm anterior to the preauricular sulcus that is parallel to the nasolabial fold (Fig. 2). The subSMAS dissection is limited in the face but extends inferiorly in a subplatysmal plane. The SMAS–platysmal flap is pulled posterosuperiorly and suture-suspended to the proximal SMAS and dense zygomatic fascia. This type of SMAS manipulation allows essentially a single vector of pull to efface jowling and to tighten the neck. There is little effect on the appearance of the nasolabial fold or midface using this technique. The SMAS is anchored securely to muscle and periosteum along the posterior margin of the zygomatic muscles. Therefore, posterior traction on the SMAS does little to elevate the malar fat pad or efface the nasolabial fold. In addition, pos-

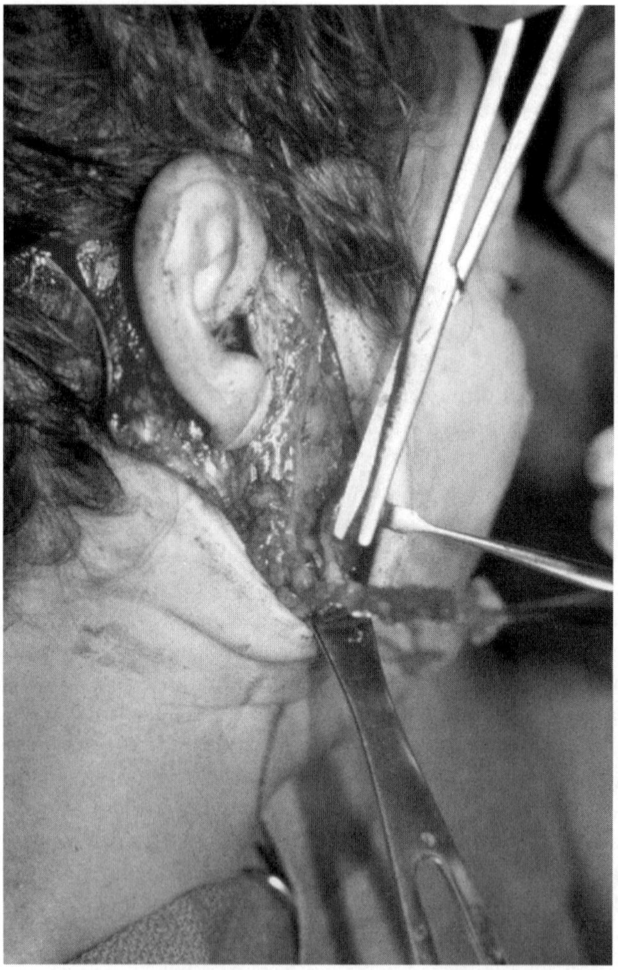

Figure 2 Patient undergoing a traditional lateral rhytidectomy in which a narrow strip of SMAS is resected over the parotid along a line 2–3 cm anterior to the preauricular sulcus that is parallel to the nasolabial fold.

terior traction on the subcutaneous flap despite extensive medial dissection cannot correct a ptotic malar fat pad.

Conventional

A conventional rhytidectomy is performed by undermining an extensive subcutaneous flap with SMAS suspension along two relatively independent vectors: posterior and superior. This is accomplished by incising the SMAS transversely under the zygomatic arch and vertically just anterior to the preauricular sulcus. A subSMAS dissection proceeds medially to the anterior border of the parotid gland and inferiorly under the platysma just beyond and inferior to the angle of the mandible. The SMAS–platysma along the vertical incision is pulled posteriorly while the SMAS along the upper transverse incision is pulled primarily in a superior direction. The SMAS is anchored with sutures and excess is trimmed. Of course, the subcutaneous flap is also pulled posterosuperiorly and the excess skin is trimmed (Fig. 3). This type of facelift, compared to lateral rhytidectomy, results in further improvements in effacement of the jowls and neck tightening. This procedure, like lateral rhytidectomy, will not result in significant improvement of midface aging. As is the case with any rhytidectomy, midline neck problems such as platysmal banding and excess submental fat should be corrected through a separate submental incision before posterior traction and suspension on the platysma is done.

Lateral and conventional rhytidectomies are the most commonly performed of all types of facelift procedures. Despite their popularity, it is obvious that these procedures do not adequately address significant midface aging and deep nasolabial folds. For patients in need of correction in these areas, further medial dissection and suspension within the midface itself is required to lift the malar fat pad and flatten the nasolabial fold. The malar fat pad has ligamentous attachments to the overlying skin and underlying zygomatic muscles. The fat pad may be lifted with the skin if the ligamentous attachments are severed directly over zygomatic muscles (extended and deep plane rhytidectomy) or if the zygomatic muscles are lifted in conjunction with the fat pad and overlying skin (composite and subperiosteal rhytidectomy). These procedures require more extensive dissection than lateral or conventional rhytidectomy and carry a higher risk of facial nerve injury and protracted facial edema and ecchymosis.

There are predominantly only anecdotal and biased reports that actually claim that significant improvements in the appearance of the midface can be had after extended medial dissection during routine rhytidectomy. Ivy et al. performed lateral and conventional rhytidectomies on one side and extended rhytidectomies on the opposite side in a series of patients (16). They found that immediately postoperatively there was indeed a significant improvement in the midface on the sides of the extended dissection. However, the differences rapidly dissolved after the postoperative edema subsided. Considering that the dissection plane for extended rhytidectomy is inherently more hazardous, an extreme medial subSMAS dissection appears unwarranted, at least to improve the appearance of the midface. Nevertheless, there are advantages to a medial subSMAS dissection in conjunction with a foreshortened subcutaneous dissection (deep plane rhytidectomy) that will be discussed shortly. It is clear that to provide meaningful improvements in the midface a deep level of dissection is required along with a more superior advancement of

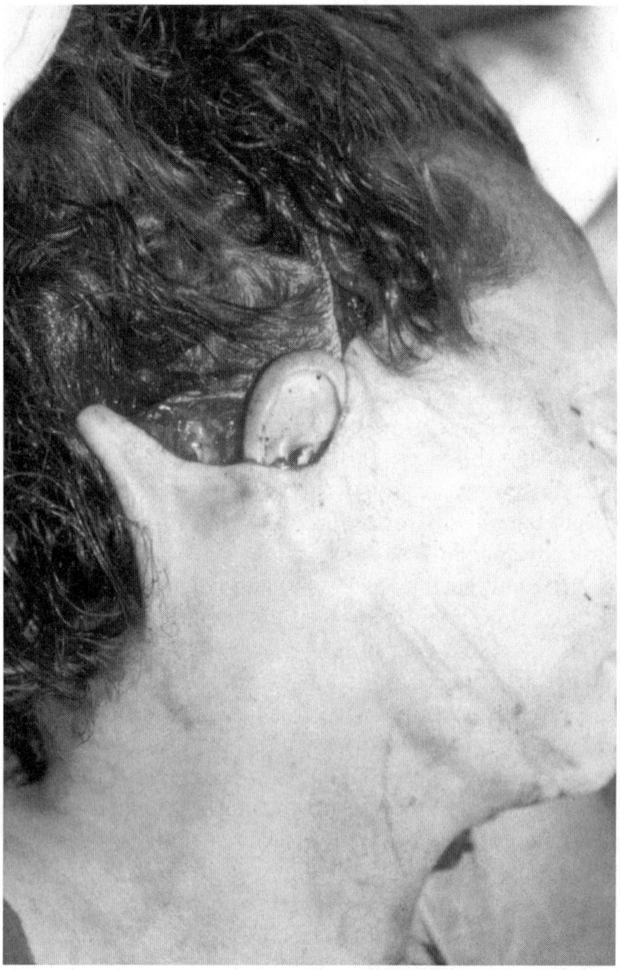

Figure 3 Typical excess skin that results after SMAS plication and gentle posterior traction on the subcutaneous flap. Excess skin is trimmed, being conservative near the lobule to prevent distortion.

tissue. This type of dissection and tissue movement is difficult, if not impossible, through the standard rhytidectomy approach. The composite and subperiosteal rhytidectomies more effectively address midface aging but require dissection and access incisions within the area of the midface.

Extended

The extended rhytidectomy is similar to the conventional type except that the sub-SMAS dissection is extended medially beyond the nasolabial fold. The plane of dissection passes over the zygomatic muscles, thereby releasing the ligaments tethering the malar fat pad and skin overlying the nasolabial fold. The SMAS layer becomes quite fragile beyond the anterior border of the parotid gland. By developing this layer independently, the ability to use the SMAS to suspend the deep tissues of the midface is compromised. However, by dividing the retaining ligaments, the fat pad can be suspended with the skin flap. Pulling the skin flap posteriorly can efface the nasolabial fold but this effect is temporary because the deep tissues of the midface remain fixed. As mentioned, extended medial dissection of the SMAS using this technique to improve midface aging is probably unwarranted considering the increased risk of injury to the facial nerve.

Deep Plane

The deep plane rhytidectomy technique also involves an extensive medial subSMAS dissection, however, it is performed through a significantly foreshortened subcutaneous flap dissection (17). The deep plane (subSMAS) is extensively dissected to release the ligamentous attachments of the SMAS to the zygomatic muscles, parotid, and masseter muscle. The resulting SMAS–platysma–skin flap is advanced posteriorly as a single unit. The initial subcutaneous dissection extends medially to a line that is tangent to the angle of the mandible to the origins of the zygomatic muscles. The incision into the SMAS follows this same line and an extensive subSMAS dissection then proceeds medially similar to that done in an extended rhytidectomy. A thick myocutaneous flap is created that contains the freed malar fat pad. This flap is then pulled posterosuperiorly along multiple vectors and secured both at the SMAS and skin levels. Although long-term improvements in the midface are debatable, Kamer found that the thicker SMAS–platysma–skin flap is hardier and less prone to marginal necrosis, which is especially advantageous for patients that smoke (18). Other advantages noted by Kamer are smoother mandibular lines, softened nasolabial folds, improved incisional healing, and fewer skin surface irregularities.

Composite

To address midface aging further, Hamra modified his deep plane technique to include dissection and elevation of the orbicularis oculi and zygomatic muscles through a separate blepharoplasty incision (19). This modified technique was dubbed composite rhytidectomy. It is a supraperiosteal technique in which, in addition to a deep plane flap, a composite deep muscle flap is developed to lift the midface. This results in elevation of the malar fat pad and periorbital rejuvenation. The original version of this rhytidectomy technique involved elevating the orbicularis muscle via a blepharoplasty incision so that this muscle could be included in the deep plane flap. This allowed a smoother transition from the lifted malar fat pad to the periorbital area. According to Hamra, although the aesthetic results were improved, it resulted in prolonged malar edema in many patients. He eventually added a subzygomatic muscle lift as well to avoid disrupting the origins of the zygomatic muscles (zygomaticus–orbicularis plane), resulting in less trauma and less postoperative edema (19). The results of this type of rhytidectomy are more favorable with regard to improving midface and periorbital aging. However, the risk of permanent injury to the facial nerve and surrounding musculature is greater. This type of lift must be reserved for patients in need of correction of significant periorbital and midface aging problems. A subperiosteal midface lift in conjunction with a more traditional rhytidectomy is an alternative.

Subperiosteal

The subperiosteal approach to periorbital lifting was introduced by Tessier in 1980 (20). A subperiosteal mobilization of the superolateral orbital rim was performed during a routine coronal lift to improve periorbital rejuvenation. Subsequent modifications by Ramirez resulted in today's periorbital and midface subperiosteal lifts, primarily performed through a temporal approach. Incorporation of a midface subperiosteal dissection through a standard rhytidectomy approach is difficult because of problems with adequate visualization and facial nerve injury. An extended temporal approach is needed (i.e., combine a rhytidectomy with a standard midface lift) or the subperiosteal plane may be entered and widely dissected using separate incisions near the malar eminence and under the cheek. Baker describes a subperiosteal rhytidectomy (triplane rhytidectomy) that uses this latter technique (20). Through a standard rhytidectomy approach, an incision is made through the SMAS near the zygomatic eminence and the subperiosteal plane is entered bluntly. Wide subperiosteal dissection proceeds over the lateral orbital rim, malar eminence, and anterior zygomatic arch. The subperiosteal midface dissection is completed through a gingivobuccal incision by undermining the periosteum over the face of the maxilla, nasal bone, pyriform aperture, infraorbital rim, and zygomatic eminence. The deep face (periosteum and SMAS) is then suture-suspended along two vectors: superior and lateral. The main advantage of using separate incisions to approach the subperiosteal plane in the midface is avoidance of crossing the plane of the facial nerve branches. Subperiosteal lifts can be dramatic in terms of midface and periocular rejuvenation. A criticism of this method is that the lifting is excessive leading to unnatural elevation and lateralization of the lateral canthus and tissues in the upper and middle face.

Midface Lifting

Although several rhytidectomy techniques have been developed to improve the midface as outlined above, in some circumstances only a midface lift is needed. This is often the case in younger patients in whom jowling is not a major problem but periocular and midface aging changes are apparent. In these cases, a temporal approach often combined with a coronal forehead lift is what is most often performed. This approach to midface lifting is quite similar to that originally described by Tessier and later modified by Ramirez (see above).

Routine Conservative SMAS Rhytidectomy: The Author's Technique

The patient is positioned supine and, after administration of adequate anesthesia, is prepped with a povidone–iodine solution and draped in a sterile manner. Draping should be performed in a way that will allow for full facial exposure and allow adequate mobility for turning the head. The incisions are then infiltrated with local anesthetic consisting of 0.5% lidocaine with epinephrine. A more dilute solution may then be used to infiltrate and hydrodissect the facial skin flaps. This will provide not only an anesthetic effect but also a hemostatic benefit by local vasoconstriction.

The skin incision starts in the temporal hair, 5 cm superior to the ear and 3–5 cm posterior to the hairline. From this point, the incision proceeds inferiorly, parallel to the hairline, toward the root of the helix. The temporal incision may be modified in revision facelift patients and male patients to avoid displacing the sideburn

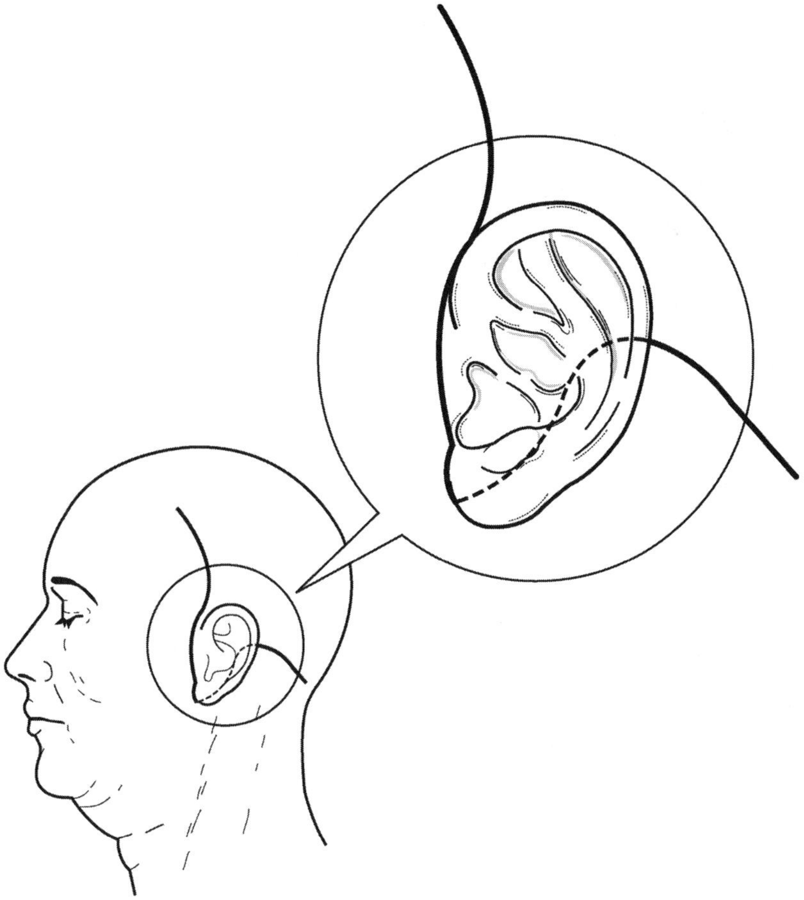

Figure 4 To ensure consistent results, the posterior incision (postauricular) should be in line with the temporal incision.

and hairline superiorly. Placement of the preauricular aspect of the incision may proceed antetragally or retrotragally. The incision then continues around the base of the lobule and onto the posterior conchal skin. The conchal incision should be placed at least 2–3 mm above the retroauricular sulcus. Proceeding superiorly, the incision is then turned posteriorly along the hairline for 3–5 cm. To ensure consistent results, the posterior incision should be in line with the temporal incision (Fig. 4).

The focus, initially, is directed to the subcutaneous dissection of the temporal skin flap. This is accomplished with a combination of electrocautery and facelift scissors. The dissection proceeds medially in the subcutaneous plane thus exposing the SMAS layer below (Fig. 5). Dissection proceeds up to 1 cm lateral to the lateral orbital rim, across the malar region, and along the nasolabial fold to a point 1 cm lateral to the oral commissure (Fig. 6). The retaining ligaments mentioned earlier will be released from their zygomatic and mandibular attachments. Careful hemostatic measures using bipolar electrocautery should be employed throughout the dissection to minimize the risk of hematoma formation postoperatively.

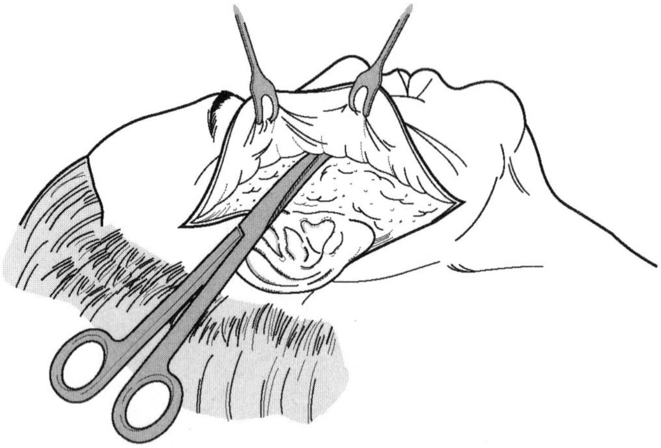

Figure 5 The skin flap subcutaneous dissection is shown using face-lift scissors. The opposite hand palpates the tip of the scissors to confirm its position within the subcutaneous plane.

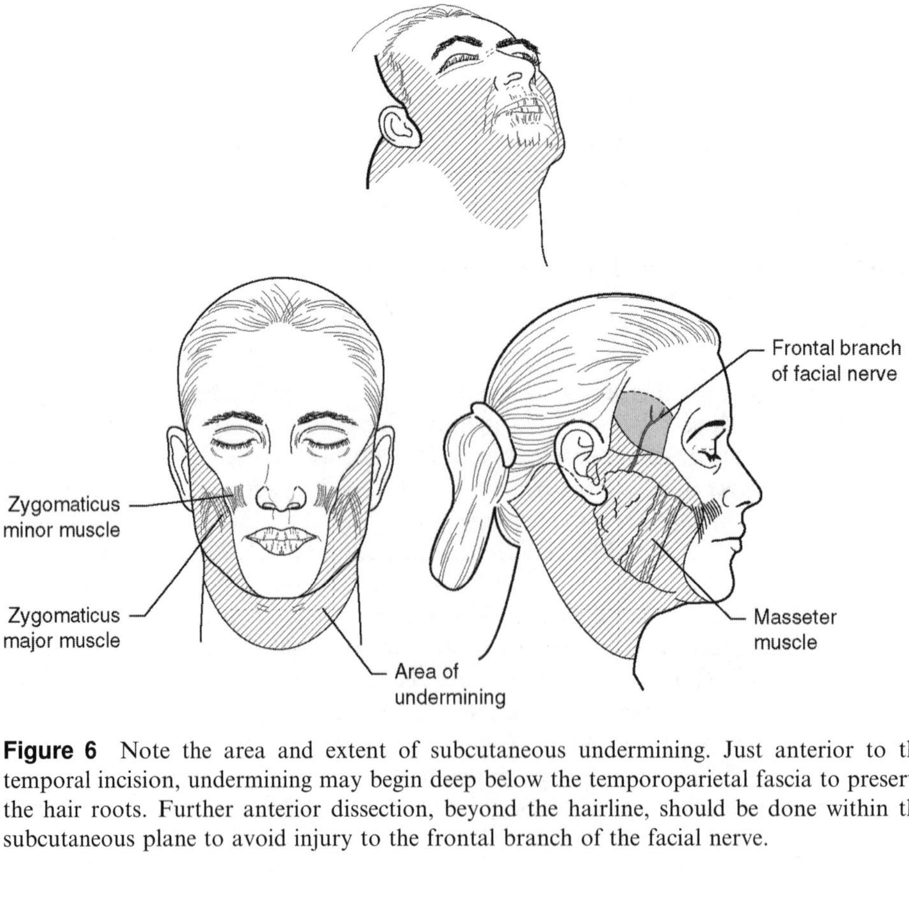

Figure 6 Note the area and extent of subcutaneous undermining. Just anterior to the temporal incision, undermining may begin deep below the temporoparietal fascia to preserve the hair roots. Further anterior dissection, beyond the hairline, should be done within the subcutaneous plane to avoid injury to the frontal branch of the facial nerve.

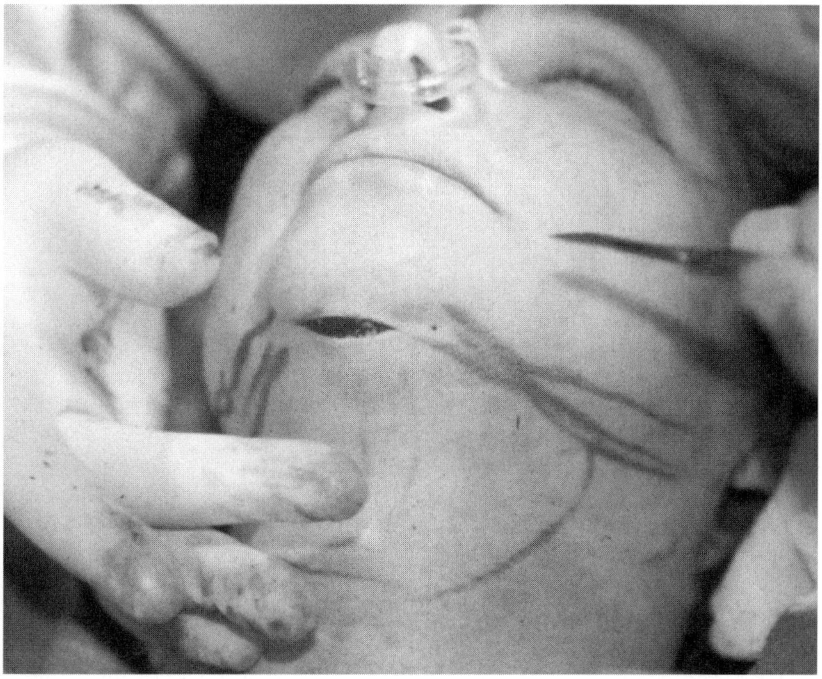

Figure 7 During rhytidectomy, if there is evidence of platysmal banding or neck lipodystrophy, a separate submental incision may be necessary to provide access for platysmal plication and submental lipectomy. These procedures should be complete prior to posterior traction on the skin flap and SMAS.

Attention is next focused on the postauricular area. These skin flaps are also dissected in a subcutaneous plane proceeding inferiorly and medially onto the neck to expose the underlying platysma. If there is evidence of platysmal banding or neck lipodystrophy preoperatively, a separate submental incision may be necessary to provide access for platysmal plication and submental lipectomy (Fig. 7). This is best accomplished before rhytidectomy. Care should be taken to avoid injury to the great auricular nerve, which may identified 6.5 cm inferior to the bony external auditory canal. The nerve usually courses across the anterior border of the sternocleidomastoid muscle with the external jugular vein. Transection of the great auricular nerve will lead to permanent loss of sensation in the ear lobule and helix (Fig. 8).

Dissection and suspension of the SMAS are the most crucial elements in ensuring a long lasting aesthetic result. Once the skin flaps have been elevated, a permanent suture (3–0 Mersilene) is used to plicate the SMAS to the zygomaticotemporal fascia, fascia of the bony external auditory canal, and the mastoid fascia. Good fascial bites will provide an adequate anchor from which to suspend the SMAS. This will allow the subcutaneous tissues in the midface to be elevated alleviating jowling, smoothing the nasolabial folds, and providing an improvement in neck contour. An identical SMAS suspension should be performed on the contralateral side before skin closure.

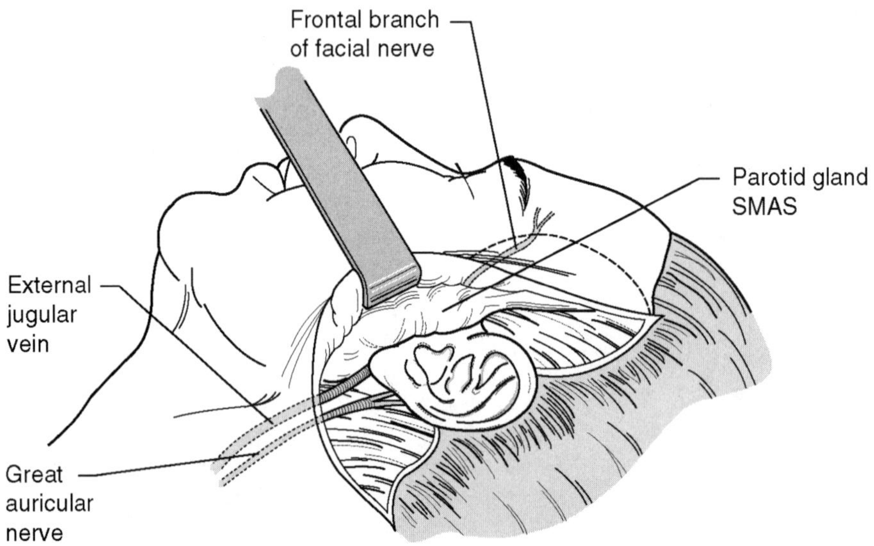

Figure 8 Note the very superficial location of the great auricular nerve: the most commonly injured nerve in facelifting.

Following SMAS suspension, skin flap redraping may proceed. The skin flaps are retracted in a superior and posterior direction along vectors determined preoperatively. Two points are then anchored using 2–0 nylon sutures: one in the temporal scalp incision 1–2 cm superior to the root of the helix and the other at the apex of the postauricular incision (Fig. 9). Excess skin in the temporal region is excised and the incision is closed with 3–0 Vicryl in the dermis followed by 3–0 Prolene or staples in the skin. Excess posterior conchal and preauricular skin is excised and

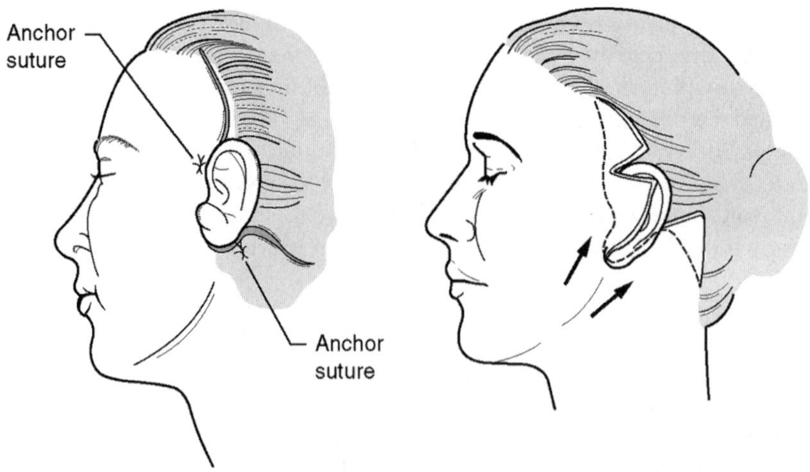

Figure 9 The skin flap is pulled along two vectors. Two points are anchored using 2–0 nylon sutures: one in the temporal scalp incision 1–2 cm superior to the root of the helix and the other at the apex of the postauricular incision.

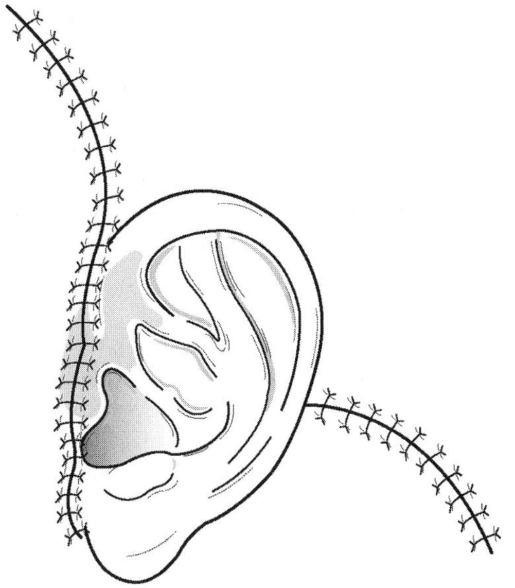

Figure 10 Final skin closure. Note the drain taken out of the postauricular incision. Trimming of skin under the earlobe should be conservative to prevent distortion.

the dermis is approximated with 4–0 Vicryl. The preauricular skin is closed with 5–0 nylon and the postauricular conchal skin is approximated with 5–0 catgut. Skin trimming under the lobule should be limited to prevent visible scar and distortion of the ear lobe (Fig. 10). Skin excess in the retroauricular area is removed and the skin flap is closed with 3–0 Vicryl dermal sutures and skin staples. Bacitracin and Xeroform dressings are placed over the incisions followed by gauze. The patient is then wrapped with gauze and an elastic bandage or a compressive facelift garment. Prior to closure of the posterior incisions, a small suction drain is placed under the neck skin flap and brought out of the posterior most aspect of the retroauricular incision.

Complications

Complications after rhytidectomy occasionally occur and should be recognized and addressed by the surgeon expeditiously. These include hematoma, skin slough, alopecia, scarring, nerve injury, and pigmentary changes. Other minor complications as defined by Baker are alopecia (1–3%), infection (1%), hypertrophic scar (1–4%), and earlobe deformity (5%) (21). Careful preoperative evaluation, meticulous surgical technique, and appropriate postoperative management are key elements of a successful rhytidectomy.

Hematoma

Hematoma is the most common complication in facelift surgery. It usually occurs within the first 24 h and can threaten skin flap survival and potentially obstruct the airway. If hematoma is suspected, the patient should be promptly evaluated. Dressings should be removed and, if a hematoma is present, sutures removed to provide immediate relief. The patient should then return to the operating room for the surgeon to evaluate the skin flaps and attempt to find the bleeding vessel. An obvious source of bleeding is rarely discovered. Small hematomas may not be apparent until after facial edema has resolved. In these cases, one should wait 1–2 weeks for the hematoma to liquefy before attempting aspiration. This may require several treatments. Untreated hematomas may lead to skin irregularity, skin induration, and ecchymotic discoloration that in some cases can leave permanent hemosiderin deposits and staining of the skin. Overall, the incidence of hematoma formation is 0.3–8.1% (22). Patients most likely to develop a hematoma are men, hypertensive patients, and those taking acetylsalicylic acid or other anticoagulants.

Skin Slough

Skin slough may be full or partial thickness. It may be seen as a result of hematoma or infection. Studies indicate that the incidence of skin slough is between 1 and 3% (23,24). It is most frequently encountered in the postauricular and mastoid areas, as a result of hematoma, intraoperative injury to the flap, elevation of an excessively thin flap, or excessive tension on the skin closure. Smokers are also at increased risk of skin necrosis due to the effects on the microcirculation of nicotine and carbon monoxide (25). Initial treatment consists of observation and dressing changes. Partial-thickness loss is allowed to re-epithelialize and contract with little noticeable scarring. After several days, small areas of skin necrosis may be excised and the skin flap readvanced.

Nerve Injury

Nerve injury is rare. Early numbness of the cheek and lower ear is due to postoperative edema and division of small sensory nerve branches. This alteration in sensation is usually transient. The nerve most commonly permanently injured is the greater auricular nerve, resulting in numbness of the ear lobe and helix. It occurs as a result of dissecting too deep over the sternocleidomastoid muscle. If recognized during the procedure, it should be repaired immediately. Permanent injury to the facial nerve occurs infrequently. Facial nerve injury can be avoided by having a thorough understanding of facial nerve anatomy and its relationship to other facial structures involved in facelift surgery. The buccal branches are the most commonly injured but, because of significant cross innervation, this injury is usually not disfiguring. Injury to the marginal mandibular and temporal branches will be obvious postoperatively. If a facial nerve injury is noted at the time of surgery, it should be repaired immediately. Facial nerve palsies should be observed, with most resolving within a year. A review of recent literature reveals that the incidence of nerve injury is reported to be between 0 and 4.3%.

BROW AND FOREHEAD LIFTING

Forehead aging is rarely improved by standard rhytidectomy techniques. Correction of brow ptosis, transverse forehead wrinkles, and glabellar creases often require direct surgical intervention. Endoscopic and traditional forehead lifting procedures have been the most effective methods for treating forehead aging. However, recently botulinum toxin type A (Botox, Allergan), a diluted form of botulinum toxin, has recently received approval by The Food and Drug Administration (FDA) for the treatment of glabellar rhytides. Although targeted injections of Botox can result in some degree of brow lifting, surgery is still required in the vast majority of patients seeking a significant change in elevation and effacement of the brow and upper eyelids.

Anatomy

Several muscles are involved in the formation of forehead rhytides. Overactivity of these muscles results in forehead and glabellar wrinkling. Natural skin aging and gravitational effects, on the other hand, are primarily responsible for forehead and brow ptosis. The primary muscles involved in wrinkle formation are the frontalis, procerus, and corrugators. The frontalis muscle is an extension of the galea aponeurotica and inserts into the dermis of the upper brow. Frontalis activity produces transverse forehead wrinkling. Procerus and corrugator muscles are primarily medial brow depressors. The procerus originates from the upper nasal bones and inserts into the glabellar dermis. Contraction of the procerus will depress the medial brow, thus causing transverse wrinkling of the nasal radix. The corrugator muscles also work to depress the medial brow. They originate on the superomedial orbital rim and insert onto the medial brow skin. When contracted, vertical and oblique glabellar wrinkles form. These muscles are the primary focus of modern forehead lifting procedures and must be adequately addressed to ensure satisfactory results (26).

Patient Evaluation

The patient should be evaluated in a well-lit examination room. The characteristics of the forehead should be assessed, including the degree of wrinkling in the forehead and glabella. Forehead height, hairline position, and hair density are also important elements in the initial examination. Brow position should be noted, including its contribution to upper eyelid fullness. In certain cases, elevation of the brow will relieve fullness in the upper eyelid, thus avoiding the need for blepharoplasty. The ideal brow position has been described by Ellenbogen (27) as follows (Fig. 11):

1. Beginning medially at a vertical line perpendicular to the alar base.
2. The lateral brow terminates at an oblique line through the nasal ala and lateral canthus.
3. The medial and lateral ends lie approximately at the same horizontal level.
4. The apex of the brow lies on a vertical line directly above the lateral limbus.
5. The brow arches above the supraorbital rim in women; it lies along the rim in men.

Techniques

Several surgical techniques have been described for forehead rejuvenation. The simplest of these is direct excision of skin along the upper eyebrow. This procedure is usually suitable for men with thicker eyebrows that can provide camouflage for the scars and for patients with alopecia that would make scars on the forehead or scalp apparent. Excision of an ellipse of skin in the midforehead may be suitable

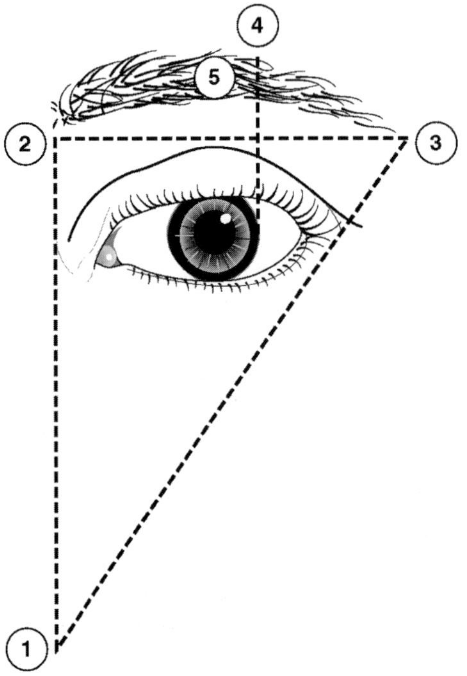

Figure 11 The ideal brow position begins medially at a vertical line perpendicular to the alar base (1–2); the lateral brow terminates at an oblique line through the nasal ala and lateral canthus (1–3); the medial and lateral ends lie approximately at the same horizontal level (2–3); the apex of the brow lies on a vertical line directly above the lateral limbus (4).

for patients with thinning eyebrows but with deep midforehead creases that can provide camouflage for the scar. A distinct advantage of the direct and midforehead brow lift is the ability to tailor the degree of elevation and shape of the eyebrow by altering the width and shape of the ellipse of skin excised (Figs. 12, 13).

The coronal incision forehead browlift is employed by most surgeons. In a patient with a high forehead (> 5 cm), an anterior hairline incision should be performed to avoid elevating the hairline further (28) (Fig. 14). When performing a standard coronal brow lift, several dissection planes are available. Subcutaneous dissection has the advantage of directly addressing forehead wrinkles without disrupting the supraorbital nerves that provide sensation to the anterior scalp. The disadvantage of the subcutaneous approach is that the vascularity of the skin flap may be compromised leading to alopecia, wound dehiscence, skin slough, and poor scarring (29). A subgaleal (supraperiosteal) dissection may be preferable because of the ease and rapidity of the dissection, allowing direct visualization of the muscles responsible for forehead wrinkling (30). The main disadvantage of the subgaleal dissection is scalp numbness posterior to the incision secondary to division of the supraorbital nerves. The subperiosteal approach is believed to produce a more effective lift of the brows. This is accomplished by allowing the forehead tissues to slide easily over the frontal bone. Scarring of the periosteum to the underlying frontal bone adds to the permanency of the lift. The theoretical disadvantage of this approach is that some bone resorption may occur because the frontal bone has been

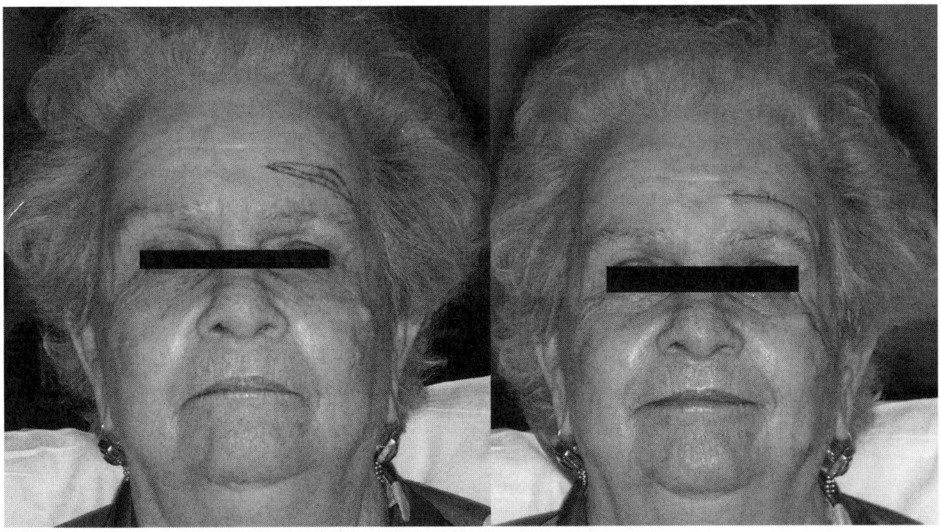

Figure 12 As noted in left photograph, this patient has age-related descent of her left brow resulting in asymmetry, heaviness, and a superior visual field cut. An ellipse of skin in the midforehead is excised, resulting in controlled correction of this deformity and elimination of the vision problems.

separated from the periosteum that provides its blood supply. The subperiosteal approach is the most common approach used in endoscopic forehead lifting (31).

Coronal Lift

The planned coronal incision is marked so that the central portion of the incision is placed at least 7 cm behind the anterior hairline. This allows, after resection of redundant skin, at least 5 cm of hair-bearing scalp to remain anterior to the incision. This marking should then be carried laterally, gently curving into the temporal scalp toward the root of the helix (Fig. 15). Once the markings are finished, the sides should be compared for symmetry. The planned incision is then infiltrated with lidocaine with epinephrine to provide anesthesia and hemostasis. The incision is then made with a scalpel beveled in the direction of the hair follicles to minimize injury and postoperative alopecia. Once the incision is complete and hemostasis achieved, a subgaleal dissection is carried down toward the supraorbital rims. As the dissection approaches the orbital rims, care should be taken to identify the supraorbital and supratrochlear neurovascular bundles. By taking the time to do so, the risk of inadvertent injury is minimized. The flap can be released from its supraorbital attachments and the dissection continued onto the nasal dorsum. The corrugators are next identified and cut, avoiding injury to the supratrochlear nerves. Complete resection of the corrugators is not recommended since doing so may lead to a soft tissue depression. The procerus muscle attachments to the glabella are released sharply under the areas of transverse glabellar creasing. At this point, the forehead flap is redraped posteriorly and fixated deeply at three points with 2–0 nylon sutures. These points include the midline and each temporal scalp: roughly in line vertically with the lateral canthus. Once fixation is accomplished, excess flap is trimmed and the

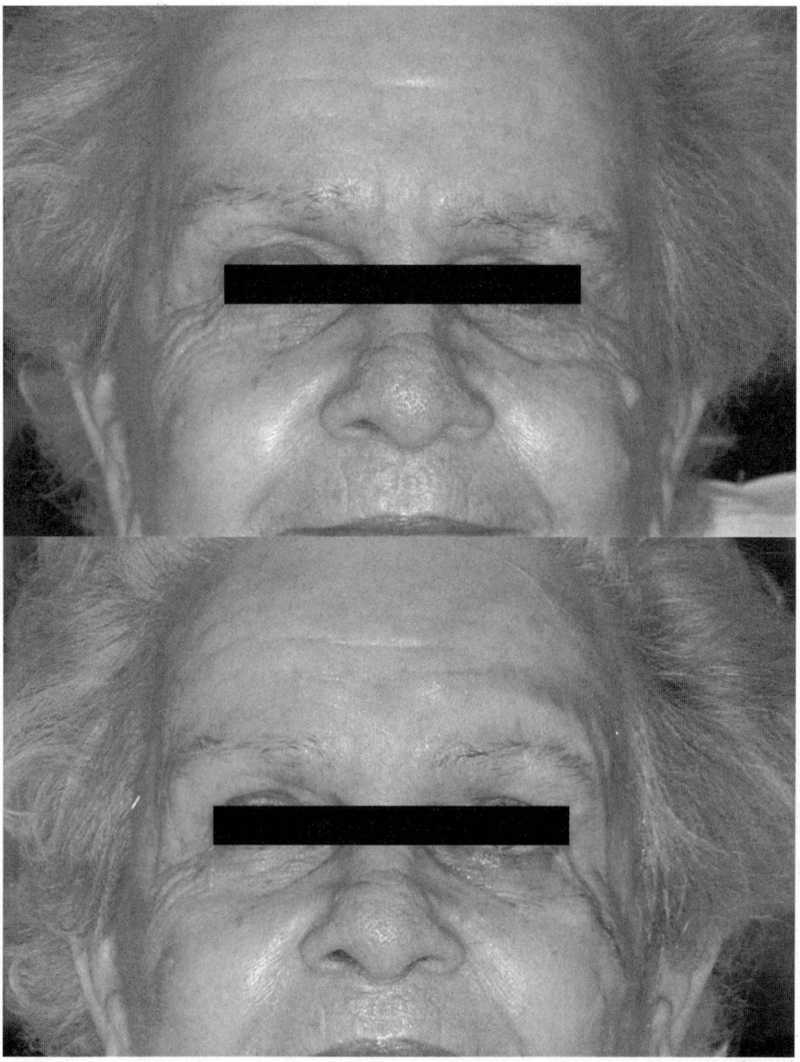

Figure 13 Same patient as in Figure 12. Preoperative photograph (above) shows brow asymmetry and postoperative result (below) shows appearance after a unilateral midforehead brow lift.

galea/ subcutaneous tissues are approximated with 2–0 and 3–0 Vicryl sutures (Fig. 16). The skin is closed with staples. Postoperatively, the patient should expect mild to moderate pain, some eyelid elevation requiring ophthalmic lubrication, swelling, and periorbital ecchymosis.

Endoscopic Forehead Lift

The increasing popularity of minimally invasive surgery has not been overlooked in the advancement of aesthetic surgery. The endoscopic brow lift is an easy, safe, and effective method of rejuvenating the forehead and lifting the eyebrows. Candidates

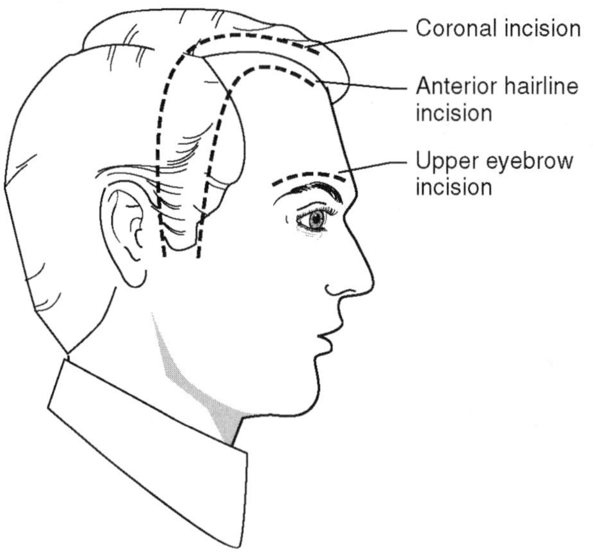

Figure 14 Different incisions used in brow and forehead lifting: anterior hairline (pretrichial), upper eyebrow, and coronal.

for endoscopic forehead lifting include those with a short forehead and balding patients to avoid placement of conspicuous coronal scars. The basic instrumentation for performing endoscopic brow elevation includes a 4–5 mm rigid 30 degree angled scope with a standard light source, one or two angled endoscopic periosteal elevators, graspers, scissors, and cautery. The procedure begins with preoperative markings at the planned incision sites. These are three to five sites through which the endoscope and instruments will gain access. Each incision is 2 cm in length and placed 3–5 cm posterior to the anterior hairline: one in the midline, two incisions each 4 cm lateral to the midline, and two incisions each in the temporal region in line with the lateral canthi. It is advisable at this point to mark the general location of the

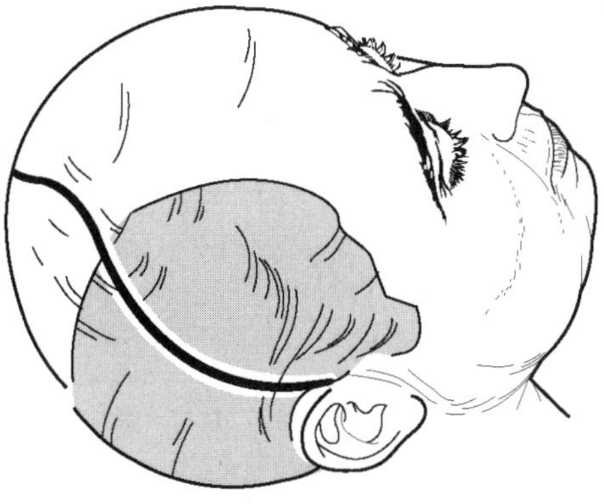

Figure 15 The coronal lift is performed by first incising the scalp across the vertex, gently curving into the temporal scalp toward the root of the helix.

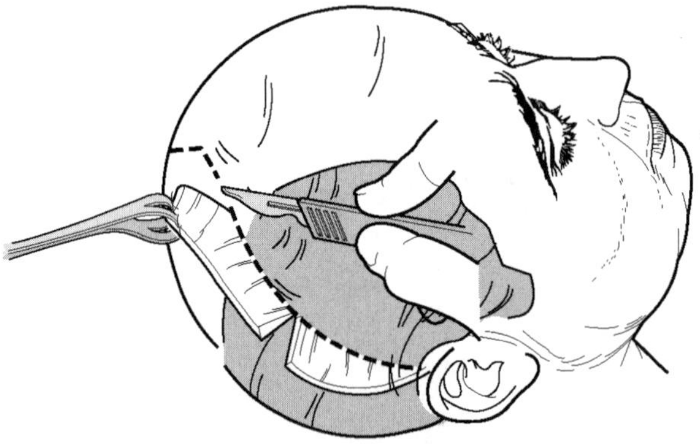

Figure 16 At the completion of the coronal lift, the flap is redraped posteriorly and fixated deeply at the midline and each temporal scalp: roughly in line vertically with the lateral canthus. Once fixation is accomplished, excess flap is trimmed and galea/subcutaneous tissues are approximated.

supraorbital and supratrochlear nerves as a reference when performing the dissection. Following administration of general anesthesia, a mixture of lidocaine and epinephrine is injected into the proposed incisions as well as into the forehead flap for hemostasis.

After the incisions are made, the dissection begins in the temporal scalp. Through the lateral incisions, the dissection proceeds through the temporoparietal fascia in a subgaleal plane over the deep temporal fascia. Using the elevators, the dissection proceeds up to the lateral orbital rims and to the anterior two-thirds of the zygomatic arch. Dissection in the region of the posterior zygomatic arch should be avoided to prevent injury to the superficial temporal vessels. Once the temporal dissections are complete the central dissection commences. This dissection is carried toward the supraorbital rims in the subperiosteal plane (Fig. 17). At the level of the orbital rims the supratrochlear and supraorbital nerves should be identified. The lateral dissection proceeds to join the temporal dissection. Upon completion of the entire dissection, the corrugators and procerus muscles are visualized, cut, and partially resected. In some cases, free fat grafting may be necessary to avoid a glabellar depression after muscle resection. Careful hemostasis should be achieved before closure.

The periosteum of the forehead flap is fixated to screws inserted directly into the frontal bone. These titanium screws are 1.5 mm in diameter and 12–18 mm in length. They are placed 4 mm into the bone through the three central incisions. The screws will suspend the forehead flap by the periosteum and are removed 10–14 days postoperatively, after the flap has sufficiently scarred into place. As an alternative, resorbable screws may be used that are placed under the skin and need not be removed. Plication of the temporoparietal fascia to the deep temporal fascia using 3–0 PDS is also useful in fixating the flap. All incisions are closed in two layers, with the final skin closure performed with staples. The patient remains on oral antibiotics for 7 days postoperatively. If a drain is used, it is usually removed on postoperative day 3. The staples and percutaneous fixation screws may be removed postoperative days 10–14.

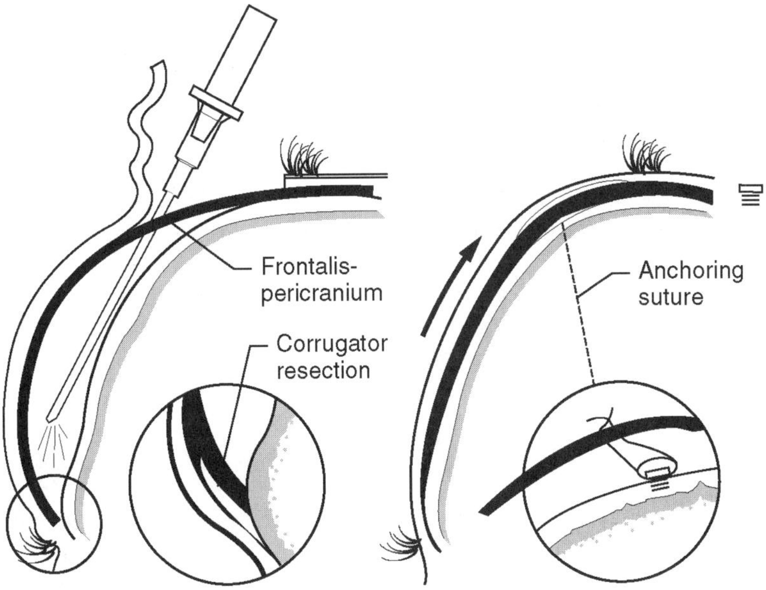

Figure 17 The endoscopic forehead lift is performed through minimal access scalp incisions with specially designed curved endoscopic scopes and surgical cutting and grasping instruments. Key parts of the procedure include corrugator resection and suture anchoring at the access incisions.

Disadvantages include the cost of equipment and training, extended operative time, and increased risk of nerve or vessel injury due to poor visualization (32). Complications include hematoma, alopecia, paralysis of the frontalis muscle, loss of sensation, scar pain and itching, and skin necrosis. Hematoma is rare but can result in flap necrosis and alopecia. If hematoma is suspected, the patient should be promptly evaluated and treated. Alopecia may also be caused by excess flap tension or hair follicle injury around the incisions. Frontalis muscle paralysis due to injury of the frontal branch of facial nerve is usually temporary, with return of function usually occurring within the first year.

Botulinum Toxin

Botulinum A toxin (Botox, Allergan) is a medical protein derived from the *C. botulinum* bacteria. When Botox is injected into a muscle, it causes temporary paralysis of that muscle. It has been safely used for many years in the treatment of eyelid spasm, eye muscle spasm causing crossed eyes, correction of facial muscle imbalance, and neck muscle spasm. The FDA has cleared Botox for the above uses and recently approval was given for its use to improve glabellar wrinkles.

Botox (botulinum toxin type A) works by blocking neuromuscular transmission by first binding to the cholinergic motor nerve terminal (via its heavy chain). The toxin molecule is internalized and its light chain is released. This light chain blocks acetylcholine release by cleaving a cytoplasmic protein on the cell membrane of the nerve terminal. The synthesis and reserves of acetylcholine within the cell remain unaffected. As a result of the toxin, the motor end-plate actually expands and there is new collateral axonal sprouting that eventually establishes a new neuromuscular junction, thereby resulting in return of motor function (33–35). The original motor terminal may also return to functionality, according to literature cited by Allergan (36).

Hyperactive facial muscles around the eyes and lower forehead may give a person an angry or tired/displeased appearance, even when they are not experiencing that emotion. Inactivating these small muscles reduces this undesirable effect and decreases the propensity to form wrinkles from these expressions. The cords or bands that protrude from the neck with the aging process may require surgery. However, certain patients can get significant improvement in these bands using Botox therapy. The cosmetic uses of botulinum A toxin include glabella frown lines (wrinkles between the eyebrows), forehead creases and horizontal forehead lines, crows feet, and platysmal bands (thick cords or bands in the neck).

Procedure

In a simple office procedure, the toxin is injected using a fine needle in the overactive muscles (Fig. 18). The muscle function becomes weakened, eliminating part or all of its function. Long standing skin creases will soften and may eventually disappear. The result is a softer, more relaxed, pleasant appearance. The procedure takes about 10 min. The patient may return to work immediately, however, he or she should avoid exercise or massaging the area for at least 4 h to limit any possible spreading of the toxin to adjacent muscles. The effects take several days to develop. Once the muscle function is impaired, the results will last 3–11 months. In some cases, the initial therapy will not be totally effective and the treatment may need to be performed again. Most patients require less frequent injections over time as the muscles retrain or weaken from disuse. Possible side effects include mild swelling at the injection site, headache, localized numbness, bruising, rash, and temporary loss of function of a nearby muscle (ptosis).

CERVICOFACIAL LIPOSUCTION

Aging, hereditary factors, and a lifetime of diet and exercise choices lead to a variety of facial and cervical contour aberrations caused by isolated excess deposits of fat that are especially evident in the neck. These fatty deposits often persist despite weight loss and exercise. Although rhytidectomy may tighten the overlying skin, and other techniques may be applied to address platysmal banding, the fat pads remain. Only surgical removal through open or closed techniques will effectively solve the problem.

Facial Analysis

Overall, the appearance of the submental–cervical region is influenced by the degree of laxity of the SMAS and platysma, lipomatosis, mandibular contour and dental configuration, and hyoid position (37). A cervicomental angle of between 90 and 120 degrees is considered youthful and attractive (37),(38),(39). A cervicomental angle of more than 120 degrees makes the neck look full and heavy. The hyoid bone

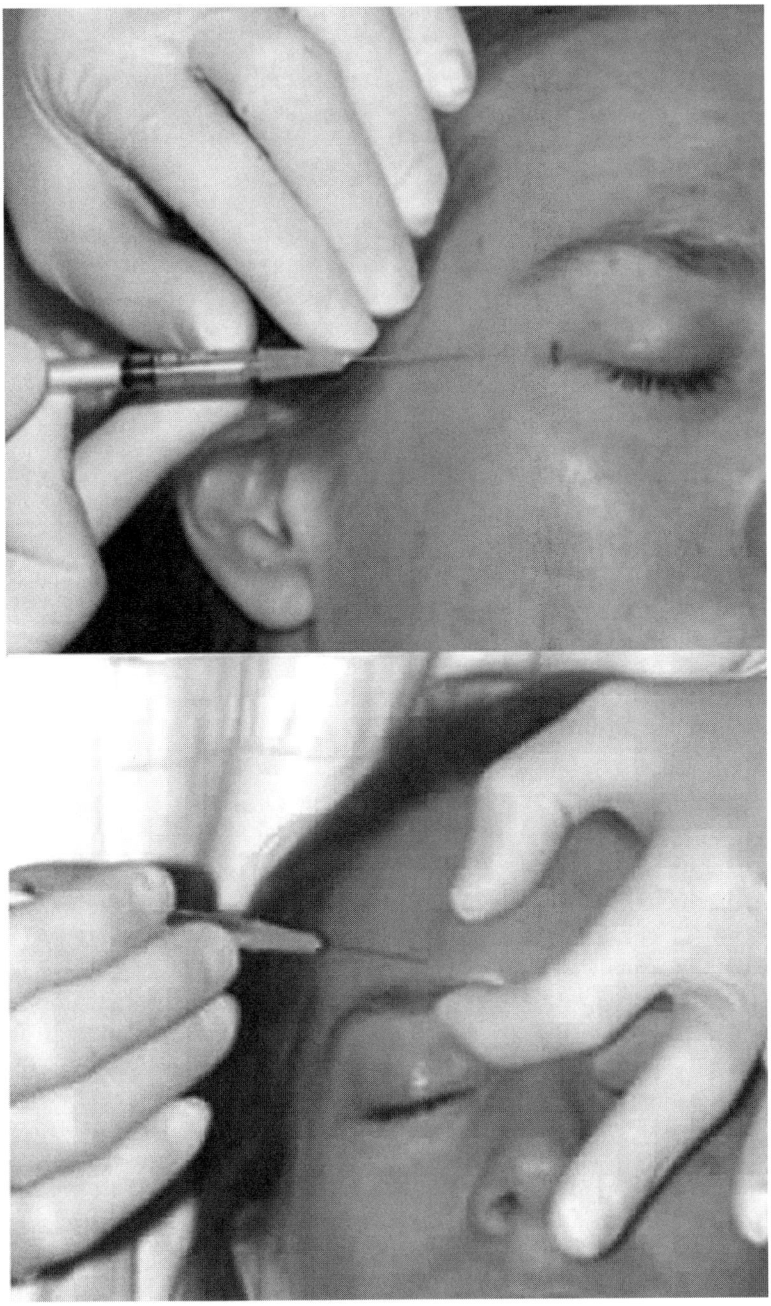

Figure 18 This patient is undergoing Botox injections for crow's feet (upper photograph) and for glabellar frown line (lower photograph). Injections for crow's feet are very superficial: just under the dermis. Injections for glabellar frown lines are performed by grasping the corrugator muscle and deeply infiltrating the muscle.

should be at the apex of this angle and the platysma should be well decussated in the midline from the mentum to the hyoid bone. Additionally, there should be a well-defined inferior border to the mandible, a distinct anterior sternocleidomastoid muscle border, a visible bulge of the thyroid cartilage, and a mild subhyoid depression. Of course, excessive fat blunts these angles and limits the degree to which anatomical borders appear distinct.

Pathophysiology

The body generates new fat cells through puberty. After puberty, the number of new fat cells formed greatly decreases. However, the fat cells present retain an ability to increase in size considerably through the deposition of additional fatty materials within their cell membranes. Isolated pockets of fat may become particularly noticeable when the fat cells increase in size. Experience has shown, however, that when the isolated pockets of fat are surgically removed in part, any future weight gain is distributed more evenly throughout the body. Therefore, a former problem area may not become as noticeable as it once was, despite the increase in weight.

Surgeons have thus striven to improve the cervicofacial appearance by resection of isolated fat pockets. Sharp surgical lipectomy was often performed at the time of rhytidectomy since wide and open exposure of the fatty deposits was necessary to achieve the desired results. Unfortunately, sharp surgical lipectomy is difficult to perform well. It is challenging to remove an even and appropriate amount of fat and leave the patient with smooth skin with subtle transitions. Furthermore, the procedure was beset with the risk of scarring and dimpling of the overlying skin (40). Fortunately, with the advent of closed techniques and suction lipectomy, more consistent and reliable results are attainable.

Liposuction

In 1983, Illouz reported on a 5 year experience with over 3000 cases of suction lipectomy (41). Liposuction can either be done open as during a rhytidectomy or closed in which only very small hidden incisions are made for access. In essence, the technique allows for a reduction of areas with excess fat by repeatedly passing a blunt-tipped cannula through the fat deposit. The cannula is connected to suction that allows for the mechanical removal of adipocytes. The matrix of bluntly dissected tunnels allows for an even removal of fat. Subsequent contraction of the tunnels permits the overlying skin to recontour in the treated areas. Liposuction provides many advantages over sharp lipectomy including more controlled and even removal of fat, decreased scarring, improved patient comfort, and lessened surgical risk.

Of course, liposuction is not a treatment for general obesity: it is most effective for isolated fat deposits. Typically, it is advisable for patients to maintain a stable weight for at least 6 months prior to the procedure. The neck is a particularly favorable area for liposuction because dramatic long-term improvements in skin laxity can occur (42). However, the techniques used in suction lipectomy have many additional applications. For example, liposuction facilitates the development of the subcutaneous flap during rhytidectomy and can be used in the treatment of benign lipomas, Madelung's disease, and human immunovirus (HIV) lipodystrophy. In addition, liposuction has been reported to improve the contour of both free and pedicled flaps (43–45).

Patient Selection

As with any surgical procedure, appropriate patient selection is important. Specifically, since closed liposuction depends upon contraction and recontouring of the overlying skin, patients with excessive skin redundancy or excessive loss of skin elasticity may be poor candidates. Of course, it has been noted "of all body sites the neck is, by far, the area where retractability after suction lipectomy is greatest" (42). The face, however, has poor retractability after liposuction. For example, liposuction of the buccal fat pads may lead to an unappealing cavernous facial appearance. Some success has been achieved with liposuction around the nasolabial folds, although the results have been inconsistent. The jowls and submental and submandibular regions fare well after liposuction. However, not all authors agree that the neck and jowls retain their ability to recontour. After 40 years of age, the skin may not contract satisfactorily and additional treatments (e.g., rhytidectomy or platysmal procedures) may be required (46).

In addition to assessing skin laxity, it is important to determine the degree to which other anatomical variables are contributing to the appearance of the neck. A low-lying hyoid bone, retrognathia, and platysmal banding will adversely affect the outcome of otherwise successful liposuction. A chin implant or advancement and platysmal plication are reasonable adjuncts in some patients. A low-lying hyoid cannot be reliably corrected and this should be pointed out to the patient. Any pre-existing scars, dimples, and imperfections of the skin should be likewise noted.

Equipment

The equipment necessary for liposuction is simple in concept. In addition to the basic instruments needed to make a small incision in the skin (scalpel blade, dissecting scissors), a liposuction cannula is needed with a source for suction.

Varieties of cannulae are available. They vary in length, shape, number, and location of holes. They may be disposable. Often, the most popular type is single-use disposable cannulae that eliminate the difficult cleaning and sterilization required for reusable cannulae of such small diameter. Regardless of the cannula selected, all should have a blunt tip for atraumatic tunneling and be smooth with a consistent diameter. Typical cannula length for neck liposuction is 25 cm with a diameter of 3–6 mm with a rounded or spatulated blunt tip. Larger liposuction cannulae allow more rapid removal of fat; however, the smaller cannulae for use in the cervicofacial area creates more tunneling and results in improved skin contraction and contour.

A variety of liposuction machines are available that provide a consistent and adjustable vacuum, an appropriate-sized collection jar, and thick-walled suction tubing that can withstand the negative pressures applied. Typically, cervicofacial liposuction is performed at around −700 mm HG suction pressure. However, suction up to −1 atm may be used. For smaller fat pockets or to obtain small volumes of fat for autologous fat injection, the suction provided by a 60 cc syringe is adequate.

Technique

One particular advantage for surgeons targeting the head and neck is that cervicofacial liposuction addresses fat deposits directly underneath the dermis (i.e., the superficial fat). This fat is in the supraplatysmal plane, well superficial to the facial nerve that lies in the subplatysmal plane. The liposuction cannula can be palpated with the thumb and index finger of the nondominant hand during liposuction, and cannula depth and fat removal can be easily noted. Therefore, intraoperative monitoring of the amount and consistency of fat removal is easier in the cervicofacial area than in other parts of the body (42).

Although not always necessary, for patients with prominent isolated fat collections preoperative marking may be a helpful reminder to the surgeon because the appearance of the neck may change once the patient is placed in a supine position. Marking, of course, should be done with the patient in a sitting or standing position. Appropriate surgical preparation is required as well.

Cervicofacial liposuction can be done under general anesthesia, with intravenous sedation, or with straight local anesthetic use. Infiltration of an anesthetic and vasoconstricting solution (e.g., 1% lidocaine with 1:100,000 epinephrine) via a long small-gauge needle is necessary. In addition to assisting with anesthesia and bleeding at the sites of incision, wide diffuse infiltration of the fatty deposits will help with bleeding and subsequent bruising, provide anesthesia, and permit a smoother removal of the fat. Some surgeons prefer to utilize techniques that have been proven helpful in body liposuction such as the infiltration of a high volume of a very dilute lidocaine solution (tumescent technique). For example, a large-bore blunt injector could place up to 500 ml of a solution of normal saline with 50 cc 1% lidocaine with 1:100,000 epinephrine (40). However, the usually limited volume of fat in the neck and the ease with which the progress and cannula position can be ascertained have obviated the need for these high-volume injections. The use of vibrating cannulae or the application of an external ultrasound device has been used with benefit in body liposuction but likewise is not necessary for cervicofacial indications.

Following injection and marking, an access incision is made. For neck liposuction, the incision can be made posterior to the lobule of the ear in the inferior aspect of the postauricular sulcus. Many surgeons prefer to use a small incision in the submental crease primarily and to use the postauricular incision only to refine the submandibular region. If the nasolabial fold is going to be targeted, a very well camouflaged incision can be made in the nasal vestibule. The incision need only be slightly larger than the diameter of the cannula. The incision in this so-called closed liposuction technique serves only to allow the cannula to enter the subcutaneous space and to be moved without excessive friction (Fig. 19). After the incision is made, a minimal amount of dissection with a scissors may be helpful to allow for easier insertion of the cannula. Following this, several passes are made with the cannula to create tunnels. This is done without suction as it permits the surgeon to familiarize him or herself with the depth and path of the cannula and to create preformed tunnels for easier cannula movement and fat evacuation.

In general, tunnels should stay anterior to the anterior border of the sternocleidomastoid muscle and posterior to the thyroid cartilage of the larynx. Superiorly, one should use liposuction on the jowls along the mandible to create a more defined mandibular border. However, caution must be exercised because excessive fat removal in this area can overly define the mandibular border and masculinize the neck. This is of particular concern when the patient is to undergo a simultaneous rhytidectomy in which the skin and SMAS draping will further define these structures.

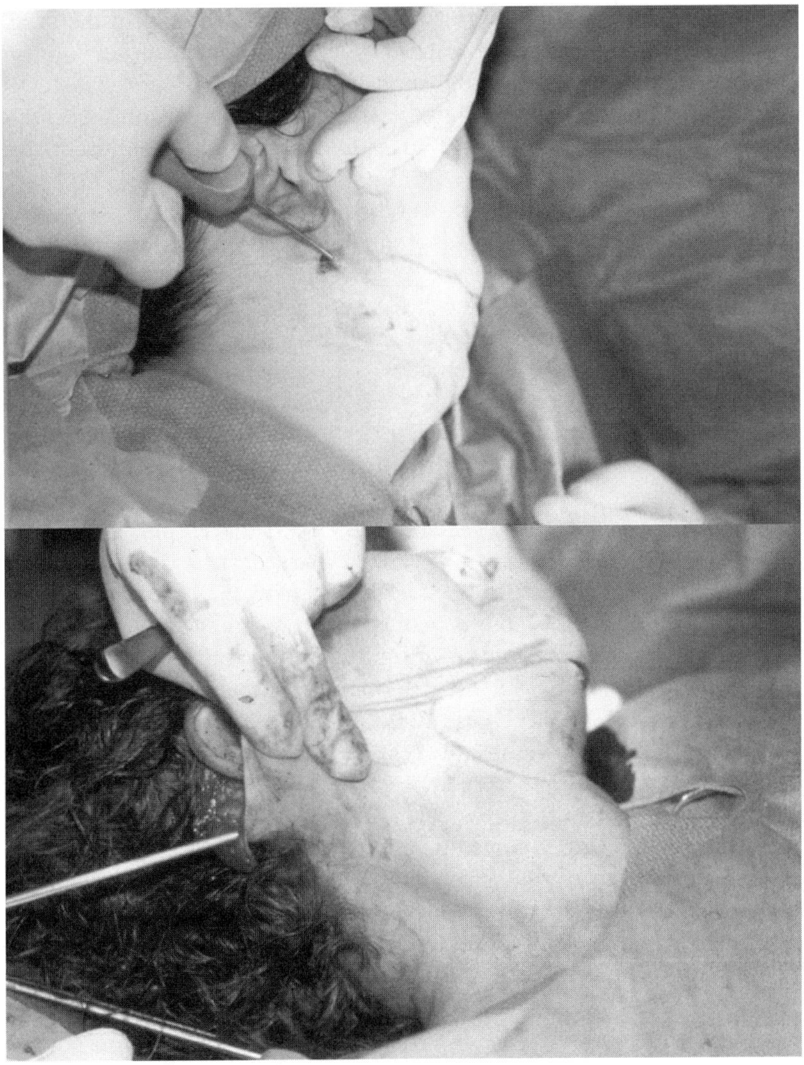

Figure 19 Liposuction via a closed technique as depicted in the upper photograph and via an open technique in the lower photograph. Although the instrumentation is similar, the closed technique is performed through a small access incision, usually near the lobule. An open technique is often performed during rhytidectomy under a widely undermined subcutaneous flap.

Passes with the cannula radiate from the incision site and the nondominant hand of the surgeon can be used to palpate the cannula beneath the skin. This allows the surgeon to know the precise location of the cannula as well as its depth from the skin surface. It is important to pay careful attention to cannula depth to ensure that a consistently thick layer of subcutaneous fat remains on the deep surface of the overlying dermis. This fat layer will prevent dimpling and scarring of the overlying skin to the platysma muscle.

After pretunneling has been done, the suction tubing is attached to the cannula and the suction is turned on. It is important to be certain that the openings to the lumen of the cannula remain oriented away from the skin during suction lipectomy. If the overlying skin were to be pulled into the suction, scarring, dimpling, and lesions could occur. In addition, an excessive amount of fat would be removed from the undersurface of the dermis.

As liposuction continues, it is important to assess regularly the amount of fat removed. This is done by palpating and pinching the skin on the neck. As fat pockets are reduced, the borders of the fat pockets should undergo liposuction to a lesser degree to allow for a smooth feathering from one area to another and more consistent redraping of the overlying skin. As mentioned, frequent assessment is necessary. Once it has been determined that an area needs additional attention, be certain not to turn the suction on until the cannula tip is in the offending fat. This will help to prevent overresection of fat elsewhere as well as injury to the underlying muscle. In some cases, areas of skin dimpling caused by fibrous fatty deposits will present themselves as the liposuction progresses. These areas can be addressed sharply or with repeated passes with the cannula.

Liposuction is a helpful adjunct to rhytidectomy. After a small amount of the flap has been raised, the liposuction cannula can be passed as in the closed technique into the neck. Fat removal can proceed as described but pretunneling can also be done inferior to the zygoma and over the cheek to the nasolabial fold. Elevation of uniform rhytidectomy flaps is greatly facilitated by the tunneling of liposuction, particularly in the neck. In typical cases, only relatively widely spaced fibrous septae remain to be divided. A spatula-shaped suction cannula can also be placed opening down directly onto the preparotid fat for sculpting.

The goal of liposuction is to remove fat so that the overlying tissues can recontour to the underlying structures and provide a more youthful defined neck. It is imperative that the overlying tissues heal smoothly. Therefore, at the completion of the procedure a light pressure dressing is applied around the neck. Several liposuction and rhytidectomy bandages are commercially available or an elastic bandage can be used. The patient is instructed to wear this dressing continuously for 1 week and then at night for an additional 1–2 weeks. The dressing improves contour, reduces edema, and helps reduce the chance of hematoma formation. Several authors stress that improvement in cervicofacial contour and appearance can be expected for up to a year postoperatively and may not be seen as rapidly as with body liposuction (40,42). In fact, the area can be hard, lumpy, edematous, or infiltrated for several months.

Complications

Complications are rare with cervicofacial liposuction as the overall volume reduction is quite low compared to body liposuction (after which shock, blood loss, fluid shifts, and deep venous thrombosis are all risks). Hematomas and seromas are the most common, although they still occur only rarely. These can be addressed with drainage, rolling, and a light pressure dressing. Poor results are often due to patient selection (e.g., patients with excessive skin laxity or low-lying hyoid bone), although inexperience can contribute to nonsymmetrical liposuction or irregularities. Scarring and facial nerve injury (usually temporary) are infrequently encountered. Small areas of fat persistence can be treated with office liposuction using a small cannula and a syringe or with periodic steroid injections.

REFERENCES

1. Lober CW, Fenske NA. Cutaneous aging: effect of intrinsic changes on surgical considerations. South Med J 1991; 84:1444–1446.
2. Uitto J. Connective tissue biochemistry of the aging dermis. Age-associated alterations in collagen and elastin. Clin Geriatr Med 1989; 5:127–147.
3. Smith L. Histopathologic characteristics and ultrastructure of aging skin. Cutis 1989; 43:414–424.
4. Kligman LH. Photoaging Manifestations, prevention, and treatment. Clin Geriatr Med 1989; 5:235–251.
5. Beighton P, Bull JC. Plastic surgery in the Ehlers-Danlos syndrome. Case report. Plast Reconstr Surg 1970; 45:606–609.
6. Beighton P, Bull JC, Edgerton MT. Plastic surgery in cutis laxa. Br J Plast Surg 1970; 23:285–290.
7. Ng AB, O'Sullivan ST, Sharpe DT. Plastic surgery and pseudoxanthoma elasticum. Br J Plast Surg 1999; 52:594–596.
8. Duvik M, Lenak NA. Werner's syndrome. Dermatol Clin 1995; 13:163.
9. Mitz V, Peyronie M. The superficial musculo-aponeurotic system (SMAS) in the parotid and cheek area. Plast Reconstr Surg 1976; 58:80–88.
10. Stuzin JM, Wagstrom L, Kawamoto HK, Wolfe SA. Anatomy of the frontal branch of the facial nerve: the significance of the temporal fat pad. Plast Reconstr Surg 1989; 83:265–271.
11. Baker DC, Conley J. Avoiding facial nerve injuries in rhytidectomy. Anatomical variations and pitfalls. Plast Reconstr Surg 1979; 64:781–795.
12. Dingman R, Grabb W. Surgical anatomy of the marginal ramus of the facial nerve based on the dissection of 100 facial halves. Plast Reconstr Surg 1962; 29:266.
13. Furnas DW. The retaining ligaments of the cheek. Plast Reconstr Surg 1989; 83:11–16.
14. Skoog T. Plastic Surgery—New Methods and Refinements. Philadelphia: WB Saunders, 1974.
15. Baker DC. Deep dissection rhytidectomy: a plea for caution. Plast Reconstr Surg 1994; 93:1498–1499.
16. Ivy EJ, Lorenc ZP, Aston SJ. Is there a difference? A prospective study comparing lateral and standard SMAS face lifts with extended SMAS and composite rhytidectomies. Plast Reconstr Surg 1996; 98:1135–1143.
17. Hamra ST. The deep-plane rhytidectomy. Plast Reconstr Surg 1990; 86:53–61.
18. Kamer FM. One hundred consecutive deep plane face-lifts. Arch Otolaryngol Head Neck Surg 1996; 122:17–22.
19. Hamra ST. The zygorbicular dissection in composite rhytidectomy: an ideal midface plane. Plast Reconstr Surg 1998; 102:1646–1657.
20. Baker SR. Triplane rhytidectomy. Combining the best of all worlds. . Arch Otolaryngol Head Neck Surg 1997; 123:1167–1172.
21. de Castro CC. The anatomy of the platysma muscle. Plast Reconstr Surg 1980; 66:680–683.
22. McDowell AJ. Effective practical steps to avoid complications in face-lifting. Review of 105 consecutive cases. Plast Reconstr Surg 1972; 50:563–572.
23. Rees TD, Aston SJ. Complications of rhytidectomy. Clin Plast Surg 1978; 5:109–119.
24. Baker DC. Complications of cervicofacial rhytidectomy. Clin Plast Surg 1983; 10:543–562.

25. Rees TD, Liverett DM, Guy CL. The effect of cigarette smoking on skin-flap survival in the face lift patient. Plast Reconstr Surg 1984; 73:911–915.
26. Knize DM. Muscles that act on glabellar skin: a closer look. Plast Reconstr Surg 2000; 105:350–361.
27. Ellenbogen R.. Transcoronal eyebrow lift with concomitant upper blepharoplasty. Plast Reconstr Surg 1983; 71:490–499.
28. McKinney P, Mossie RD, Zukowski ML. Criteria for the forehead lift. Aesthetic Plast Surg 1991; 15:141–147.
29. Ortiz-Monasterio F, Barrera G, Olmedo A. The coronal incision in rhytidectomy—the brow lift. Clin Plast Surg 1978; 5:167–179.
30. Connell BF, Marten TJ. The male foreheadplasty. Recognizing and treating aging in the upper face. Clin Plast Surg 1991; 18:653–687.
31. de la PR, de la CLCan some facial rejuvenation techniques cause iatrogenia? Aesthetic Plast Surg 1994; 18:205–209.
32. Ramirez OM. Endoscopic subperiosteal browlift and facelift. Clin Plast Surg 1995; 22:639–660.
33. Alderson K, Holds JB, Anderson RL. Botulinum-induced alteration of nerve-muscle interactions in the human orbicularis oculi following treatment for blepharospasm. Neurology 1991; 41:1800–1805.
34. Coffield JA, Bakry N, Zhang RD, Carlson J, Gomella LG, Simpson LL. In vitro characterization of botulinum toxin types A, C and D action on human tissues: combined electrophysiologic, pharmacologic and molecular biologic approaches. J Pharmacol Exp Ther 1997; 280:1489–1498.
35. Blasi J, Chapman ER, Link E, Binz T, Yamasaki S, De Camilli P et al. Botulinum neurotoxin A selectively cleaves the synaptic protein SNAP-25. Nature 1993; 365:160–163.
36. de Paiva A, Meunier FA, Molgo J, Aoki KR, Dolly JO. Functional repair of motor endplates after botulinum neurotoxin type A poisoning: biphasic switch of synaptic activity between nerve sprouts and their parent terminals. Proc Natl Acad Sci USA 1999; 96:3200–3205.
37. Moreno A, Bell WH, You ZH. Esthetic contour analysis of the submental cervical region: a study based on ideal subjects and surgical patients. J Oral Maxillofac Surg 1994; 52:704–713.
38. Ellenbogen R, Karlin JV. Visual criteria for success in restoring the youthful neck. Plast Reconstr Surg 1980; 66:826–837.
39. Vistnes LM, Souther SG. The anatomical basis for common cosmetic anterior neck deformities. Ann Plast Surg 1979; 2:381–388.
40. Adamson PA, Cormier R, Tropper GJ, McGraw BL. Cervicofacial liposuction: results and controversies. J Otolaryngol 1990; 19:267–273.
41. Illouz YG. Body contouring by lipolysis: a 5-year experience with over 3000 cases. Plast Reconstr Surg 1983; 72:591–597.
42. Goddio AS. Suction lipectomy: the gold triangle at the neck. Aesthetic Plast Surg 1992; 16:27–32.
43. Coleman WP, III.. Noncosmetic applications of liposuction. J Dermatol Surg Oncol 1988; 14:1085–1890.
44. Field LM. Adjunctive liposurgical debulking and flap dissection in neck reconstruction. J Dermatol Surg Oncol 1986; 12:917–920.
45. Hallock GG. Liposuction for debulking free flaps. J Reconstr Microsurg 1986; 2:235–239.
46. Dedo DD. Management of the platysma muscle after open and closed liposuction of the neck in facelift surgery. Facial Plast Surg 1986; 4:45–56.

Index

Cash-in on Collecting

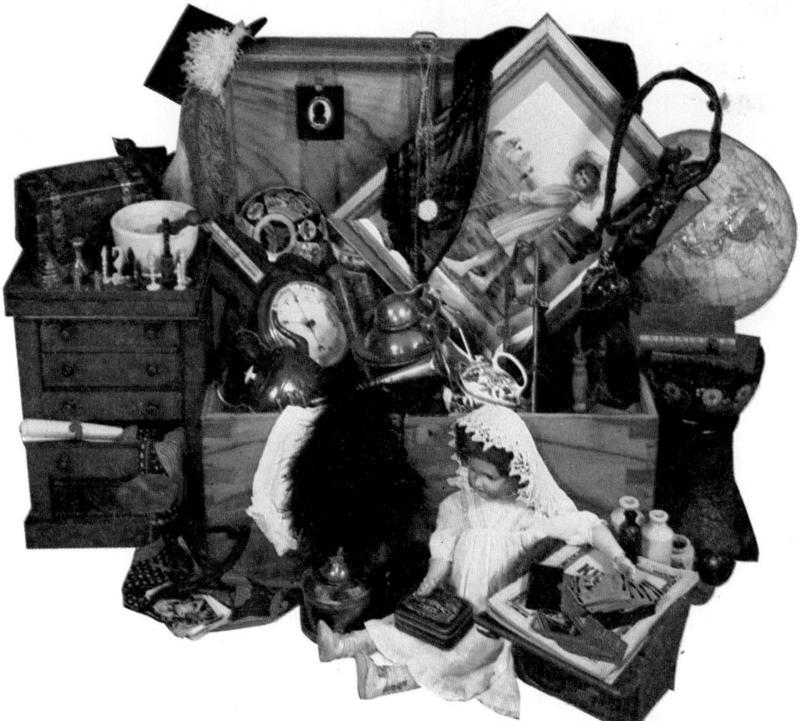

While every care has been taken in the compiling of information contained in this volume the publishers cannot accept any liability for loss, financial or otherwise, incurred by reliance placed on the information herein.

The publishers wish to express their sincere thanks to the following for their involvement and assistance in the production of this volume:–

TEXT BY LIZ TAYLOR AND ANNETTE CURTIS
EDITED BY TONY CURTIS

JANICE MONCRIEFF
KAREN DOUGLASS
NICHOLA FAIRBURN
TANYA FAIRBAIRN
SALLY DALGLIESH
FRANK BURRELL
ROBERT NISBET
EILEEN BURRELL
MARGARET ANDERSON
SHELLEY CURTIS
DAVID BOLAND

Additional photographs by

KEVIN COLE
J. HAYCOCK
JACK HICKES
GORDON LOCKIE
ALAN McEWEN
DAVID MARCHANT
BRIAN THATCHER

British Library Cataloguing in Publication Data

Cash in on collecting.
1. Antiques – Purchasing 2. Selling – Antiques
I. Curtis, Tony, 1939-
745.1 NK1125

ISBN 0-86248-055-8

Printed by Hazell Watson & Viney Limited, Aylesbury, Bucks.
Bound by Dorstel Press Limited, Harlow, Essex.

INTRODUCTION

Collecting is a passion that can become a way of life. The lure of the chase, the search for the elusive treasure, the fascination of knowing almost, but not quite, everything about some out-of-the-ordinary subject are what makes a collector's adrenalin surge.

Collectors thrive most of all on the teasing certainty that fortunes can be made out of their hobbies and that around the next corner they could find the one thing that will make their collection complete and unique.

This book contains the stories of many fascinating and successful collectors. They are men and women of all ages and from all walks of life who have been bitten by the collecting bug. Their specialities range from old bank notes to cigarette lighters, from dolls to picture postcards.

From their own experience they give first hand tips on collecting including how to start, where to go and, most interesting of all for the would be collector, what to start specialising in now so that your hobby can be turned into money.

The astute collector picks an area of the market that is unexploited and develops it. Two young men who tell their collecting story in the book introduced the words 'street jewellery' to the Oxford English Dictionary because that was what they called the enamel signs, manhole covers and street direction boards which they began to collect only a few years ago. Street jewellery is now a large and thriving area for other collectors.

Everything and anything can be collected from 18th century prints to today's throwaway beer cans. In this book you learn how to build up your collection and also how to add an unexpected pleasure to your life for collecting can not only be a cure for boredom and the blues but it carries with it the very real possibility of turning a modest outlay of money into a considerable nest egg.

The sky is the limit for the successful collector. Read how it can be done.

Tony Curtis

ACKNOWLEDGEMENTS

Michael Akeroyd – Motoring Signs
Ian Allen – Nursey Rhyme Collectibles
Margaret Anderson – Fairings
Brenda & Bob Beecroft – Brewery Badges
Alan Blakeman – British Bottle Review
Christine Blackmore – Eye Baths
Duncan Bray – Banknotes
John Brooks – Youth Hostel Memorabilia
Peter Brooks – Cigarette Lighters
Patricia Cockrell – Royal Memorabilia
Peter F. Cook – Cheese Labels
David Cope – Doulton Figures
Harry Cope – Red Cross Postal Covers
Alan Cunningham – Football Memorabilia
Shelley Curtis – Dolls & Toys
Trevor Edwards – Pencils
Lembit Eha – Dolls
David Ellison – Cream Pots
Ken Everett – Smoothing Irons
Jock Farquharson – Car Mascots
Clifford Frewin – Shaving Cream Pot Lids
David Fulton – Disney Films
John 'Paddy' Furniss – Golfing Books
Michael Gosling – Baden Powell Memorabilia
Gerald & Joan Gurney – Racketana
Melvin Hatcher – Advertising Memorabilia
Peter Haworth – Shaving Mugs
Jane Henery & Charles Garvie – An Ad Man In Your Larder
Rosemary Hill – Cookery Books
Tonie & Valmai Holt – Bairnsfather Ware
Jones Family – Mechanical Music & Dolls
Margaret Jones – Oriental Pottery & Porcelain
Michael Jones – Beer Bottle Labels
Graham Keene – Rubber Tyre Ashtrays
Trevor King – Anchovy Pot Lids
Michael Knight – Match Strikers
Ruth Lambert – Gramophone Needle Boxes
Bert Latham – Reform Flasks
Jenny Lees – Elephant Items
Danny Loftus – Woodworking Tools
Ronald Lucibell – Ceramic Inhalers
John Luker – Match Boxes
Alan McEwen – 'Quack' Medicine Bottles
Roger & Pauline Martin – Soda Syphons
Jamie Maxtone-Graham – Piscatorial Items
Richard May – Crown Cork Bottle Openers
Janice Moncrieff – Trade Catalogues
Somerset Moore – Sardine Boxes
Nigel Morter – Jaguar Model Cars
Christopher & Marion Nunn – Rural Memorabilia
Keith Osborne – Beer Bottle Labels
Joyce Palmer – Gladys Cooper Postcards
Neville Peakall – Postcards of Lighthouses
Lynda Pine – Goss China
Nicholas J. Pine – Goss Cottages
Geoff & Linda Price – Model Buses & Trams
John Roberts – Masonic Items
Alan Roman – Shell Memorabilia
Paul Sheppard – Postcards
Jonathan Sneath – Horse Brasses
Mark Stafford-Lovatt – Auctioneering Items
Street Jewellery (Christopher Baglee & Andrew Morley) – Enamel Signs
Brian Swann – Car Club Badges
Merlyn Tancock – Miner's Lamps
Liz Taylor – Books About The British in India
Brian Thatcher – Poison Bottles
Ken Tomlinson – Cigarette Paper Packets
Ray & Iris Tunnicliff – Fairground Memorabilia
Brian Wain – Veterinary Items
Raymond Walls – Petrol Pump Globes
Simon Warden – Advertising Inserts
Bob Warner – Wirelesses
Ruth Warner – Perfume Bottles
Nick Waters – Ink Bottles
Dr. Bernard Watney – Guinness Stout Bottles
Neil Wayne – Razors
Geoffrey Wellsteed – Cricketing Pubs
Fred Wheatcroft – Beer Mugs
Michael Whitbread – Ginger Beer Bottles
Denis Wilkins – Cigarette Lighters & Holders
Keith Wilson – Breweriana
Ian Wright – Railwayana
Bleddyn Wynn-Jones – Mineral Water Bottles
Dennis Yates – Wireless Equipment
Mick Yewman – Doulton Character Jugs
Dr. Anne Young – Medical Items

If you wish to contact any of the collectors please write to them c/o Lyle Publications, Glenmayne, Galashiels, TD1 3NR, and we will undertake to foreward the letters on.

CONTENTS

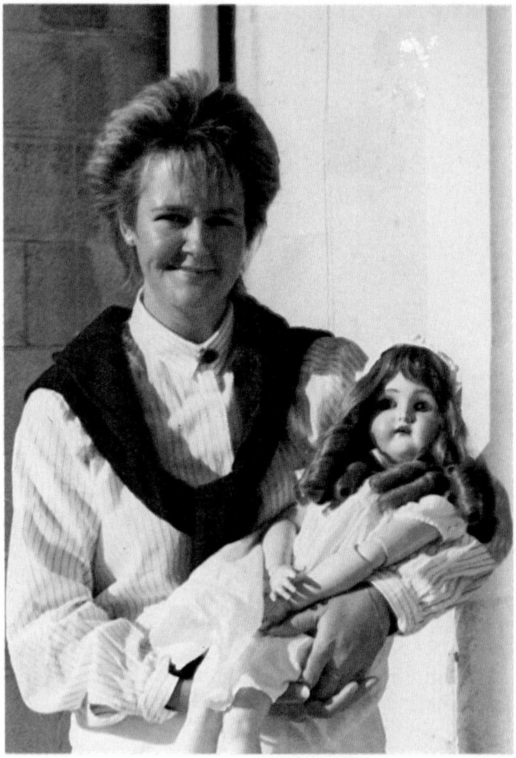

Shelley Curtis is a graduate of Edinburgh University and she collects dolls and toys.

"I began collecting when I was young, probably because from an early age I was surrounded by antiques and, being a little girl, it was the dolls and toys that interested me most of all.

"My collection is not restricted solely to antique toys although it has to be said that apart from having a greater appeal they do represent an excellent investment potential, with some actually doubling or tripling in value since I bought them. For example the few bears I managed to collect before they started rising in price are much cherished and now quite valuable and the very old ones are like gold-dust to find.

"It's odd to think that from about the 17th to early 19th century ownership of fine dolls was generally the exclusive privilege of the fashionable ladies and children just didn't get a look-in.

"Recent trends show that it is well worth looking at modern toys and dolls and I have a few which I consider to be quite speculative. In particular an American cloth doll which a friend brought from New York. This is an adult doll, very glam' with bright red hair and wearing roller skates and half a ton of sequins. She cost around $100 from a specialist 5th Avenue store who are no longer trading and I think it is going to prove to be a good investment. I discovered early on that dolls and toys still in their original packaging are worth more and I have kept almost every toy and game I've ever had together with their boxes. There are toys being produced today which will be of interest and value to collectors in the future; like the Cabbage Patch dolls and the new and originally designed handicapped dolls. I am only twenty four now and yet some of the toys I enjoyed playing with as a child are already of interest to collectors so the message is, providing you can commandeer a large cupboard space, everything is worth consideration!"

The doll Shelley would most like to own is an autoperipatetic doll — which simply means walking around and talking — "especially an old Victorian one by Simon & Halbig or a Bebe Bru because they have such delightful faces but, we are talking about thousands of pounds for one of these".

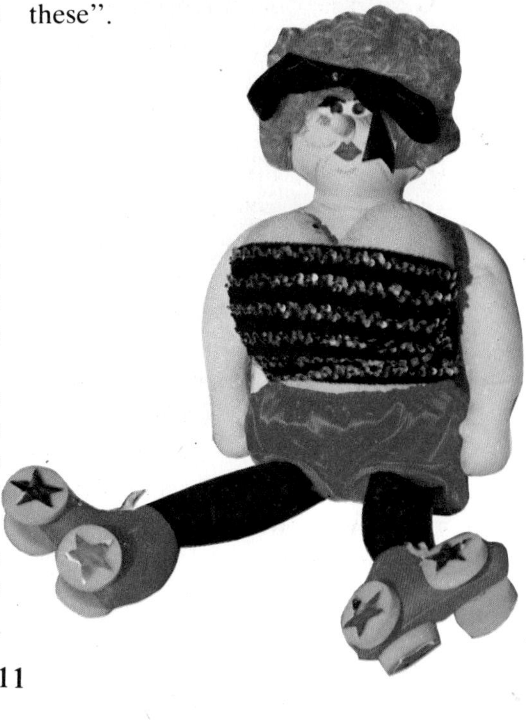

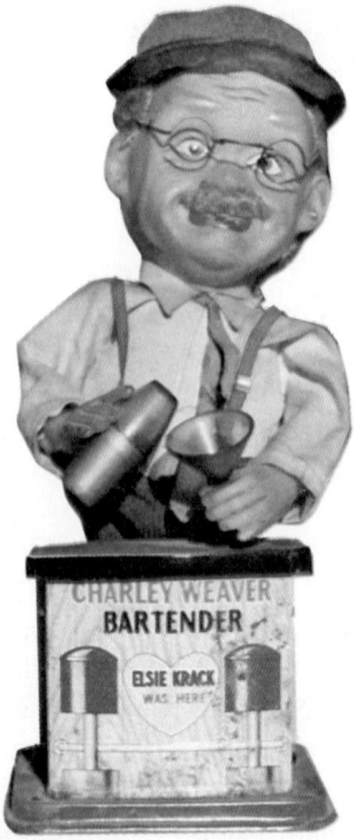

Charley Weaver the Bartender, an early battery operated, all metal, automaton toy, 12in. high. £80

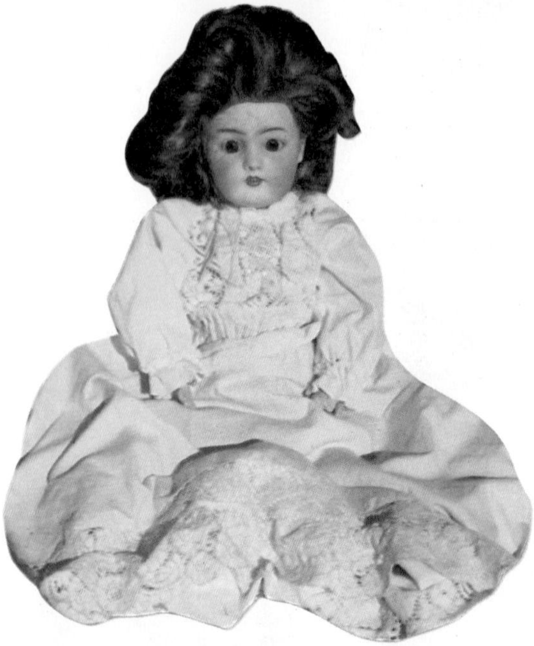

A small German doll by Simon & Halbig, with porcelain head and hands, 15½in. high. £175

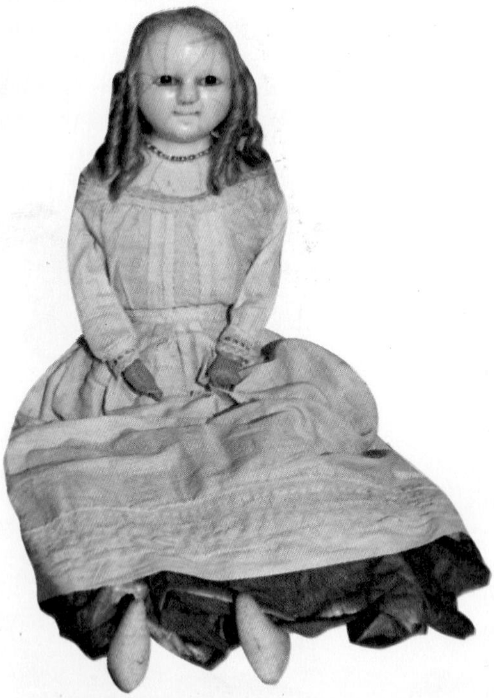

Late 19th century, wax head and shoulder doll with kid body and eye mechanism at the waist, original clothes, 24in. high. £150

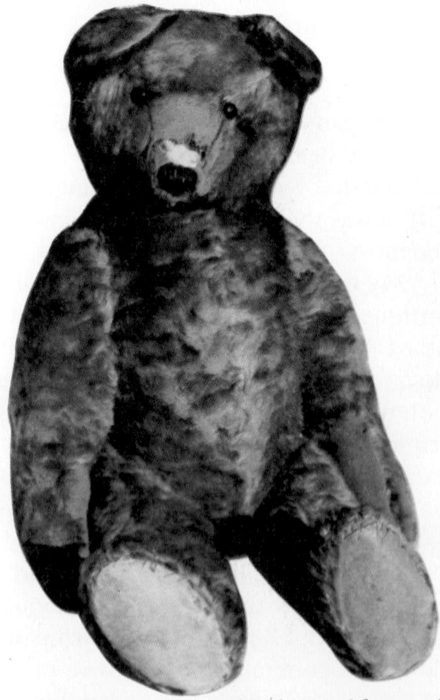

An early 19th century teddy bear with round ears, button eyes, pronounced hump and long paws, complete with growl, 28in. high, well loved. £300

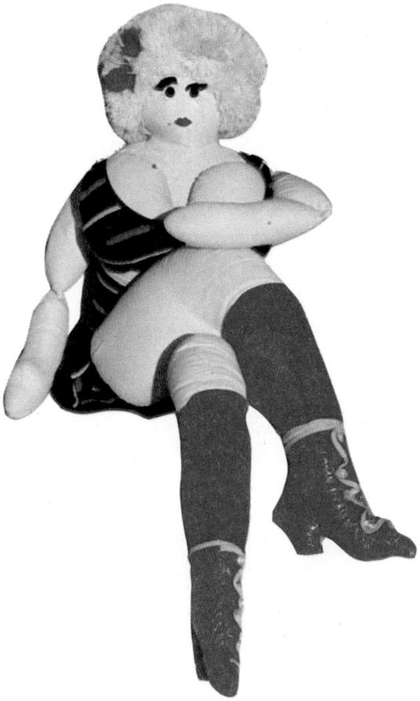

Late 1970's, American limited edition, glamour doll, 35in. high. £100

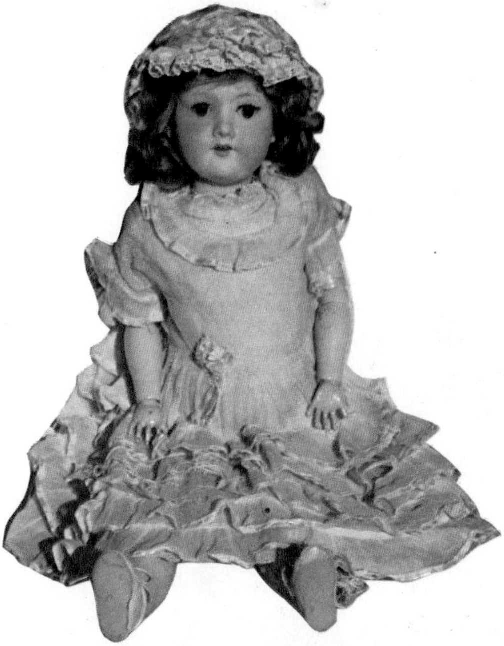

A pretty German doll by Armand Marseille with original clothes and hair, 21in. high. £200

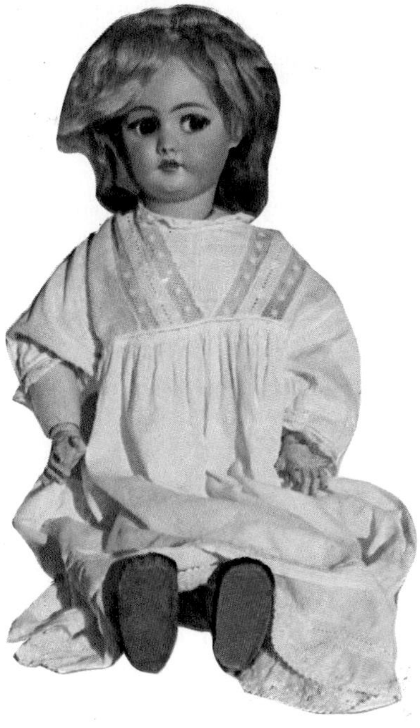

An interesting German doll by Simon & Halbig, 20in. high. £275

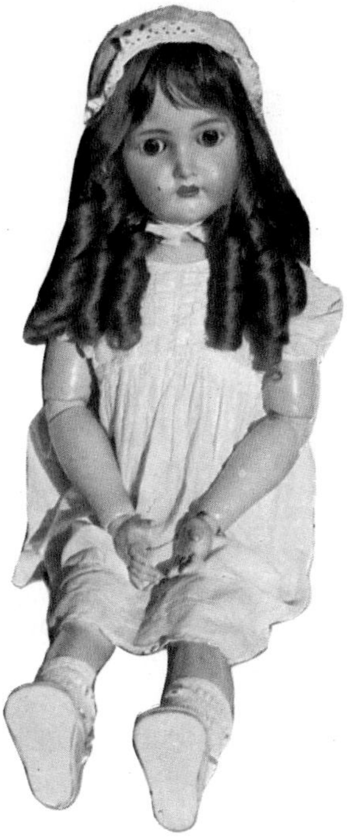

Late 19th century German doll by Simon & Halbig, 26in. high. £225

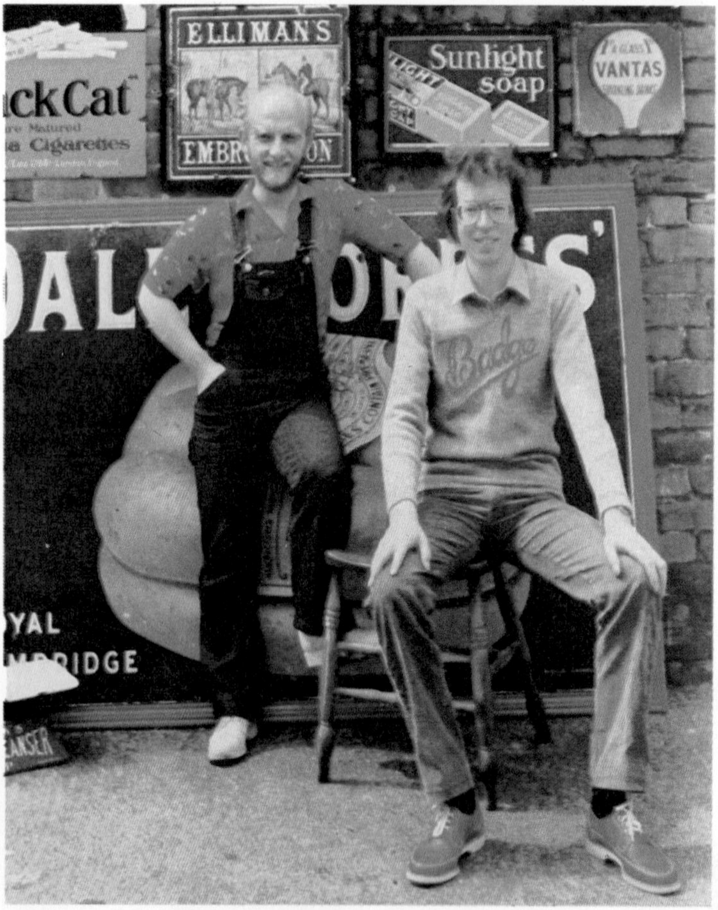

Christopher Baglee and Andrew Morley are writers and leading collectors who have established enamel advertising signs as a highly desirable form of specialist collecting. Their comprehensive collection of 'Street Jewellery' is on permanent display in the Linden Pub in the grounds of Linden Hall Hotel, Longhorsley, Northumberland.

Andrew said: "We coined the term 'Street Jewellery" and it's a pleasure to see that it's recently been included in the Oxford English Dictionary Supplement as a recognised description for enamelled advertising signs. We first used the term in our books about signs — 'Street Jewellery' and 'More Street Jewellery' which we wrote in the late '70's and early '80's.

"Christopher and I started collecting independently of each other in the 1960's but we joined forces in 1975 and since then interest in enamelled signs has simply exploded.

"In 1977 we were asked to mount an exhibition in Newcastle on Tyne of 150 of our best signs and it was an instant success for it later toured the country, visiting 18 other cities. The catalogue for the exhibition formed the basis of our first book which went into various European and USA editions. In 1983 we founded the Street Jewellery Society which now has over 100 members."

Christopher is a graphic designer and his special interest is enamel finger plates which were found as push plates on shop doors and advertised a wide range of products from Shell petrol to Colman's Mustard. Andrew likes and is always looking for the more illustrative enamel signs — "the more detailed the better."

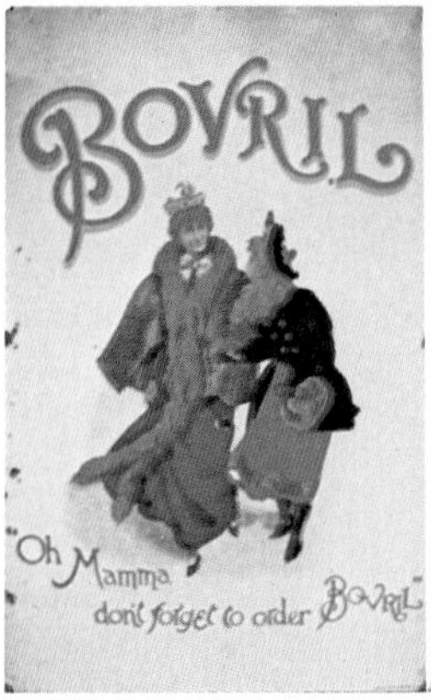

Bovril, 'Oh Mama don't forget to order Bovril'. £400

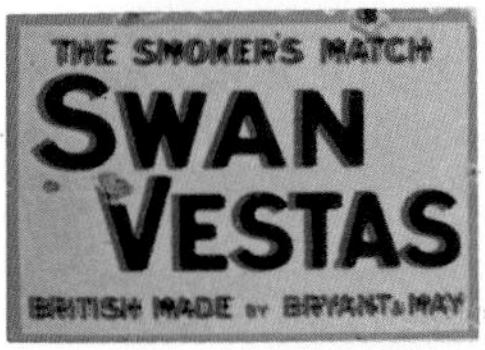

The Smoker's Match, Swan Vestas. £40

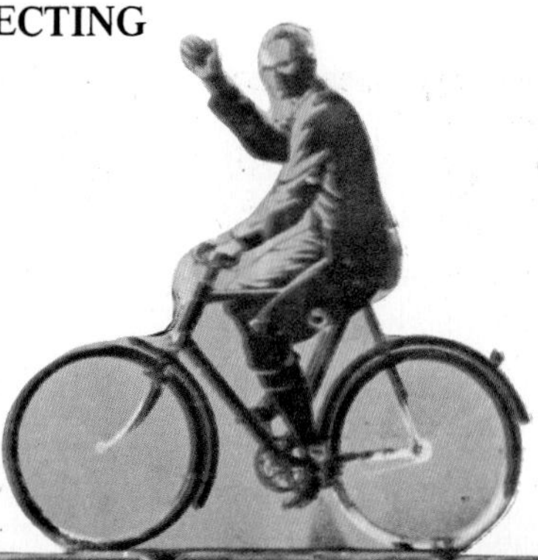
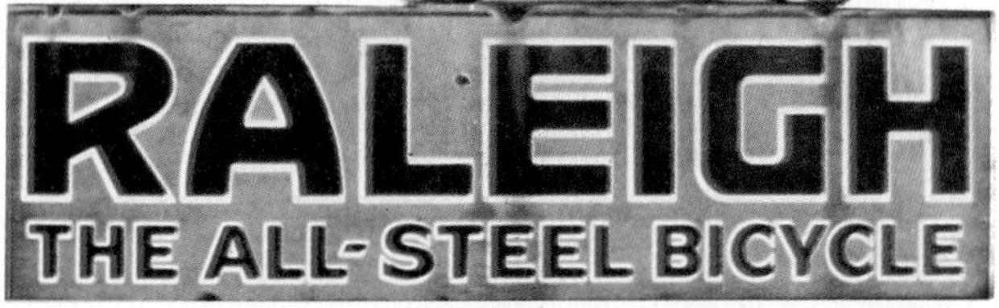

Raleigh, The All-Steel Bicycle. £120

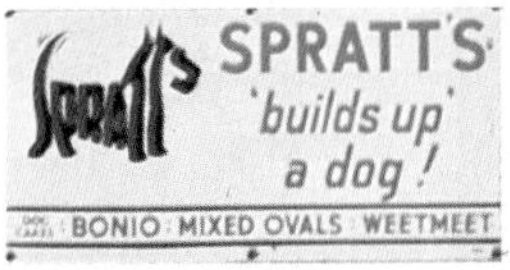

Spratt's 'builds up' a dog! £45

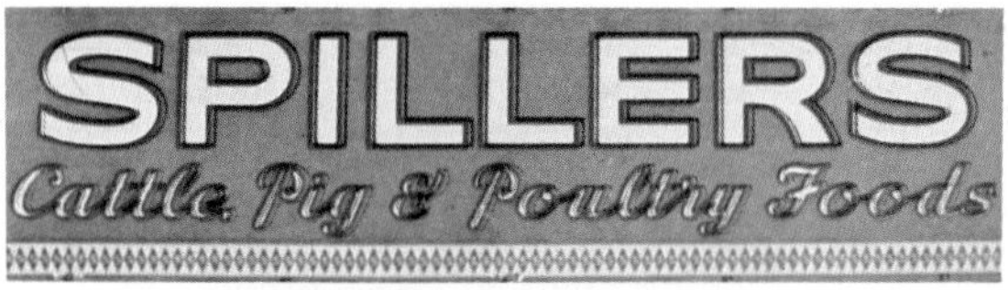

Spillers Cattle, Pig & Poultry Foods. £40

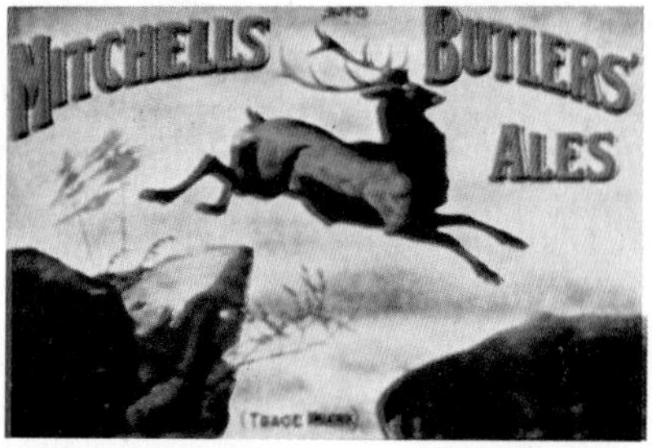

'Mitchells And Butlers' Ales. £200

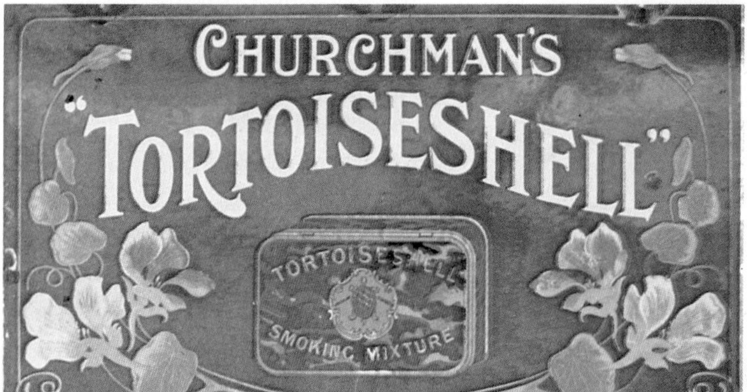

Churchman's 'Tortoiseshell' Smoking Mixture. £175

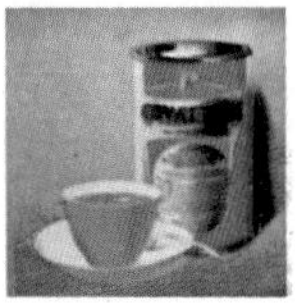

Ovaltine. £80

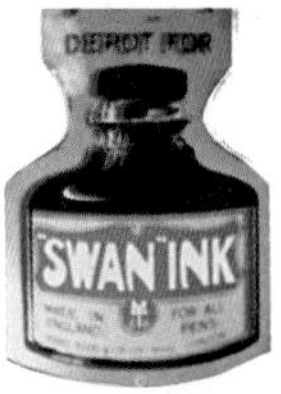

Depot for 'Swan' Ink. £85

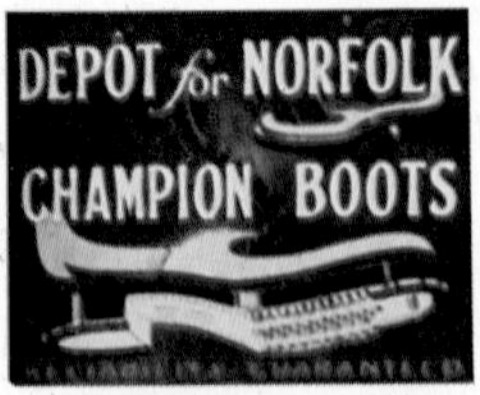

Depot for Norfolk Champion Boots. £75

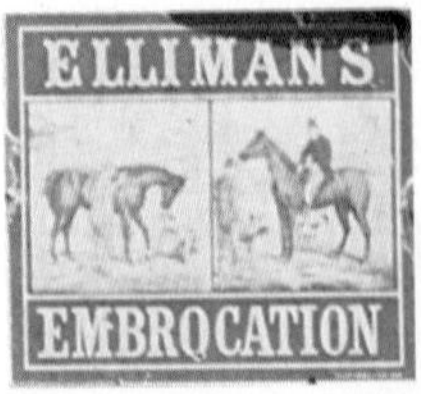

Elliman's Embrocation. £250

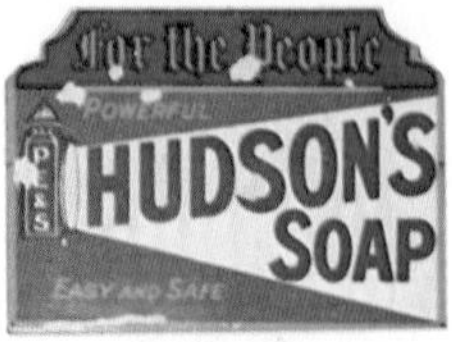

For the People, 'Hudson's Soap'. £50

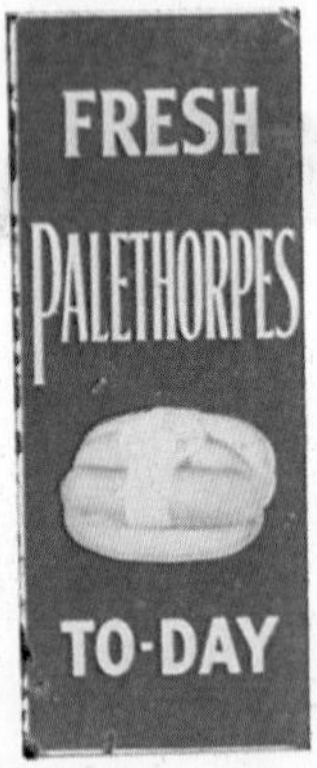

Fresh Palethorpes Today. £60

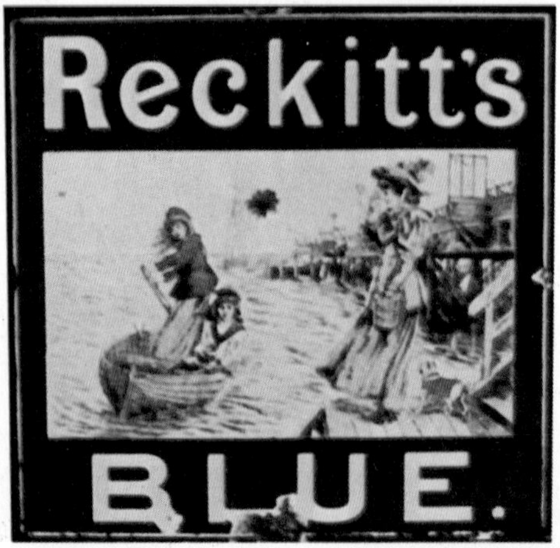

Reckitt's Blue. £300

Wills's Star Cigarettes. £80

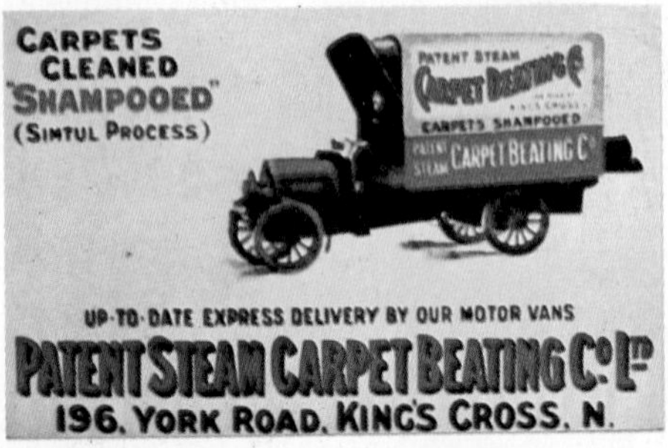

Patent Steam Carpet Beating Co Ltd. £250

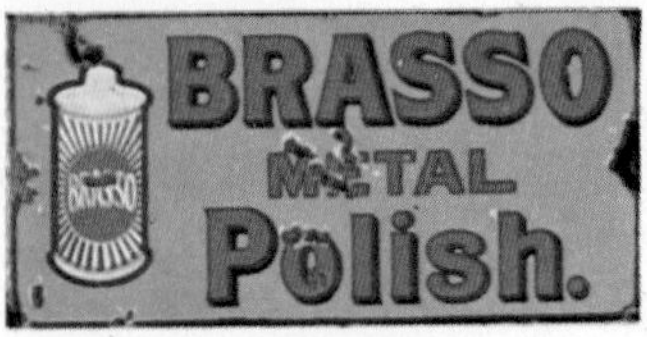

Brasso Metal Polish. £50

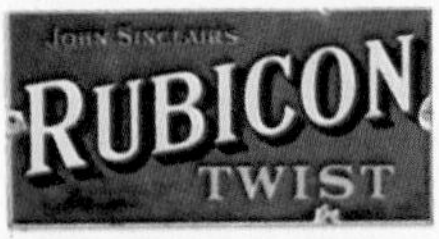

John Sinclair's Rubicon Twist. £40

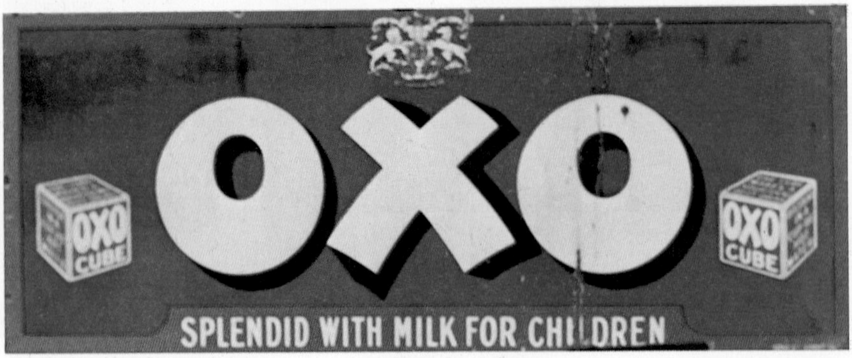

Oxo, Splendid With Milk For Children. £50

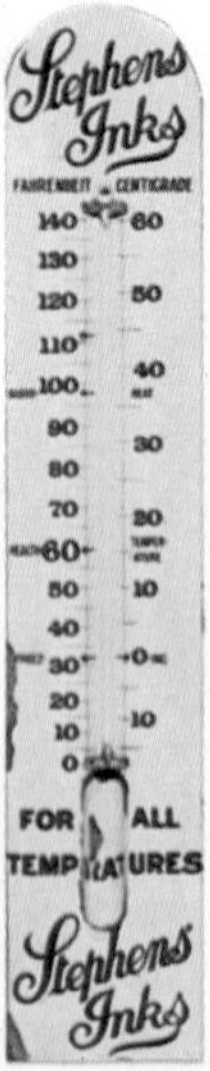

Stephens Inks, For All Temperatures. £85

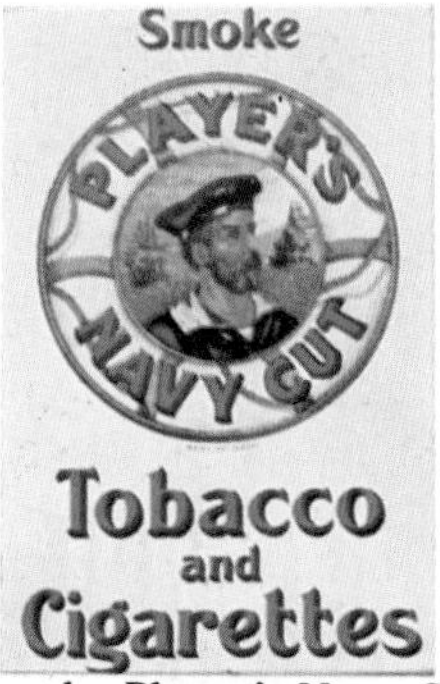

Smoke Player's Navy Cut, Tobacco and Cigarettes. £75

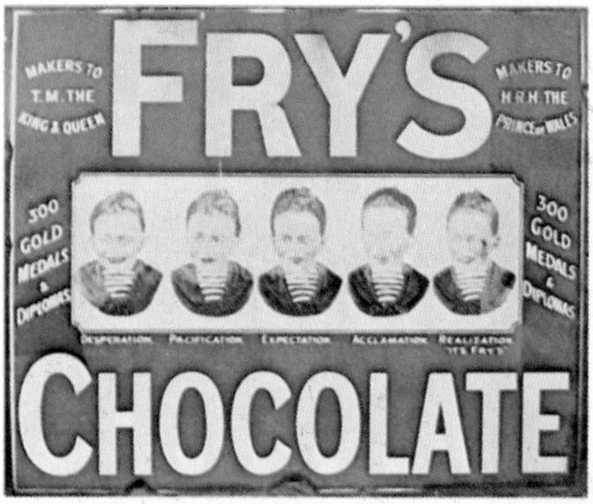

Fry's Chocolate - Five Boys. £200

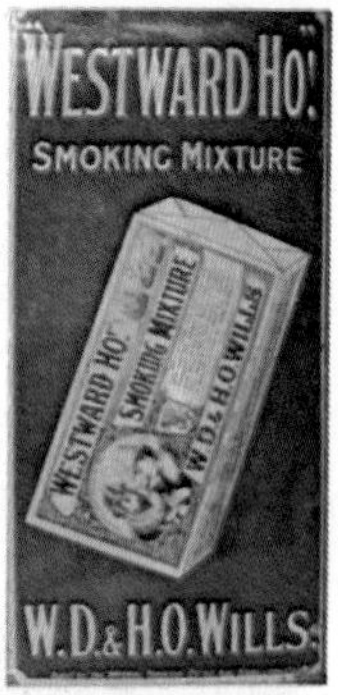

'Westward Ho!' Smoking Mixture. £75

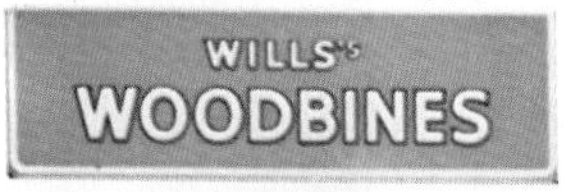

Wills's Woodbines. £30

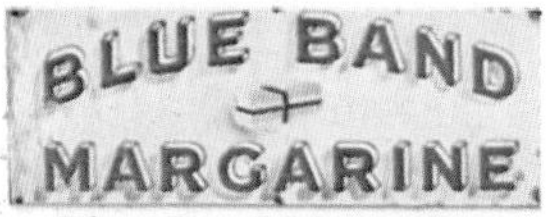

Blue Band Margarine. £45

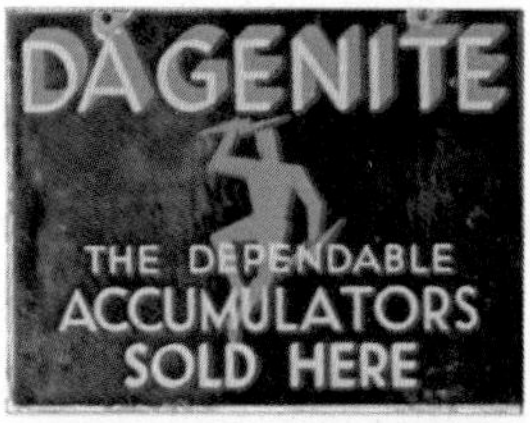

Dagenite, The Dependable Accumulators Sold Here. £40

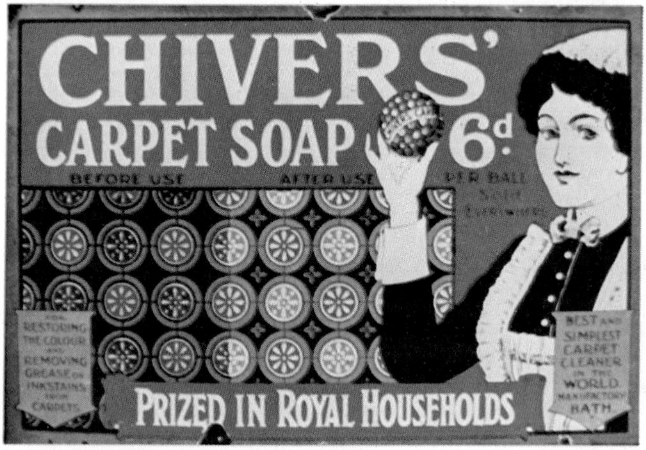

Chivers' Carpet Soap, Prized In Royal Households. £200

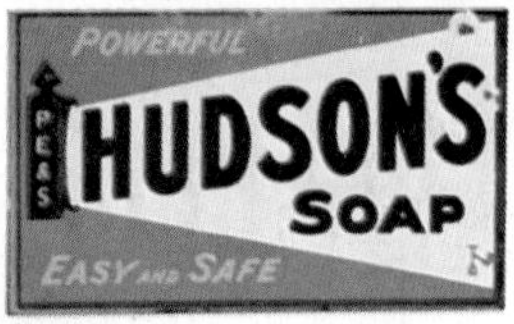

Hudson's Soap, Powerful Easy And Safe. £50

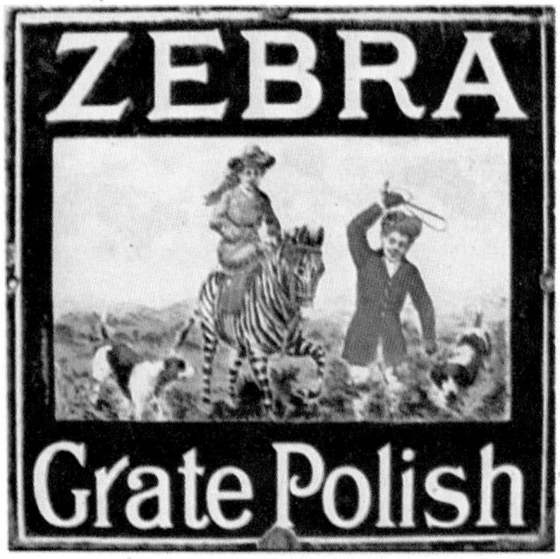

Zebra Grate Polish. £300

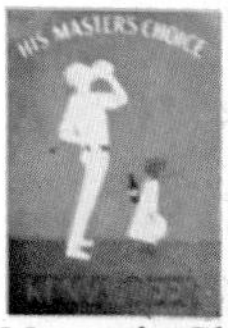

His Master's Choice, Kenya Beer. £100

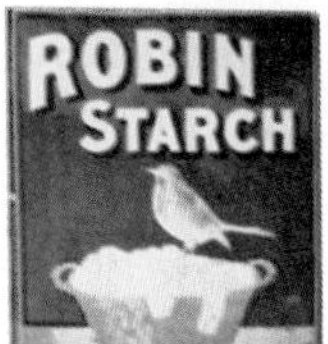

Robin Starch. £175

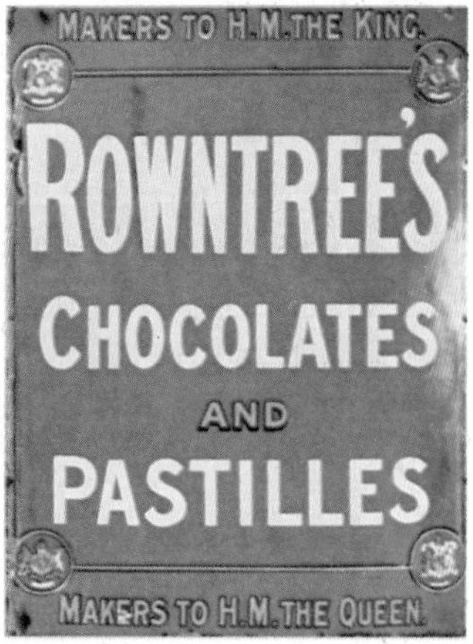

Rowntree's Chocolates and Pastilles. £45

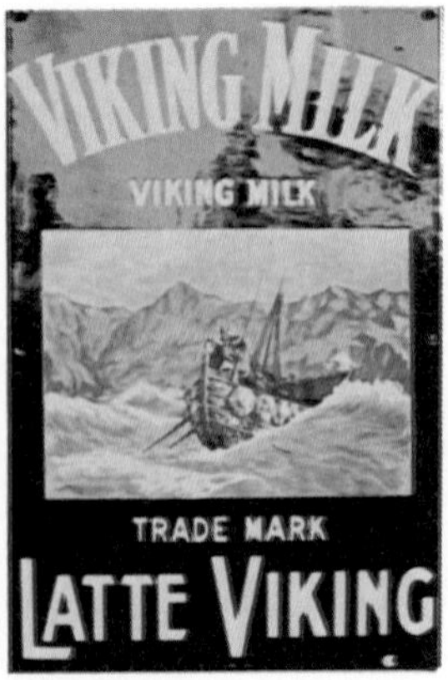

Viking Milk, 'Latte Viking'. £175

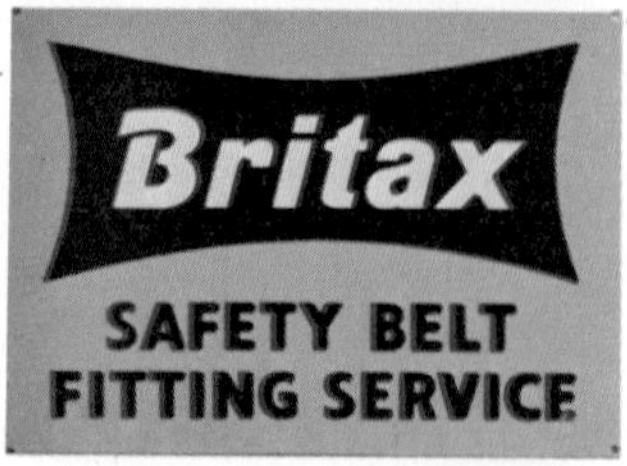

Britax, Safety Belt Fitting Service. £20

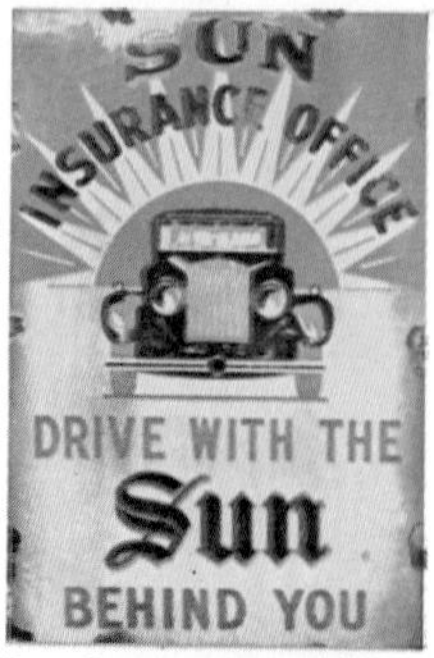

Sun Insurance Office. £150

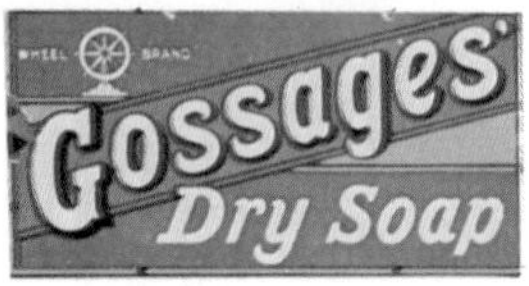

'Gossages', Dry Soap. £75

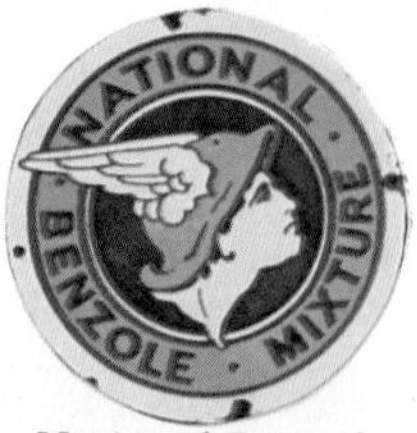

National Benzole Mixture. £75

Player's Please, 'Its the Tobacco that Counts'. £75

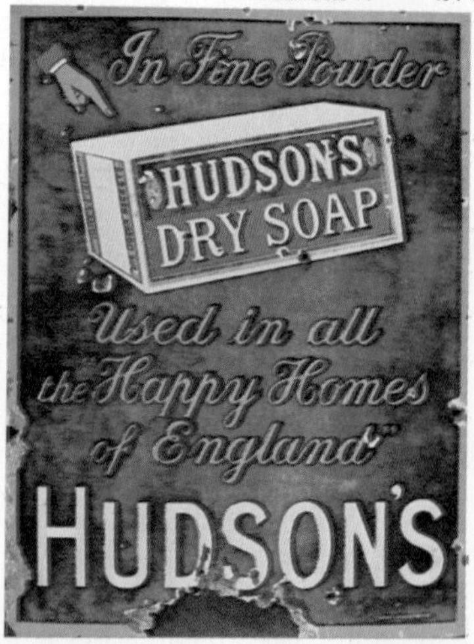

Hudson's Dry Soap, In Fine Powder. £45

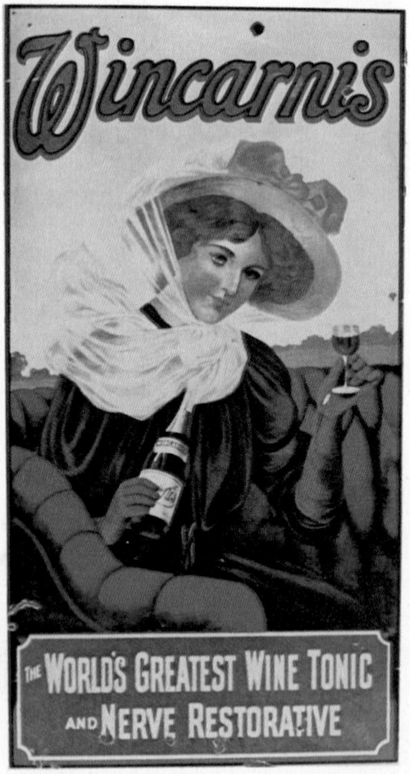

Wincarnis, 'The World's Greatest Wine Tonic'. £450

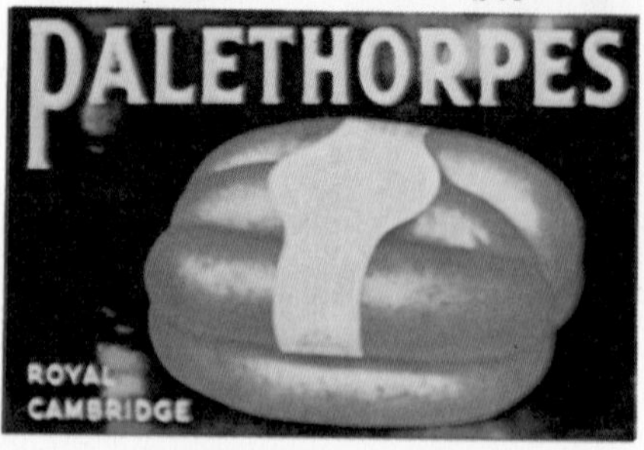

Palethorpes, 'Royal Cambridge' Sausages. £75

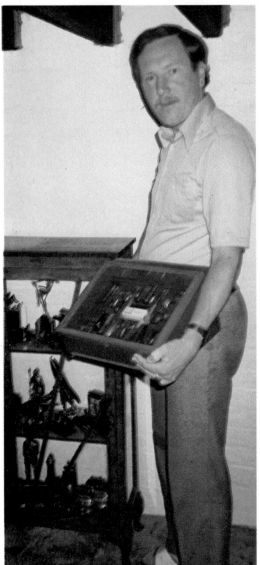

Peter Brooks is retail controller for a firm of newsagents and collects cigarette lighters.

"My collection consists of 250 table lighters and around 300 pocket ones. I'm adding to them all the time because my brother is in the antiques trade and he keeps an eye open for the sort of thing I want as he goes round the country.

"I also write away for copies of old catalogues from the various manufacturers all over the world, and there were lots of them, to look through and familiarise myself with the sort of lighters that were made. That way you find out what there is available and what you haven't got in your own collection yet."

Perhaps the most widely collected lighters are those made by Dunhill but some of them are very expensive today. The one Peter is most fond of in his collection is a Dunhill but it is quite unusual because it's in the shape of a hunting horn with the lighter in its base.

One of the lighters which has so far eluded him is an early Ronson called the 'Banjo lighter' which was made in the 1920's. He said: "I've seen one in someone else's collection but it wasn't for sale. If I was able to find one I expect it would cost something in the region of £100."

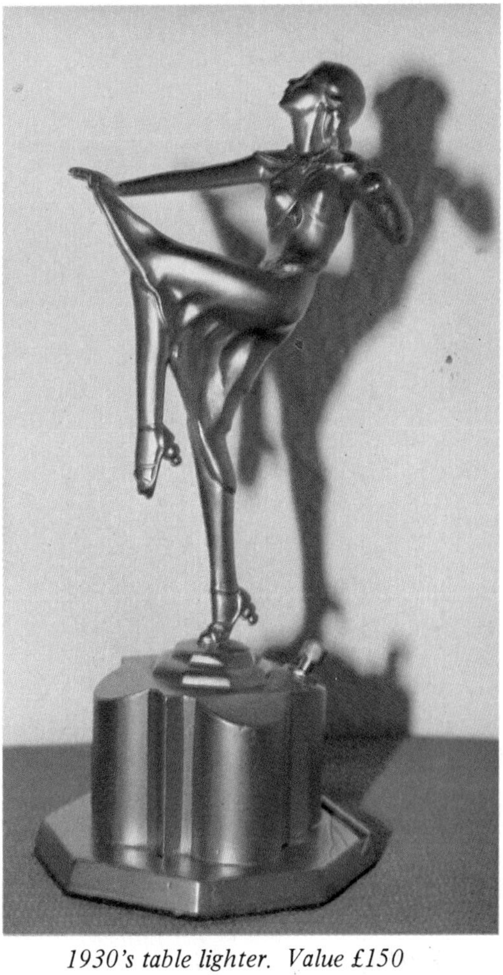

1930's table lighter. Value £150

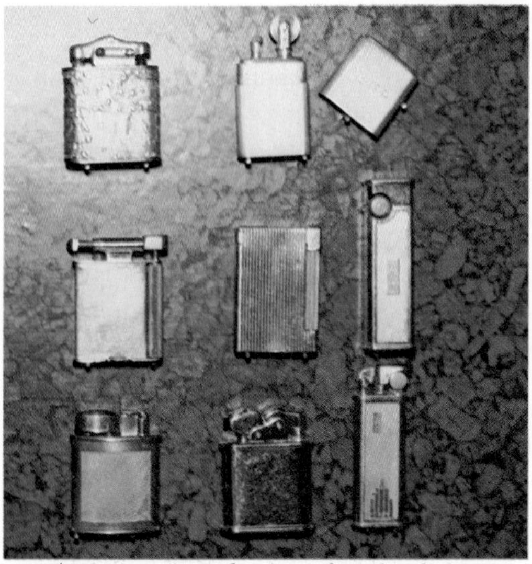

An interesting selection of pocket lighters including a Howitt (top right), a Parker Beacon (centre left), a Polo (right centre), and on the bottom row an Imco 3000, a Thorens Oriflam and a Beney 666.
Value £7 – £15, except the Howitt £75

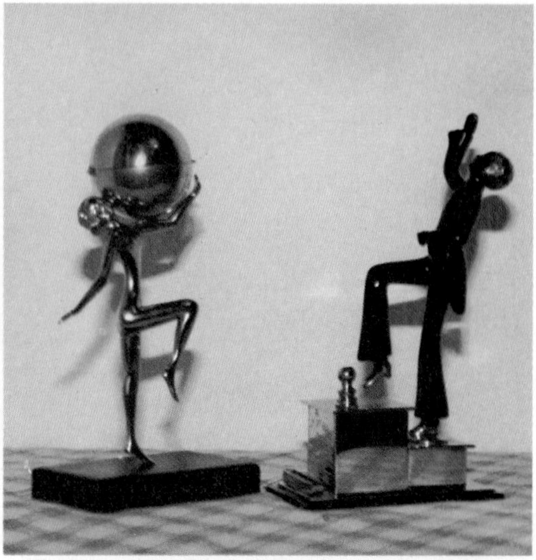

Fashionable table lighters from the 1920's, in the form of dancing figures, the one on the right being a strike lighter where a torch is withdrawn from the fuel tank forming the base and struck on a strip of cerium to produce a flame. *Value £30 – £50*

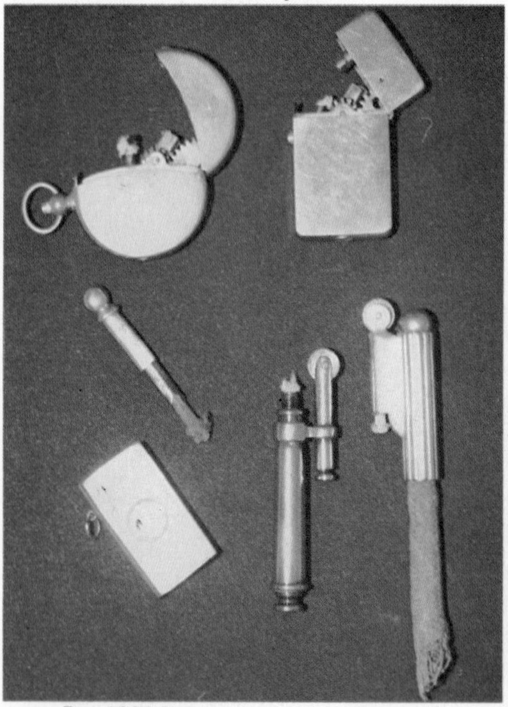

Pre 1920 lighters including two semi-automatic models (top), an interesting Cerium, strike lighter (left), and two 1910 lighters (bottom right), one of which is an Orlik. *Value £7 – £20*

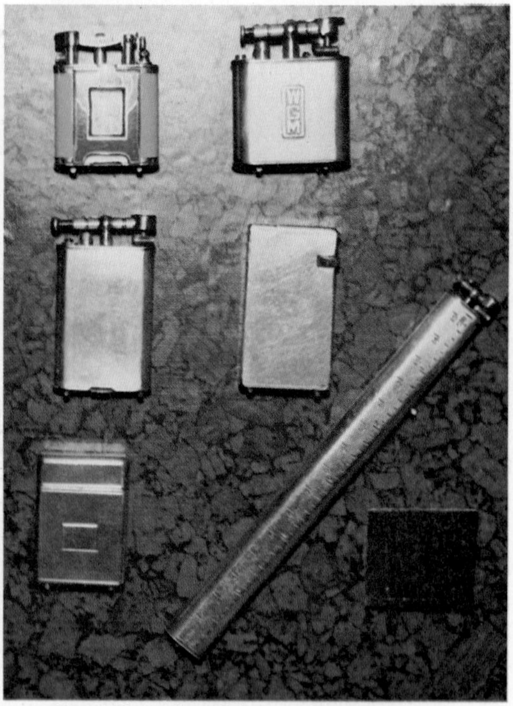

Dunhill pocket lighters including 'two 1930's', double wheel versions (top), a Unique and a Broadway (middle), a London Rollalite and a 6in Sylph Rule from the 50's (bottom). Value £30 upwards.

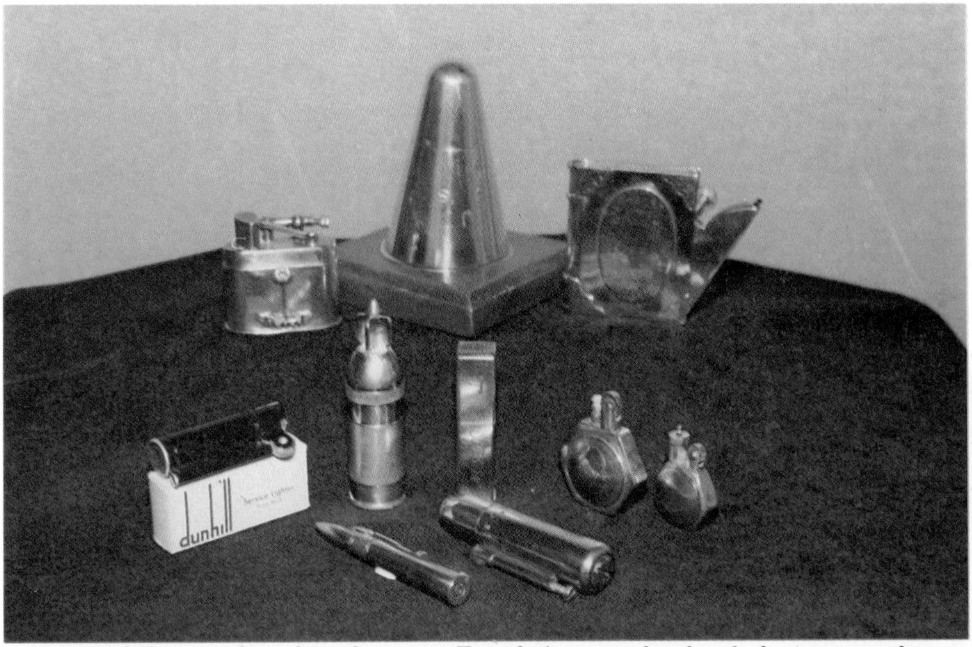

Wartime lighters such as these, known as Trench Art, were handmade from scraps of brass, coins, bullets and shell cases, while the later Dunhill is an economy model made for the services. *Value £5 – £25*

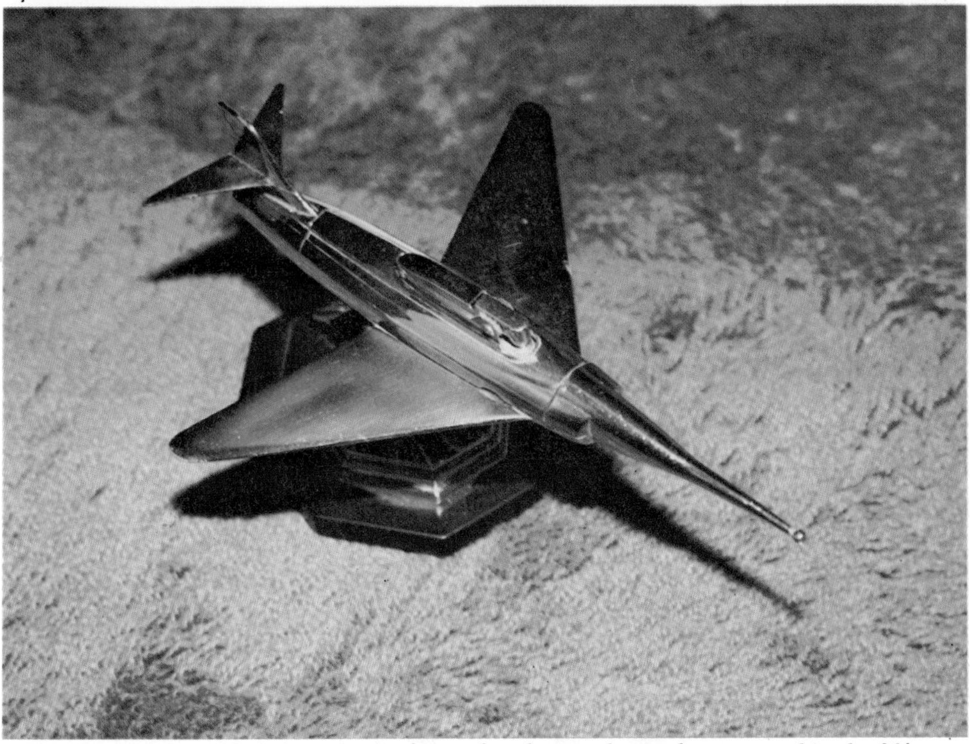

The demand for table lighters in the form of rockets and aeroplanes started in the 30's with the fashionable interest in technology and has continued with this stylish chrome plated example. *Value £70*

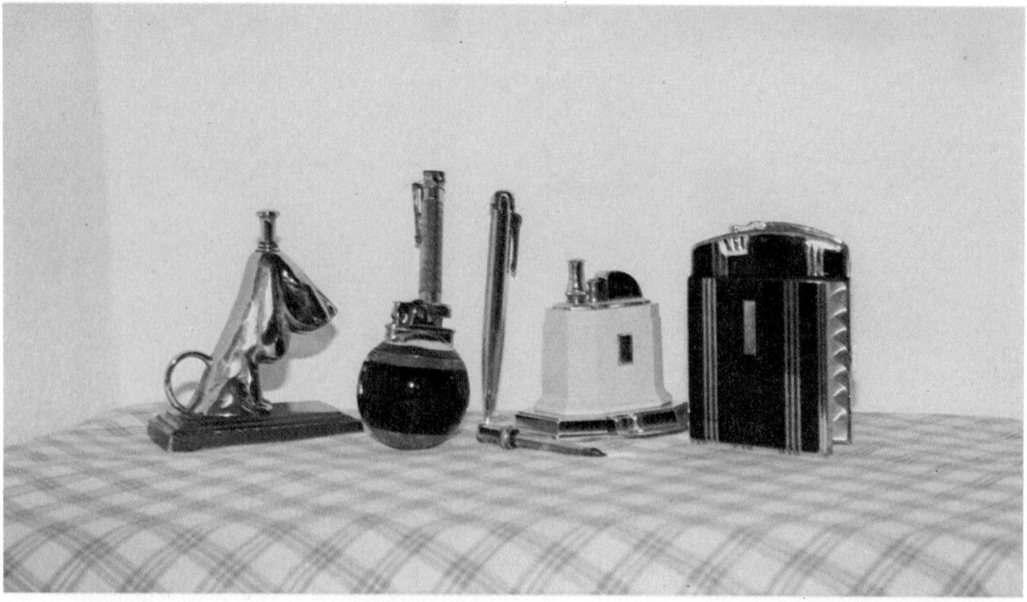

Stylish Ronson lighters including a dog strike lighter 1935, a Rondilight 1937, Pencil lighters 1930, 1947, a Touch Tip 1930's and a Twentycase 1930's. Value £40 – £100

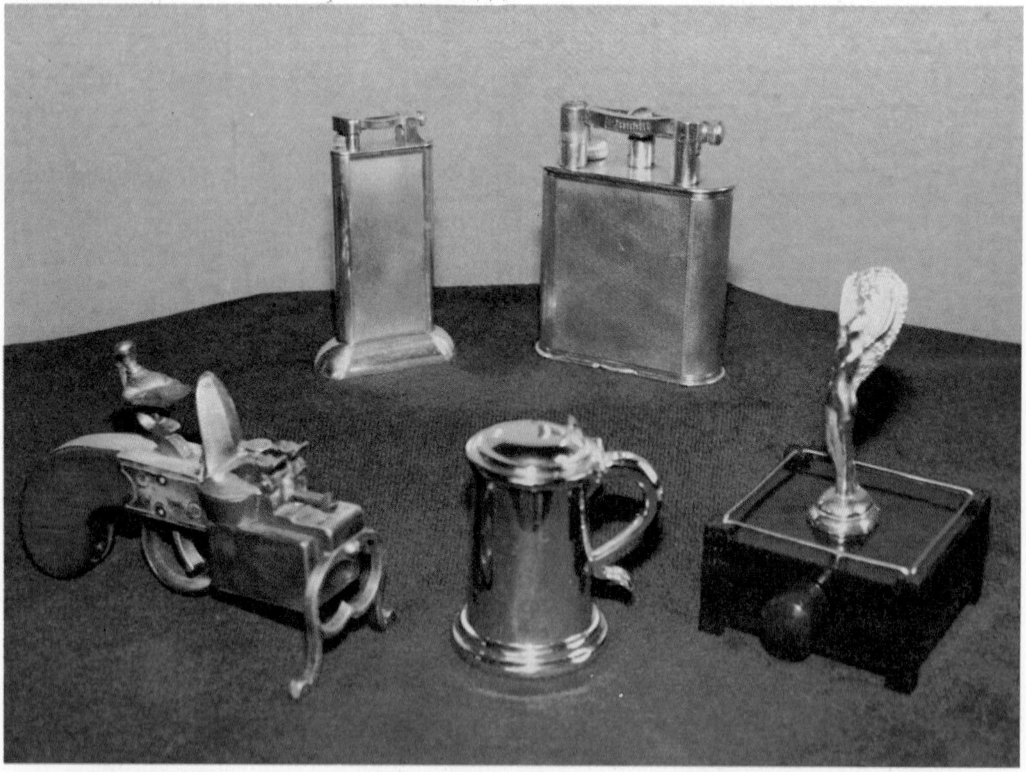

Dunhill table lighters including a Standard 1948, (top left) a giant 1930 (top right), a Tinder Pistol 1934, a Tankard 1950 and a rare electric Dunhill made in America (front right). Value £50 to over £200 for the pistol.

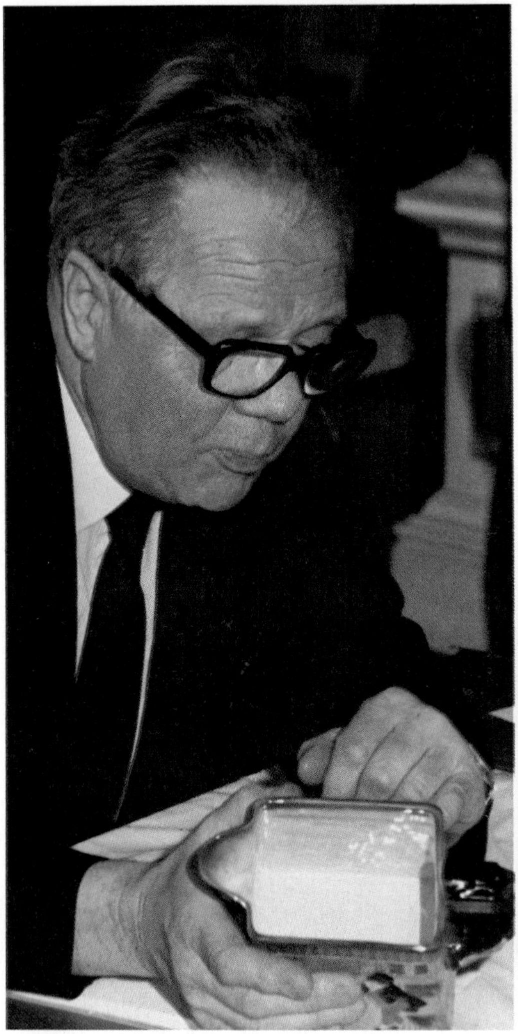

Mick Yewman is an auctioneer who runs his own saleroom in Abridge, Essex. He is an international expert on Doulton china and collects character jugs.

"I started collecting character jugs because of my granny, my father's mother, who lived in Bethnal Green when I was small. She was a Doulton collector and though I was born in Essex I used to visit with her and we'd go round all the retail shops in London that sold Doulton products. When she died in 1937 some of her stuff was left to me because I'd always liked it and that was what started me off really.

"I didn't go into the auction business at first but did war time service in the Royal Navy and was an amateur boxer also. Then I did a bit of car dealing but all the time I was collecting Doulton pieces and in 1967 I took a gamble and opened the Abridge Auction Rooms, specialising in Doulton sales. I've got a little museum beside the saleroom where I keep my own collection. Collectors from all over the world come here to buy and we turn over more than 5,000 lots of Doulton every year."

Mick's collection includes a large number of the finest Doulton character jugs including his most recent acquisitions, a pair of the very rare Blue Pearly Boy and Girl. They are both three and a half inches high and though they have hairline cracks, the pair cost him £3,500.

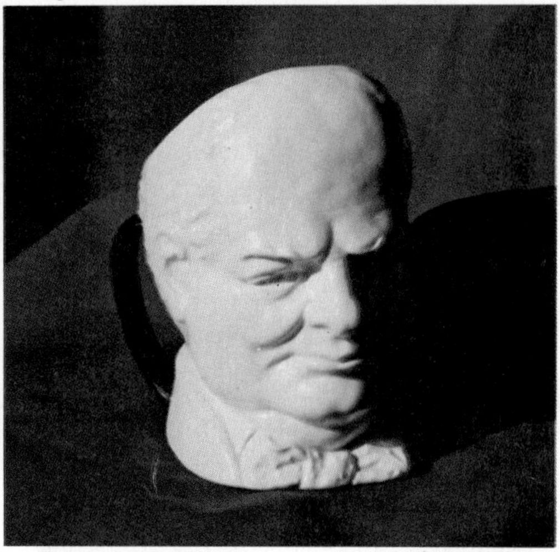

He is always looking out for copies of the White Churchill character jug which was withdrawn from production after only 18 months because Churchill did not consider it a good likeness. The price of the jug in auction can range between £5,000 and £10,000 today.

Character jugs which Mick would most like to find include three prototypes which are very rarely seen. One is of a Maori, produced in 1938, of which only two pilot copies were ever recorded and which is worth $10,000 at auction in America; another is of Buffalo Bill of which only one copy is known and the third is a Baseball Player.

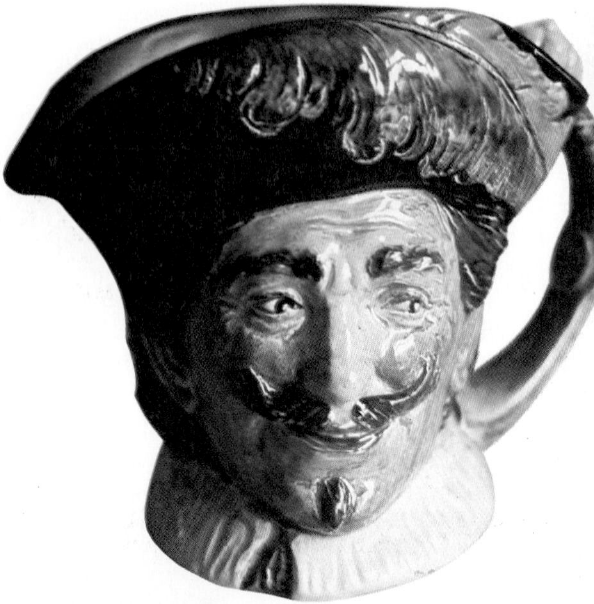

'Cavalier' D6114, designed by H. Fenton, issued 1940-42, large, with goatee beard. £1,200

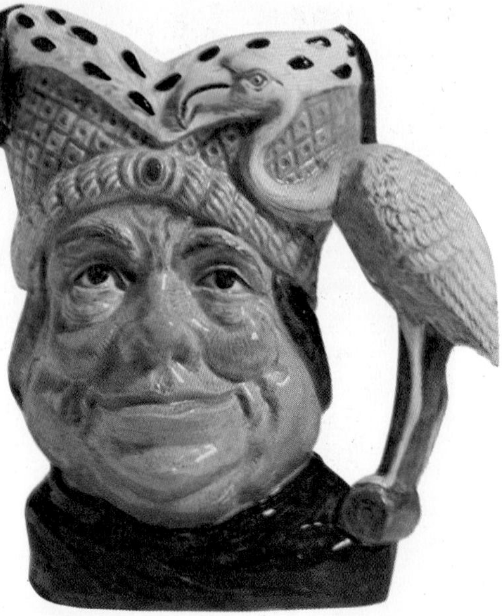

'Ugly Duchess' D6599, designed by M. Henk, issued 1965-73, large. £230

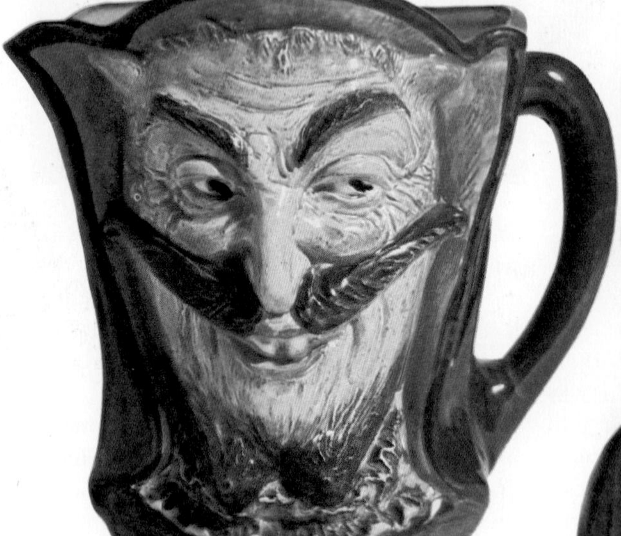

'Mephistopheles' D5757, designed by H. Fenton, issued 1937-48, large. £900

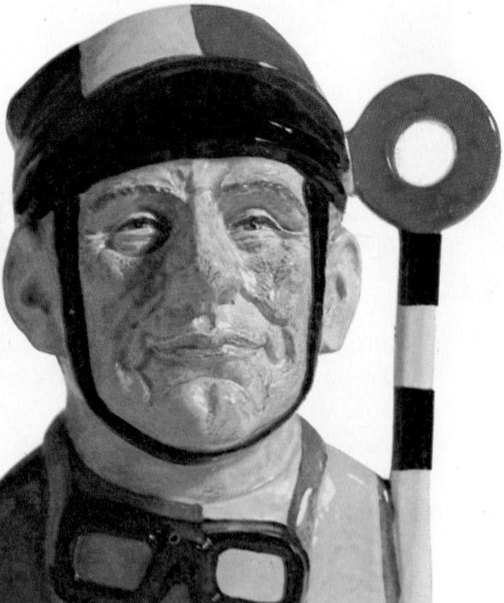

'Jockey' D6625, designed by D. Biggs, issued 1971-75, large. £170

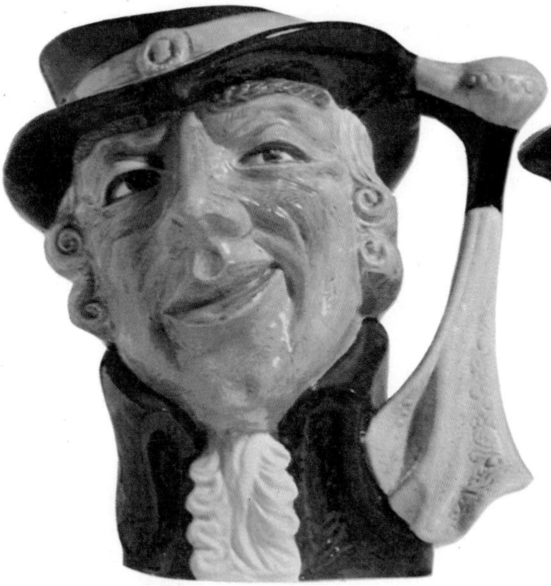

'Regency Beau' D6559, Designed by D. Biggs, issued 1962-67, large. £450

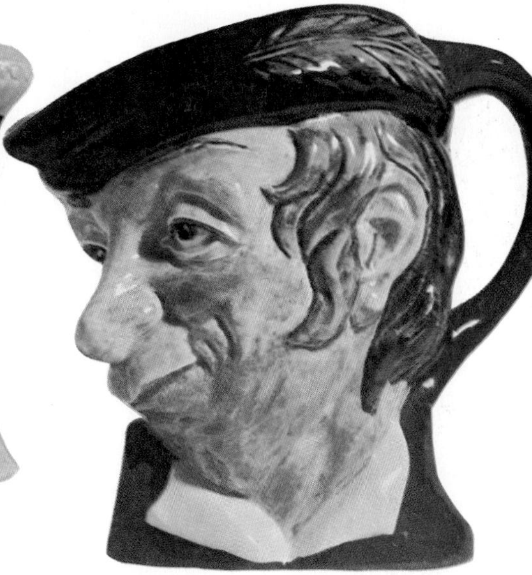

'Simple Simon' D6374, designed by G. Blower, issued 1953-60, large. £260

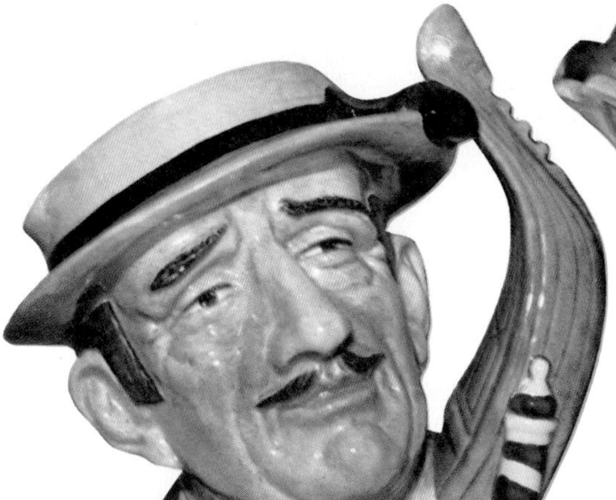

'Gondolier' D6589, designed by D. Briggs, issued 1964-69, large. £230

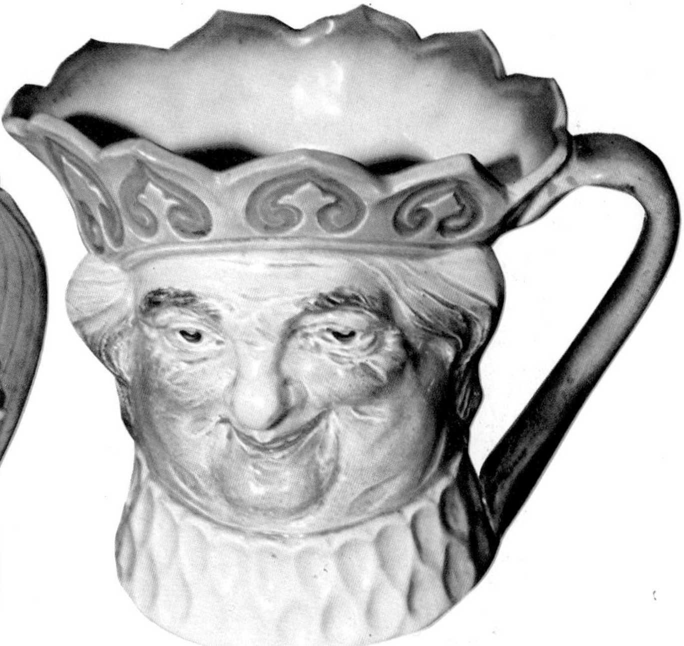

'Old King Cole' D6036, designed by H. Fenton, issued 1939-40, large, yellow crown. £800

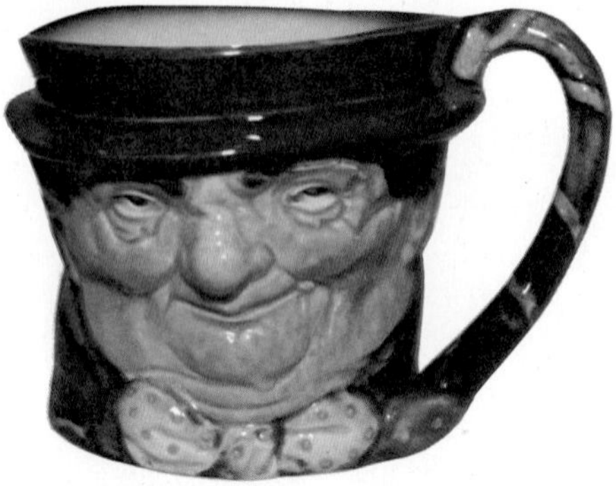

'Tony Weller' D5530, designed by L. Harradine and H. Fenton, issued 1936-60, small. £38

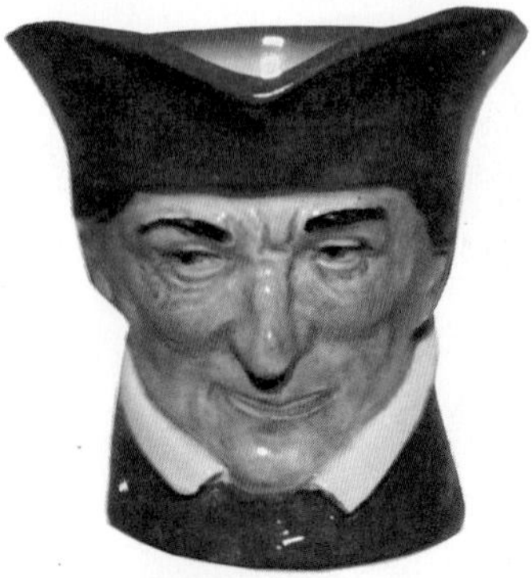

'Cardinal' D6033, designed by C. Noke, issued 1939-60, small. £38

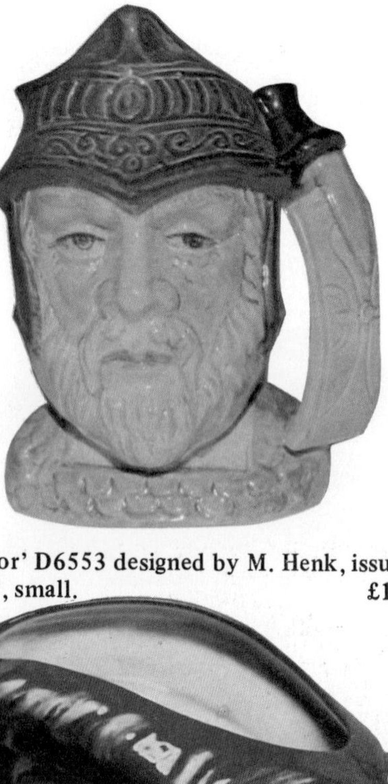

'Gladiator' D6553 designed by M. Henk, issued 1961-67, small. £180

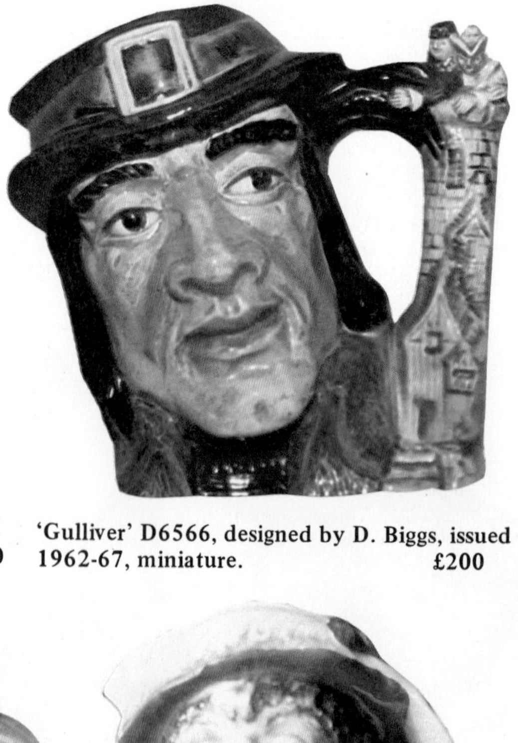

'Gulliver' D6566, designed by D. Biggs, issued 1962-67, miniature. £200

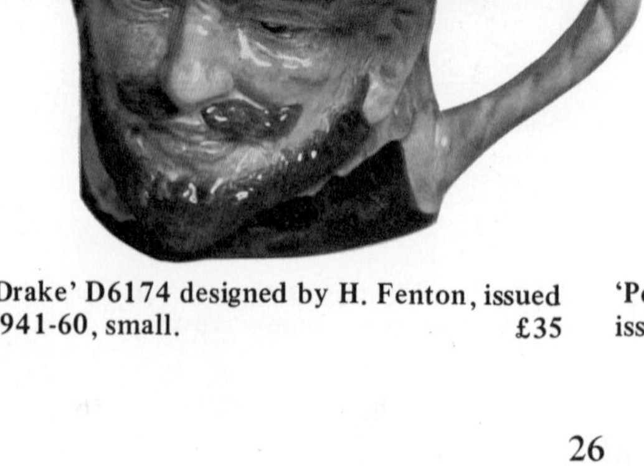

'Drake' D6174 designed by H. Fenton, issued 1941-60, small. £35

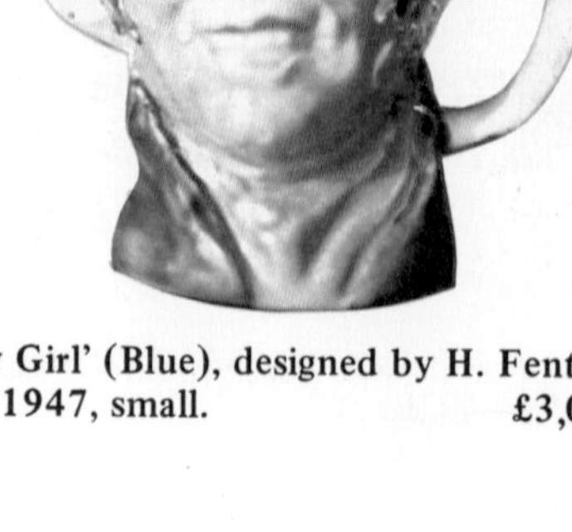

'Pearly Girl' (Blue), designed by H. Fenton, issued 1947, small. £3,000

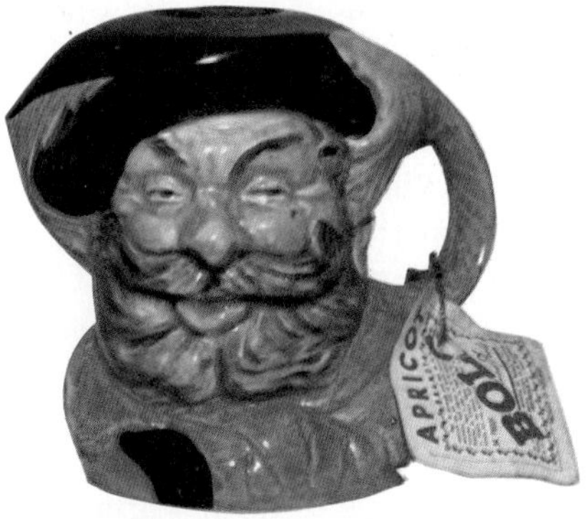

'Falstaff' D6385, designed by H. Fenton, issued as a small liquer flask in the 1960's. £40

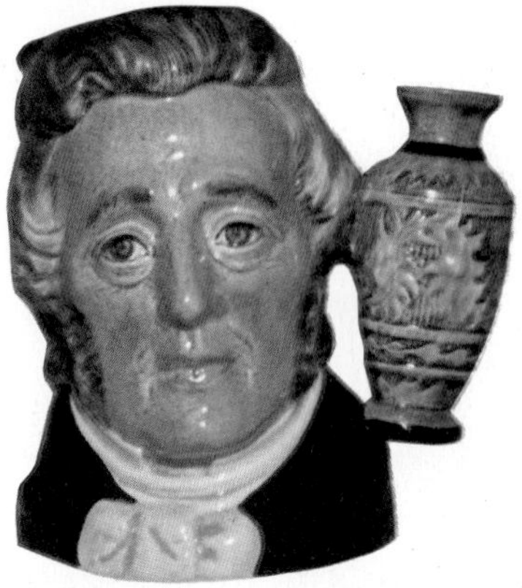

'Sir Henry Doulton' D6703 designed by E. Griffiths, issued 1984, small. £30

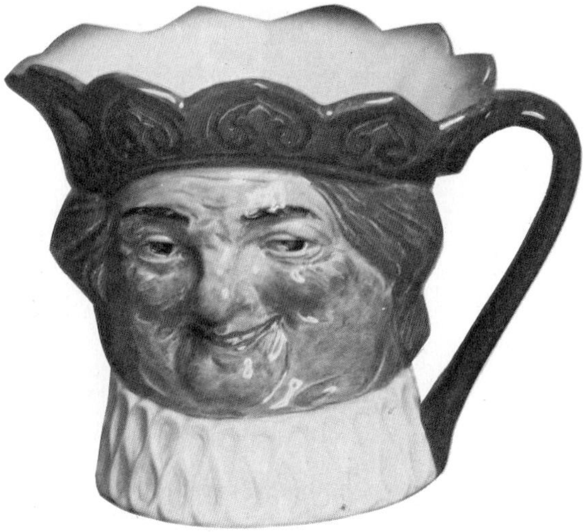

'Old King Cole' D6037, designed by H. Fenton, issued 1939-60, small. £50

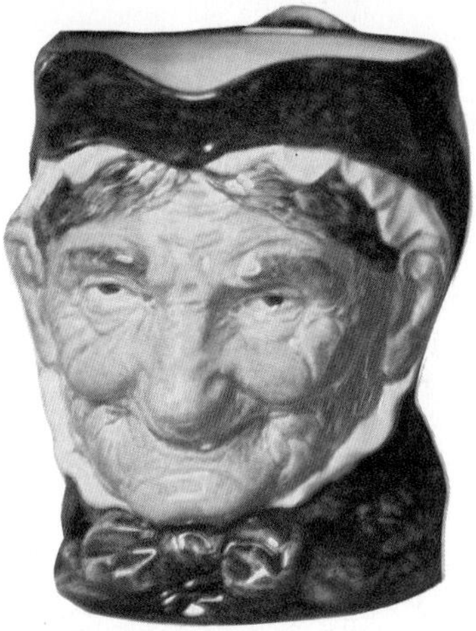

'Granny' D6384 designed by H. Fenton and M. Henk, issued 1953-83, small. £20

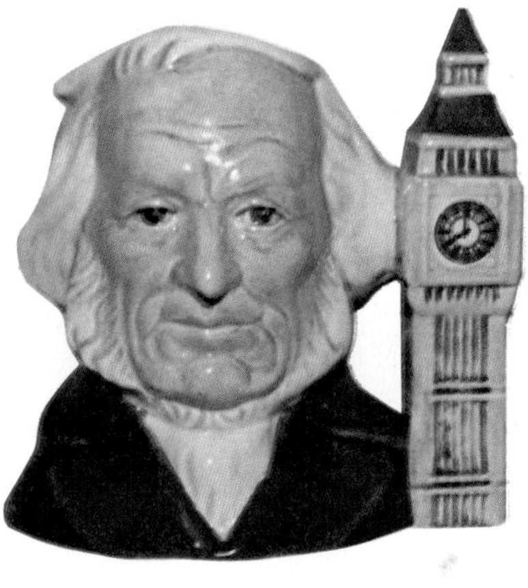

'John Doulton' D6656 designed by E. Griffiths, issued 1980, small. £38

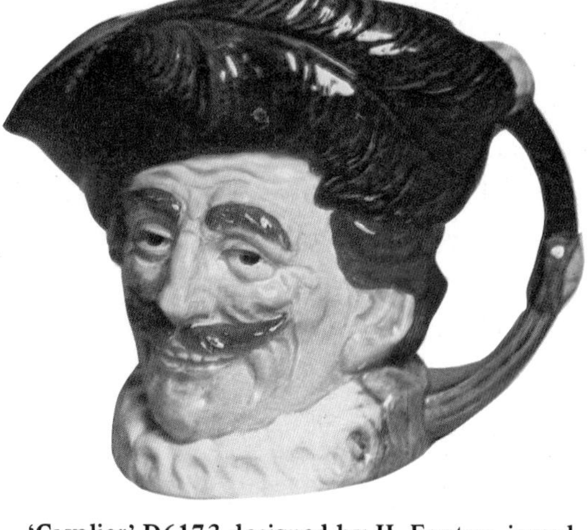

'Cavalier' D6173 designed by H. Fenton, issued 1941-60, small. £35

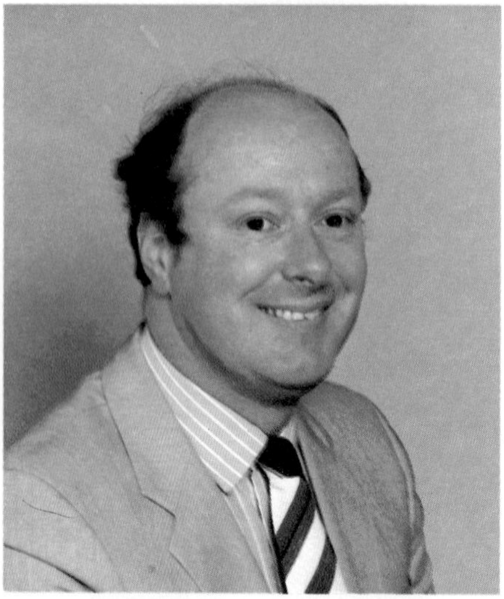

Nicholas Pine first became interested in Goss china when he discovered a few pieces nestling in a friend's living room cabinet. This began an involvement which has become his life's work.

Originally trained as a surveyor, he ran his own building business before giving up this career in 1970 to develop his growing interest in Goss china, which could be bought from junk shops for 3d and 6d a piece at that time.

Quickly realising that little was known or published about Goss china, he set about researching the subject and in 1978 published *The Price Guide to Goss China,* now in its fourth edition.

Nicholas is considered as being largely responsible for re-popularising heraldic china in recent years after its 30 year decline from 1940.

The leading authority in his chosen field for some twenty years, he founded Goss & Crested China Ltd, the leading dealers, who have maintained an orderly market in Goss china for many years.

Constantly researching the subject at which he works tirelessly to publicise, he is a frequent contributor to antique journals and columns, has appeared on television and radio and frequently lectures on Goss china.

Nicholas, who is in his mid-thirties, lives in South Hampshire with his wife, Lynda and their three young children.

There is little in the way of Goss china Nicholas Pine has not seen but recently some shards of a coloured version of Massachusetts Hall, Harvard University, Boston, Massachusetts, have come to light in the factory spoil heap. The version currently known is white glazed but somewhere there could be a fully coloured variety, and that could be worth a great deal of money.

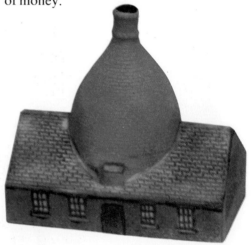

The Goss Oven, orange chimney version, 75mm. long. £185

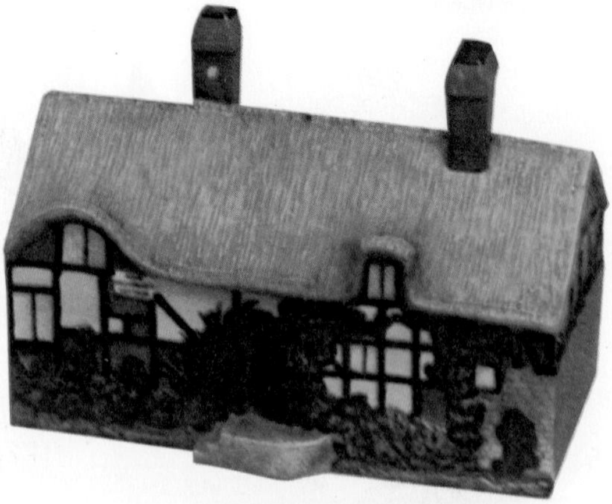

Ann Hathaway's Cottage, Shottery, at Stratford-on-Avon. Nightlight version, 148mm. long. £225

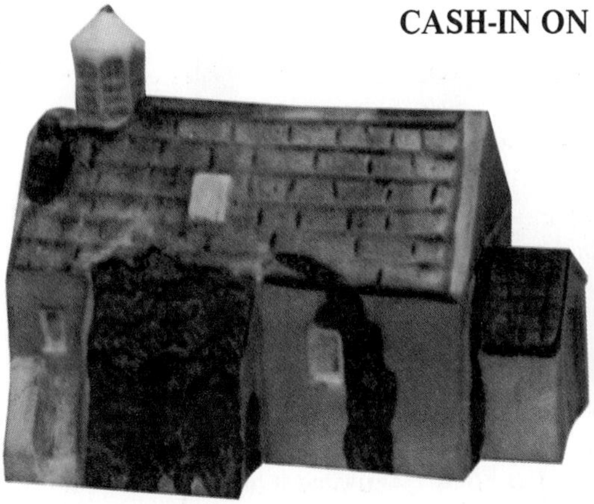

St. Nicholas Chapel, Lantern Hill, Ilfracombe, 74mm. high. £145

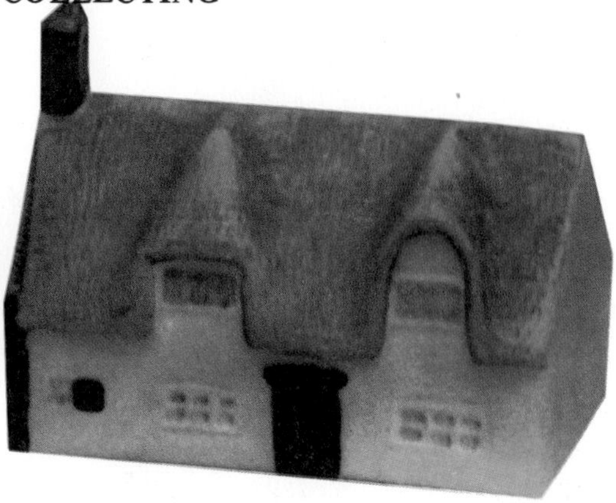

The Old Thatched Cottage, Poole, 68mm. long. £350

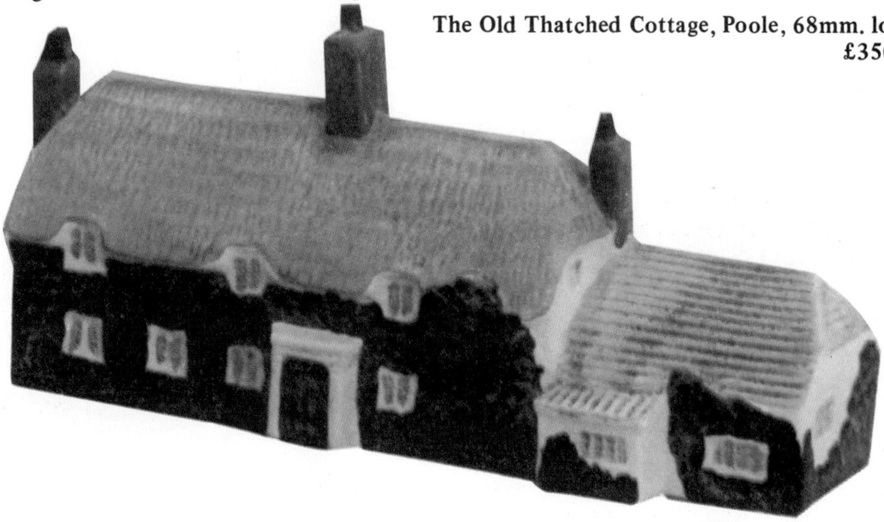

Thomas Hardy's Birthplace, Dorchester, 100mm. long. £325

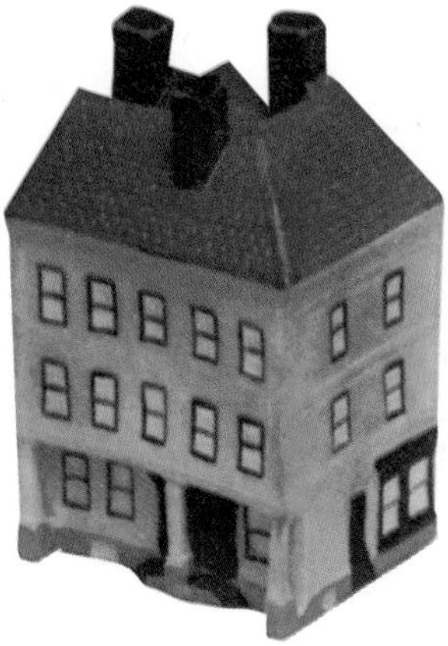

Dr. Samuel Johnson's House, Lichfield, 75mm. high. £140

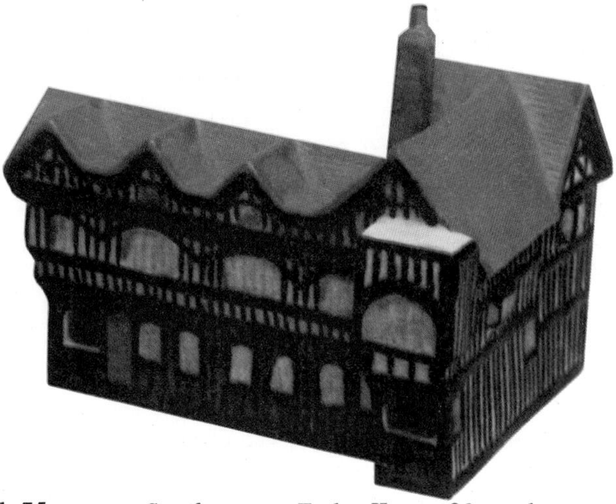

Southampton Tudor House, 83mm. long. £265

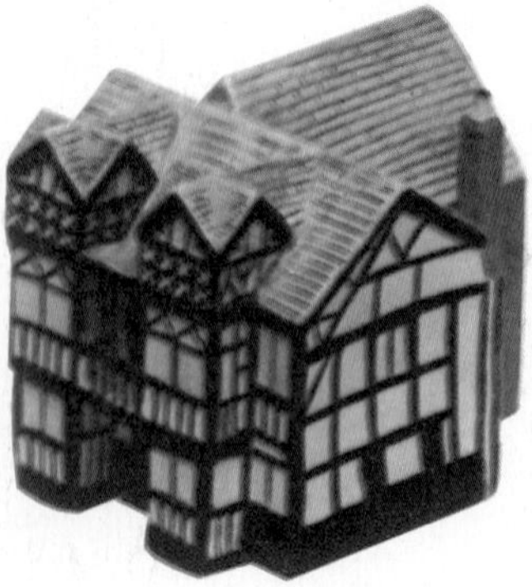

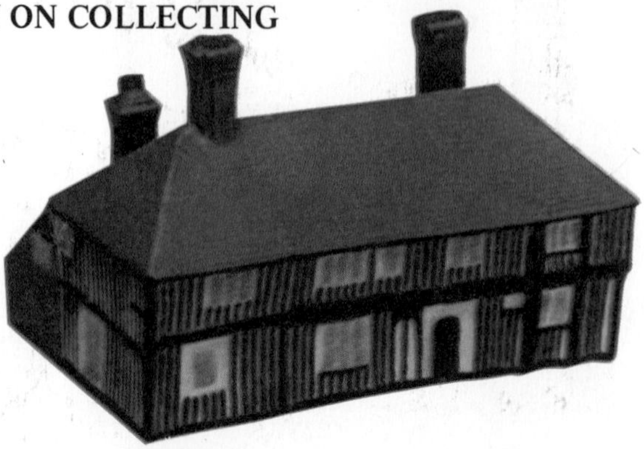

Miss Ellen Terry's Farm near Tenterden in Kent, 70mm. long. £290

Priest's House, Prestbury, 90mm. long. £900

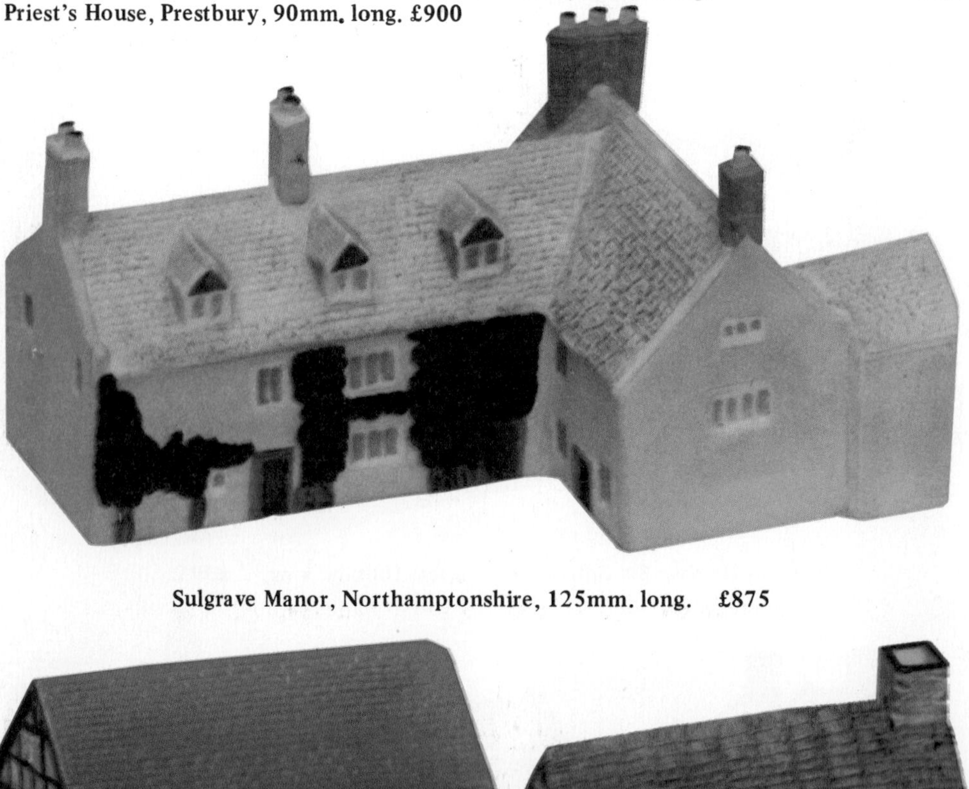

Sulgrave Manor, Northamptonshire, 125mm. long. £875

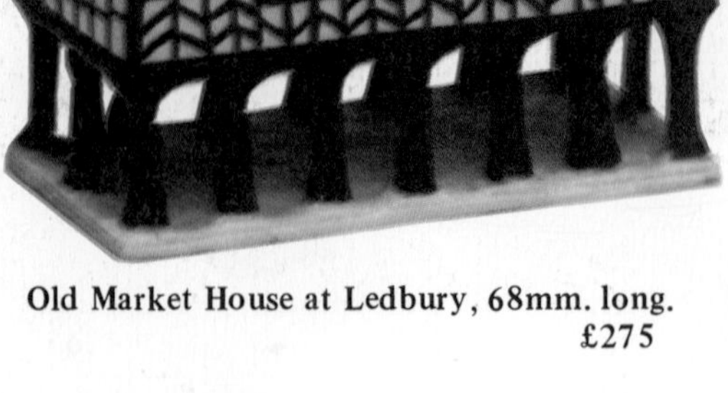

Old Market House at Ledbury, 68mm. long. £275

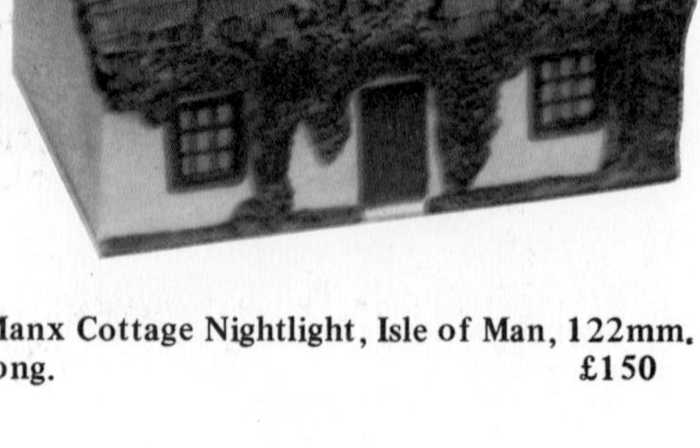

Manx Cottage Nightlight, Isle of Man, 122mm. long. £150

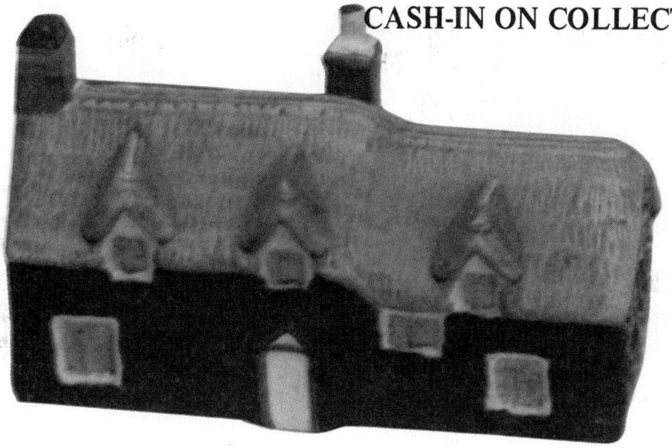

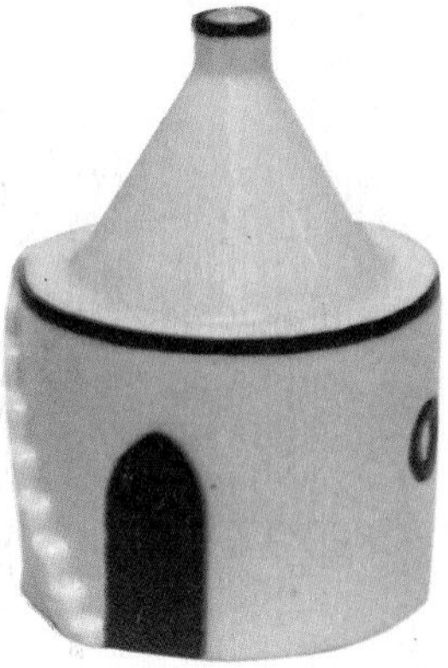

Old Maids Cottage, Lee, Devon, 73mm. long.
£115

Look-out House at Newquay, 65mm. high.
£85

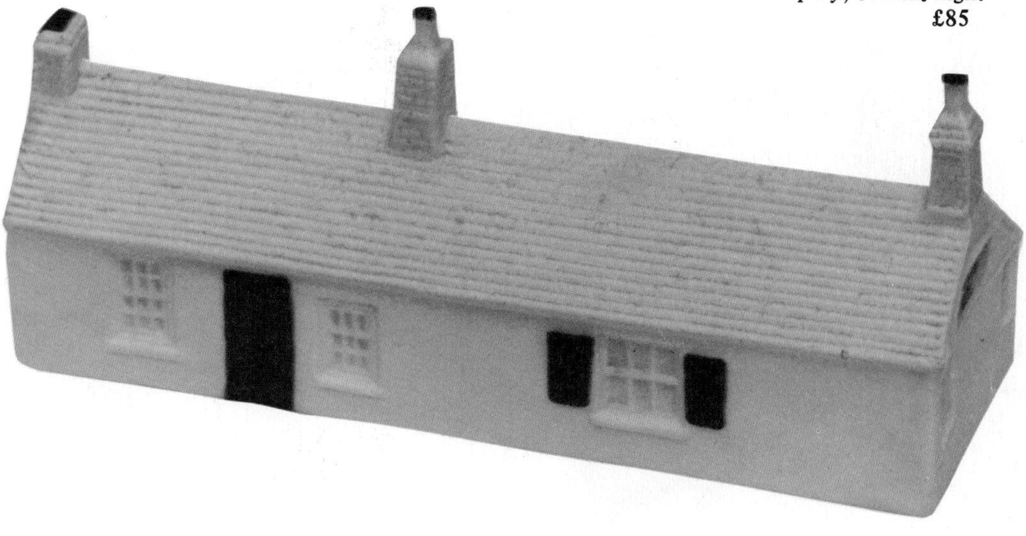

First and Last House in England, with annexe 140mm. long. £650

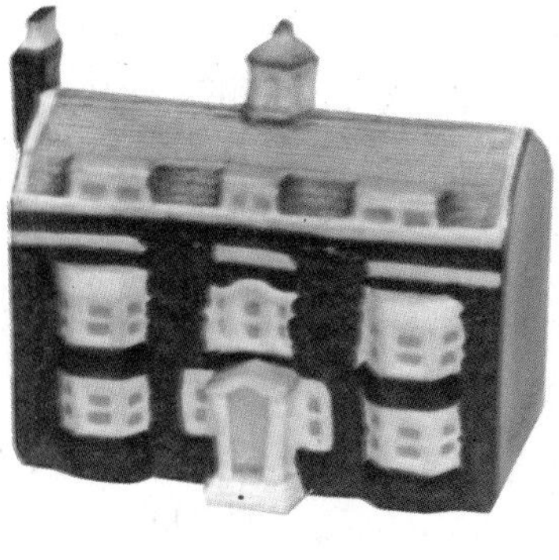

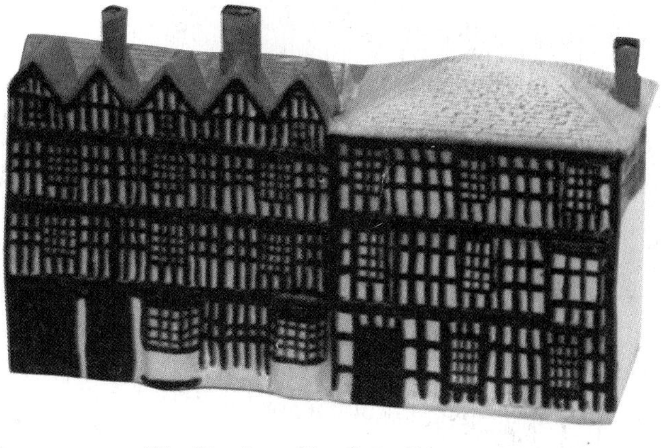

Charles Dickens House at Gads Hill, near Rochester. £115

The Feathers Hotel, Ledbury, 114mm. long.
£700

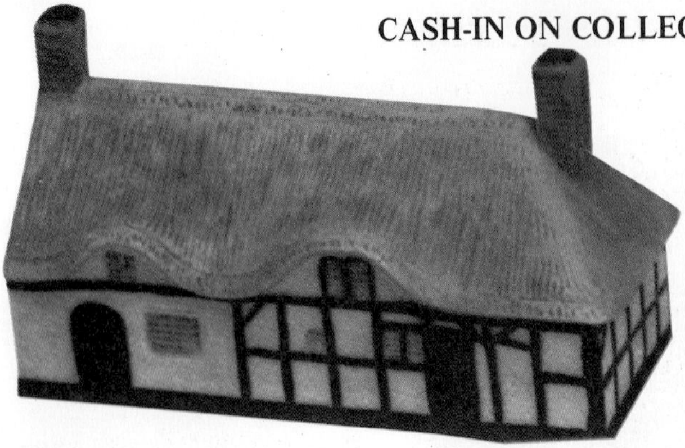

Isaac Walton's Birthplace, Shallowford, 86mm. long. £325

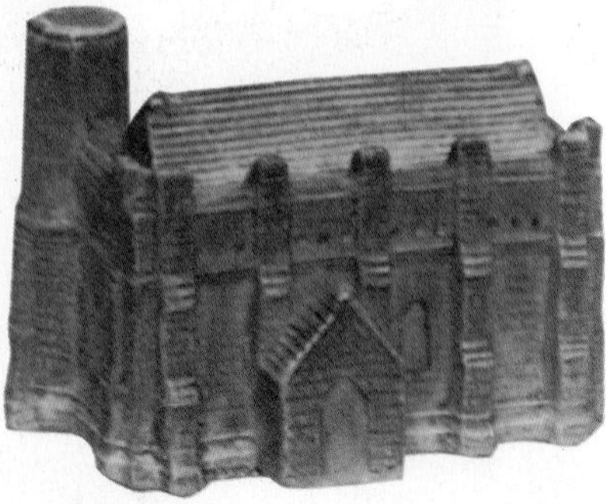

St. Catherine's Chapel, Abbotsbury, 87mm. long. £400

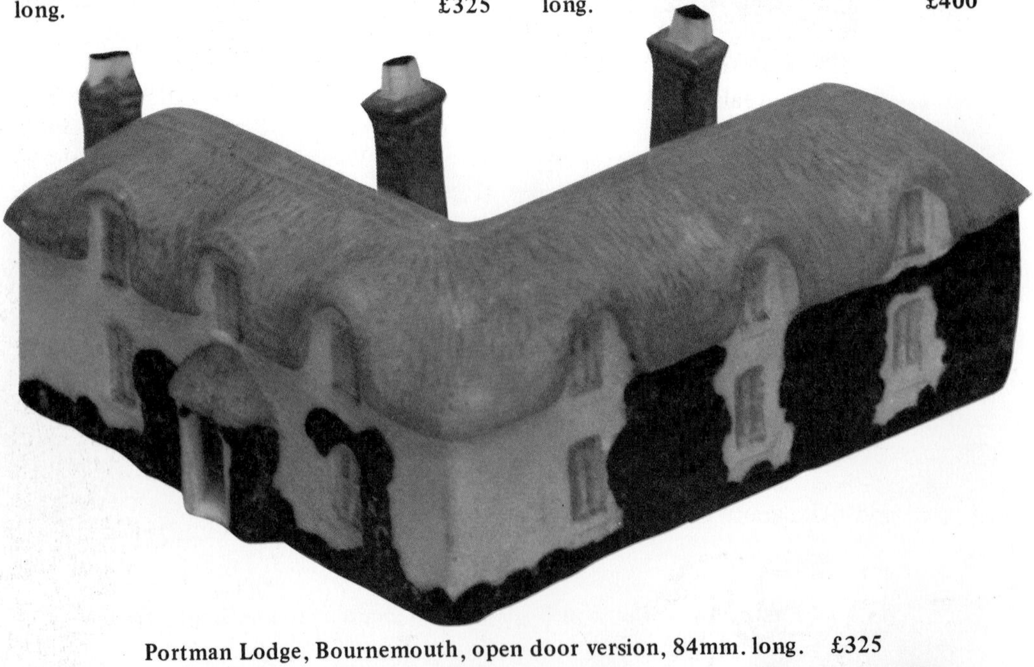

Portman Lodge, Bournemouth, open door version, 84mm. long. £325

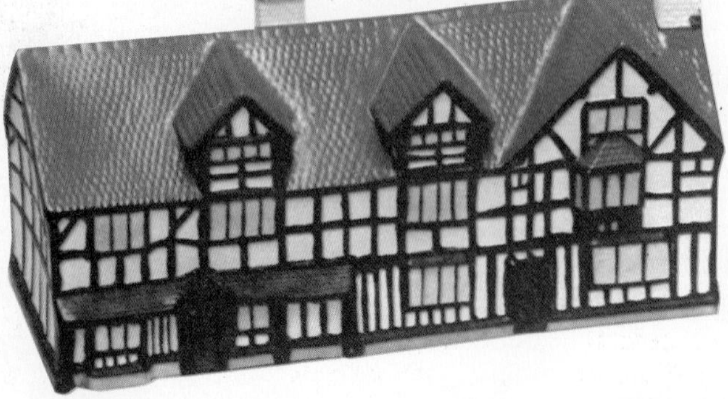

Shakespeare's Cottage, Stratford-on-Avon, 65mm. long. £65

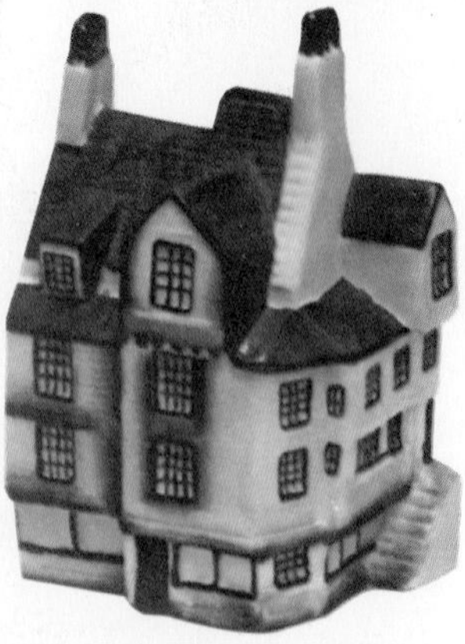

John Knox's House at Edinburgh, 102mm. high. £350

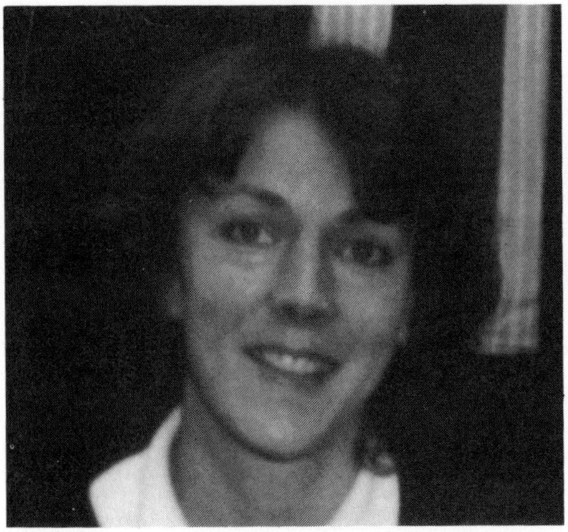

Little did Lynda realise when she first met her future husband, Nicholas Pine, that Goss china was to play such a large part in her life. His house was full of miniature Goss artefacts each decorated with coats of arms of towns, abbeys, schools, colleges etc, and she soon became just as interested in heraldic china as Nicholas.

Born in Bournemouth, Dorset, Lynda taught Physical education in a Hampshire Comprehensive before leaving to have a family of three children and deal in, research and write about Goss china.

W.H.GOSS

Such is the excitement of the Goss world, with the telephone ringing all day, mountains of post connected with heraldic china pouring in weekly, with a growing demand for questions to be answered, problems of pricing and buying and selling to be sorted out, how could Lynda sit back and leave her husband to cope alone?

Although her husband Nicholas did not realise it at the time, he had started collecting a type of china which the world had forgotten about for the last few decades since production finally ceased in 1940.

Goss and crested china was not old enough then to be antique and at least three-quarters of that in Edwardian homes was thrown out during the forties, fifties and sixties.

Lynda and Nicholas Pine's research has led to the publication of the family biography and factory history *WILLIAM HENRY GOSS. The Story of The Staffordshire Family of Potters Who Invented Heraldic Porcelain.* (Milestone Publications, Murray Road, Horndean, Hampshire £15.00).

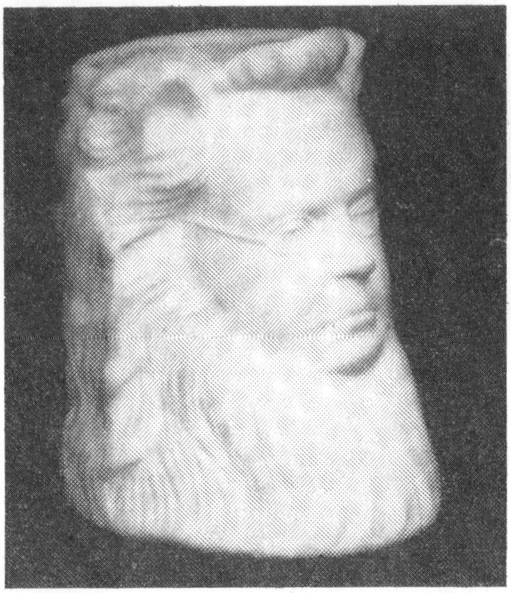

A piece Lynda has always been keen to acquire is the Goss model of a spill holder featuring Edward Kenealy, the Victorian lawyer who defended the infamous Tichborne claimant, and who was so heartily disliked by W. H. Goss that he made no less than three varieties of Kenealy spill-holder, so depicted as to show an empty head!

CASH-IN ON COLLECTING

Every generation has its new hobby, and almost a century ago heraldic china collecting became a craze which swept the country.

It began in the 1870's when William Henry Goss of Stoke on Trent began supplying the Oxford and Cambridge Colleges and notable public schools of the day, with white porcelain ornaments bearing their own coats of arms. This led to his eldest son, Adolphus, decorating shapes modelled after a variety of elegant ancient artefacts to be found in various museums across the country. These bore the arms of their locality and were only supplied in their own area via selected agencies, which could vary from a station bookstall, pharmacy, library, sweet shop to the best china shop in town. To obtain a particular crest, one had to journey to that place to buy one. In this way, Adolphus built up a network of agencies all over the country, and eventually overseas too.

By the turn of the century, the smaller crested shapes were retailing new for between sixpence and a shilling, with the fonts and cottages half-a-crown. By the middle of the First World War in 1916, sales plummeted and the Goss factory was eventually sold by the family in 1929, production ceasing finally around 1939.

The last ten years has seen a keen interest in collecting Goss and prices have soared. In his *Price Guide to Goss China* Nicholas Pine has listed every known shape made and its correct value, and explains why a white Shakespeare's font is worth £28, whilst a brown Hereford Cathedral Font fetches £285. The St. Buryan Cross is £100 but a similar looking shape, the grey Hambledon Cricket stone is valued at £830.

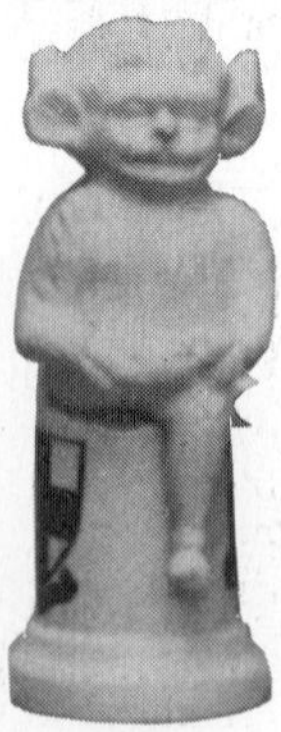

Lincoln Imp on pedestal, unglazed figure seated on glazed plinth. £85

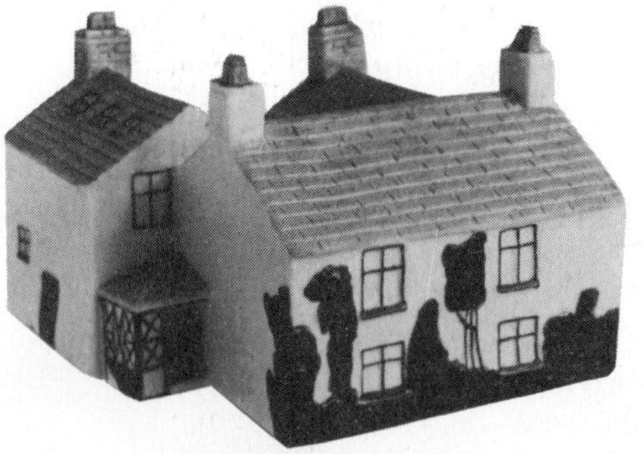

Dove Cottage, William Wordsworth's home in Grasmere; a lot of cottage for £375.

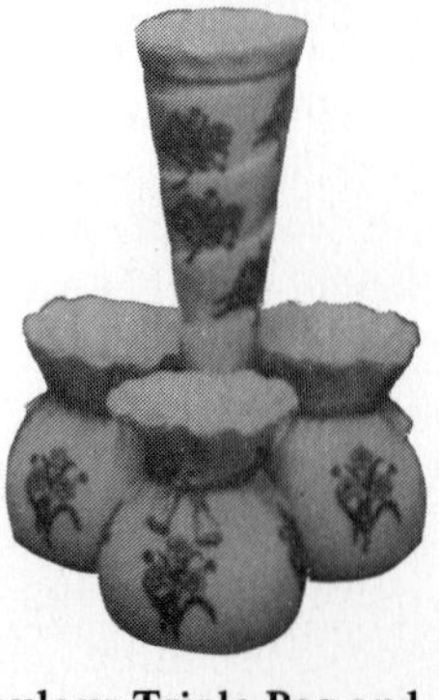

Fabulous Triple Bag and Shell Centrepiece, 160mm. high. It is decorated with sprays of blue and green forget-me-nots. £130

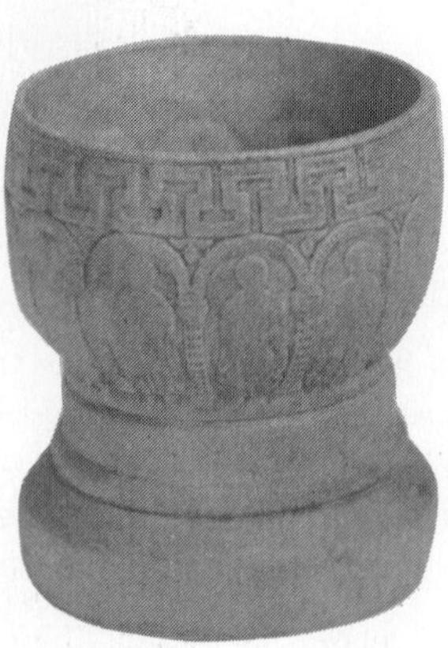

Brown Hereford Cathedral Font. £285

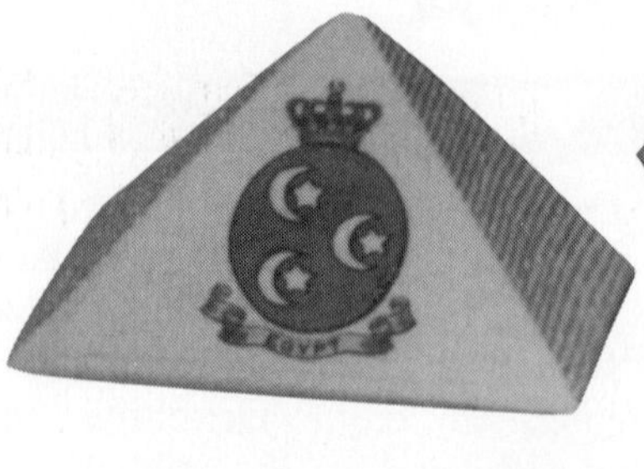

Egyptian Pyramid with arms of Egypt. The brickwork is beautifully moulded. £80

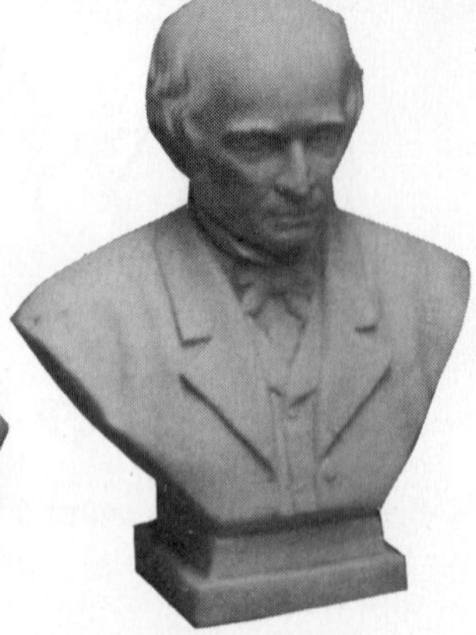

'Wordsworth', white parian bust, unglazed on square base. £125

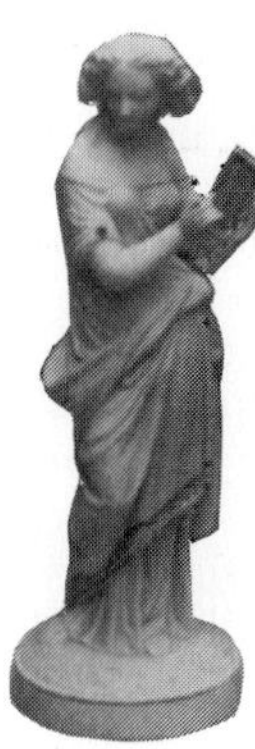

White unglazed parian figurine playing lyre, tastefully trimmed with gold and blue. £275

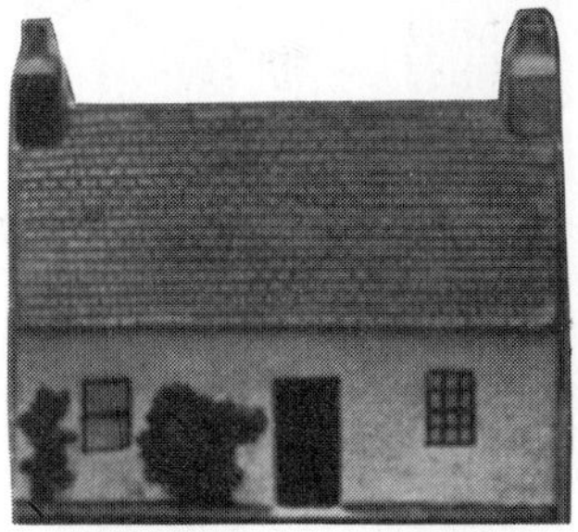

'A Window In Thrums', nightlight. £220
This cottage in Kirriemuir was the subject of a novel by author J. M. Barrie.

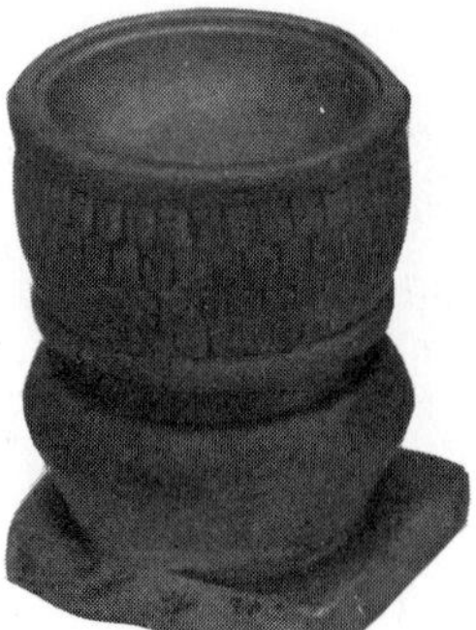

A rare brown font, The St. Iltyd's at Llantwit Major now worth £435.

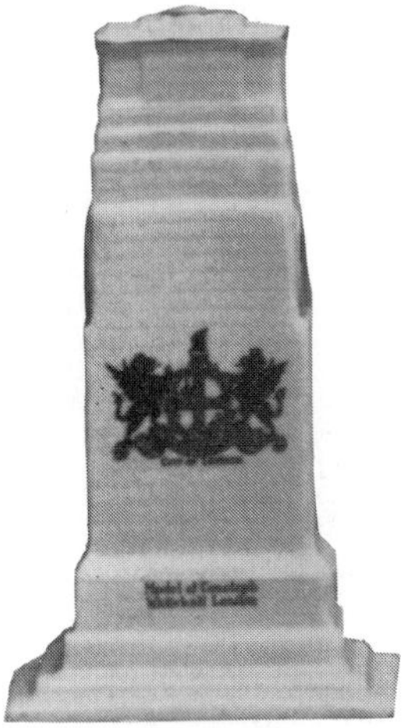

Cenotaph, the later version. £35
Similar examples made by other factories only fetch one fifth of this value.

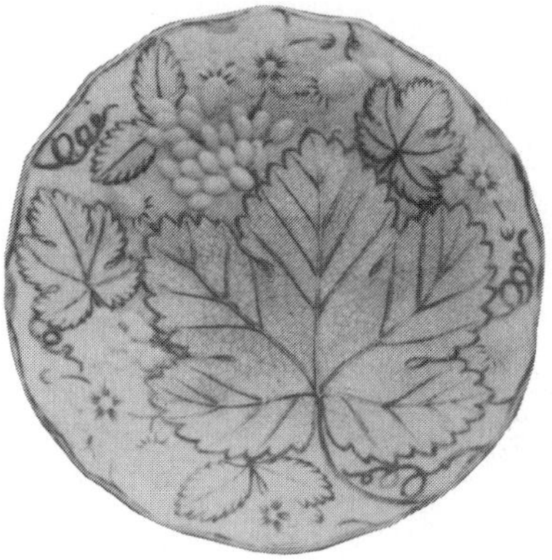

Parian unglazed plate with grapevine decoration in relief, highlighted in gold. £100

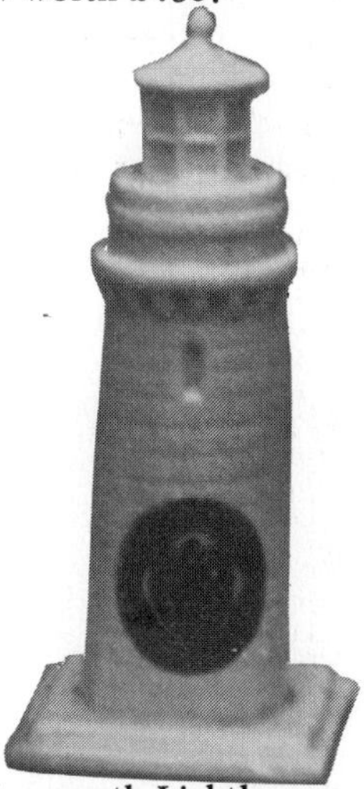

Teignmouth Lighthouse. £37
There is a range of lighthouses to collect.

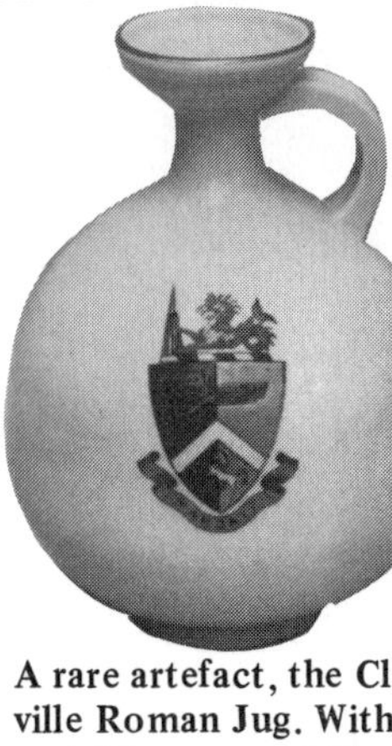

A rare artefact, the Cliftonville Roman Jug. With the matching arms of Margate it can fetch £220.

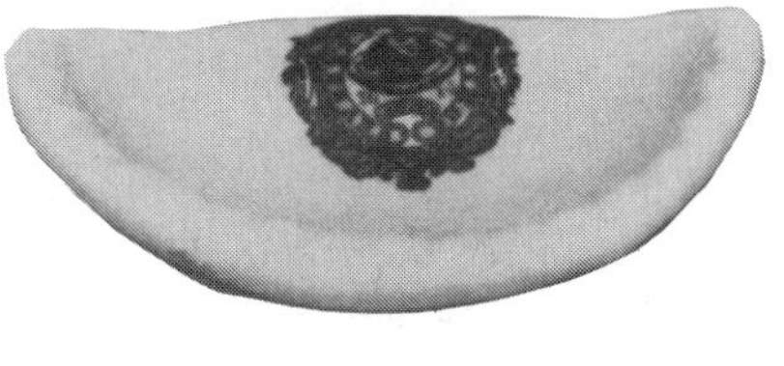

Cornish Pasty, coloured yellow – £95 and white – £80.

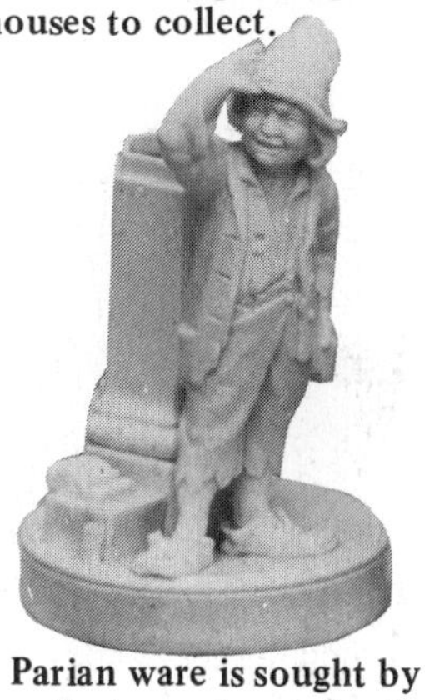

Parian ware is sought by collectors who prefer the earlier Goss made 1860 to 1900. This is the Bootblack spill holder, worth £350.

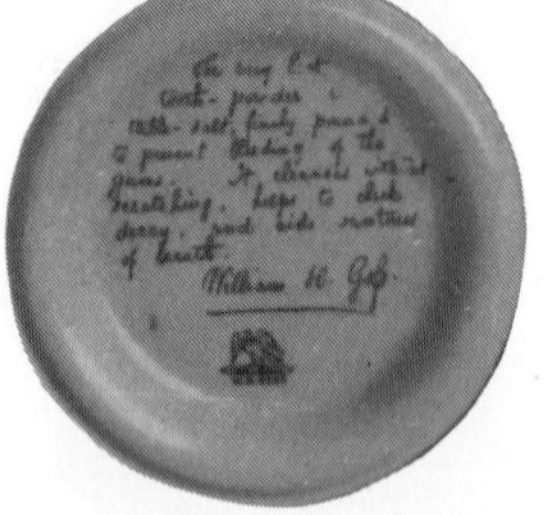

Toilet Salt Mortar in Gothic script in William Henry Goss' own handwriting. With pestle, it can fetch up to £75.

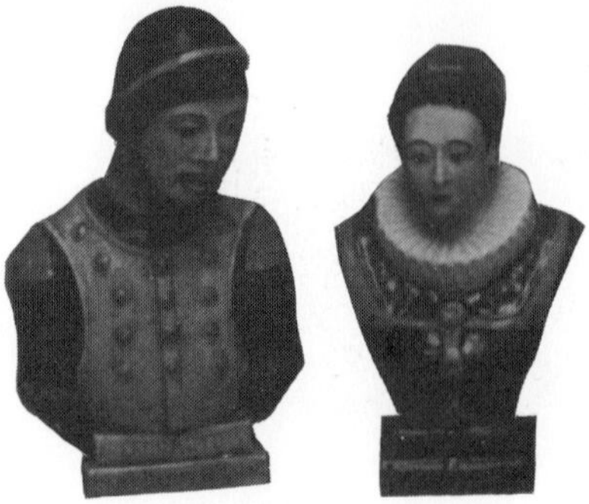

Peeping Tom and Ann Hathaway, coloured busts. £145 and £175
These would have been sold in Coventry and Stratford upon Avon.

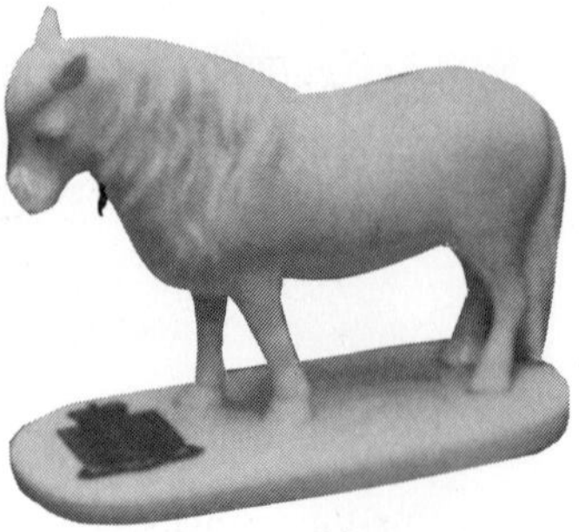

The Shetland Pony, length 103mm., and valued at £175.

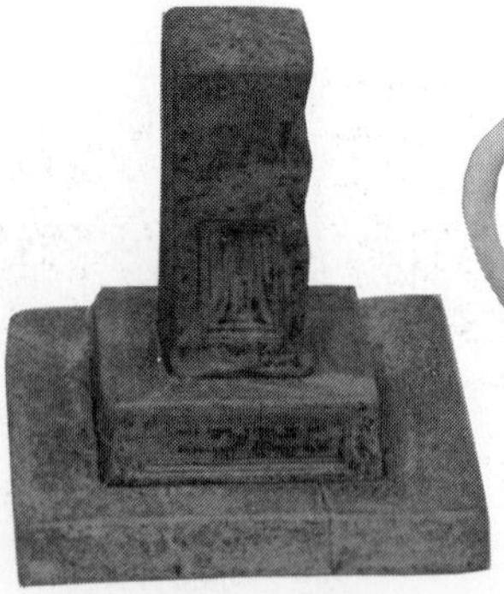

Hambledon Cricket Stone in grey. £830
Examples have changed hands for as much as £1,500 each.

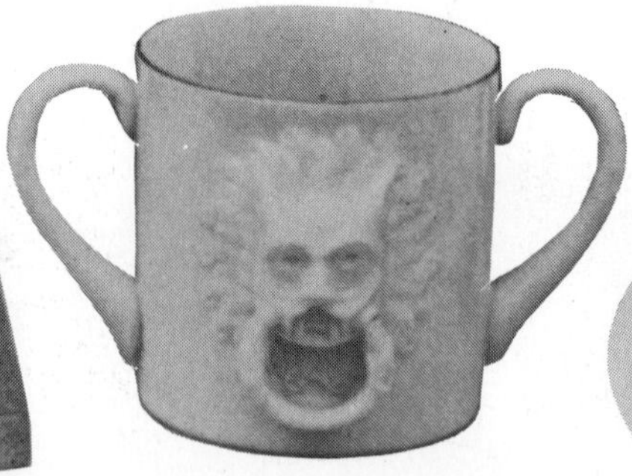

Durham Sanctuary Knocker Mug with gargoyle in relief, arms of Durham on reverse. £82

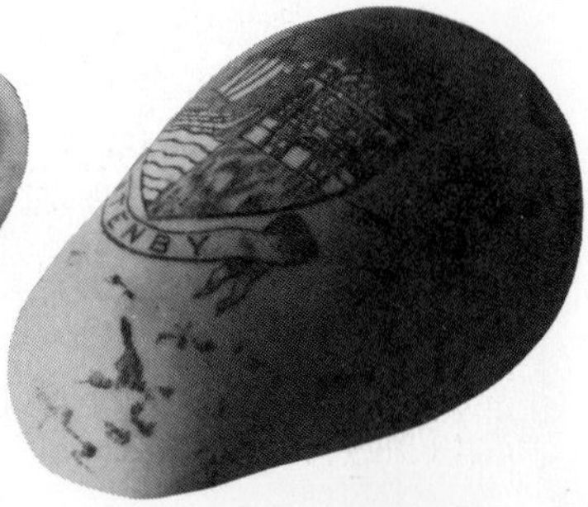

Guillemot Egg wall ornament. The pale green speckled wafer thin porcelain is deceptively strong. £50

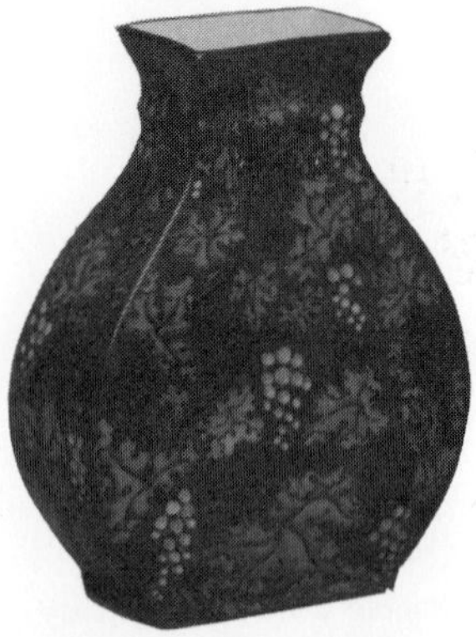

Flame coloured pear-shaped vase with grapevine decoration. £175

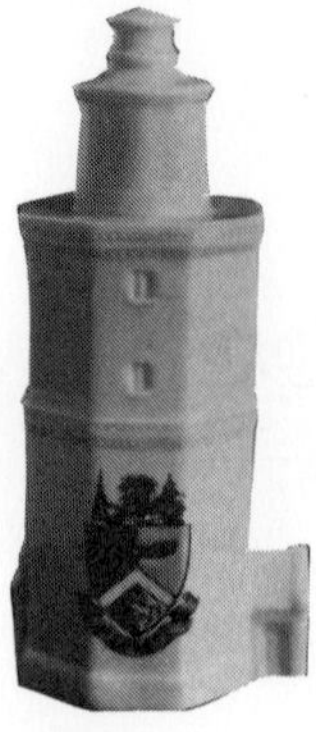

North Foreland Lighthouse, 108mm. high. This tiny porcelain replica is worth £50.

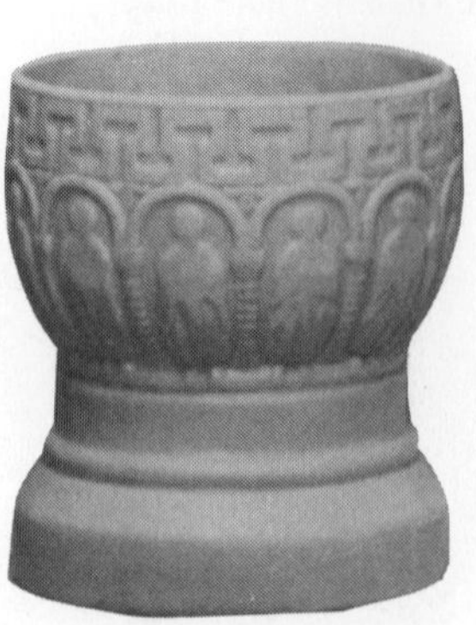

The Hereford Cathedral Font in white glazed parian. £145

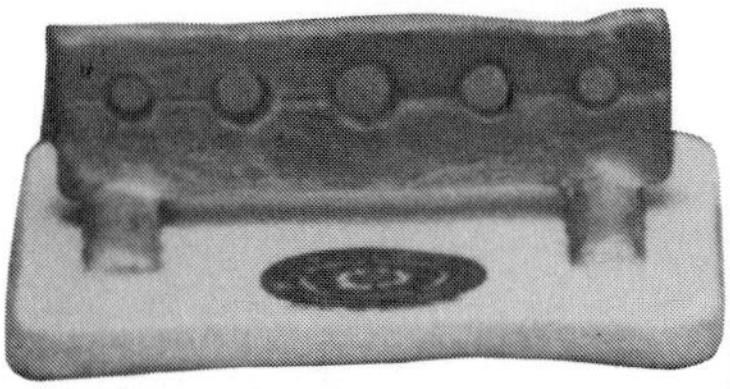

The Brading Stocks,
I.O.W. £160
The originals, like many Goss subjects, are still in existence.

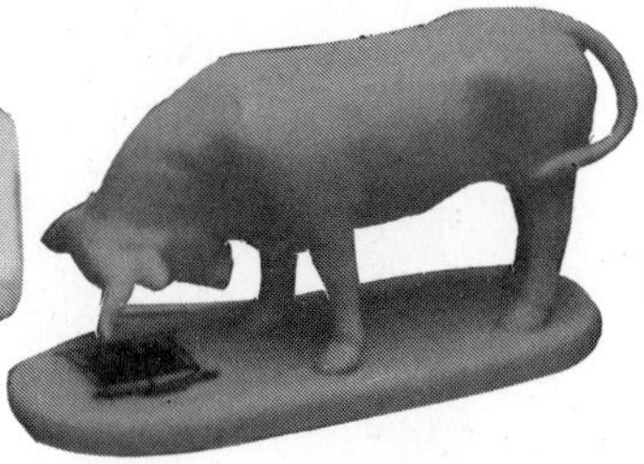

The Spanish Bull on oval plinth. £400

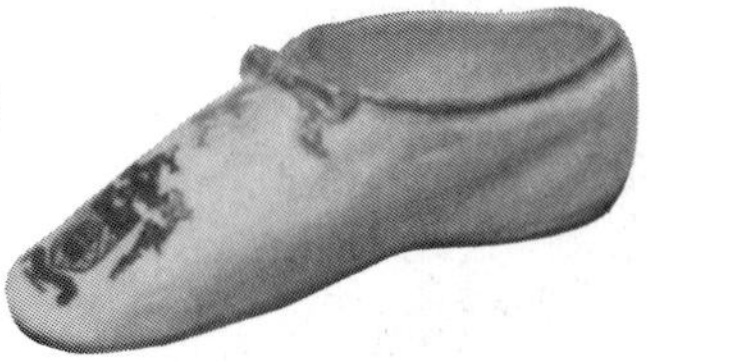

Queen Victoria's First Shoe, with beige sole and turquoise blue ribbon. £26

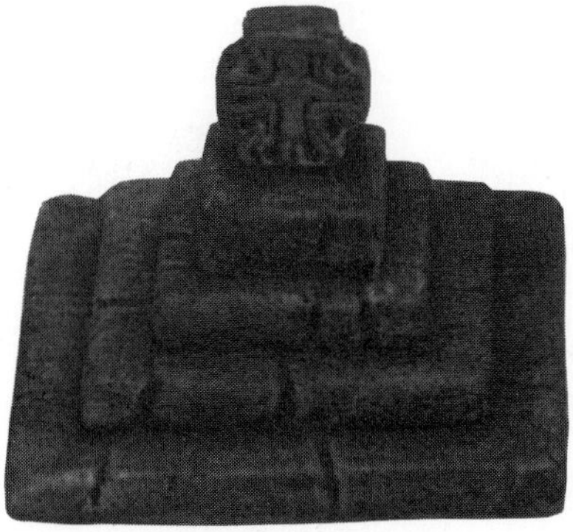

St. Buryan Cross in brown, tinged with green to represent stone. £100

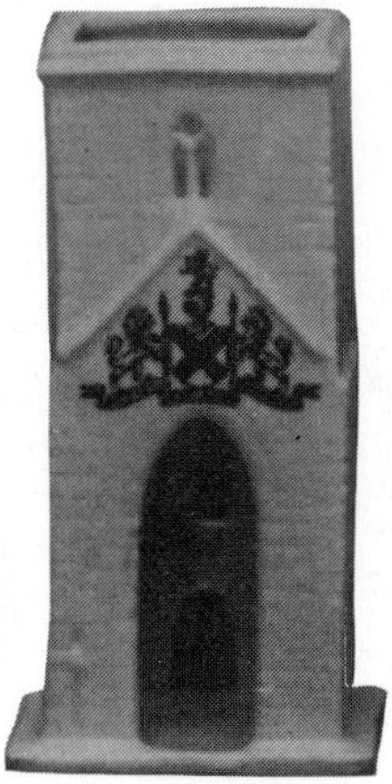

Windleshaw Chantry, a souvenir of the 1920 Church Bazaar, St. Helens, Lancashire. £145

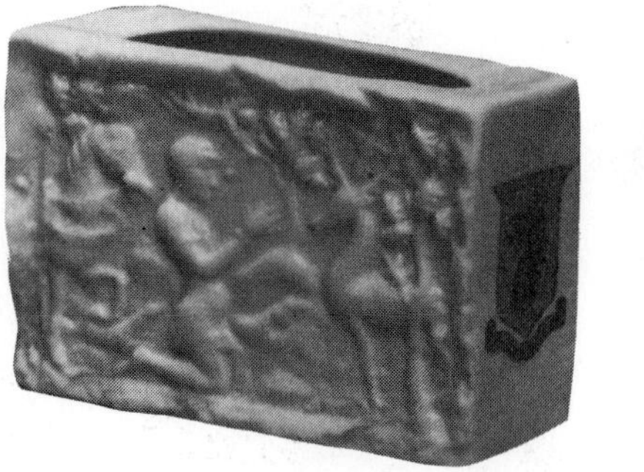

This is no ordinary brick but the Goss Denbigh Brick, white glazed with coats of arms of Barmouth and Denbigh. £88

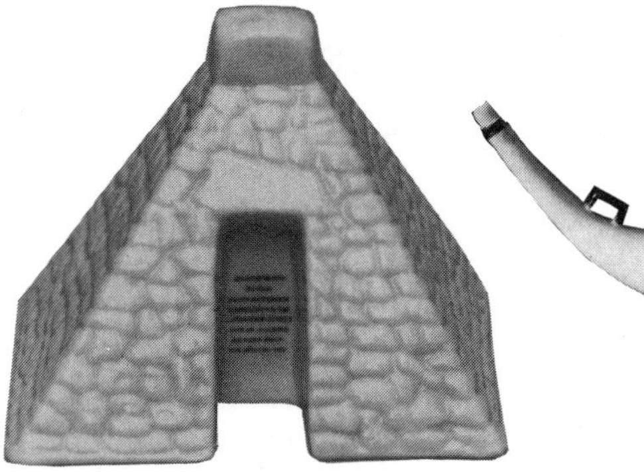

King Richard's Well Cover.
£215
One of the more elusive crested buildings.

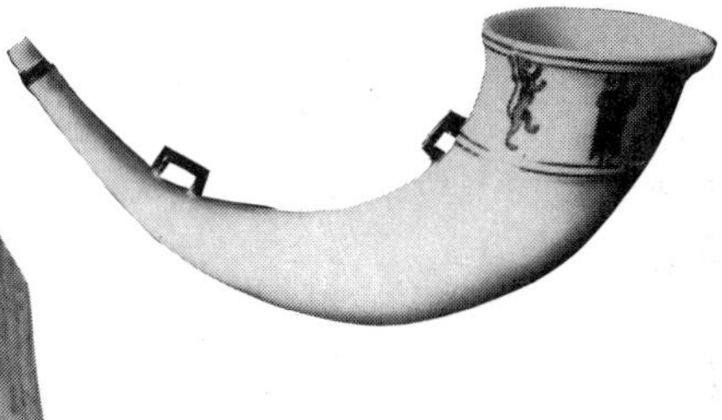

Winchester Castle Warden's Horn. A slim, delicate piece only 152mm. long.
£175

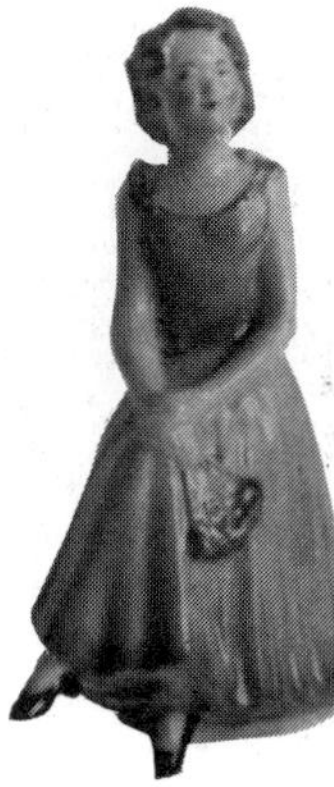

1930's Flower Girl 'Daisy', in yellow and green flapper dress, valued at £160.

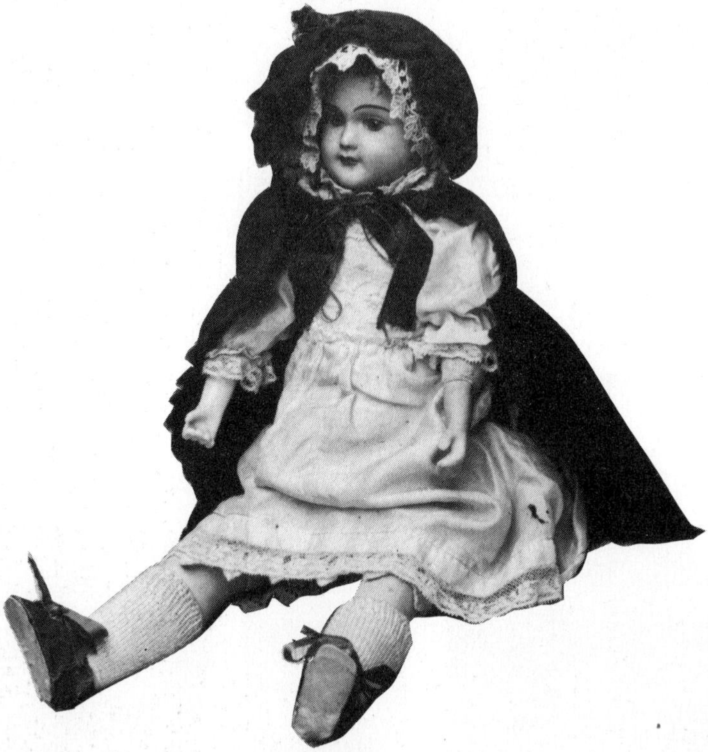

Little girl Goss doll with real hair, porcelain arms, head and legs. £400

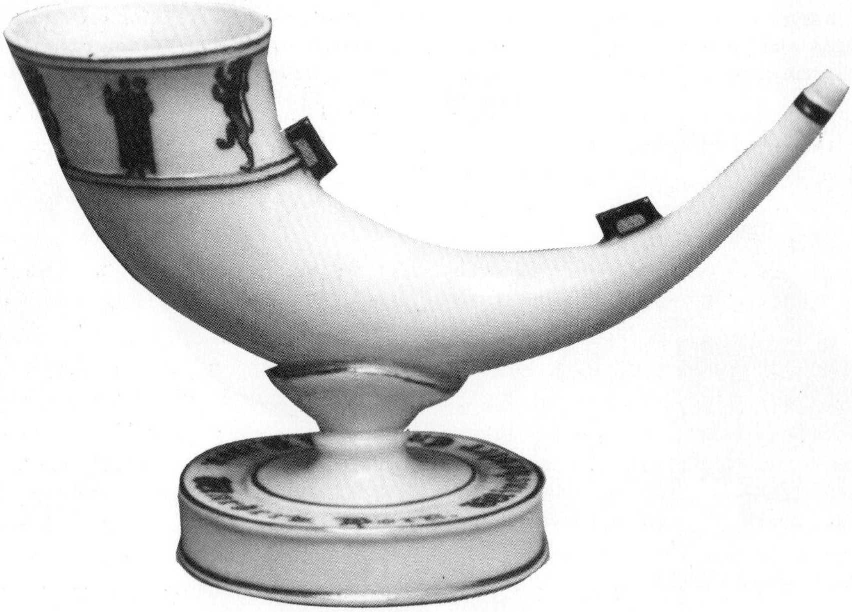

Winchester Castle Warden's Horn on plinth. £300

CASH-IN ON COLLECTING

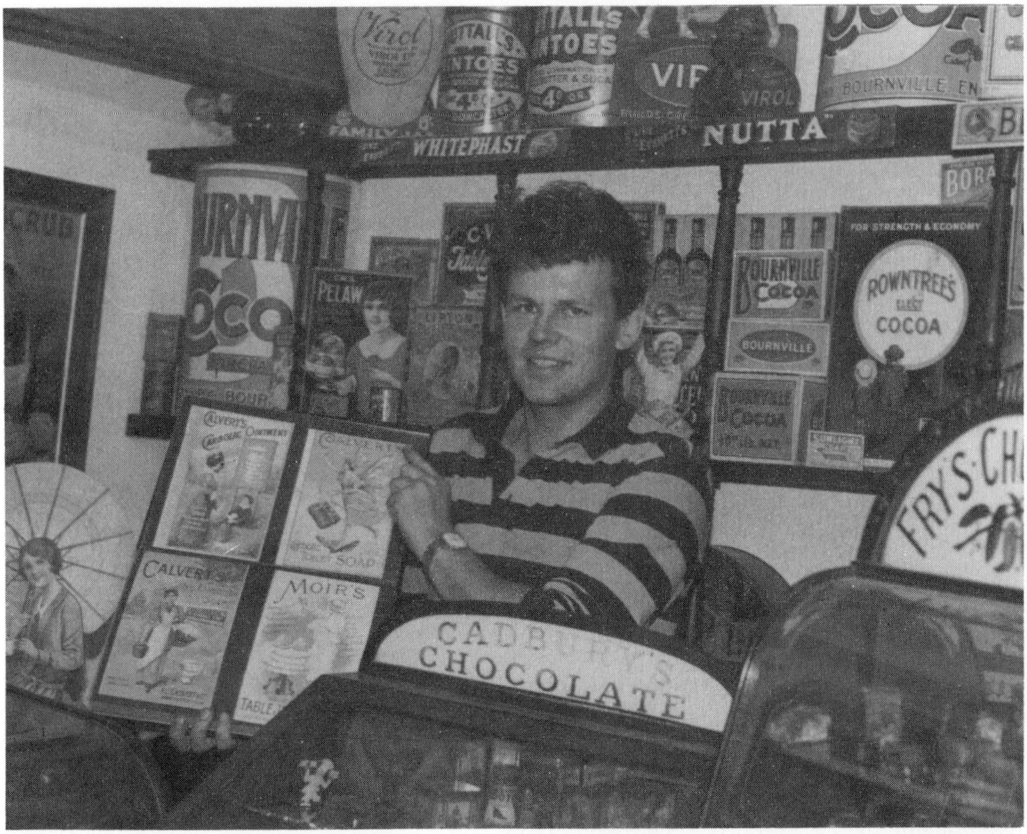

Simon Warden lives in Darlington and collects old advertising inserts.

"I got into collecting old advertising items first because I used to go digging for bottles and I extended my interest into collecting advertising for the things I found.

"I have enamel signs from the front of shops, showcards, cutouts and advertising packaging but the magazine inserts are a collection in their own right and I now have over 200 of them.

"My particular interest is chromolitho printing which was used for many of the inserts but is too expensive to be used today. It gave a very wide range and intensity of colour that modern printing cannot match.

"My collection covers the period between the 1880's and the 1920's for that was the start of the really big consumer boom and manufacturers started to be aware of the value of advertising. Many companies had their own commercial artists, men like Tom Brown, Will Owen and John Hassell. The inserts they designed were glued between the pages of magazines like 'The Strand', 'Chambers' Journal' and 'The Handyman'. The strange thing is that most of the inserts advertised soap but I have also got some for paints and carpets."

There has been little research into Simon's speciality and he says that is part of the excitement — 'not knowing what's going to turn up'. It is a fairly inexpensive category of collecting because an insert can cost between £2 and £6 depending on its condition and its subject matter. Inserts featuring children or black people are most sought after. Simon said that part of the enjoyment he gets from his collection is seeing the change in social attitudes reflected in the methods of advertising in the past.

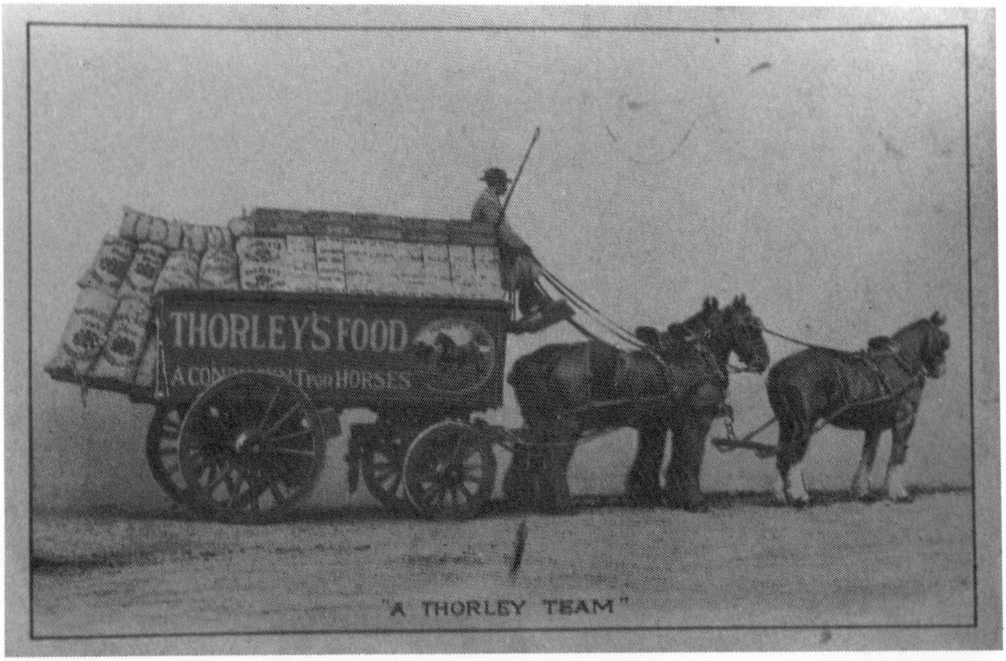

'A Thorley Team', Thorley's Food. £3 – £5

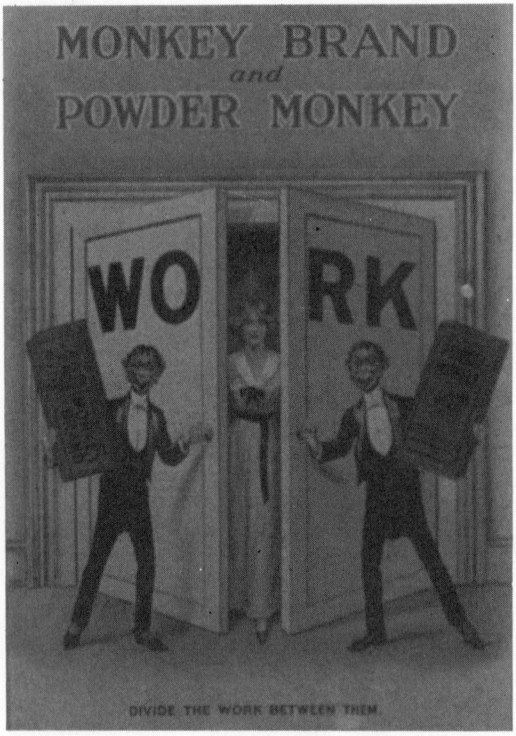

Monkey Brand and Powder Money, Divide The Work Between Them. £3 – £5

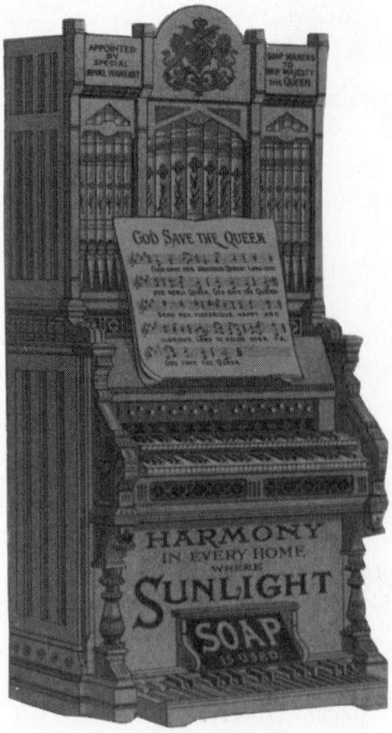

Harmony in Every Home Where Sunlight Soap Is Used, organ circa 1890. £5 – £8

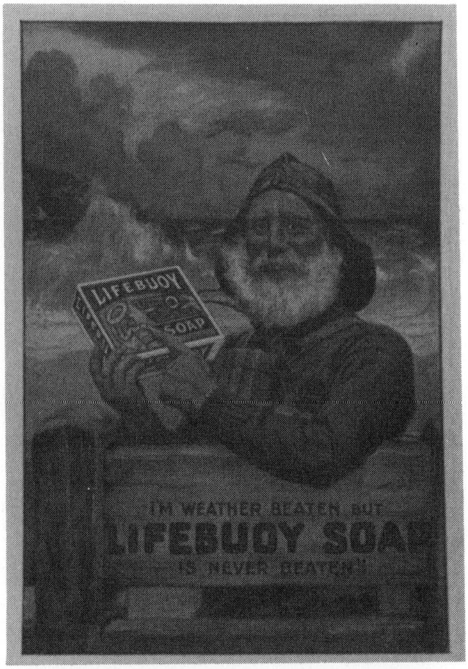

I'm Weather Beaten But Lifebuoy Soap Is Never Beaten, illustrator G. E. Robinson. £2.50 – £5

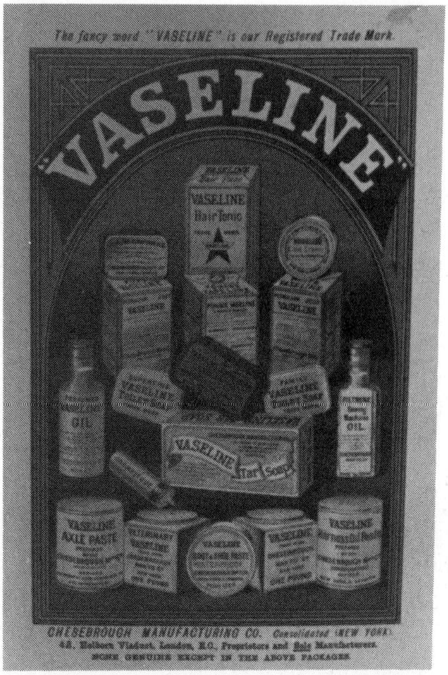

The fancy word 'Vaseline' is our Registered Trade Mark, 1889. £5

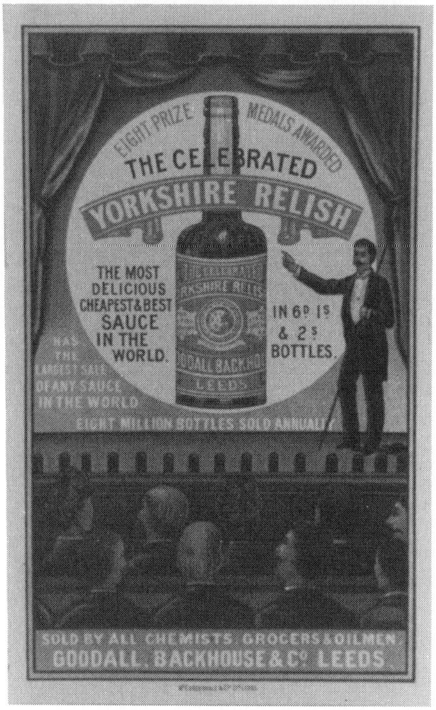

The Celebrated 'Yorkshire Relish', late Victorian four page insert. £4 – £7

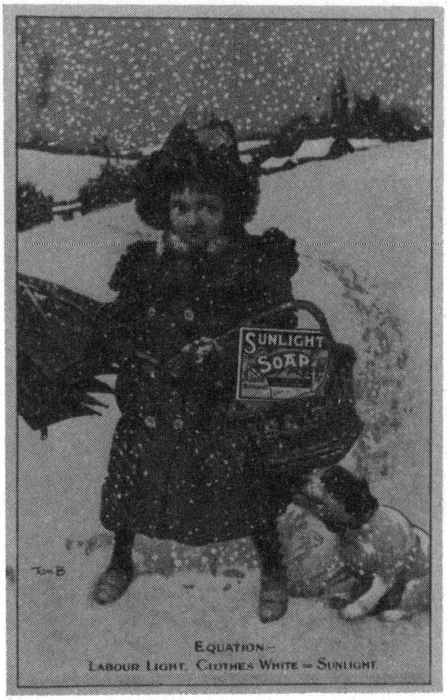

'Sunlight Soap' Equation – Labour Light, Clothes White – Sunlight, illustrator Tom Browne. £2.50 – £5

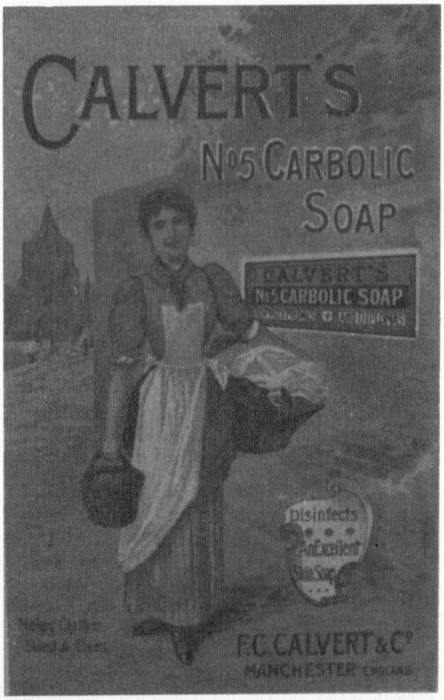

'Calvert's Carbolic Soap', Makes Clothes Sweet & Clean, late Victorian insert. £5 – £7

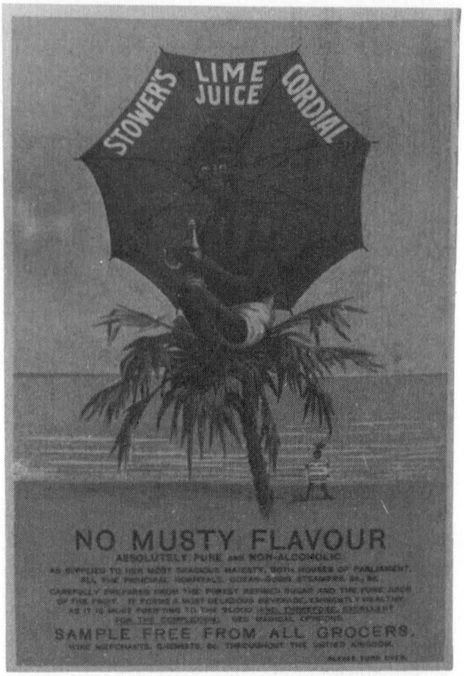

Stower's Lime Juice Cordial, illustrates the change in social attitudes and this advert would not be accepted today. £3 – £5

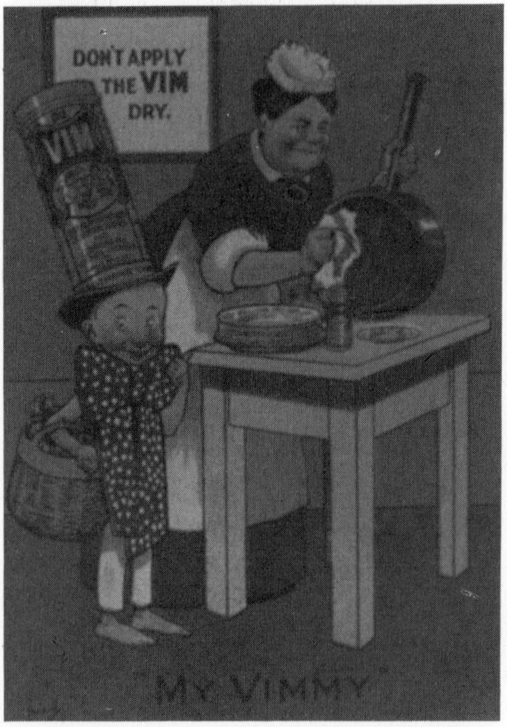

'My Vimmy', Don't Apply the Vim Dry, illustrator John Hassall, 1912. £3 – £5

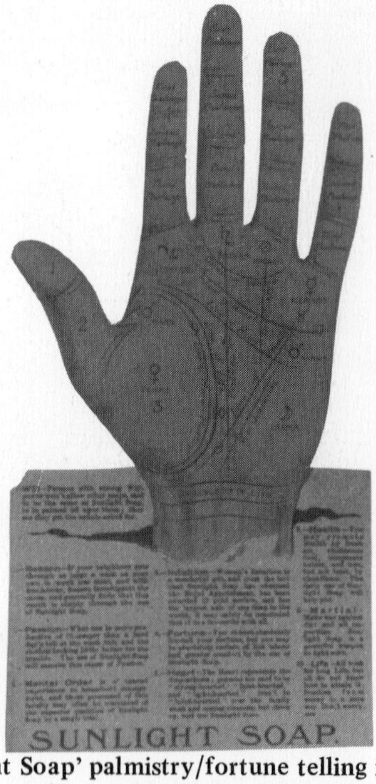

'Sunlight Soap' palmistry/fortune telling insert 1890, one of a number of Lever Bros. cut-outs. £5 – £8

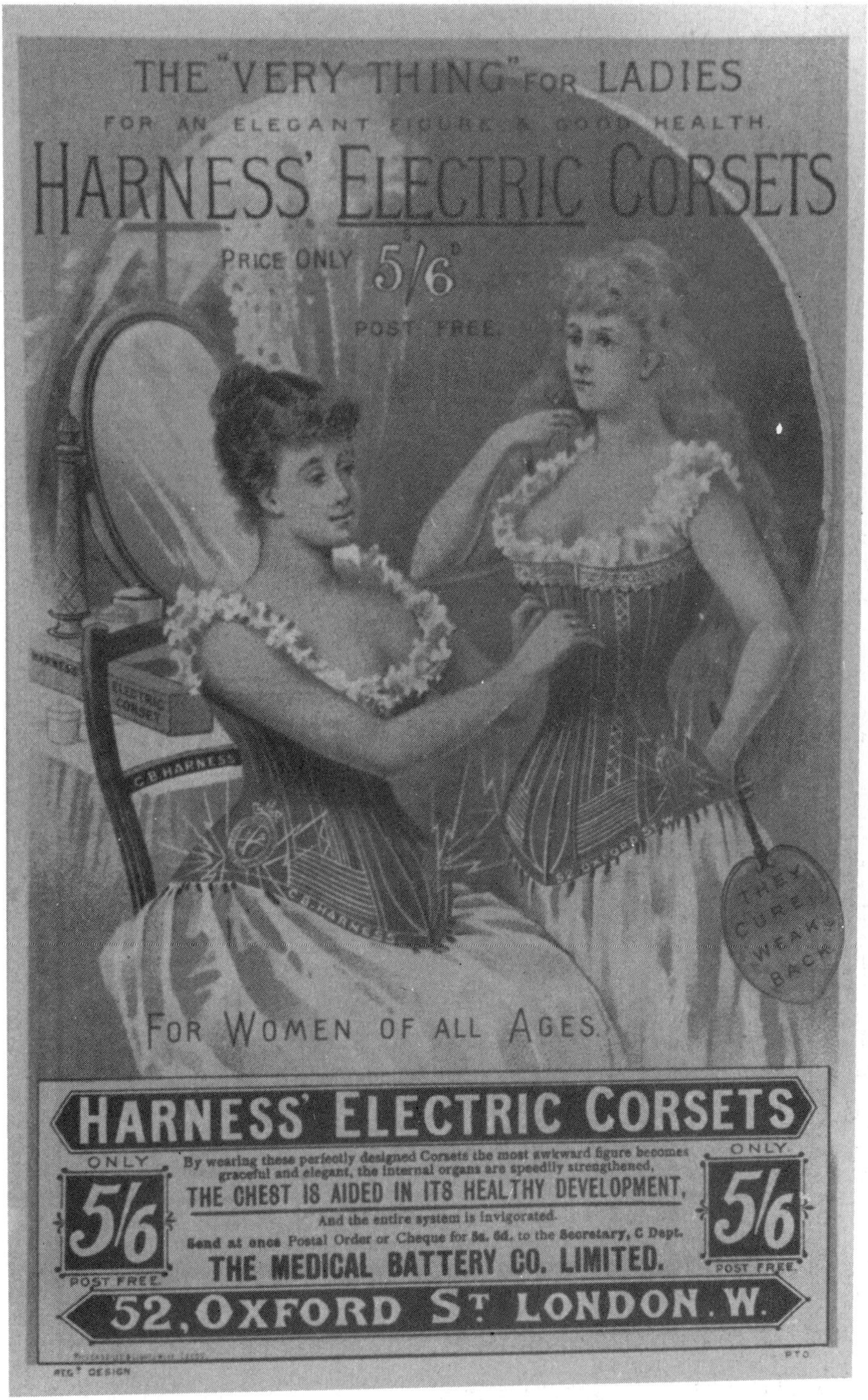

The 'Very Thing' for Ladies 'Harness' Electric Corsets, circa 1905. £3 – £5

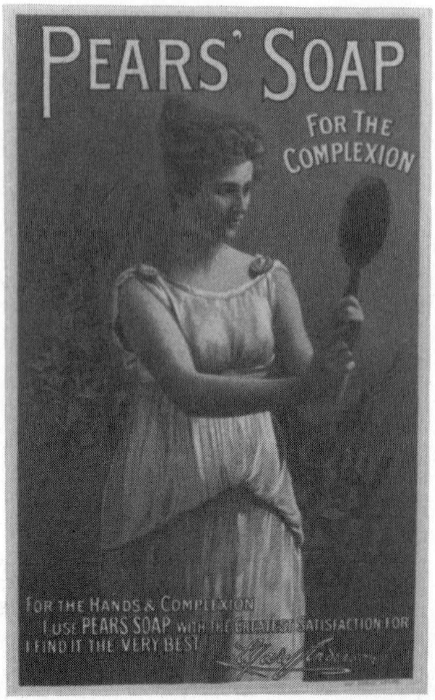

'Pear's Soap' For the Complexion. £4 – £7

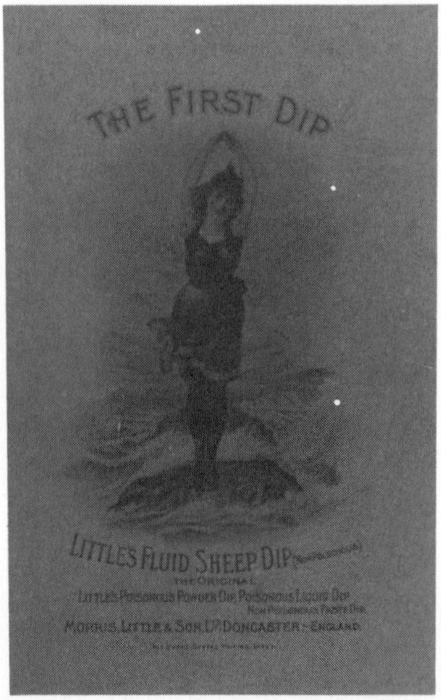

Little's Fluid Sheep Dip, delightful farming insert with regional appeal to S. Yorkshire. £4

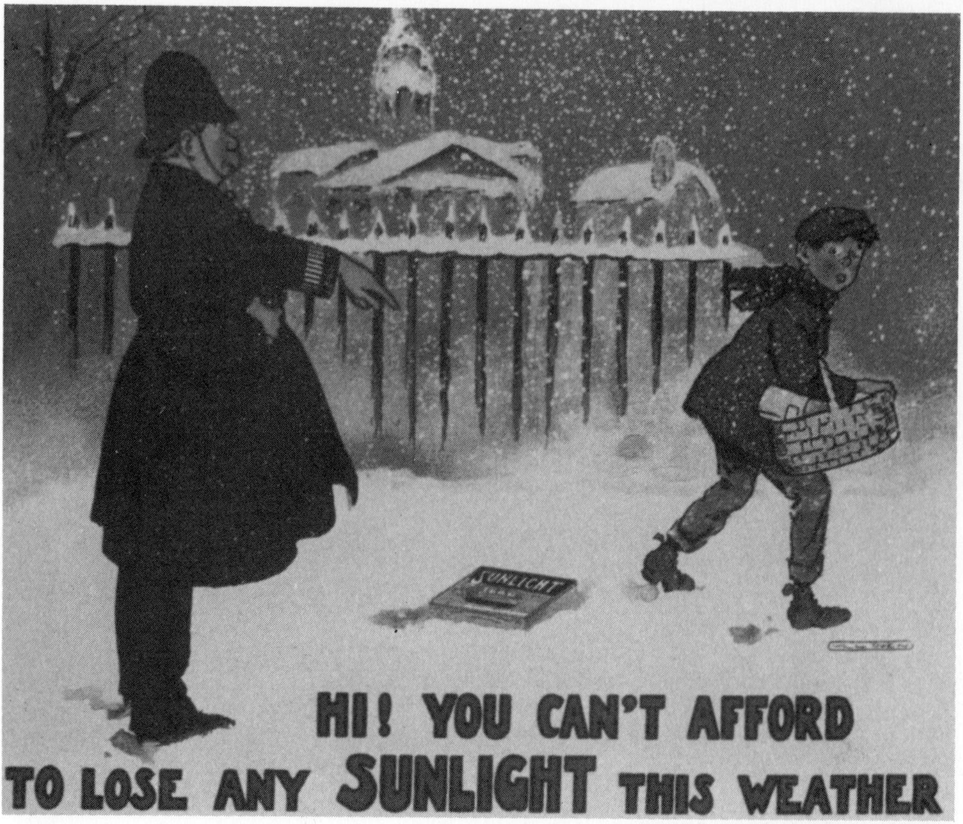

Hi! You Can't Afford To Lose Any Sunlight This Weather, illustrator Will Owen. £2.50 – £5

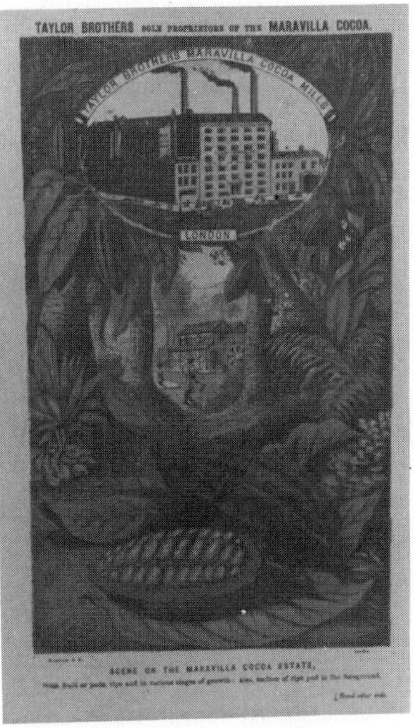

'Maravilla Cocoa', scene on the Maravilla Cocoa Estate, circa 1868. £5

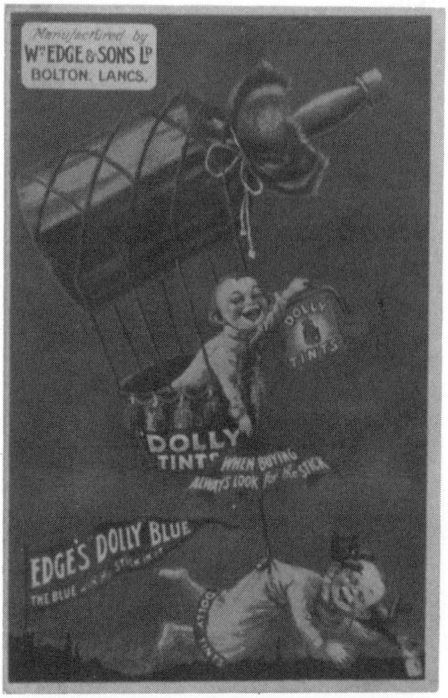

'Dolly Tints', Manufactured by Wm. Edge & Sons Ltd., Bolton, Lancs., circa 1910. £4 – £6

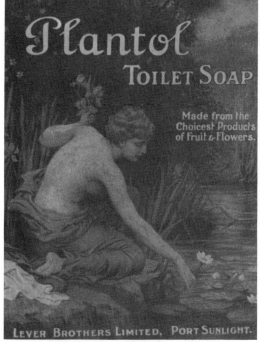

'Plantol' Toilet Soap, Made from the Choicest Products of Fruit & Flowers, circa 1905. £2.50 – £5

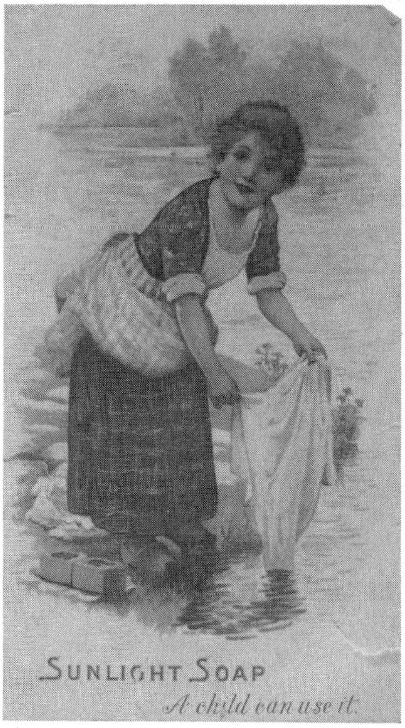

'Sunlight Soap', A child can use it. £5 – £8

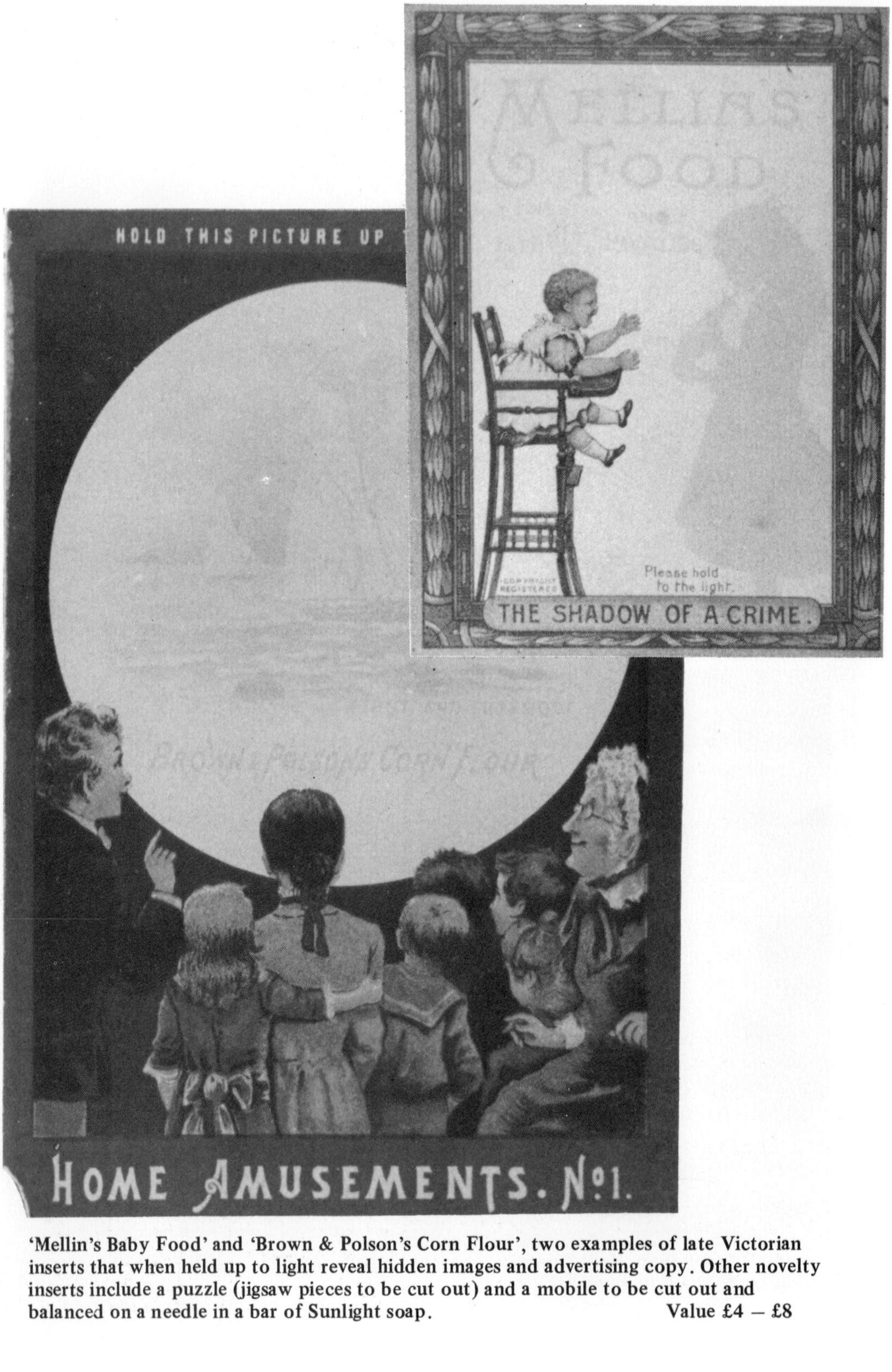

'Mellin's Baby Food' and 'Brown & Polson's Corn Flour', two examples of late Victorian inserts that when held up to light reveal hidden images and advertising copy. Other novelty inserts include a puzzle (jigsaw pieces to be cut out) and a mobile to be cut out and balanced on a needle in a bar of Sunlight soap. Value £4 – £8

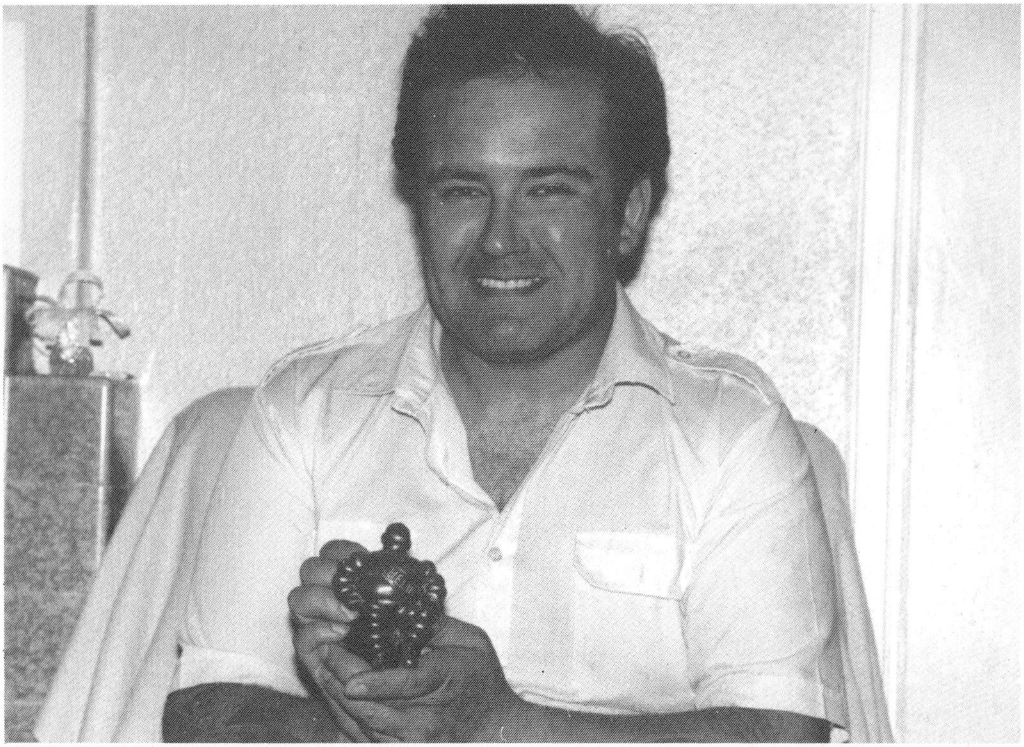

Graham Keene works as an aircraft plumber and collects rubber tyre type ashtrays.

"It all started when I was a young lad and used to have my hair cut at a local barber's where there was one of those ashtrays. I was very interested in everything to do with motoring and the ashtray in the barber's shop was a real miniature tyre, made with every attention to detail. It fascinated me and I always remembered it.

"Then about five years ago, in a street market in Devon I bought a rubber tyre ashtray and my wife suggested that I should start collecting them."

Now he has over 90 different types of rubber tyre ashtrays which were originally issued by tyre making companies as advertising material. His collection includes tyres from all over the world — Korea, Poland, Czechoslovakia, USA and Japan.

The price range can vary from 10p for an ashtray bought in a car boot sale to £8 which Graham paid for an 1920's Indian tyre . . . "the price was high because it was of sentimental value to the man who owned it. It came from the family of Raymond Mays who developed Ford car engines for racing."

He is keen to contact other collectors who would want to swap examples because, as he says, "I've lots of spare tyres!"

The type of ashtray Graham would most want to add to his collection is a Michelin which is uncommon.

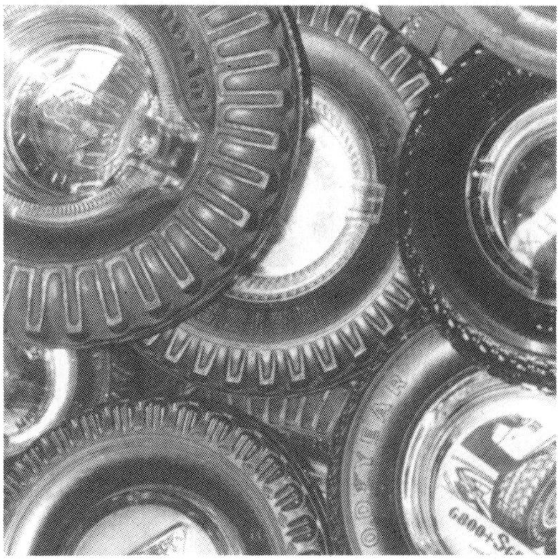

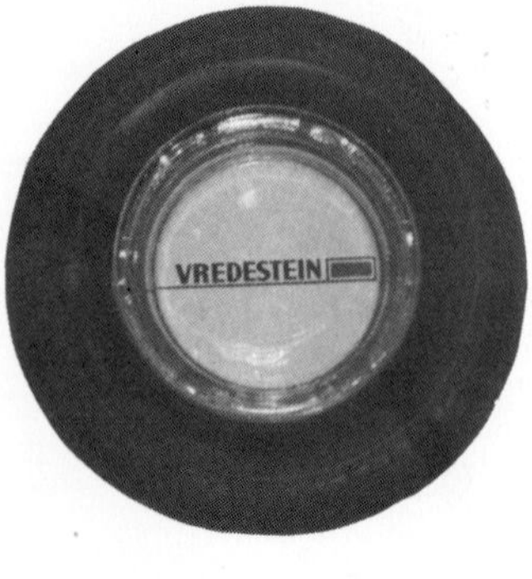

A Vredestein economy radial tyre, in current production. £2 – £3

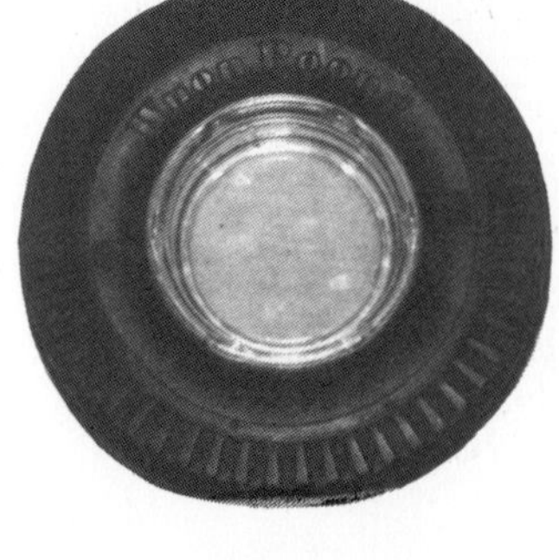

An ashtray advertising 'Wuon-Poong' from Korea, rare. £10

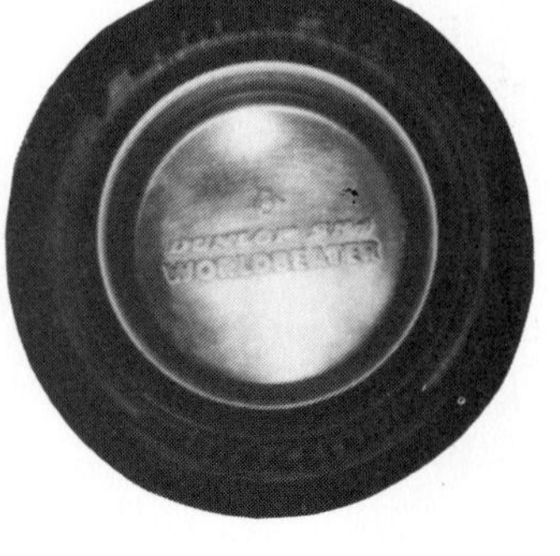

Modern Dunlop SP4 with embossed aluminium insert, £4 – £5

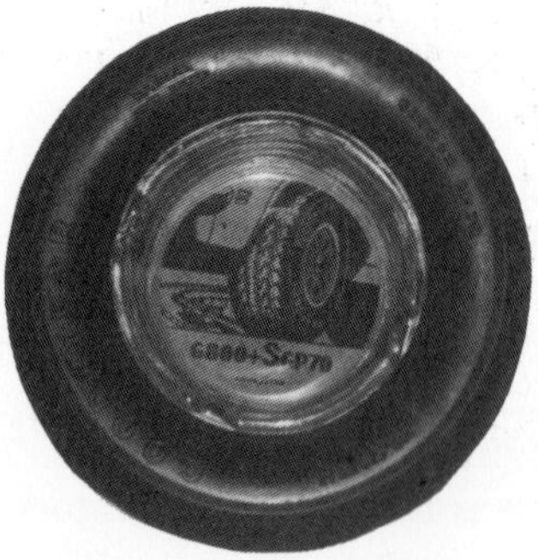

Goodyear G800 + SGP70, 1970's, radial with pictorial insert. £4

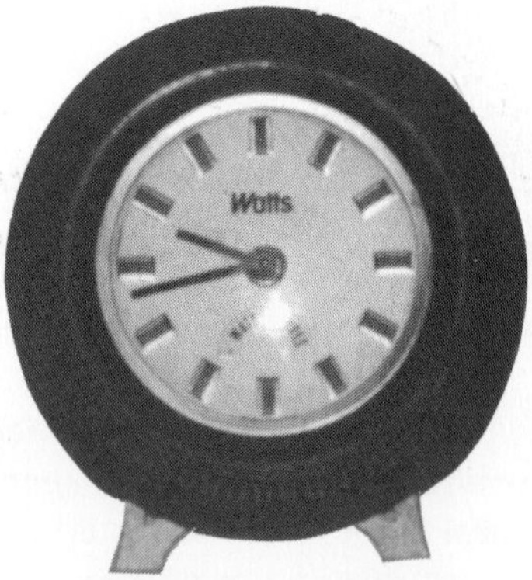

A desk clock from Watts Tyre & Rubber Co. of Gloucestershire, in working order. £15

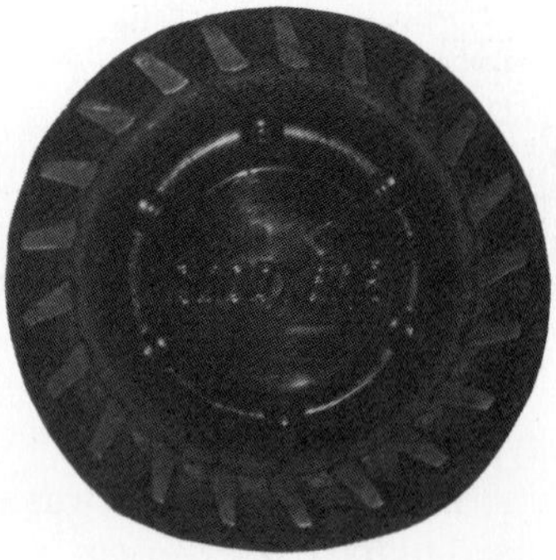

A Goodyear tractor tyre with amber glass insert, circa 1950. £6

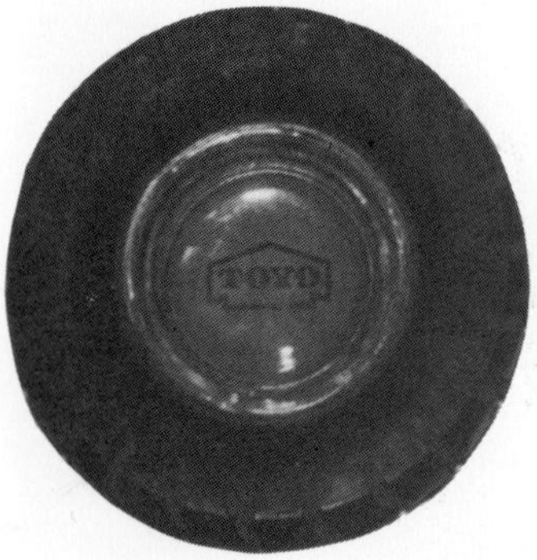

A 'Toyo' off-the-road commercial tyre from Japan, rare. £10

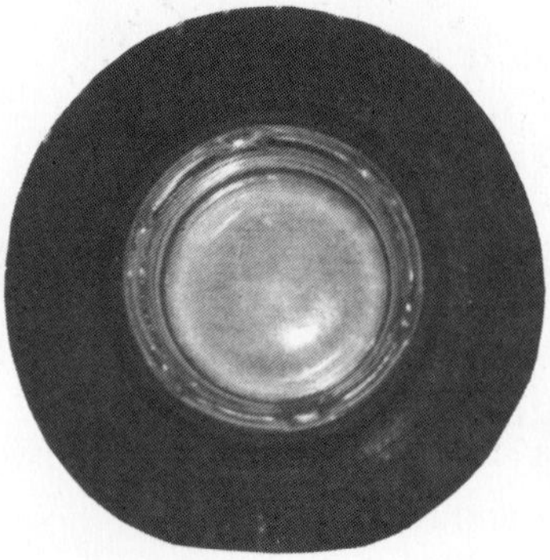

A Watts 'monomatic' ashtray, these tyres are used on forklift trucks. £3.50

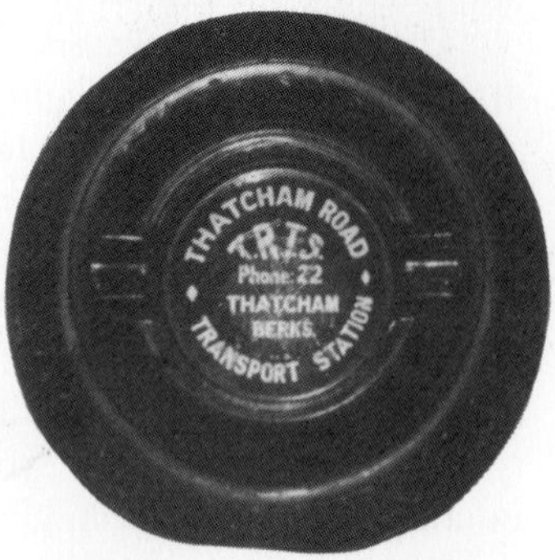

An early 'Firestone' ashtray, advertising the Thatcham Road Transport Station. £6

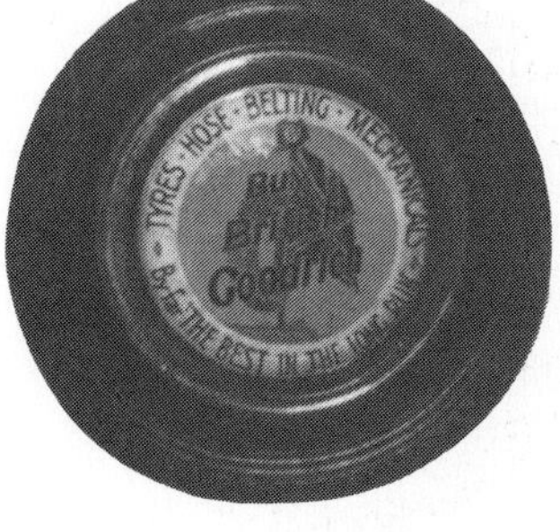

Buy British Goodrich, from Leyland in Lancashire, circa 1920's. £8 – £10

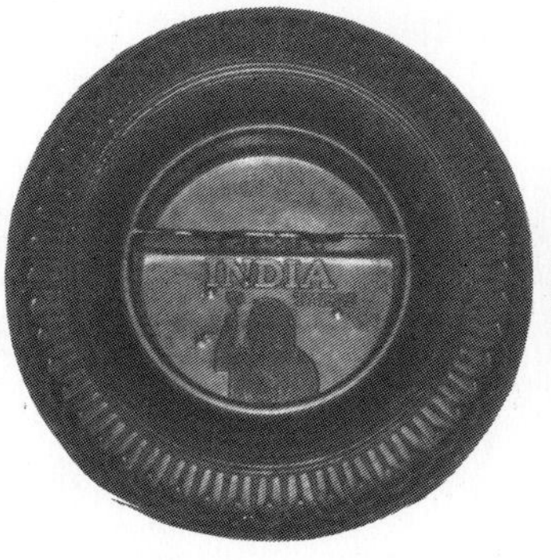

An India called 'Britannia', she is embossed on the insert, made of bakelite, 1930's. £8 – £10

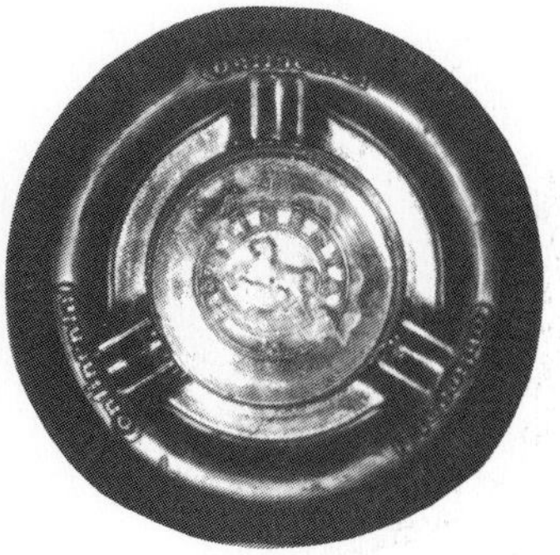

An exceptionally large Continental tyre ashtray, 9½in. diam. The standard size is approx. 5½in. £7 – £8

A Goodyear 'NCT' rally tyre, in current production. £3.75

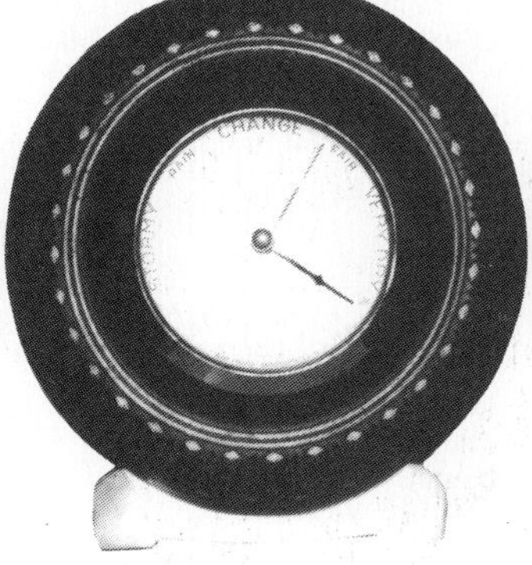

Goodyear barometer, fitted with one variety of Goodyear 'Eagle' tyre. £10

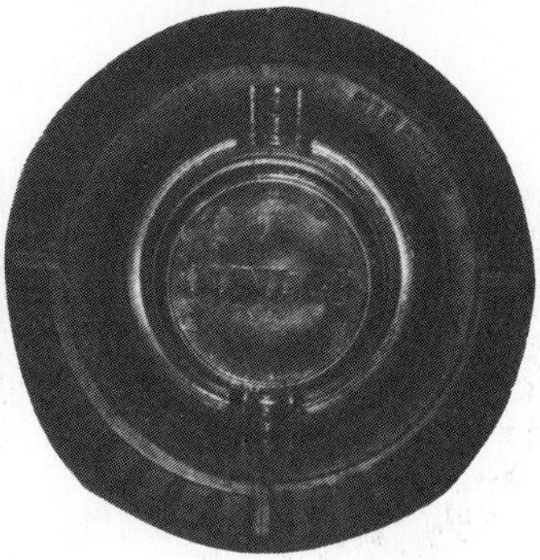

An unusual four in one Dunlop ashtray, circa 1940/50. £10

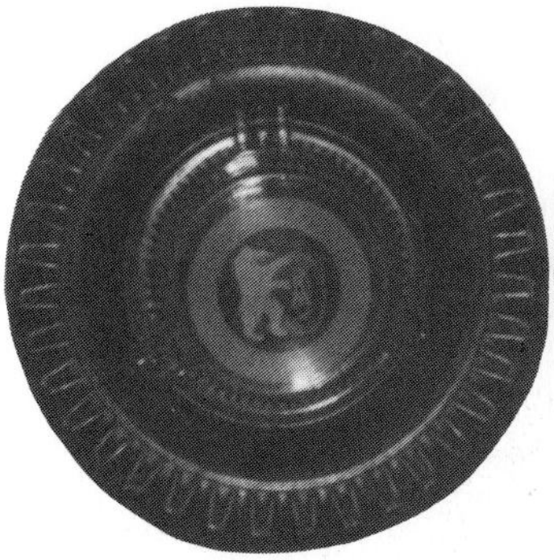

A Metzler from West Germany showing their prancing animal logo, in colour. £5

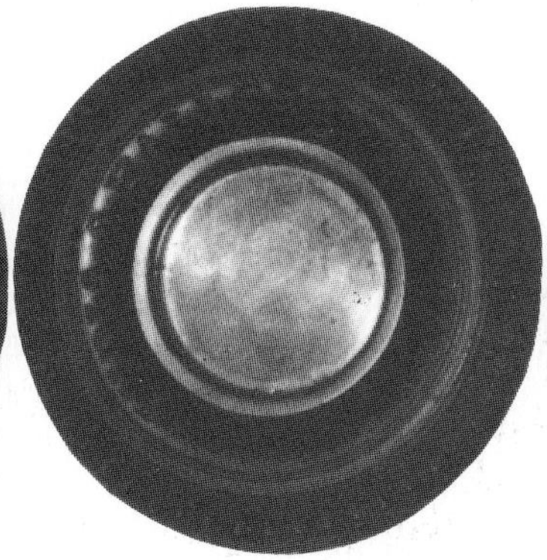

An India 'balloon' with a red band on the side wall and fitted with a copper insert, 1920's. £10

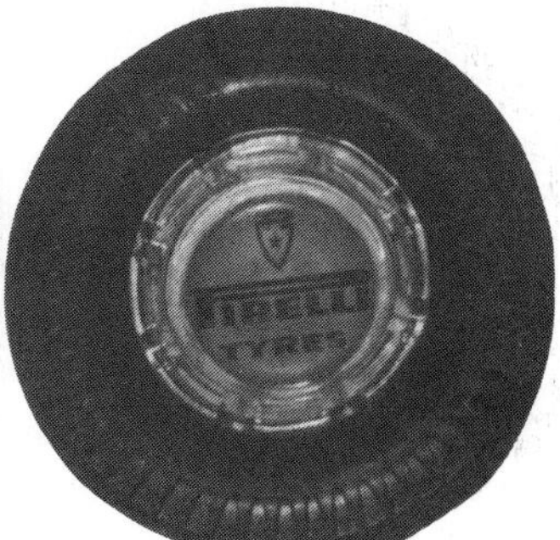

A pictorial 'Pirelli' of the late 1950's and 1960's. £5

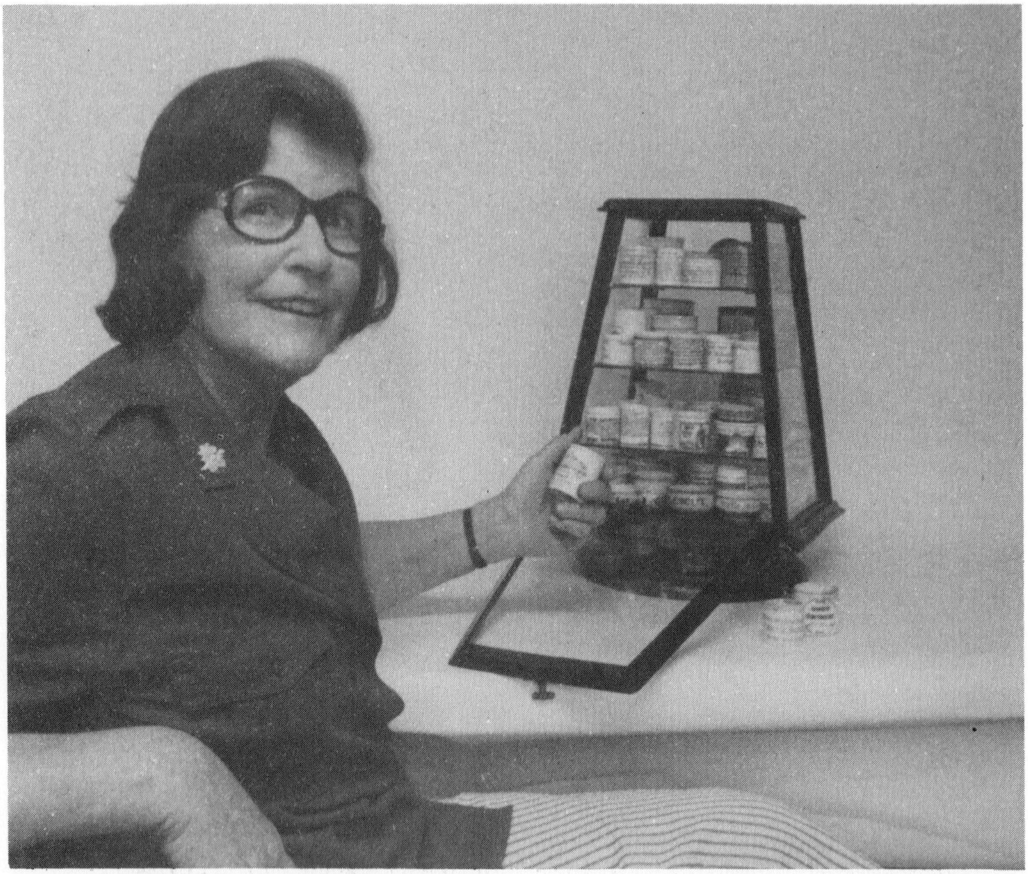

Dr Anne Young is a retired psychiatrist and collects medical items.

"I started by collecting early domestic medicine chests. Some people describe them wrongly as apothecaries' chests but they were really the precursors of our modern bathroom cabinets and held bottles of medicines or their constituents and a mortar and pestle etc. Families used to travel with them and they vary in style a good deal but they are all beautifully made. The majority are made in wood, mahogany or walnut, but there are some 18th century ones which are covered in fish skin. Some are bound with brass or silver. They went out of use at the end of the 19th century when specific cures came along and tablets were invented.

"My interest began because when I was a medical student my father gave me a little medicine chest as a present and I used it for keeping cosmetics in but one day I wrote to the Arthur Negus radio programme about my little box and he told me what it was. He said on the radio: 'Now this would be a splendid subject for you as a doctor to collect'.

"This was all very well but I soon found that although one can find tiny homeopathic boxes from around £20, the orthodox or allopathic ones start at around £200 and can cost up to £1,000.

"So I cast around in the medical and quasi-medical fields and hit upon ointment pots which are small, easy to display, and cheap. In contrast to other countries we produced masses of them in Victorian times and they are found, all over the country, by energetic dump diggers. Some became nationally or even internationally famous like Holloway's ointment, others were made and sold in very restricted geographical areas. This means that one stands a good chance of finding a rare — even unique — example.

"Medicine chests were owned by the well-to-do and a lot is known already about medical facilities for the rich in pre-N.H.S. days. Much less is known about the poor, and one learns a bit about how the poorer people coped — or were conned — by studying these little pots."

Her ointment pots range from 16th century Delft ones to pots used for Holloway's ointment or Singleton's eye ointment in the 1920's.

The claims for cures printed on the pots are fascinating and in fact they are sometimes known as 'cure alls' but their downfall came when legislation was brought in making it necessary for all the constituents to be named on the receptacles. Also people became more informed and less gullible. They didn't believe what the cure alls said any longer.

"The favourite piece in my collection is an 18th century Delft 'ointment' with DELESCOT written on it in dark blue. Delescot was an apothecary who lived at 19 Duke Street, Pall Mall, London and he patented his 'Conserve of Myrtle Opiate' in 1749. Today the pot is worth about £200."

The advent of tubes for ointment in the 1920's meant that the use of the more expensive pots gradually disappeared. The item which Dr Young would most like to find for her collection is a one inch tall Delft pot with the picture of a bear on it. It held 'Bear's grease' and dates from the 17th century. An example of this pot was recently sold at auction for £700 though the majority of ointment pots cost less than £30. There are two less exotic pots she covets also, both with elaborate underglaze transfer lettering — "The Electrical Herbal" and "The Star Carbolic" ointments.

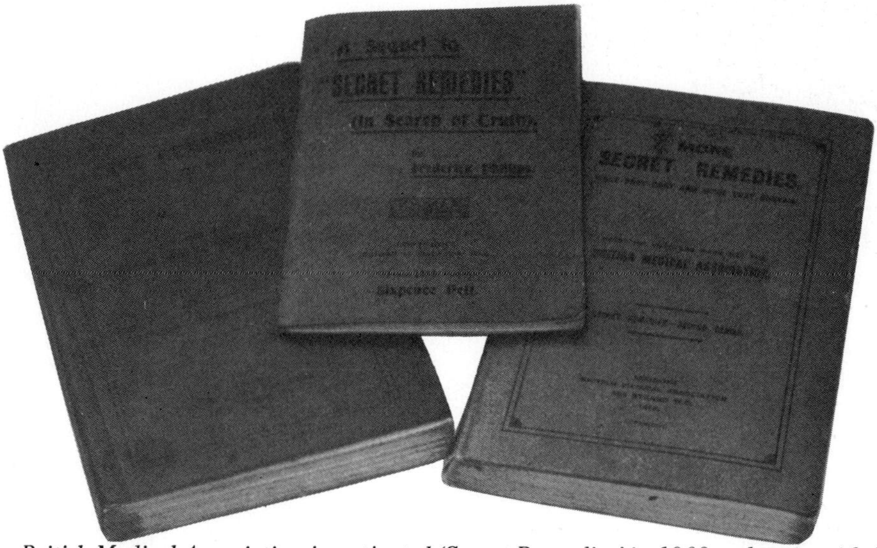

The British Medical Association investigated 'Secret Remedies' in 1909 and again with 'More Secret Remedies' in 1912. They analysed hosts of 'quack' cures, mainly draughts, pills and a few ointments. Their aim was to make the public aware of the unrealistic claims and also the enormous profits made by the vendors.
Singleton's for example, was found to contain 7.4% by weight of red mercuric oxide and cost, they estimated, 1/9th of a penny to produce, while it sold for two shillings.
'A Sequel to Secret Remedies', sub-titled 'In Search of Truth', written in 1910 by Frederick Phillips, a lecturer in Maths and Chemistry, rebuffed the B.M.A. findings however. He pointed out that the analysis of Singelton's was incomplete and anyway the medics used mercurial ointments for eye infections.

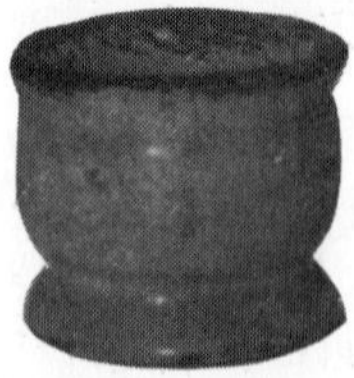

Pinkish tin glaze ointment pot, possibly 17th century, 1.1/8in. tall. £45

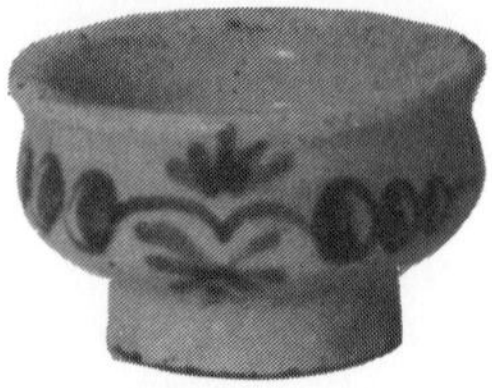

An early bluish glaze ointment pot with dark blue decoration, circa 1730. £70

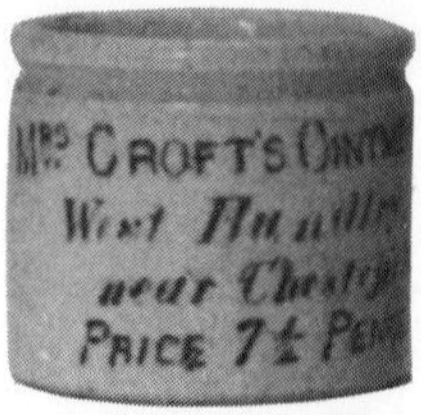

Mrs. Croft's Ointment, West Hanley, near Chesterfield. £15

Sturton's Poor Man's Cerate, Peterborough. £30

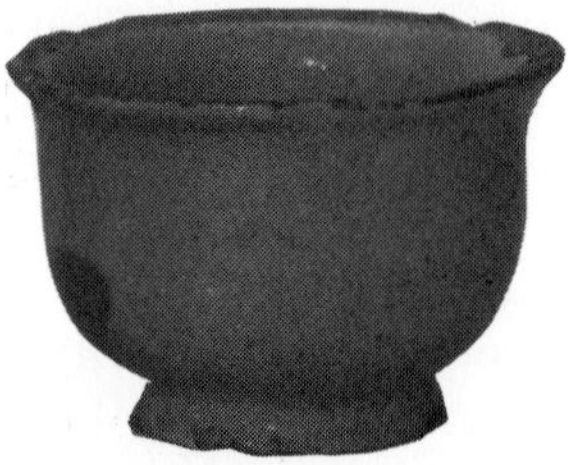

Bluish grey glaze ointment pot, circa 1730, 1.5/8in. high. £25

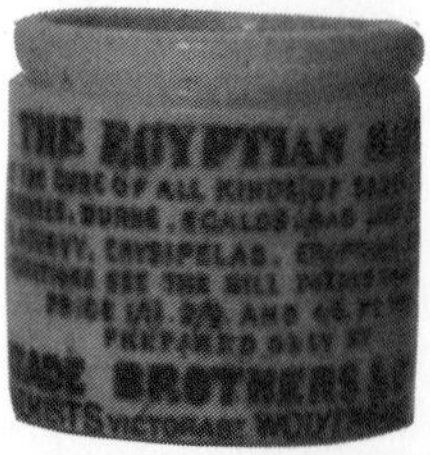

The Egyptian Salve, Wolverhampton, based on a recipe first recorded in the Ebers Papyrus in 1500 B.C., 1½in. high. £8

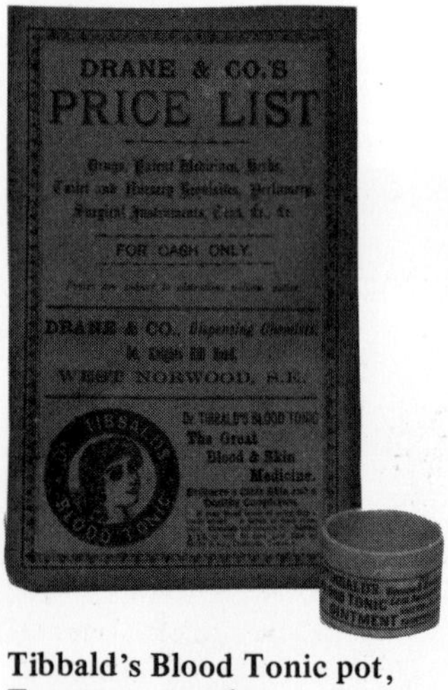

Tibbald's Blood Tonic pot, Taunton, complete with its advert, 1¼in. high. £25

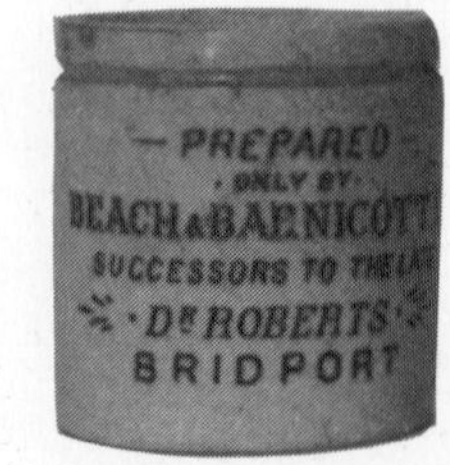

'Poor Man's Friend', sold by Beach & Barnicott, Bridport, circa 1840, 1¾in. high. £15

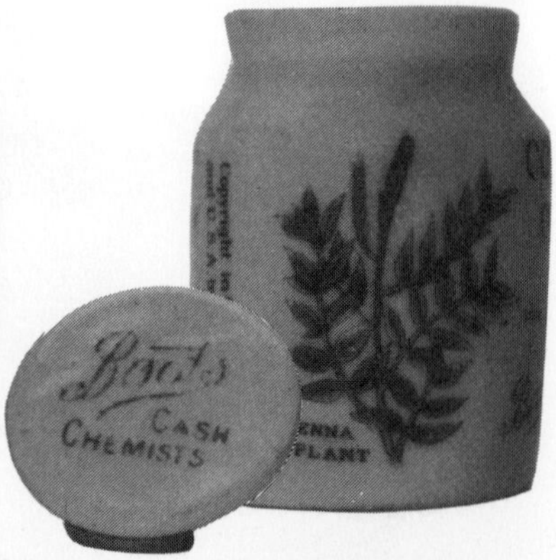

Boots 'Confection of Senna' pot with attractive fern decoration, 3¼in. high. £10

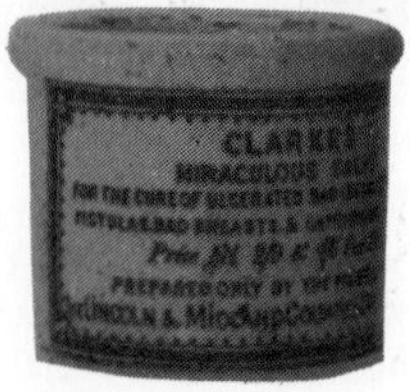

Clarke's Miraculous Salve, Lincoln, 'For the Cure of . . . , 1½in. high. £4

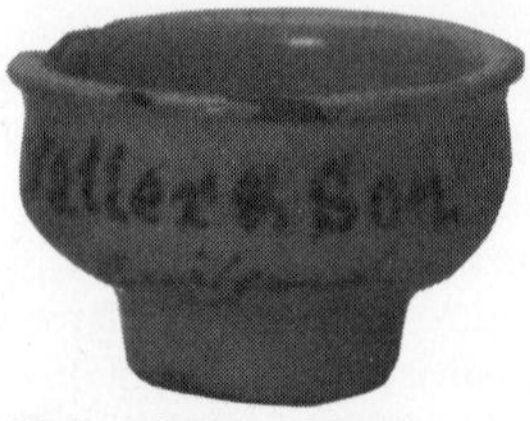

Waller & Son, bluish tin glaze pot, Guildford, Surrey, late 18th century. £150

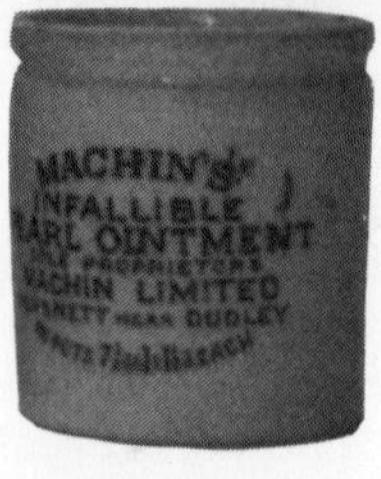

Machin's Infallible Pearl Ointment, Dudley. £20

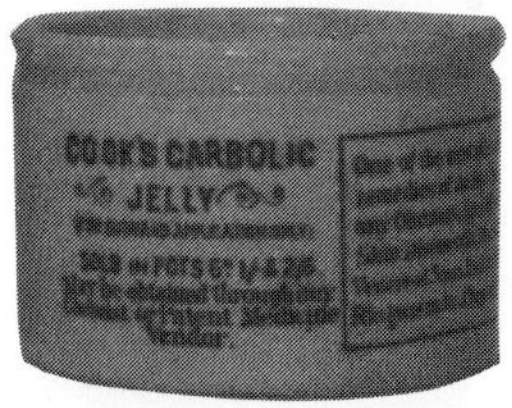

Cook's Carbolic Jelly, Nottingham, 1.1/8in. high. £40

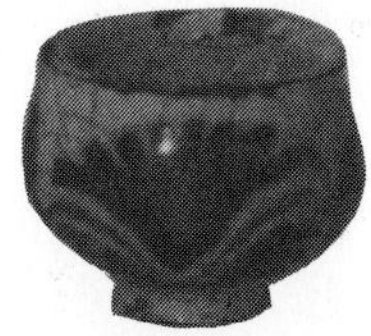

Small bluish glaze pot with dark blue decoration, circa 1700. £90

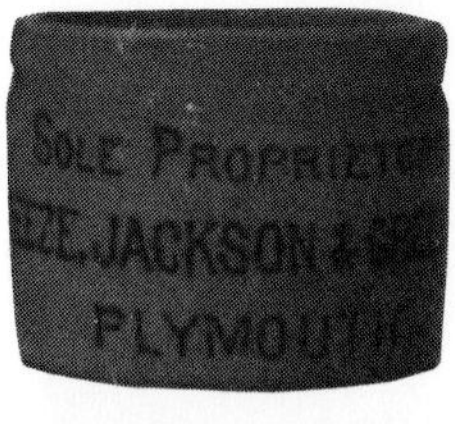

Handall's Celebrated Ointment, Plymouth. £25

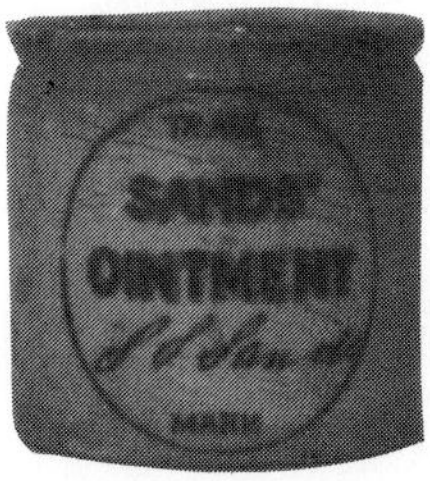

Sands' Ointment, 1½in. high. £35

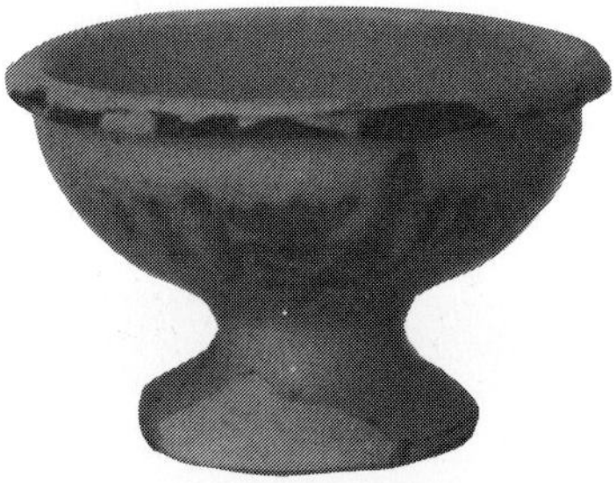

An early bluish glaze pot with dark blue decoration, circa 1780. £55

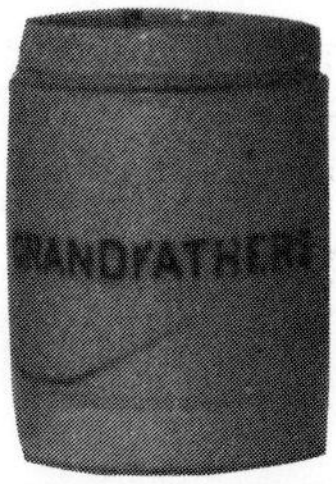

Grandfather's Ointment. £30

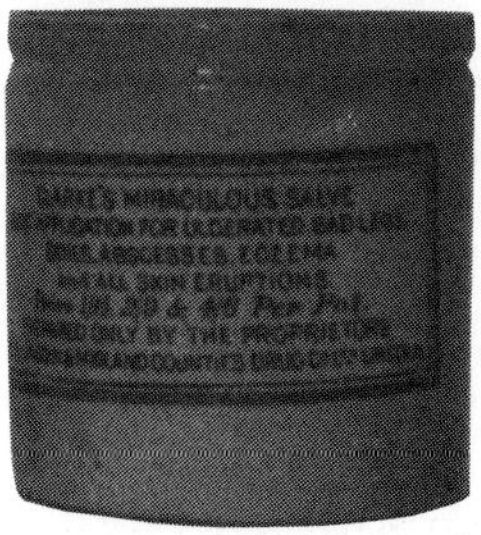

Clarke's Miraculous Salve 'Best Application For . . . , 2.5/8in. high. £8

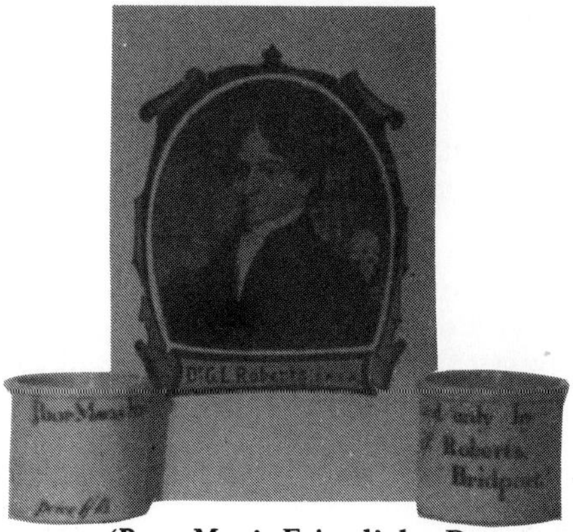

'Poor Man's Friend', by Dr. Giles Roberts, on sale from late 1700's, to early 1900's, 1.5/16in. high, by courtesy of Bridport Museum. £40

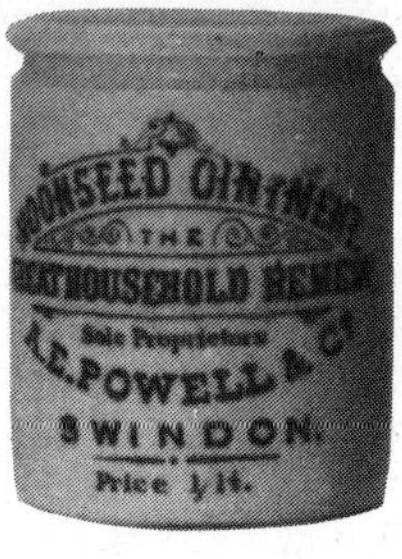

Moonseed Ointment, The Great Household Remedy, Swindon, 2in. high. £25

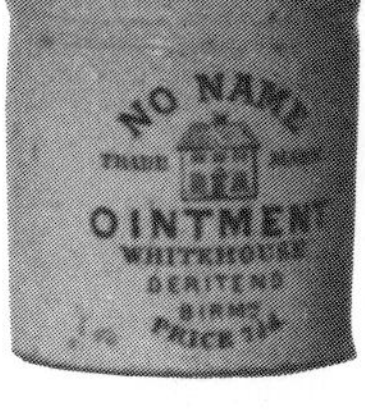

No Name Ointment, Birmingham. £20

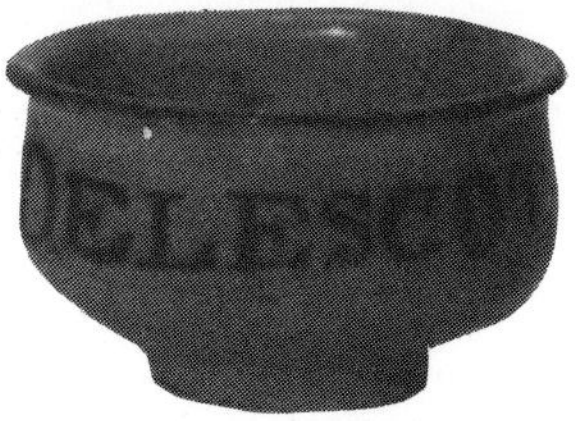

'Delescot', bluish tin glaze pot, Duke St., London, 1749. £150

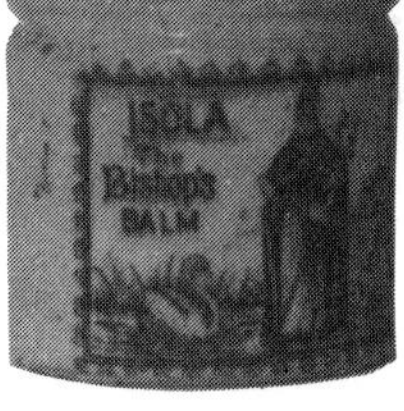

Isola 'The Bishop's Balm', 1¼in. high. £80

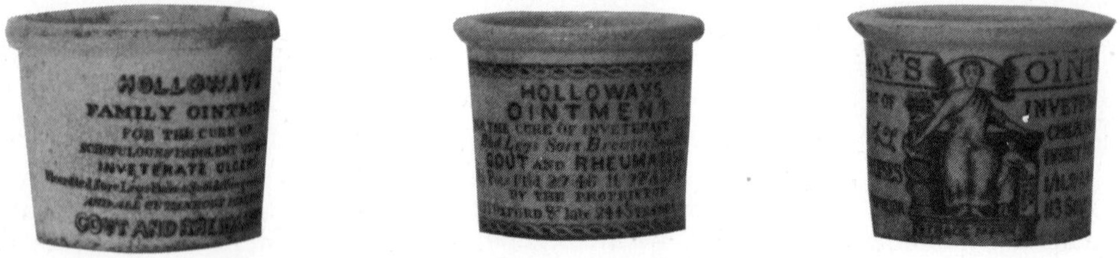

'Professor" Holloway's Ointment was sold world-wide because of brilliant promotion. (Over £26,000 per annum was spent on advertising in 1850). Holloway became very rich and a great philanthropist with an estate valued at 15 million pounds on his death in 1883.
The earliest non-pictorial pots are worth £7, the later pictorial example £3.

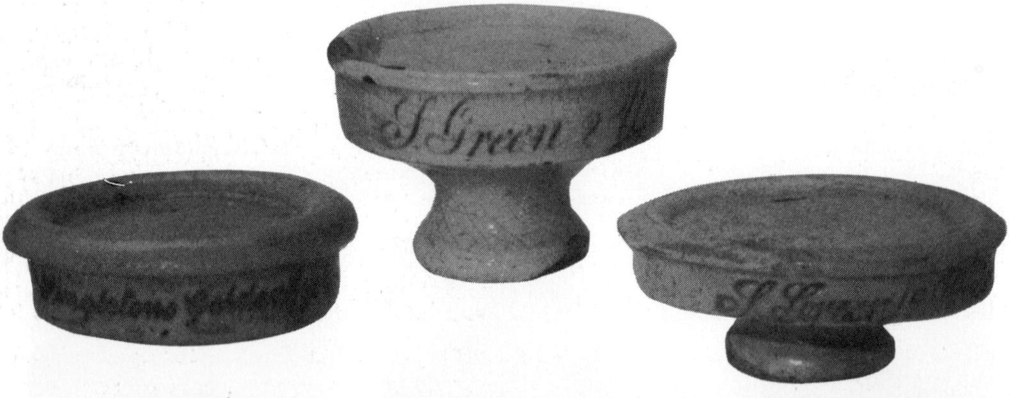

The propriety ointment with the longest history – Singleton's Eye Ointment, on sale from late 1700's until 1949, was based on a recipe 'invented' by Dr. Thomas Johnson in 1596. The pots contained a thin layer of ointment, covered by parchment and later foil, which was designed to be held against the eye. Early pots were bulky with a large pedestal foot and unglazed examples are extremely rare. From 1780-1825 they were signed Fulgham, from 1826-1858 they were signed Green, then reverted to Singleton. Early examples are worth £25 – £45, while later 19th century and 20th century examples are very common and worth only £1.

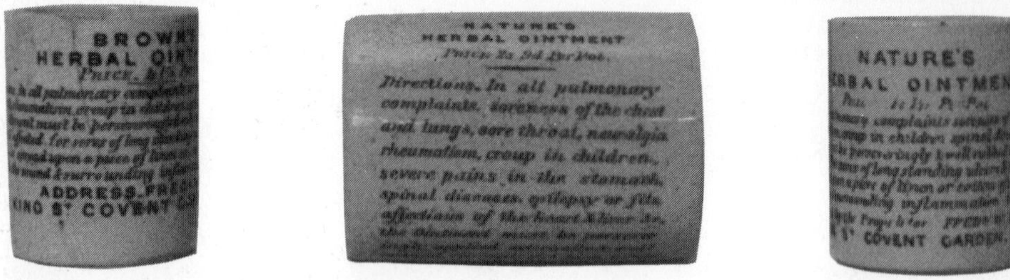

Brown's Herbal ointment, later Nature's, inscribed 'In all pulmonary complaints, soreness of the chest and lungs, sore throat, neuralgia, rheumatism, croup in children, severe pains in the stomach, spinal diseases, epilepsy or fits, affections of the heart and liver, for corrupt sores of long standing such as ulcers and tumours of a scrofulous character'. Hence 'cure-alls'. Small 1¾in. high – £5, large 2¾in. high – £15.

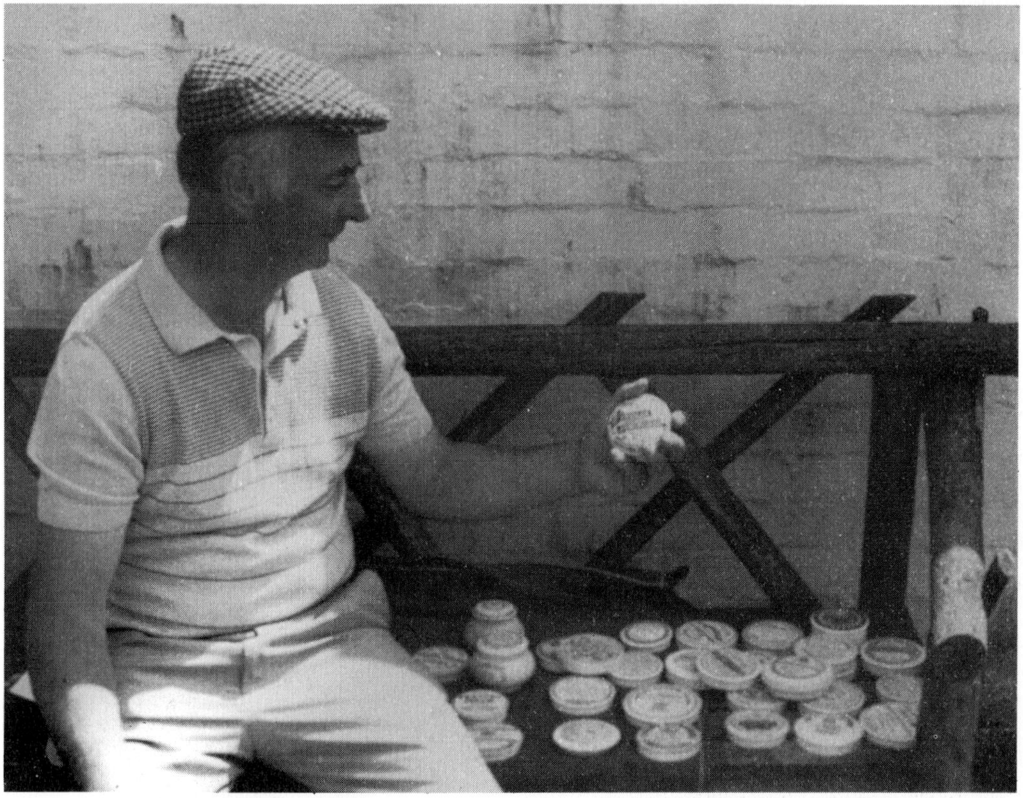

Clifford Frewin collects shaving cream pot lids.

"When I was bottle digging in the early 70's I found three shaving cream pot lids and thought they would be nice to collect as many of them are pictorial and attractive.

"I have around 100 lids and I buy or swap them with other collectors now that there are so few dumps left.

"They date from the early Victorian period and petered out around 1920. One of the earliest that I have was issued by a firm that claimed their product was used by Prince Albert.

"The majority of the lids are large size, bearing the name of the product, the name of the maker or barber, and sometimes instructions for use. One of mine comes from a London Hotel and is decorated with little lions. Most lids are black print on white, but I have a few in green and brown. Although most have no pottery marks, they were made by about half a dozen major firms in the Potteries during the 20th century; some fancy decorated pots were made by Doulton."

Clifford said he is still keen to acquire more of these shaving cream lids which can sell for prices between £5 for a Boots's lid to £300 for a rare pictorial lid.

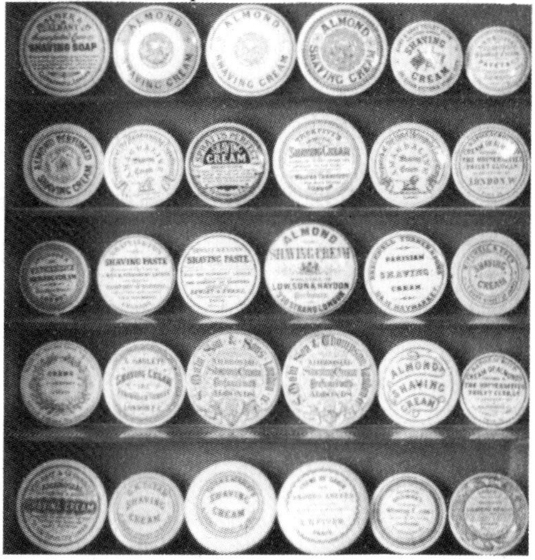

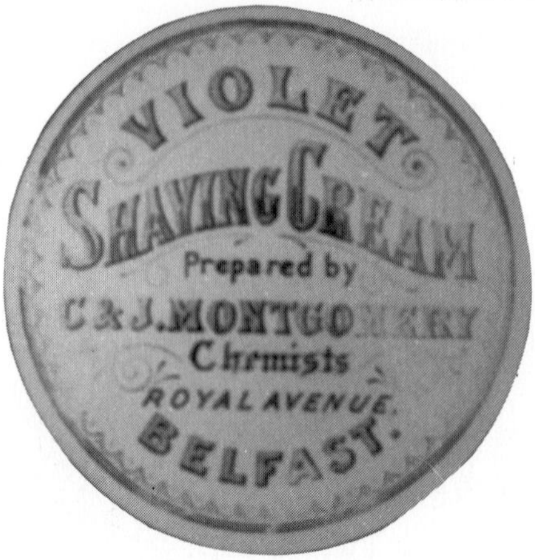

Violet Shaving Cream, Prepared by C. & J. Montgomery of Belfast, a rare Irish lid. £25

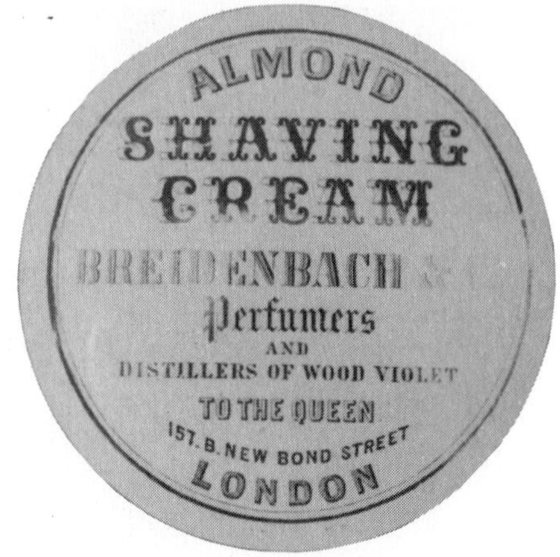

Breidenbach & Co. Almond Shaving Cream, New Bond St., London, large sige. £20

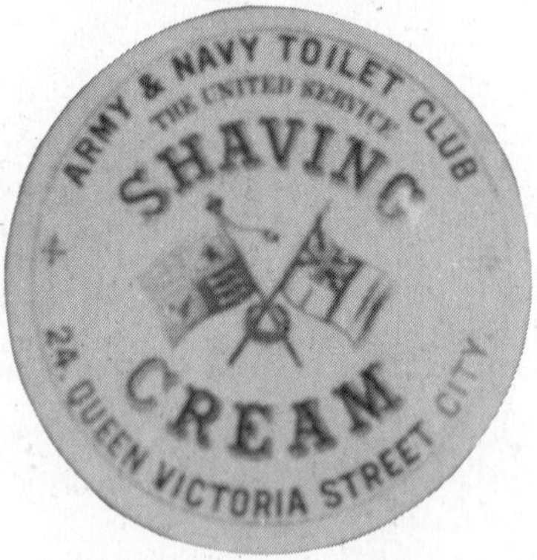

Army & Navy Toilet Club, The United Service Shaving Cream. £25

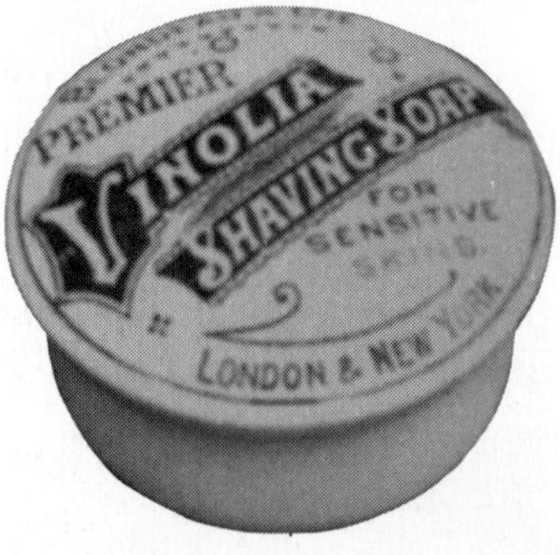

Blondeay & Cie, Premier Vinolia Shaving Cream for Sensitive Skins, circa 1920. £25

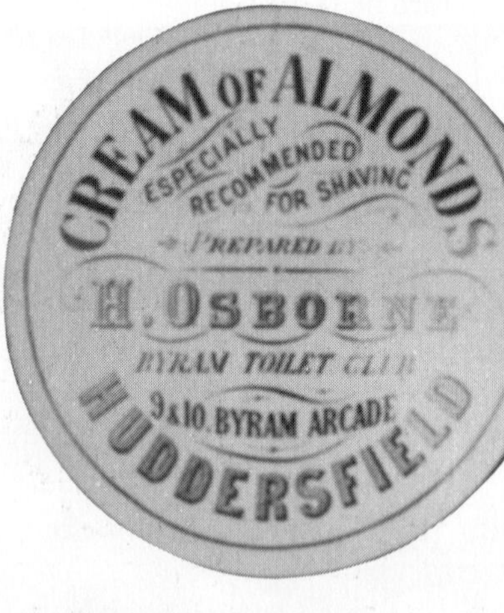

H. Osborne, Cream of Almonds, Byram Toilet Club, Huddersfield. £18

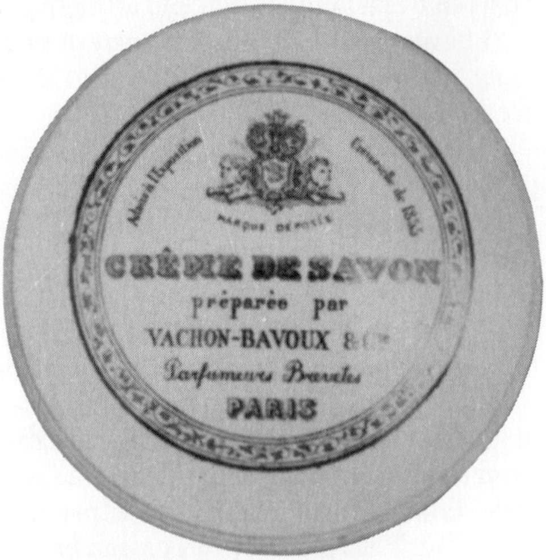

Vachon -Bavoux & Cie, 'Creme de Savon', a French lid possibly only sold in France. £35

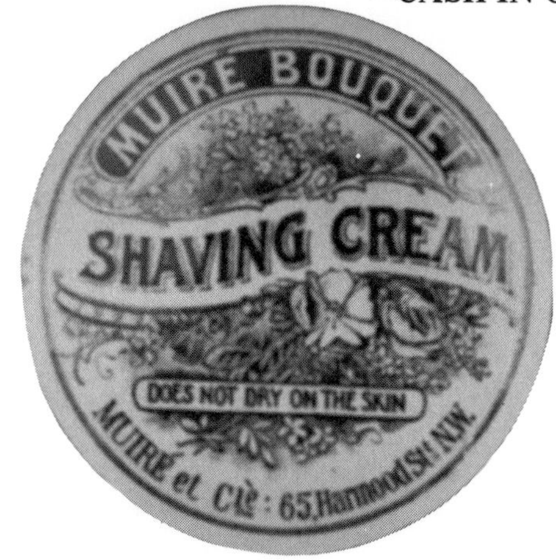

Muire Bouquet Shaving Cream, 'Does not dry on the skin', the French name had sales appeal. £35

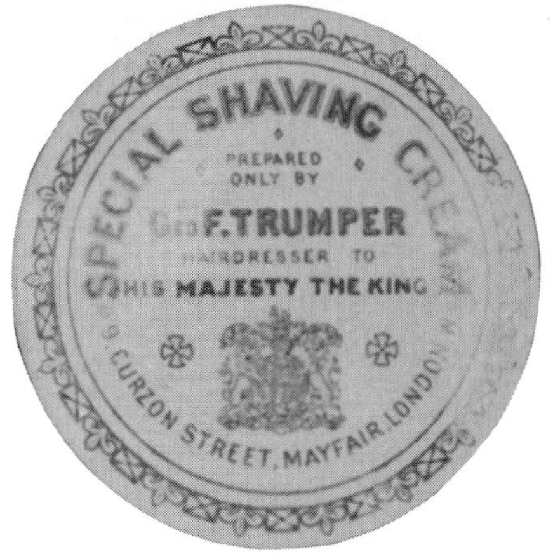

Geo. F. Trumper Special Shaving Cream, a large lid, circa 1921. £30

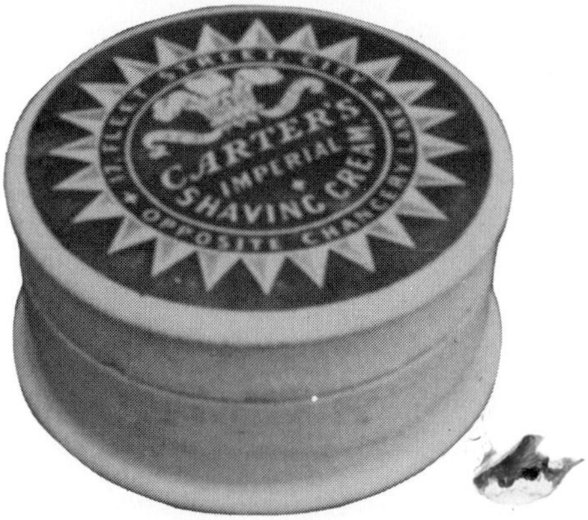

Carter's Imperial Shaving Cream, an unusual lid with white lettering in a black background. £40

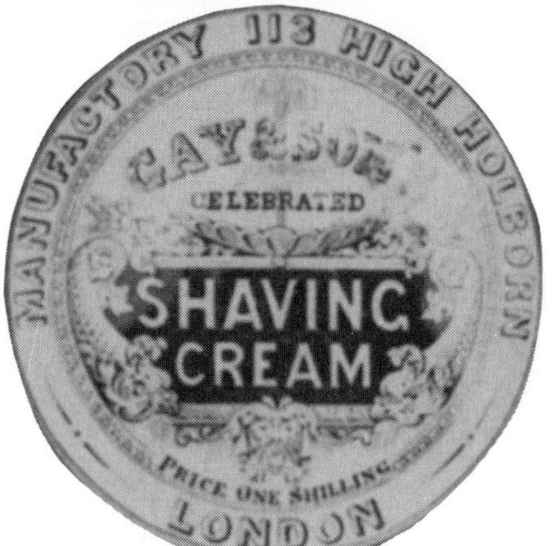

Gay & Sons Celebrated Shaving Cream, London. £35

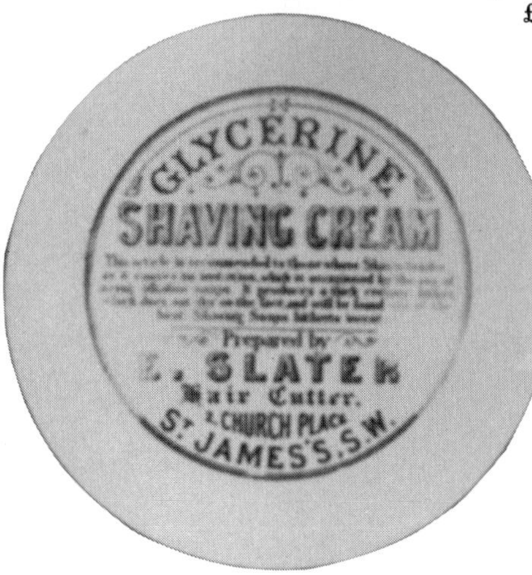

Glycerine Shaving Cream, by E. Slater, Hair Cutter, St. James's, London. £25

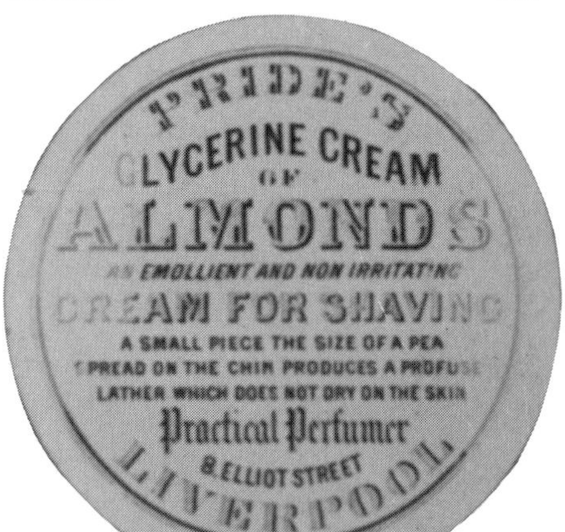

Pride's Glycerine Cream of Almonds, An Emollient and Non Irritating Cream for Shaving, Liverpool. £30

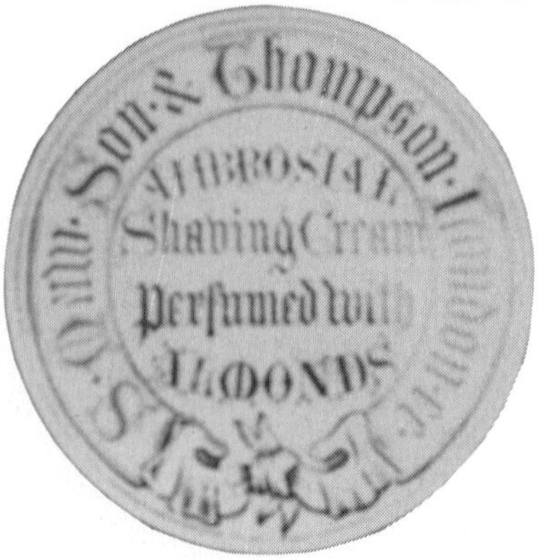

S. Maw, Son & Thompson, Ambrosial Shaving Cream, Perfumed with Almonds, small size. £25

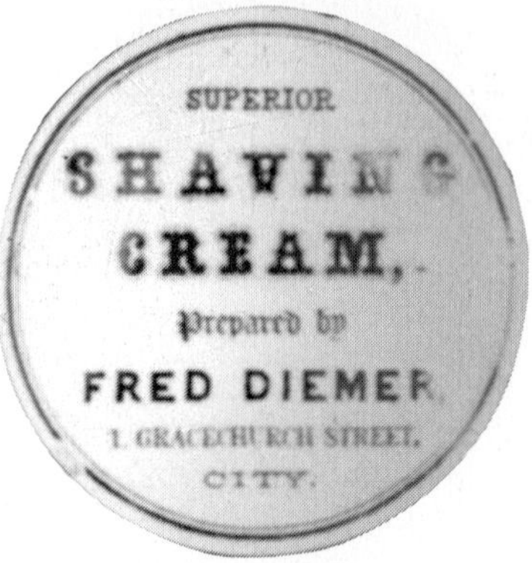

Fred Diemer, Superior Shaving Cream, an old lid from the City of London. £18

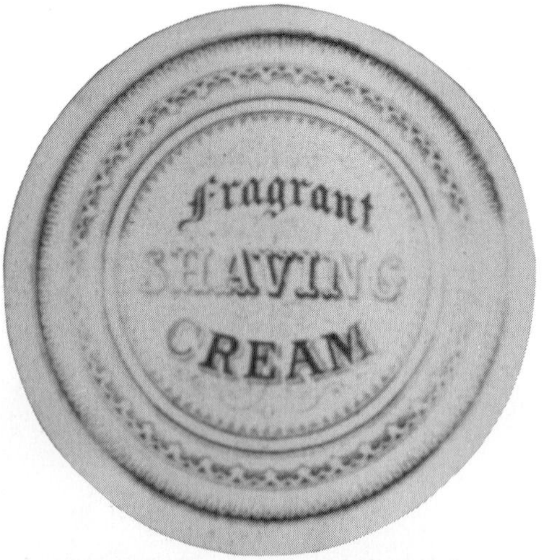

Fragrant Shaving Cream, this lid was illustrated in the Wholesale Chemist's Catalogue of 1890. £20

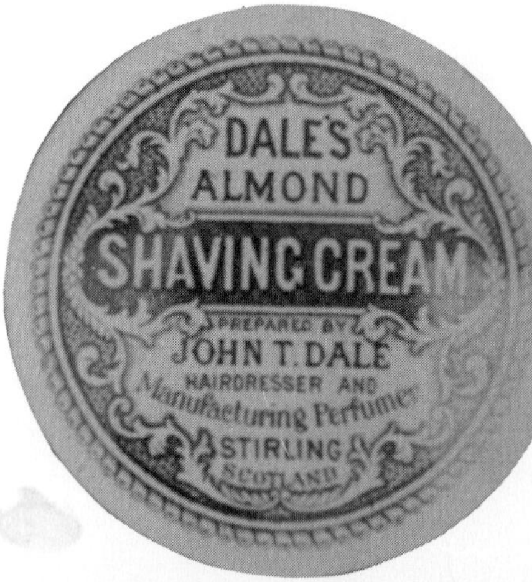

Dale's Almond Shaving Cream, Prepared by John T. Dale, Stirling, Scotland. £25

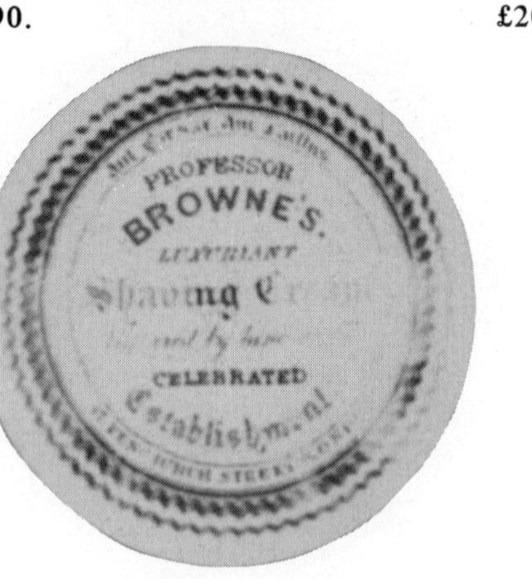

Professor Browne's Luxuriant Shaving Cream, Fenchurch Street, London. £25

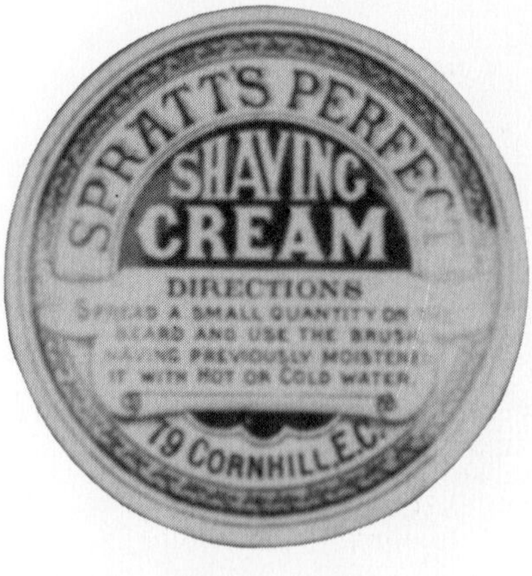

Spratt's Perfect Shaving Cream, a small London lid complete with directions. £20

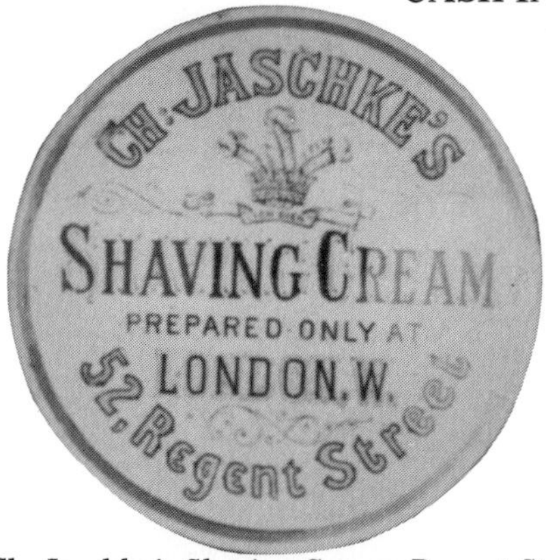

Ch. Jaschke's Shaving Cream, Regent St., London, decorated with a gold band. £20

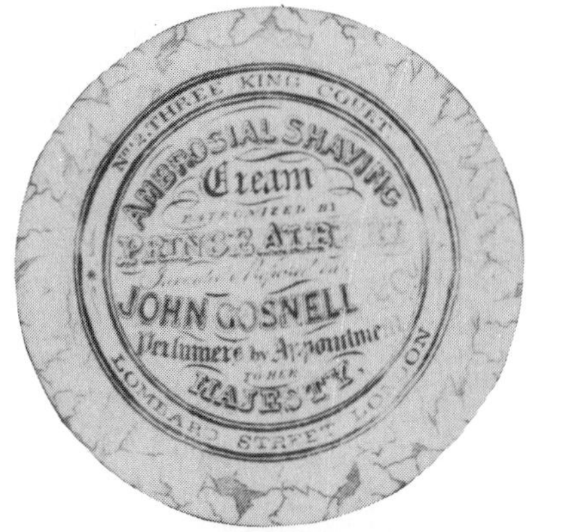

John Gosnell & Co. Ambrosial Shaving Cream, an early lid which changed the reference to Prince Albert after his death in 1861 to 'Patronized by the Nobility'. £50

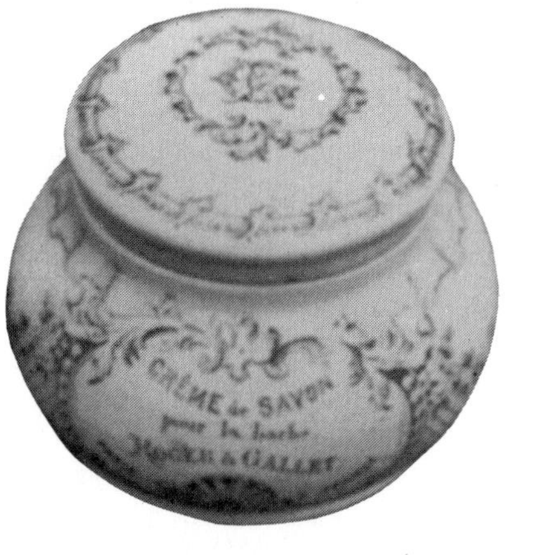

Roger & Gallet, Creme de Savon, a French lid and pot printed in green. £15

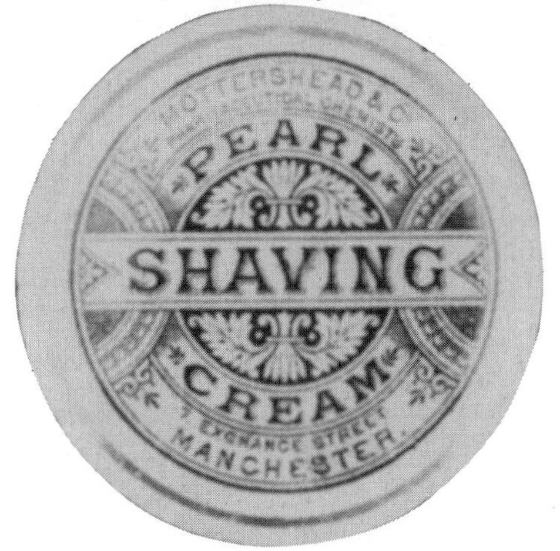

Mottershead & Co. Pearl Shaving Cream, a large early lid from Manchester with gilt edging. £30

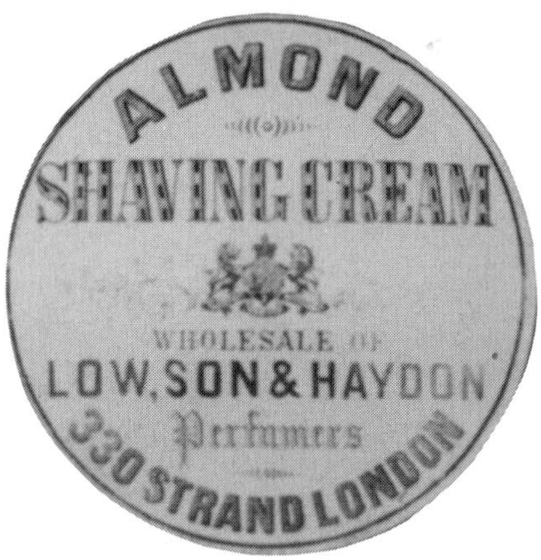

Low, Son & Haydon, Almond Shaving Cream, Strand, London. £30

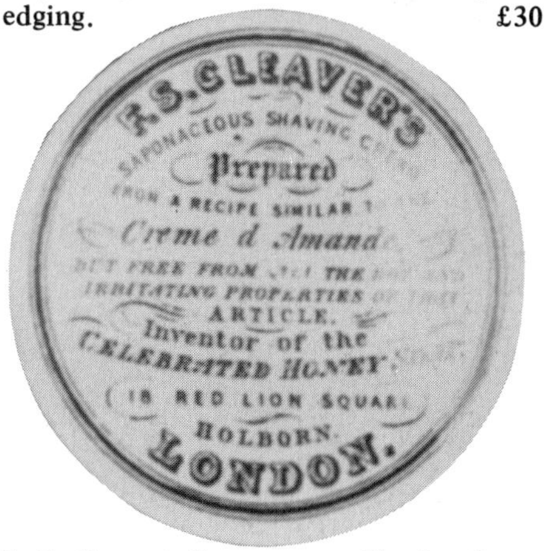

F. S. Cleaver's Saponaceous Shaving Cream, from the 'Inventor of the Celebrated Honey Soap', London. £40

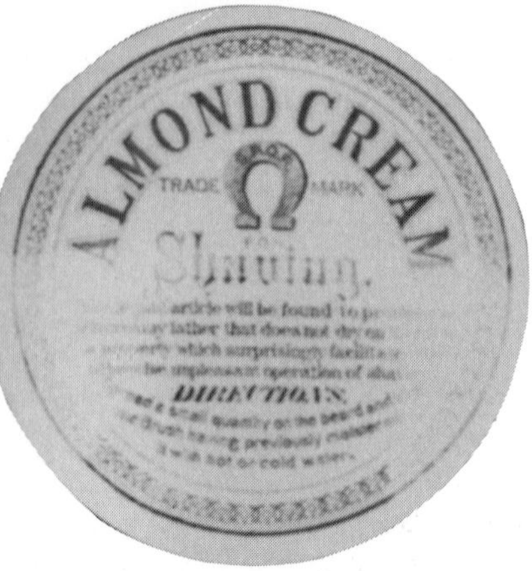

S.P.Q.R. Almond Cream, a rare lid. £30

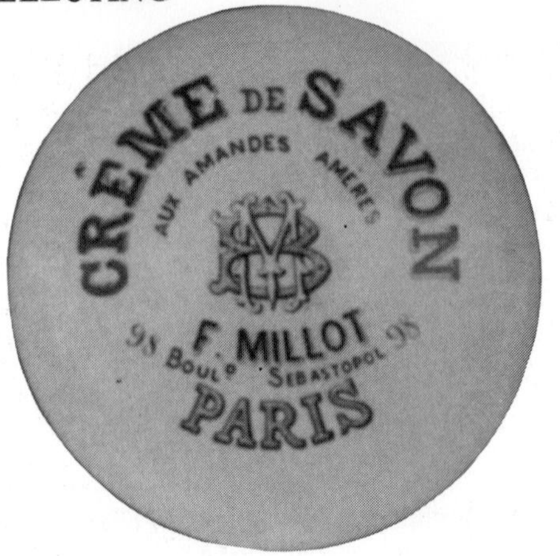

Creme de Savon, by F. Millot of Paris, a plain but rare French lid. £20

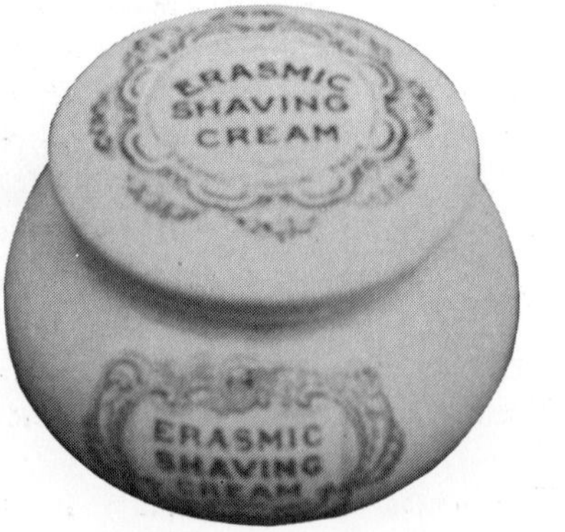

Erasmic Shaving Cream, lid complete with matching pot. £25

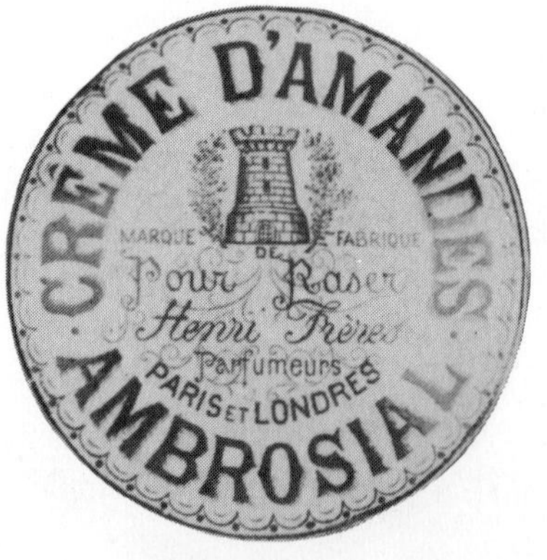

Henri Freres, Creme D'Amandes, Ambrosial, a French style lid with an attractive trade mark. £35

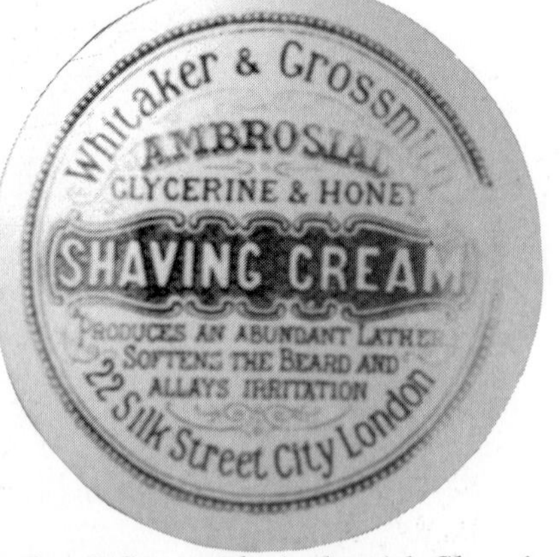

Whitaker & Grossmith, Ambrosial, Glycerine & Honey Shaving Cream, a large lid from the City of London. £25

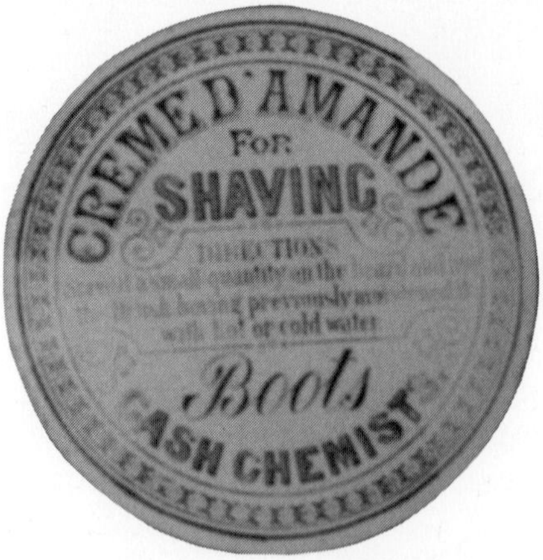

Boots Creme D'Amande for Shaving, probably the most commond shaving cream lid. £8

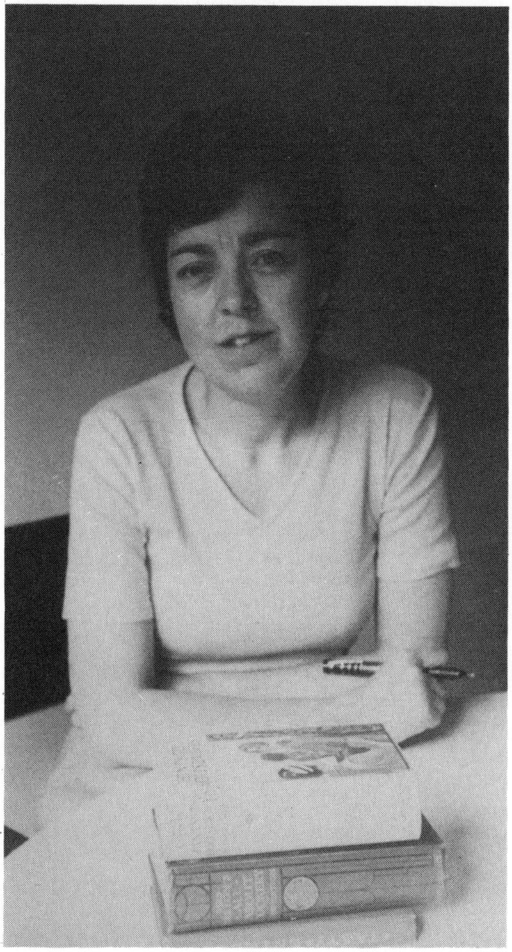

Rosemary Hill is a secretary in the City of London and collects cookery books.

"The first one I bought 12 years ago was a 1913 edition of Mrs Beeton for £1.50 and it started from there.

"I restrict myself to books published after 1880 and also I only buy books that I think are socially important, they have to mark some change in our way of living. For example I've bought some modern books on Nouvelle Cuisine because I think people will look back and realise that marked a watershed in our ideas about food.

"One of the authors I like who is writing today is Glyn Christian because his recipes are so fresh and original but I've also got books by people like Elizabeth David because she writes so beautifully. I can read her like a novel though I don't much like the sort of dishes she recommends.

"A good deal of my collection is recipe leaflets and one of the treasures is a very, very tiny booklet, only three inches by two inches, issued by McDougall's Flour. It was given to me by an old lady who got it when she was at school around 1912. It advertises self raising flour and I think it must be one of the first recipe books for that kind of flour.

"I like advertising booklets because it will be very interesting to look back and see the social changes. I've got booklets for low fat cheese and things like that for instance."

Rosemary will only buy a cookery book if it has some historical interest and one of her treasures is a booklet for Tunbridge Wells wafers which were very popular at the time of Queen Victoria but which no longer exist. She is also proud of a 1930's booklet advertising Colman's Mustard which she bought for 10p and has since been priced at £4.

"It has lovely illustrations of women with bobbed hair and cigarette holders," she said.

The books she would like to add to her collection are a cookery book illustrated by Mabel Lucy Attwell and one edited on behalf of a charity by Wallis, the late Duchess of Windsor.

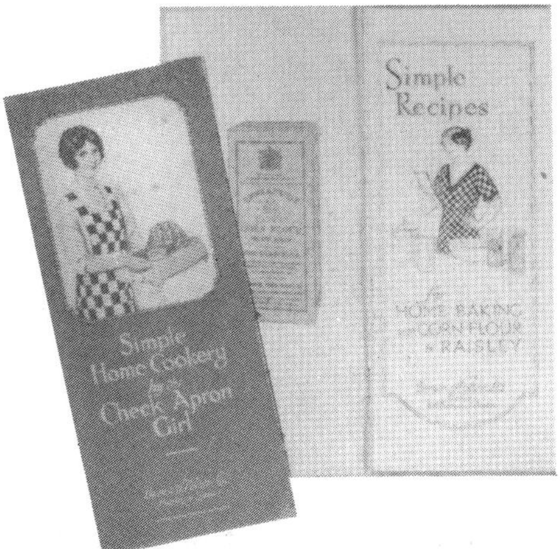

'Simple Home Cookery' by the Check Apron Girl. *£2.50*

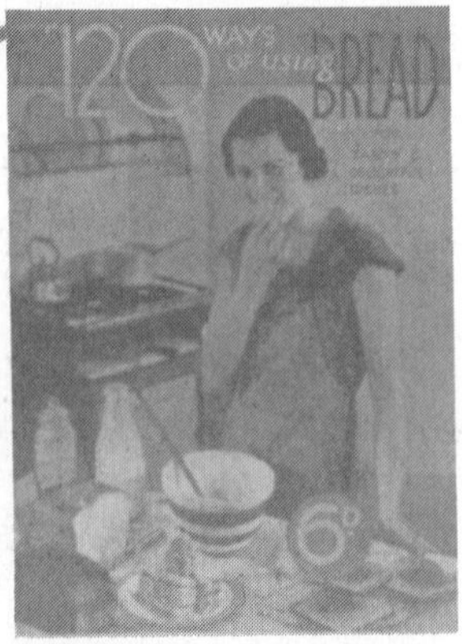

'120 Ways of Using Bread for Tasty and Delightful Dishes'. £1

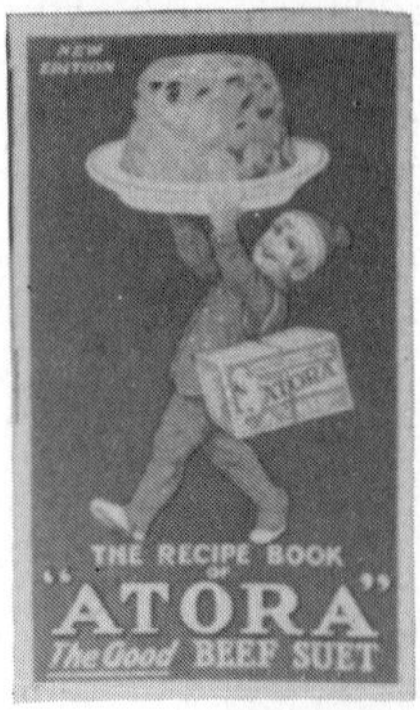

The Recipe Book of 'Atora', The Good Beef Suet, circa 1900. £2

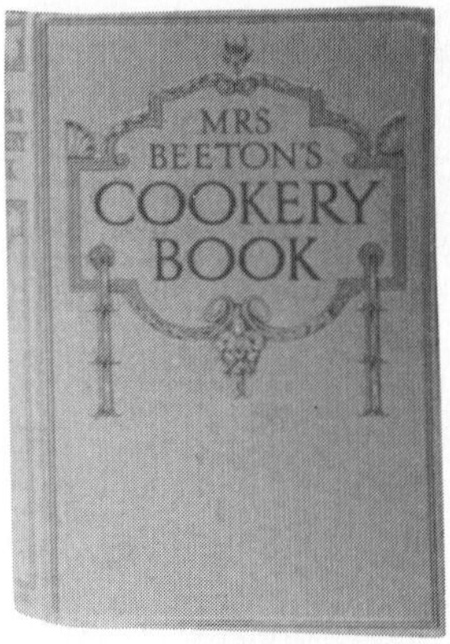

Mrs. Beeton's 'Cookery Book', 1930's. £2

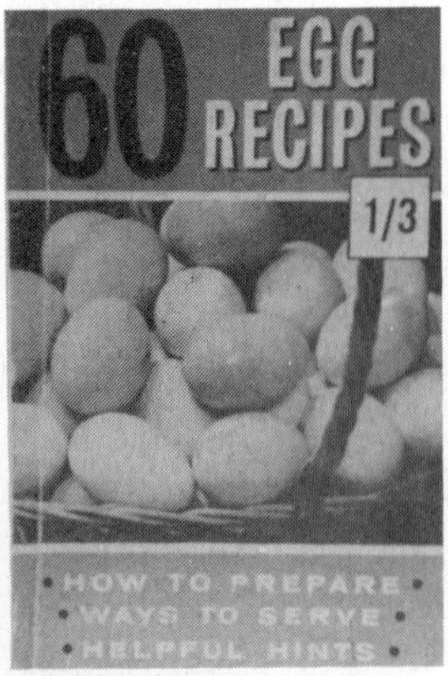

'60 Egg Recipes, How to Prepare, Ways to Serve, Helpful Hints', by the Egg Marketing Board. 75p

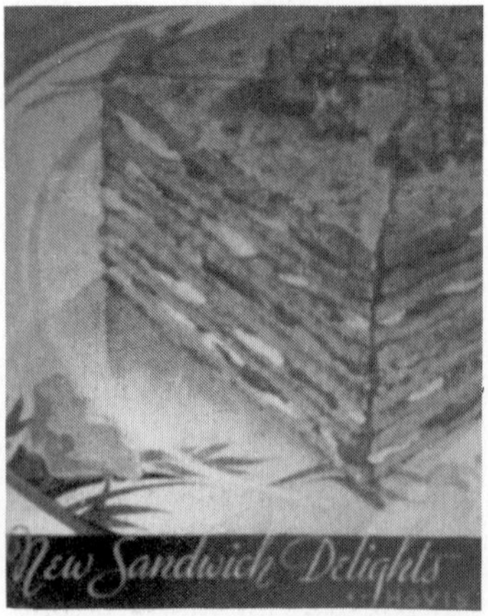

'New Sandwich Delights', by Hovis. 75p

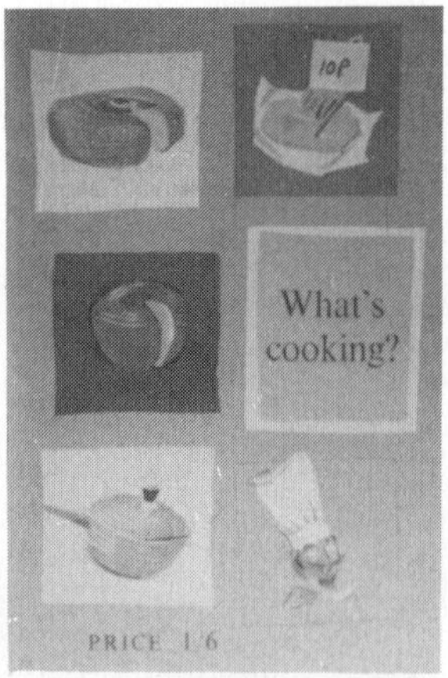

'What's cooking?' Dutch. 75p

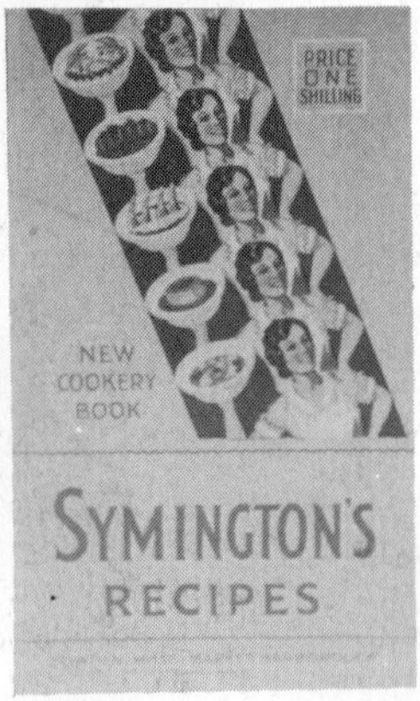

'Symington's Recipes, New Cookery Book', 1930's. £1

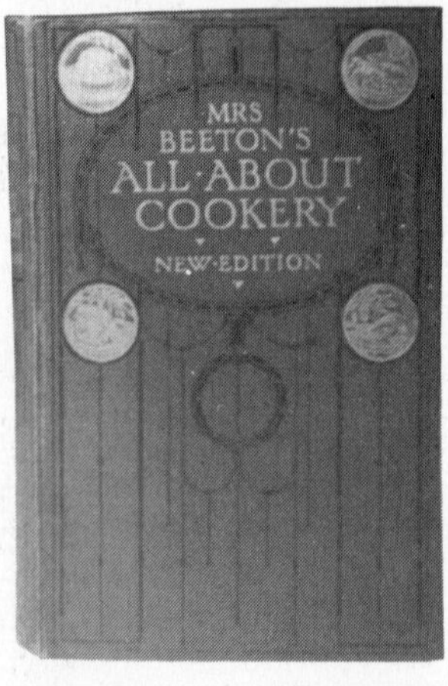

Mrs. Beeton's 'All-About Cookery', New Edition, 1913. £10

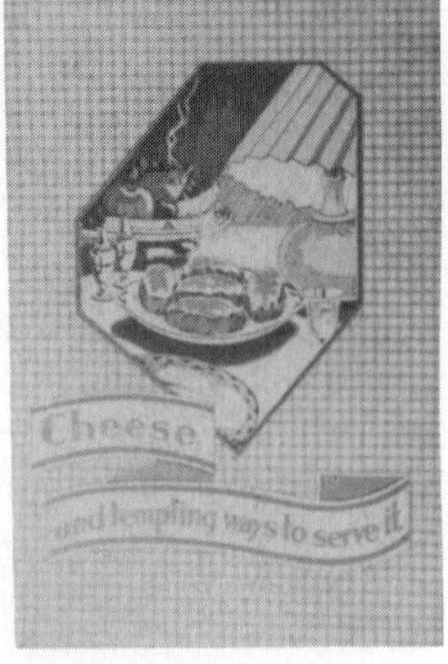

'Kraft Cheese and Tempting Ways to Serve it', 1930's. £1

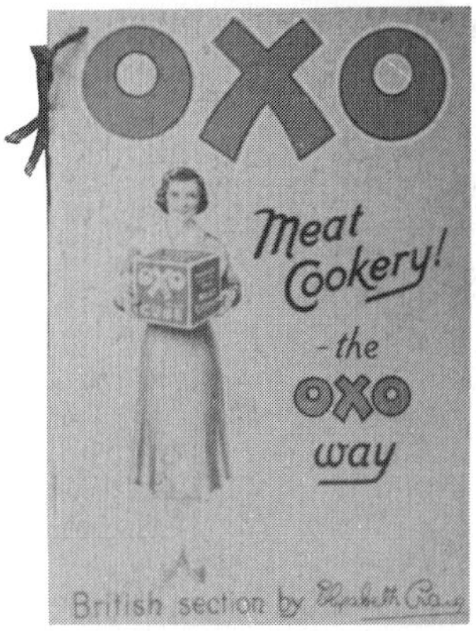

'Oxo Meat Cookery! – the Oxo way', by Elizabeth Craig, 1930's. £1

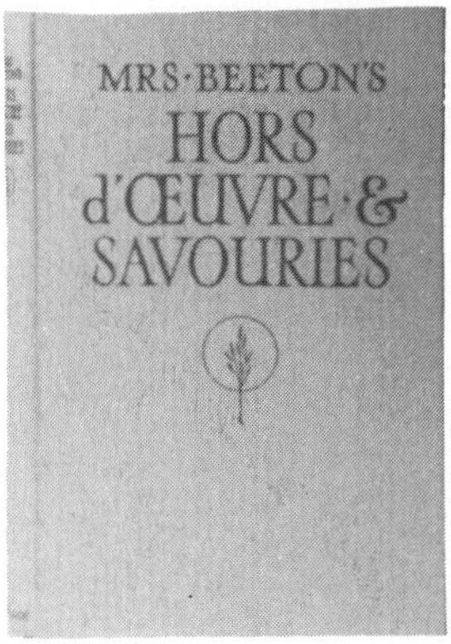

Mrs. Beeton's 'Hors d'Oeuvre & Savouries', 1930's. £3

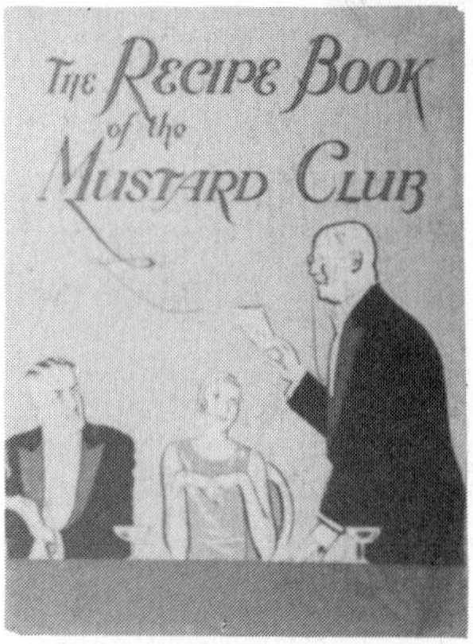

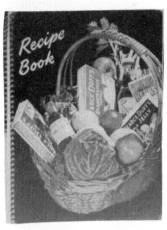

'The Recipe Book of the Mustard Club', by Colman's, 1930's. £4

'Recipe Book', by Pearce Duff, 1950's. £1

'Spillers Party Cook Book', 1950's. £1

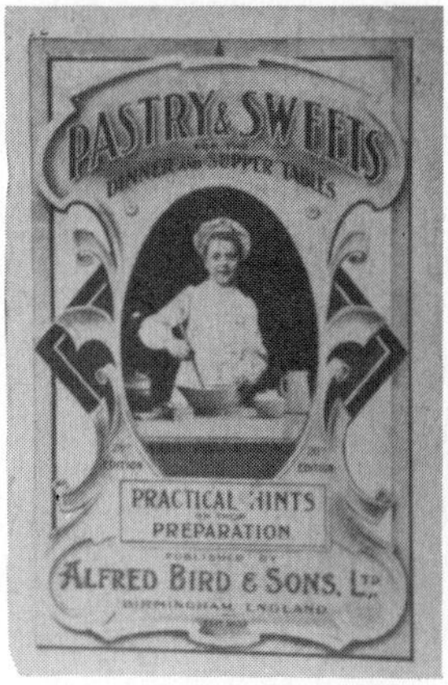

'Pastry & Sweets For The Dinner and Supper Tables', by Alfred Bird & Sons Ltd., circa 1900. £2

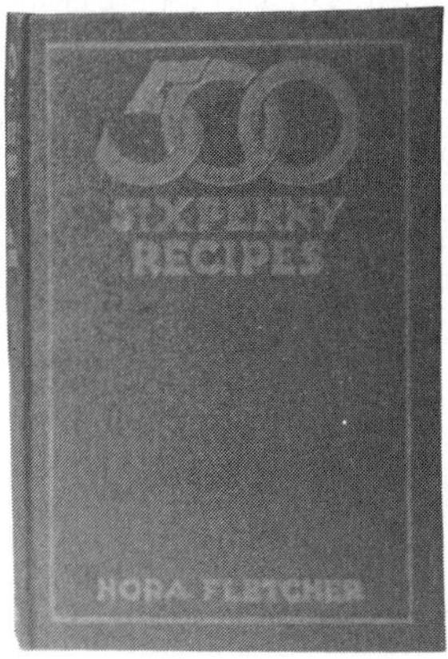

'500 Sixpenny Recipes', by Nora Fletcher, 1934. £2

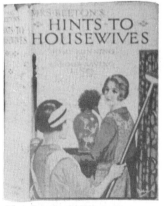

Mrs. Beeton's 'Hints to Housewifes', 'Home Running on Labour Saving Lines', by Ward Lock & Co. Ltd., 1930's. £5

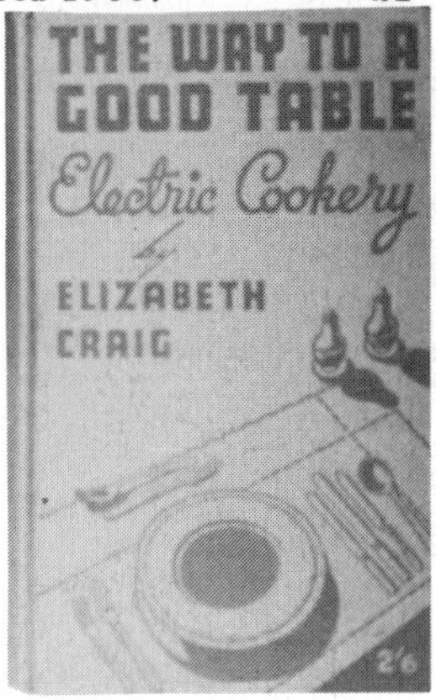

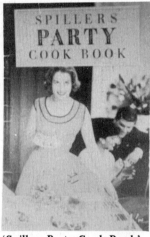

'The Way To A Good Table, Electric Cookery', by Elizabeth Craig, 1930's. £1.50

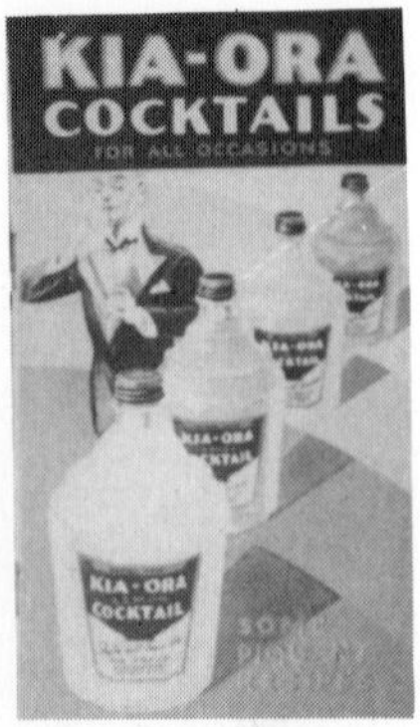

'Kia-Ora Cocktails For All Occasions', Some Piquant Recipes, 1930's. £1

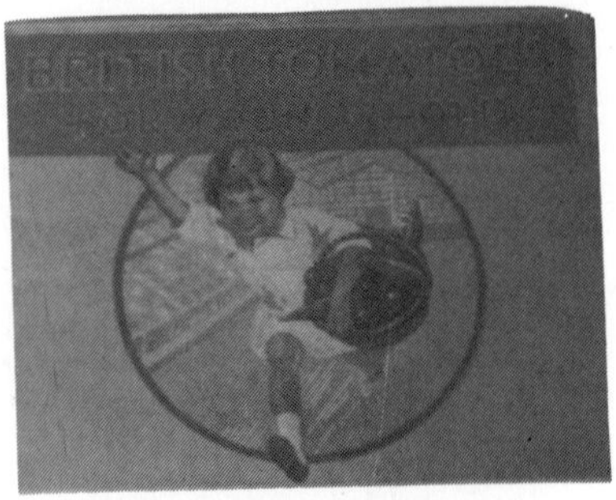

'British Tomatoes For Young & Old'. 25p

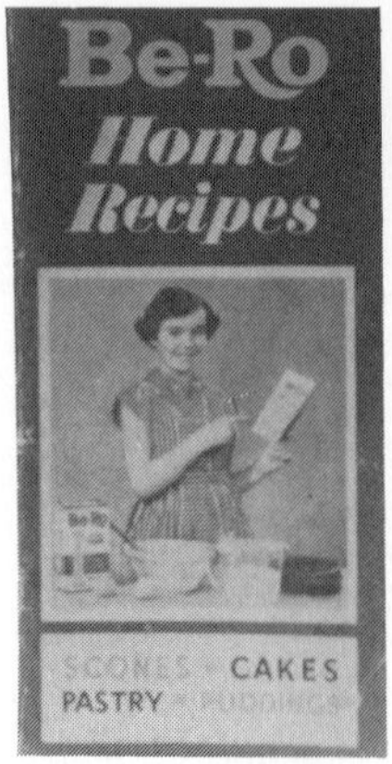

'Be-Ro Home Recipes, Scones, Cakes, Pastry, Puddings'. 50p

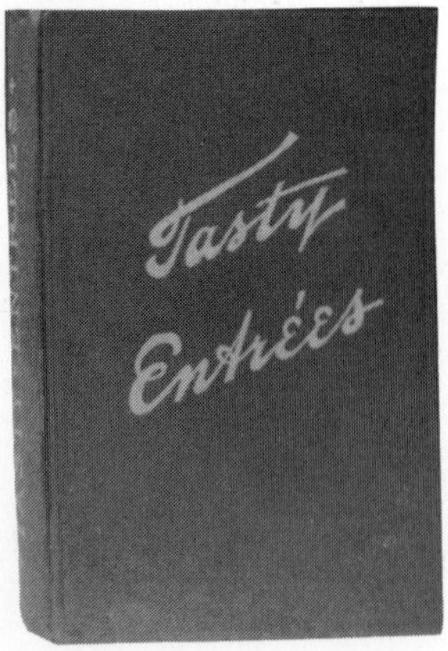

'Tasty Entrees', by Miss C. L. Howland, circa 1900. £3

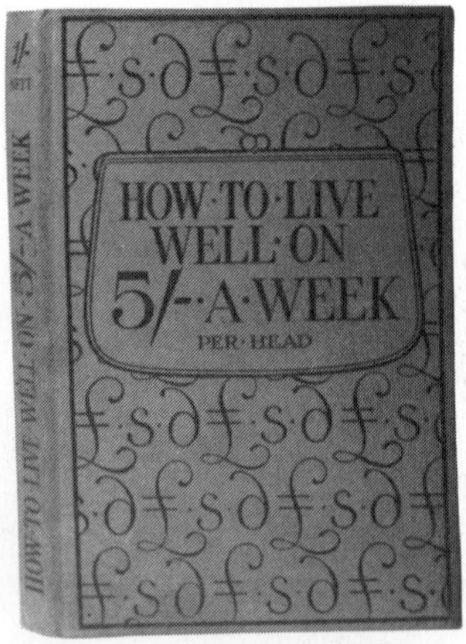

'How to Live Well on 5/- a Week Per Head', by L. Rutherford Skey, 1910. £3

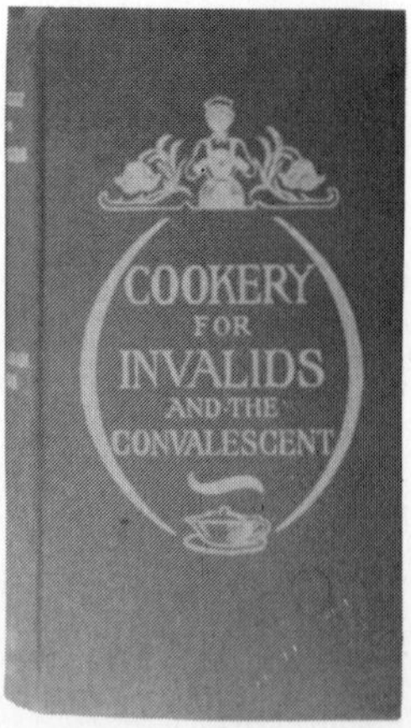

'Cookery for Invalids and the Convalescent', by Herman-Senn, 1910. £2

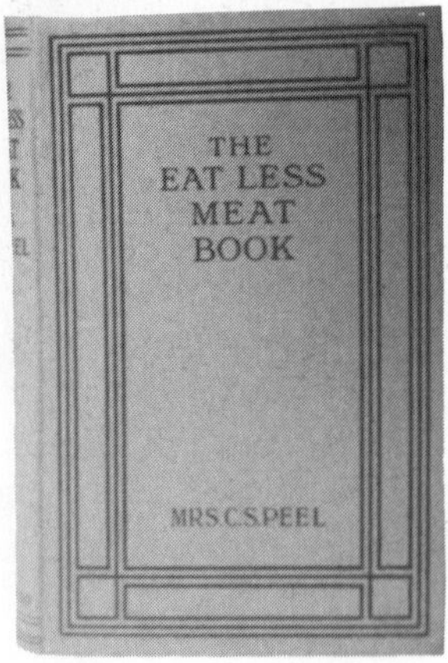

'The Eat Less Meat Book', by Mrs. C. S. Peel, 1914-18. £3

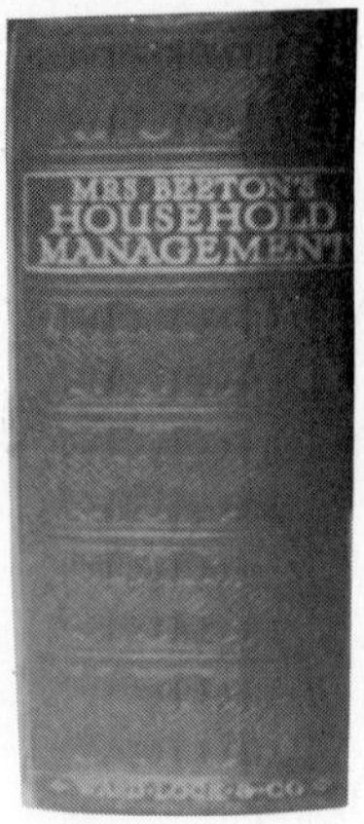

Mrs. Beeton's Household Management, by Ward Lock & Co., 1936. £20

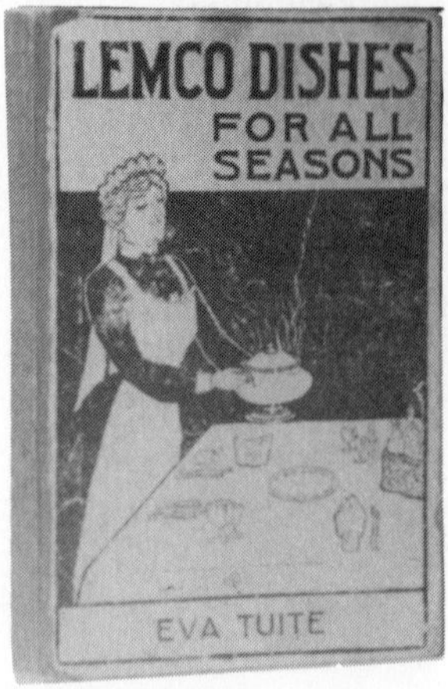

'Lemco Dishes For All Seasons', by Eva Tuite, circa 1900. £3

Ronald Lucibell is a photographer and collects ceramic inhalers.

"During the Victorian period the wealthy middle classes were very health conscious and that's why manufacturers could sell them all sorts of bizarre things which were meant to aid bronchial trouble.

"These ceramic inhalers were produced in different shapes and sizes but they were basically pot things which you filled with boiling water, added something like Friars' Balsam and breathed in the fumes through special tubes. They come in various sizes ranging from little ones for travellers to big ones that held two pints of water.

"I've got two dozen different examples but I didn't know anything about them till my wife dug one up on a Victorian tip one day in the mid '70's. I liked it because it was very decorative and had a pretty transfer printed label."

Some of Ron's collection of inhalers are printed all over with designs of flowers or humming birds and they are sepia, blue or multi coloured. He has researched the history of the ceramic inhaler in old medical catalogues and has found that the earlier ones were basically jam jar shaped with two inhaling tubes while the later ones had more efficient lids and the tubes were often set at right angles to the body. Most modern ones were bulbous in shape with an outlet at the back and the mouthpiece in a cork. They went on being produced by firms like Maw's and Dr Nelson's till the late 1930's. Inhalers range in price from £5 to over £100 for a rare example in good condition and with its original lid.

Ron's favourites in his collection are the Westminster inhaler printed in sepia, the Alexander which is multi coloured or the Acme inhaler made by Hockins which is covered with multi coloured flower prints.

The inhaler Ron would most like to find is one he has only seen illustrated in catalogues called the Bournemouth inhaler. It dates from the 1880's and was printed in sepia.

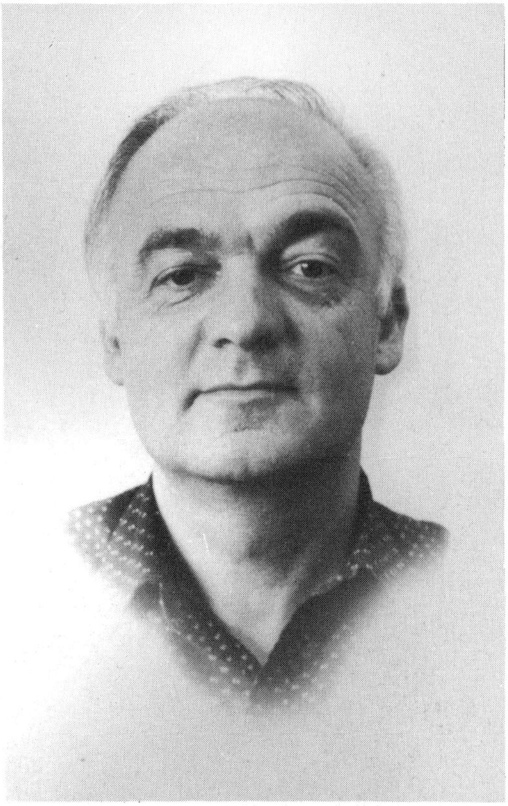

Ronald Lucibell, keen collector of ceramic inhalers.

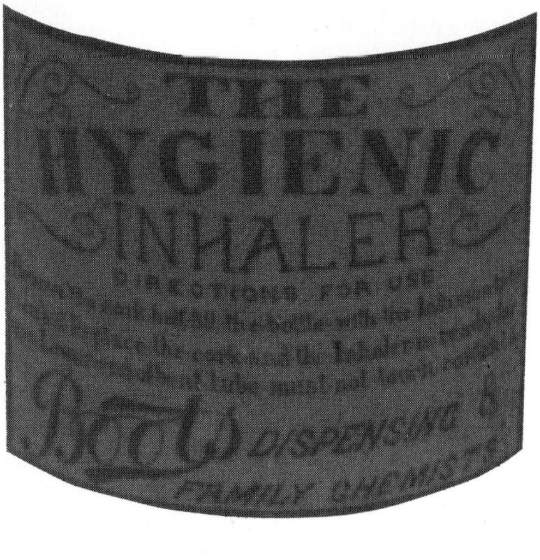

All inhalers come complete with their 'Directions for Use'.

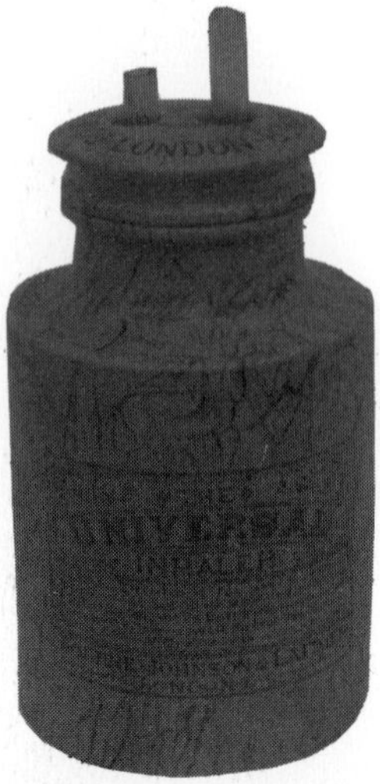

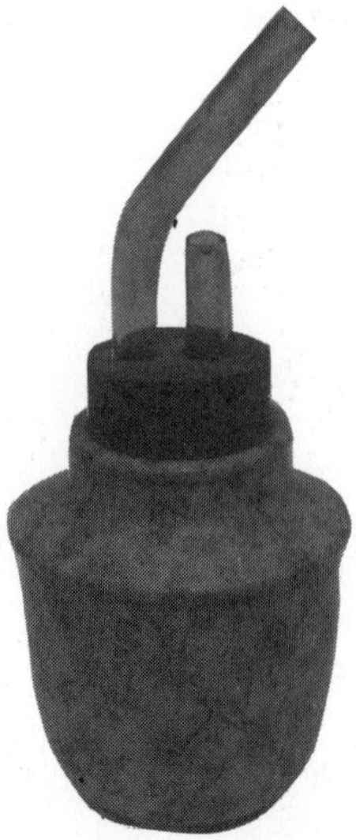

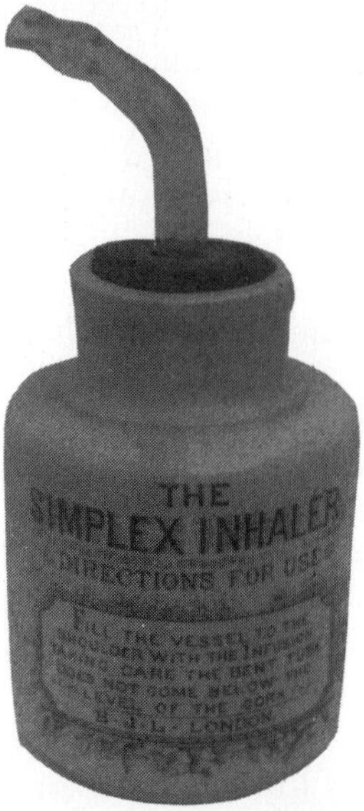

A rarer version of 'The Universal', an all over light blue colouring, veined in black. £60

Small inhalers for use when travelling. Nice specimens can be found in dark blue, or sepia floral prints. £15

The 'Simplex', in white, over printed in black. £40

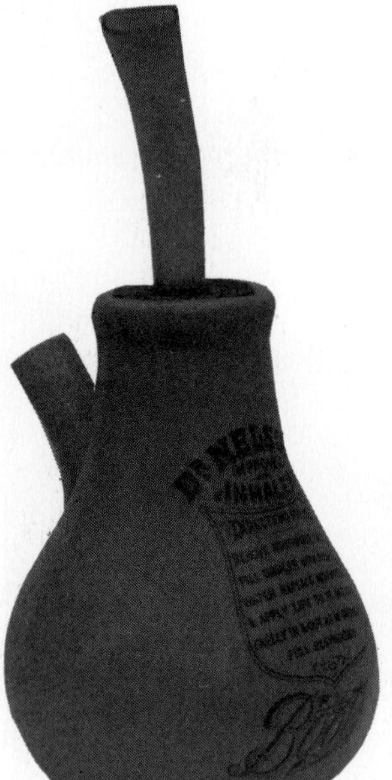

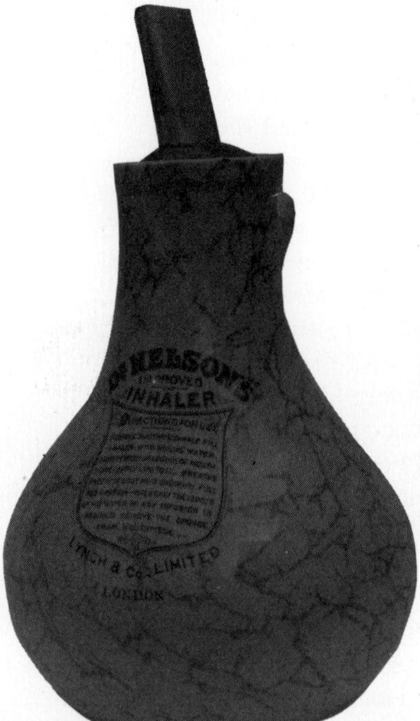

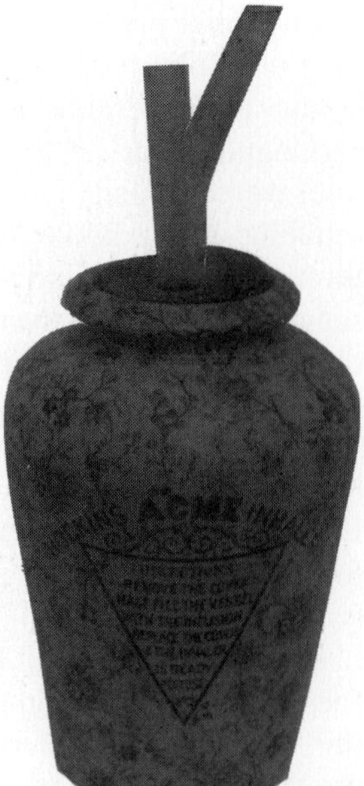

The 'Dr. Nelson's were as widely available as the Maws. The bulbous white version was distributed by Boots, a larger blue veined version had nationwide availability. £10 and £25 respectively.

Hockins marketed 'The Acme', in similar prints as the portables, but over printed with the company's name and with the directions for use. £50

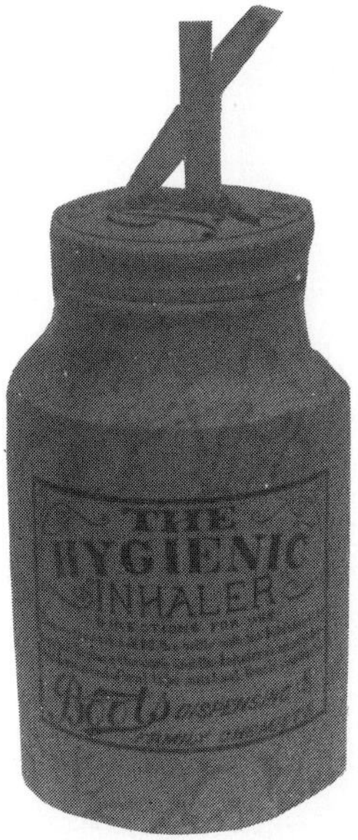

One of the earlier jar shaped inhalers 'The Hygienic', sold by Boots, is attractively veined in blue. £30

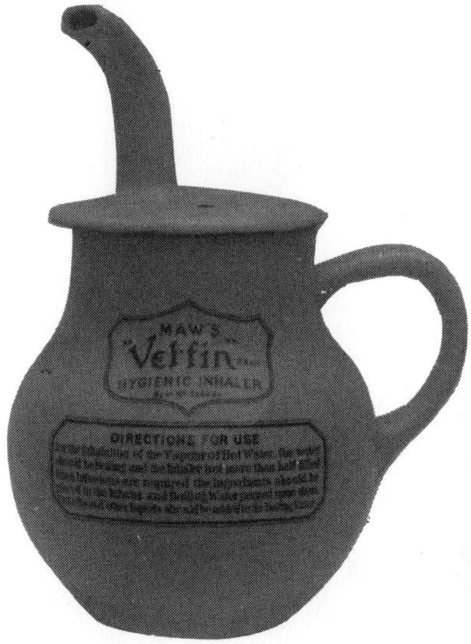

Manufacturers S. Maw & Son, later incorporating Thompsons, created interesting variations. The 'Vel-fin' is jug shaped, with the mouth-piece incorporated into the lid. £30

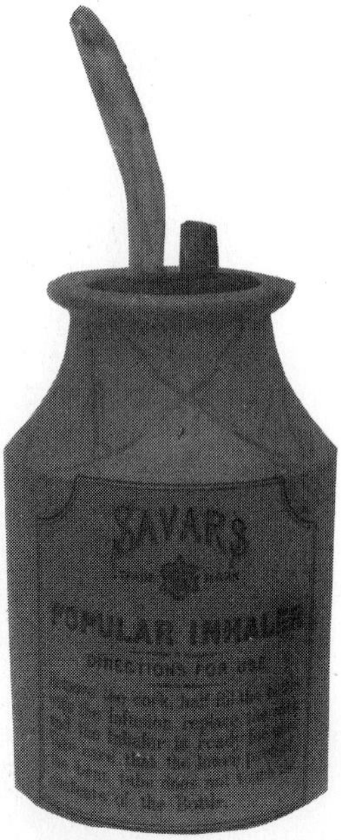

The Savars 'Popular' is mottled in pink. £50

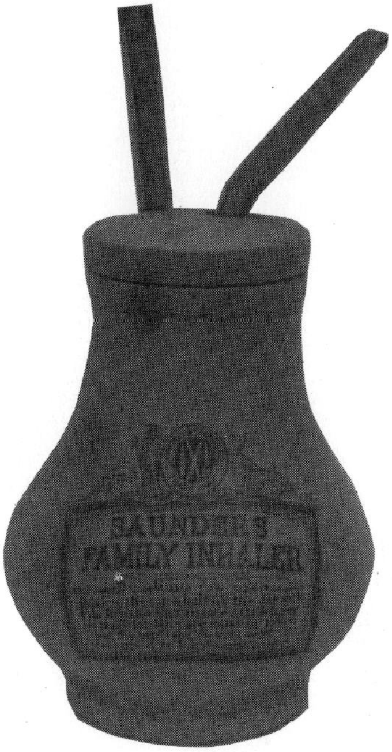

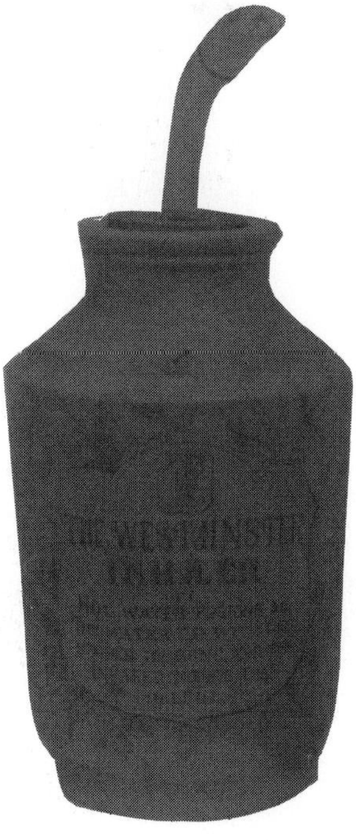

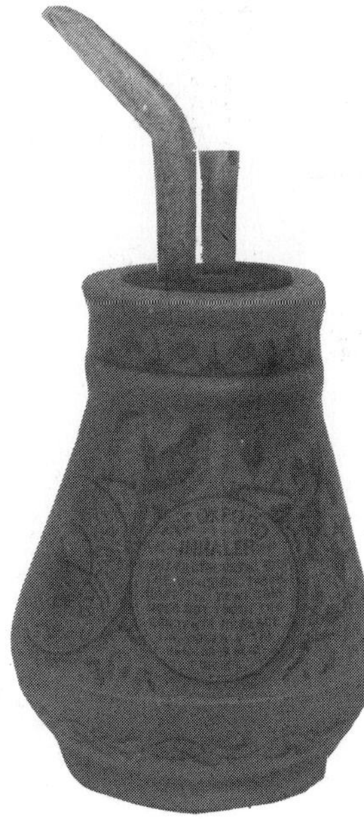

'The Saunders Family Inhaler' was a fore-runner of later inhalers to be produced in a bulbous shape. White, with blue. £40

There was a tendency to produce very decorative examples named for places. Desirable rarities are sepia printed 'The Westminster' and 'The Oxford'. £60

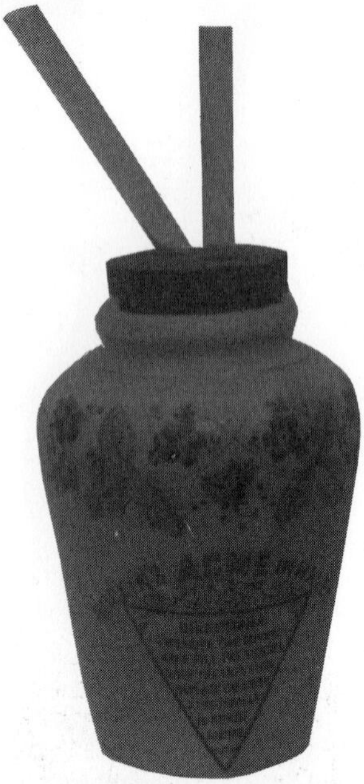

An attractive variation of 'The Acme' is in white, with grey leaves and orange flowers decorating the shoulders. £50

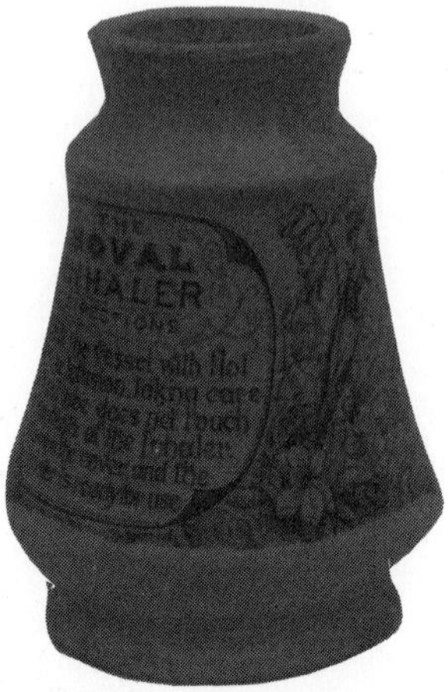

'The Boval' is nicely fluted and decorated in sepia print of blue-bells, daisies, etc. £60

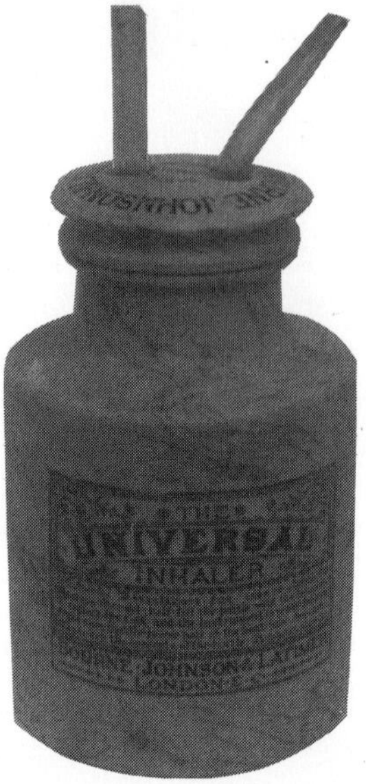

Bourne, Johnson & Latimer, of London, distributed 'The Universal', white, mottled in lavender. £40

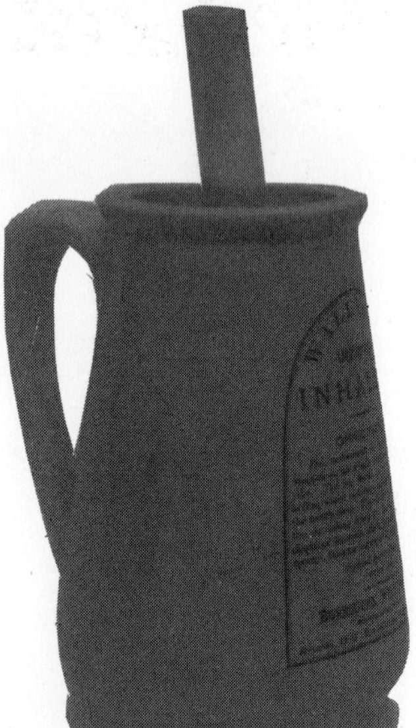

The company of Burroughs & Wellcome distributed the 'Wallich's Improved Inhaler', an unusual jug shaped vessel, complete with handle. £40

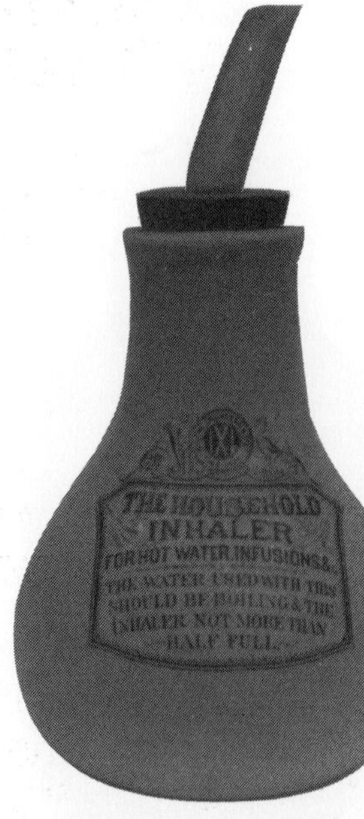

Manufacturers eventually replaced the the two glass tubes – the air intake and the mouthpiece to look more professional. The intake was moulded into the container, while the mouth-piece was delicately shaped. A good example is Ayrton & Saunders 'Household'. £25

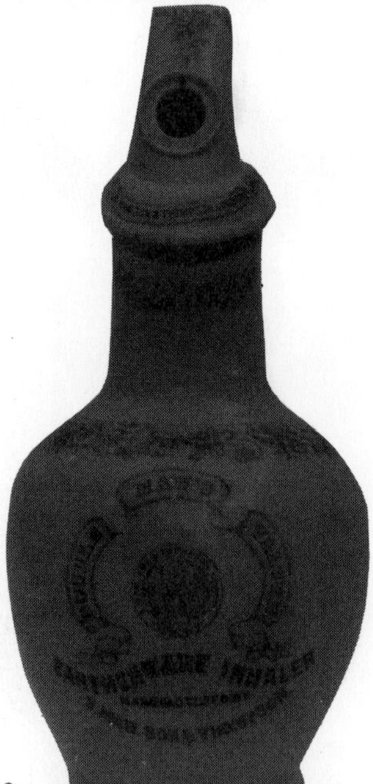

The 'Double Valve', conventially had the mouth-piece situated in the cork. A pretty blue leaf print decorates this example. £60

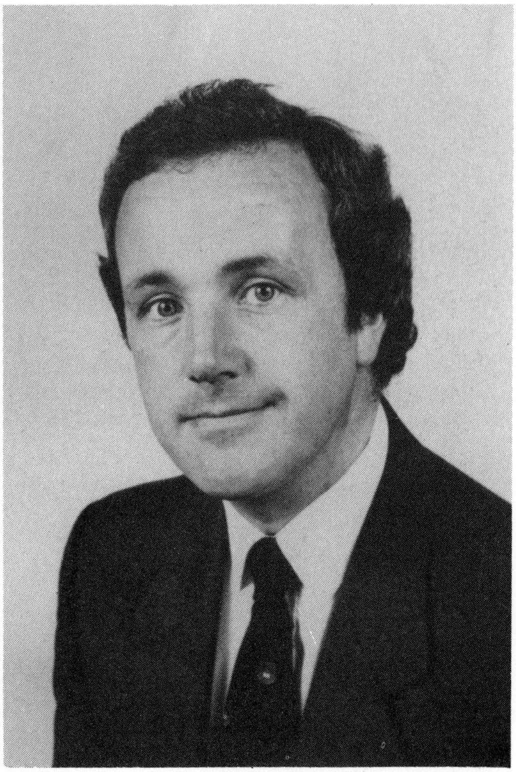

Michael Knight

Michael Knight works as a university caretaker and collects match strikers.

"There are only a handful of people in the country who collect match strikers but I have been doing it for several years and now have over 50 of them. They are basically round ceramic match holders with a serrated edge for striking the matches on and they were given away as promotional advertising by tobacco and mineral water firms as well as beer and spirit companies.

"They date from the late Victorian through the Edwardian period but generally went into disuse after the First World War.

"They were made in different shapes — animals, figures and bottles sometimes — and the advertising ones are the most collectible."

Michael finds his match strikers in bottle shows and jumble sales or antique shops. Often people do not know what they are. When he started collecting prices were low with a maximum of around £7 for a very good example but recently they have escalated and now a good match striker can fetch between £30 and £40.

The sort of match striker that Michael is most interested in finding now are the ones with printed slogans on them — but they have to be unchipped and in good condition.

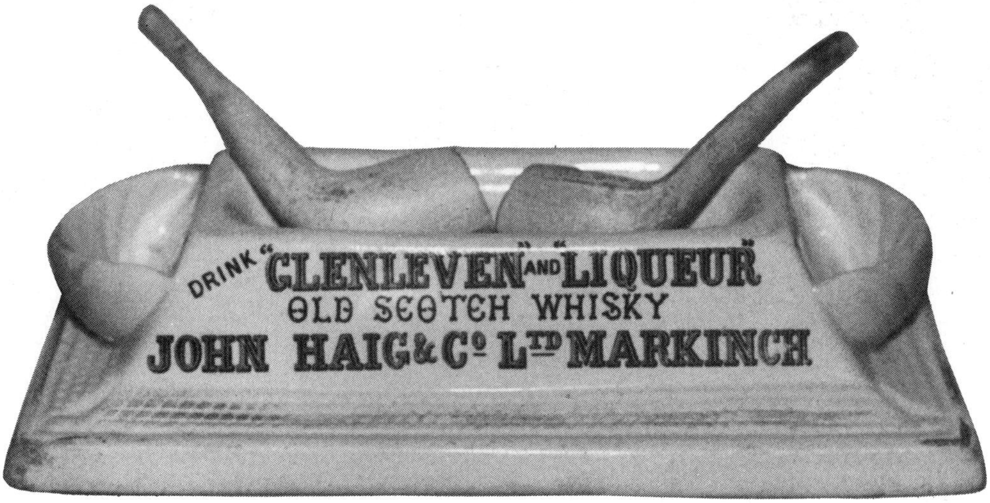

Combined striker/ashtray produced for John Haig & Co. Ltd., Markinch, to advertise Glenleven Old Scotch Whisky, by Ralph Hammersley of Burslem, circa 1895.   £60

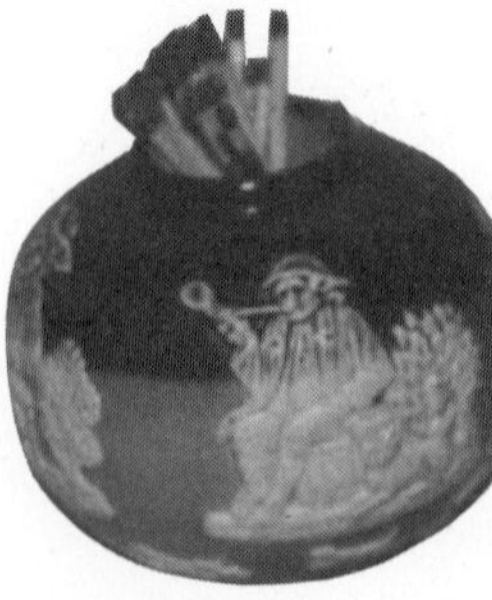

Doulton's of Lambeth match striker with impressed date, 1885. £35

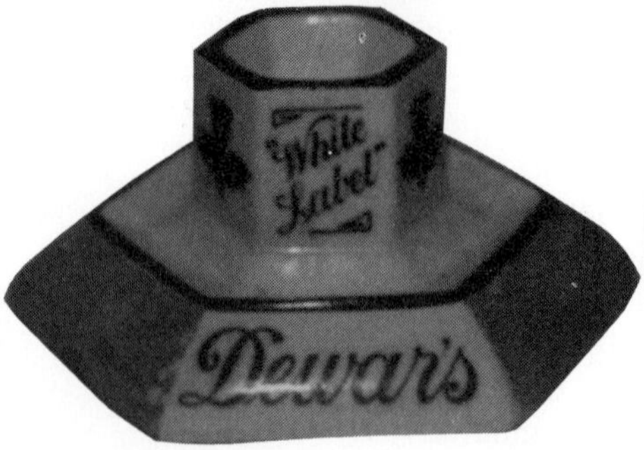

Royal Doulton Dewar's White Label whisky striker/ashtray, circa 1905. £40

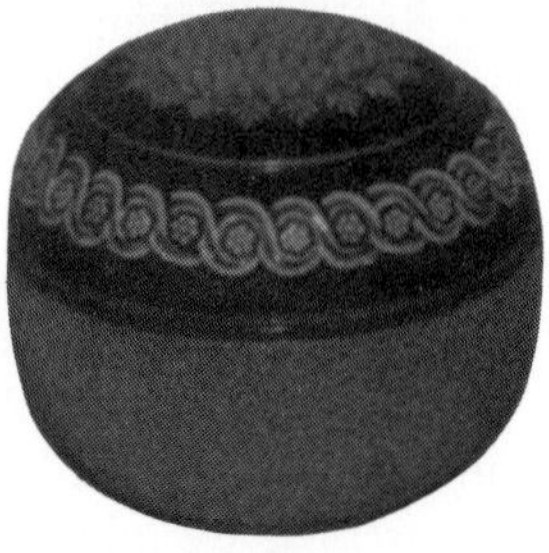

Doulton of Lambeth striker with impressed mark, 1918. £40

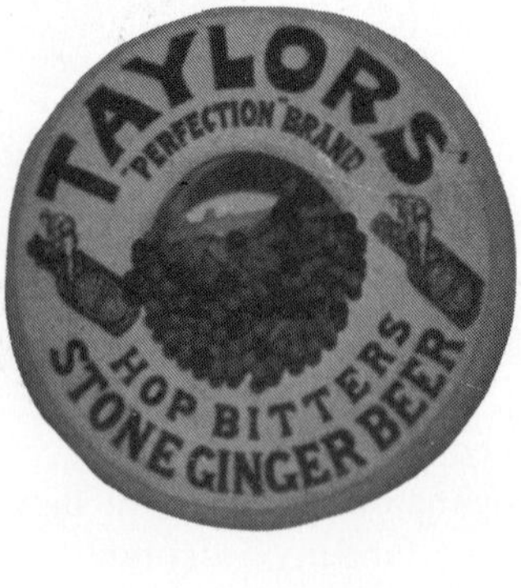

Taylors' 'Stone Ginger Beer' match striker made by Wiedekind & Co., circa 1890. £25

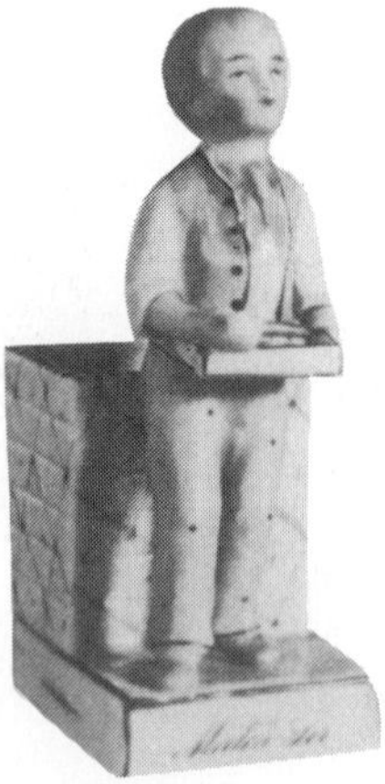

German fairing match striker 'Match Sir', circa 1890. £75

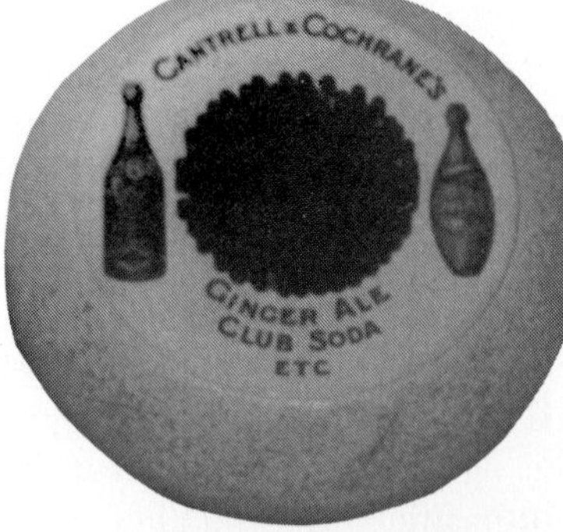

Cantrell & Cochrane's Ginger Ale, Club Soda striker, circa 1895. £50

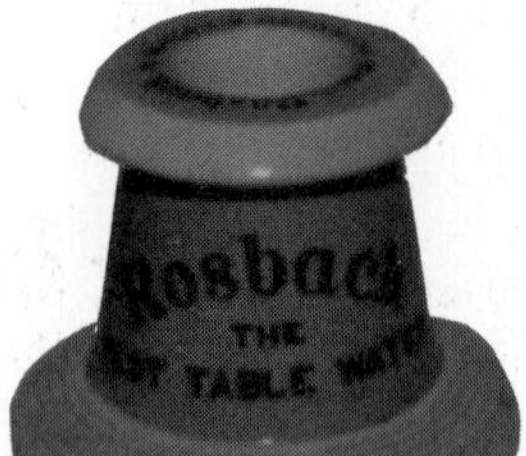

Rosbach Table Waters striker made by Wardle of England, circa 1890. £25

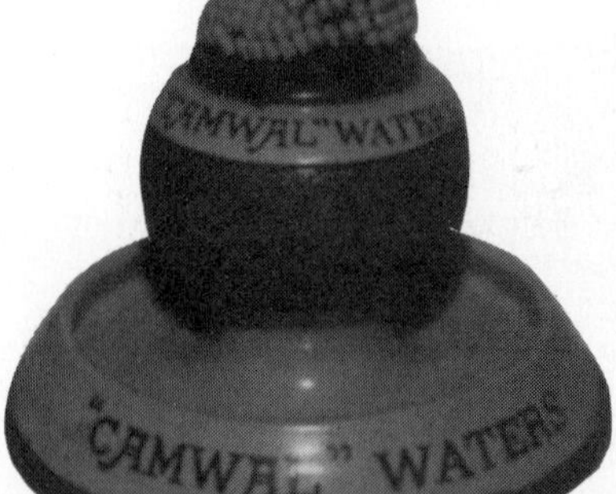

'Camwal' Waters combined striker and ashtray, circa 1900. £30

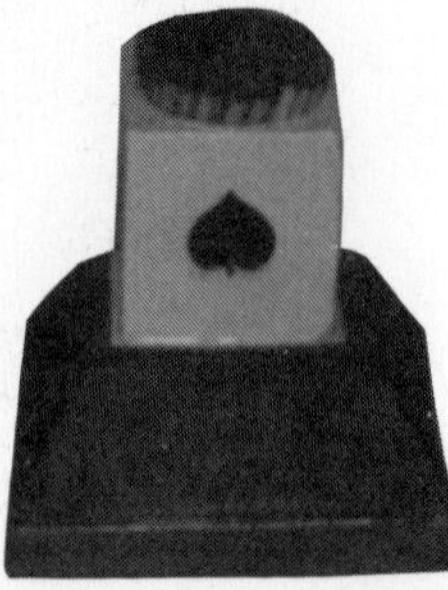

Match striker for use on a card table showing Diamonds, Hearts, Spades and Clubs on each of the four sides, circa 1895. £40

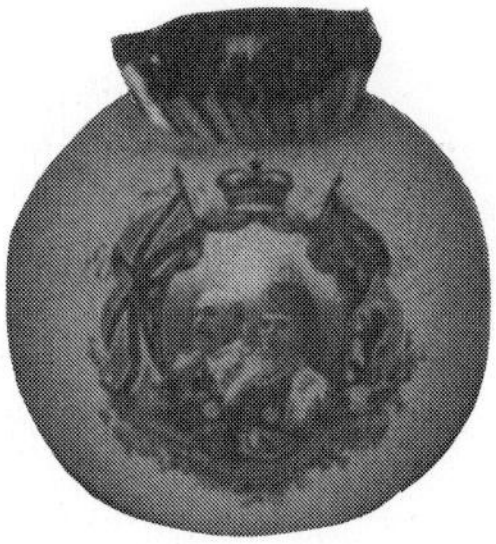

Commemorative striker for the Coronation of Edward VII, 1902. £35

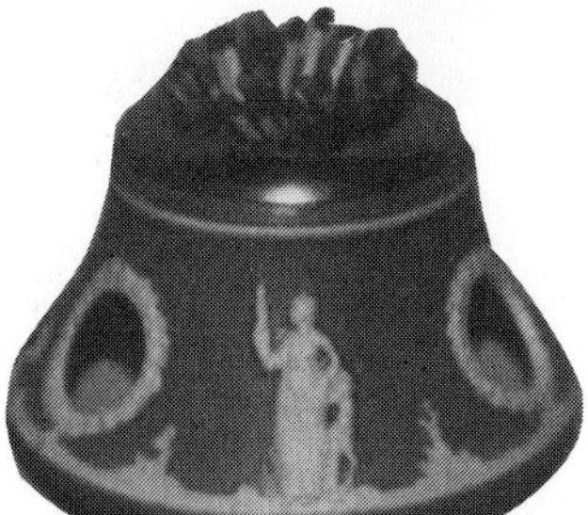

Wedgwood jasper ware striker, circa 1900. £40

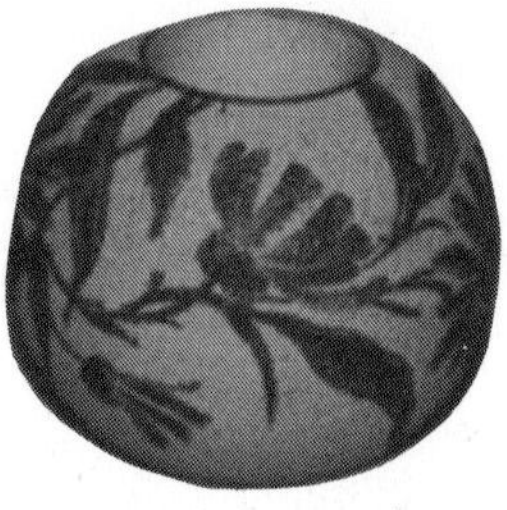

Floral design striker by Taylor Tunncliff, circa 1900. £30

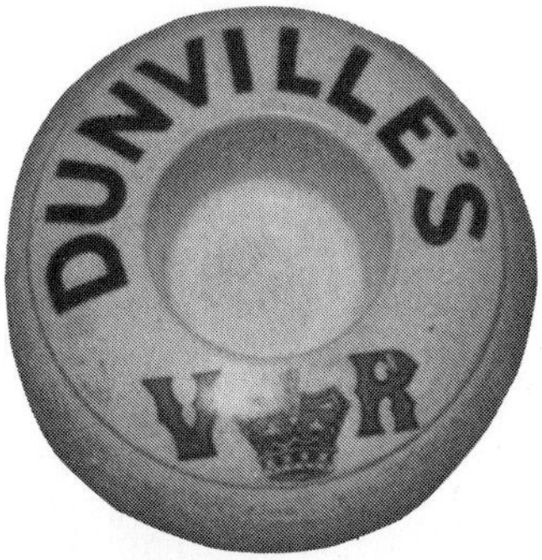

Dunville's striker made by Richard Patterson, circa 1890. £25

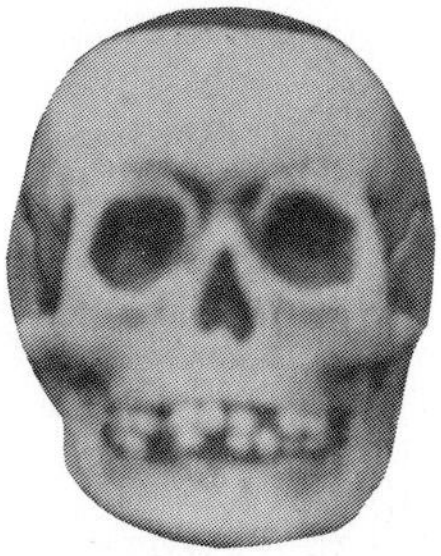

Porcelain skull match striker, circa 1900. £45

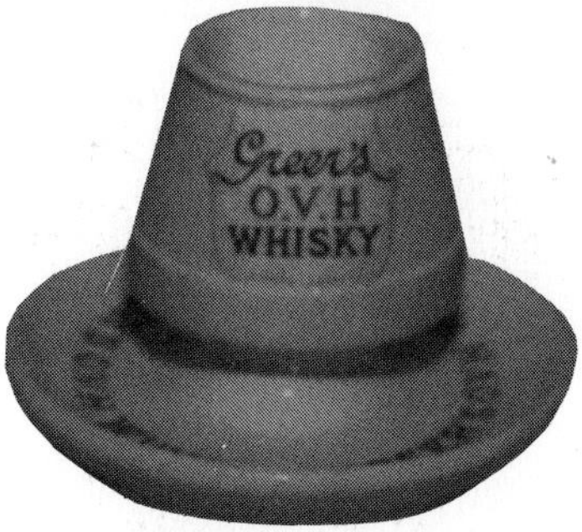

Greer's O.V.H. whisky match striker made by Fieldings, circa 1895. £30

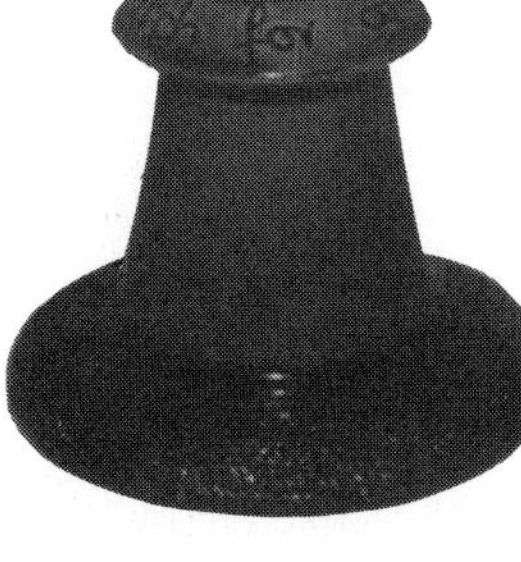

'A match for any man', made in Devon, circa 1930. £15

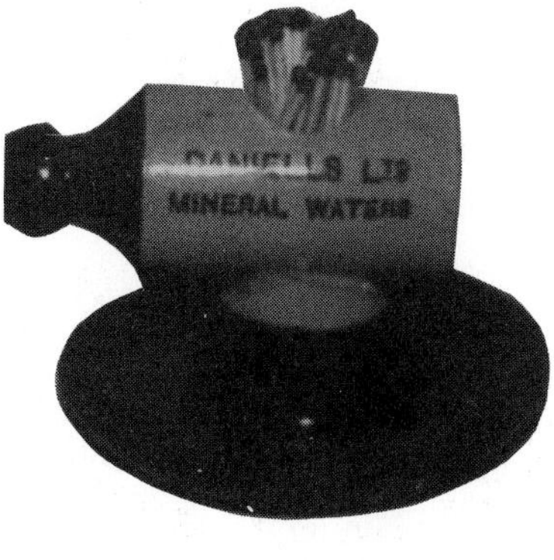

Daniells Ltd. Mineral Waters striker in the shape of a bottle, circa 1900. £60

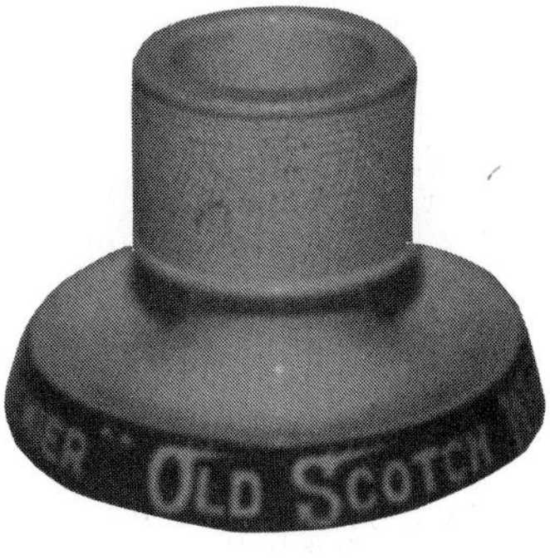

Wright & Greig's Premier Old Scotch striker, circa 1885. £25

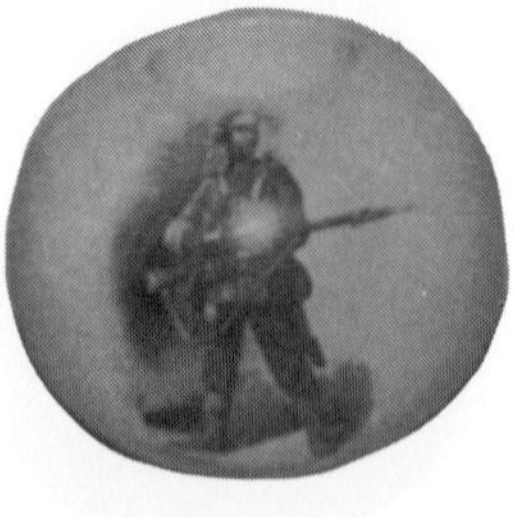

'Gentleman in Khaki' striker made by McIntyre, circa 1890. £40

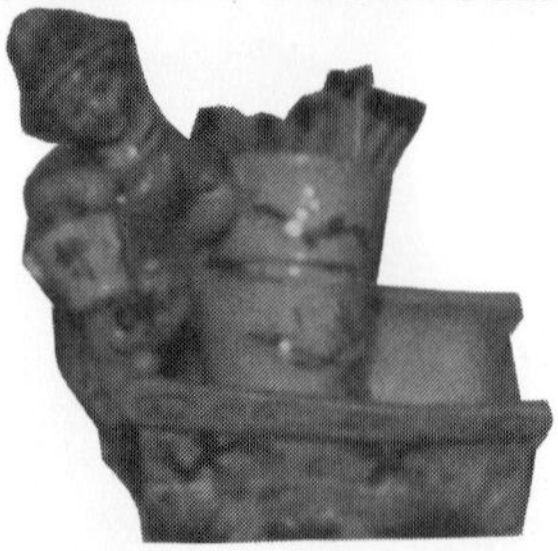

German fairing match striker, circa 1890. £50

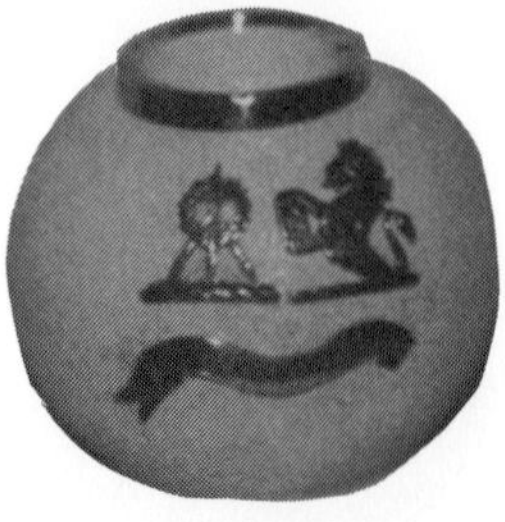

Ship's striker with hallmarked silver decoration London 1889. £60

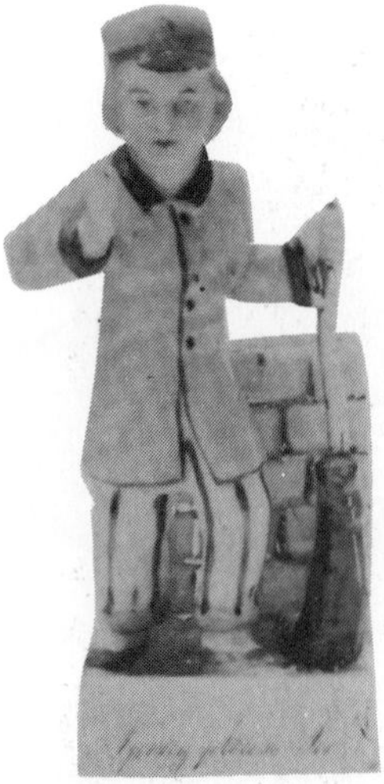

German match striker 'Penny Please, Sir?', circa 1890. £75

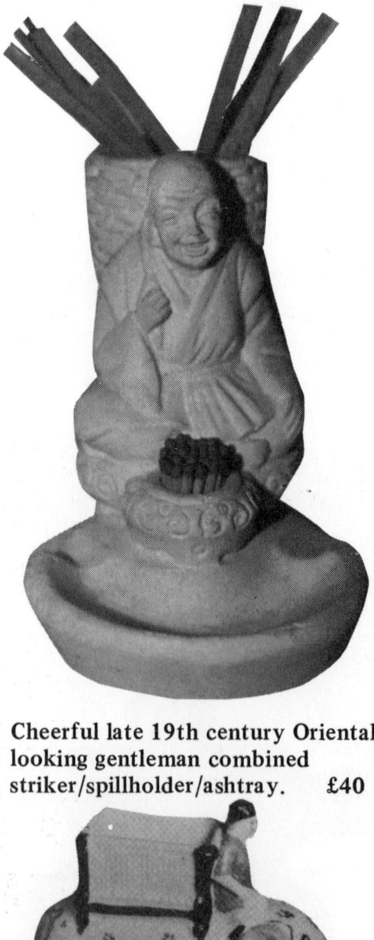

Cheerful late 19th century Oriental looking gentleman combined striker/spillholder/ashtray. £40

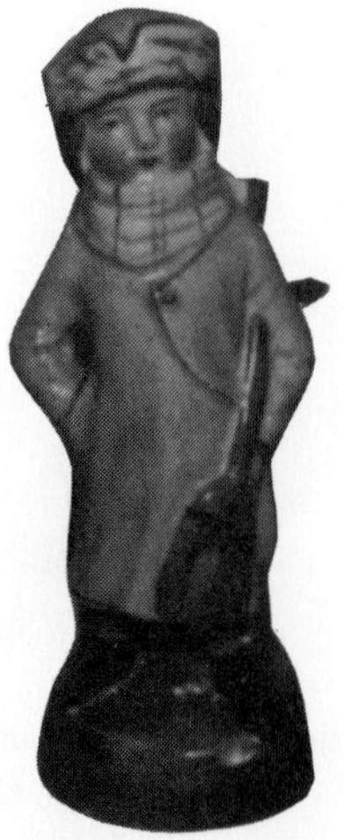

China match striker figurine of a young girl, circa 1890. £50

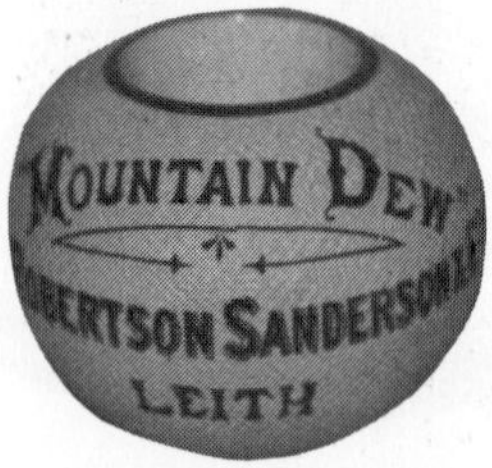

'Mountain Dew' whisky by Robertson Sanderson & Co., Leith, circa 1882. £30

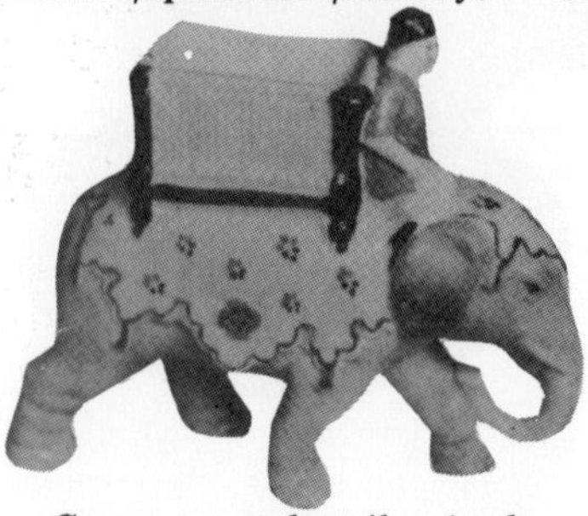

German match striker in the form of an elephant, circa 1890. £35

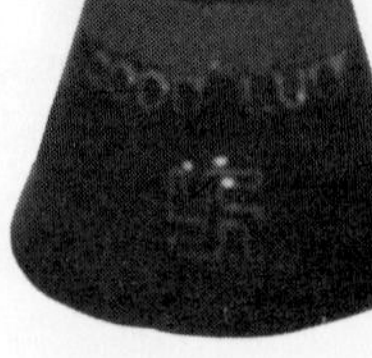

Striker with old 'good luck' symbol by Royal Doulton, circa 1905. £40

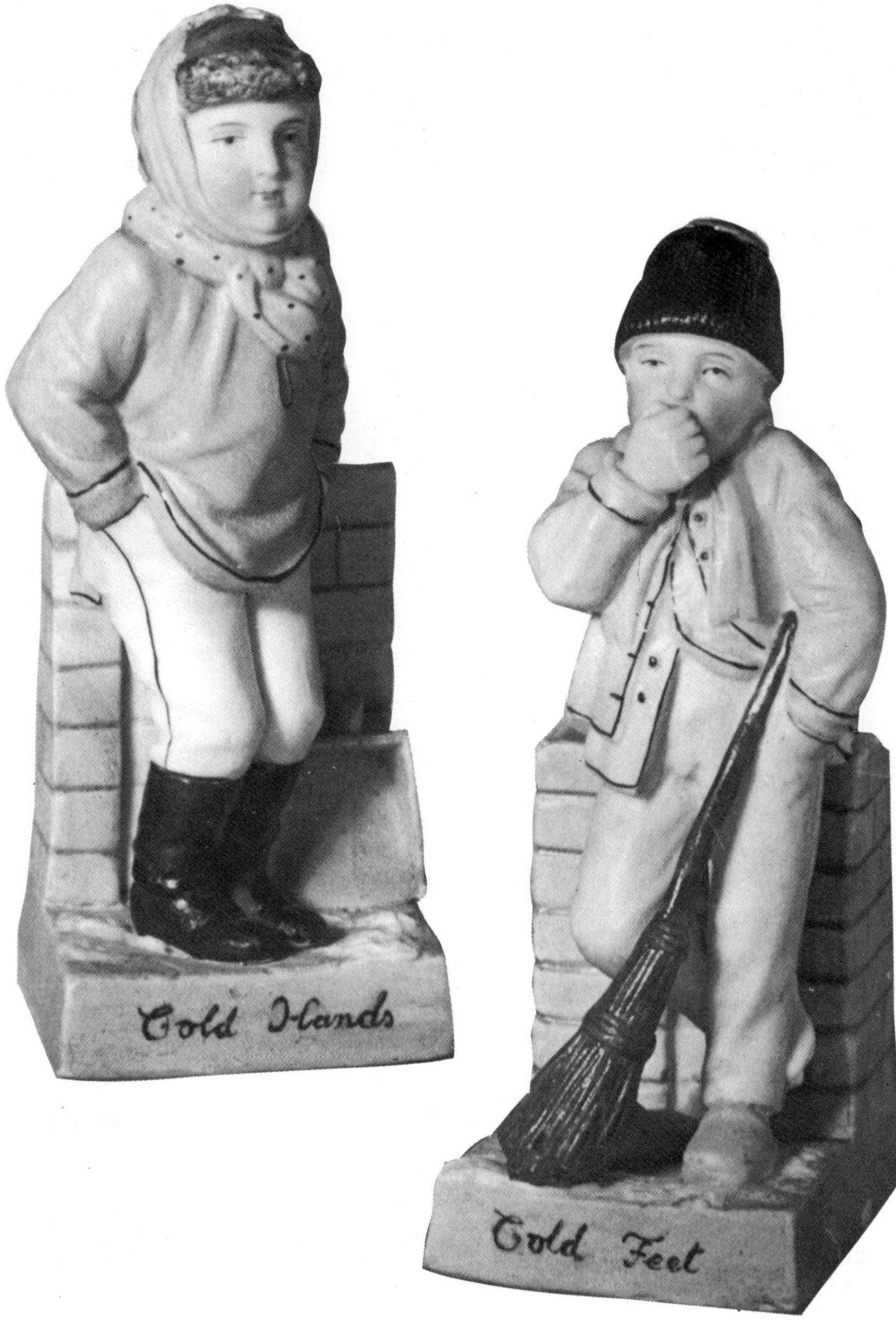

A fine pair of Victorian match strikers entitled 'Cold Hands and Cold Feet'. £125

Ian Allen is the creator of the popular Thames TV puppet series 'Button Moon' and collects tins with fairy tale characters on them.

"I started my career doing window displays and I'd got very interested in old advertising when I was at art school. The first decorated tin I bought had Red Riding Hood on it and that became the inspiration for my first solo puppet show. It was so successful that Red Riding Hood has become a sort of lucky charm for me and anything I see with her on it, I buy.

Nursery rhyme decorated tins are quite difficult to find but I've got some for Mazzawattee Tea decorated with pictures of Red Riding Hood and custard tins with Tom, Tom The Piper's Son and Four and Twenty Blackbirds — in fact almost all the popular nursery rhymes are represented in my collection.

I like old advertising because it helps me in my work though there's nothing nostalgic about Button Moon — quite the opposite.

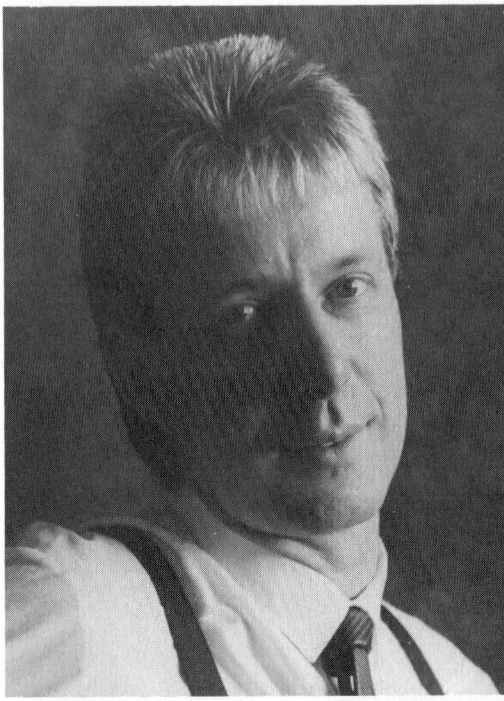

Ian Allen known for the T.V. Series 'Button Moon'.

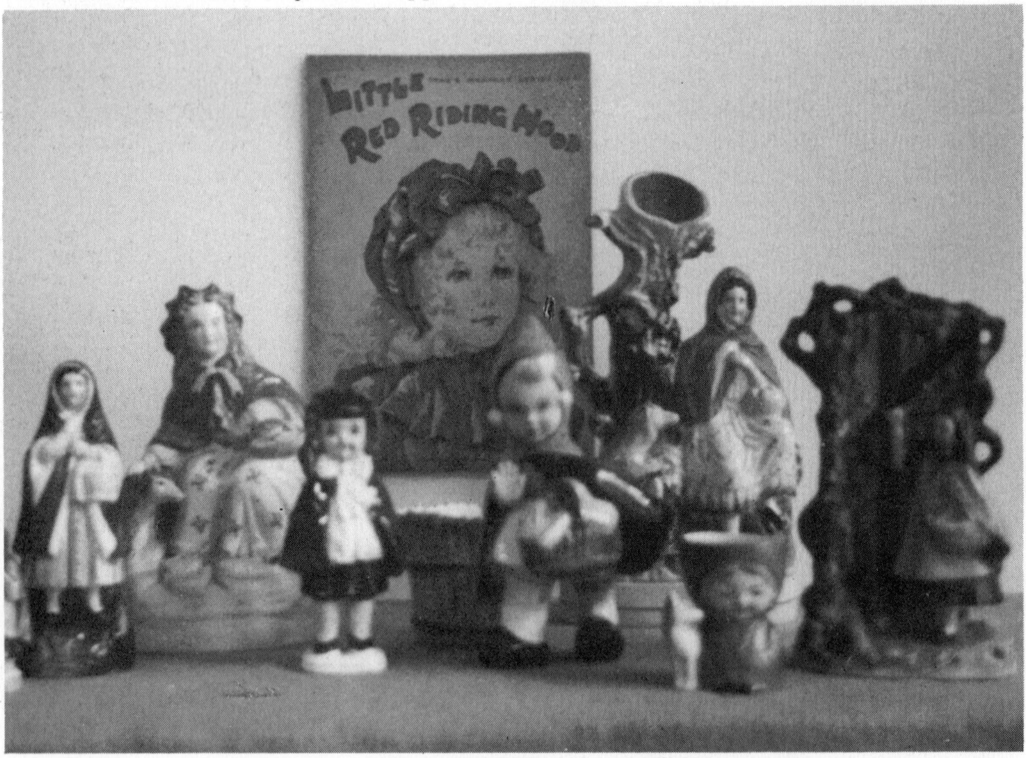

Part of Ian's Red Riding Hood collection.

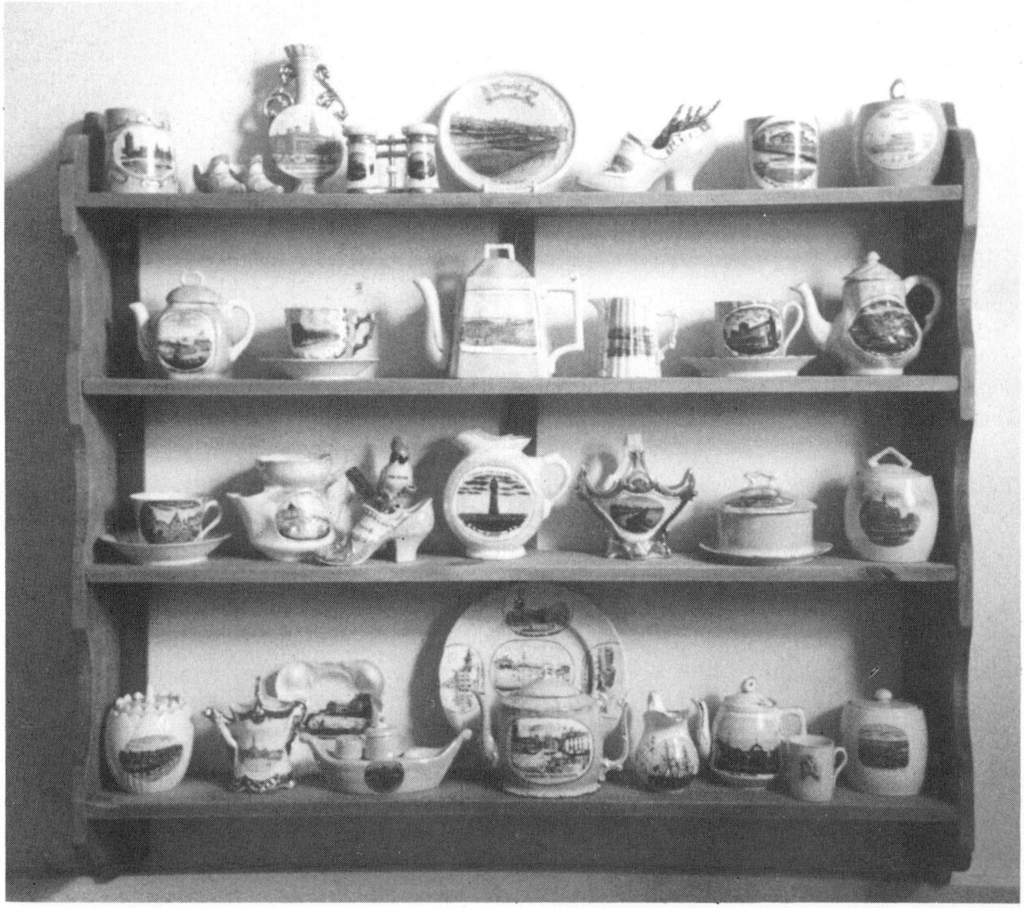

Another of Ian's interests is collecting Souvenir China, mostly made in Germany.

Thc tins show mc how idcas havc changcd and I think Red Riding Hood used to have much more fun in Victorian times than she did later because they allowed her to get into bed with the wolf!"

Ian's collections includes tin handbags that were made to contain biscuits and also several children's tea sets painted with nursery rhyme characters. He said that when he started collecting, tins were cheap but they have gone up recently and it is now common to be asked around £100 for one.

The items he would like to find for his collection include a Fry's chocolate tin with a picture of Red Riding Hood taking chocolates to her granny and a booklet on Red Riding Hood produced in the 1890's by Colman's mustard.

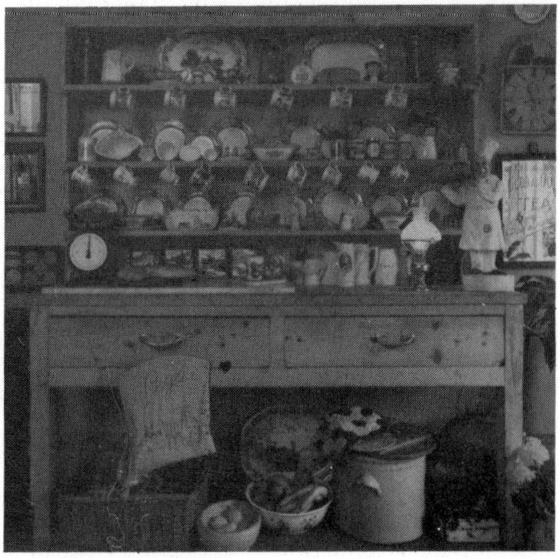

An attractive display in Ian's kitchen.

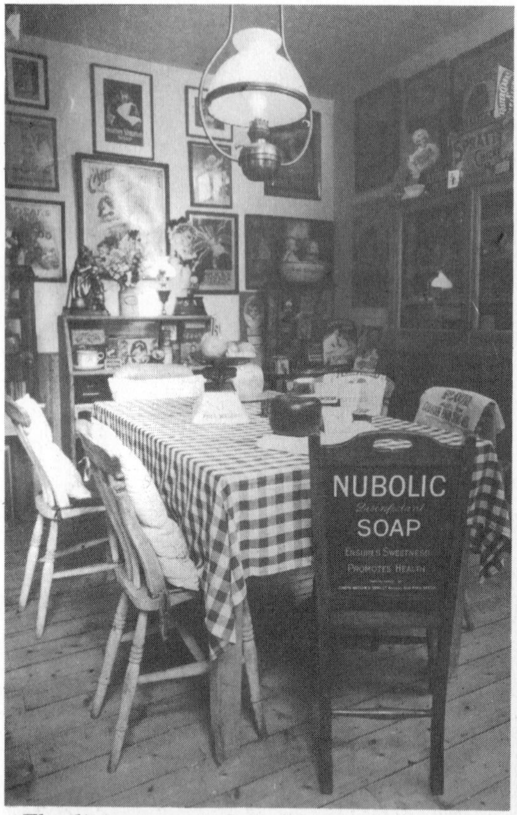

The dining room in Ian's house well illustrates his creative flair.

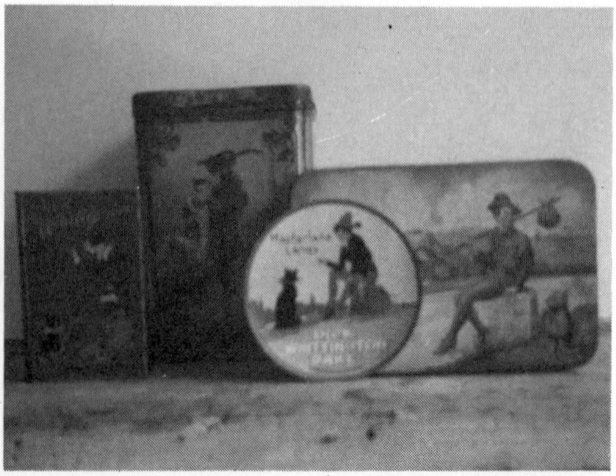

Colourful tins decorated with Dick Whittington.

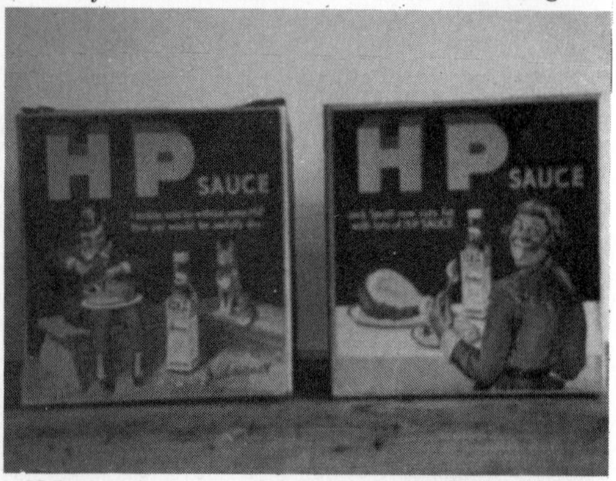

H.P. Sauce boxes depicting Little Jack Horner and Jack Spratt.

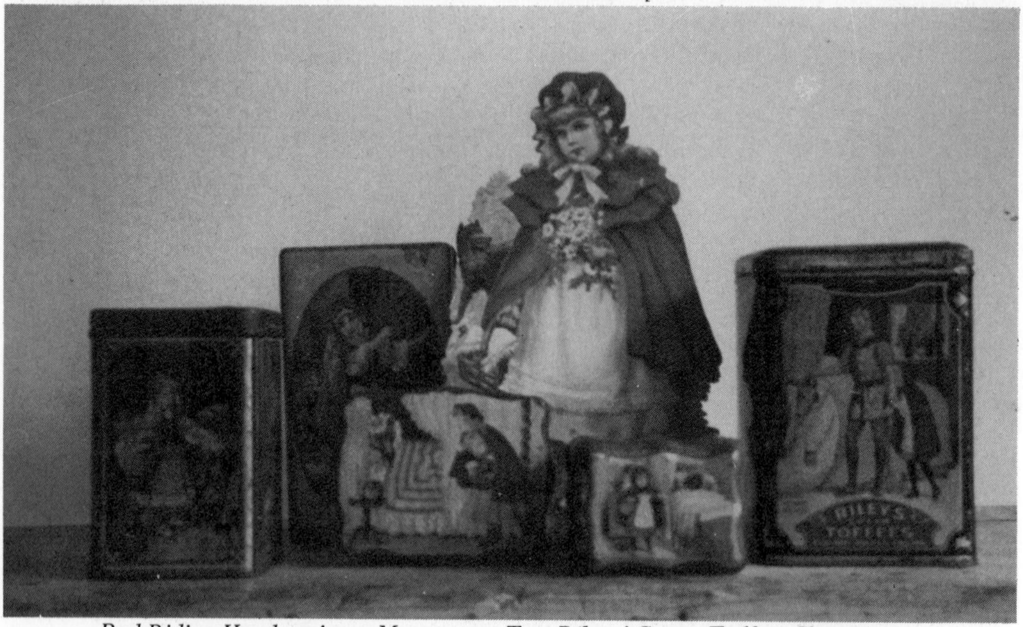

Red Riding Hood again on Mazawattee Tea, Rileys' Cream Toffee, Champions Mustard Tins and Raphael Tuck cut-out.

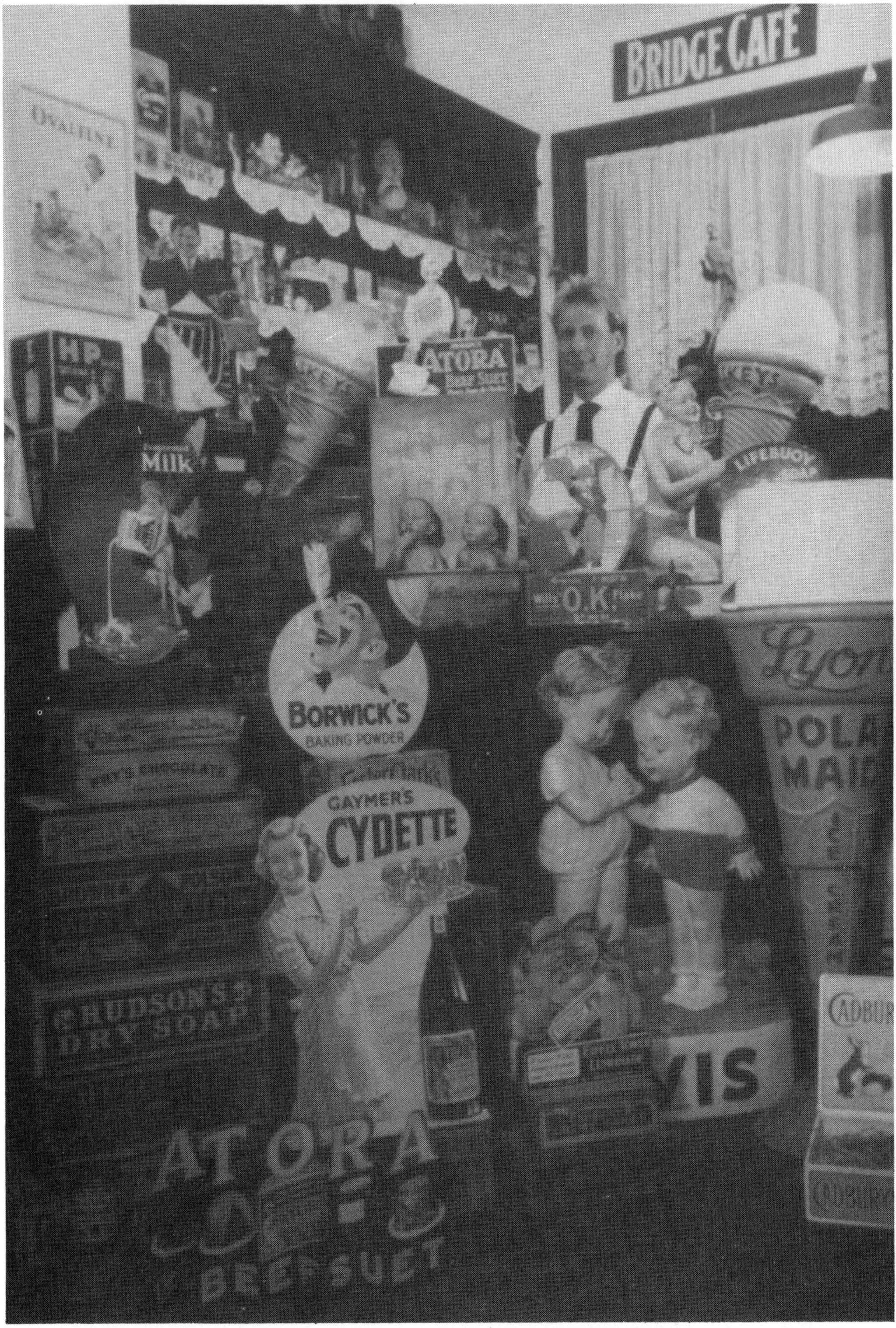

Ian with his amazing collection of Victorian and Edwardian advertisements.

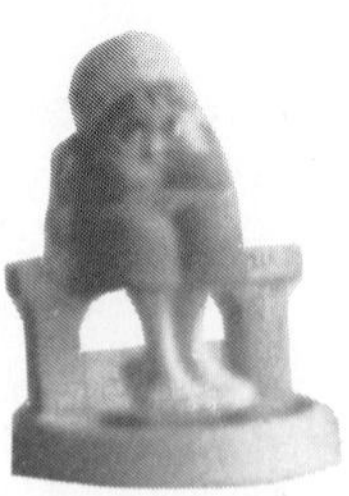

Lady in bathing outfit nodding figure £50

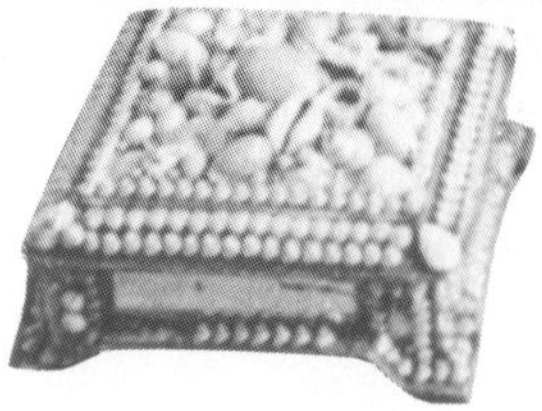

Shell art box. £20

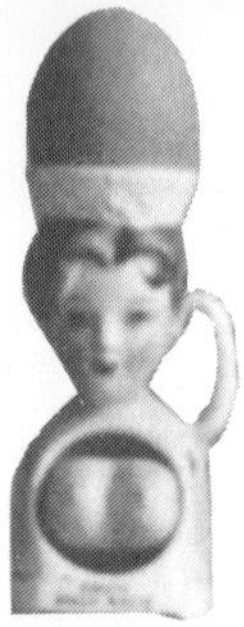

1950's 'Chaste Makes Waste' egg cup £6

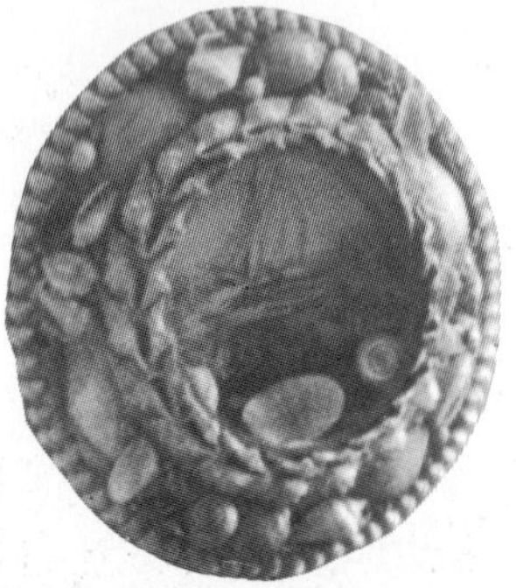

Shell art picture fame. £24

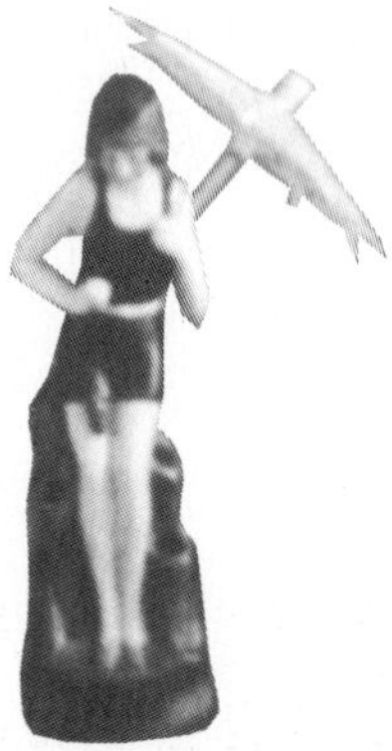

1930's 'Bathing Beauty' figure £55

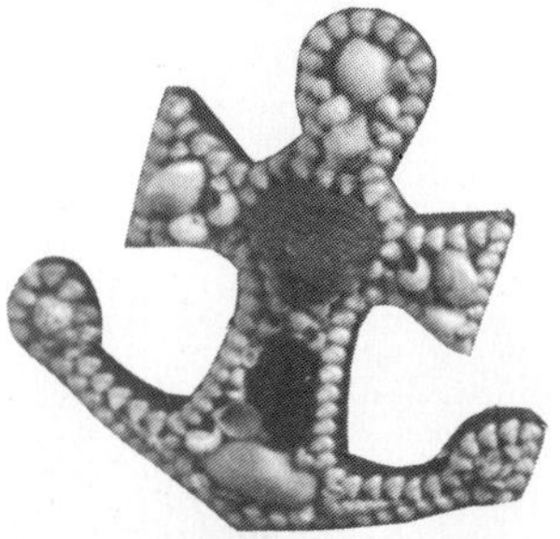

Shell art anchor pin cushion. £14

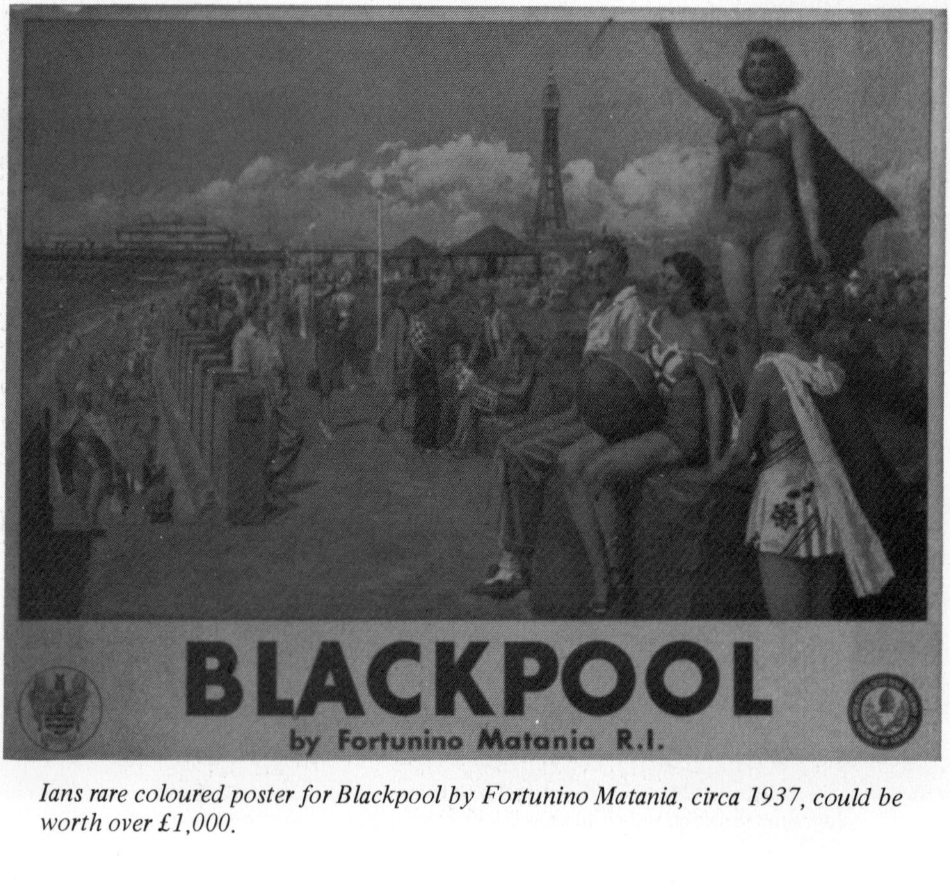

Ians rare coloured poster for Blackpool by Fortunino Matania, circa 1937, could be worth over £1,000.

Richard May is an electronics engineer and collects crown cork bottle openers.

"Since childhood I've been a collector and one day I was having a glass of beer with a friend and he said something about crown top bottle openers being a good thing to collect, so I started and now I've got over 1,000 of them.

"The most collectible come from breweries that have gone out of business and the best ones are made of cast iron. Most were for beer but some were made for mineral water bottles and some foundries made them as advertising items. The later ones are made of pressed steel and are not so desirable. I only collect the ones with trade names on them and ideally British. I don't have the kind that say 'A Present From Blackpool' or anything like that.

"Some date from before the First World War but they are difficult to date unless you can trace the firm.

"The rarest one I've got is worth about £25 and was made in the shape of a face with the mouth being the opening part. It advertised a brewery called Thomson, Wooton of Ramsgate."

Prices for crown top bottle openers can range from 10p to £5 for the ordinary variety but rarer ones cost more. The one that Mr May wants to add to his collection was made for Bugle Brand Guinness Stout of Woolwich and is shaped like a bugle. 'I'd go up to £5 for that,' he said.

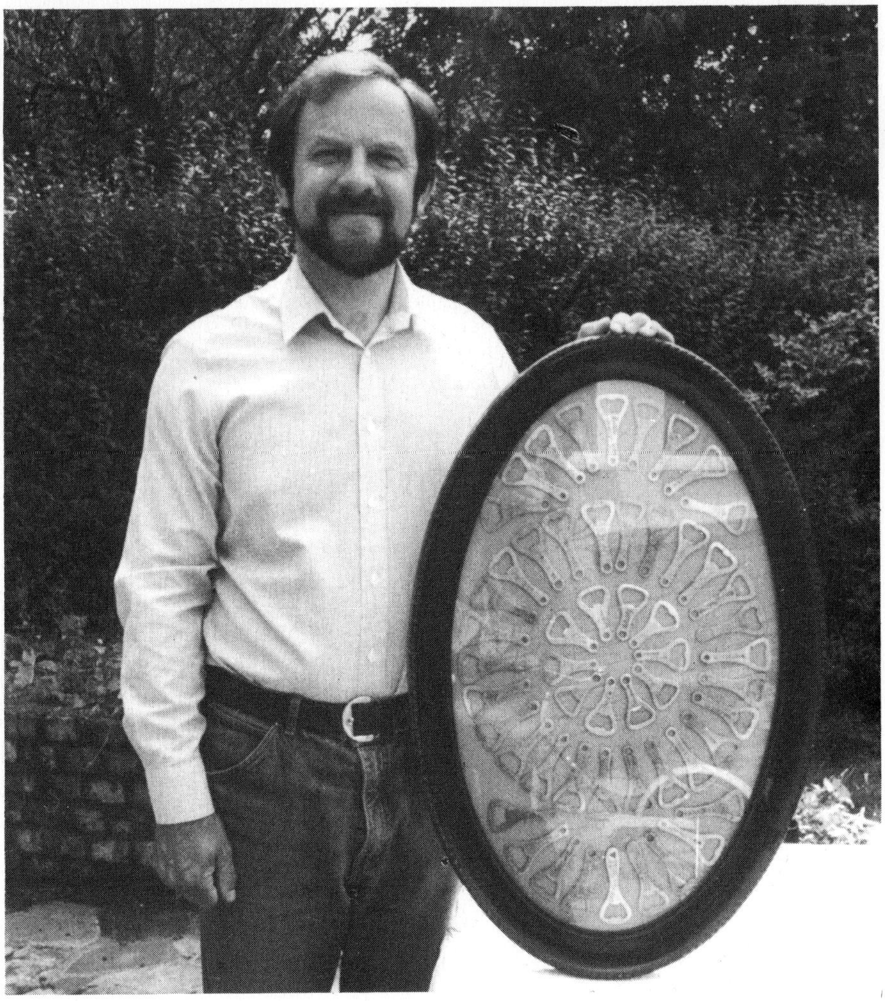

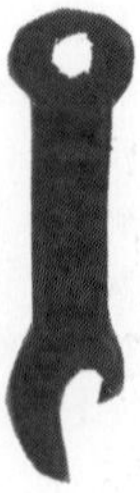

'Try Ehrets Extra', U.S. pressed steel opener. £3

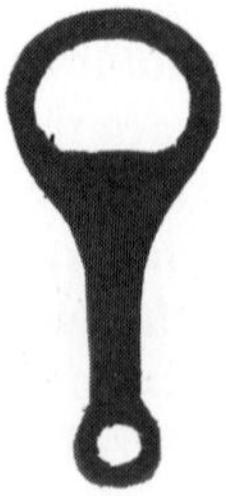

Imperial cork seal. £2

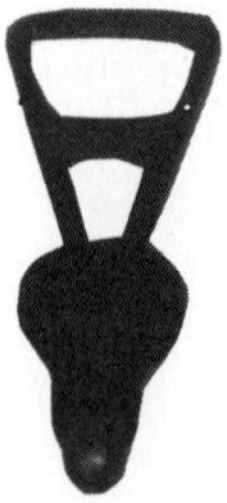

Perrier opener with screw stopper. £3

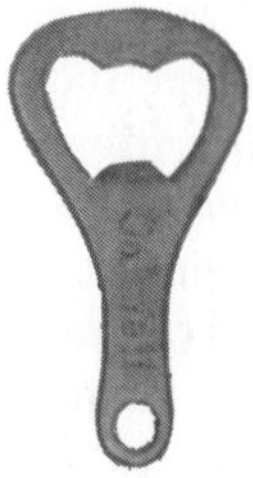

Barnsley Brewery opener 'Oakwell S.P. (Strong & Pure)'. 50p

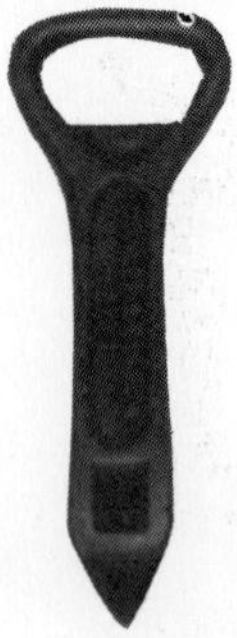

Dunlop & Ranken of Leeds. £1

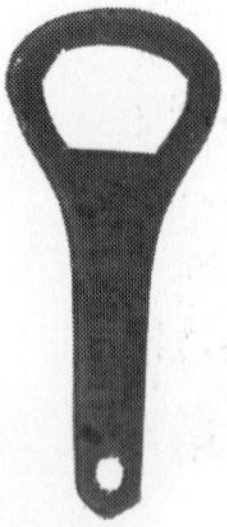

An early pattern opener Prize Medal Allbright. £1

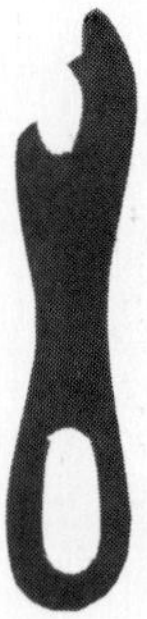

Schweppes pressed steel opener with spanner for screw stoppers. £1

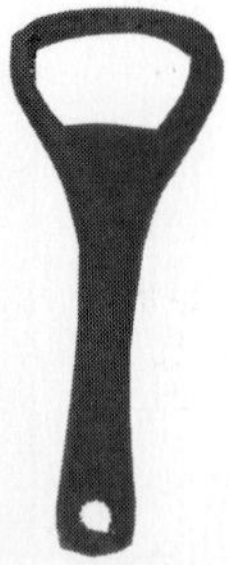

Mackintosh, Plumstead opener. £1

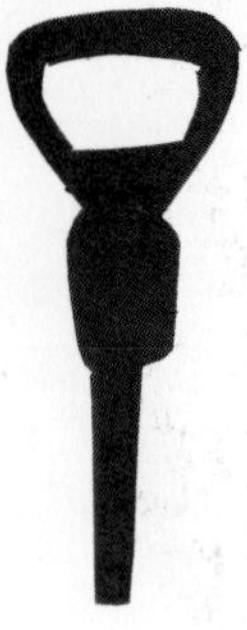

Courage opener with bung. £2

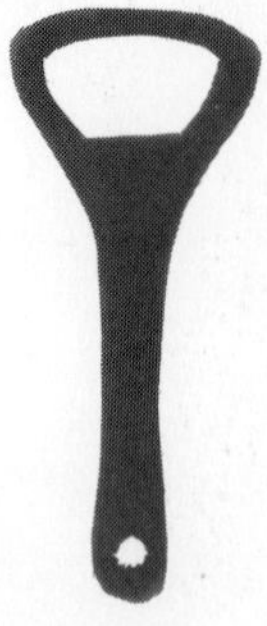

H & G Simonds Ltd., Reading. 50p

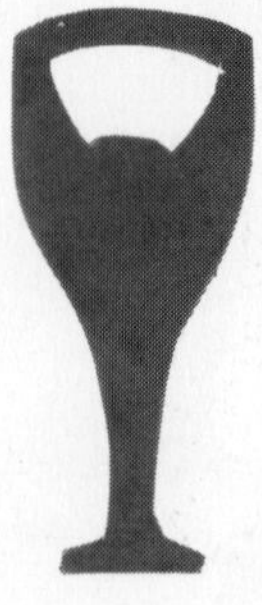

Jacobs Lager drinking glass opener. £2

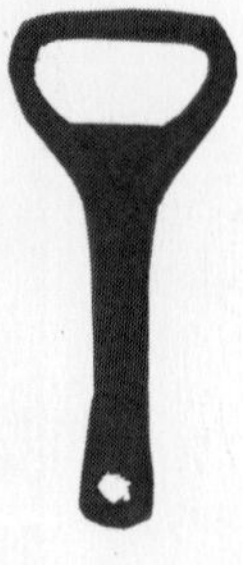

Starkeys 'Prize Ales' cast iron opener. £1

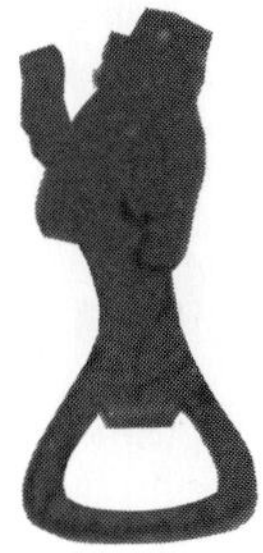

'Get Younger Every Day' opener featuring Father William. £2

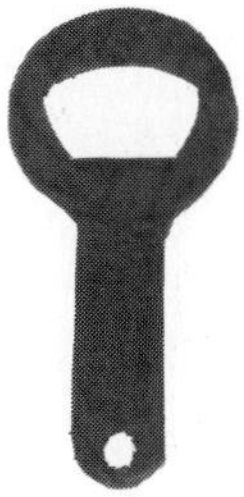

Bentley & Shaw's Town Ales, a football shaped opener. £1

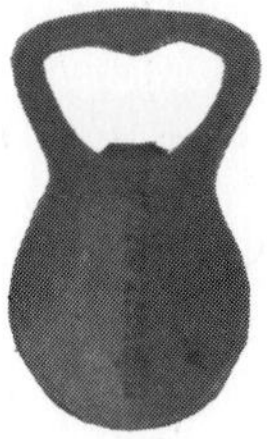

Air New Zealand shoe horn opener. £1

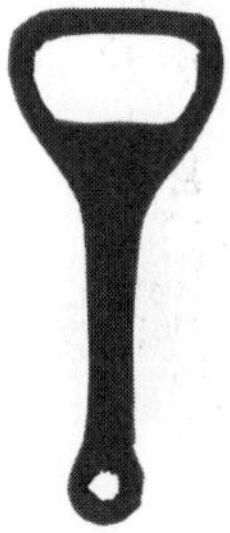

Scotts Lemonade cast iron opener. £1

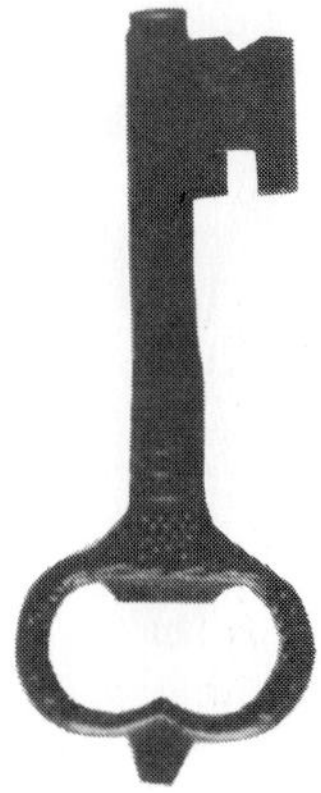

Unusual key-shaped bottle opener. £5

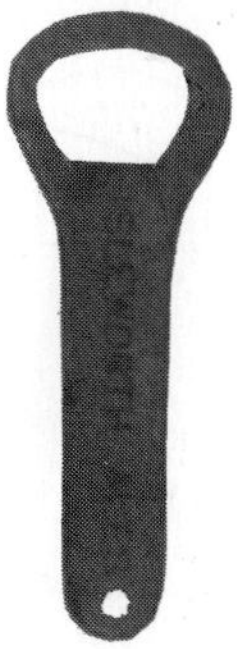

Isleworth Ales, early design, opener. £1

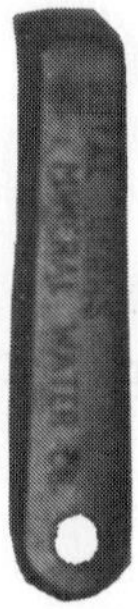

Royal Berks Mineral Water Co. cap lifter. £1

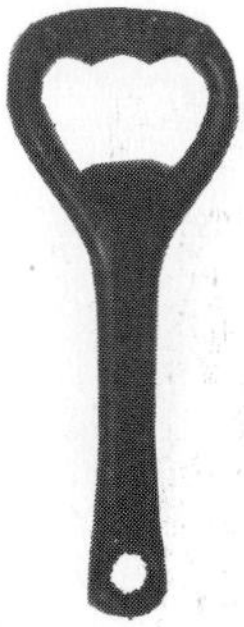

Barnsley Bry, Oakwell opener Rd. 811274. £1

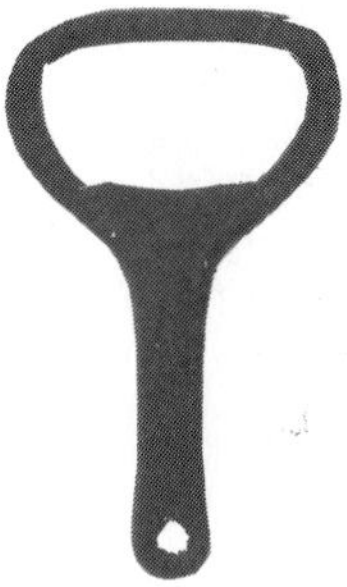

W.U.D. Ltd., Moonraker. £1

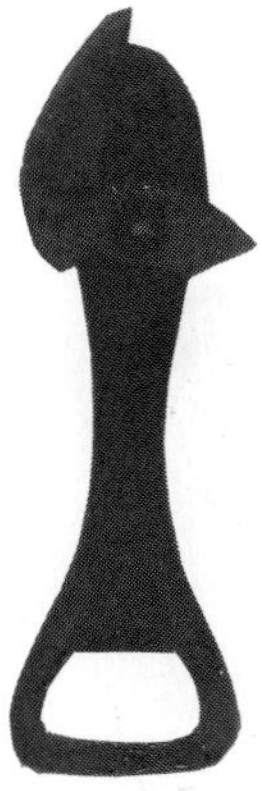

Cast iron combined can and bottle opener. £1

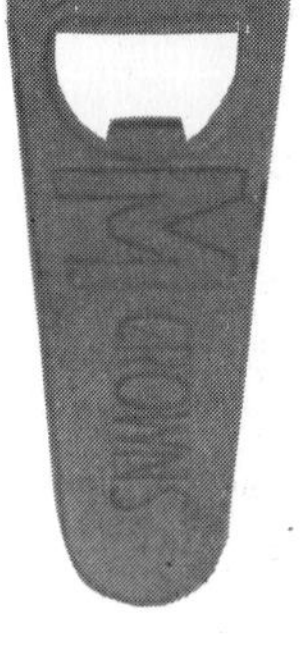

R.D.M. Crowns opener. £1

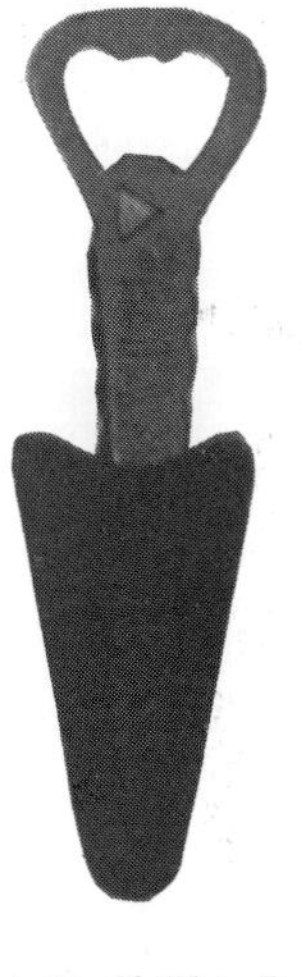

Great Stuff This Bass pipe reamer with leather case. £2

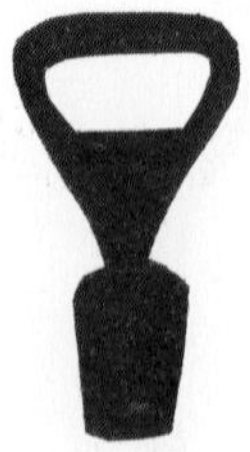

M & B opener with bung. 50p

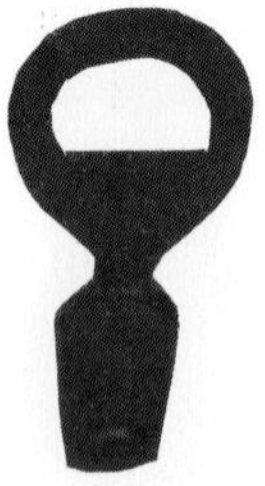

The Circle Brand opener with bung. £3

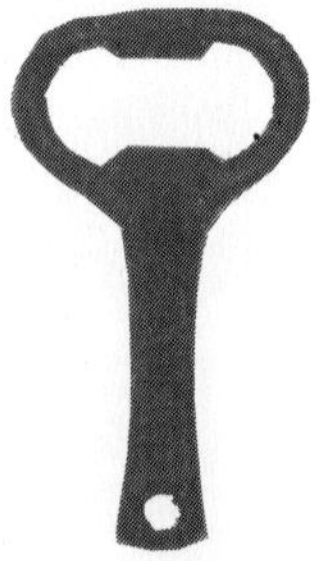

Co-op Milk Is Best. £1

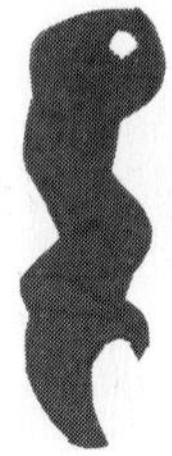

Dares Ales of Birmingham nude pressed steel opener. £3

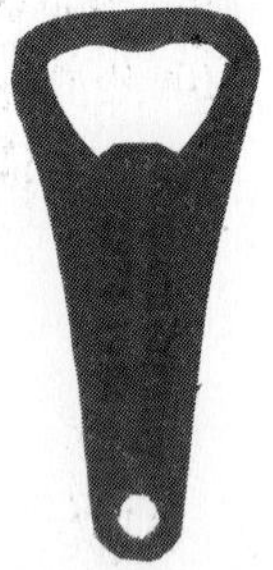

Bass Runcorn Brewery commemorative opener. £1

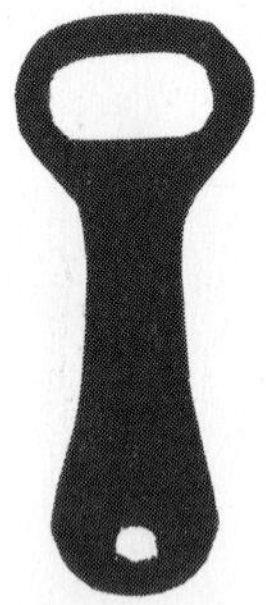

An unusual painted metal opener, City. £1

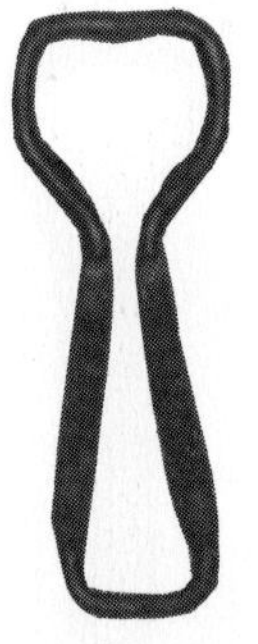

'Put Eastside Inside', U.S. wire opener. £1

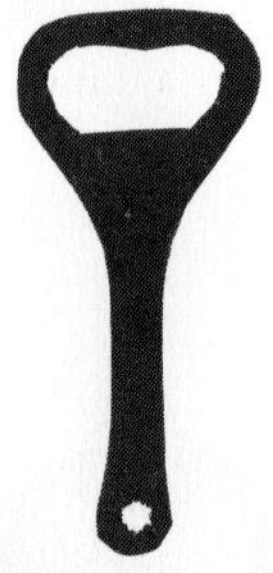

Rawlings Lemonade cast iron opener. £1

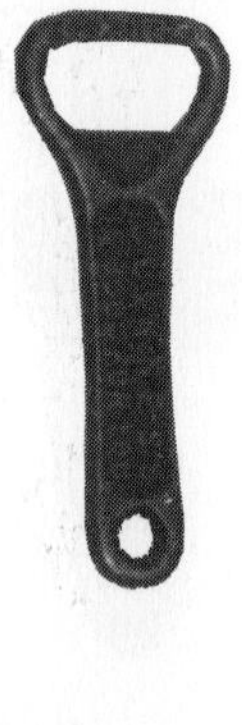

'Guinness is Good for You'. £1

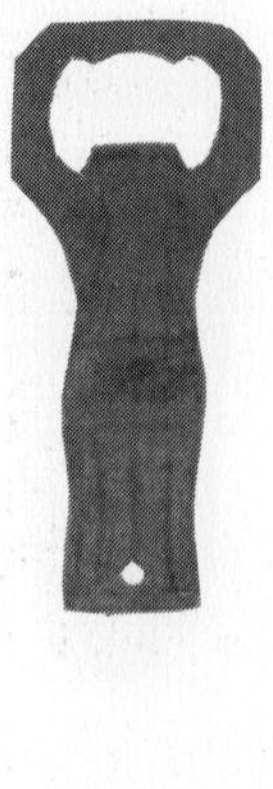

Coca Cola bottle profile opener. £2

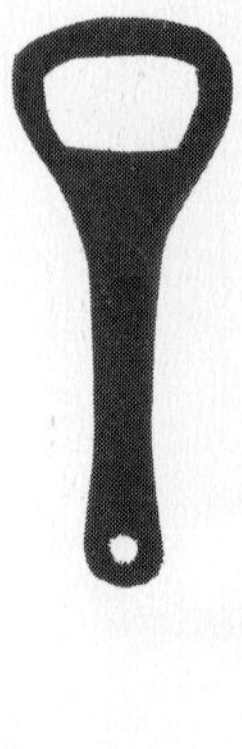

Barrnett & Foster opener, London. £1

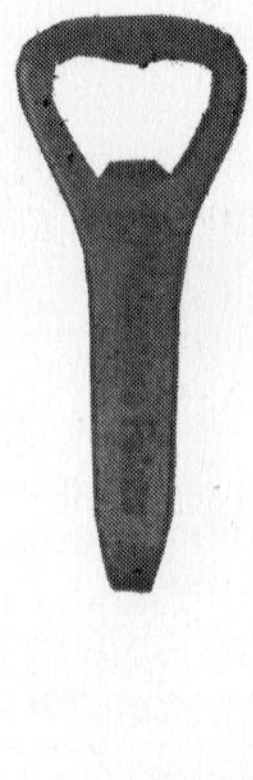

Valentine Paints with can lid lever. 50p

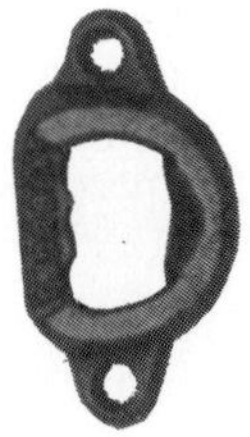

Thorben opener with mounting holes. £2

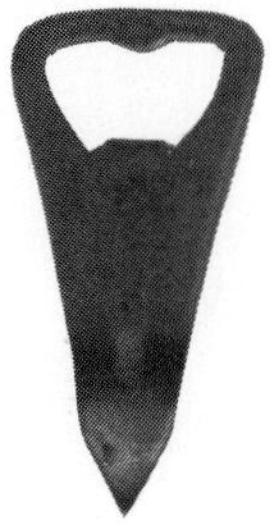

United Caledonian Breweries Ltd. bottle opener/can piercer. 50p

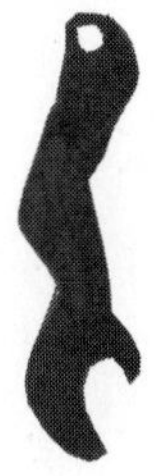

Ask for Garsides Soda Water, Bathing Belle opener. £3

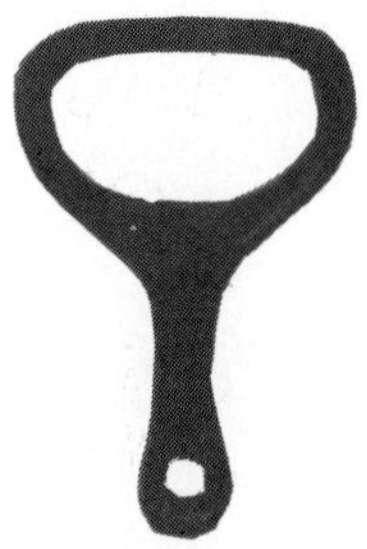

Emerson, Chanin opener. £1

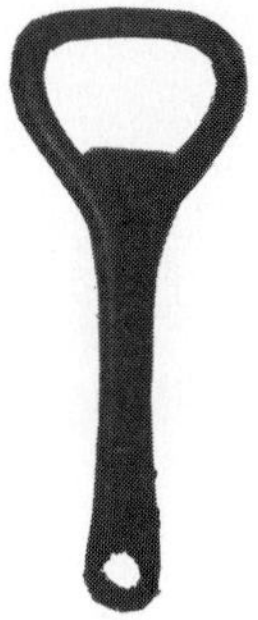

Grattans Mineral Waters opener, Belfast. £1

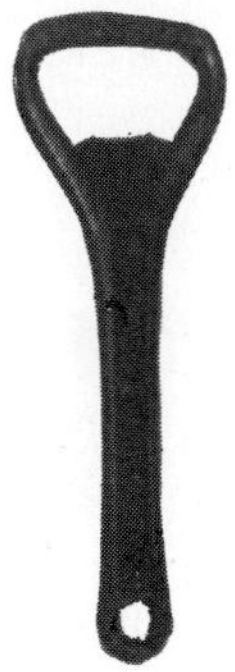

Backus & Johnston opener Rd. 702661. £1

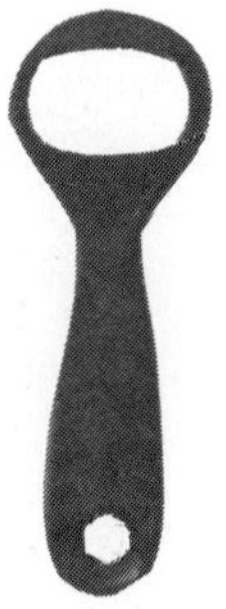

Farrow & Jackson, cork screw makers. £1

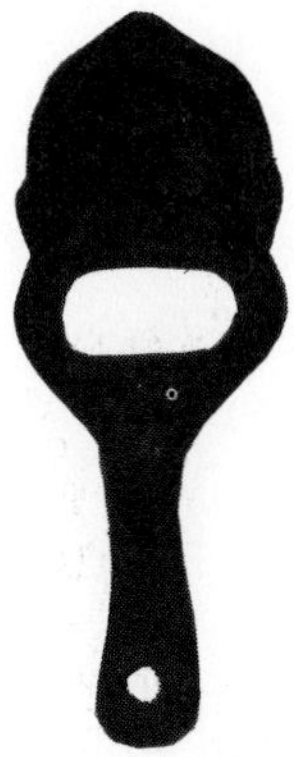

Face shaped opener by Allbright, Wooton & Thomson of Ramsgate. £10

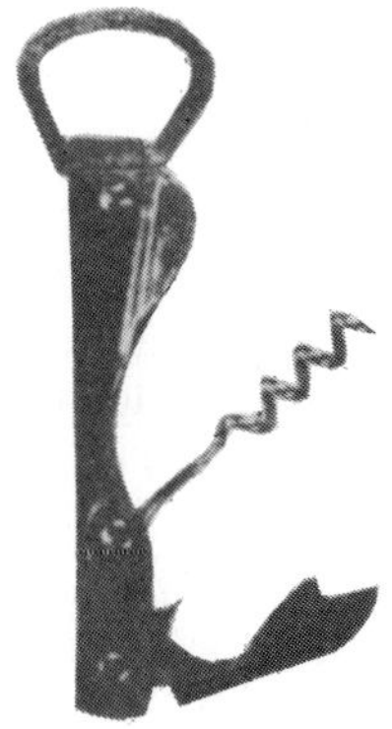

Sky-line Bottle Boy, an all chrome Crown cork opener combined with corkscrew. £2

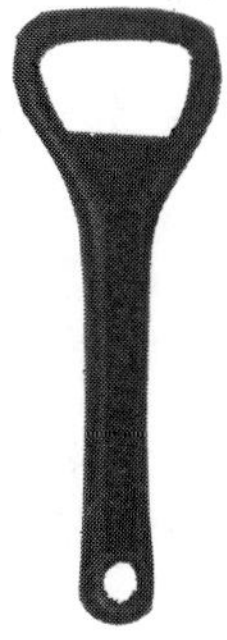

'Dog's Head Guinness' opener. £1

Lowenbrau 'Brewed and Bottled in Munich' opener. £1

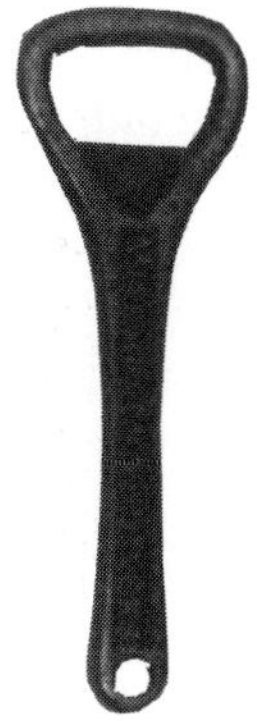

Mitchells & Butlers Extra Stout. £1

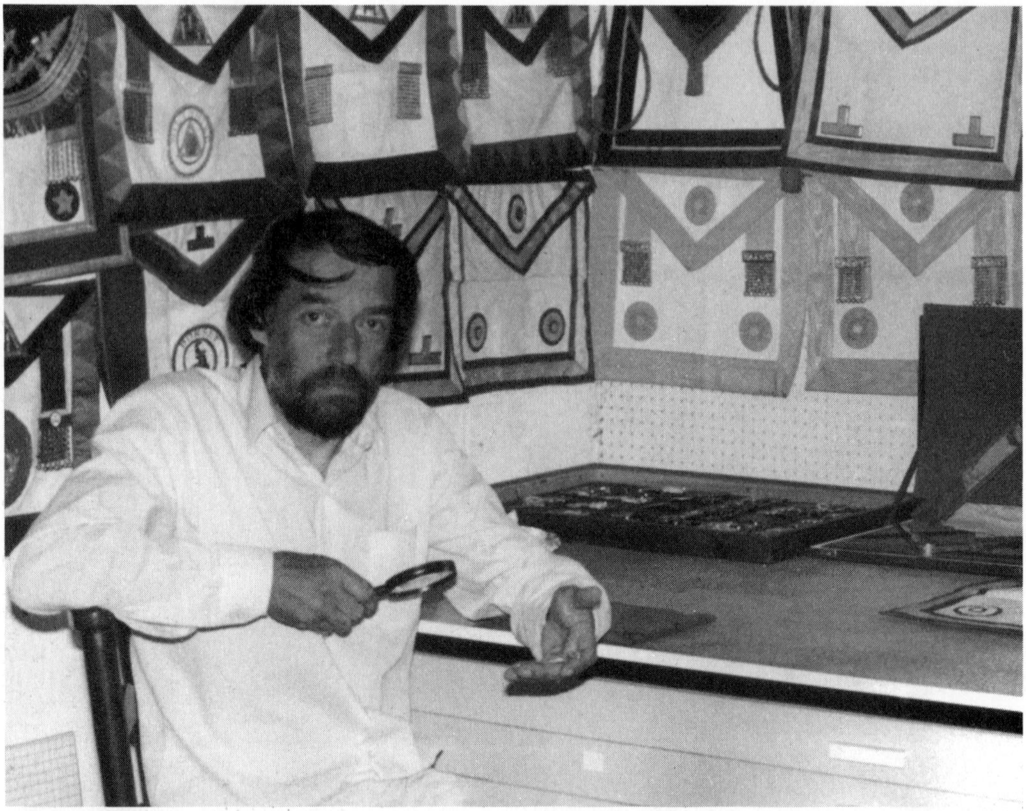

John Roberts is the Director of a Zoological and Adventure Park and collects Masonic related items.

"My collection started some years ago with a few jewels and items of regalia and has expanded to include postal covers, glassware and even furniture. The history of many pieces goes back to the 18th century, several of which originate from Scotland.

"The collection is now vast and would be sufficient to fill an entire room. I am aiming to build up enough to start a Museum perhaps associated with a specific Lodge — until then all of the rare and valuable items must remain in the bank vaults for safe keeping. The Museum of the Grand Lodge in London is the finest in the world and boasts many unique pieces."

Freemasonry is universal and John has found a number of pieces in bric-a-brac shops all over Europe. Books and manuscripts figure largely in the collection, but the bulk of it is the regalia and jewels of the several degrees of Freemasonry and those struck to commemorate the extensive charitable work of Freemasons.

John's favourite pieces include a 6 ft. × 4 ft. Hebrew parchment mounted on canvas showing the building of King Solomon's Temple, but the star of his collection is a snuff box that may once have belonged to Napoleon. It has a secret compartment, which when opened, shows the symbols of the Royal Arch. It is thought that Napoleon may have been a Freemason, although the movement was proscribed during his time.

One item John would like to add to his collection is the Freemasons' Hall medal of 1780 of which only a very limited number were struck.

There is always the chance that this and many other equally uncommon pieces may turn up in a bric-a-brac shop or at a sale and be purchased for only a few pounds.

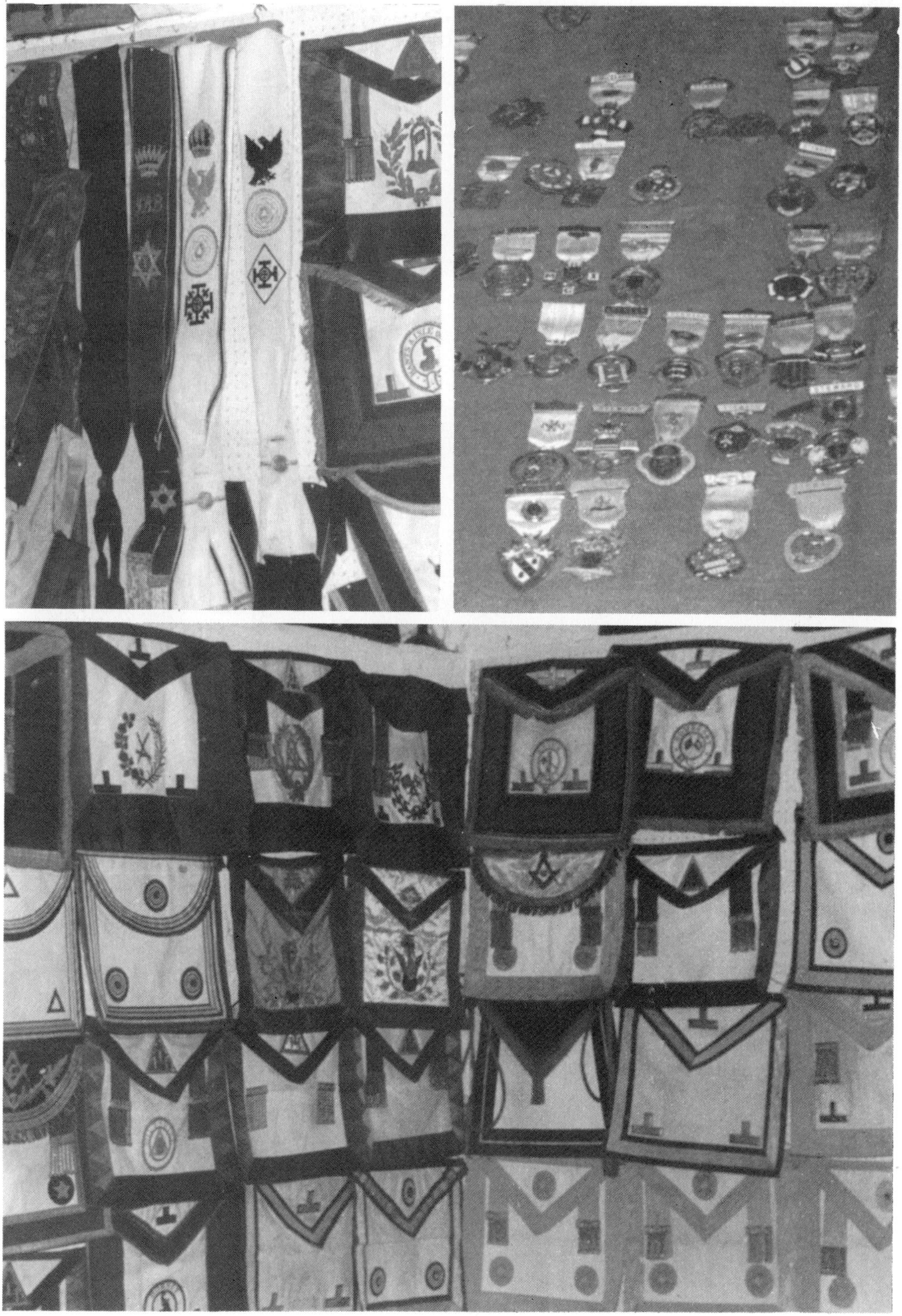

Part of John's vast collection of Masonic items.

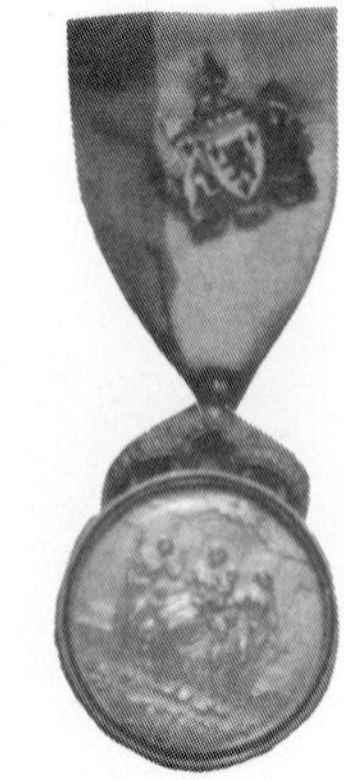

Masonic Grand Charity jewel.

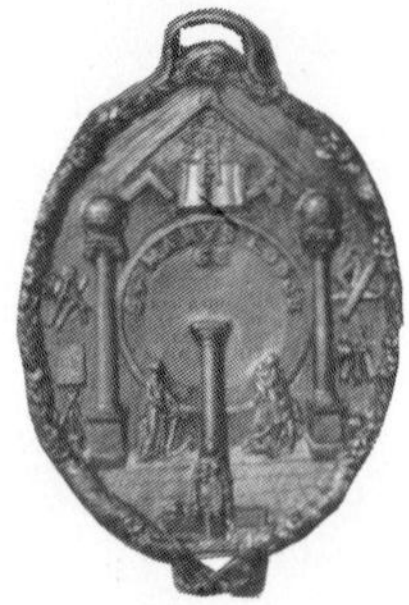

Past Master's jewel, St. Mary's Lodge No. 63, 1867.

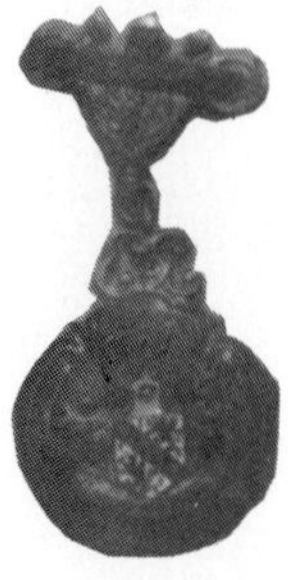

Charity jewel, Royal Masonic Benevolent Institution.

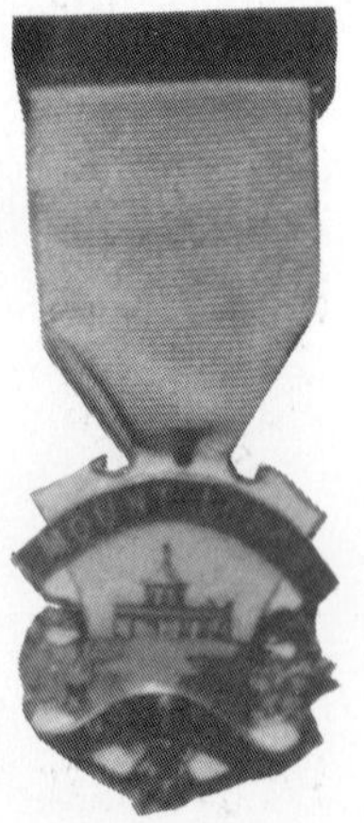

Lodge Founders jewel, Mount Lodge No. 65.

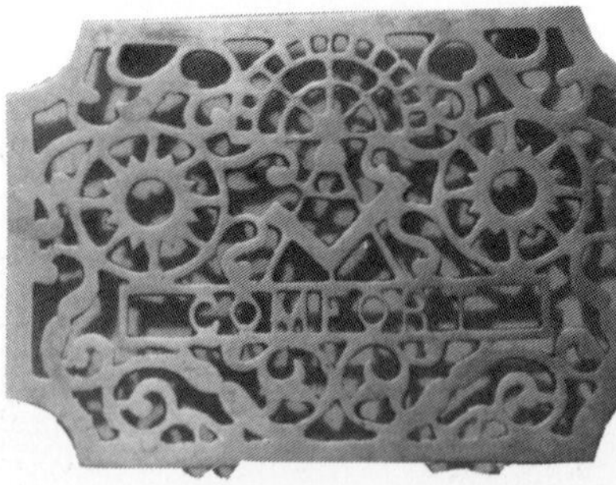

Brass trivet with Masonic emblems.

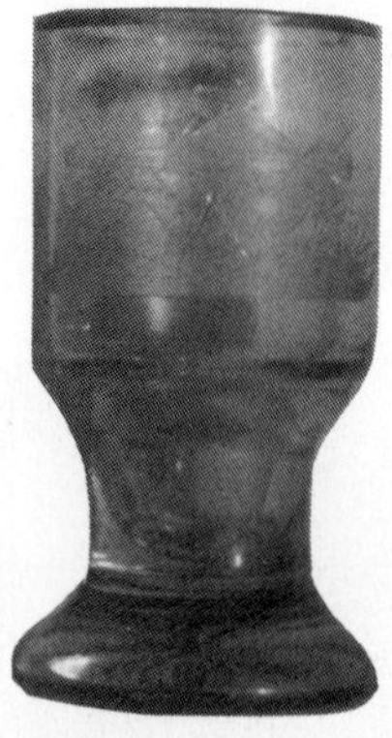

A Masonic firing glass.

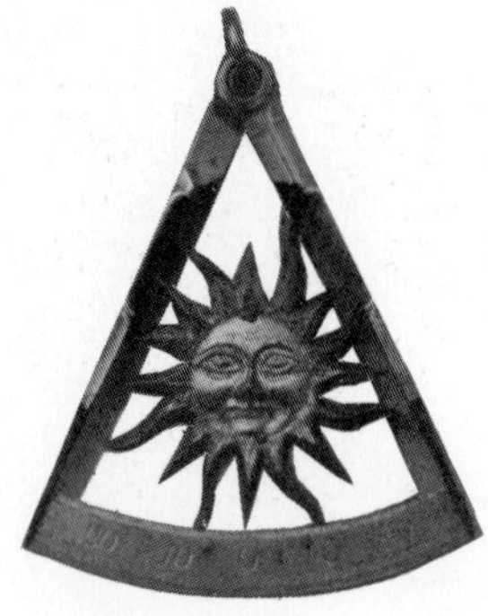

Masonic collar jewel, early 1800's.

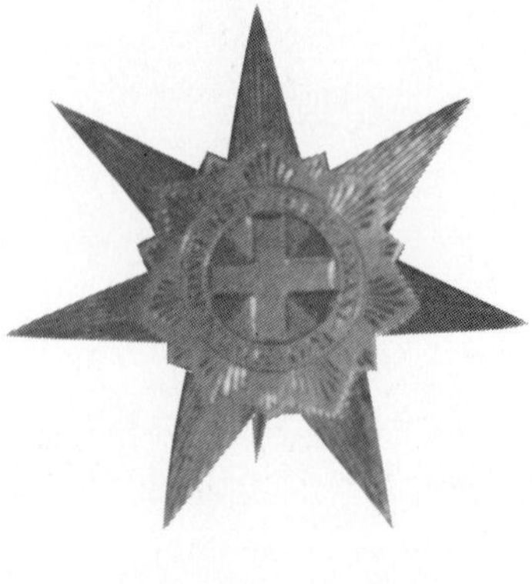

Knight's Templar plate jewel, early 1800's.

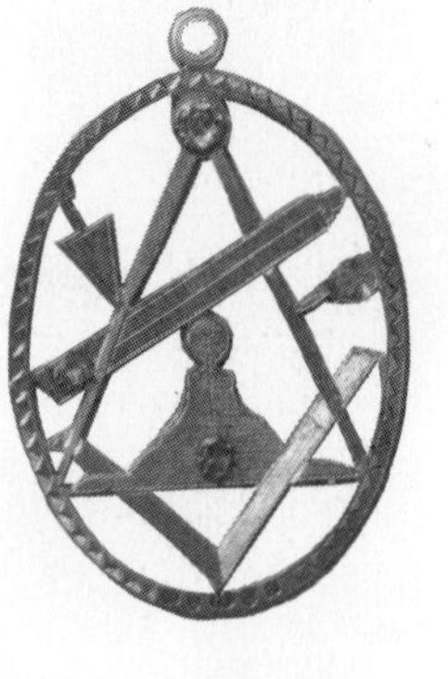

Silver collar jewel, early 1800's.

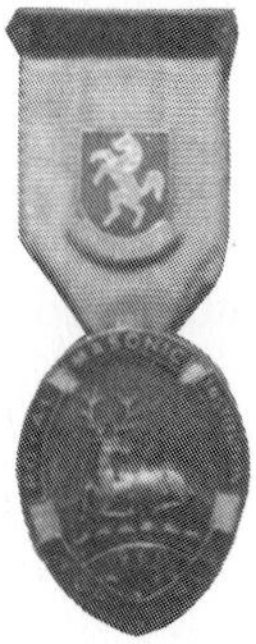

Charity jewel, Royal Masonic Institute For Girls.

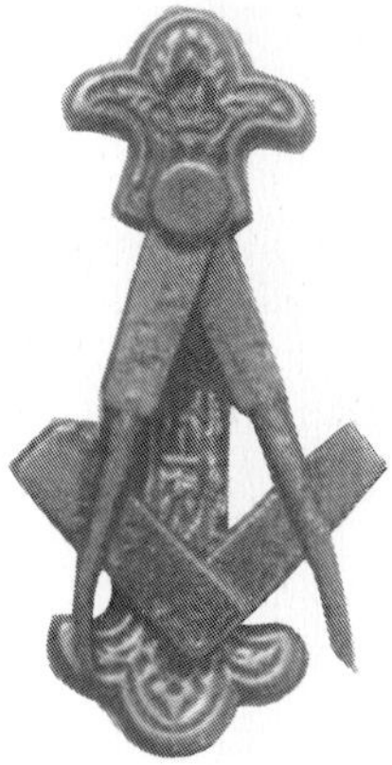

Brass door knocker with Masonic emblems.

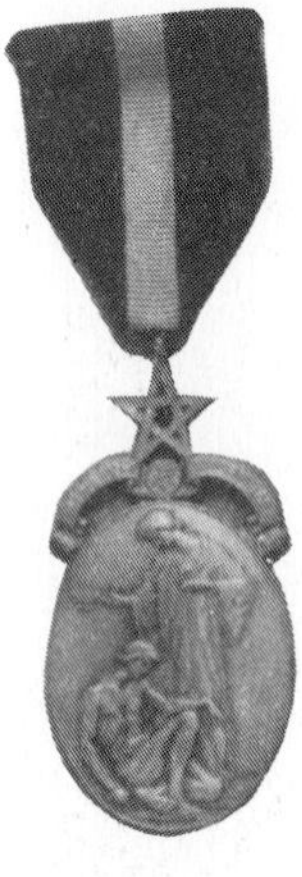

Charity jewel, Royal Masonic Hospital.

Past Master's jewel, Thomas Lockitt Lodge.

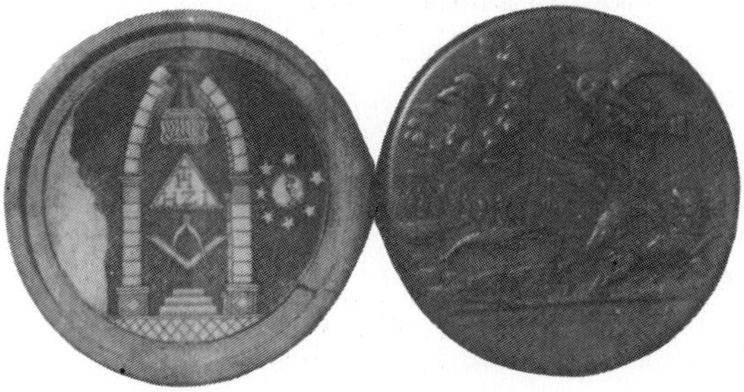

Napoleonic snuff box with secret compartment concealing Masonic emblems.

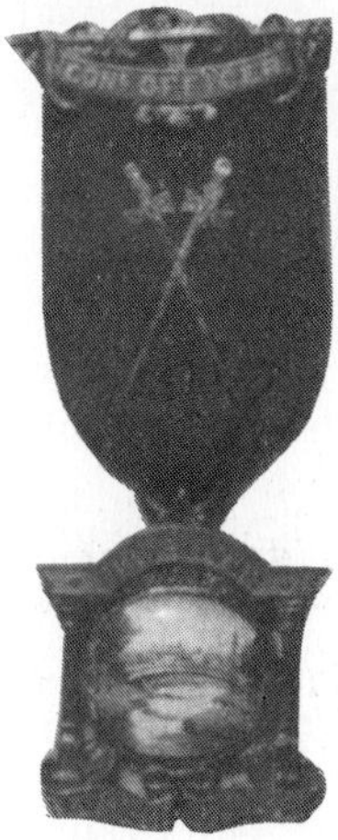

Consecration Officer's jewel, New River Lodge.

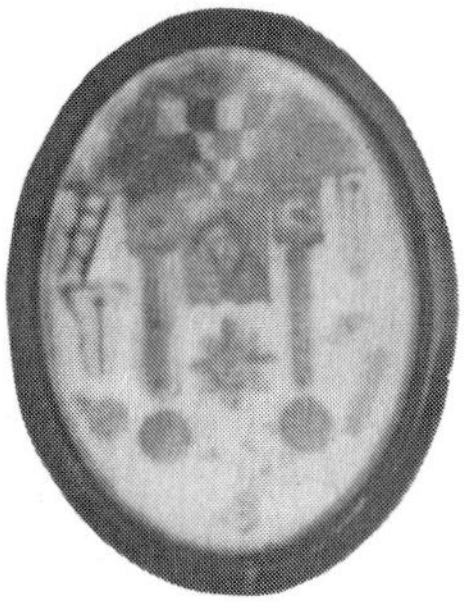

French prisoner-of-war locket with Masonic emblems.

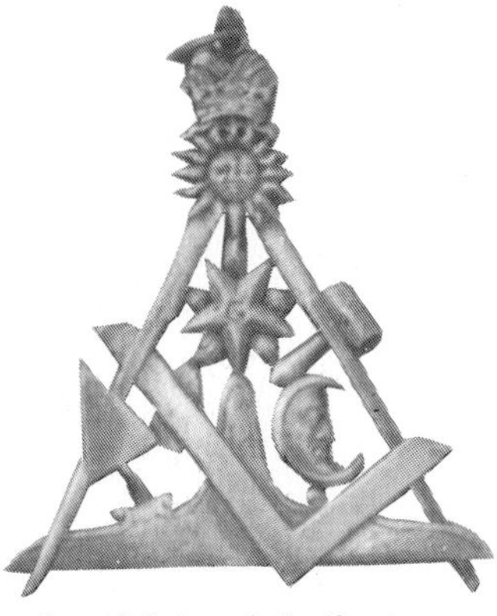

Scottish jewel similar to the Master jewel used by the Mother Kilwinning Lodge No. O, circa 1750.

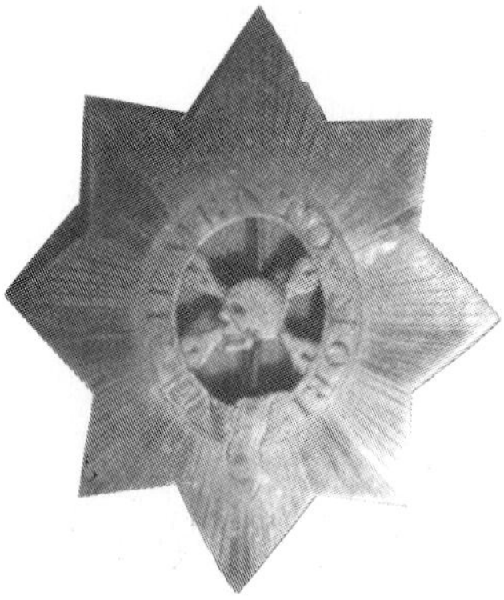

Knight's Templar plate jewel, early 1800's, hallmarked.

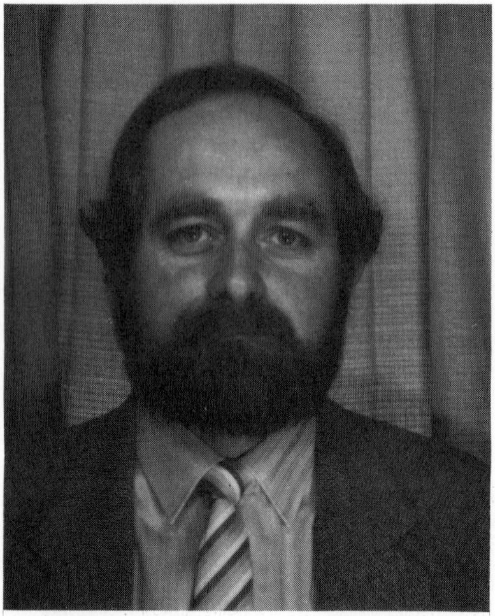

Nick Waters is the headmaster of a school in South London and collects ink bottles.

"There's a very tenuous link between my job and my collection which began when my sister in law was appointed head of a private school in Bath and discovered a lot of old Victorian things in the cellar. She gave me an old stone ink bottle with Stephens Ink written on it and that was the first item in the collection.

"Later I was on a school trip to the Isle of Wight and one of the boys was a keen collector of bus tickets so I went with him to a shop which sold them and there I saw some ink bottles. The man who kept the shop told me about them and after that I began collecting.

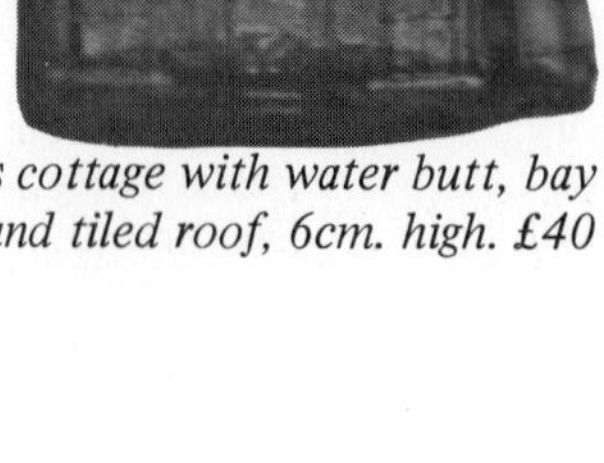

Aqua glass cottage with water butt, bay windows and tiled roof, 6cm. high. £40 – £70

"I collected hundreds of every possible variation but I've had to discipline myself now because of space and I've kept about 100 of the extra rare and colourful ones which make a wonderful display.

"The ones I am most interested in are sheered lip bottles which means that the glass was just broken off and not polished on the rim. The bottle was then sealed with a cork and sealing wax. They did this because ink was expensive so bottles had to be kept as cheap as possible. I have some sheered lip inks going back to 1840 but this is such a specialised area that I'm lucky if I find a rare sheered lip bottle once a year now.

However I also have salt glaze and porcelain inks. One of my most valuable pieces is a cottage shaped bottle in the form of a thatched farm cottage. It is about two and a half inches high and is worth in excess of £250. I have another called a turtle ink which may be French. The Australians call them sunflower inks because they look like a flower head seen from above and the spout is on the side. They can be bought in aqua or clear glass but mine is a lovely green and it is the only example in that colour that I have seen in ten years. It is worth around £200."

It is difficult to get hold of good examples of ink bottles and what Nick would most like to find is a bottle shaped like a locomotive. He has one already but it is unfortunately damaged. If it was perfect it would be worth £500.

Americans are very interested in ink bottles and Nick buys from a dealer in Philadelphia who holds auctions for which he accepts overseas bids.

Bottles with embossing on them make it possible to trace the history of the company that sold the ink and Nick is currently interested in three companies called W. Chandler and Co.; C. Chandler and Co. and Chandler and Chalo. These names have turned up on cottage inks which he owns and he feels the companies must have been connected in some way.

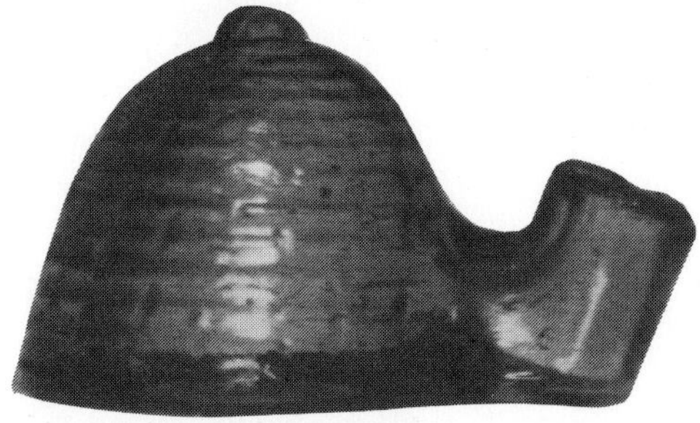

Aqua glass inkwell in the form of an igloo embossed with tiny blocks and with U.K. Registration Diamond on the base. £120

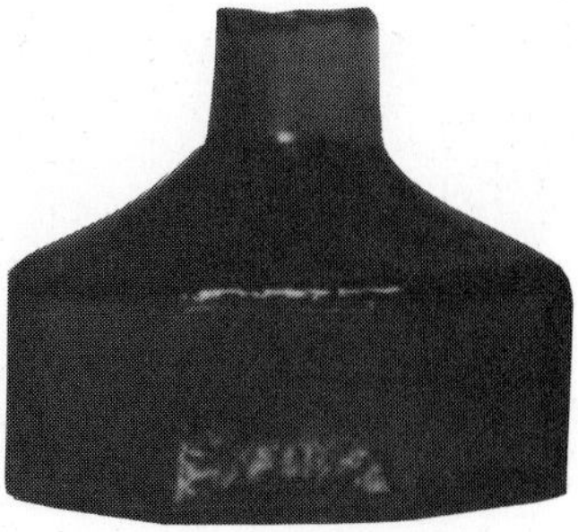

A rare cobalt blue glass tent inkwell. £50

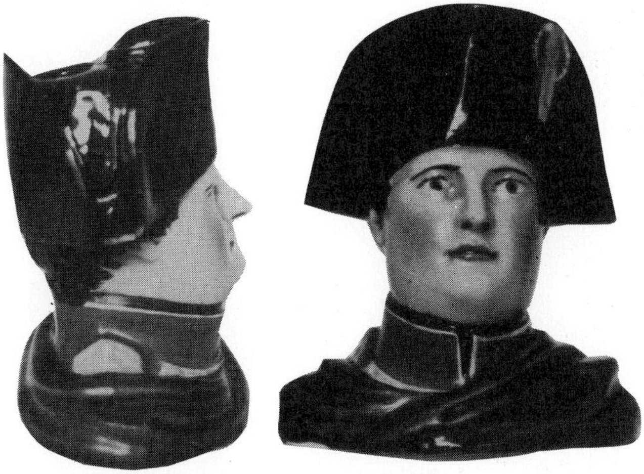

Mid 19th century 'Bonaparte' ink bottle, the hollow body forming the reservoir while the front hole acts as a quill holder and the rear hole as access to the ink. £150

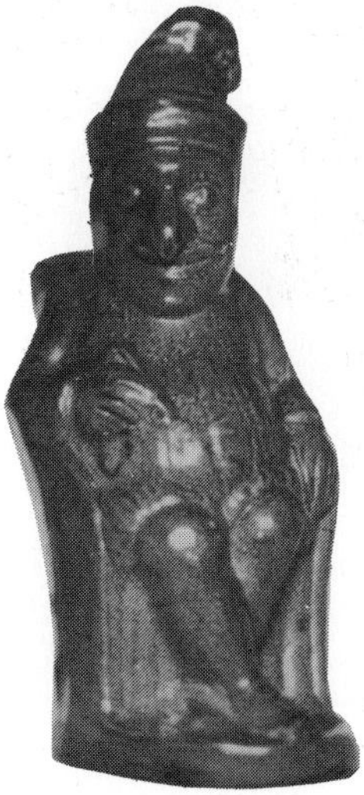

'Mr. Punch', one of the most sought after salt-glaze ink bottle, incised on the back 'Gardeners Ink Works, Lower White Cross St., London', together with the U.K. Registration Diamond mark for 1851, 4½in. high. £120 plus

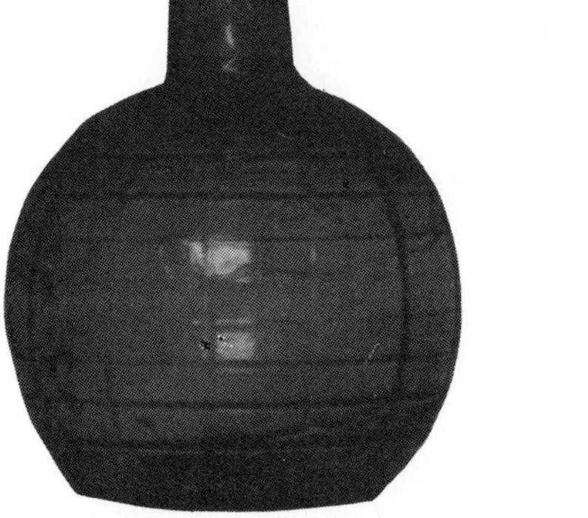

Very rare green glass globe inkwell embossed with lines of longitude and latitude as a representation of the world. £100 plus

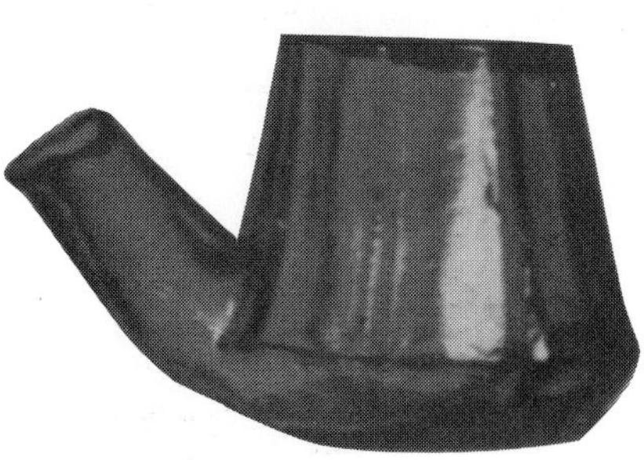

An aqua glass tea kettle. £50
Coloured ornate varieties can make up to £300.

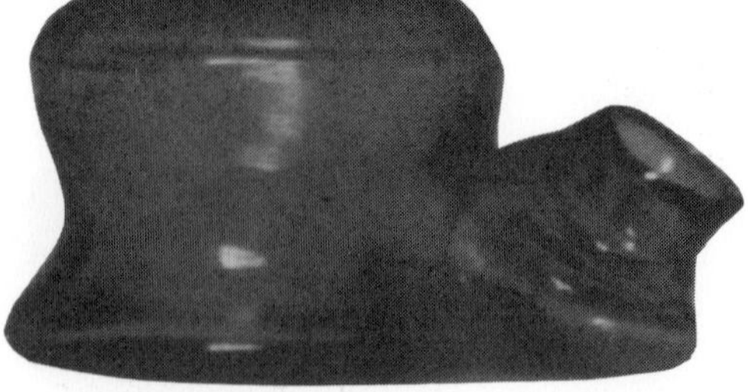

An aqua glass snail inkwell. £50

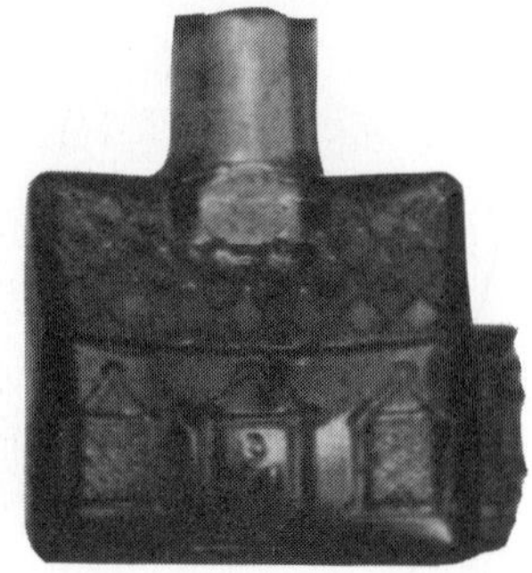

Rare cottage inkwell with water butt in green glass embossed C. Chandler & Co., 6cm. high.
£100

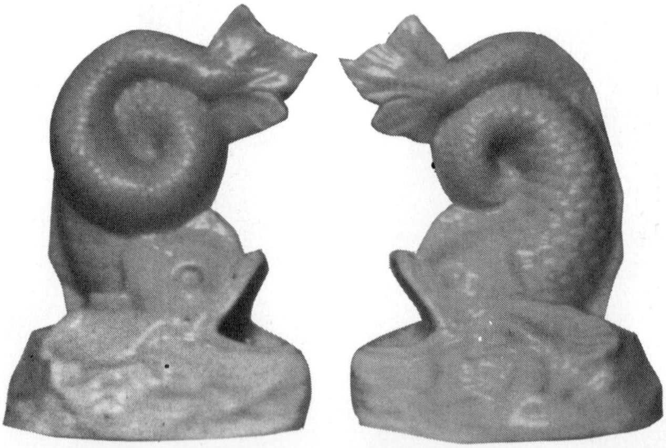

A fine pair of white china inkwells in the form of dolphins, the open mouth providing access to the reservoir, with Registry of Designs diamond mark for July 16th 1874 and Perry & Co., London, printed on the base.
£150 – £200

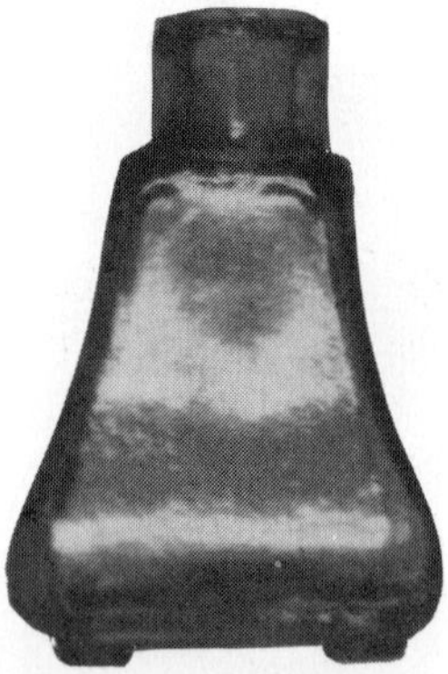

Plain aqua glass inkwell of bulbous conical shape, 6cm. high. £6

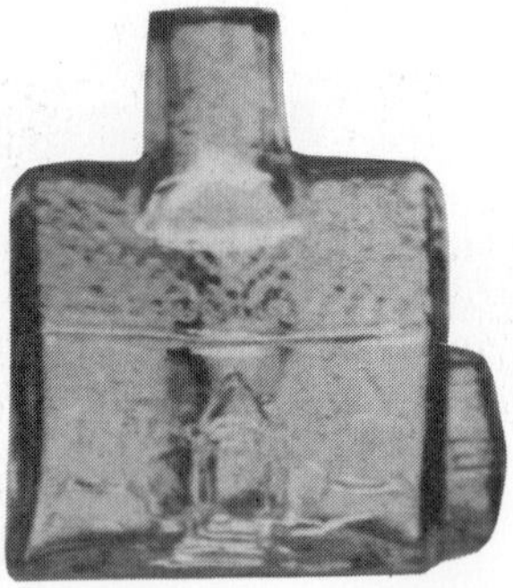

Aqua glass cottage inkwell with water butt and stippled roof decoration, 6cm. high.
£40 – £70

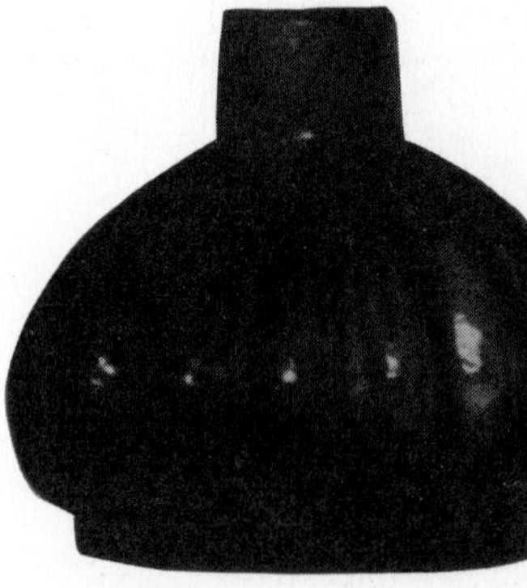

A rare dark green glass pumpkin inkwell embossed with F. M. & Co. (F. Mordant). £60

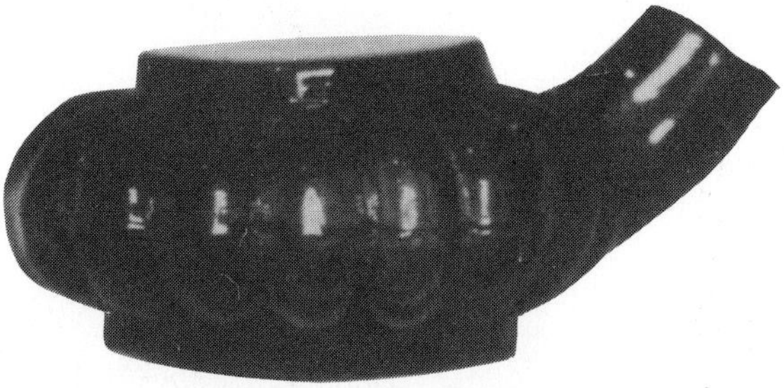

An extremely rare deep green glass turtle or sunflower inkwell, possibly French. £200

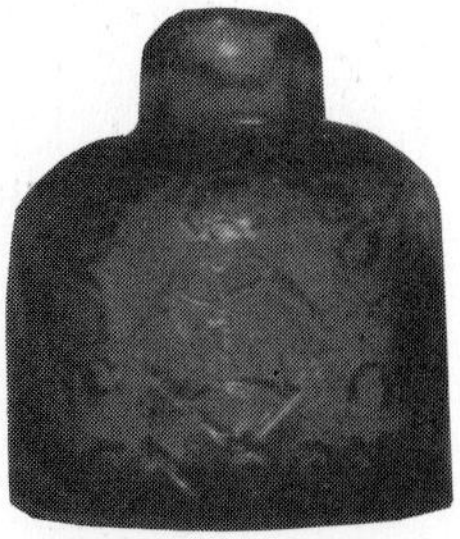

Blackwoods of London, aqua glass igloo inkwell with embossed Registry of Designs diamond. £15

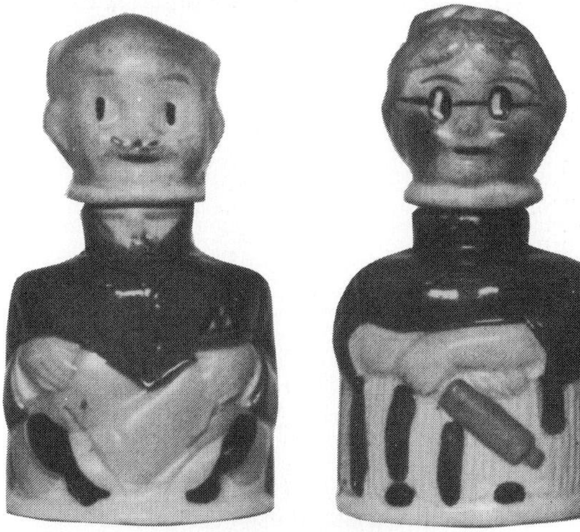

American red and blue ceramic bottles known as 'MA' and 'PA' with removable heads forming the cork stoppers. The 'Mr. & Mrs. Carter's Ink' were patented by C. H. Henkels of Philadelphia for Carter's Ink Co. of Boston and were made in Germany prior to World War I and later in the U.S.A. From 1914-16 they were offered in a National magazine for 25 cents together with a coupon from the magazine and as a result over 50,000 coupons were received. £100

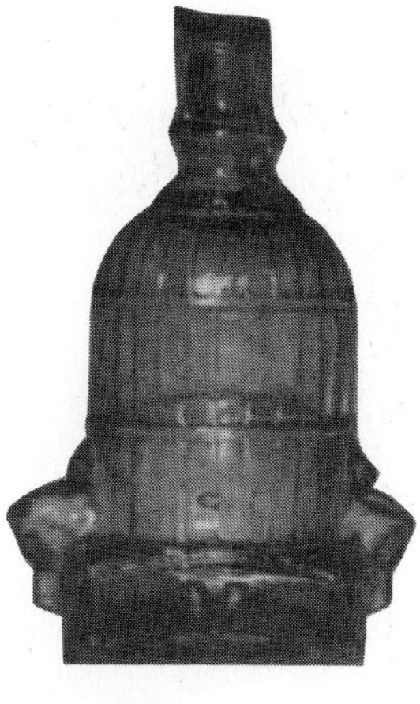

Aqua glass birdcage inkwell embossed with bars, a door and two feeders. £25

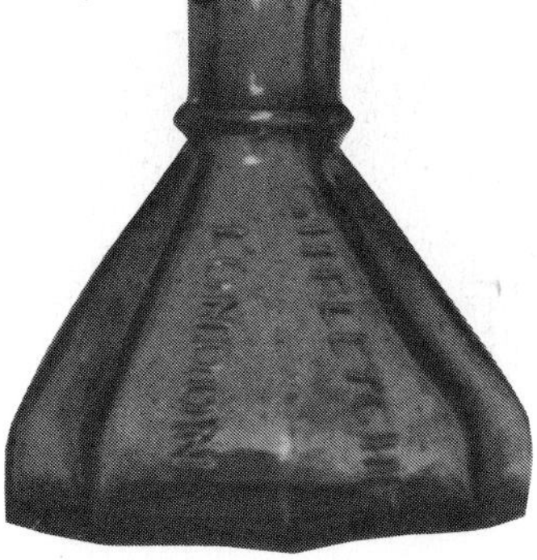

Aqua glass umbrella inkwell embossed with G. H. Fletcher, London. £25

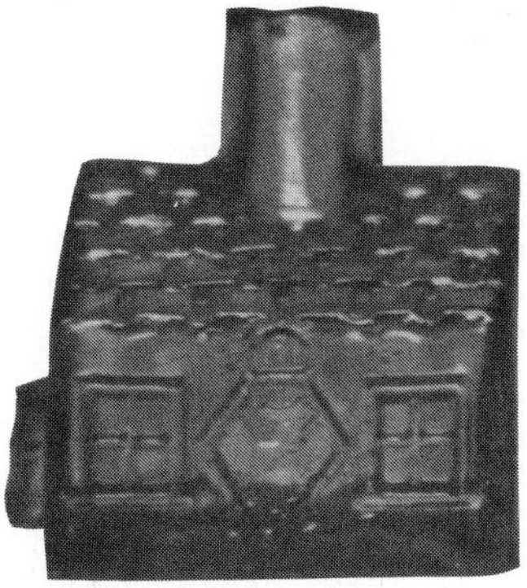

A rare cottage inkwell in aqua glass with Registry of Designs diamond embossed on the front for April 5th 1869, 5½cm. high. £100 plus

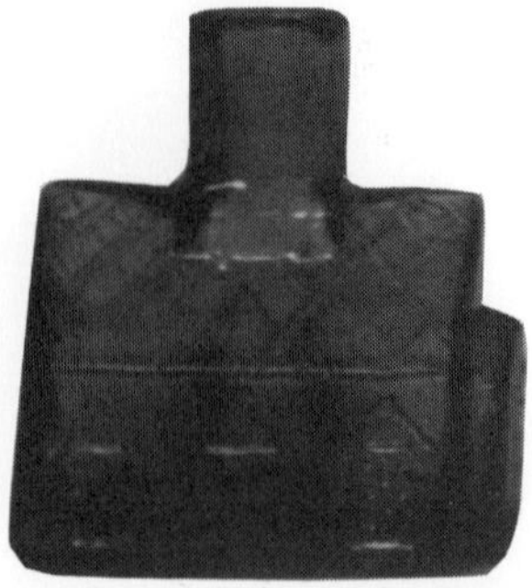

Green glass cottage inkwell with vertical cavity at the rear to hold a free nib, 6cm. high. £100

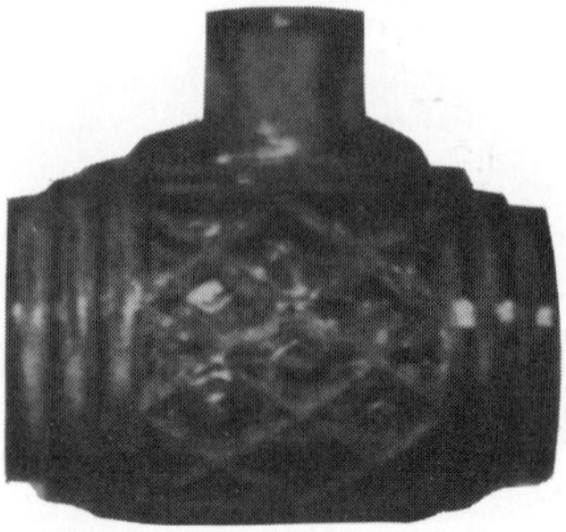

Barrel shaped glass inkwell with cross hatched body. £12

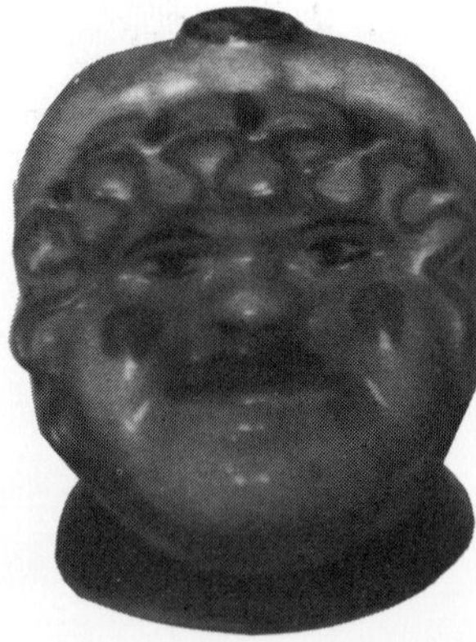

Staffordshire ceramic face ink bottle in the form of Sairey Gamp with the open mouth providing access to the ink reservoir and with the quill holder on top. This can also be found in saltglaze stoneware. £60

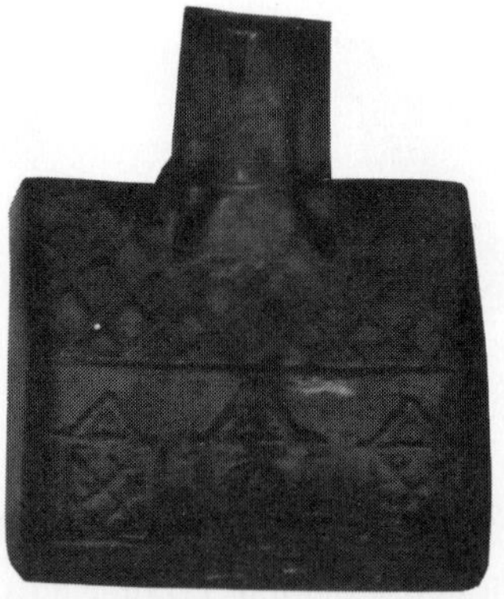

Aqua glass cottage inkwell with cross hatched roof and no side embossing, 6cm. high. £40 – £70

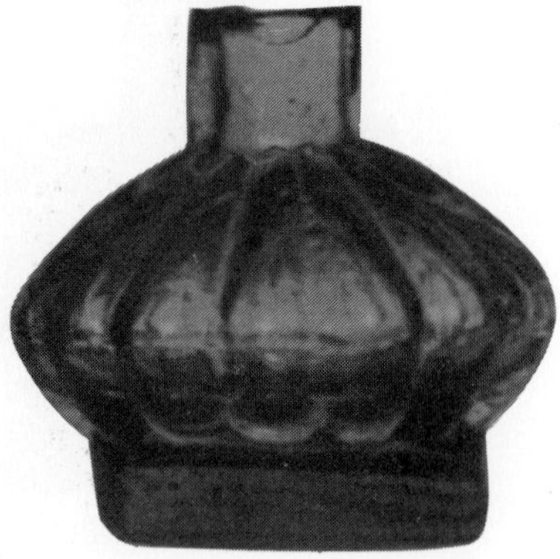

An aqua glass segmented inkwell. £10

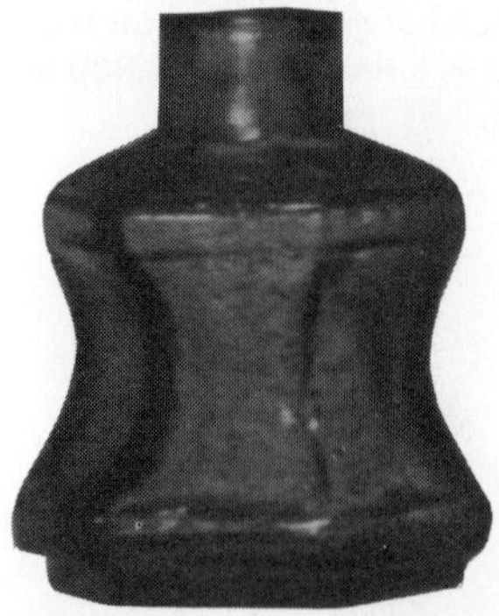

Capstan shaped glass inkwell with concave sides, 5cm. high. £10

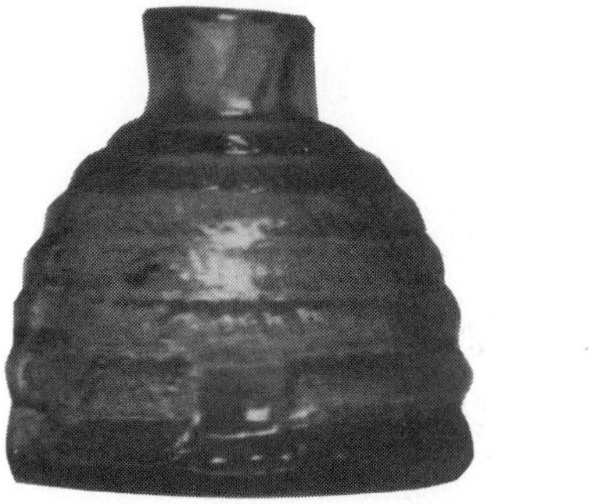

Aqua glass inkwell in the form of a beehive made from coiled straw with opening at the base. £100

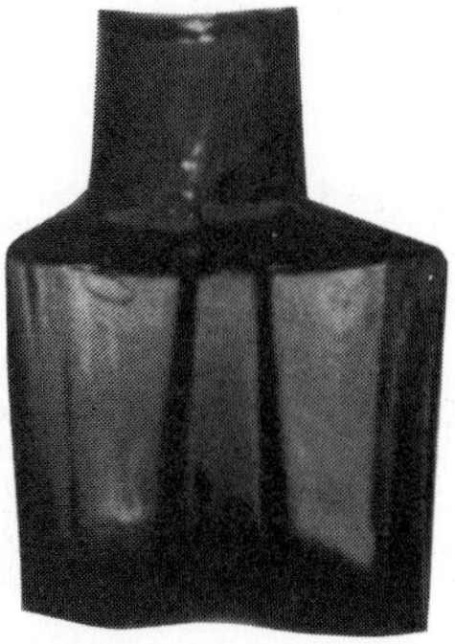

A cobalt blue glass square shaped inkwell with cavity for free pen nib. £20

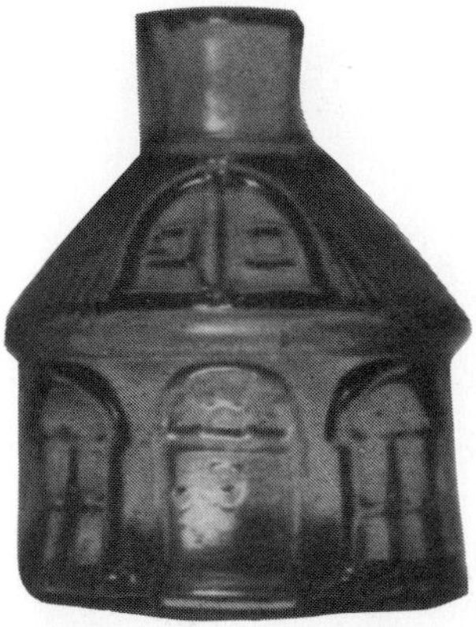

An extremely rare circular cottage inkwell in aqua glass with Registry of Designs diamond embossed on the base for August 1868, 6cm. high. £150 – £200

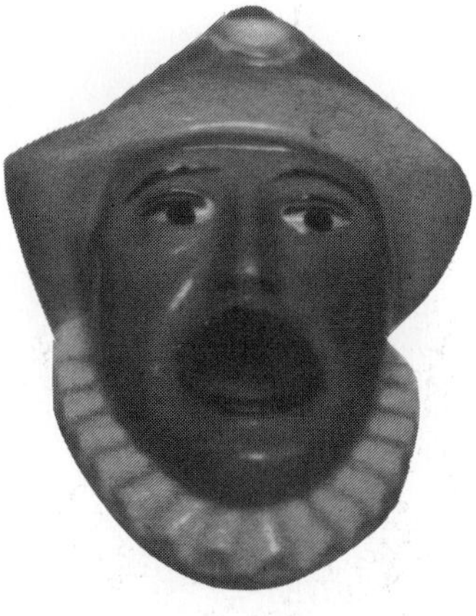

Staffordshire ceramic clown head ink bottle, the open mouth providing access to the ink reservoir and with a quill holder on top of the head. £60

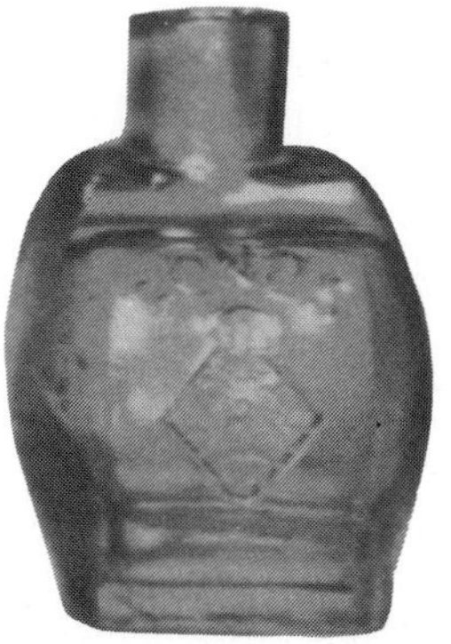

Bonds aqua glass inkwell embossed with Registry of Designs diamond and pen rest, 6cm. high. £30

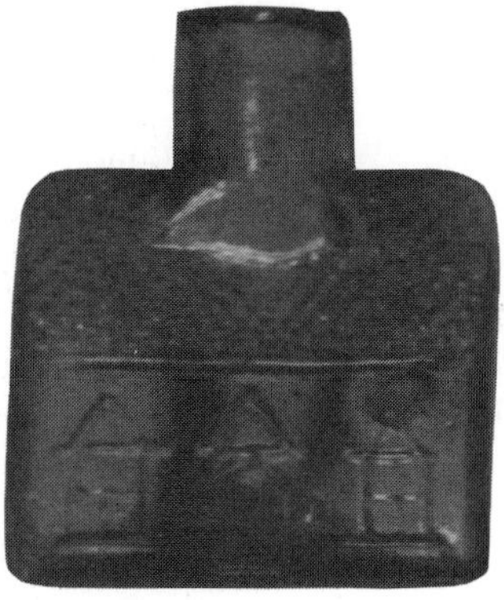

Aqua glass cottage inkwell with stippled roof and no side embossing, 6cm. high. £40 – £70

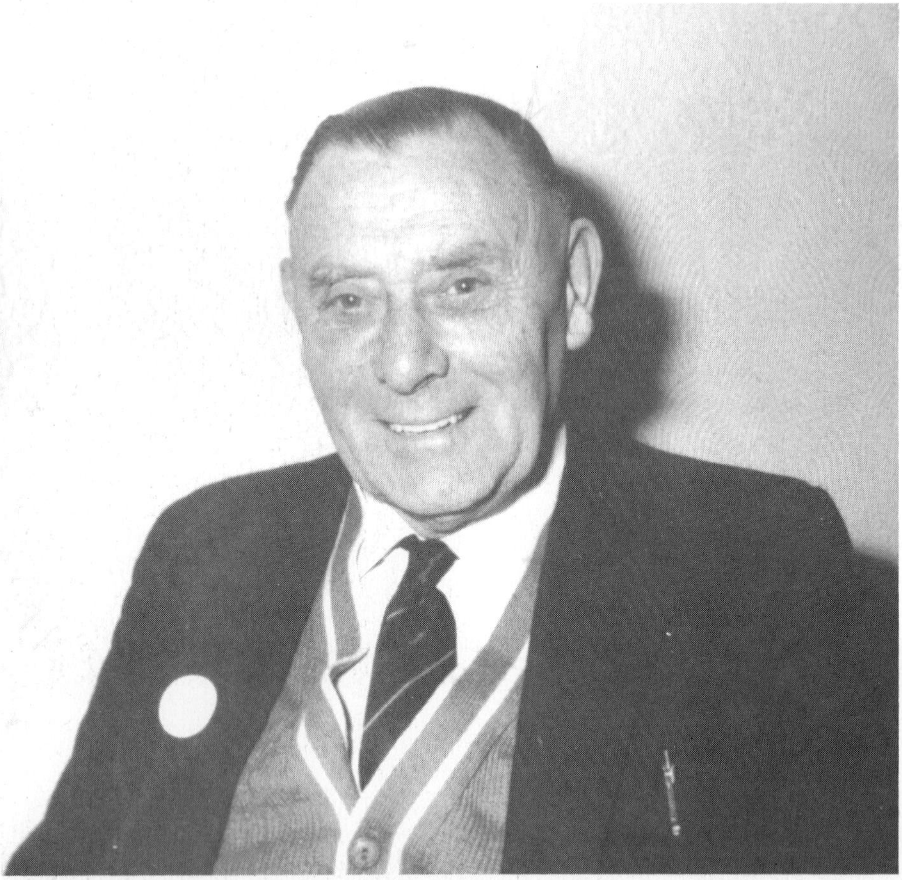

Harry Cope is a retired taxi driver who collects postal covers connected with the International Red Cross.

"Because I'm the secretary of the Forces' Postal History Society I got interested in war mail and that developed into the whole of the mail system and charity labels of the Red Cross.

"Items in my collection date back to the Boer War and the Boxer Rebellion because the Red Cross began in 1867 and its history mirrors all the wars, rebellions, insurrections, earthquakes and volcanic disasters since then.

"I've got several items from prisoners of war in the First World War, from Russians in Germany and Germans in Imperial Russia. One of the most interesting sections are bogus charity stamps which were put out during the First World War by a Frenchman called De Landre who pocketed the money that people thought they were giving to the Red Cross. I've got around 80 of these and each is worth in the region of £7 today.

"I've got lots of items from the Second World War including message sheets from the Channel Islands and the collection extends to the present day with items from the Arab Israeli War, all in different languages."

Harry is one of the leading collectors in this field in the world and he has 800 sheets of mounted printed material . . . 'I'm very choosey about what I buy' he said.

His star lot is the only known cover from Madagascar dating from the period of the Second World War before the Free French moved in. What he still wants to find are covers from the Spanish Civil War and from the Falklands campaign.

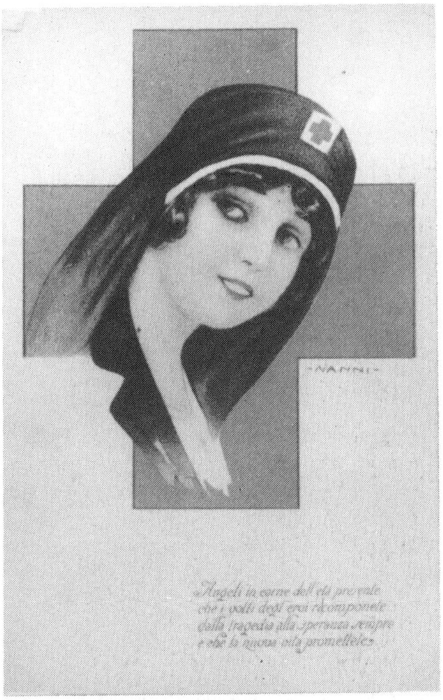

Italian First World War series of 'Pretty Girls' in Red Cross headgear drawn by Nanni in order to raise funds.

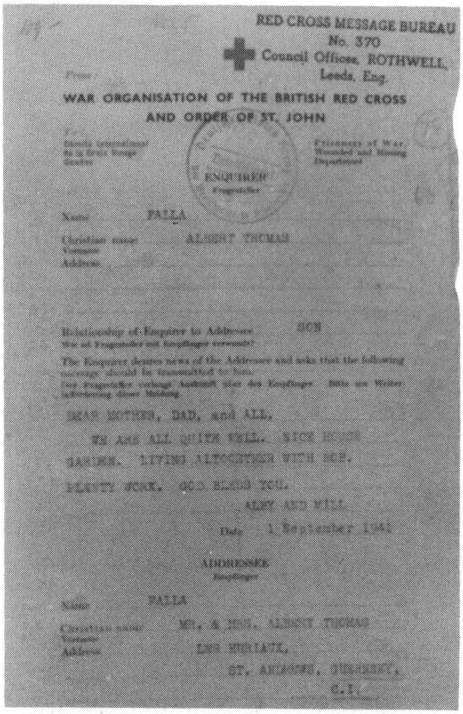

RED CROSS MESSAGE BUREAU
No. 370
Council Offices, ROTHWELL,
Leeds, Eng.

WAR ORGANISATION OF THE BRITISH RED CROSS
AND ORDER OF ST. JOHN

ENQUIRER

Name FALLA

Christian name ALBERT THOMAS

Address

Relationship of Enquirer to Addressee SON

The Enquirer desires news of the Addressee and asks that the following message should be transmitted to him.

DEAR MOTHER, DAD, and ALL,

WE ARE ALL QUITE WELL. NICE HOUSE [illegible] GARDEN. LIVING ALTOGETHER WITH BOB. PLENTY WORK. GOD BLESS YOU.

ALFY AND [illegible]

Date 1 September 1941

ADDRESSEE

Name FALLA

Christian name MR. & MRS. ALBERT THOMAS

Address LES HURIAUX, ST. ANDREWS, GUERNSEY, C.I.

Second World War message for correspondence between the Channel Islands and anywhere in the world.

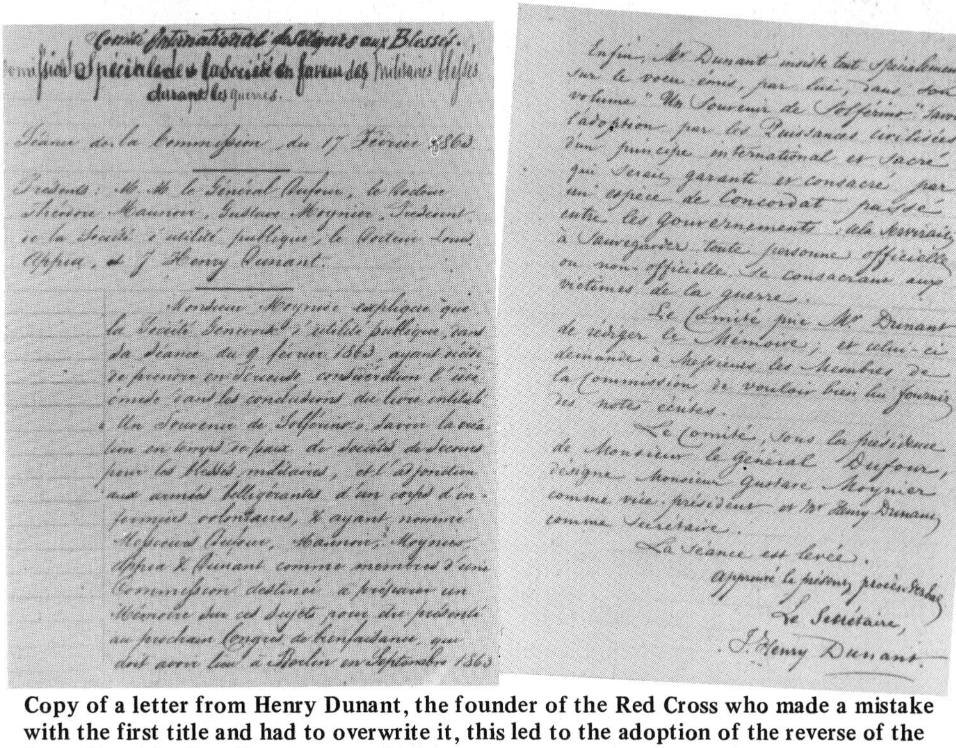

Comité International de Secours aux Blessés.
Commission Spéciale de la Société en faveur des militaires blessés durant les guerres.

Séance de la Commission du 17 Février 1863.

Présents: MM. le Général Dufour, le Docteur Théodore Maunoir, Gustave Moynier, Président de la Société d'utilité publique, le Docteur Louis Appia, et J. Henry Dunant.

Monsieur Moynier explique que la Société Genevoise d'utilité publique, dans sa séance du 9 février 1863, ayant résolu de prendre en sérieuse considération l'idée émise dans les conclusions du livre intitulé « Un Souvenir de Solférino », savoir la création en temps de paix de sociétés de secours pour les blessés militaires, et l'adjonction aux armées belligérantes d'un corps d'infirmiers volontaires, & ayant nommé Messieurs Dufour, Maunoir, Moynier, Appia & Dunant comme membres d'une Commission destinée à préparer un Mémoire sur ces sujets pour être présenté au prochain Congrès de bienfaisance, qui doit avoir lieu à Berlin en Septembre 1863

Enfin, Mr Dunant insiste tout spécialement sur le voeu émis, par lui, dans son volume "Un Souvenir de Solférino" savoir l'adoption par les Puissances civilisées d'un principe international et sacré qui serait garanti et consacré par une espèce de Concordat passé entre les Gouvernements; cela servirait à sauvegarder toute personne officielle ou non-officielle se consacrant aux victimes de la guerre.

Le Comité prie Mr Dunant de rédiger le Mémoire, et celui-ci demande à Messieurs les Membres de la Commission de vouloir bien lui fournir des notes écrites.

Le Comité, sous la présidence de Monsieur le Général Dufour, désigne Monsieur Gustave Moynier comme vice-président et Mr Henry Dunant comme Secrétaire.

La séance est levée.

Approuvé le présent procès-verbal
Le Secrétaire,
J. Henry Dunant.

Copy of a letter from Henry Dunant, the founder of the Red Cross who made a mistake with the first title and had to overwrite it, this led to the adoption of the reverse of the Swiss flag, 'the Red Cross' as a symbol.

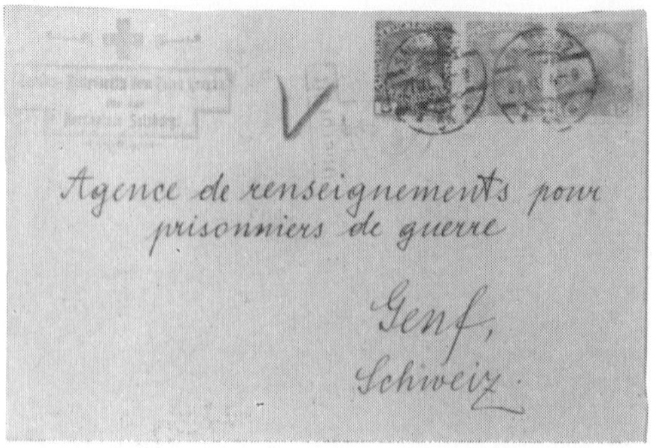

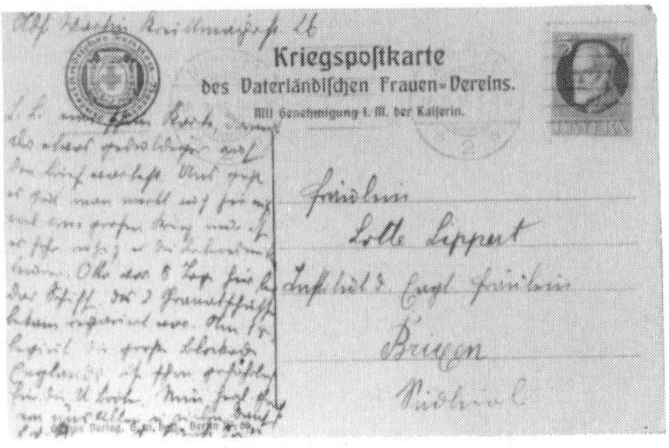

Austrian Help Committee handstamp from the First World War, Salzburg area.

First World War Bavarian fund raising card.

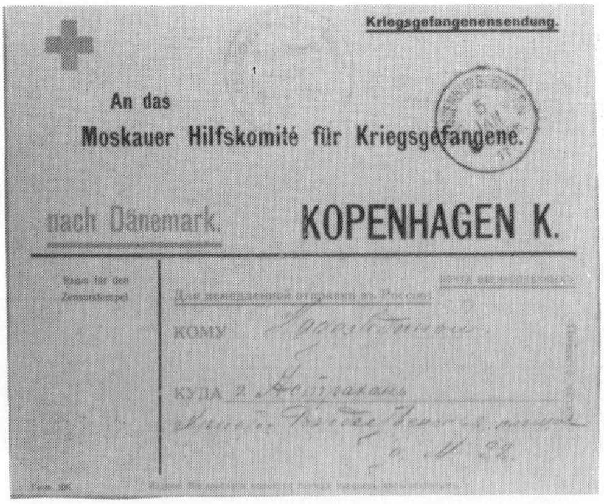

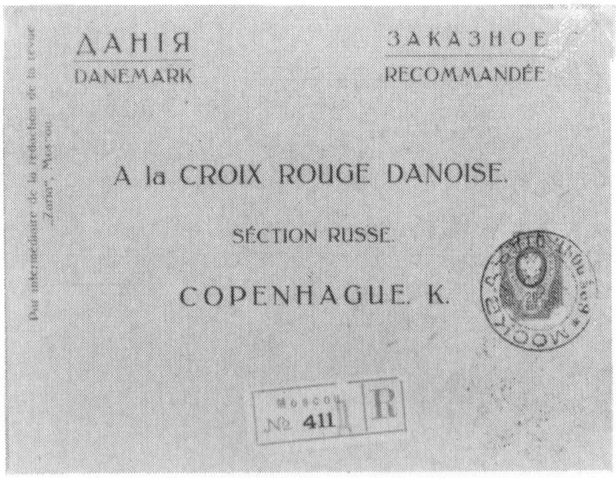

Envelope to the Moscow Help Committee in Copenhagen which dealt with Russian prisoners of war in Germany, Austria and Hungary.

An envelope addressed to the Danish Red Cross from a prisoner of war in Russia, First World War.

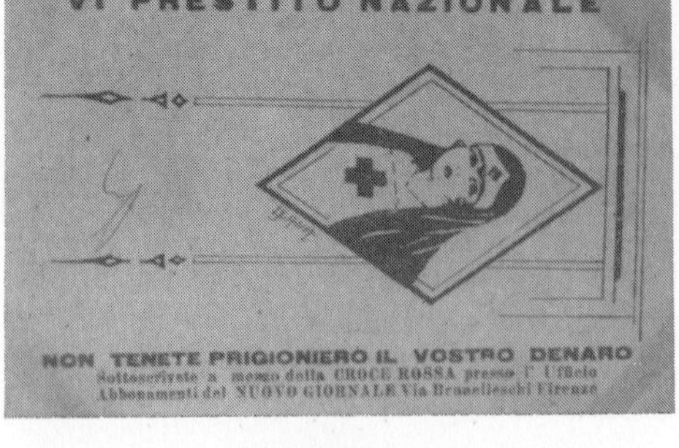

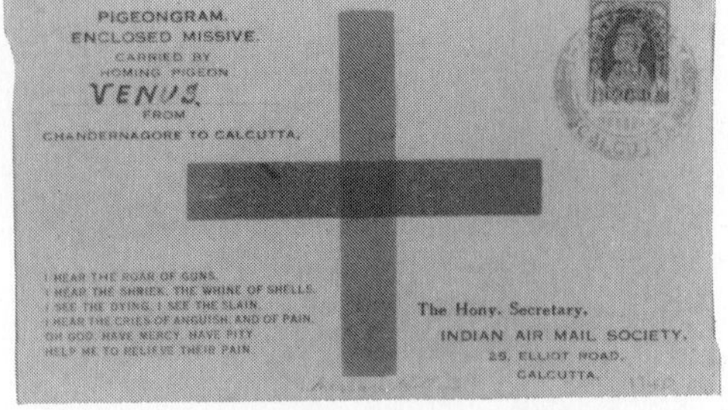

Italian First World War card.

A second World War fund raising card, enclosing a small message slip.

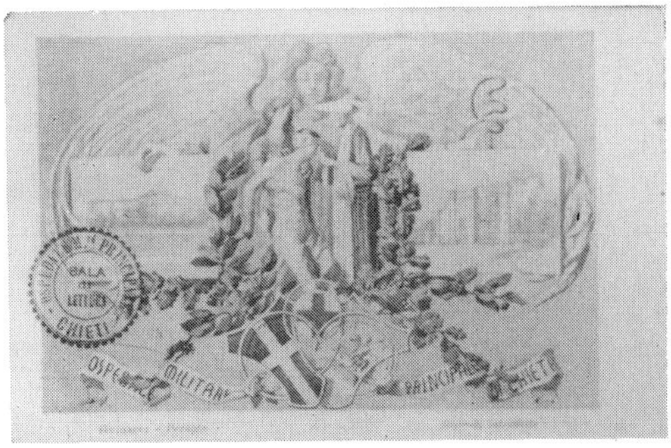

Fund raising card from the early 1900's, which continued until after the Italo-Turkish War.

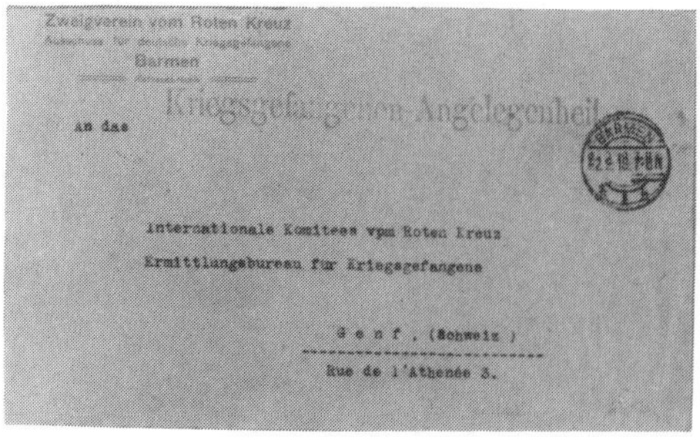

German International Red Cross cover from Barmen camp which housed Belgium, French, French Colonial and some British Infantry.

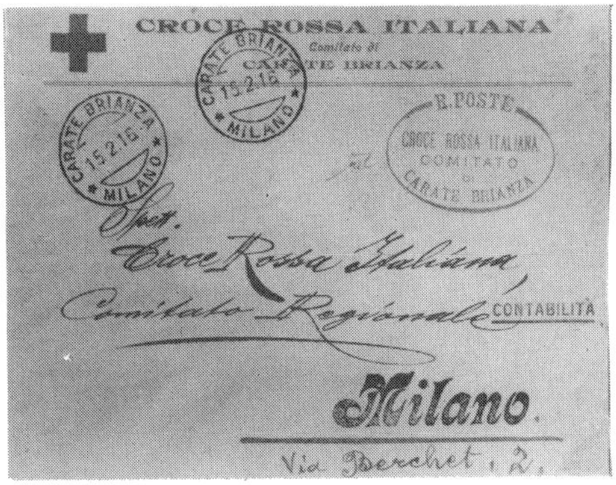

Italian First World War envelope from the local committee Carate Brianza.

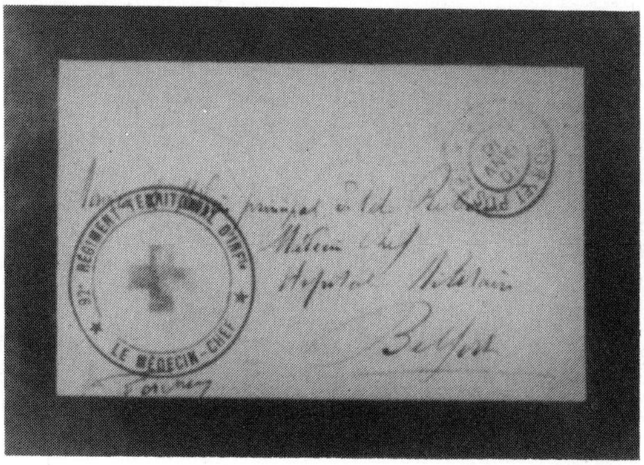

French First World War Mourning envelope.

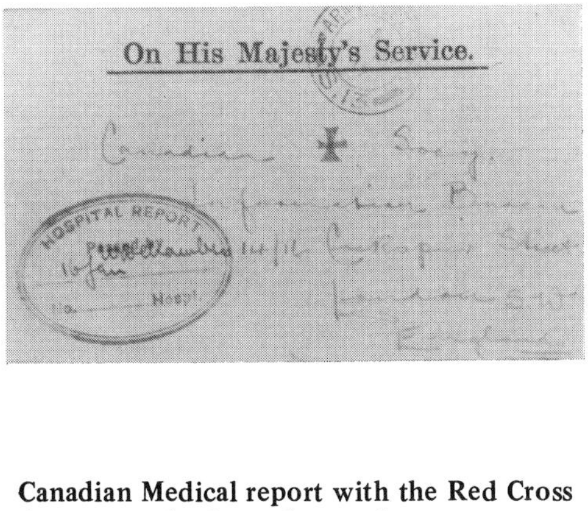

Canadian Medical report with the Red Cross drawn in red ink on the envelope.

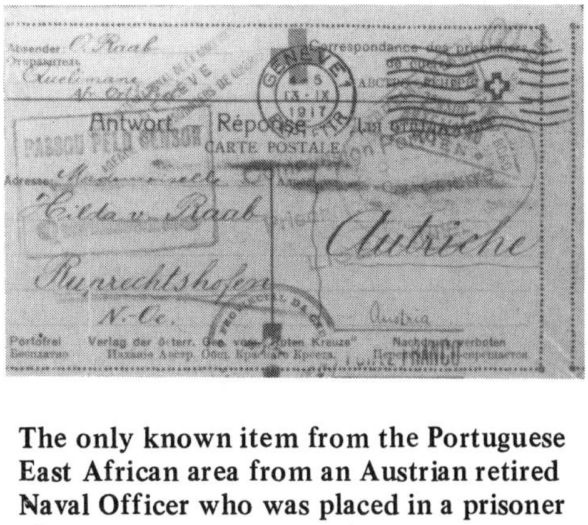

The only known item from the Portuguese East African area from an Austrian retired Naval Officer who was placed in a prisoner of war camp.

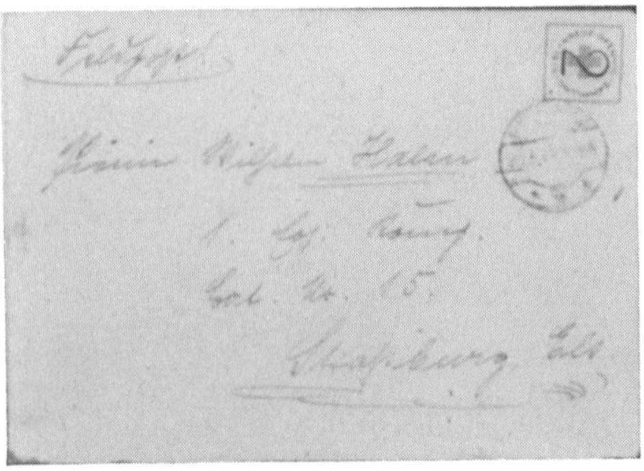

German First World War charity stamp envelope for Red Cross funds.

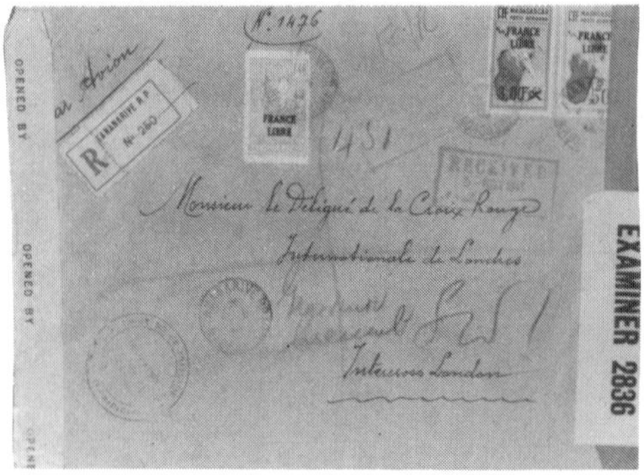

A cover from the Free French Red Cross which were the only French unit to be present in the first stage of the occupation of Madegascar.

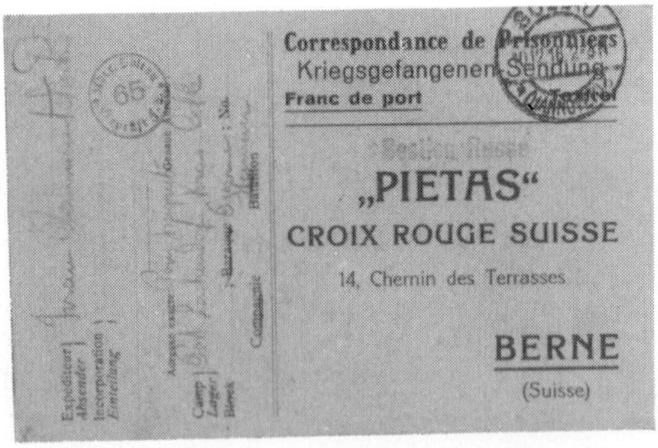

A prisoner of war parcel acknowledged card sent in a parcel from the Swiss National Red Cross 'Section Russe' and redirected to England.

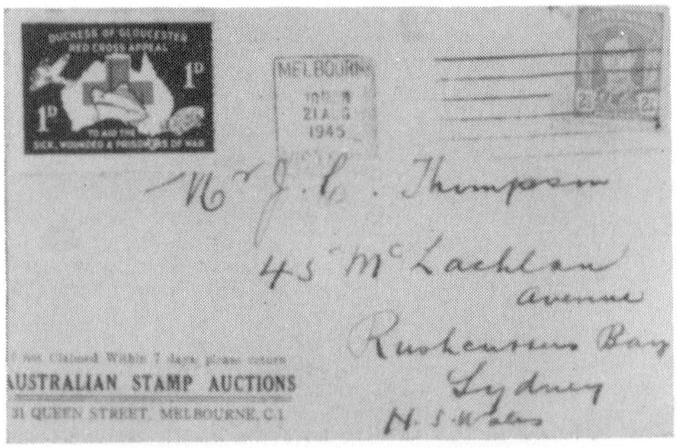

2nd World War Australian charity label, 1945.

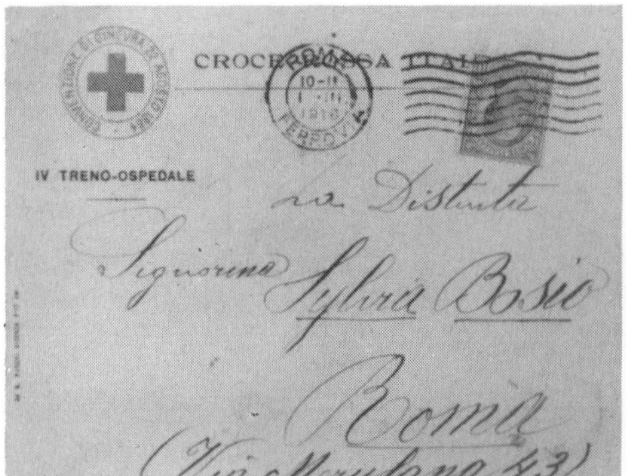

Envelope from an Italian Hospital Train.

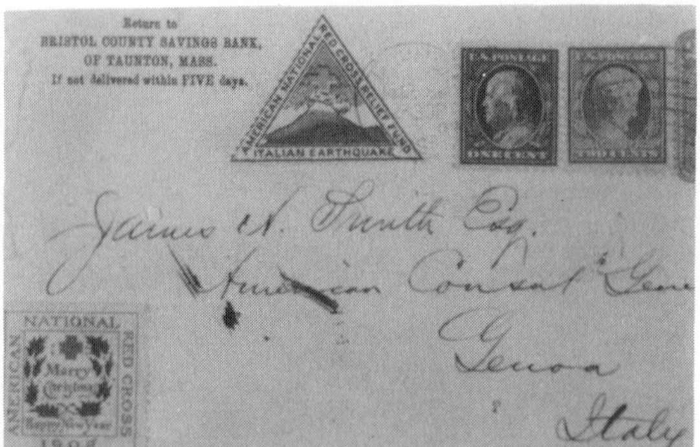

Fund raising label from the U.S.A. for victims of the Messina earthquake, 1908.

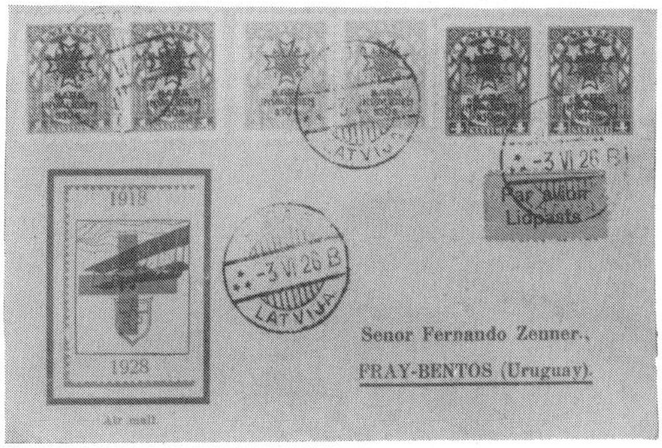

A bogus cover purporting to be airmailed from Latvia to Uraguay , concocted by a stamp dealer in Switzerland named Sekula who was sent to prison for producing them.

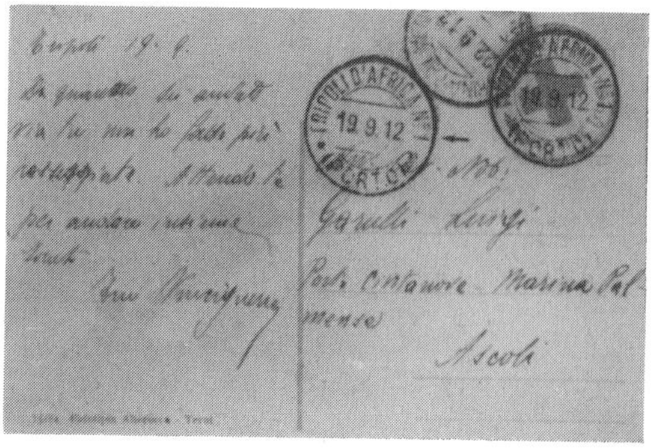

Card used in North Africa during the Italo-Turkish War.

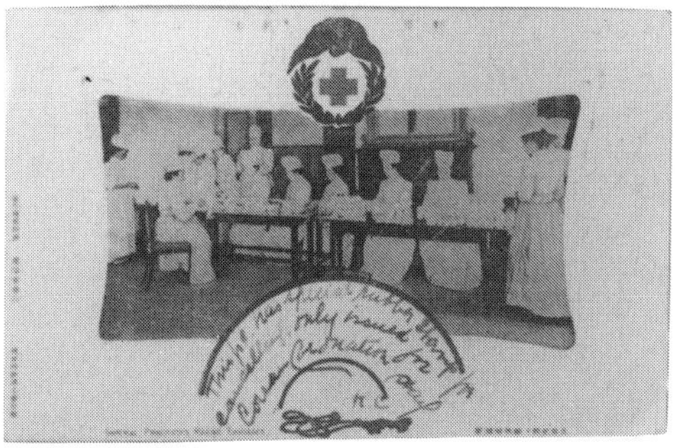

Card from the period of the 1st Japanese-Korean War.

Fund raising card issued for and after the Russo-Japanese War, 1904-05.

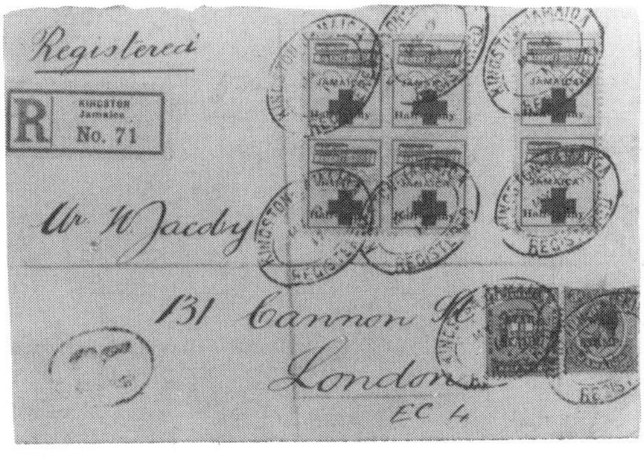

First World War Jamaican cover with six Red Cross charity stamps.

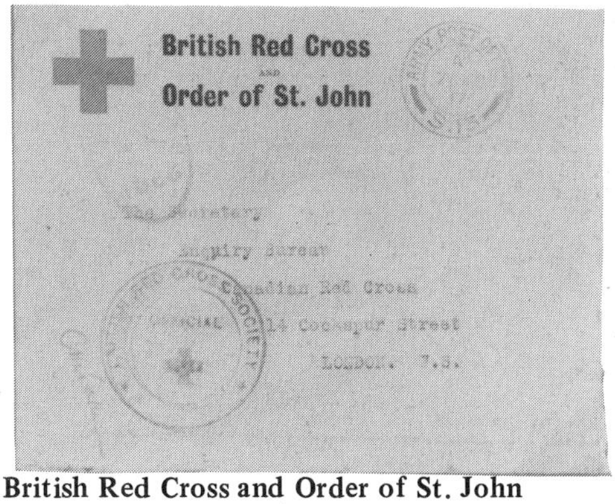

British Red Cross and Order of St. John envelope for use by the Joint Committee, after the combining of the British Red Cross, St. Andrews Society and St. Johns Ambulance Brigade.

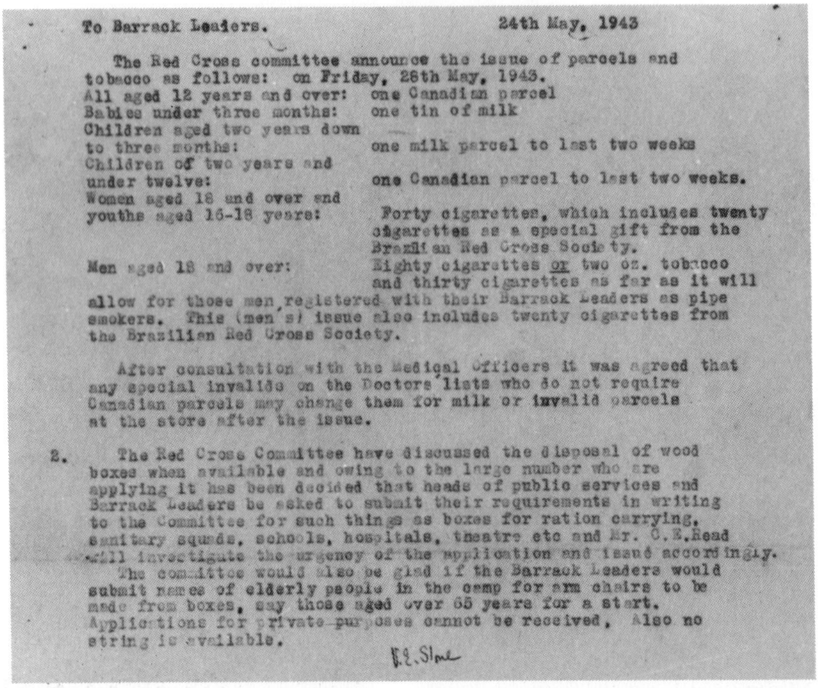

To Barrack Leaders. 24th May, 1943

The Red Cross committee announce the issue of parcels and tobacco as follows: on Friday, 28th May, 1943.

All aged 12 years and over:	one Canadian parcel
Babies under three months:	one tin of milk
Children aged two years down to three months:	one milk parcel to last two weeks
Children of two years and under twelve:	one Canadian parcel to last two weeks.
Women aged 18 and over and youths aged 16-18 years:	Forty cigarettes, which includes twenty cigarettes as a special gift from the Brazilian Red Cross Society.
Men aged 18 and over:	Eighty cigarettes or two oz. tobacco and thirty cigarettes as far as it will

allow for those men registered with their Barrack Leaders as pipe smokers. This (men's) issue also includes twenty cigarettes from the Brazilian Red Cross Society.

After consultation with the Medical Officers it was agreed that any special invalids on the Doctors' lists who do not require Canadian parcels may change them for milk or invalid parcels at the store after the issue.

2. The Red Cross Committee have discussed the disposal of wood boxes when available and owing to the large number who are applying it has been decided that heads of public services and Barrack Leaders be asked to submit their requirements in writing to the Committee for such things as boxes for ration carrying, sanitary squads, schools, hospitals, theatre etc and Mr. C.E.Read will investigate the urgency of the application and issue accordingly.

The committee would also be glad if the Barrack Leaders would submit names of elderly people in the camp for arm chairs to be made from boxes, say those aged over 65 years for a start. Applications for private purposes cannot be received. Also no string is available.

E.E.Sloane

Letter or notice from the Second World War regarding distribution of Contents of Parcels to Channel Islanders interned at Biebeuach Internment Camp.

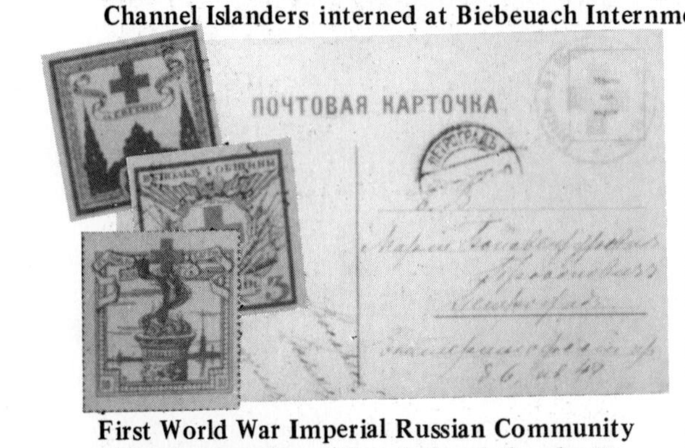

First World War Imperial Russian Community of St. Eugenie No. 2 Hospital and the charity stamps of the Society.

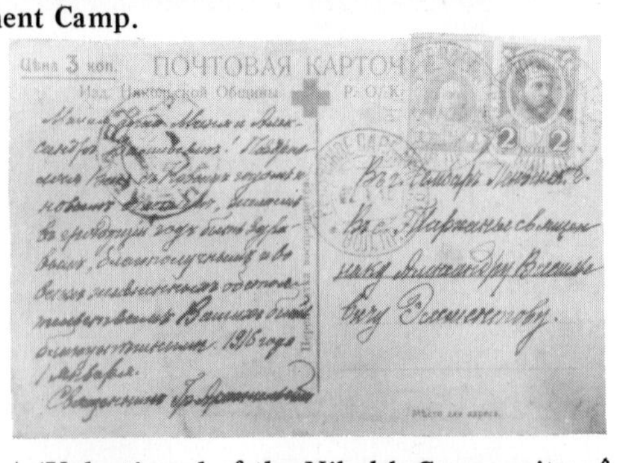

A 'Volost' card of the Nikolsk Community of the Russian Red Cross. (Volost was a group of villages).

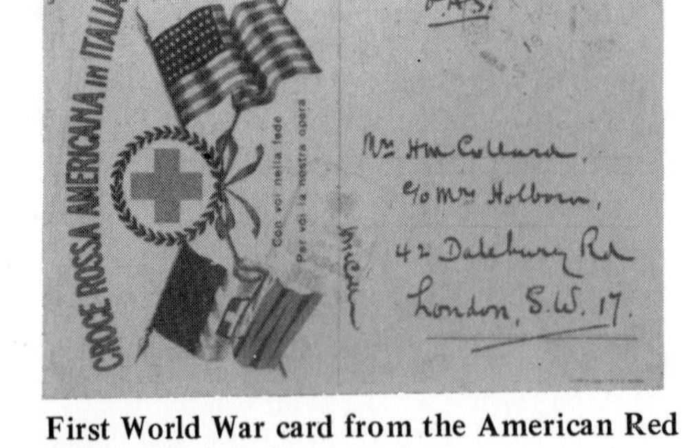

First World War card from the American Red Cross in Italy.

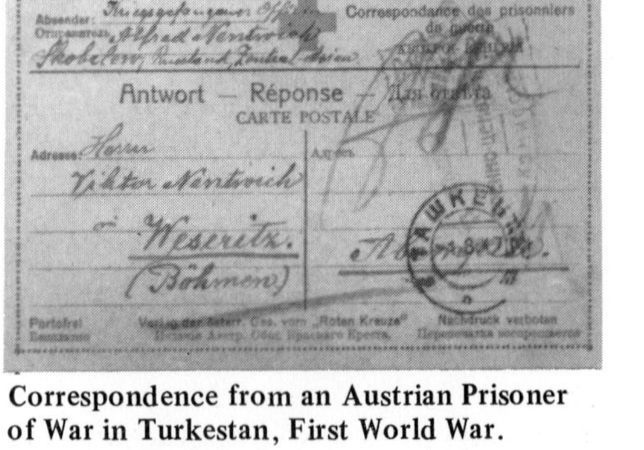

Correspondence from an Austrian Prisoner of War in Turkestan, First World War.

While the majority of Red Cross postal covers can be bought for as little as £2 – £3, rare examples can be worth as much as £50.

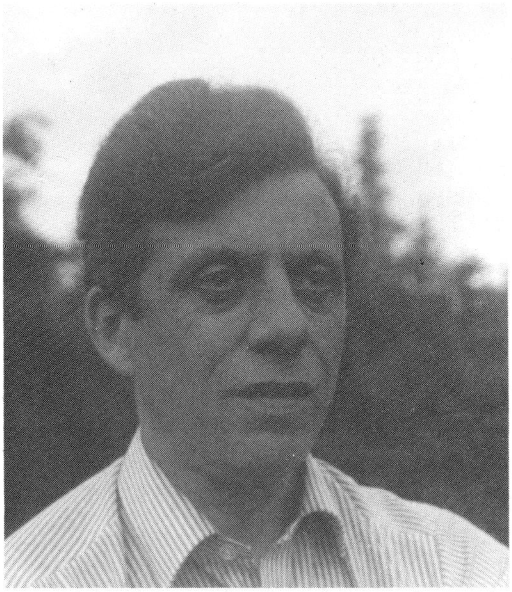

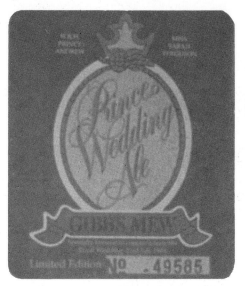

Michael Jones works in computing and collects old beer bottle labels.

"I didn't have any idea there were so many different types of beer before I started collecting but now I've got over 26,000 different labels and they're only from the British Isles.

"I began collecting around 1976 because a landlord of a pub I called into one day offered me a bottle of special beer which was brewed by Harveys of Lewes. It had such an attractive label that I took the bottle home and soaked the label off.

"Then I began writing to breweries asking if they would supply me with some of their labels and several sent me old ones as well. That was how I got hooked.

"Beer bottle labels go back to 1850 and one of the oldest I've got is a label for Tennent's Lager from Scotland. Before 1900 there were little breweries in almost every town and village and they all used their own labels. A lot of the items I have are unique because they are the only known examples used by particular breweries.

"The older labels are the most attractive because modern ones are more functional. They have to declare all the contents and too much writing spoils a label. The shapes have changed too because today most of them are rectangular but before the 1950's you got lots of oval ones. The rectangular shape is used because of high speed bottling techniques. Beer used to be bottled by hand up to the 1920's and it was called "flogging". The flogger put in the corks and there was someone beside him who stuck on the labels."

Michael's favourite label is one issued about 1910 by the Bournemouth Brewery which is unique. The first ever commemorative label celebrated the Antarctic Expedition of Franklyn in the 1850's. It was followed by labels for Queen Victoria's Jubilee in 1897 and the Coronations between 1902 and 1953. There was a big upsurge in commemorative labels at the time of the Silver Jubilee in 1977.

Pricing of labels is difficult because it depends on the rarity and age of a label and

also how much it is wanted by a collector. In general they are bought for between 5p and 25p although £20 might be asked for the Bournemouth Brewery label.

The one that Michael would most like to find was issued by Salt's Brewery of Burton-on-Trent to commemorate Queen Victoria's Diamond Jubilee.

Anyone with old labels are invited to contact him on 0376-512568.

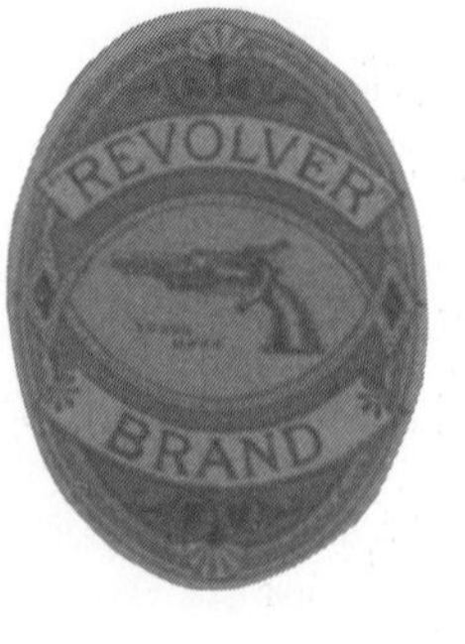

Revolver Brand, label in red, pale green and black on white. £3

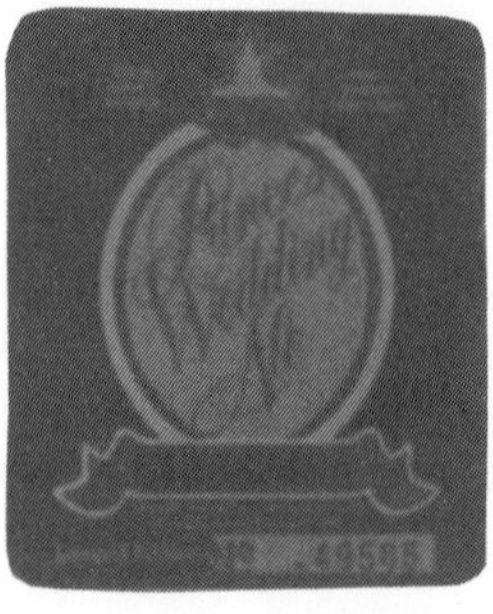

Princes Wedding Ale, by Gibbs Mew, purple pink and gold. 5p

Light Dinner Ale, a unique label from the Army & Navy Co-operative Brewery 1896. £25

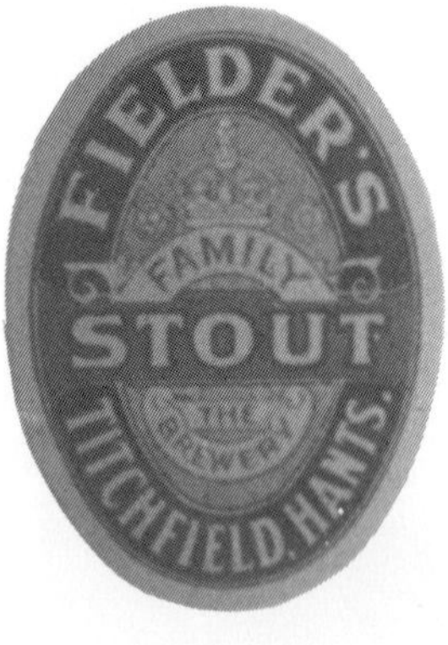

Fielder's Stout, Titchfield, Hants, black and brown on buff, 1950's. £1

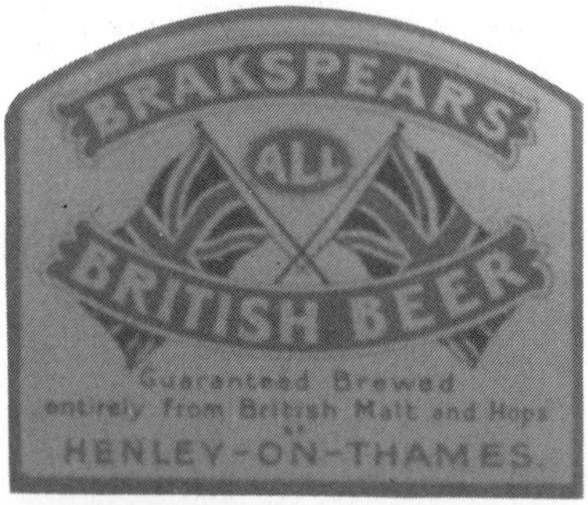

Brakspears All British Beer, Henley on Thames, in red, white and blue, 1930's. 75p

Harman's Stout, a classic label from the 1950's, in blue and brown on white. £1.50

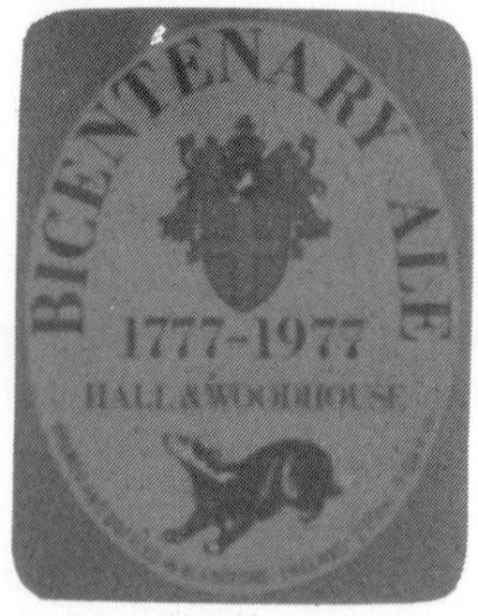

Bicentenary Ale, 1777-1977, Hall & Woodhouse, an old established family brewery in Dorset. 10p

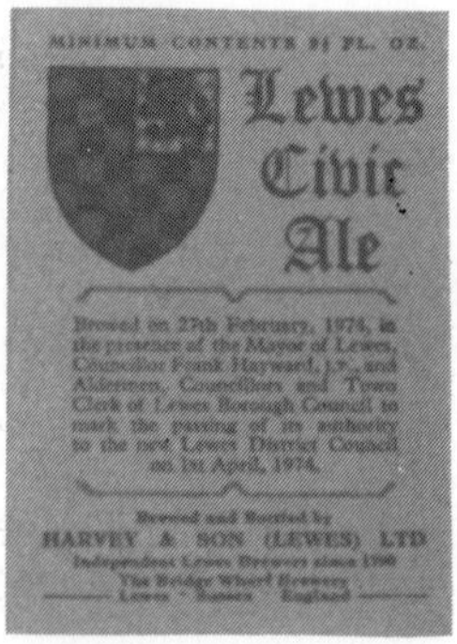

Lewes Civic Ale, by Harvey & Son, issued April 1974, blue, black, red and gold on white. 20p

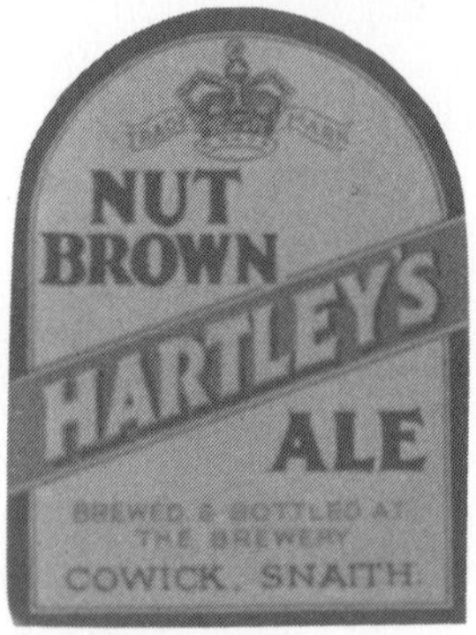

Hartley's Nut Brown Ale, Cowick, Snaith, brown and red on white, 1930's. £2

'Pale Ale', by Blair's, Edinburgh, a common Victorian label in red and black on white. 50p

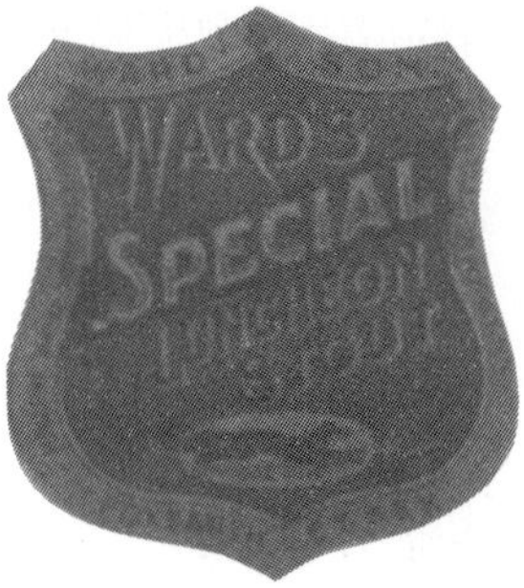

Shield shaped label for Ward's Special Luncheon Stout, brown and purple on buff, 1930's. £1.50

Bitter Beer, by Bell & Co. Ltd., Stockport, blue and red on white. 50p

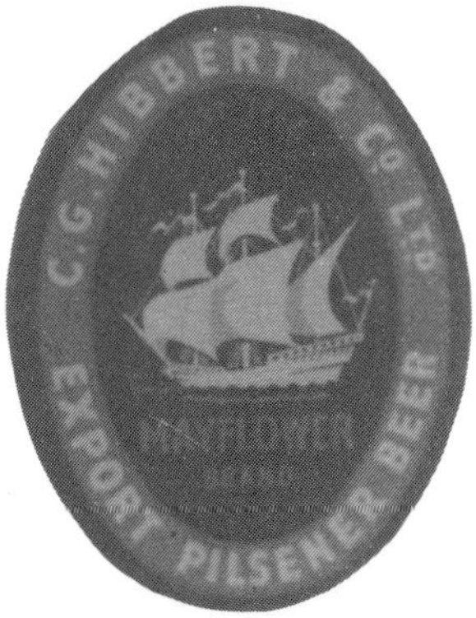

C. G. Hibbert & Co., Mayflower Brand, served on liners operating from Southampton in the 1940's. 15p

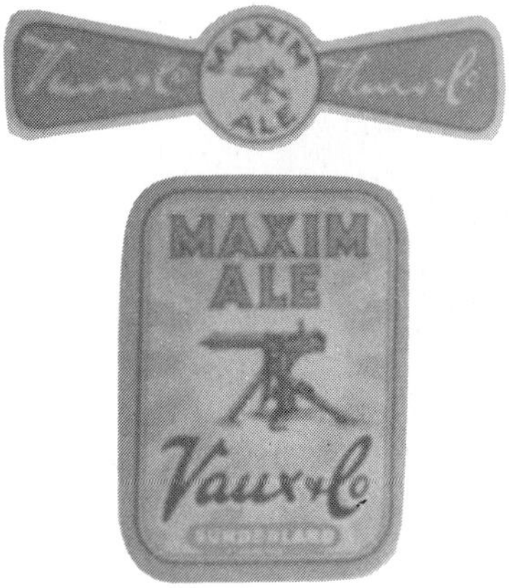

Maxim Ale, by Vaux & Co., Sunderland, in yellow, blue, black and gold, 1920's. £1

Offilers' of Derby, Nut Brown Ale, 1950's. 75p

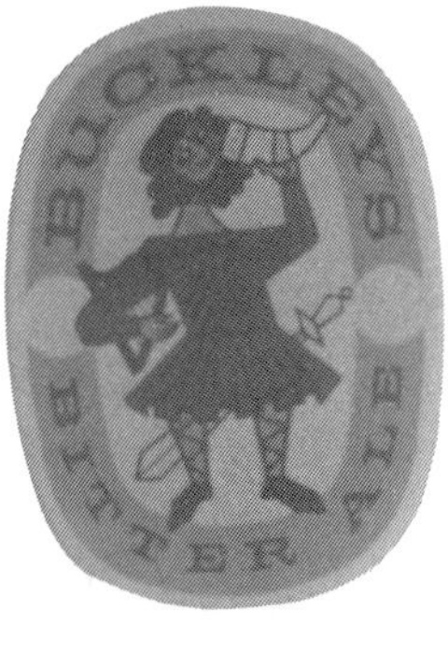

Buckleys Bitter Ale, a Welsh label from the mid 1950's, brown and purple on white. 20p

Royal Oak, a current issue label in natural colours. 1p

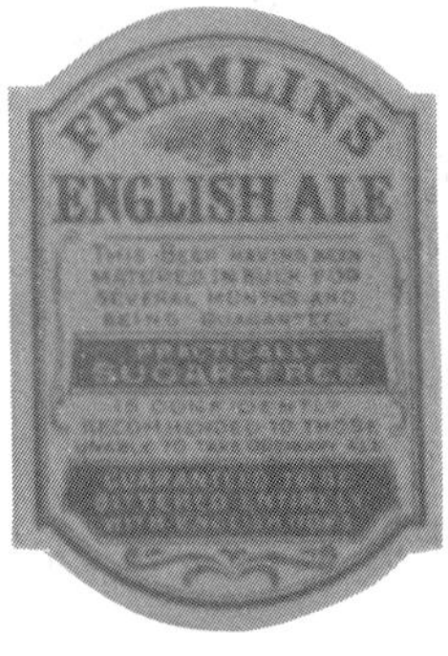

Fremlins English Ale with guarantee, red on white, 1930's. 75p

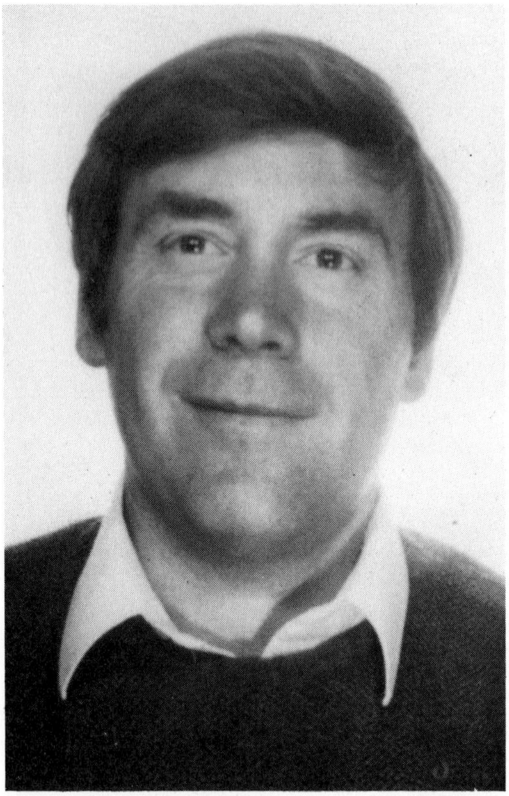

Brian Thatcher is a member of the Metropolitan Police and collects old poison bottles.

"It's quite funny how it started because in 1976 I went to arrest a car breaker and tripped over an old bottle in his yard. I picked it up and later found out that it was a Victorian poison bottle and my interest started from there.

"The first English poison bottle was patented in 1859 and from then on manufacturers came out with bottles in more and more unusual shapes and designs because those were the days when people often had to dose themselves in the dark and they had to be sure that they weren't taking something poisonous. That's why poison bottles were ridged or peculiarly shaped — just so that people could tell as soon as they touched them that they contained poison.

"In those days poison covered all sorts of things from carbolic acid which was used as a disinfectant to lip salve.

"Some of the bottles were also coloured in bright shades of cobalt blue, green or amber. Cobalt glass was last used for domestic bottles about 1956. Blue plastic was then used, as it was cheaper."

Brian has a magnificent display of over 1,000 poison bottles in his home and he is also Chairman of the Kent Bottle Club.

He is not interested in bottles with labels but has some embossed with names of local chemists, hospitals, and borough councils. The stars of his collection include the only bottle known in Britain, shaped like a pair of binoculars, valued at around £800; a submarine shaped bottle worth around £150 and a wasp waisted bottle which can sell for around £400.

The bottle Brian would most like to find is shaped like a skull and was made in USA. Its price is about £400.

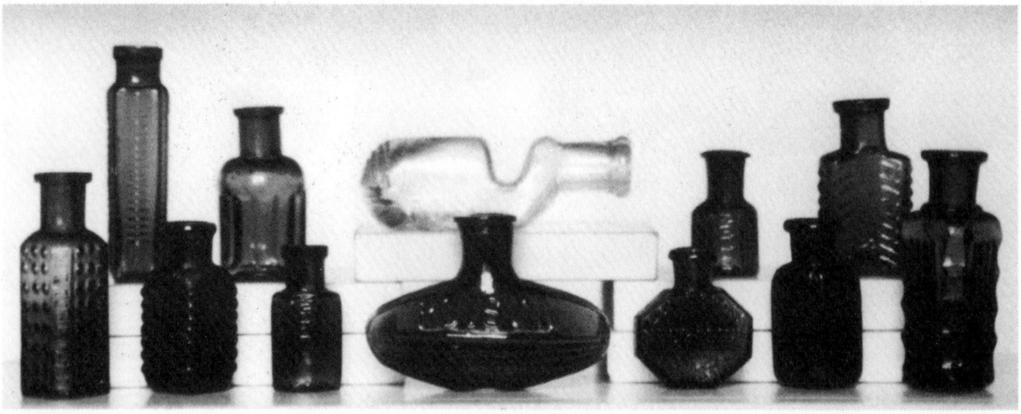

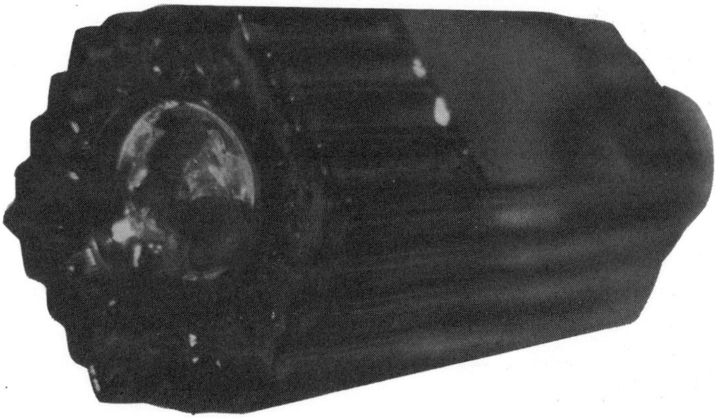

This illustration shows the base view of a six sided poison bottle in cobalt blue, embossed with Savory's Patent and bearing a Pontil mark. It was patented by John Savory and William Barker in January 1859 and from this patent all forms of six sided poison bottles evolved. This particular bottle, with the base embossing and Pontil mark, is the only one known to exist and could be valued up to £500.

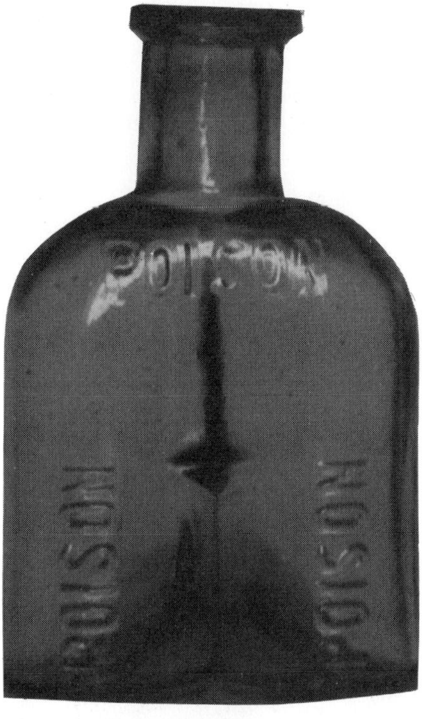

O'Reilly's Patent, known as Binoculars Poison. Bottle is ice blue, has 'Poison' across shoulder and embossed on cylinder bottom sections, and is also embossed on the base 'O'Reillys Patent 1905'. Only two of these bottles are known, the other bottle is in an American collection. £800 plus

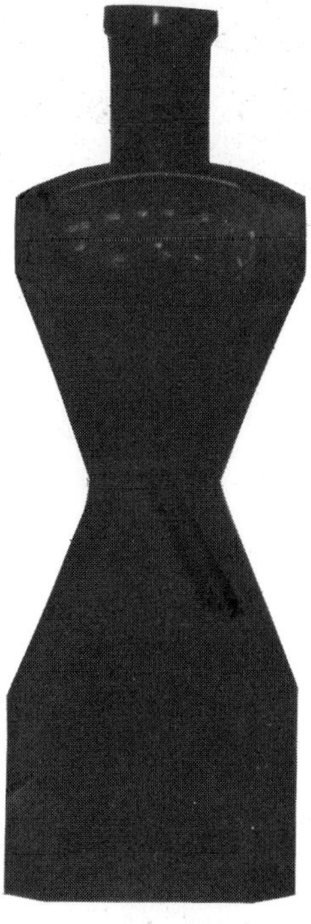

Very rare 'Wasp Waist' Poison, of which various sizes exist, with rows of diamond points embossed on the front and side panels and the Reg. No. 460944 at the foot of the back panel, cobalt blue only, Patented 1894. £450 plus

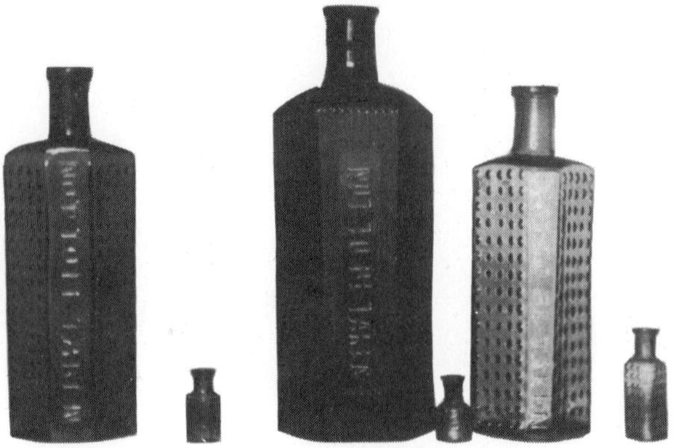

Poisons, large and small, bottles range in size from 1 dram (bottle third from right) to 40oz. (large centre bottle).

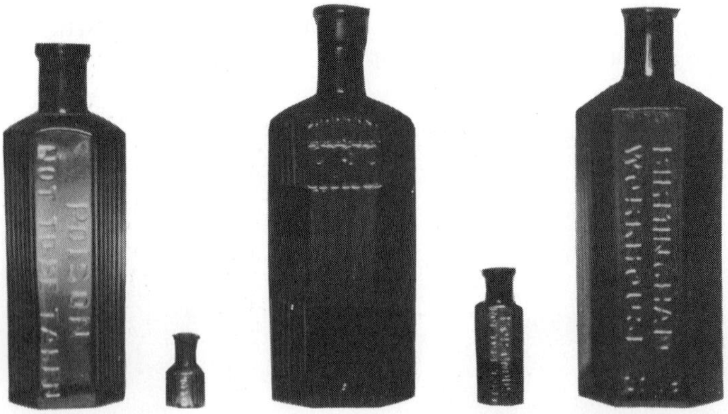

Six sided bottles in green, amber and blue with various embossing. The large bottle on the right is embossed 'Birmingham Workhouse'. Valued between £3 and £15

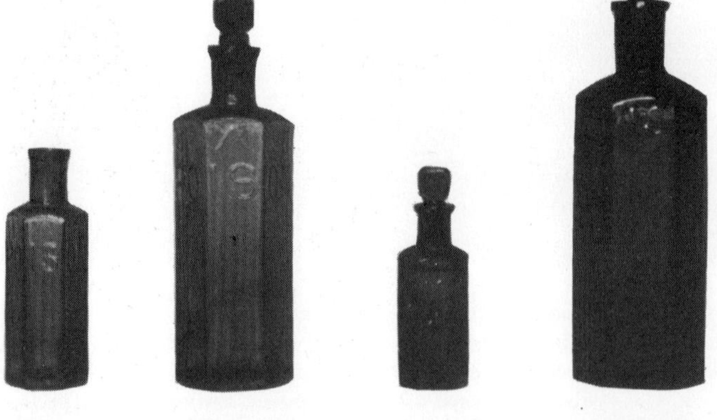

Cobalt blue six sided poisons, Po/is/on and embossed arrow on rear three panels, all the other panels vertical ribbed, some with ground in blue glass stoppers. £10 to £20 depending on size.

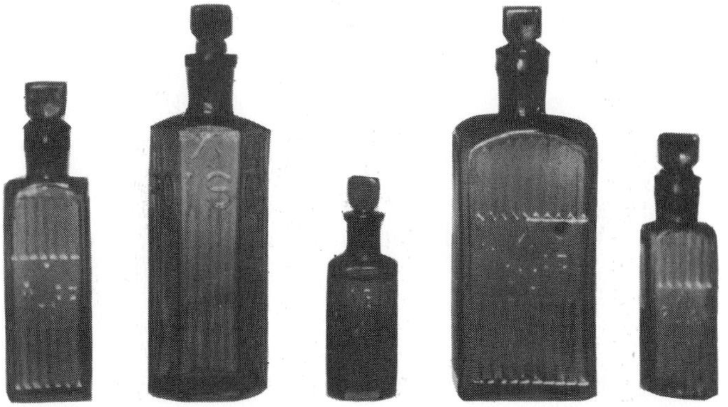

A mixture of six sided and square bodied poison bottles known as Admiralty. The front panel with an embossed arrow, capacity and the letter N, the remainder being vertical ribbed. These bottles range in size from 1oz. up to 24oz. Value £10 to £40 according to bottle and type.

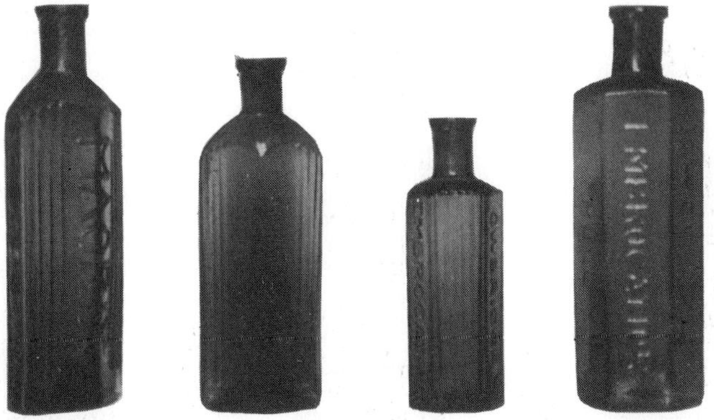

The two green bottles on the left are embossed 'Maorix' and 'Not To Be Taken', both are rare. Value up to £30.
The cobalt blue bottles on the right are embossed 'Owbridges Embrocation' and 'Owbridges Embrocation Hull'. Value £5 to £10

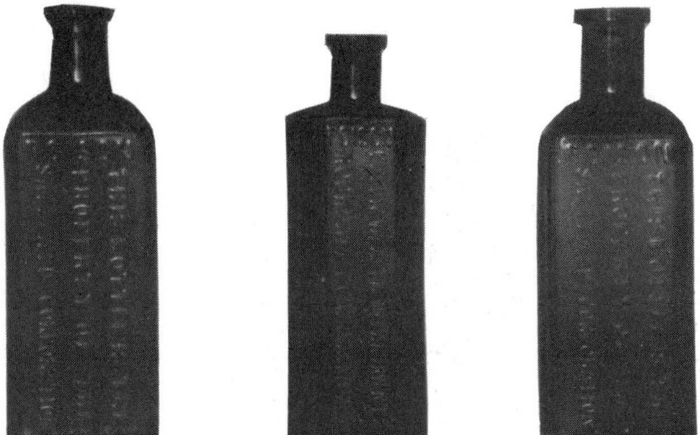

The bottle in the centre is embossed 'Poison' at the top and bottom of front panel, and 'Public Health Department, Rochdale Corporation', cobalt blue, extremly rare. Value £25. Flanking bottles are cobalt blue and emerald green embossed 'Poison' at the top and bottom of front panel, and 'This bottle is the property of the Sheffield Corporation'. Value £40.

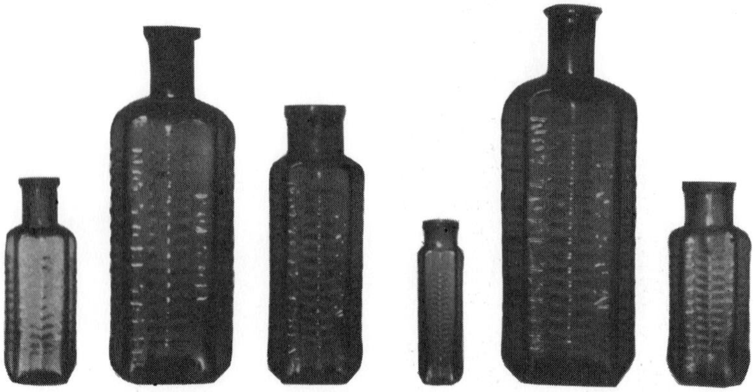

Known as 'Star' poison bottles (star shaped cross section), they are embossed 'Not To Be Taken' and 'Poison' in the two front panel depressions and Reg. No. 716057 embossed at the foot of the back panel. The bottles range from 1oz. to 16oz., are cobalt blue, green and amber glass with wide and narrow mouth types. Value ranging between £35 to £70, cobalt blue bottles command higher prices.

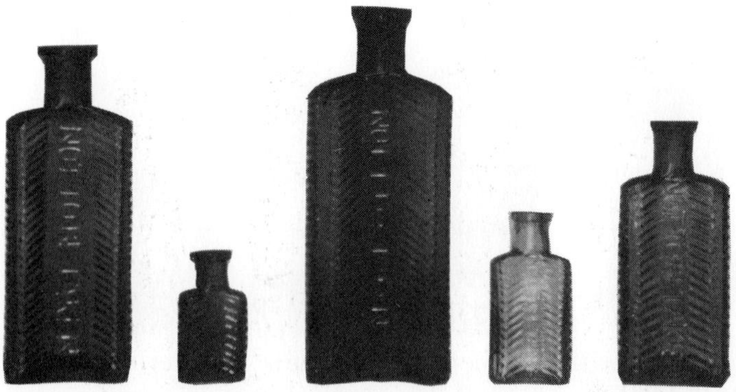

Known as 'Crescent' poison bottles, Registered in 1905, (crescent shaped in cross section) they have 'Not To Be Taken' down front panel or, and much rarer, 'Poison'. Found in cobalt blue, copper blue, emerald green, and aqua glass. Value £10 to £20

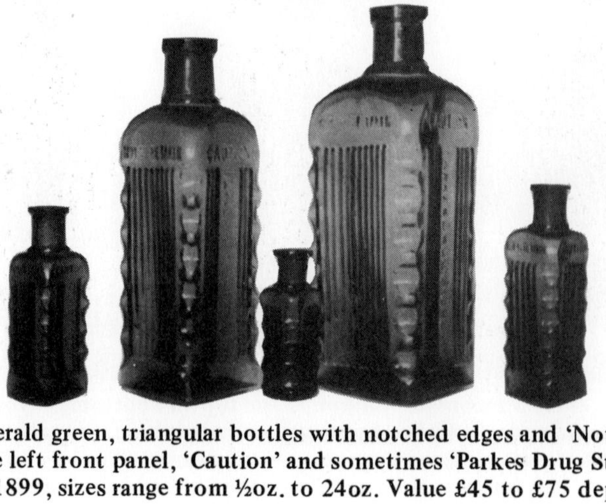

Wilsons Patent emerald green, triangular bottles with notched edges and 'Not To Be Taken' and 'Patent' on the left front panel, 'Caution' and sometimes 'Parkes Drug Stores' on the right, Patented in 1899, sizes range from ½oz. to 24oz. Value £45 to £75 depending on size.

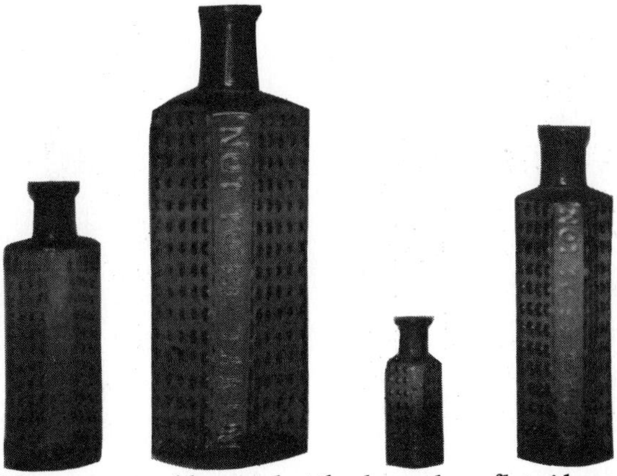

Taylors Liverpool Patent, emerald green bottles have three flat sides and a curved back, with embossed 'Caution' at top of rear panel, Reg. No. 409210 at the foot and 'Not To Be Taken' down front panel. The base is embossed 'Taylor Liverpool' and with capacity. Patented 1905 – it also has rows of bumps on the front panels. Value £15 to £40 depending on size. (Very small and large sizes in most Patents are often the rarest and are worth more.)

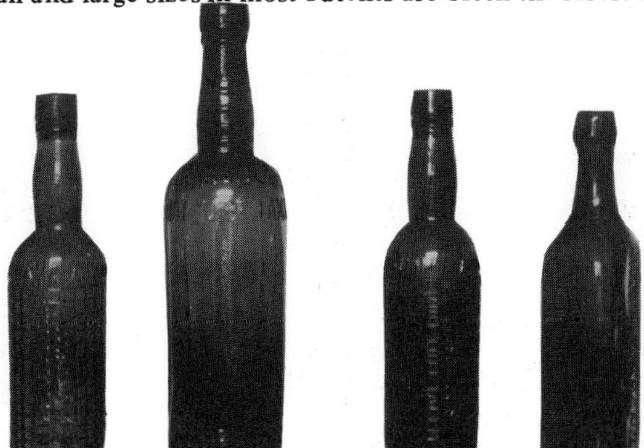

Four Ammonia Poisons in shades of green and brown. Bottle second from right is of rare triangular shape, is embossed with 'Sharpes Ammonia' and 'Not To Be Taken'. Value £50. Other bottles £5 to £15.

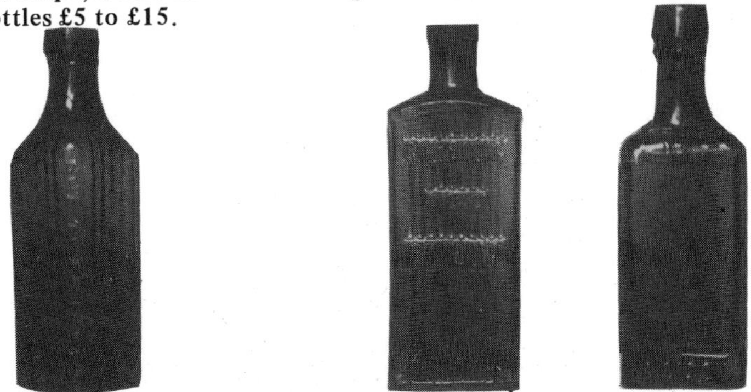

Three shaped Poisons – left, triangular shape with curved back, 'Not To Be Taken' down front and vertical ribbing on adjacent panels, shades of green and black. Value £5.
Middle – 'Carbolic Acid Poison' on front panel, this bottle is rectangular shaped in amber glass. Rare £25.
Right – cobalt blue bottle with 'Poison' at the foot of the front panel, 'Ossidine' on the left and 'Coles Patent England' on the right panel. Very rare, only three known. Value £70 plus.

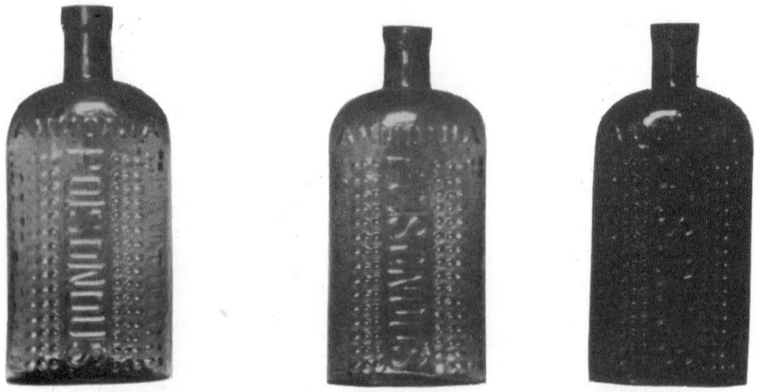

Ammonia Poisons, three identical bottles, from left in amber, green and cobalt glass, embossed 'Ammonia' across top and 'Caution', 'Poisonous', 'Not To Be Taken' down front panel. Value £10 to £25 depending on colours.

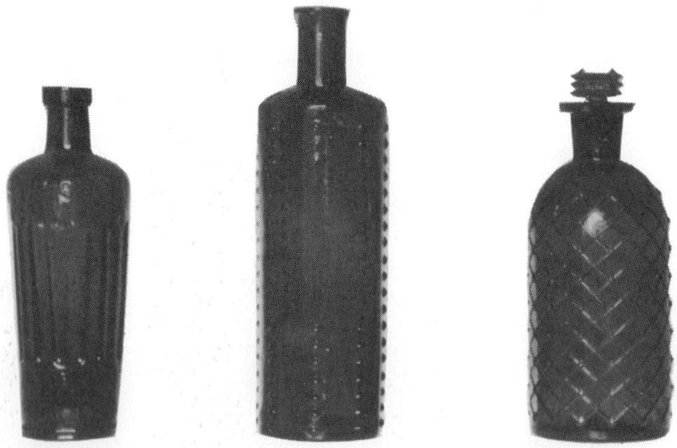

Three rare Poisons in cobalt blue glass – left, Tippers Poison bottle which tapers from shoulder to base and has 'Poison' embossed across the top of the front, 'Tippers Animal Medicines' at foot, Patented 1904. Value £100 plus.
The middle bottle has 'Poison' on the shoulder, rows of diamond points on the sides, and the base has 'Patent' embossed on the rim, and L. and T. Co. embossed in the centre. Value £75.
The bottle on the right is American, known as 'Quilt Poison', has cross hatching around the sides of the bottle and has a stopper with sharp points and embossed 'Poison' at side and top. Value £100

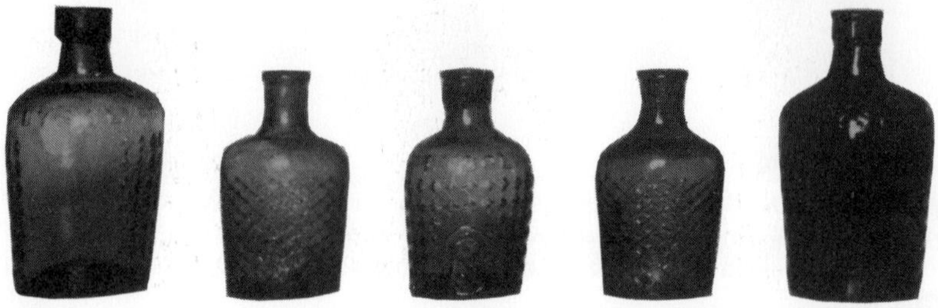

Lysol Disinfectant bottles in a range of sizes with various embossings, in blue, green, amber and black glass. Value 50p to £10. Black and blue being much rarer.

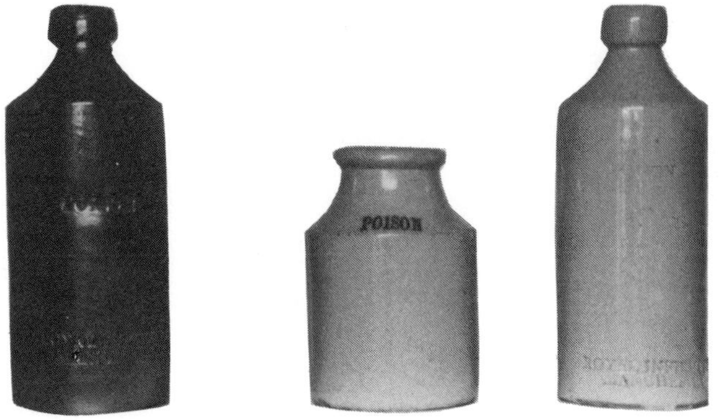

Three stoneware Poisons with the outer bottles stamped 'Poison', 'Royal Infirmary Manchester'. Value £10 to £15.

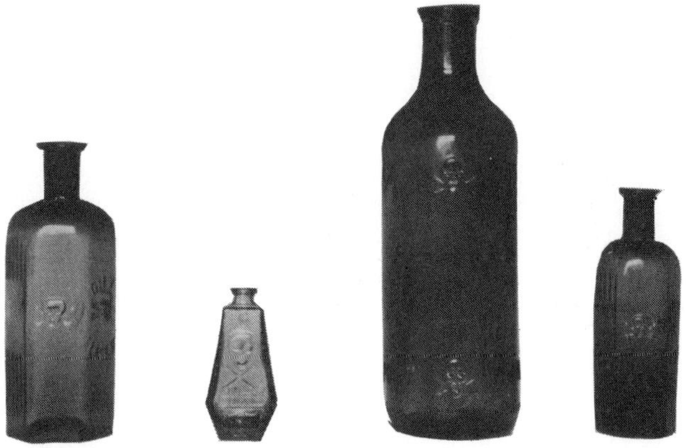

Poison bottles with skulls – the three larger bottles illustrated are all emerald green, of German origin, and have embossed skull and cross bones and also embossed 'Gift Flasche' which translated indicates 'Poison Bottle'.
The bottle second from left is of American origin, is coffin shaped and has a skull and cross bones embossed on front with the rear embossed R.I.P. £125

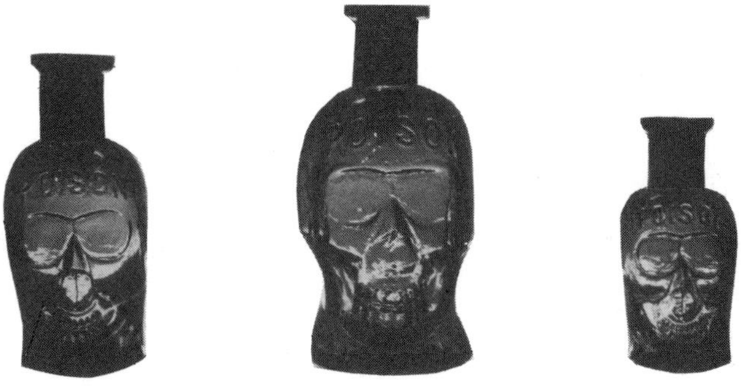

Skull Poisons, Patented by Carlton H. Lee, 1894, in America, are rare and come in three sizes of cobalt blue glass. Value £350 plus.

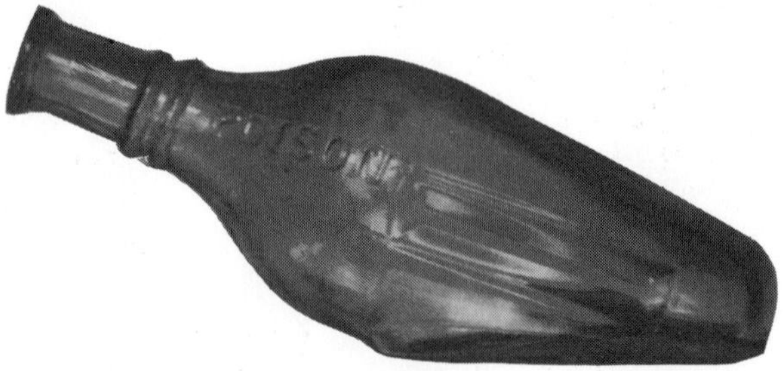

Quine's Patent, aqua glass bottle with 'Poison' embossed on the side or back, and capacity embossed on belly, Patented 1893. Various sizes exist, all rare. £75 plus.

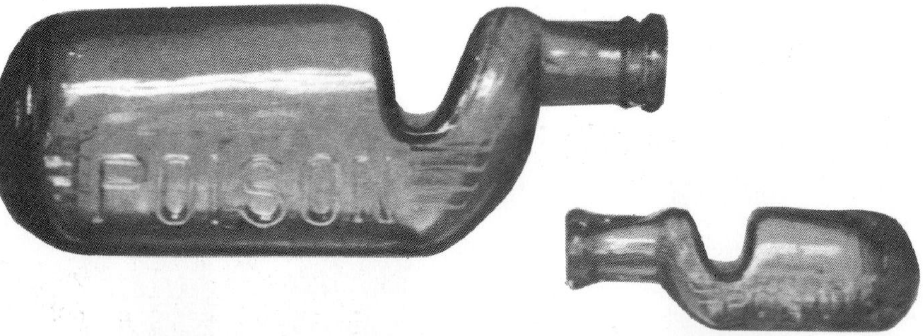

Martins Patent bottle 1902. The bottle stands as shown, the U bend is believed to act as a trap to prevent spilling the contents. Various sizes and embossings exist with the rare types having 'Poison', 'Not To Be Taken' embossed on side, with others just 'Poison', also embossed 'The Martin Poison Bottle'. Can be found in aqua and ice blue glass and are thought to exist in amber and cobalt blue. For very small and large sizes prices increase £75 up to £150.

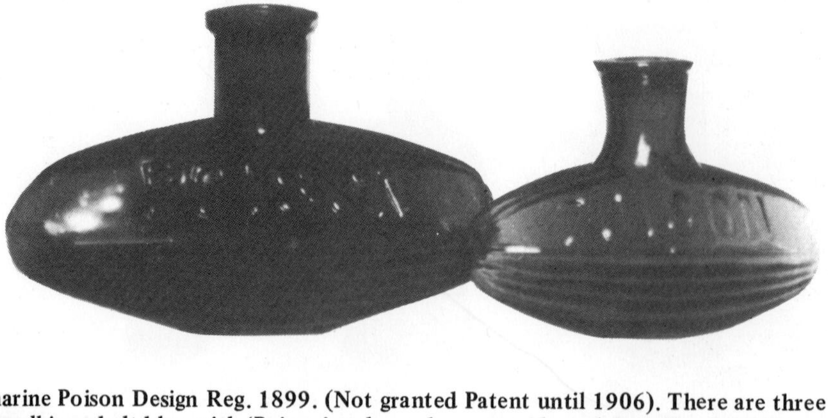

Submarine Poison Design Reg. 1899. (Not granted Patent until 1906). There are three sizes known all in cobalt blue with 'Poison' embossed on one side and Reg. No. 336907 on the base. Rare in all sizes and highly sought after by collectors. £100 – £150 depending on size.

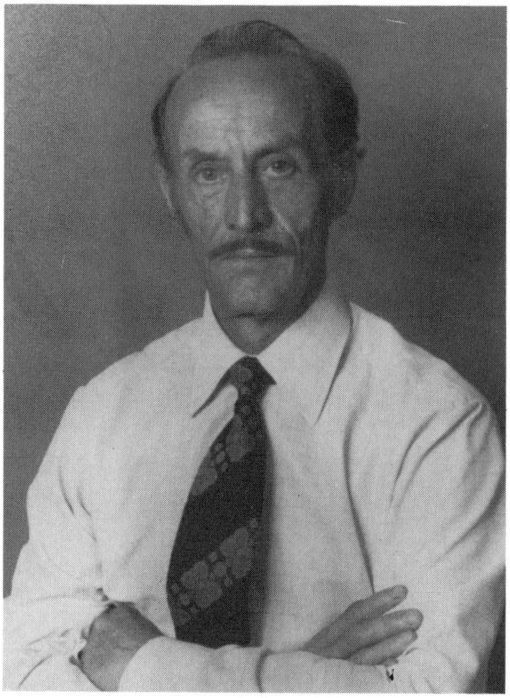

Peter Haworth is retired and collects shaving mugs.

"Until recently I had 250 big shaving mugs but I've weeded out the best of them and now I'm down to 80 with an extra collection of 150 miniature crested mugs which has taken me a long time to collect. When you start collecting you buy all you see but later on you become more discriminating.

"I've been collecting for 12 years and have had to pick up information as I go along because there's a shortage of literature on shaving mugs.

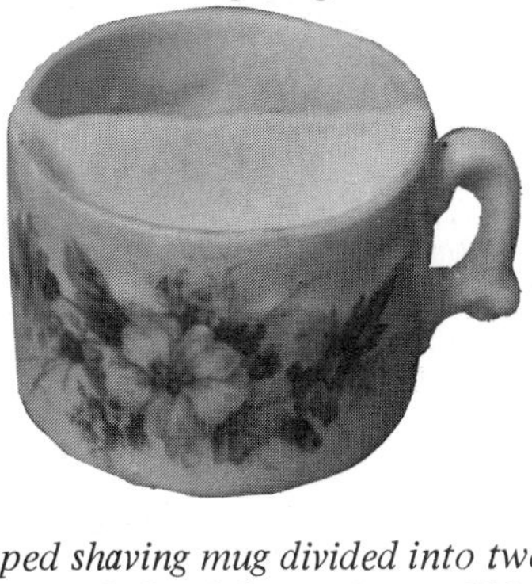

Cup shaped shaving mug divided into two compartments with floral decoration. £18-£25

"They seemed to have appeared first as bowls and beakers in the 15th century but shaving mugs as we know them today were produced from the early 19th century until the late 1930's when electric razors arrived on the scene. Some are decorated with pictures, numbers or have a man's name on them and they can be made in a wide range of materials including pottery, brass, copper or silver as well as porcelain.

"Some of the rarest are the 'four in ones' with holders for water, soap, a brush and a razor and there are also 'three in ones' and French brush vases which are taller and thinner than ordinary shaving mugs. Recently I bought a pair of French brush vases for £4."

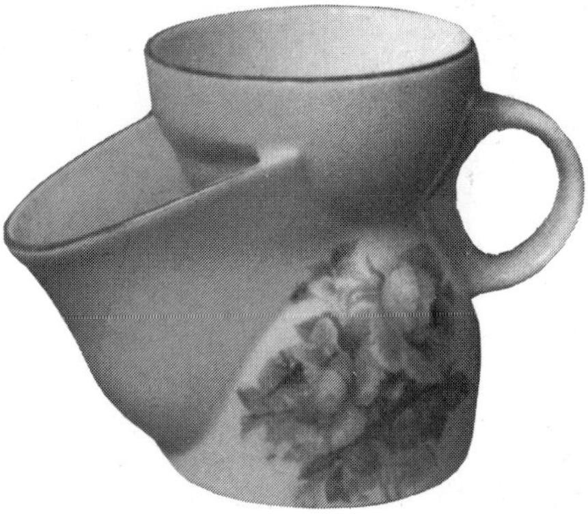

Edwardian white shaving mug decorated with floral sprays and gilt edging. £7-£14

Peter said that there are dozens of shaving mugs still to be found but look for ones that are unchipped. Amateur collectors can be fooled by reproductions but a good mug should feel heavy in the hand and be worn at the bottom. They can be picked up for between £4 and £20 on market stalls but in antique shops prices tend to go up to £50 and over. Crested mugs made by Goss are more expensive with prices of around £60 being not uncommon.

He would love to find an American 'four in one' shaving mug called the Utility of Boston.

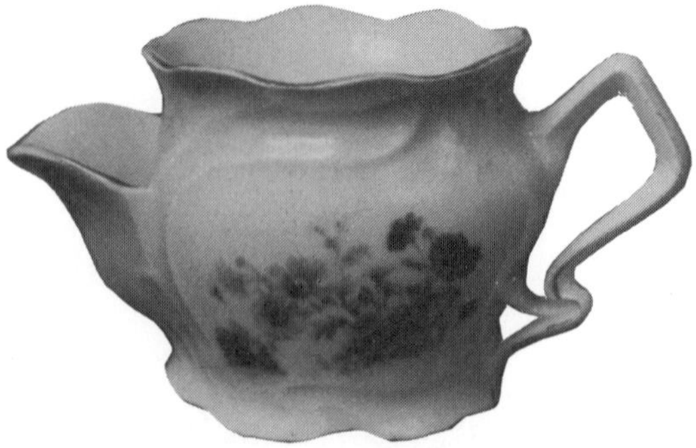

Large late 19th century bowl shaped shaving mug with floral decoration and shaped handle. £15 – £25

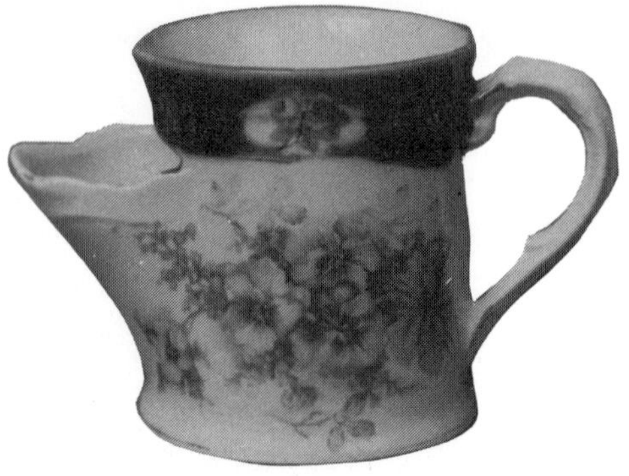

Late Victorian shaving mug with fine floral decoration and dark blue frieze. £25 – £35

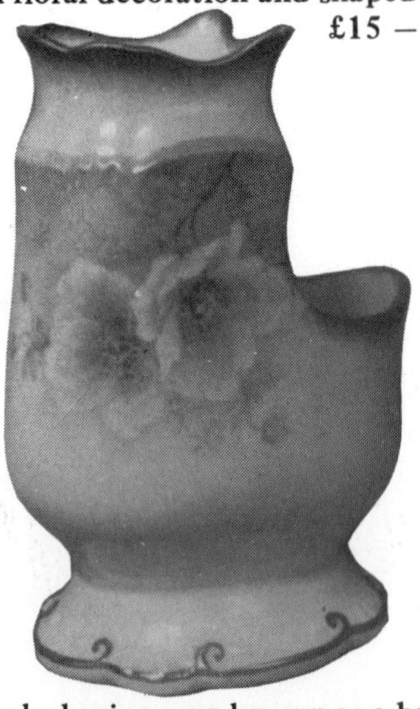

Tall French shaving mug known as a brush vase with gilt and floral decoration, circa 1890. £20 – £40

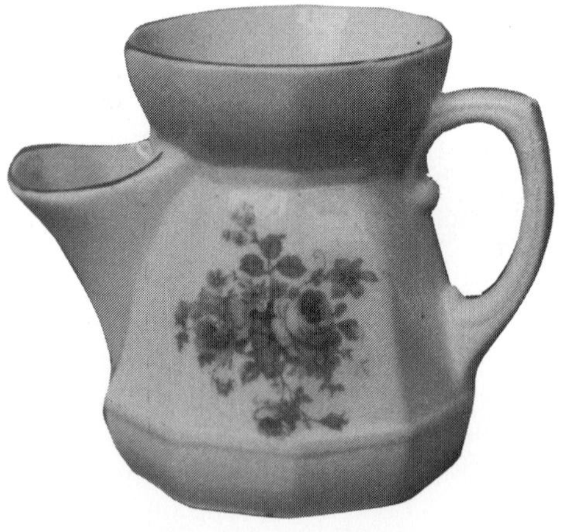

Large, late 19th century, shaving mug with floral decoration and gilt edging. £15 – £25

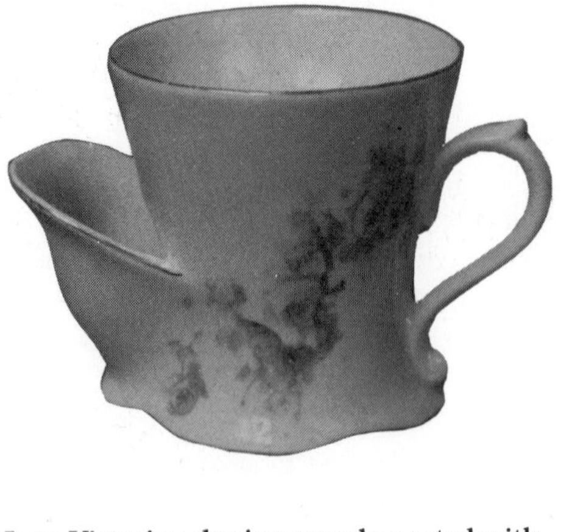

Late Victorian shaving mug decorated with floral sprays. £14 – £20

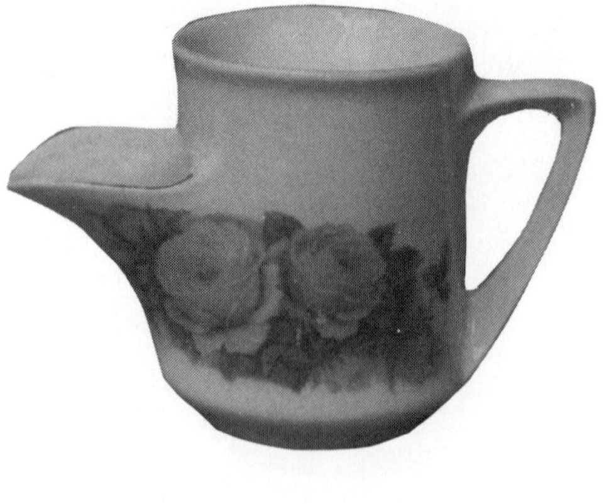

Elegantly shaped white shaving mug decorated with pink floral sprays. £12 – £20

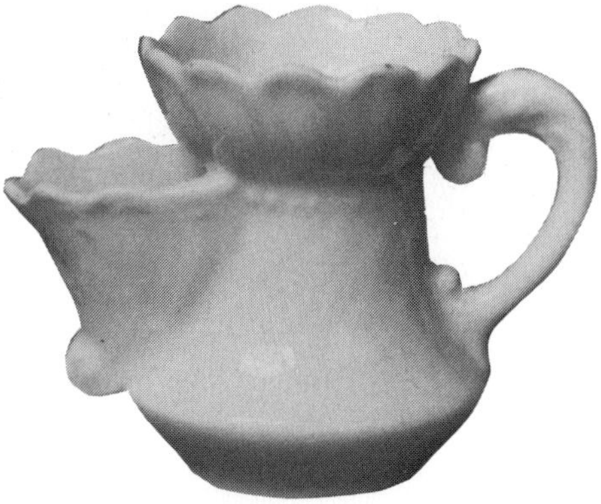

Heavy Victorian plain white shaving mug.
£14 – £20

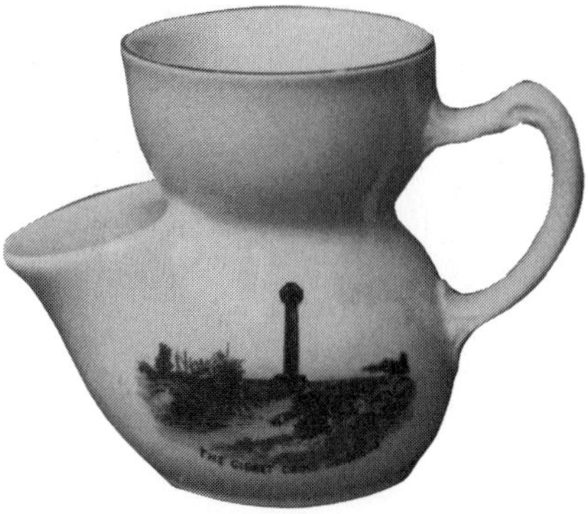

Goss shaving mug with colour transfer of 'The Gibbet Cross, Minehead'. £40

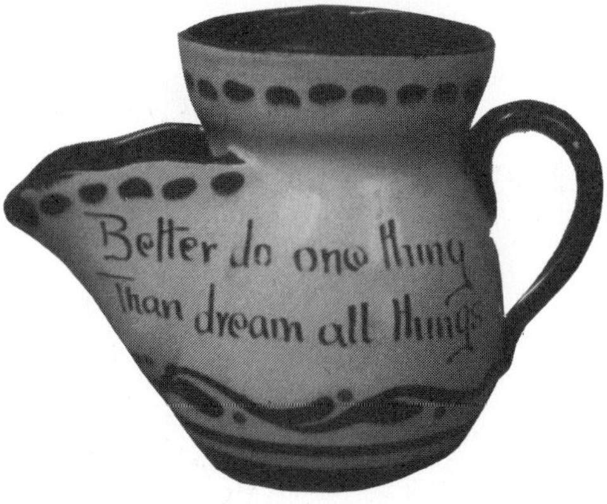

Torquay Ware shaving mug in brown and cream bearing the motto 'Better do one thing, Than dream all things!'. £15 – £30

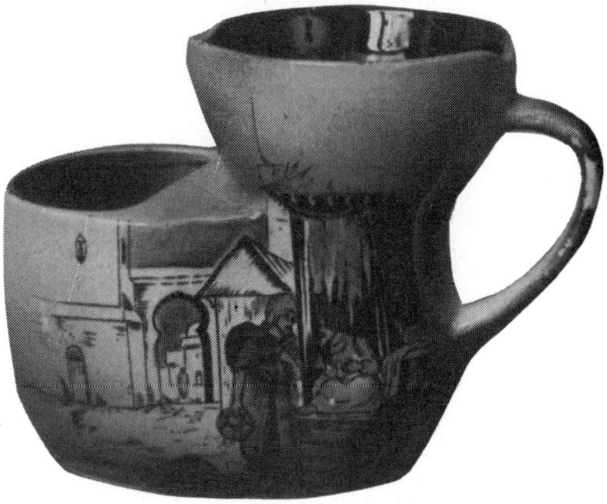

'Glimpses of the East', a multi-coloured shaving mug, circa 1920's. £15 – £25

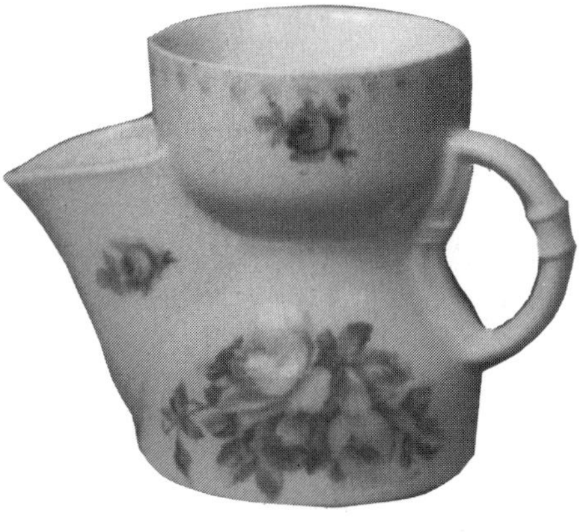

An interesting signed shaving mug, G. Wiegand, with floral decoration. £30 – £45

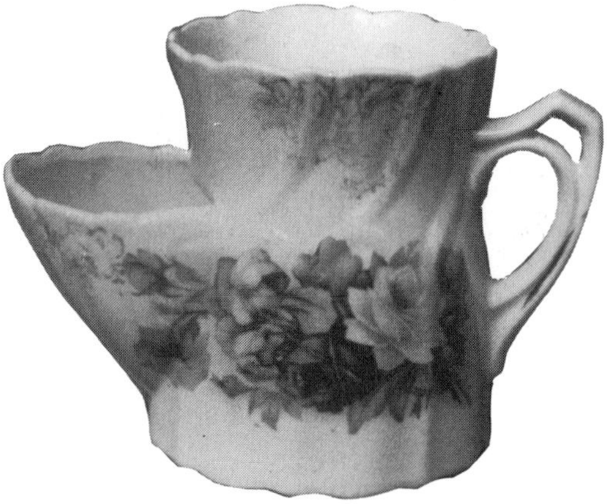

Large, late 19th century, shaving mug with floral decoration and unusual double handle.
£25 – £40

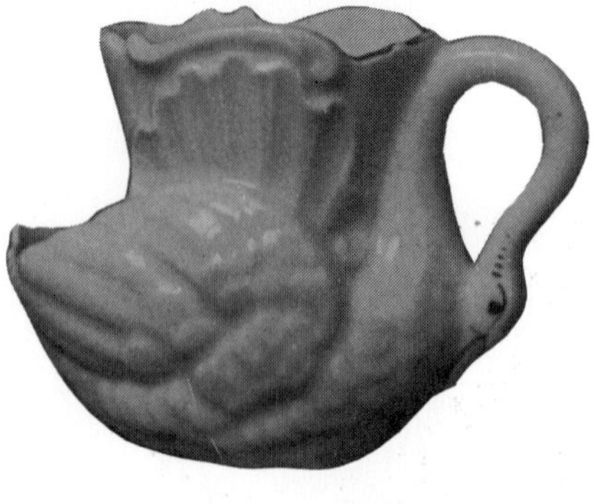

Swan shaped shaving mug with gilt edging, circa 1900. £20 – £30

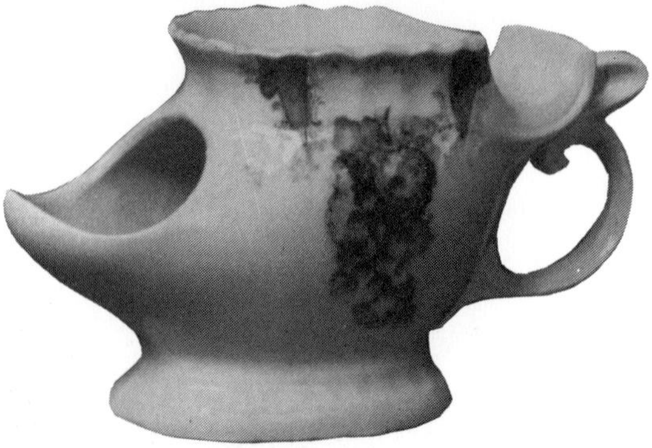

Three in one shaving mug with a place for water, the soap and a brush, circa 1900. £18 – £30

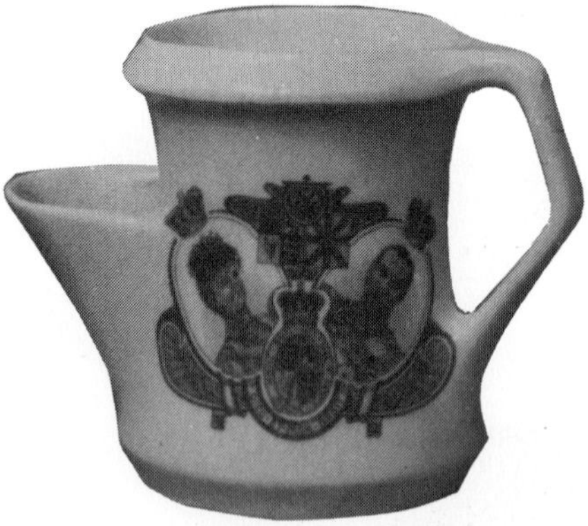

Souvenir Coronation shaving mug for George V and Queen Mary. £15 – £25

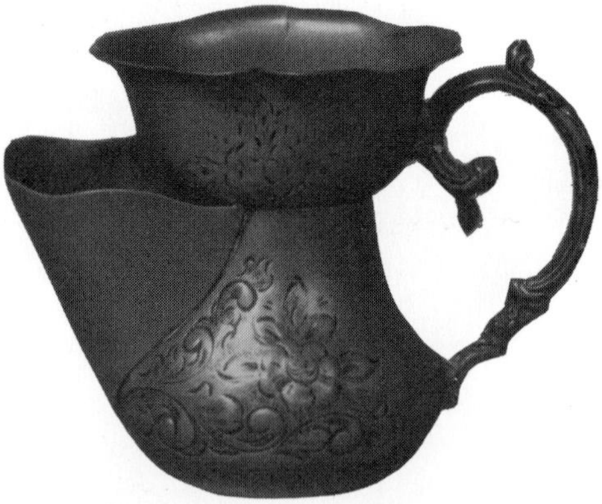

Late Victorian pewter shaving mug with embossed floral decoration. £35 – £55

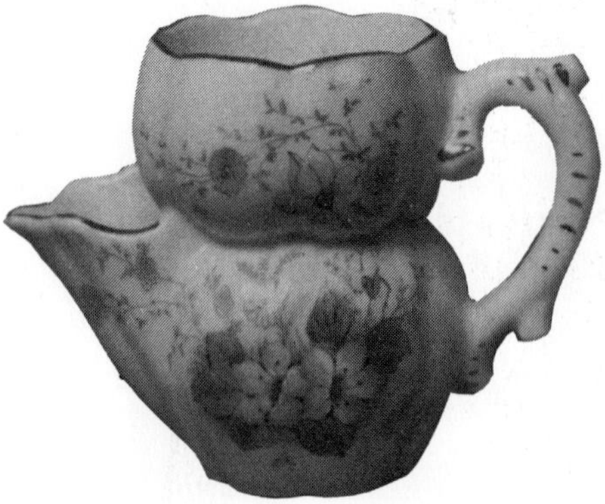

Victorian shaving mug with hand-painted floral decoration and gilt edging. £25 – £40

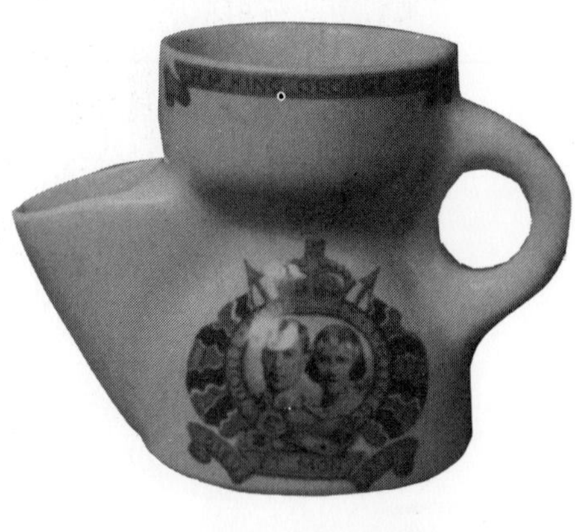

Souvenir Coronation shaving mug for H.M. King George VI and Queen Elizabeth. £15 – £25

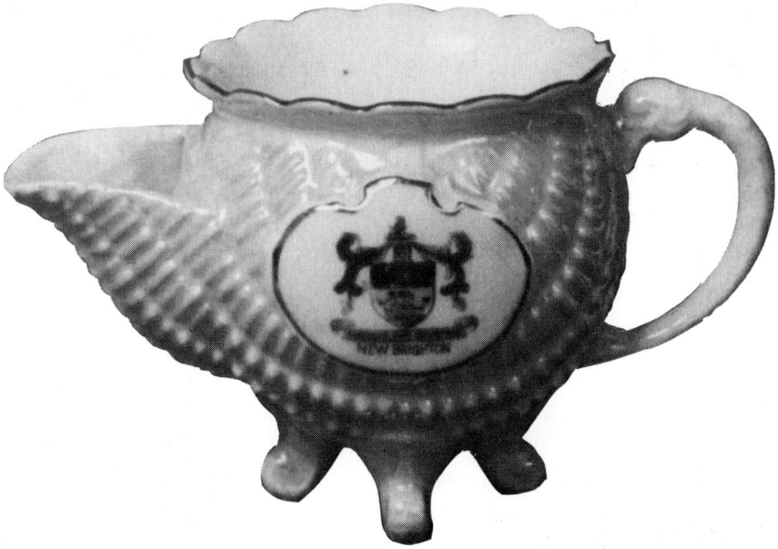

Pearl lustre shaving mug, on four scroll feet, bearing the crest of New Brighton. £14 – £20

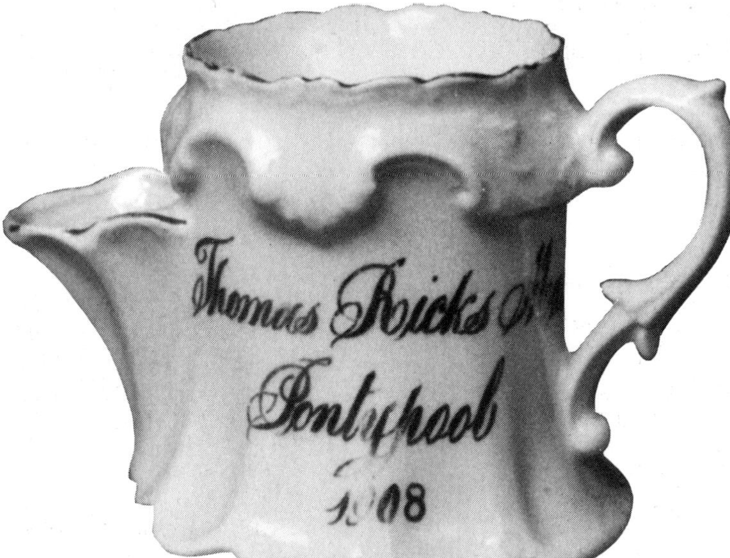

Personalised shaving mug in white with gold lettering, 'Thomas Ricks, Maskelyne, Pontypool, 1908'. £50

David Fulton owns a toolshop and collects Disney films and movie stills.

"When I was a boy I was very keen on the movies and actually tried making some cartoon films myself using an 8mm and later a 16mm cine camera. When I was eleven in 1946, I was given a hand turned cine projector for Christmas and gave shows to the local kids. I made a room in my home into a cinema with me sitting in a chair on top of a table and shining the film through a screen with a hole in it. It was just like the real thing!

"A lot of people collect films but not so many concentrate on just Disney films as I do. Video killed cine films in general and you can buy them now in collectors' fairs but the market is in a state of flux because a few people are cottoning onto the idea that they are going to become very collectible just because they are obsolescent.

"At the moment a cartoon film lasting seven or eight minutes will cost around £12 but that price could go up. I have around 100 Disney cartoons as well as posters and front-of-house stills. I also have some cartoons by animators who left Disney's Burbank Studios and set up on their own but they were never as popular as Disney. He was a genius of innovation".

David's ambition is to own a full length feature film such as 'Snow White and The Seven Dwarfs' which is however unobtainable legally because Disney has never released the copyright for narrow-gauge prints of their full length films. Copies can be bought on the black market and they cost around £800 but people who own them are liable to prosecution if they are found out. When Disney released the film 'Dumbo' on video David wrote to them in California and asked when and if they would be releasing this and other features in 8mm format but so far he has received no reply. "It seems the cine film people who have been faithful to them for years have been given a bit of a raw deal", said David.

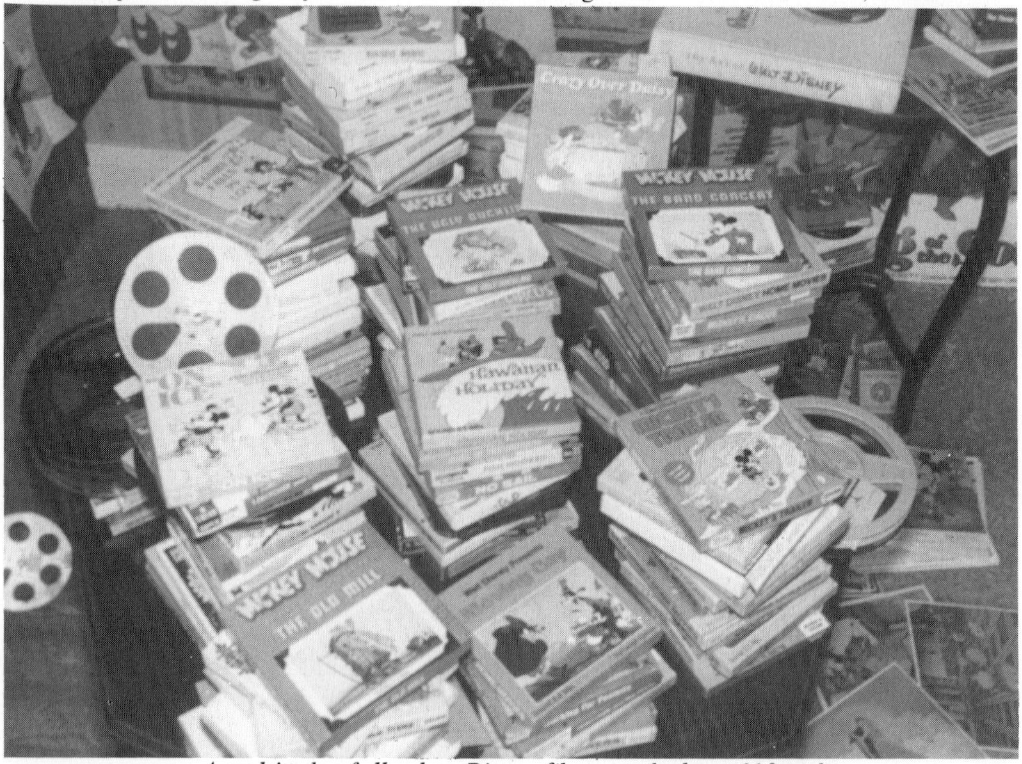

A multitude of all colour Disney films worth about £10 each.

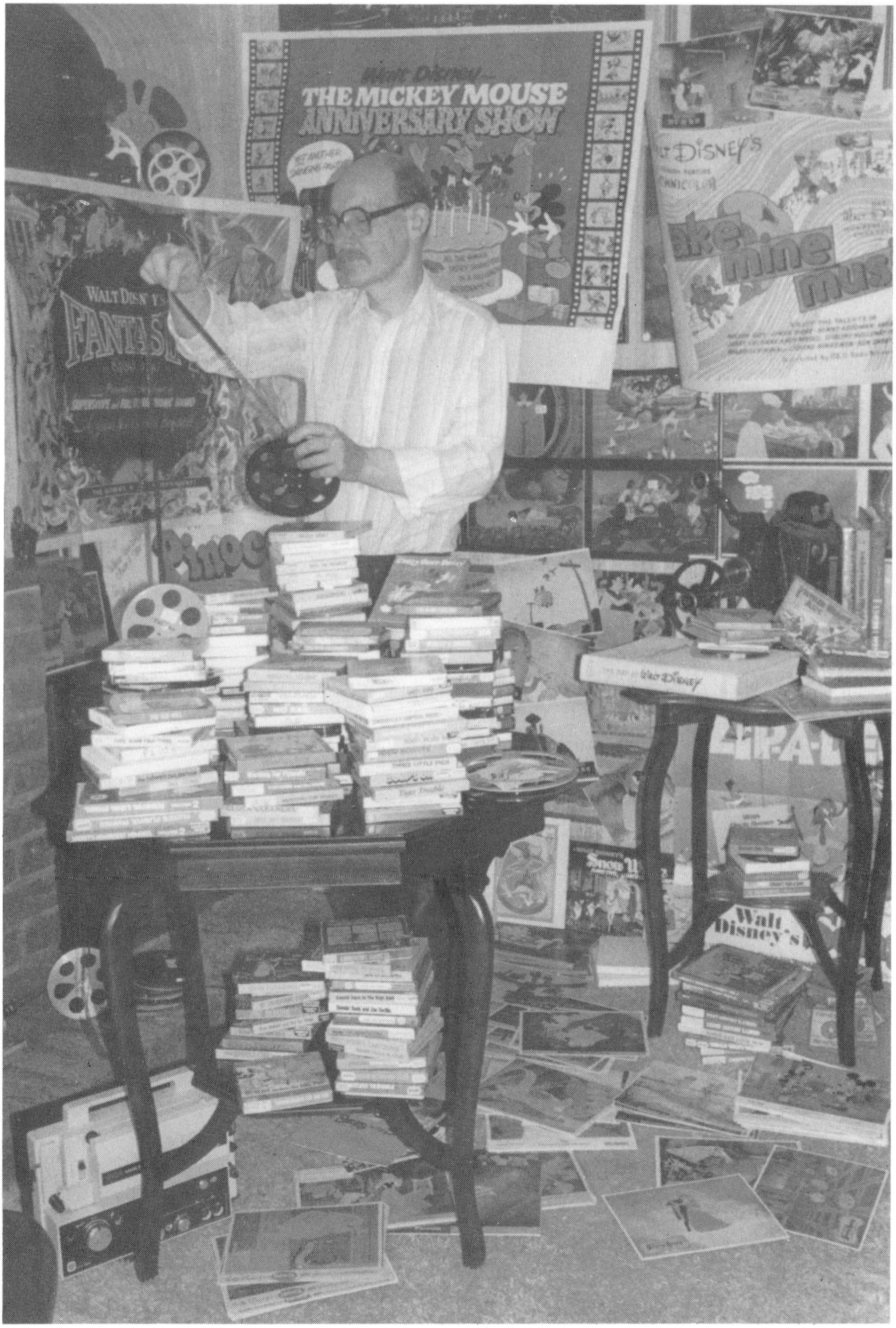

David amid an assortment of Disney films, movie posters and front-of-house stills.

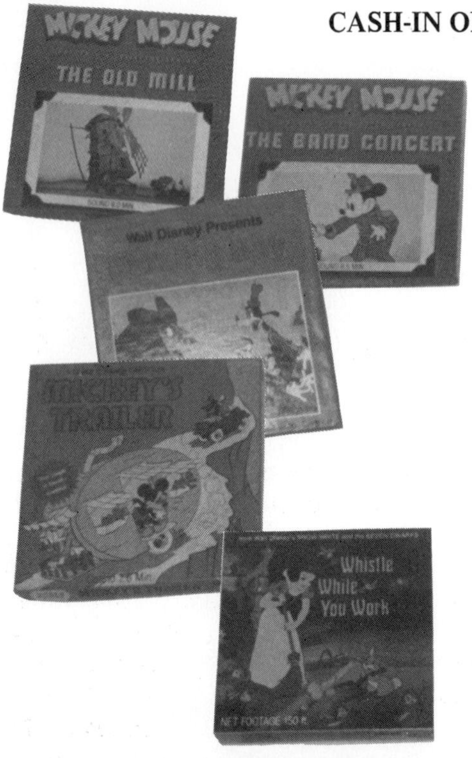

All colour/sound films in 'super 8' guage, roughly 200 ft. in length with a screening time of about seven minutes, value about £10 each.

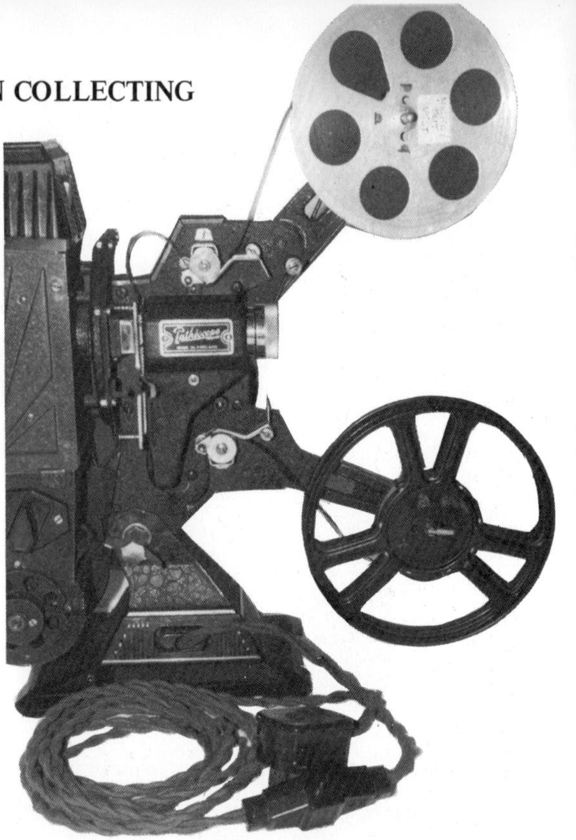

Pathescope 'Ace' 9.5 mm silent projector, circa 1940, value £40.

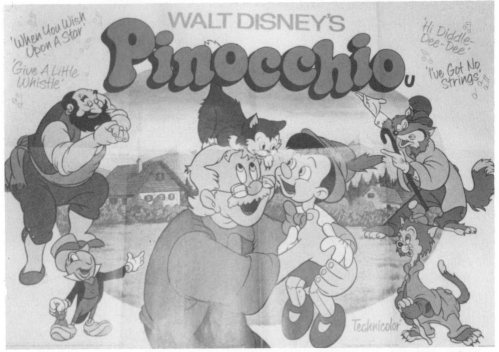

Movie poster for Walt Disney's Pinocchio for display outside the cinema, 'Copyright Walt Disney Productions'. Value about £5 but rare posters are worth £10 or more.

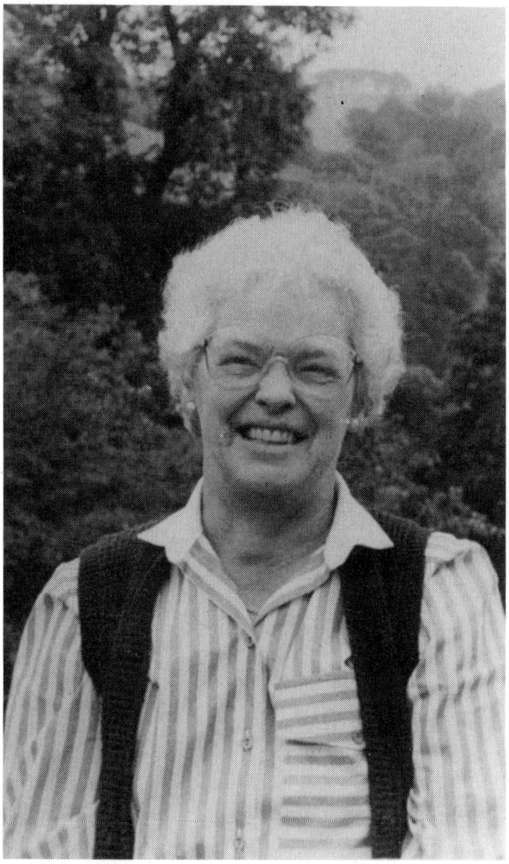

Margaret Anderson is a housewife who collects fairings.

"Everywhere I go I have to visit the local antique shops and my eyes go round and round the stock looking for fairings. It's a surprise to me that even many dealers cannot recognise fairings but that's a good thing too because it means you can still pick up bargains. I've found them in places as far apart as Newcastle and Worthing and I even picked one up in the Paris Flea Market. That was 'A Mouse, A Mouse' and it cost me £30.

"I began collecting about ten years ago and the first one I got was 'The Last In Bed To Put Out The Light' which was given to me as a present. Now I've quite a few and they're displayed in my sitting room. They're very attractive because they are so small and neat and are painted in lovely soft colours.

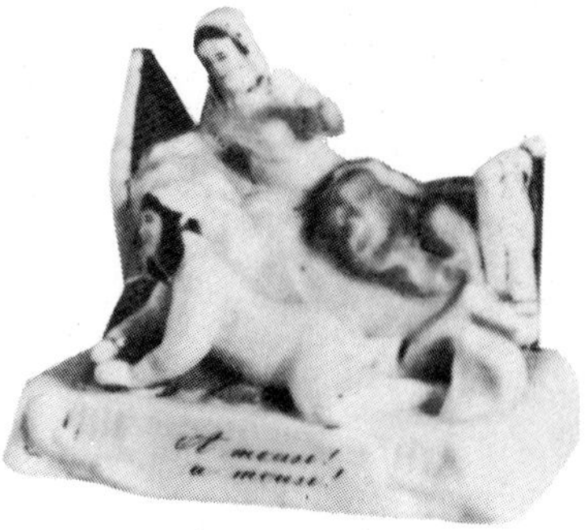

A Mouse, A Mouse

"The favourites in my collection are 'One O'Clock In The Morning' and 'Waiting For A Bus' which were bought for £13 each in Newcastle and must be worth well over £80 each. The one I'd most like to find however is 'To Epsom, To Epsom' showing people riding in a bicycle taxi. It's very rare and its value is well into four figures."

Fairings were given away as prizes at fairs and sideshows from the 1860's till the early years of this century. Earlier ones are generally of better quality than later examples. Over 400 different varieties depicting risque jokes or dealing with politics, war or children were mass produced in Germany by Conte and Boehme of Possneck. In recent years some counterfeit fairings have appeared on the market but the real ones are numbered and most have flat bases.

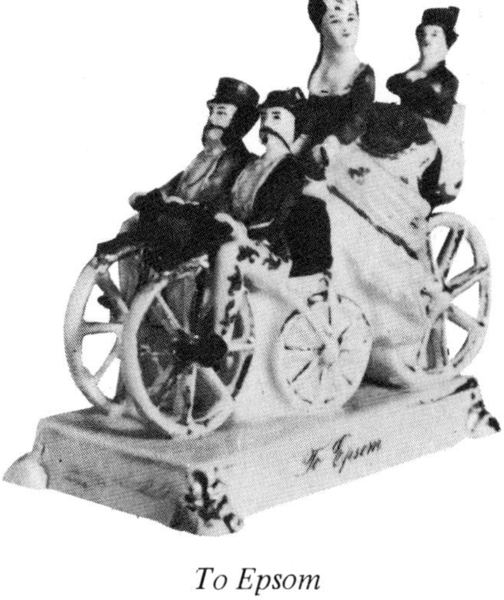

To Epsom

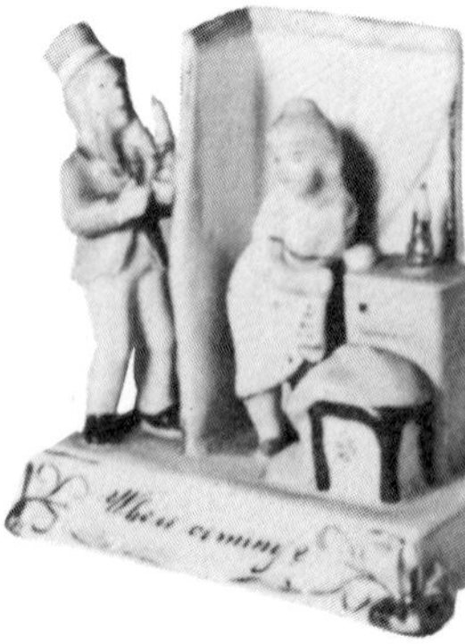

Who Is Coming? £70-£90

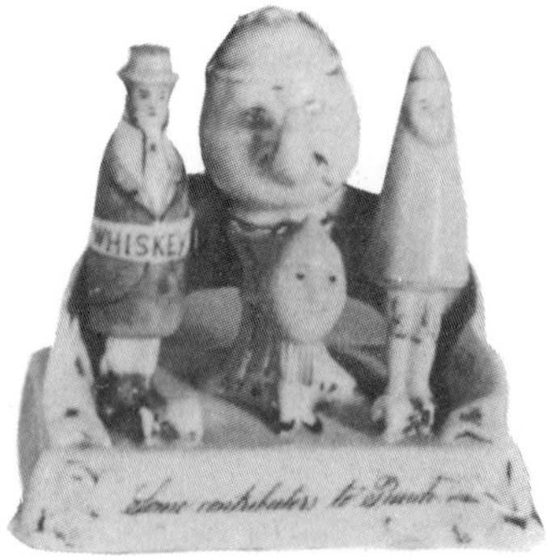

Some Contributors To Punch £300-£500

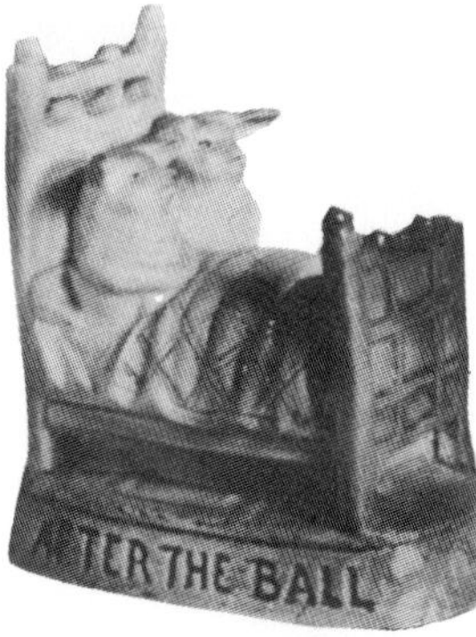

After The Ball £70-£90

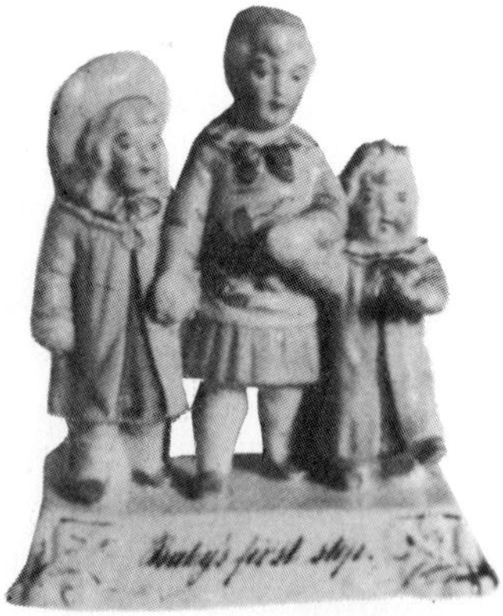

Baby's First Step £40-£60

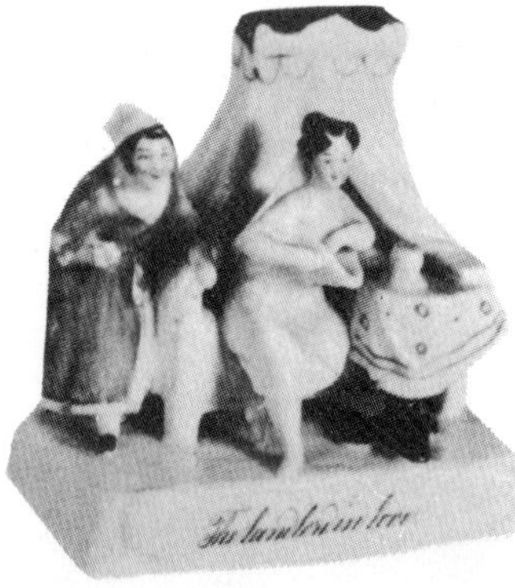

The Landlord In Love £150-£200

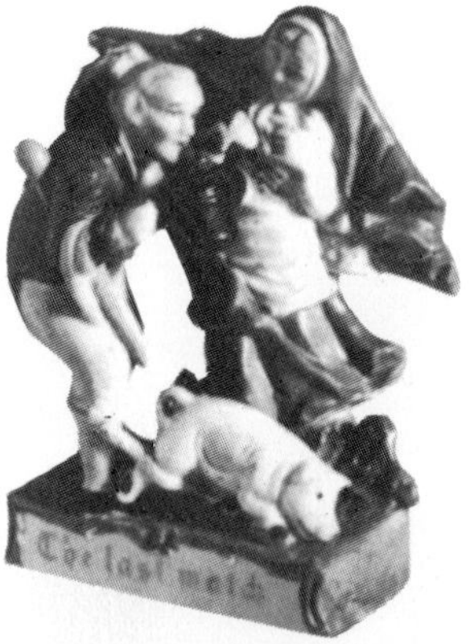

The Last Match £40-£60

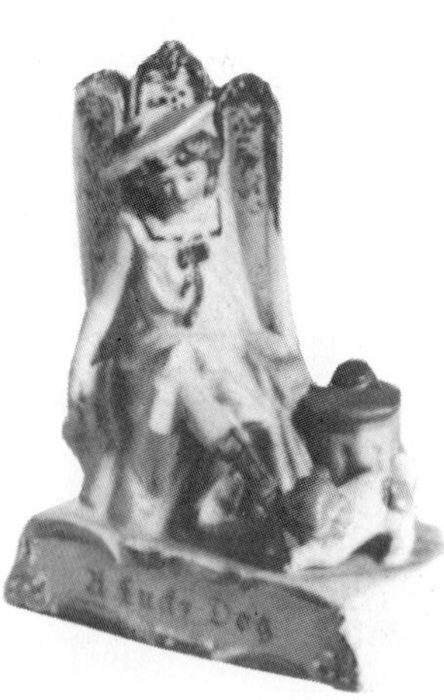

A Lucky Dog £40-£60

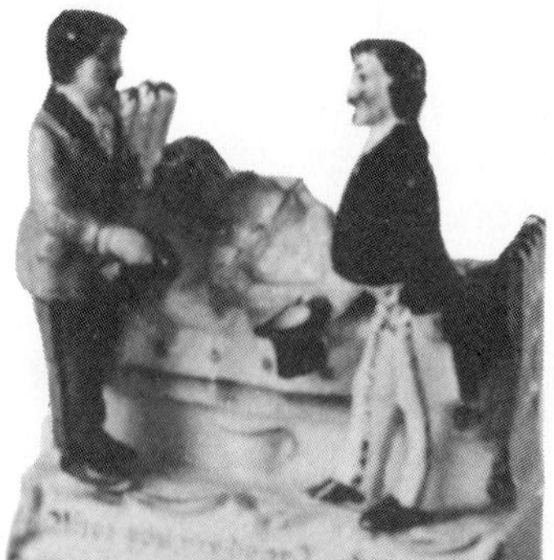

After You My Dear Alphonso £100-£150

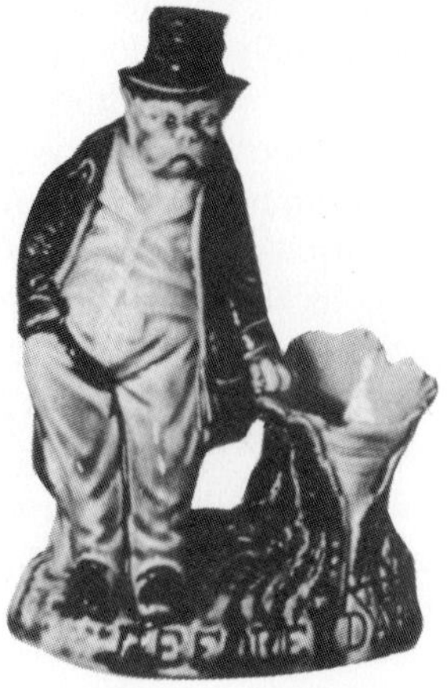

Before Darwin £20-£30

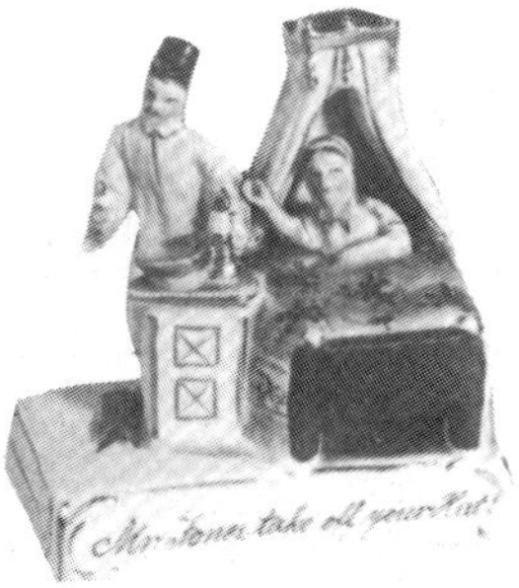

Mr Jones Take Off Your Hat £70-£90

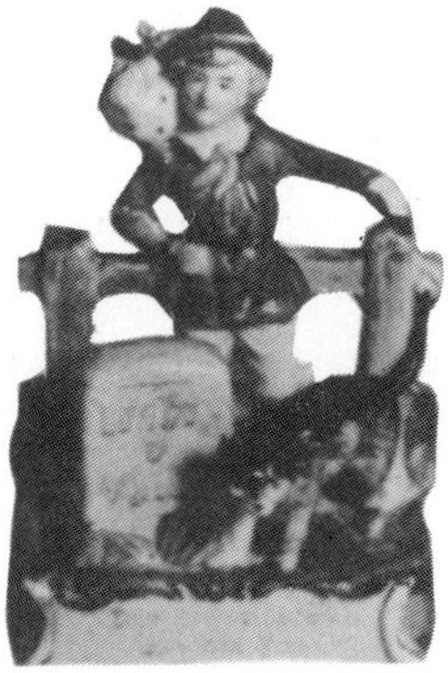

Dick Whittington And His Cat £20-£30

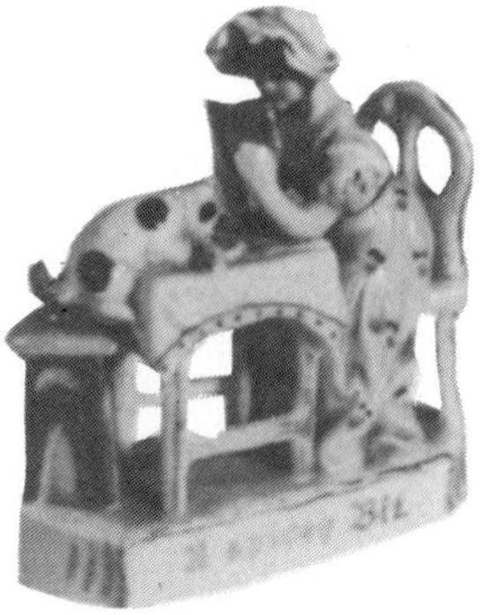

A Spicey Bit £40-£60

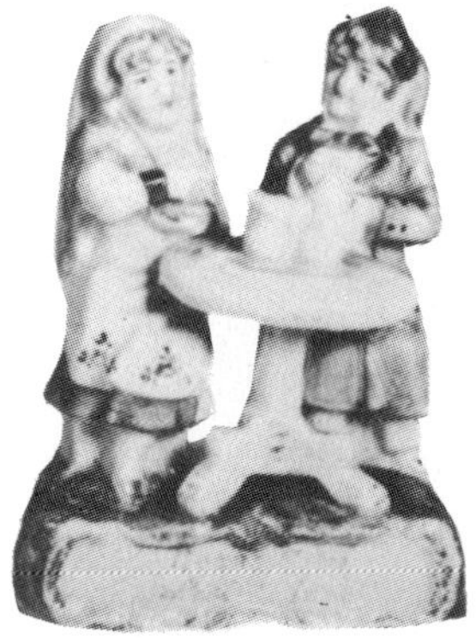

Young Cups And Old Cups £40-£60

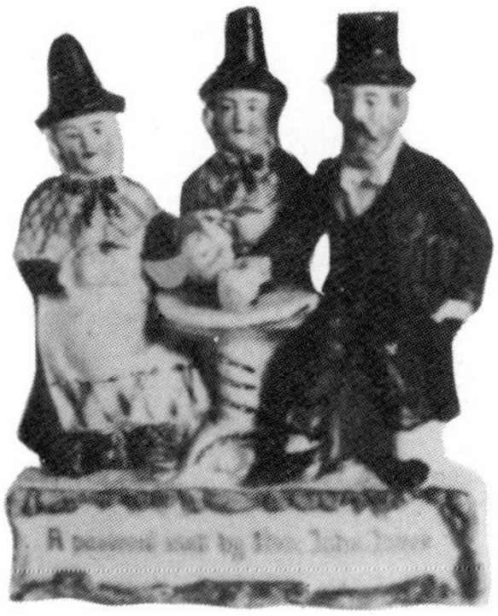

A Pastoral Visit By Rev. John Jones £20-£30

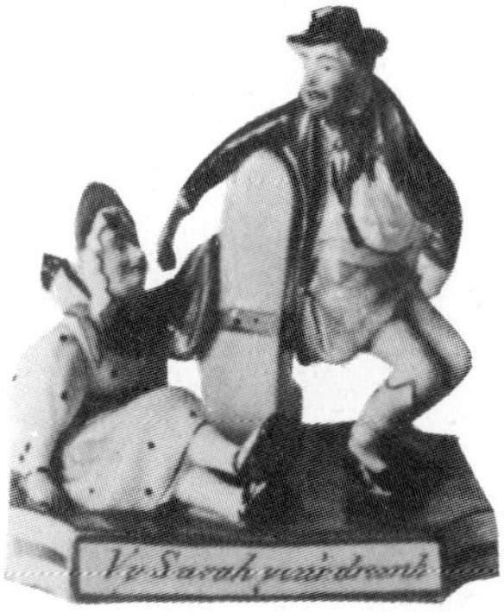

Vy Sarah You're Drunk £70-£90

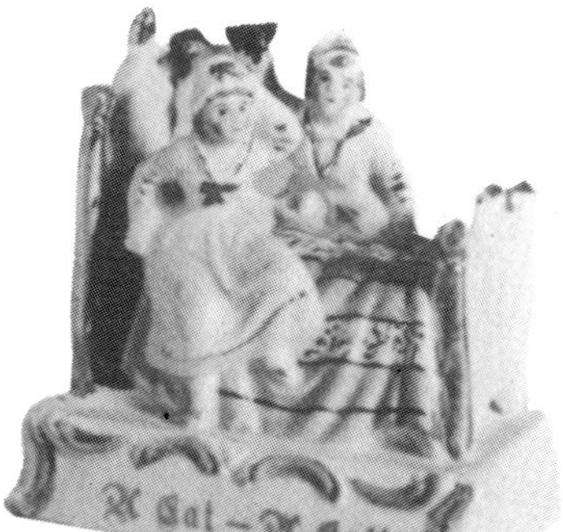

A Cat, A Cat £40-£60

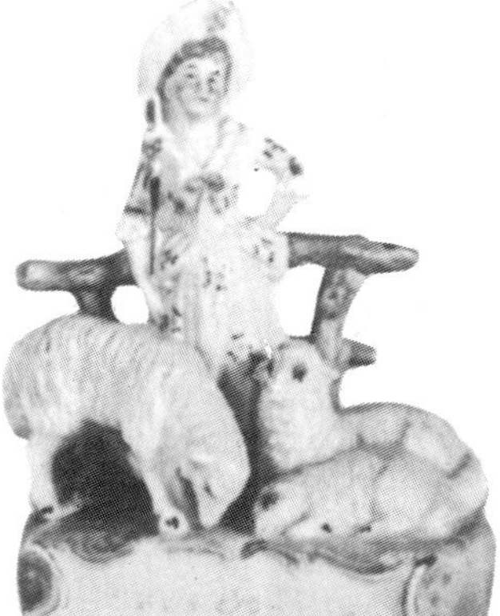

Little Bo Peep £20-£30

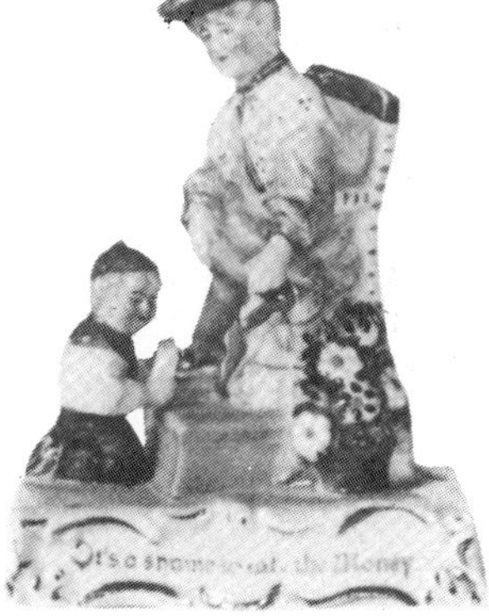

It's A Shame To Take The Money. £70-£90

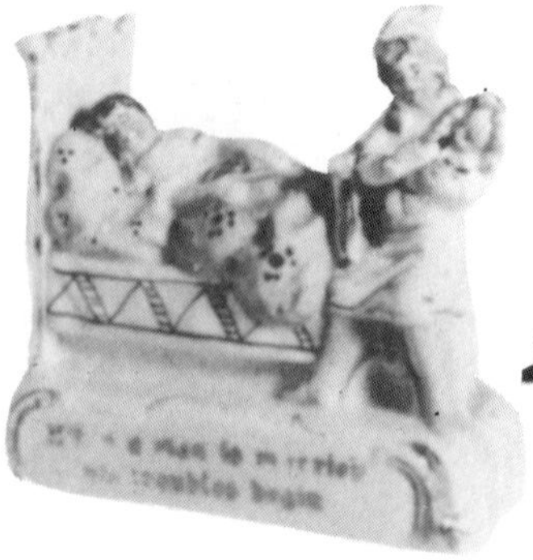

When A Man's Married His Troubles Begin £20-£30

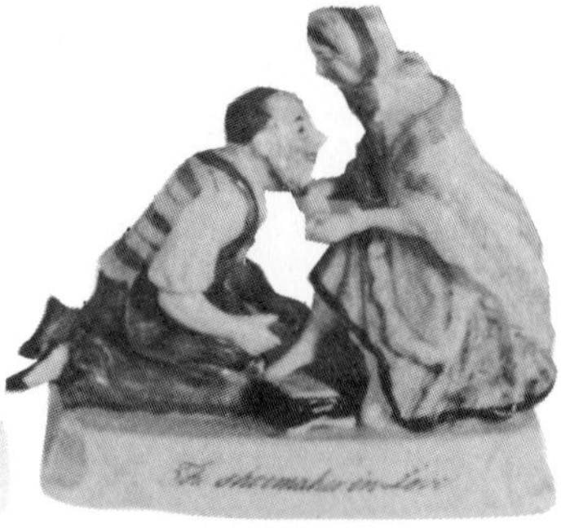

The Shoemaker In Love £300-£500

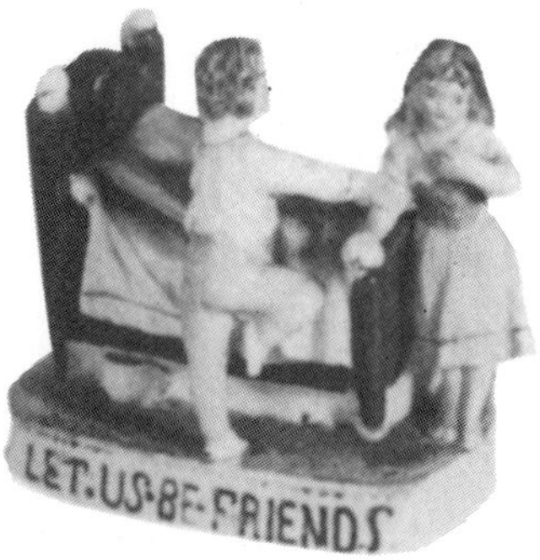

Let Us Be Friends £70-£90

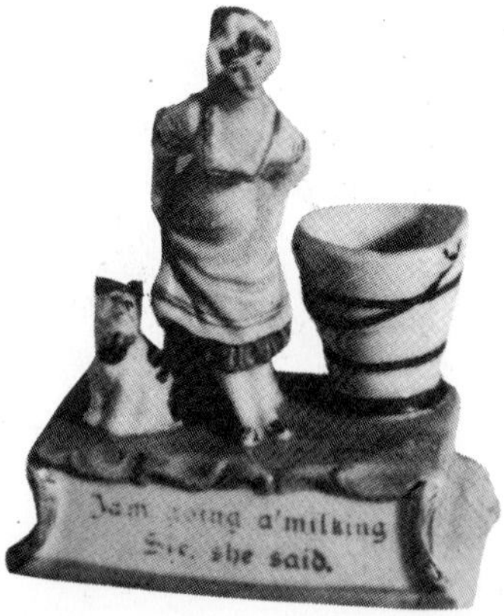

I Am Going A-Milking Sir, She Said £70-£90

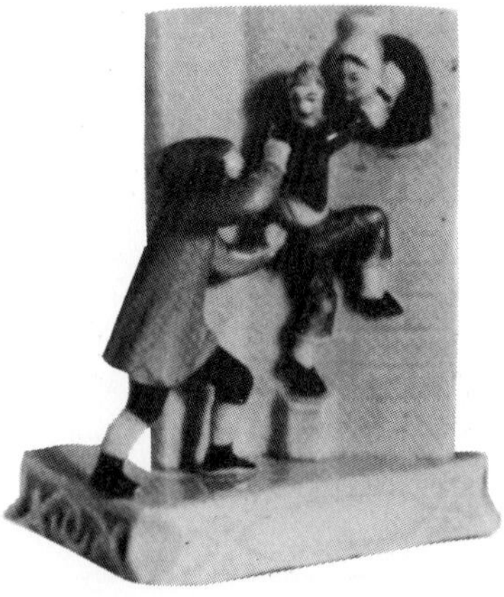

Caught In The Act £150-£200

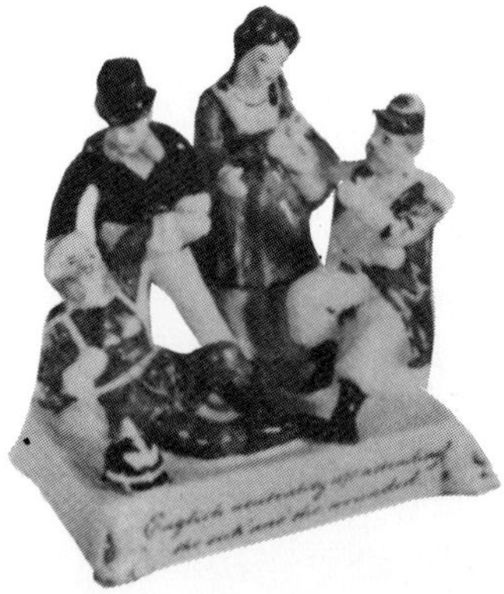

English Neutrality 1870/71 Attending The Sick And Wounded £300-£500

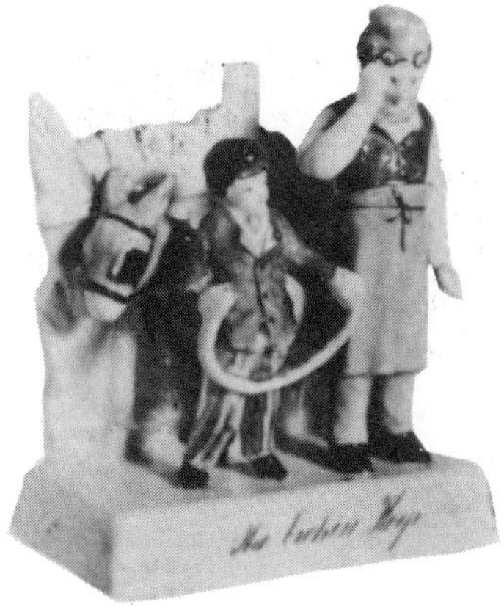

The Broken Hoop £100-£150

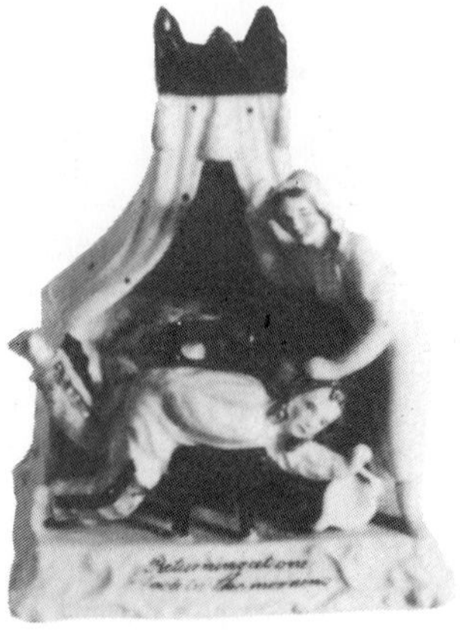

Returning At One O'Clock In The Morning £40-£60

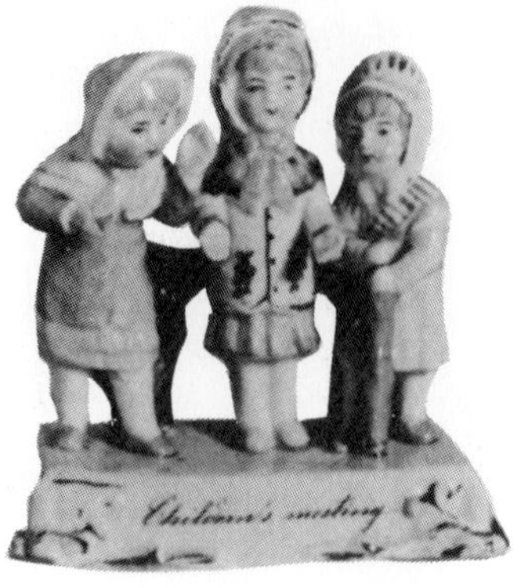

Children's Meeting £40-£60

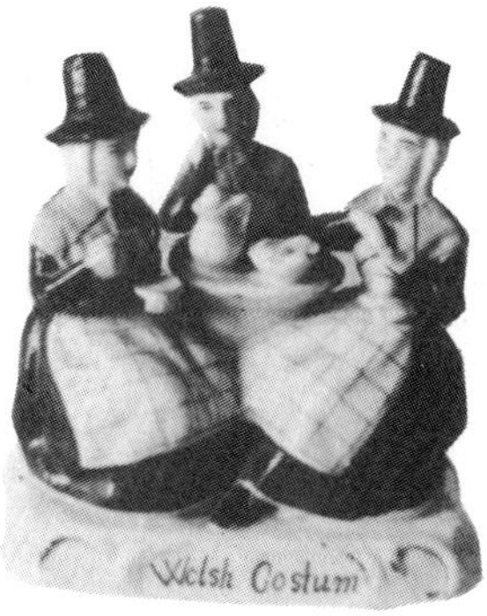

Welsh Costume £20-£30

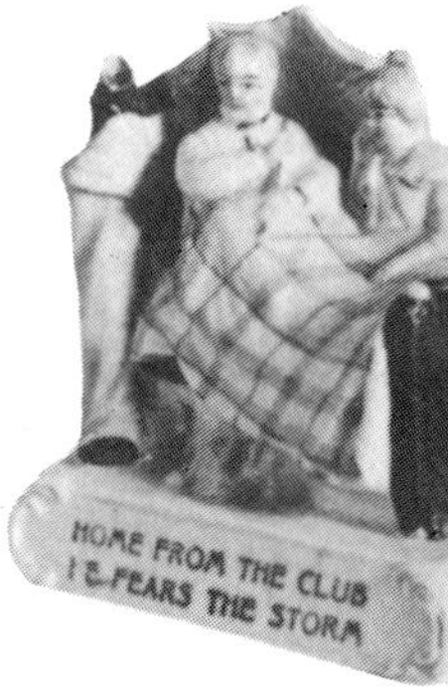

Home From The Club He Fears The Storm £100-£150

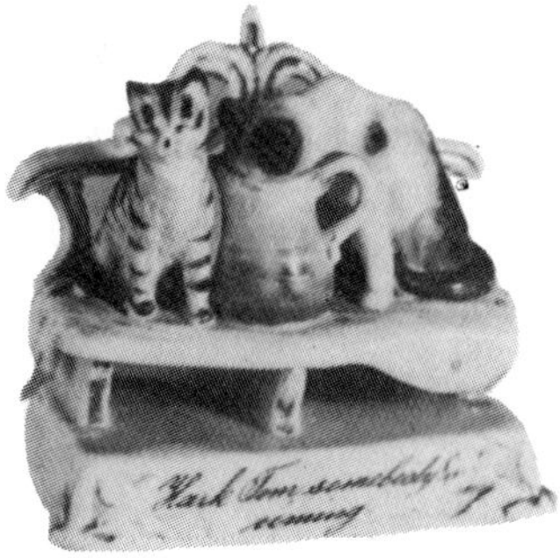

Hark Tom Somebody's Coming £70-£90

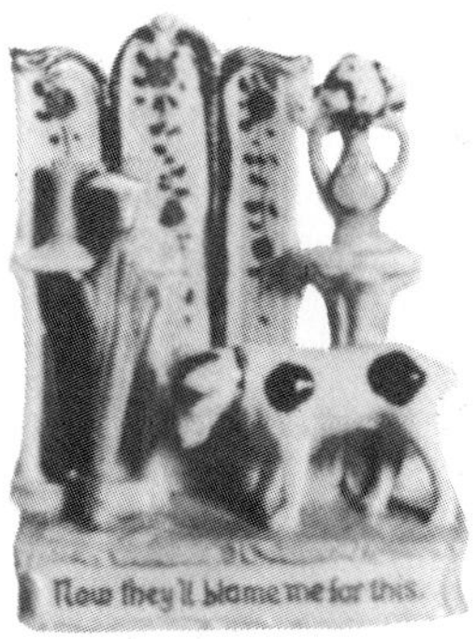

Now They'll Blame Me For This £70-£90

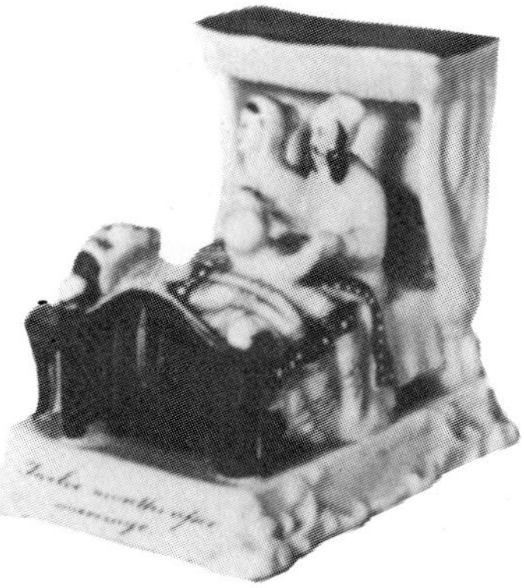

Twelve Months After Marriage £40-£60

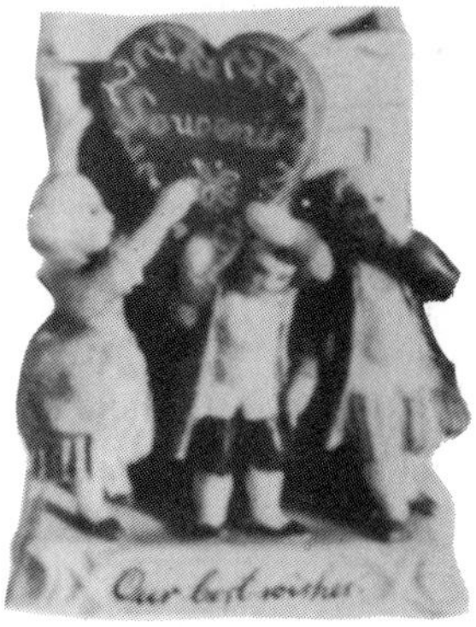

Our Best Wishes £150-£200

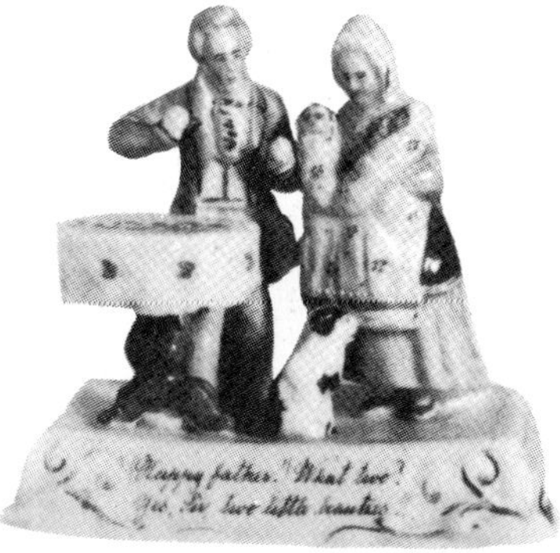

(Happy Father) What Two? Yes Sir. Two Little Beauties!! £40-£60

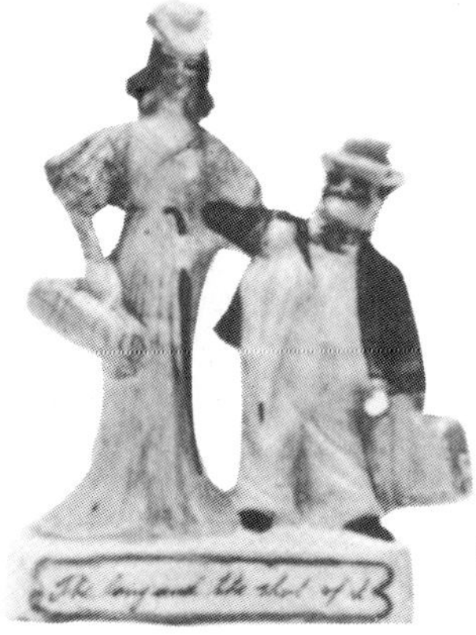

The Long And Short Of It £100-£150

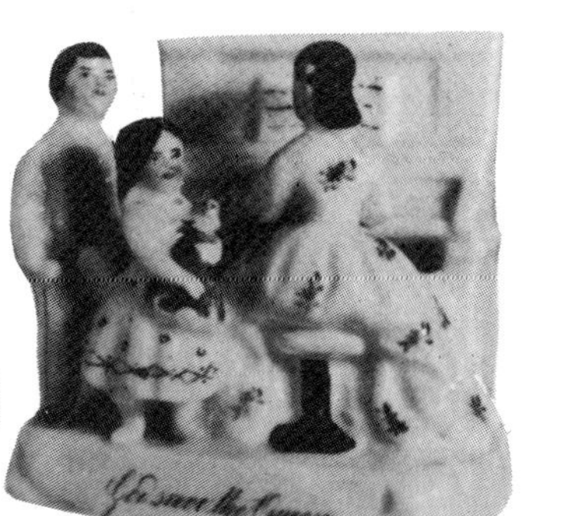

God Save The Queen £70-£90

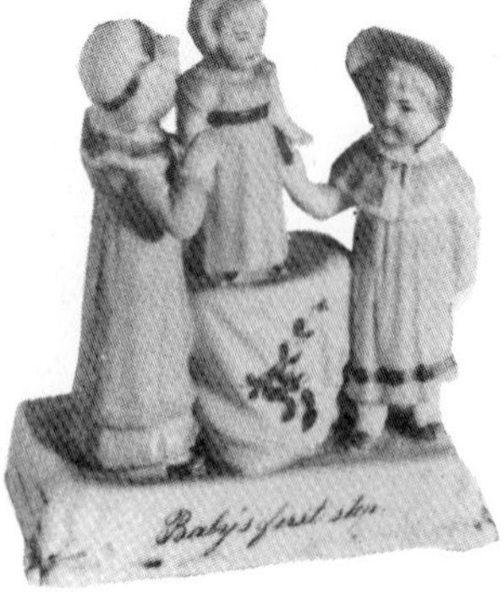

Baby's First Steps.
£40 – £60

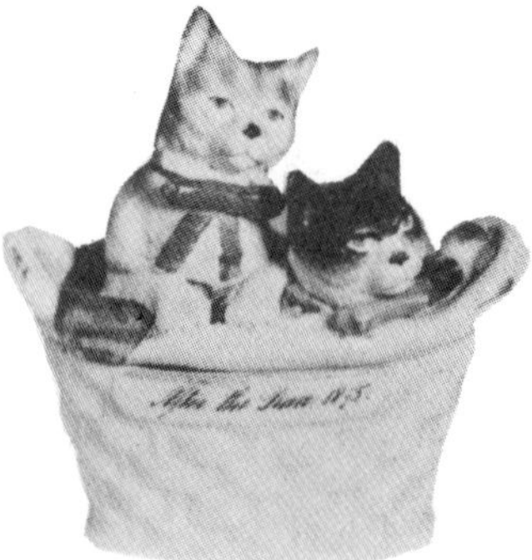

After The Race, 1875.
£20 – £30

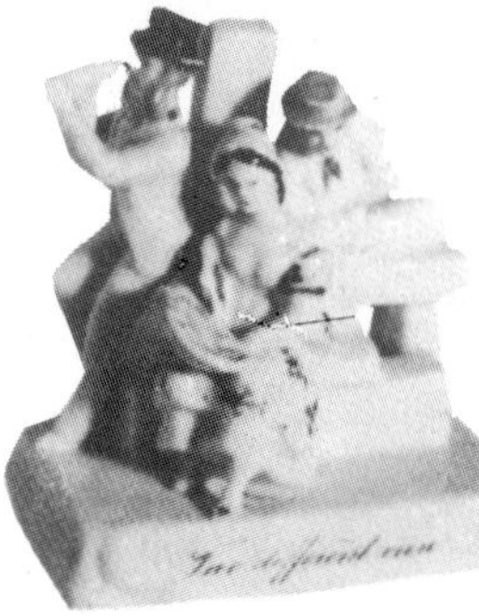

Two Different Views.
£150 – £200

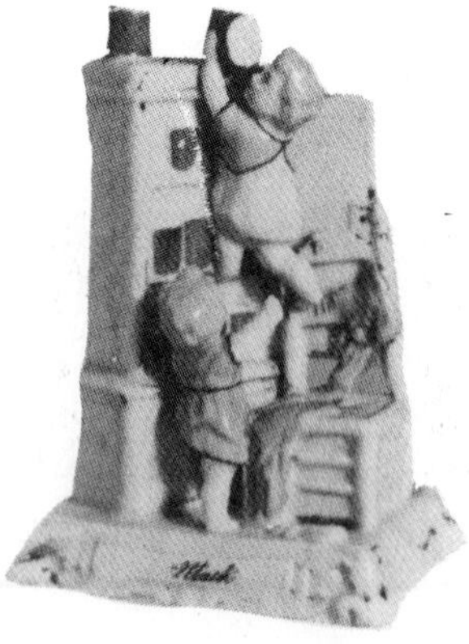

Attack. £70 – £90

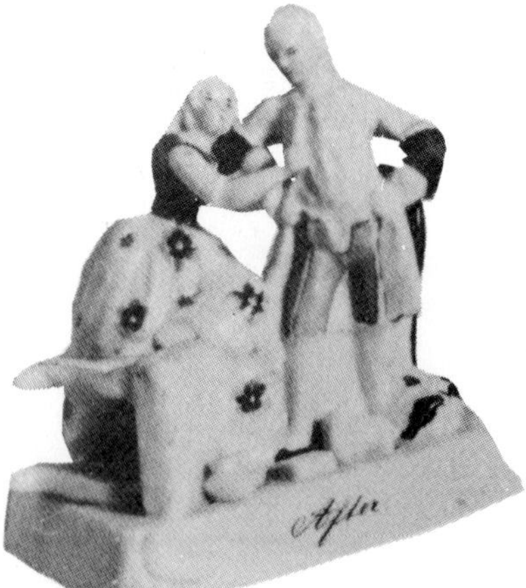

After. £70 – £90

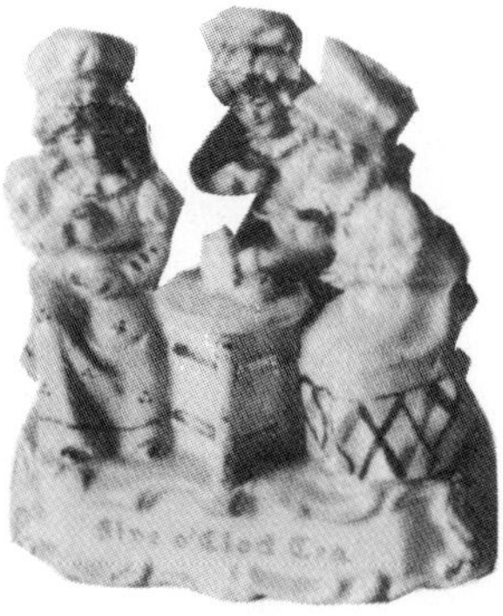

Five O'Clock Tea.
£40 – £60

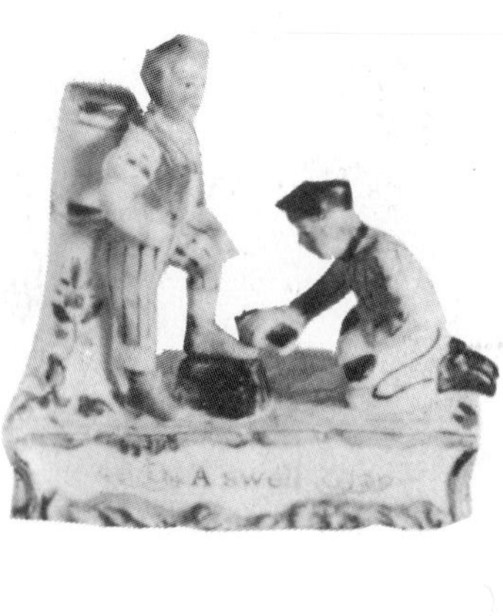

A Swell. £40 – £60

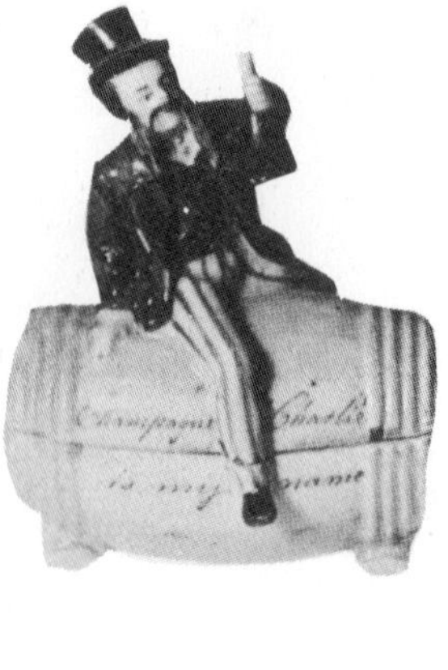

Champagne Charlie Is My Name. £100 – £150

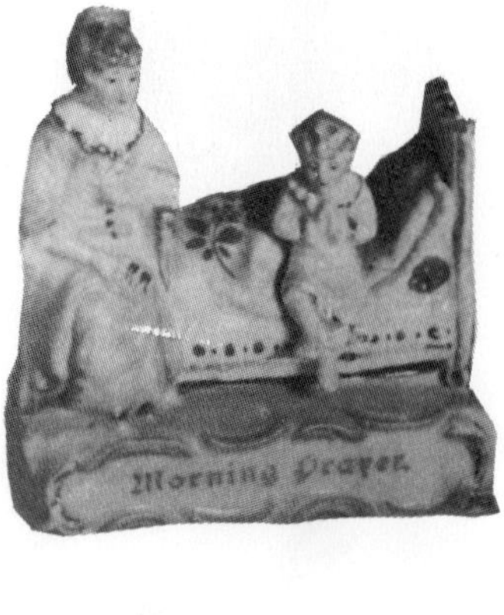

Morning Prayer. £20 – £30

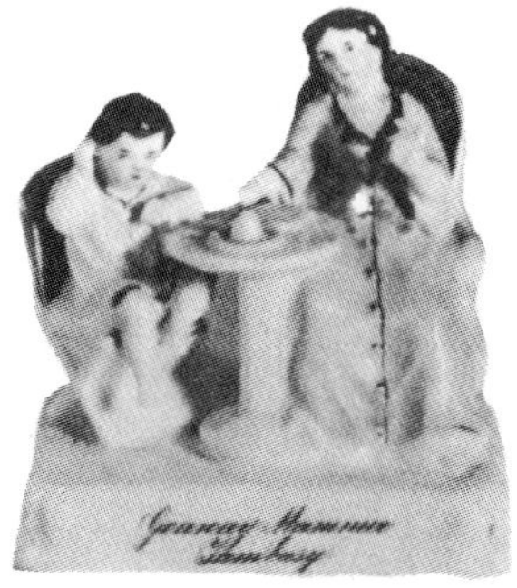

Go Away Mamma I Am Busy. £70 – £90

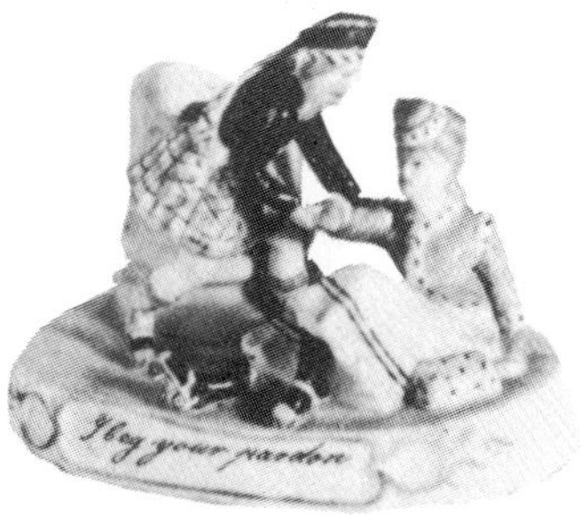

I Beg Your Pardon. £100 – £150

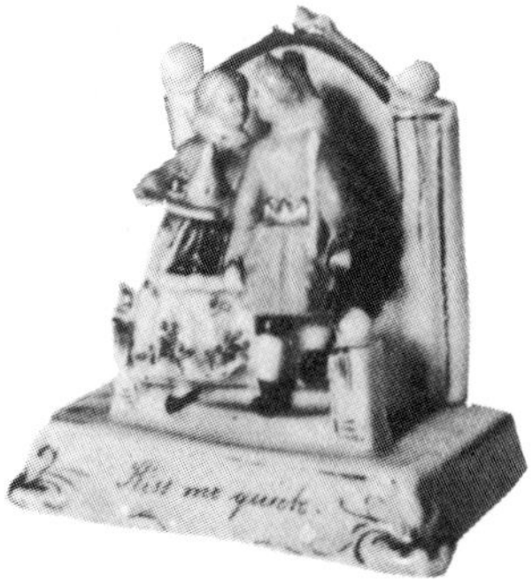

Kiss Me Quick. £40 – £60

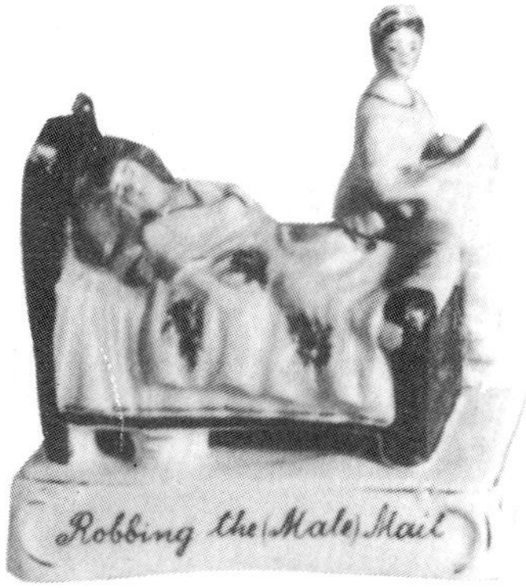

Robbing The (Male) Mail. £70 – £90

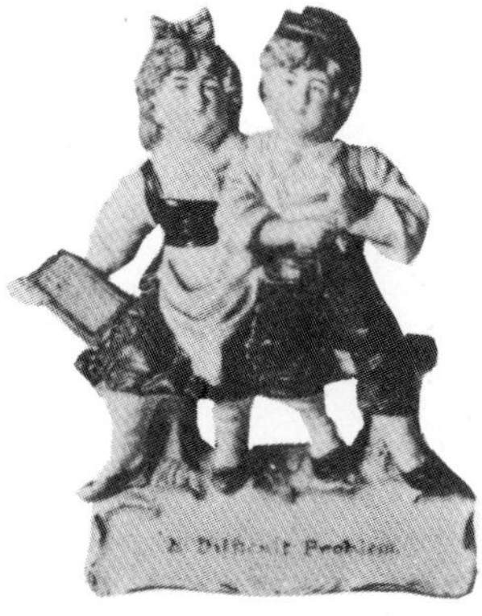

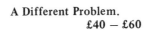

A Different Problem. £40 – £60

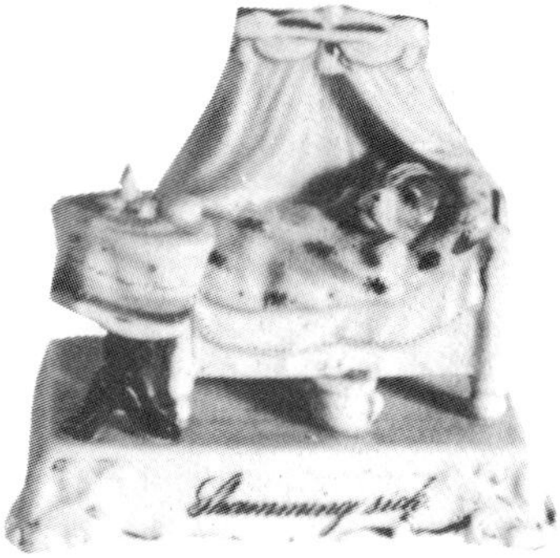

Shamming Sick. £70 – £90

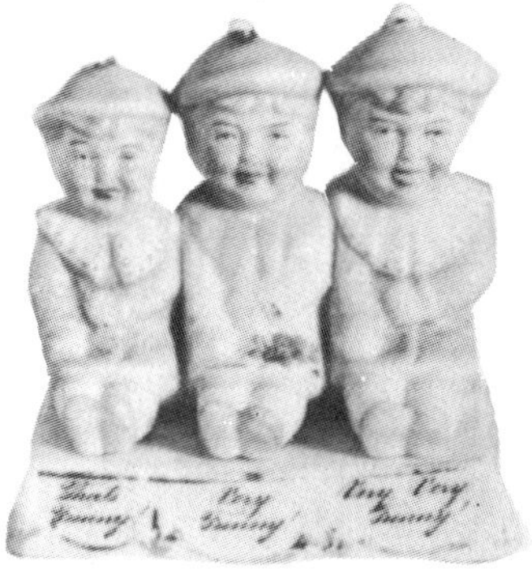

That's Funny, Very Funny! Very, Very Funny! £70 – £90

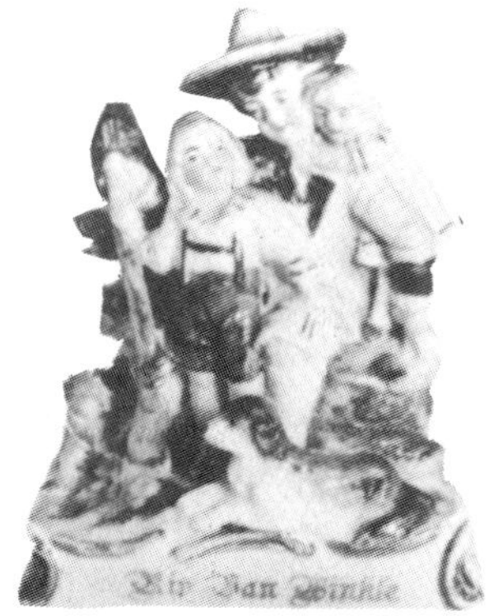

Rip Van Winkle. £20 – £30

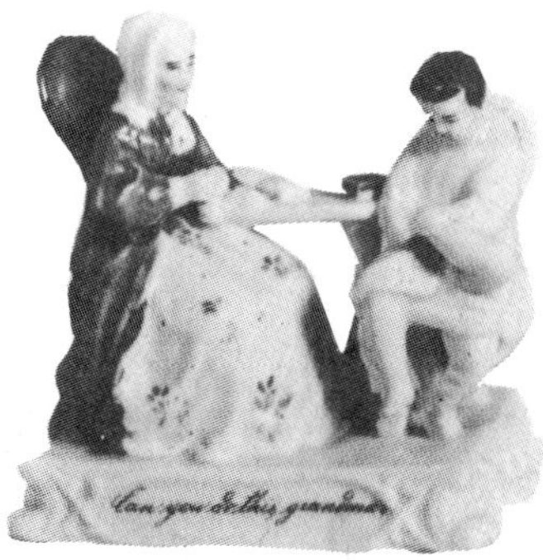

Can You Do This Grandma? £100 – £150

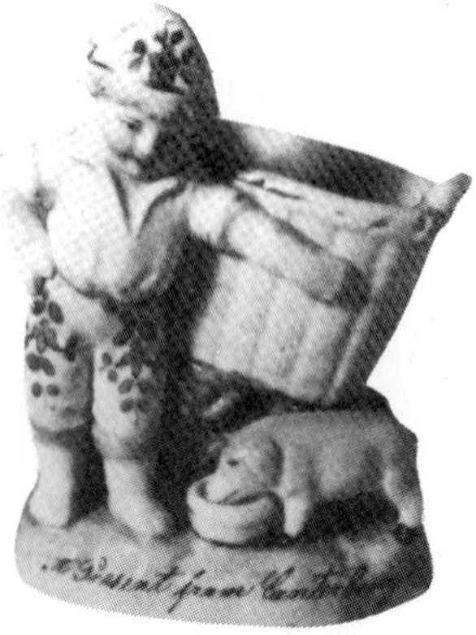

Present From Canterbury £20-£30

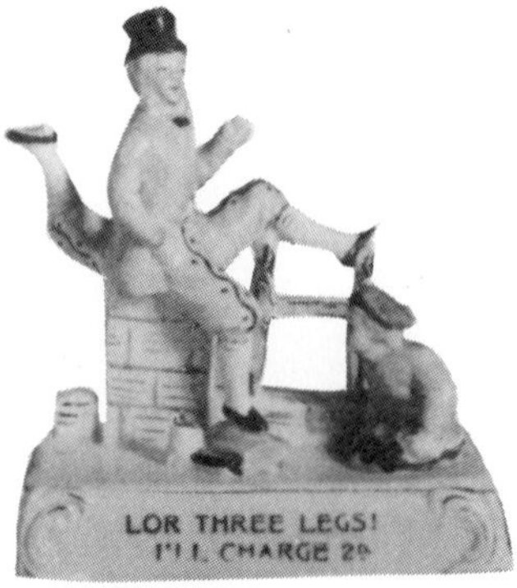

Lor Three Legs! I'll Charge 2d. £40-£60

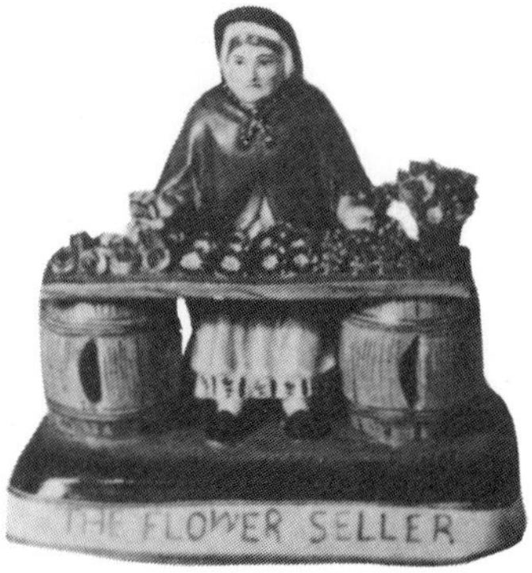

The Flower Seller £40-£60

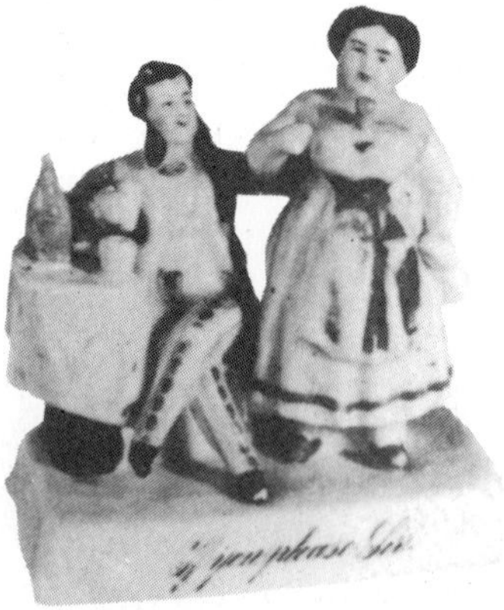

If You Please Sir £150-£200

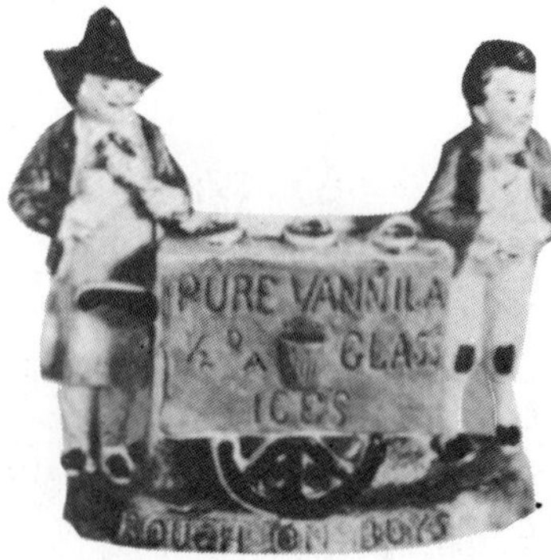

Rough On Boys £20-£30

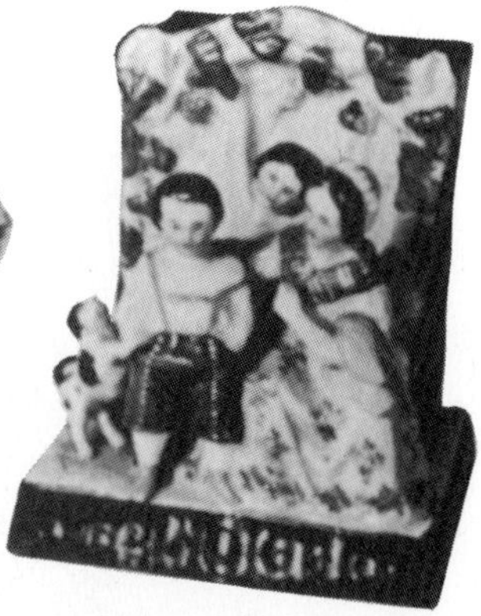

His First Pair £70-£90

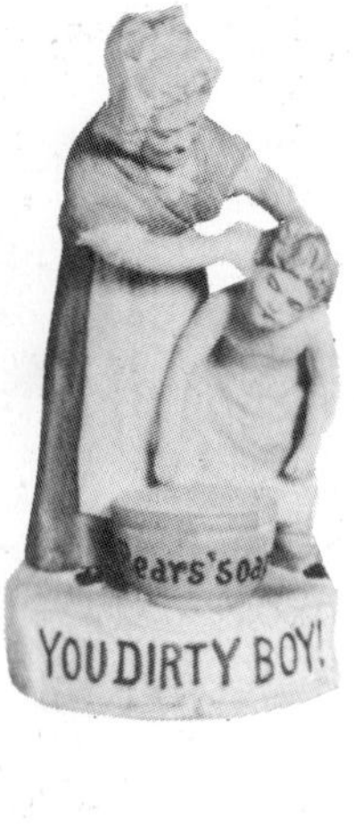

You Dirty Boy £40-£60

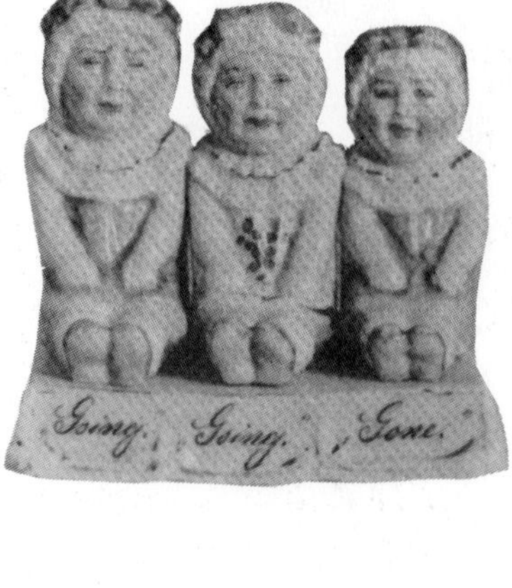

Going, Going, Gone £40-£60

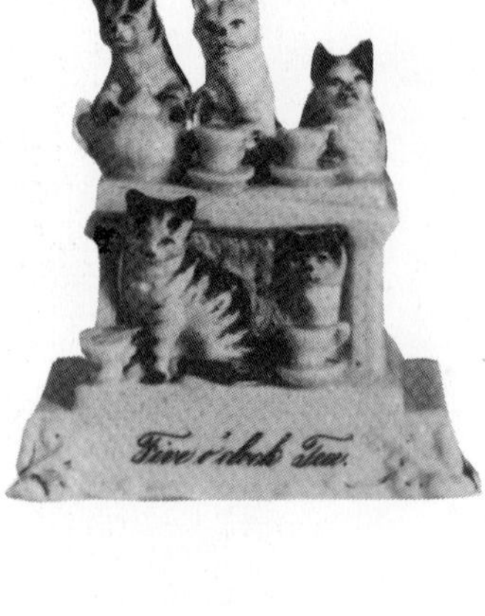

Five O'Clock Tea £40-£60

Michael Akeroyd is a civil servant who collects enamel signs connected with motoring.

"I've got all my signs hanging on the walls of my garage and they make a magnificent show. The favourite ones I've got are connected with Morris because I own two Morris cars. One of the signs is for Morrisol Oil and is like a wastepaper basket to be attached to the wall. I've also got two in the shape of radiators for Morris trucks and Morris cars. Signs are being reproduced now but when I started collecting there was not a great deal of interest and you could pick them up in situ. However the reproductions are usually of the more common ones and are generally smaller than the originals because of the expense of making them.

My rarest sign is for BP petrol and has a racing car on it and I've another rarity advertising Dominion Insurance for car coverage.

Another sign you don't see around much is for 'The Order Of The Road' motoring organisation. You see motor car badges for it but I've never seen another sign."

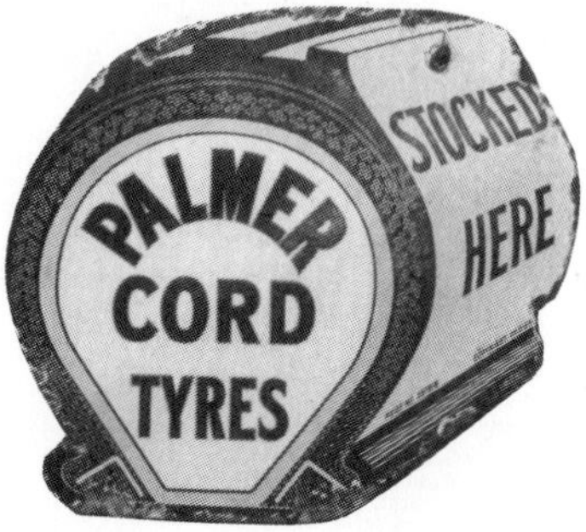

Michael has a sign for Palmer Cord tyres showing a section of a car tyre and another for Michelin tyres which has a coat of arms on it and the statement that they were used by 'His Late Majesty King Edward VII'. The sign Michael would still like to find is from the 1920's and advertised Shell Petrol. It is in the shape of an arrow pointing towards a petrol station.

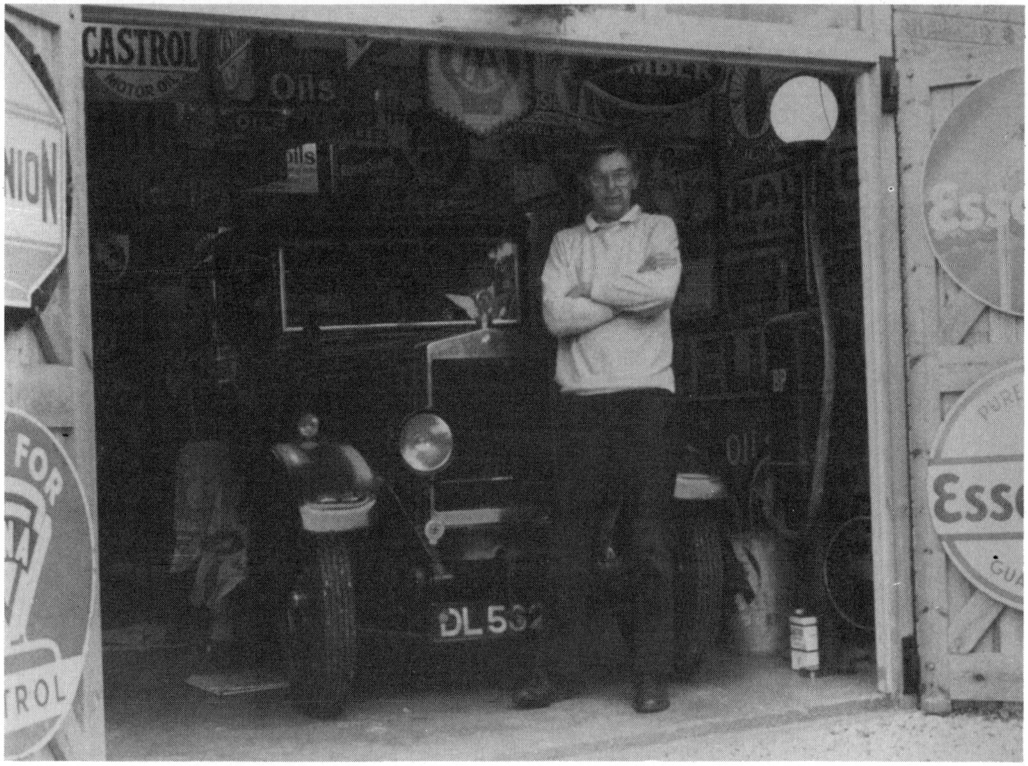

Michael Akeroyd with his amazing collection of motoring signs.

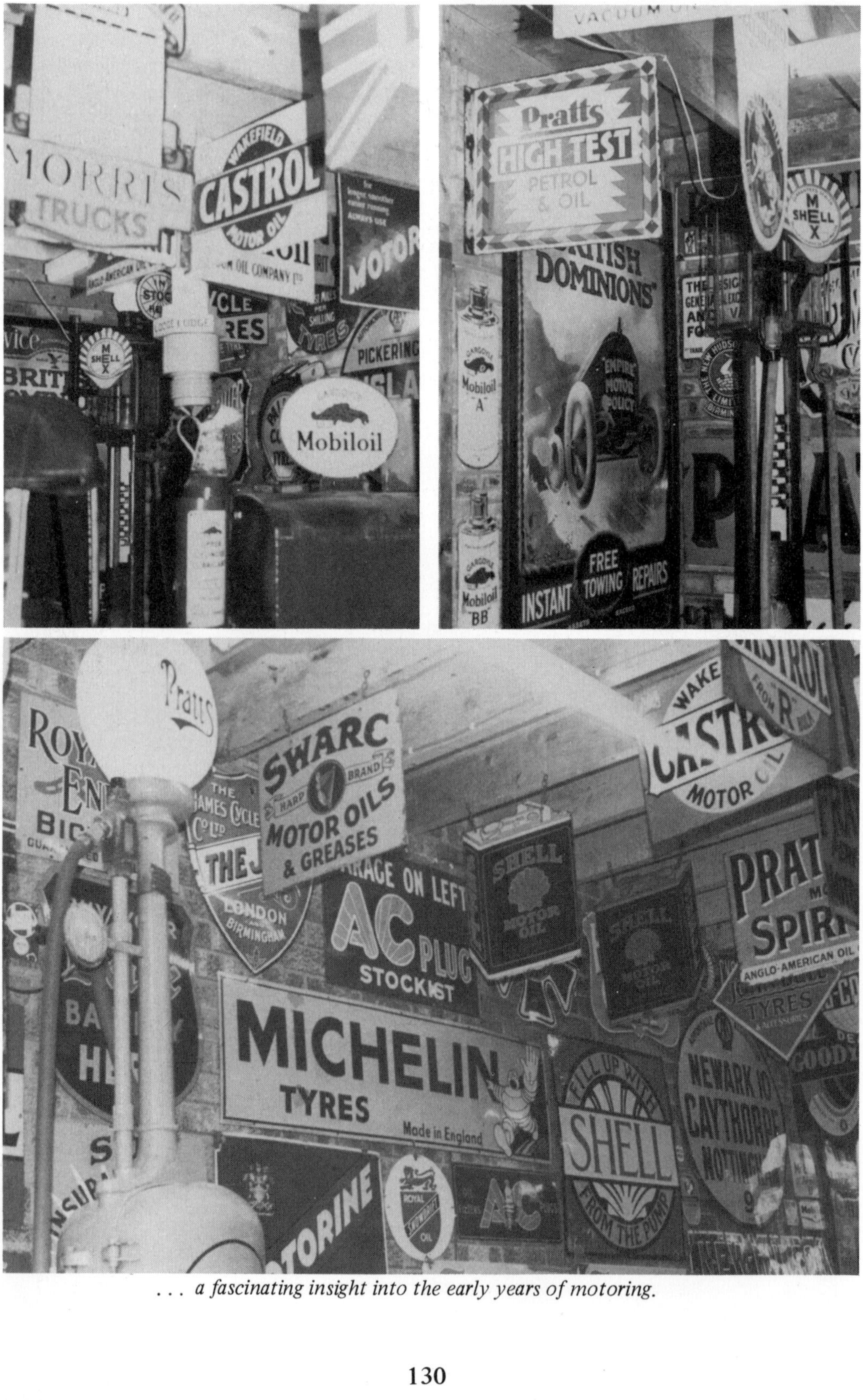

. . . a fascinating insight into the early years of motoring.

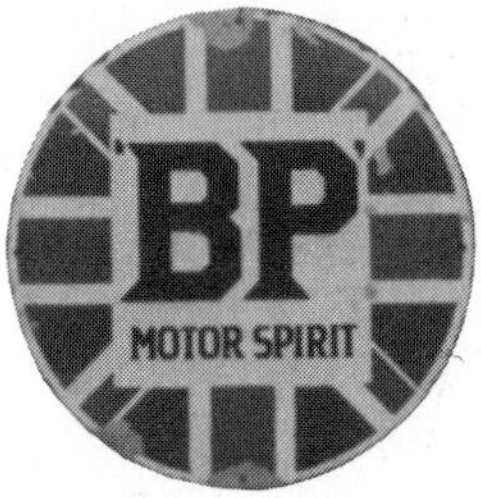

Small round B.P. motor spirit enamel sign. £35

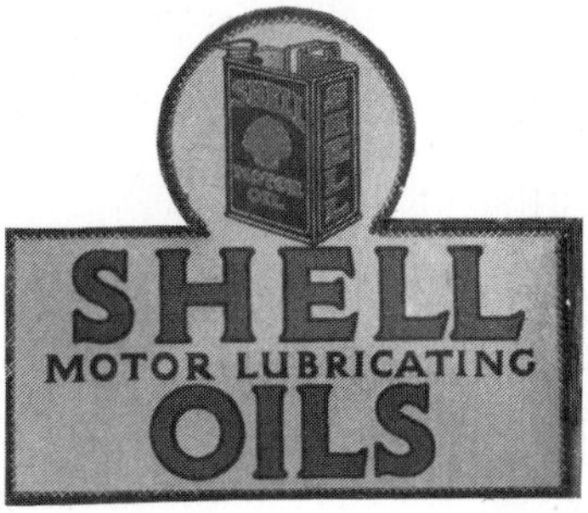

Double-sided Shell Oils pictorial sign dated 1922. £100

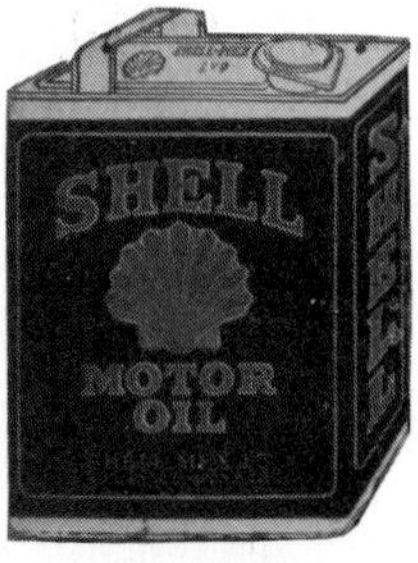

Cut out Shell Motor Oil sign in the form of a can. £120

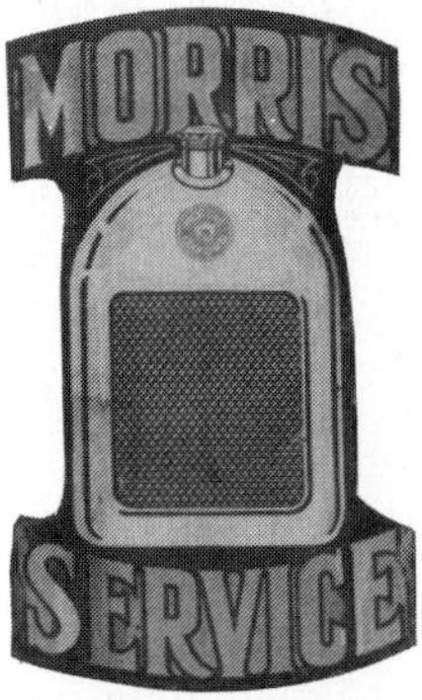

'Bullnose' Morris Service sign, dated 1926. £300

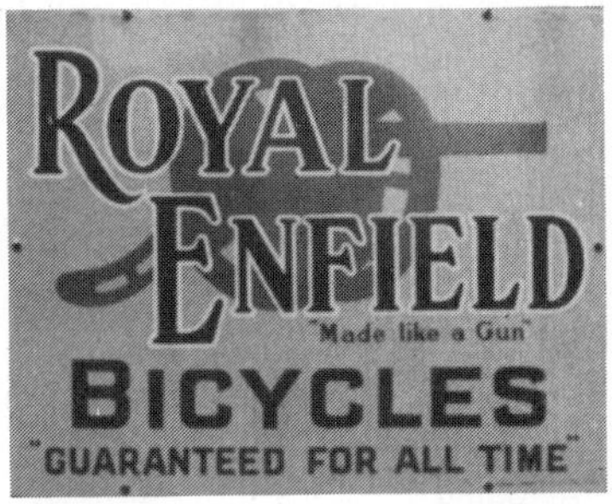

Royal Enfield Bicycles sign 'Made like a Gun'. £40

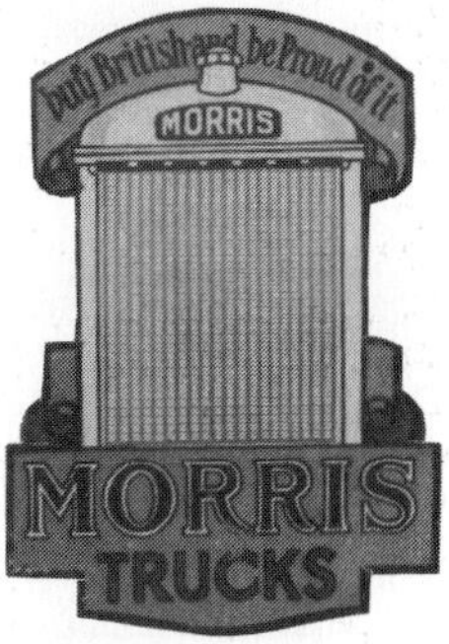

Morris Trucks sign 'Buy British and be Proud of it', pre 1927. £250

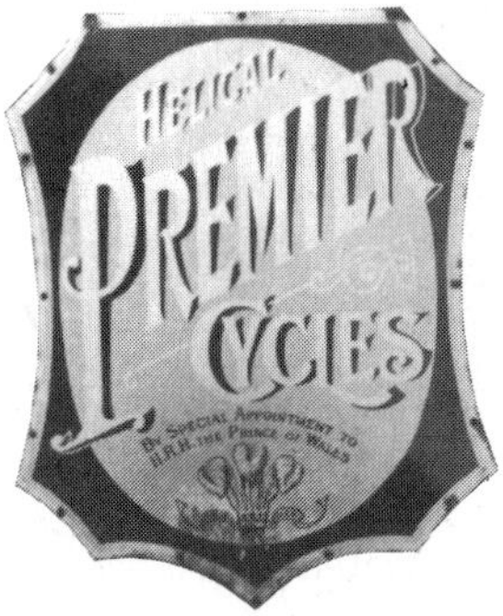

Premier Cycles shaped enamel sign, circa 1907. £75

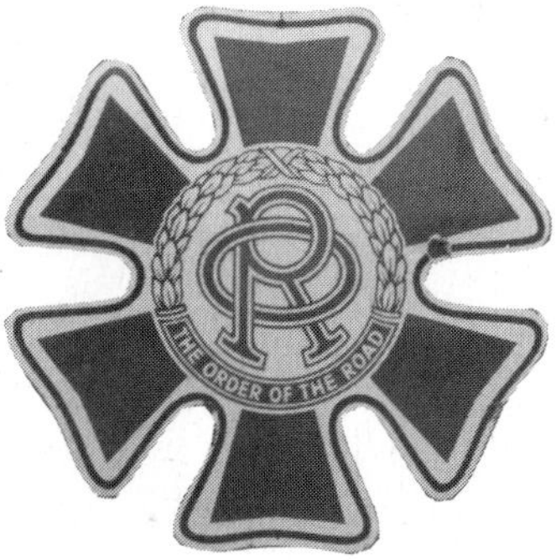

Large enamel sign 'The Order of the Road', normally seen as a car badge. £50

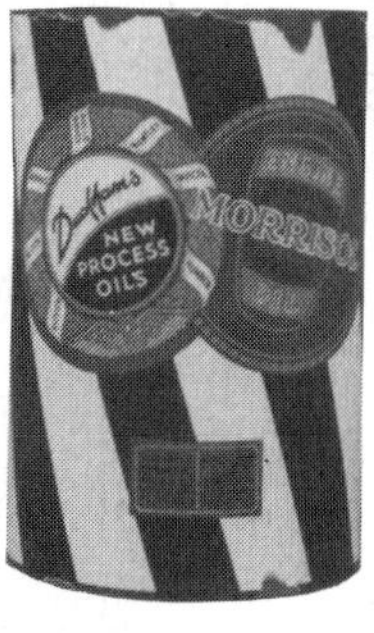

Duckham's curved Morrisol enamel sign, probably the front of a wastepaper basket. £70

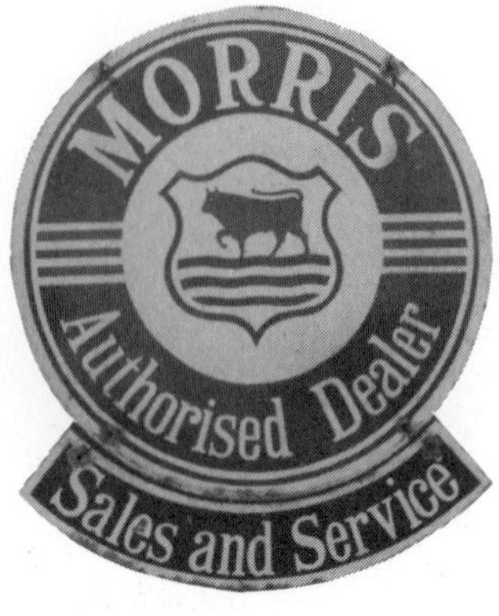

Morris Authorised Dealer enamel sign, 1930's. £120

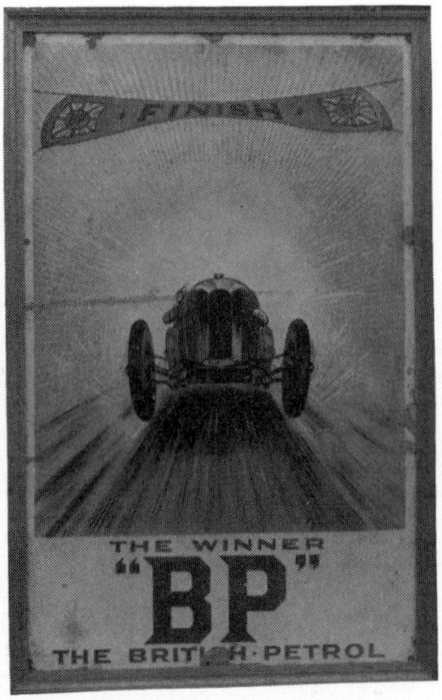

'The Winner' racing car enamel sign for B.P. Petrol. £400

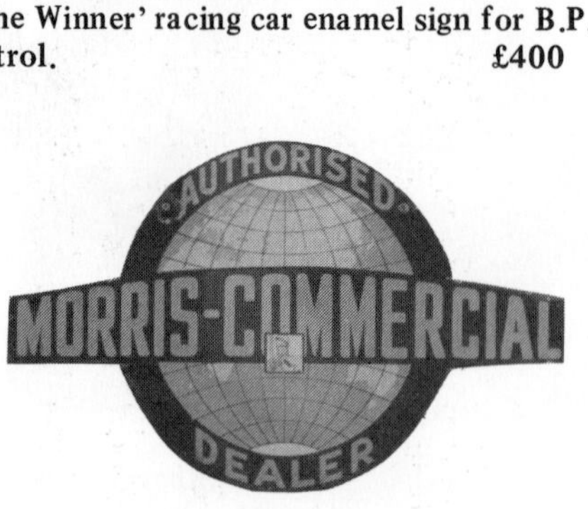

'Authorised Morris-Commercial Dealer' enamel sign. £175

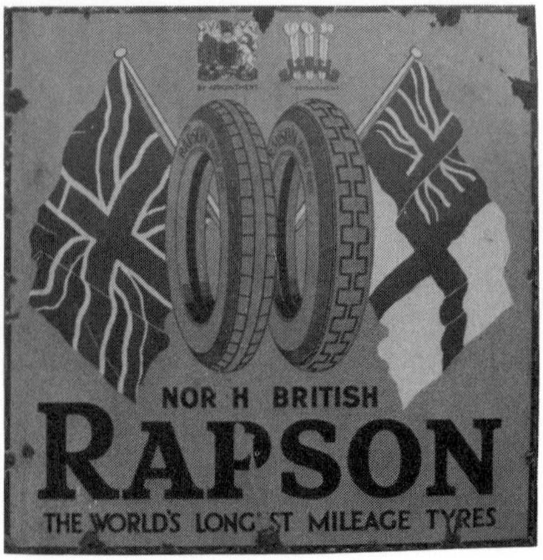

Rapson Tyres pictorial enamel sign 'The World's Longest Mileage Tyres'. £100

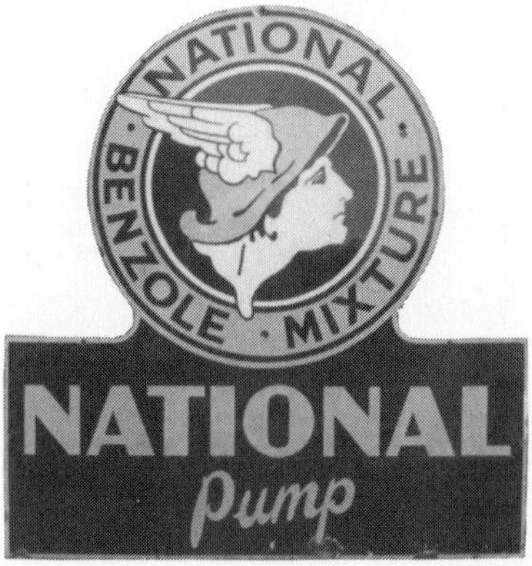

National Benzole pump sign. £50

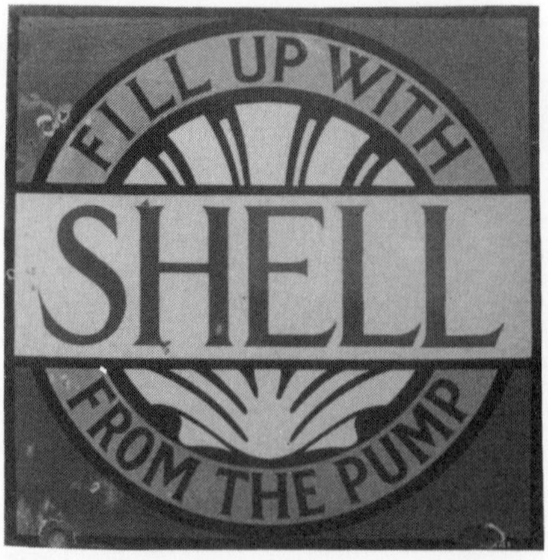

Shell 'From the Pump' sign dated 1921, previously petrol had been bought in two gallon cans. £75

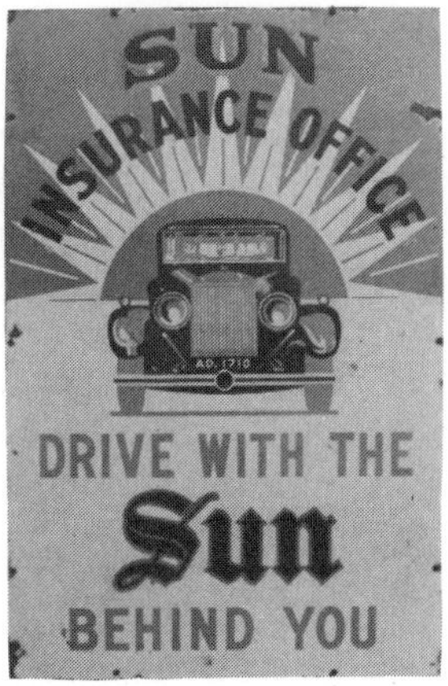

Sun Insurance enamel sign 'Drive with the Sun behind you', circa 1930. £150

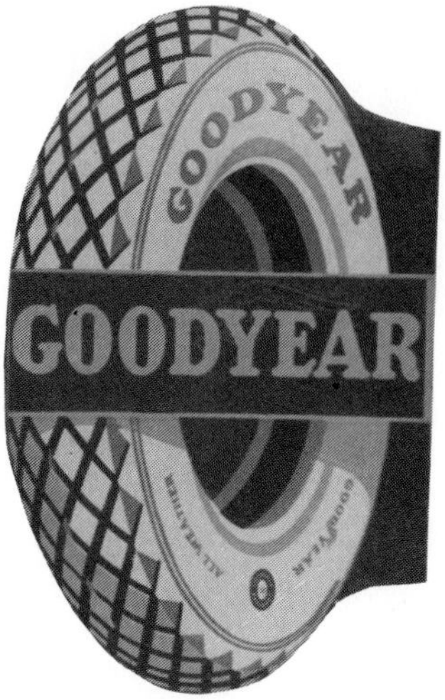

Goodyear cut out tyre sign of German manufacture. £80

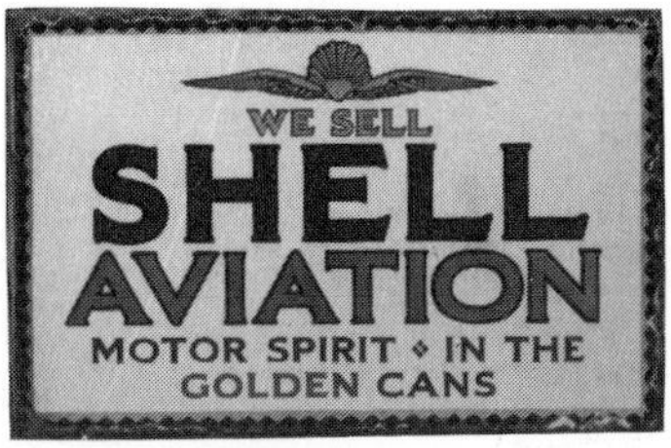

A double-sided sign for Shell Aviation Motor Spirit In The Golden Cans. £160

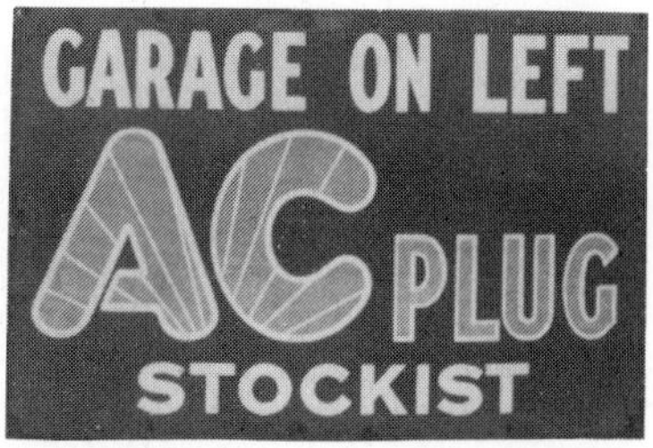

Garage enamel sign incorporating an AC Plug advertisement. £55

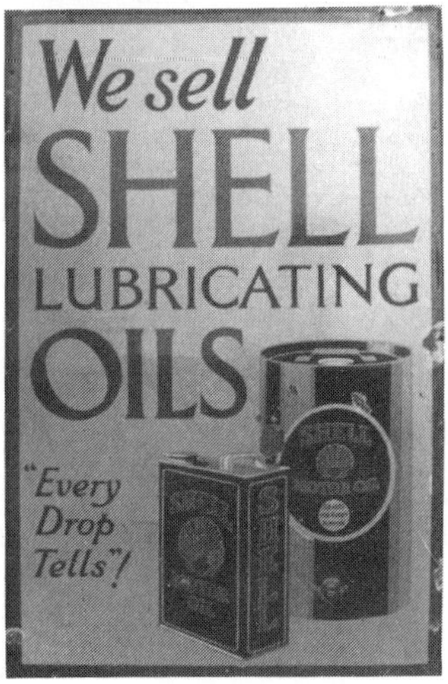

Pictorial 'We sell Shell Lubricating Oils' enamel sign, dated 1927. £85

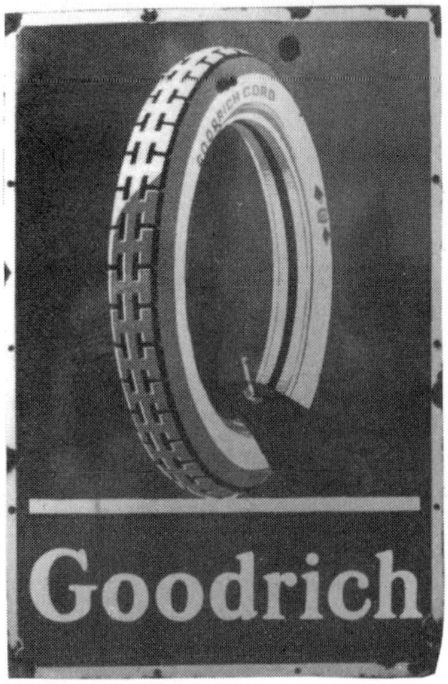

'Goodrich Tyres' sign illustrating an early tyre with tube. £60

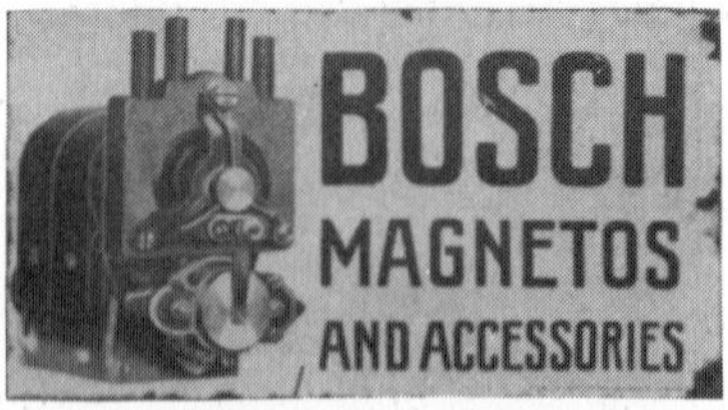

Very early 20's Bosch Magnetos enamel sign. £100

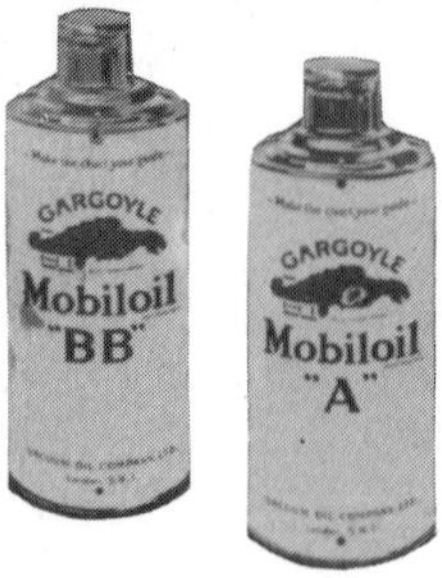

Small cut out enamel signs for Mobiloil. £100 each

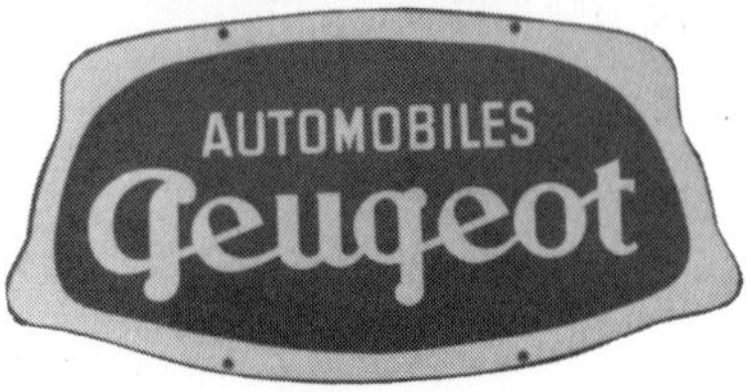

Peugeot enamel sign in the shape of a radiator badge by Art France-Touraine. £75

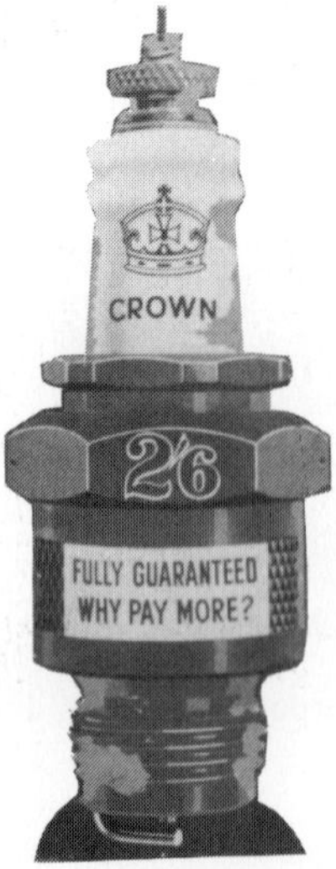

Cut out enamel sign for Crown Spark Plug dated 1933. £60

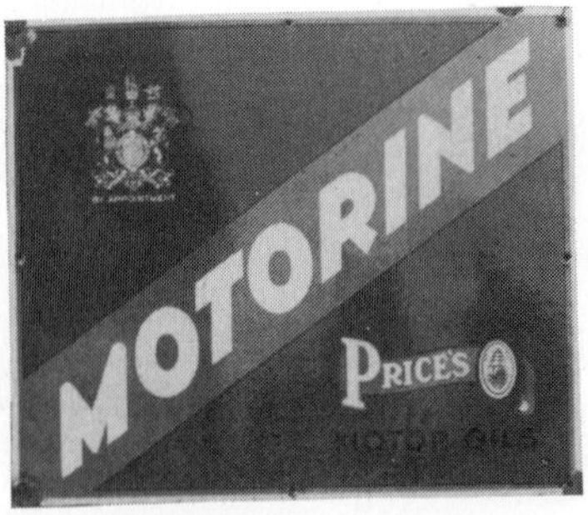

Motorine Oil sign with detailed Coat of Arms. £55

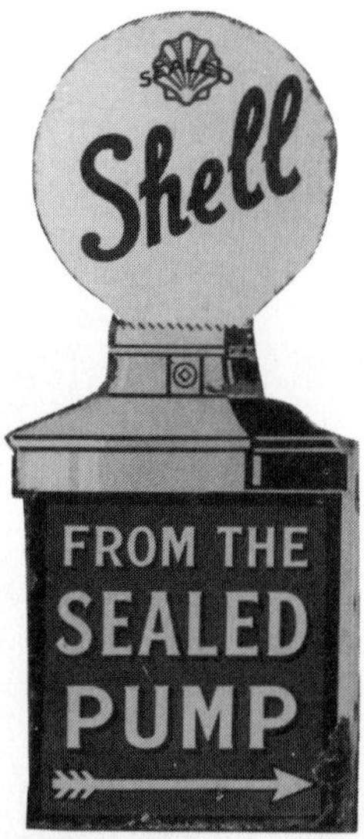

Shell from the Sealed Pump, an early sign encouraging motorists to use the new pumps. £250

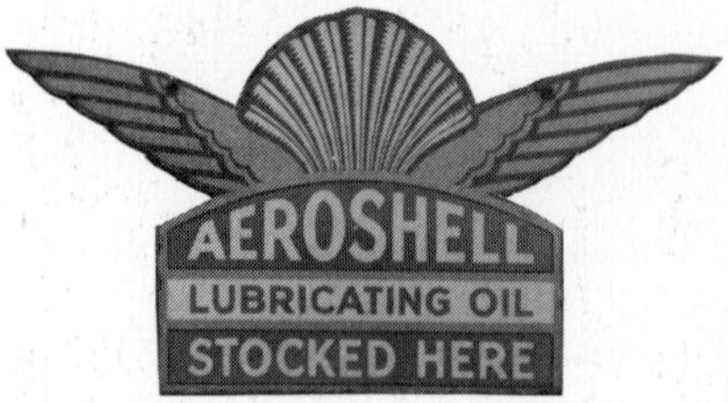

'Aeroshell Lubricating Oil', a quality oil for motor-cycles and racing engines. £80

An early R.A.C. enamel sign. £35

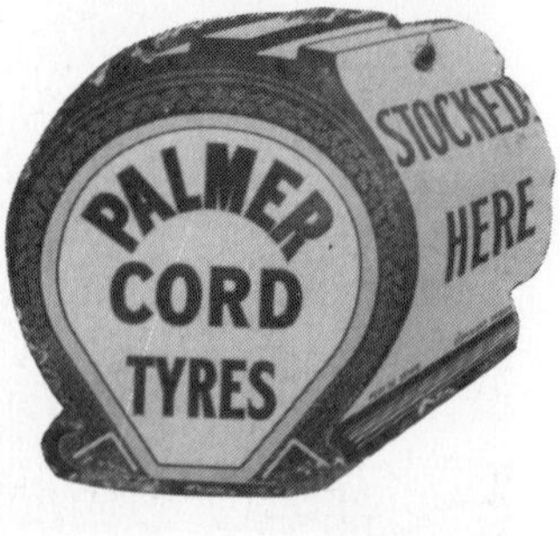

Palmer Cord Tyres sign in the form of a cut out cross section. £100

Michael Whitbread collects Galtee More ginger beer bottles.

"Galtee More is the name of a patent bottle which had the corks held in by a metal pin through the neck. They had a short life span because they were only produced between 1900 and 1918 but they were made all over the country so you never know where they are going to turn up. A couple of my nicest ones come from Cornwall. They were usually coloured either white, dark or light brown but the rarest ones have blue or green shoulders and they're the ones that make the most money.

"I found my first one when I was diving in the Thames and I still find the occasional one there but most turn up now in bottle fairs."

Galtee More bottles are usually transfer printed with the name of the ginger beer supplier and they were made by a range of manufacturers including Price's and Doulton's. Prices range from £2.50 for ordinary examples in car boot sales or junk shops to around £12 from antique shops but a rarer blue top bottle was recently sold for £75.

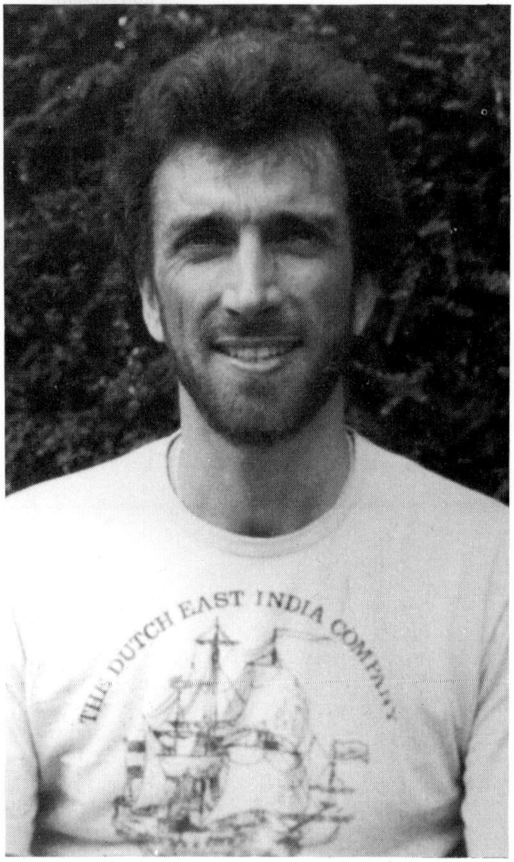

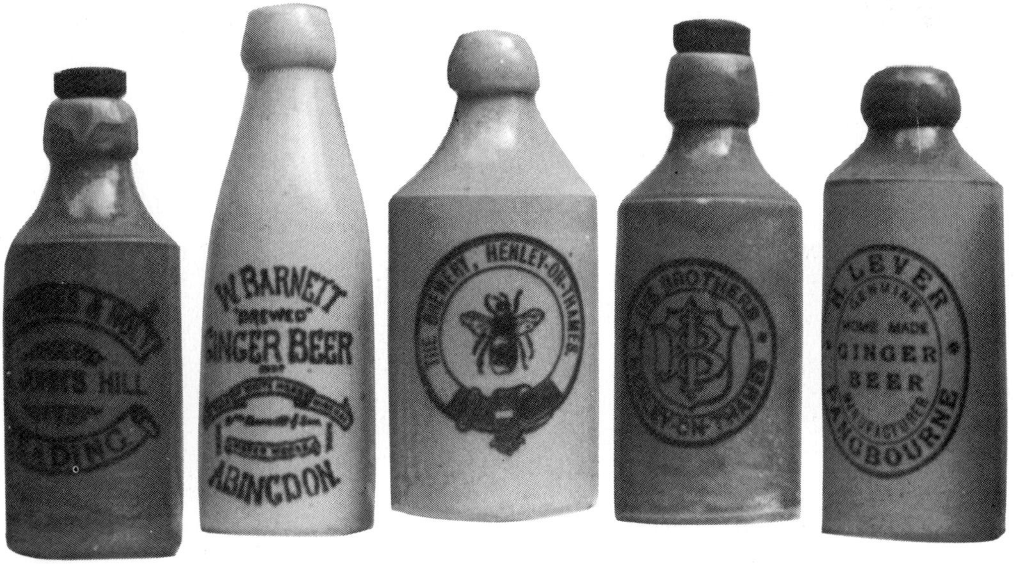

All these bottles were recovered from the River Thames at various locations.

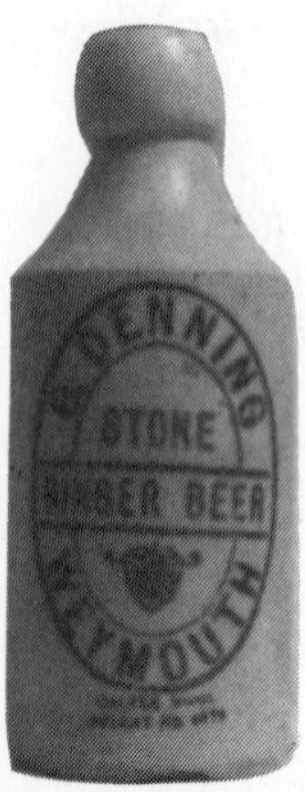

'Stone Ginger Beer' bottle by G. Denning, Weymouth. £12

Ginger Beer bottle from Gibb's Pure Mineral Water Co., Wootton Bassett. £8

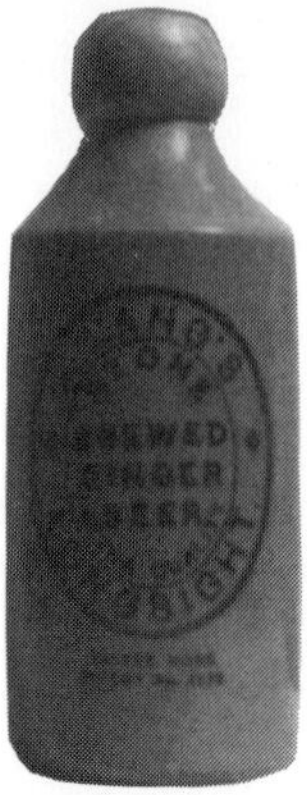

Stone Brewed Ginger Beer bottle by J. Lang's, Longsight. £8

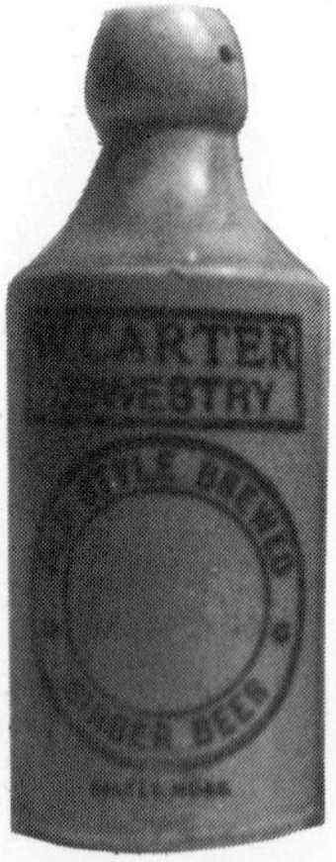

'Old Style Brewed Ginger Beer' bottle by W. Carter, Oswestry, honey colour with black printing. £10

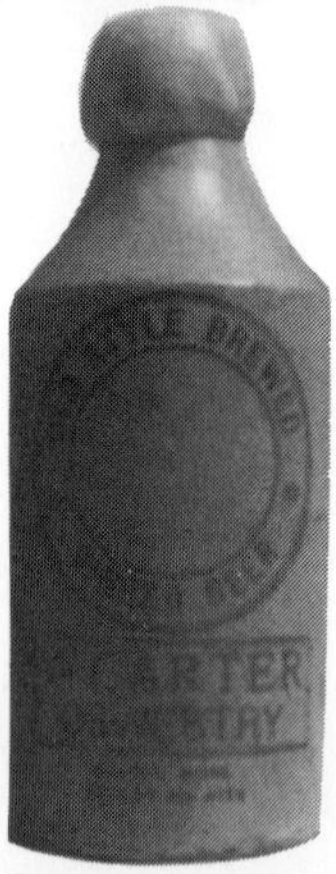

W. Carter, Oswestry, 'Old Style Ginger Beer', in honey coloured bottle with black printing. £10

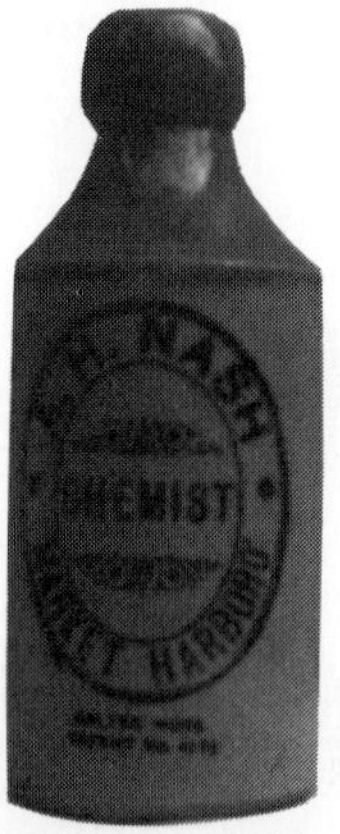

Honeynecked Ginger Beer bottle from A. H. Nash, Market Harboro', Chemist. £10

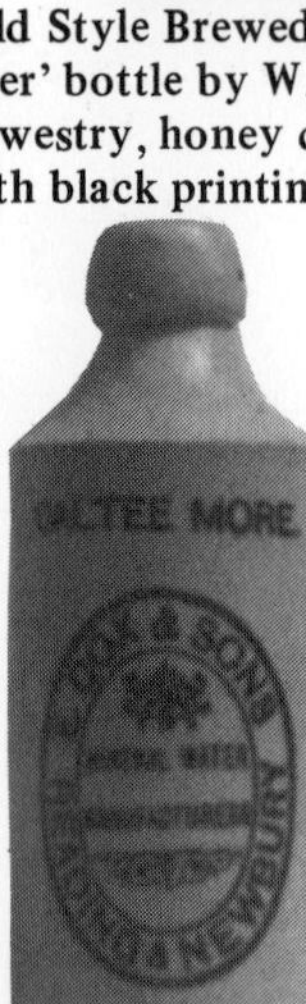

Galtee More bottle from E. Cox & Sons, Reading and Newbury, Mineral Water Manufacturers.£10

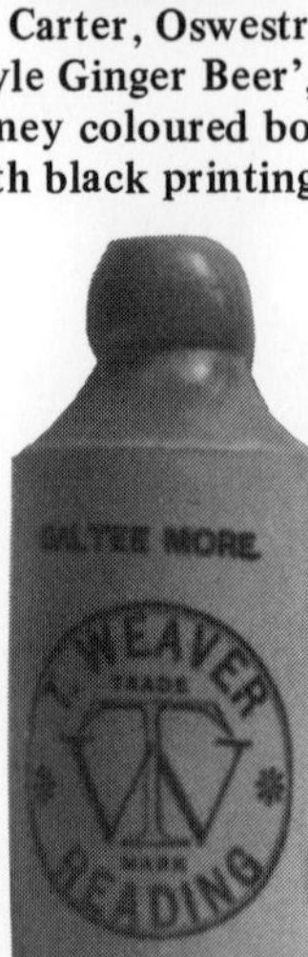

Ginger Beer bottle from T. Weaver, Reading, honeyneck with white base. £12

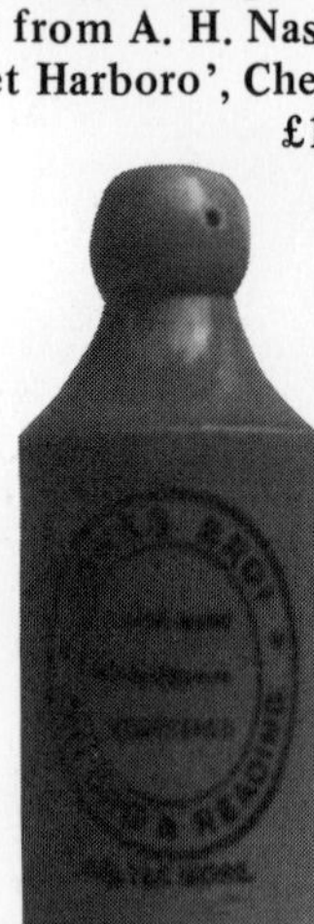

Galtee More honey coloured Ginger Beer bottle, by Jones Bros., Oxford and Reading. £25

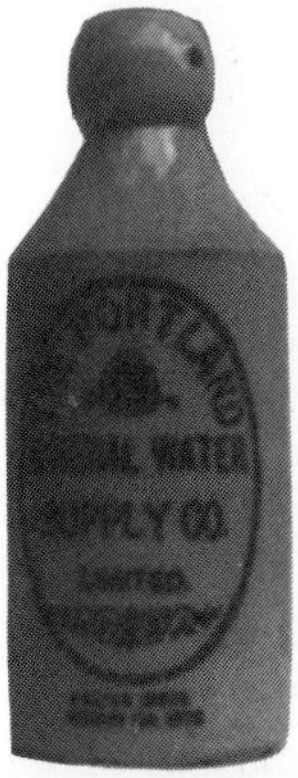

Stoneware Ginger Beer bottle from The Portland Mineral Water Supply Co., white with black lettering. £12

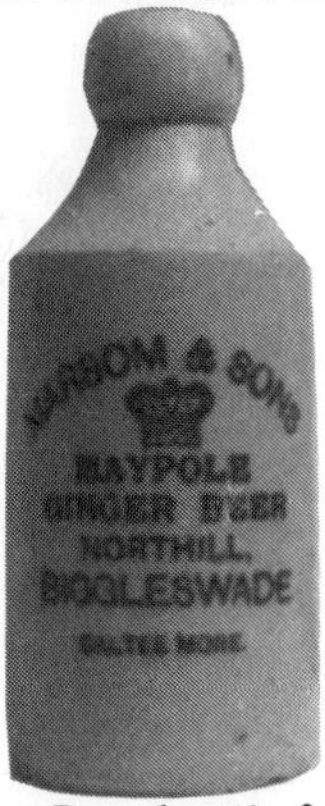

Ginger Beer bottle from Marsom & Sons, Northill, Biggleswade, white with black printing. £6

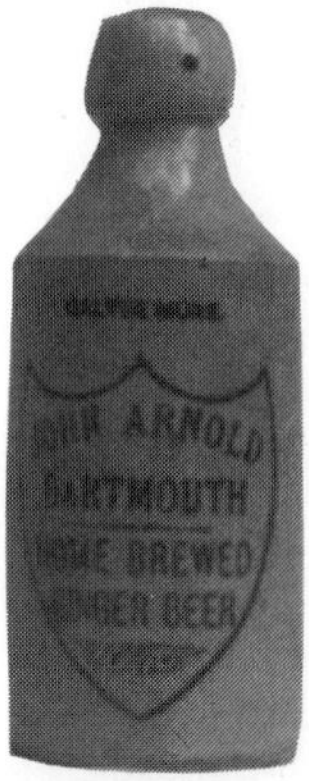

'Home Brewed Ginger Beer. by John Arnold, Dartmouth, in shield shaped label. £8

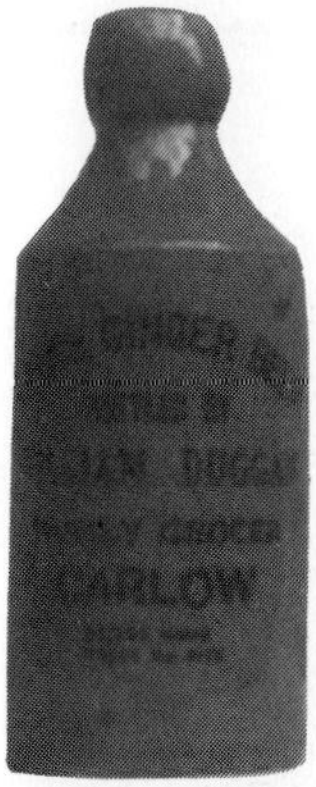

'Stone Ginger Beer', by Wm. Duggan, Family Grocer, Carlow, honey coloured with black lettering. £12

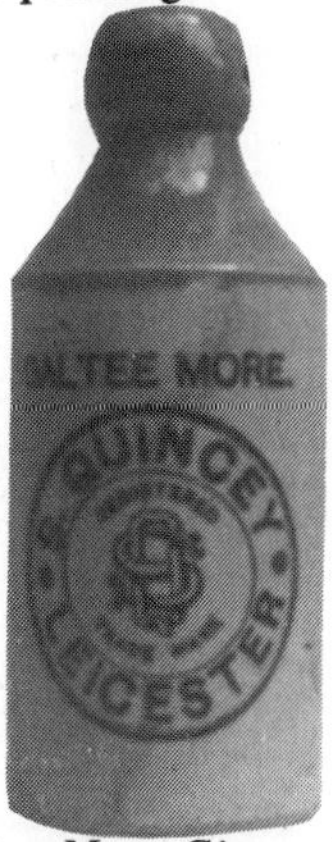

Galtee More Ginger Beer bottle by S. Quincey, Leicester, honeyneck with white body. £12

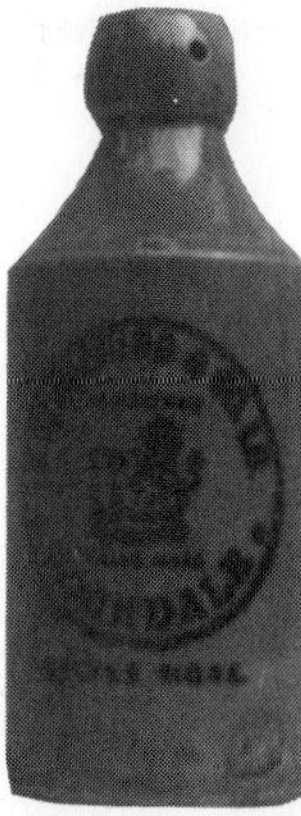

Galtee More Ginger Beer bottle from L. Standring & Co., Rochdale, honey colour with black lettering. £10

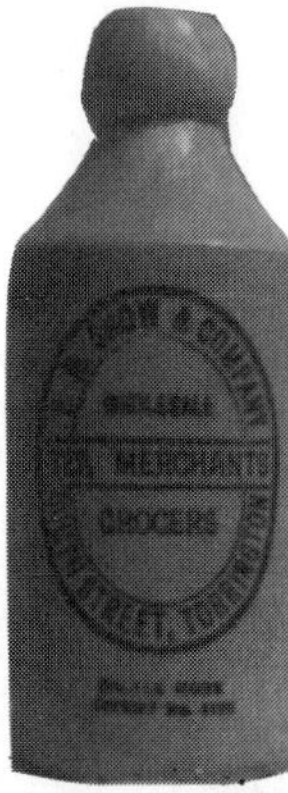

Ginger Beer bottle from R. M. Snow & Company, Tea Merchants, South St., Torrington, white with black printing. £10

Ginger Beer bottle by The Scarborough & Whitby Breweries Ltd., honey coloured. £12

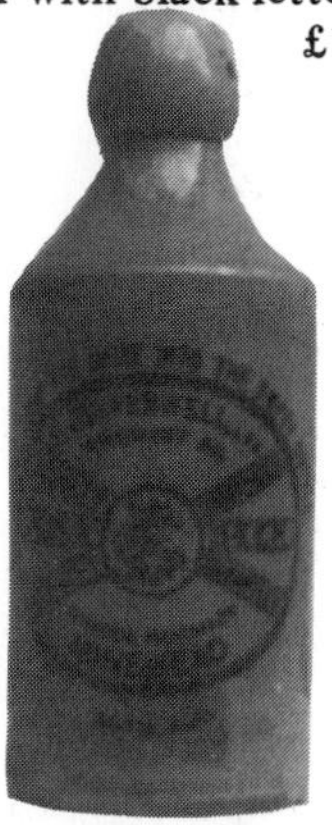

Ginger Beer bottle from E. Culverwell A.P.S. Chemist, Exmoor Pharmacy, Minehead, honey coloured, black lettering. £10

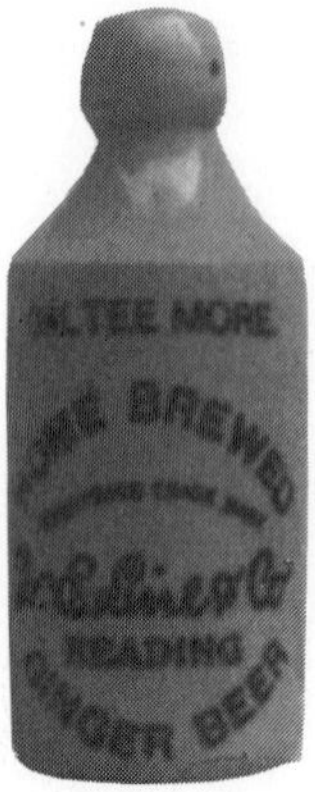

Galtee More Ginger Beer, by E. Line & Co., Reading. £15

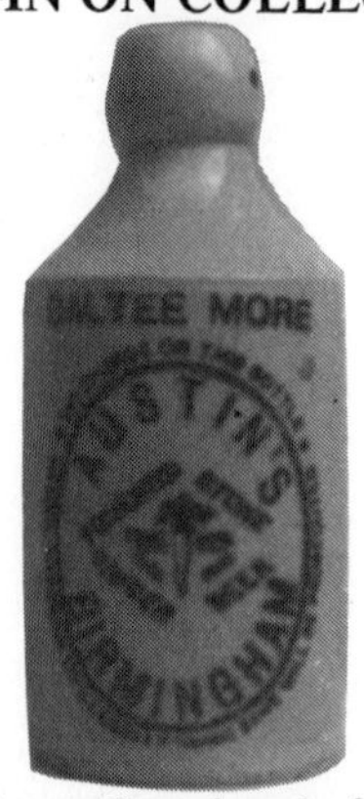

Ginger Beer bottle from Austins, Birmingham, with ginger root in the design. £10

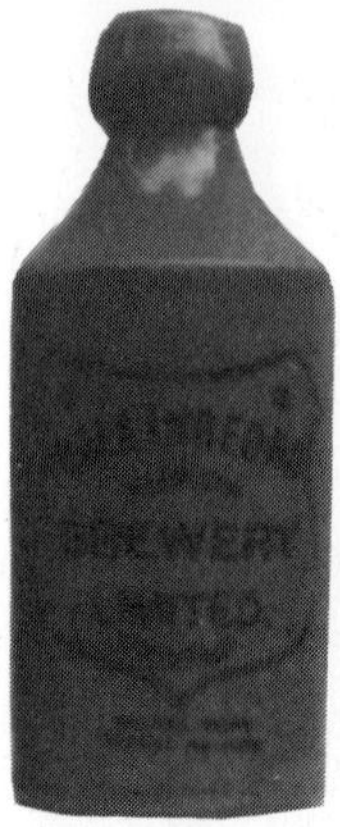

Wallingford Brewery Ltd. Ginger Beer bottle. £10

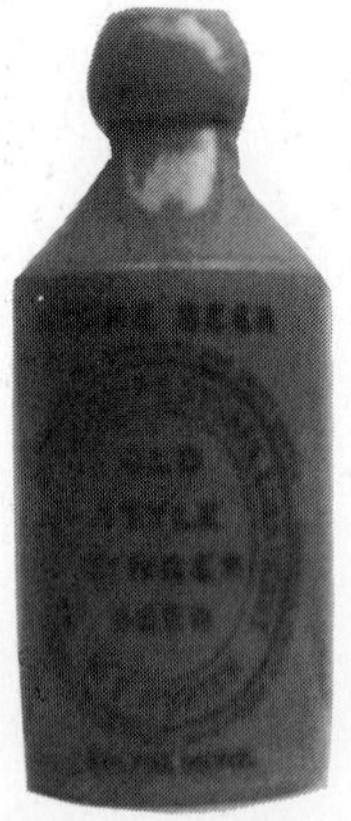

'Old Style Ginger Beer' bottle from M. P. O'Brien Universal Providing Stores, Edenderry, honey colour with black printing. £8

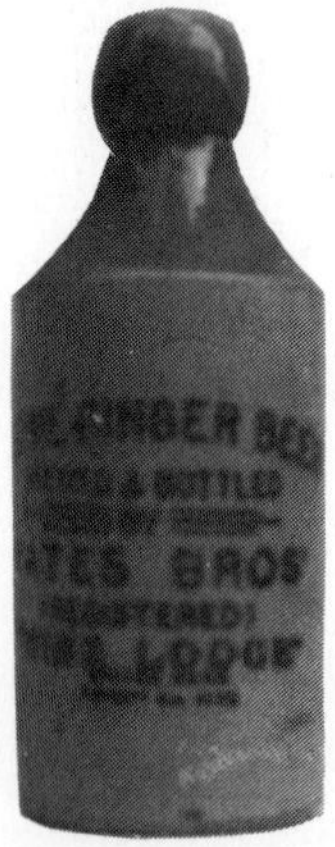

Ginger Beer brewed and bottled by Yates Bros., honeyneck with white body. £12

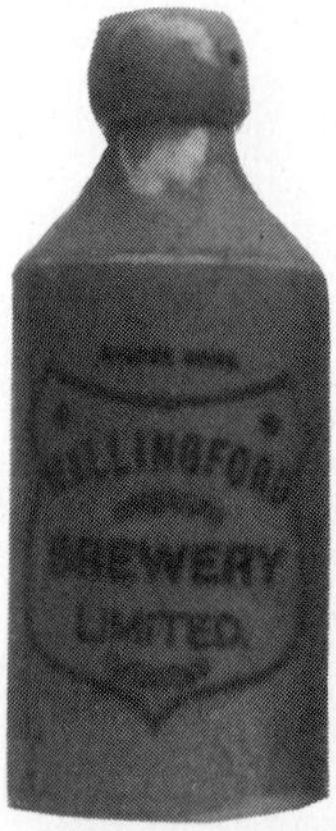

Galtee More Ginger Beer bottle from Wallingford Brewery Ltd. £10

Galtee Patent Ginger Beer bottle of honey colour impressed Lewis Evans, Dolgelly, Wales. £10

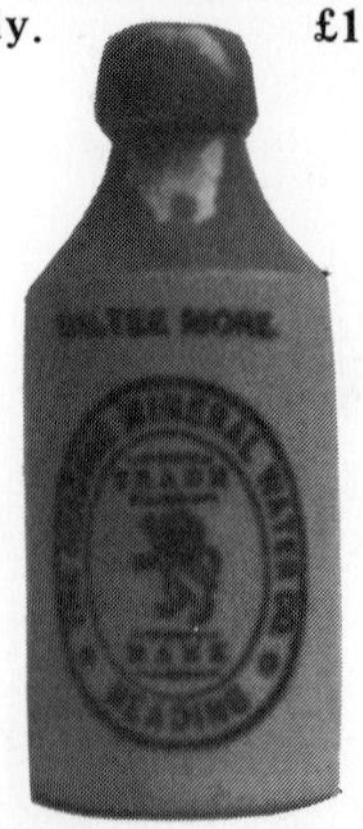

Galtee More honeyneck Ginger Beer bottle from The Reading Mineral Water Co. with the lion trade mark. £10

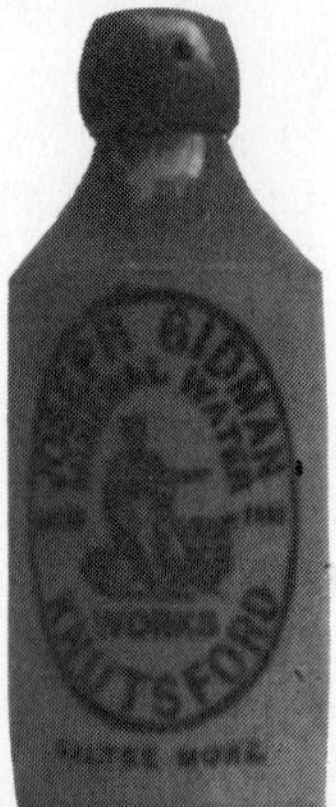

A rare honeyneck Ginger Beer bottle by Joseph Gidman, Mineral Water Works, Knutsford. £75

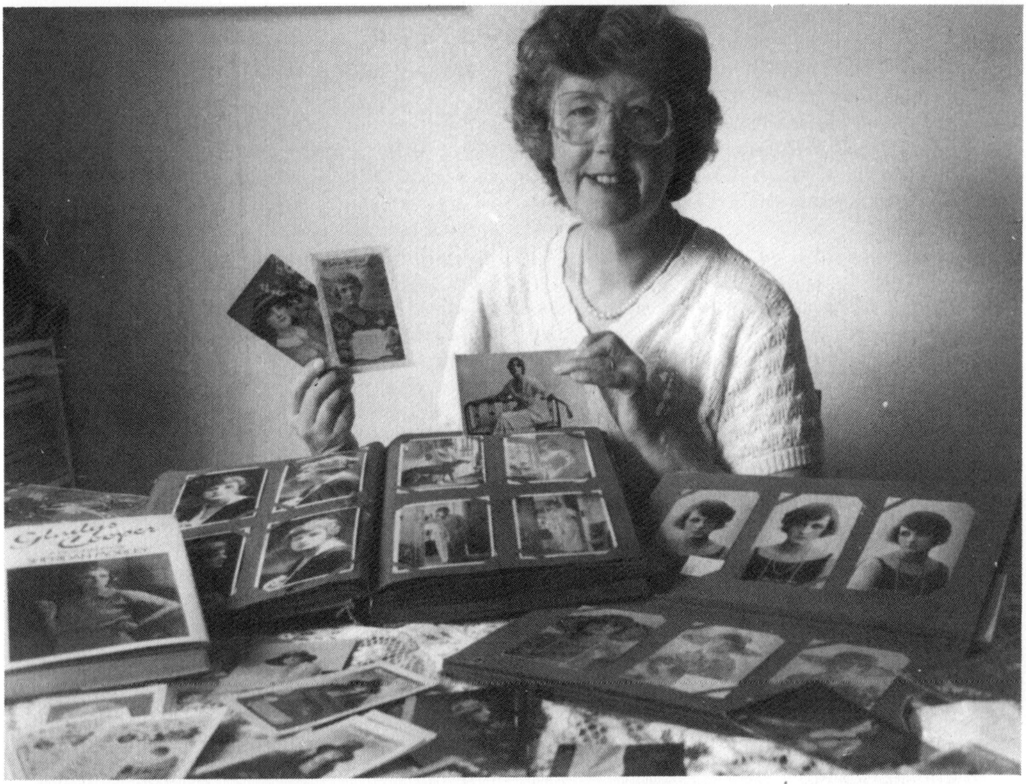

Joyce Palmer is a housewife who shares her husband's hobby of collecting postcards. Joyce's special subject is the actress Gladys Cooper.

"I've always admired her so much because she was extremely beautiful and also a very fine actress. I sort of grew up with her because she was in many radio plays that I listened to as a child.

"In my family we had some postcards of her and I decided that I was going to collect as many as possible. As a child, Gladys was a photographic model and I have a card taken when she was very young with an older girl who was a famous pin up of her day and took Gladys under her wing. It's interesting that you rarely see a card of her smiling because she's meant to have had not very good teeth.

"She was born in Lewisham and had a very glamorous life. She had three husbands and her children went on the stage. Her daughter married Robert Morley. Gladys was in the film of 'My Fair Lady' playing Rex Harrison's mother and died in her eighties not long after that."

Joyce said that several people share her collecting passion for Gladys Cooper and 'we are all quite fanatical'. She finds her postcards in fairs and through swapping and now has over 1,000. All are different but some were re-issued as coloured postcards after having been out in black and white first. Many were put out in sets of six and Joyce has discovered that they are really only three different photographs reversed. Prices for glossy, embossed cards of the actress are around £1 but those showing her in stage productions cost £3.

Joyce's favourite card is of Gladys Cooper in a full length 1920 style evening dress with long beads and satin shoes. It was taken by court photographer Dorothy Wilding.

Although the actress appeared in many films Joyce has no postcards of her in those roles. If there are any in existence she would very much like to find them.

Gladys Cooper, born, Lewisham, London 1888, had a very varied career spanning seventy-five years. She became Dame Gladys in 1967 and died on tour in 1971.

In 1894, chaperoned by the lovely photographic model Miss Marie Studholme, Gladys was taken to the Court photographers W. & D. Downey and subsequently became 'the most photographed child in London'. Many Downey and other photographs were later issued as picture postcards. By 1908, Gladys was earning £200 a year from one major postcard company alone – Messrs. Rotary Photographic. The enormous number of her cards is still untotalled. She was a major 'pin-up' of World War I, and many greetings cards, including midget postcards given free with 'Red Letter' magazine have her portrait with suitable verses and patriotic symbols. These, and many of her other cards were coloured by hand. Hundreds of all-occasion greetings cards were issued, many with portraits 'lifted' and miniaturised from the non-greetings types, which were usually issued in sets of six. These are especially interesting, because one or more portrait is issued as a mirror image, coloured differently, but given away by the fact that things like Gladys' wedding ring appear to have jumped from left to right hand! Very few pictures show her smiling – teeth were not a strong point.

Sets are not easily completed – a fact which should, ideally, be reflected in catalogues.

Gladys' stage career began in 1905, and play advertisement and stills cards are fairly uncommon, as are pictures of her as a Gaiety Girl, and midget postcards. Still more difficult to find are the multi-mini-portrait cards, perforated like sheets of stamps and gummed on the back.

Advertising by Gladys on cards have escaped the catalogues and are therefore difficult to value. She also loved to be photographed with her children – Joan, who married Robert Morley, John, and Sally, who married Robert Hardy. No catalogue yet has caught up with the rare 'Sally' card, nor pictures taken with the first of Gladys' three husbands 'Buck' Buckmaster. Her life was extraordinarily hard-working. She was a radio actress, star of silent films, then 'Talkies' and made forty-five altogether, here and in America.

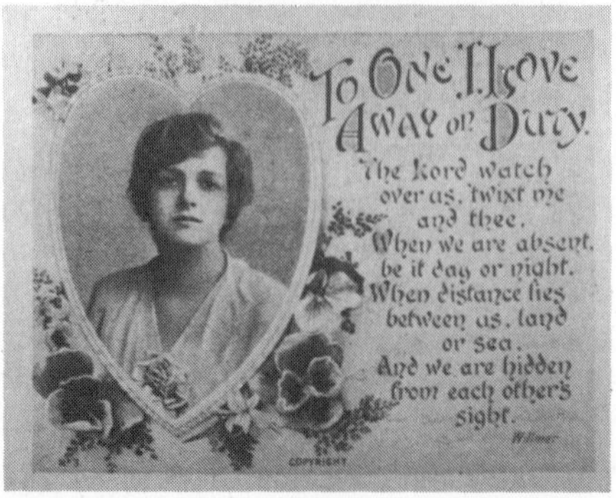

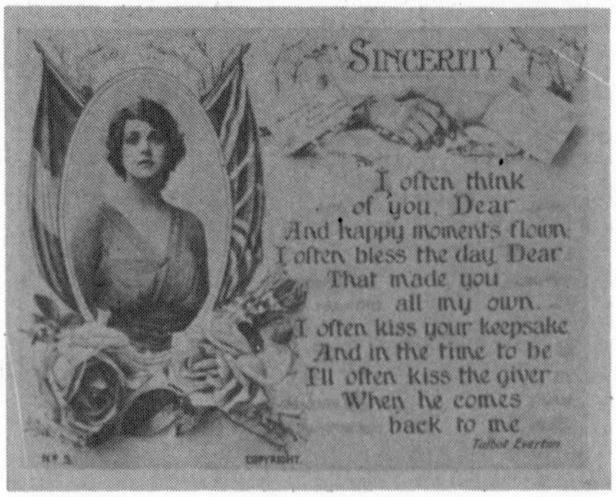

Two patriotic midget cards given away with 'Red Letter' World War I, Nos. 3 and 5. 75p – £1

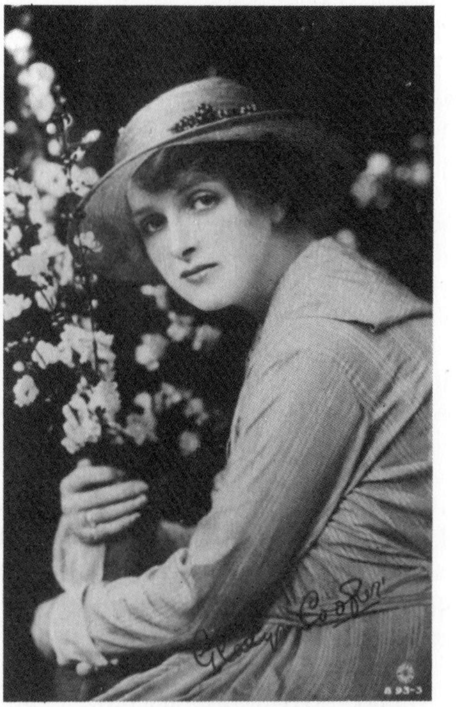

Example of 'mirror image' photo, Rotary Photo set B93, No. 5. 40p

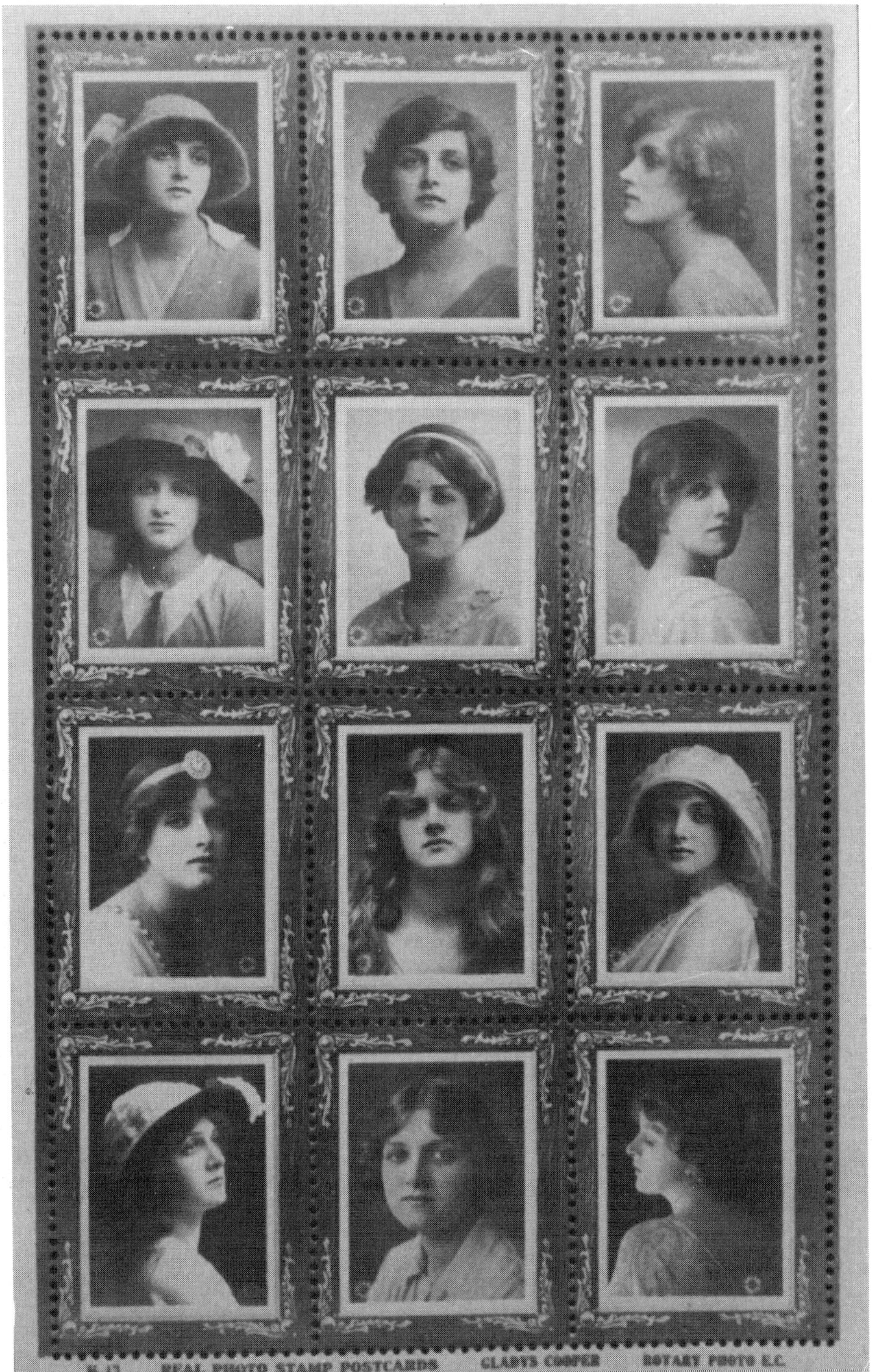

Twelve portraits with perforations and gummed back, Rotary Photographic C
K13. £5 – £7

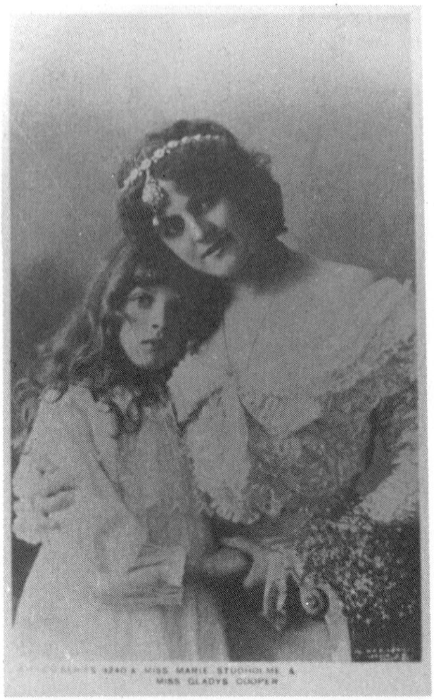

Gladys with 'aunt' Marie Studholme, portrait by Downey, circa 1895. Later a postcard by Philco 3240A. £1.50

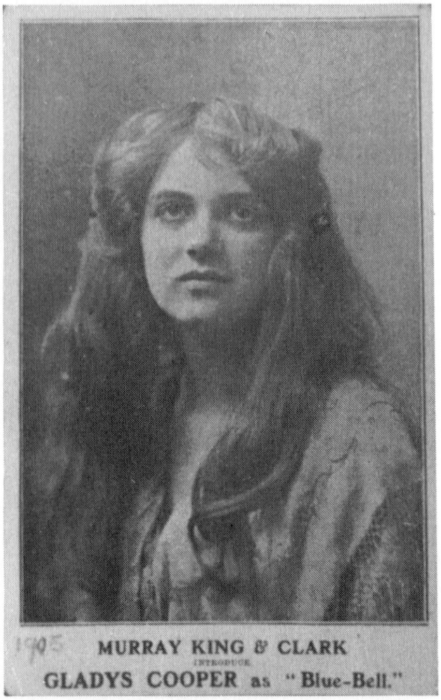

Theatre Advertisement card for her debut in 1905, at Colchester. £2.50

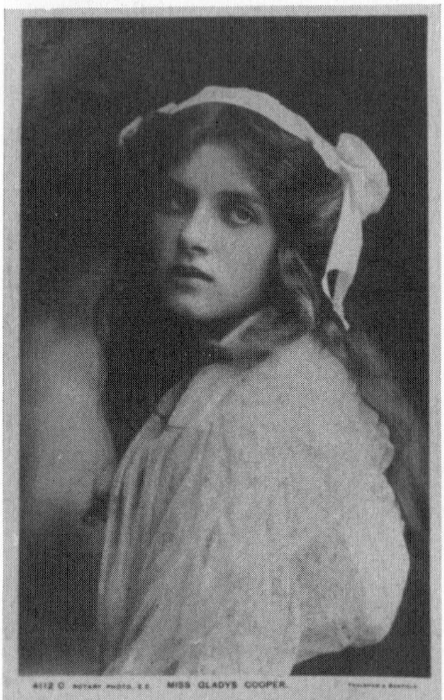

'Most photographed child in London', circa 1902, by Foulsham & Banfield/Rotary Photo 4112C. £1,50

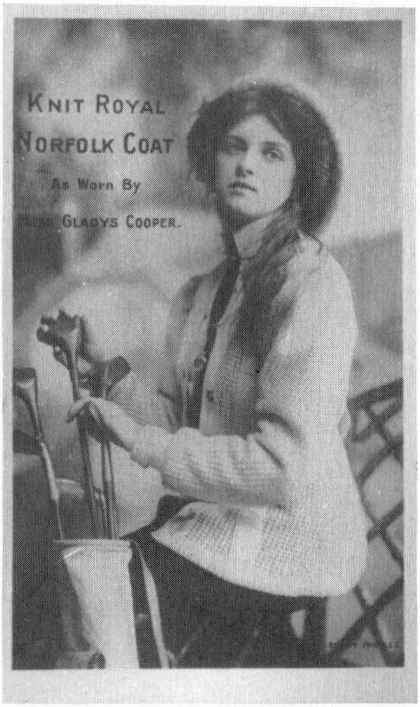

Advertising knitwear, circa 1912, Rotary Photo. £3.50

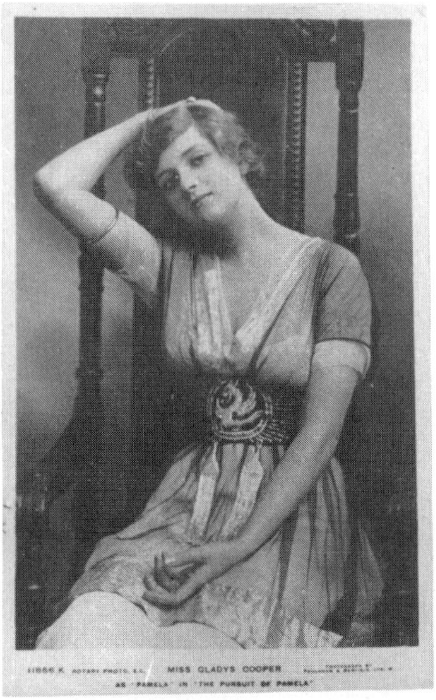

As Pamela, in 'The Pursuit of Pamela', a play, 1913, Rotary Photo 11856K. £1.50 – £2

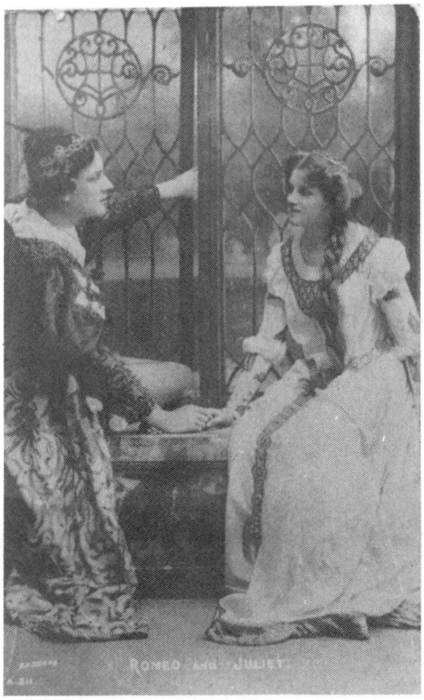

As Juliet, with Johnston Forbes-Robertson, P.mk 1911, Rotary A311. £1.50 – £2

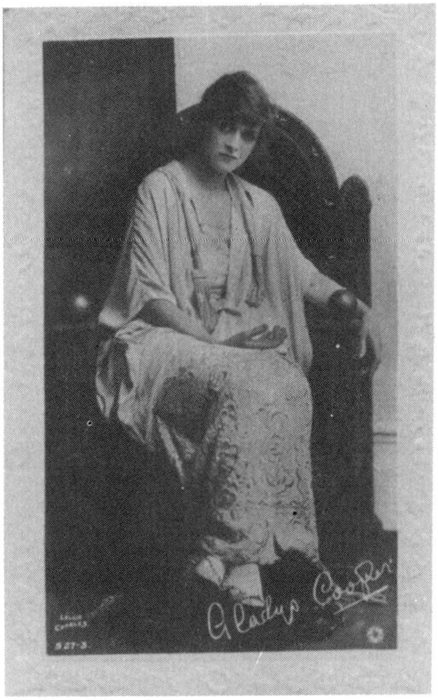

Portrait in theatrical costume by Lallie Charles, facsimile, signed, hand-coloured, Rotary Photo, S27-3, 1915. 40p

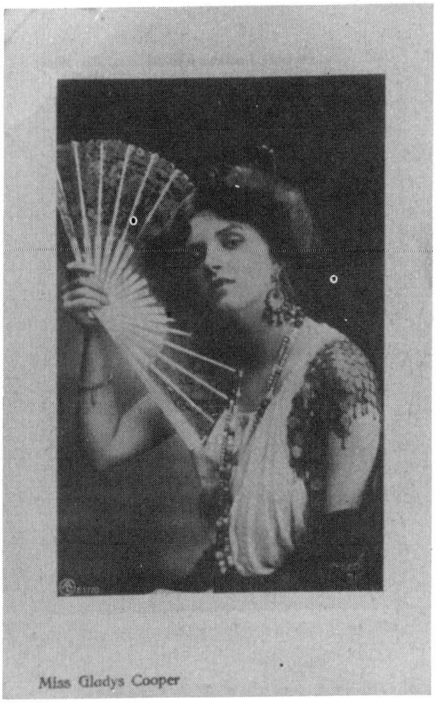

Dressed in Spanish costume, Aristophot Co. Ltd., 1910, coloured. 40p

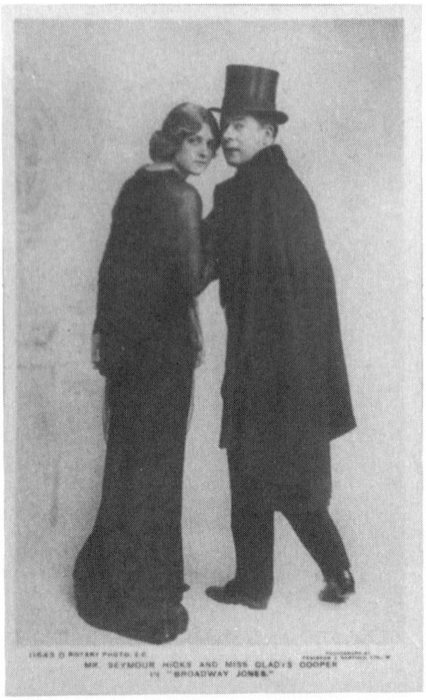

With Seymour Hicks in 'Broadway Jones', Theatre Royal, Bradford, 1913. Foulsham & Banfield photo/Rotary Photo 11643D.
£1,50 – £2

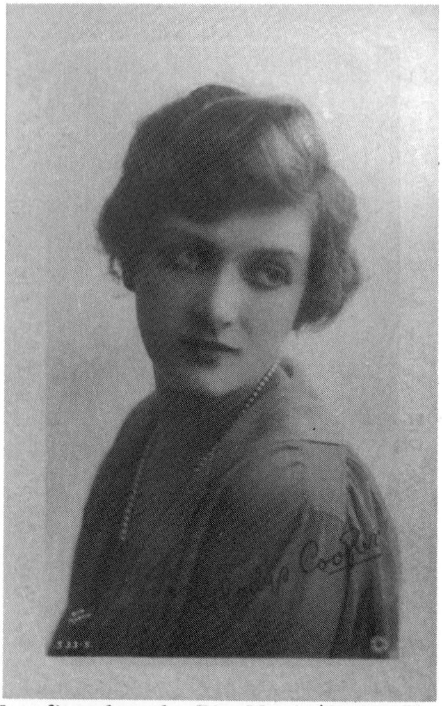

Very fine photo by Rita Martin/Rotary Photo S33-5, coloured. 40p

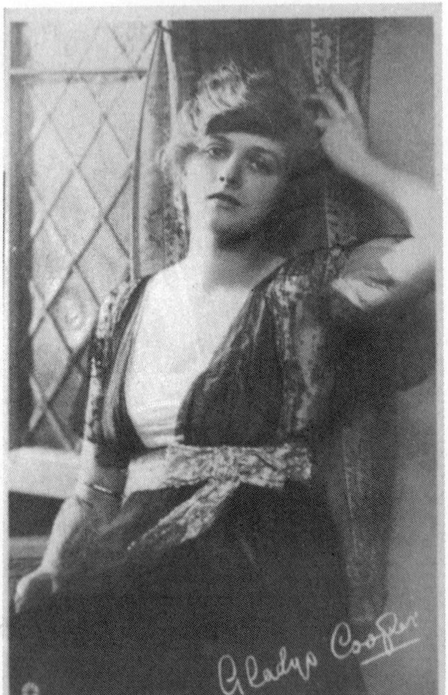

Striking a glamorous pose, one of a set of six by Rotary Photographic B137-2, hand-coloured.
40p

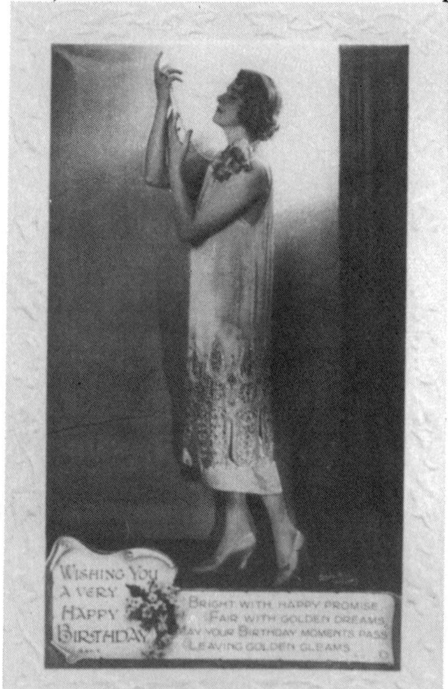

'Fashion' portrait by court photographer Dorothy Wilding, circa 1926, issued as a birthday card, Rotary Photo B841-6, coloured.
£1.50

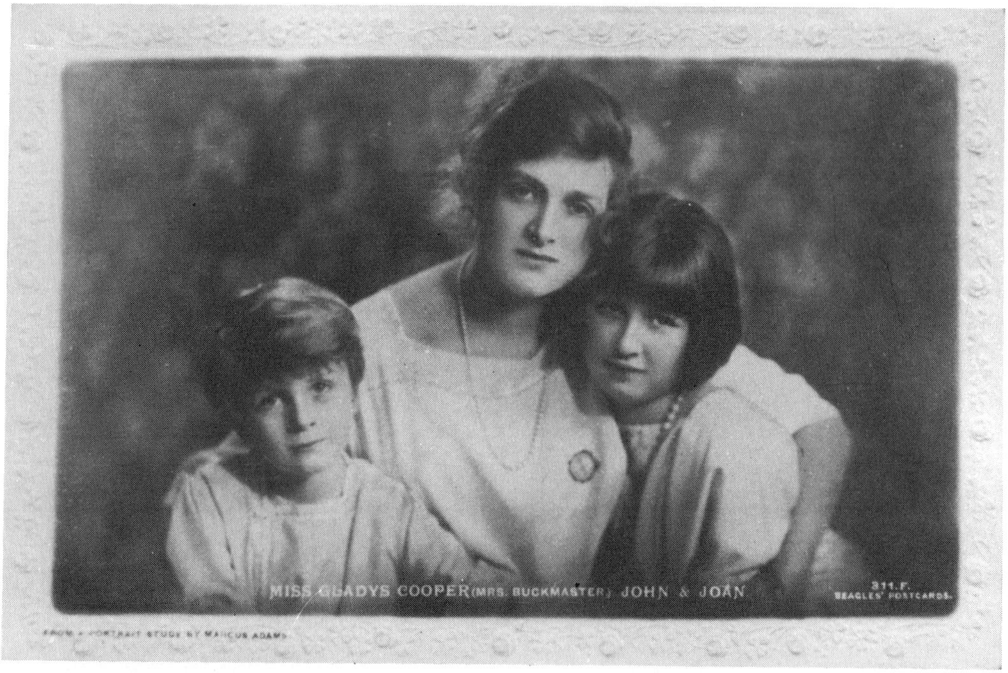

Gladys, John and Joan, by court photographer Marcus Adams, Beagles 311-F, coloured, P.mk 1921. £1.50

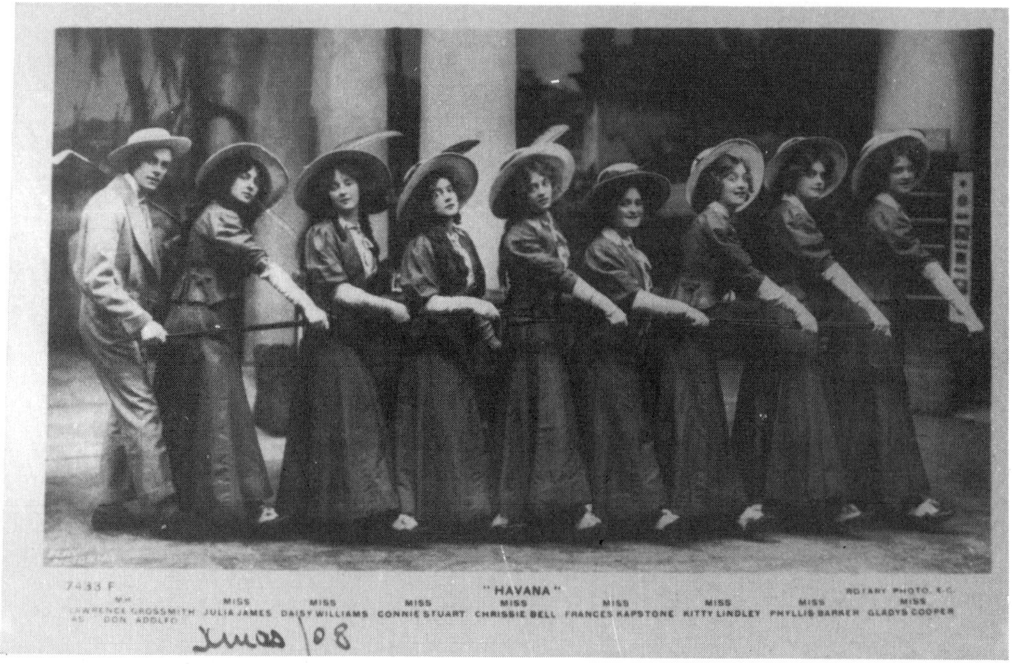

At far right in 'Havana', Gaiety Theatre 1908. Play Pictorial photo/Rotary Photographic 7433F. £1

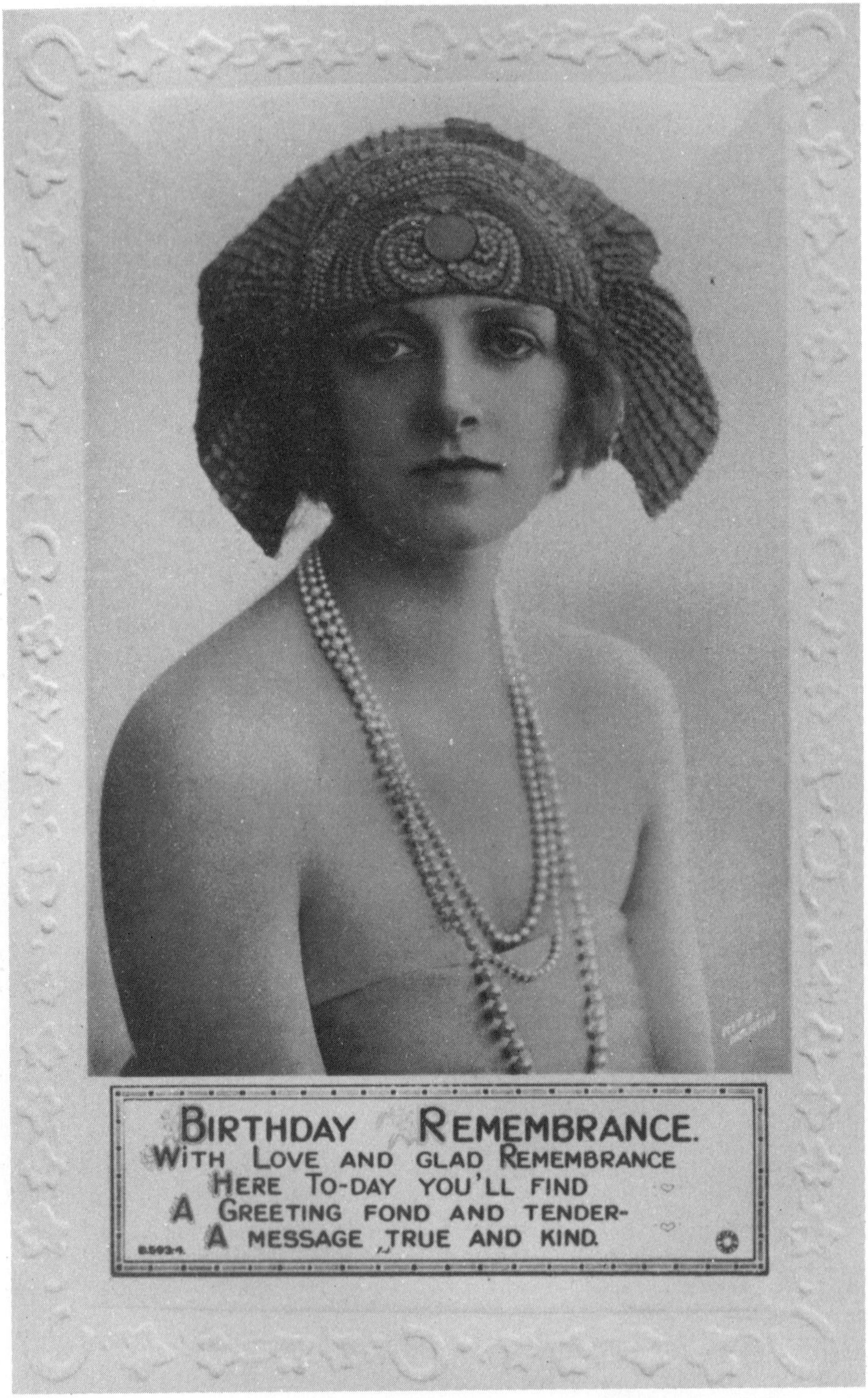
BIRTHDAY REMEMBRANCE.
WITH LOVE AND GLAD REMEMBRANCE
HERE TO-DAY YOU'LL FIND
A GREETING FOND AND TENDER-
A MESSAGE TRUE AND KIND.

Birthday greetings, Egyptian-style headdress. (The discovery of Tutankhamen's tomb influenced all the arts in the later 1920's). Rita Martin photo/Rotary Photo, hand-coloured. 40p

Roger and Pauline Martin collect both soda syphons and "uglies", which are foreign-made, bisque figures from around the time of the First World War. The figures, all bearing distinctive expressions, some grotesque, some comic, were probably made as match or taper holders, and possibly some as pomanders. The Martins have been collecting them over the past 8 years. They are difficult to find and Roger considers himself lucky to pick up one or two a year.

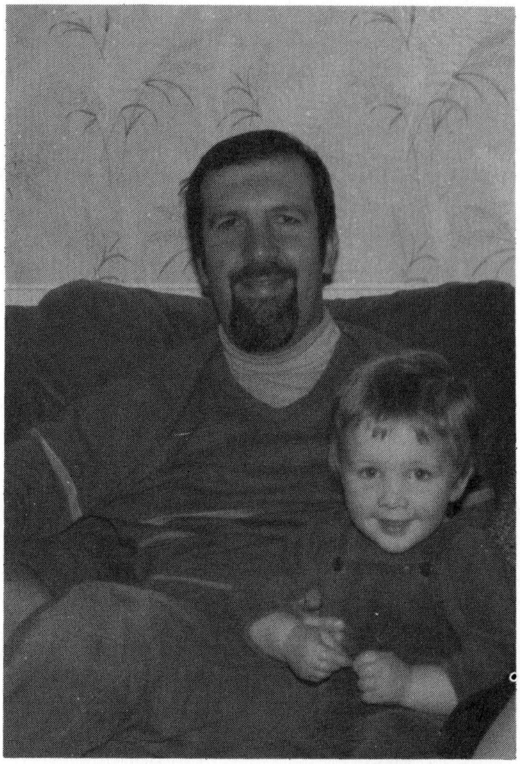

Roger Martin with his son Andrew.

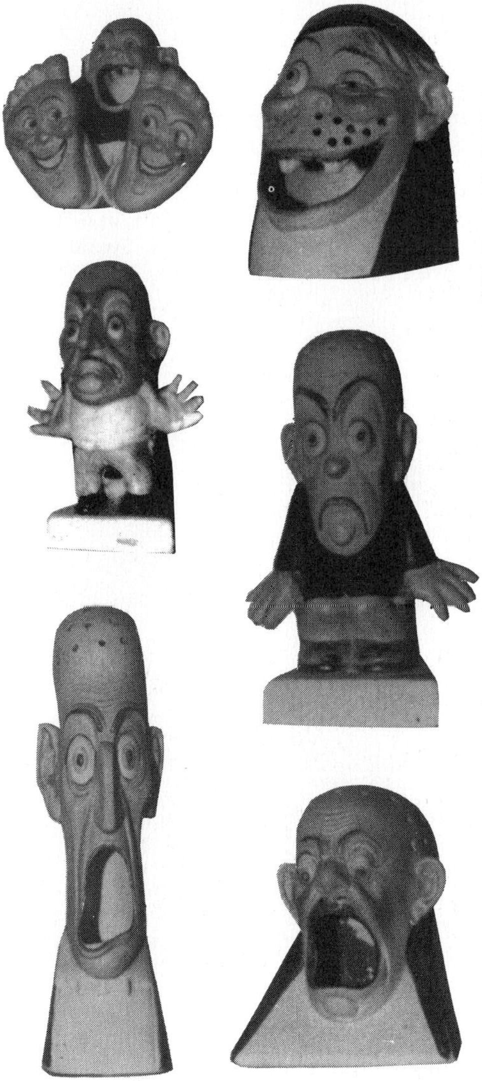

A selection of 'Uglies' worth between £10 and £35.

The Martin soda syphon collection includes items with coloured vases in pink, green, blue, yellow, brown and amber. The collection has some very early patents and includes Gazateur and Seltzogenes (some French) with wire or basket-weave covering. Its purpose was to guard against the possibility of explosion caused by the gas pressure of the syphon's contents.

The classic soda syphon shape was developed in the second half of the 19th century. Syphon tops, though, have changed with early ones being made of tin or pewter, then becoming porcelain-lined and chrome-plated and nowadays they are made of plastic.

It is possible to pay between £2 and £30 for a syphon depending on age and condition.

One syphon has so far eluded Roger. It is a Mayo syphon, made in the 1860's, with a porcelain body. He has read about it but has never yet seen one for sale.

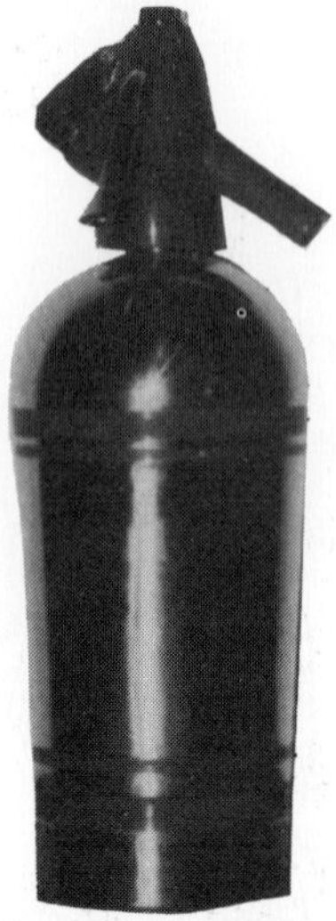

Art Deco style plated Sparklets type syphon, 29cm. high. £4

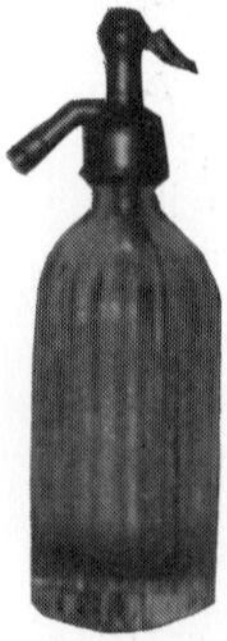

A clear glass Schweppes sample syphon, 16cm. high. £20

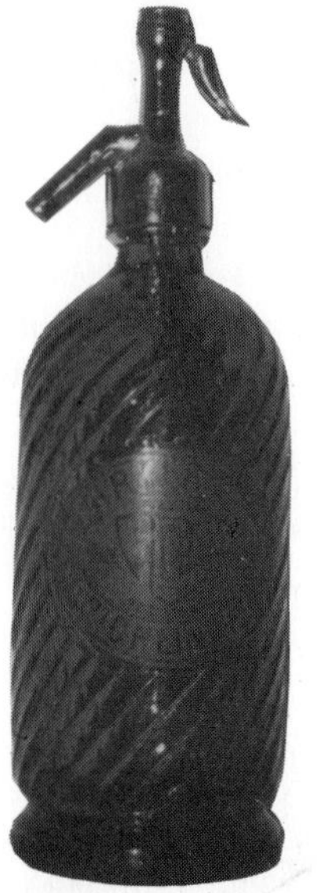

Amber glass writhened syphon by Parker Bros. of Drighlington, 31cm. high. £25

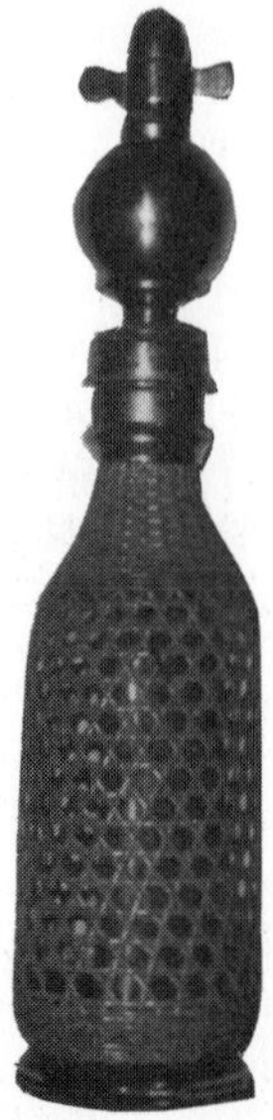

One shot, basket covered, Sparklets type syphon, 32cm. high. £8

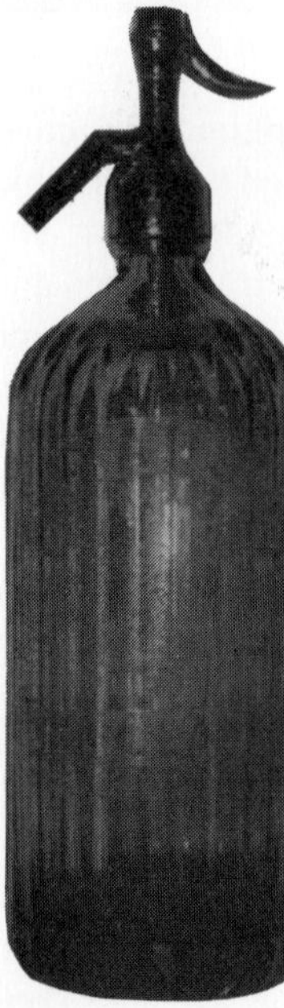

Pink faceted glass syphon by Maps, illustrated with a figure of a man, 33cm. high. £18

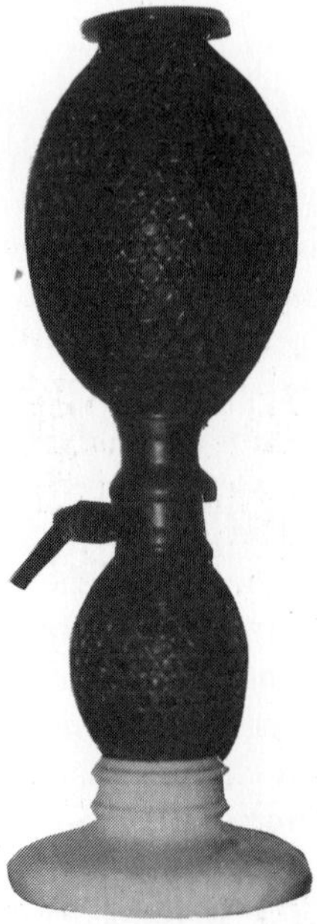

Basket covered Gazateur syphon with a porcelain base, 45cm. high. £50

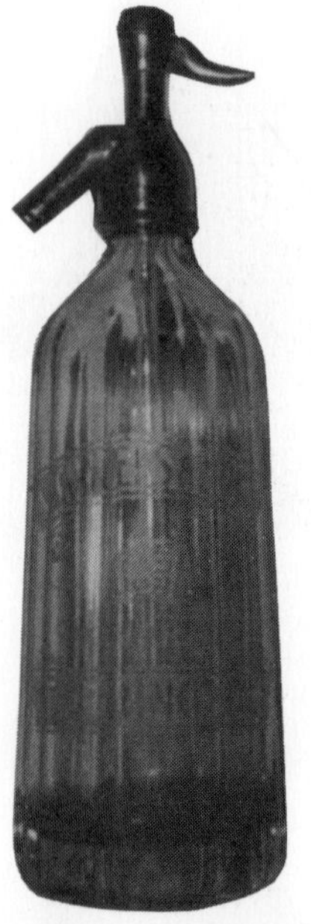

Yellow glass syphon by L. G. Weeks & Sons of Torrington, 33cm. high. £16

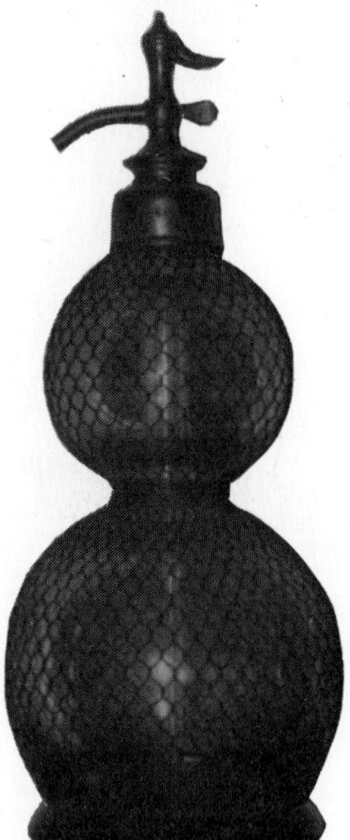

Seltzogene twin bulbed syphon made by D. Fevre, Paris, 45cm. high. £30

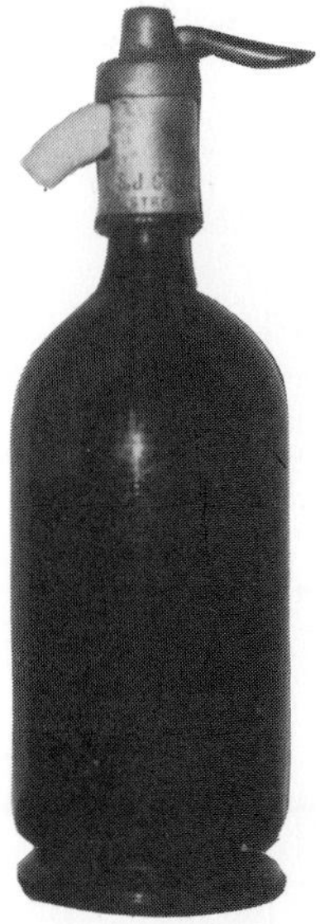

Early cobalt blue syphon by S. J. Coley of Stroud with patented porcelain top, 30cm. high. £25

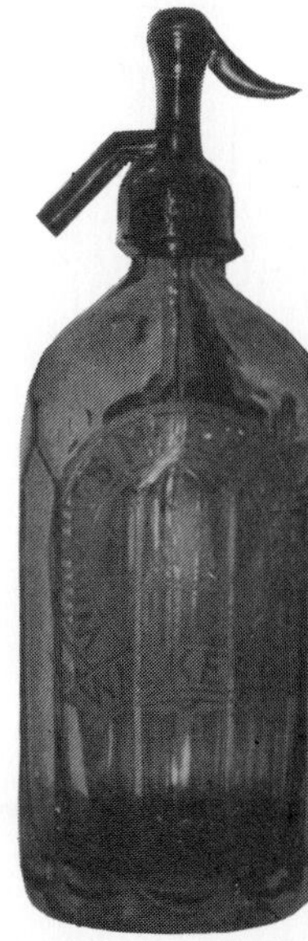

Faceted clear glass syphon by Wrights of Walkery, 31cm. high. £16

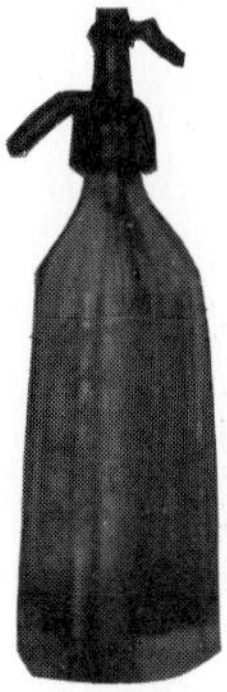

Miniature blue/green glass syphon by the Dorset Mineral Water Co. of Poole, 17½cm. high. £30

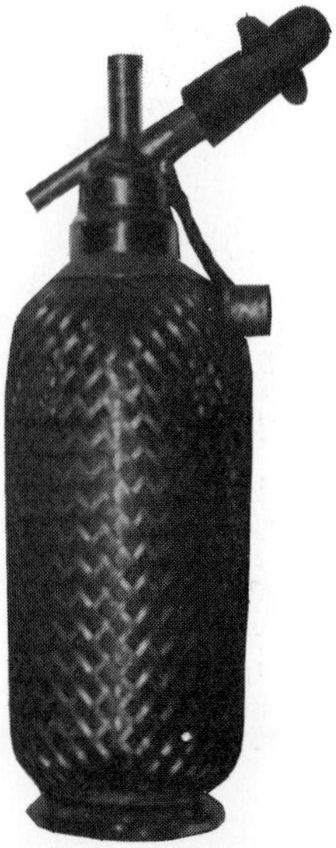

Sparklet clear glass, mesh covered syphon, circa 1925, 37cm. high. £3

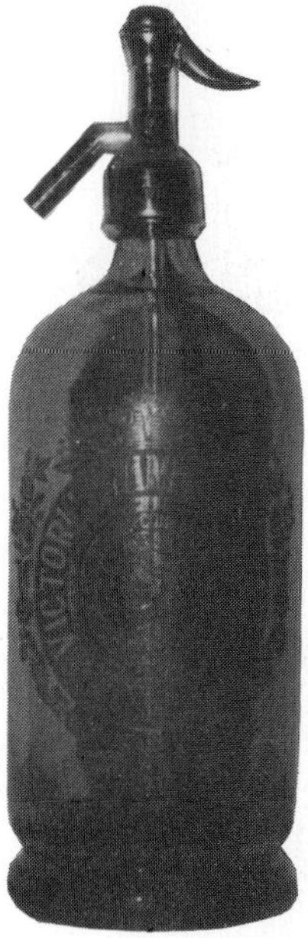

Green glass syphon by the Victoria Wine Co. illustrated with a picture of Queen Victoria, 33cm. high. £16

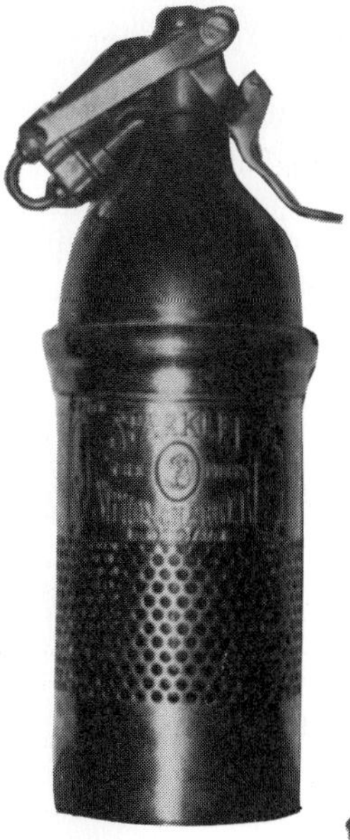

Sparklet syphon charger used by hotels to refill syphons, 39cm. high. £35

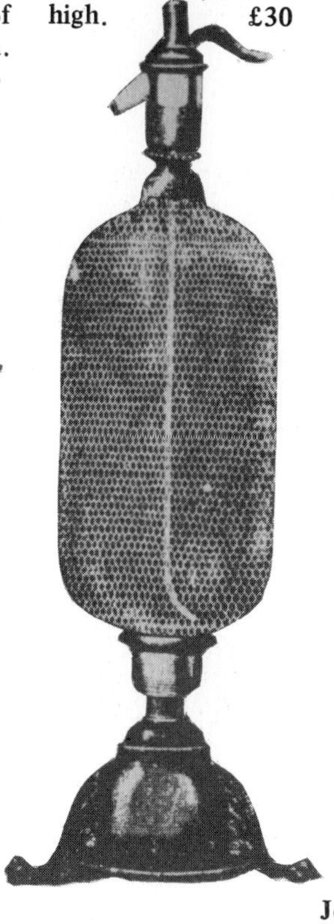

Loze's patent Seltzogene mesh covered syphon, circa 1900, 45cm. high. £50

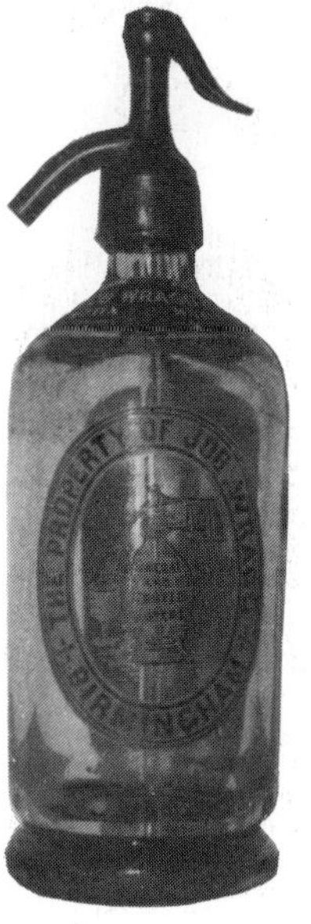

Job Wragg of Birmingham clear glass syphon illustrated with a picture of the syphon in use in red print, 31cm. high. £10

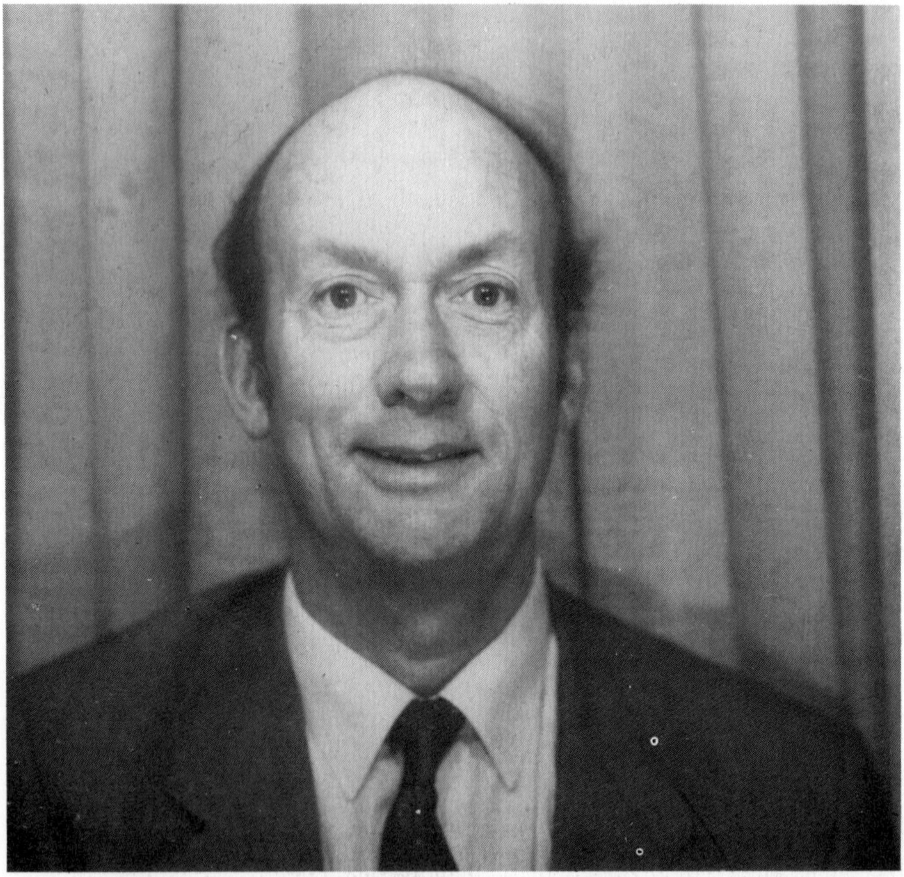

Alan Roman collects material connected with the Shell Motor Oil Co. because he works for them.

"I'm interested in everything to do with the company's advertising from a series of postcards of Shell advertisements issued in 1908 to lapel badges, posters, books and toys.

"The posters were carried on fuel delivery lorries and were designed by famous artists of the 1930's like McKnight Kauffer, David Gentleman and Paul Nash. Today an original poster in good condition is worth £200."

Alan's collection includes petrol cans with the Shell logo which were once strapped to the outsides of cars; enamel signs advertising the products and a pull-out tin toy that speaks the message 'Crikey – That's Shell That Was!'. It was a giveaway in the 1930's but today is worth between £40 and £50.

The books in his collection include some of the first Shell guides dating from the 1930's.

What Alan would still like to find are original postcards of Shell advertisements published between 1908 and 1920 and more of the Art Deco posters designed by McKnight Kauffer.

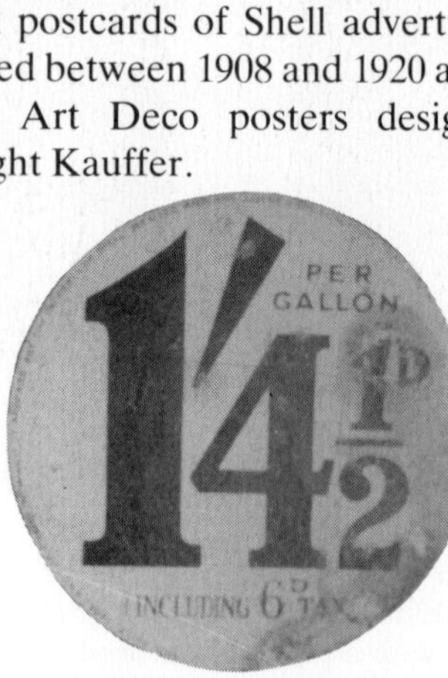

Metal sign used on 'Shell' pumps.

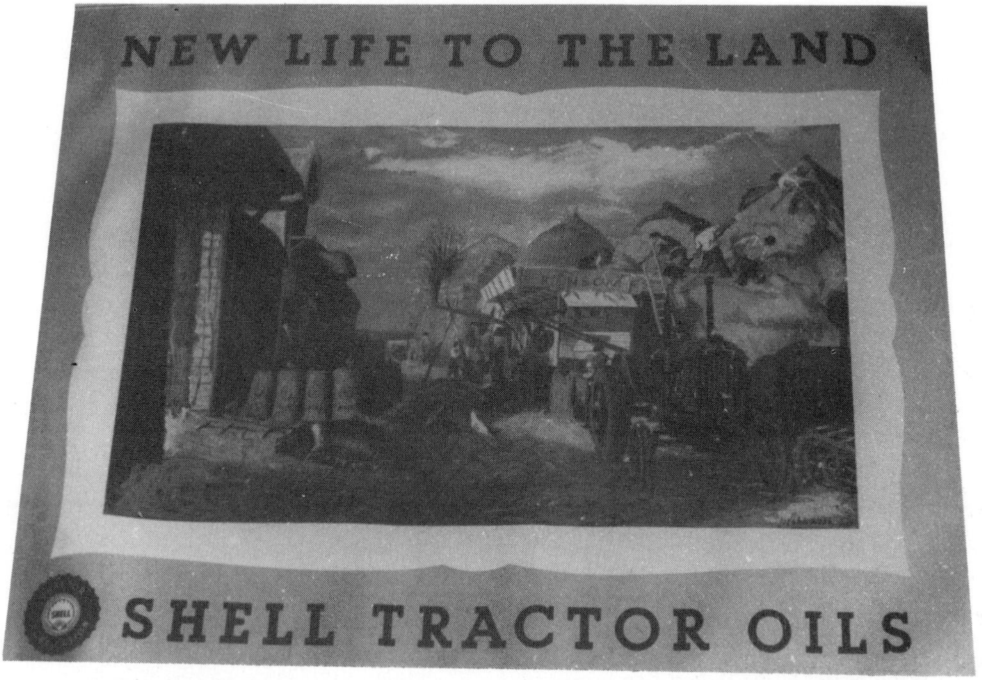

Shell Tractor Oil 'Now Life to the Land' designed by Joseph Webb, circa 1951.
£30

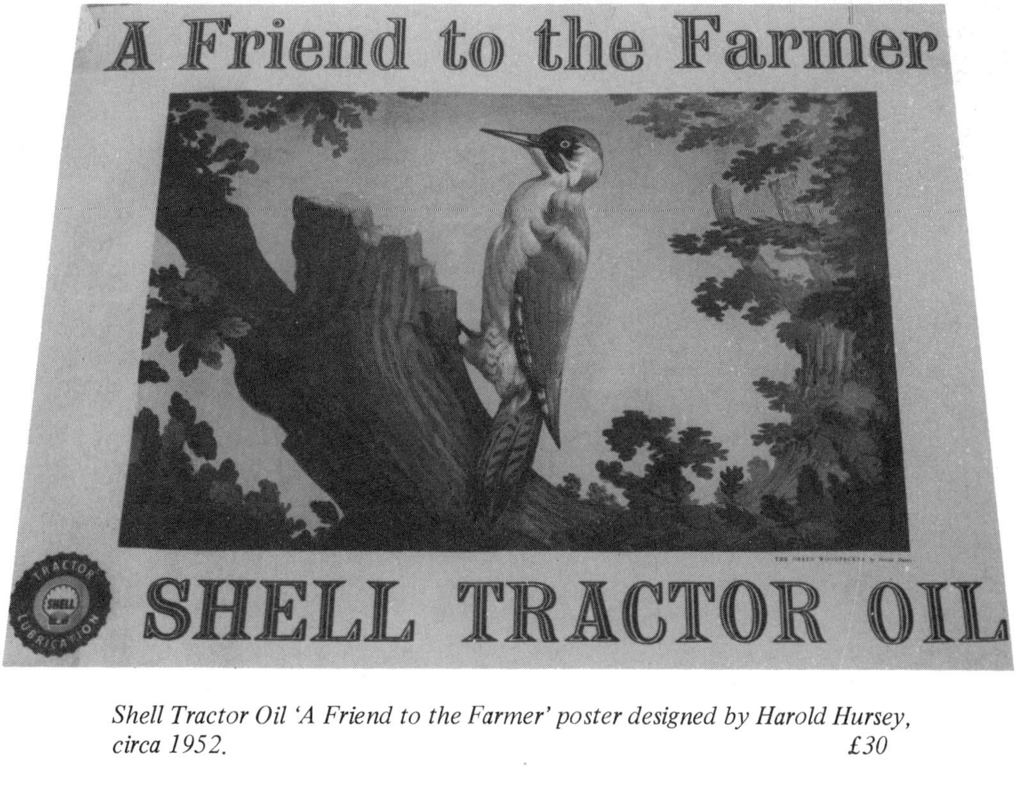

Shell Tractor Oil 'A Friend to the Farmer' poster designed by Harold Hursey, circa 1952. *£30*

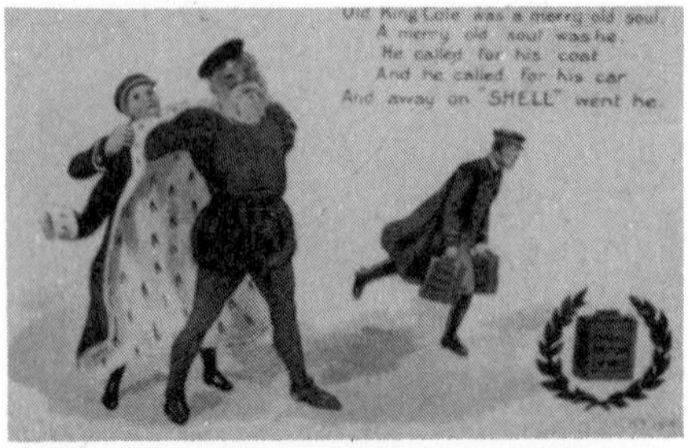

Old King Cole was a Merry Old Soul . . . and away on Shell went he.

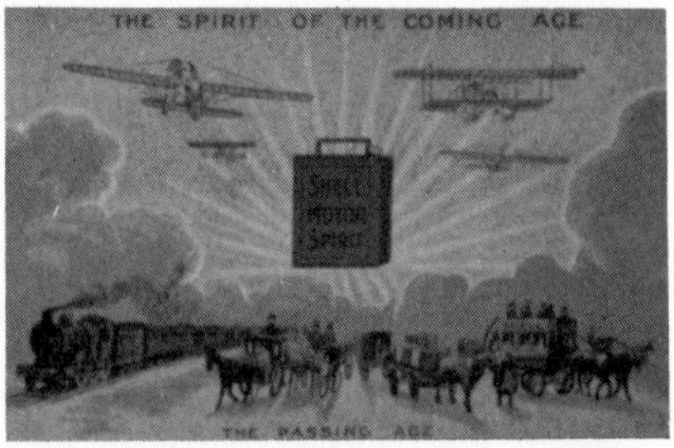

The Spirit of the coming age, 'Shell' Motor Spirit.

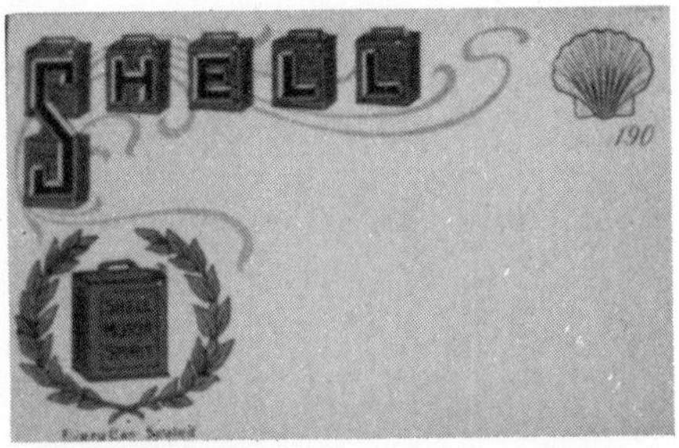

Shell Motor Spirit, Every Can Sealed.

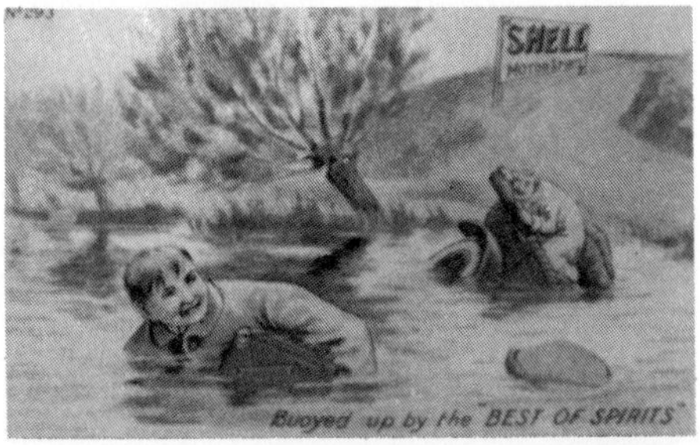

'Shell', Buoyed up by the 'Best of Spirits'.

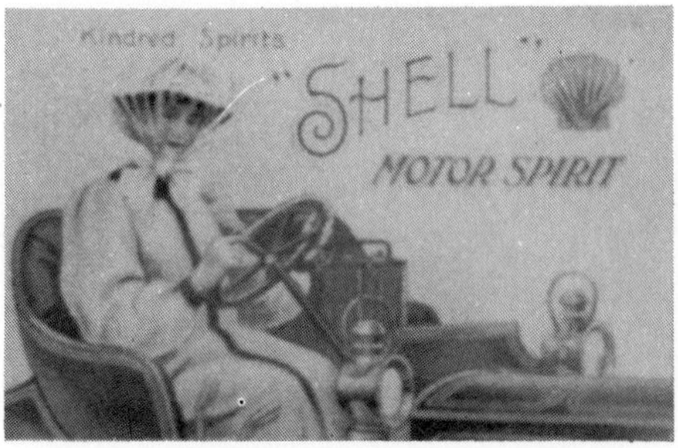

Kindred Spirits 'Shell' Motor Spirit.

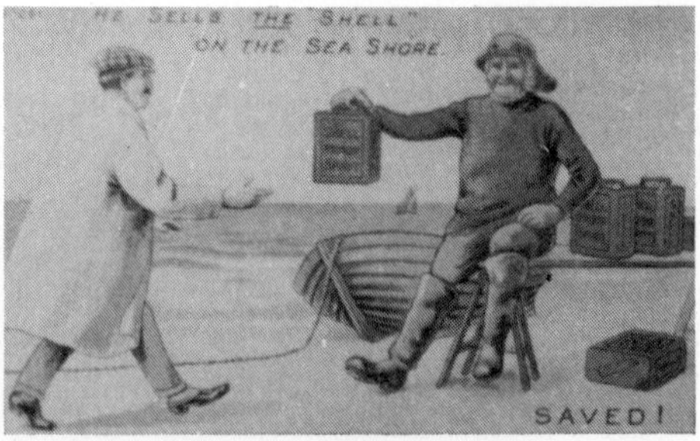

He sells the 'Shell' on the sea shore – Saved!

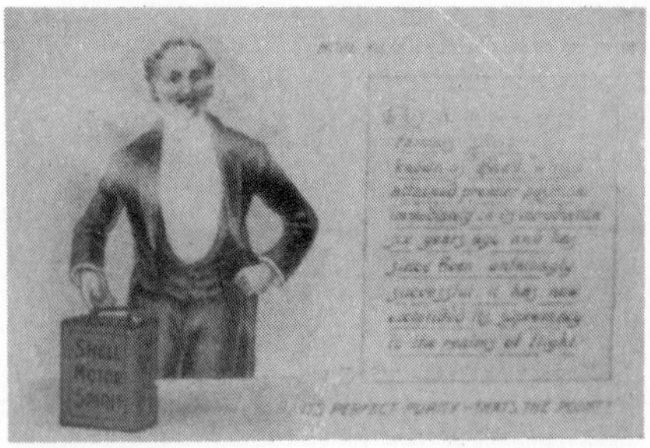

'Shell' Motor Spirit, Its Perfect Purity – That's The Point.

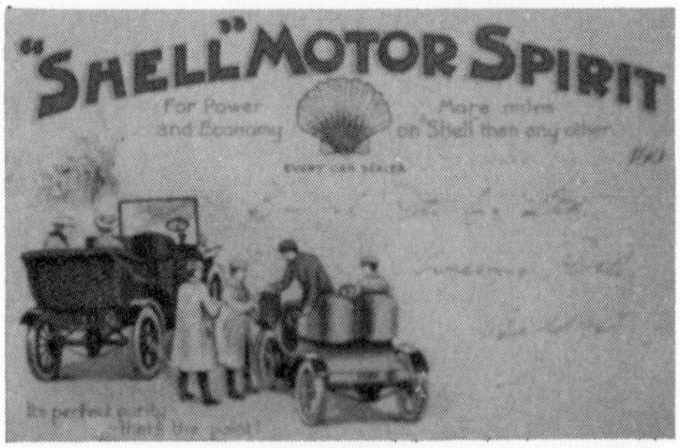

'Shell' Motor Spirit, For Power and Economy.

Postcards featuring 'Shell' from 1905 to 1920. £25 – £35 each

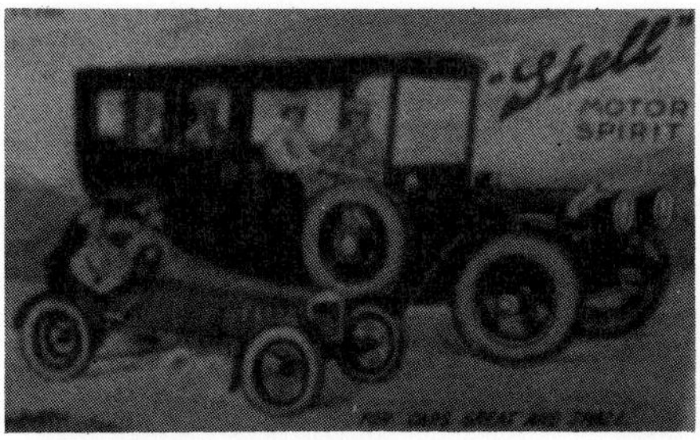

'Shell' Motor Spirit, For Cars Great And Small.

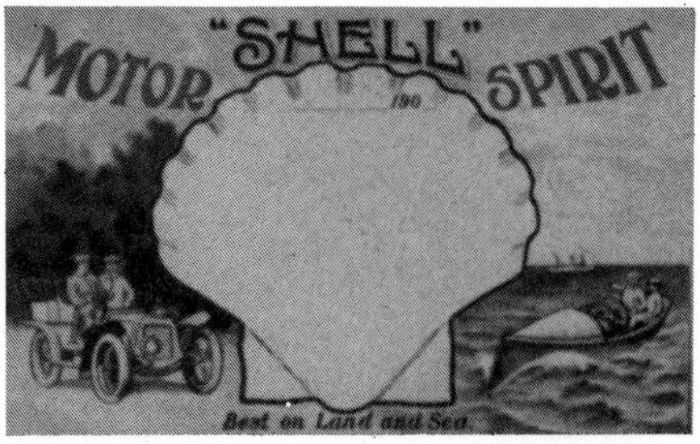

'Shell' Motor Spirit, Best on Land and Sea.

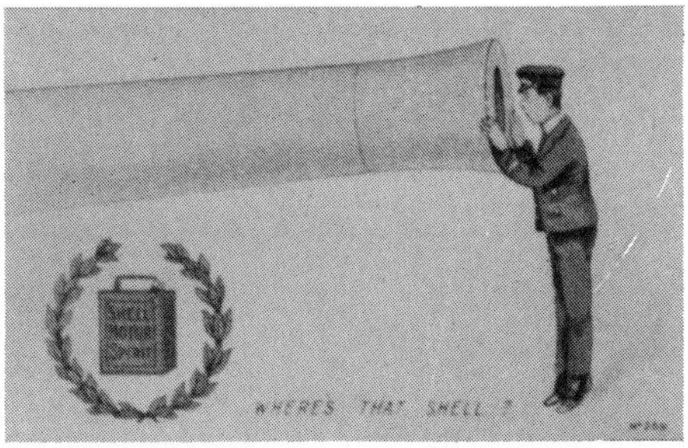

Where's that Shell?, 'Shell' Motor Spirit.

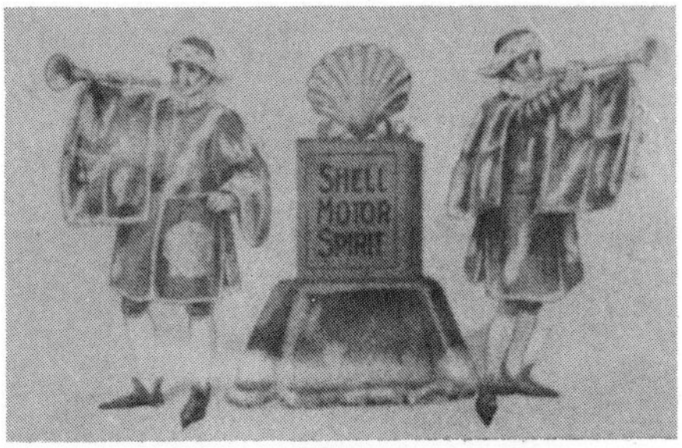

Shell Motor Spirit, Fanfare.

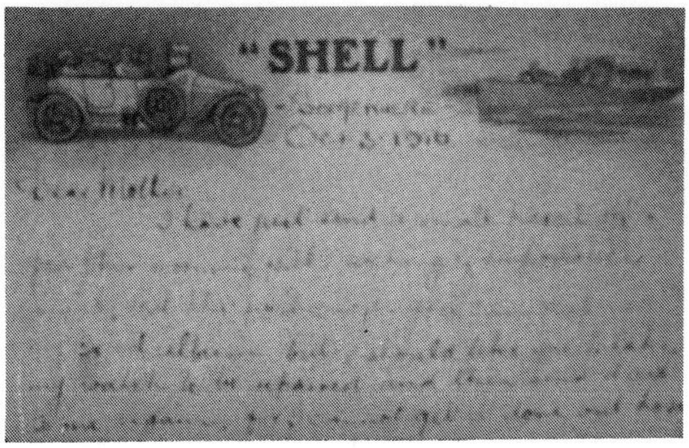

'Shell' postcard October 3rd 1916.

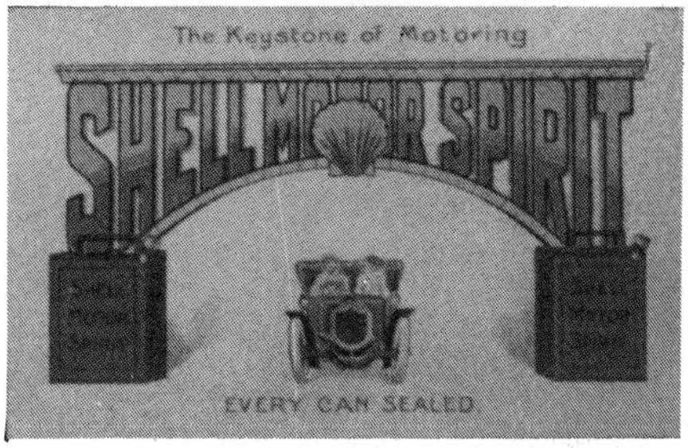

The Keystone of Motoring, Every Can Sealed.

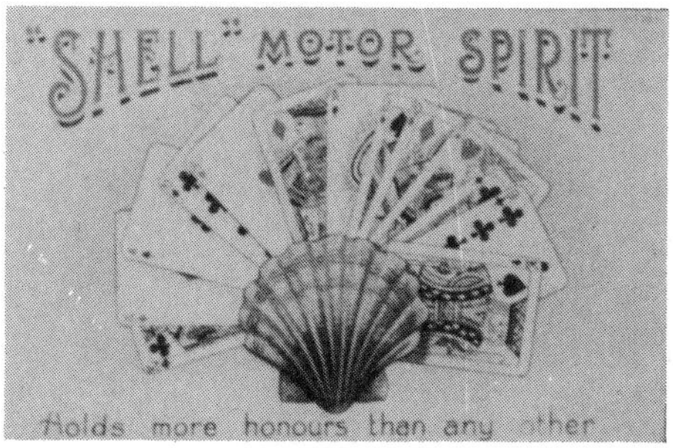

'Shell' Motor Spirit, Holds more honours than any other.

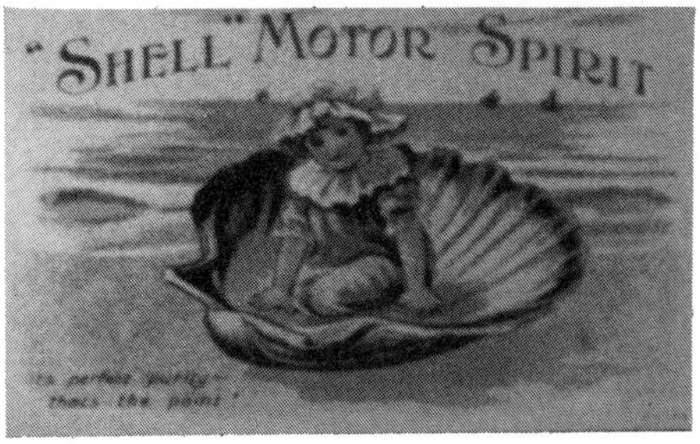

'Shell' Motor Spirit, It's perfect purity – that's the point.

Postcards featuring 'Shell' from 1905 to 1920.   £25 – £35 each

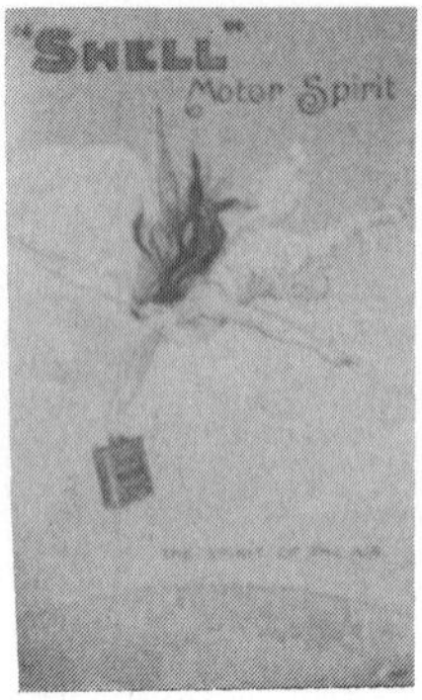

'Shell' Motor Spirit, The Spirit of the Air.

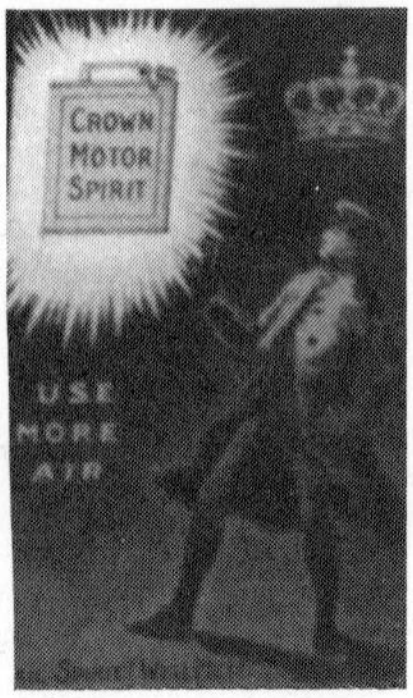

Crown Motor Spirit, Use More Air, Hail Spirit! Well Met!

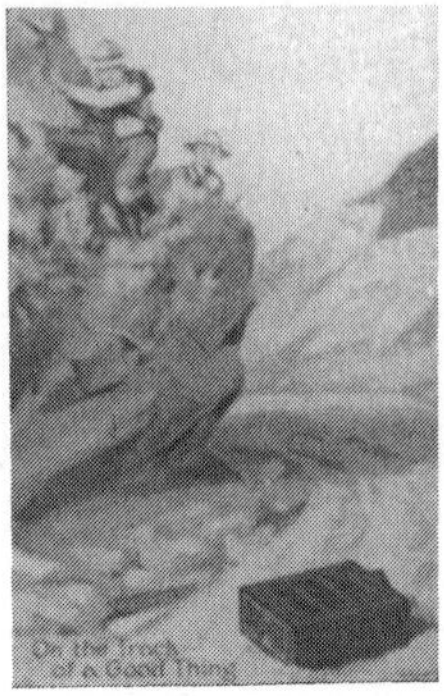

On the Track of a Good Thing.

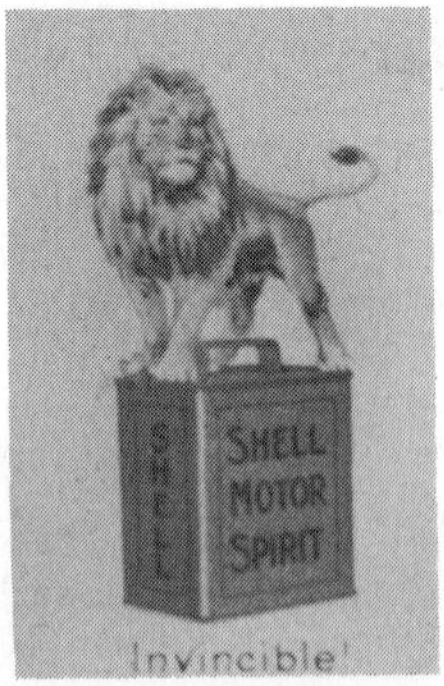

Shell Motor Spirit, 'Invincible'.

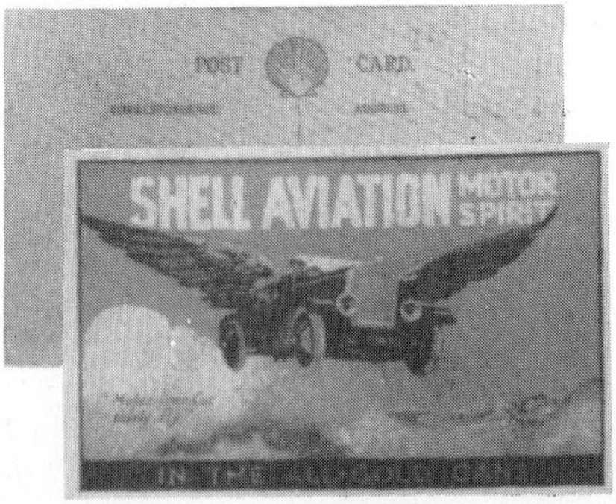

Shell Aviation Motor Spirit, In the All-Gold Cans.

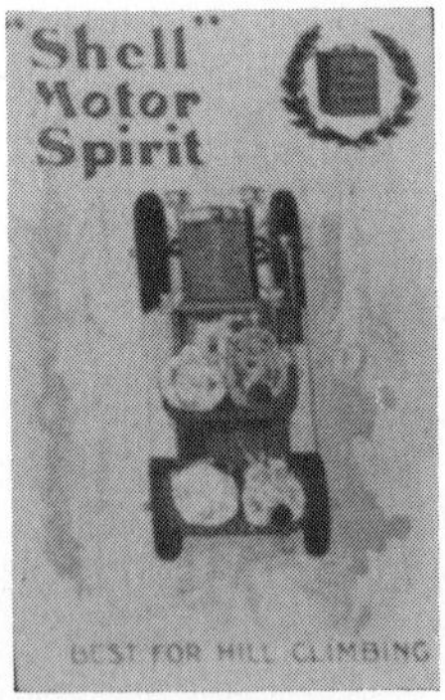

Best for hill climbing, 'Shell' Motor Spirit.

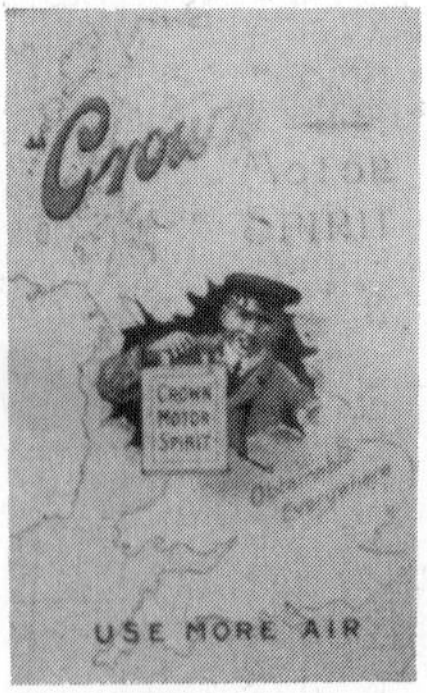

'Crown' Motor Spirit, Obtainable Everywhere.

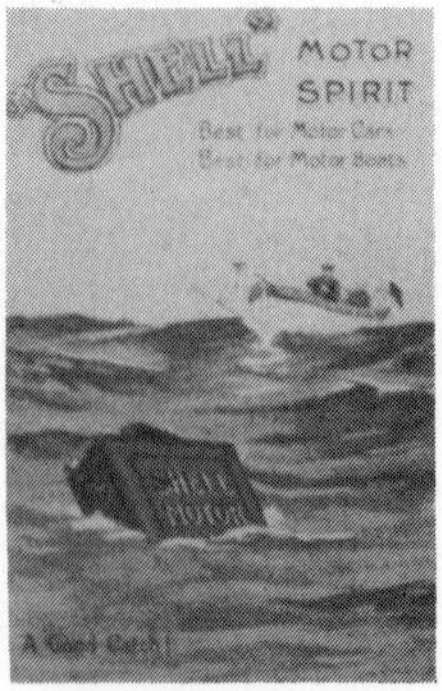

Best for Motor Cars, Best for Motor Boats, 'Shell' Motor Spirit.

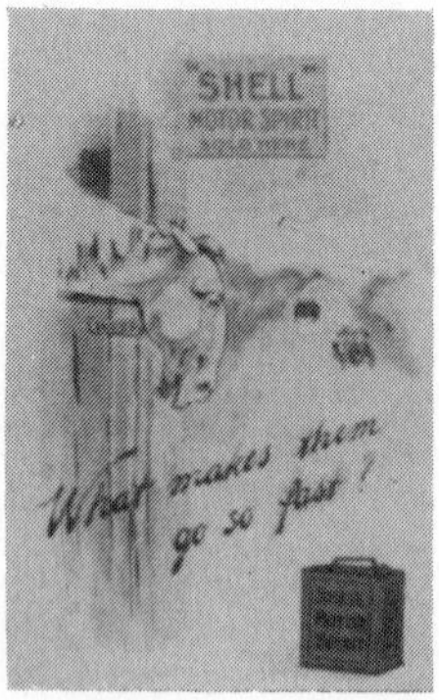

What makes them go so fast? 'Shell' Motor Spirit.

Postcards featuring 'Shell' from 1905 to 1920. *£25 – £35 each*

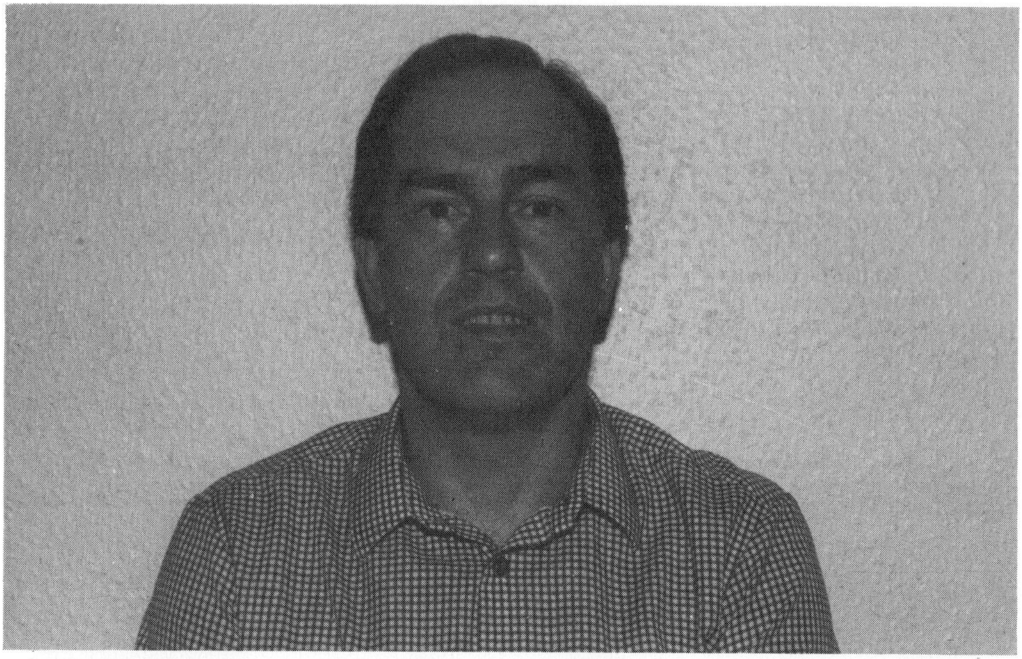

David Ellison, a civil servant, collects Victorian/Edwardian cream pots as well as "dairyana" and ginger beer bottles.

"I have always been fascinated by objects from the past and discovered my first cream pot while excavating a Victorian refuse tip.

"The pots date from the 1880's to the 1920's and were used to hold the cream sold by independent dairies. The interesting ones have printed labels underneath the glaze and some have coloured lips and shoulders in green, blue or brown.

"Most collectors seek examples with attractive printed pictorial labels illustrating milkmaids, dairy scenes, cows or milk churns.

"Cream pots, jars and jugs can be found all over the UK particularly in Scotland and the North of England. They were made by most of the major potteries of the time such as Port Dundas of Glasgow and Price of Bristol. Most were used just once before being thrown away — hence their appearance in old refuse tips."

David has a collection of over 40 pots as well as other dairy artefacts like the illustrated milk pail, butter crocks, pots and dairy invoices.

He feels that collectors should collect what appeals to them which might include those from a particular area or illustrating a particular theme.

Prices range from around £2 for common simple labelled types to over £200 for rare examples with pictorial labels and coloured glazed necks and shoulders.

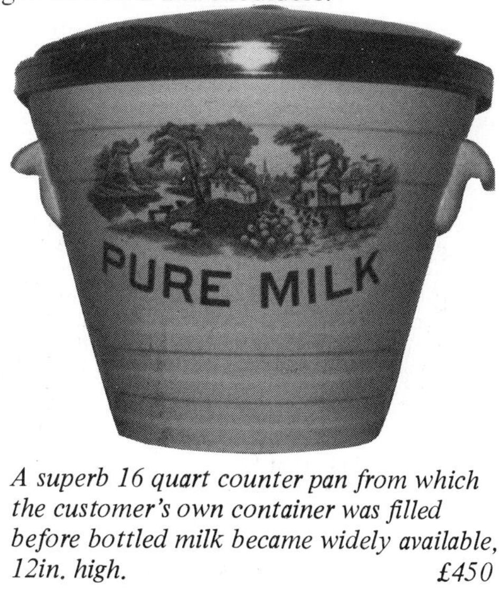

A superb 16 quart counter pan from which the customer's own container was filled before bottled milk became widely available, 12in. high. *£450*

CASH-IN ON COLLECTING

Cream pots, jars and jugs were used between 1880 and the 1920's for vending different forms of the product including "thick", "clotted", "pure" and "thin" cream. Those of particular interest to collectors still retain the original label printed on the pot – either with an inked rubber stamp or a paper transfer taken from an inked engraved copper plate – before application of the glaze. When fired in a kiln the design was absorbed by the clay and protected by the glaze to give it permanence.

These stoneware containers vary in size from 2in. to 6in. but average about 4in. and were usually rendered airtight by inserting a cork or disc in the mouth of the pot and covering it with a tinfoil seal.

The growth of railways coupled with the development of a preservative allowed this perishable product to be transported from farm to table in almost perfect condition.

Though the most satisfying way to acquire one of these pots is to find it whilst digging in a long forgotten refuse tip the less energetic might best be advised to visit a bottle show. Here you will meet other collectors and make useful contacts who will probably know the name and address of your local club secretary.

Other promising hunting grounds include antique shops, flea markets, car-boot sales, bric-a-brac stalls and local auctions.

For further details of this fascinating hobby subscribe to the quarterly magazine 'British Bottle Review' which is available from Alan Blakeman, 2 Strafford Avenue. Elsecar, Barnsley, South Yorkshire, S74 8AA – currently £4 per year.

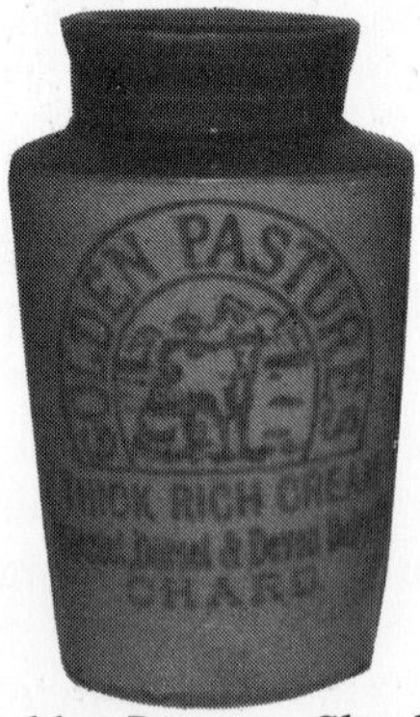

Golden Pastures, Chard, a crudely made pot with blue printed label and blue glazed lip and shoulder. £18 – £25

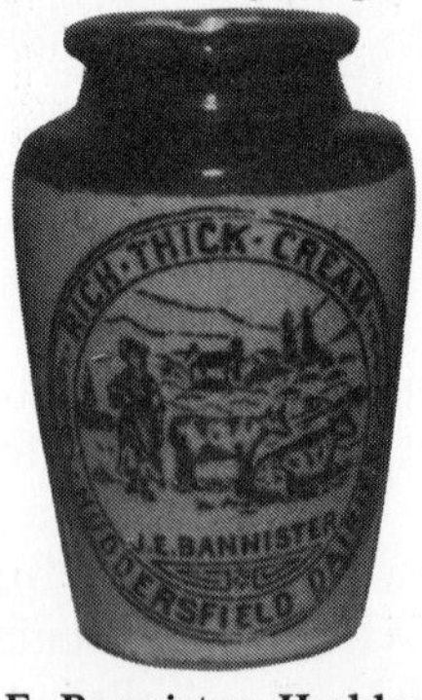

J. E. Bannister, Huddersfield, a cream jug with pouring lip and handle, brown top and black printed label. £15 – £20

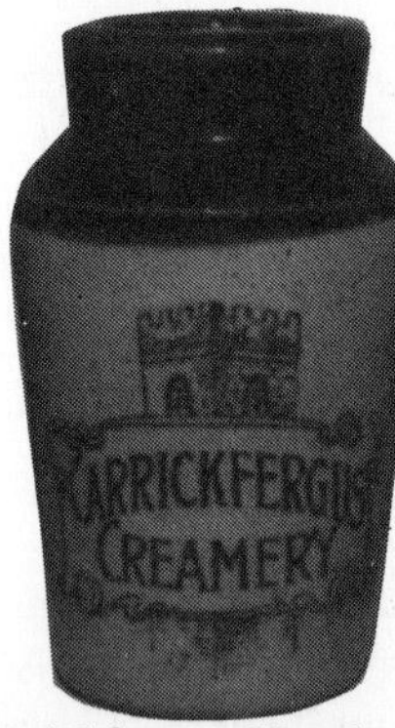

Carrickfergus, Northern Ireland, a rare pot with black label and brown top. £65

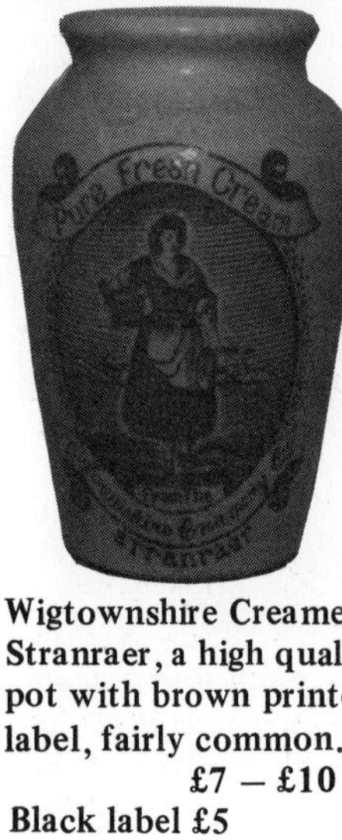

Wigtownshire Creamery, Stranraer, a high quality pot with brown printed label, fairly common. £7 – £10
Black label £5

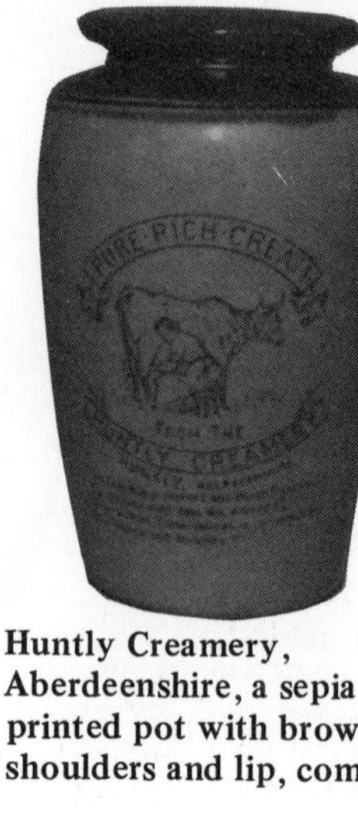

Huntly Creamery, Aberdeenshire, a sepia printed pot with brown shoulders and lip, common. £8

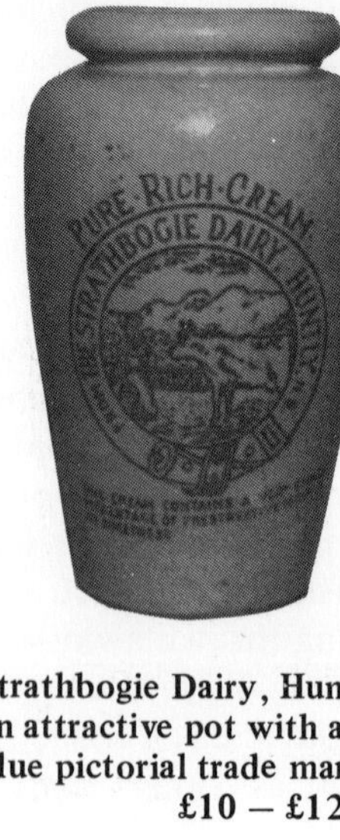

Strathbogie Dairy, Huntly, an attractive pot with a blue pictorial trade mark. £10 – £12

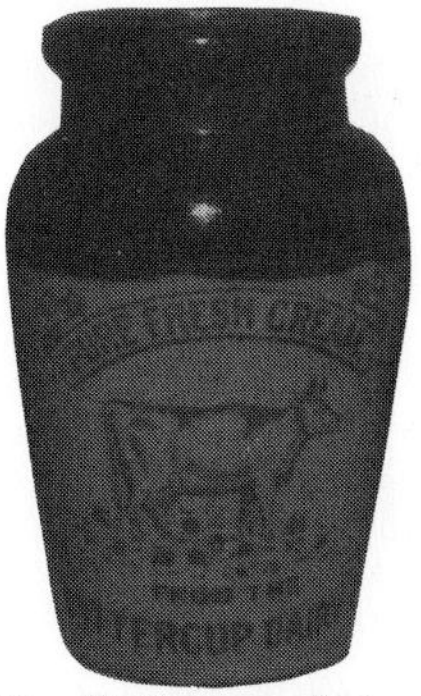

The Buttercup Dairy, Scotland, a fine jar with blue label and cobalt blue lip and shoulders.
£40 – £45

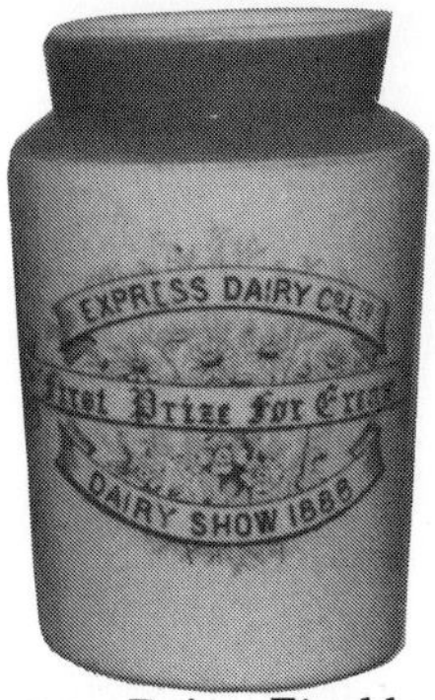

Express Dairy, Finchley, a white earthenware pot with blue top and label. £25 – £35

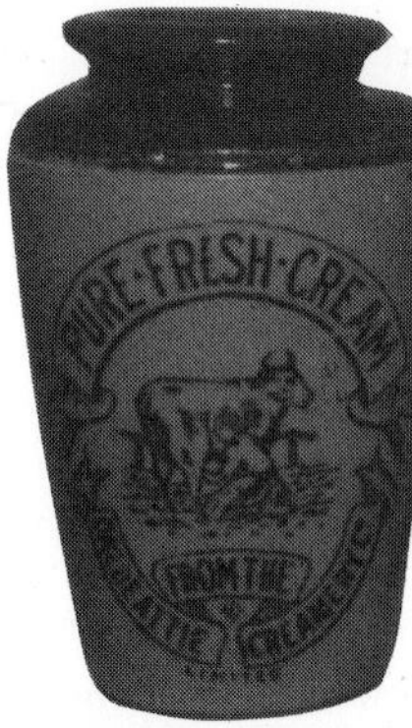

Dalbeattie Creamery, a nice pictorial Scottish pot with black label and brown top.
£35

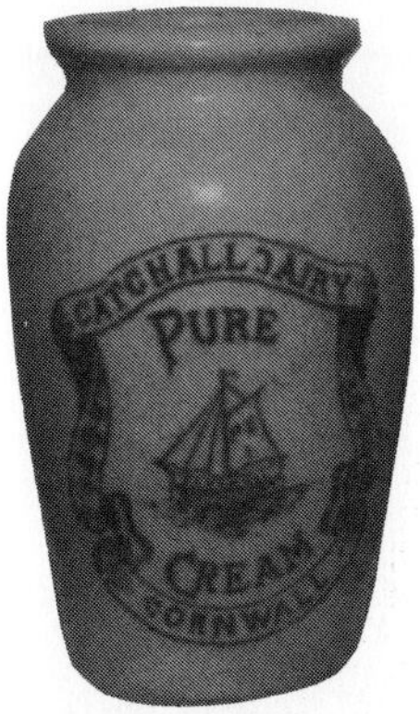

Catchall Dairy, Cornwall, a rare pot made in two sizes with the pottery mark for Kennedy Pottery, Glasgow.
£65 (small) £80 – £100 (large)

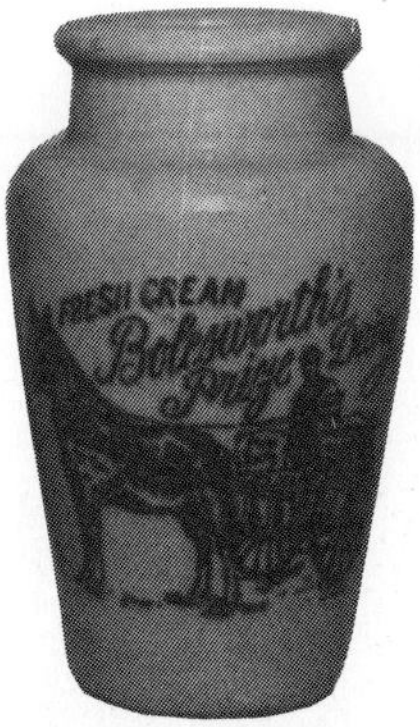

Bolesworth's Prize Dairy, Loughborough, Leicestershire, an extremely rare pot with a striking black label, although there is a slightly less rare example with a green top.
£250 plus (black)
£200 (green)

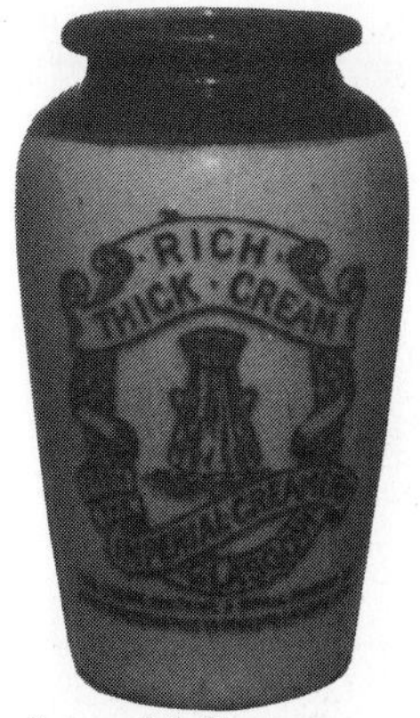

The Imperial Creamery, Glasgow, a rare jar with green glazed top and black label with a pictorial trade mark. £120 – £150

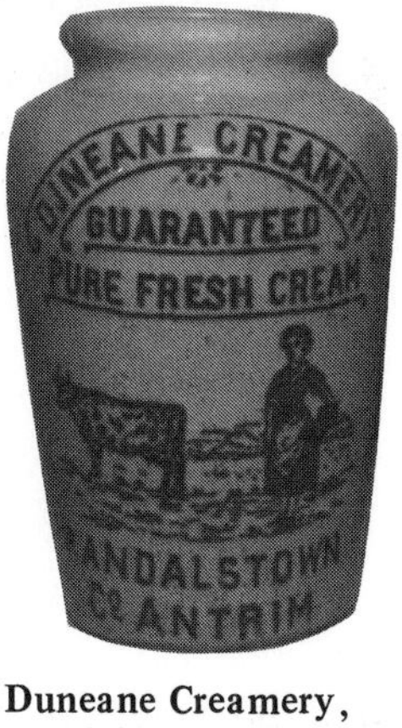

Duneane Creamery, Randalstown, Co. Antrim, a black printed pictorial pot. £25 – £30

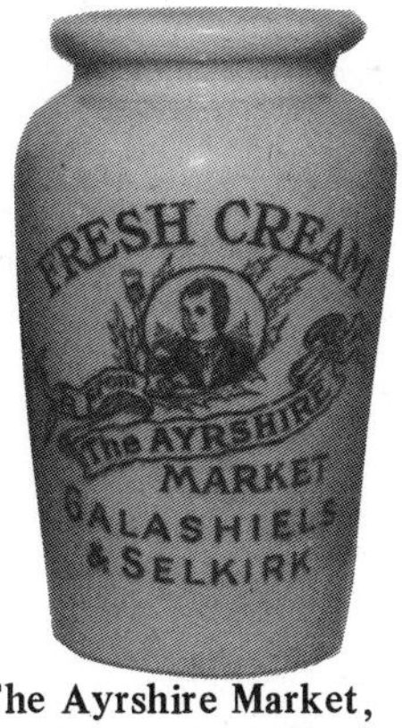

The Ayrshire Market, Galashiels and Selkirk, a grey pot with black printed label of Robbie Burns. £25

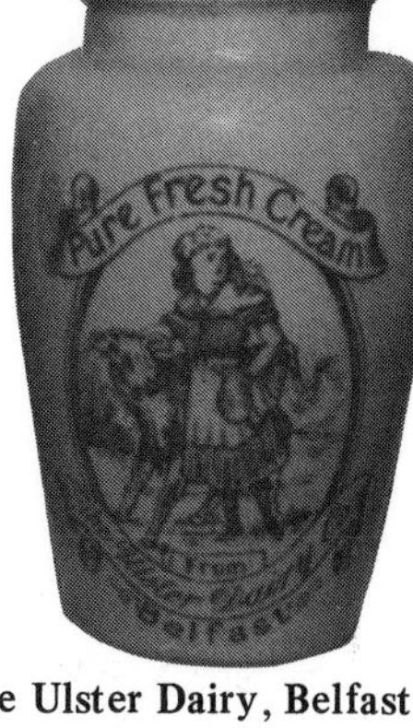

The Ulster Dairy, Belfast, an attractive and desirable pot with sharp sepia pictorial label and high glaze.
£100

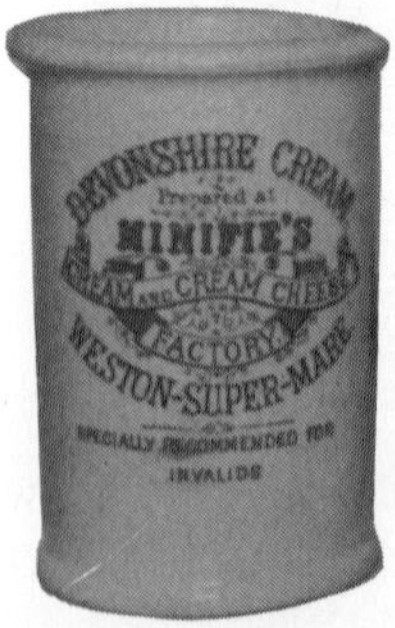

Minifie's, Weston-Super-Mare, a small cylindrical white pot made by C. T. Maling, Newcastle, 3¼in. high. £40 – £60

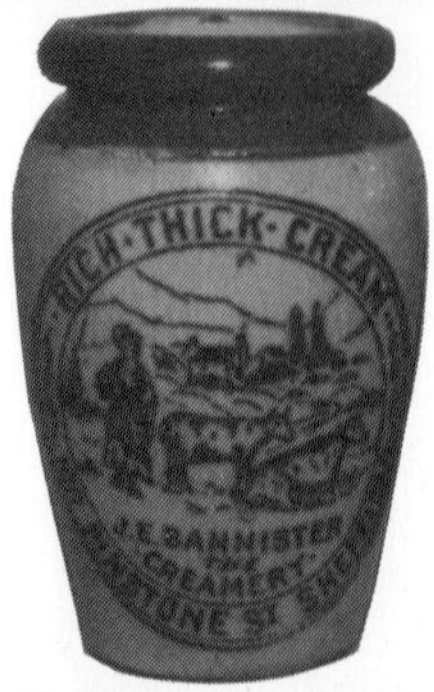

J. E. Bannister, Sheffield, an extremely rare pot with a green glazed lip and shoulder as opposed to the normal brown. £175

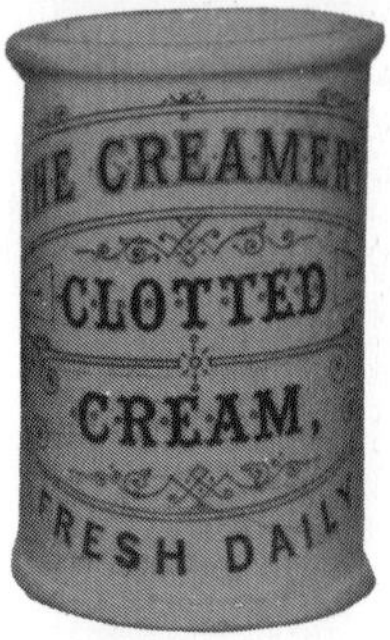

The Creamery, a small white cylindrical pot with black printed label, 3¼in. high. £40 – £60

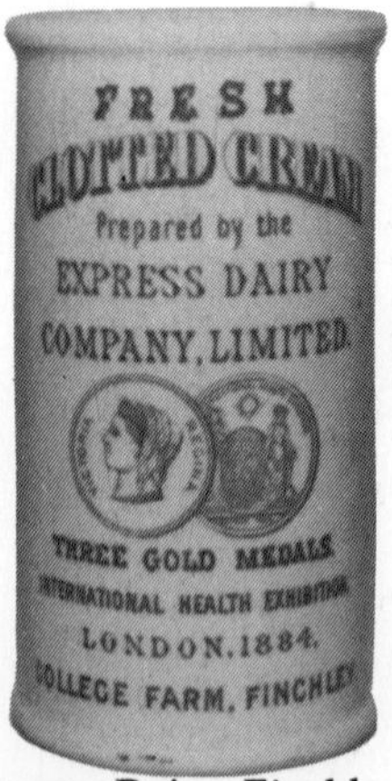

Express Dairy, Finchley, a white earthenware pot with dark blue label. Cylindrically shaped pots were tradtionally used for clotted cream. £115 – £140

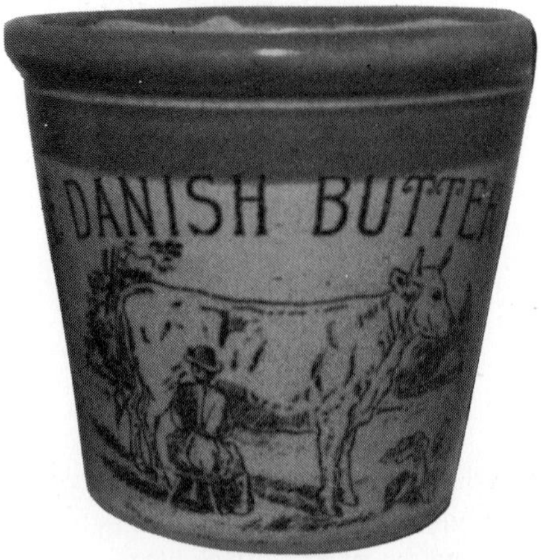

An attractive butter crock manufactured by The Caledonian Pottery, Rutherglen, 5in. high. £150

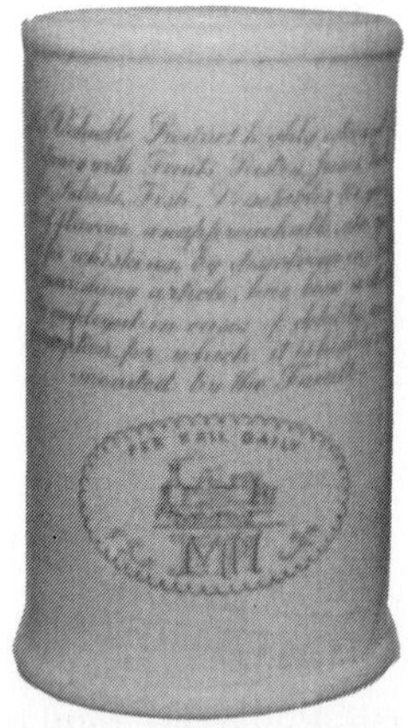

A mauve printed white pot thought to be an early version of Harris's Original Clotted Cream, 5in. high, circa 1880. £65

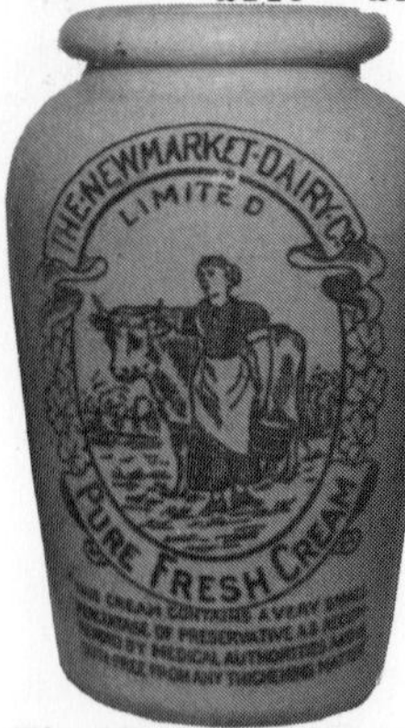

The Newmarket Dairy Co., a rare Irish pot with fine transfer printed label. £80 – £100

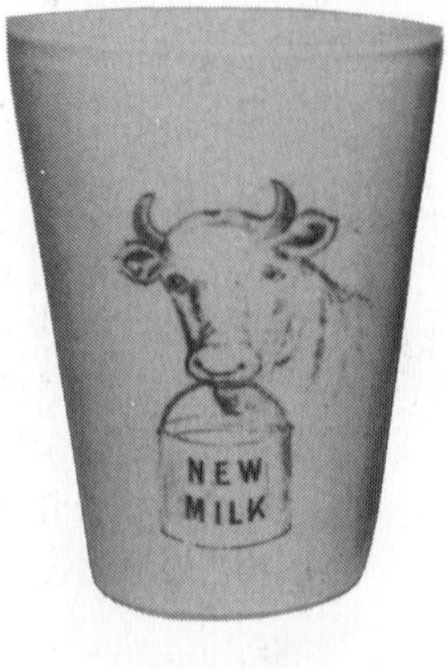

Promotional beaker from The Dairy Supply Co., 4in. high. £45

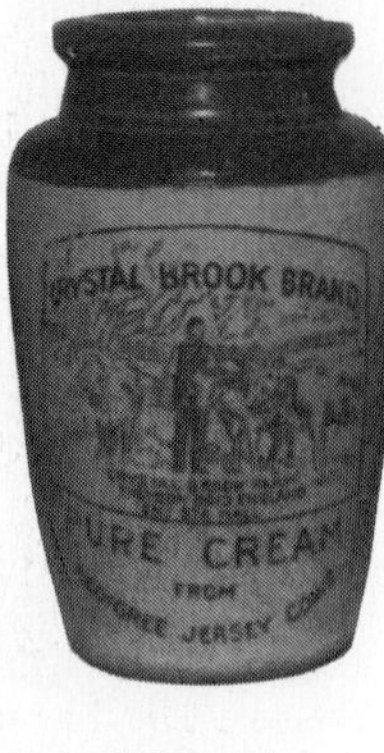

Crystal Brook Brand, Theydon Bois, a rare pot with green top and label. £80 – £100

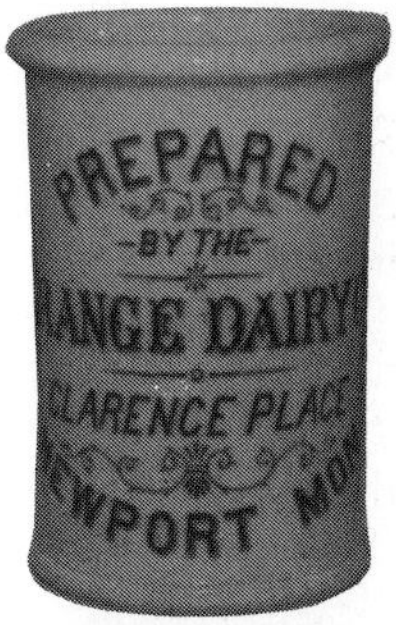

A small cylindrical Welsh pot in white with black printed label, 3¼in. high. £40 – £60

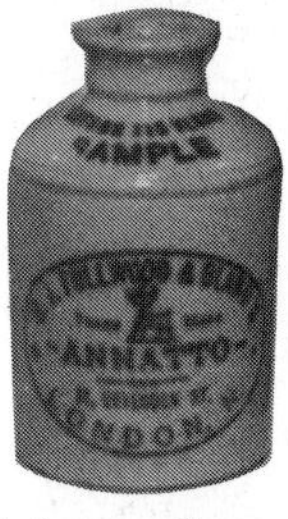

A miniature flagon which contained a free sample of Fullwoods Annatto, a colouring agent for butter, 2½in. high. £30

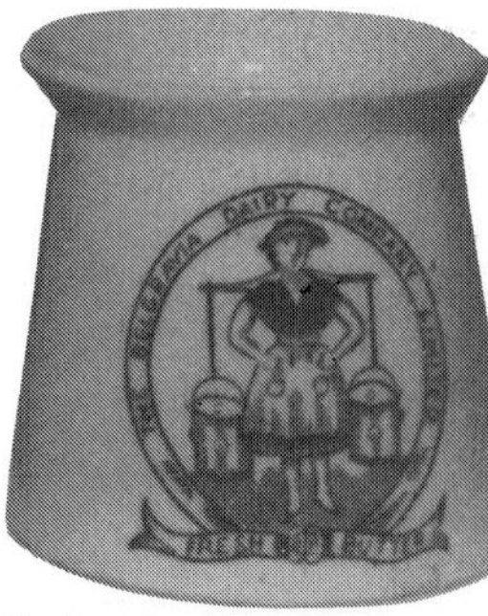

Belgravia Dairy butter pot made by Belleek Pottery, Fermanagh, N. Ireland, with green transfer printed label, post 1890, 2¼in. high. £165

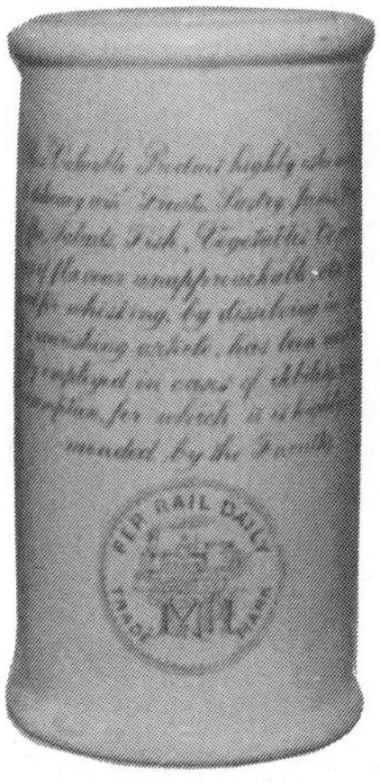

Harris's Original Clotted Cream, Devon, a cylindrical white pot with mauve printed label, 5in. high, circa 1880. £50

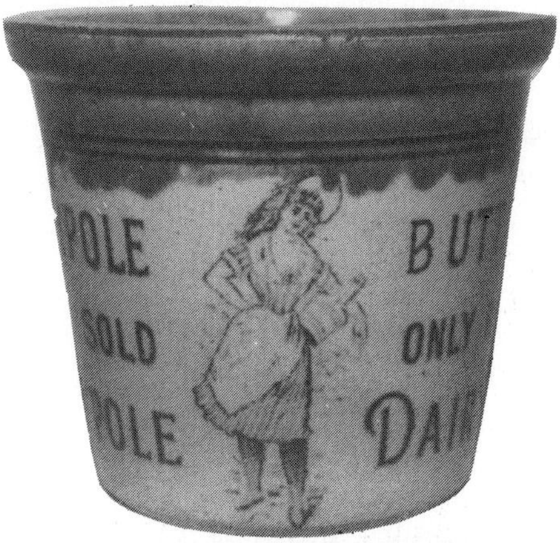

Maybole butter crock for transporting butter in the same way as cream. This rare example in grey stoneware has a tan coloured glazed top and black printed label, made by The Port Dundas Pottery, Glasgow, 5in. high. £150

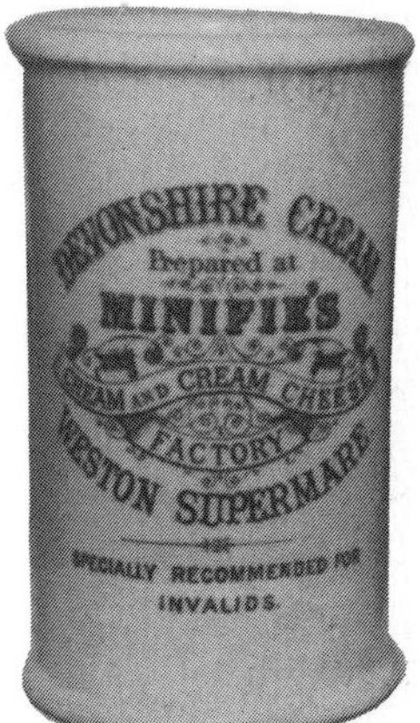

Minifie's, Weston-Super-Mare, a cylindrical white pot with black transfer, 5in. high. £60

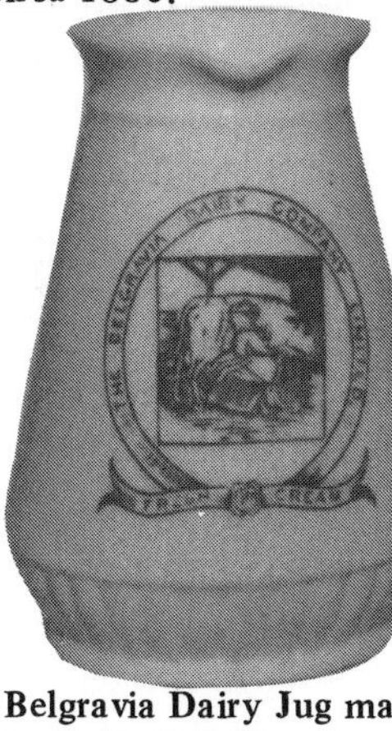

Belgravia Dairy Jug made by Belleek Pottery, Fermanagh, Northern Ireland, with green label 1880 – 1890. £80

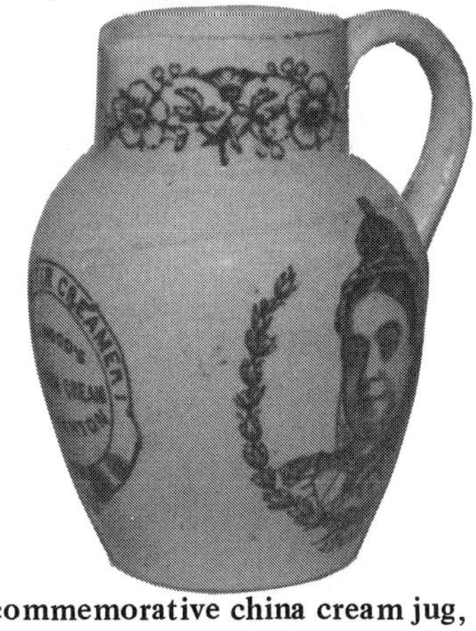

A commemorative china cream jug, by Hailwood's, made for Queen Victoria's Royal Jubilee Exhibition, Old Trafford, Manchester, 1887, with black label. £150

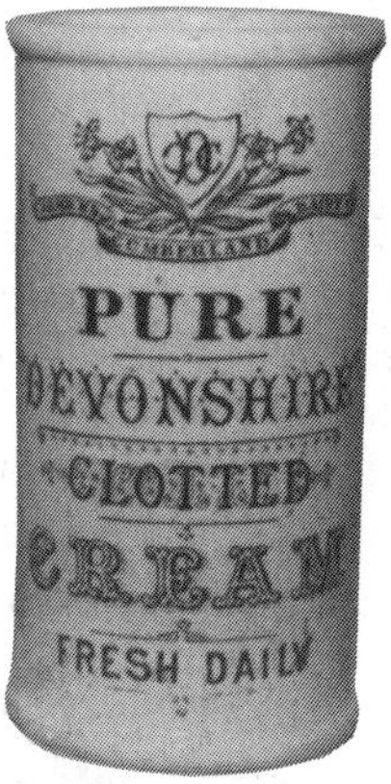

Carrick's Dairy, Cumberland, a cylindrical white pot with black label, 5in. high. £100

Tonie and Valmai Holt run a Battlefields Tour Company taking parties to sites of historical military interest in Europe, North Africa and the USA. They are also leading authorities on picture postcards which they collect and write about. Their special interest is the work of Bruce Bairnsfather.

Tonie Holt said: "Bruce Bairnsfather came into our lives almost by mistake because while we were researching for our book 'When The Boys Come Home' on the First World War depicted through postcards, the importance of Bairnfather's cartoons in raising the morale of the troops became very obvious. There was very little known about him however and my wife Valmai and I started to piece together fragments of information about his life.

"Valmai used to teach history and I was at Sandhurst and in the Army so our previous experience helped us a lot in our researches. Bairnsfather took over our lives for four years and we found links in the chain of his story in places as far apart as the British Legion Club in Colwall and the Library of Congress in Washington. He was a most interesting and complex man and finally we wrote our book about him "In Search of the Better 'Ole'. I think it was a help that a husband and wife team could assess Bairnsfather from both a male and a female, a military and a civilian point of view."

Bairnsfather created 'Old Bill', the best known cartoon character of the First World War, and he was the first officially appointed British Officer Cartoonist. His work appeared on playing cards, postcards, jig saw puzzles, plates, cups, mugs, car mascots and ashtrays. The Holts have collected the whole series of 48 postcards by him entitled 'Fragments From France' with the help of their son Gareth but they say that the Bairnsfather spectrum is so large that they do not expect ever to fully complete their collection — there will always be something they are looking for.

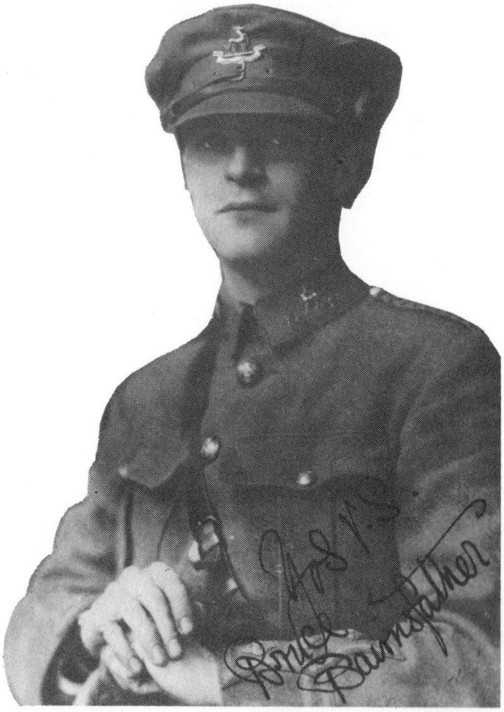

Captain Bruce Bairnsfather

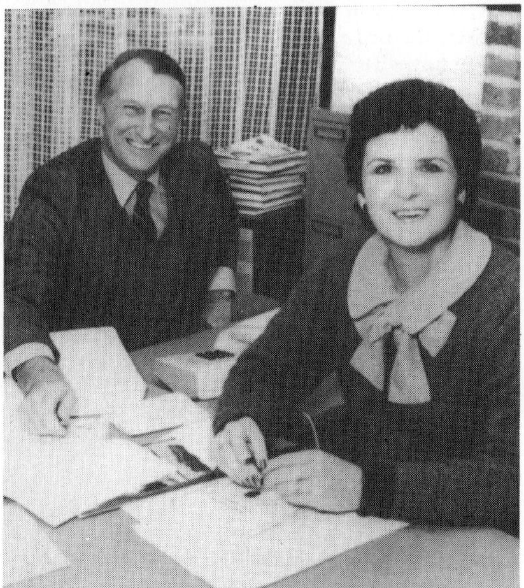

Tonie and Valmai Holt

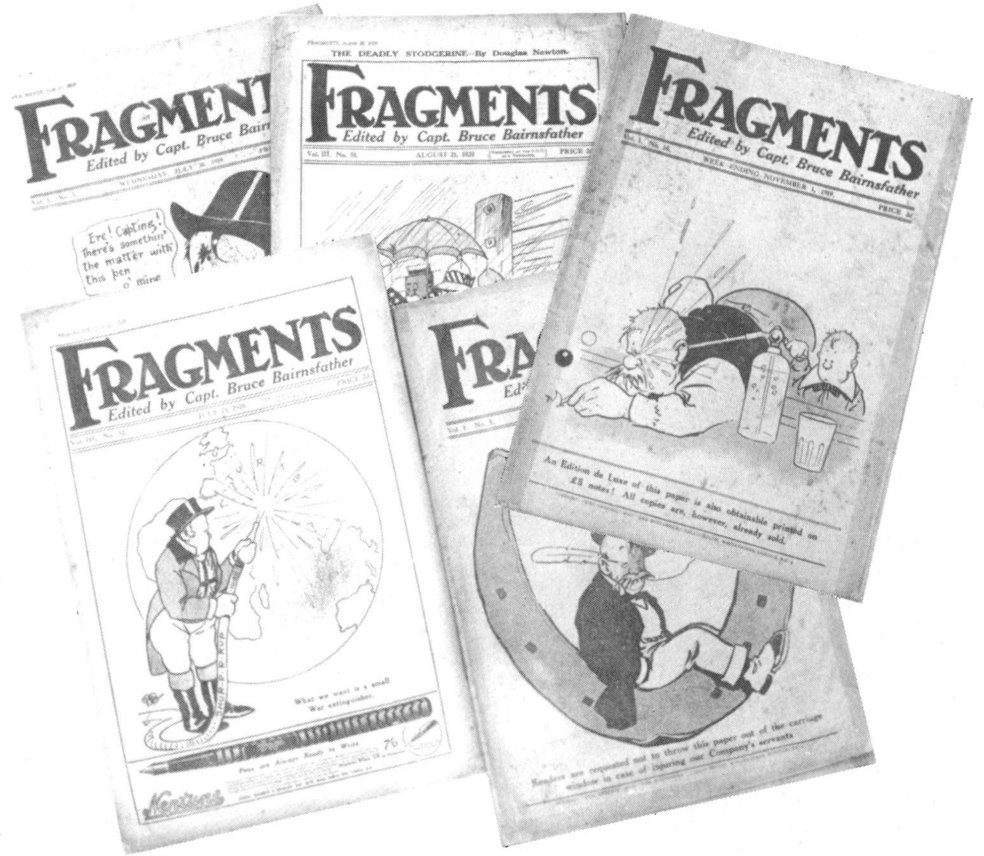

'Fragments' magazines edited by Bruce Bairnsfather. £5 – £10

Bruce Bairnsfather was the war artist who created the famous cartoon character 'Old Bill'. The long-suffering archetypal 'Tommy' of World War I. During and after the war, a vast range of 'Bairnsfather ware' was produced.
These wares fall into seven main categories:

Original paintings, drawings, sketches and letters by Bairnsfather.

Pottery items bearing 'Fragments from France' cartoons and models of Old Bill's head.

Bystander Products. Original 'Fragments from France' cartoons, postcards, (there are fifty-six available in a complete set), jigsaws and prints.

Metal ware. Car Mascots of Old Bill, ash trays, etc.

Theatre and Cinema ephemera including posters, advertising postcards, magazines and photographs of the various plays and films made about Old Bill or by Bairnsfather.

Books and Magazines about or by Bairnsfather.

Miscellaneous: dolls, hankies, badges, glass slides.

The market is still in its infancy and these wares are currently largely overlooked and inexpensive. A boost to the market is assured, however, by publication of the first priced and illustrated catalogue to Bairnsfather ware 'In Search of the Better 'Ole', (Milestone Publications, 62 Murray Road, Horndean, Hampshire PO8 9JL). £11.95

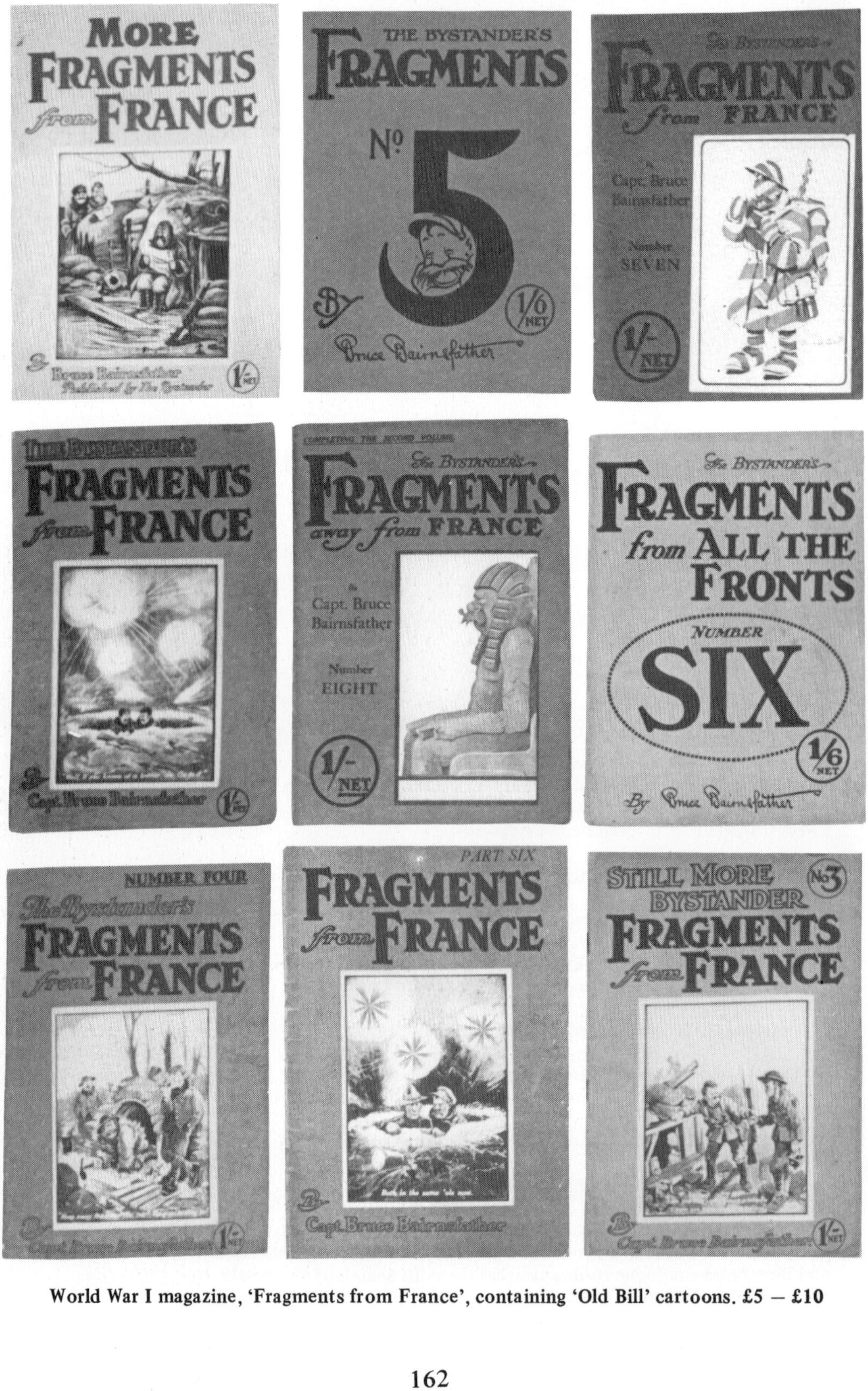

World War I magazine, 'Fragments from France', containing 'Old Bill' cartoons. £5 – £10

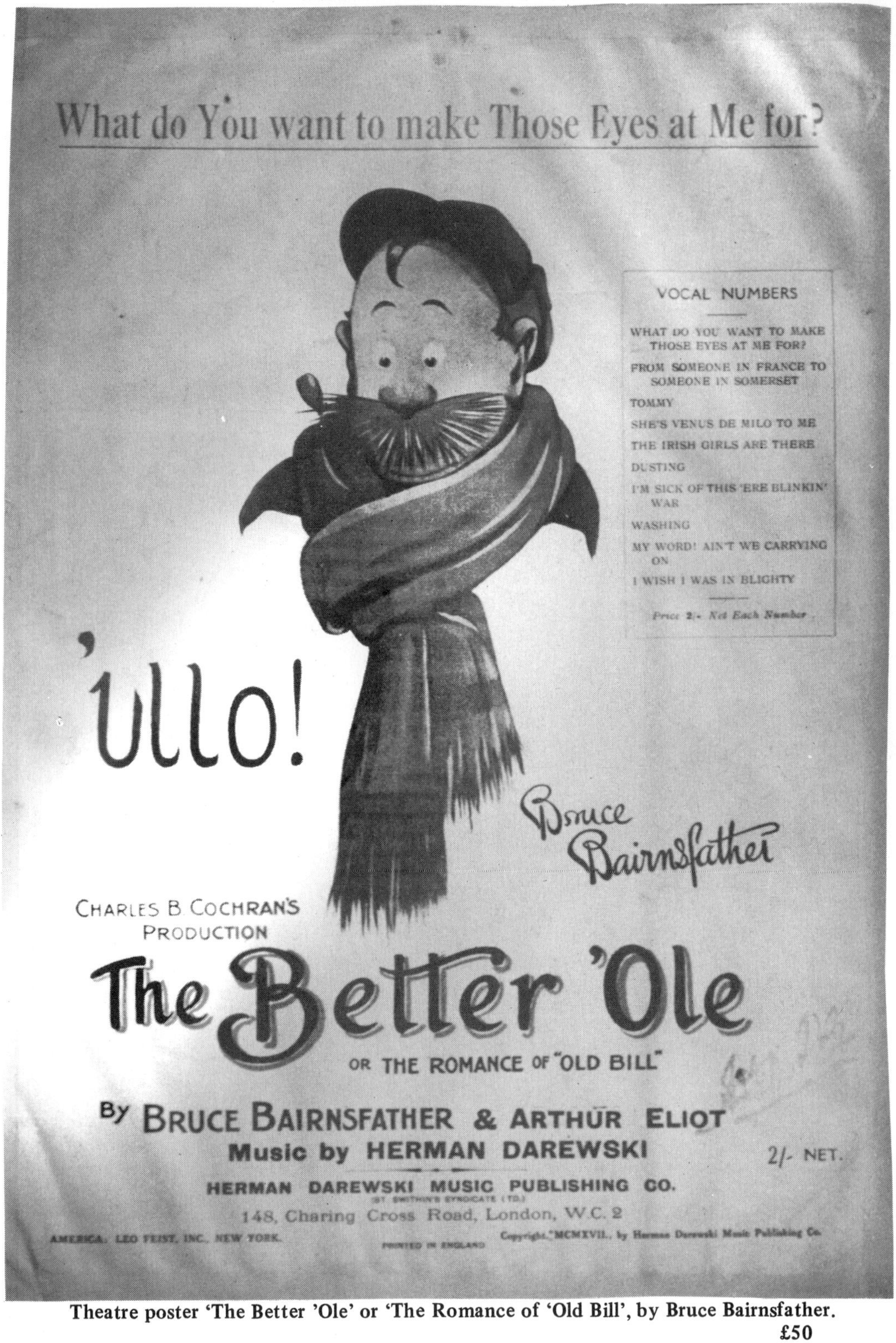

Theatre poster 'The Better 'Ole' or 'The Romance of 'Old Bill', by Bruce Bairnsfather.
£50

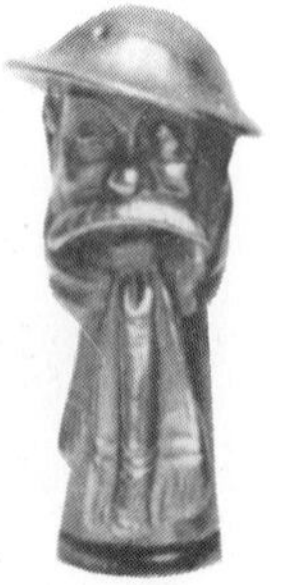

A small 'Old Bill' brass motor cycle mascot. £100

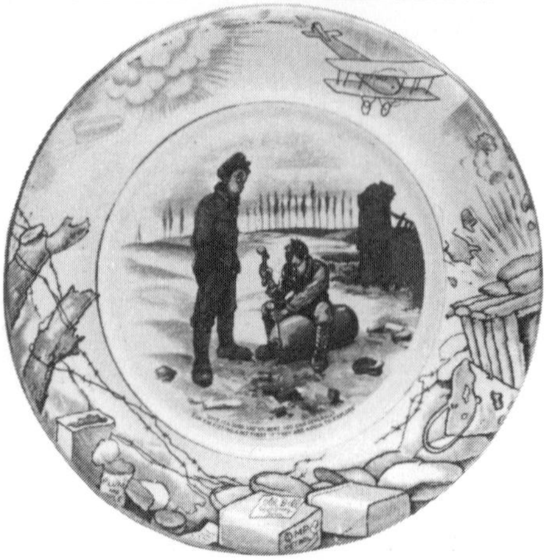

Grimwade plate 'Give it a good 'ard 'un Bert, you can generally 'ear 'em fizzing a bit first if they are agoin to explode!' £40

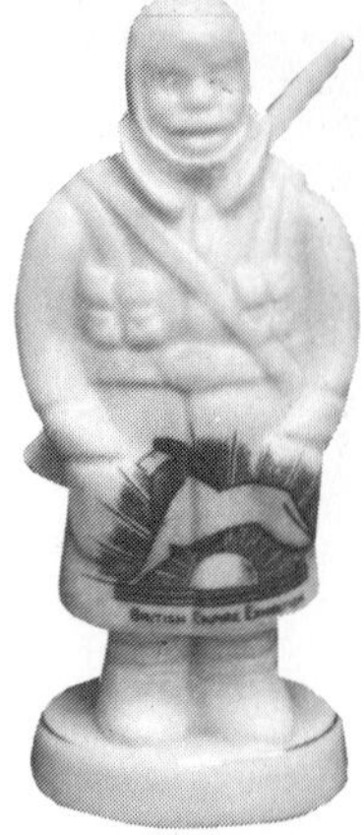

Carlton ware standing figure of 'Old Bill', 'British Empire Exhibition'. £75

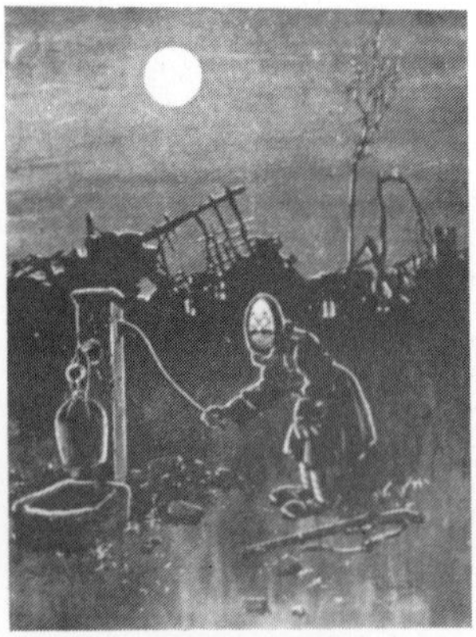

Glass slide 'The Fatalist', 'I'm sure they'll 'ear this damn thing squeakin'. £5

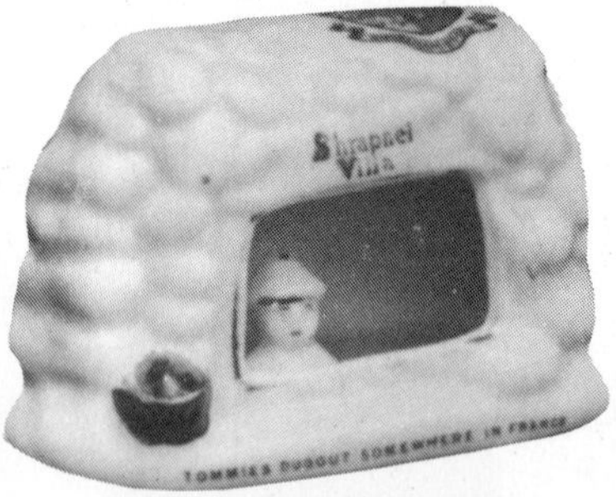

Carlton ware 'Shrapnel Villa', 'Tommies Dugout Somewhere in France!' £30

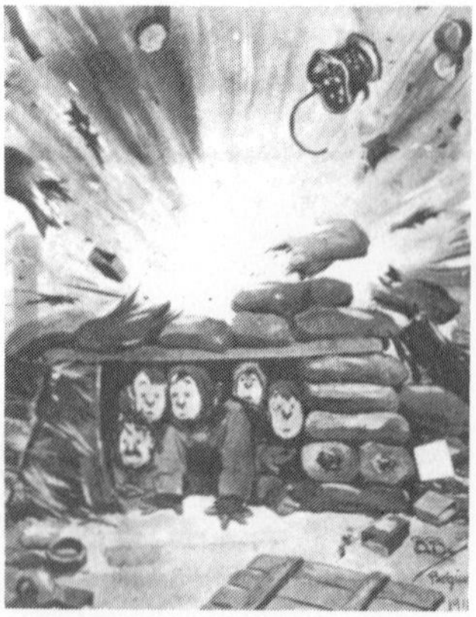

Glass slide 'Where did that one go to?' £5

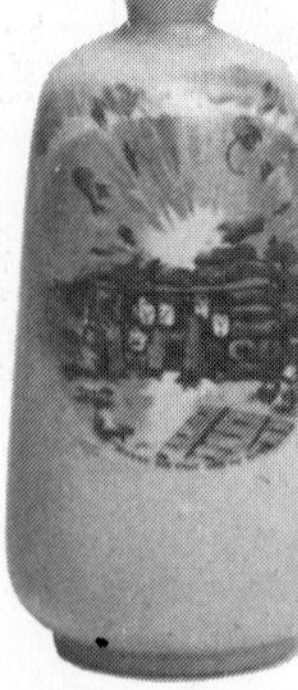

Small shouldered Grimwade vase, 'Where did that one go?' £40

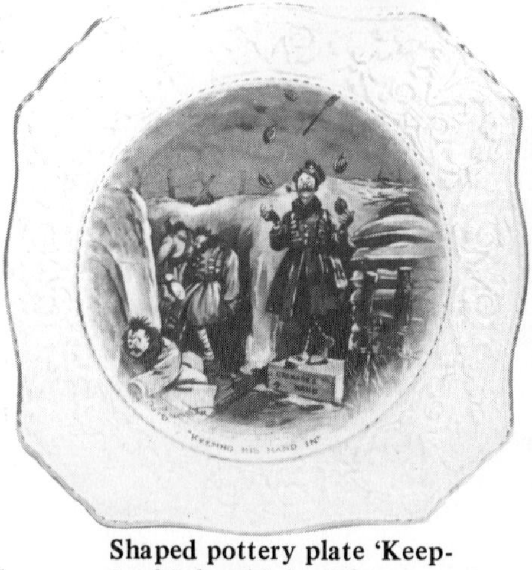

Shaped pottery plate 'Keeping his hand in', with a decorative border in relief. £35

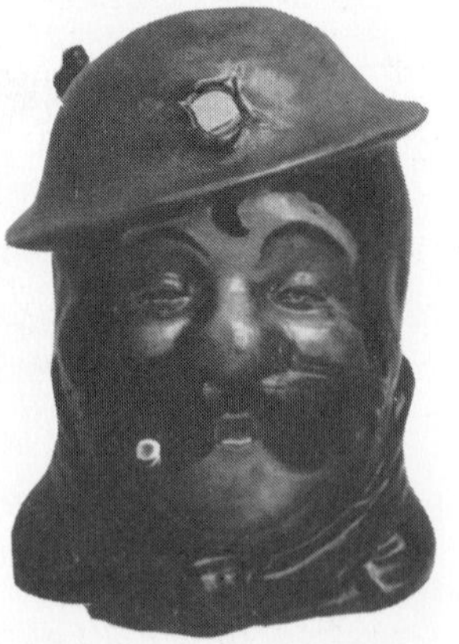

'Old Bill' coloured pottery head. £45

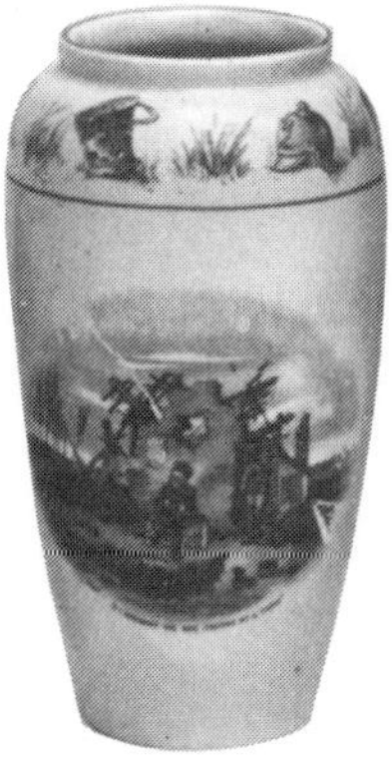

Grimwade vase depicting 'Old Bill', 'At present we are staying at a farm'. £40

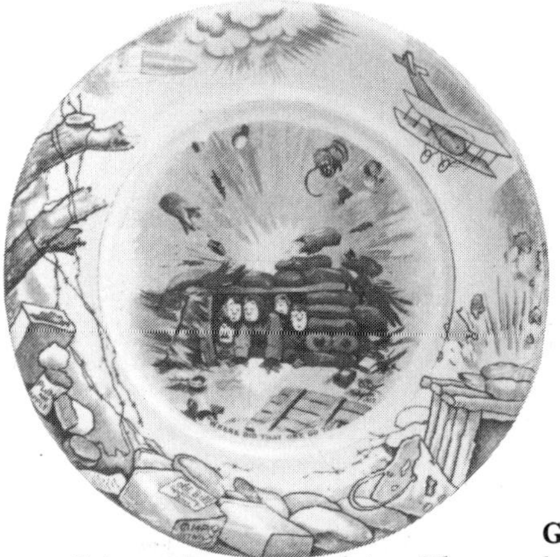

Grimwade pottery plate with decorative edging 'Where did that one go to?' £40

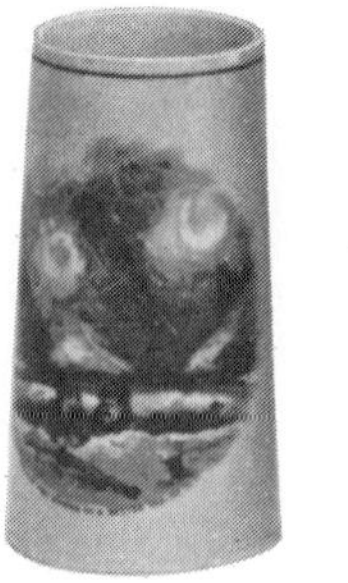

Grimwade vase 'Well if you knows of a better 'ole, go to it'. £40

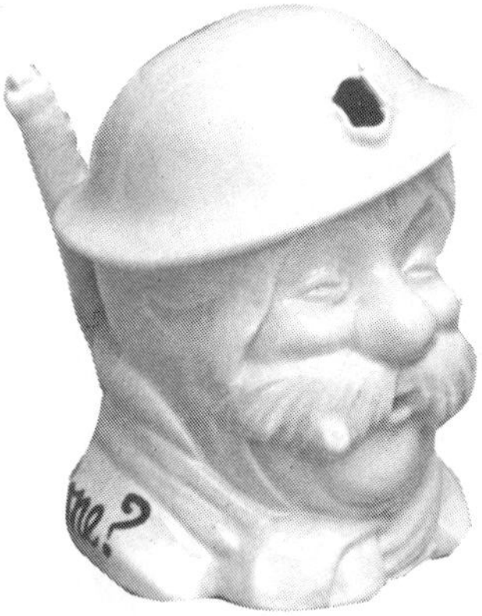

'Old Bill' pottery head in white. £40

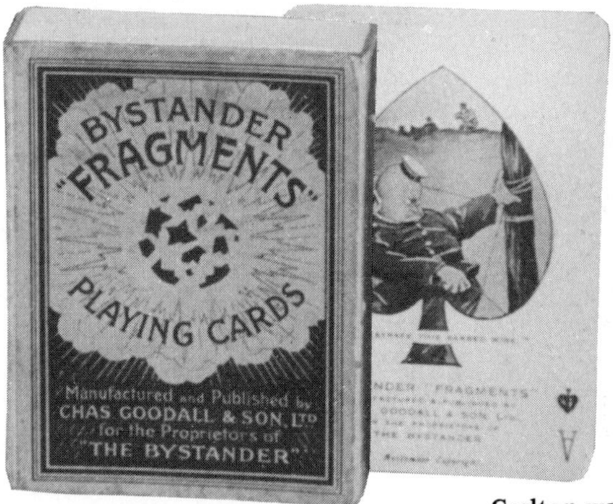

Bystander 'Fragments' Playing Cards, by Chas. Goodall & Son Ltd. £25

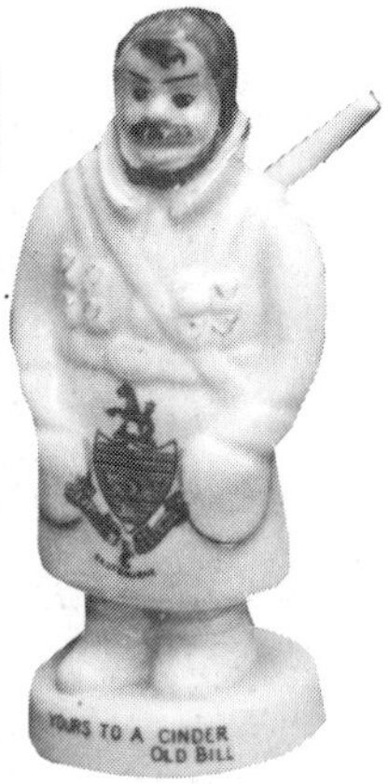

Carlton ware standing figure of 'Old Bill', with coloured face and balaclava, 'Yours to a cinder Old Bill'. £95

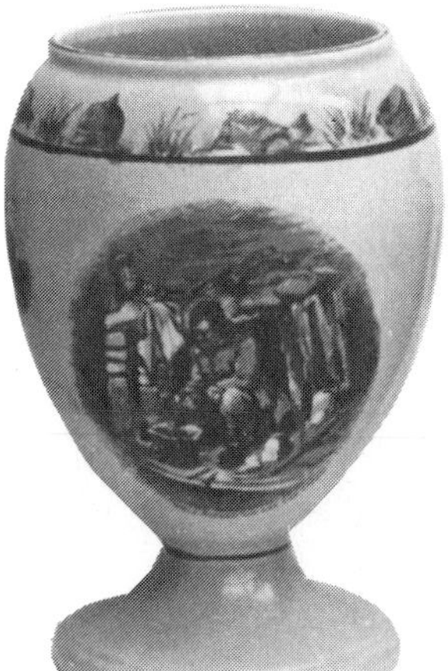

Grimwade vase 'Well Alfred, 'ow are the cakes'. £50

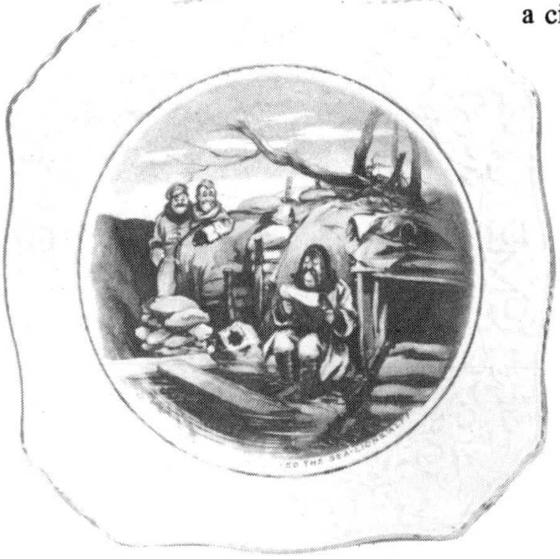

Shaped pottery plate with decorative border in relief 'What time do they feed the sea lions Alf?' £35

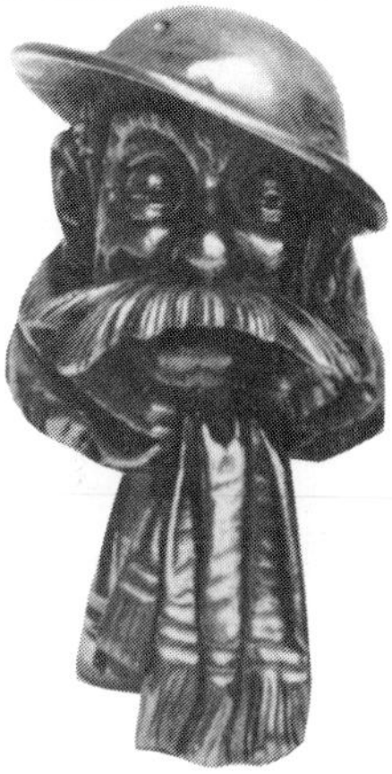

'Old Bill' brass car mascot. £100

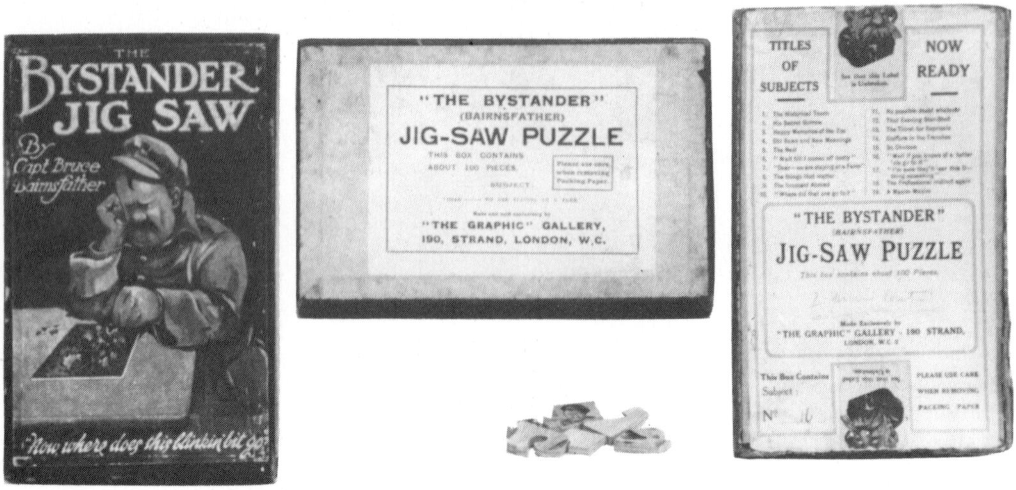

The Bystander Jigsaw Puzzle, 'Now where does this blinkin bit go'. £30

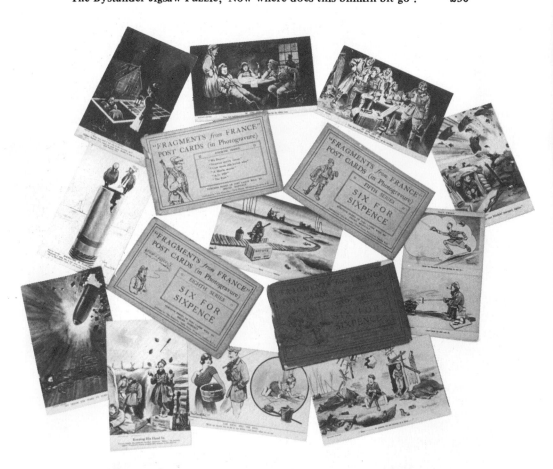

A selection of Bruce Bairnsfather postcards – £2 each. Sets of six in special envelopes £15

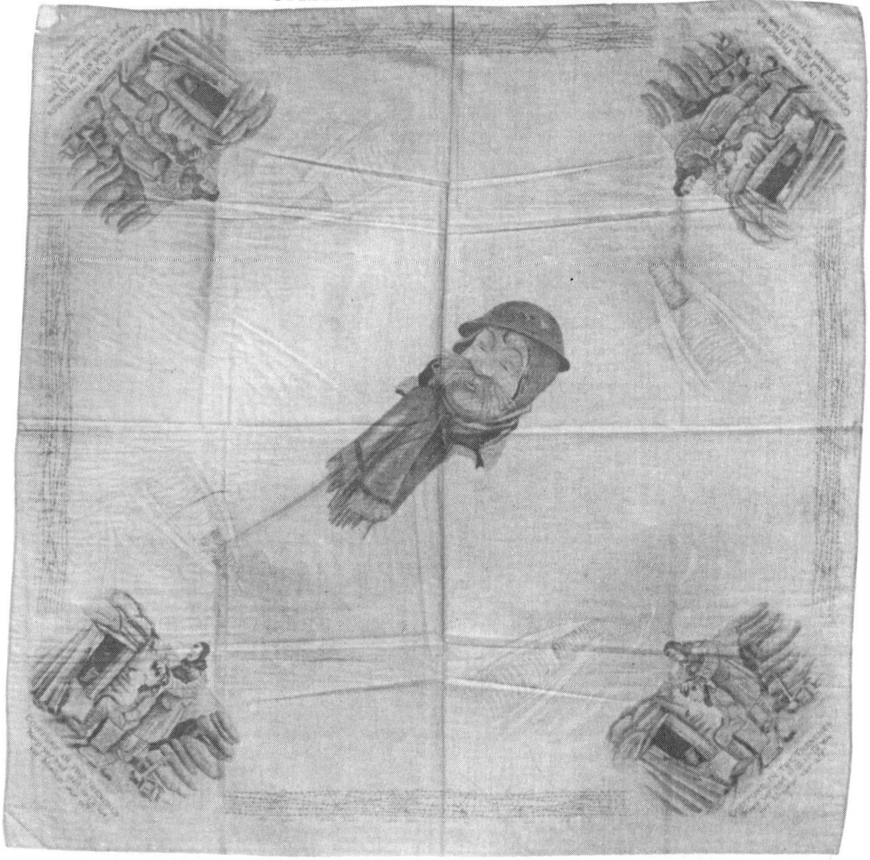

'Old Bill', lady's headscarf, 'Coiffure in the Trenches, Keep Yer 'ead Still or I'll Have Your Blinkin 'ear Off'. £20

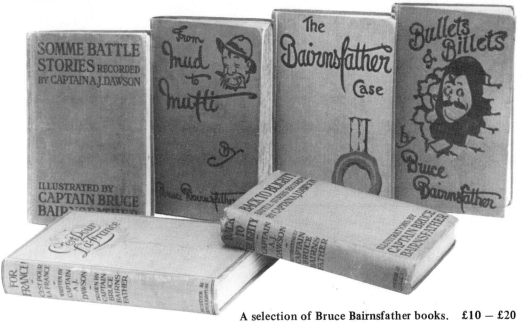

A selection of Bruce Bairnsfather books. £10 – £20

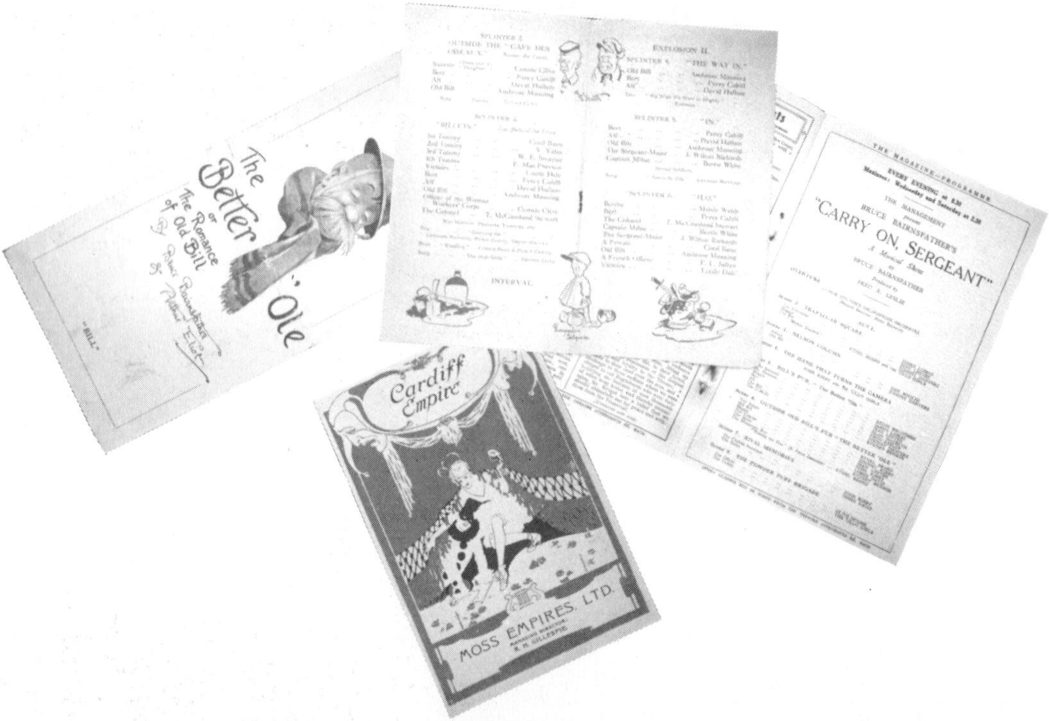

Bruce Bairnsfather theatre programmes. £20

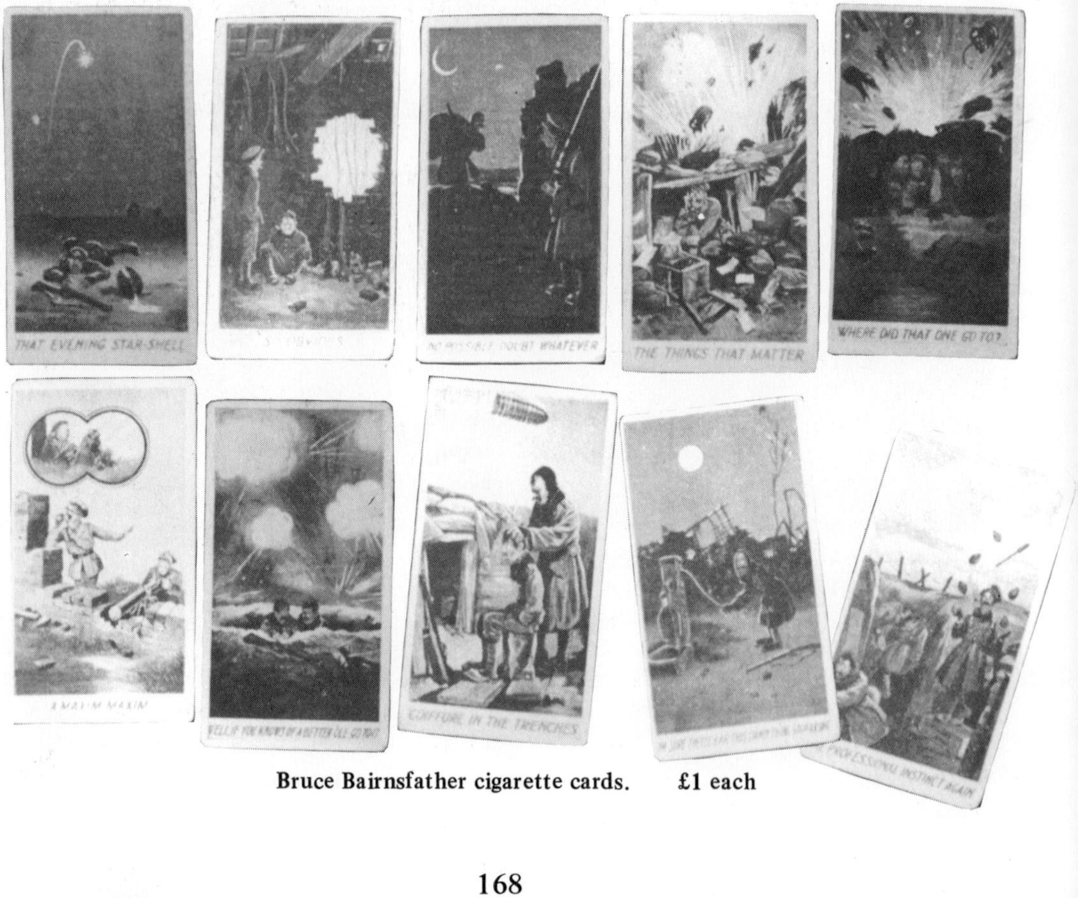

Bruce Bairnsfather cigarette cards. £1 each

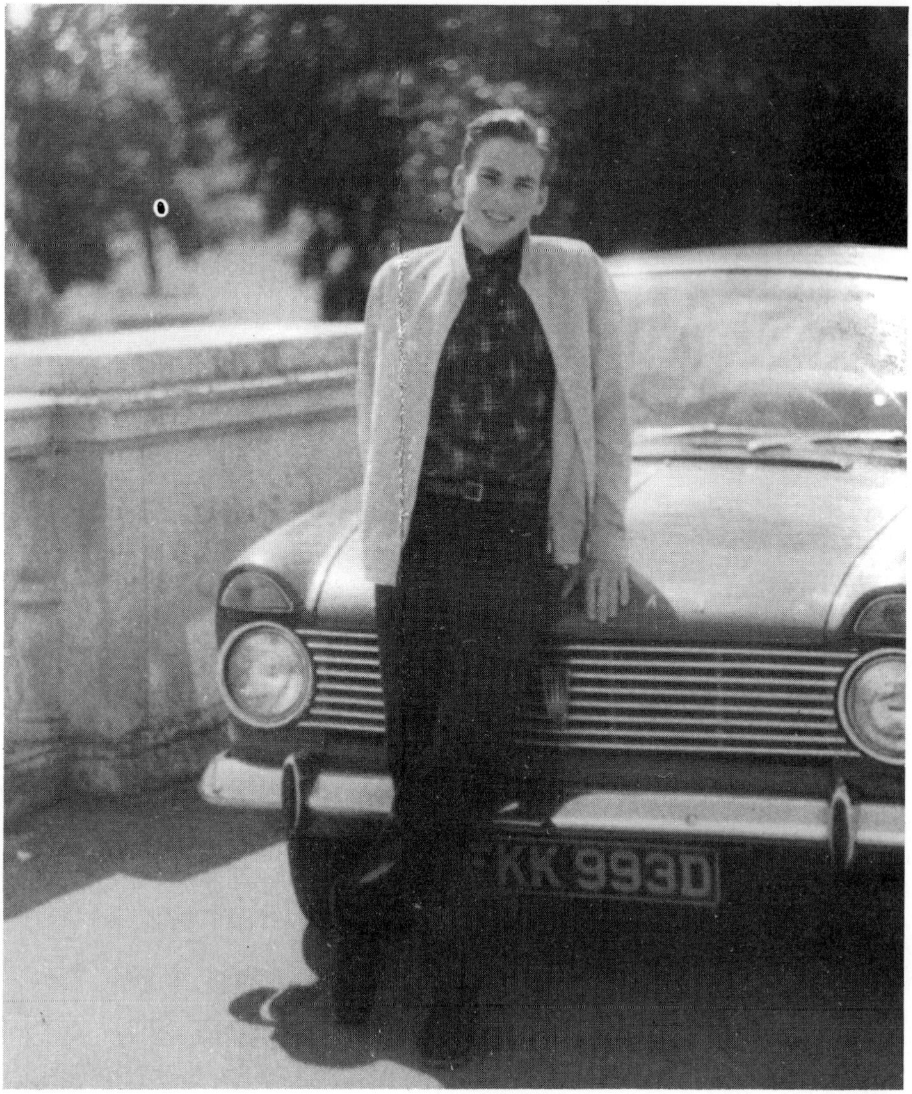

Nigel Morter deals in antiques and collects models of Jaguar cars.

"I collect Jaguar models because that's the car I'd like to be able to drive and can't afford yet. It began about four years ago and I've got 150 different ones, all diecast models. The Jaguar car first came out in 1935 and I've got all the early models but not all subsequent models have been diecast. Dinky started making them in 1946 and I've also got models by Spot On, Corgi, Matchbox and also in white metal made by smaller companies like Bellini, Mark 43 and Western Models . . . these are of very high quality. I haven't got a favourite however because I like them all, they're very decorative."

White metal models range in price from £35 to £200 but the price of Dinky Jaguars rises from £10 to £100 according to the scarcity of the model. For other makes of cars Dinky prices can go up to £500 but Jaguars are not so pricy because they were made in larger quantities than many other marques.

Nigel wants to find a Spot On Jaguar XKSS from around 1962. It should cost him around £70.

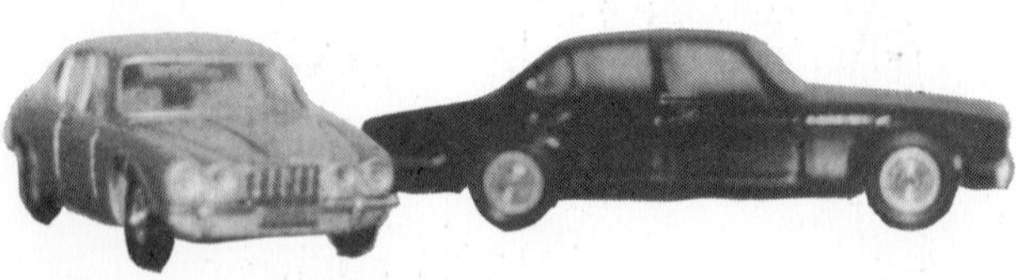

Solido XJ12's, now ceased production.
£5 – £10

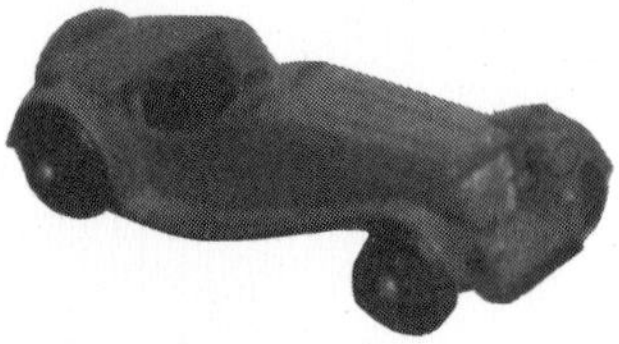

Dinky Toys, SS100 Jaguar, produced 1946-50. £15 – £25

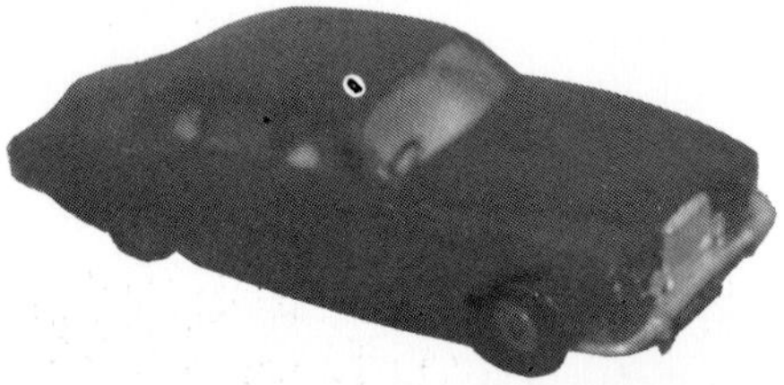

Spot-On Mark X with turning wheel and opening boot, 1963-64. £15 – £30

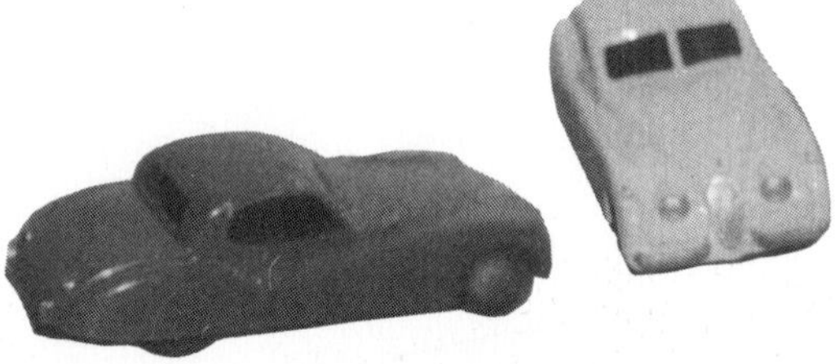

Dinky Toys, XK120 model, produced 1954-62.
£15 – £25

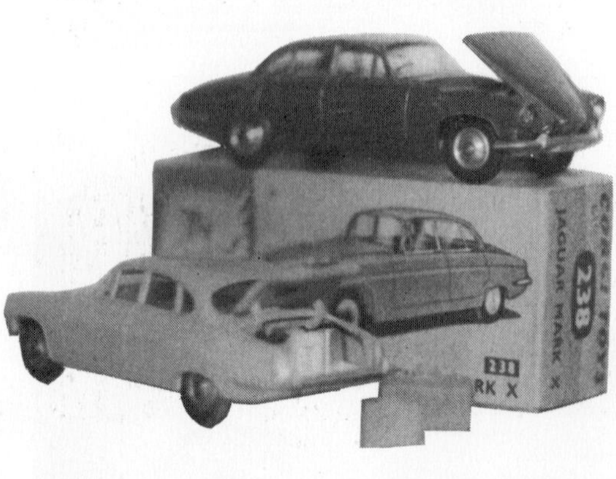

Corgi Toys, Mark X with opening boot and bonnet, 1962-67. £10

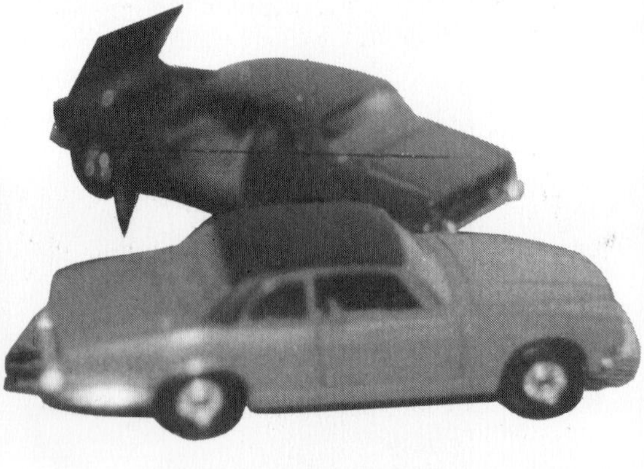

Corgi Toys, XJ Coupe, with opening doors and bonnet. £4

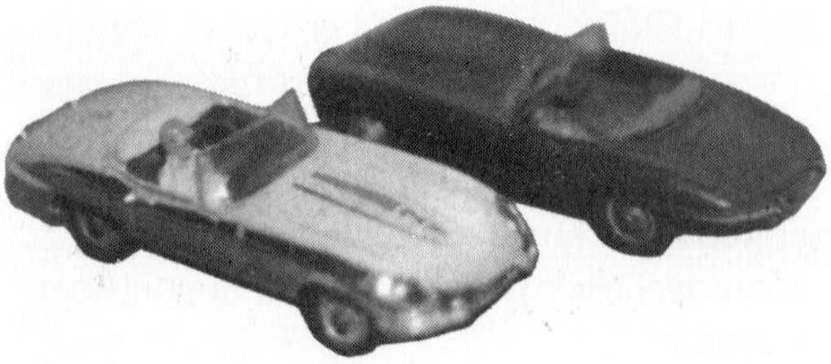

Corgi Toys, E type with racer in the foreground, production car behind, 1962-64. £15 – £25

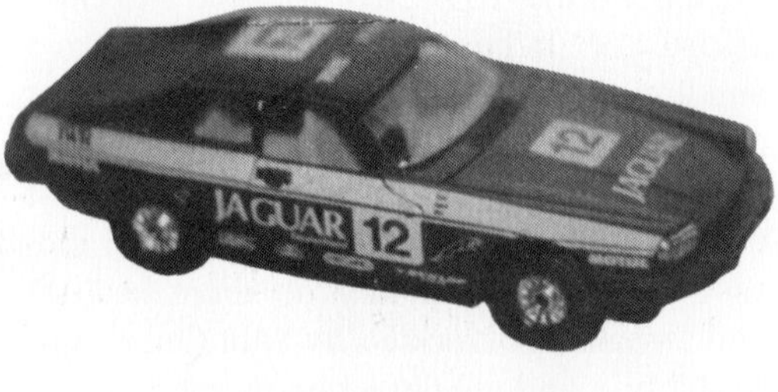

Corgi Toys, Jaguar XJS racer with good detail, current model. £3.50

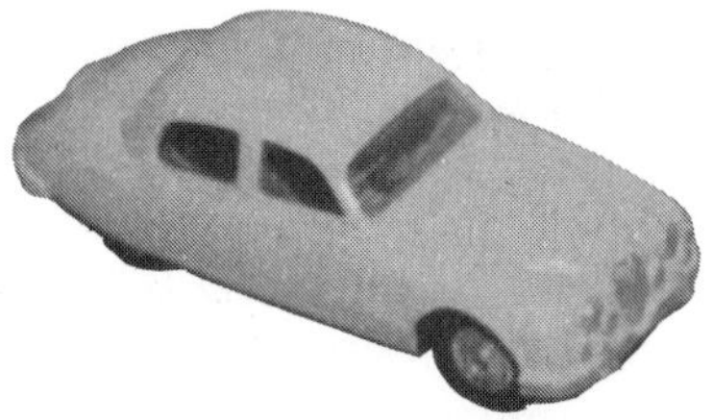

Corgi Toys, MK1 Jaguar, in yellow trim, 1960-63. £15 – £25

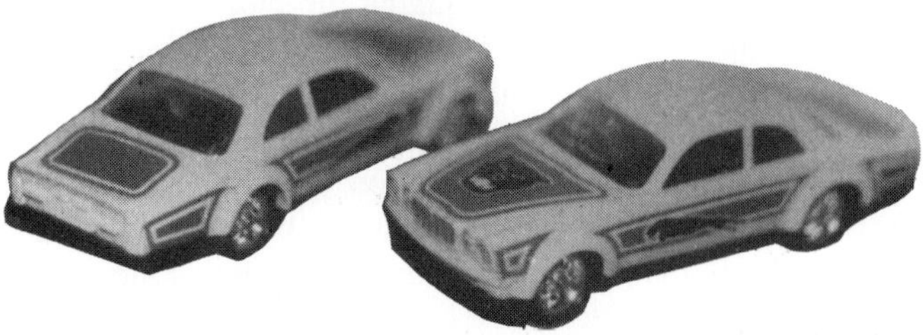

Dinky Toys, XJ Coupe B roadspeed, limited production in the 1970's, no box issued. £3 – £5

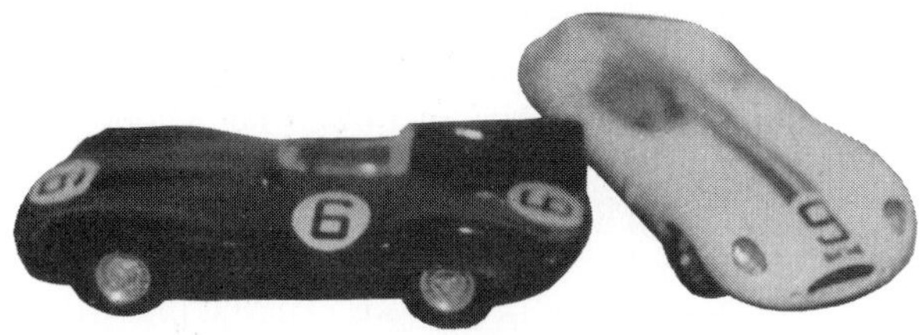

Western Models, D types, (No. 6 Hawthorns 1955 Le Mans Winner). £15 – £25

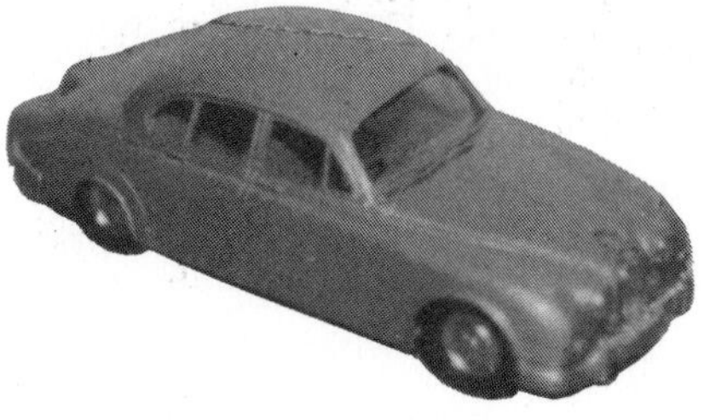

Western Models, MK11, 3.8 Jaguar, current model. £26

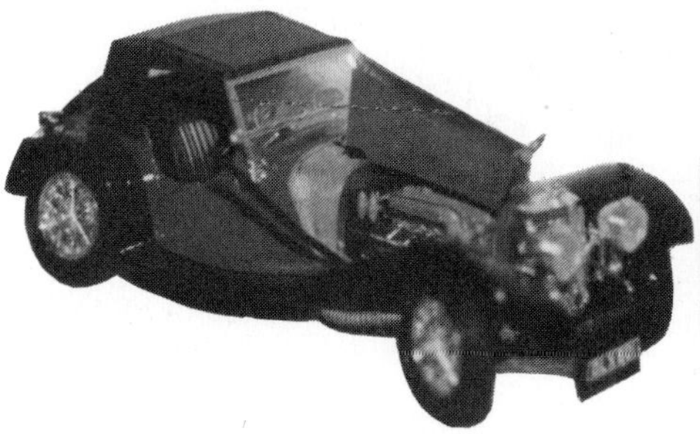

Burago SS100, well detailed current model showing engine components, exhaust and suspension. £9.95

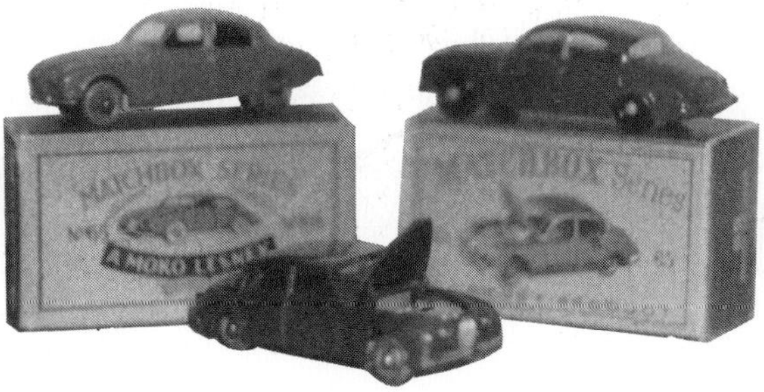

Matchbox Series, 3.8 MK11, complete with original box, 1959-67. £5 – £10

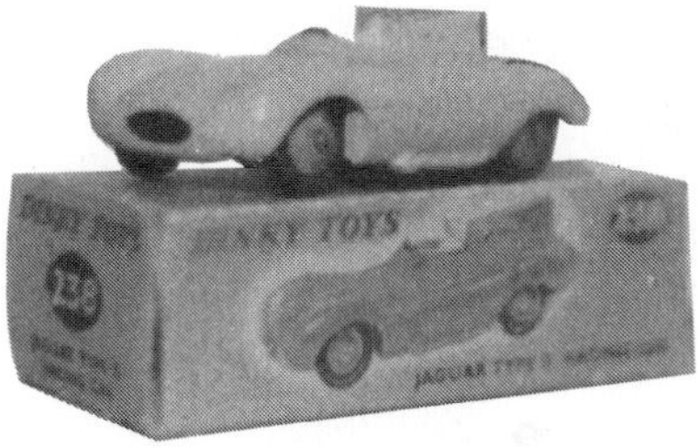

Dinky Toys D type Jaguar in light green, complete with original box, 1957-62. £15 – £30

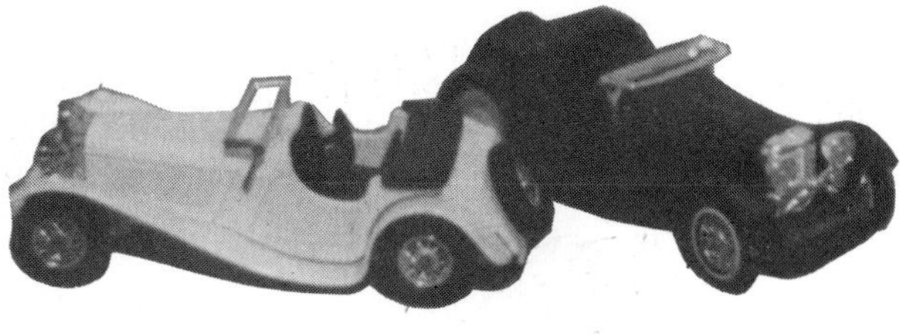

Matchbox Model of yesteryear, SS100, current model. £3

Alan McEwen is the managing director of his family engineering company and is a dedicated collector of quack medicine bottles.

"My collection concentrates on quality rather than quantity and consists of about 80 quack medicines, many being extremely rare "one-offs" which have not been noted elsewhere.

"History has always fascinated me from being a small boy, and in 1982 I was elected a member of the Newcomen Society, the learned body that studies the history of engineering technology. Back in the early '70s while watching Arthur Negus discussing the merits of the then new hobby of bottle collecting on the Pebble Mill television programme, I became so fascinated that within a few weeks I was well and truly bitten by the bottle collecting bug.

"Subsequently while clearing out rubbish from the cellar of our engineering premises (a former Midland Railway Warehouse built in 1869) I found some old blob-top, embossed beer bottles dating from 1880 and my interest was further heightened.

"I started to specialise in quack medicine bottle collecting in 1974 following a meeting with some American collectors who had shown me some splendid bottles embossed with the most curious and amusing claims.

"There are basically two categories in my collection — pre-1850 'pontilled' bottles, usually made of lead or flint glass and extremely rare, and the post-1850 quack bottles in various shades of aqua — some being of coloured glass — ambers, greens, blues and browns.

"I have a few beautiful 'pontilled' bottles embossed with interesting wording such as 'Dr Sibley's Solar Tincture by His Majesty's Royal Letters Patent', 'Dr McMunn's Elixir of Opium' and 'Dr Solomon's Cordial Balm of Gilead'.

The bottles in my collection made after 1850 include, William Radam's Microbe Killer, Warner's Safe Cure, Dr Kilmer's Swamp Root, Kidney, Liver and Bladder Cure, Benbows Dog Mixture, Mouse-Ear Syrup, Holden's Tommy bottle for Sprains and many others.

Some of my quack cures can command prices up to £200, but the price is usually

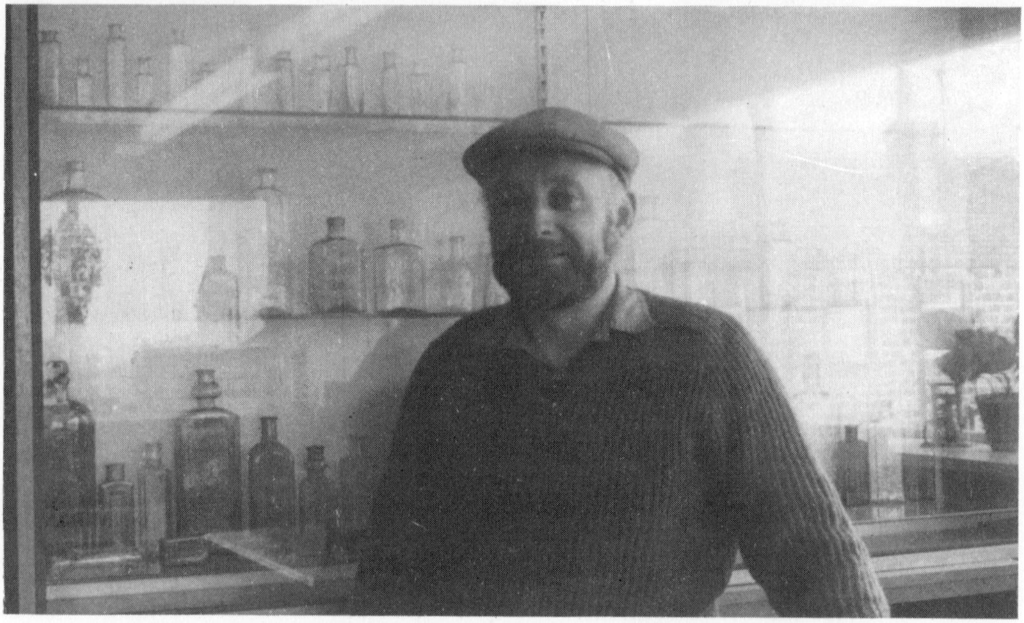

Alan McEwen with his back-lit glass shelved display case which shows his 'Quack' Medicine bottles to their best advantage.

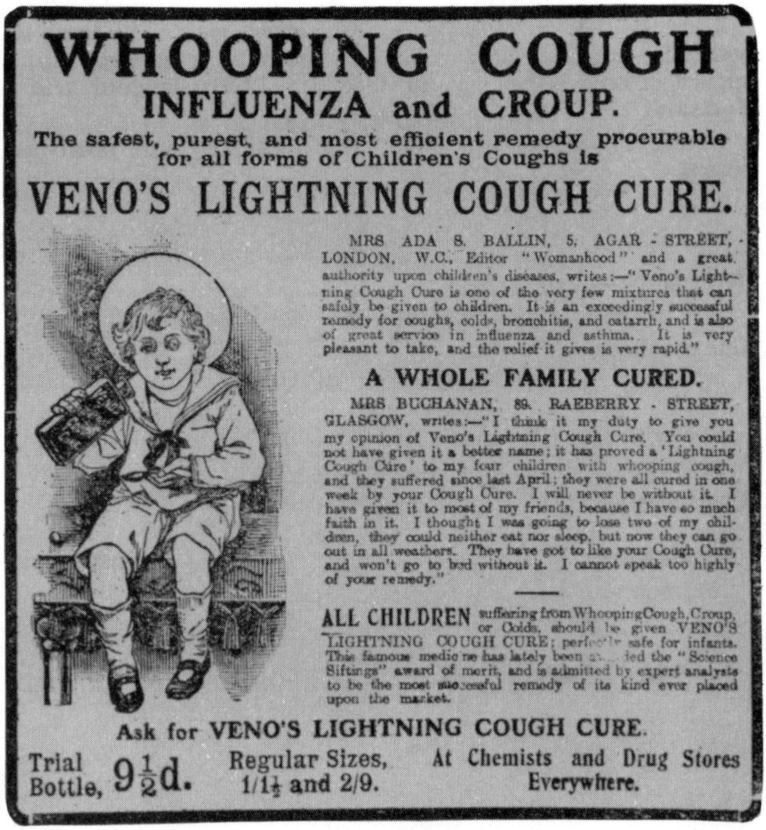
WHOOPING COUGH
INFLUENZA and CROUP.
The safest, purest, and most efficient remedy procurable for all forms of Children's Coughs is
VENO'S LIGHTNING COUGH CURE.
MRS ADA S. BALLIN, 5, AGAR - STREET, LONDON, W.C., Editor "Womanhood" and a great authority upon children's diseases, writes:—"Veno's Lightning Cough Cure is one of the very few mixtures that can safely be given to children. It is an exceedingly successful remedy for coughs, colds, bronchitis, and catarrh, and is also of great service in influenza and asthma. It is very pleasant to take, and the relief it gives is very rapid."
A WHOLE FAMILY CURED.
MRS BUCHANAN, 89, RAEBERRY - STREET, GLASGOW, writes:—"I think it my duty to give you my opinion of Veno's Lightning Cough Cure. You could not have given it a better name; it has proved a 'Lightning Cough Cure' to my four children with whooping cough, and they suffered since last April; they were all cured in one week by your Cough Cure. I will never be without it. I have given it to most of my friends, because I have so much faith in it. I thought I was going to lose two of my children, they could neither eat nor sleep, but now they can go out in all weathers. They have got to like your Cough Cure, and won't go to bed without it. I cannot speak too highly of your remedy."
ALL CHILDREN suffering from Whooping Cough, Croup, or Colds, should be given VENO'S LIGHTNING COUGH CURE; perfectly safe for infants. This famous medicine has lately been the "Science Siftings" award of merit, and is admitted by expert analysts to be the most successful remedy of its kind ever placed upon the market.
Ask for VENO'S LIGHTNING COUGH CURE.
Trial Bottle, 9½d.
Regular Sizes, 1/1½ and 2/9.
At Chemists and Drug Stores Everywhere.

"by negotiation" because there are as yet only a handful of serious collectors in the U.K."

Alan was undoubtedly the driving force behind the collecting of quack cures in the U.K. and in 1977, compiled and published, the only book on the hobby in Britain called, "Collecting Quack Cures" and is currently completing a much more comprehensive volume of British Quack Medicines.

The item he would most like to find to complete his collection is a bottle embossed with 'Extract of Mistletoe — The Druid Cure'. It dates from around 1880 and only two examples have ever been found but both were broken. It is amber glass, about six inches high, and is embossed with the head of a Celtic Druid wearing a crown of mistletoe.

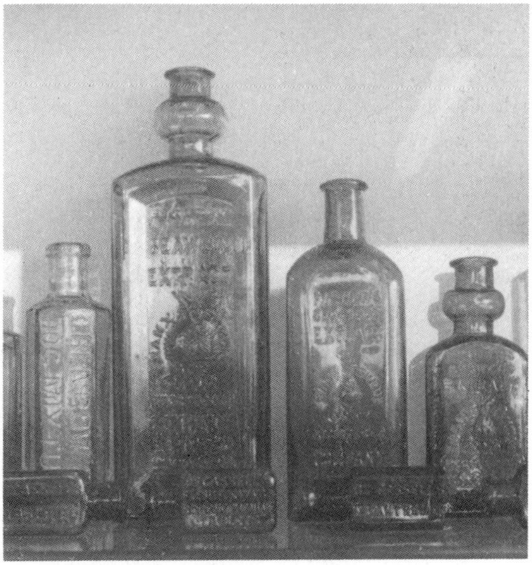

A fine display including the rare, large size, Fisher's Seaweed Extract , in emerald green glass worth £150.

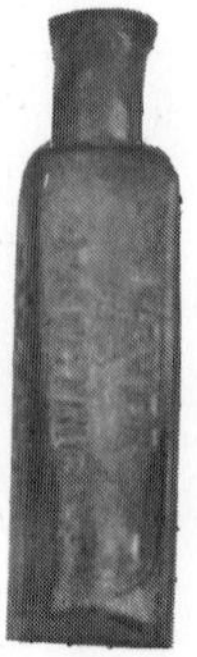

J. Cropper's 'Never Failing Gout Mixture', in aqua coloured glass bottle, circa 1850. £20

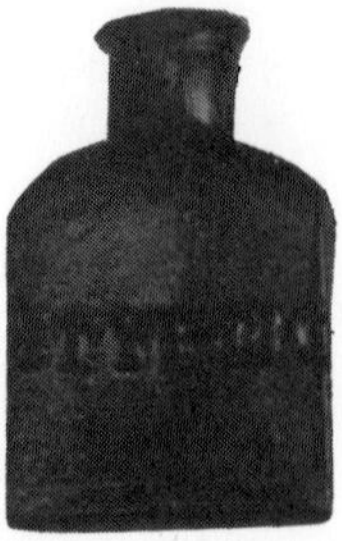

Pre 1850 Ruspinis Styptic in cobalt blue pontilled bottle. £100

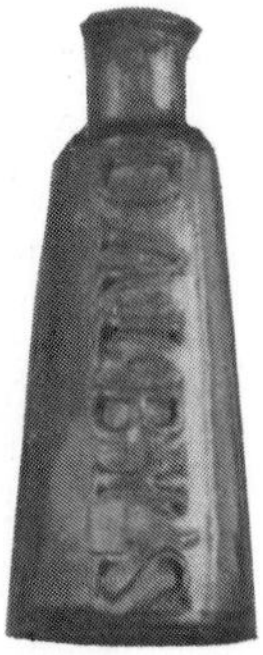

Dalby's Carminative, in a cone-shaped aqua bottle. £30

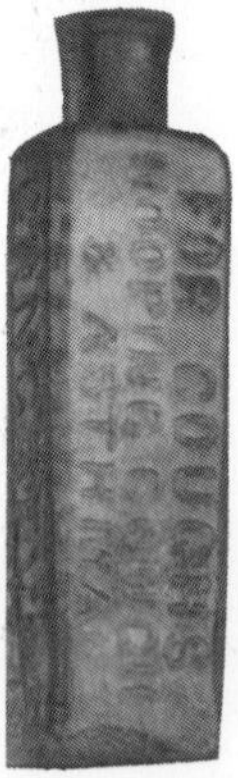

Large size, clear glass Congreaves Balsamic Elixir for (W)Looping Cough and Asthma. £30

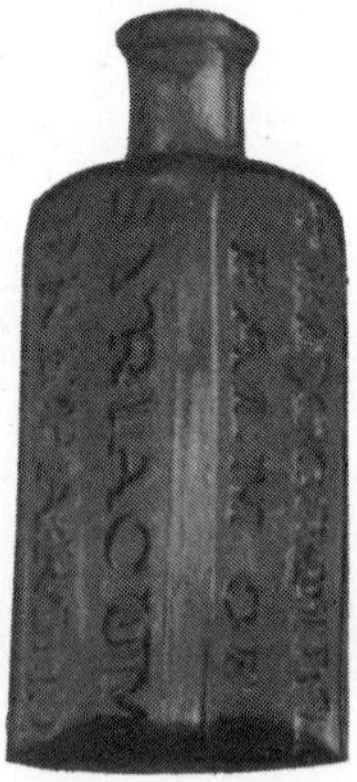

Cordial Balm of Syriacum, in aqua glass bottle. £100

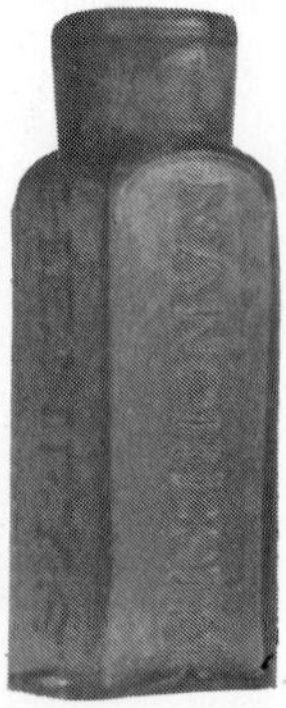

Henry's Calcined Magnesia, Manchester, in a lead glass pontilled bottle. £30

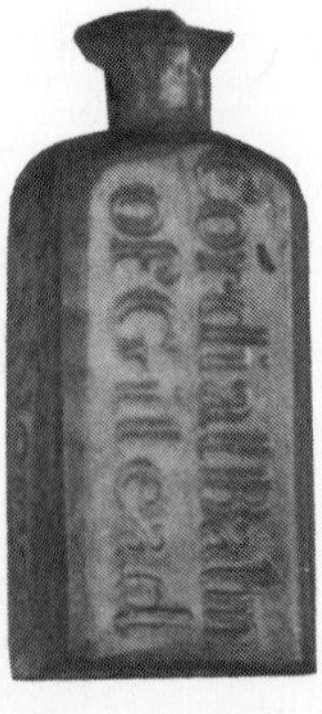

Dr. Solomon's Cordial Balm of Gilead, in moulded aqua glass bottle. £150

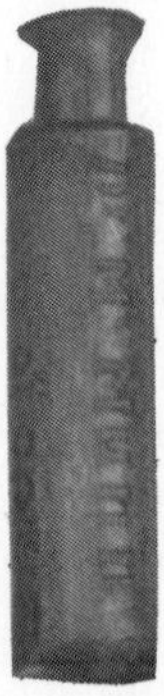

Dr. McMunn's Elixir of Opium, in aqua glass pontilled bottle. £40

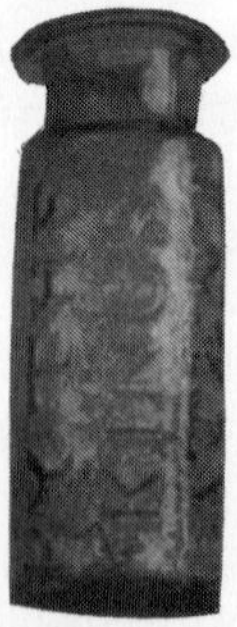

'By the King's Patent', True Cephalic Snuff, in a crudely blown pontilled bottle of light green glass. £100

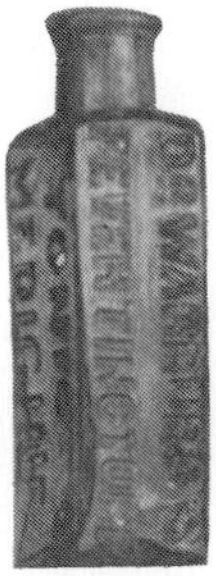

Dr. Wartburg's Fever Tincture, Tonic Medicine, in aqua moulded bottle. £50

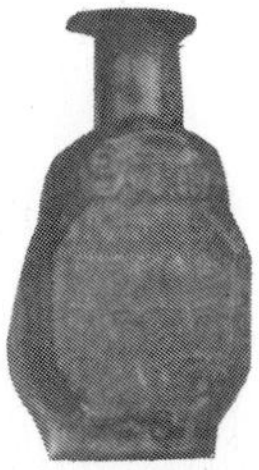

Violin shaped clear glass pontilled bottle, 'By the King's Patent Granted to Robt. Turlington – For His Invented Balsam of Life – Jan. 26th 1754. £100

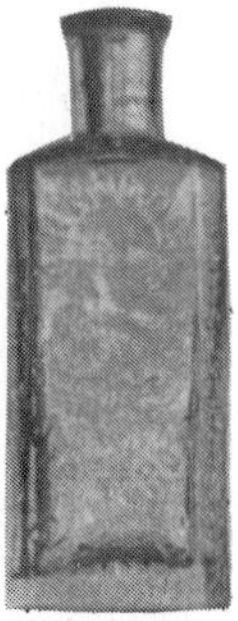

Holden's 'Tommy' bottle, 7½ pence size, Cures Sprains and Sore Throats, aqua glass. £30

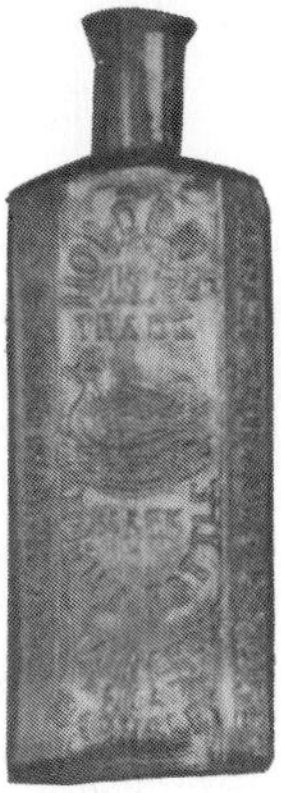

Holden's 'Tommy' bottle, 13½ pence size, Cure for Sprains, Bruises, Rheumatism, Sore Throats and Sciatica, rare aqua glass. £40

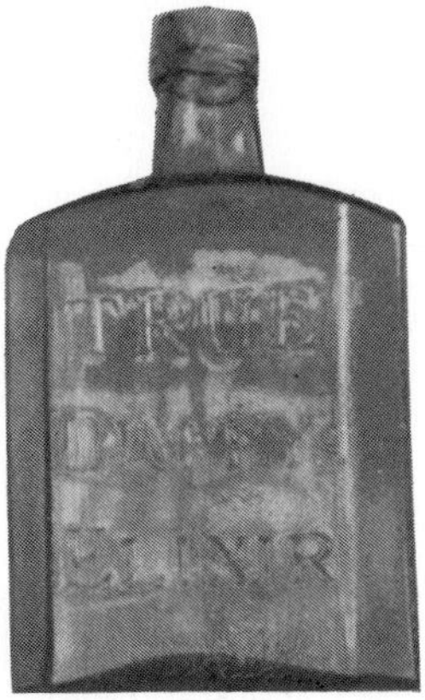

True Daffys Elixir, in a lime green pontilled bottle. £100

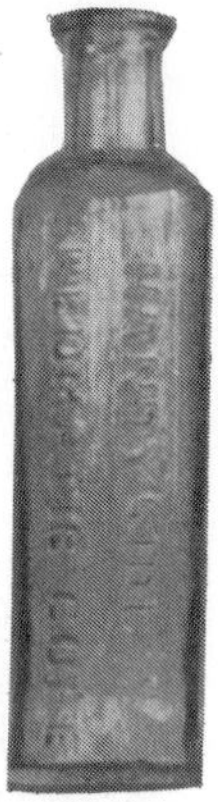

George Handyside's 'Rheumatic Cure', in clear glass, rare. £30

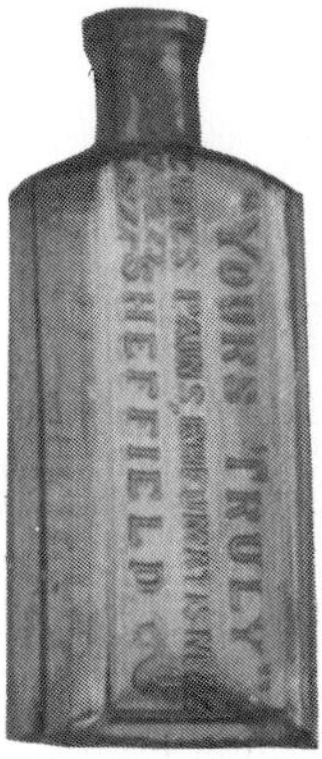

'Yours truly' cures pains, rheumatism, Sheffield, rare aqua glass. £30

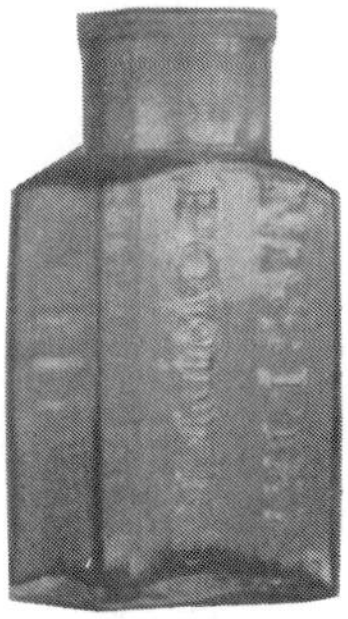

Miss Pikes Powders for Fits and Nervous Complaints, in a lead glass bottle, circa 1800. £100

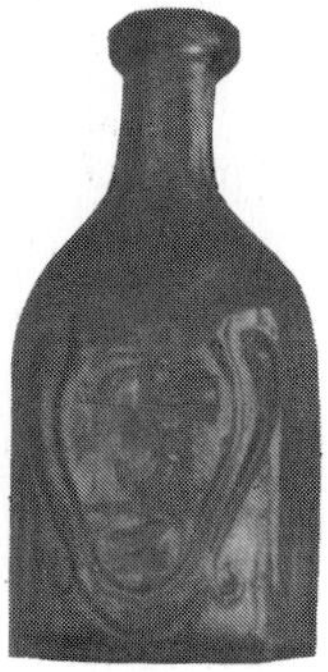

Dr. Lobb's Blob Lipped, cylindrical clear glass bottle with an embossed humanoid face on the reverse. £140

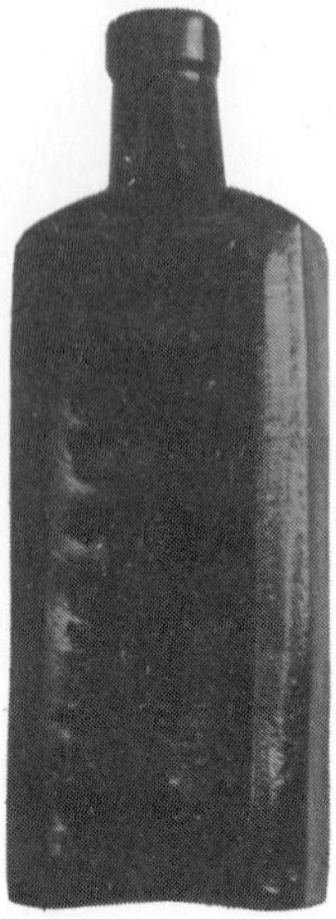

George Handyside's 'Blood Purifier', in black glass, rare. £80

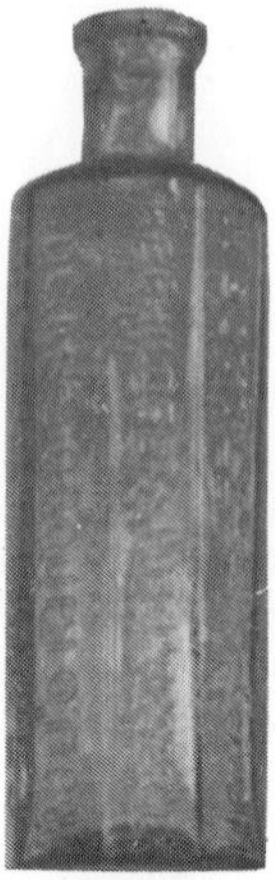

Edgar's Group Lotion, 'The Children's Life Preserver', in octagonal aqua glass bottle. £30

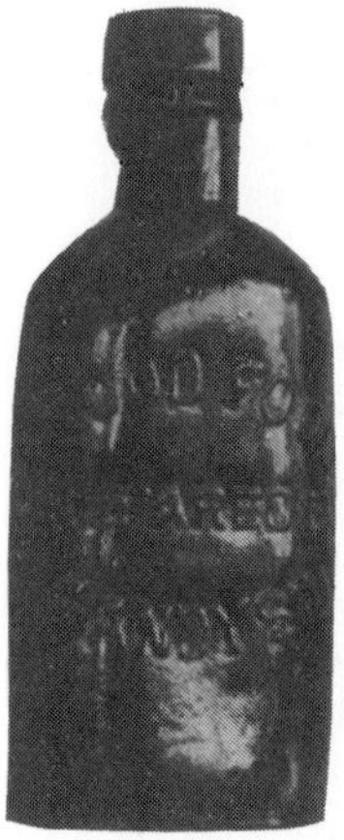

George Handyside's small 'Blood Food' in black glass full of attractive yellow bubbles, rare. £50

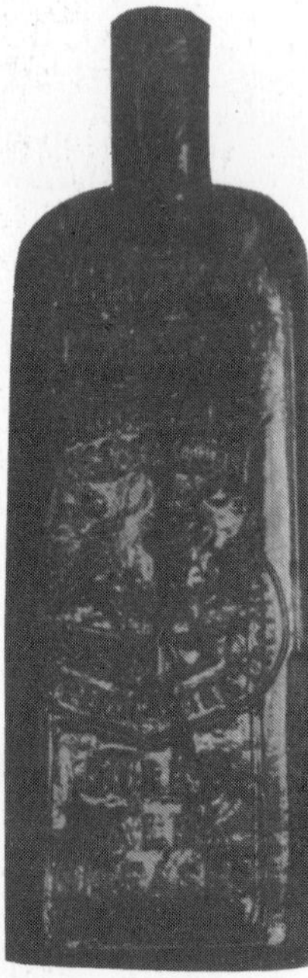

William Radam's Microbe Killer, a beautifully embossed rare amber glass bottle. £80

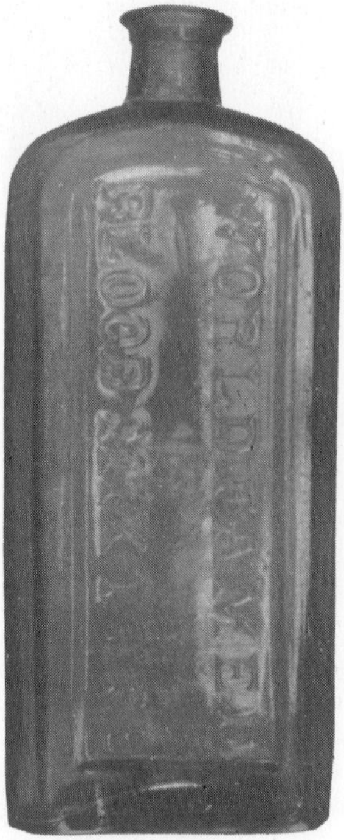

A rare, large size, copper blue Clarke's 'World Famed Blood Mixture'. £35

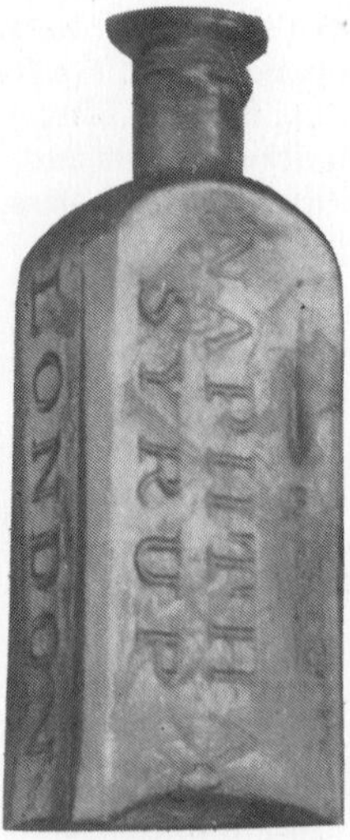

Dr. Hasting's Naphtha Syrup in rectangular shaped aqua glass pontilled bottle. £80

Brenda and Bob Beecroft collect brewery badges.

Bob said: "The badge collection is really Brenda's but she has been ill recently and I've been going round buying things she hasn't already got in the collection. She now has 120 badges in all and it's the biggest collection that I know of.

"Some of the badges go back 60 years and there are very nice ones among them like the Tetley of Leeds' huntsman; John Smith's cockerel; Whitbread's hind and Scottish and Newcastle's old man with a beard.

"People who worked in the various breweries used to wear those badges in their lapels. We've even got one made for the members of Guinness's bowling club which was in existence in the 1950's.

"Quite a few of the badges represent breweries that are no longer in existence or have been taken over by others. We write to breweries and some send us free badges but it is difficult to find a few of them — Guinness badges in particular are hard to come by. The majority turn up in antique fairs and the most we've had to pay is £15 for a rare badge."

The badges are very colourful and show a wide range of emblems from Fremlin's elephant to the Guinness toucan. One of the rarest in the collection is a Bass bottle and another of a Guinness bottle on the end of a tie pin. The badge that Brenda and Bob would like to find is one from William Younger's showing a white bearded old man in the act of throwing a dart. Bob has only ever seen one and it was unfortunately not for sale.

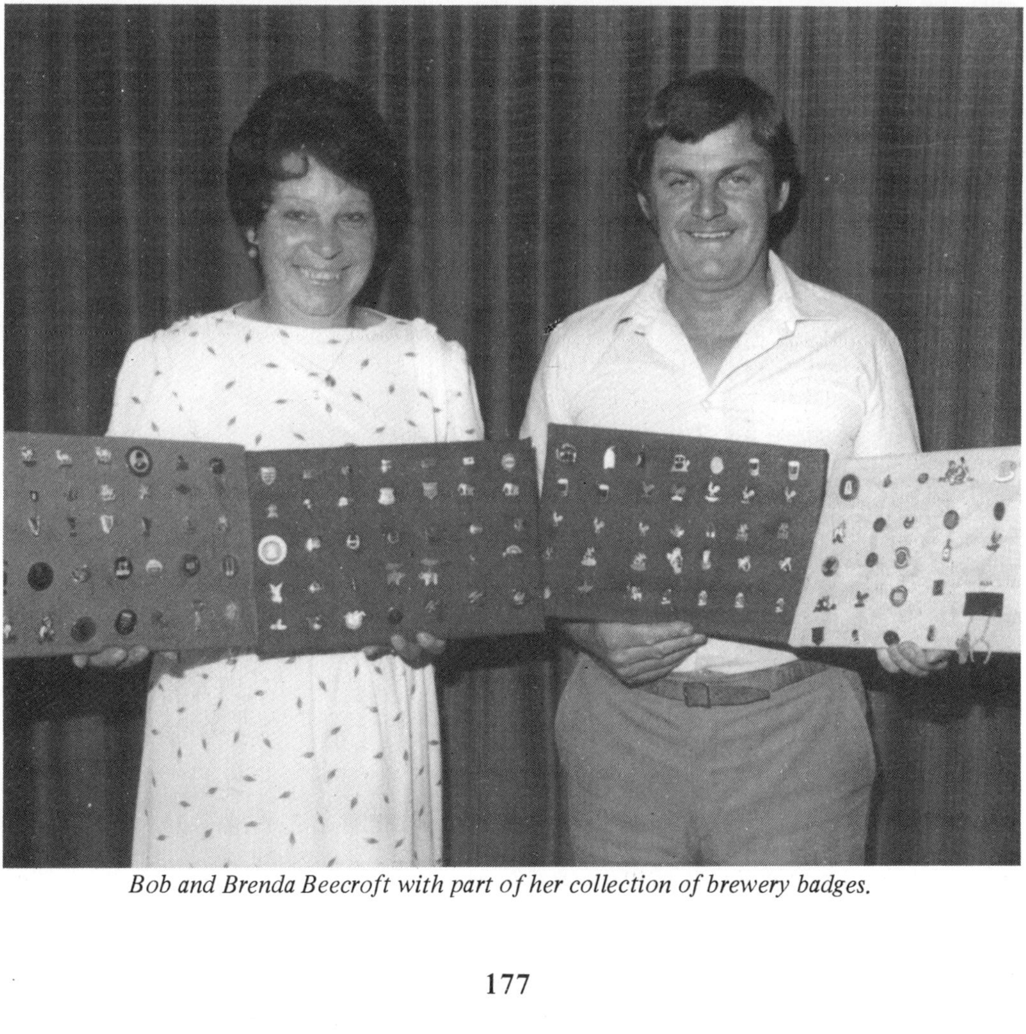

Bob and Brenda Beecroft with part of her collection of brewery badges.

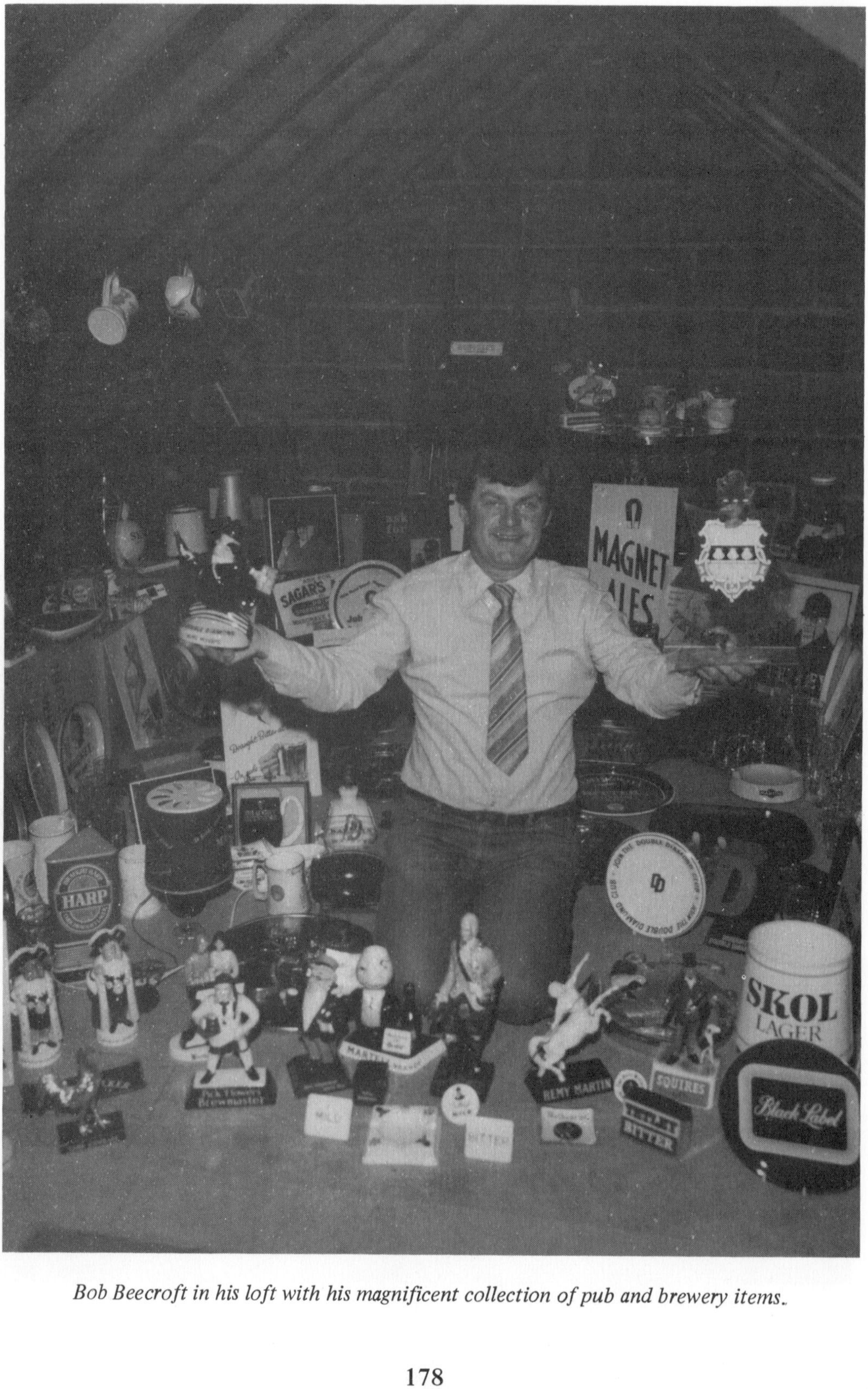

Bob Beecroft in his loft with his magnificent collection of pub and brewery items.

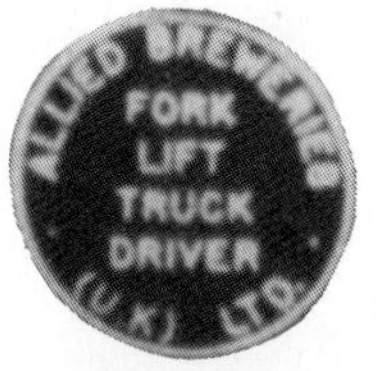

Allied Breweries (UK) Ltd.
£1

Campaign For Real Ale.
£1

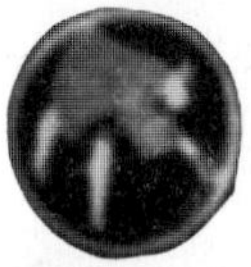

An extremely rare badge from the 'Melbourne Brewery', a Leeds firm now ceased trading. £10

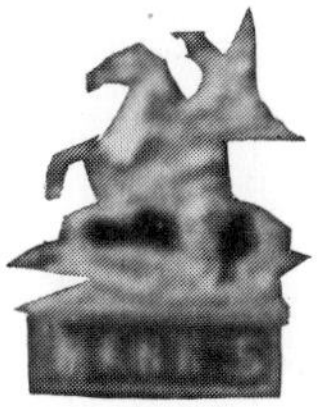

Manns enamel badge. £2

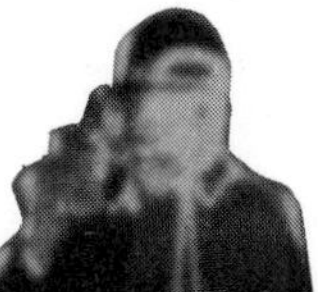

Tetley of Leeds Huntsman.
£5

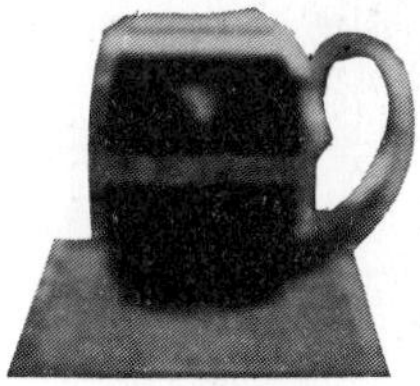

Guinness badge. £3

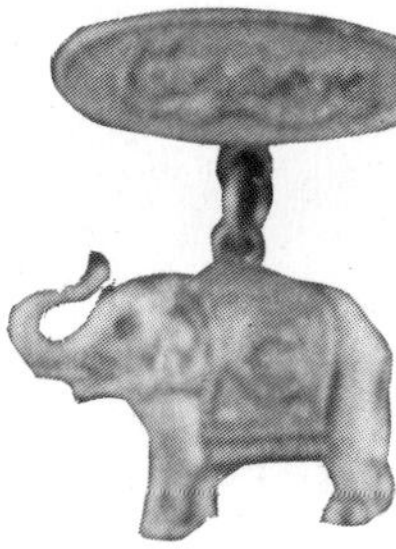

Carlsberg Elephant badge.
£2

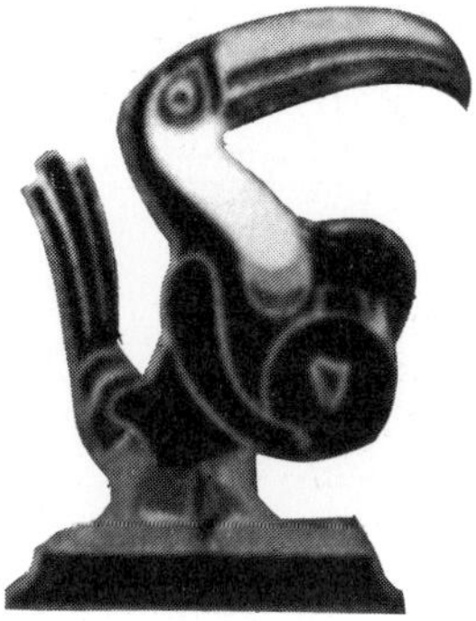

Very rare Guinness Toucan bowling club badge. £15

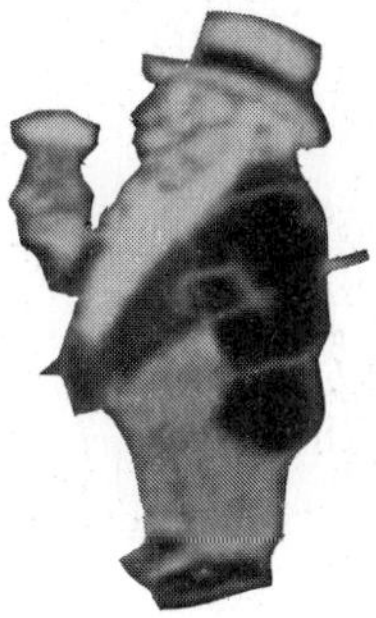

William Youngers 'little old man holding a pint'. £5

Holts Traditional Ales.
£1

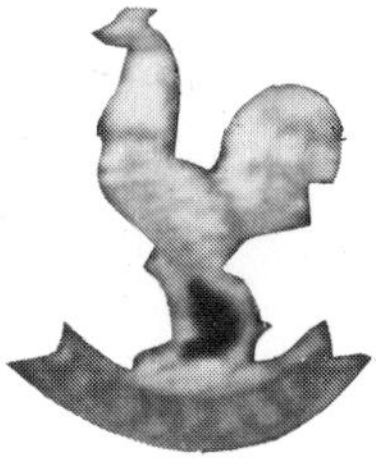

Courage Cockerel. £2

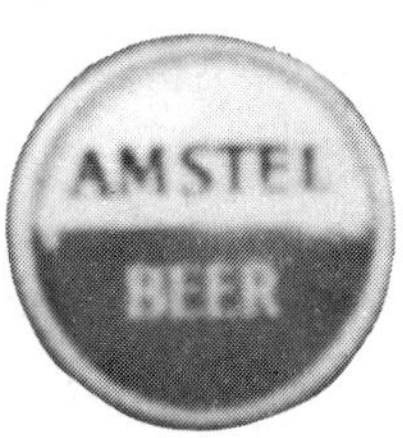

Amstel Beer. £1

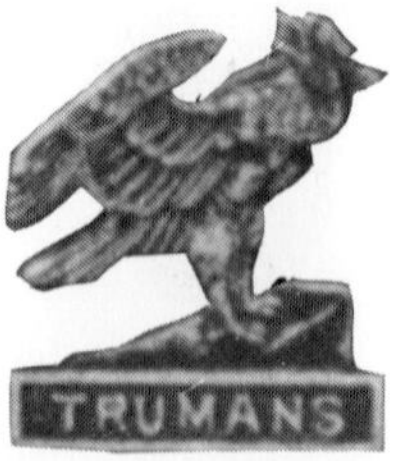

Trumans Eagle badge. £2

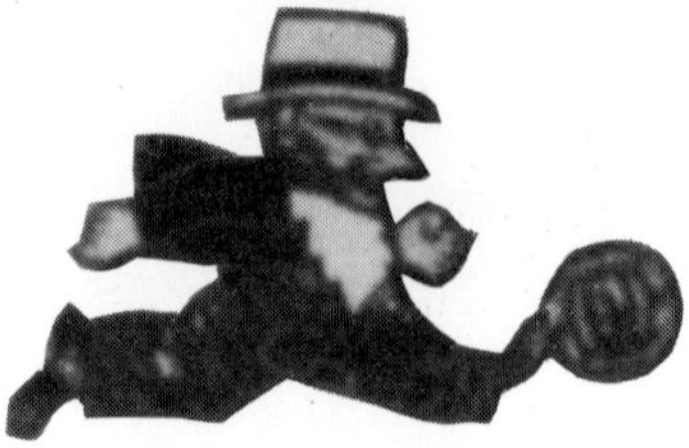

Rare badge depicting Father William, footballer. £10

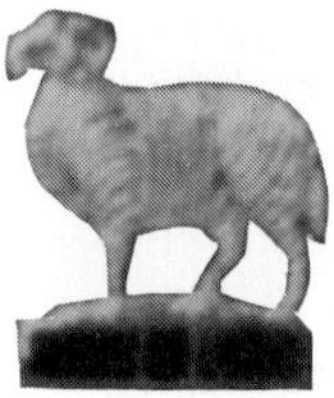

Young's Ram badge. £5

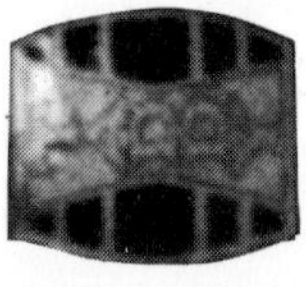

Very rare Samuel Smith's Taddy Barrel badge. £10

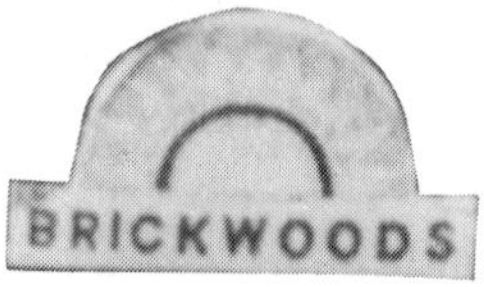

Brickwoods enamel badge. £1

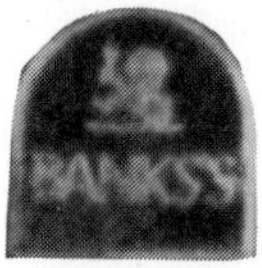

Banks's badge. £1

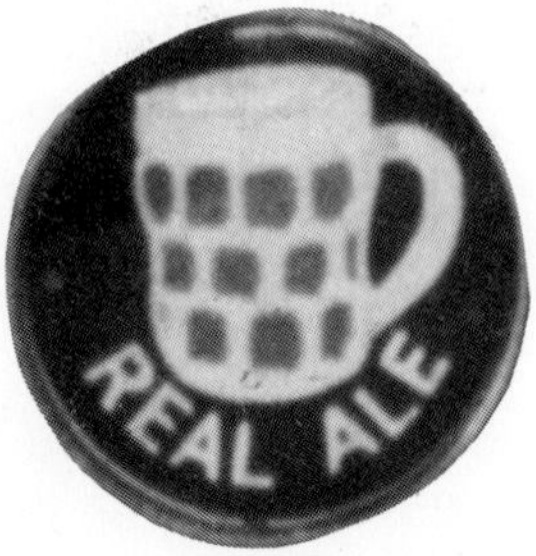

Real Ale badge. £1

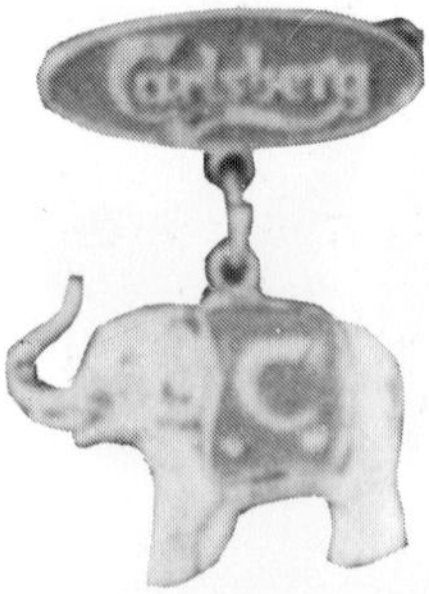

Carlsberg Elephant badge. £2

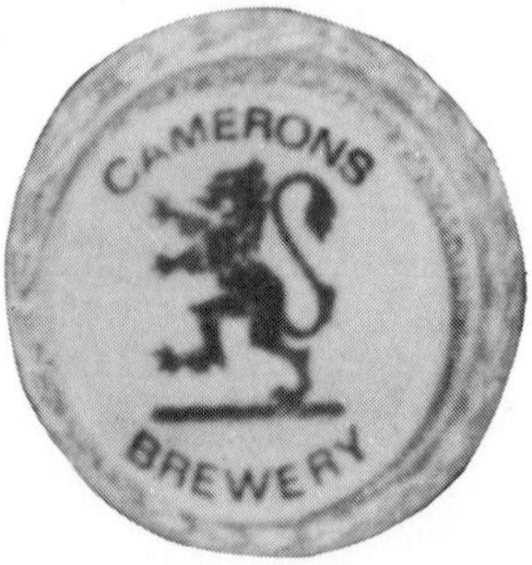

Camerons Brewery. £1

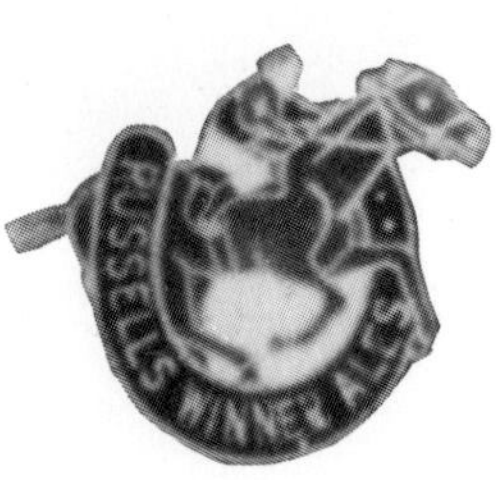

Russells Winner Ales, a rare badge. £10

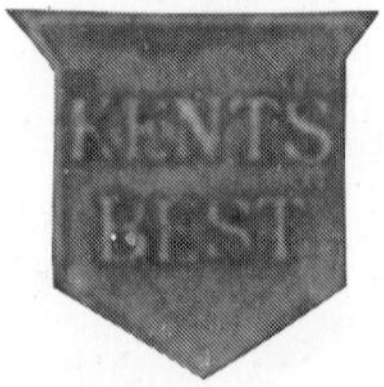

Kents Best. £1

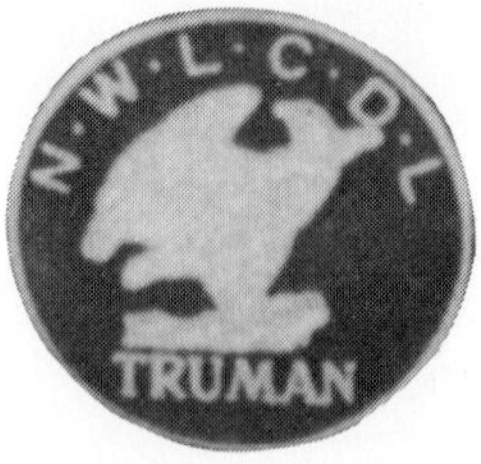

N.W.L.C.D.L. Truman. £1

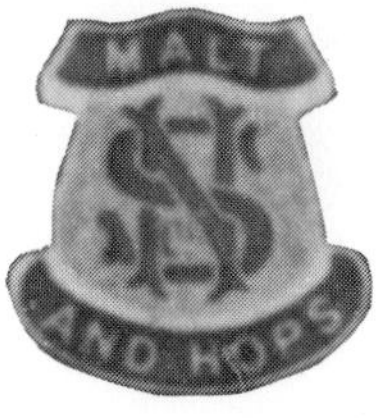

Malt and Hops. £2

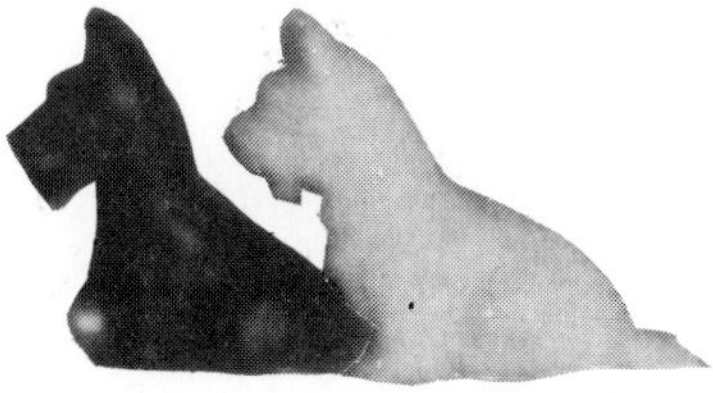

Black & White Whisky badge. £2

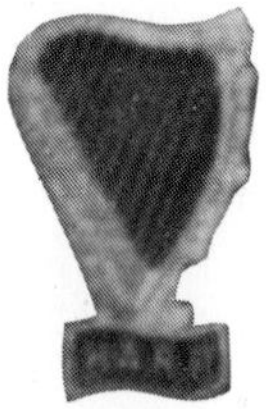

Harp badge. £2

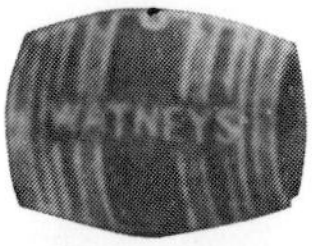

Watneys 'Red Barrel' badge. £1

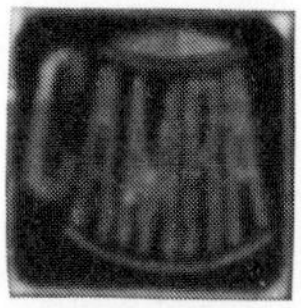

Camra badge. £1

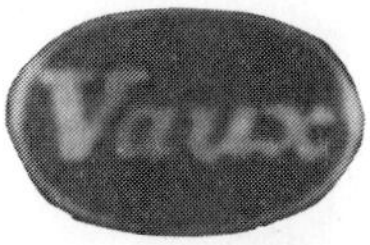

Vaux badge. £1

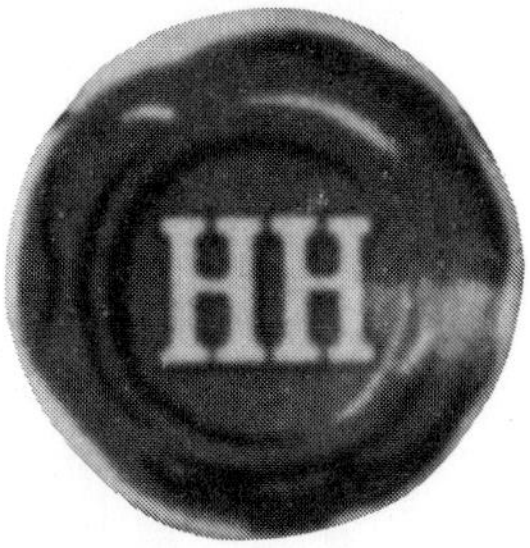

Hey and Humphries badge, a bottling firm in Leeds now ceased trading. £10

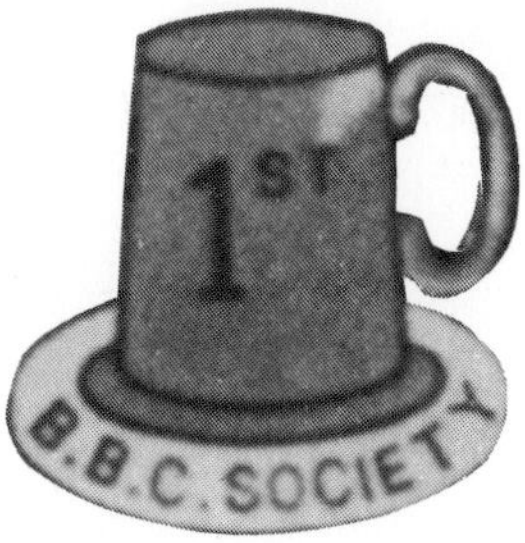

B.B.C. Society badge. £2

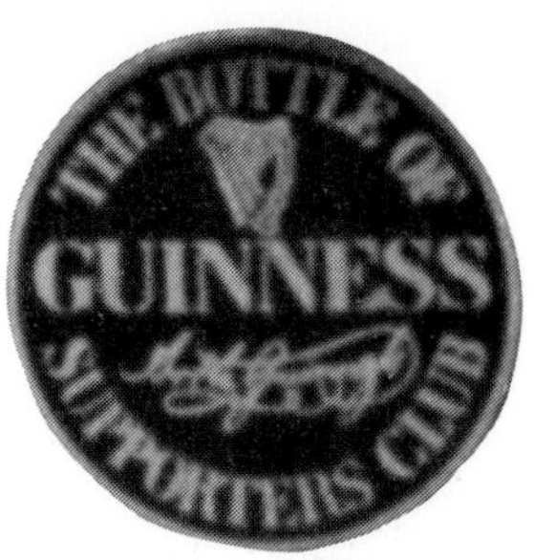

The Bottle of Guinness Supporters Club. £2

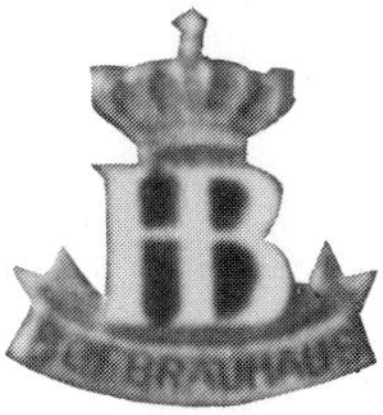

'HB' enamel badge. £2

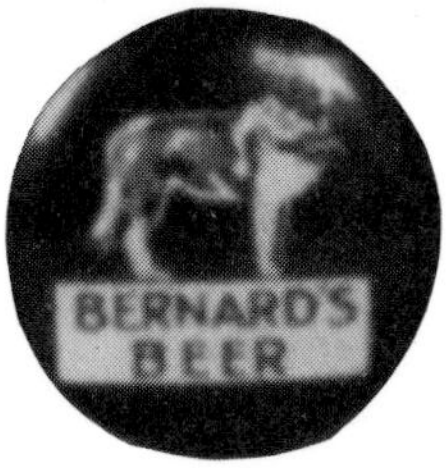

Bernard's Beer. £1

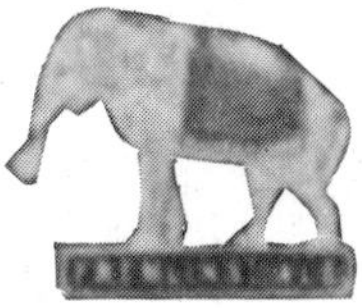

Fremlin's Elephant badge. £2

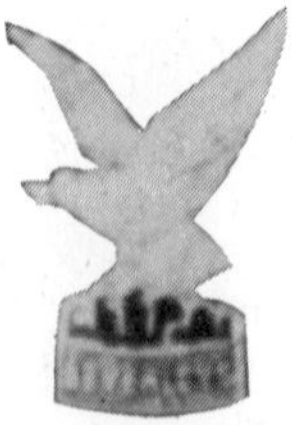

Beverley! Eagle badge. £5

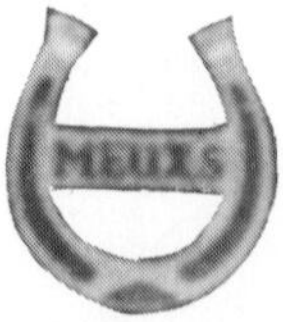

Meux's badge. £1

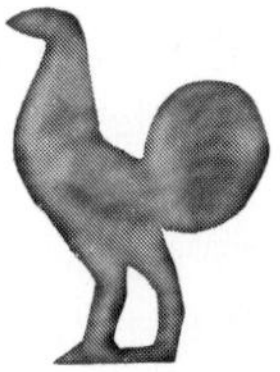

John Smith's cockerel. £3

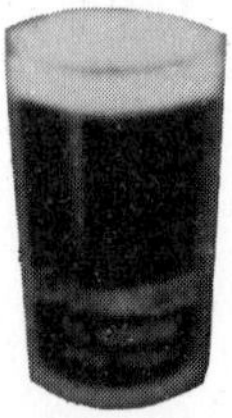

Guinness is Good For You. £3

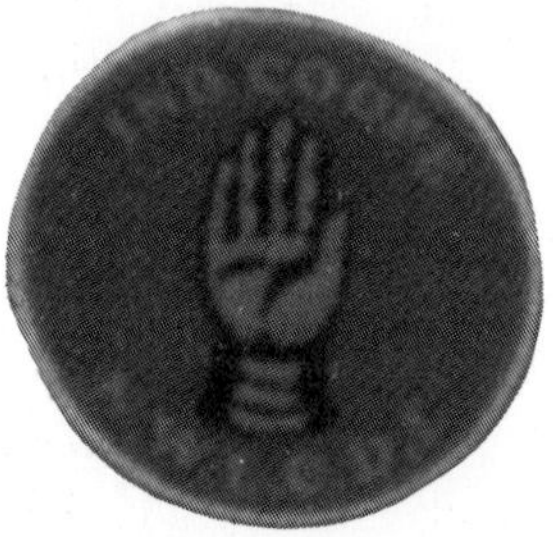

Ind Coope N.W.L.C.D.L. £1

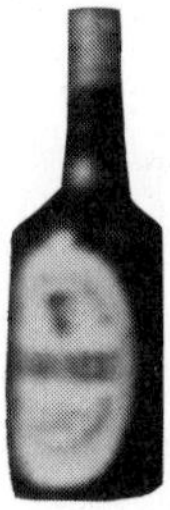

Very rare Guinness miniature bottle, 1950's. £5

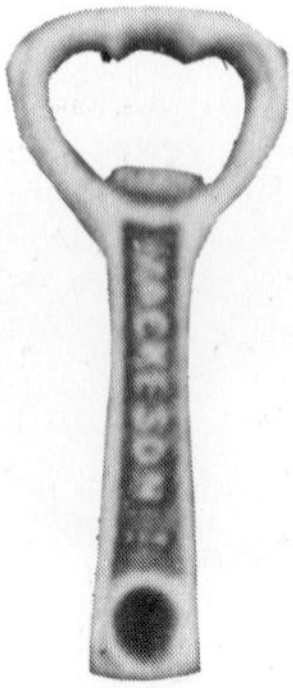

Mackeson bottle opener badge. £2

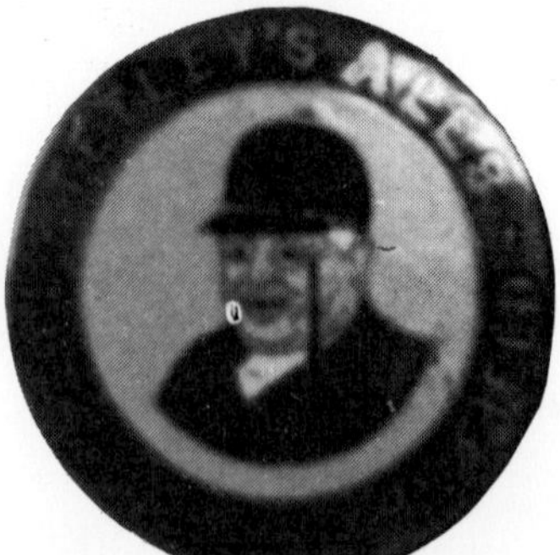

Tetley enamel badge from an ash tray. £5

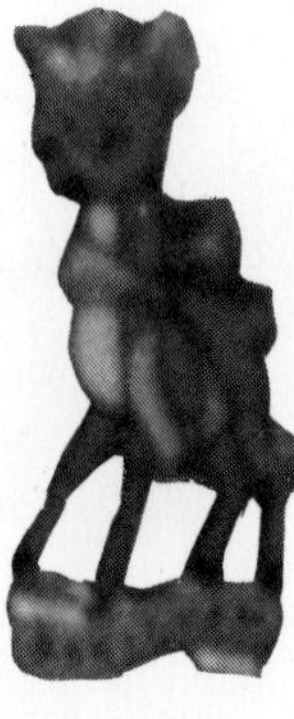

Babycham badge. £2

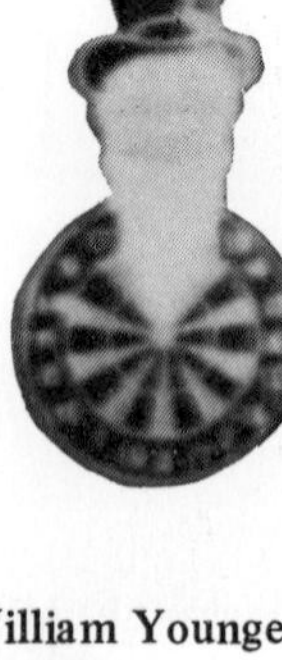

William Youngers 'Dartboard'. £5

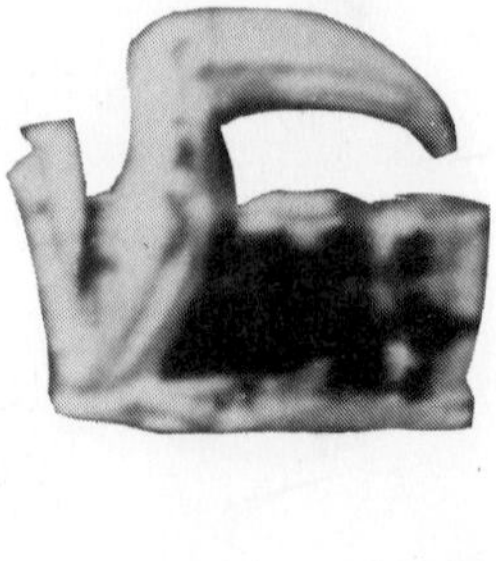

Very rare Guinness Toucan with glasses. £10

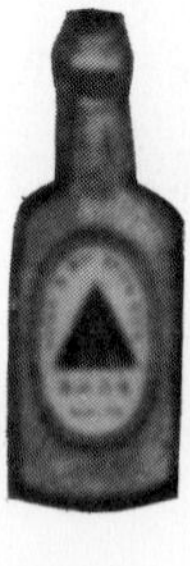

Very rare bottle badge by Bass. £15

Patricia Cockrell is a housewife with a spare time job selling Avon cosmetics who also collects magazines and all kinds of printed matter connected with British royalty.

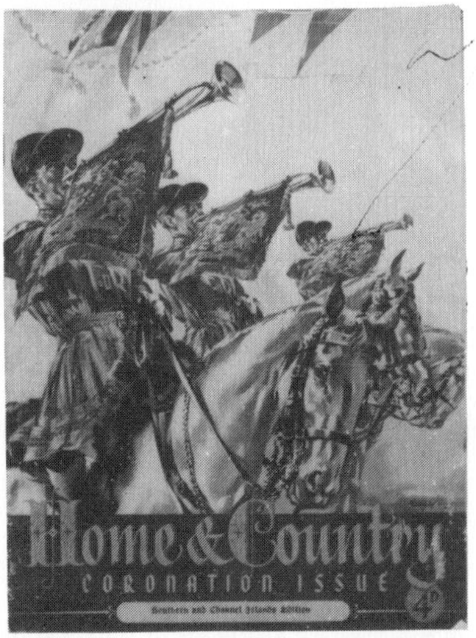

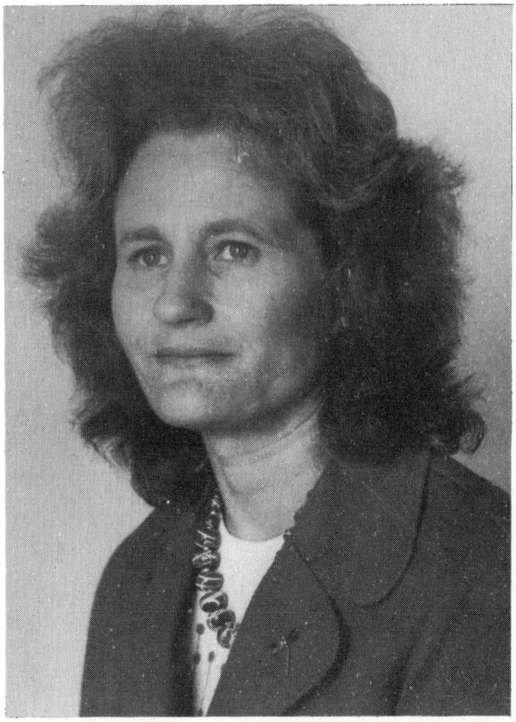

"The whole thing started when I was ten years old in 1953. At the time of the Queen's coronation I became very interested in the Royal Family and my mother suggested that I start a scrapbook about them. I've been collecting ever since and now my material goes back to the days of Queen Victoria and fills 1,200 separate albums not to mention boxes and paper bags all over the house. I've also got over 160 tins printed with pictures of royalty which are on display in my sitting room and more than 2,500 magazines about the British royal family. If there is a large section in a magazine, I don't cut it out but keep the magazine intact. My most recent acquisitions are pages from the copies of the Illustrated London News of the 1880's with articles about members of Queen Victoria's family."

Patricia's collection also includes spoons, thimbles and china with pictures of royalty on them but as she says, the newspaper cuttings are her first love. This summer has been a busy one because she has bought all the newspapers carrying pictures and reports of the courtship and wedding of the Duke and Duchess of York. She says she will look back on 1986 as a vintage year — not only the Royal wedding but also the Queen's 60th birthday gave her a bonanza time for collecting. Her only regret is that she is so busy keeping her collection up to date that she has no time to go out to see members of the Royal family in the flesh.

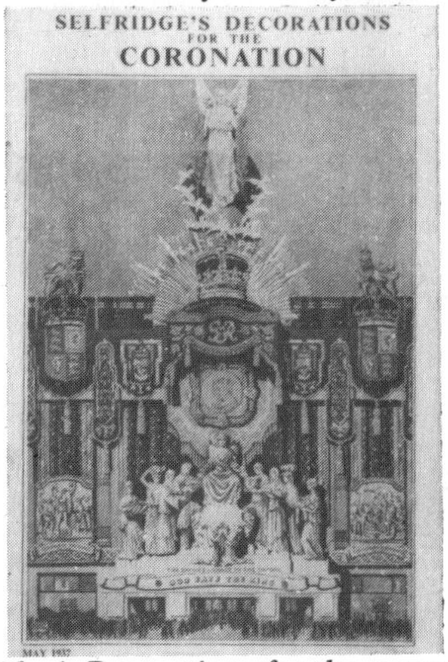

Selfridge's Decorations for the coronation, 1937. £3

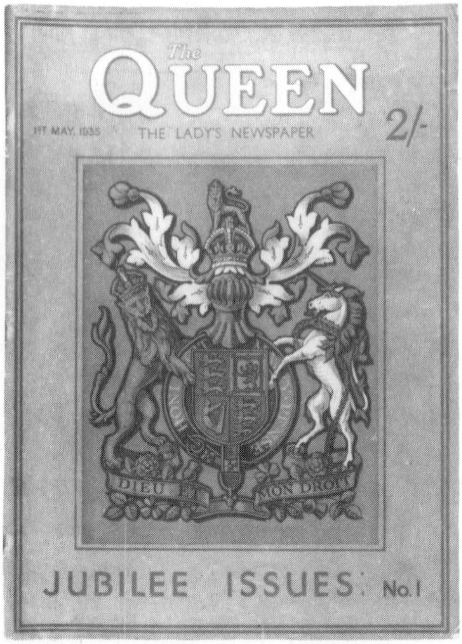

The Queen – Jubilee Issues No. 1, 1935. £4

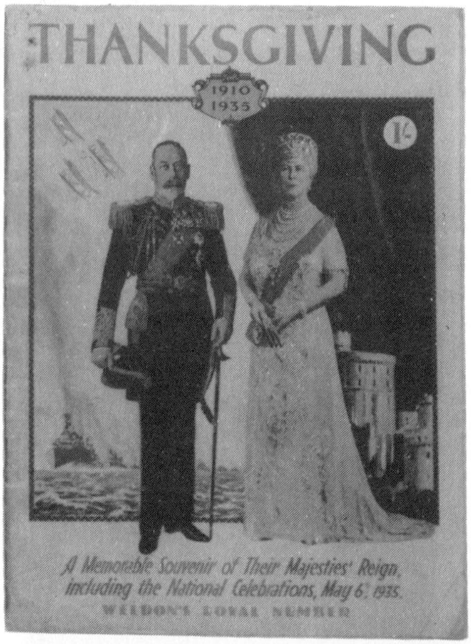

Weldon's – Jubilee Souvenir of Their Majestie's Reign, 1935. £3.50

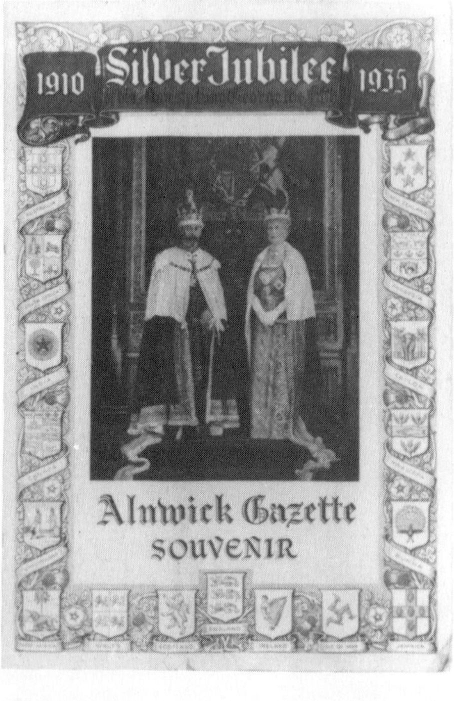

Alnwick Gazette – Silver Jubilee – George V, 1935. £3

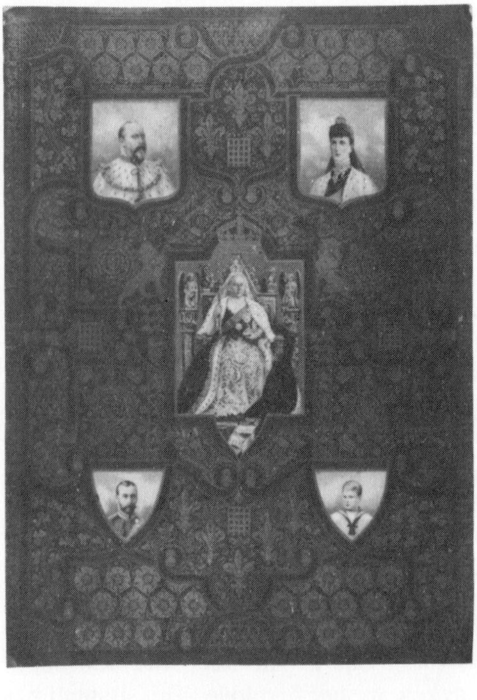

Illustrated London News – Record of Reign of Queen Victoria, 1901. £15

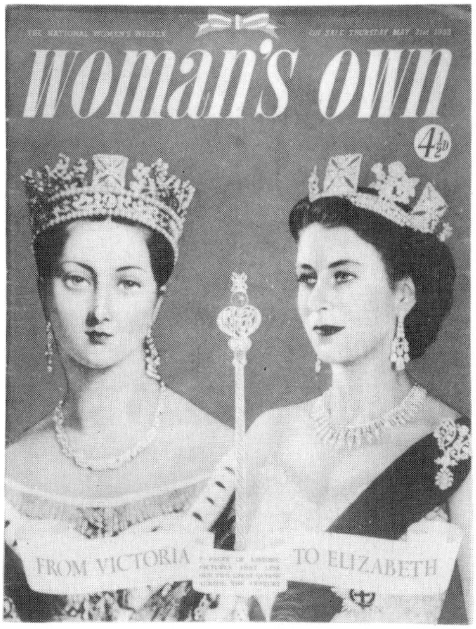

Woman's Own – Historic Pictures that link Victoria to Elizabeth, 1953. £1.50

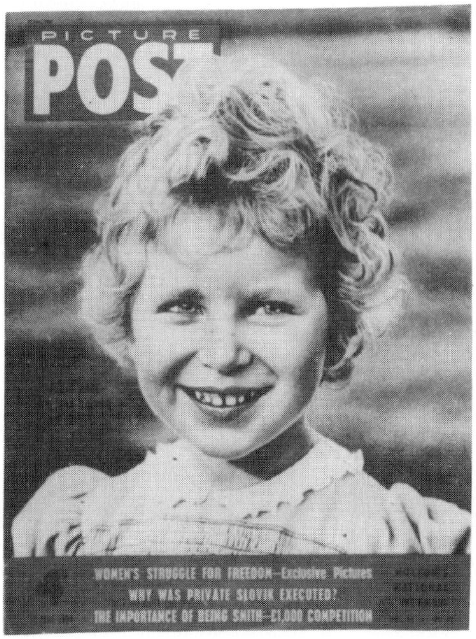

Picture Post – Colour Pages of Royal Children, 1954. £1

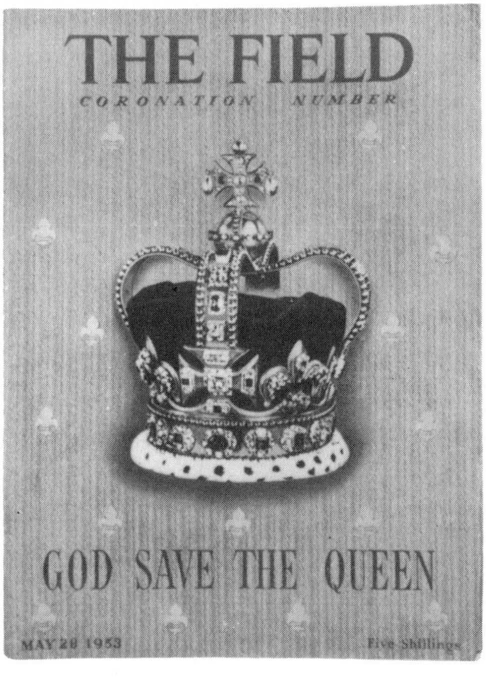

The Field – Coronation Number, 1953. £3

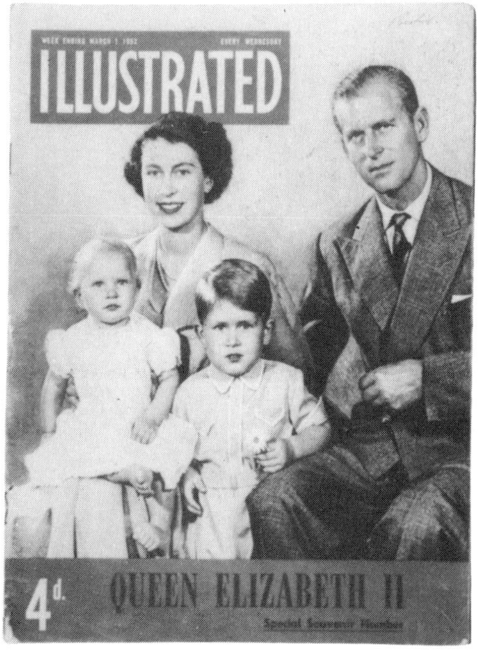

Illustrated – Queen Elizabeth II Special Souvenir Number, 1952. £2

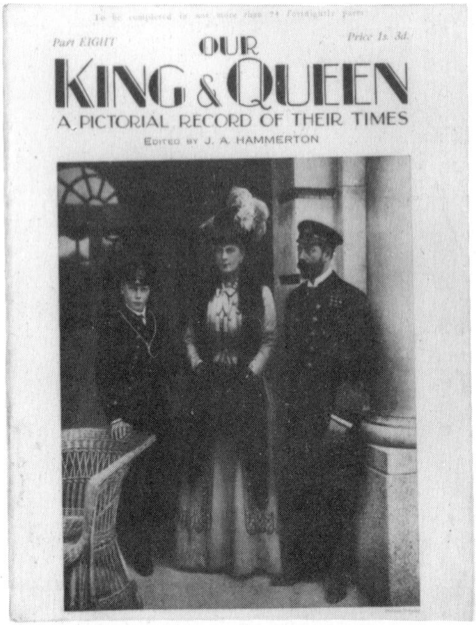

Our King and Queen – A Pictorial Record of their Times, 1929. £2

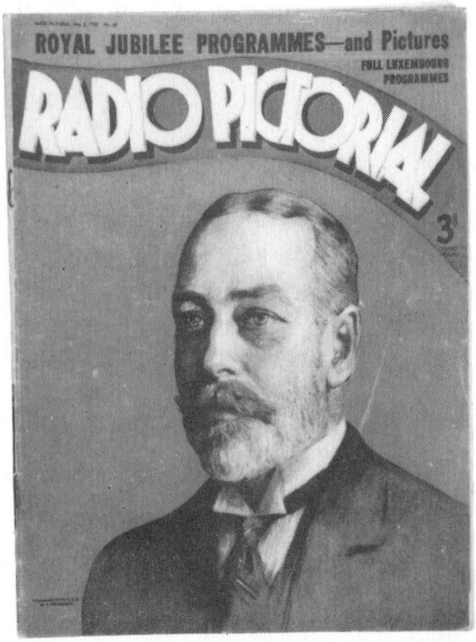

Radio Pictorial – Royal Jubilee Programmes, 1935. £1.50

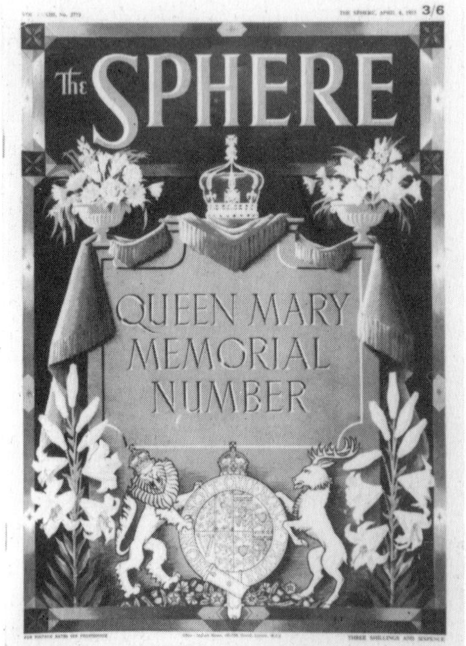

The Sphere – Queen Mary Memorial Number, 1953. £4

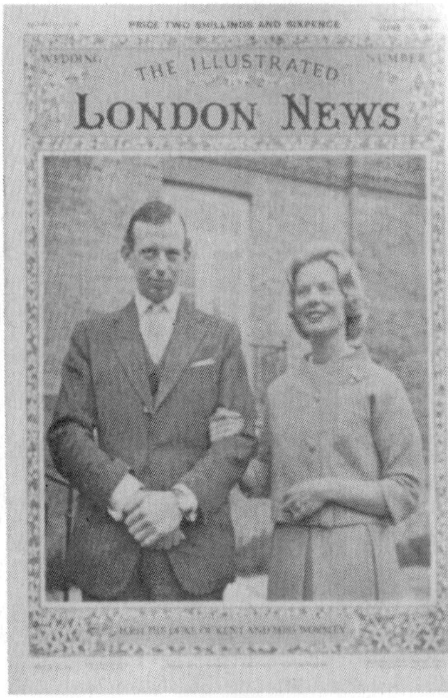

The Illustrated London News, 1961. £1.50

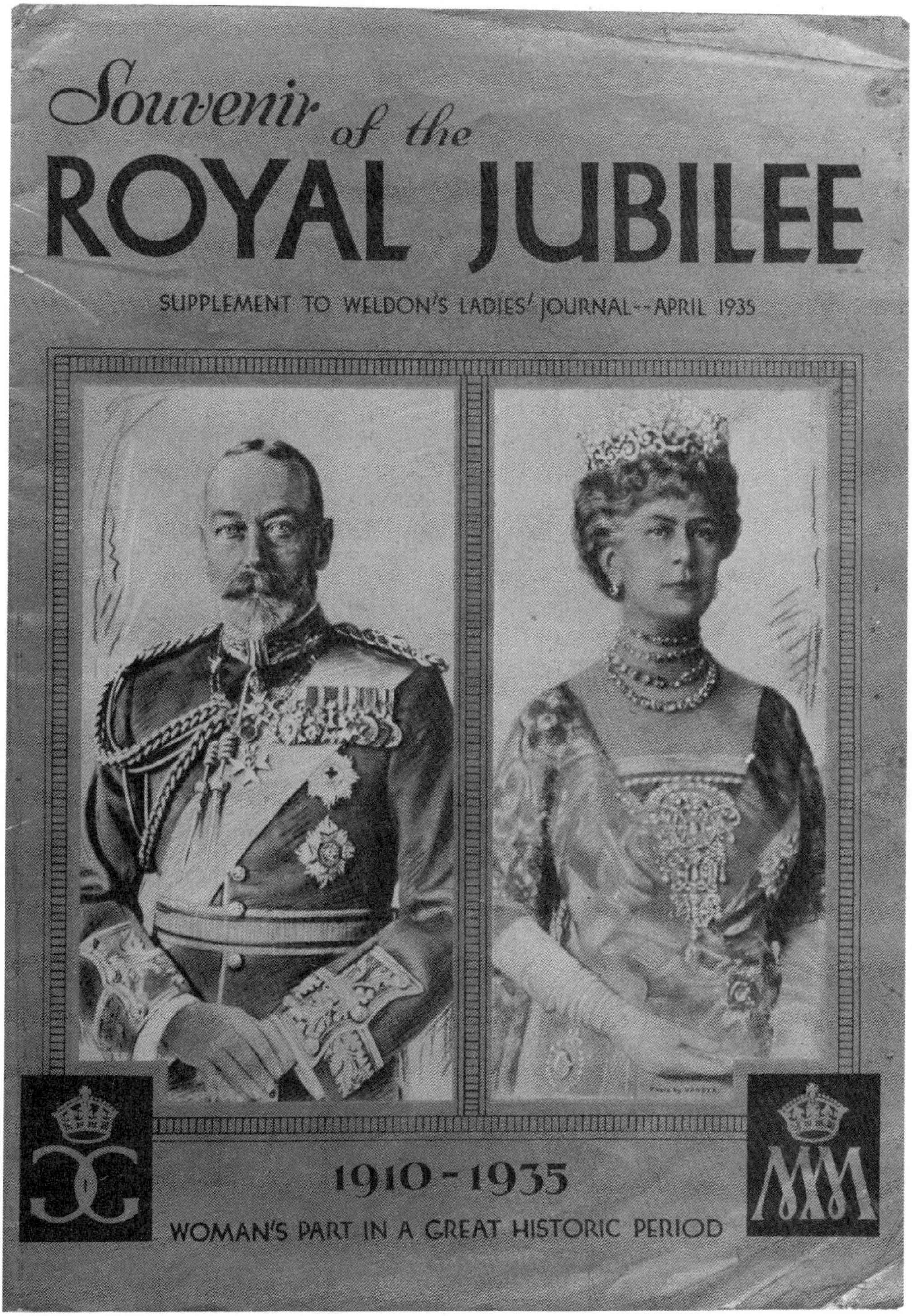

Souvenir of the Royal Jubilee 1910-1935, supplement to Weldon's Ladies Journal, April 1935. £3.50

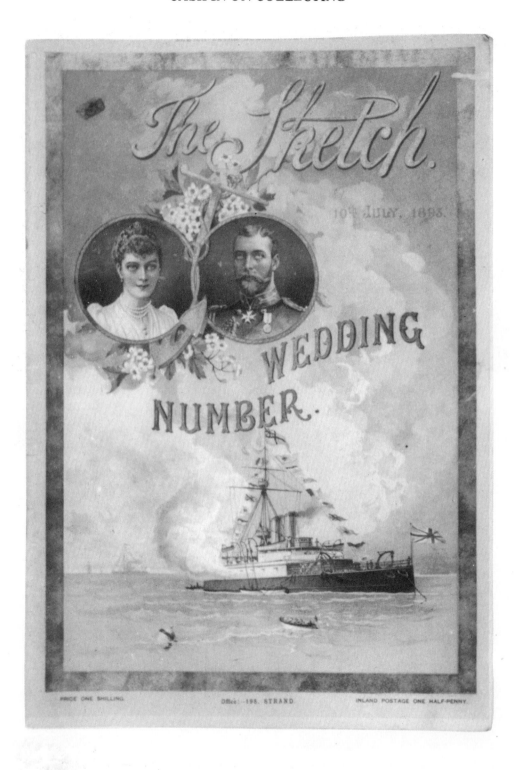

The Sketch, Wedding Number, Duke of York, 1893. £8

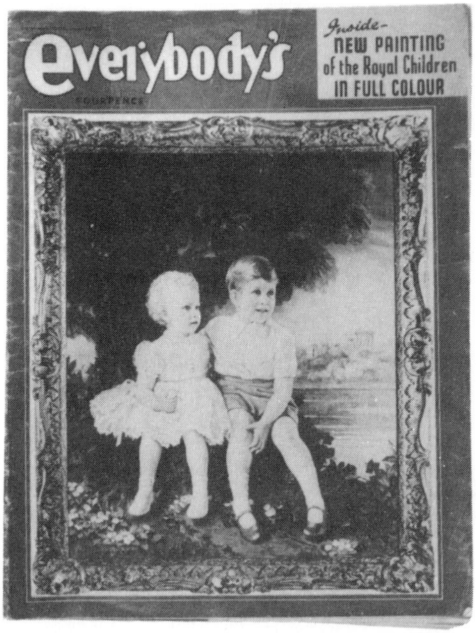

Everybody's – Paintings of the Royal Children, 1953. £1.50

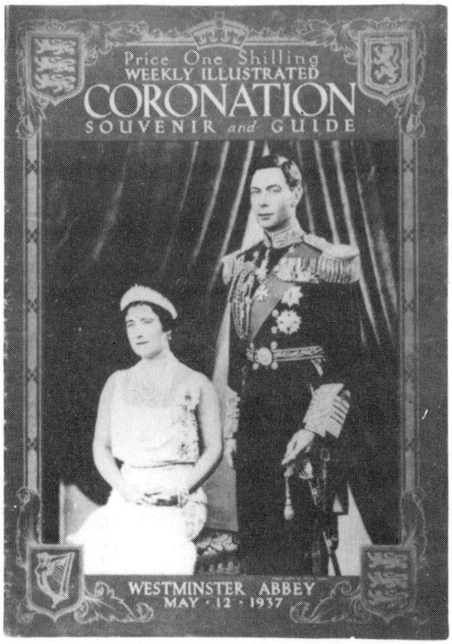

Weekly Illustrated – Coronation Souvenir and Guide, 1937. £4

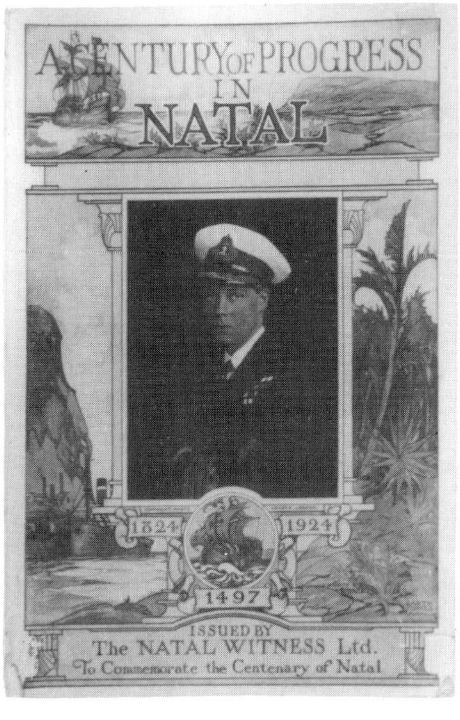

The Natal Witness – A Century of Progress in Natal, 1924. £3

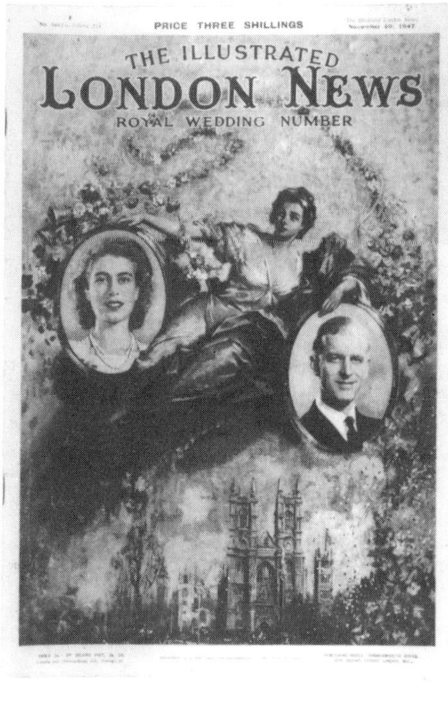

Illustrated London News – Royal Wedding Number, 1947. £4

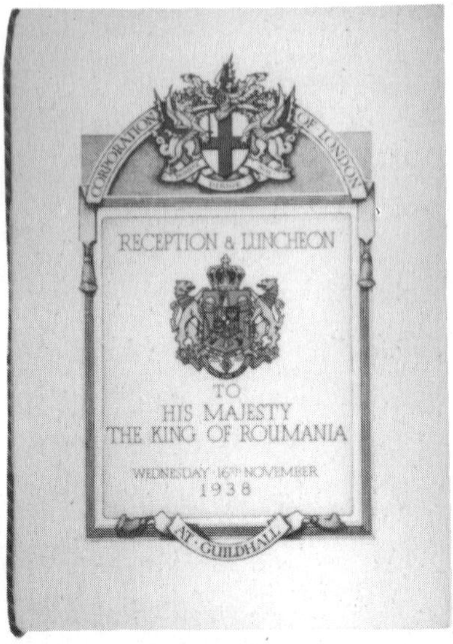

Menu – Reception and Luncheon to King of Roumania, 1938. £8

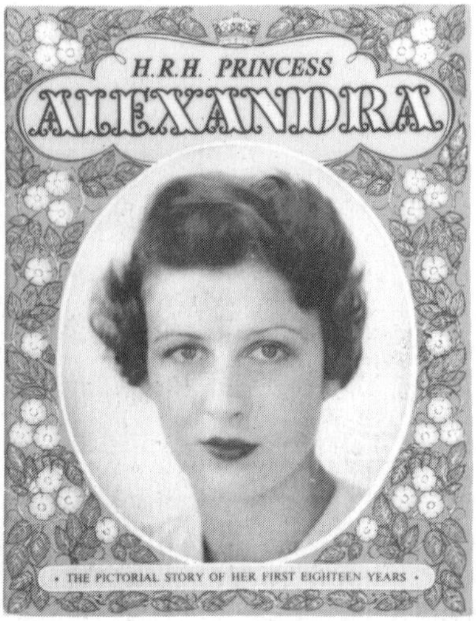

Pitkins – Princess Alexandra – Her First Eighteen Years, 1955. £1.50

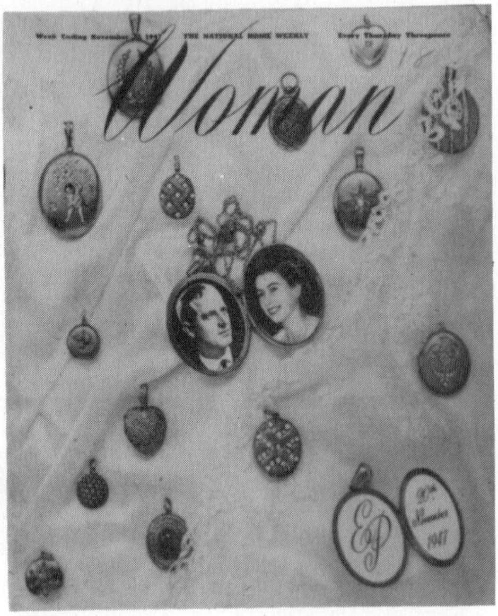

Woman – Pre-Wedding Issue, 1947. £1

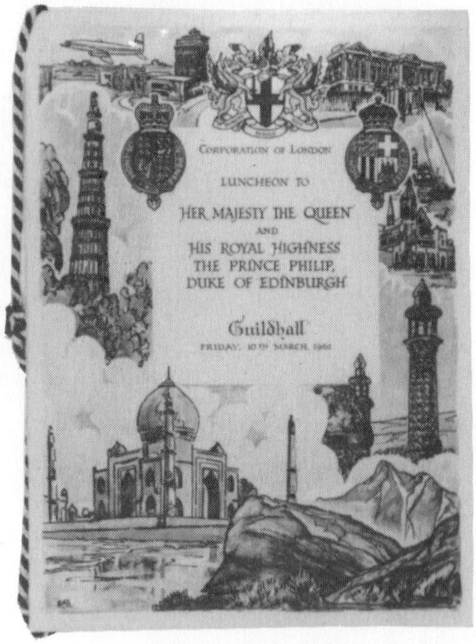

Menu – Luncheon to the Queen and Prince Philip, 1961. £3

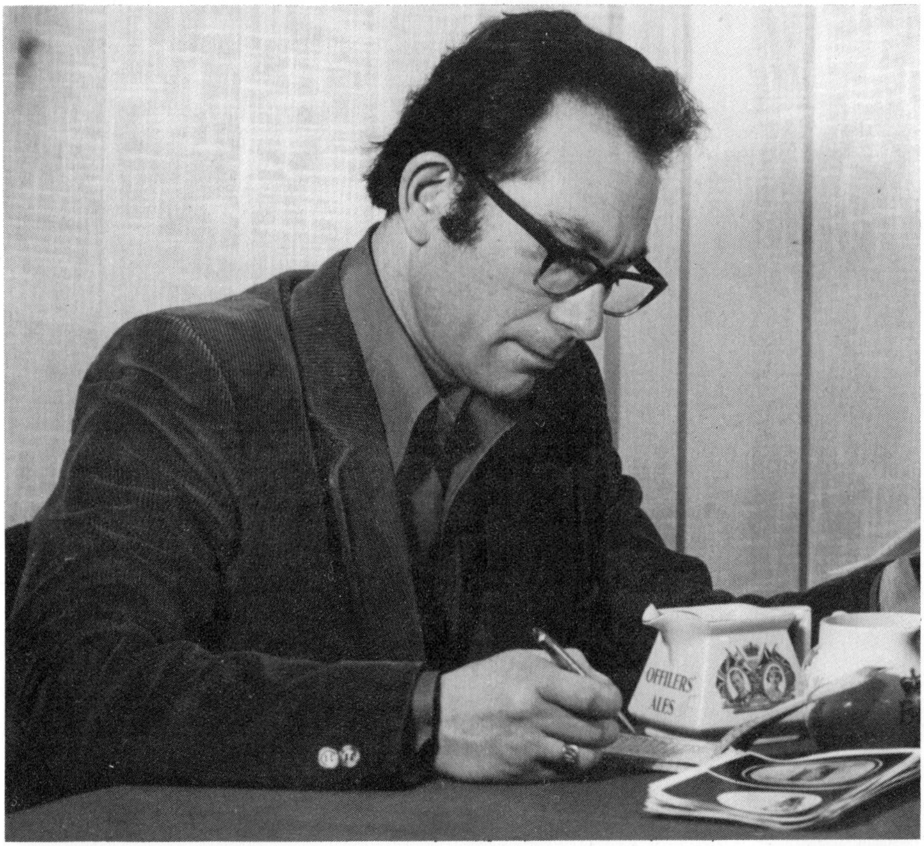

Keith Wilson is a dealer in items connected with pubs and breweries and has written two books on the subject — 'An Introduction to Breweriana' and 'Commemorative Breweriana'. His personal collection, however, is of beer mats.

"My passion for collecting started about 30 years ago when I was at school. I'd collect anything at all in those days, but eventually I settled on beer mats. Now I've got more than 14,500 of them, from British breweries only.

"A collection of beer mats has no intrinsic value except to beer mat collectors, which makes the tracking down of old and previously unknown issues all the more exciting.

"Beer mats were unknown in British pubs until after the First World War. It is thought that the idea was introduced by servicemen returning from the Continent, where mats had been in use since before the turn of the century. At that time there were more than 4,000 breweries in England, the majority of which are now obsolete; and it is the mats from these companies which are most eagerly sought. Another challenge has been set by the numerous recently formed "small breweries" who issue mats, often in very limited editions.

"With the exception of the Offilers mat which is the only known copy and star of my collection, the illustrations show a few of the rarities issued by obsolete companies within an approximate 30 mile radius of my home town."

Keith's business is called 'Brewtique' and he buys and sells everything related to brewery advertising. His customers come from all over the world but especially from places where there is still nostalgia for anything British — 'the old English pub captures the imagination of people of British descent abroad' said Keith.

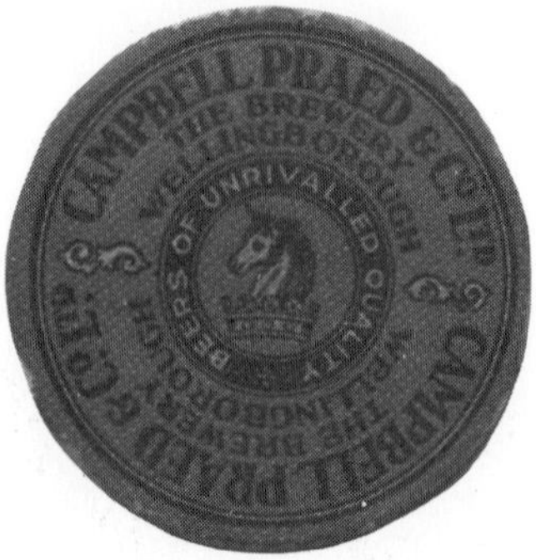

Pre war issue from Campbell Praed & Co. Ltd. of Wellingborough.

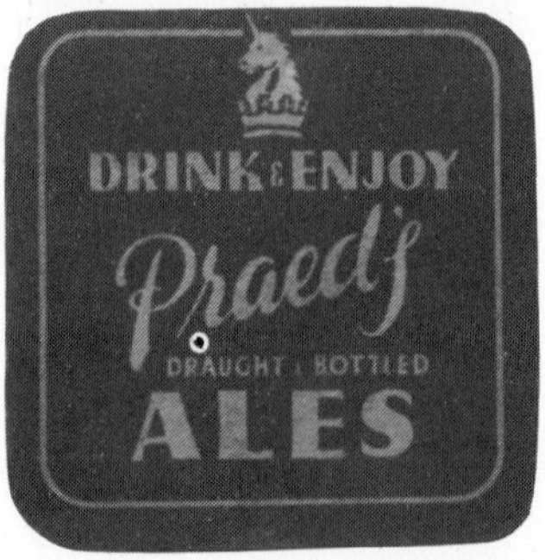

Post war issue from Campbell Praed & Co. Ltd. of Wellingborough.

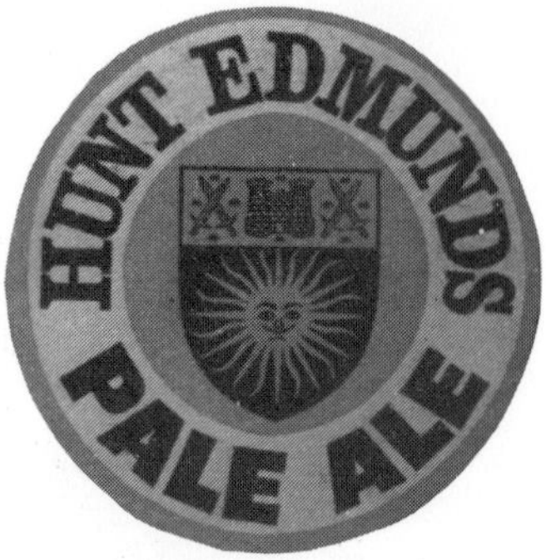

The only Hunt Edmunds mat not to incorporate their trademark 'Banbury Cross'.

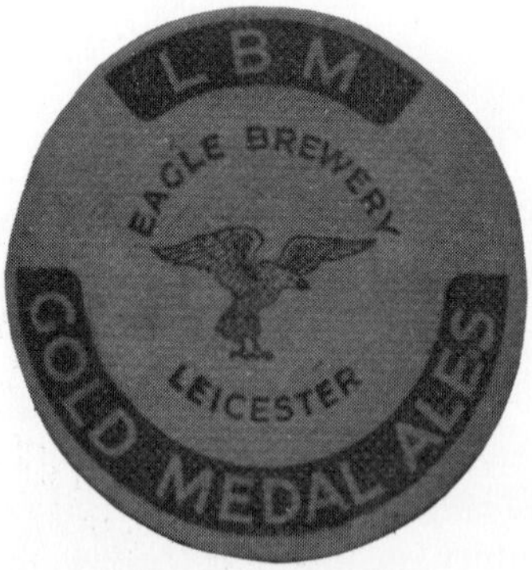

'L.B.M. Gold Medal Ales' from the Leicester Brewing & Malting Co.

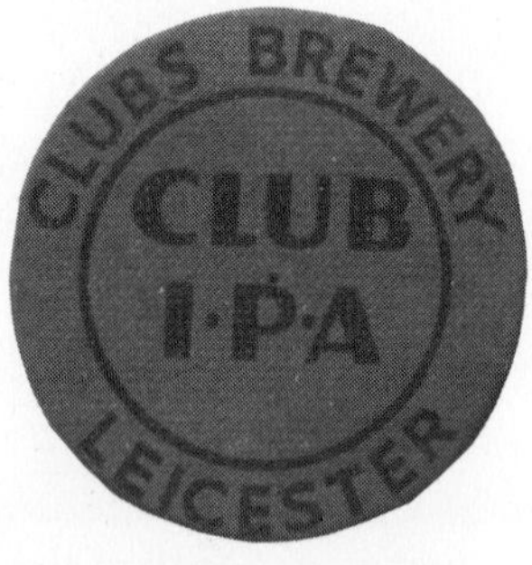

Post war mat from the Northants & Leicestershire Clubs Co-operative Brewery Ltd.

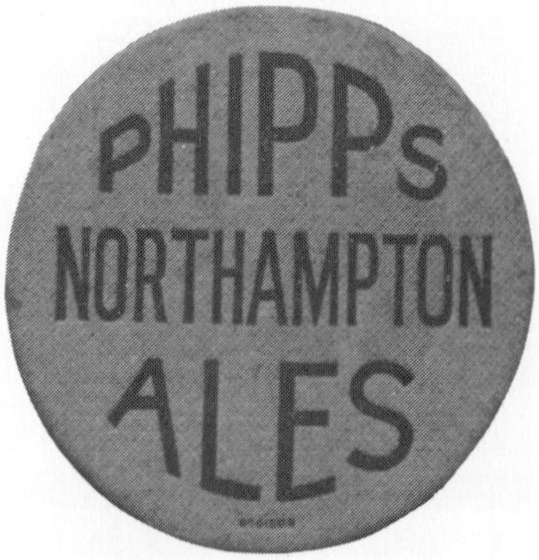

Pre war issue from Phipps of Northampton.

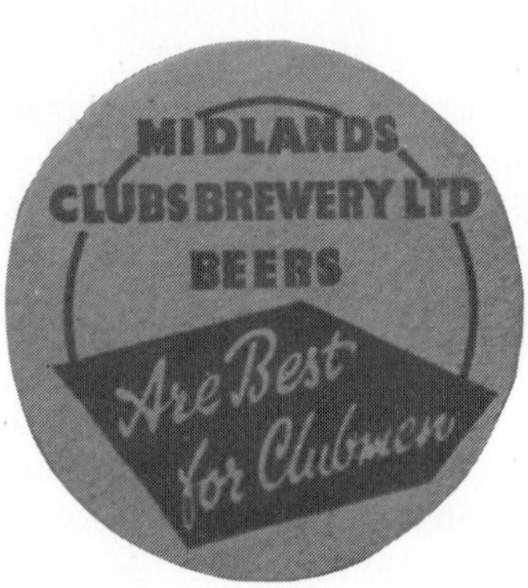

First issue from the Midlands Clubs Brewery Ltd.

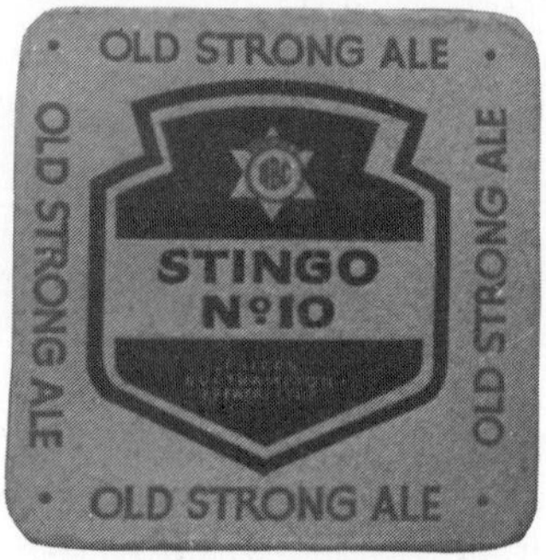

Stingo No. 10, first issue from the amalgamation of Phipps and Northampton Brewery Co.

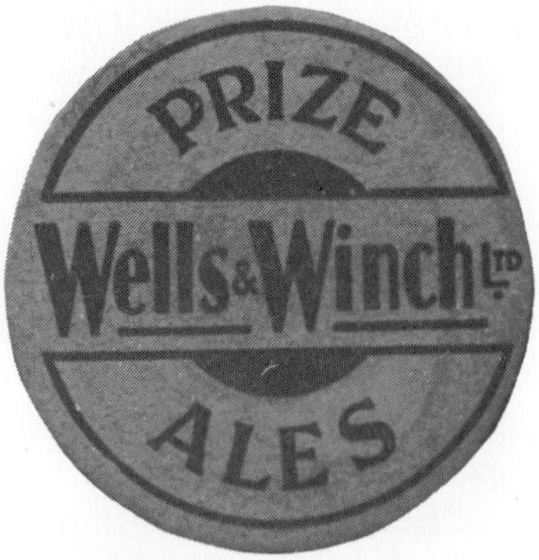

An early post war mat from Wells & Winch Ltd. of Biggleswade, 'Prize Ales'.

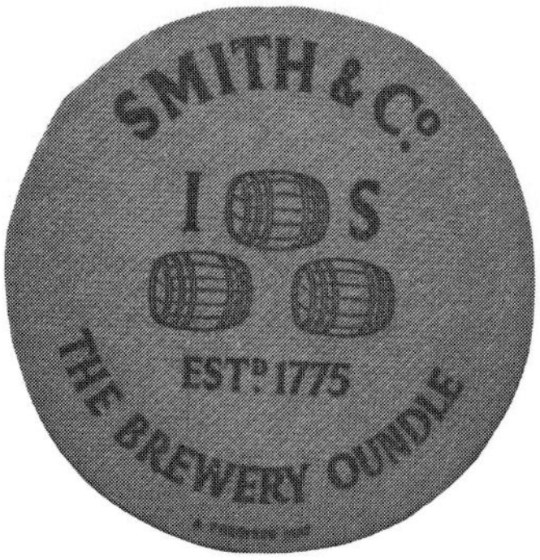

The only issue from Smith & Co., The Brewery, Oundle.

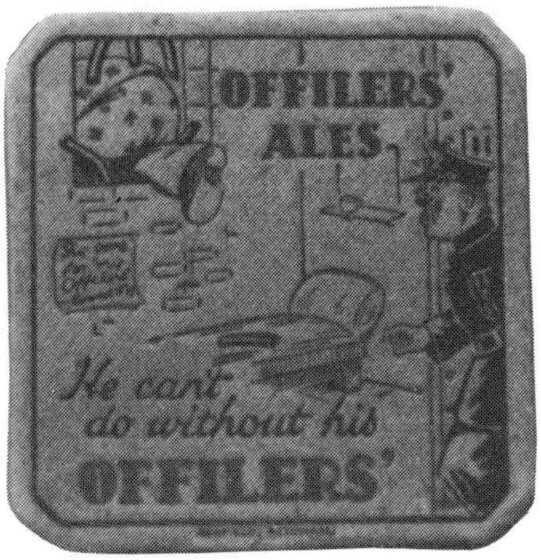

The only known example of this Offilers mat, 'He can't do without his Offilers'.

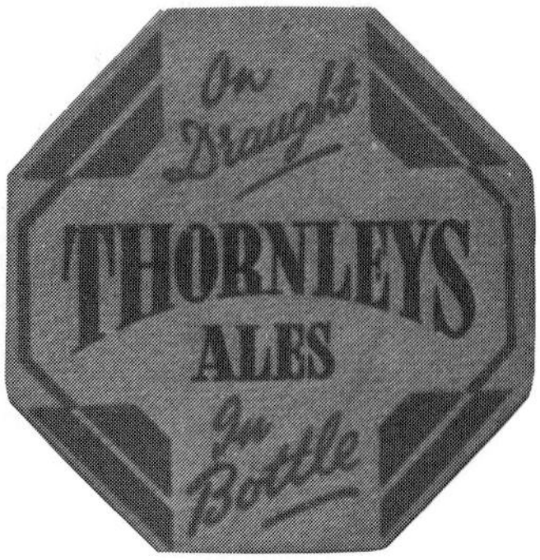

'On Draught, In Bottle', an octagonal mat issued by Thornley Kelsey of Leamington Spa.

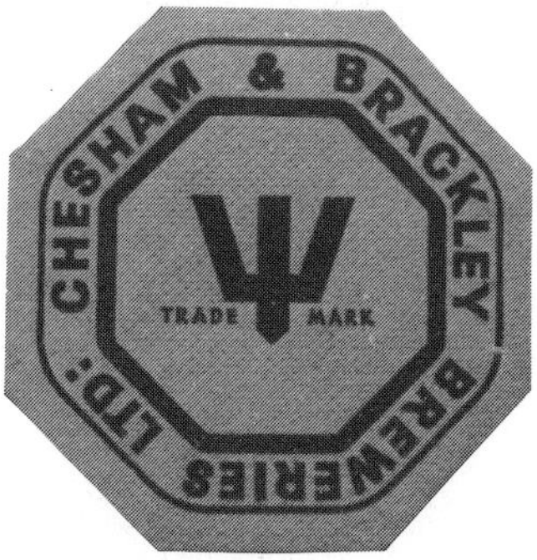

One of only two issues by Chesham & Brackley Breweries of Brackley.

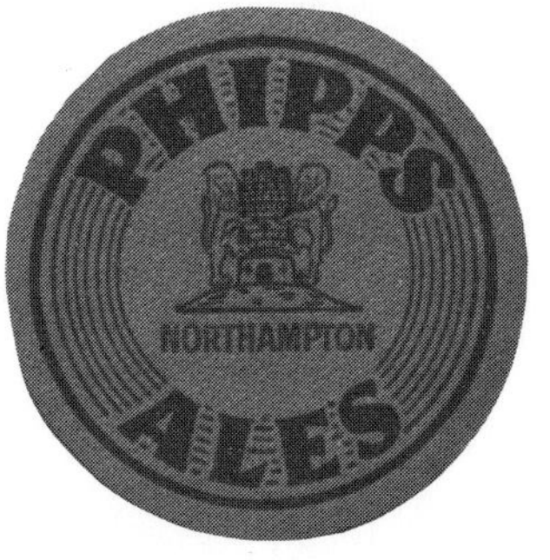

Post war issue from Phipps of Northampton.

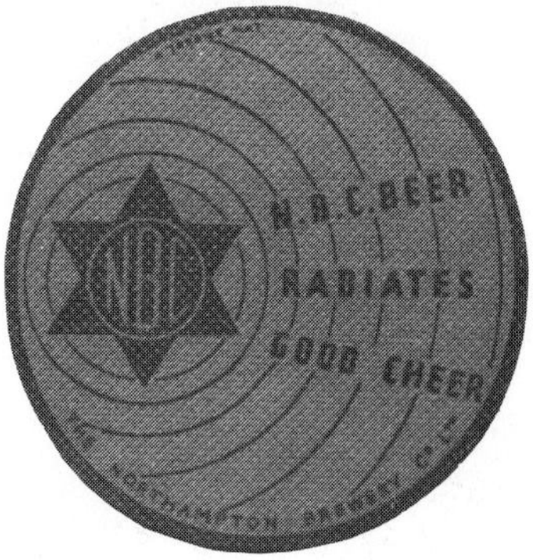

N.B.C. Beer Radiates Good Cheer, an early issue from The Northampton Brewery Co. Ltd.

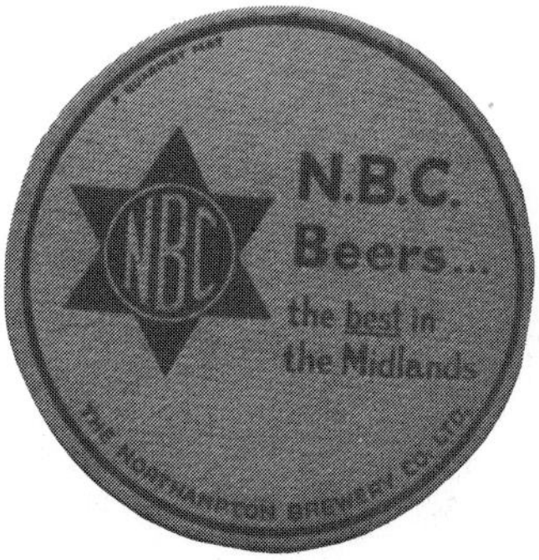

N.B.C. Beers, the best in the Midlands, an early issue from The Northampton Brewery Co. Ltd.

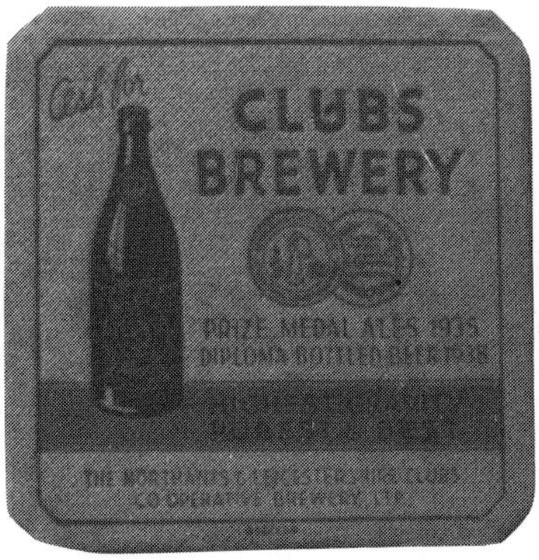

Pre war issue from the Northants & Leicestershire Clubs Co-operative Brewery Ltd.

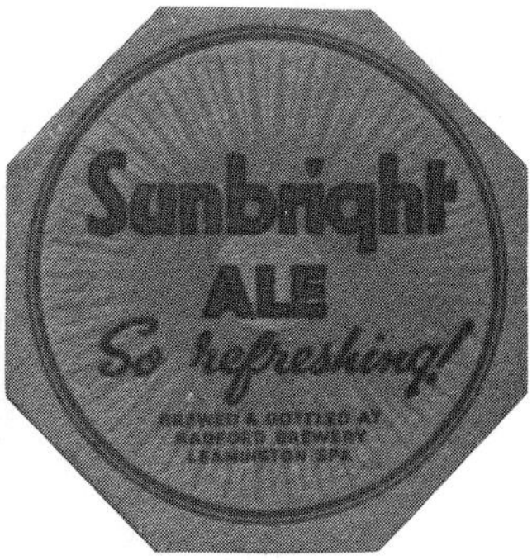

'Sunbright Ale, So Refreshing', an octagonal mat issued by Thornley Kelsey of Leamington Spa.

Ray and Iris Tunnicliff are collectors of fairground memorabilia and run their own Fairground Museum. Ray, a retired police officer, is the Chairman of the Fairground Society.

Ray said: "I hate to see everything from the past being dispersed and I suppose that's why I began collecting things from old fashioned fairgrounds about thirty years ago when it became obvious that they were all going to disappear forever quite soon. In fact the first thing I ever bought was an old music box and it grew from there.

"In four large buildings on the farm steading where we live we house and display the collection we have built up over the years as well as a few items on loan from other members of the Fairground Society. They range from music boxes to fairground organs and Tiller's Royal Marionettes which is a marionette show said to have been put on before Queen Victoria's children.

"I retired from the police after being badly injured in a riot 11 years ago and then we bought this place. It took nine furniture vans to move the collection here and it has gone on growing ever since."

The Rutland Cottage Music Museum is located on the B1165 road between Spalding and Wisbech and it is open every week-end between April and September. A tour of the museum takes around one and a half hours because it is vast comprising old fashioned fairground horses and figure carvings; a bioscope front; 7,000 photographs of fairgrounds going back to 1830; 200 circus posters going back to 1891; old gramophones and 10,000 old 78 rpm records dating from between 1890 and 1950. Admission to the museum is £1 for adults and 50p for children or OAPs.

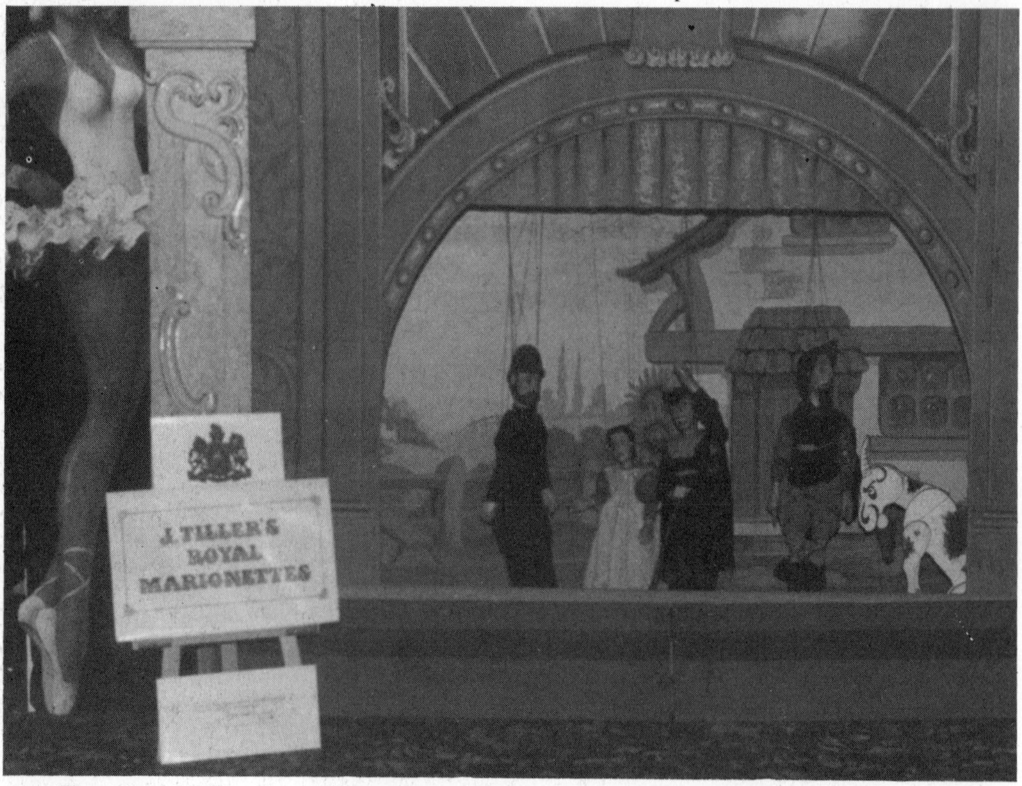

The original Tillers Royal Marionettes which travelled the fairs in the early 19th century, comprising over thirty Marionettes, stage, scenery and props.

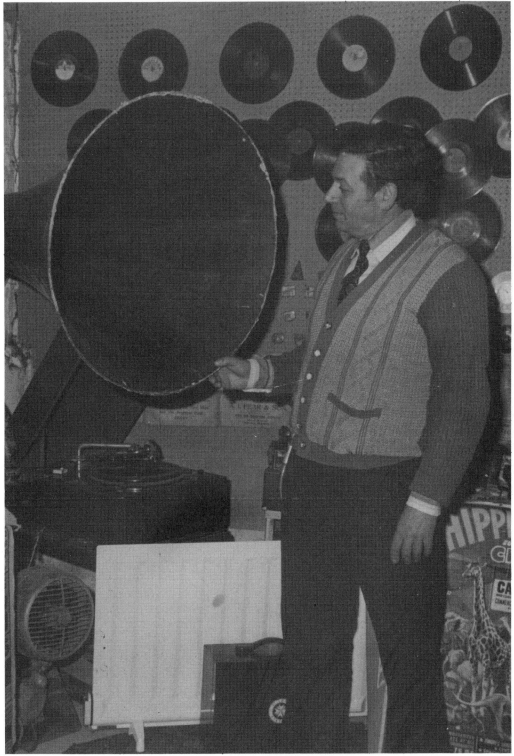

Ray Tunnicliff in his Music Museum.

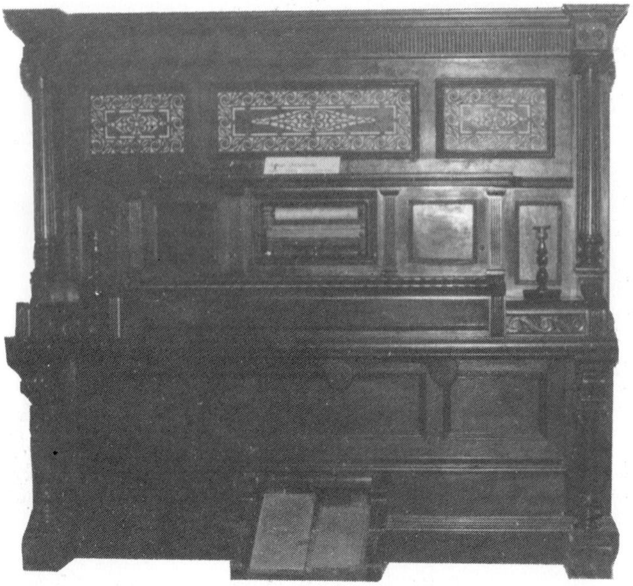

Aeolian Orchestrelle Model V (1890-1900), plays 58 note rolls. £1,000

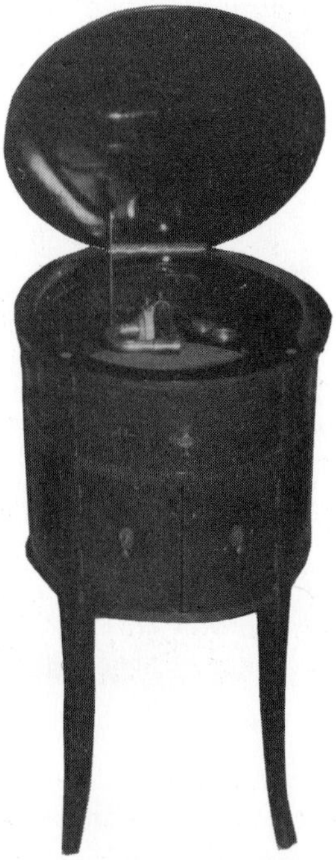

An unusual circular gramophone by E. F. Tyler, the oval cabinet in the Sheraton style made between 1922 and 1927. £160

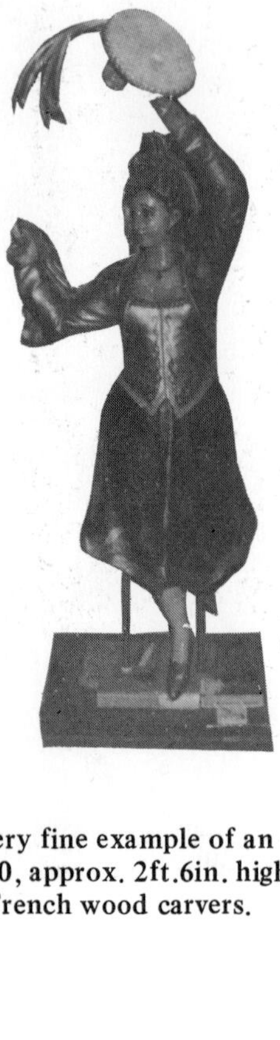

A very fine example of an organ figure, circa 1900, approx. 2ft.6in. high, probably the work of French wood carvers. £600

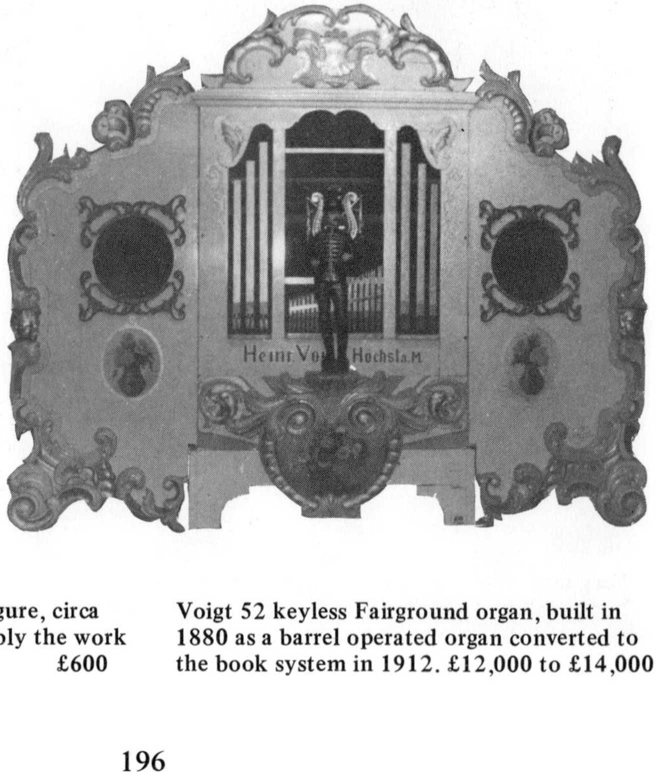

Voigt 52 keyless Fairground organ, built in 1880 as a barrel operated organ converted to the book system in 1912. £12,000 to £14,000

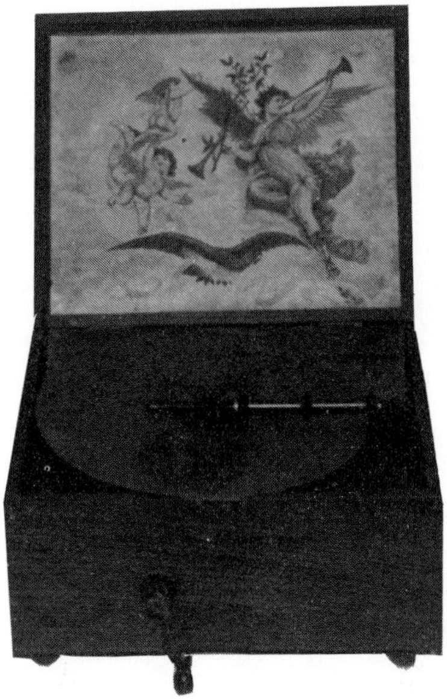

Fortuna disc music box, made by Jules Heinrich Zimmermann, Leipzig, Germany, with 21cm. discs, circa 1903. £120

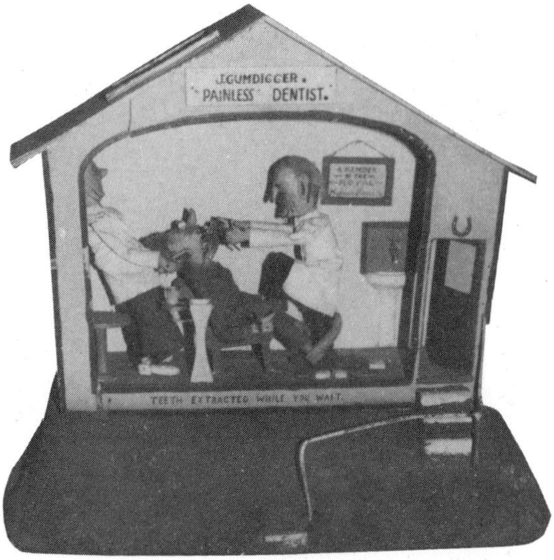

Fairground Automata Dentist, circa 1900, part of a much larger show which travelled. £200

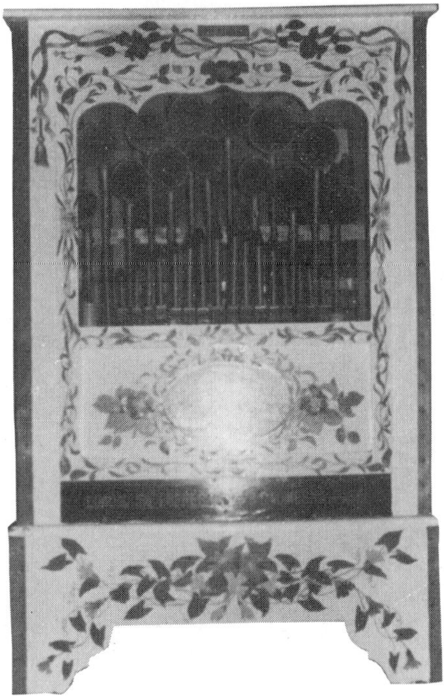

Very rare playing example of a Limonaire Trumpet barrel key Fairground organ, with two barrels, nine tunes on each barrel, circa 1890. £8,000

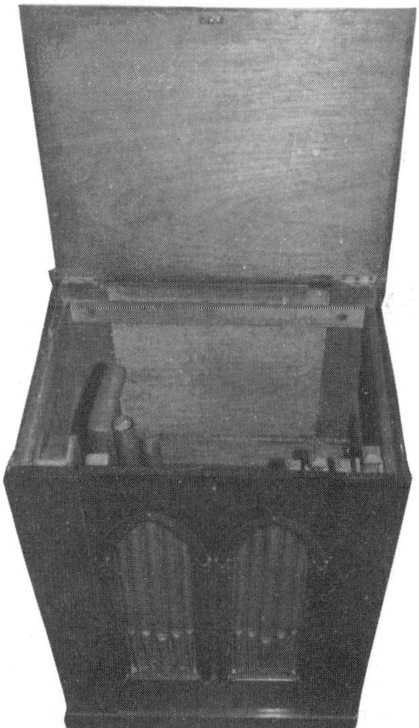

Church barrel organ or chamber organ, playing ten hymns with three ranks of pipes, circa 1845. £1,200

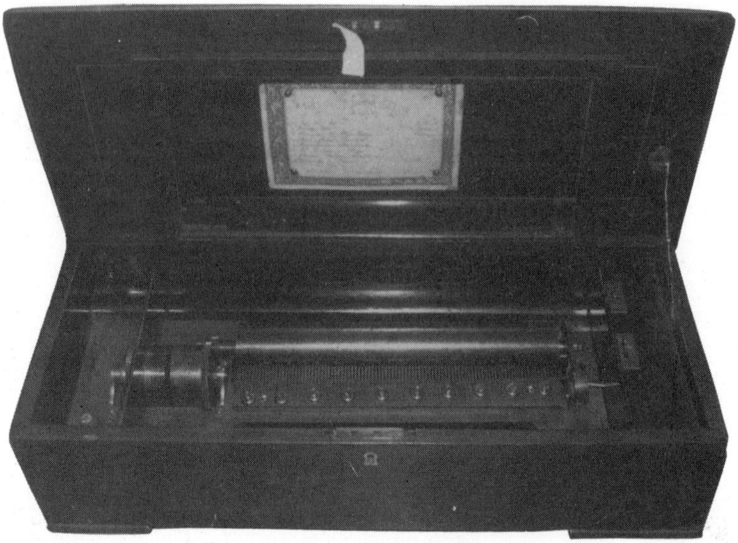

Large music box by Nicole Freres, playing 8 tunes, with double sprung movement giving about 30 minutes playing. £1,000

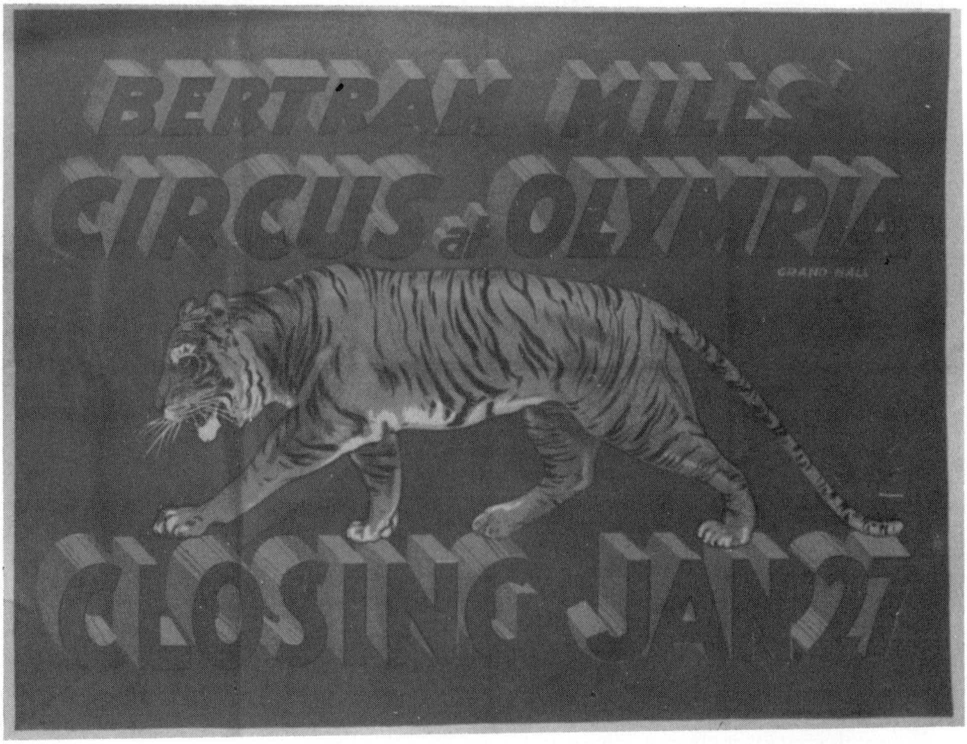

Circus Poster Bertram Mills Circus, circa 1937. £30

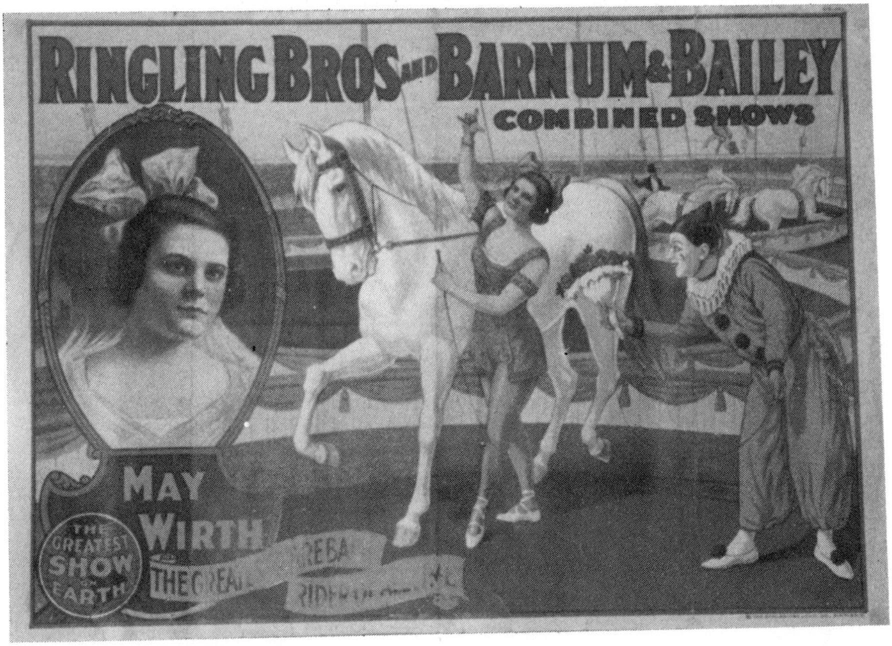

Circus Poster Barnhum and Bailey's Circus, circa 1930. £50

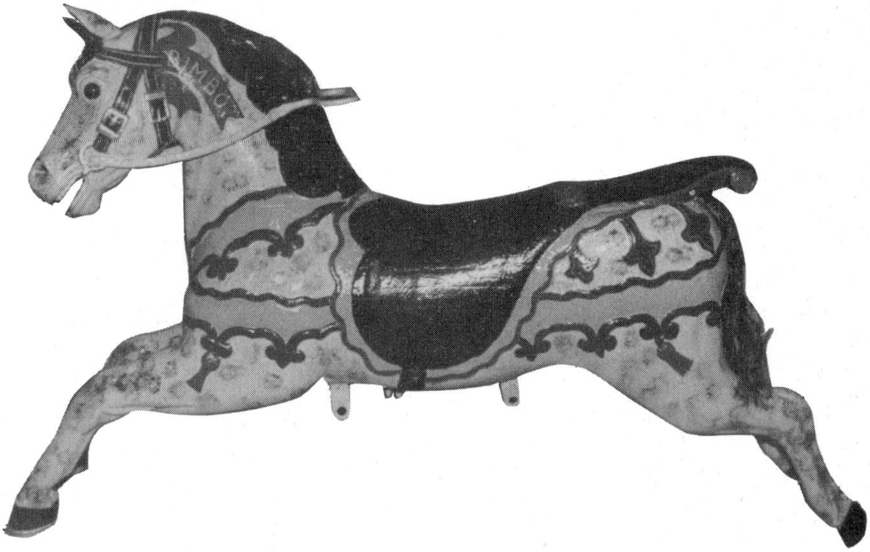

Large Fairground horse from a set of Gallopers, made by Savages of Kings Lynn, 1893. £900

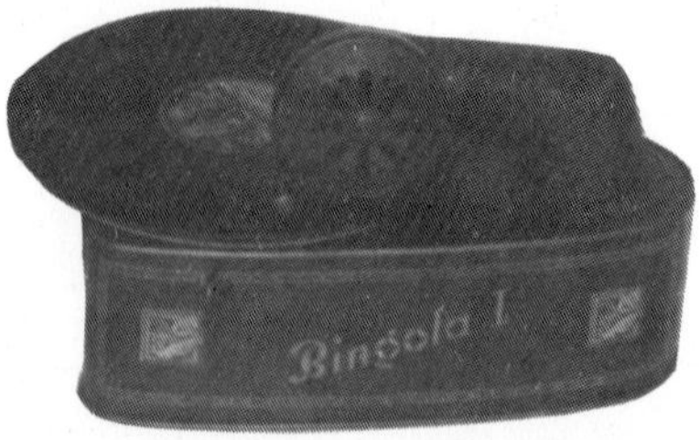

Bingola I child's gramophone, simple clockwork action key wind, circa 1920. £60

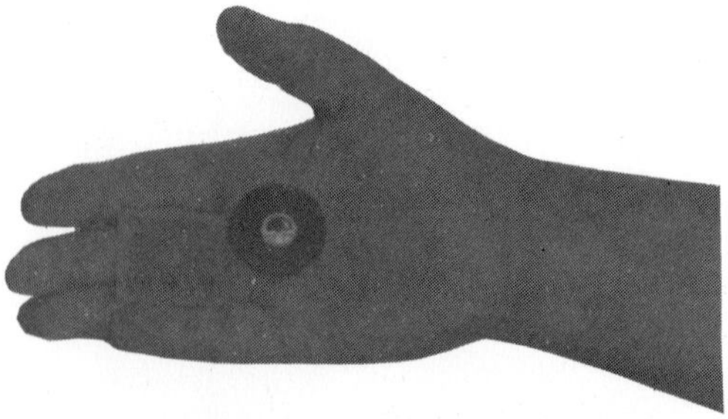

Smallest gramophone record and cover, made in 1924 for Queen Mary's Dolls' House, plays God Save the King. £110

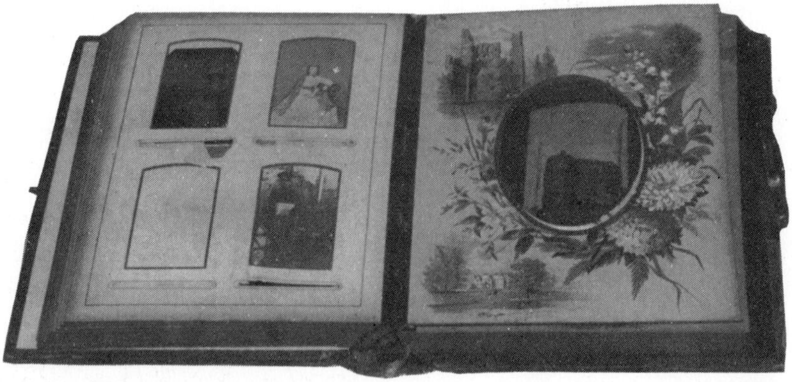

Victorian photo album with music box movement, circa 1890. £40

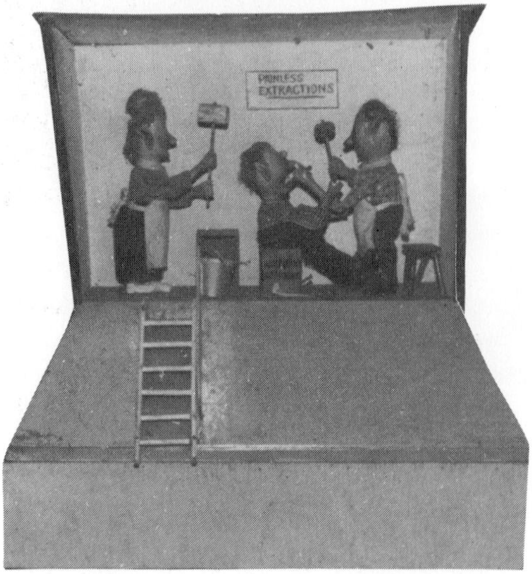

Fairground Automata Dentist, cira 1900, part of a much larger show which travelled. £200

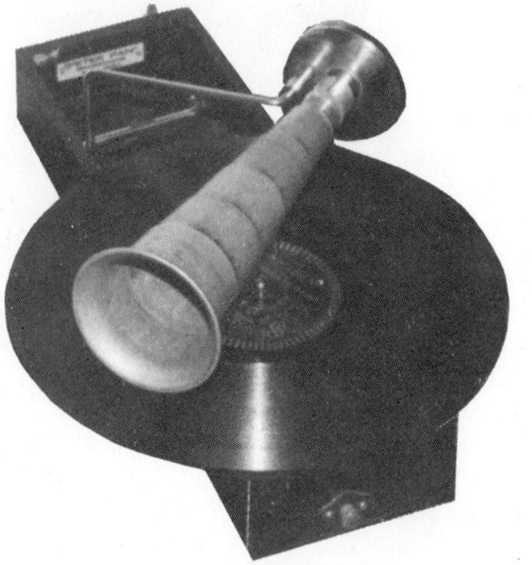

Portable gramophone by Peter Pan now much sought after by collectors, circa 1920. £120

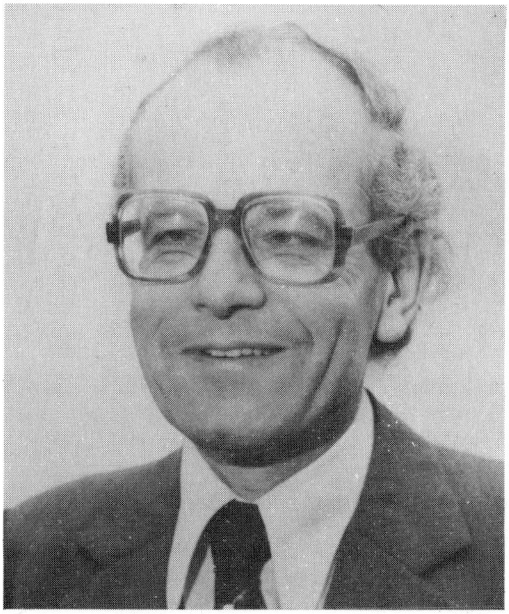

Dr Bernard Watney is a medical practitioner who collects old stout bottles, particularly Guinness bottles.

"I used to work as a medical officer for Guinness and when I joined the firm in 1971 I became interested in their early stone bottles. A man I met in Ireland told me they used to call those bottles "yellow necks' which I thought was a nice name.

"One of the first ones I bought is still full of Guinness and there's a paper label on it saying 'Donnelly, Ritz Bar, Waterside, Derry'. It dates from the turn of the century but the Guinness will be off now, I'm afraid.

"Some of the earliest stout bottles were made in London by the Stephen Green Pottery of Lambeth which pre-dated Doulton and they are impressed with the mark 'glass lined' which meant not porous.

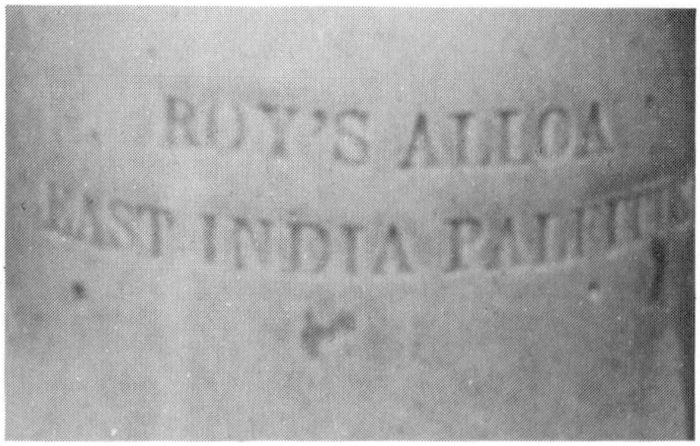

They made some fine bottles for Browning of Lewes impressed with names like Brown Stout and Porter. Yet another good bottle I have of theirs is stamped with the name 'Roy's Alloa East India Palfitt' — it's very rare. My favourites are the ones with impressed wording and you can find the name Guinness spelt in many different ways, sometimes as Guineas. They are getting very hard to find and one of my best is a yellow neck impressed with 'Guinness' XX Stout' from George Gordon of Strabane."

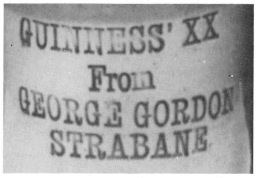

Dr Watney finds that Durham is a good area to go looking for Guinness bottles because people up there seem to have drunk a great deal of it at the turn of the century. Prices used to be as low as 50p for a bottle but they have now risen to around £25 for an average example and can go as high as £250 for special impressed ones.

In the Guinness museum Dr Watney saw what he describes as 'a lovely early shape bottle dating from around 1840 which is coloured creamy white all over.' He would like to find another similar for his collection.

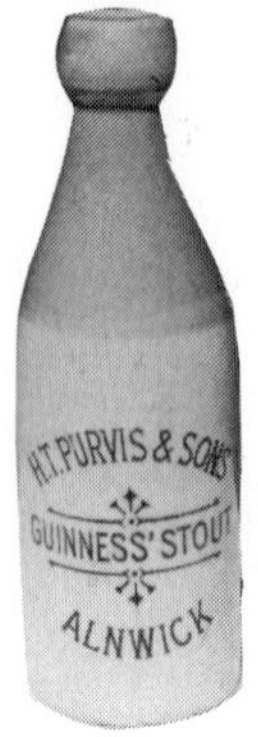

Guinness' Stout by H. T. Purvis & Sons, Alnwick. £30

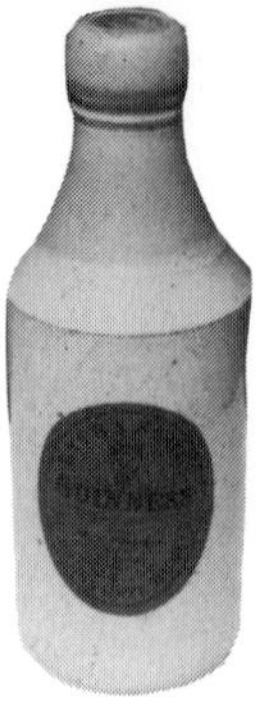

Stoneware stout bottle with Guinness Extra Stout, W. J. Donnelly, Derry. £30

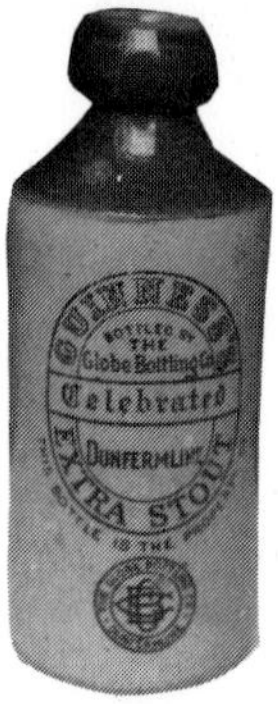

Guinness's Extra Stout, bottled by Globe Bottling Co., Dunfermline. £40

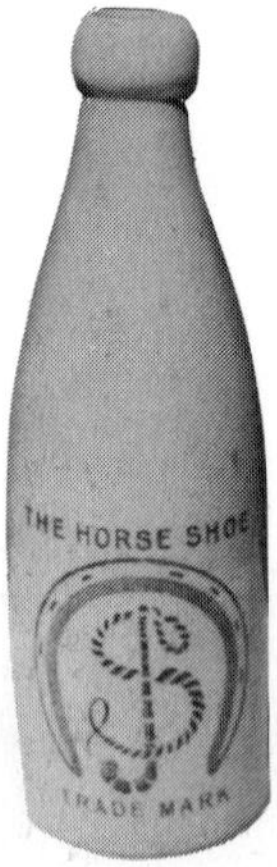

Stout bottle by The Horse Shoe. £50

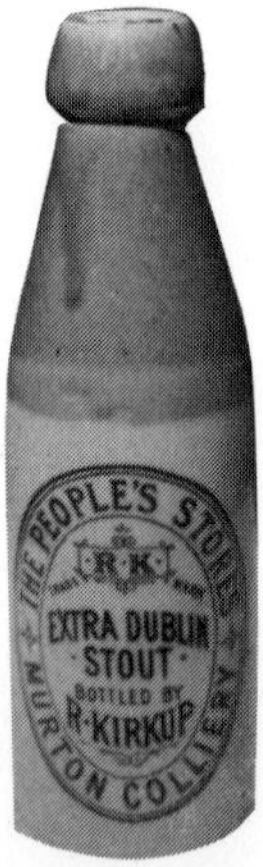

Extra Dublin Stout, bottled by R. Kirkup. The People's Stores, Murton Colliery. £40

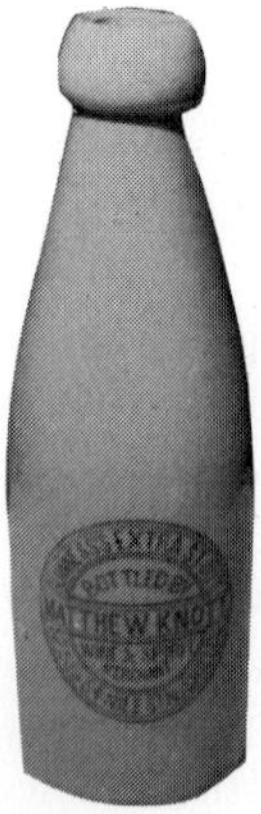

Guinness's Extra Stout, bottled by Matthew Knott, Wine & Spirit Merchant. £30

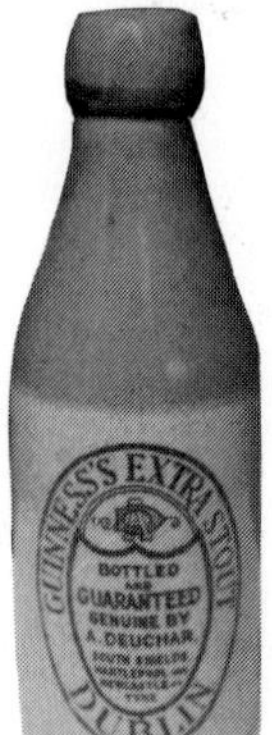

Guinness's Extra Stout, bottled and guaranteed genuine by A. Deuchar, Newcastle-upon-Tyne.£30

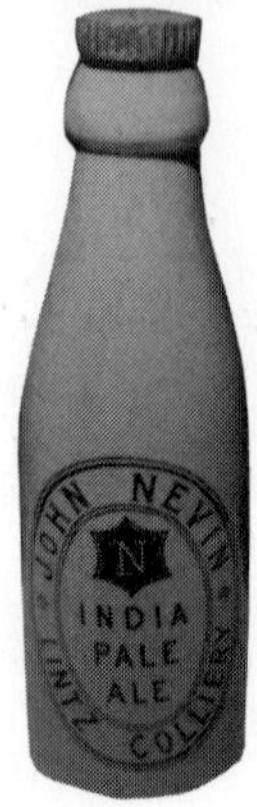

India Pale Ale by John Nevin, Lintz Colliery. £30

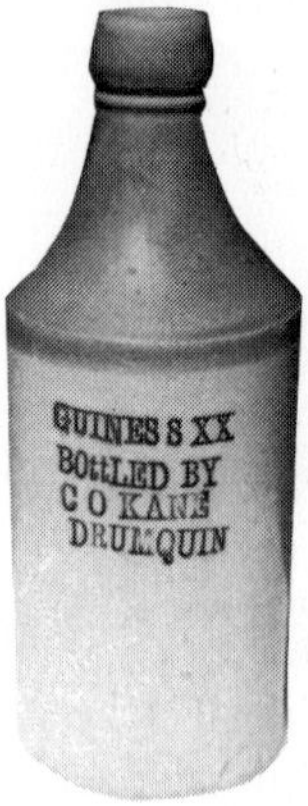

Guiness XX, Bottled by C. O. Kane, Drumquin. £50

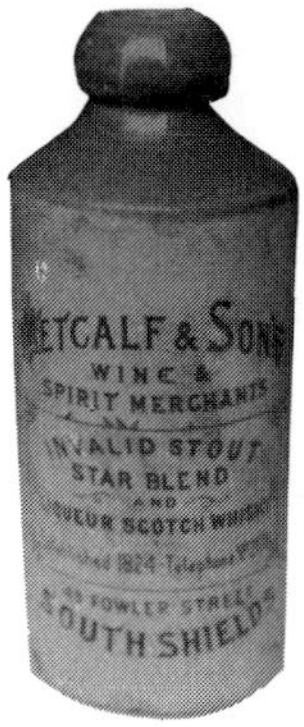

Metcalf & Sons, Invalid Stout, Star Blend, South Shields. £30

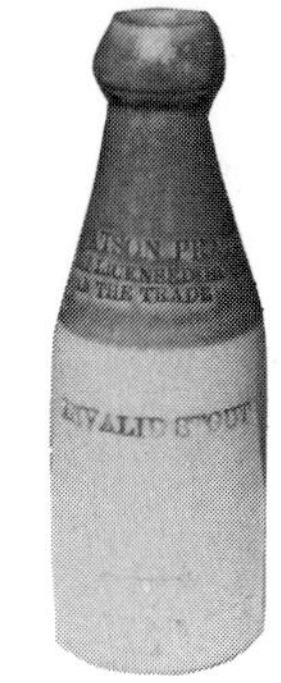

Watson Pratt 'Best Licensed House in the Trade', Invalid Stout. £40

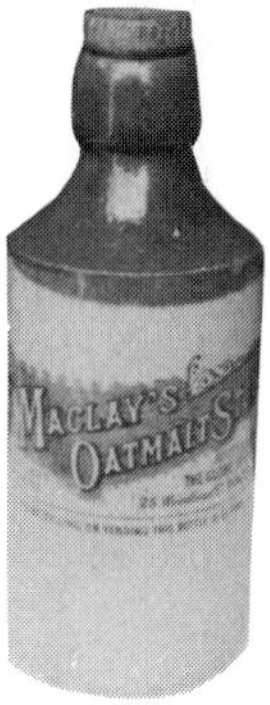

Maclay's Oatmalt Stout. £40

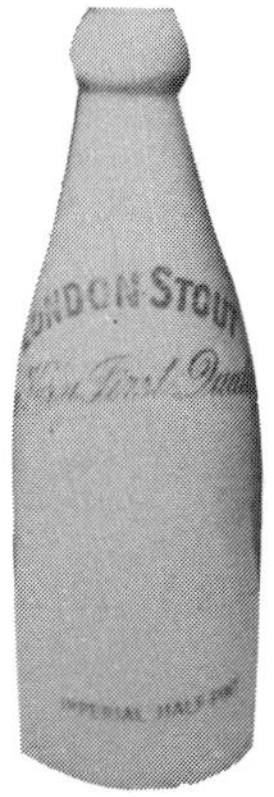

London Stout, 'The Very First Quality', Imperial Half-Pint. £50

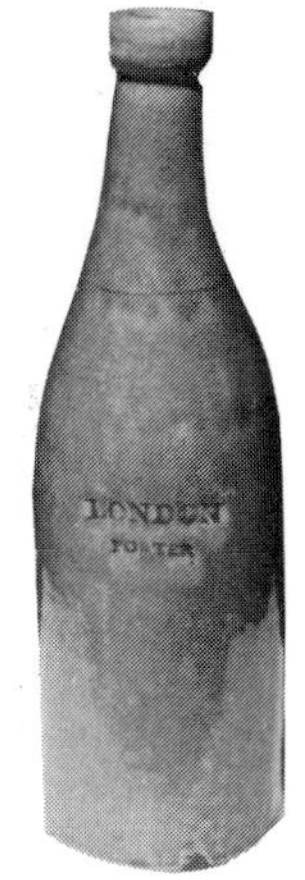

Stoneware stout bottle impressed 'London Porter'. £20

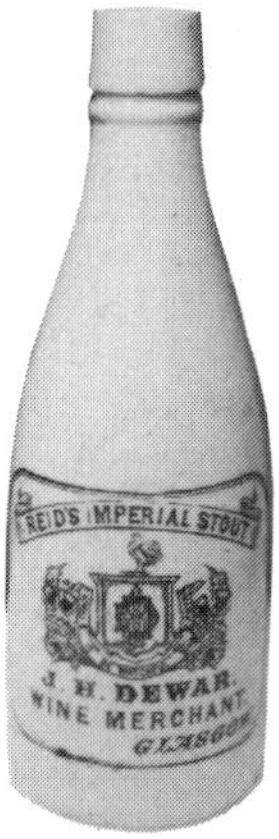

Reid's Imperial Stout by J. H. Dewar, Wine Merchant, Glasgow. £30

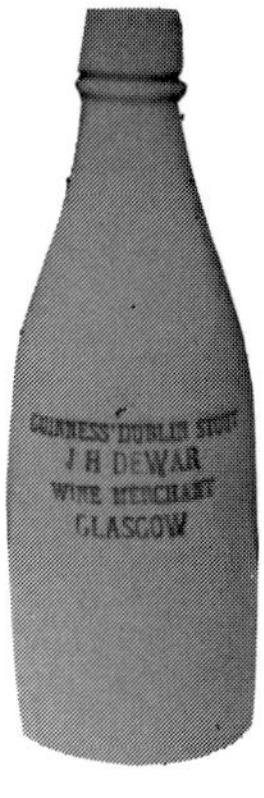

Guinness' Dublin Stout by J. H. Dewar, Wine Merchant, Glasgow. £30

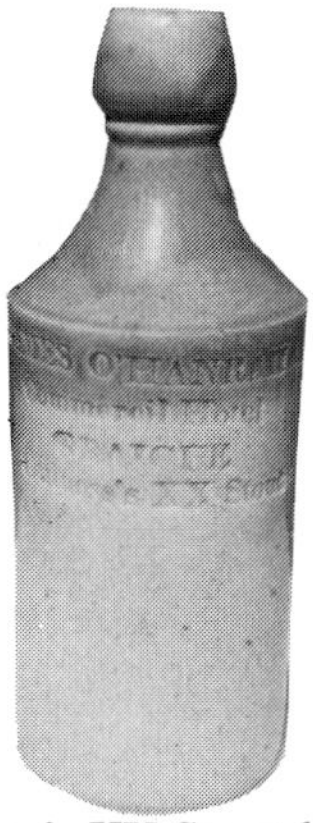

Guiness's XX Stout by James O'Hanrahan, Commercil Hotel, Graigue. £50

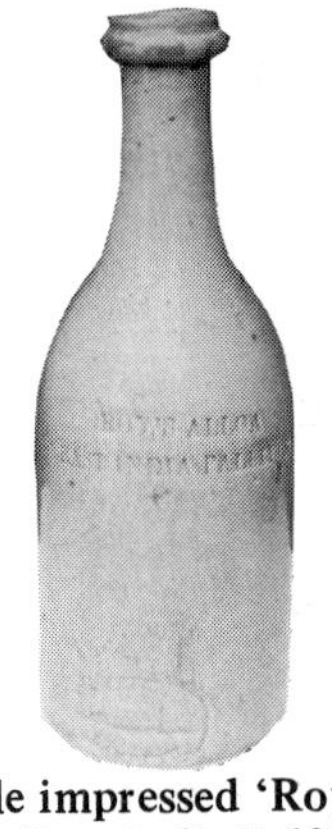

Bottle impressed 'Roy's Alloa East India Palfitte by Stephen Greens, Lambeth', 'Glass Lined Inside'. £150

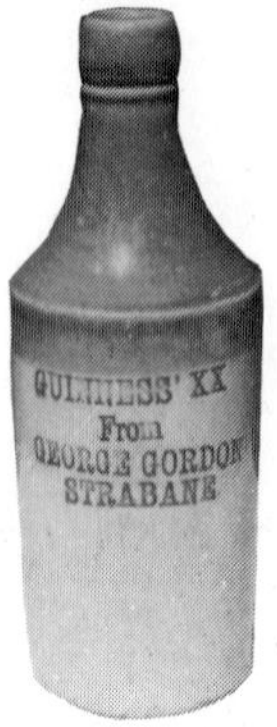

A very rare bottle impressed 'Guinness'XX from George Gordon, Strabane'. £150

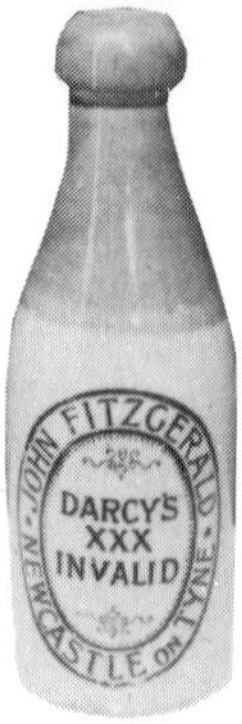

Darcy's XXX Invalid Stout by John Fitzgerald, Newcastle on Tyne. £30

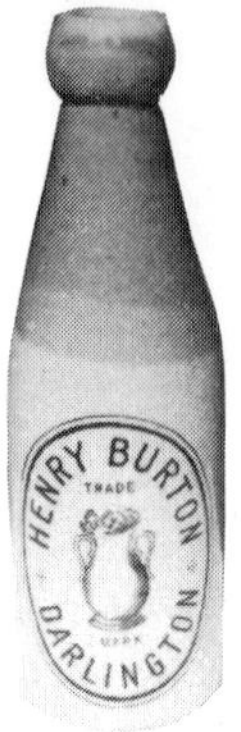

Stout bottle by Henry Burton, Darlington. £50

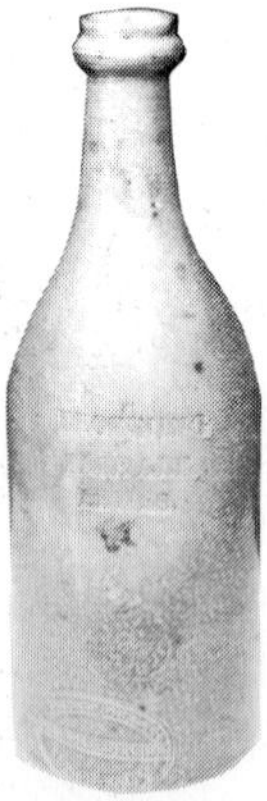

Bottle impressed 'Browning Pale Ale Lewes by Stephen Greens, Lambeth,' 'Glass Lined Inside'. £150

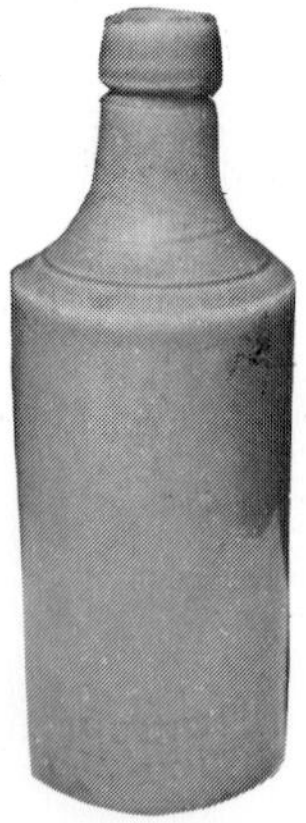

Stoneware stout bottle, incised 'Guineas, Dublin Porter'. £30

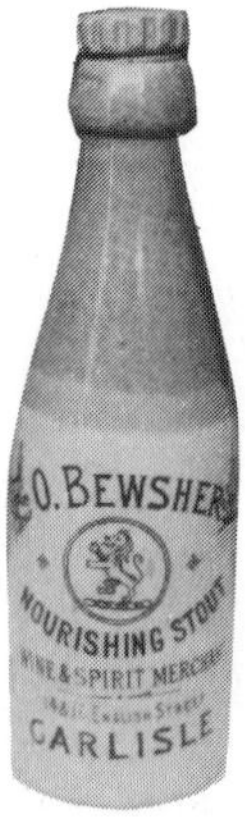

Nourishing Stout by O. Bewsher's, Wine & Spirit Merchant, Carlisle. £30

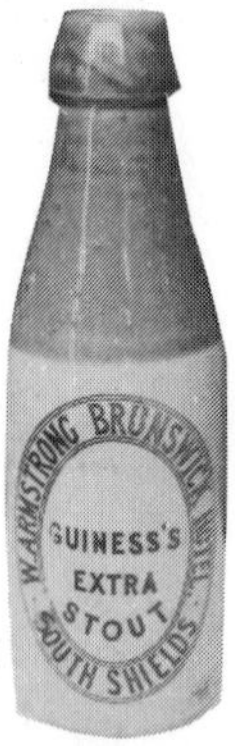

Guiness's Extra Stout by W. Armstrong, Brunswick Hotel, South Shields. £30

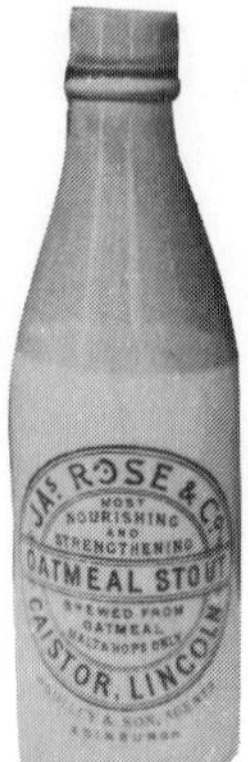

Oatmeal Stout by Jas. Rose & Co., Caistor, Lincoln. £30

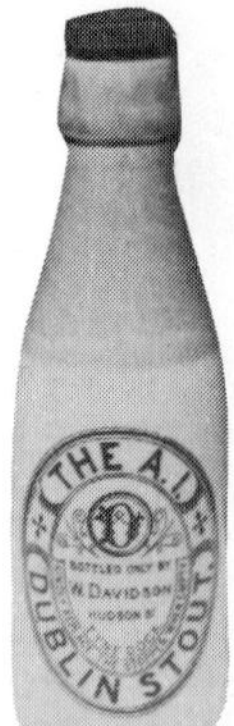

The A.I. Dublin Stout bottled only by W. Davidson, Hudson St., Tyne Dock. £30

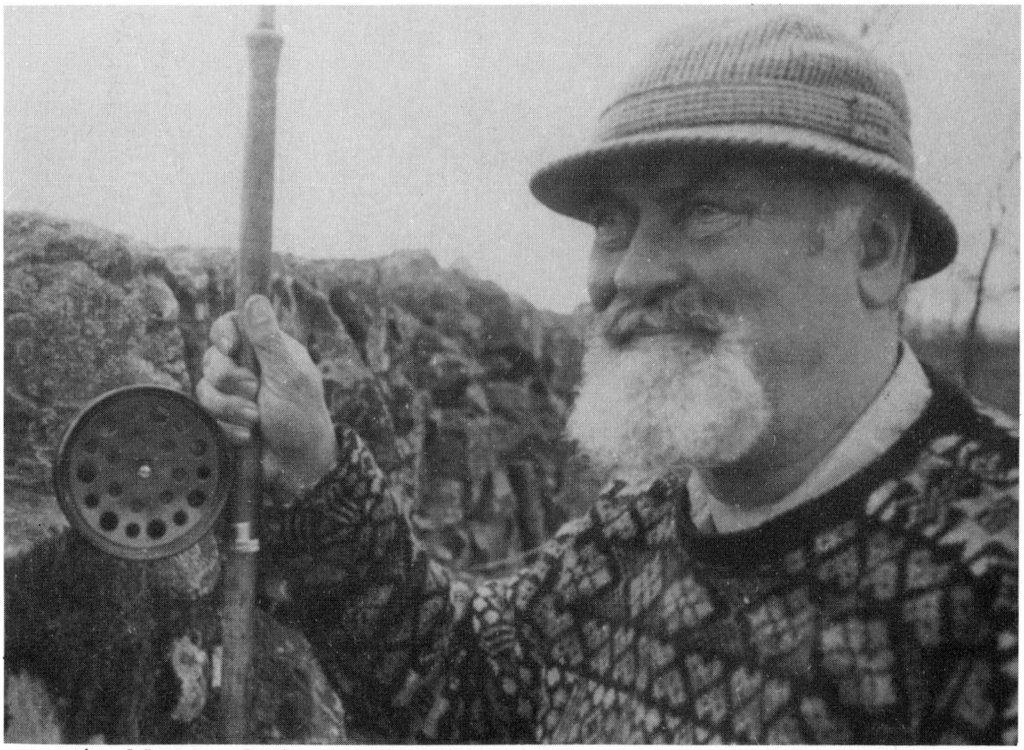

Jamie Maxtone-Graham collects and deals in items connected with fishing.

"I love doing this because you never know what's going to turn up, there's so little known about piscatorial items.

"Fishing is a very popular pastime all over the world and I've got 400 customers in 25 different countries from USA to Japan.

"I began dealing because I've always been a keen fisherman myself and one day by accident in the Scottish Borders I met a German acquaintance who I'd previously met while fishing in Yugoslavia. He was looking for an old fashioned brass reel and I happened to have one made by Malloch of Perth which I sold to him and from there on I was in business.

"Now I've got over 500 examples for collecting old reels is a big hobby both in this country and in America. I've also got 150 rods and literally thousands of flies, landing nets, gaffs etc. Many of the items in my catalogue are unique."

His most unusual items at the moment include two pieces of wood, about 5 inches by 2 and a half inches by two inches, with large lead weights inset in them. They were used for 'harling' on the River Tay. Harling means that the fishermen is rowed out into the middle of the river by a ghillie and the line is then wrapped round the piece of wood 'so you can see when something happens'.

Also rare are two 18th century Scottish 'pirns' which were used to run line around before fishing reels were invented. They are worth £200 each.

The item he would most like to find is what he describes as 'the Rolls Royce of fishing reels'. It is a Silex Rex made by Hardy's of Alnwick in the 1930's and is a level wind reel which does not get tangled. It costs around £1,000.

Jamie Maxtone-Graham is the author of two books about fishing — 'The Best of Hardy's Anglers' Guides' and 'To Catch a Fisherman' which describes all the fishing tackle patents taken out between 1857 and 1950.

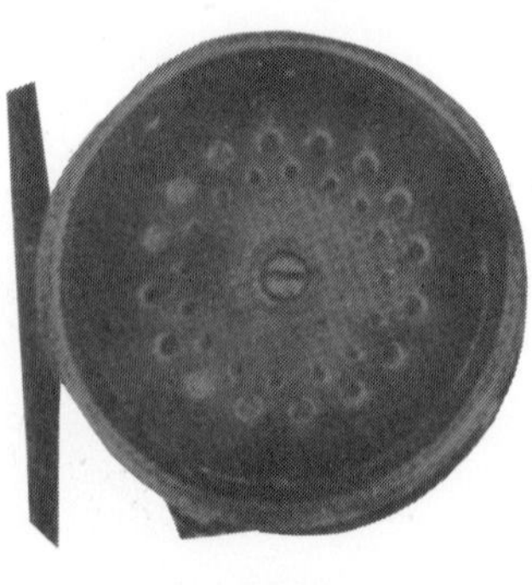

4in. Hardy 'Perfect' aluminium salmon reel with trademark, ivorine handle and leather case.£100 – £120

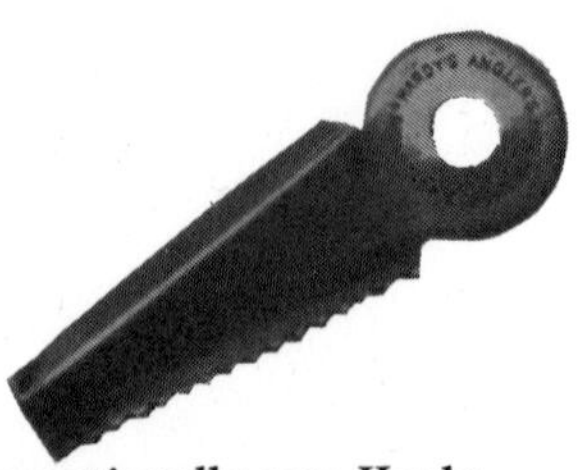

Exceptionally rare Hardy accessory, the reamer made to clear the bowl of the 'Hardy's Angler's and Sportsman's Pipe'. £8 – £12

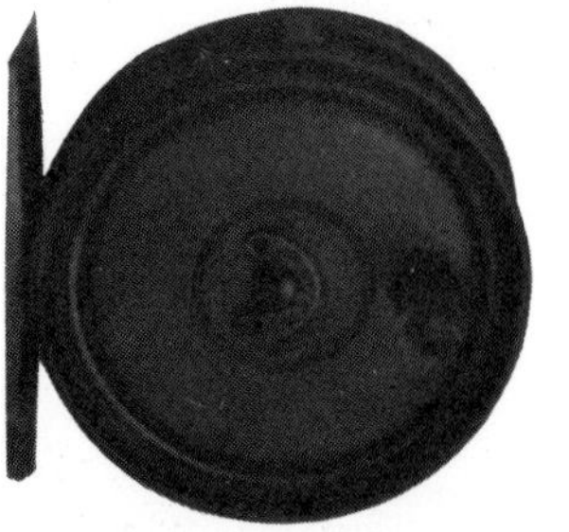

3.1/8in. Hardy 'Uniqua' narrow-drum trout fly reel, with ivorine handle, horse-shoe drum latch, 1918 check, stamped Mk I Duplicated.
£25 – £40

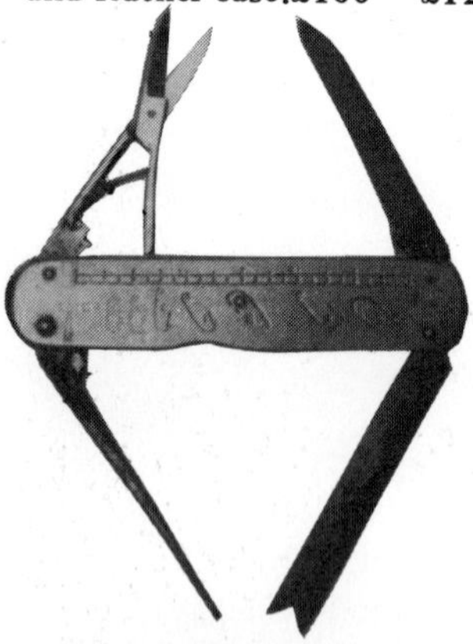

Unnamed angler's knife (pattern originally devised by casting champion Fred Shaw), with selection of useful angling tools, one nickel-silver side engraved with 3in. scale, and seven hook sizes. £8 – £12

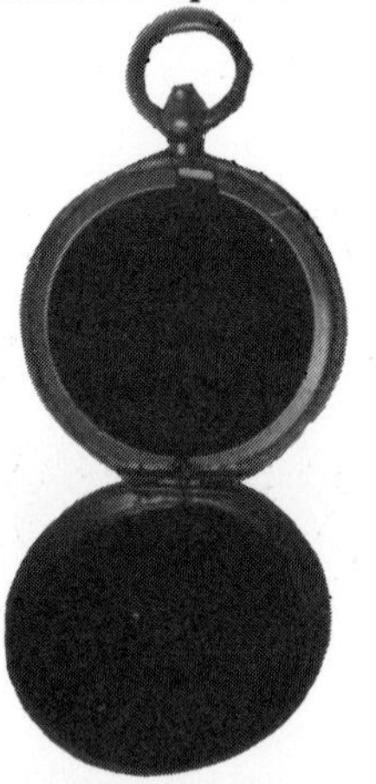

Hardy 'Drianoil' nickel silver fly dresser, one side of amadou for drying a soaked fly, the other of oiled felt for making it float again, in a watch case.
£8 – £12

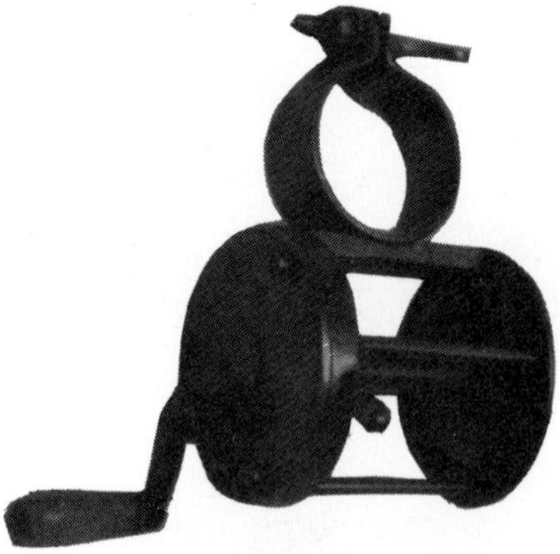

1.5/8in. Haywood of Birmingham brass multiplying reel, with drum lock and screwed collar attachment to rod, circa 1840-60.
£50 – £80

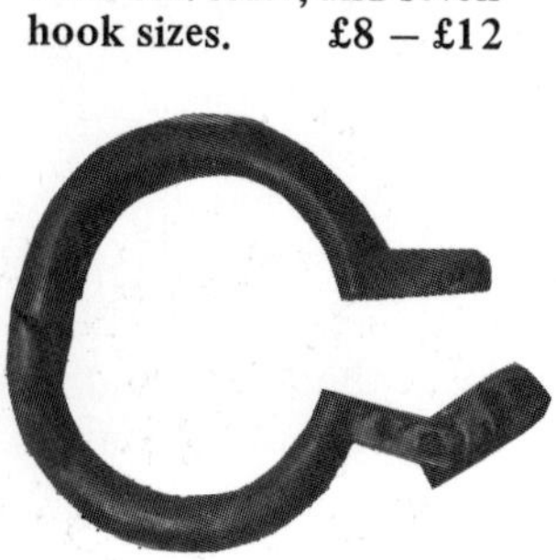

19th century brass clearing ring, heavy enough to slide down a fishing line with a strong string attached, to release a snagged bait.
£10 – £15

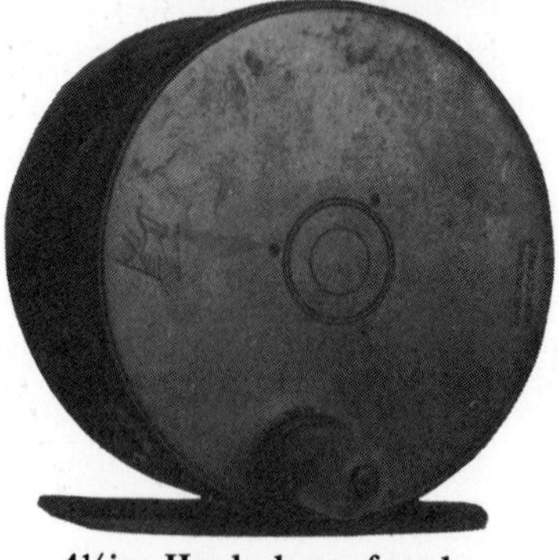

4¼in. Hardy brass-faced 'Perfect' salmon reel, with ivorine handle, rod-in-hand trademark on face, turk's head locking nut over tension regulator, 1906 check mechanism. £60 – £80

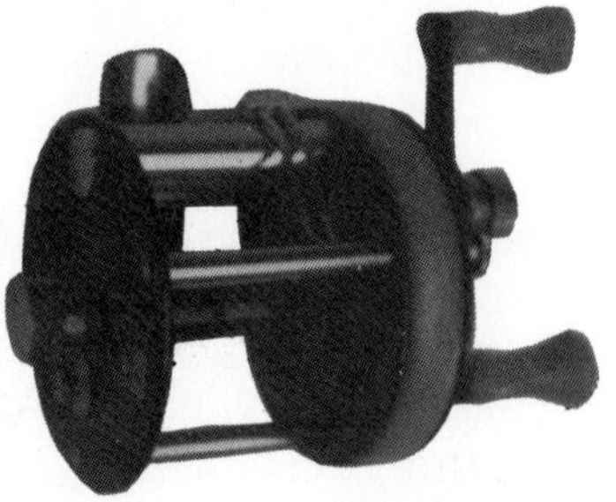

Rare level-wind bait-casting reel by ABU of Sweden, No. 1750A (an export-only number), with fine red anodised finish, imitation mother-of-pearl rim, catalogued only 1964/65.
£15 – £20

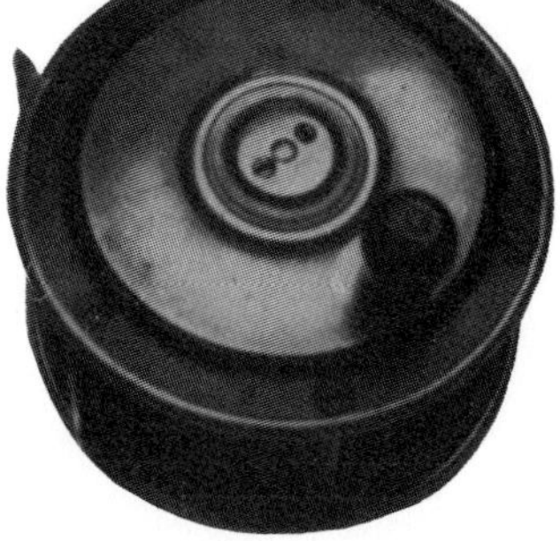

4¼in. brass and rosewood general purpose reel, probably made in Perth in the last half of the 19th century, with handsome brass rims and bridges and loud click. £30 – £50

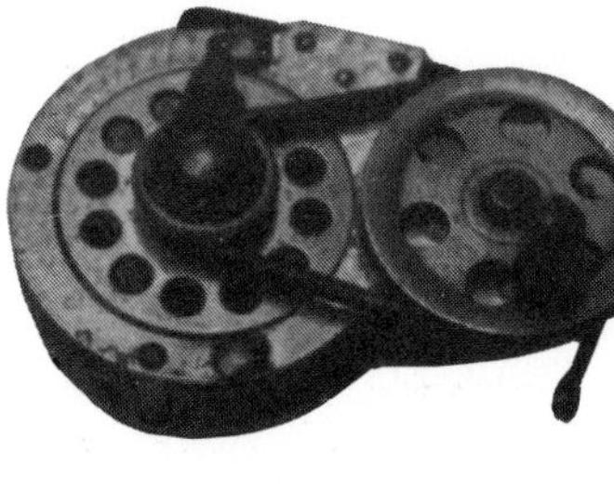

3in. 'Kitchen's Patent', only known example of a belt driven multiplier, with worm-gearing line distributor. £100 – £200

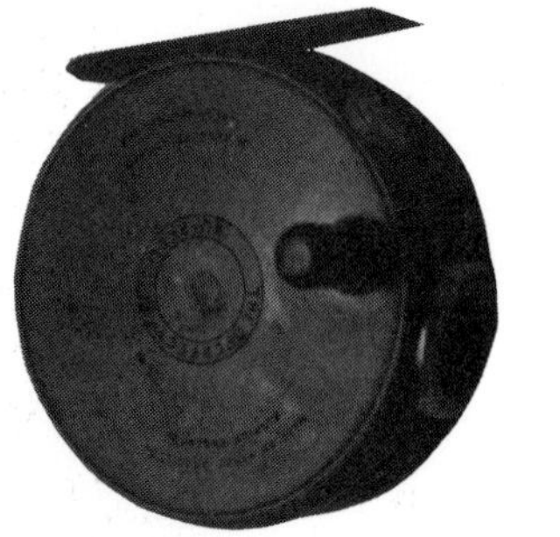

2.7/8in. Hardy 'Perfect' trout fly reel, with black ebonite handle, Duplicated Mk II check, agate line guard, notched brass foot, from the 1930's. (2.7/8in. size is rare). £50 – £80

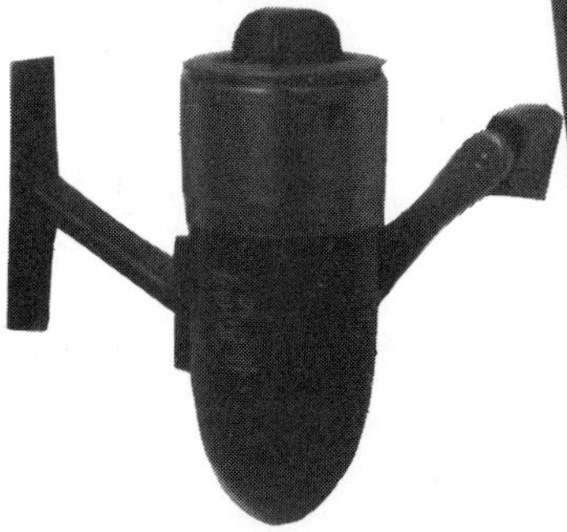

American 'Holliday 30' fixed-spool spinning reel from the 1960's with smart brass spool and rich dark green case, and ingenious slot which is supposed to pick up the line after casting but doesn't. £5

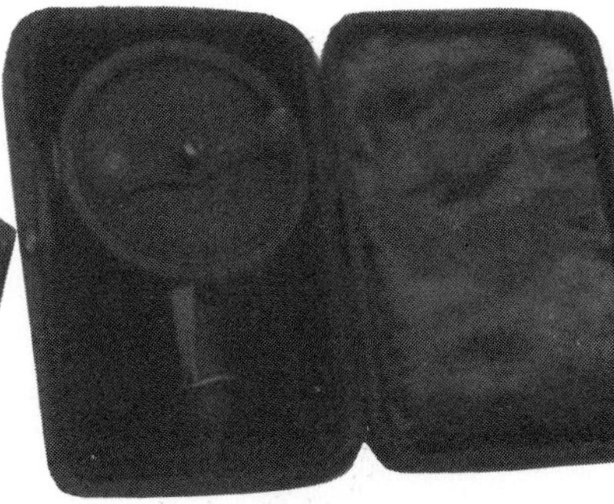

First model Illingworth spinning reel, with reciprocating spool giving distribution of the line, marked 'Patent 9338-1905', in blue plush-lined leather case. £70 – £100

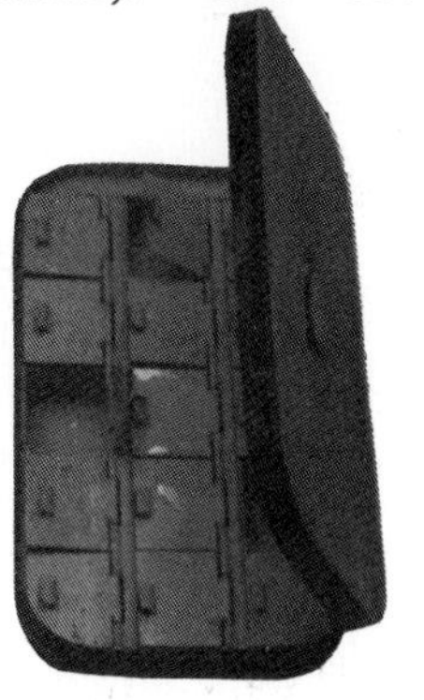

Hardy 'Girodon Pralon' (name of French nobleman inventor) black japanned dry fly compartment box, 15 compartments with hinged lids, internal cream finish. £10 – £15

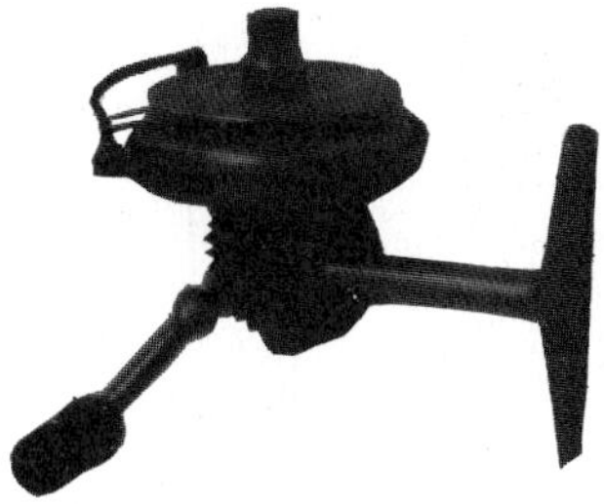

Arthur Allan of Glasgow 'Spinet' fixed-spool spinning reel, with 3/16in. width of drum, half bail-arm, and knurled brass drag regulator, circa 1920's. £12 – £20

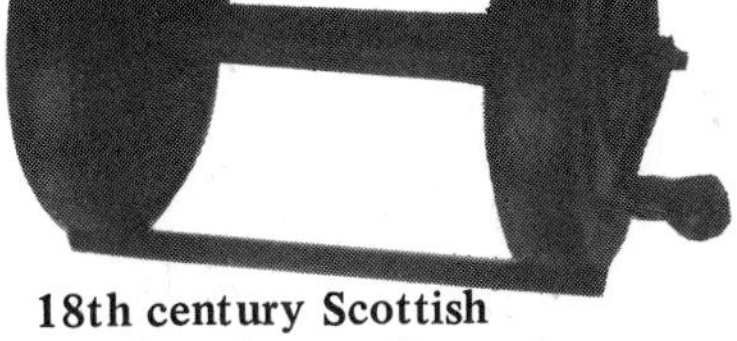

18th century Scottish wooden pirn, made specifically for trolling and harling, with oak board whose hole jams onto the rod butt, walnut case and spool, iron crank and turned wooden handle, extremely rare. £70 – £100

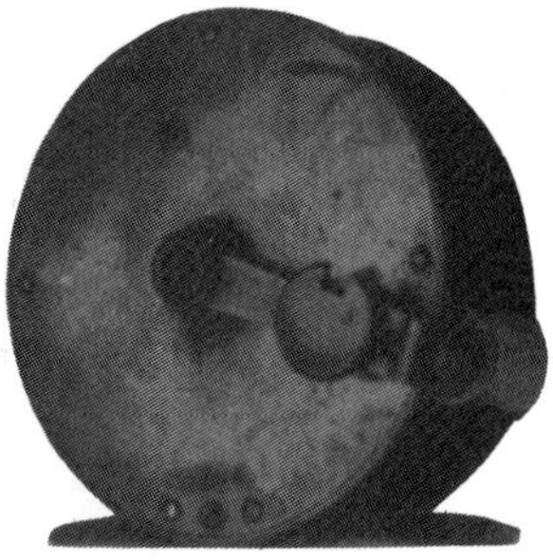

3¼in. unnamed brass fly reel, circa 1860-90, with protective folding handle and brass rim lock. £30 – £40

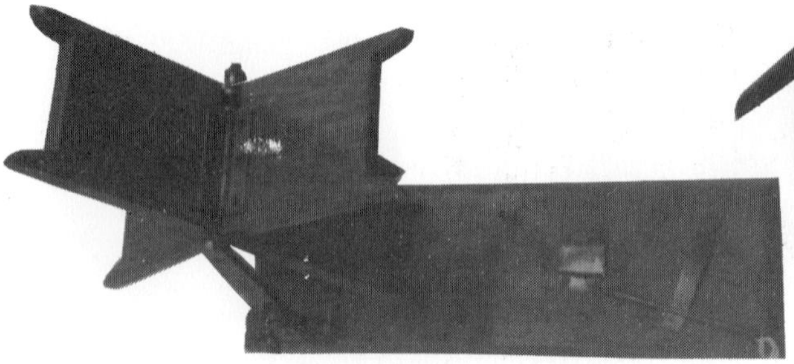

Hardy 1911 model line drier, with oak base and four folding oak vanes and brass reel fittings.
£20 – £30

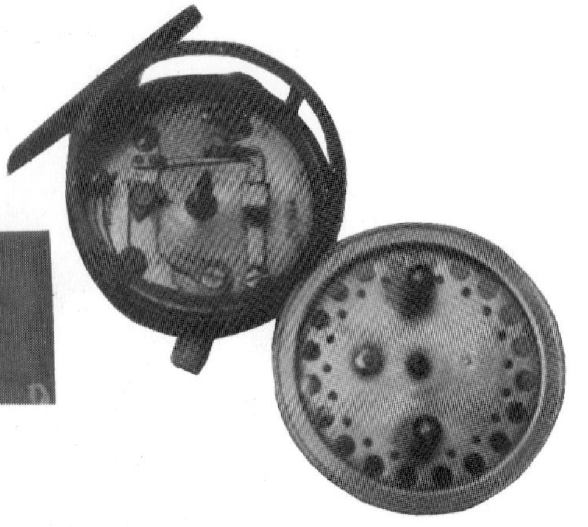

3¾in. Hardy 'Super Silex' centre-pin casting reel, with bright finish drum and overlapping drum giving easy finger control, high quality internal mechanism, jewelled bearing, circa 1930's. £60 – £80

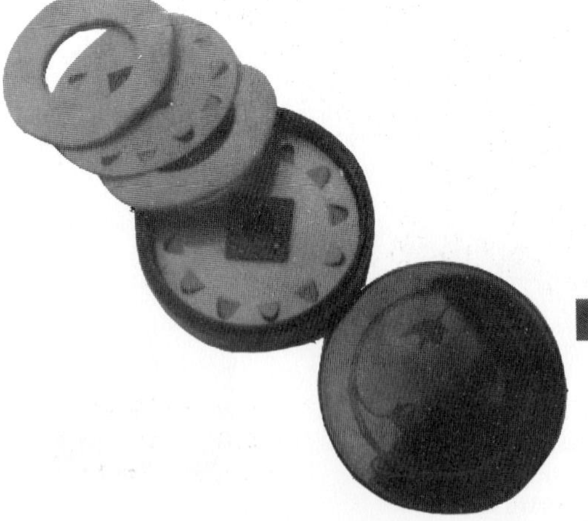

Hardy 'Album' cast box, of imitation tortoiseshell flecked bakelite, slightly domed lid with embossed cast and three flies each with a touch of colour, the interior holding two xylonite cork-fitted rings each fitted for winding on two casts. £10 – £15

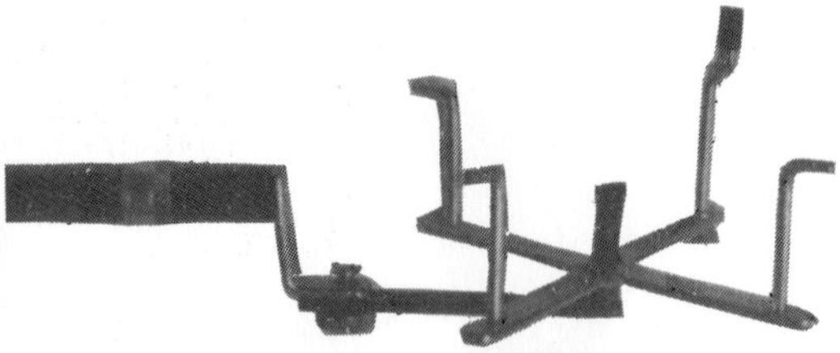

Hardy 'Compact' line drier, second model with vulcanite handle. £12 – £20

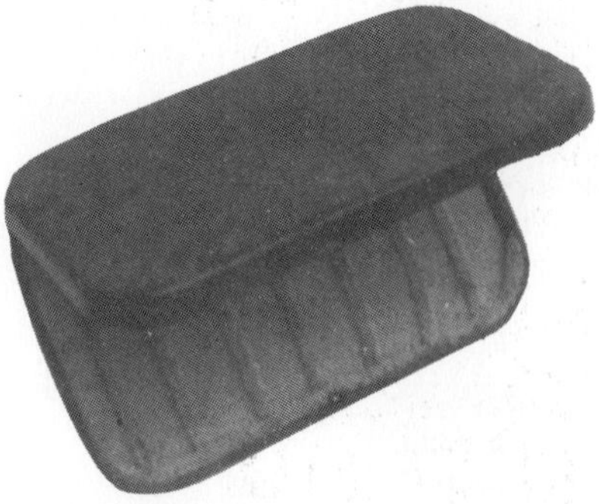

Hardy 'Neroda' fly box of attractive imitation tortoiseshell flecked bakelite, interior fitted with chenille bars to hold flies, created 1934.
£10 – £15

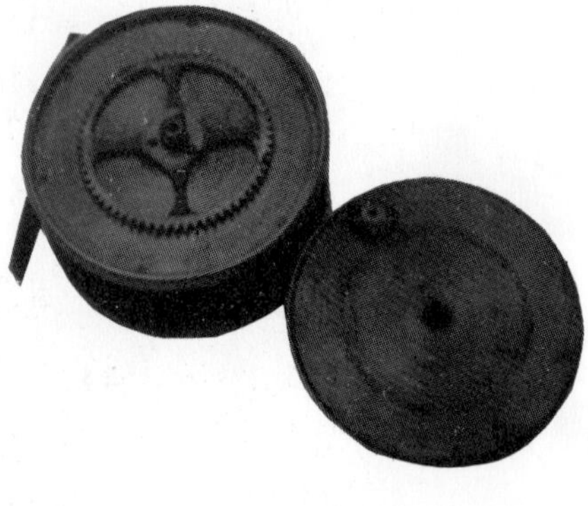

4in. Malloch 'Sun & Planet' brass and ebonite reel, with internal gearing connecting drum and handle so that when a fish runs only the knob turns on its own spindle, bulbous 12-sided ebonite handle, patented 1880.
£40 – £60

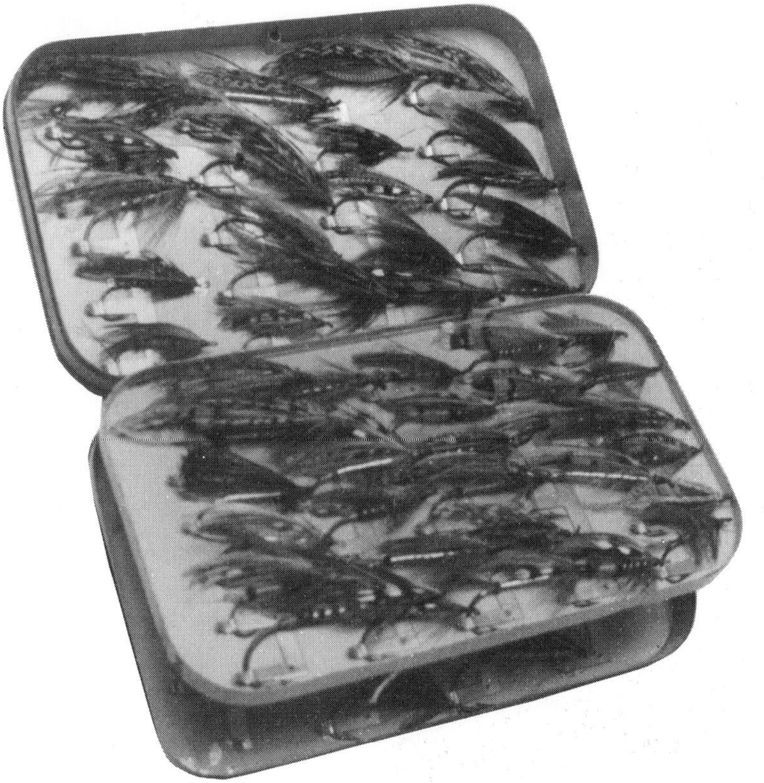

Black japanned salmon fly box, with 100 spring clips (patented by Malloch in 1886) to hold the hooks, central swing leaf, containing many historic flies. Box £10 – £15
Flies 25p – £1 each

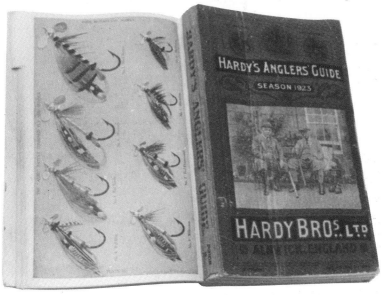

Hardy's Anglers' Guide 45th edition C 1 1923, green cover with picture of Hardy directors, 388pp., with illustrations of most Hardy tackle. £15 – £20

Fred Wheatcroft works for the Local Authority and collects beer mugs, jugs and glasses.

"I started collecting when I was with the Army in Germany and bought a very attractive beer glass with a green handle called a Falcon Brau. My collection now consists of over 1,000 glasses and they are all photographed and catalogued. I'm not really interested in what they're worth because I'd never want to sell any of them. If I parted with any one of them I'd have to part with the whole collection.

"The thing about them that interests me most is the names printed on them and how good they look. I send away all over the world for special glasses and recently sent to America for a glass made for Hurricane beer. I also write to brewers for their special glasses and most of them are prepared to sell one to me.

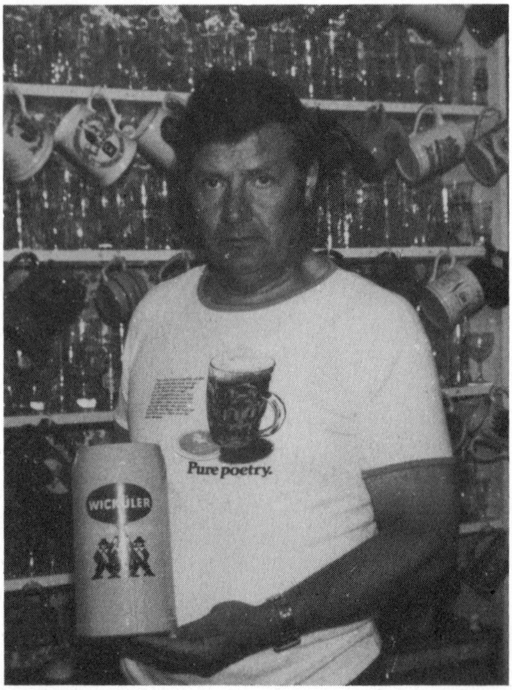

Fred Wheatcroft holding a two litre Wickuler Beerstein.

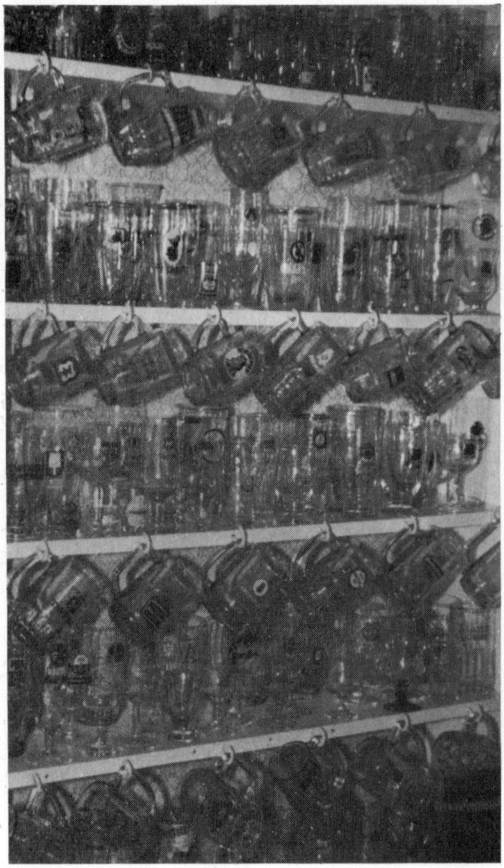

"The rarest one I've got is a Mocha mug which has the name of a country club in Torquay on it. My research found out that the club operated in the 1850's and the house is still there but today it is a pub.

"My next favourite is a half pint tumbler made for John Smith's Tadcaster Gold Medal Award ale which won the prize at Amsterdam in 1883."

The price of glasses depends on their age and appearance. Fred owns a German frog stein, also a German harvest stein which he paid £10 for but has since seen the same item advertised at £80.

The glass he would most like to add to his collection is a Pickwick mug issued by Bass in the 1960's at the time they took over Worthington. They brought out a set decorated with different Pickwick characters, two with pink designs, two with green and two with blue. Fred needs one blue one to make up his set and he has not been able to find it. Even Bass have none left.

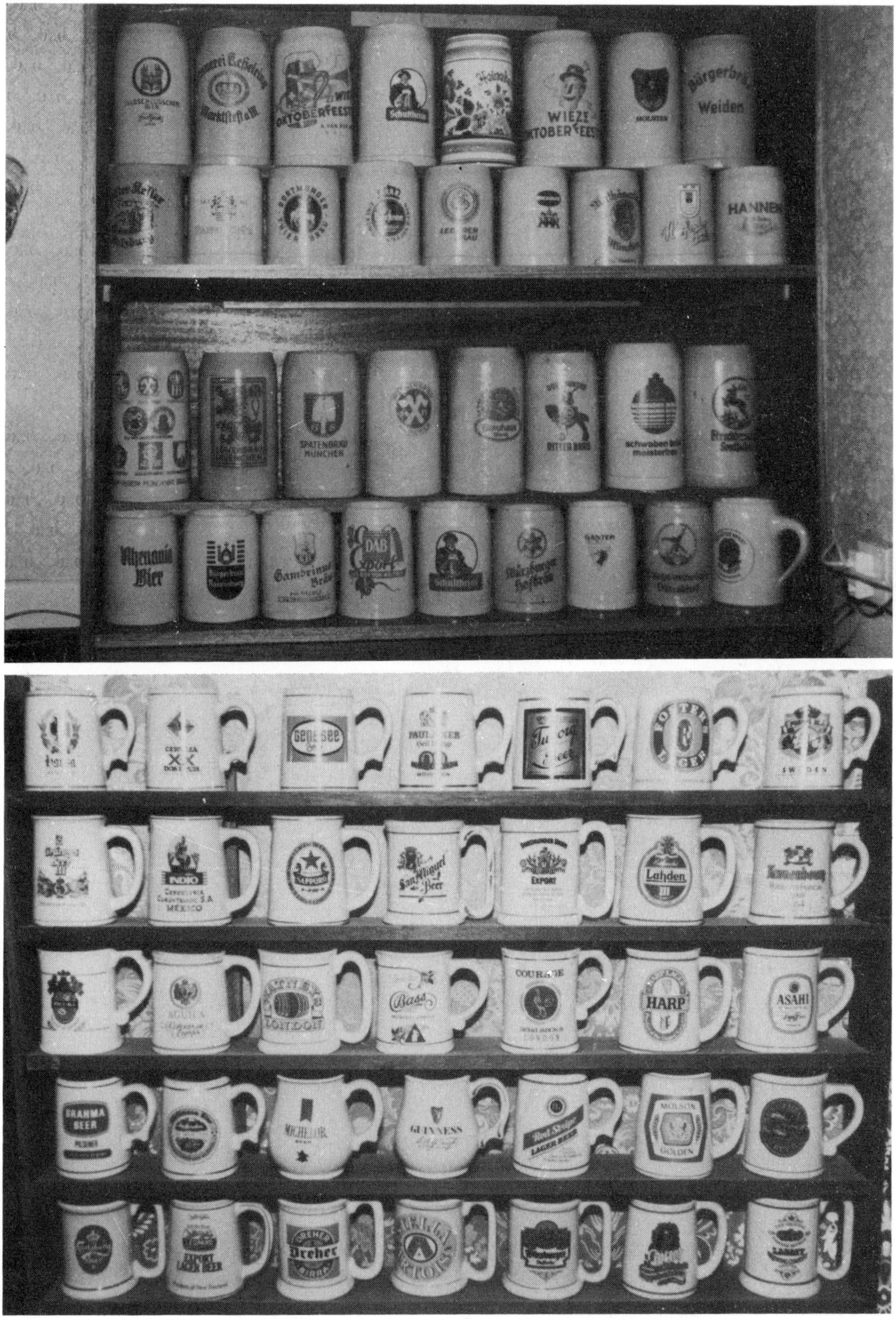

Part of Fred's amazing collection of over 1000 beer mugs.

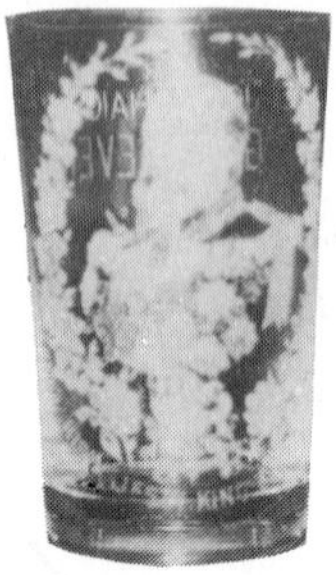

A Glenlivet Scotch whisky glass on the back of which is a picture of King Edward VII, which would date the glass to 1901-10.

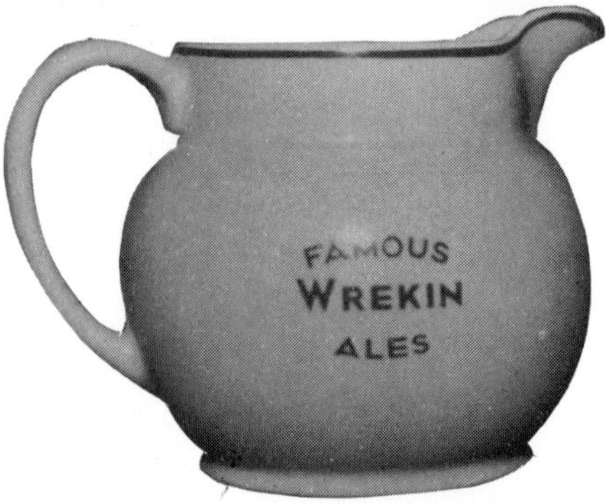

A green ½ pint water jug 'Famous Wrekin Ales' produced by Wade's, 1954-69.

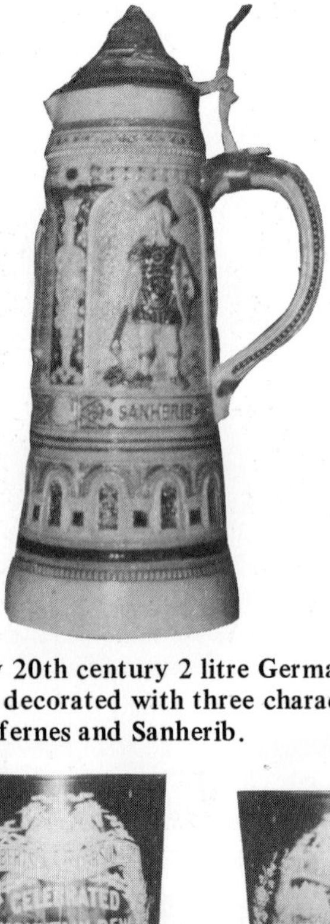

Early 20th century 2 litre German harvest stein decorated with three characters, Saul, Holofernes and Sanherib.

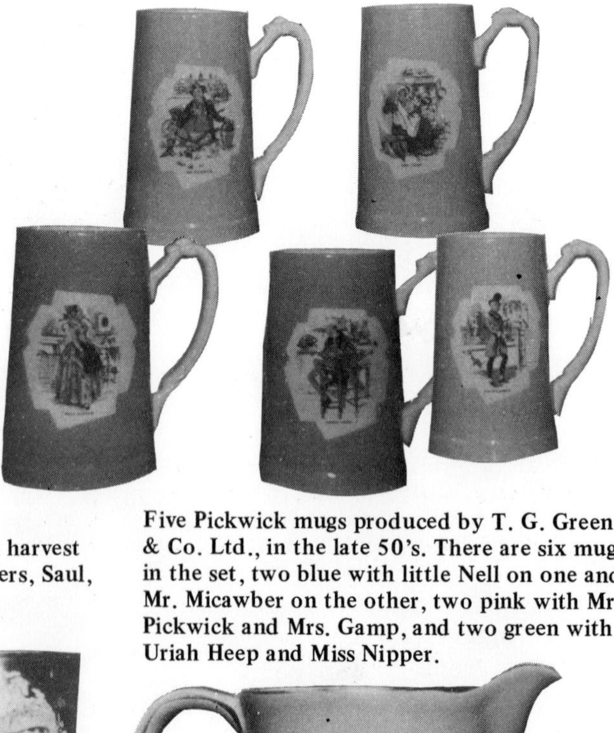

Five Pickwick mugs produced by T. G. Green & Co. Ltd., in the late 50's. There are six mugs in the set, two blue with little Nell on one and Mr. Micawber on the other, two pink with Mr. Pickwick and Mrs. Gamp, and two green with Uriah Heep and Miss Nipper.

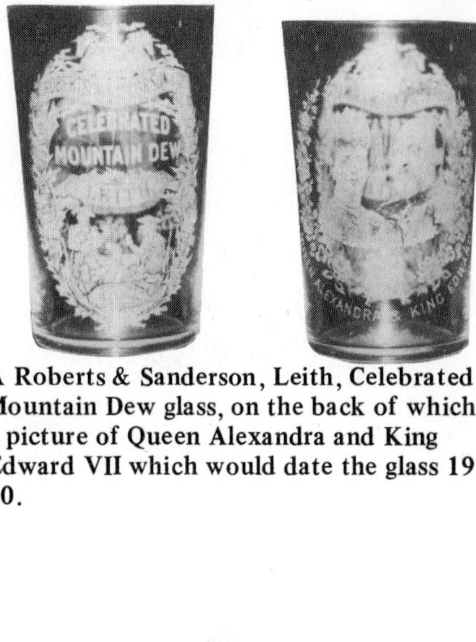

A Roberts & Sanderson, Leith, Celebrated Mountain Dew glass, on the back of which is a picture of Queen Alexandra and King Edward VII which would date the glass 1901-10.

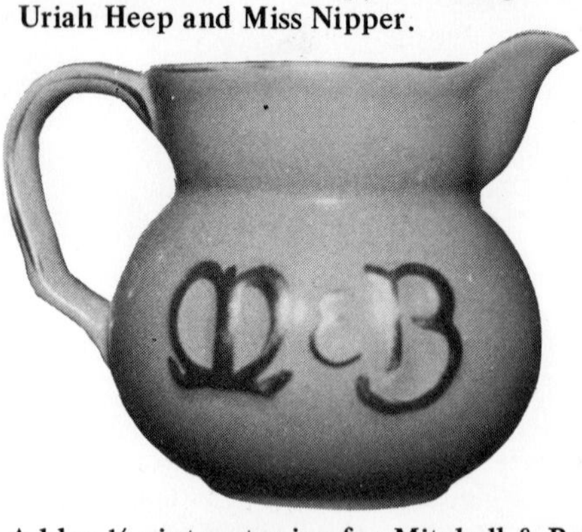

A blue ½ pint water jug for Mitchell & Butler's, produced by Wade's between 1954-69.

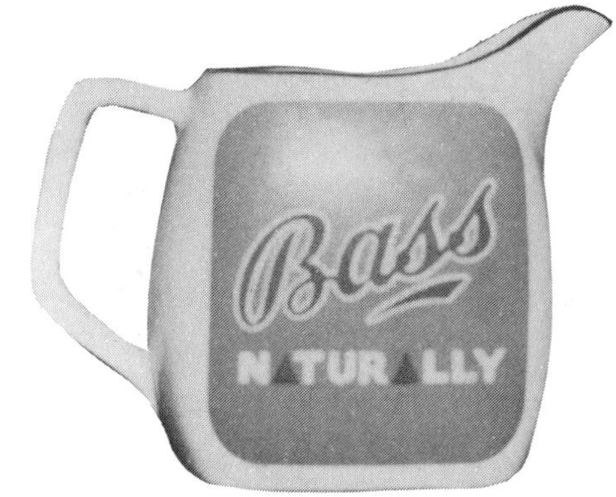

A white one pint water jug 'Bass Naturally', produced by Hancock, Corfield & Waller Ltd., circa 1950.

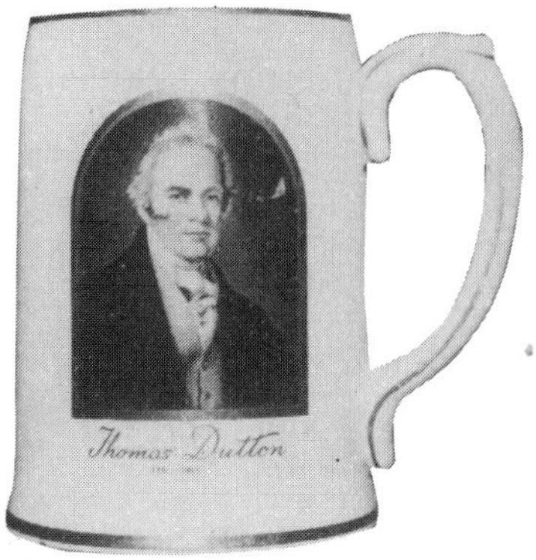

A white 1 pint mug for Thos. Dutton Brewery, on the front of which is T. Dutton, 1751-1815, on the back is the name Dutton's. The base is printed 'Produced for Henry Milner Ltd., Manchester II by Empire Porcelain Co., Stoke-on-Trent', also the numbers 7 – 62 which would would date it July 1962.

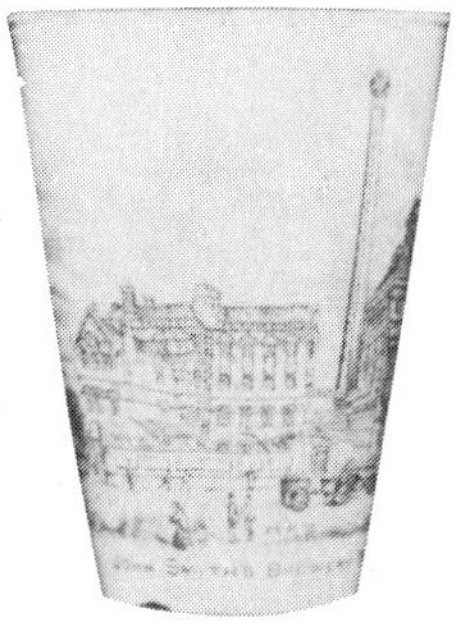

A white and brown tumbler for John Smith's of Tadcaster, gold medal award, Amsterdam 1883. On the base is printed a greyhound dog, trade mark E.M. & Co. with the letter B under it.

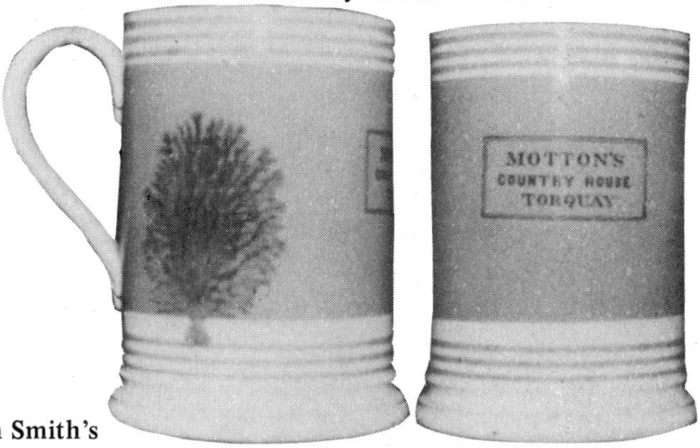

A 1 pint Mocha mug produced for Motton's Country House, in Ellacombe Road, Torquay. Mr. Motton was the landlord of the country house between 1879-97, there is no maker's name or mark.

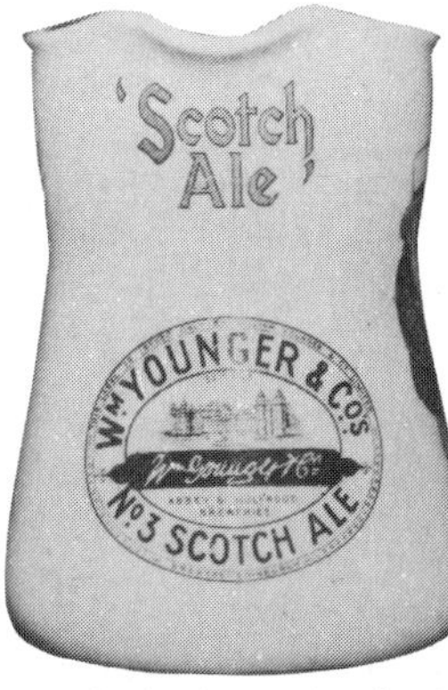

A white and black ½ pint jug for Wm. Younger's No. 3 Scotch ale, produced by the Royal Doulton Co., the number 246 is printed on the base and a figure 2.

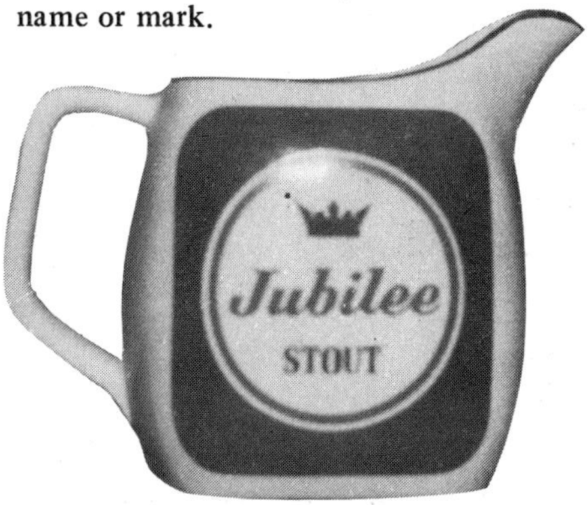

A white 1 pint water jug 'Jubilee Stout', produced by Hancock, Corfield & Waller Ltd., mid 1950's.

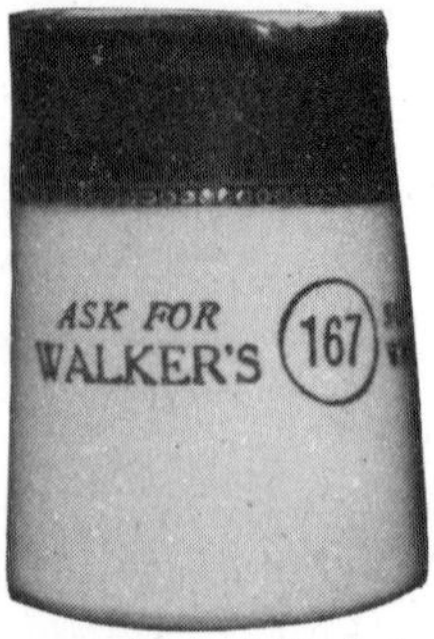

A blue and stone coloured ½ pint water jug from the Peter Walker Brewery, Warrington. The number 167 is the number of the site the brewery was built on in 1846 so the jug could be early 1900. The base impressed Price 3 Bristol.

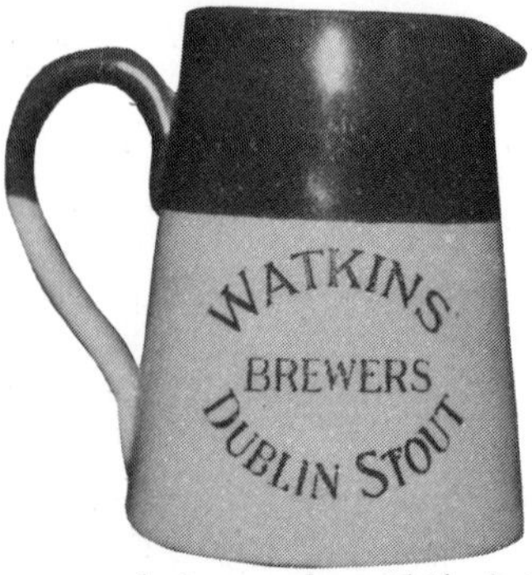

A brown and stone coloured ½ pint water jug for Watkins Brewers Dublin Stout, possibly by Thos. Watkins of Llandovery and if so it would be dated before 1927. Printed on the base is Hancock, Corfield & Waller Ltd. Imperial Work's Mitcham and also letter A.

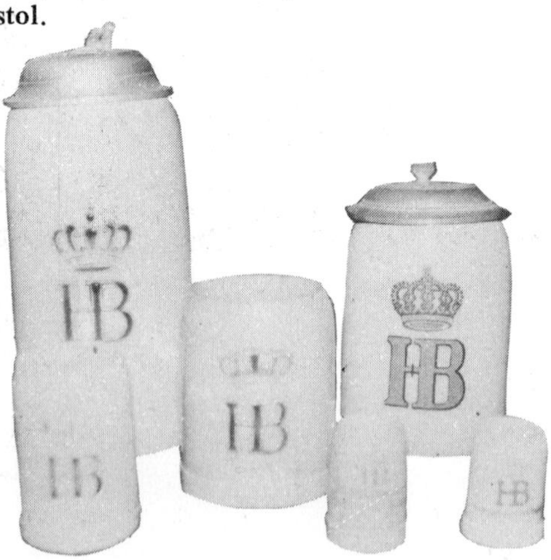

An assortment of Hofbrauhaus beer steins, the two with pewter lids early 1950's.

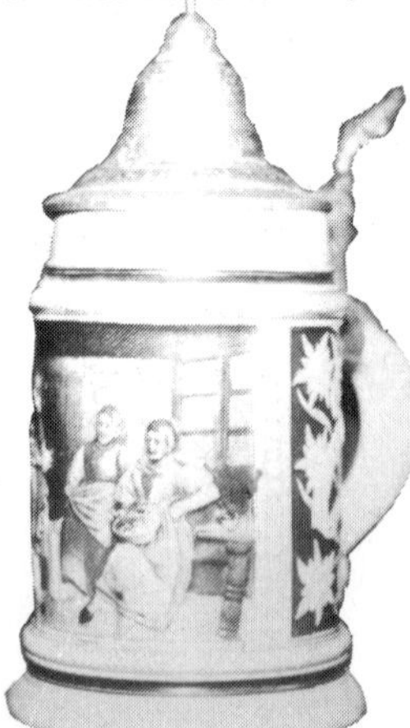

A 5 litre German frog stein produced in the early 1900's, with the name Germany and number 1244 impressed on the base.

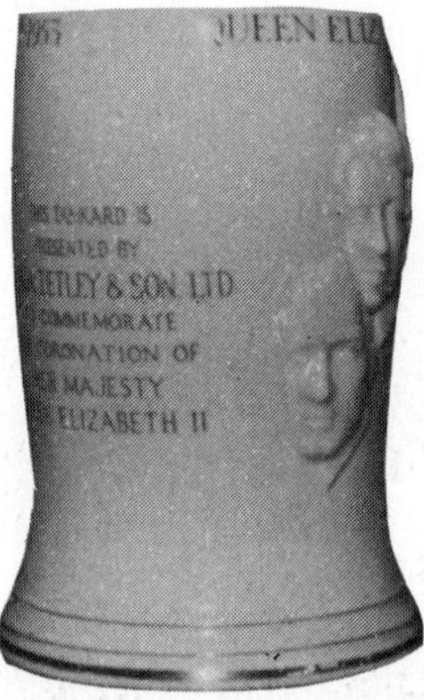

A cream coloured 1 pint mug issued by Joshua Tetley & Son Ltd., to celebrate the Coronation of Queen Elizabeth II in 1953. The mug was produced by H. G. Stephenson Ltd., A 518 is impressed on the base.

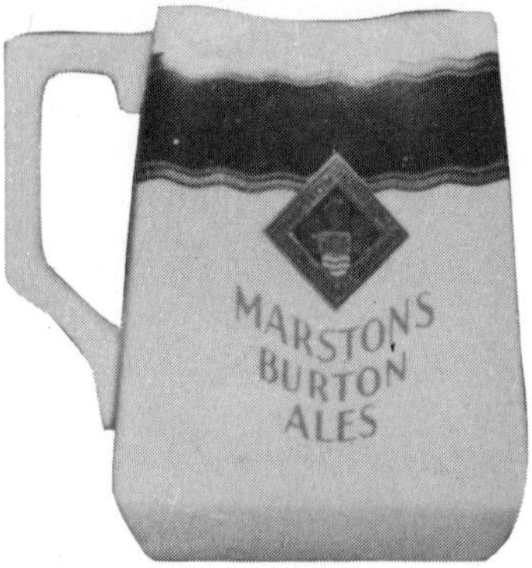

A cream coloured ½ pint water jug 'Marstons Burton Ales', produced by Royal Doulton in 1935.

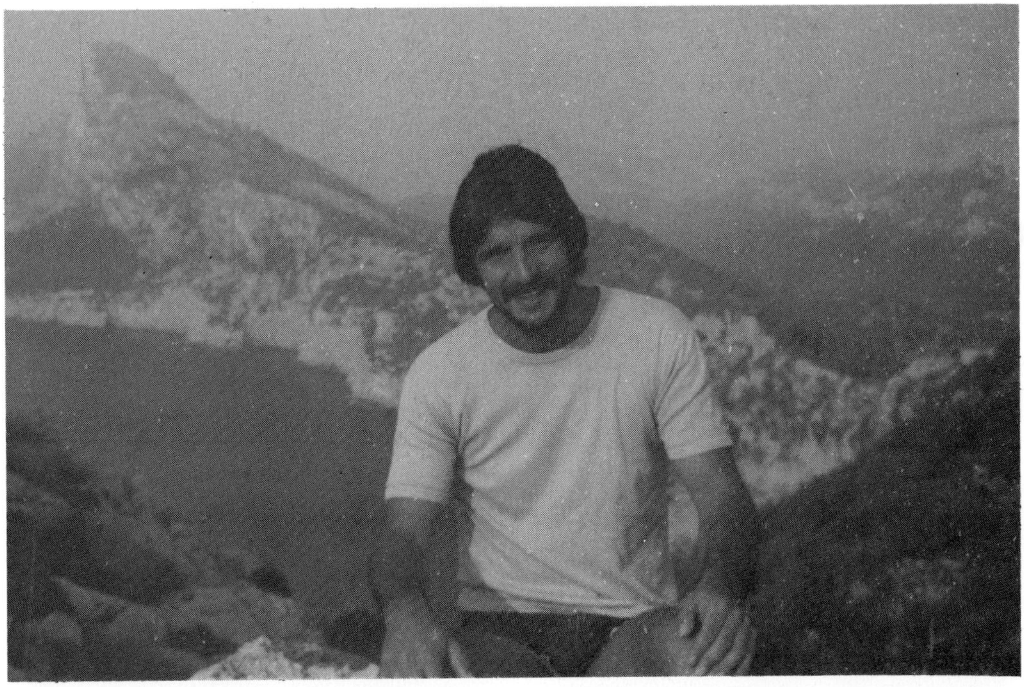

Ken Tomlinson is a teacher and collects cigarette paper packets.

"Cigarette papers are something that have been missed by other collectors until now but they are becoming increasingly collectible just because of that. I know of two other serious collectors in Britain, Peter Emmens and Owen Thomas of West Ealing.

"The trouble is that, because they are a real throwaway item, cigarette papers are hard to find and a collection cannot be built up on British papers alone. Other countries like France, Holland, Portugal, USA and Italy yield more and much of my collection has been obtained by people finding me packets abroad. There are places in the world where cigarettes are so cheap that hand rolling does not exist.

"I started collecting them five years ago and now have 1,000 packets worldwide, some of them pre-1900. Packets of cigarette papers blend in nicely with pictorial tobacco tins, cigarette packets, showcards and tobacco labels, which I also collect.

The first people to roll their own cigarettes were Turkish soldiers in the Siege of Acre during the 1850's, who rolled their own and put them in used cartridge cases. Cigarette papers were first produced by Jean Lacroix in France in the latter part of the 19th century. Lacroix Fils still produce them today in different flavours and sizes which make interesting items for Ken's collection.

He is particularly keen on the older packets which are often very colourful. Recently he obtained a highly prized 'Proclamation de la Republica' packet from Spain, a very rare and appealing packet with papers intact.

Individual prices range from 50p-£25.

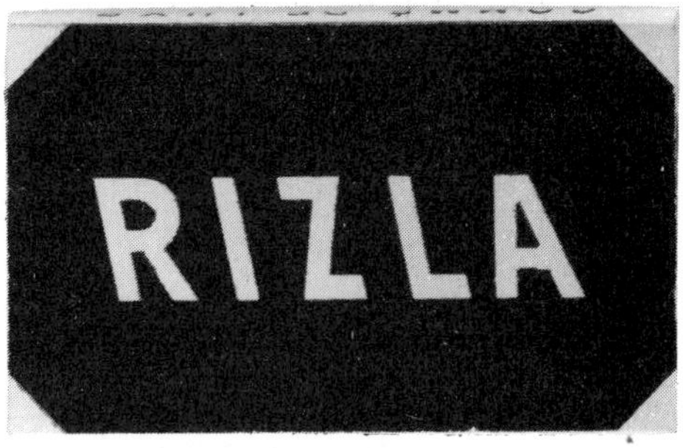

Rizla, double booklet, 1980's on sale in Belgium.

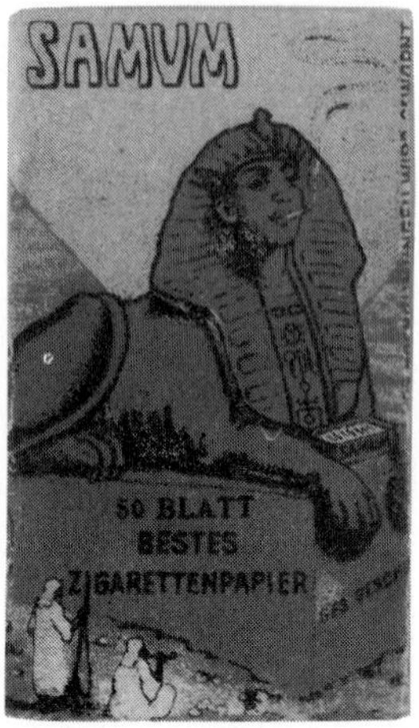

Samum, 50 leaves, folder, 1980's, Austria.

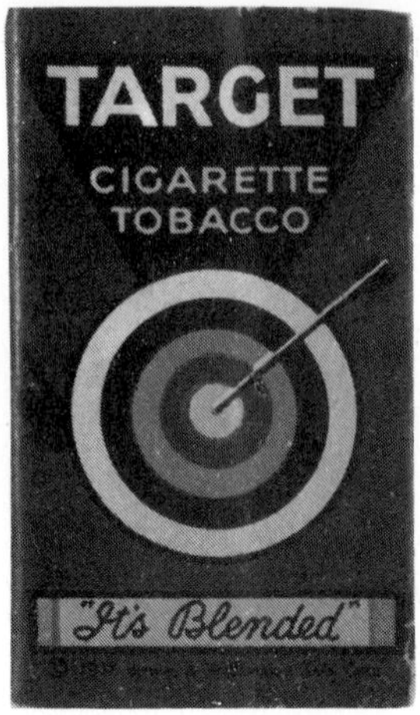

Target, 15 leaves, U.S.A., 1930's.

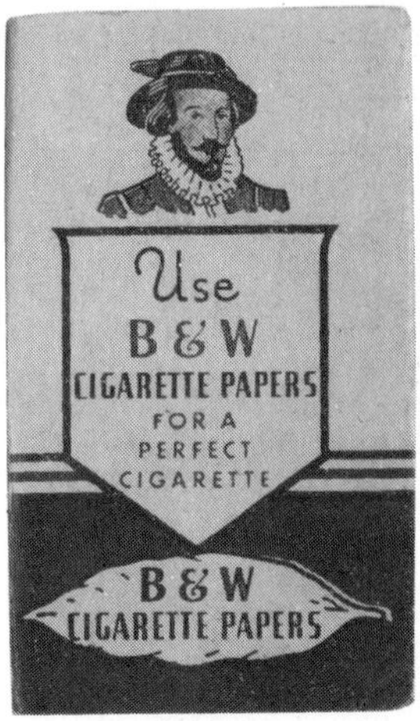

B & W Cigarette Papers, 15 leaves, U.S.A., 1930's.

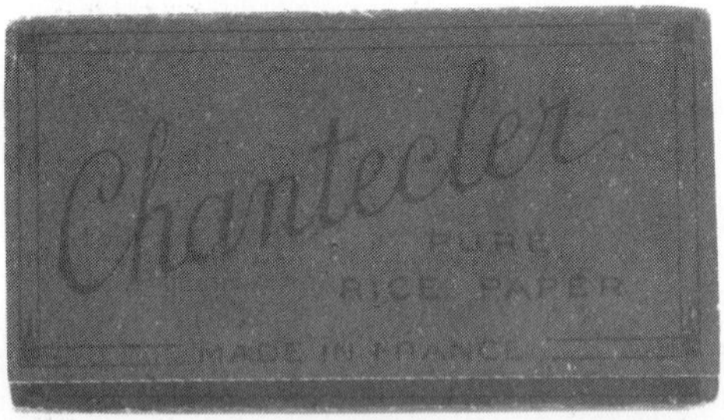

Chantecler, made as a give-away with tobacco, French, 1920's.

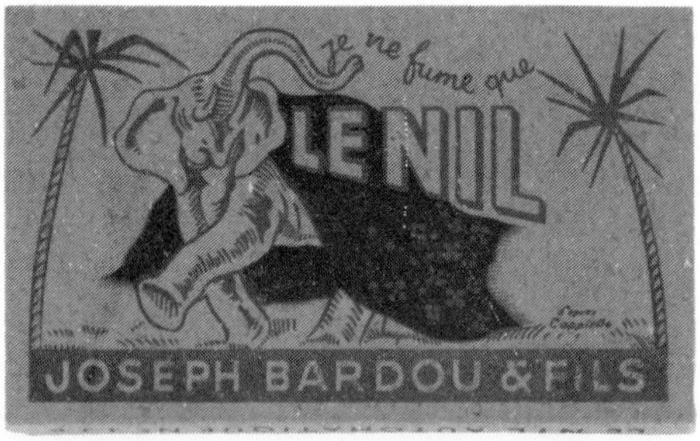

Le Nil, 100 leaves, French, 1970's.

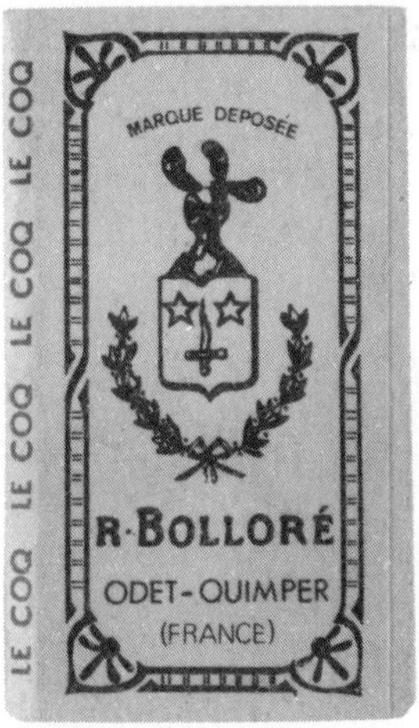

Le Coq, 1970's, Made in France, for Portuguese market.

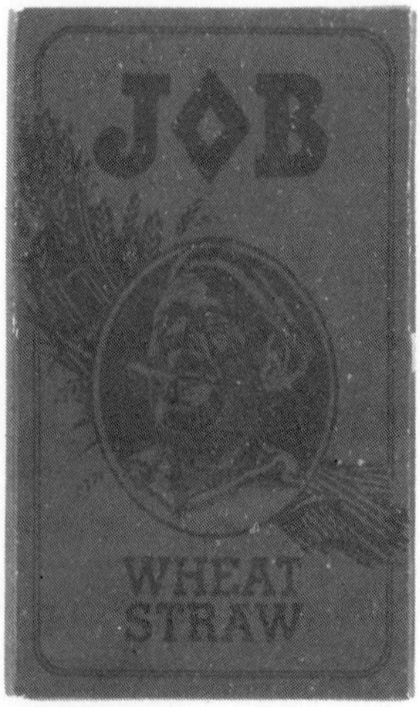

Job Wheat Straw, red double booklet for U.S. market.

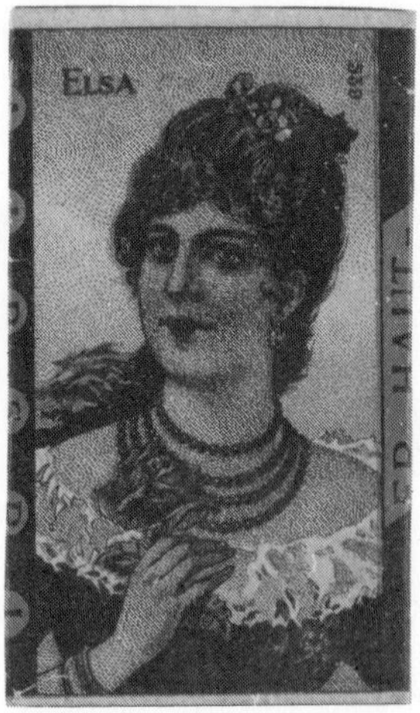

Elsa, 20 leaves, folder, 1940's, Egypt.

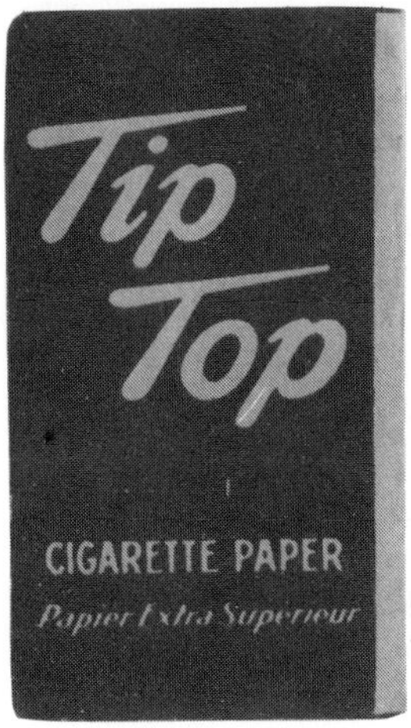

Tip Top, 15 leaves, 1930's, U.S.A.

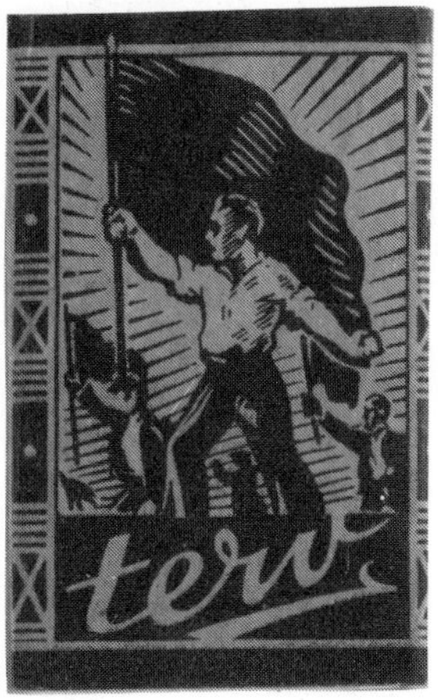

Terv, 20 leaves, folder, 1940's, Hungary.

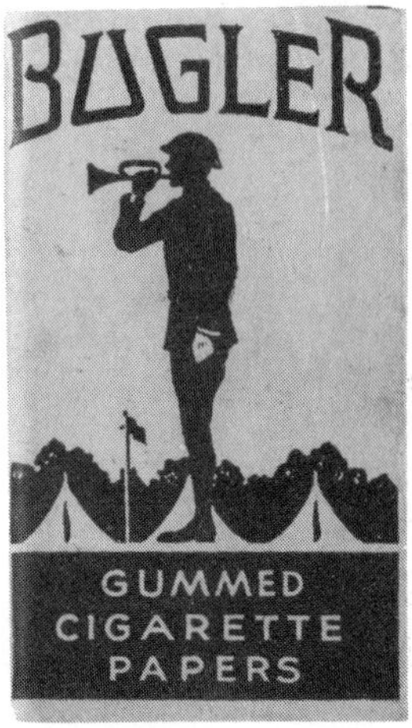

Bugler, 15 leaves, 1930's, U.S.A.

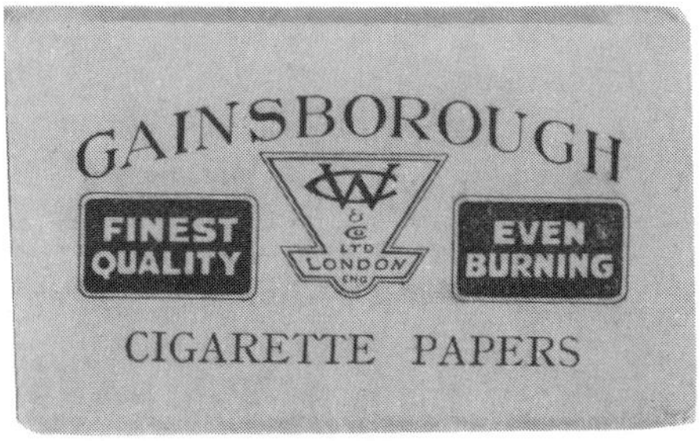

Gainsborough, 20 leaves, issued free with tobacco, 1930's, British.

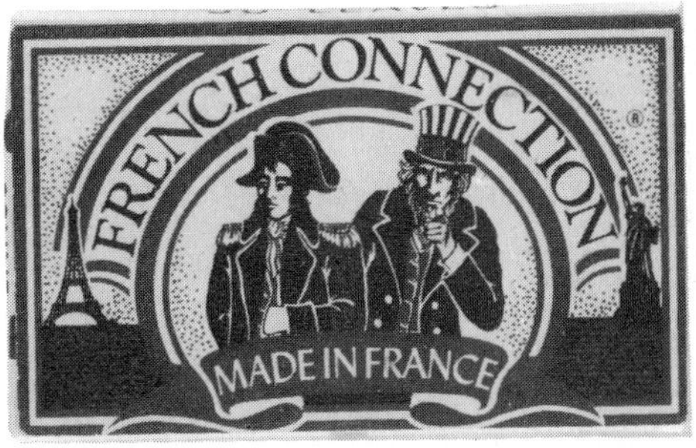

French Connection, 1980's, Made in France for U.S.A. market.

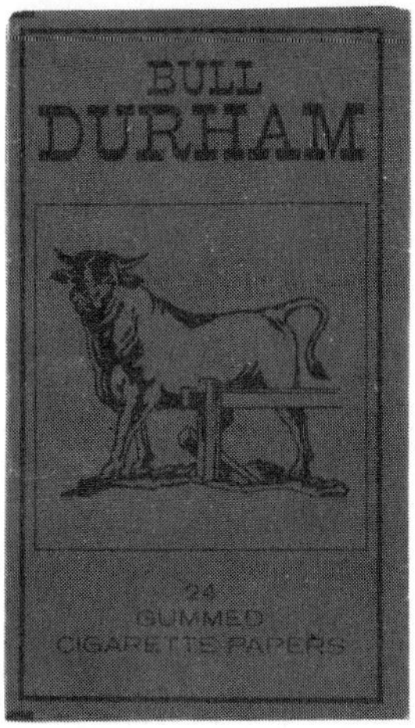

Bull Durham, 24 leaves, 1970's, U.S.A.

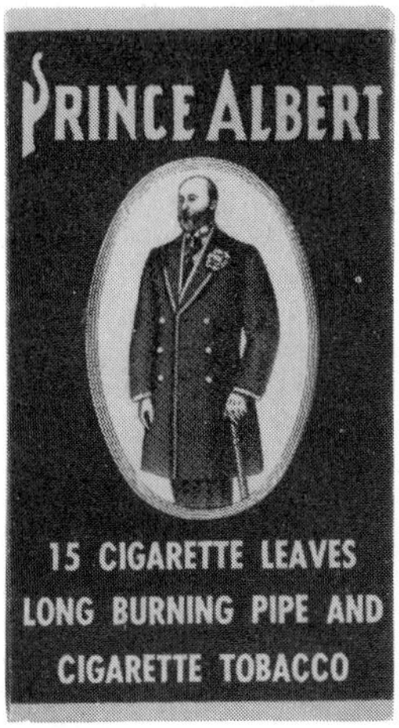

Prince Albert, 15 leaves, 1970's, U.S.A.

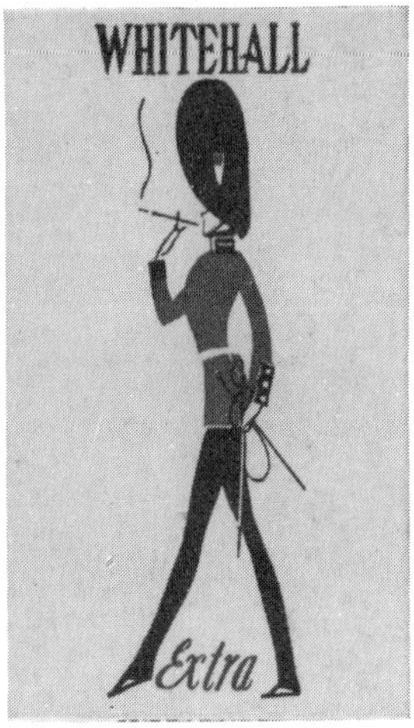

Whitehall, booklet, 100 leaves, sold in Malta, 1960's, British.

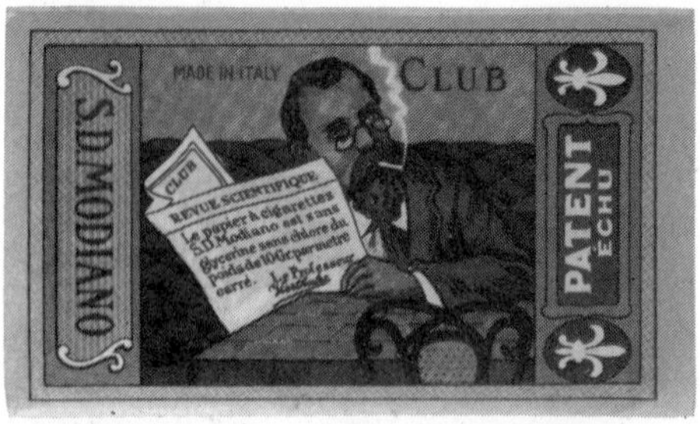

Club, 40 leaves, folder, 1980's, Italy.

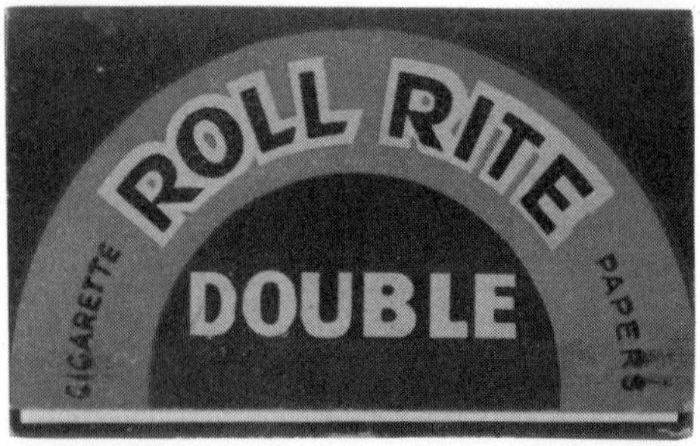

Roll Rite, 100 leaves, automatic, 1950's, New Zealand.

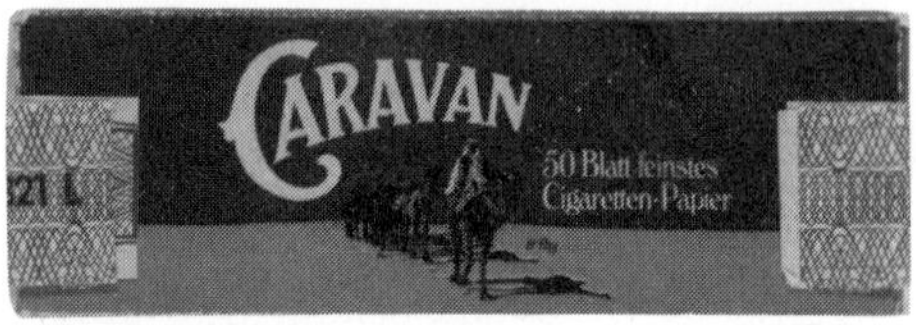

Caravan, 50 leaves, packet, 1980's, West Germany.

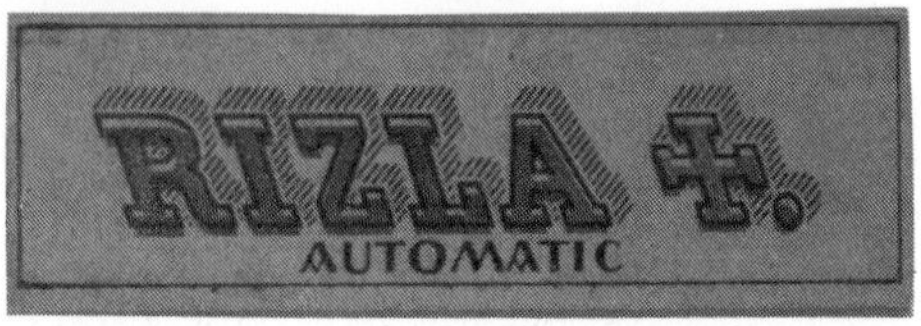

Rizla, wax tipped, 50 leaves, 1960's, British.

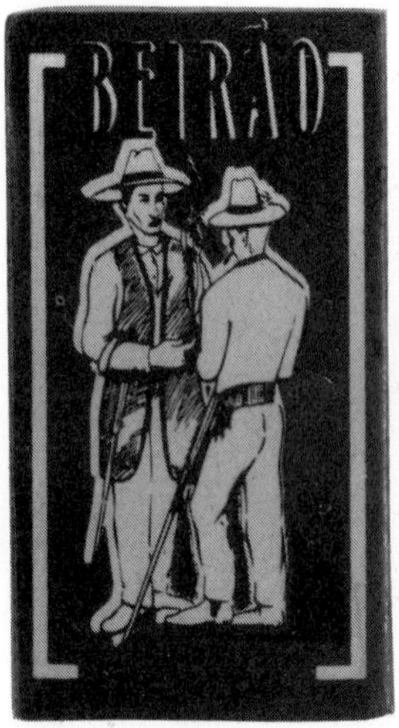

Beirao, folder, 30 leaves, Portugal.

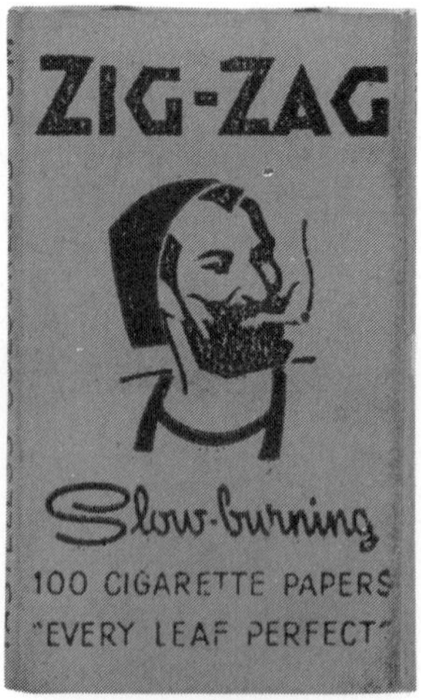

Zig-Zag, 100 leaves, copy of French design, 1950's, New Zealand.

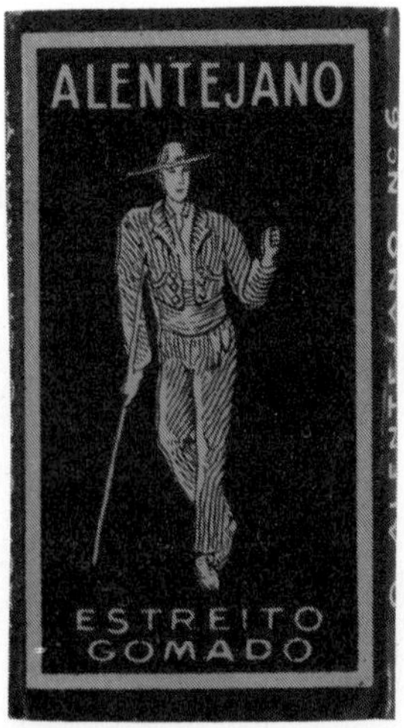

Alentejano, folder, 40 leaves, Portugal.

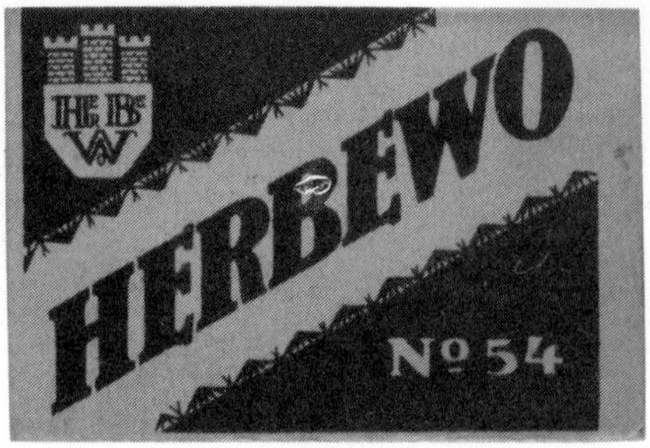

Herbewo, 20 leaves, folder, 1940's, Poland.

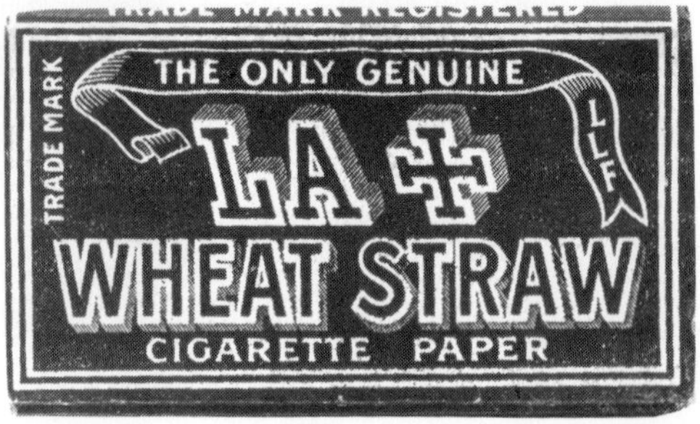

La + Wheat Straw, hard backed folder, 1905, French.

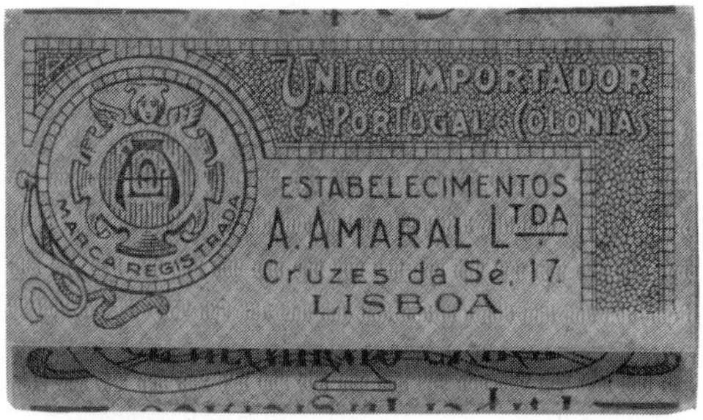

Unico Importador, early folder, 40 leaves, Portugal.

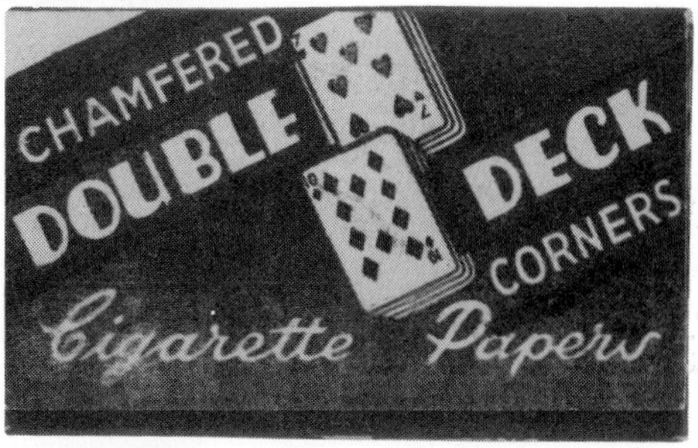

Double Deck, 100 leaves, automatic, 1950's, New Zealand.

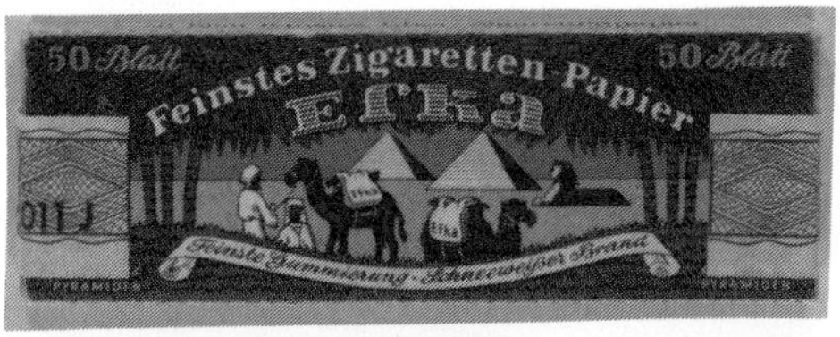

Efka, 50 leaves, packet, 1980's, West Germany.

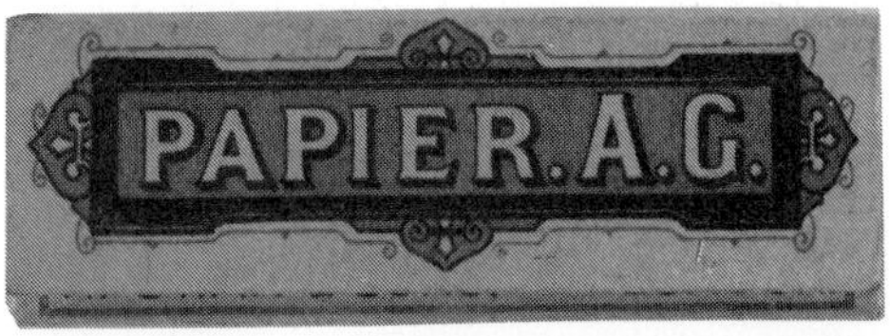

Papier. A.G., H. Swan, copy of French design, 1930's, British.

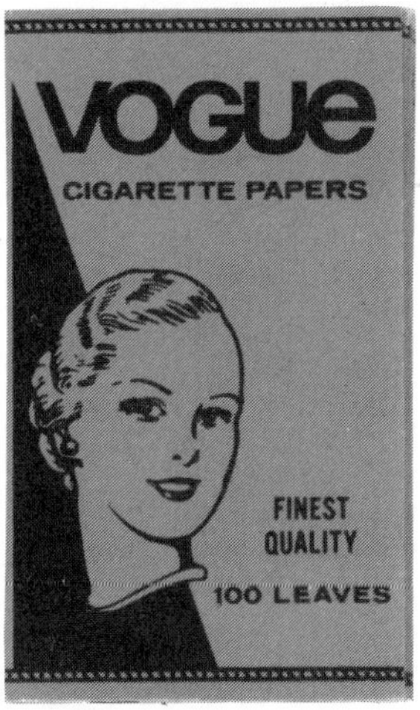

Vogue, 100 leaves, double booklet, 1980's, Canada.

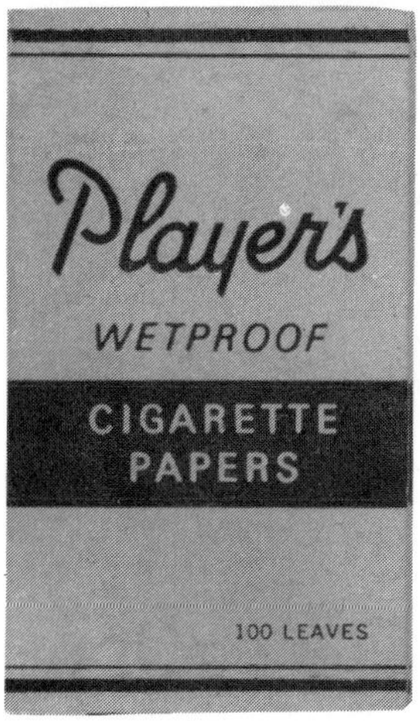

Player's, 100 leaves, double booklet, 1960's, Canada.

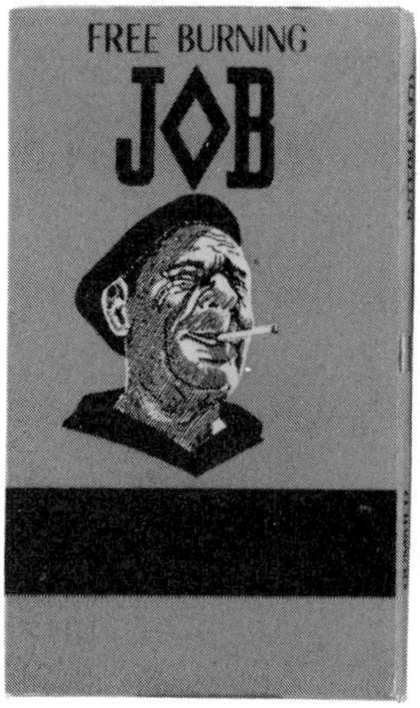

Job, blue, double booklet for U.S.A. market.

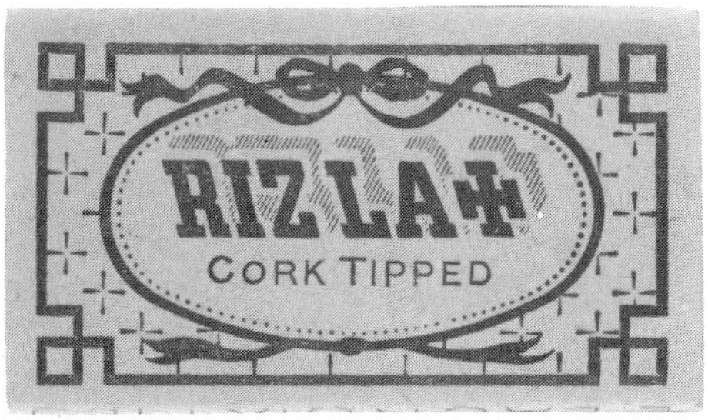

Rizla, cork tipped, 30 leaves, 1950's, French.

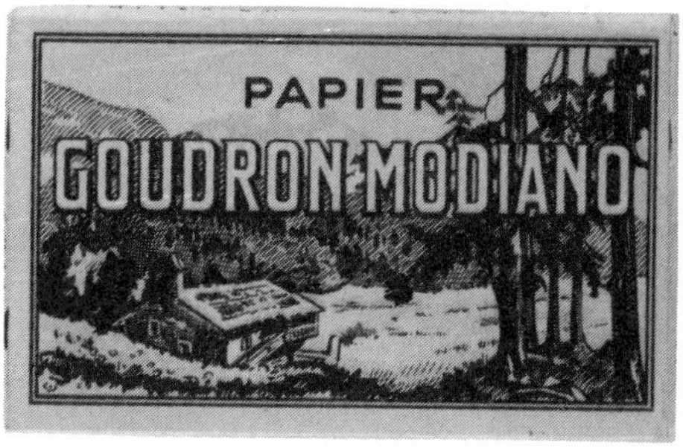

Papier Goudron Modiano, 100 leaves, double booklet, 1950's, Italy.

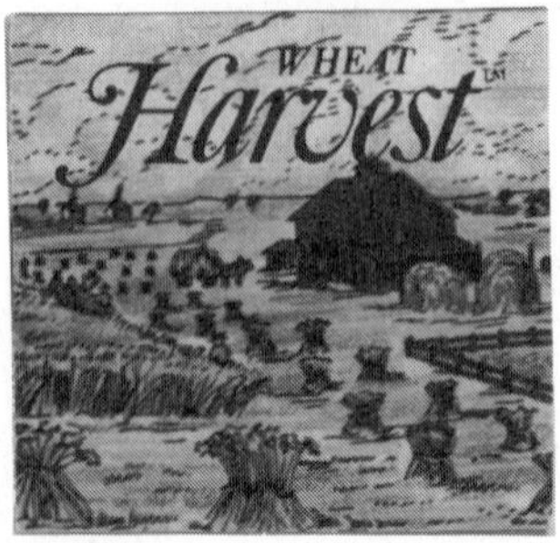

Wheat Harvest, wheat paper, 1980's, Spain.

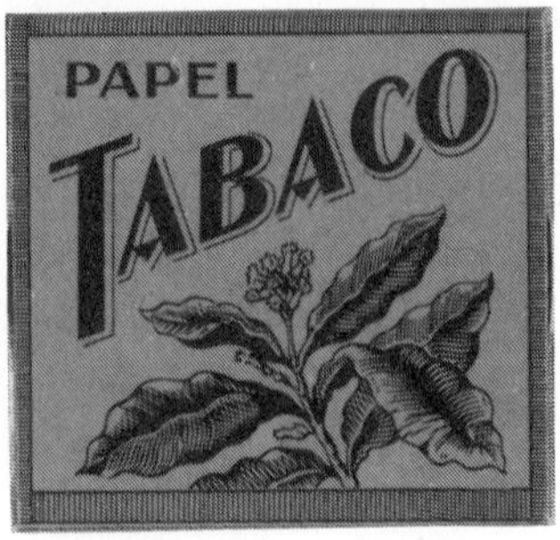

Papel Tabaco, Licquorice, 1980's, Spain.

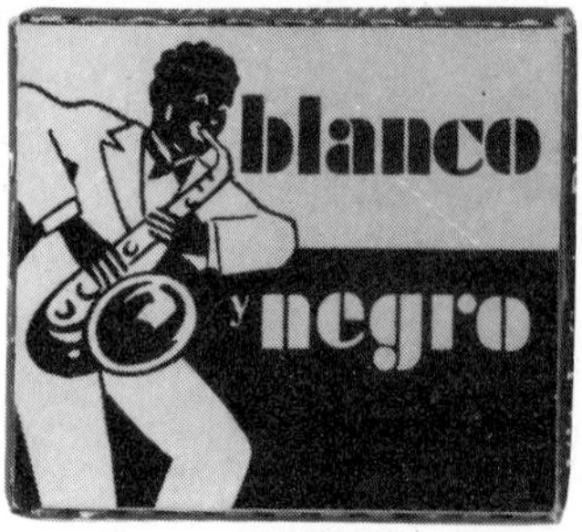

Blanco y Negro, 1980's, Spain.

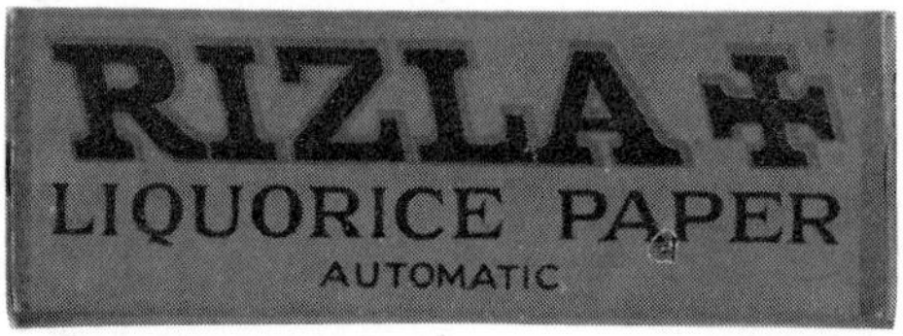

Rizla + Liquorice Paper, 1950's, British.

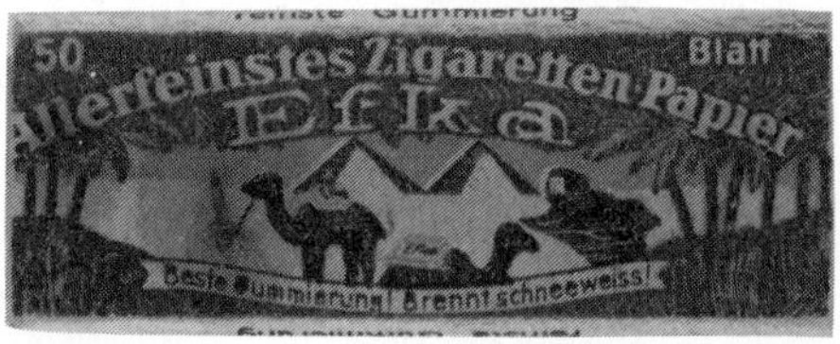

Efka, 50 leaves, packet, 1950's, West Germany.

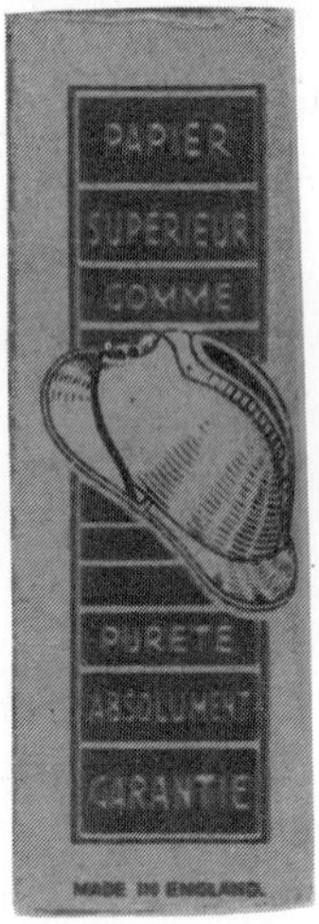

Papiers a Cigarettes F.F.L., made for French market, U.K.

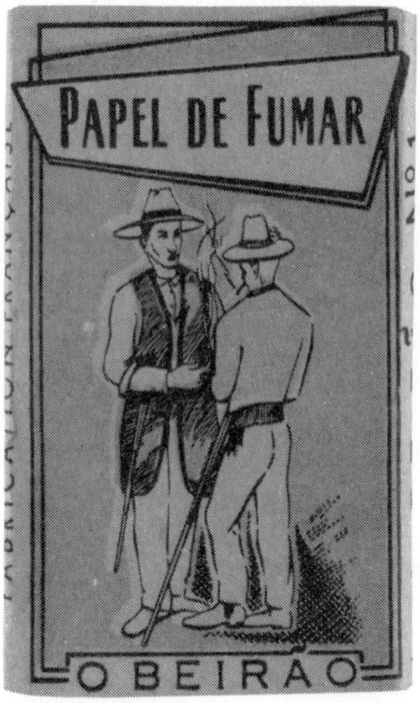

Papel De Fumar, folder, 50 leaves, Portugal.

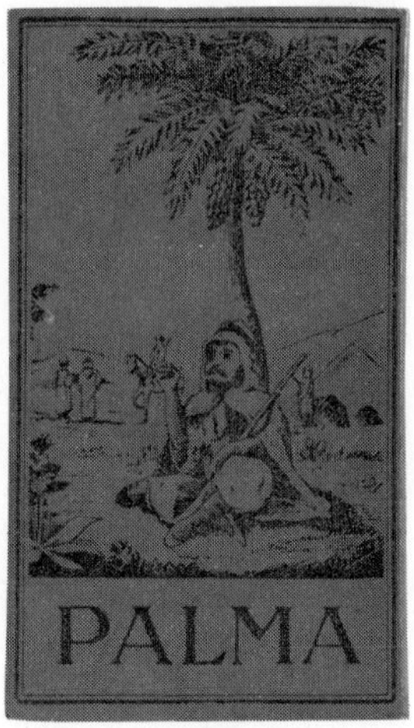

Palma, 40 leaves, folder, 1970's, Saudi Arabia.

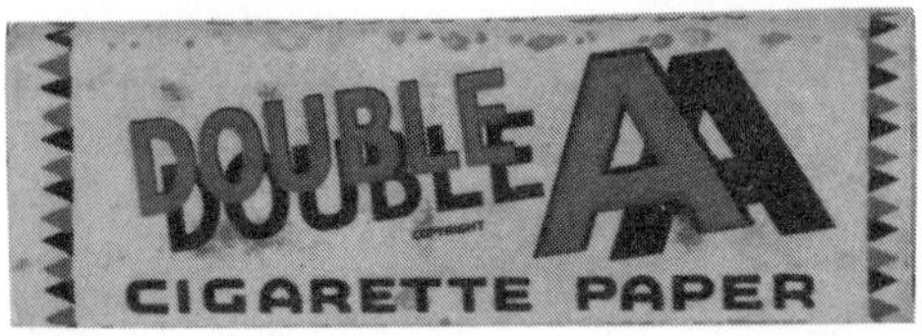

Double A.A., wrap around folder, 1940's, London.

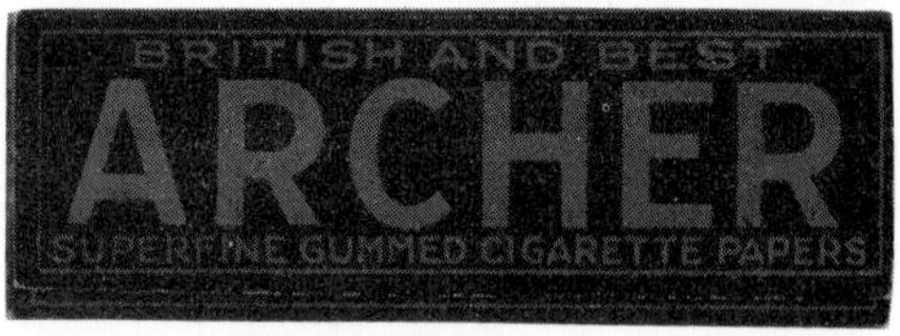

Archer, 60 leaves, red single packet, 1940's, British.

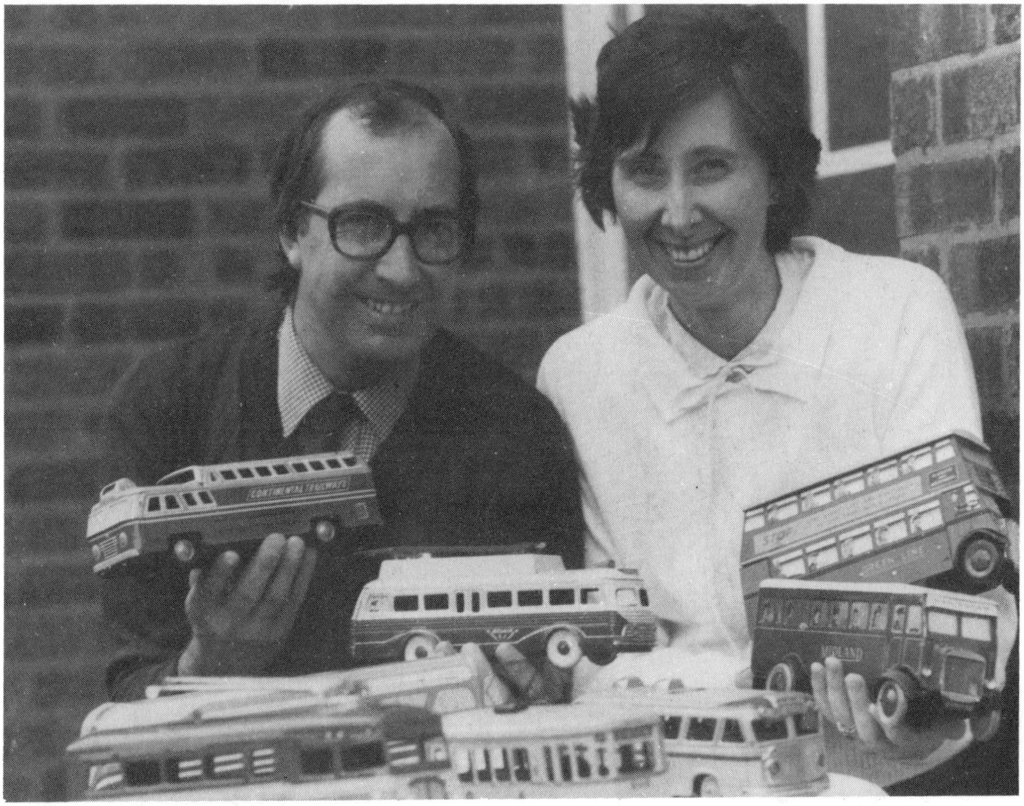

Geoff and Linda Price have a collection of model buses and trams worth well over £25,000. Geoff is the manager of a shoe shop and Linda works as a secretary for a local authority.

Geoff said: "Like so many other people, I began as a child collecting Dinky toys but I soon decided that buses and trams were my favourites and when Linda and I married, she got interested too and now she's as keen as I am. We've even had to build an extension onto our house to display the larger models because they range in size from one inch long to over 8 feet.

"We've got 2,830 different models dating back to 1903 and they come from all different parts of the world. They are in tinplate, die cast, plastic or wood and I've also got a collection of crested china charabancs.

"We have two big items — a 1949 miniature coach with a motor cycle engine which can seat two children. It was made in 1949 by Harrington's the coach builders as a scale model advertisement and it's more than 8 feet long. The second one is a 1945 French fairground coach from Lyons, it's 8 feet long too but it's not motorised. I reckon that each of these must be worth over £3,000 today."

As well as travelling all over Britain and Europe in search of special models, Geoff and Linda also buy all current models that are produced so that they can keep their collection up to date. Geoff's favourites are tin models made by Chad Valley in the 1930's but they are difficult to find in good condition.

The things he still wants to find include a Carr's biscuit tin in the shape of a bus which was produced around 1948 and a crested china model of a tram made by Willow China. He has all the china buses and double deckers but the sole example of a china tram has still eluded him.

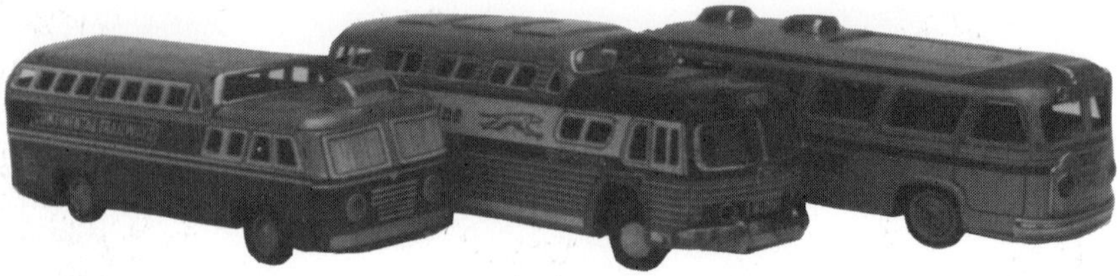

Trailways Greyhound Eagle, Made in Japan, 1960's tinplates. £15 – £40

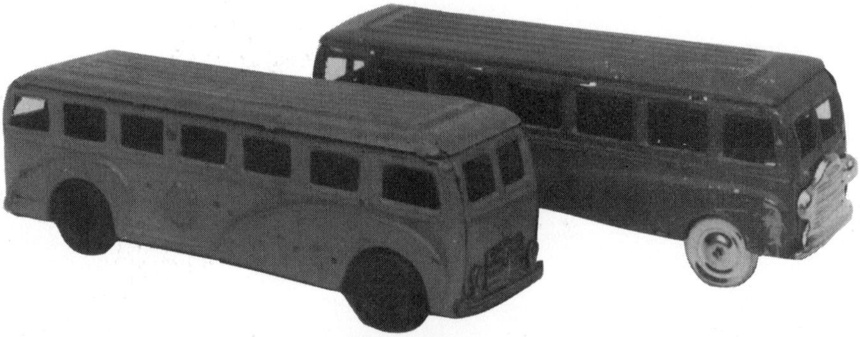

Tinplate coaches by Jaj, Portugal, circa 1960. £15 – £20

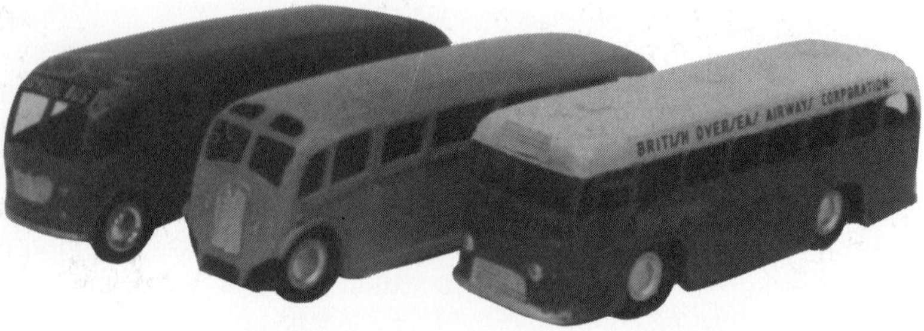

Three plastic Dinky copies of the 1960's, by Maks, Hong Kong. £8 – £10

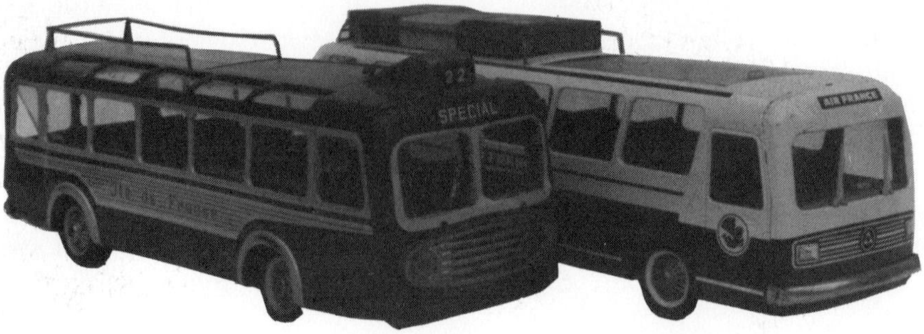

Tinplate coaches by Joustra, France, one 1950's – £65, the other 1960's – £35.

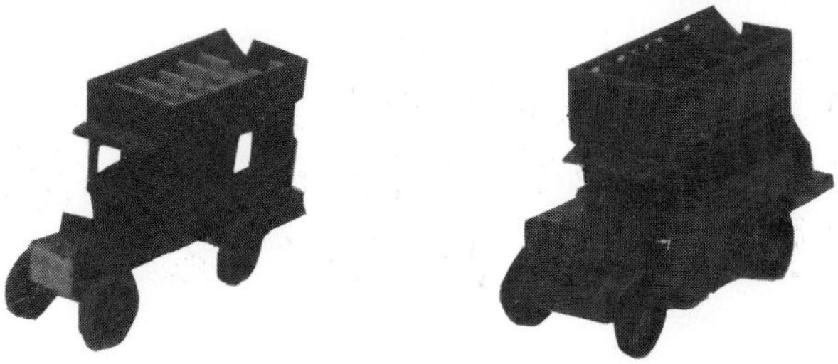

Three small double deck, by Charbens, U.K., 1955 and 1958. £25 – £30

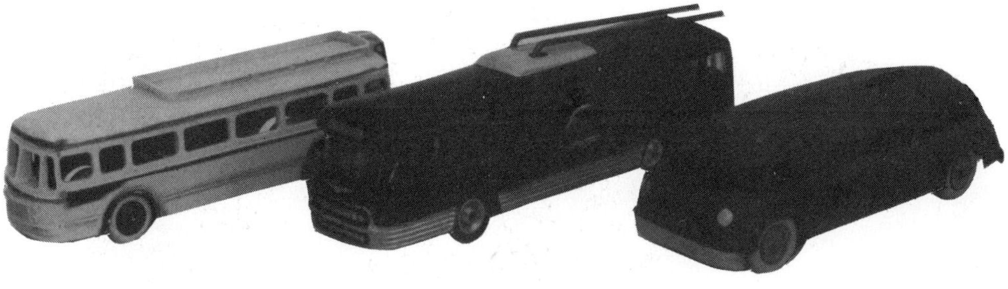

CIJ Renault coach, diecast, 1953 – £35, a trolley, 1960 and a Solido coach, diecast. £18 – £35

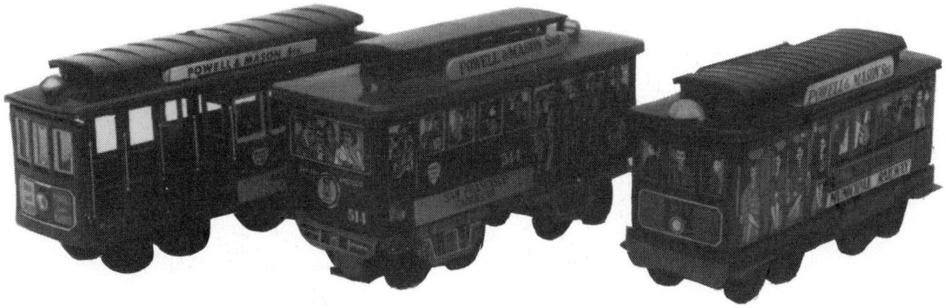

Tinplate San Francisco trams, Made in Japan, 1950's/1970's. £15 – £20

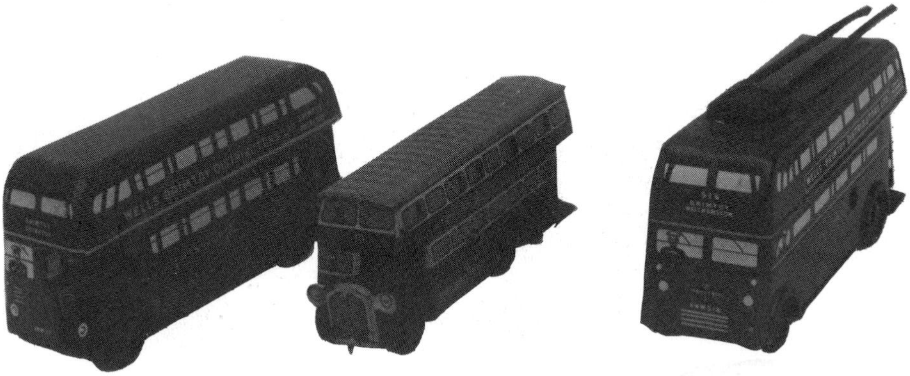

Two double decks and trolleybus, by Wells Brimtoys, U.K., 1950's. £30 – £45

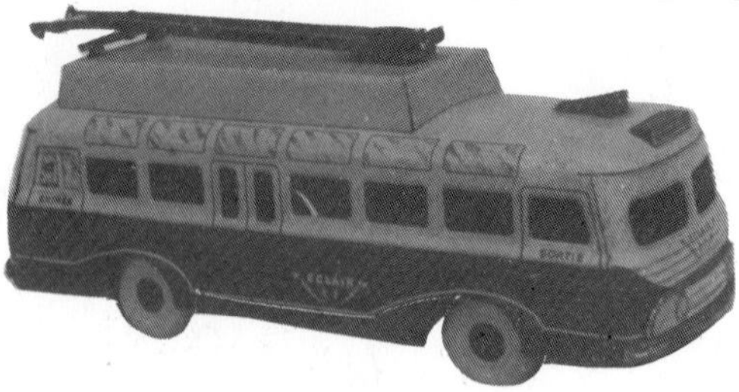

A trolleybus, by C.R., France, 1950. £50

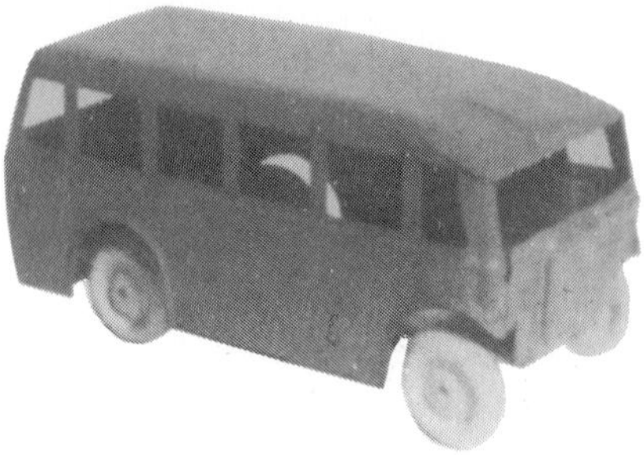

A pre-war tinplate bus with white rubber wheels, by Triang, U.K. £40

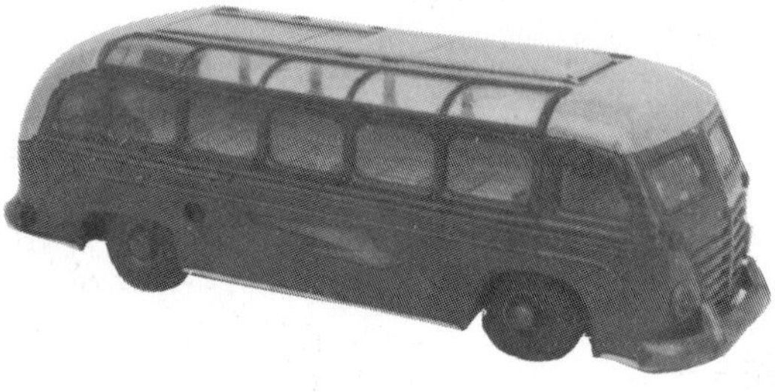

Tinplate coach, by Guntermann, Germany, map on base, 1948. £60

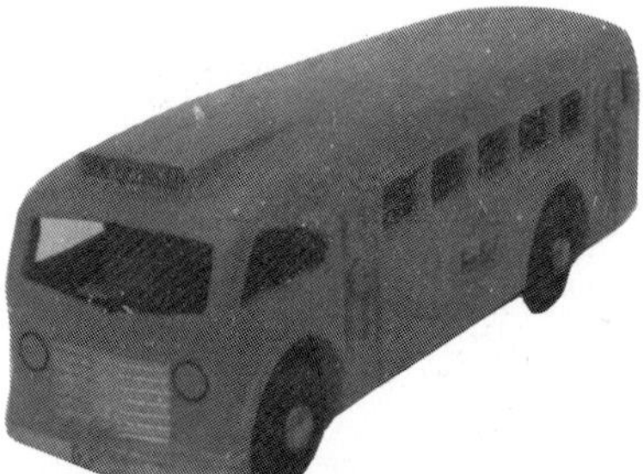

Large Bedford coach, by Fun Ho, New Zealand, cast aluminium, 1965. £18

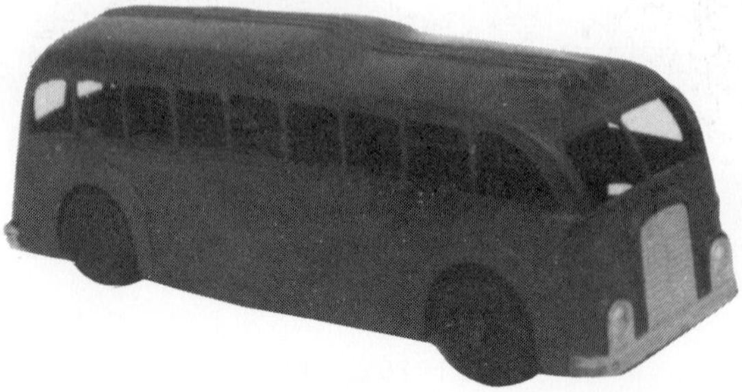

Guy Arab coach, by Mettoy, U.K. (predecessors of Corgie Toys), diecast, 1950. £45

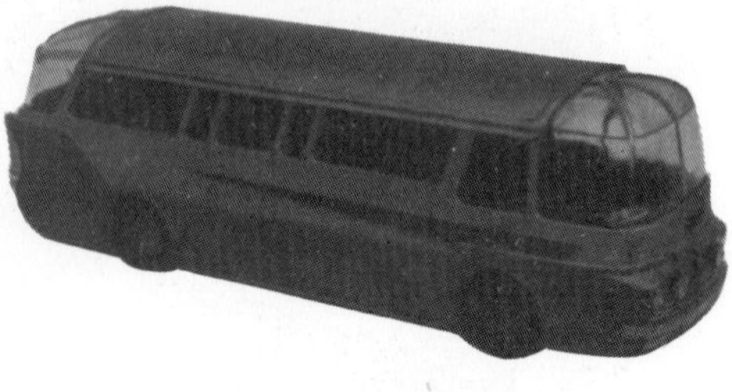

Mulliner Coach, by Spot-On, U.K., 1963. £150

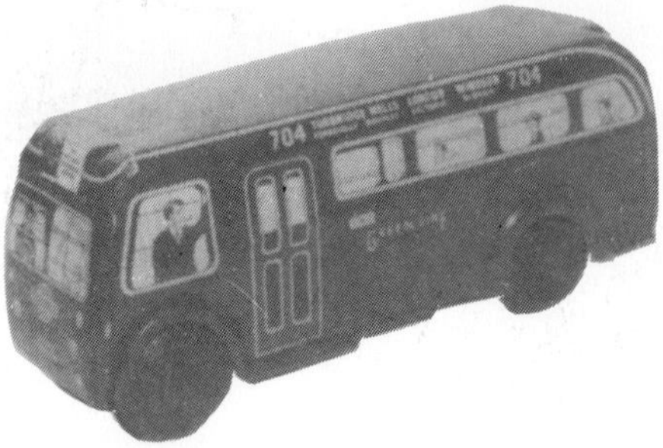

Greenline tinplate coach, by Wells Brimtoys, U.K., 1950's. £50

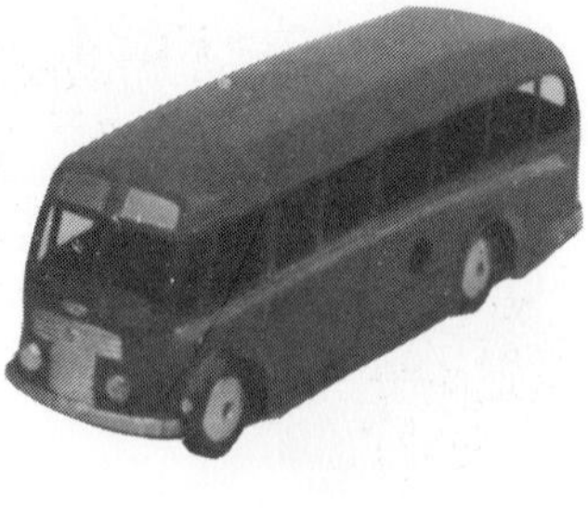

A Commer Avenger coach, by Chad Valley, U.K., 1954. £60

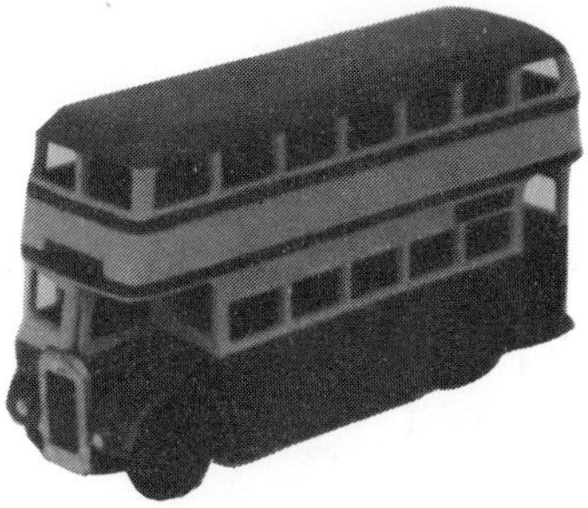

A double deck, by Chad Valley, U.K., 1949. £85

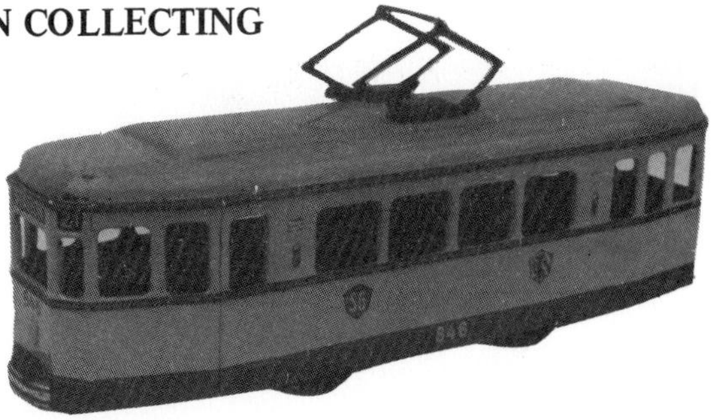

A tramcar, No. 846, by Guntermann, Germany, 1955. £65

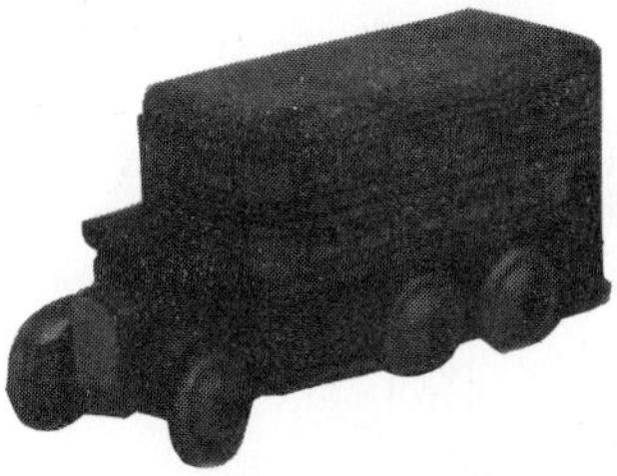

German Penny toys, 1930's. £40

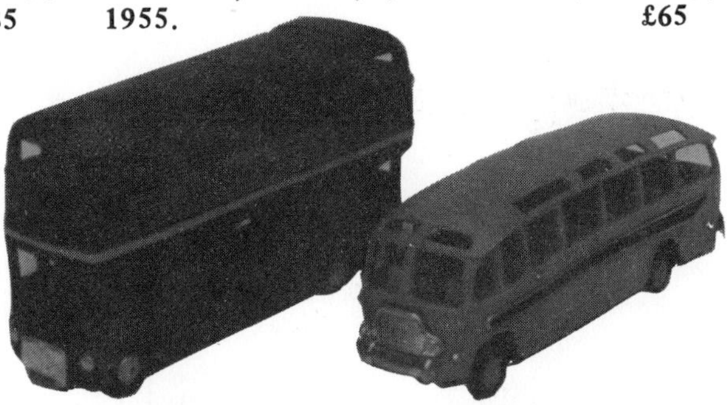

Minic Motorways double decker and coach, by Triang, U.K., 1960's. £18 – £35

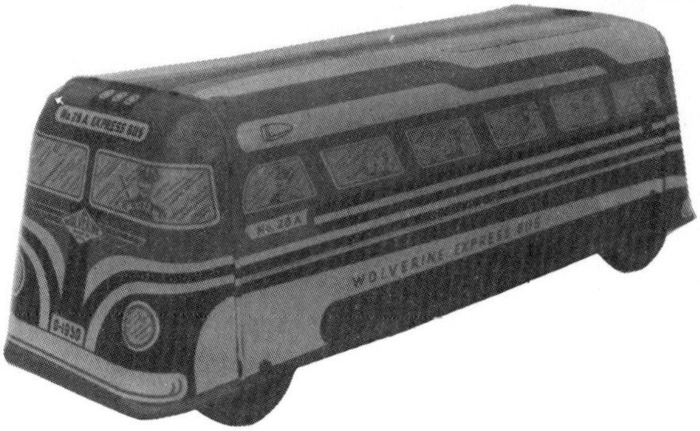

A 1950 tinplate Express bus, by Wolverine, U.S.A. £60

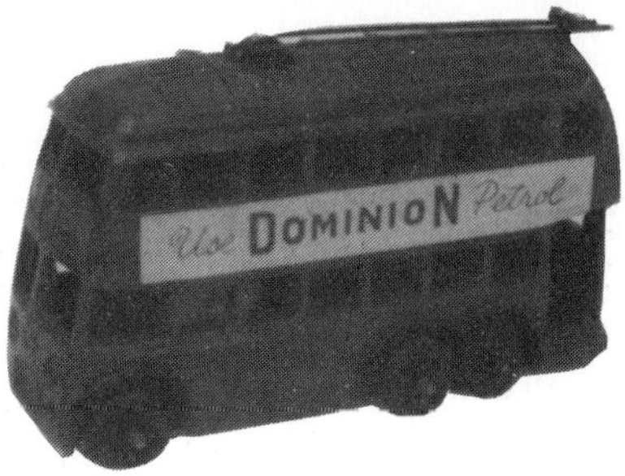

A diecast trolleybus, by Taylor & Barrett, U.K., 1936. £40

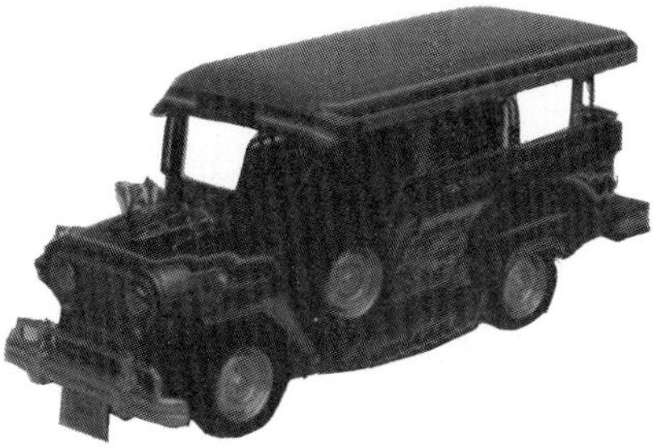

Jitney Bus, Made in Phillipines, 1970's/80's. £15

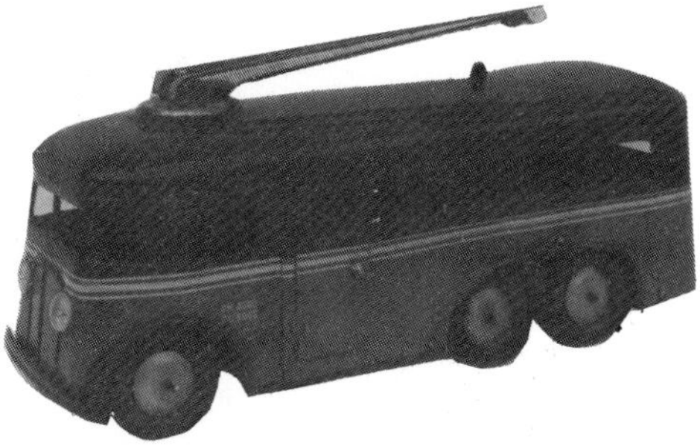

Six-wheeled trolleybus, by Joustra, France, tinplate, battery operated lights, 1952. £95

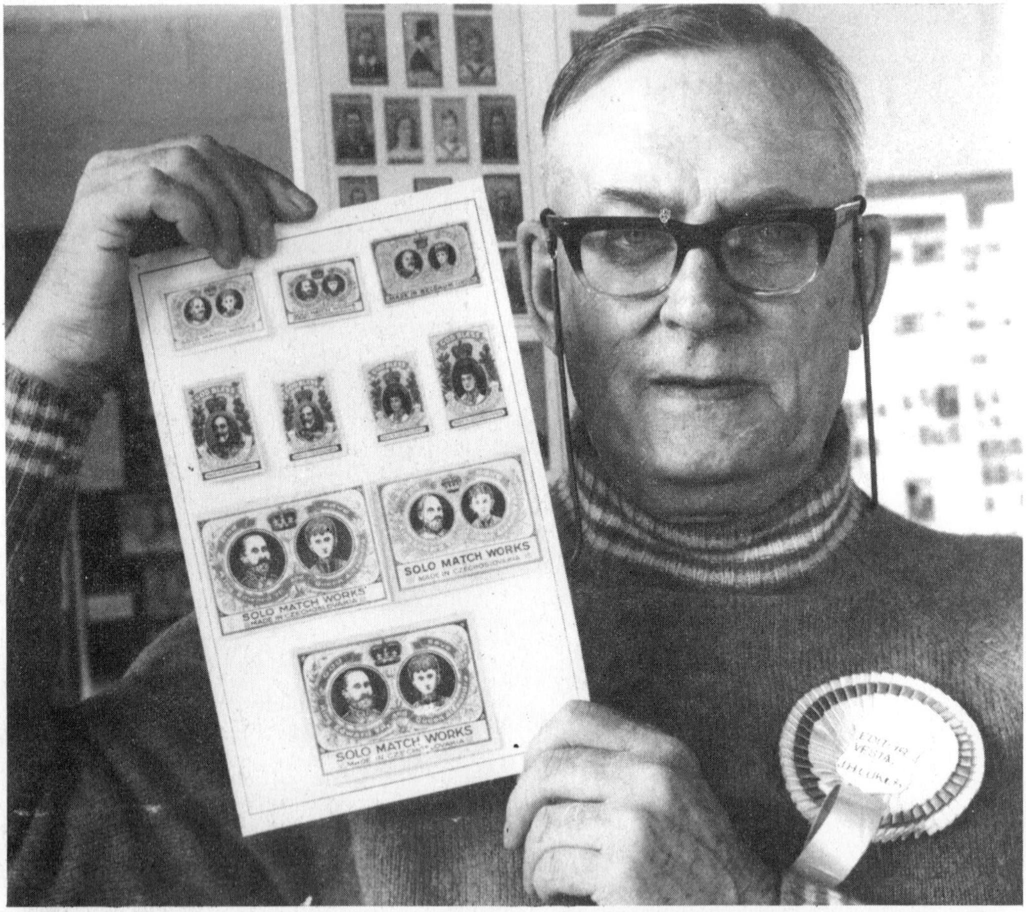

John Luker is retired but continues to publish 'Vesta' magazine and to deal in matchboxes, tins and labels which he collects.

"What I call hardware are match tins and their story goes back to the 1860's when matches were first put into tins. In my collection I have some that are more than a hundred years old.

"The rarest is a Vesta tin of 1871 which is worth £25. Some of the tins I've got are decorated with pictures of Queen Victoria or Bismark. I also have an early Vesta black japanned tin with a gold design on it which was made by a Reading firm called Huntley, Bourne and Stevens around 1870.

"Other things that I'm particularly fond of and would not want to sell are two stands made by Bryant & Mays in 1886 in the form of a donkey and a turtle. They are in cast iron and held matchboxes on their backs. The donkey must be worth £25 and the turtle between £40 and £50.

"Matchboxes were made from 1826 onwards. They were bigger than they are today and because they were made of chipboard were very fragile. It is rare to find early ones. If it was possible to find one I'd like an 1826 match box for my collection."

Mr Luker is very knowledgeable about the history of the match industry and has written several books and articles on the subject. In his collection he has some of the long square matches that were produced in Victorian times. Their heads were heavily impregnated with sulphur and the girls who manufactured them suffered from a disease of the gums brought about by breathing in the fumes.

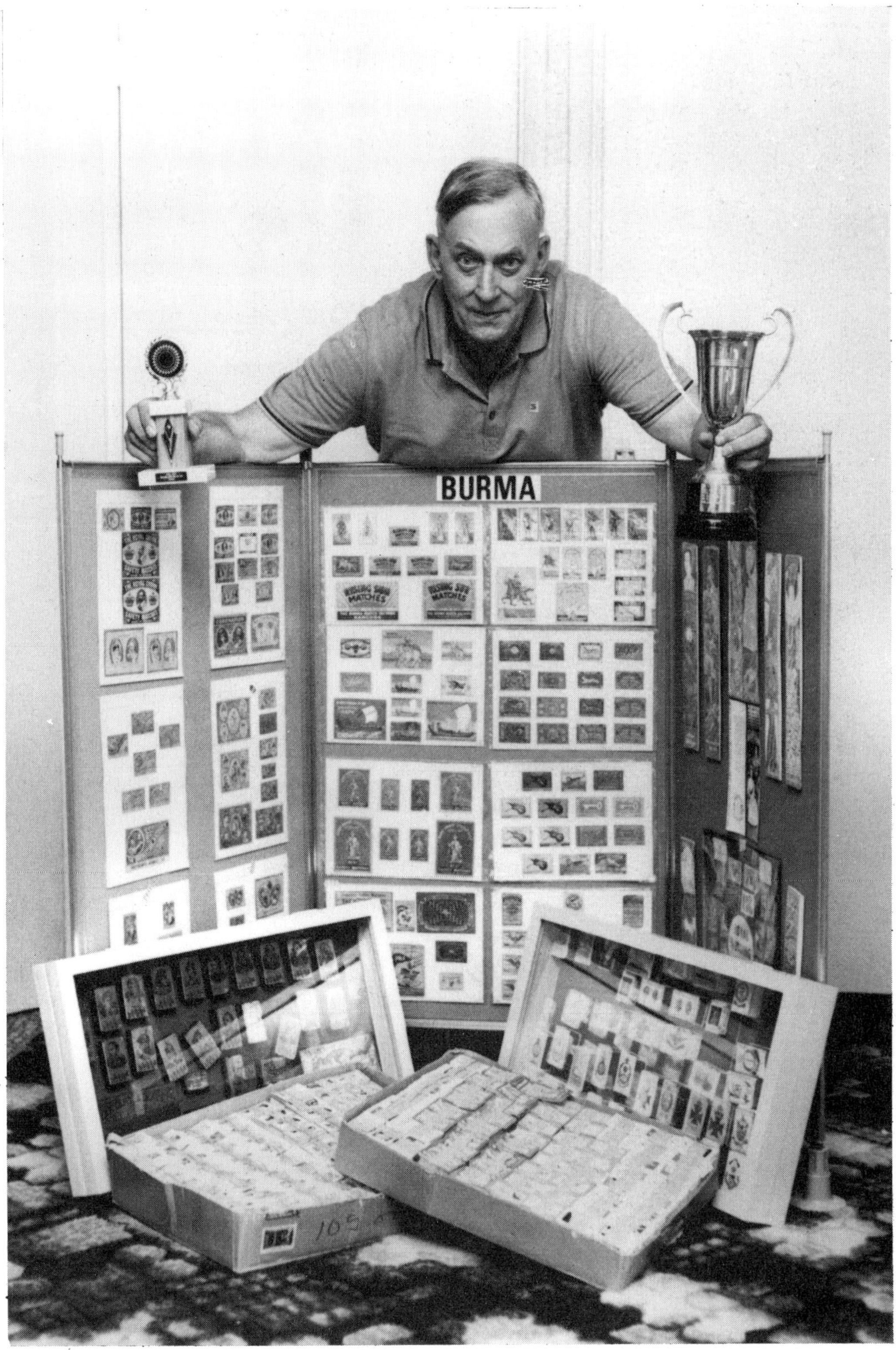
BURMA
RISING SUN MATCHES
RISING SUN MATCHES

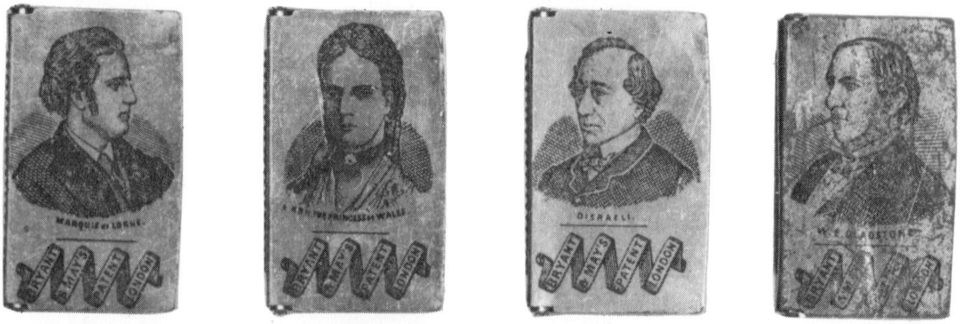

Vesta container, circa 1876 featuring the Marquis of Lorne, HRH The Princess of Wales, Disraeli and Gladstone.

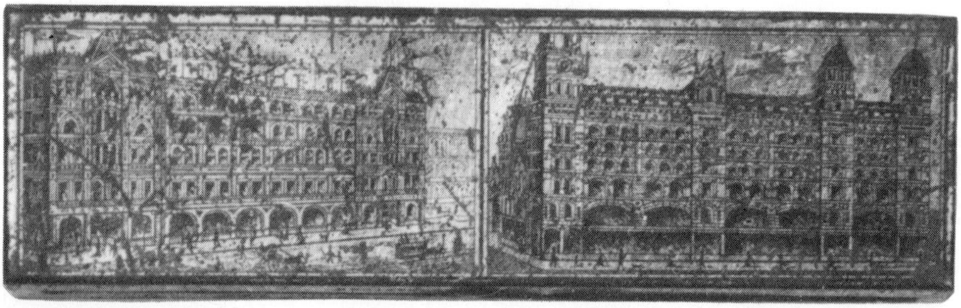

Match container for Lewis Stores, 1884.

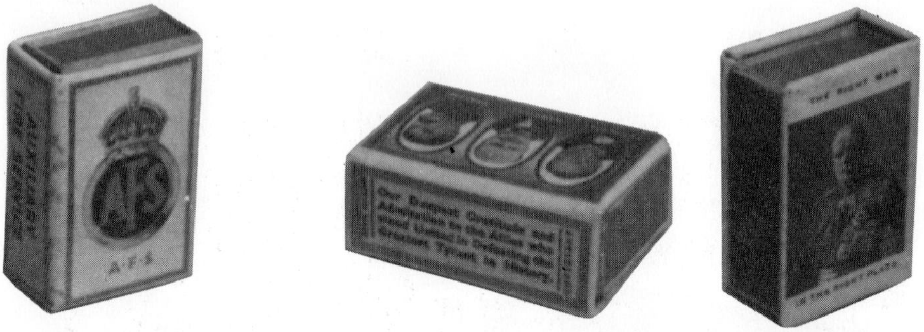

Three patriotic grips from the 2nd World War.

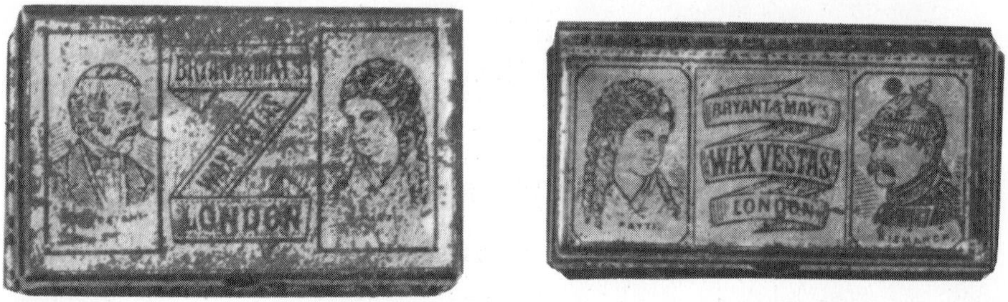

Bryant & Mays, London, Wax Vestas containers.

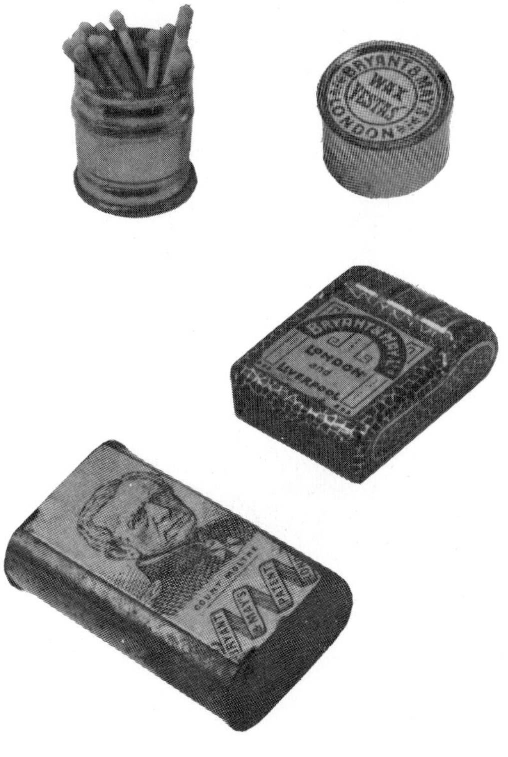

Early Vesta containers from Bryant & Mays.

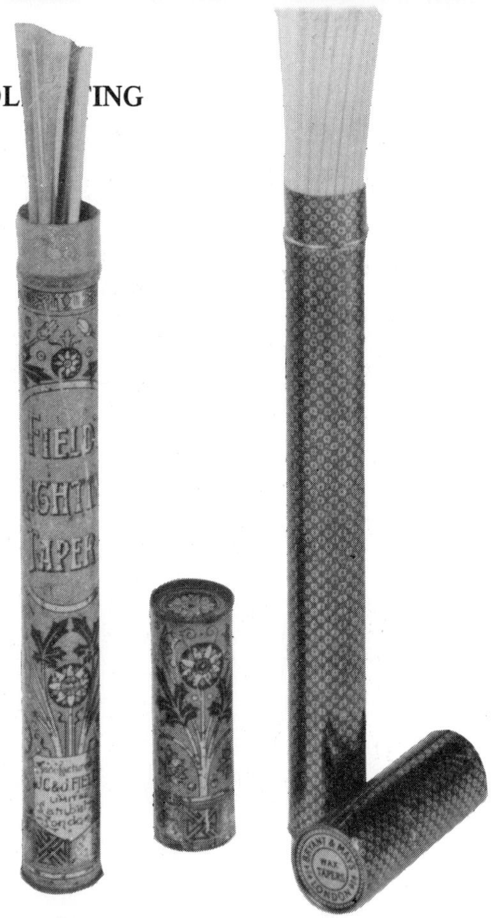

Interesting wax taper containers by W. C. & J. Field and Bryant & Mays.

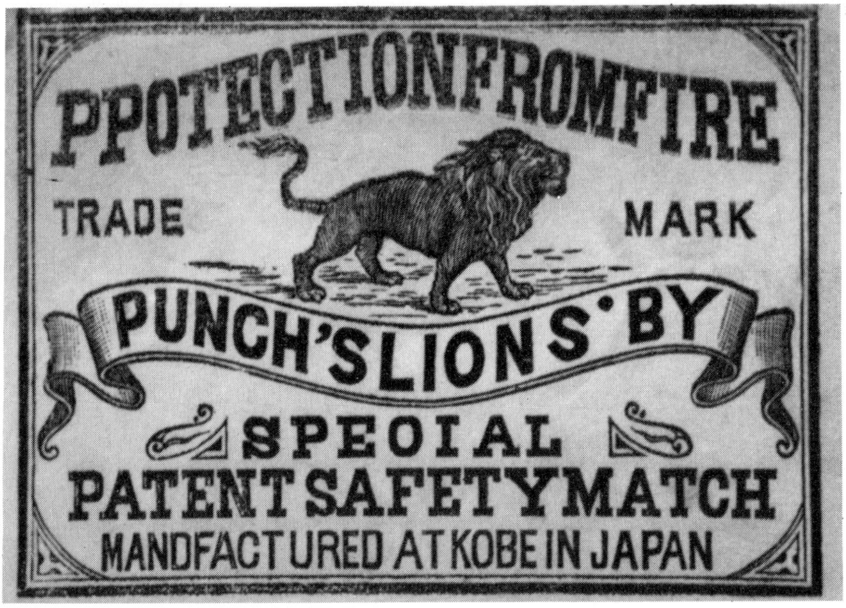

An interesting Japanese label, with a host of spelling mistakes.

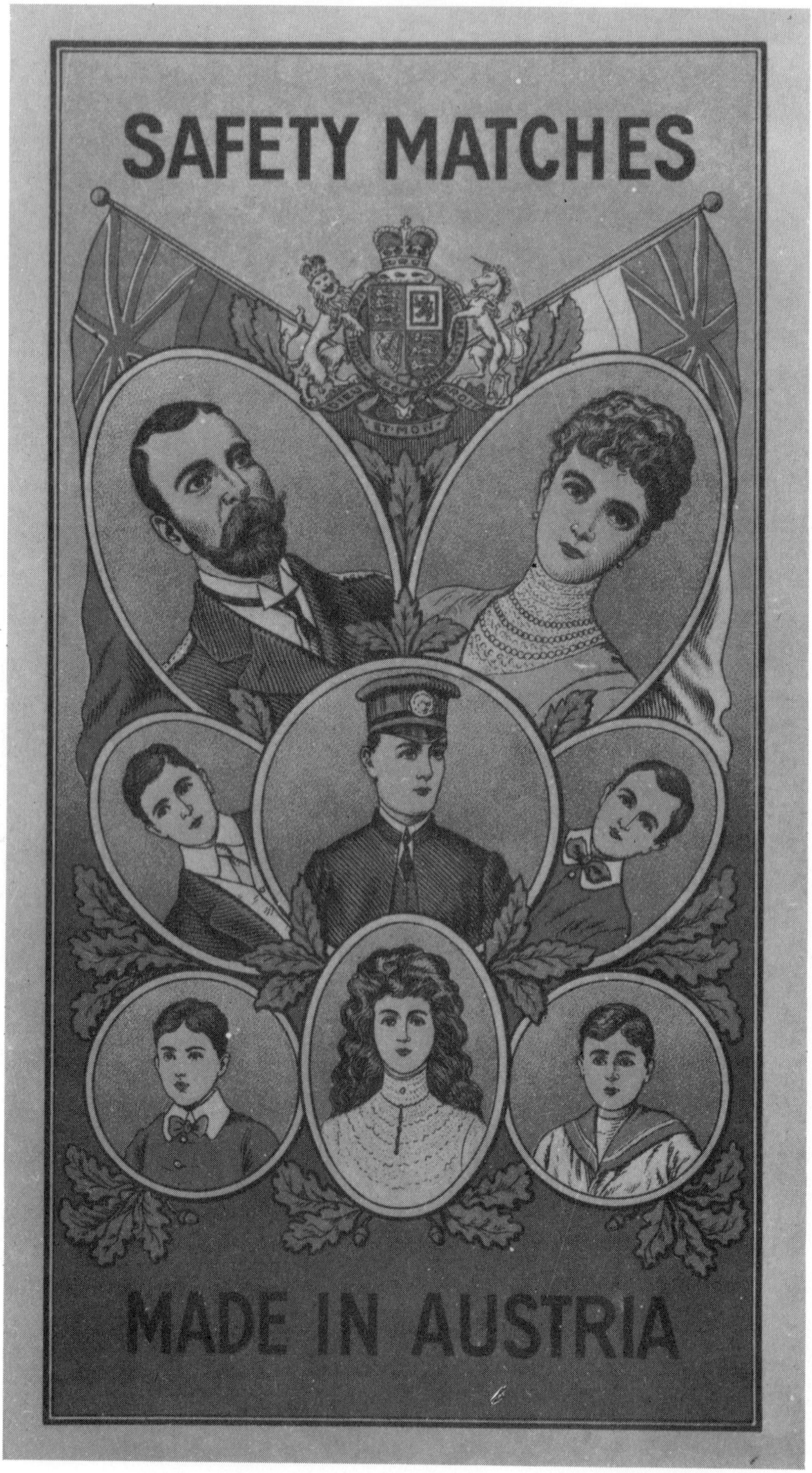

Austrian packet label featuring the Royal Family.

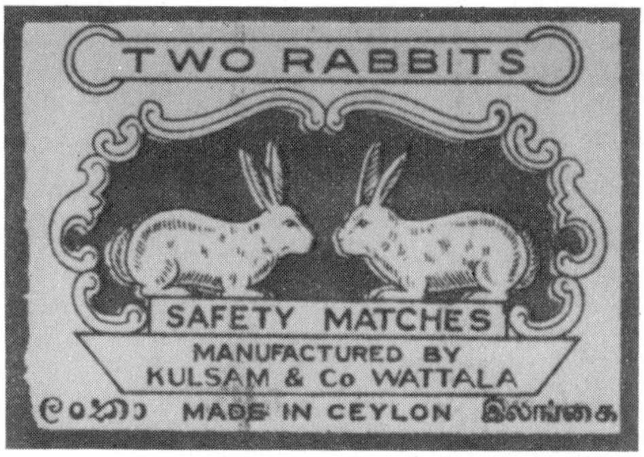

'Two Rabbits' safety matches made in Ceylon.

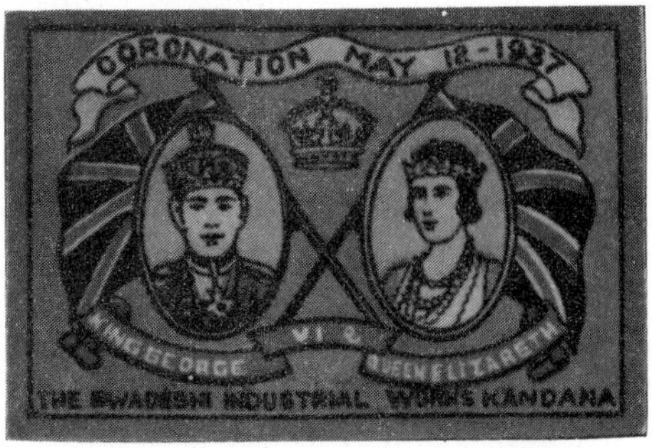

Commemorative label made in Ceylon for the Coronation 1937.

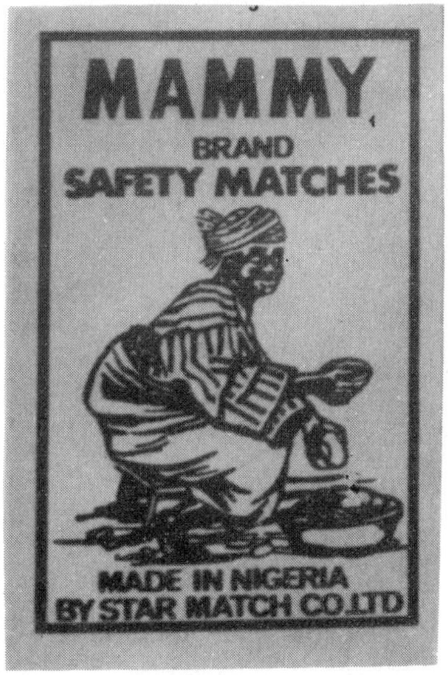

'Mammy' brand safety matches made in Nigeria.

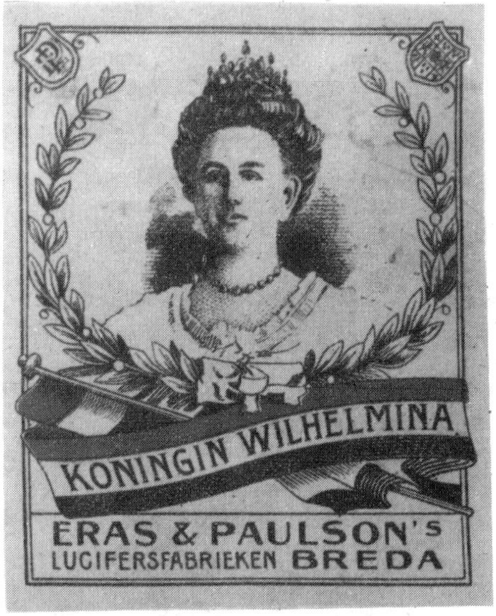

'Koningin Wilhelmina' matches by Eras & Paulson, Holland.

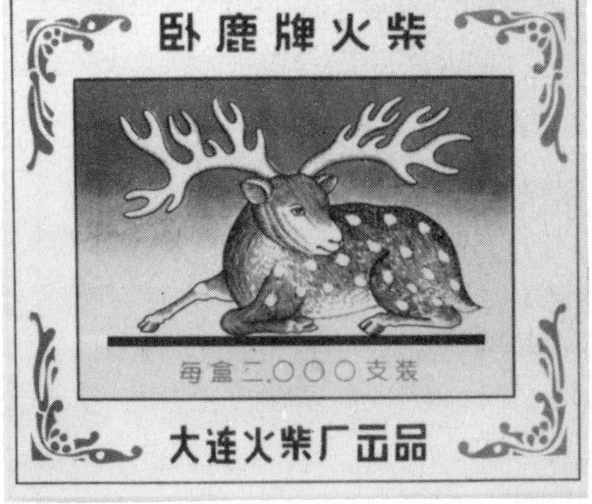

Chinese matchbox label with 2000 contents.

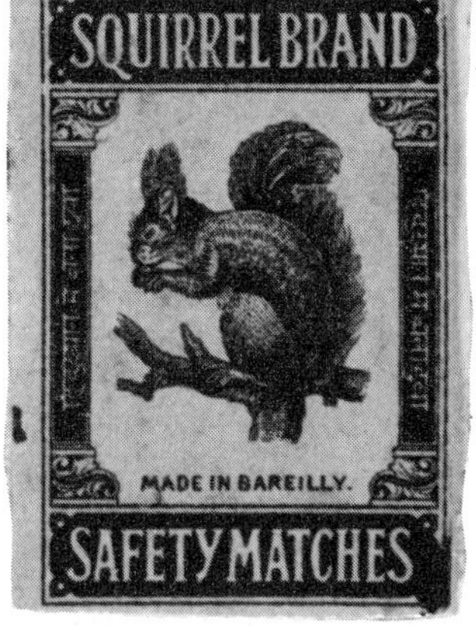

Squirrel Brand matches made in India 1923.

BRYANT & MAY'S

PILLAR-BOX WAX VESTAS.

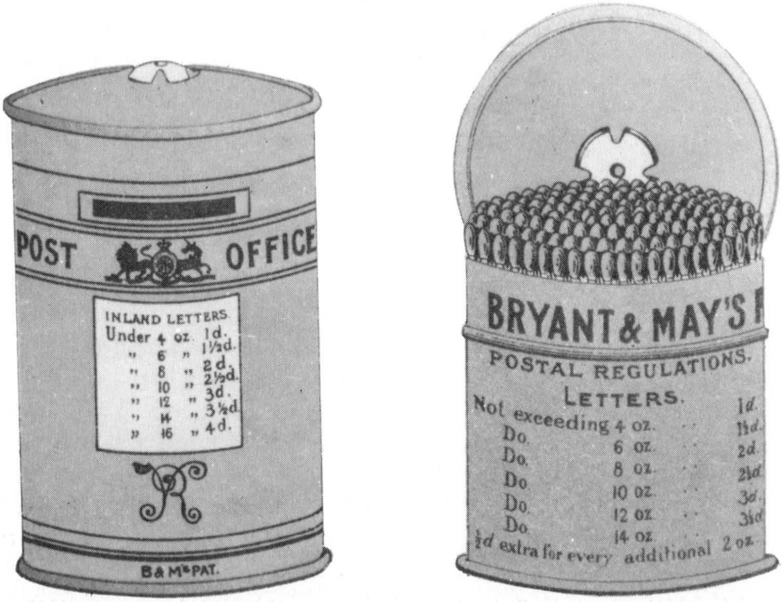

No. 35.

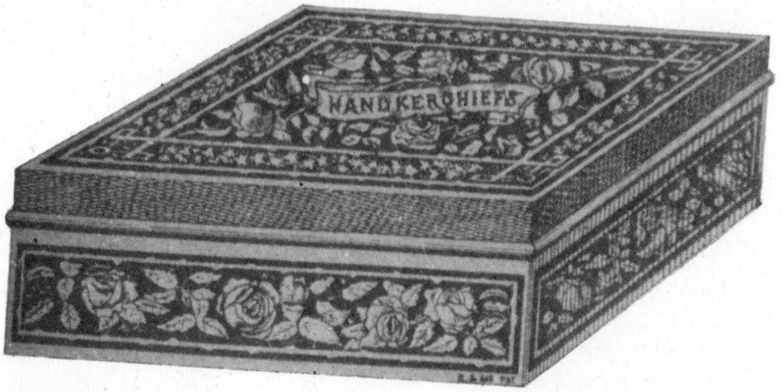

DECORATED TIN HANDKERCHIEF BOX TO CONTAIN ONE DOZEN POST OFFICE PILLAR VESTA BOXES.

BRYANT & MAY, Fairfield Works, Bow, London, E.

An interesting page from an early Bryant & Mays catalogue for Pillar-Box Wax Vestas.

Alan Cunningham owns a shop called 'Football Crazy' selling all sorts of football memorabilia and collects soccer programmes for his own interest.

"In the late '50's I used to go to football matches as a kid and I kept all the programmes and my father, who went to the big matches in the West of Scotland, brought his programmes back for me. The collection started then and now it's grown to the stage that it takes up an entire room.

"I'm mainly concerned with football in Scotland and the game started up here in 1867 when Queen's Park were formed. My collection goes back to before 1900 and as well as programmes I've got a lot of books, statistical information, photographs and annuals. I've a full set going back to the 1930's of the 'Wee Red Book' issued by the 'Glasgow Evening Times' every autumn.

"I'm a Partick Thistle supporter myself although I live in Edinburgh and it's a Glasgow team. One of my proudest possessions is the programme for the 1971 Scottish League Cup Final when Partick played against Celtic. They beat Celtic 4-1.

"If I had a wish for a special programme I'd want another Partick Thistle programme — the one for the 1921 Scottish Cup Final in which they played against Rangers. Partick Thistle won 1-0 and they scored the winning goal while the Rangers centre half was off having his shorts changed. That caused a lot of protest from Rangers supporters."

The price range for soccer memorabilia ranges from a few pence to several pounds according to what the collector is looking for but it is a hobby that need not be expensive. It is still possible for example to pick up pre First World War cigarette cards of famous footballers for £1 each.

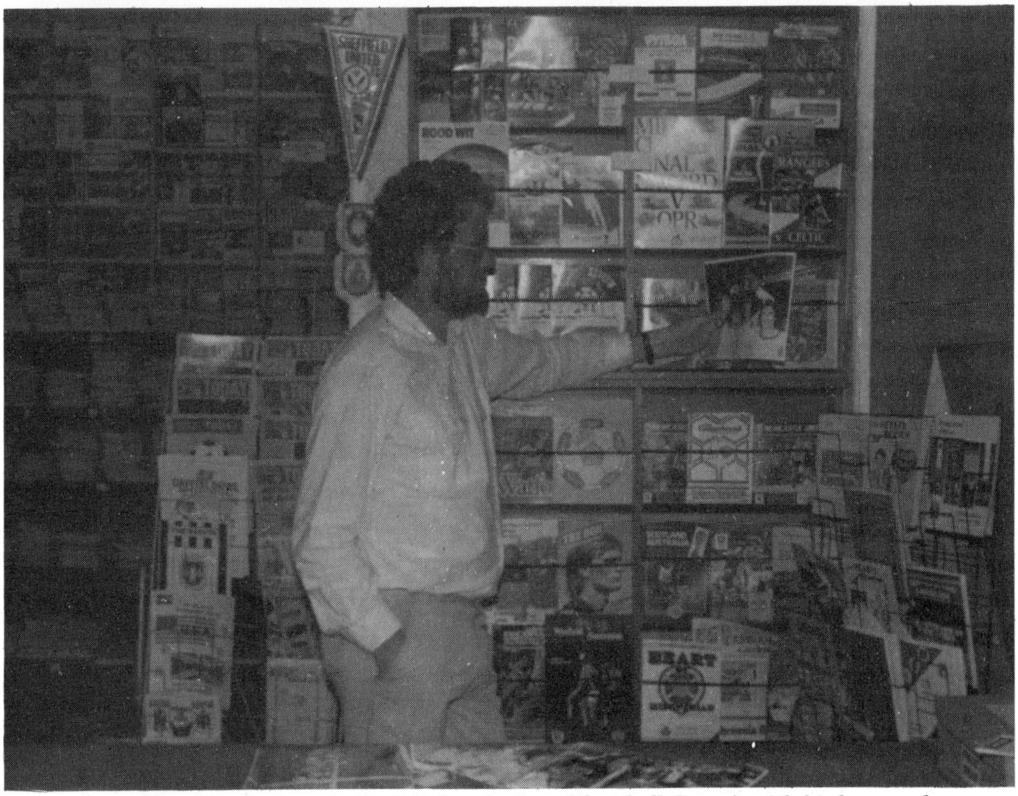

Alan Cunningham in his Edinburgh shop, 'Football Crazy', with his large and varied stock.

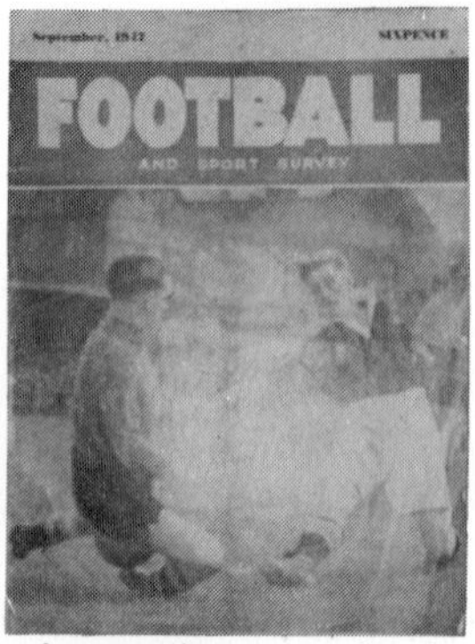

An interesting magazine issued by the Scottish Players Union, 'Football and Sport Survey, September 1947' with interesting social comment as well as football news. £2

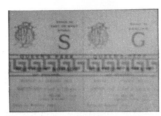

Match ticket for Queen's Park v. Northern Nomads, 1911/12. £3

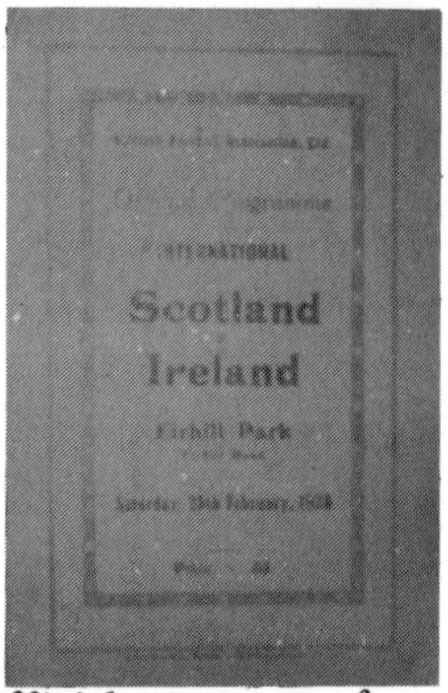

Official programme for the 1928 Scotland v. Ireland International played at Firhill where it attracted the record attendance of 52,000 fans. £30

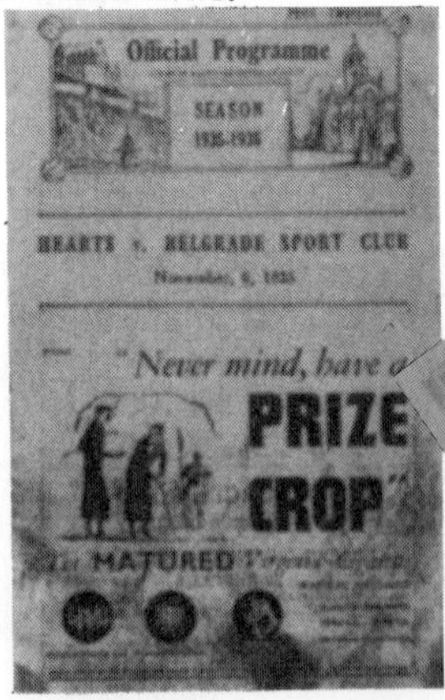

1935/36 Hearts v. Belgrade Sport Club, a very rare pre war issue. £35

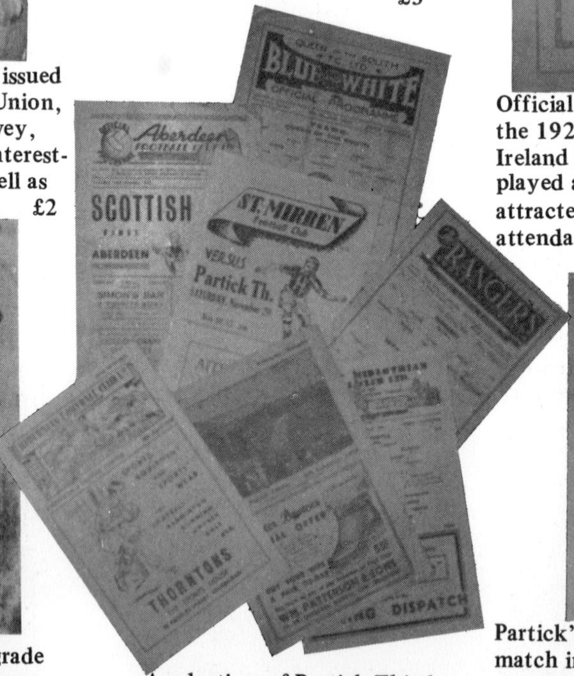

A selection of Partick Thistle away programmes from the 1940's. £2 – £5 each

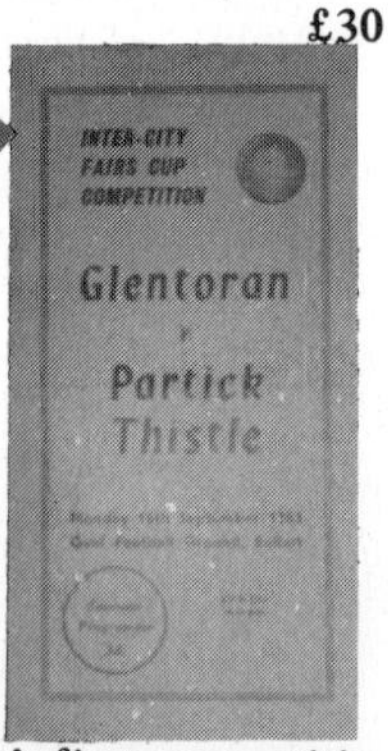

Partick's first competitive match in Europe was in the 1963/64 Fairs Cup against Glentoran in Belfast. £15

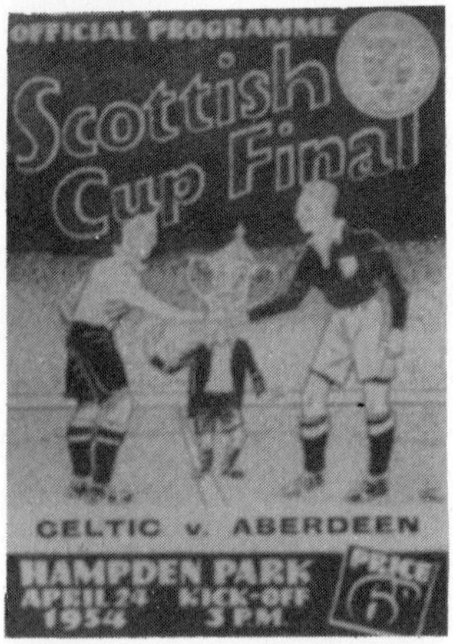

1953/54 Celtic v. Aberdeen Scottish Cup Final and Celtic win 2-1. £8

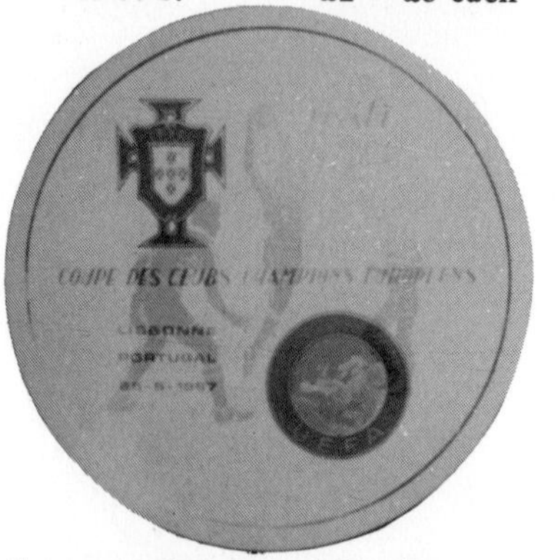

Souvenir plate issued for the 1967 European Cup Final when Celtic became the first British team to win this premier competition. £15

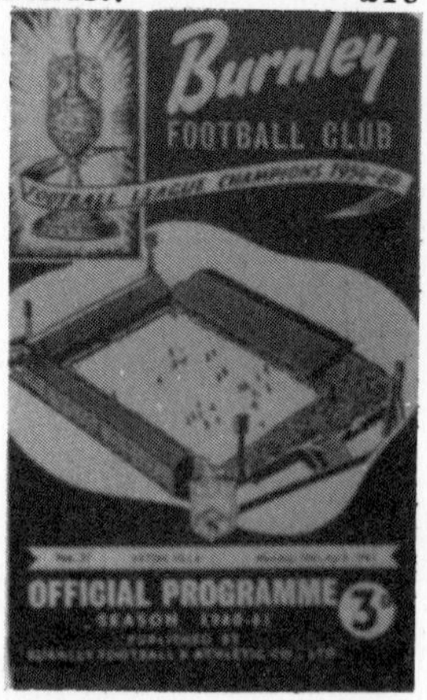

1960/61 Burnley v. Aston Villa League Cup Semi Final. £6.50

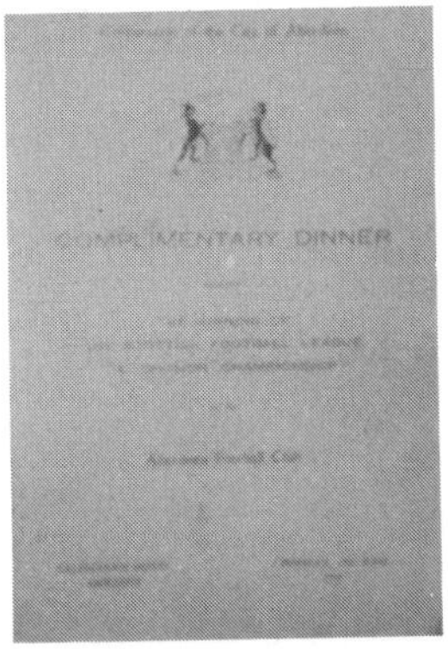

Celebration Dinner Menu for Aberdeen winning the Championship in 1954, fully autographed by the Don's team. £10

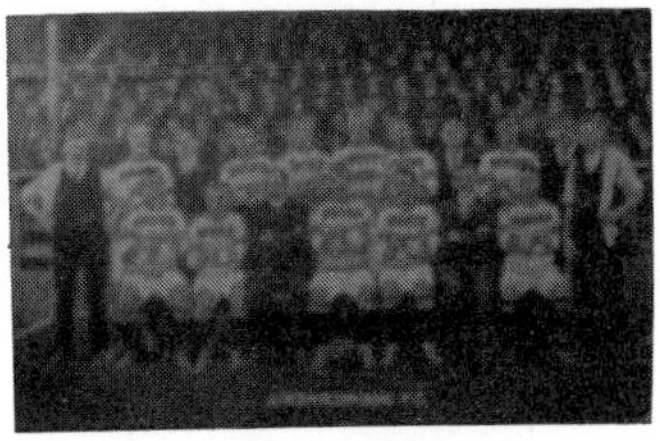

Postcard of Airdrieonians F.C. circa 1900. £6

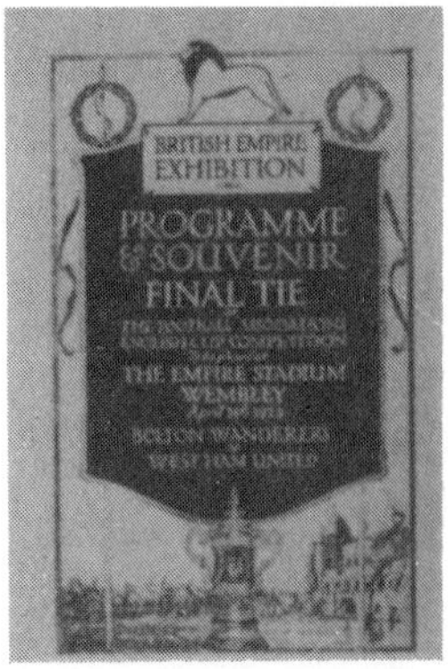

1922/23 FAC Final between West Ham Utd. and Bolton was the first Wembley Final. £140

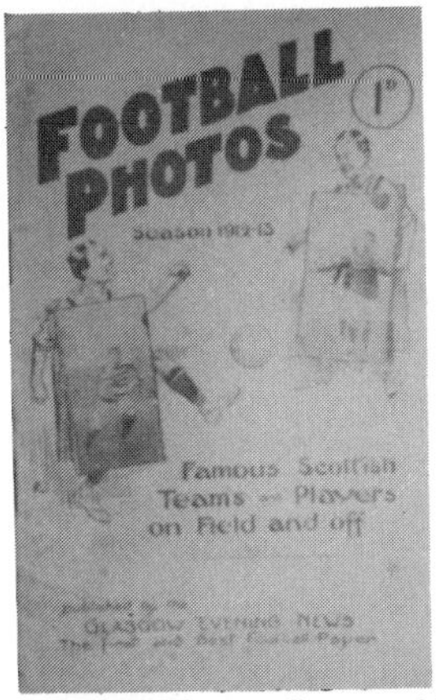

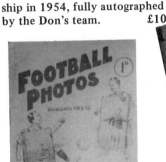

'Football Photos Season 1912-13' published by the Glasgow Evening News, which contains action photographs and team groups. £10

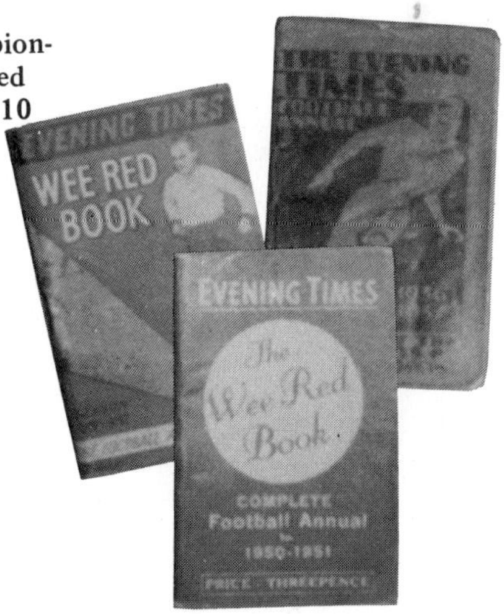

The name 'Wee Red Book' was first used by the publishers, The Glasgow Evening Times, in the 37/38 season although the annual had been produced prior to 1928/29.

Pre War	£10
1940's	£5
Early 1950's	£3

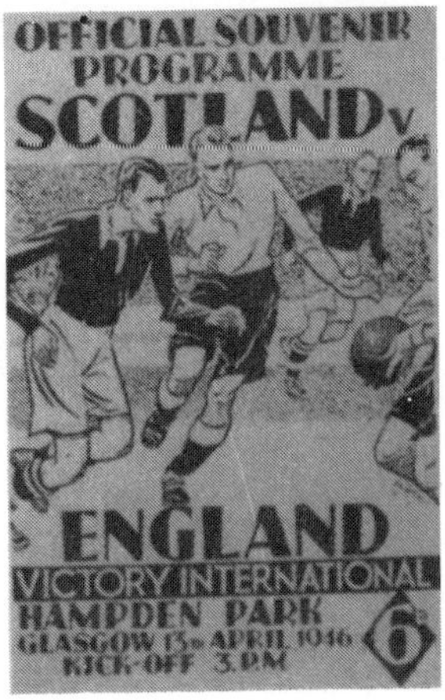

1945/46 Scotland v. England (Victory International). £12.50

1974/75 Meadowbank v. Alloa. Meadowbank's first league match. £2.50

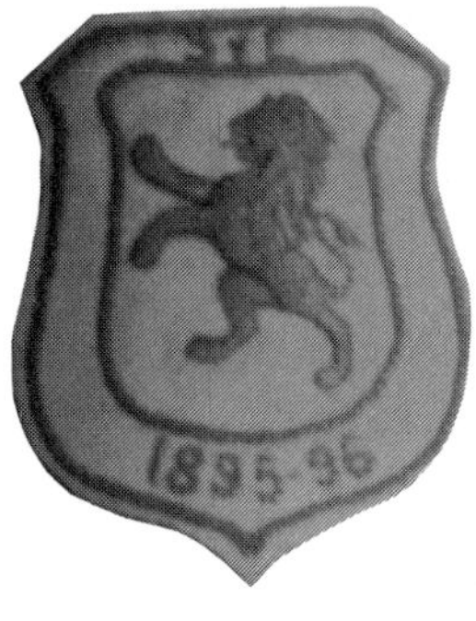

Jersey badge from the Scotland v. England match 1895/96 season. £10

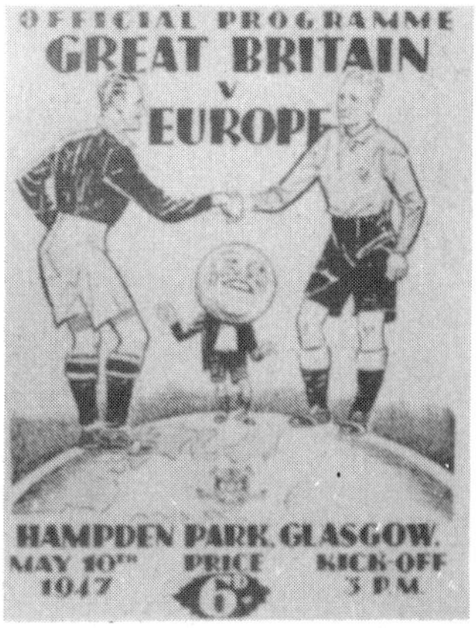

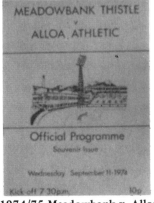

1946/47 Great Britain v. Europe rated as one of the great games of all time. £6.50

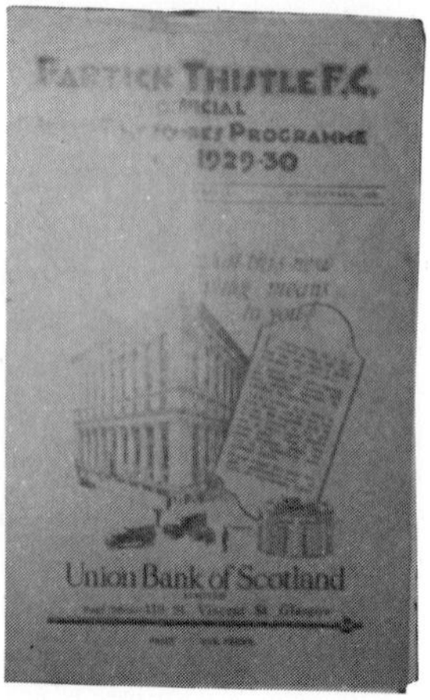

All Scottish pre war club programmes are difficult to obtain which is why this 1929/30 Partick Thistle v. Motherwell example is worth £25.

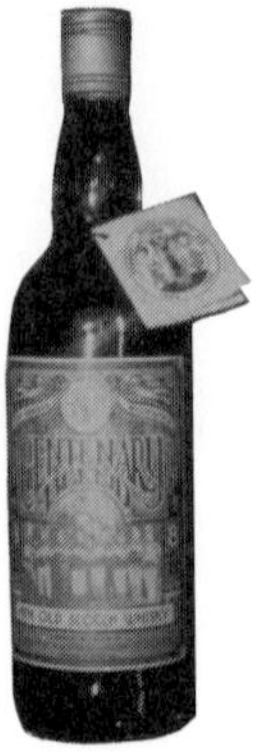

Centenary souvenir whisky bottled for Highland League team Forres Mechanics. £9

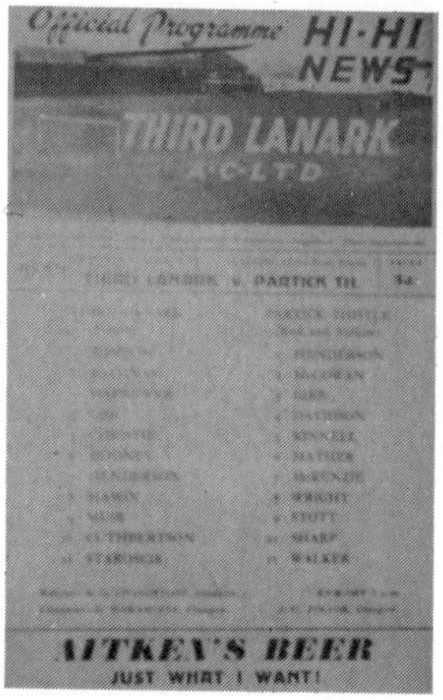

Programmes from defunct clubs are always eagerly sought by collectors. Third Lanark v. Partick Thistle in the '49/50 Glasgow Cup. £5

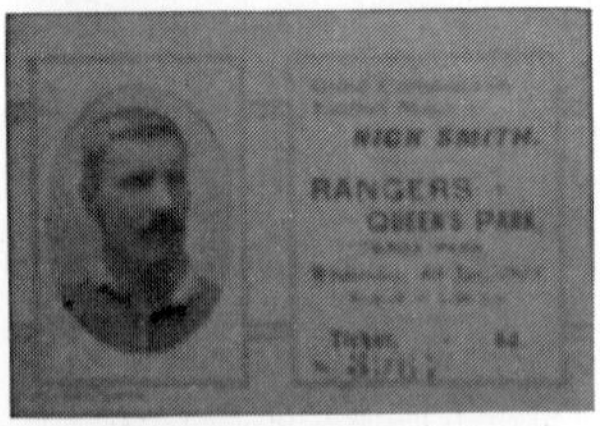

Nick Smith's Testimonial, Rangers v. Queen's Park 1904/05. £3

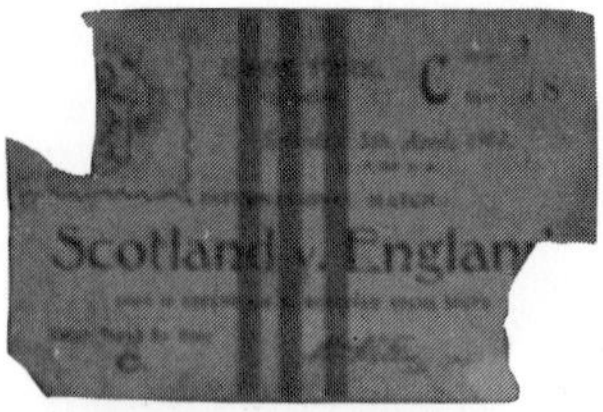

Match ticket for Scotland v. England 1901/02, the first Ibrox disaster. £3

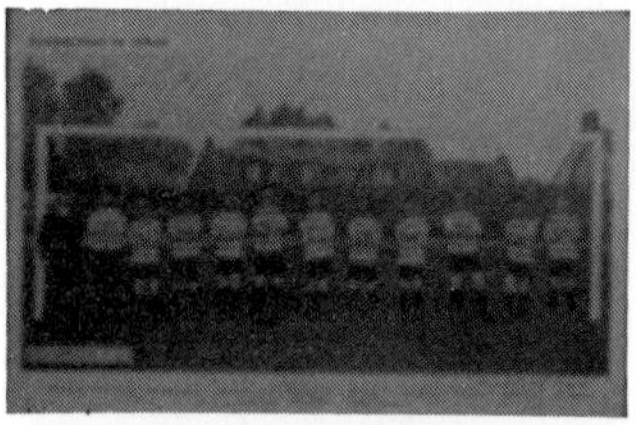

Postcard of Kilmarnock F.C. 1905. £6

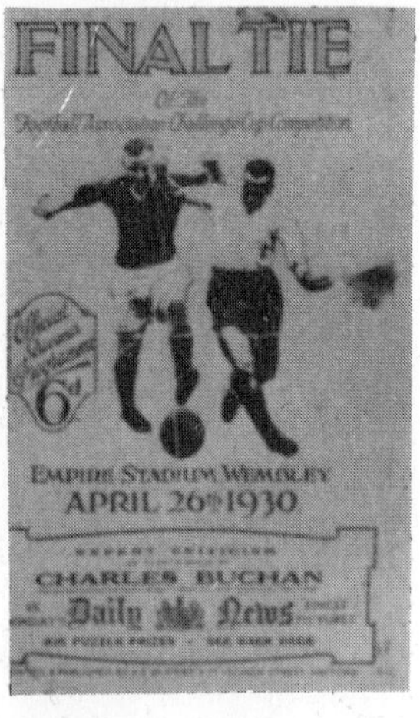

1929/30 FAC Final, Arsenal v. Huddersfield, pre war FAC Finals are amongst the most eagerly sought programmes. £60

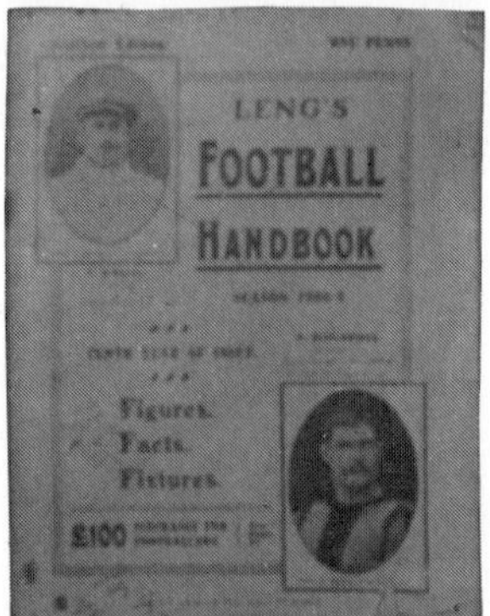

John Lengs, a Dundee based printer taken over by D. C. Thompson, published their first annual in the 1899/1900 season. The annuals contain a wealth of information on Scottish football including many minor competitions. £15

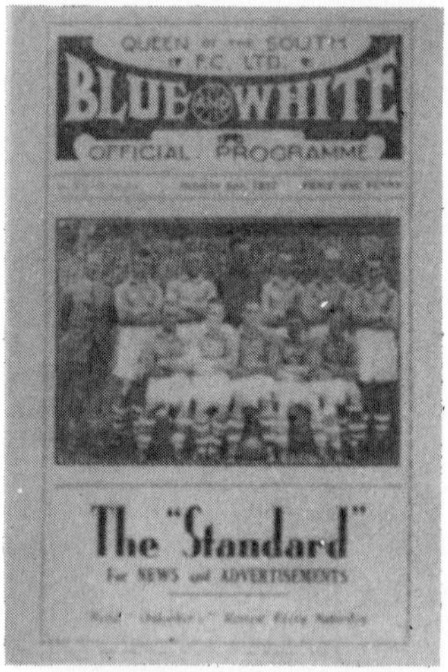

1937/38 Queen of the South Reserves v. Falkirk Reserves. Pre war Scottish programmes are very rare. £10

Jock Farquharson is a farmer who collects car mascots.

"I'm a compulsive collector and my interest in mascots began as an arm to my collection of vintage cars. I've got 130 mascots but it's difficult to buy them now because there are so many fakes around. The Rolls Royce mascot in particular is being faked basically because it's very simple.

"I've got 9 Rolls Royce mascots designed by Charles Sykes and I know they're genuine because I bought most of them from an undertaker whose fleet of hearses went back to 1910.

"My collection is valuable but what I appreciate about them most are the stories that attach to them. I remember where and when I bought each one and they've all got particular memories.

"For instance I've got a very rare German car mascot in the shape of an officer's helmet with a crown which came off the staff car of Rommel's adjutant. I bought it in 1972 from a chap who claimed to be the last Wandering Jew left in the world and it cost me £5 and a brass jelly pan."

The boom era of the car mascot was between the wars and most of Mr Farquharson's collection dates from that period. Perhaps the star is a very rare Austin mascot which is only one of three or four in the world; in rarity it is closely followed by a J. Grose mascot made for an Austin 7 in the early 1930's and a Desmo one for a 1930's MG in the shape of a dragonfly of brass and chrome with mother of pearl wings.

He also has a mascot in the shape of Bruce Bairnsfather's 'Old Bill'; an unusual lucky mascot called 'Touch Wud' and another in the shape of the Gas Board's Mr Therm. One of the mascots he is most fond of is a winged scarab in laminated aluminium made by Voison, a company which manufactured aeroplanes during the First World War and began mascot making when the war was over.

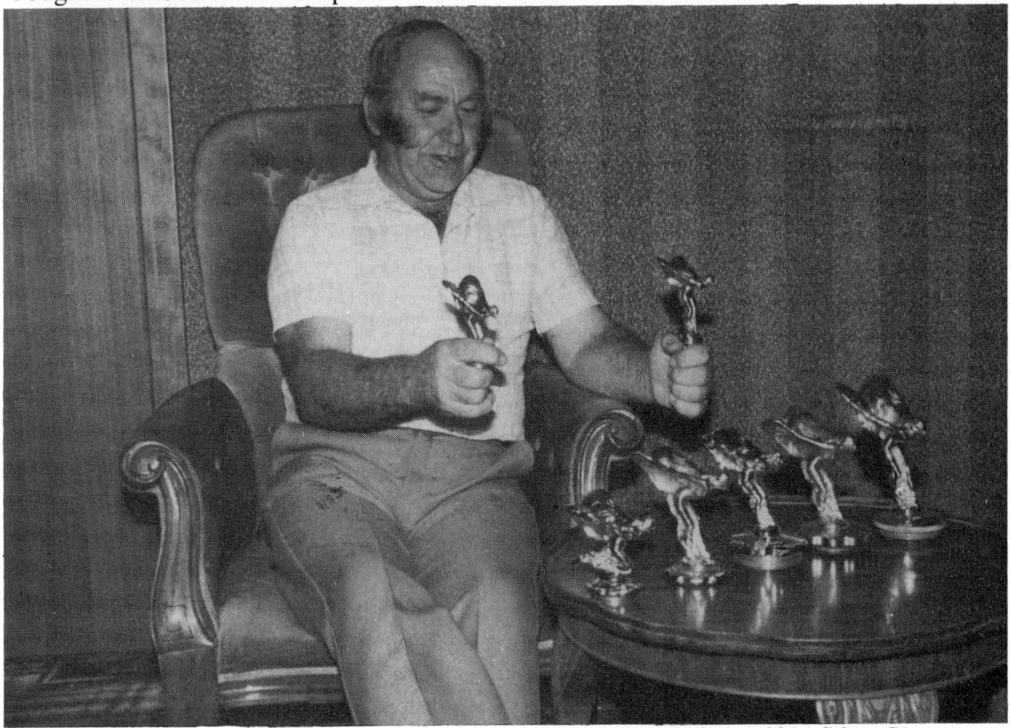

Jock Farquharson with a series of Rolls Royce mascots including a 1911 Silver Ghost.

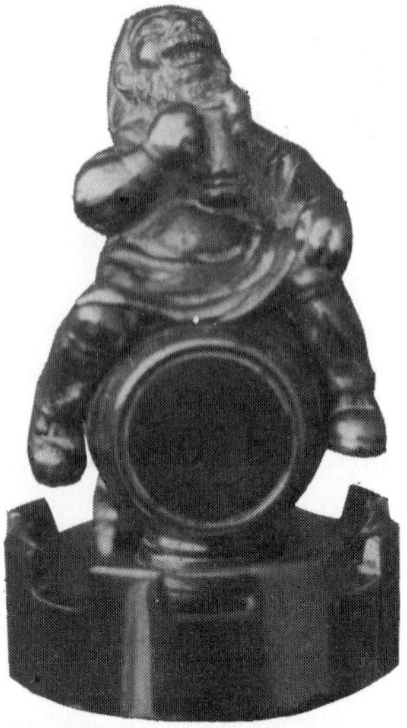

'A.O.F.B.', Antediluvian Order of Froth Blowers, depicting a gnome drinking beer astride a barrel. On the back of the barrel it is inscribed 'No Heel Taps', Birmingham Medal Co., Summerhill Terrace, Birmingham. Nickel plated, late 1920's. £80

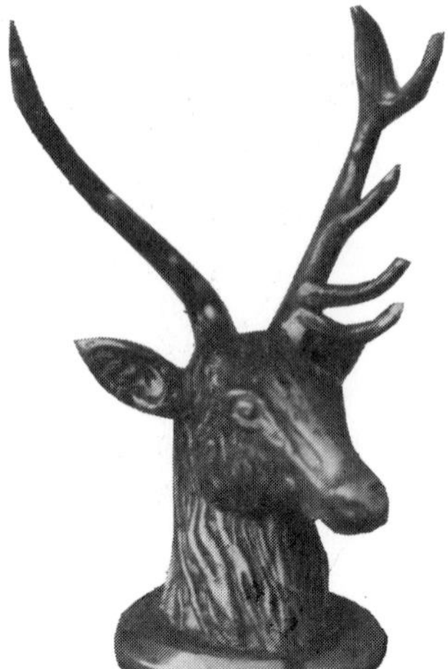

'Stag's Head', an accessory mascot, produced in the 1920's by A.E.L., nickel plated brass. £80

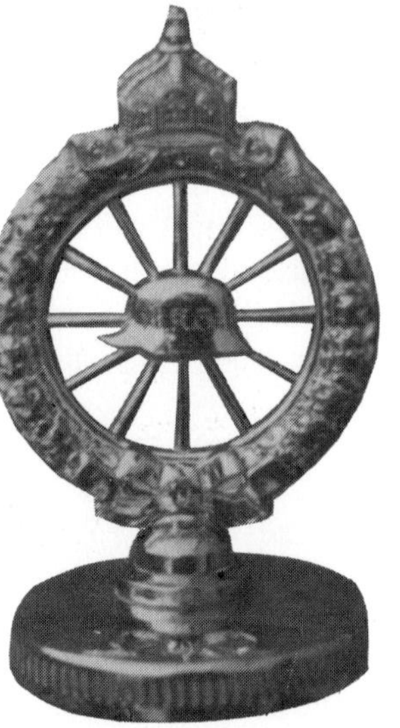

German Officer's mascot of chrome plated brass, reputed to have originally been the property of one Richter Kurler, an officer attached to Rommel's personal staff in the North African Campaign during World War II. Very rare. £500

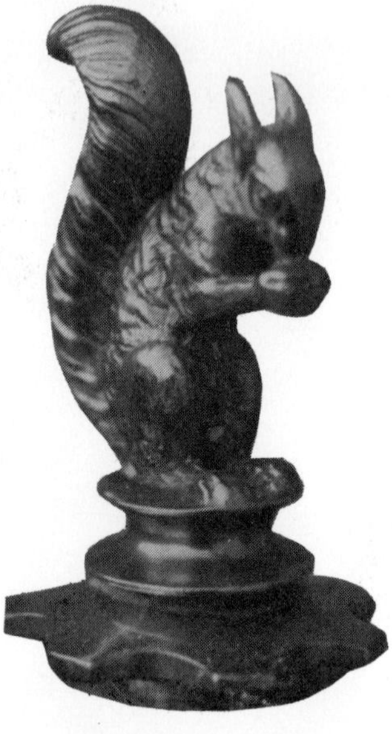

'Squirrel', this was a mascot of the Squirrel Horn Toffee Co. and was fitted to one of their delivery vans, a Model T Ford. £60

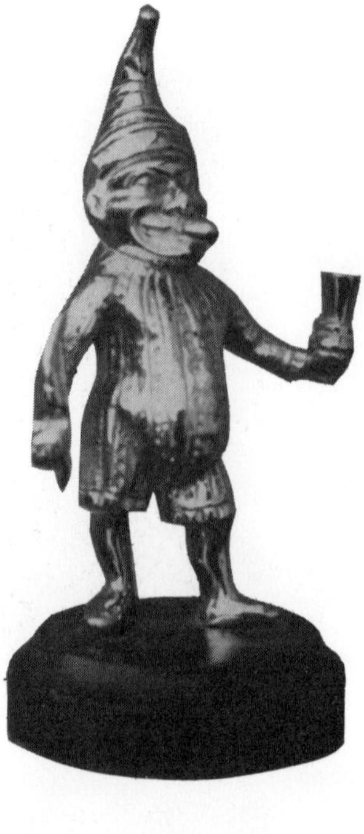

'Punch', British Made, chrome plated mascot, early 1930's, no markings or indication of the manufacturer. £50

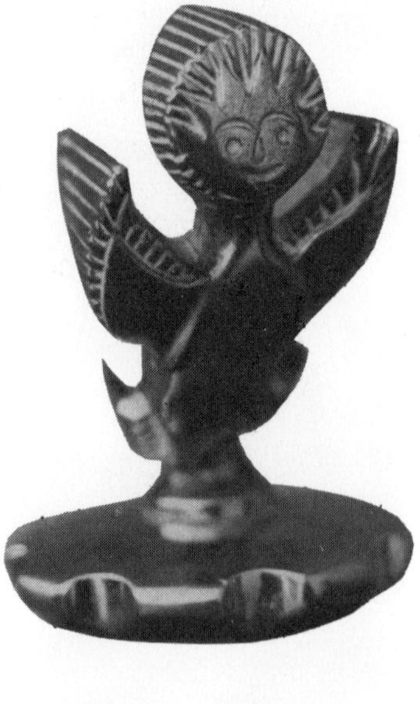

'Mr. Therm', British Made, nickel plated brass mascot of stylised flame depicting the well-known Mr. Therm the Gas Man, rare. £60

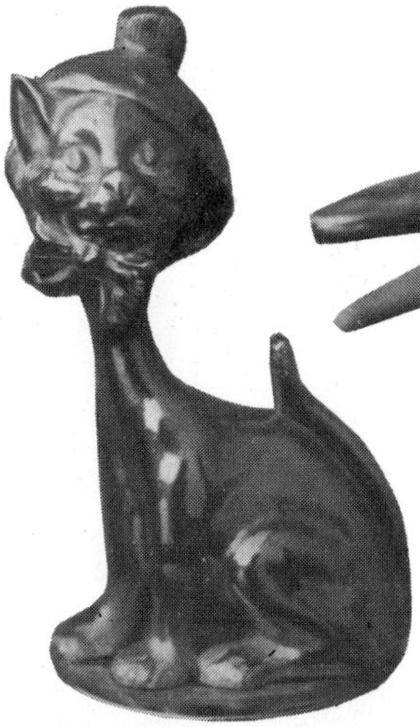

'Louis Wain Cat', this mascot is pre World War I, nickel plated. Louis Wain was an artist specialising in cats and this mascot was an example of his work. £100

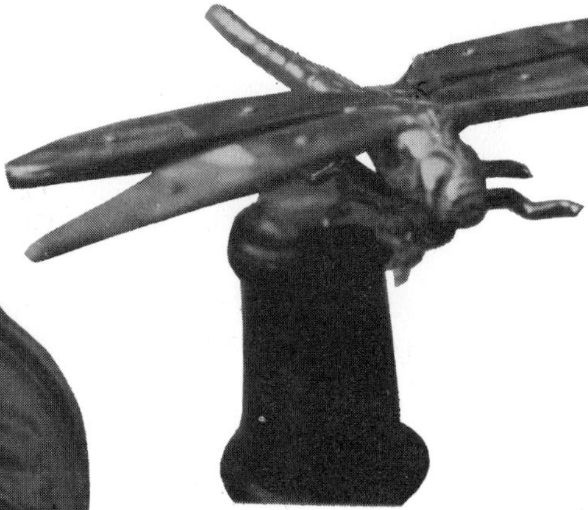

'Dragonfly', chrome plate with mother-of-pearl wings. British Made by Desmo. This mascot was used on the M.G. Midgets of the early 1930's. £250

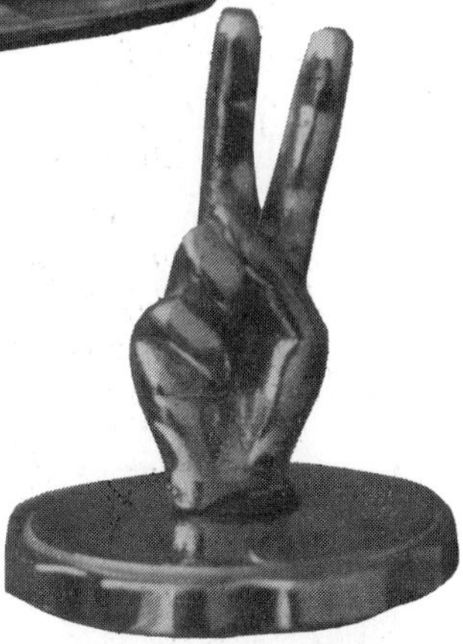

'The Two Fingers', chrome plated mascot from the 1930's, too early for Churchill's famous 'V' sign, British Made. £50

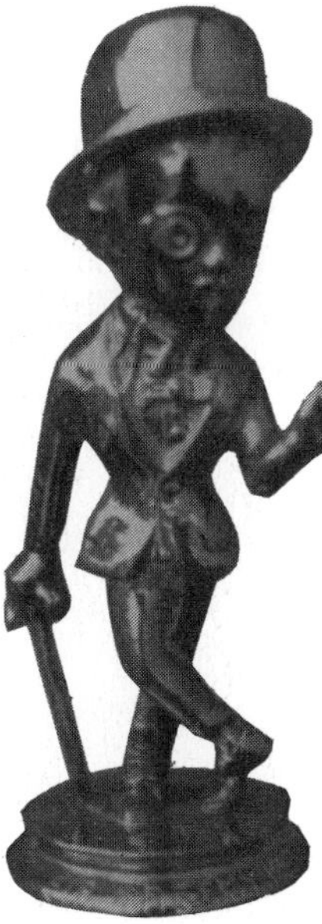

'Sir Kreemy Knut', chrome plated mascot of Sir Kreemy was the trade mark and Company mascot of Sharp's Toffee Co. £100

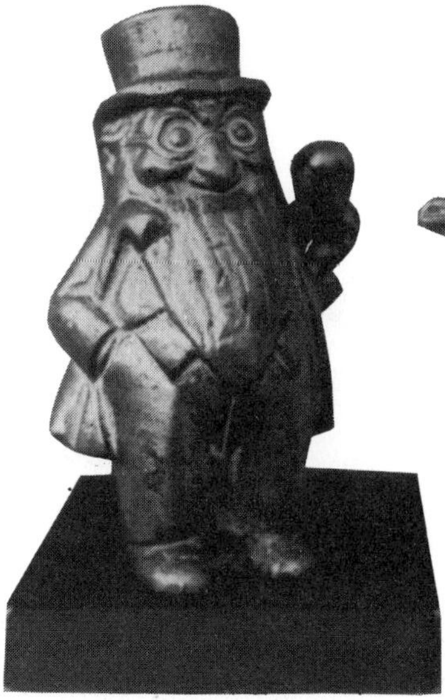

'Wm. Younger', nickel plated brass mascot of Sir Wm. Younger, the house mascot of the famous Younger's Ales Brewing Firm, extremely rare. £90

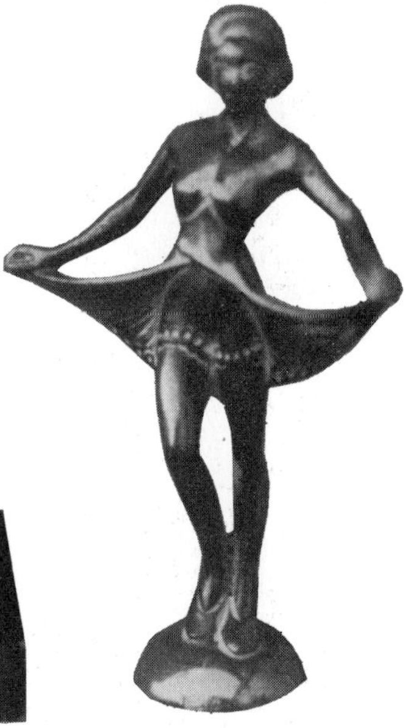

'Dancing Girl', this mascot is nickel plated brass and made by Desmo, the hair-style and clothing verify the date as late 1920's early 1930's. £35

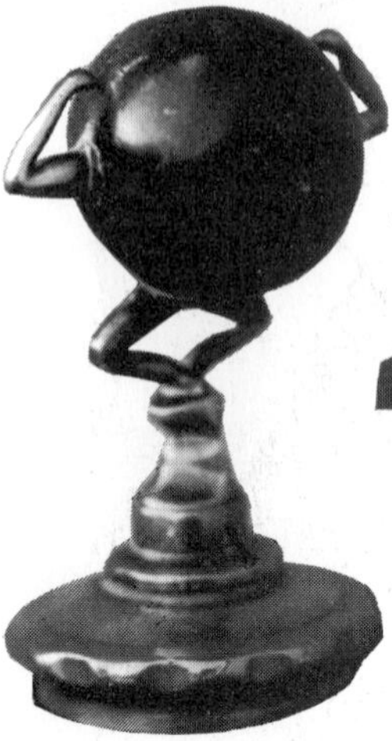

'Touch Wud', this good luck charm mascot has an oversized leather head with glass eyes, all other parts are unplated brass, circa 1908. £100

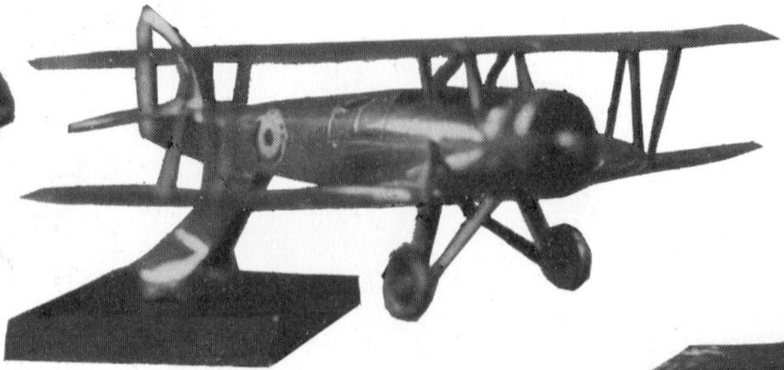

'Avro Tutor', this model aeroplane was manufactured in Britain and only given out to pilots who had trained on this particular type of aircraft. Chrome plate with the proper red, white and blue markings. £250

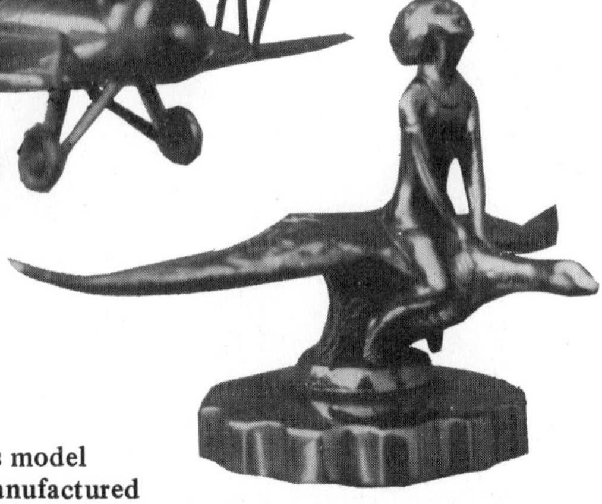

'Girl on a Goose', nickel plated, British Made, signed 'LL', Louis Lejaune. £80

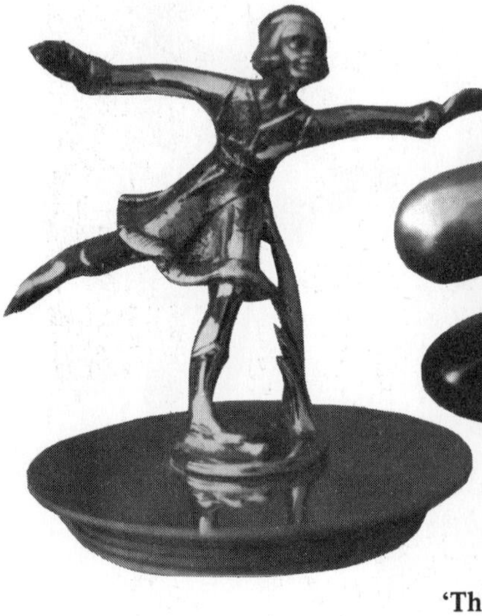

'Lady Skater', chrome plated Desmo mascot from the 1930's was for skating enthusiasts. £60

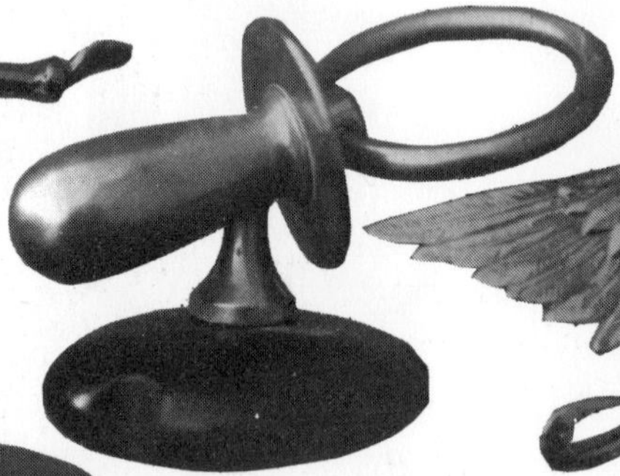

'The Dummy Teat', nickel plated mascot was manufactured by J. Grose & Co., for a few shillings in the 1920's and specially manufactured for attaching to the Austin 7, fondly known in these days as the Baby Austin, hence the dummy teat. £75

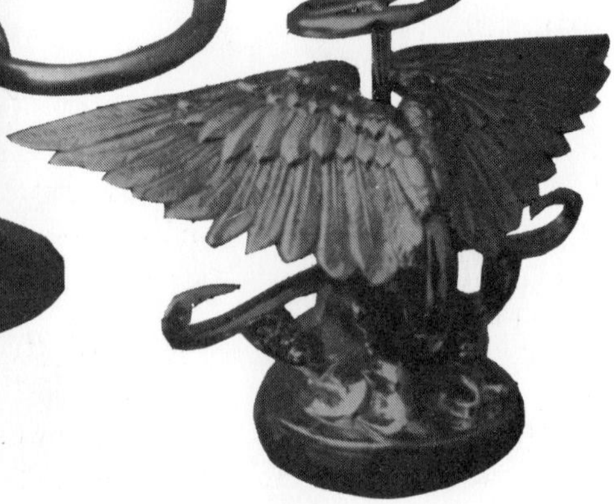

'Austin', rarest of all mascots, only three known to survive, nickel plated, 1920's. £500

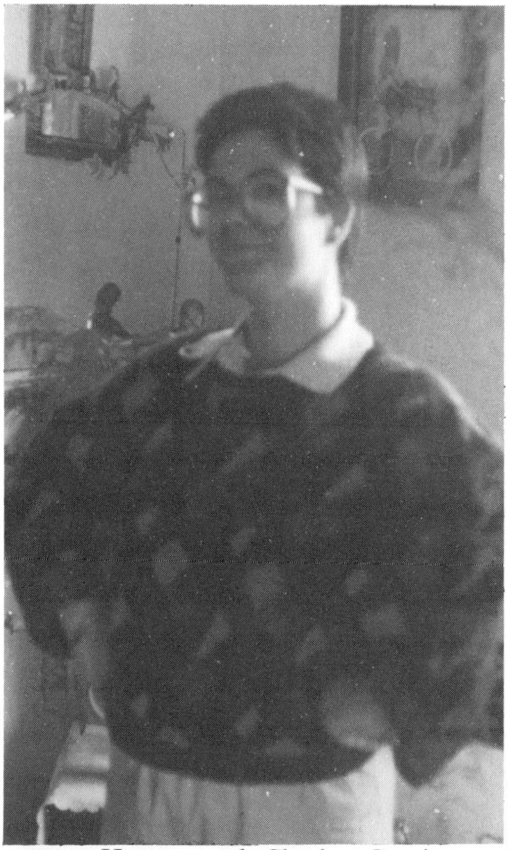

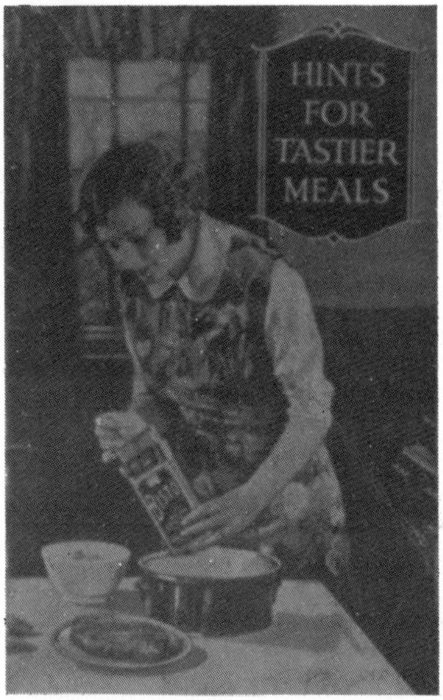

Jane Henery and Charles Garvie are freelance writers who collect anything to do with food advertising.

Charles said: "This all started by accident about ten ycars ago in Glasgow when we bought a copy of Aunt Kate's Old Time Recipes (presented with 'People's Friend') from an Oxfam shop. Originally we bought it for the recipes but we got interested in the advertising and bit by bit we started accumulating other food company give-aways.

"Now we collect books, booklets, trade cards and leaflets, both old and new. Our only criterion is that they must carry a recipe."

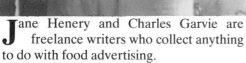

Charles and Jane track down their quarry by going round sales and junk shops as well as writing to food companies. They now have well over 1,000 items and Jane's interest is in the historical side of their collection while Charles specialises in the pictorial aspect. They call their collection 'An Ad Man in Your Larder'. Spanning over a century of advertising which begins in 1879, it follows the kitchens of Britain through the Jazz Age to Austerity and rationing up to the present day.

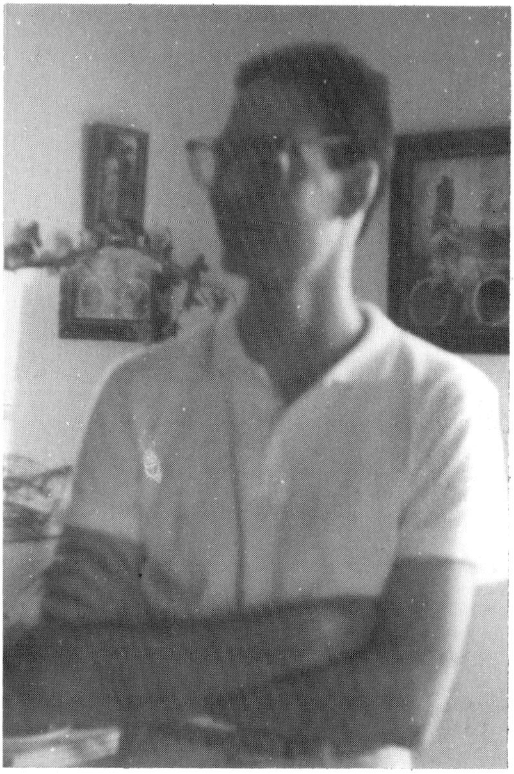

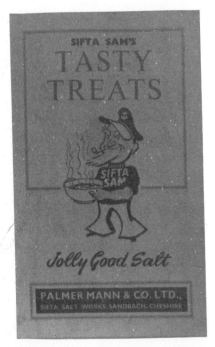

Sifta Sam's Tasty Treats (Sifta Salt), circa 1955. Value 30p.

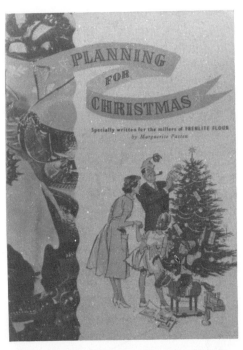

Planning For Christmas (Frenlite Flour), circa 1956, illustrated. Value 40p.

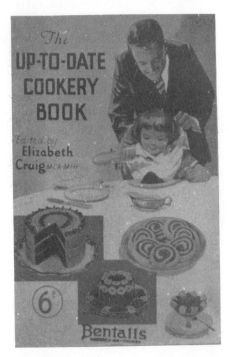

The Up-To-Date Cookery Book (Cadbury's), circa 1932, illustrated. Value 75p.

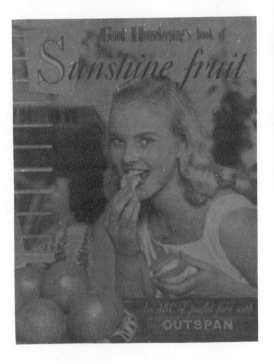

Sunshine Fruit (Outspan Oranges), circa 1954, illustrated. Value 35p.

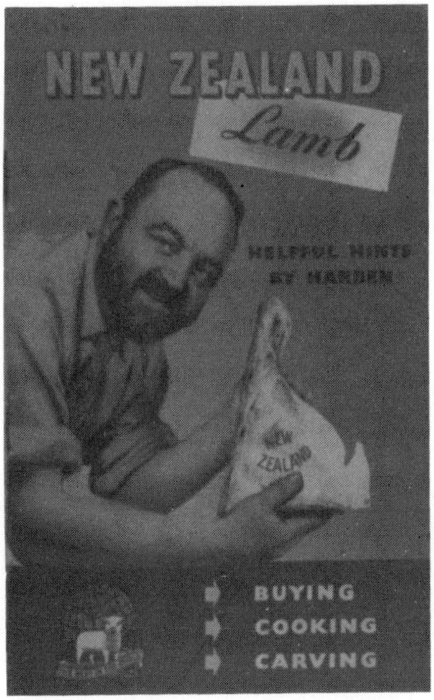

New Zealand Lamb - Helpful Hints By Harben, circa 1954. Value 50p.

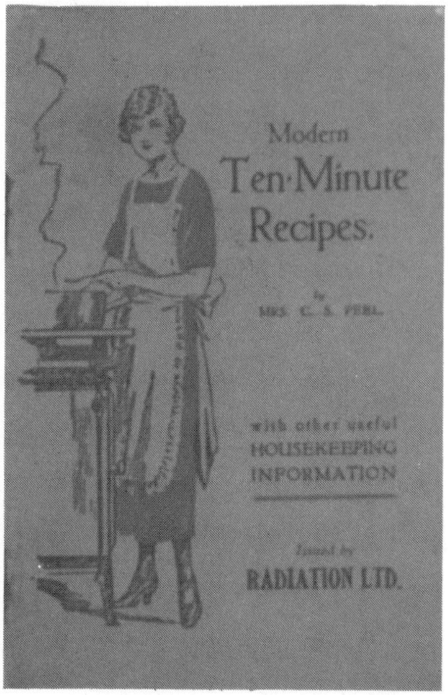

Modern Ten-Minute Recipes (Radiation Cookers), circa 1924, illustrated. Value 75p.

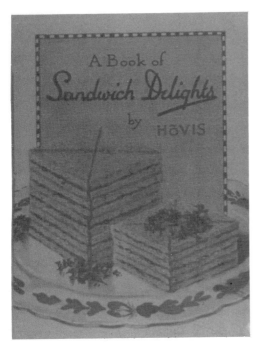

A Book of Sandwich Delights (Hovis), circa 1926, illustrated. Value 75p.

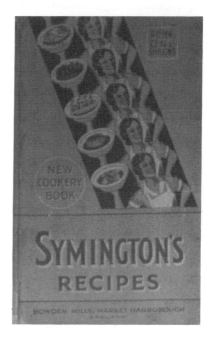

Symington's Recipes 'New Cookery Book' circa 1934, illustrated. Value £1.50 – £2.

Fowlers Treacle - Recipes for the Home circa 1955, illustrated. Value 75p – £1.

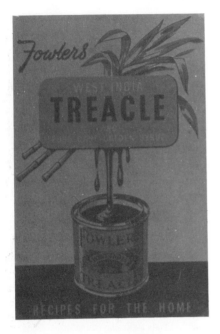

Tasty Tit-Bits ('People's Friend'), circa 1933. Value 40p.

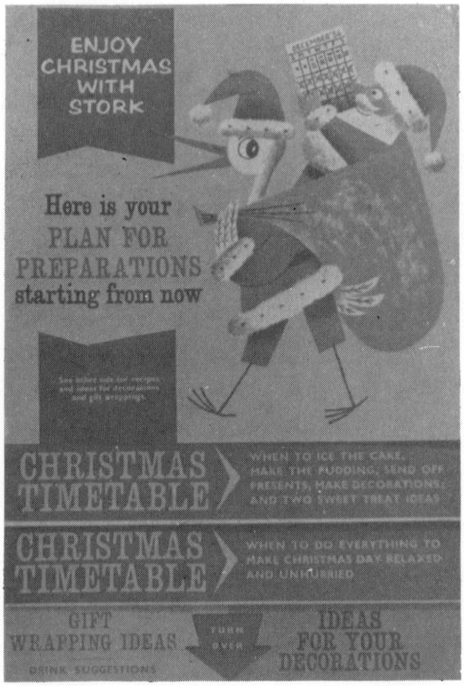

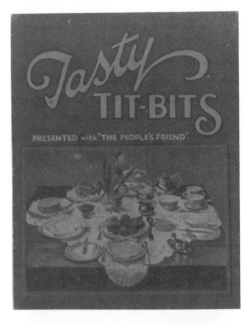

Enjoy Christmas With Stork, circa 1956, illustrated. Value 30p.

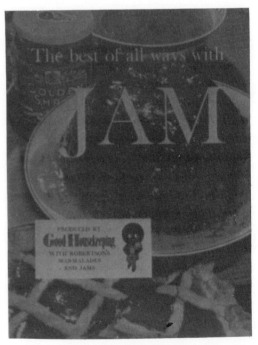

The Best of All Ways With Jam (Robertson's Preserves), circa 1954, illustrated. Value 35p.

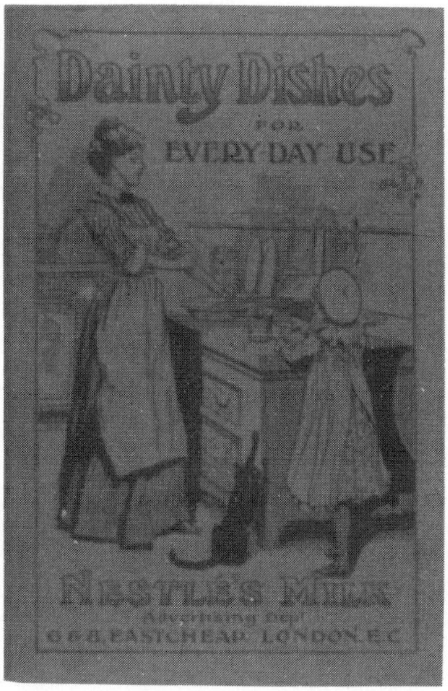

Dainty Dishes for Every-Day Use (Nestle's Milk). circa 1900, illustrated.
Value £1.50 – £2

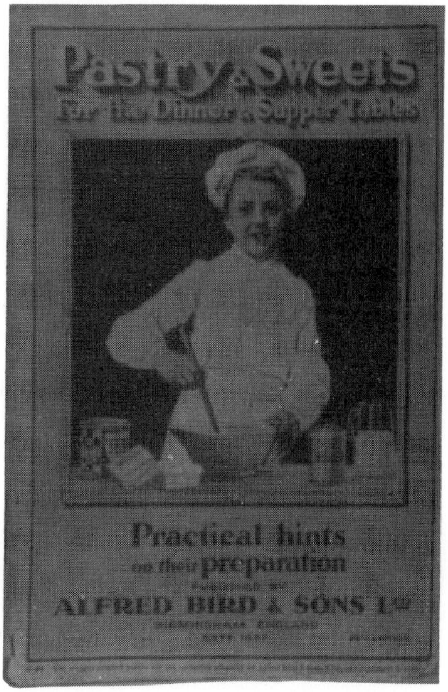

Pastry & Sweets for the Dinner & Supper Tables (Alfred Bird & Sons), circa 1915.
Value 75p – £1.

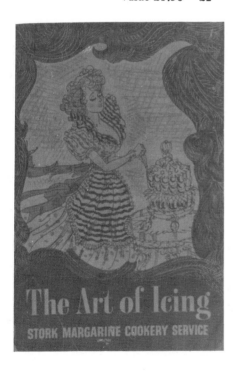

The Art of Icing (Stork), circa 1951, illustrated. Value 30p.

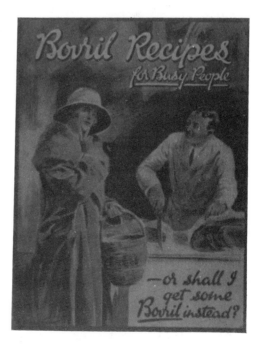

Bovril Recipes For Busy People, circa 1926, illustrated. Value 75p.

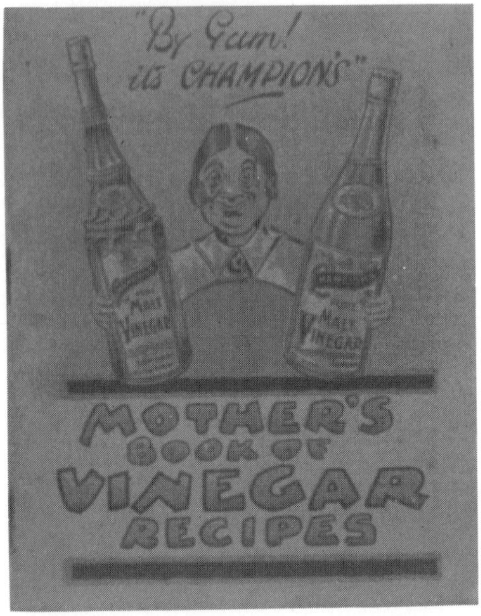

Mother's Book of Vinegar Recipes (Champion's Vinegar), circa 1918, illustrated.
Value £1.50 – £2.

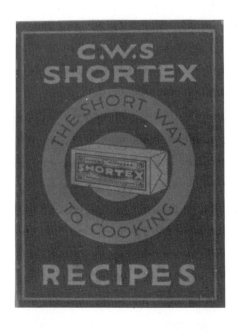

Shortex Recipes (C. W. S.), circa 1920.
Value 75p.

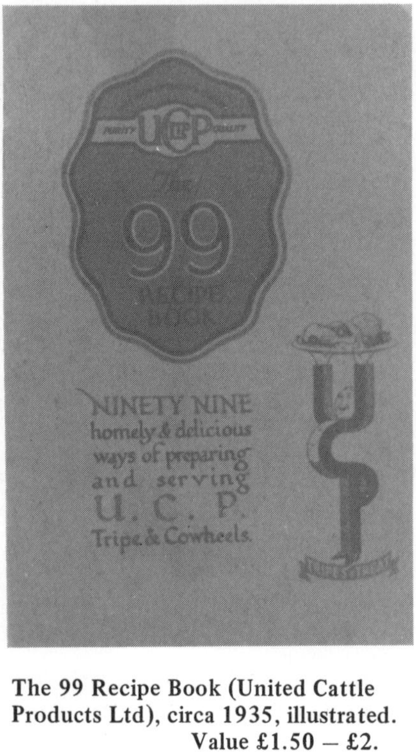

The 99 Recipe Book (United Cattle Products Ltd), circa 1935, illustrated.
Value £1.50 – £2.

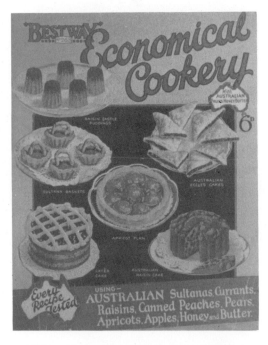

Bestway Economical Cookery (Sponsored by Australian Trade Publicity), circa 1919, illustrated.
Value £1.

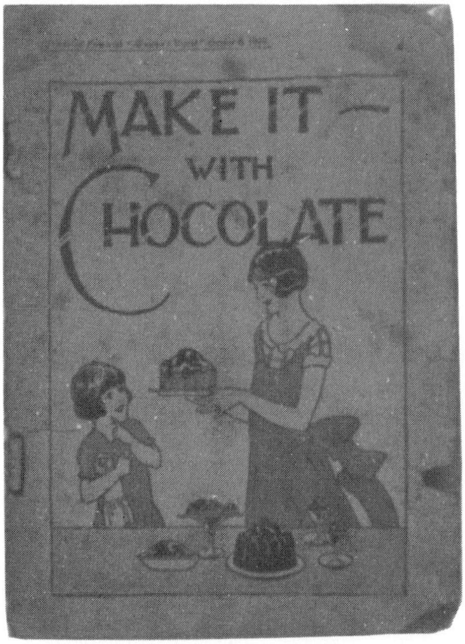

Make It With Chocolate (Cadbury's), circa 1928, illustrated. Value 50p.

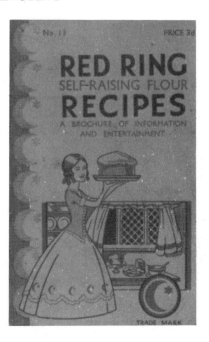

Red Ring Recipes (Red Ring Flour), circa 1918-22. Value £1.

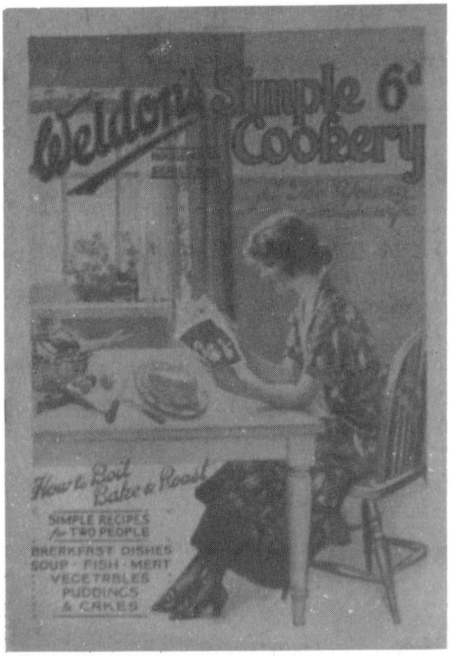

Weldon's Simple Cookery for the young housewife, circa 1922, illustrated. Value £1.

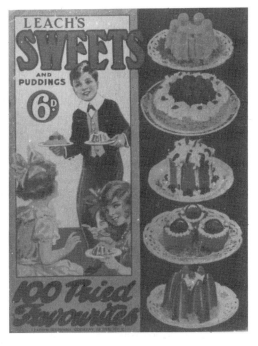

Leach's Sweets & Puddings '100 Tried Favourites', circa 1919, illustrated. Value £1 – £1.50.

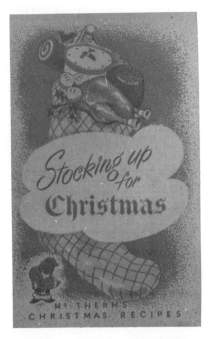

Stocking Up For Christmas (The Gas Council), circa 1953, illustrated.
Value 30p.

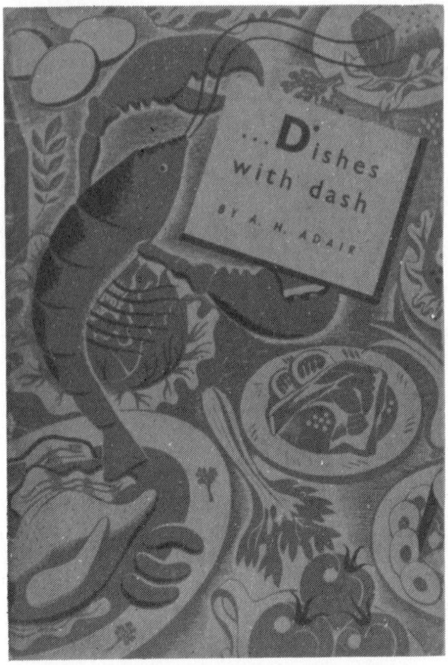

Dishes With Dash (Heinz) by A. H. Adair, circa 1935, illustrated by Eric Fraser.
Value £1 – £1.50.

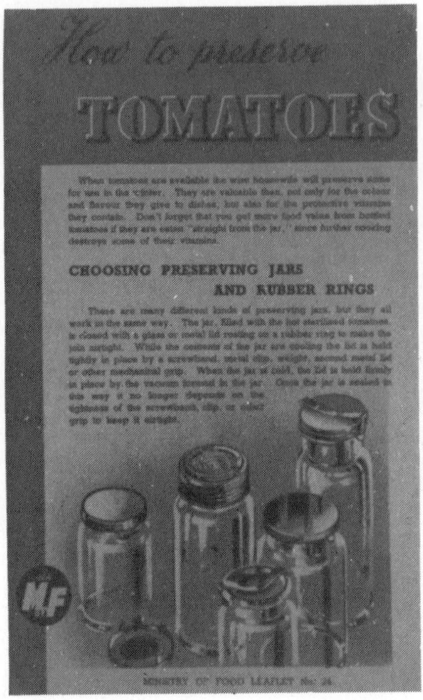

How to Preserve Tomatoes (M. O. F.) circa 1947, illustrated. Value 30p.

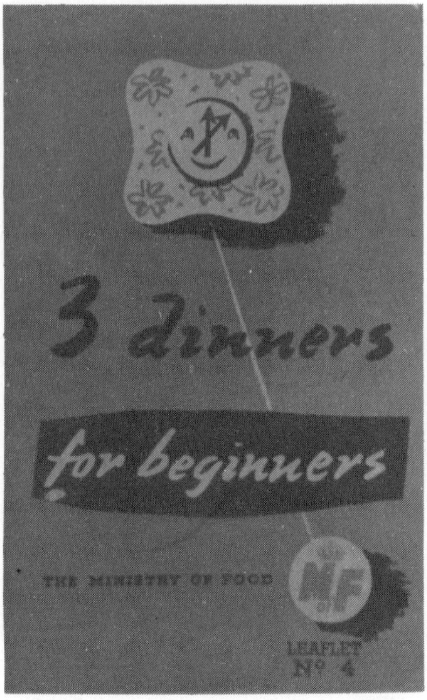

3 Dinners For Beginners (M. O. F.) circa 1945, illustrated. Value 30p.

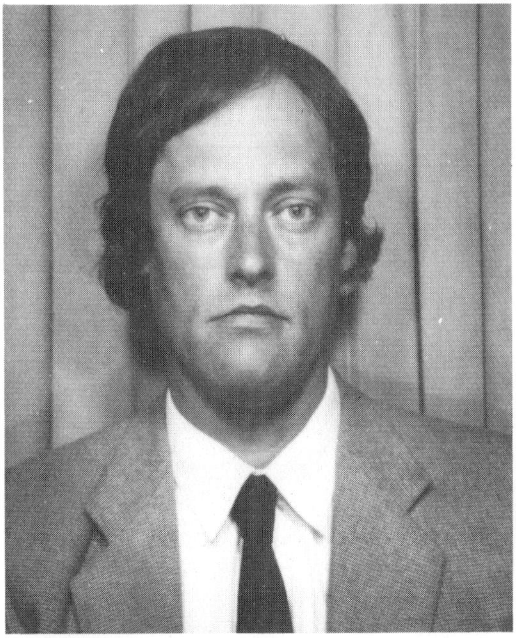

Dennis Yates collects early wireless equipment.

"My mother's brother had a wireless shop in Derby and in 1922 he was making his own sets. I used to go along to watch him though when I was a lad my main interest was breaking sets up, not building them. It makes me shudder to think of how many sets I must have ruined.

"My interest is in the really early stuff and it ends about 1925. Most collectors tend to specialise in unusual shaped sets from the 1930's — but my interest goes back to 1889 when the first commercial sets were installed on ships. In 1899 Queen Victoria sent a message via a submarine set transmitter to the Royal Navy."

Dennis has over 150 sets, all of which work, and his collection spends ten months out of each year on display to schools, colleges, building societies and other wireless collectors' clubs. Last summer it spent five months in Holland in a display for the Dutch Wireless Society.

Learning to recognise old sets takes a long time because they are often regarded as pieces of old junk.

"I also collect old televisions and they usually don't look like TV's at all," said Dennis. "The mirror drum spiral television just looks like a wooden box with a hole in it but it is worth £5,000 to collectors."

He finds his sets through advertising and the one wireless set which has so far evaded him is a coherer receiver used in ships like the Berengaria and the Titanic . . . "I would pay around £2,000 for one of those sets in good condition," he said.

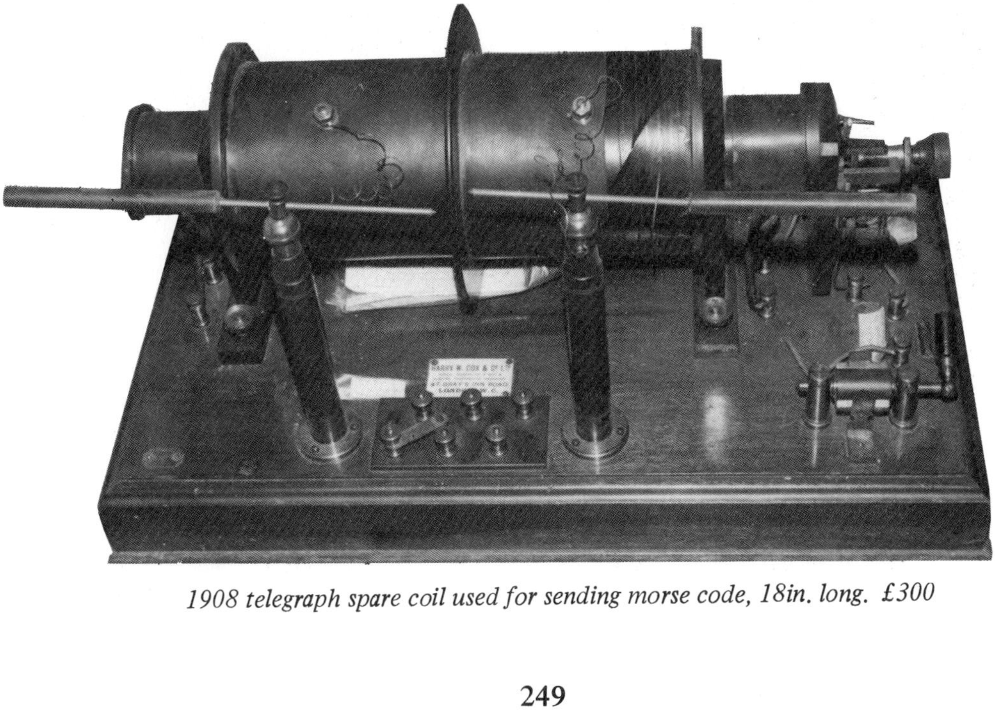

1908 telegraph spare coil used for sending morse code, 18in. long. £300

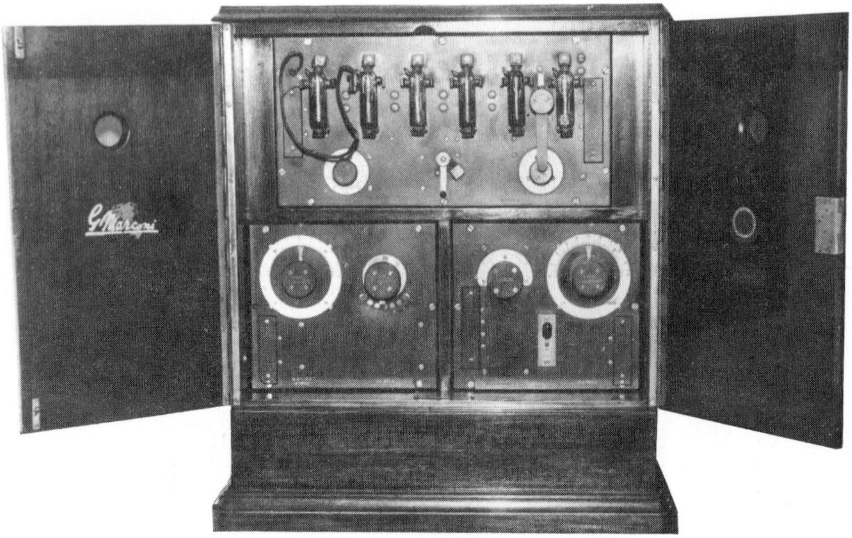

1922, Marconiphone, multi valve RB7, 1ft.8in. high, 1ft.7in. wide, a scientific type of set probably used by wealthy amateurs. £1,500

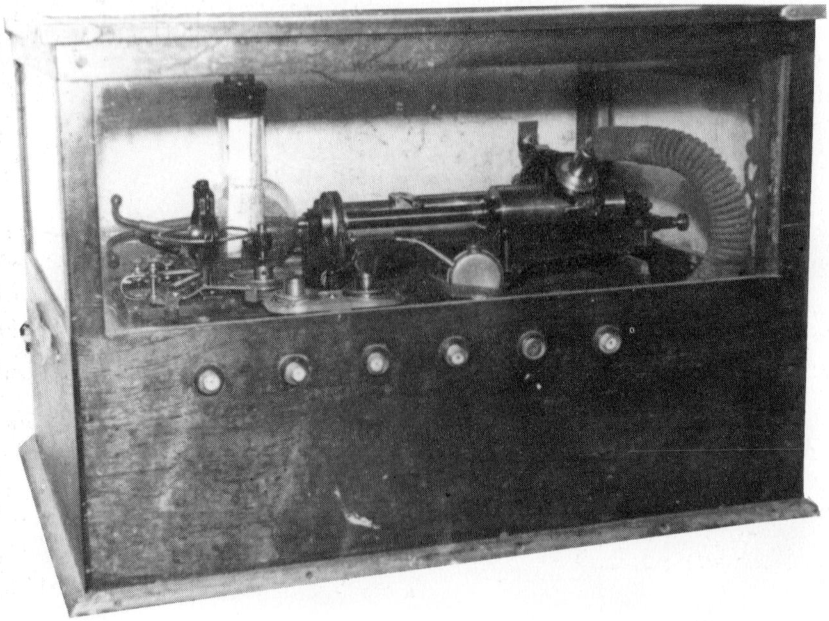

An 1898 Eddison class M electric coin-operated phonograph with listening tubes at the front, in an oak case, 18in. by 12in. £2,000

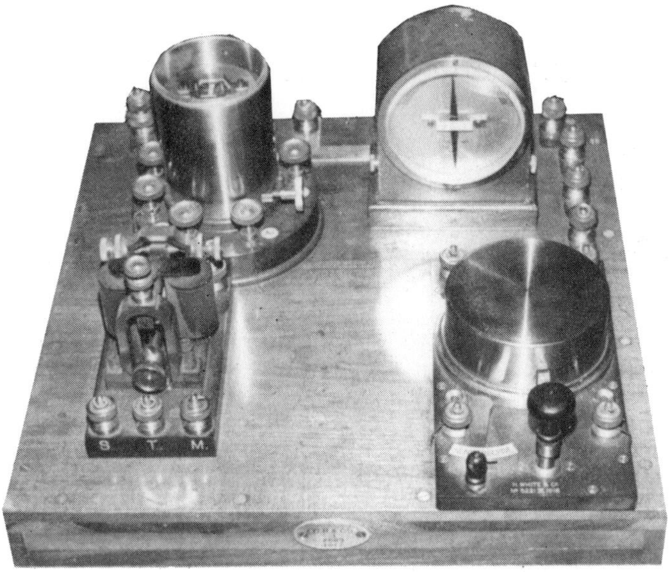

1917 submarine telegraphic land station, 1ft.5in. wide, 1ft. high. £750

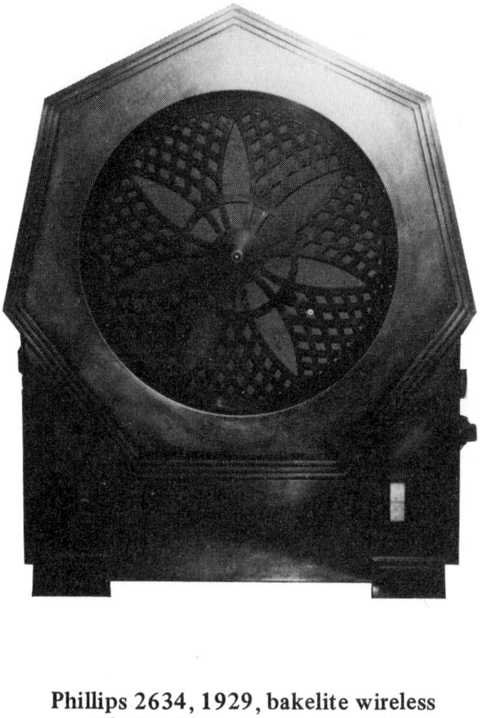

Phillips 2634, 1929, bakelite wireless set, 1ft.7in. high. £350

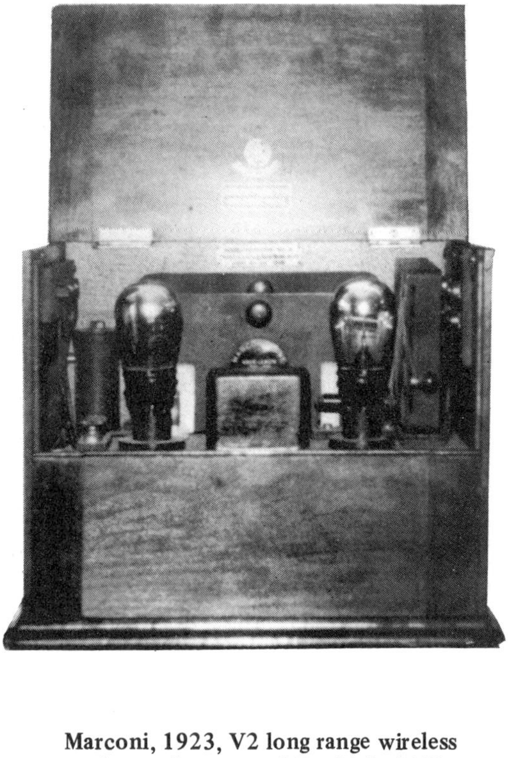

Marconi, 1923, V2 long range wireless set in a walnut case, 10in. high. £450

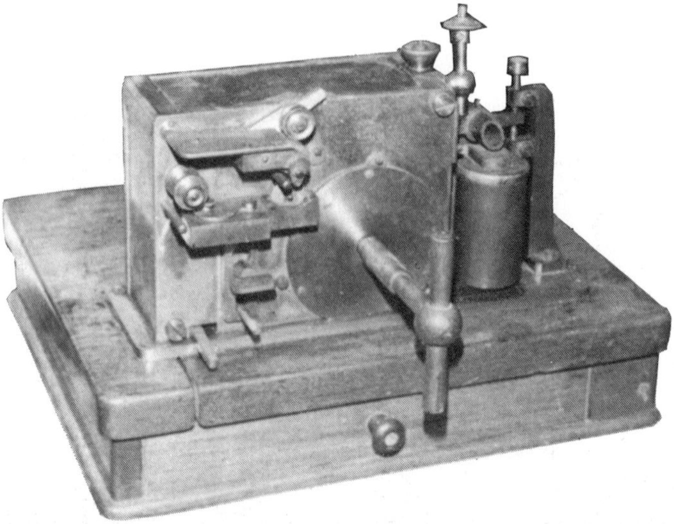

1915 telegraphic inker base station used by the Royal Flying Corps for receiving morse code, 1ft.6in. wide, 9in. high. £350

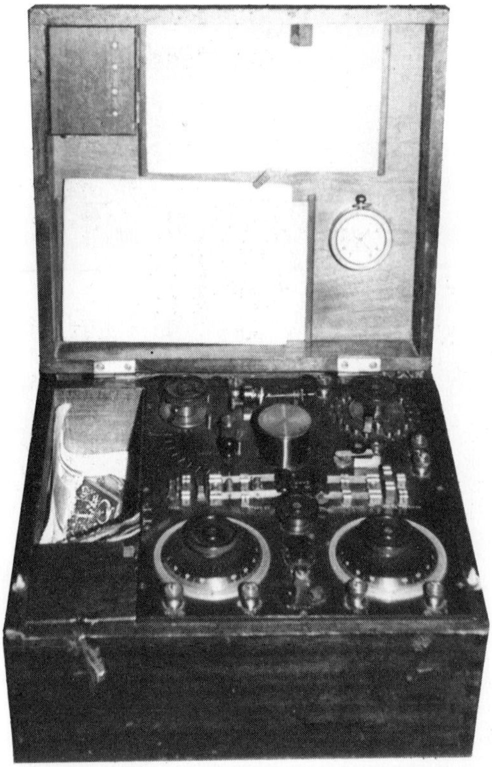

A 1917 MK3 Tuner used in communication between the front lines and headquarters, cannot transmit only receive, 12in. wide. £500

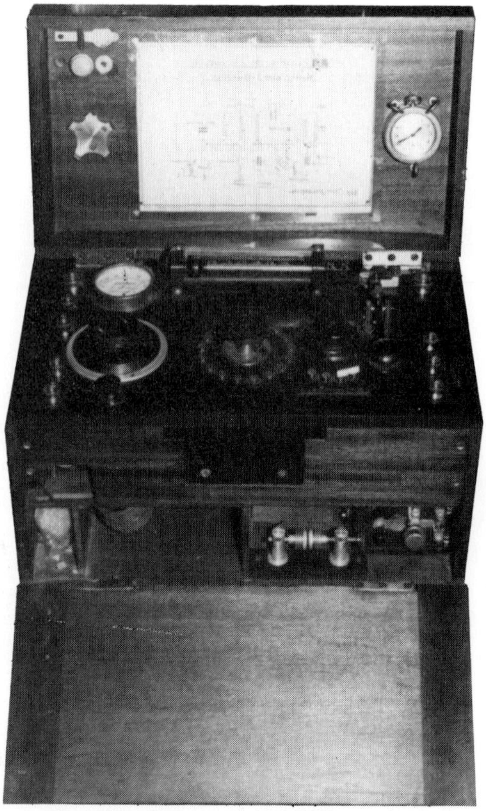

A mahogany cased 1915 Marconi Trench Spark transmitter and receiver used in communication between aircraft and gun barreries, 15in. wide, 14in. high. £800

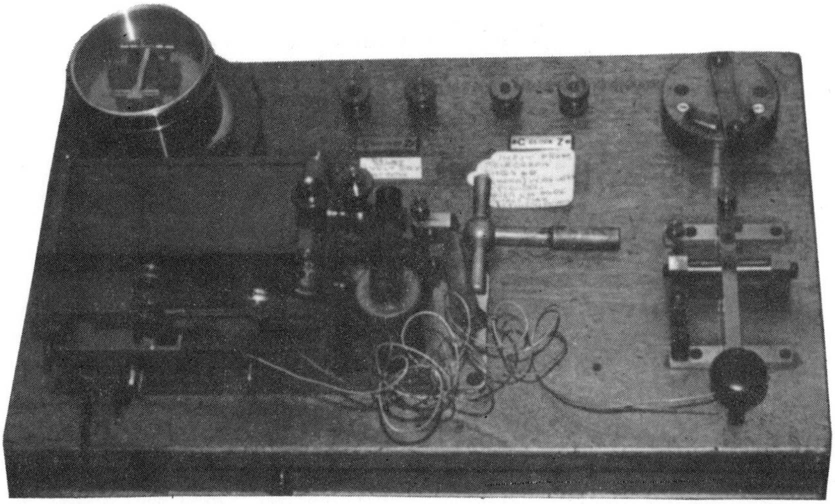

1914 combined telegraphic inker and sounder used in the trenches. £500

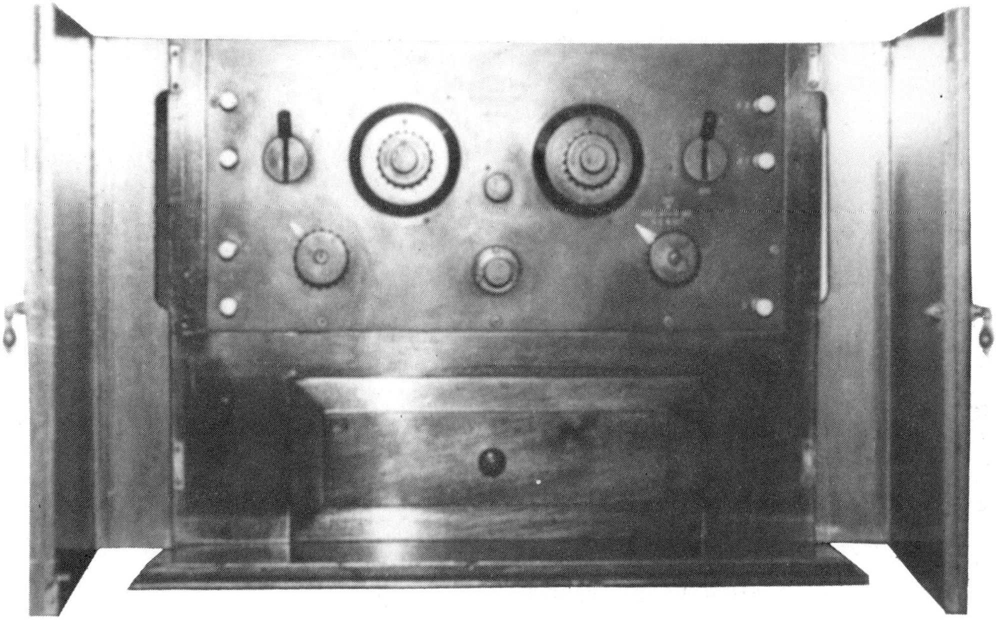

Pye 740, 1923, four valve cabinet deluxe wireless set, 14in. high. £750

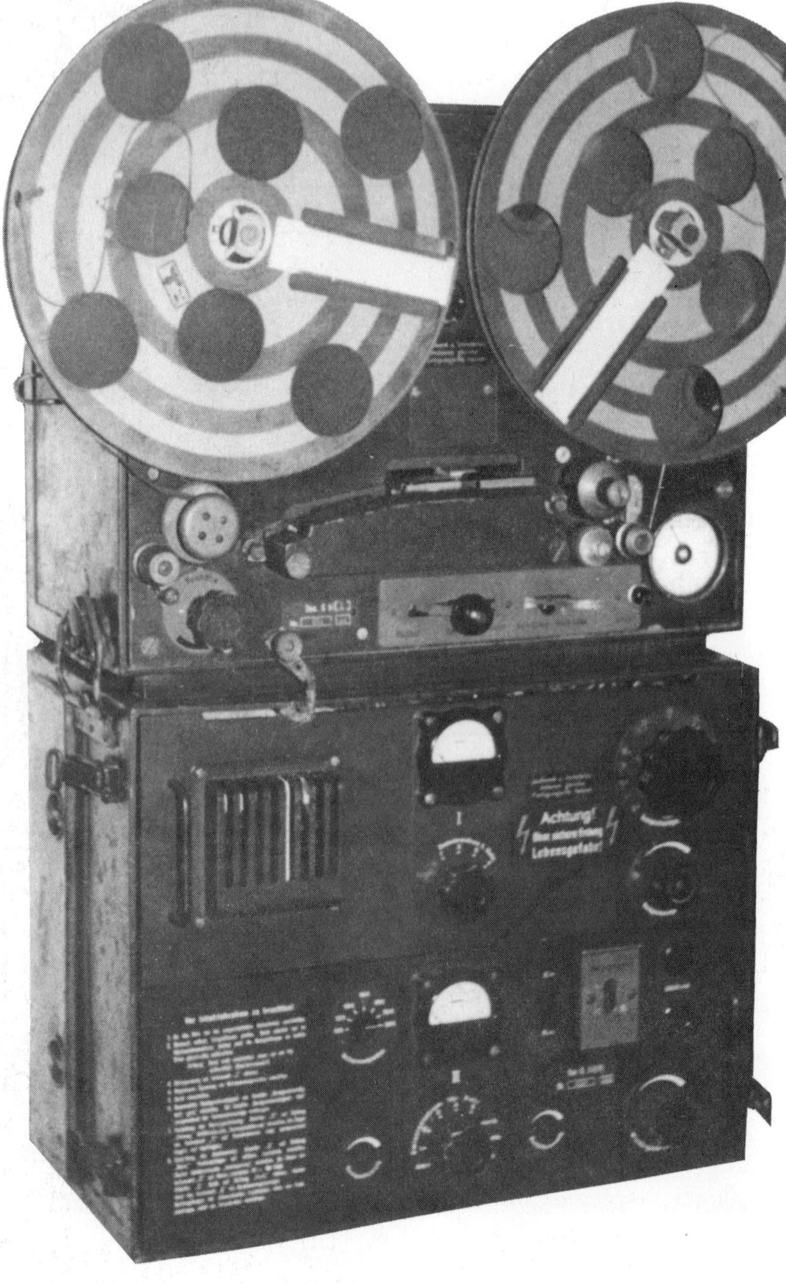

German 2nd World War tape recorder used for propaganda purposes. £2,000

Raymond Walls is a building contractor and collects petrol pump glass globes.

"In four years I've collected 130 different globes and it all began because I've a 1930 Austin 16 and my interest in old things connected with motoring began with it.

"The first one I bought was a Shell globe and now I've a full series of all the types they produced from the 1920's on. I've got globes that Shell themselves have forgotten ever existed.

"The hunt for the globes has taken me thousands of miles from the far North of Scotland to Hampshire and all over Ireland. Old garages are a good source of supply and so are auto auctions but I also advertise for globes in the 'Exchange and Mart'.

"The roof space of my house has been turned into a showroom for the globes and for my other collections of enamel signs, two gallon petrol cans and oil cans."

Raymond's collection includes some very unusual globes including one he bought at Perth in Scotland in the shape of a thistle and advertising Scotch petrol which operated in the 1920's.

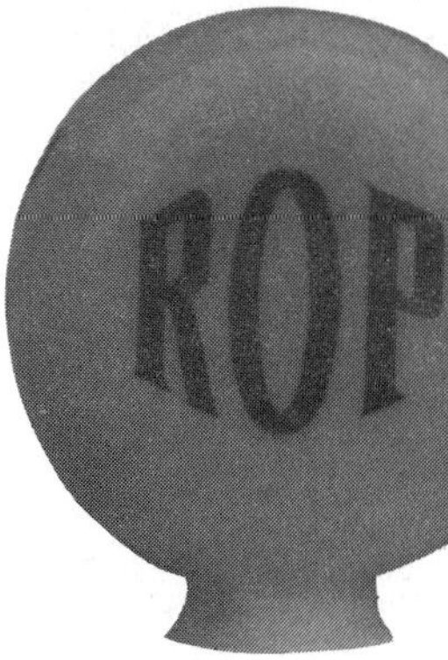

He has globes for ROP — Russian Oil Products — of the 1930's and Pratt's High Test globe also from the '30's. His favourite globe is in the shape of a shamrock which was used by the Shamrock Petrol Company in the 1920's and 1930's. Later its name changed to Lobitos and in the 1950's it was bought over by Burmah.

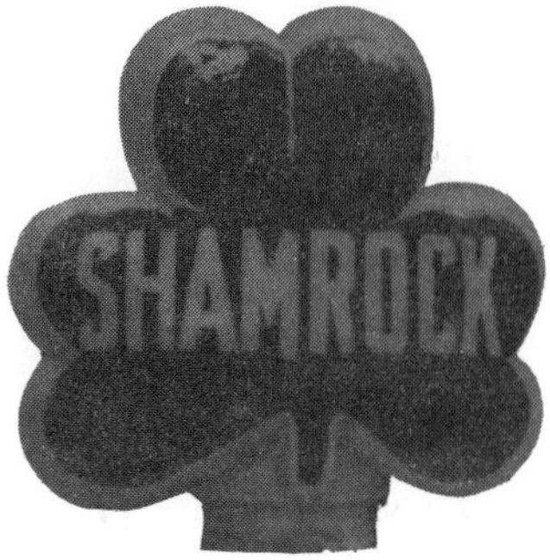

Petrol globes went out of use with the introduction of new style pumps and because of vandalism. They are becoming expensive to buy and range in price from around £20 to £40 for globes in pristine condition. Recently a Shell globe similar to one which Raymond has in his collection, sold at Sotheby's for over £200, but this is quite a rare occurrence.

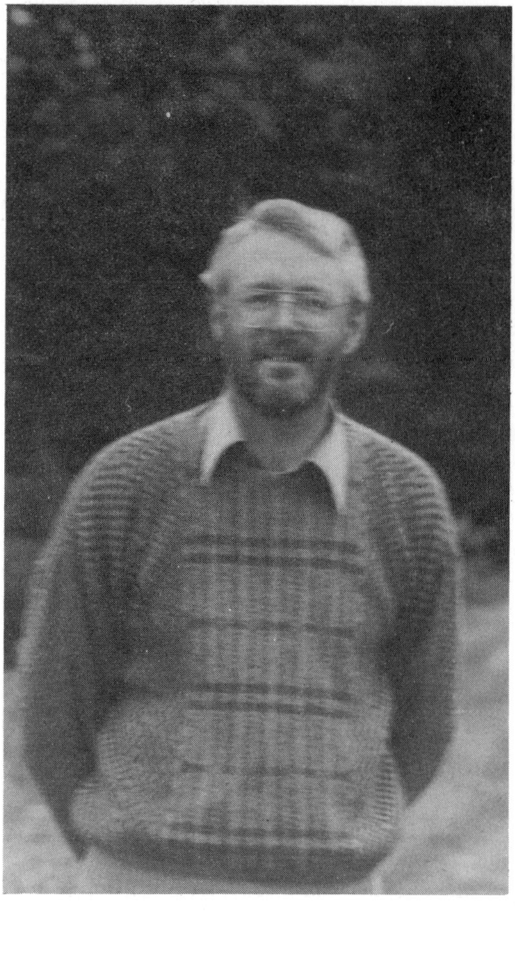

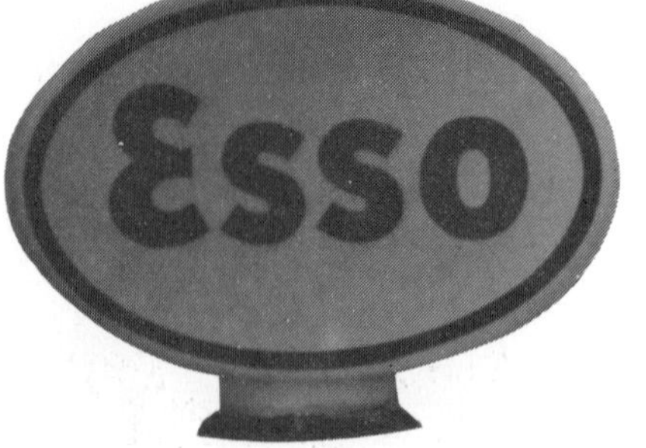

'Esso', oval shape used in the 1940's, 50's and 60's.

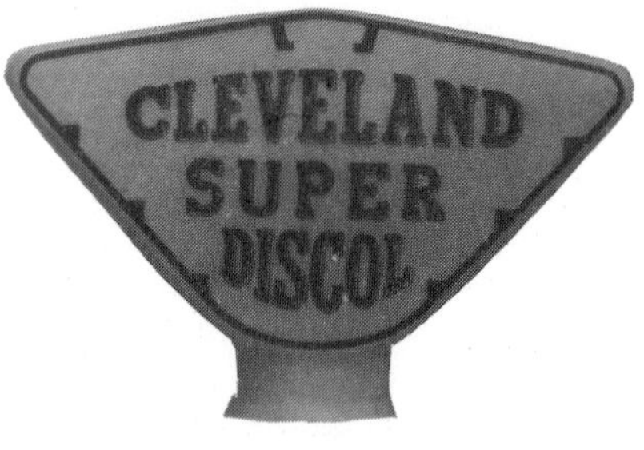

'Cleveland Super Discol', wing shape used in the 1950's.

In the early years of motoring, automobile owners bought their petrol from hotels, hardware stores, bicycle shops and chemists. A few readers may be familiar with the once-common sight of a gaily painted two gallon petrol cans fitted onto the running board of vintage cars.

The inspiration for the petrol pump came from America, and were in use in that country for at least ten years prior to their adoption in Britain. Early American brands included Gilbert & Barker, Bowser and Hammond.

Ironically, the first petrol pump in England was not introduced by a petrol company, but instead by the A.A. It was the Hon. Treasurer, Ludwig Schlentheim who proposed that the A.A. instal petrol pumps with their ubiquitous colourful globes such as the ones he had been so impressed with on his travels in the U.S.A.. It seems that the petrol and Benzole companies objected strenuously to the A.A.'s commercial venture and heavily criticised the Association for 'going into trade'. The A.A. stood their ground, arguing that the intention was to benefit its members and that the small mark-up on the price of petrol was to cover costs.

In spite of the early controversy, petrol pumps were soon adopted by wholesalers to facilitate the sale of their own brands. Following the example of their American inspirators, the petrol companies introduced colourful globes which they hoped would attract customers to their pumps. Some of the first globes that glowed brightly beside British roads bore the names of Shell, B.P., Pratts, Dominion, Redline, B.O.P. and Cleveland.

Most companies initially supplied only one grade of petrol, though pumps soon began dispensing a variety of fuel types, including 'Perfection Spirit', Ethyl petrol and High Test.

The shape of globes on top of petrol pumps went through significant change in the early years. When Pratts, which was owned by Anglo-American Oil Co., changed its name in 1935 to Standard Oil, the legend on the globe changed to Esso – a clever acronym for S.O. . The characteristic pill-shaped globe of Pratts changed to the now-familiar oval shape of Esso.

Shell globes also evolved. The early Shell globe was globular, dating from the 1930's, but this soon changed to the shell-shaped globe with which we are now familiar. In the 1950's its size was reduced though it retained its distinctive shape.

Local petrol companies retained their own brands. In Ireland the Shamrock brand actually used a globe fashioned in the shape of Ireland's lucky leaf. Scotland's most popular petrol pump globe went by the name of Scotch. Curiously, the globe was not shaped like a whisky bottle but a thistle.

Some other distinctive globes advertised brands such as National Benzole, V.I.P., Texaco, Regent, Caltex, Lobitos, Mex, Cawoods, M.S., Jet, Globe, Gulf, Mobil and Fina.

The globes that once appeared on the top of the nation's petrol pumps provide a valuable link with our motoring heritage. Unfortunately, these vulnerable objects began to be phased out in the 1960's due to increased vandalism. Nevertheless, the enthusiast can still find them in rural areas, as well as in established transport depots.

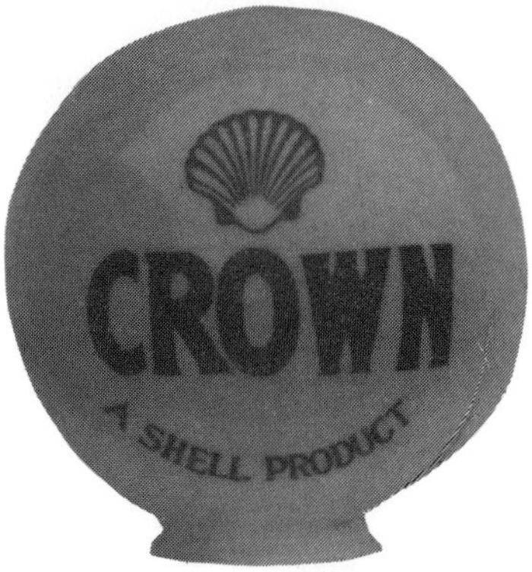

'Crown' A Shell Product, round type used in the 1920's.

'BP Super', shield shape used in the 1950's.

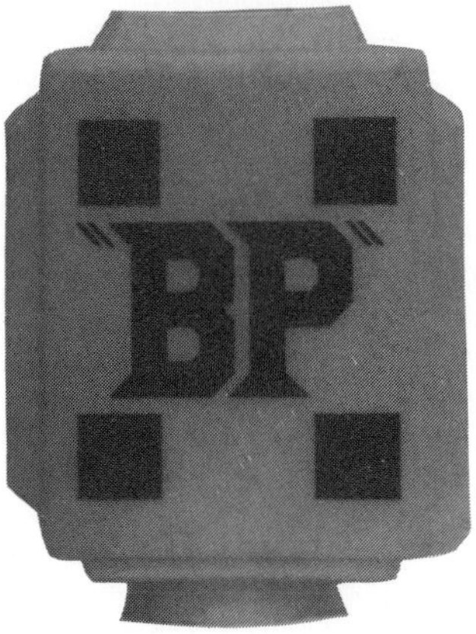

'BP' square type used in the 1940's and 50's.

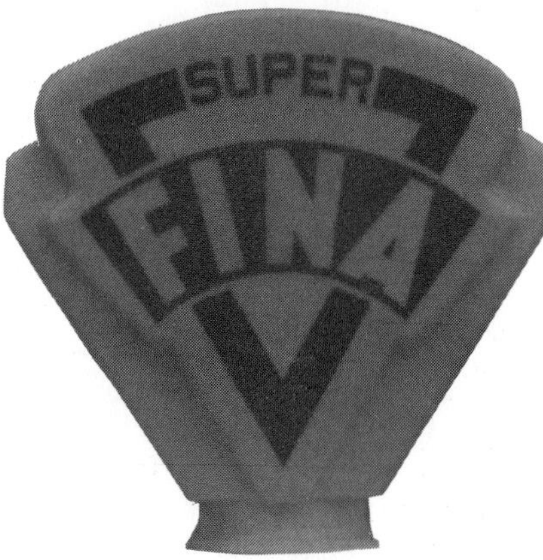

'Super Fina' used in the 1950's.

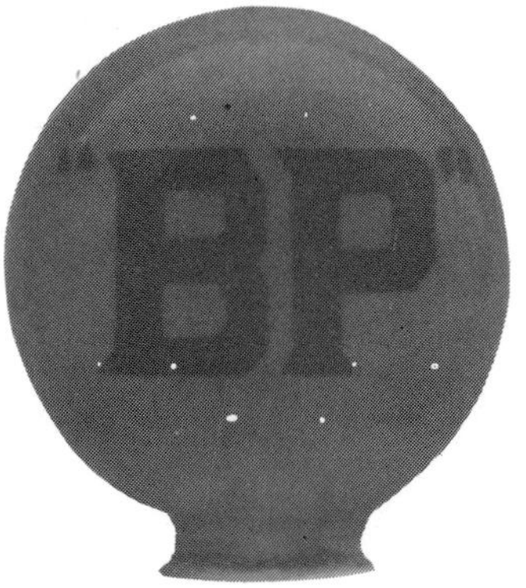

'BP' round type used in the 1920's and 30's.

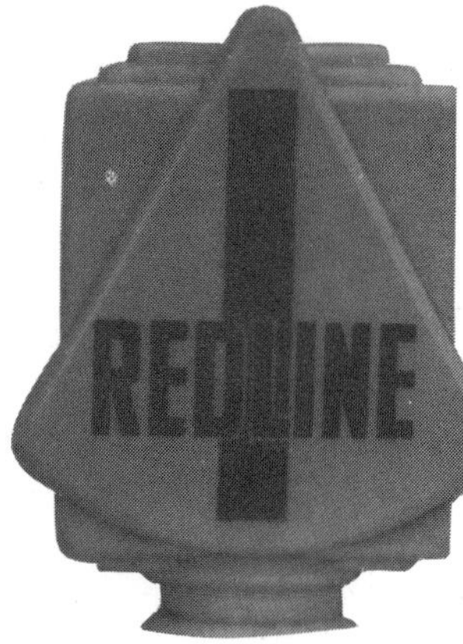

'Redline', used in the 1930's and 40's.

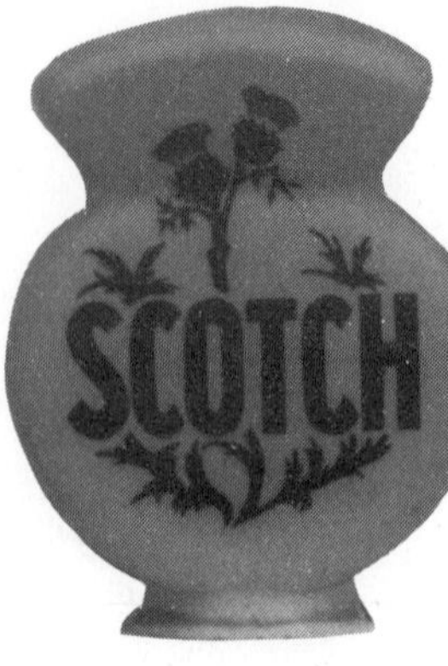

'Scotch', thistle-shape used in the 1930's.

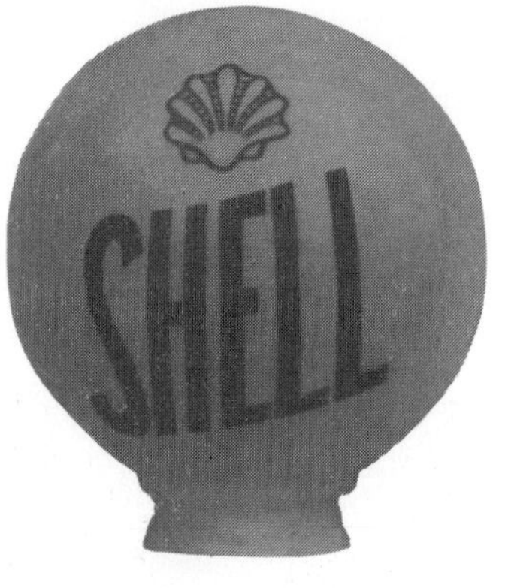

'Shell', round shape used in the 1920's.

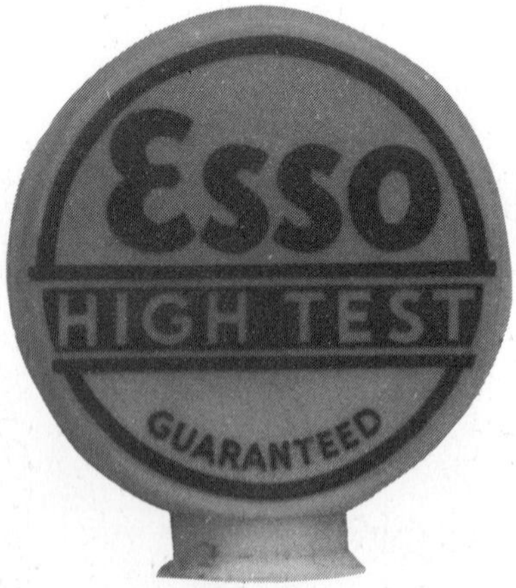

'Esso High Test Guaranteed', pill shape used in the late 1920's.

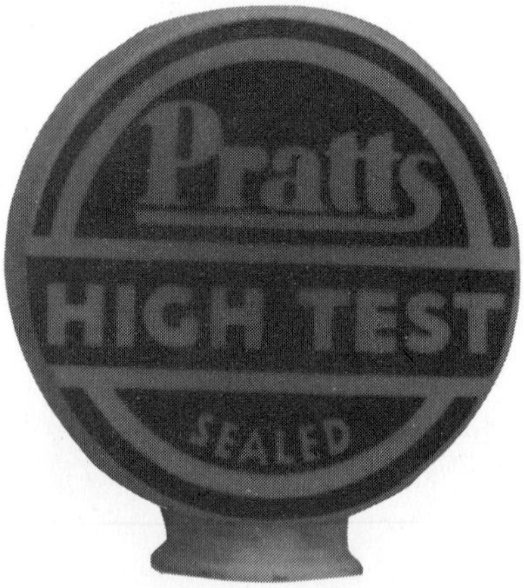

'Pratts High Test Sealed', pill shape used in the early 1930's.

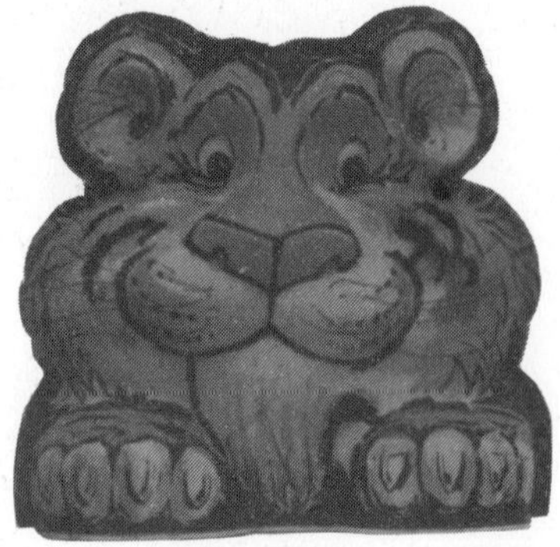

'Esso', plastic tiger sign used in the 1950's.

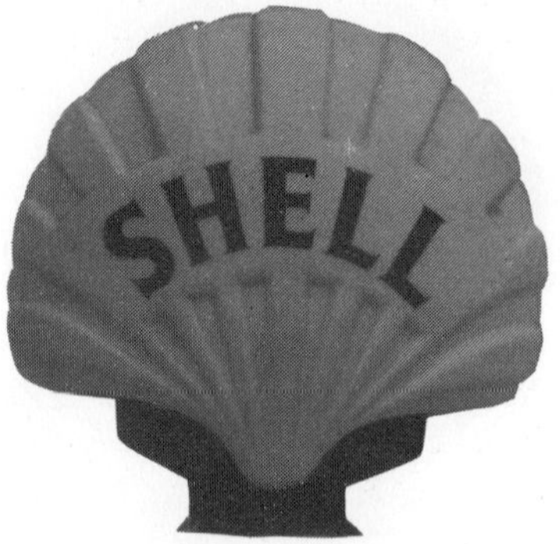

'Shell', a fat shaped sign used in the 1930's, 40's and early 50's.

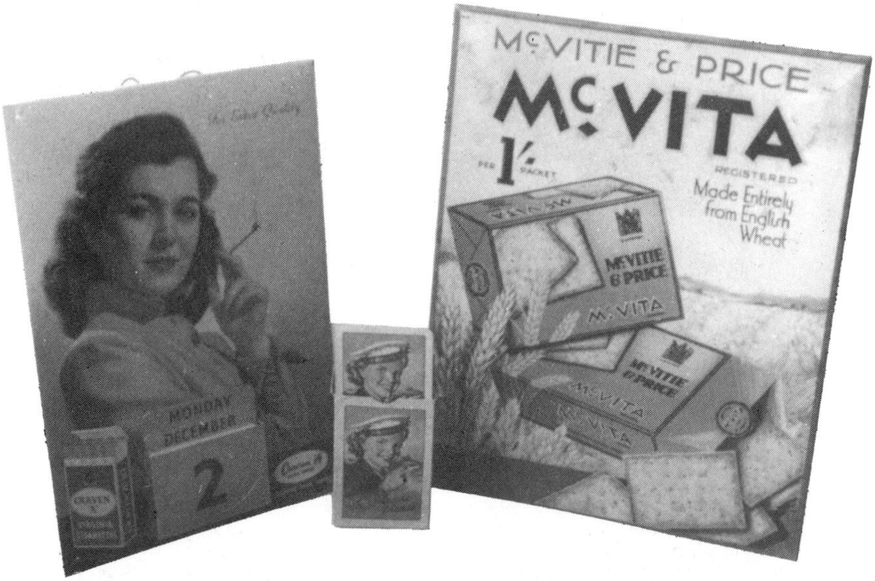

Melvin Hatcher is a graphic artist and collects everything connected with early advertising.

"I like anything that's attractive and I've got over 2,000 bits and pieces spread all over the house. Fortunately we live in a pretty large one so there's plenty of room.

"Things turn up nearly every day because a lot of it is ephemera really. The range extends from Golly brooches to gramophone needle tins and I'm particularly fond of Pears Soap prints because the art work that went into them is amazing and their printing was always impeccable.

"I've got some eye-catching enamel signs, and those that I'm particularly fond of are the ones featuring animals, such as "Black Cat" Virginia Cigarettes enamel.

"What strikes me in card advertising is how good the printing was, the high standard is not kept up today unfortunately."

Melvin's enamel signs have cost between £10 and £200 each but a good deal of his collection has cost very little because value is not his chief criterion. It has been appreciation of the art work involved . . . "The things I like are nice and bright and clean. I buy what pleases me as an artist," he said.

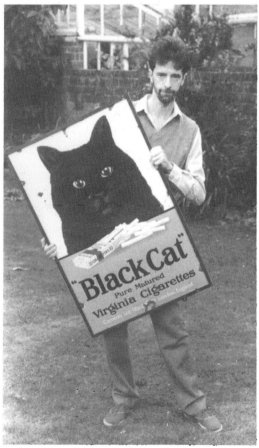

Melvin Hatcher holding an enamel sign for Black Cat cigarettes valued at £150.

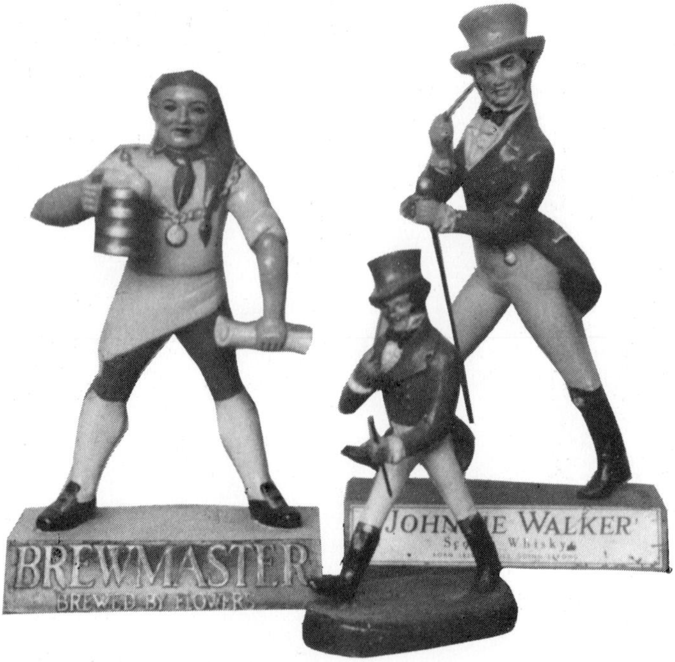

Pub advertising figures for Brewmaster, value £40, Johnnie Walker, large £30, and a small round base Johnnie Walker, value £15.

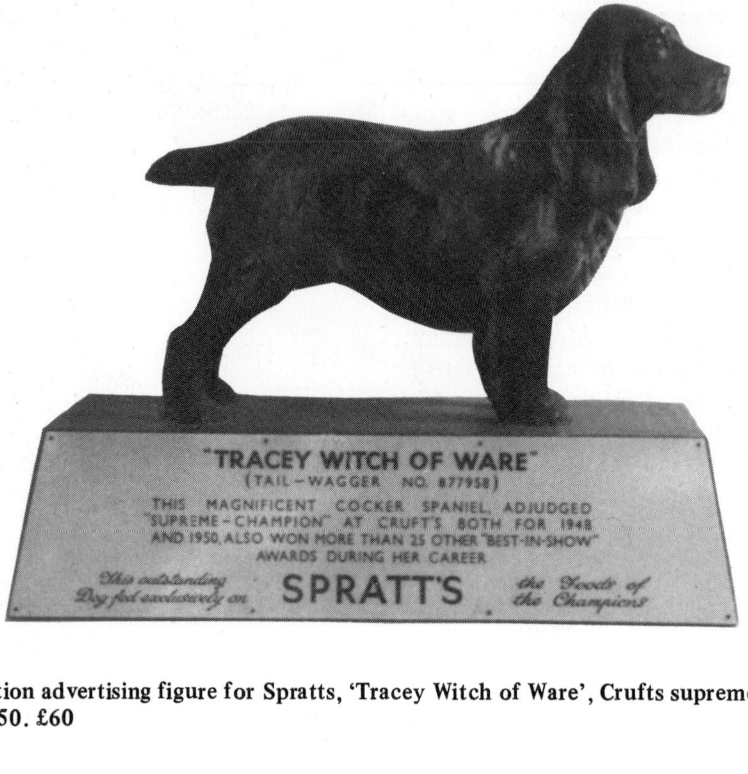

Composition advertising figure for Spratts, 'Tracey Witch of Ware', Crufts supreme champion 1948, 1950. £60

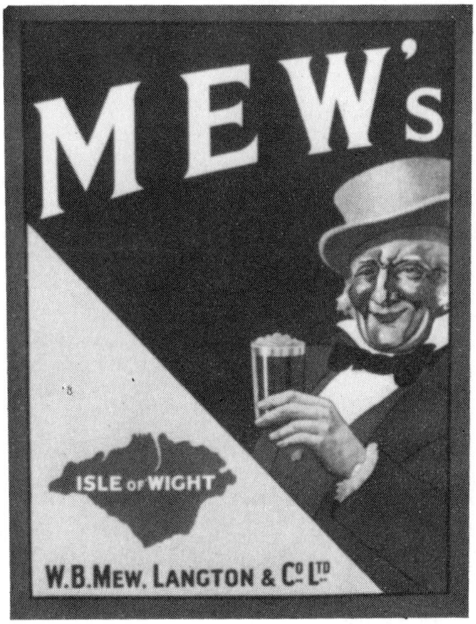

Mew's enamel sign, Isle of Wight. £75

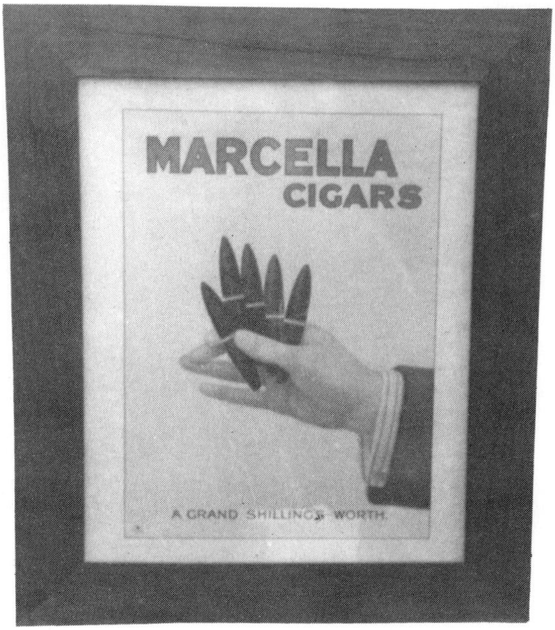

Framed advertising card for Marcella Cigars. £80

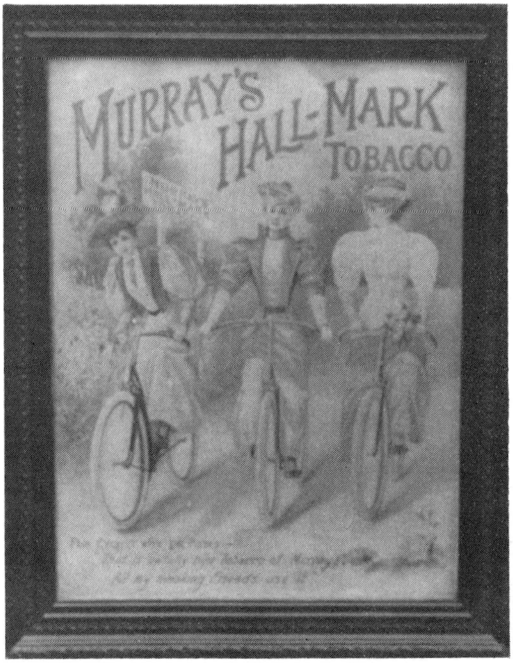

Framed print of Murray's Hall-Mark Tobacco. £60

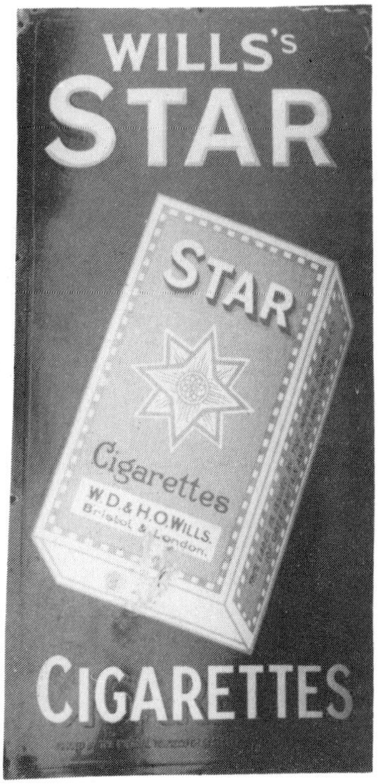

Wills's Star Cigarettes enamel sign. £70

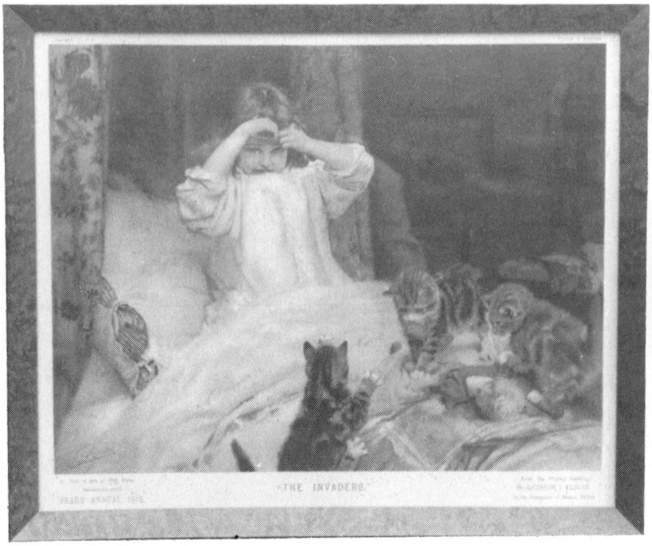

Pears print 'The Invaders'. £65

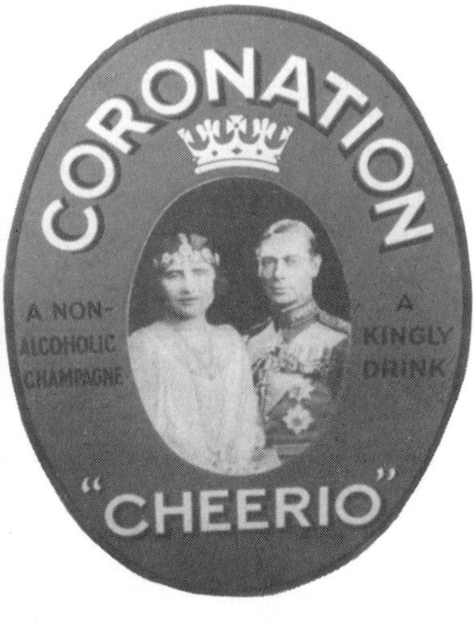

Card advertisement for Coronation 'Cheerio'. £15

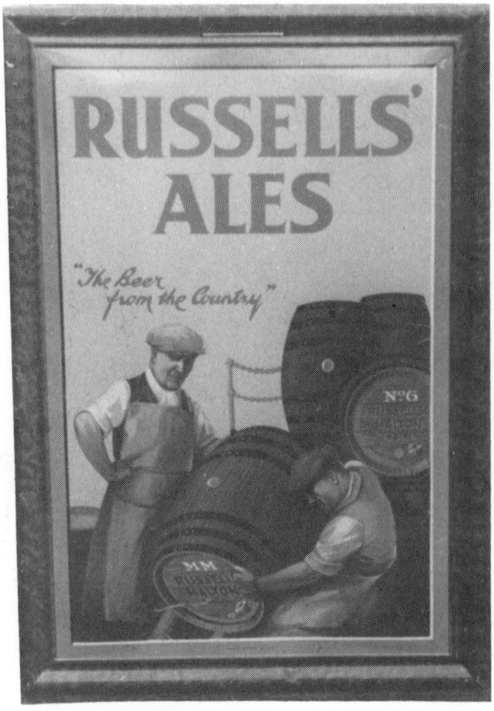

Pressed tin sign for Russells' Ales. £50

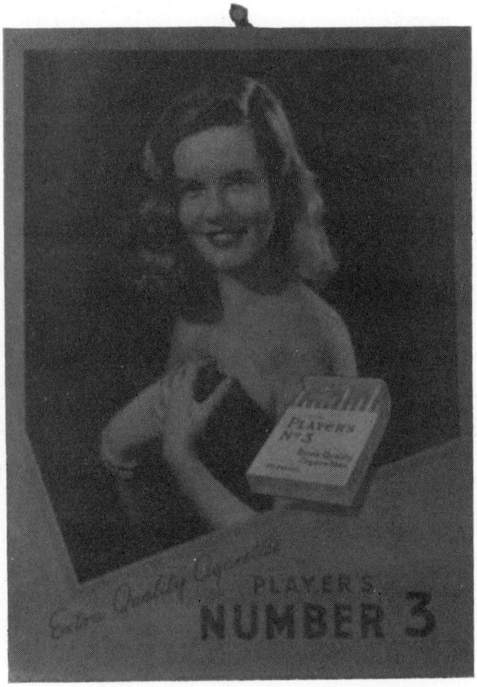

Card advertisement for Players Number 3. £15

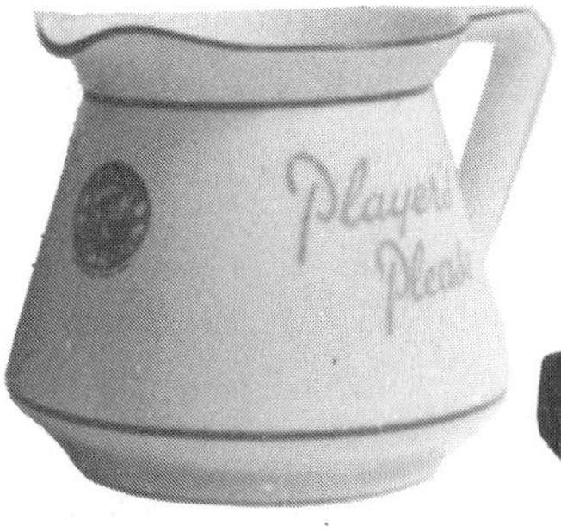

Player's Please water jug. £15

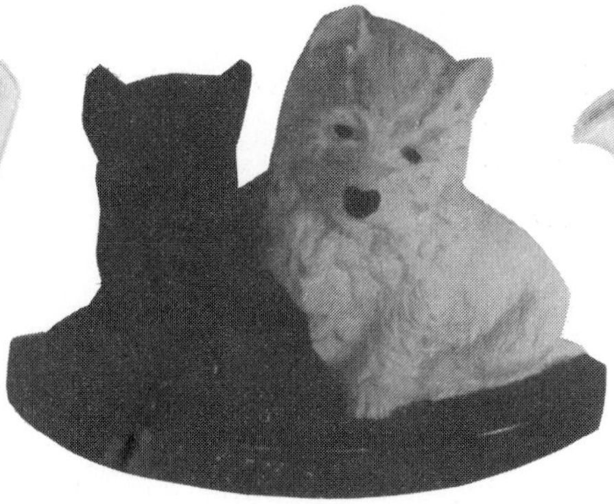

Black & White rubber flat back model. £16

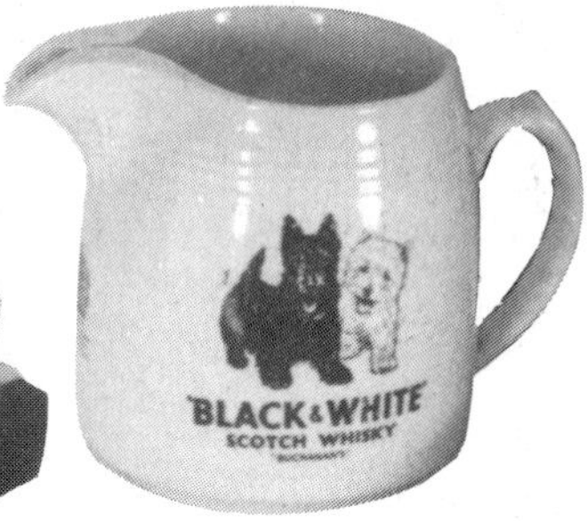

Black & White Scotch Whisky water jug. £10

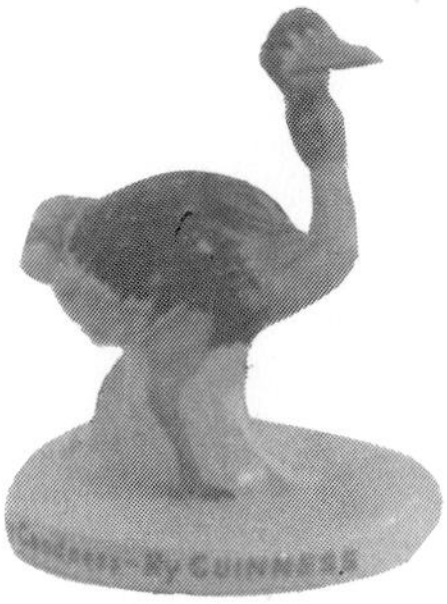

My Goodness, My Guinness statuette, 4in. high. £25

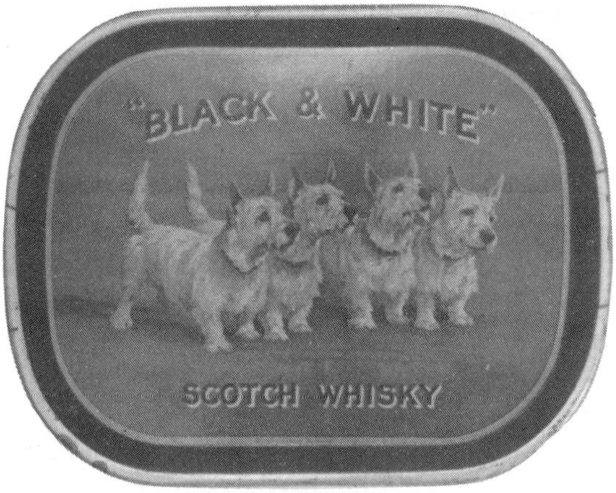

Black & White Scotch Whisky tray. £30

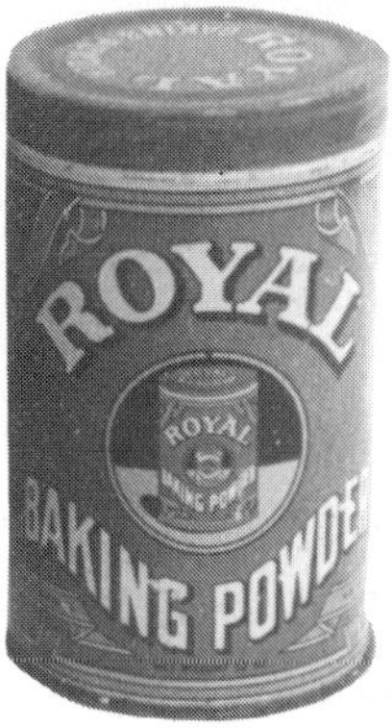

Royal Baking Powder tin. £5

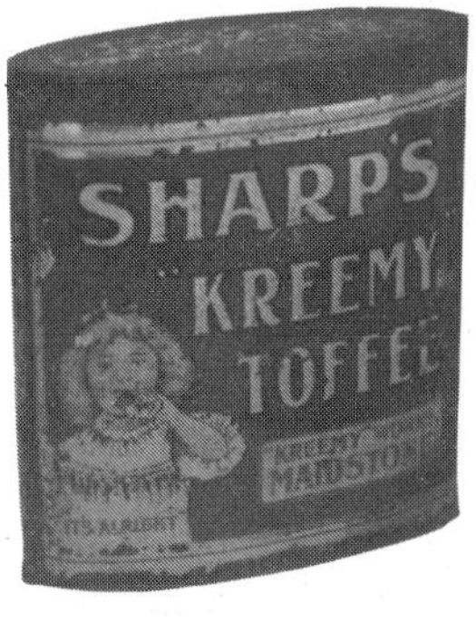

Sharp's 'Kreemy' Toffee tin. £10

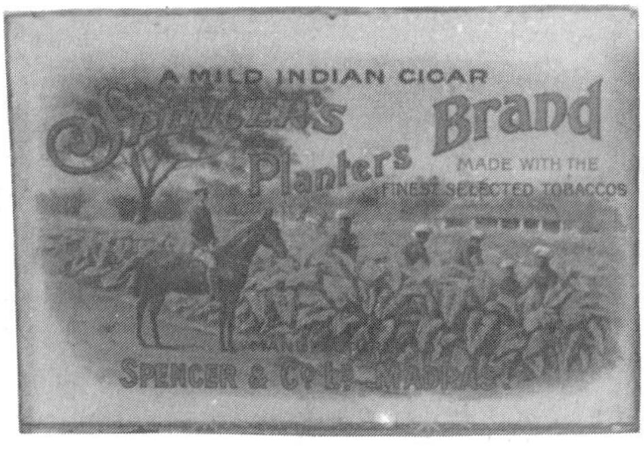

Spencers Planters Brand cigar box lid. £5

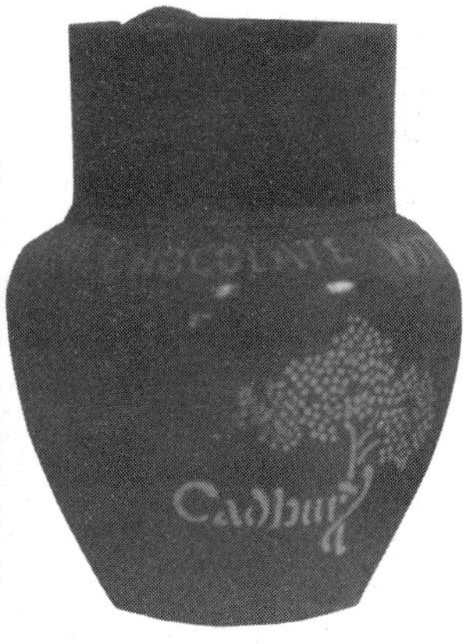

Cadbury's Drinking Chocolate milk jug. £15

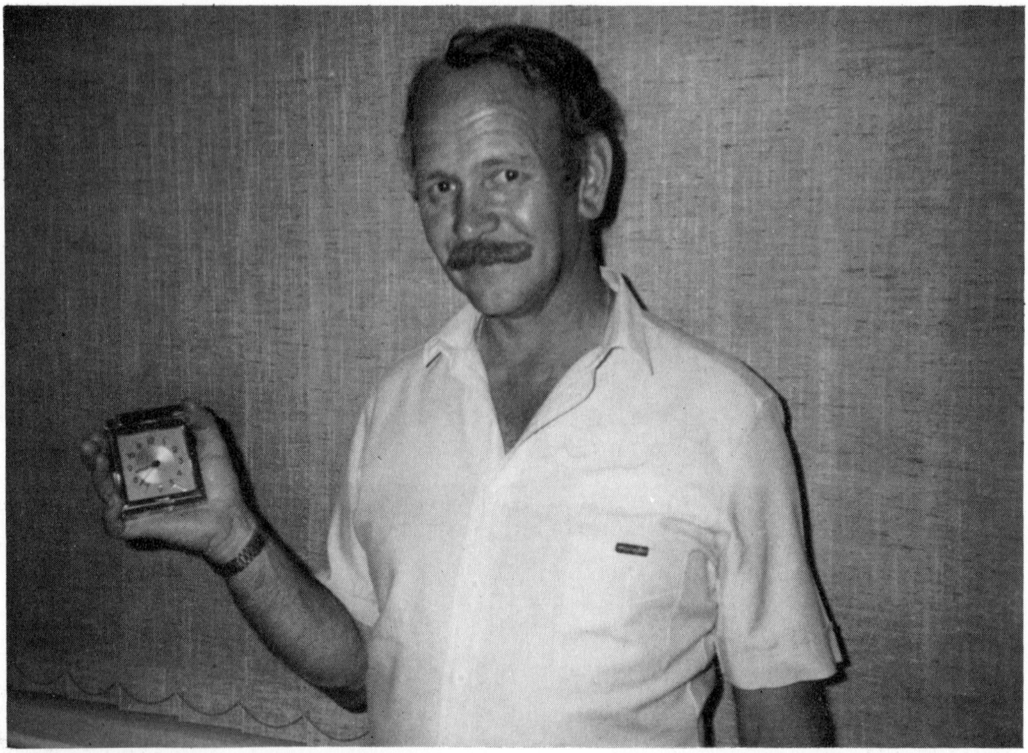

Denis Wilkins was a long distance lorry driver but is now unemployed. He collects cigarette lighters and cigarette holders.

"The funny thing is that I don't smoke myself but I've always been fascinated by anything mechanical and even when I was a kid at school people used to give me old cigarette lighters to repair. Now I've more than 200 in my collection and they all work. They've mostly cost me between 25p and 50p but today prices can go as high as £50 and it is rare to find a nice lighter below £2.

"Mine range from table lighters to the little Art Deco ones that women used to carry in their handbags. In cigarette holders, I've got about 60 ranging from little white ones like pencils to miniature meerschaums.

"I always try to buy anything that looks unusual and has an unusual mechanism and I've got some lighters which were made by soldiers in the First World War from bits of brass and small coins as well as others made by German prisoners during World War Two. They're very good and look like conventional lighters till you examine them closely and see they're handmade from scraps of aluminium and brass.

"The collection is continually growing because I keep adding more modern varieties, even throwaway plastic ones. I want to keep it up to date."

One of the more unusual items in Denis's collection is a solid brass lighter with a clock set in it. It was broken when he bought it for 50p but now the clock and the lighter are working. He still regrets missing a lighter which another collector bought under his nose. It looked like a egg shaped brass pocket watch but when a spring in the side was pressed, it opened in two parts. It had a German inscription and dated from the 1940's.

The lighter that he would most like to add to his collection is one he saw recently which is both a musical box and a cigarette case as well as a lighter. When opened it plays a tune and the contents spread out like a fan. Denis thinks it also dates from the 1940's.

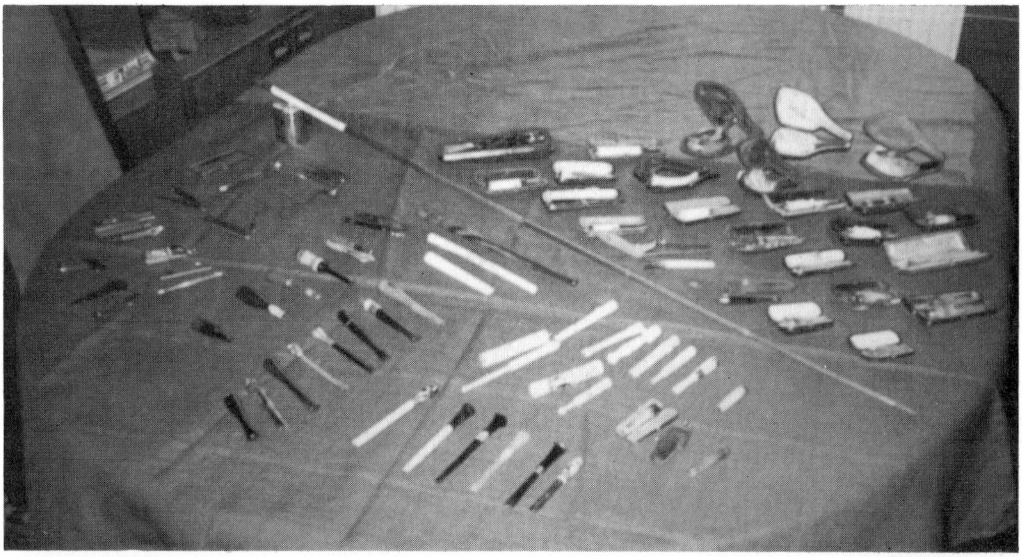

Part of Denis's collection of cigar and cigarette holders including many with gold and silver ferruls, together with some Meerschaum holders in the form of a birds claw holding an egg, a sheep dog and a mountain goat.

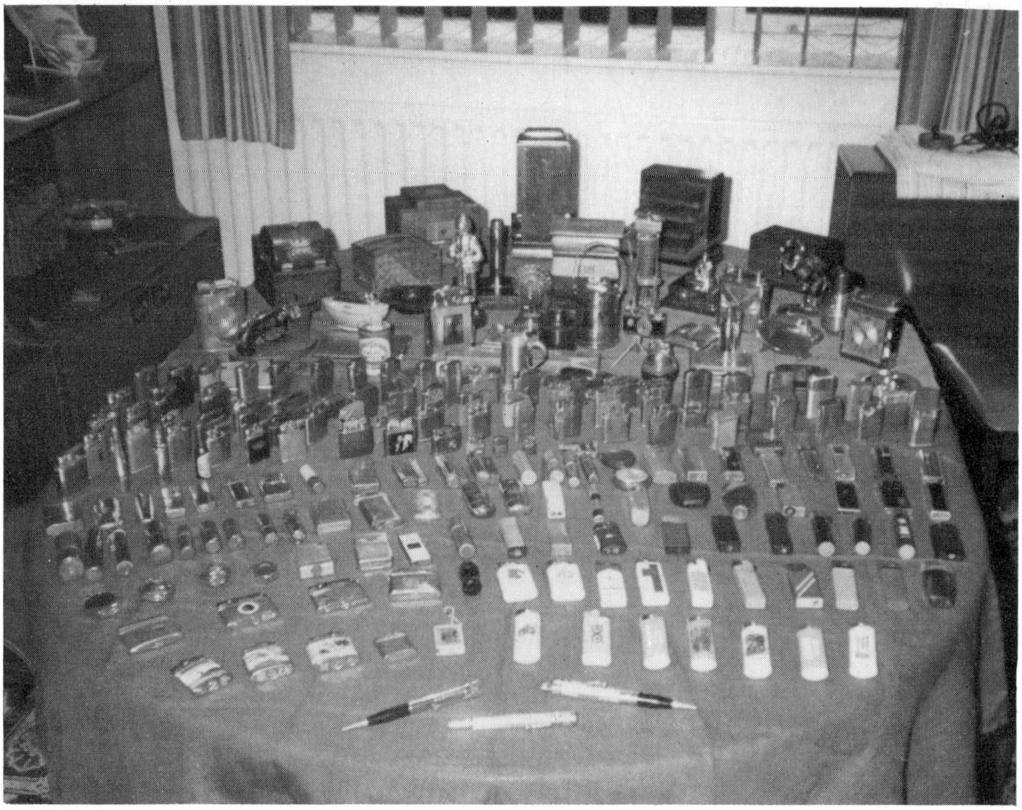

Nearly two hundred lighters from early petrol Dunhills and Ronson Pencils to ingenious Trench Art examples and even one made from the top of an incendiary bomb.

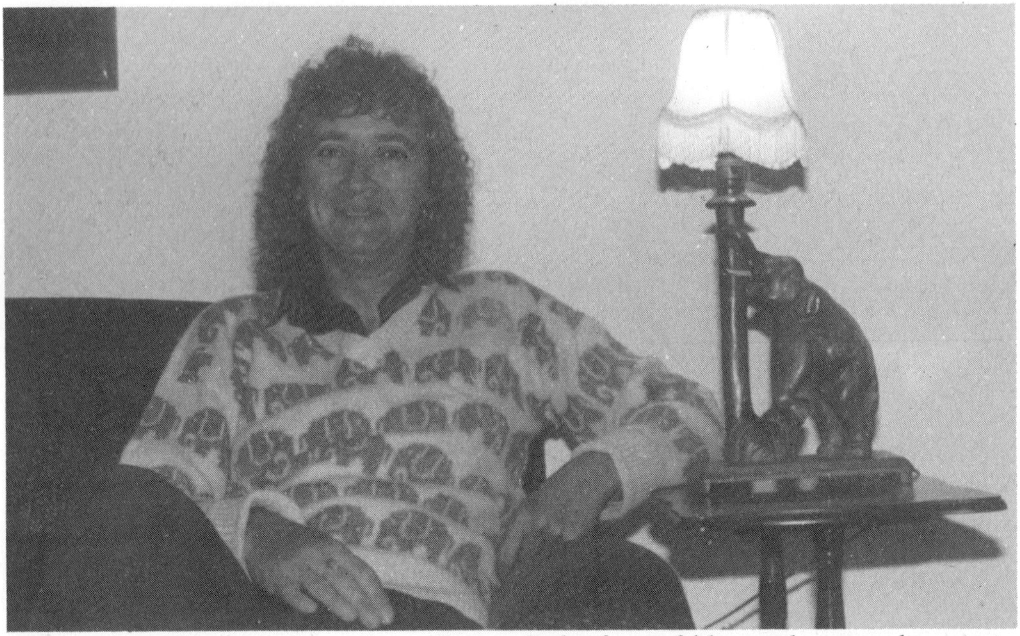

Jenny Lees is a teacher who collects anything to do with elephants.

"I'm interested in conservation and organised a sponsored walk to Save The Elephant, I think I've got a sort of affinity with them.

"The very first thing I bought was a carved figure of an elephant that was sold to me in Port Grimaud in the South of France by a Sengalese who said it was ivory. I wouldn't have bought it if it was, but of course it was really resin.

"That started me off and wherever I go I look for things depicting elephants. They mustn't just be decorative but also must serve some sort of function. I don't particularly like those lines of black elephant ornaments you see because they're not useful. I've got tables, lamps, letter openers, nutcrackers and ashtrays, plant holders, a clock with an elephant on top and a pin cushion — all to do with elephants.

"I've also got printed metal signs that were used to advertise Fremlins beer because the firm's sign was an elephant."

In her collection Jenny has a coffee table with elephants supporting it that was swapped with a Burmese seaman in Tilbury docks for a fridge and among her most treasured pieces is a moulded glass Victorian ink well in the shape of an elephant with a brass-lined howdah for holding the ink and a lead elephants' head for hanging on the wall with a pipe rack beneath it.

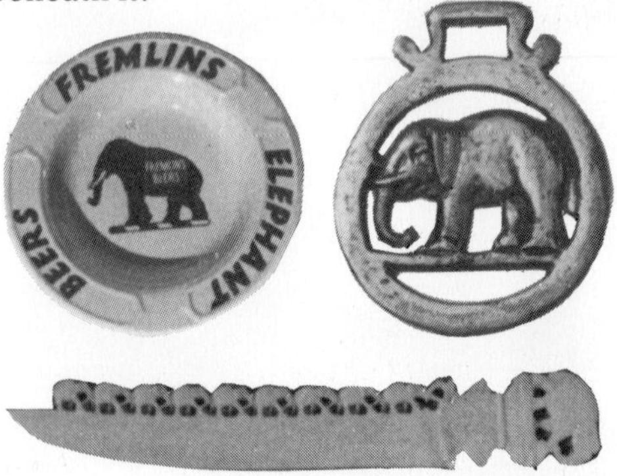

It is very difficult to find anything out about most of the pieces she collects and pricing them is also a hard task because she picks many of them up in antique fairs and car boot sales. One of her bargain buys was a table lamp with the bulb held up by an elephant which she bought for £5. Most of the things she has, with the exception of the printed metal signs for Fremlin's Beer, seem to be unique.

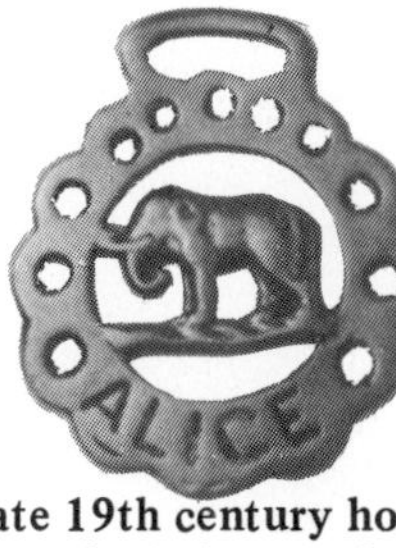

Late 19th century horse brass depicting an elephant called Alice. (Alice was a female African elephant bought by London Zoological Gardens on Sept. 9th 1865 for £550 where she was housed next to the famous Jumbo). £12

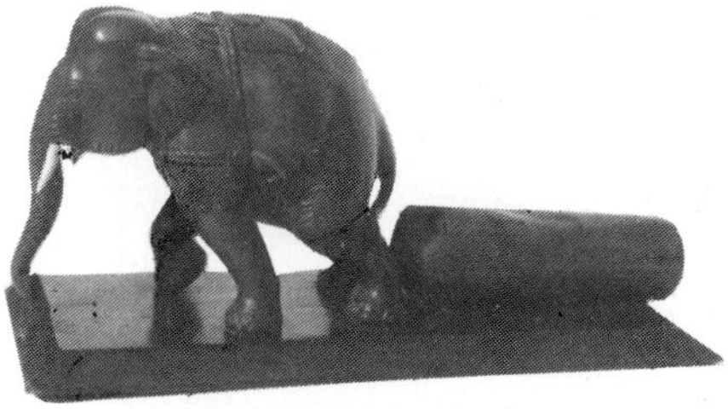

A finely carved Ceylonese elephant pulling a log in honey-coloured wood, 12½in. long. £15

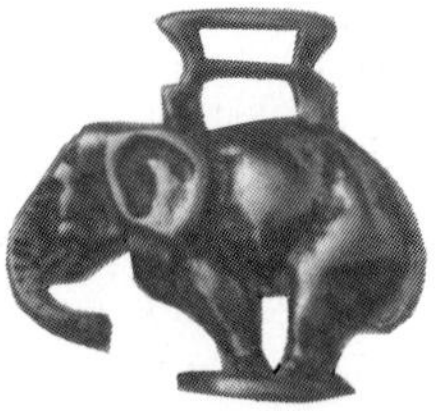

Late 19th century elephant horse brass, possibly Jumbo. £10

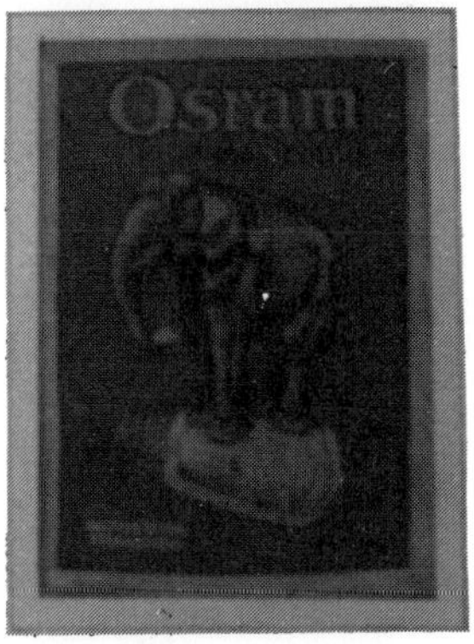

Osram silk pin cushion cover, 2¾ x 3¾in. £2.50

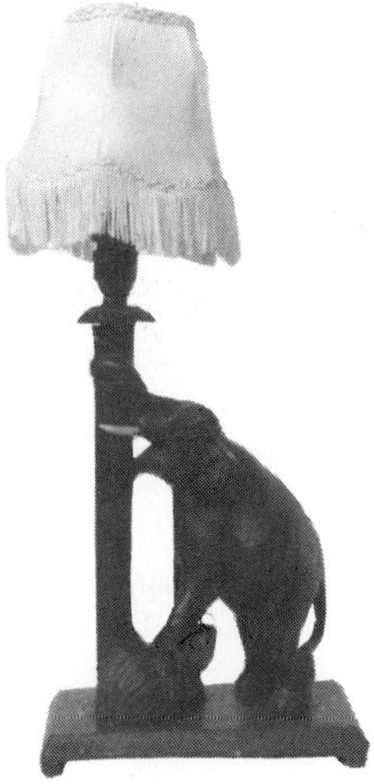

A finely carved elephant lamp, complete with fittings, 11½in. tall. £10

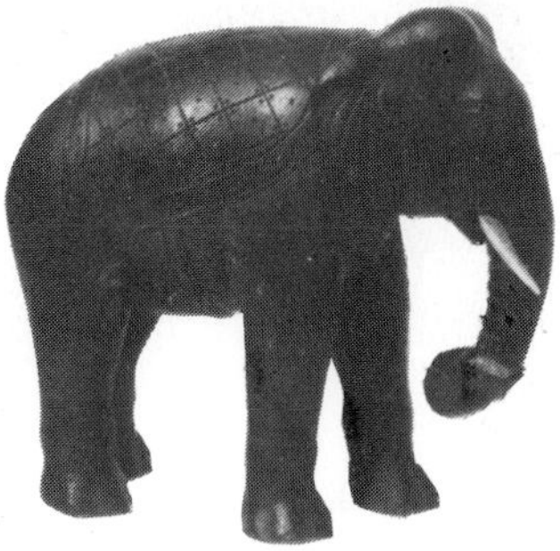

Late 19th century carved wood elephant of attractive proportions, 10in. high. £15

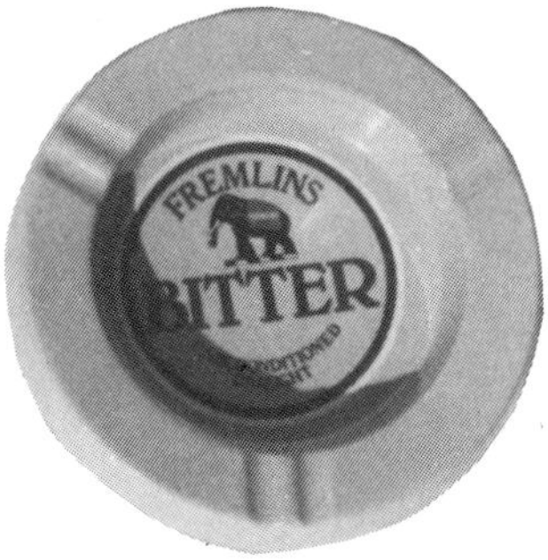

A recent Fremlins beige plastic ashtray. 50p

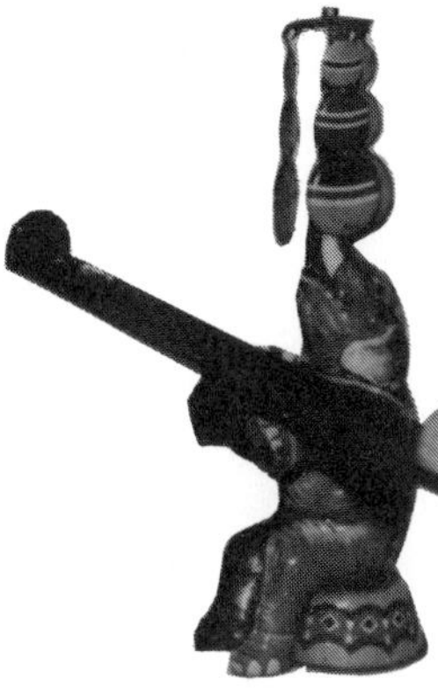

A toy tin 'balancing ball' elephant, marked 'U.S. Zone Germany', 1950's. £35

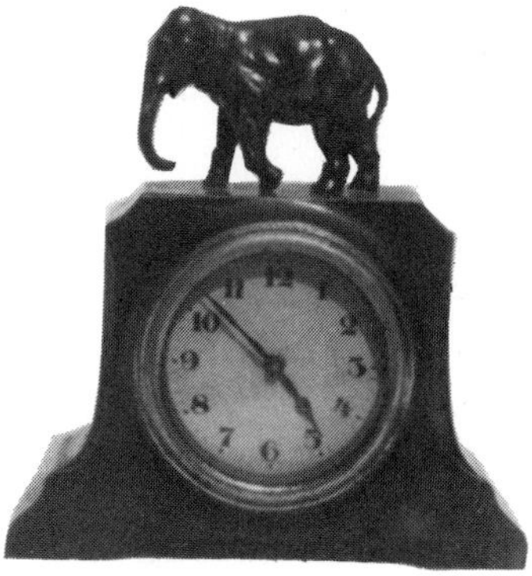

A small German metallic mantel clock, marked 'Made in Wurtemberg and Foreign', 4¾in. high. £25

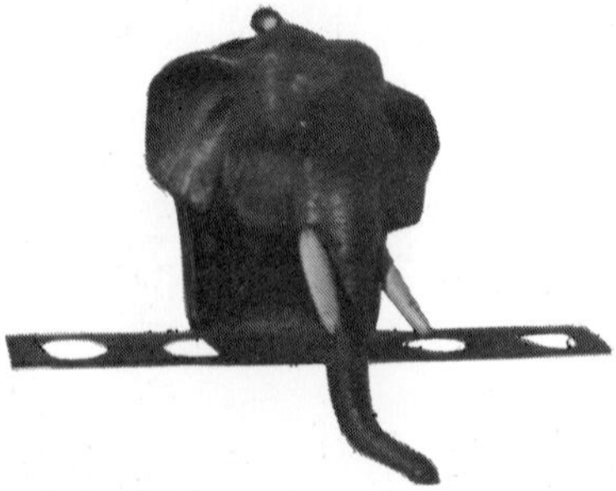

Late 19th century pipe rack in the form of a finely detailed and coloured elephant's head, 6in. wide. £5

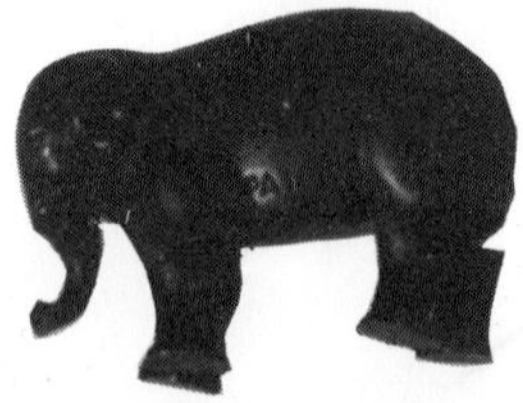

An unusual American cast metal walking elephant marked Patent 1873, 2½in. high. £35

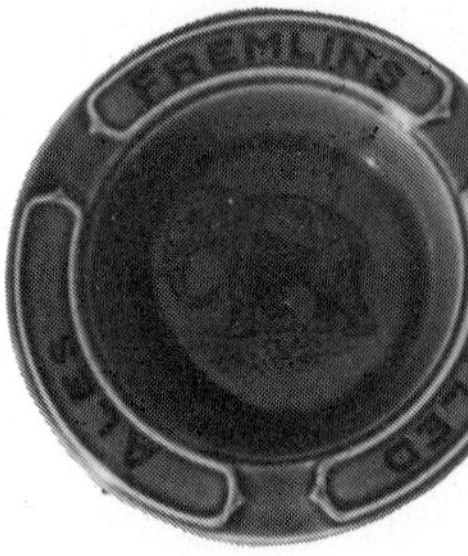

Fremlins Ales, brown ceramic ashtray, depicting their trade mark, 1930's, made by T. G. Green & Co. Ltd. £5

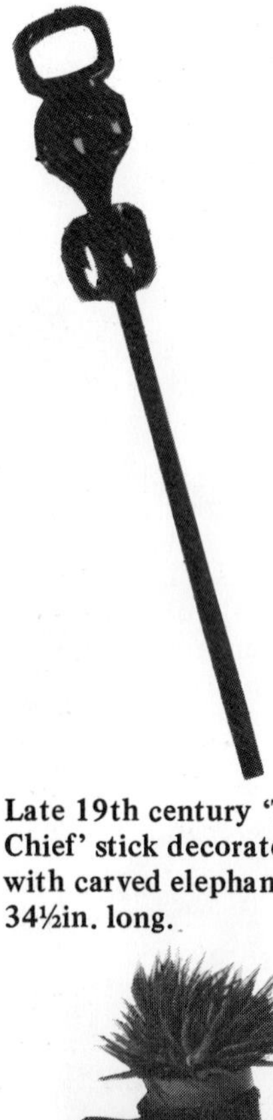

Late 19th century 'Tribal Chief' stick decorated with carved elephants, 34½in. long. £15

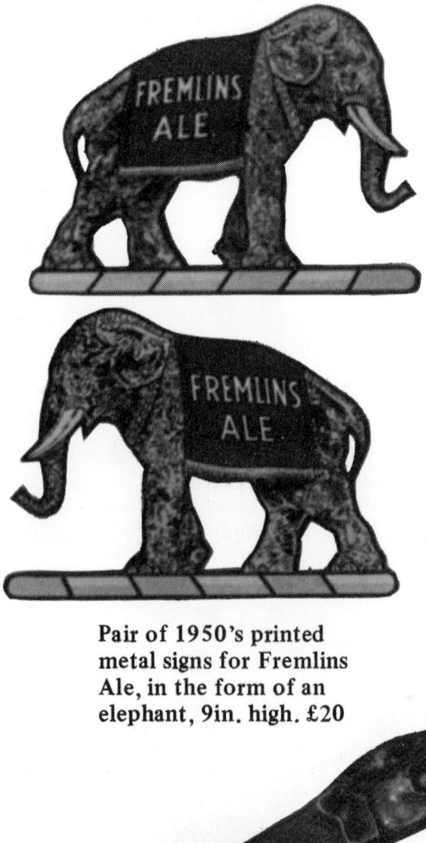

Pair of 1950's printed metal signs for Fremlins Ale, in the form of an elephant, 9in. high. £20

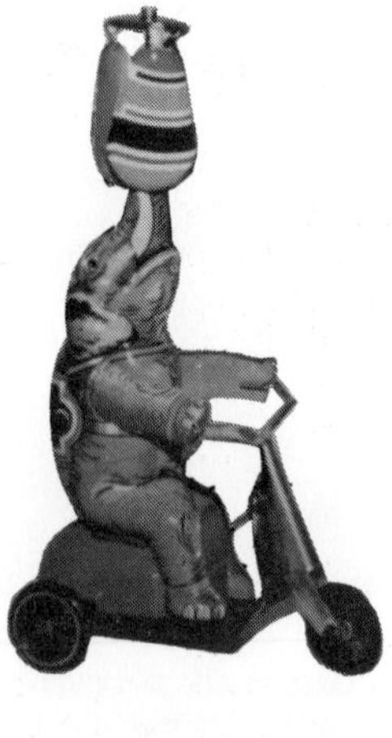

Toy tin elephant, riding a scooter and balancing an object on it's trunk, marked 'U.S. Zone, Germany', circa 1950's. £20

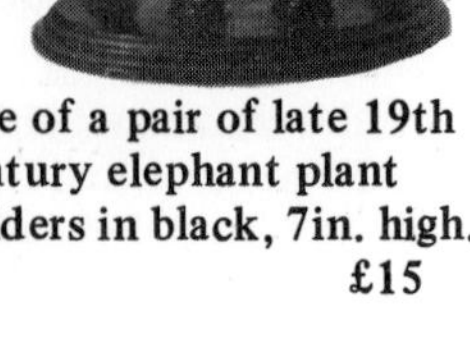

One of a pair of late 19th century elephant plant holders in black, 7in. high. £15

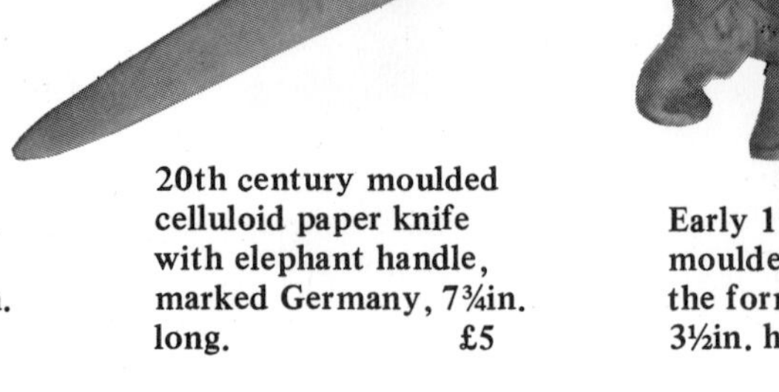

20th century moulded celluloid paper knife with elephant handle, marked Germany, 7¾in. long. £5

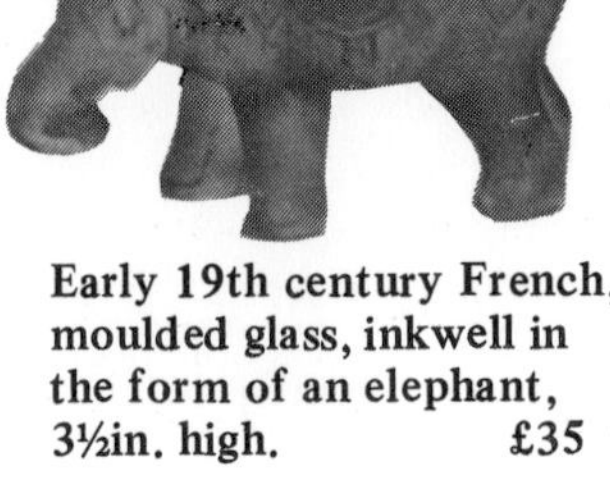

Early 19th century French, moulded glass, inkwell in the form of an elephant, 3½in. high. £35

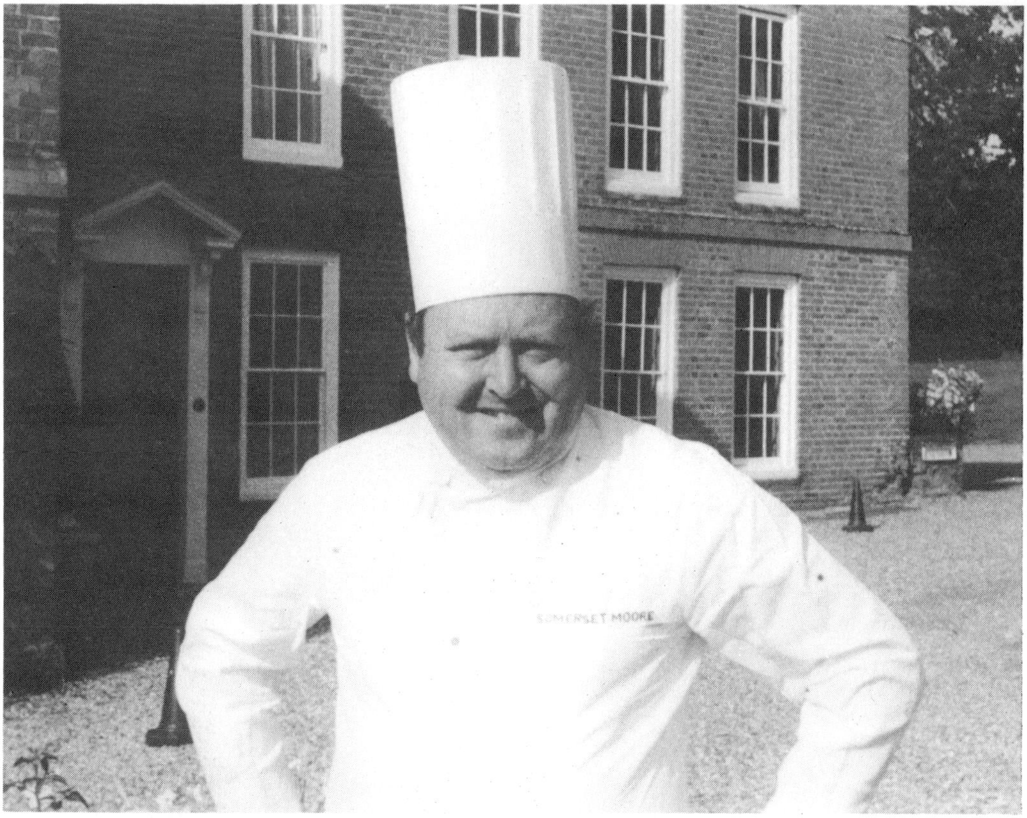

Somerset Moore is a hotelier at Flitwick Manor, Bedfordshire, who collects porcelain sardine boxes.

"I used to collect enamel signs but I dispersed most of the collection and now I'm collecting porcelain sardine boxes which are a suitable choice for this hotel because our restaurant specialises in fish dishes. The boxes are on display in the hotel for customers to see.

"At the moment I've got 40 of them and they're made in porcelain or cut glass and some have silver tops. The thing that is common with them all is that they always have a fish on the lid.

"They were used in Edwardian times by the middle classes because in those 'refined' days, when people took several meals during the day including afternoon tea and early supper, they disguised the fact that sardines arrived in tins by putting them in those very pretty porcelain boxes.

"The major British potteries made them but some of the nicest ones come from Czechoslovakia and are very beautifully painted. In my collection I have examples of fluted and chequered boxes and there's a blue and white one patterned like a tea set. I've got a very nice one painted with blackberries."

Somerset's favourite sardine box is the one with the blackberries because he thinks the connection between that fruit and fish is very unusual. It is dated 1903 and probably comes from Germany or Czechoslovakia.

Prices for the boxes vary between £12 for an ordinary one to between £250 and £450 for a fine example by Spode or Minton. Mr Moore says he will buy any that he can lay his hands on. "I like collecting in large quantities and my ambition is to own lots of them, then I can keep the good ones and sell the ones that I've already got or the ones of poorer quality."

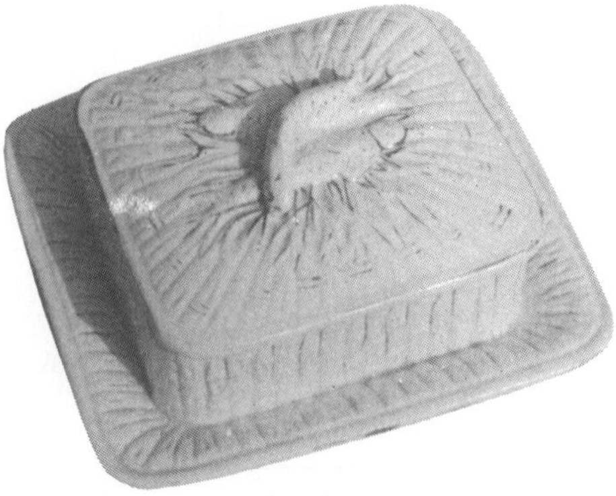

Pottery bamboo design sardine box with woven pattern on lid, made in Alloa, Scotland by Waverley. £70

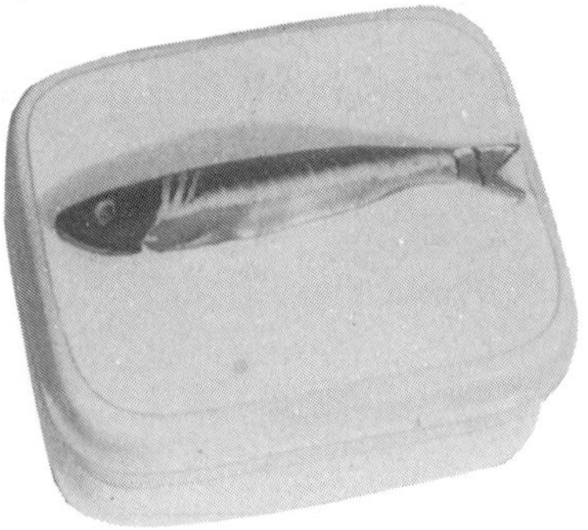

White opalescent porcelain sardine box made in Czechoslovakia decorated with a blue band. £140

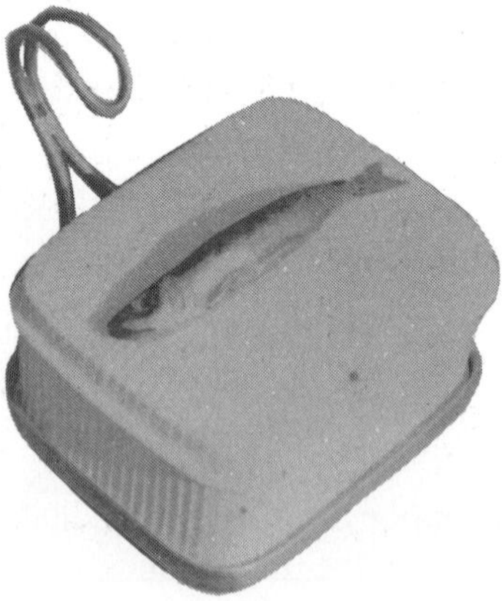

Fluted white porcelain sardine box with a finely painted fish, marked with an eagle, on plated stand. £250

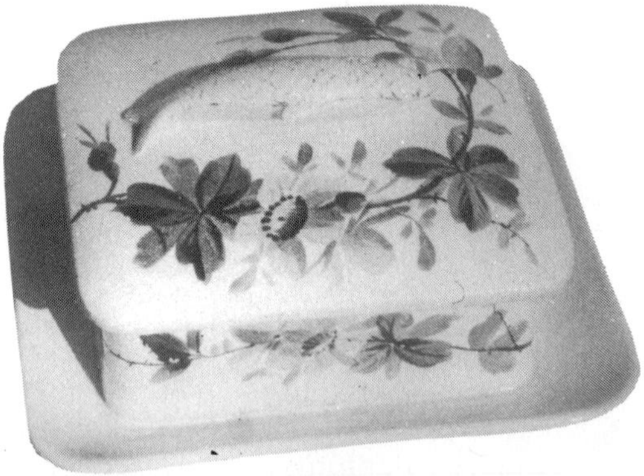

China sardine box of plain design with painted roses and a gilded scaled fish, dated 1886, marked MKK. £60

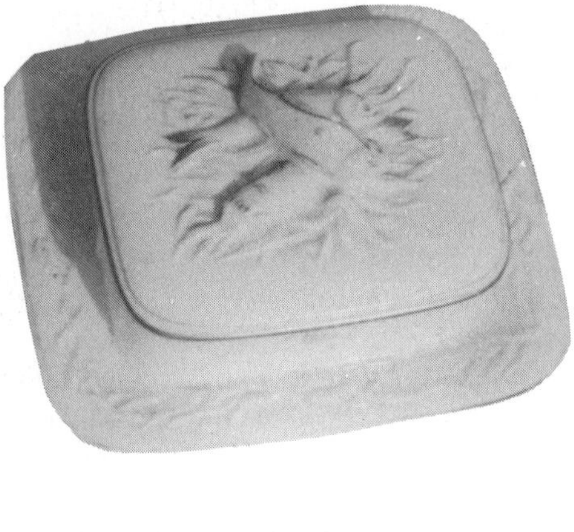

Gilded porcelain sardine box with water weed pattern, English, unmarked. £60

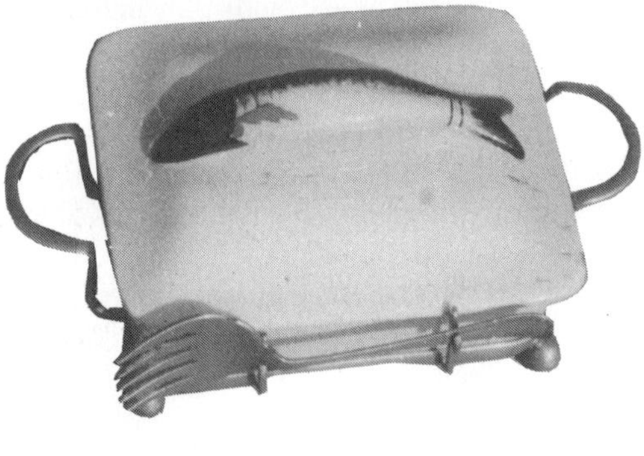

English porcelain sardine box with a finely painted fish with red fins, complete with silver plated stand and fork. £140

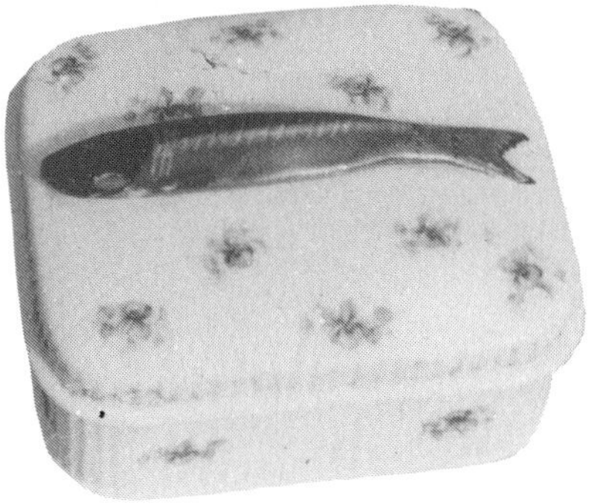

Fluted porcelain sardine box decorated with violets and gilding with a finely painted fish. £65

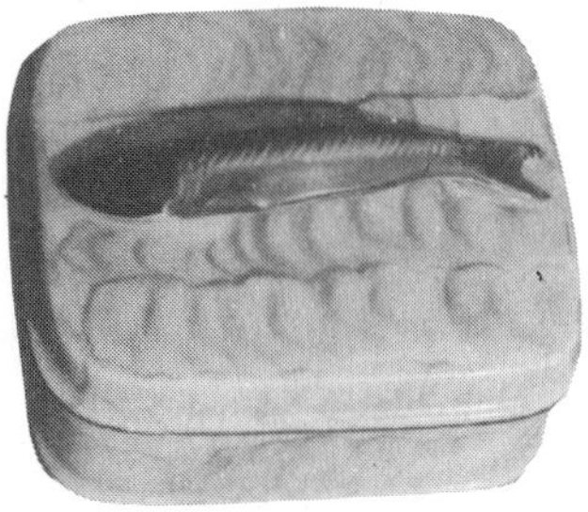

Czechoslovakian porcelain sardine box with a green marbleized effect and a good painted fish. £160

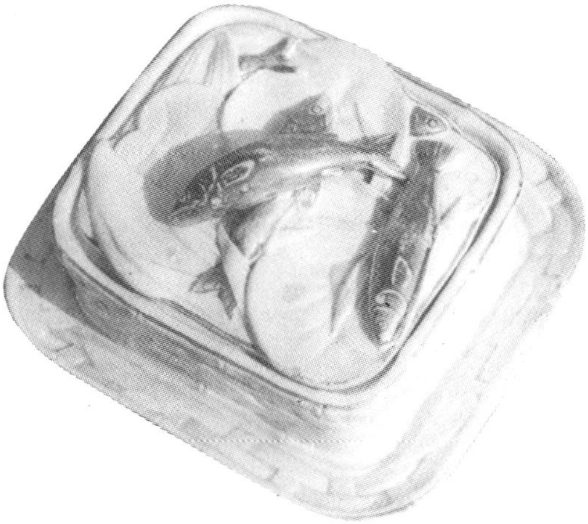

Gilded pottery sardine box with woven sides and decorated lid embellished with water lilies and reeds, unmarked probably English. £70

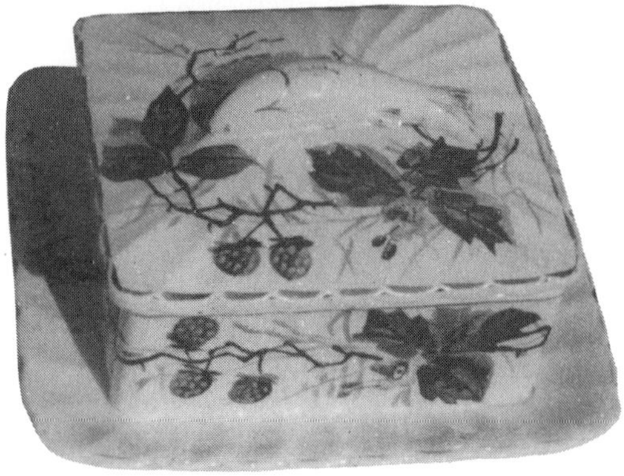

An unusual German porcelain sardine box decorated with gilding and brambles in flower and fruit by Mehlem. £130

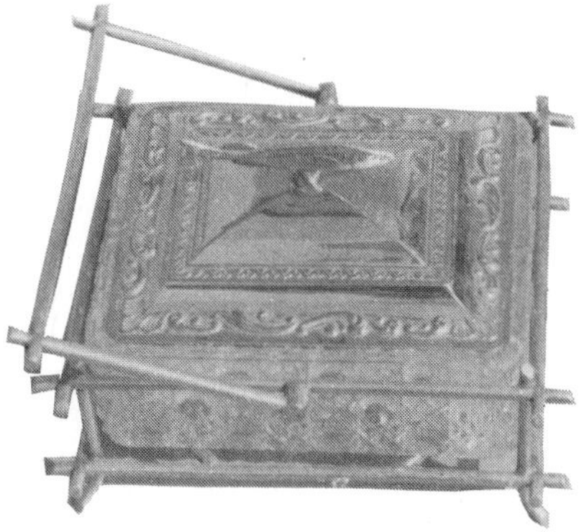

Cut glass sardine box with silver plated stand and lid, unmarked. £100

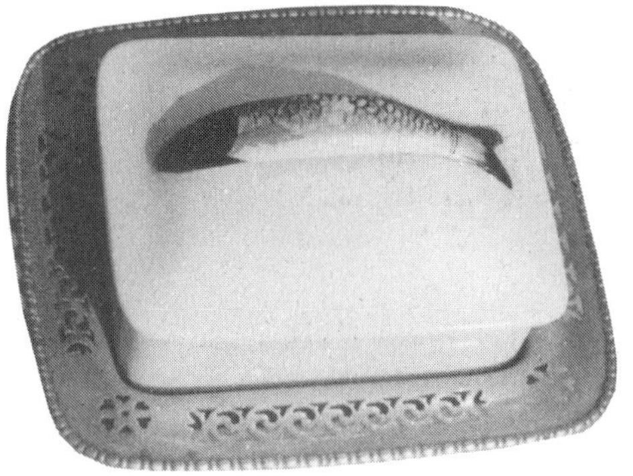

Apricot glaze sardine box marked Flos Maron, with pierced silver plated stand. £140

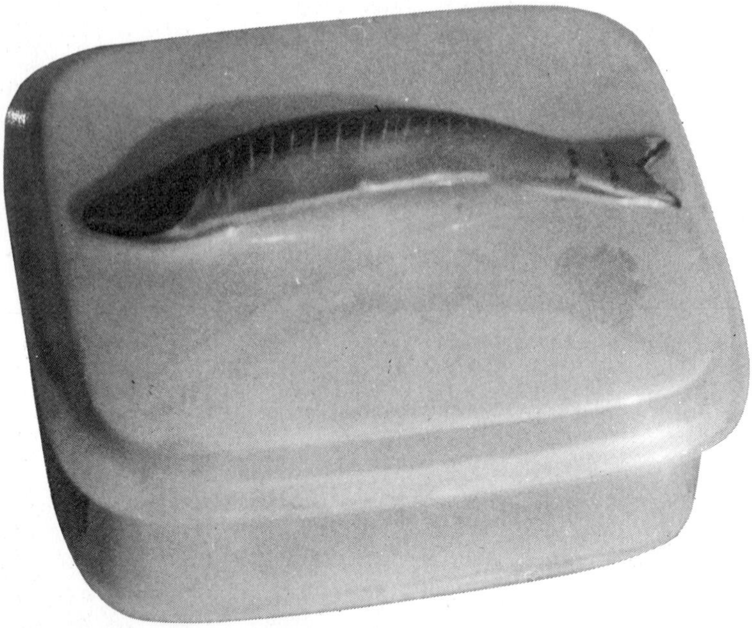

Blue porcelain sardine box with opalescent glaze and well modelled fish, made in Czechoslovakia, numbered 4641. £75

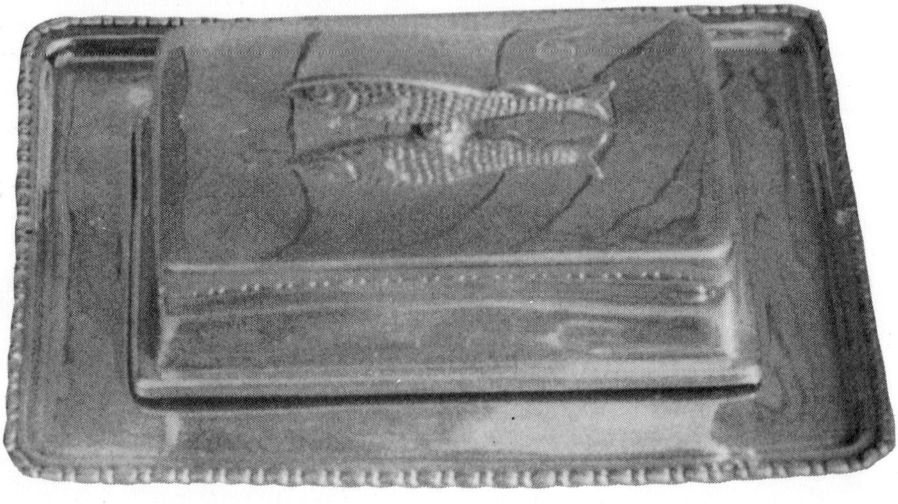

An English silver plated sardine box with cut glass liner, made by DBAS. £95

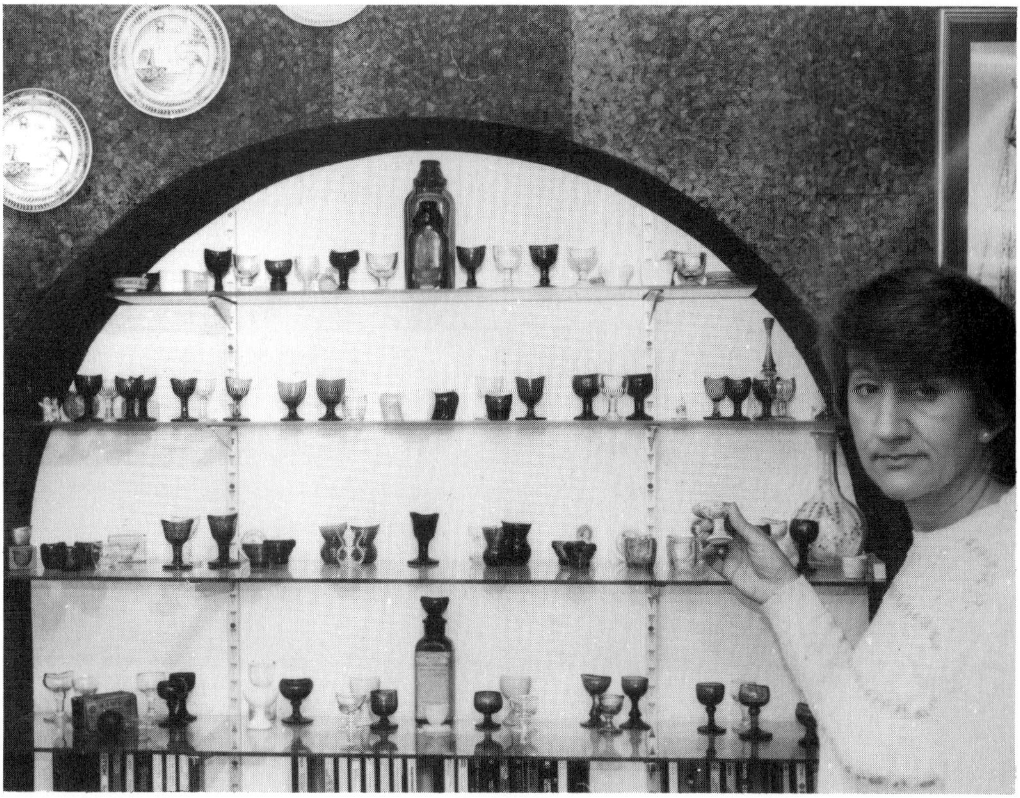

Christine Blackmore collects eye baths.

"My husband is a keen bottle collector and it makes life easier if I collect as well. About six years ago at a bottle sale, I bought my first blue glass eyebath and now I've got over 100 of them in all colours and all sorts of materials including glass, pottery, lignum vitae, celluloid, bakelite, ivory, pewter, aluminium and rubber. The only type that has evaded me so far is a silver eyebath and they do exist for one sold recently in auction for £700. It was Georgian silver and was bought by an overseas collector."

Christine's collection has been bought for prices ranging between 50p and £60. The last price was paid for a blue glass reservoir eyebath in a cottage loaf shape. Her husband keeps a photographic record of her pieces and carries it with him when he goes on his bottle buying expeditions in case he comes across something not yet represented in her collection which is displayed in backlighted glass shelves in their home.

The first detailed description of an eyebath dates from 1641 but they were little known until the late 17th century. The earliest ones are most valuable and the price also varies according to the material used. Christine would like to find a silver eyebath and also one issued in the 1920's by a chemist called Dan Davies which has an eye painted on it. The price for a Davies eyebath today is around £15

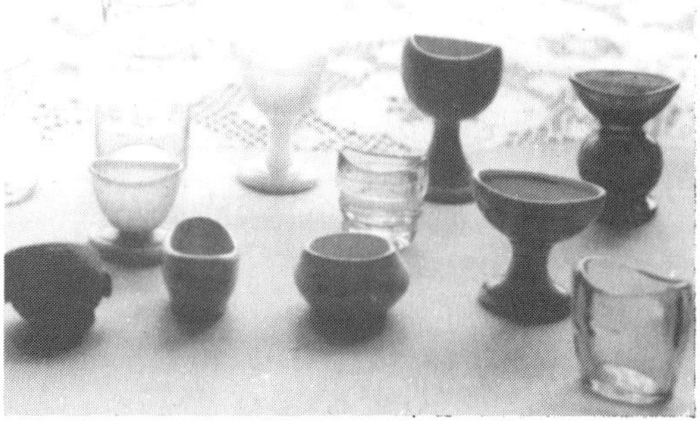

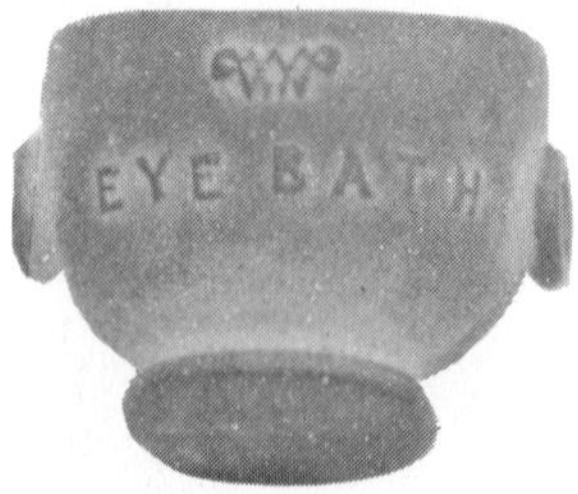

Rubber eye bath advertised as suitable for motorists. £8-£12

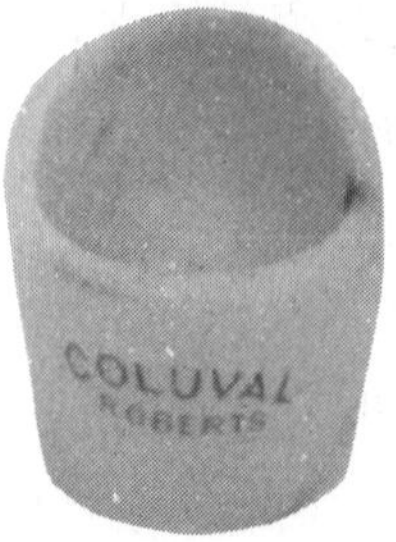

Squat white stoneware eye bath, Culuval Roberts. £10-£12

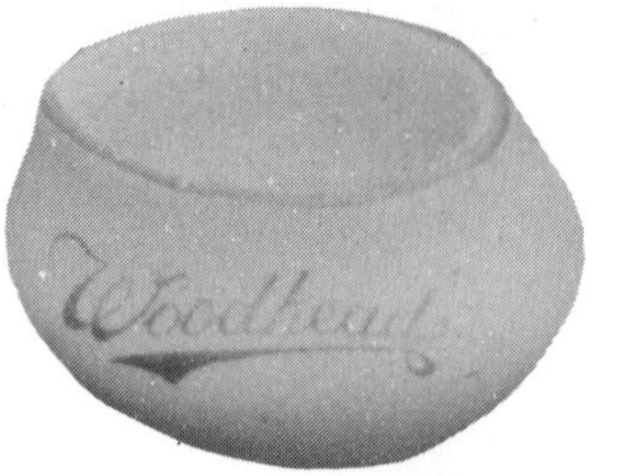

Squat white stoneware eye bath with 'Woodheads' in green print. £12-£15

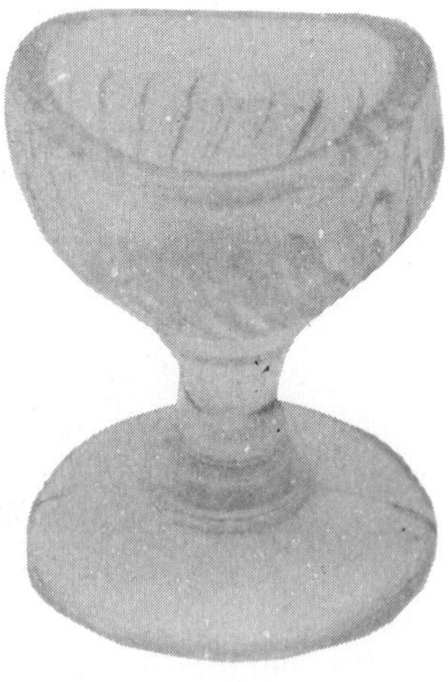

Clear glass stemmed eye bath with wrythened bowl. £6-£8

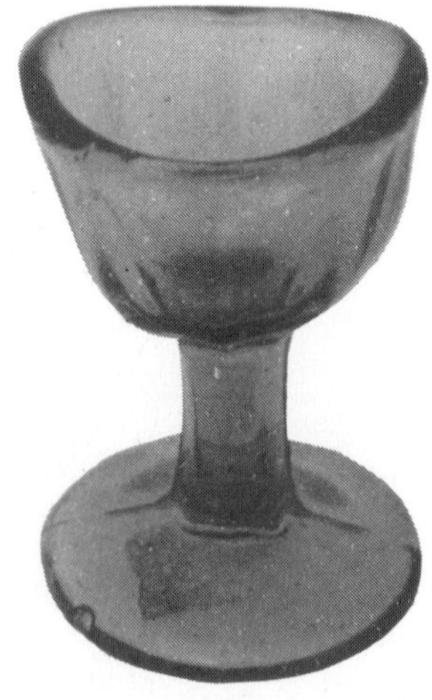

Pedestal moulded green glass eye bath. £2.50-£5

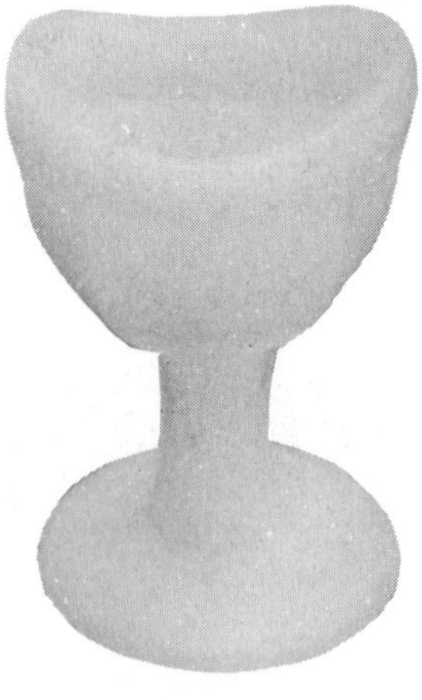

Milkglass stemmed eye bath. £8-£10

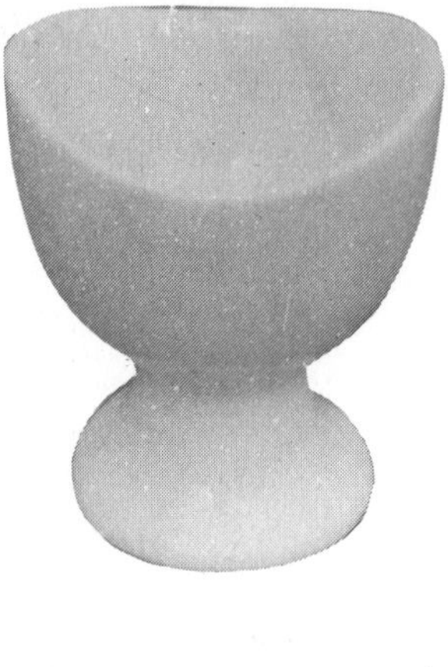

White stoneware stemmed eye bath. £12

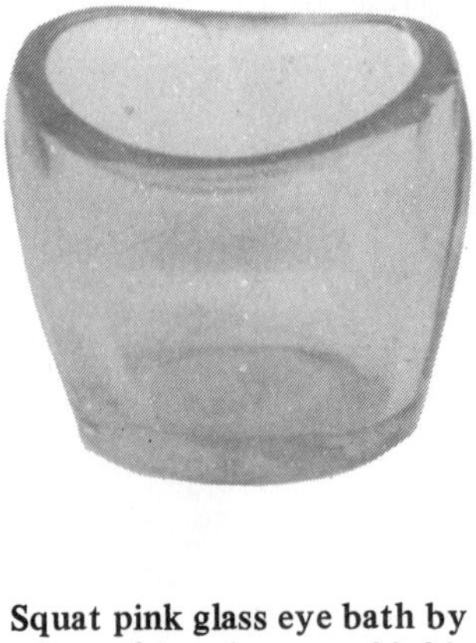

Squat pink glass eye bath by Maws of London. £3-£4

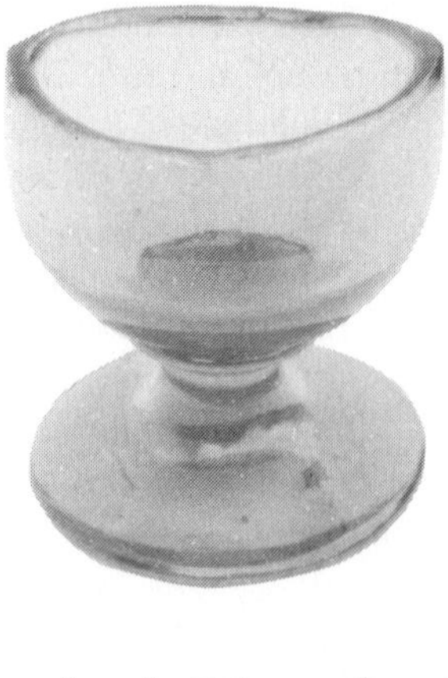

Blue glass short stemmed freeblown eye bath. £15-£20

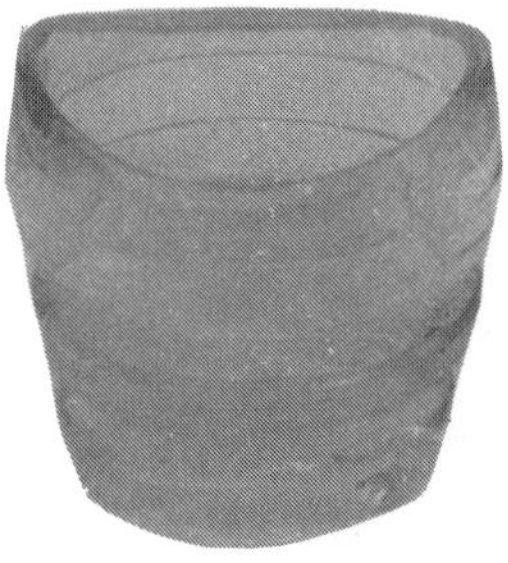

Clear glass squat ribbed eye bath. £3-£5

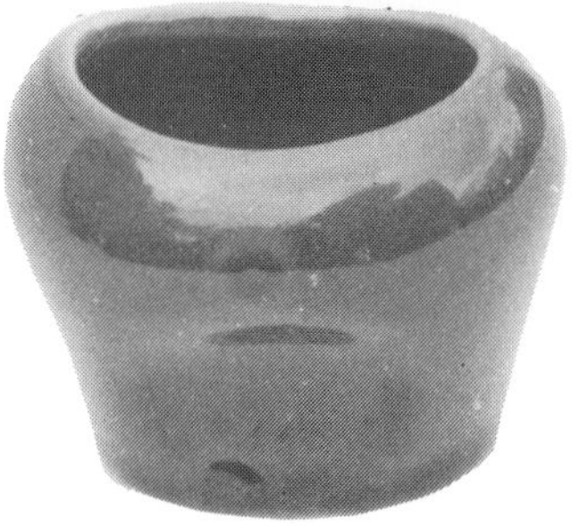

Squat blue stoneware eye bath. £3

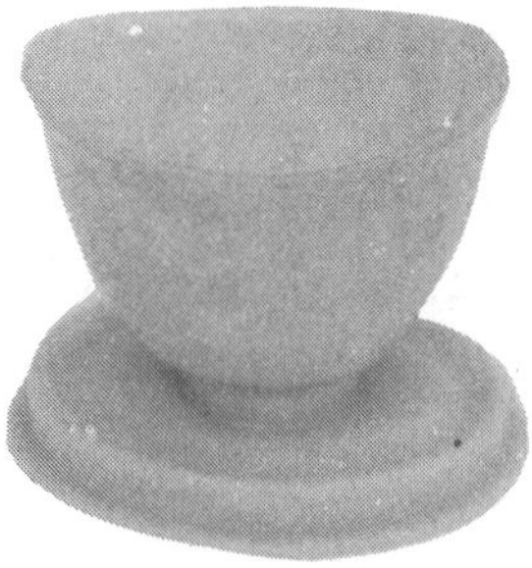

Squat bakelite eye bath with foot. £8-£10

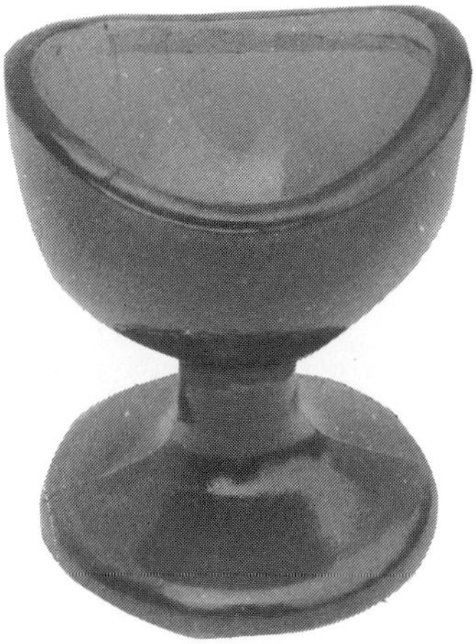

Stemmed moulded amber glass eye bath. £15

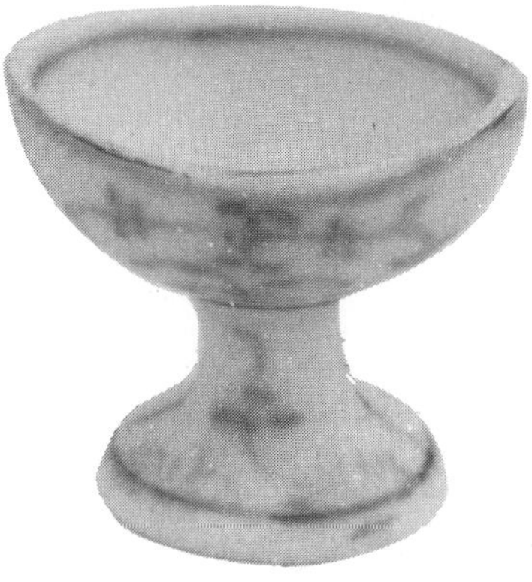

Blue and white Meissen porcelain eye bath with gold rim. £45-£55

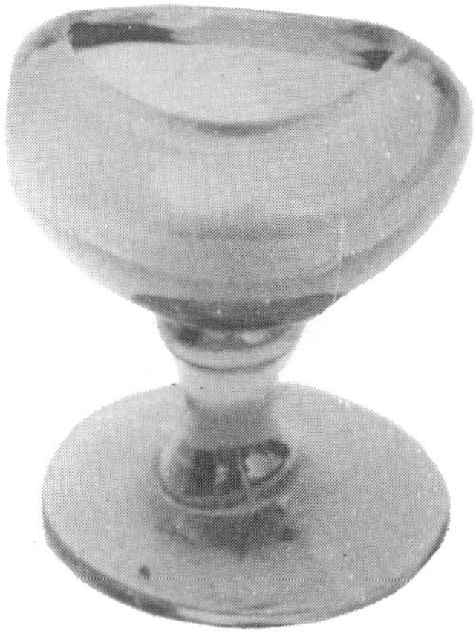

A large bowled blue freeblown eye bath. £15-£20

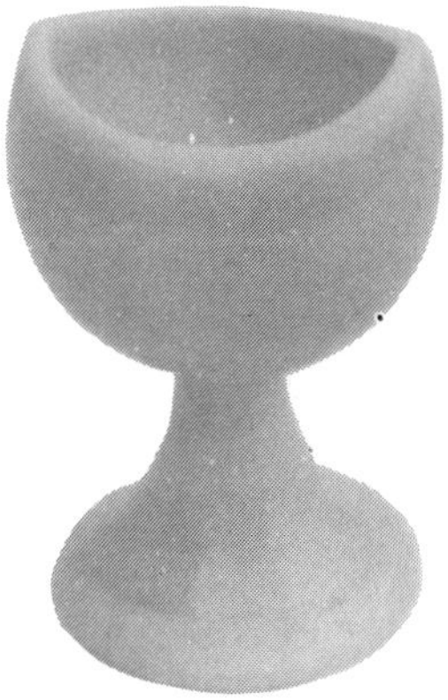

Yellow stemmed stoneware eye bath. £12-£15

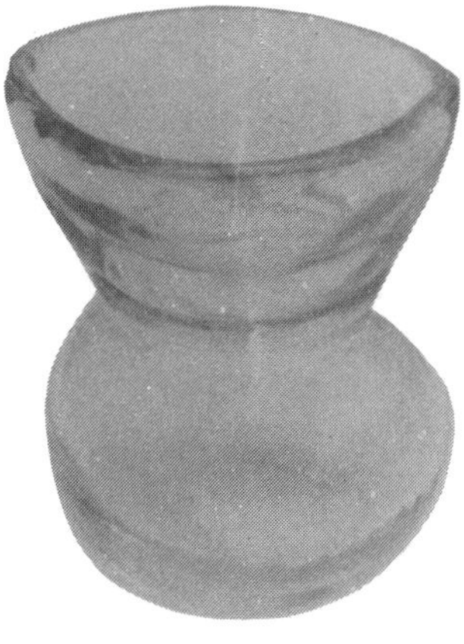

Clear glass cottage-loaf eye bath with reservoir. £2.50-£3

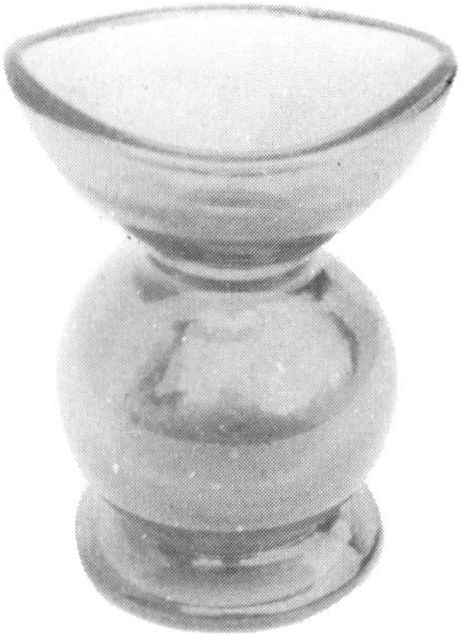

Blue glass eye bath with reservoir and foot. £25-£30

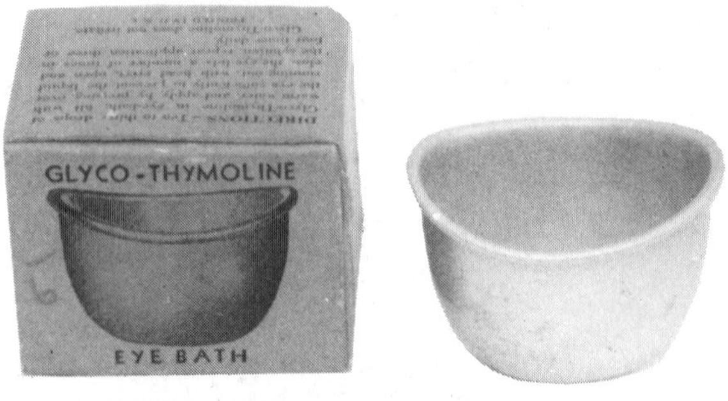

Aluminium squat eye bath by Kress & Owen, with original box. £8-£12

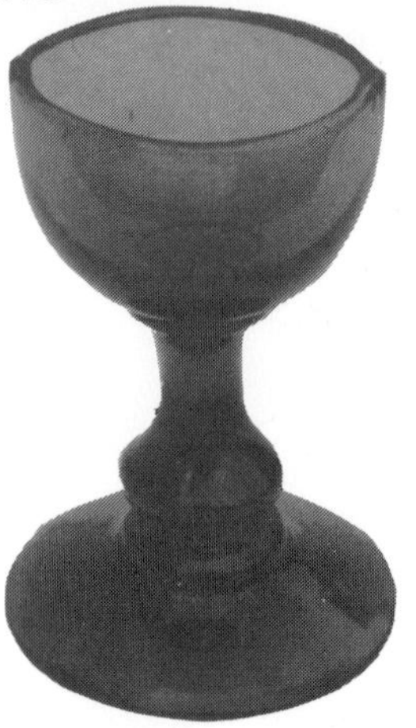

An early green freeblown eye bath with embellished stem. £20

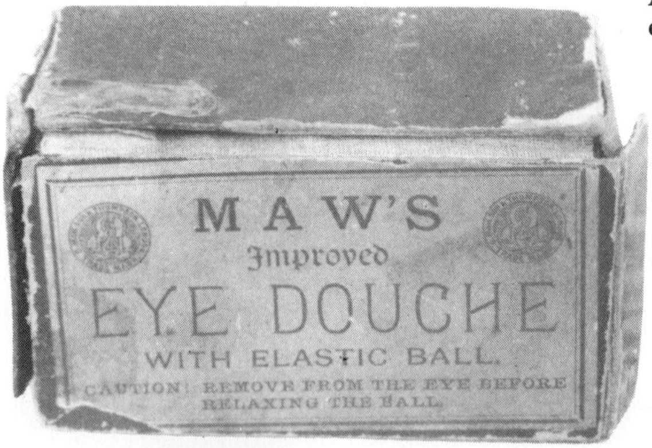

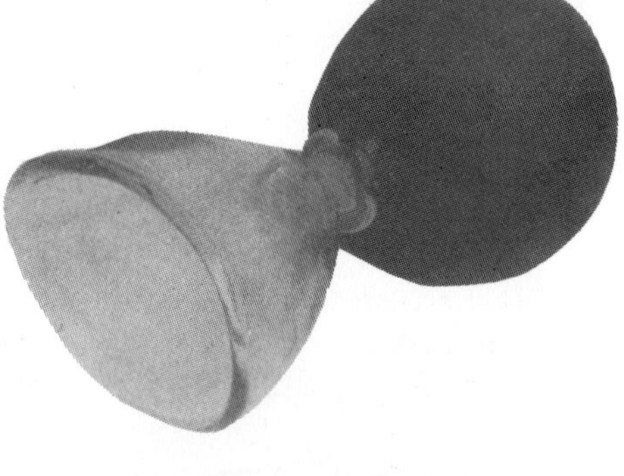

Maw's Eye Douche with rubber ball. £15-£20

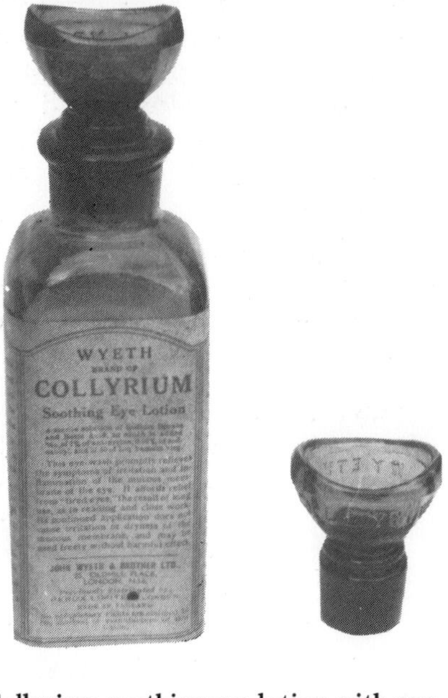

Wyeth Collyrium soothing eye lotion with eye bath stopper. £25-£30

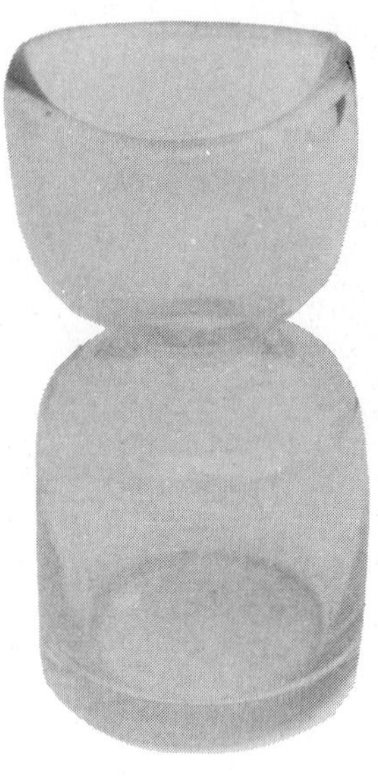

Clear waisted glass eye bath. £5

Peter F. Cook is the director of a building company and collects cheese labels.

"There are now only about a dozen people in this country collecting cheese labels seriously although it was very popular in the '50's. After that interest declined but it has recently been showing signs of reviving. However it's a very popular hobby abroad, particularly in Poland and Czechoslovakia.

"We call cheese label collecting Fromology and I got the craze at school in the 1950's — I began swapping with other collectors and spent all my pocket money buying cheese.

"Now I specialise in triangular cheese labels because I think they're more attractive than other shapes and I like to collect a specific item. My collection of 10,500 labels are kept in loose leafed albums and they date back to pre-war times.

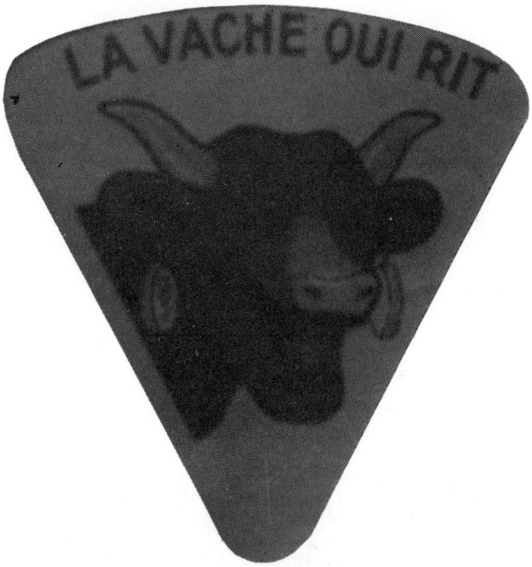

French 'BEL' laughing cow label with a red head on a white background, produced in the 1950's.

"I began with Swiss Tiger labels and now my collection covers 30 countries. A lot of them are from Switzerland but I also have labels from New Zealand and Australia, USA, Canada, Israel, Turkey, quite a lot from Russia and some from Italy where labels are particularly attractive. It's difficult to date them but many of mine go back to pre-war times and if you show them to older housewives they are able to remember buying them in chain stores."

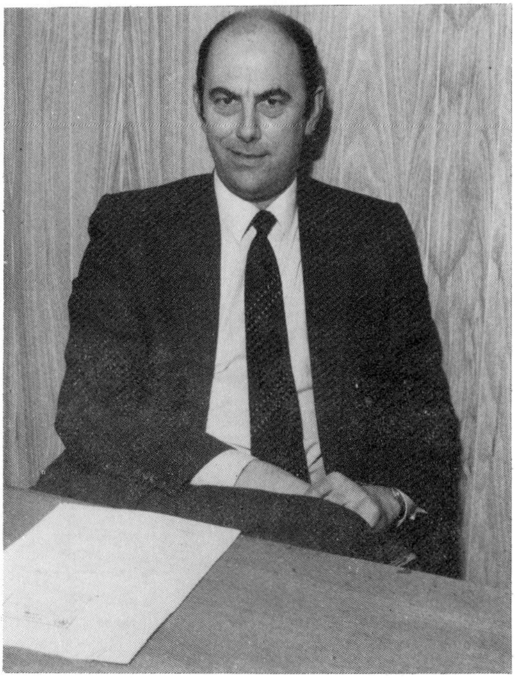

Among the interesting examples Peter owns are Italian labels with insets of animals and insects which were issued in the late 1940's and a number of sets issued by a Swiss firm called Tiger which had a sales promotion drive in the 1950's. Some of these Tiger label sets are very rare today. It is difficult to put a price on labels but on average they range between 10p and £5 each according to rarity.

Peter corresponds and swaps with 20 other collectors in Europe including a man in Switzerland who has 92,000 labels. What he is most anxious to find are labels to complete his collection of an Italian series which shows members of the national football team. Each one had a photo of a different player and there were 3 sets of 13. Peter has ten of one set and is looking for the missing three.

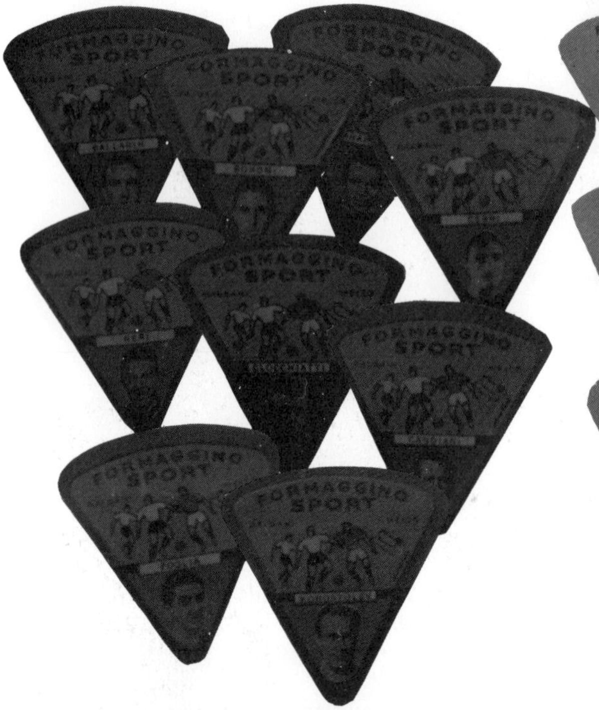

Part of three Italian sets of early post war labels possibly depicting the national side in red, green and blue with a yellow central panel.
£2 each label

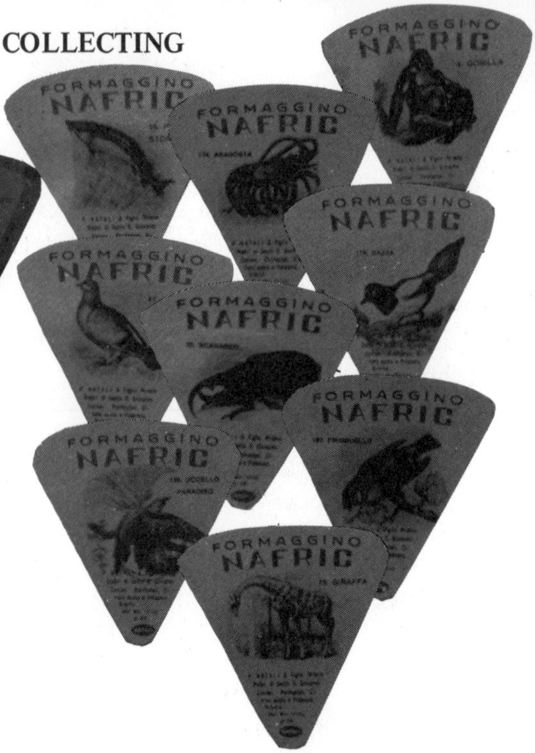

Part of a set of Italian early post war labels depicting animals and insects in full colour.
£2 each label

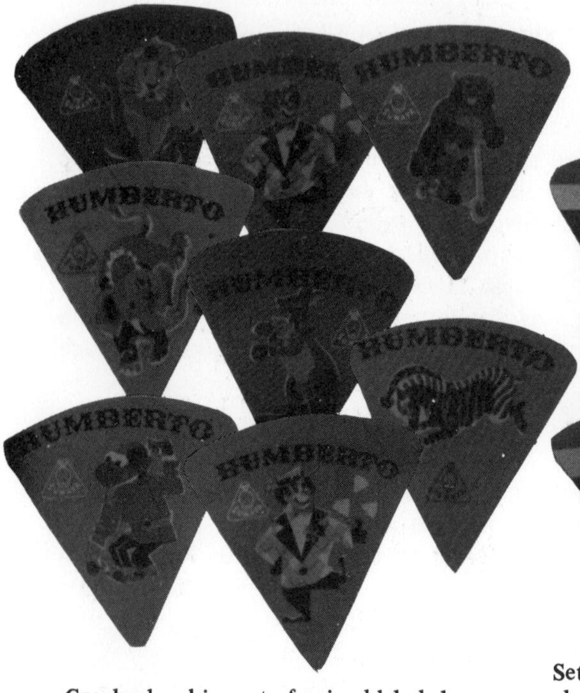

Czechoslovakian set of animal labels by Humberto.
20p per label

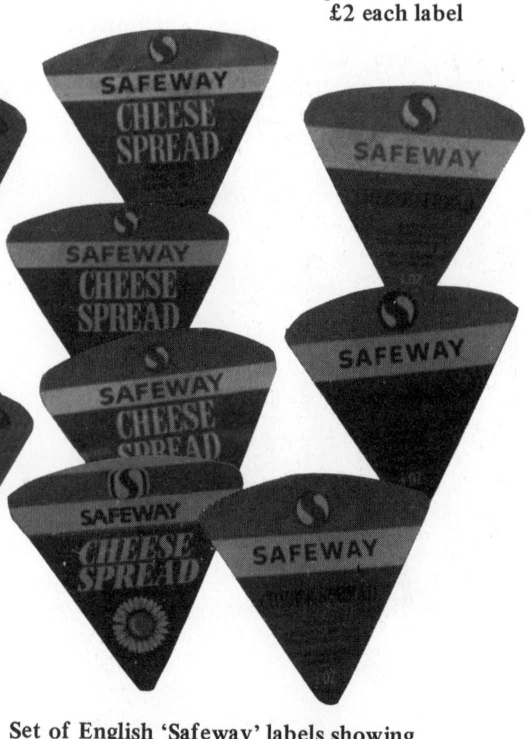

Set of English 'Safeway' labels showing changes of presentation, weight and description over the years.
10p – 50p per label

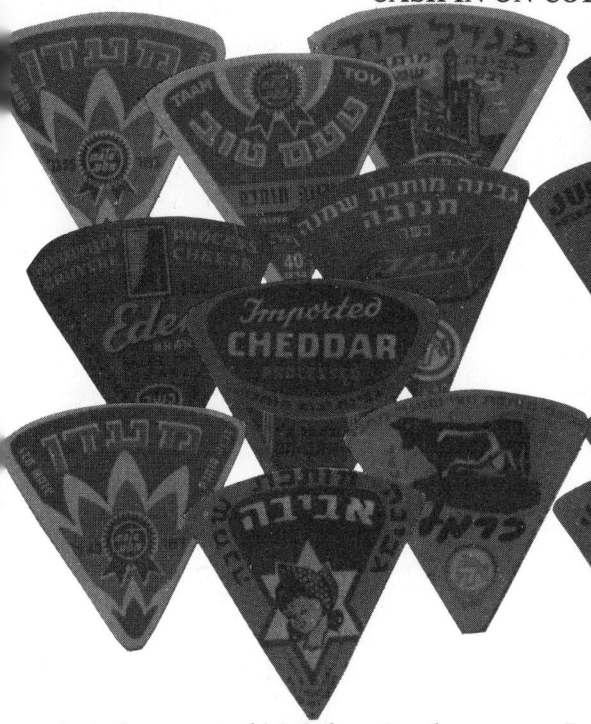

Part of a rare set of labels from Israel.
£1 per label

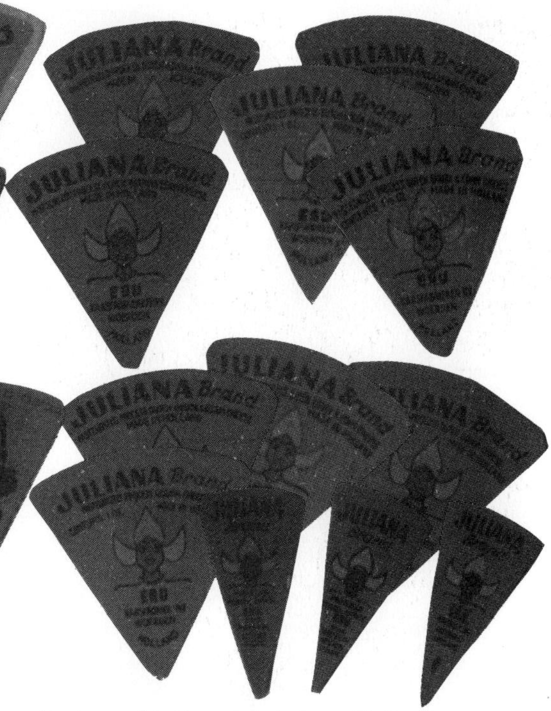

Part set of Juliana labels from Holland.
10p – 50p per label

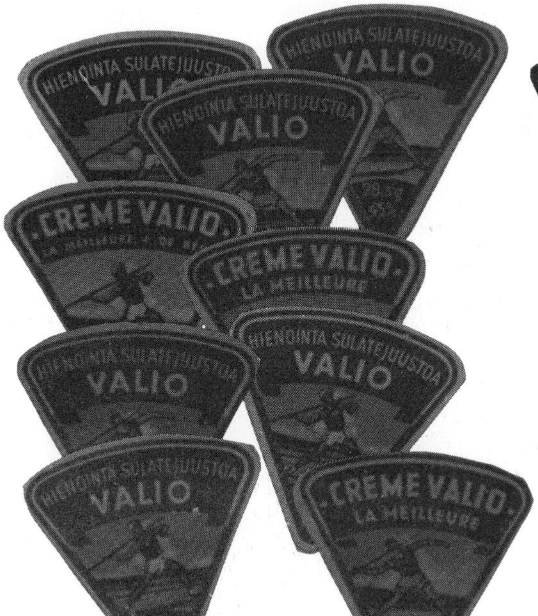

Part set of 'Valio' labels from Finland showing minor changes of weight, printing and design, over the years. 10p – 50p per label

Part set of 'Swiss Knight' cheese labels of 12 portion size, labels are generally of 6 portion size but some manufacturers produce 8 and 12 portion boxes. 10p – 20p per label

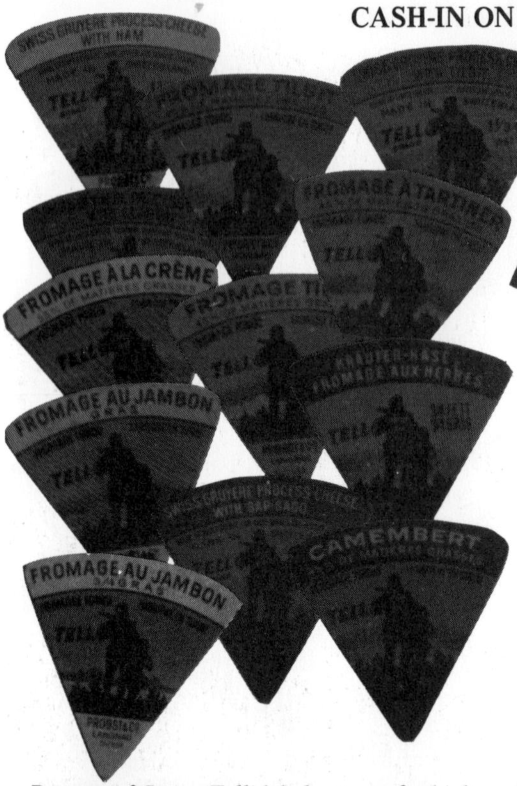

Part set of Swiss 'Tell' labels most of which were produced in the 1940's and 50's.
20p – 50p per label

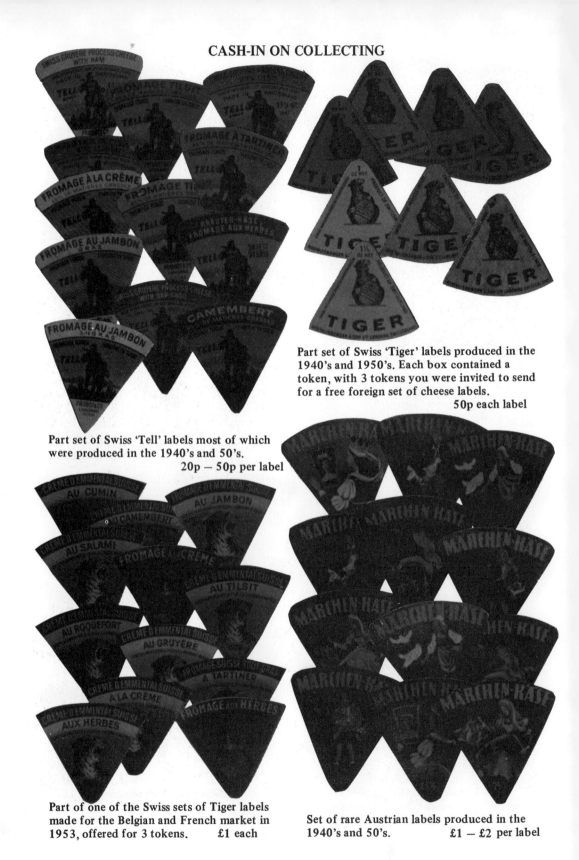

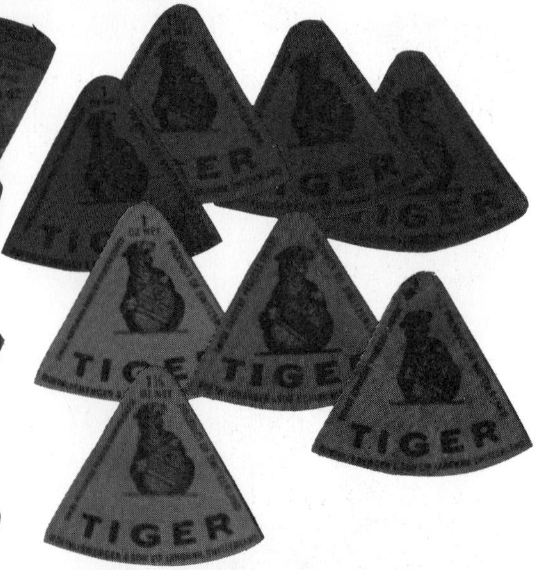

Part set of Swiss 'Tiger' labels produced in the 1940's and 1950's. Each box contained a token, with 3 tokens you were invited to send for a free foreign set of cheese labels.
50p each label

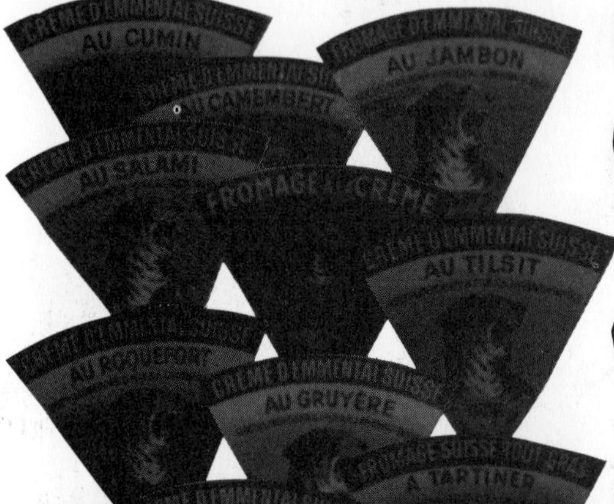

Part of one of the Swiss sets of Tiger labels made for the Belgian and French market in 1953, offered for 3 tokens. £1 each

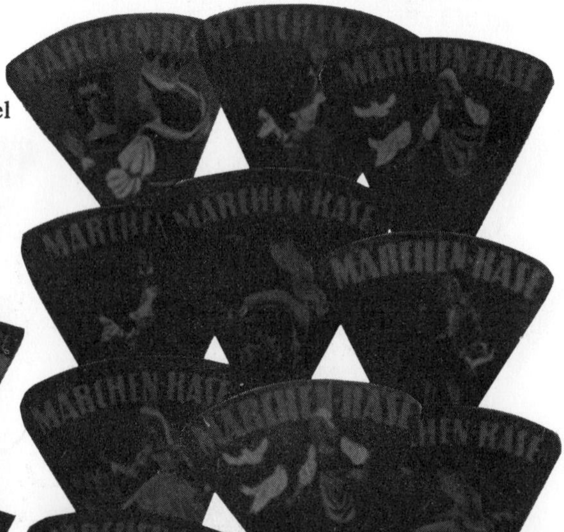

Set of rare Austrian labels produced in the 1940's and 50's. £1 – £2 per label

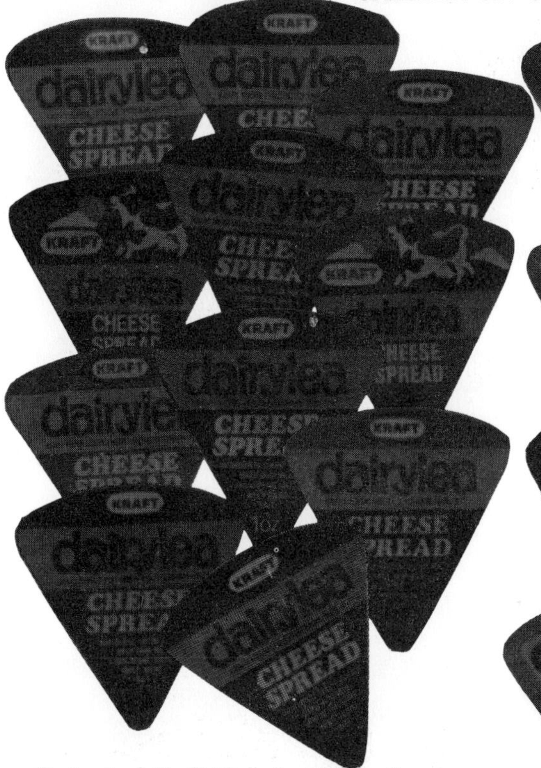

Part set of Kraft 'Dairylea' labels showing changes in design over the years.
10p – 20p per label

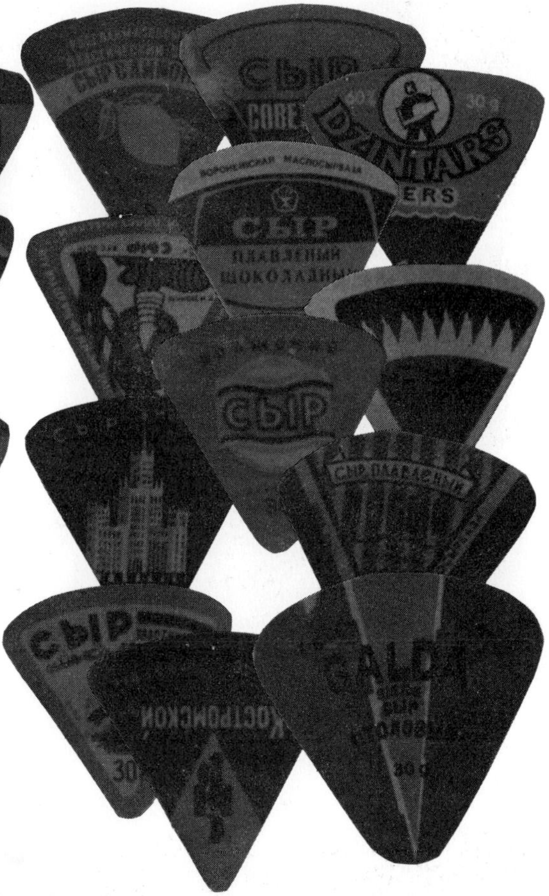

Set of mixed Russian labels, some quite rare.
50p – £2 per label

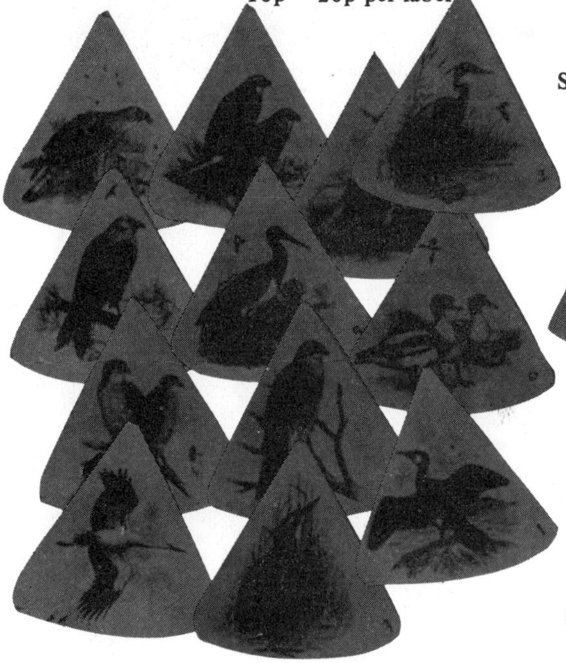

Part set of fifty Belgian animal labels from the 1980's. 20p each label

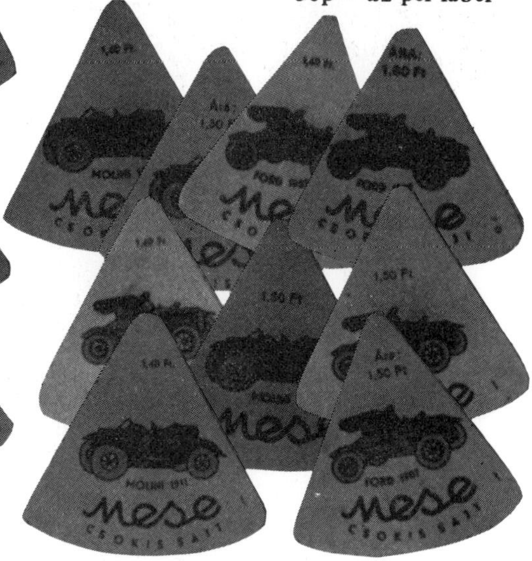

Part set of Hungarian car labels with a variety of weights and designs. 20p – 50p each

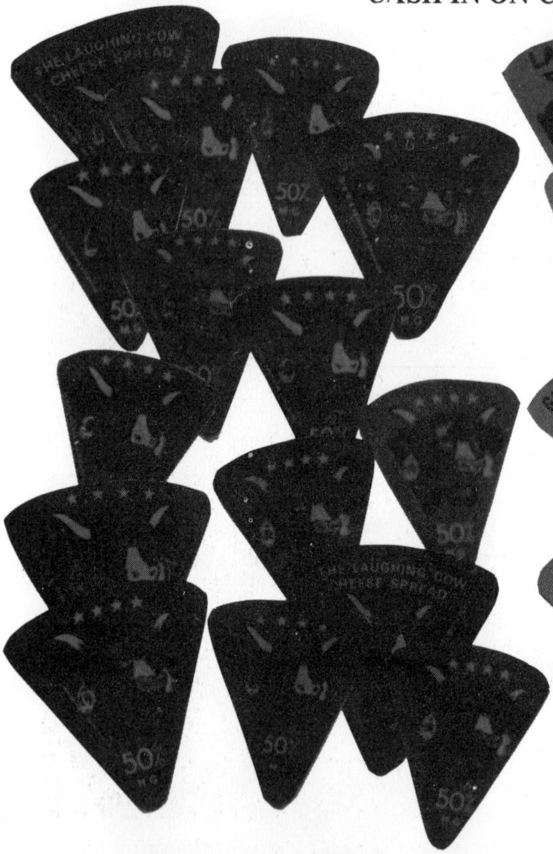

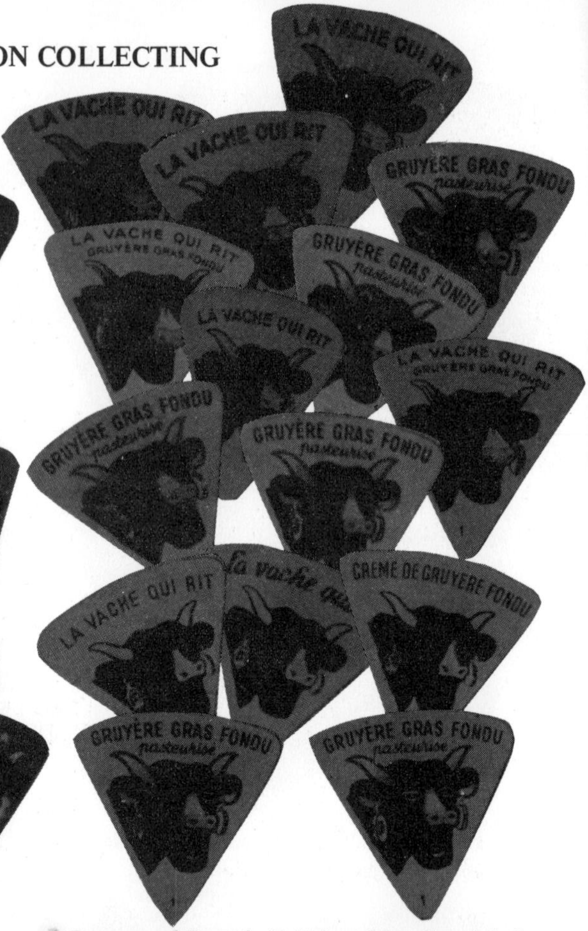

Part set of French 'Bel' Laughing Cow labels produced in the 1940's and 50's showing a variety of weights and designs with red head on a blue background. 50p – £2 per label

Part set of French 'Bel' Laughing Cow labels produced in the 1940's and 50's, with a red head on a white background. £1 – £5 per label

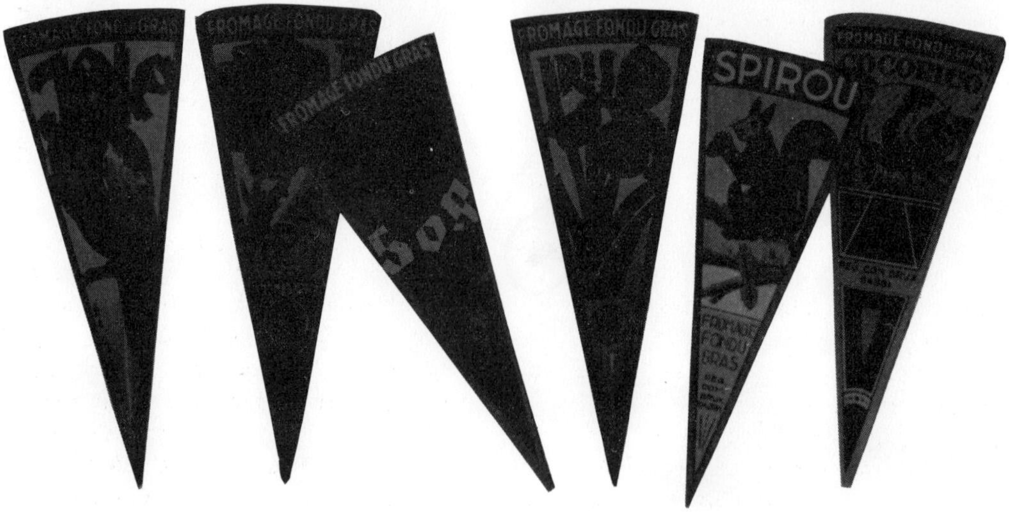

Set of colourful large labels produced in Belgium and France. £1 – £4 per label

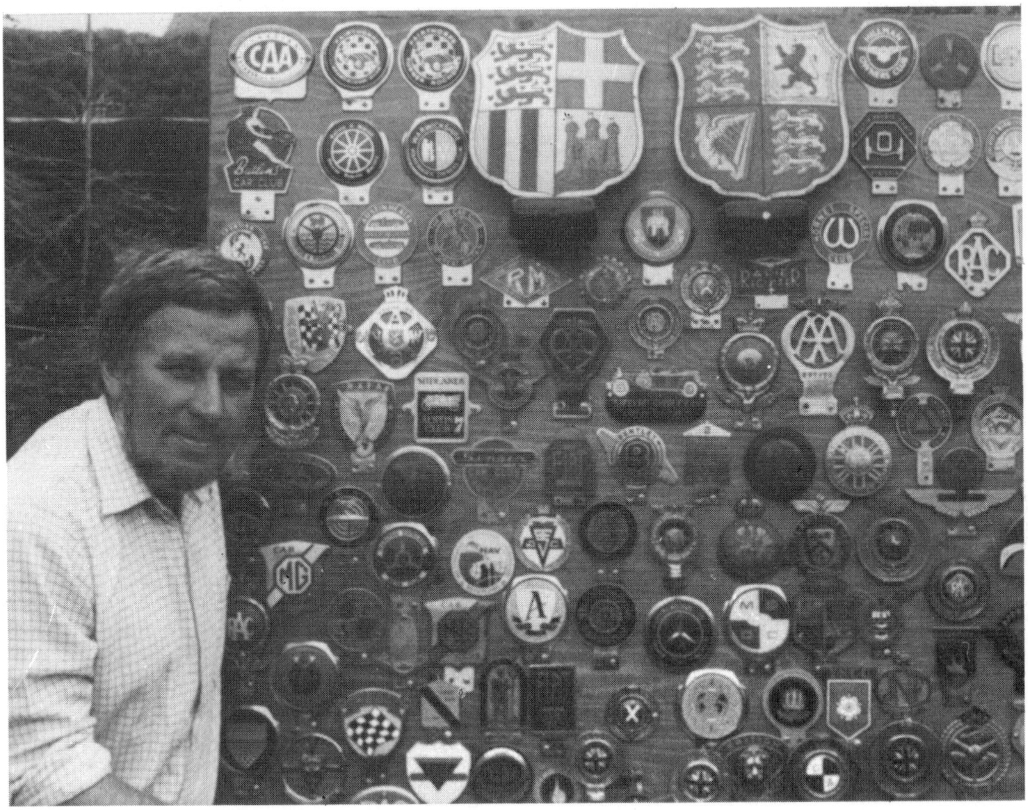

Brian Swann works as a maintenance electrician at the Peugeot Talbot Works and collects car club badges.

"What people don't realise, and what I didn't realise myself when I started, is that there were hundreds of car clubs, especially in the period between 1930 and the 1950's when there were clubs for almost every make of car; towns had their own motoring clubs and universities and different firms had them as well.

"I've got 260 different examples and now I restrict myself to British ones because there were so many clubs on the Continent and in America that the field would be too vast.

"It began with me because I was interested in vintage cars — I still run a 1934 Singer in fact — and paid 10p for an old car badge that I thought would look good on the bumper. No one wanted them at that time but recently there's been a big upsurge because of the interest in collecting vintage cars and people buy them to decorate their cars."

One of the oldest car clubs is the AA which began in 1905 and which has produced many different designs of badges since 1911. The RAC goes back to 1907 when their badges first appeared. The early ones were made of brass or nickel, chrome plated and enamelled. A 1911 AA badge costs between £45 and £50 — though Brian bought his for £5 a few years ago.

The favourite badge in his collection is a rare one issued by the Brooklands Automobile Racing Club in the 1920's which is now worth around £300. For a Singer badge for his car, Brian searched for ten years before he succeeded in finding one which cost £60. His ambition is to own a badge for every motoring club in England and he estimates that around 200 of the clubs which were in existence before the war have now disappeared.

The Motor Club Badge is as old as the Motor Car itself. From those early days, the motorist wanted to be identified as belonging to an elite band of priviledged people.

Among the very first motoring clubs to be formed were: The Liverpool Automobile Club 1896 and The Manchester Automobile Club 1899.

During the 1920's and 1930's, hundreds of motoring clubs were formed and it is mainly these club badges that are collected today. Apart from the various car clubs, almost every city, town, country, factory and various other organisations formed their own Motor Club and nearly all of these badges are made from chrome plate and enamel. Find one in good condition today and you have found a badge that is worth considerably more than an example which is chipped and pitted.

The two most popular themes in badge collecting are the A.A. and R.A.C. types. The earliest style of A.A. badge was produced in either brass or nickel and is worth approximately £100 plus. Fifteen different types of A.A. badges exist today.

R.A.C. badges are available in a variety of different metals and in quite a considerable number of different designs but generally, the earlier the badge, the higher the price it commands. The very first badge produced in 1907 is a very rare badge indeed – now worth approximately £300.

Today the choice for the collector is wide and varied with a few themes listed below:

A.A., R.A.C., Car Clubs, Factory Clubs, Caravan Clubs, Regimental Associations and Sporting Clubs.

The pleasure in searching for that elusive Motor Club Badge is beyond words. The difficulty begins when trying to put a price on that badge. Obviously, there already is a market value on Motor Club Badges, but price can vary considerably. A £100 badge in one part of the country may be worth double or even treble in another part.

The collector must really decide whether to collect all that is offered or to specialise. Obviously the more general the badge, the lower the price with specialised badges costing well into three figures. In this group belong the most desirable badges, mainly those associated with the Brooklands Race Track. A few examples are shown below:

1930's Brooklands Automobile Racing Club £250 plus
1930's Brooklands Automobile Racing Club with 120 M.P.H. Badge £700
1930's Brooklands Automobile Racing Club with 130 M.P.H. Badge £900
1930's Brooklands Flying Club £700
1930's Brooklands Aero Club £900
1930's Junior Car Club £50 plus

It is interesting to note that all these badges could be bought some years ago for considerably less!

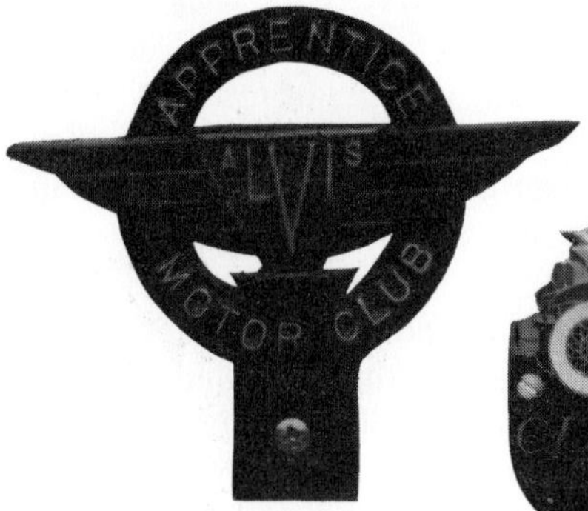

'Alvis Apprentice Motor Club', pressed aluminium, 1950's badge from The Alvis Car Co., Coventry, scarce. £15

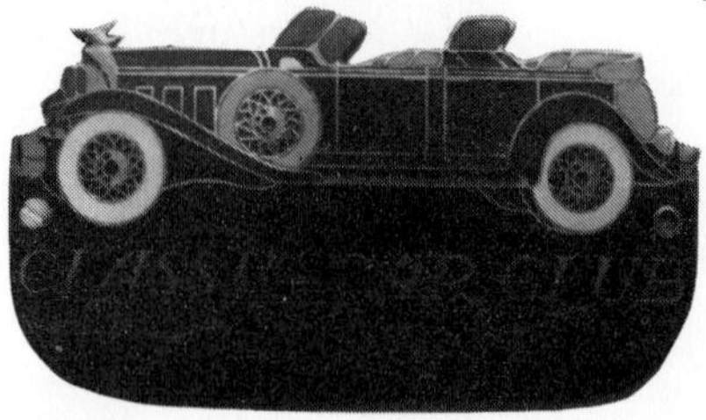

'Classic Car Club of America', Preservation Club from America, chrome and enamel, sought after, modern badge. £30

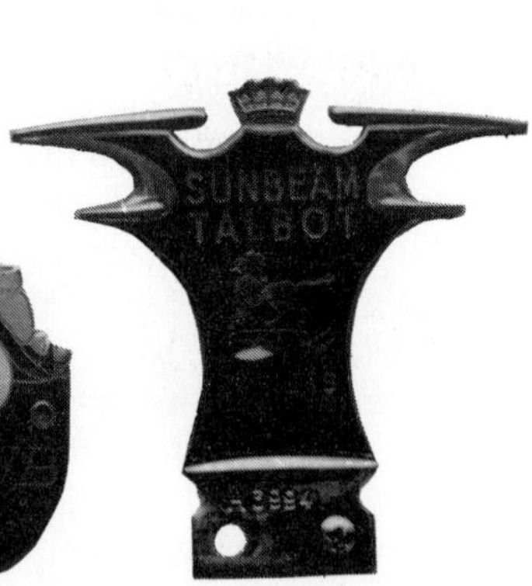

'Sunbeam Talbot Owners Club', works organised owners club, 1950's, chrome/enamel. £20

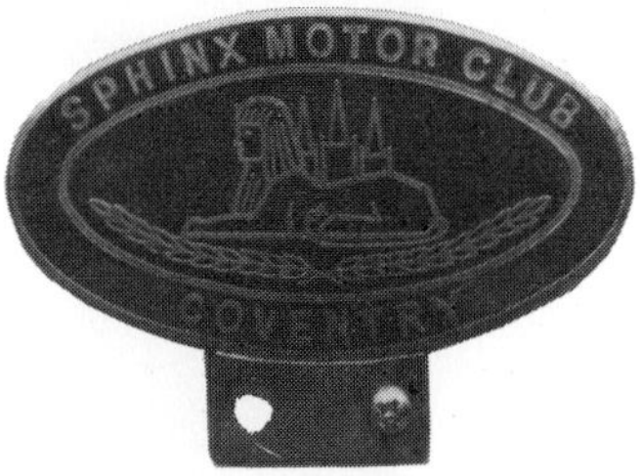

'Sphinx Motor Club', 1950's, Social Club belonging to Armstrong Siddeley Motor Works, Coventry, chrome and enamel, very scarce. £25

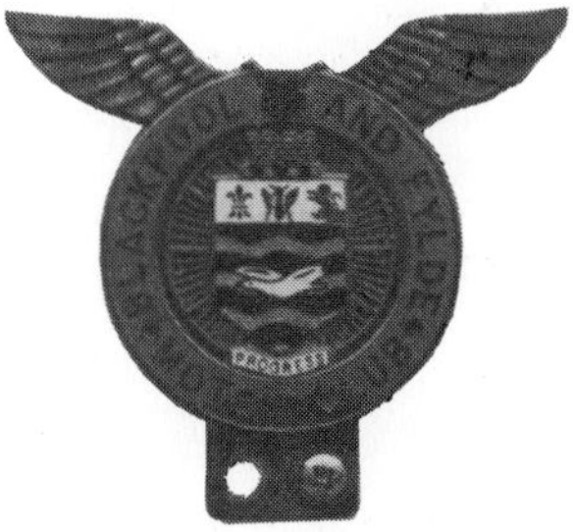

'Blackpool & Fylde Motor Club', very scarce, chrome/enamel, 1930's. £30

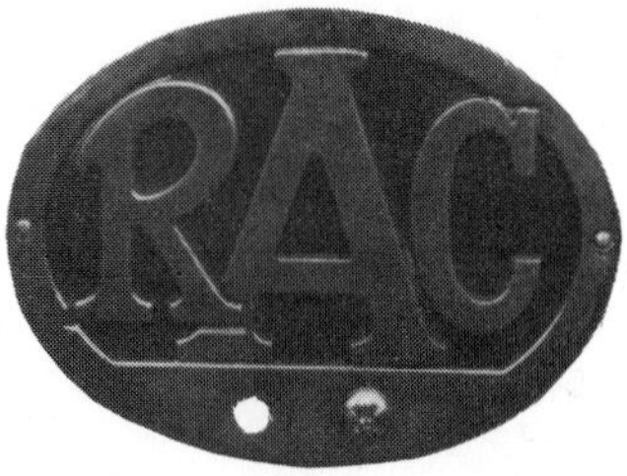

R.A.C. oval shaped, chrome plated, used on private light goods vehicles, 1940's to 1960's, rare. £30

R.A.C. Full Member's badge, flat backed, chrome plated, fairly common, 1950's/1960's. £25

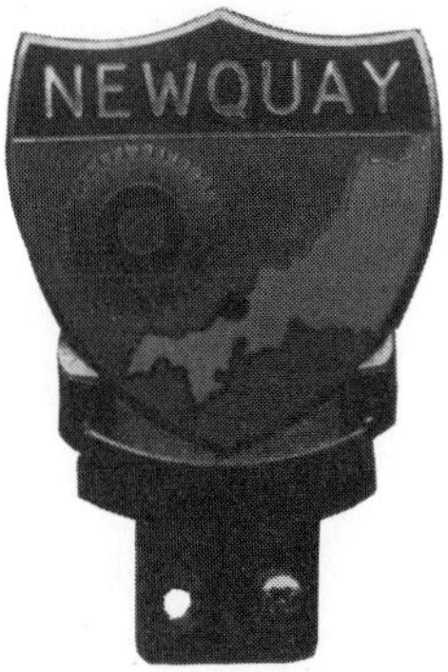

'Newquay Motor Club', modern chrome/enamel badge. £15

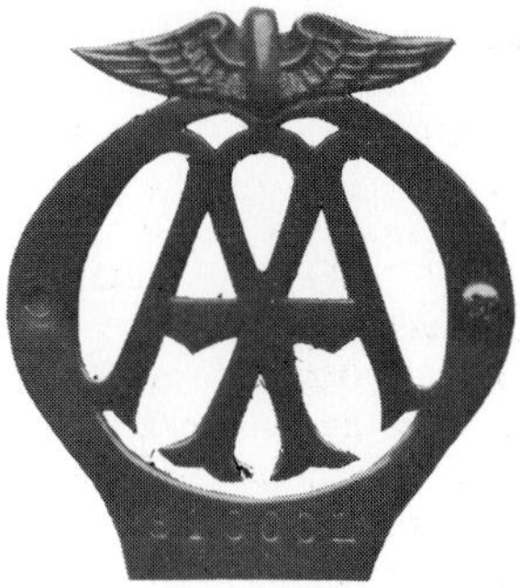

'A.A.', thin type, radiator mounting, fairly common, 1930 to 1939. £20

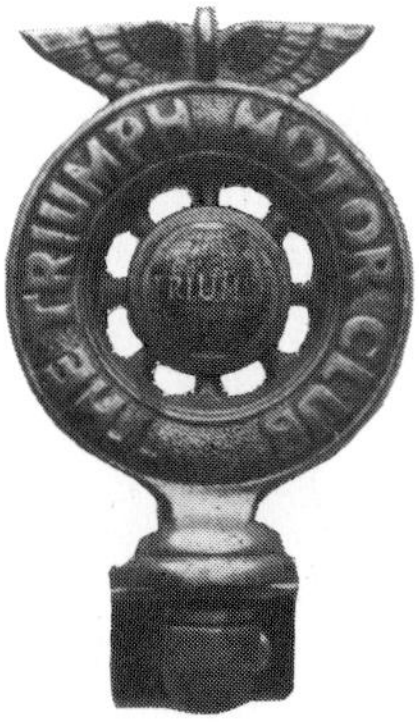

'Triumph Motor Club' very rare chromed 1930's/40's badge, sought after club badge. £50

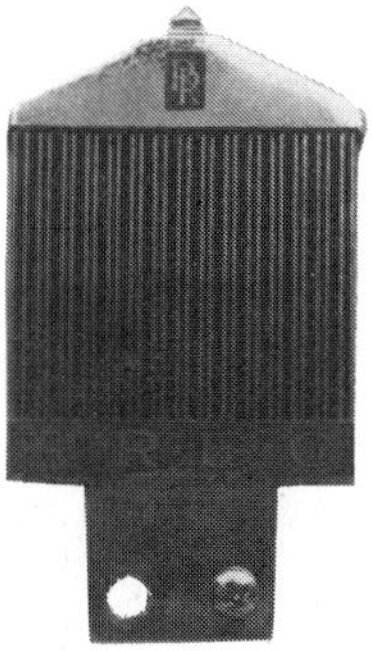

'Rolls Royce Enthusiasts Club', modern club badge, chrome/enamel. £25

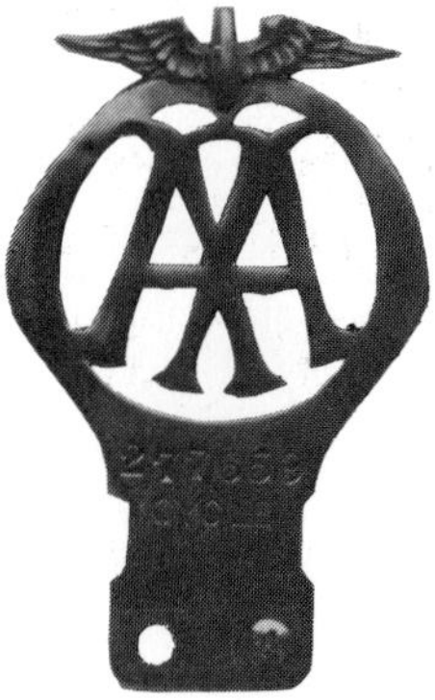

'A.A.' small type, stamped 'Cycle', rare, made 1916 to 1927. £45

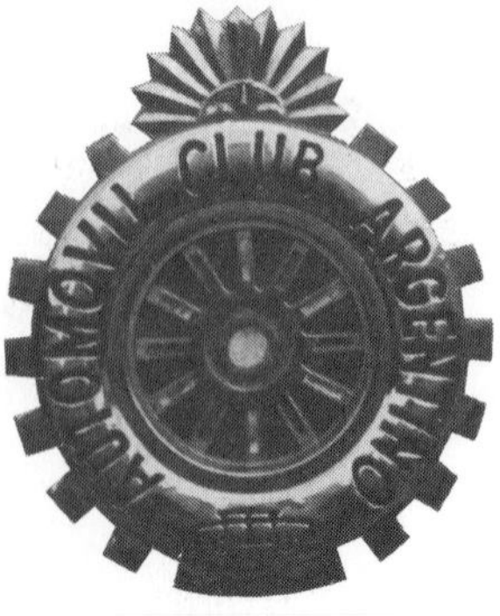

'Automovil Club Argentino' modern brass and chrome badge, National Club of Argentina. £15

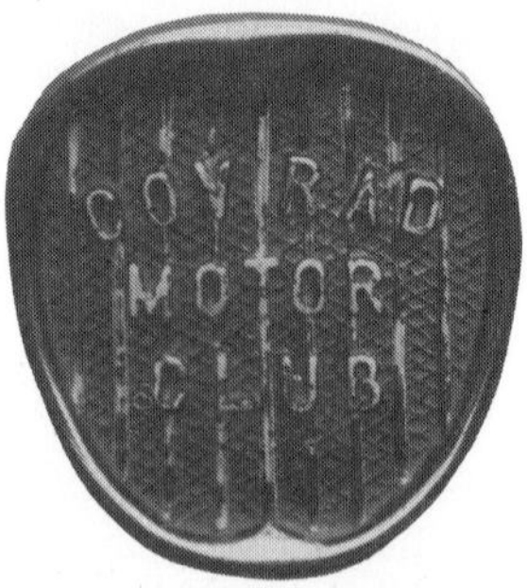

'Cov. Rad. Motor Club', 1950's, chrome badge from the Coventry Radiator Motor Co., Coventry, very rare. £25

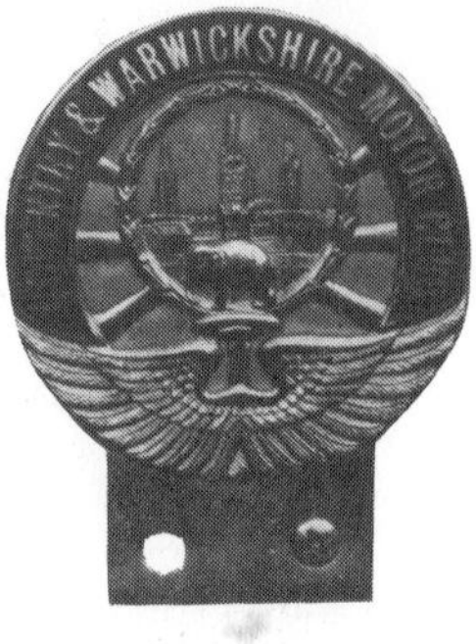
'Coventry & Warwickshire Motor Club', modern badge of an Old Motor Club, chrome/enamel. £15

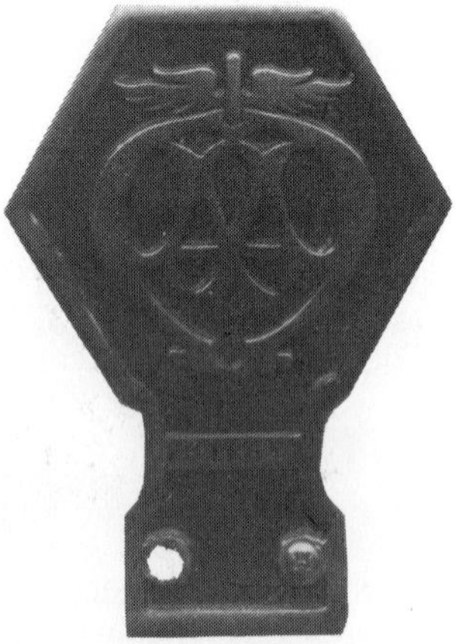
'A.A. Commercial', scarce badge, made between 1911 and 1930, three variations known. £40 – £50

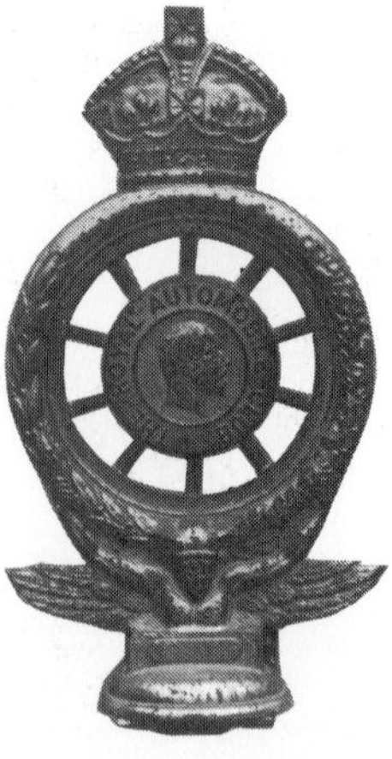
R.A.C. Full Member's badge, King's head to front, Union Jack centre on reverse, scarce, 1930's/1940's. £35

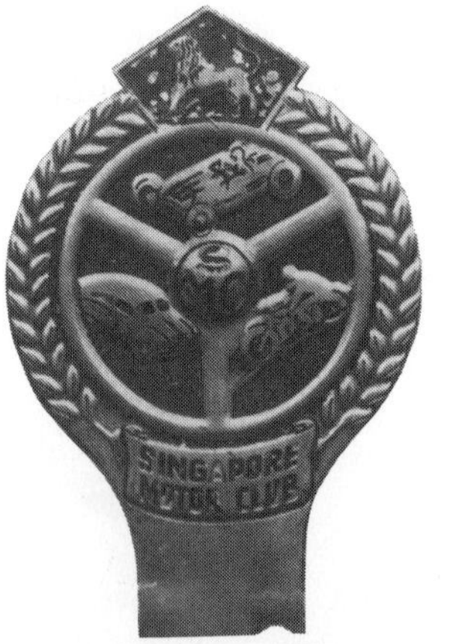

'Singapore Motor Club', 1940's badge, chrome plated, scarce. £35 – £40

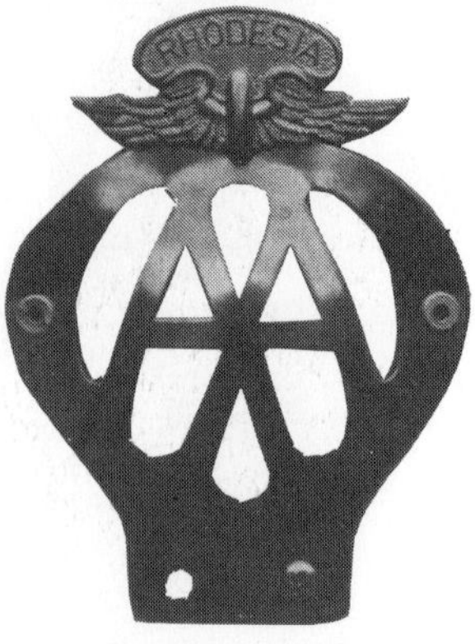

'A.A.', 'Rhodesia', only one badge from a Set of the Commonwealth 1945 to 1967. £20

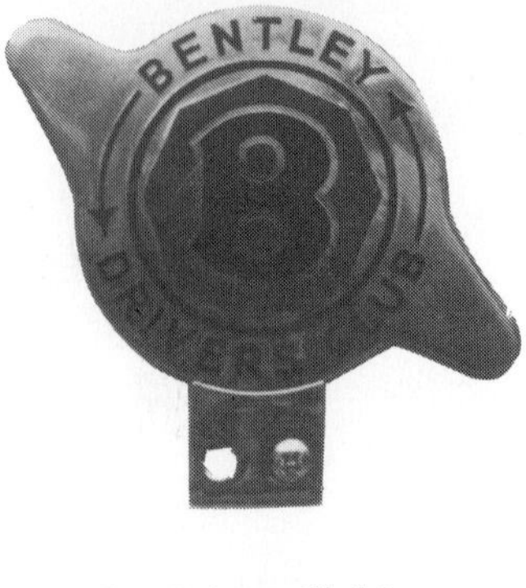

'Bentley Drivers Club', modern club badge, chrome/enamel. £25

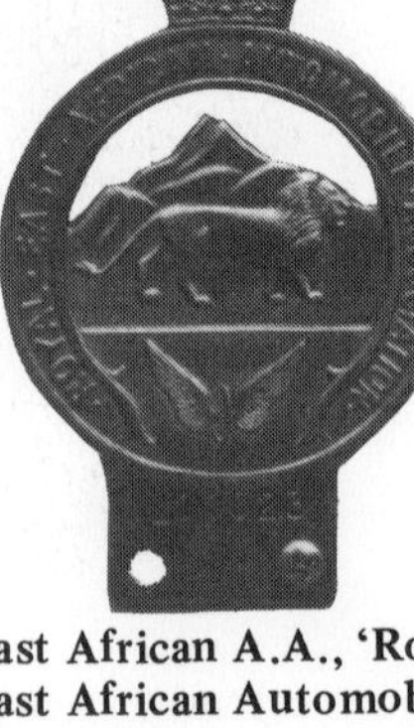
East African A.A., 'Royal East African Automobile Association', chromed 1940's badge, very scarce. £35

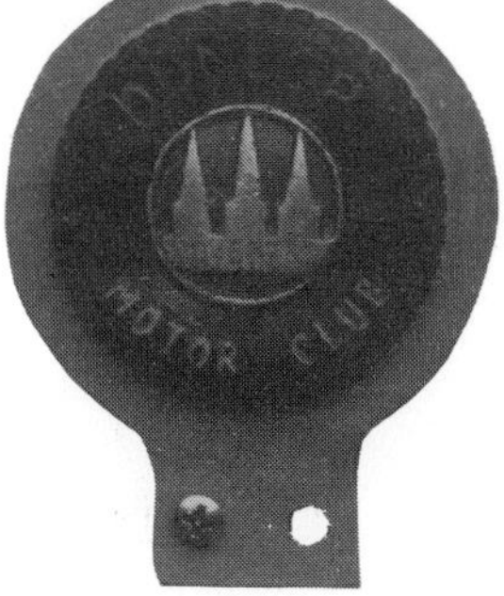

'Dunlop Motor Club', 1950's, Social Club belonging to Dunlop Tyre Co., Coventry, pressed aluminium, rare. £20

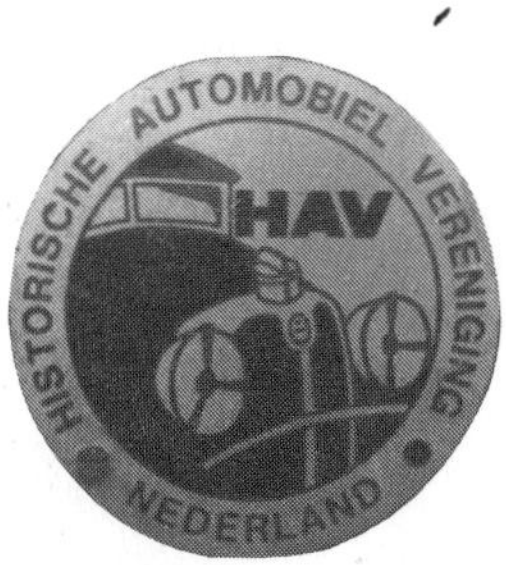

'Historische Automobiel Vereniging Nederland', modern badge, enamel and chrome, Preservation Club from Holland. £25

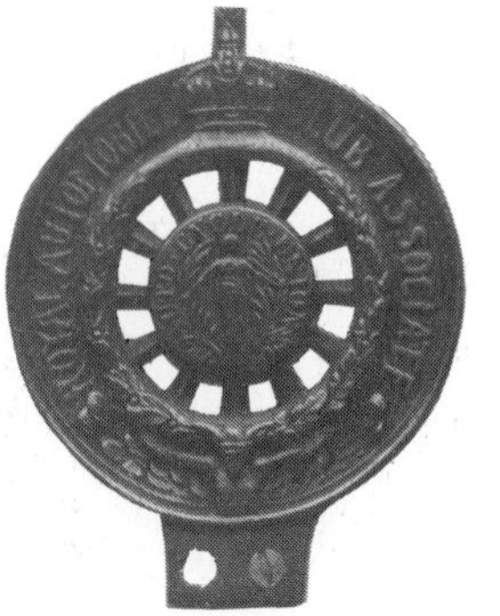

'R.A.C. Associate' small type badge, auto-cycle union centre, nickel plated, very rare. £30

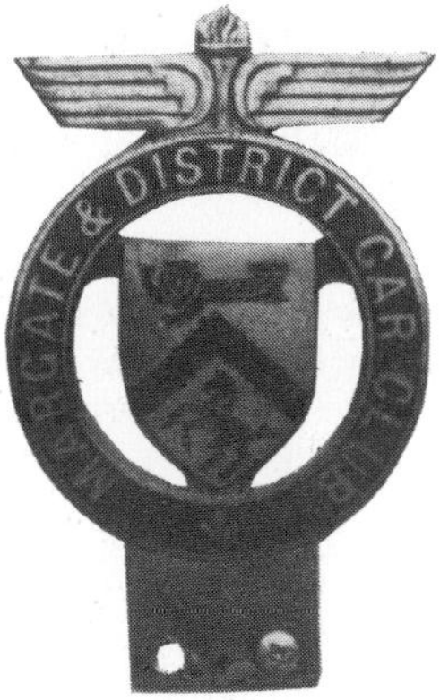

'Margate & District Car Club', very scarce, chrome badge, 1930's. £30

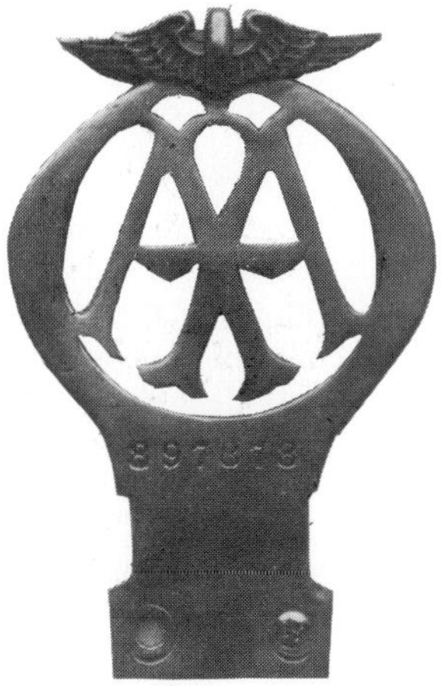

'A.A.' large type, scarce and sought after, made 1911 to 1922. £40 – £50

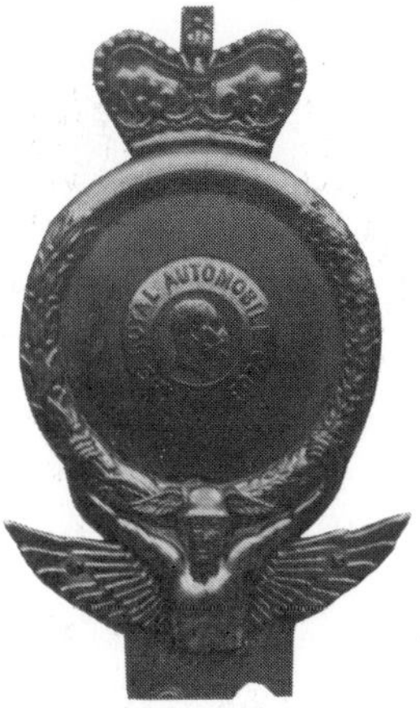

R.A.C. Full Member's badge from the 1960's, blue centre. £20

'A.A. Commercial', fairly common, 1930 to 1967. £15

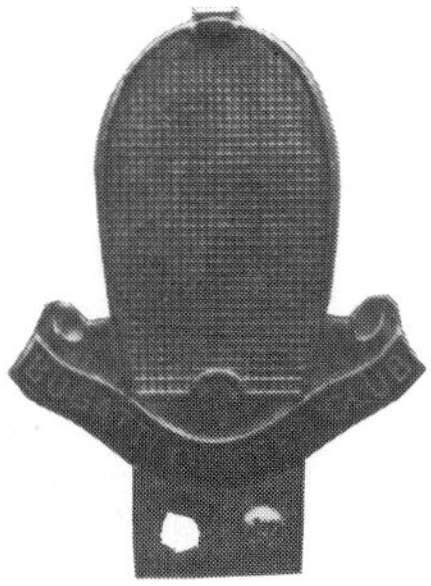

'Bugatti Owner Club', modern club badge, chrome/enamel. £30

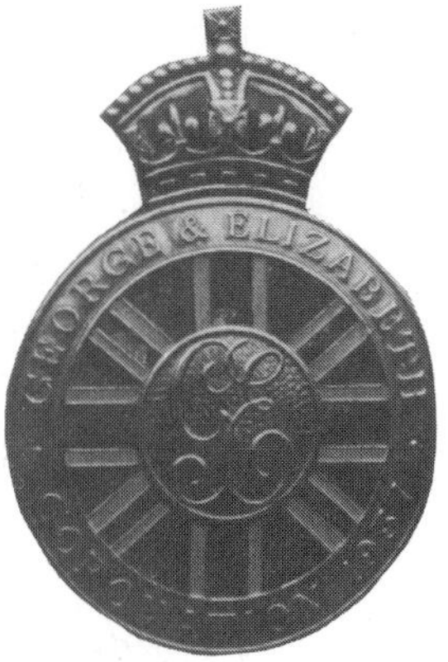

George and Elizabeth, 1937 Coronation badge, chrome/painted, scarce. £20

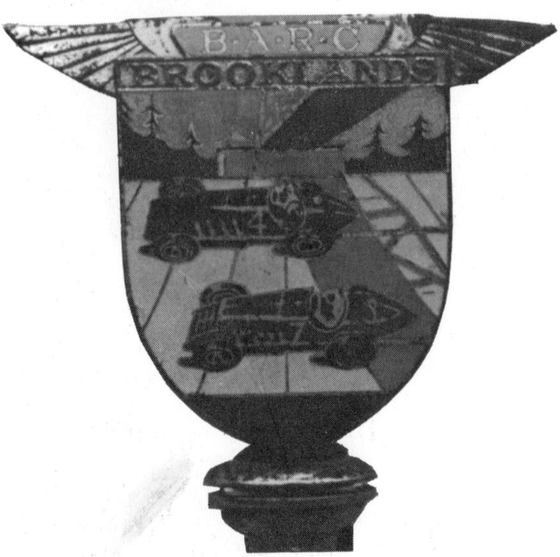

B.A.R.C. 'Brooklands Automobile Racing Club', very rare and sought after 1930's badge, chrome/enamel, all numbered. £250 plus

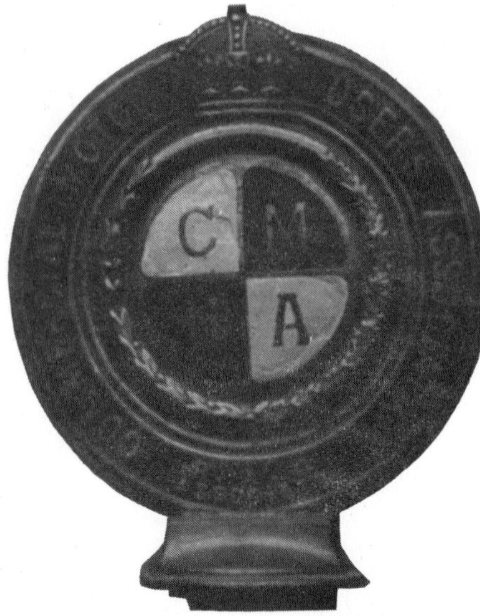

C.M.U.A. 'Commercial Motor Users Association', (RAC Associate Club), 2 types available, very scarce, sought after by owners of commercial vehicles, circa 1919. £50

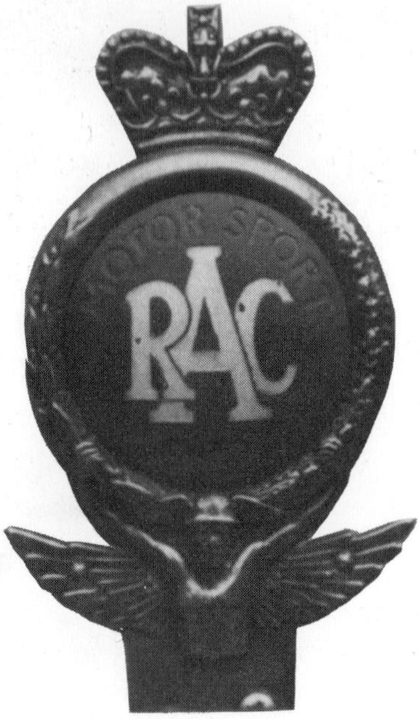

RAC 'Motor Sports Member', 1930's, scarce badge, sought after. £40

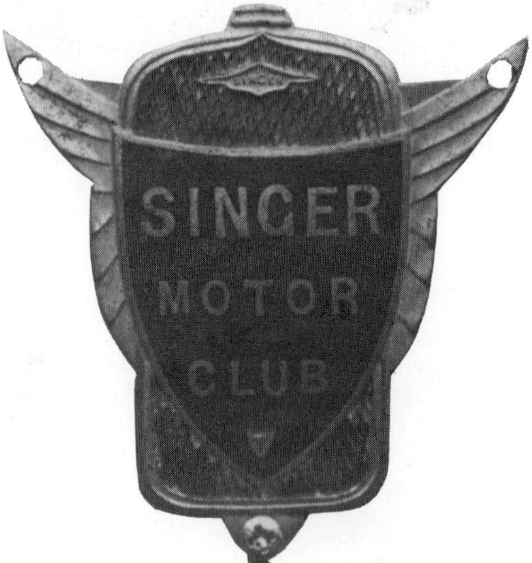

'Singer Motor Club', very rare badge, from 1934/35, less than 10 known. £90

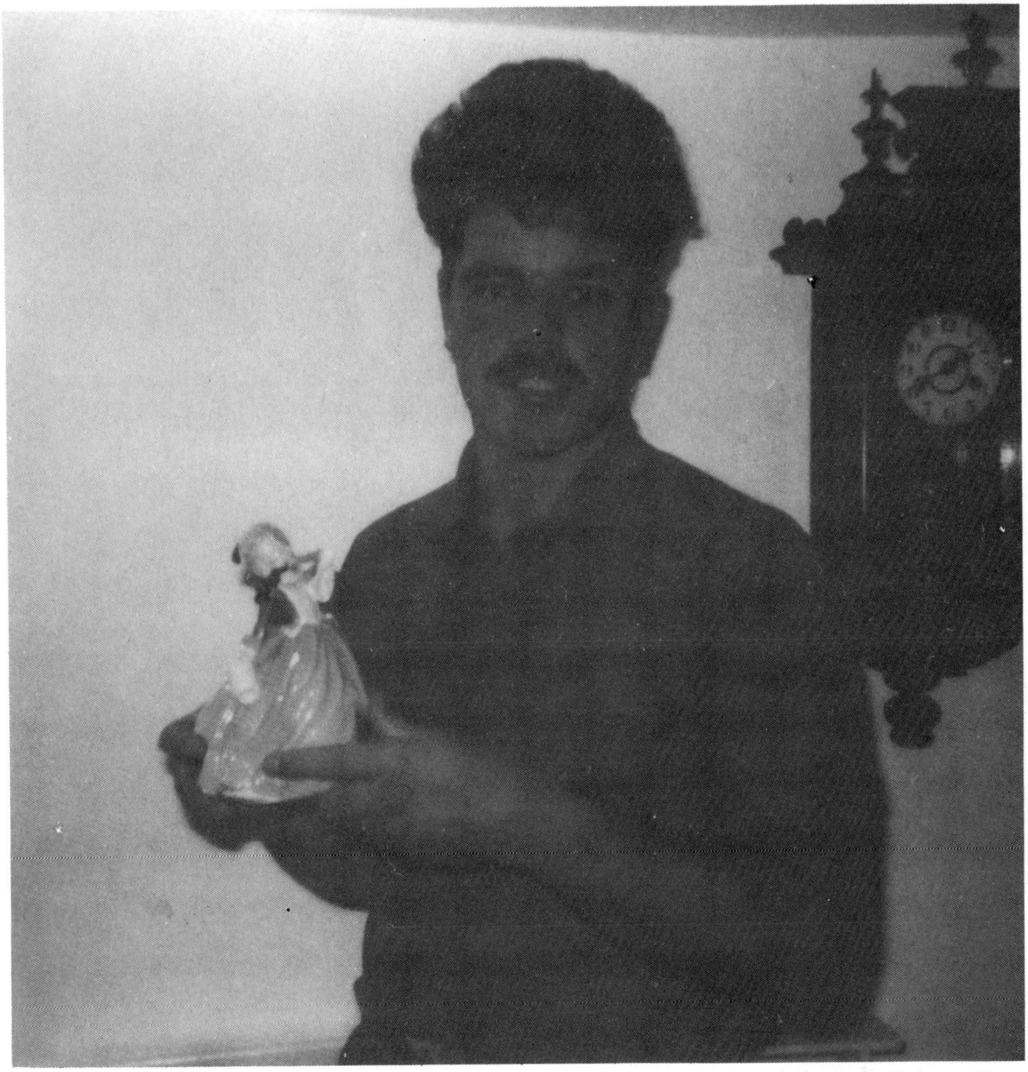

David Cope is a dealer in Doulton and has a fine private collection of Doulton figures.

"One of the presents we got when we were married was a book about the Doulton firm and that started me off really. It began as a hobby and it has become a full time job that takes up at least 70 hours a week.

"A great number of the people who come to me are Americans or Australians and they are now looking for pieces from the Art Deco period up to the 1930's, things such as masks and figures like Harlequinade.

"For myself I also like the wall masks but I'm especially fond of character figures like 'In The Stocks' and 'The Modern Piper'.

"Doulton is still an erratic market because American buyers are out in force when the dollar is standing high against the pound but they are not so eager when it drops. I was recently in New Jersey and was surprised to find that I could buy figurines there cheaper than I can buy them in this country so there is a trend to buy back from America and sell in Britain.

"I would most like to find some of the very rare pilot figures that never went into production. They change hands for prices up to £1,000."

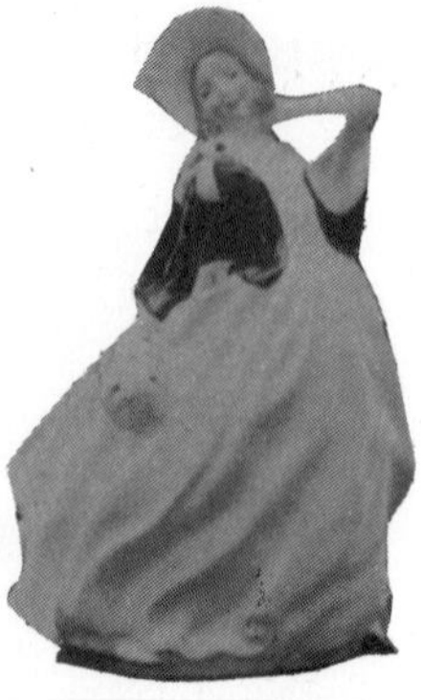

'Autumn Breezes' HN2147, designed by L. Harradine, issued 1955-71, 7½in. high. £125

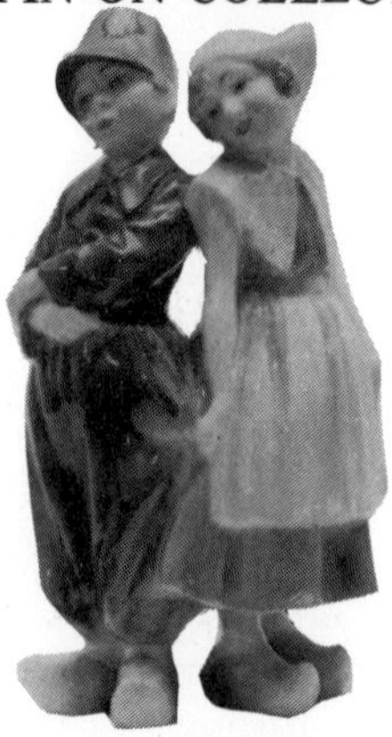

'Willy Won't He' HN1584, designed by L. Harradine, issued 1933-49, 6in. high. £140

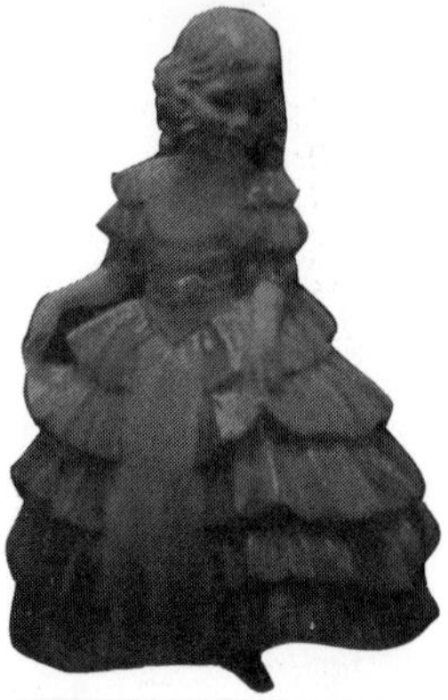

'Rose' HN1368, designed by L. Harradine, issued 1930, 4½in. high. £28

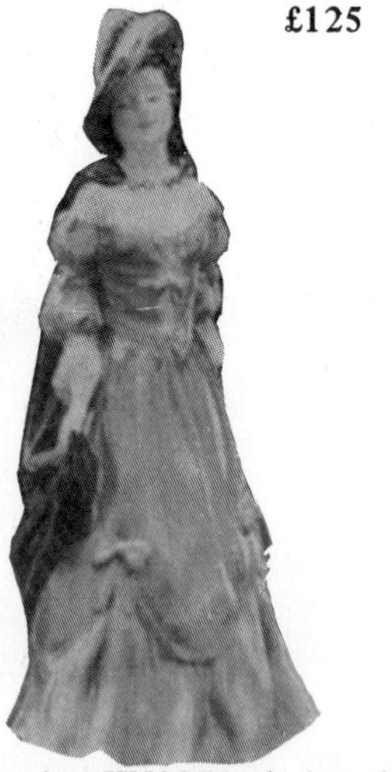

'Bernice' HN2071, designed by M. Davies, issued 1951-53, 7¾in. high. £275

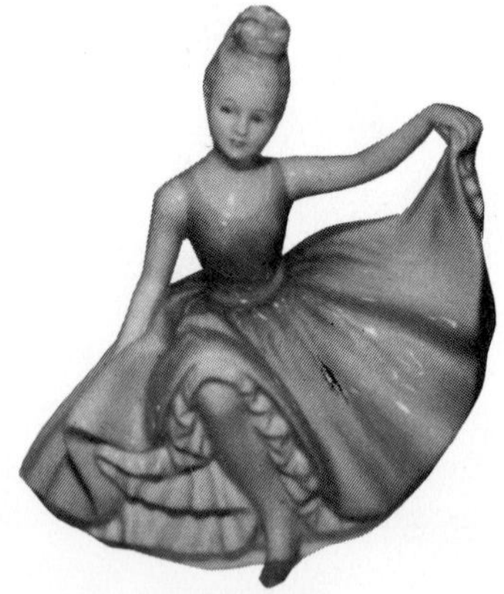

'Dancing Years' HN2235, designed by M. Davies, issued 1965-71, 6¾in. high. £120

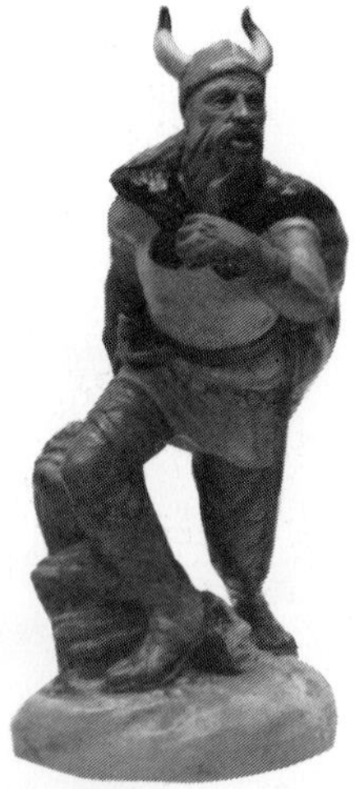

'Viking' HN2375, designed by J. Bromley, issued 1973-76, 8¾in. high. £95

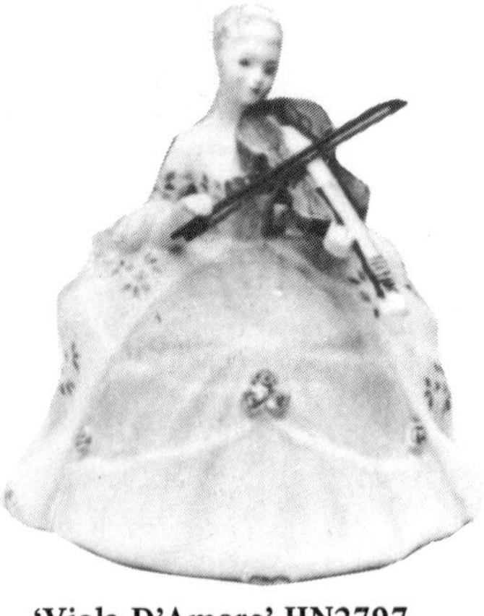

'Viola D'Amore' HN2797, designed by L. Harradine, issued 1976, 6in. high. £300

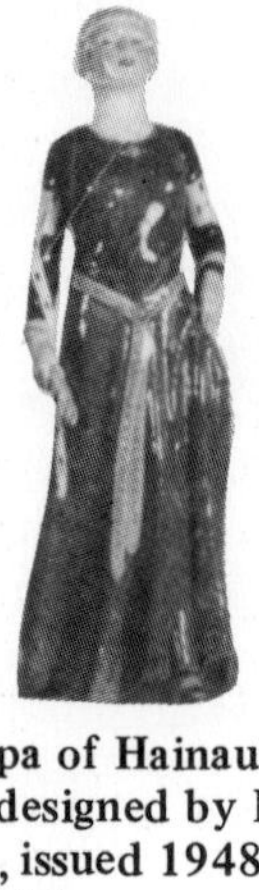

'Philippa of Hainault', HN 2008, designed by M. Davies, issued 1948-53, 9¾in. high. £350

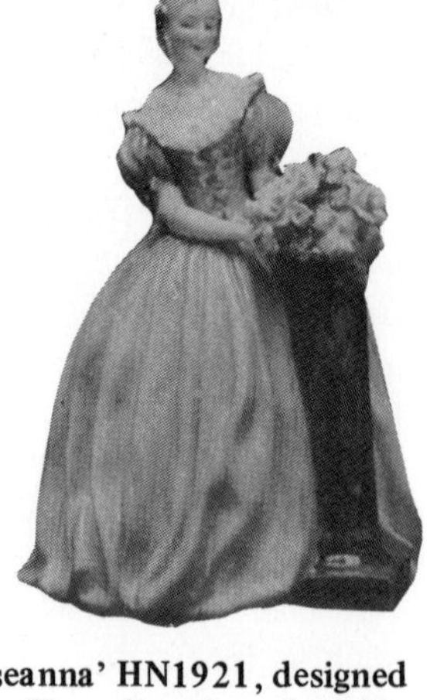

'Roseanna' HN1921, designed by L. Harradine, issued 1940-49, 8in. high. £180

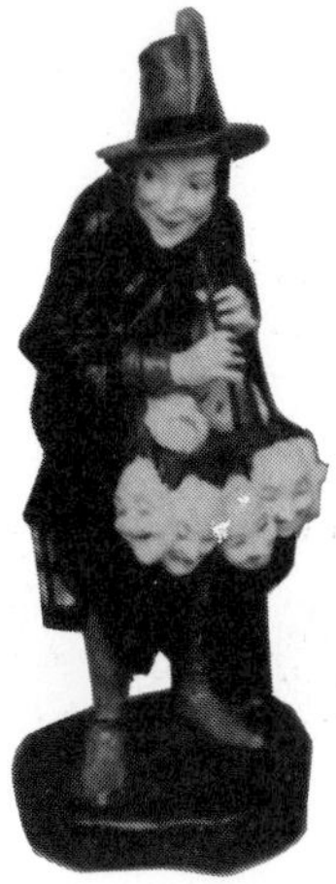

'Mask Seller' HN1361, designed by L. Harradine, issued 1929-38, 8½in. high. £350

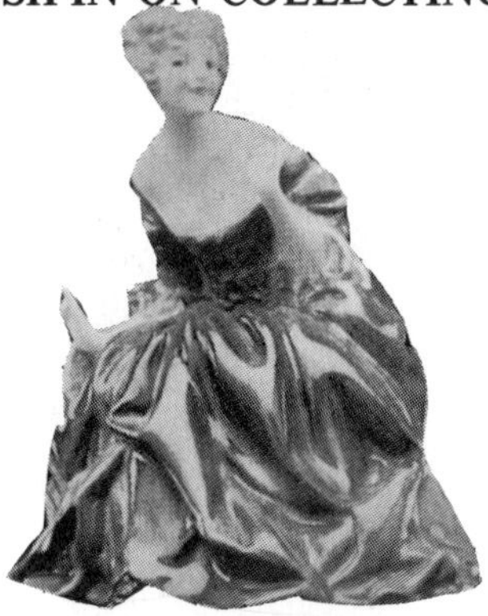

'Lady Fayre' HN1265, designed by L. Harradine, issued 1928-38, 5¼in. high. £225

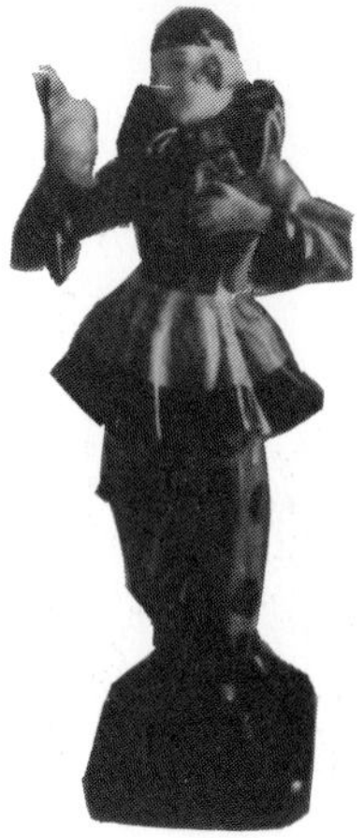

'Mask' HN785, designed by L. Harradine, issued 1926-38, 6¾in. high. £600

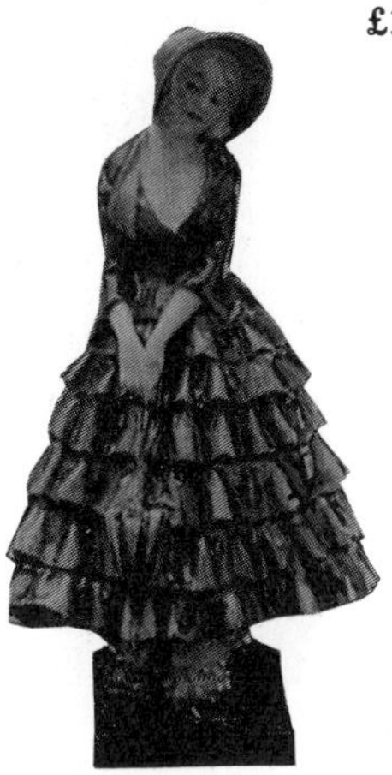

'Priscilla' HN1340, designed by L. Harradine, issued 1929-49, 8in. high. £135

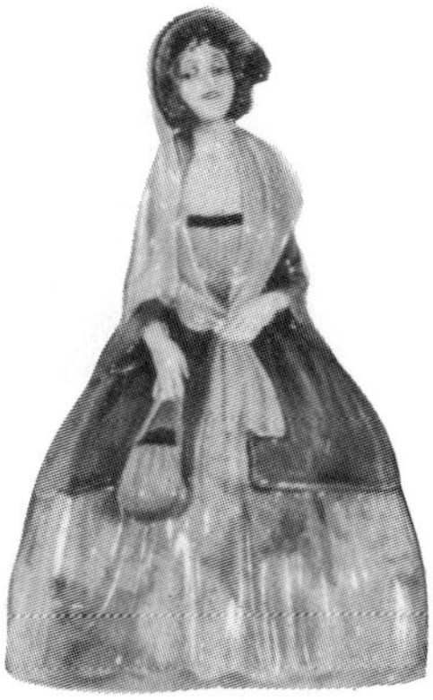

'Sylvia', HN 1478, designed by L. Harradine, issued 1931-38, 10½in. high. £180

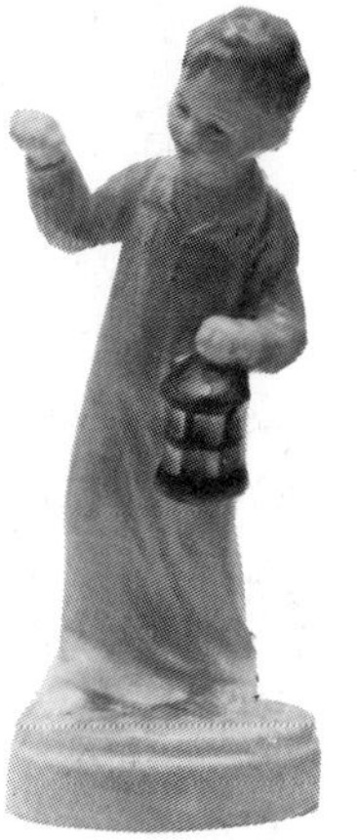

'Wee Willie Winkie' HN2050, designed by M. Davies, issued 1949-53, 5¼in. high. £130

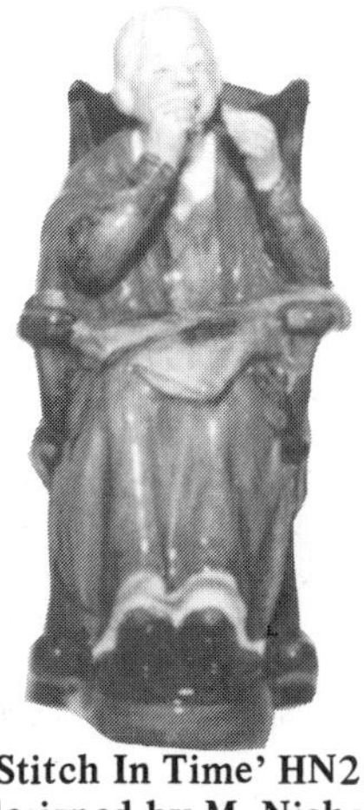

'Stitch In Time' HN2352, designed by M. Nicholl, issued 1966-80, 6¼in. high. £60

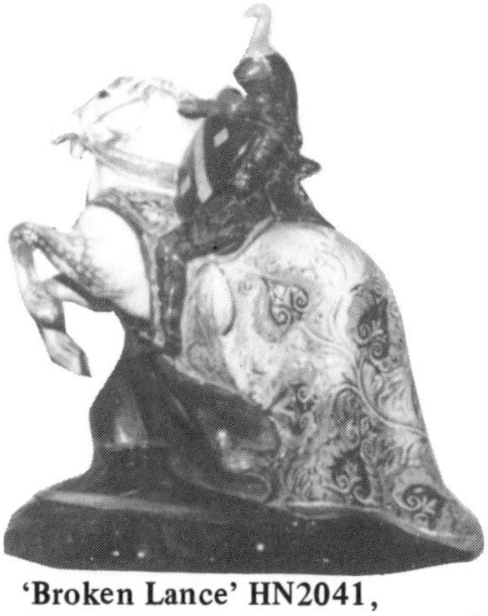

'Broken Lance' HN2041, designed by M. Davies, issued 1949-75, 8¾in. high. £180

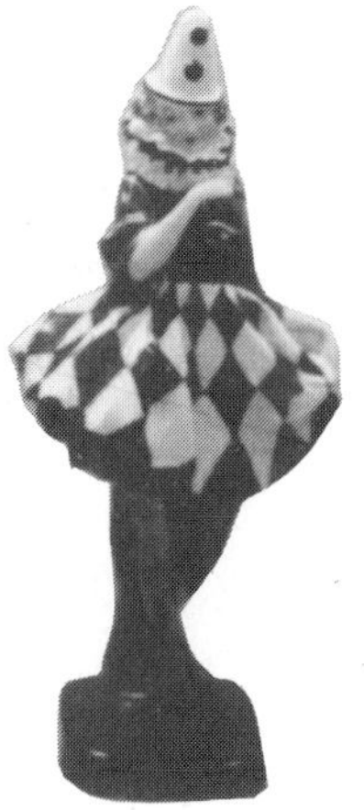

'Pierette' HN643 designed by L. Harradine, issued 1924-38, 7¼in. high. £350

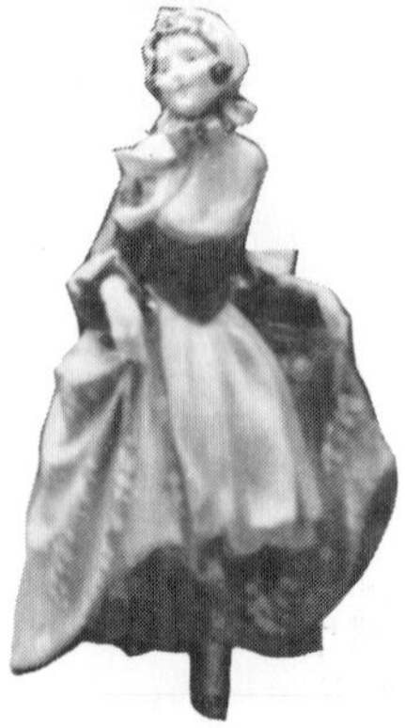

'Suzette' HN1487, designed, by L. Harradine, issued 1931-50, 7½in. high. £120

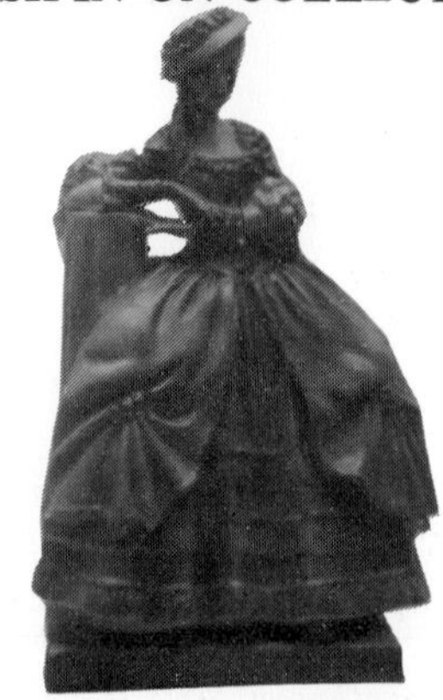

'Kate Hardcastle' HN1718, designed by L. Harradine, issued 1935-49, 8in. high. £185

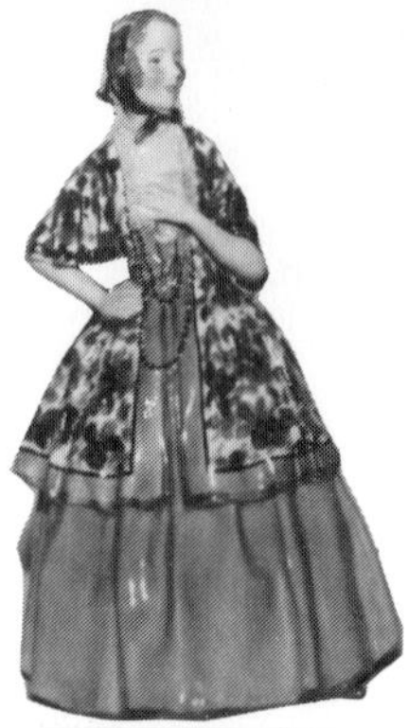

'Jasmine' HN1862, designed by L. Harradine, issued 1938-49, 7¼in. high. £195

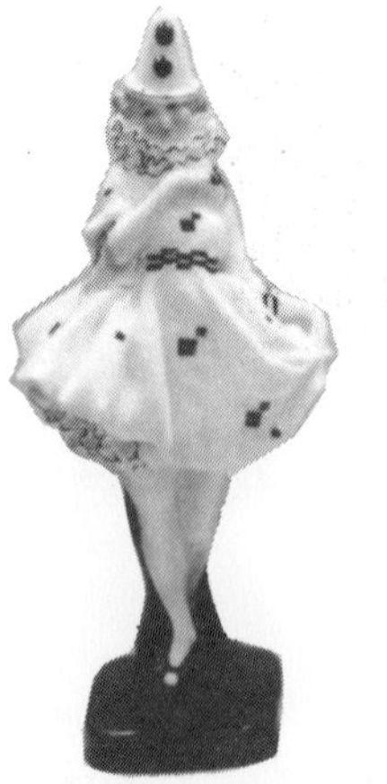

'Pierette' HN644, designed by L. Harradine, issued 1924-38, 7¼in. high. £300

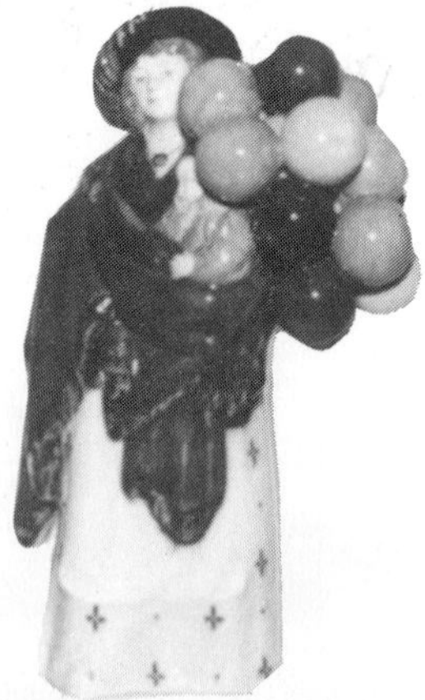

'Balloon Seller' HN583, designed by L. Harradine, issued 1923-49, 9in. high. £125

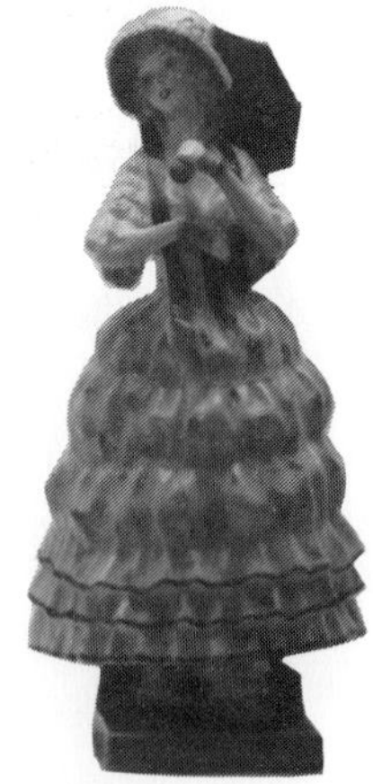

'Helen' HN1509, designed by L. Harradine, issued 1932-38, 8in. high. £295

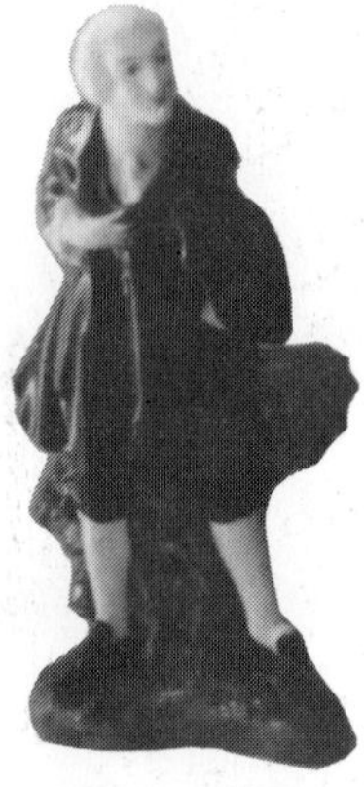

'Masquerade' HN599, designed by L. Harradine, issued 1924-49, 6¾in. high. £350

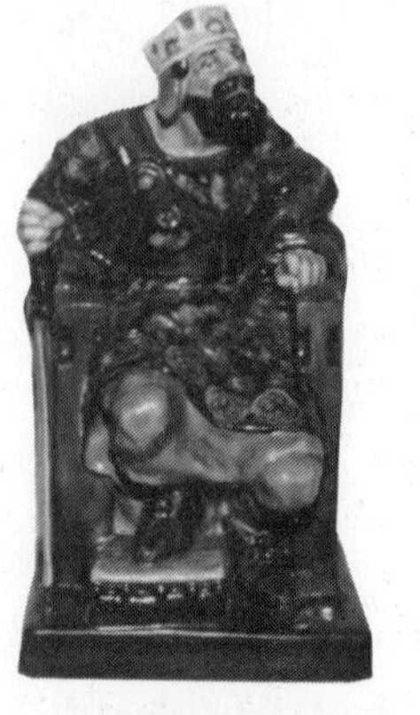

'Old King' HN2134, designed by C. J. Noke, issued 1954, 10¾in. high. £199

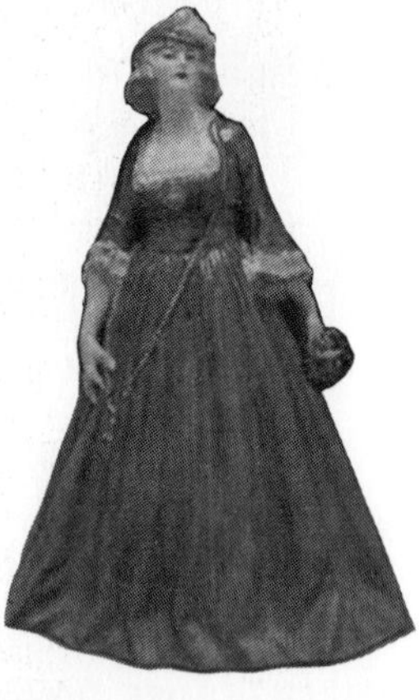

'Rosamund' HN1497, designed by L. Harradine, issued 1932-38, 8½in. high. £400

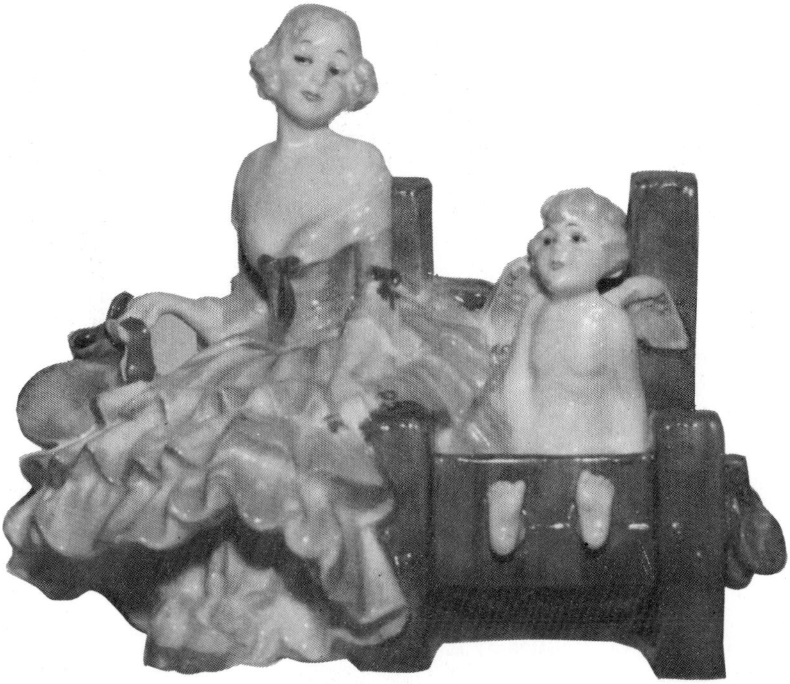

'In The Stocks', HN 1475, designed by L. Harradine, issued 1931-38, 5¼in. high. £800

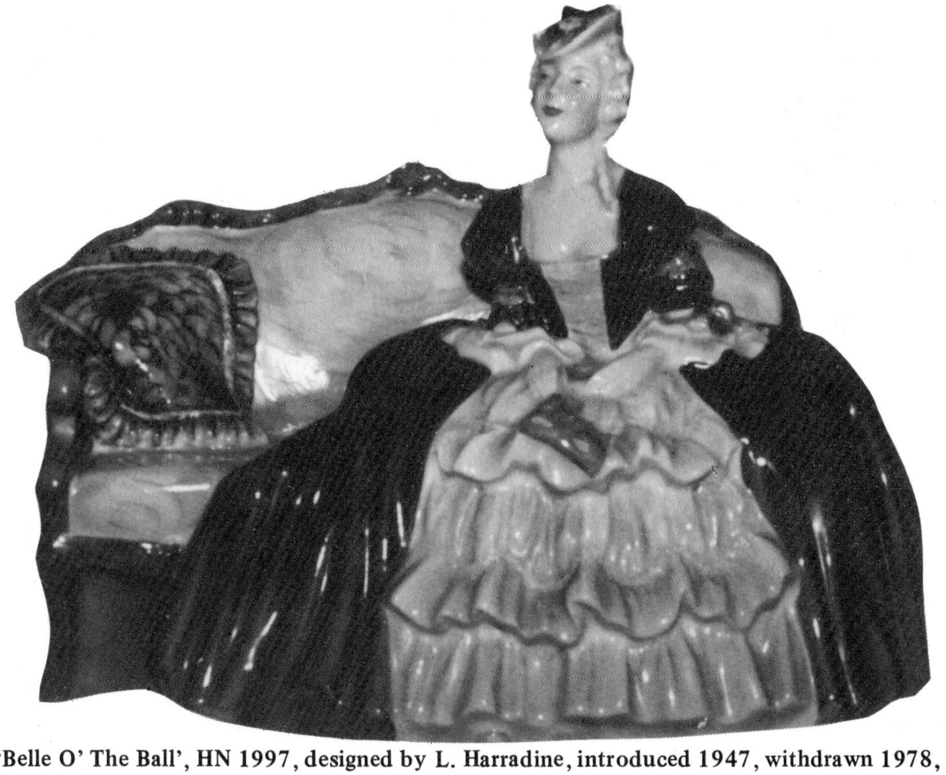

'Belle O' The Ball', HN 1997, designed by L. Harradine, introduced 1947, withdrawn 1978, 6in. high. £90

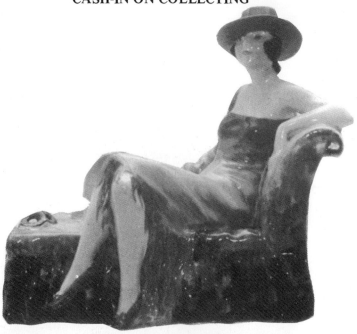

'Dulcinia', HN 1343, designed by L. Harradine, issued 1929-38, 5½in. high. £900

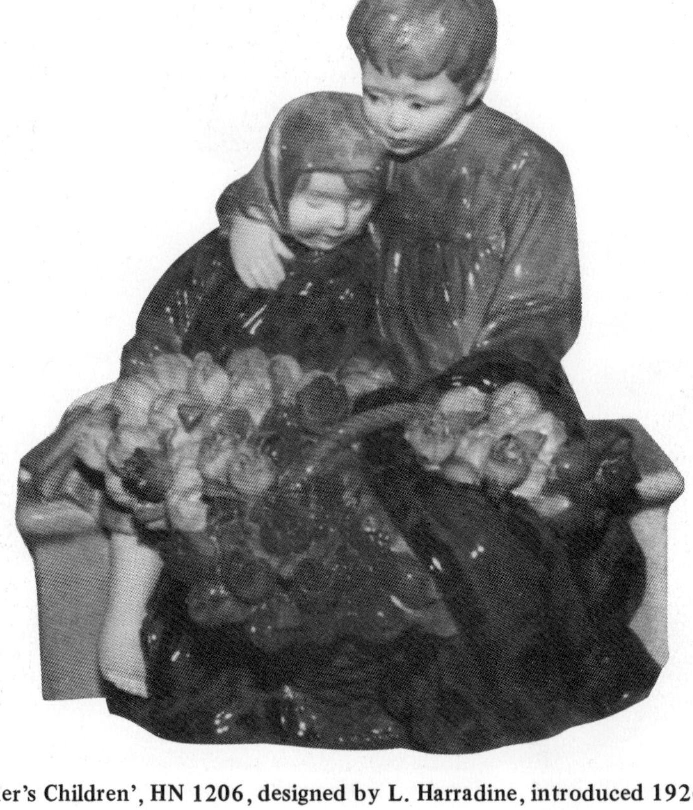

'Flower Seller's Children', HN 1206, designed by L. Harradine, introduced 1926, withdrawn 1949. £250

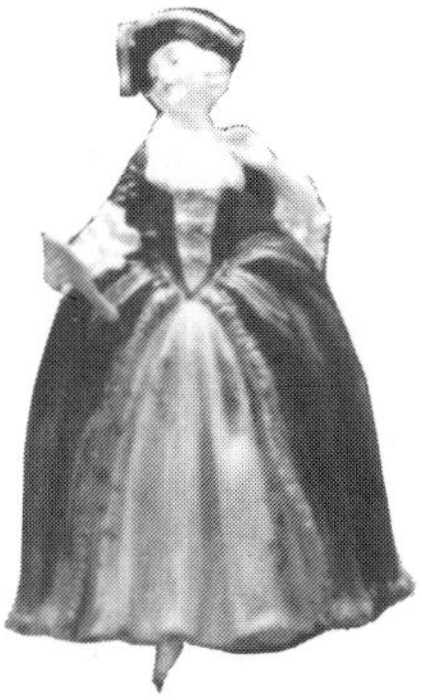

'Camille' HN1586, designed, by L. Harradine, issued 1933-49, 6½in. high. £180

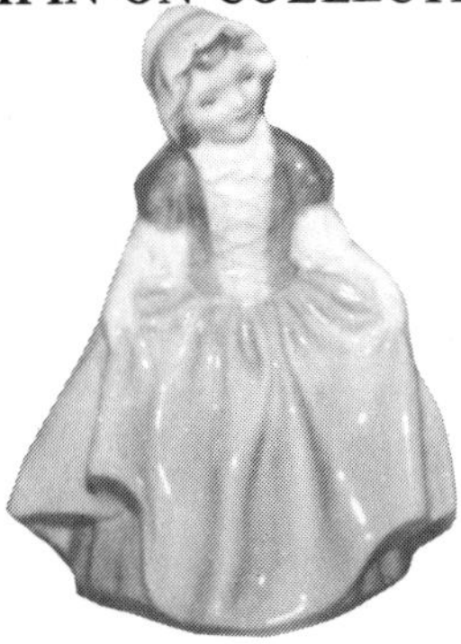

'Dinky Do' HN1678, designed by L. Harradine, issued 1934, 4¾in. high. £28

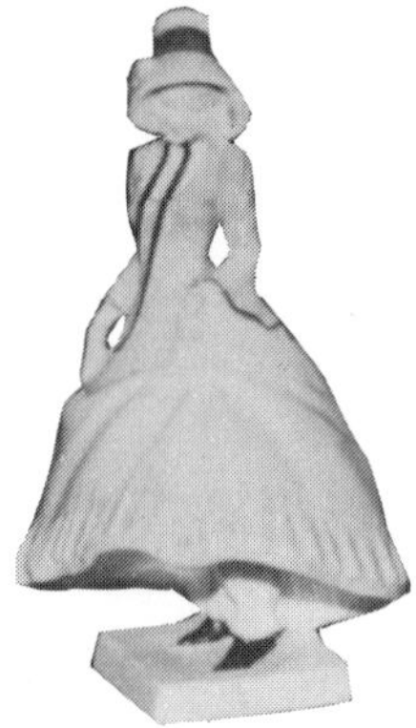

'Pantalettes' HN1709, designed by L. Harradine, issued 1935-38, 8in. high. £145

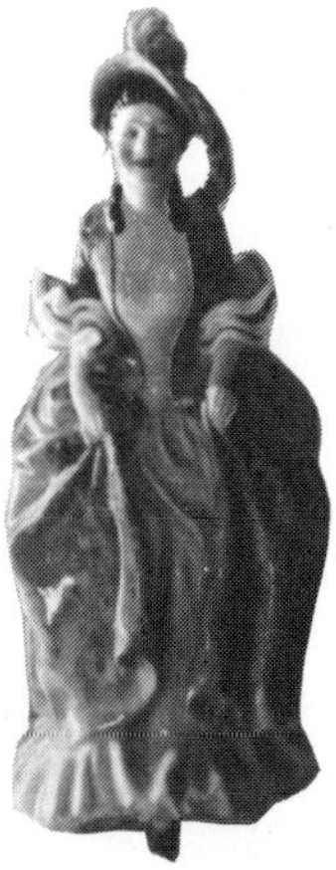

'Verena' HN1835, designed by L. Harradine, issued 1938-49, 8¼in. high. £250

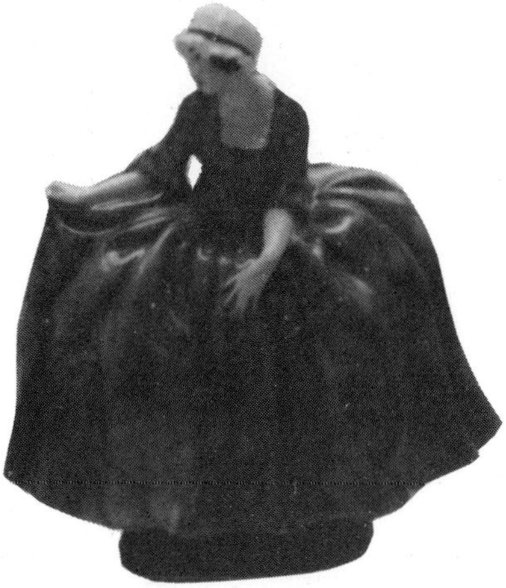

'Polly Peachum' HN550, designed by L. Harradine, issued 1922-49, 6½in. high. £150

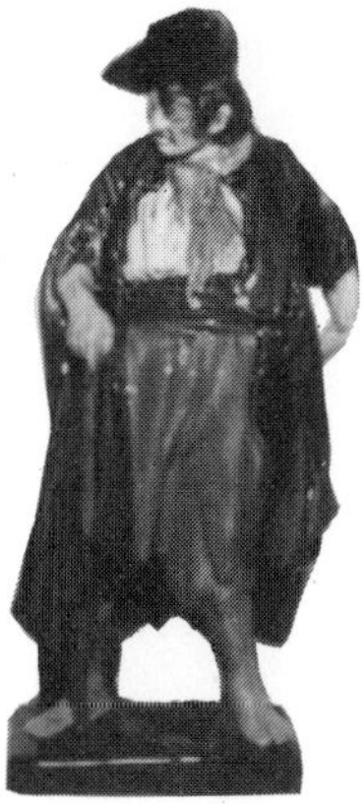

'Beggar' HN2175, designed by L. Harradine, issued 1956- 72, 6¾in. high. £180

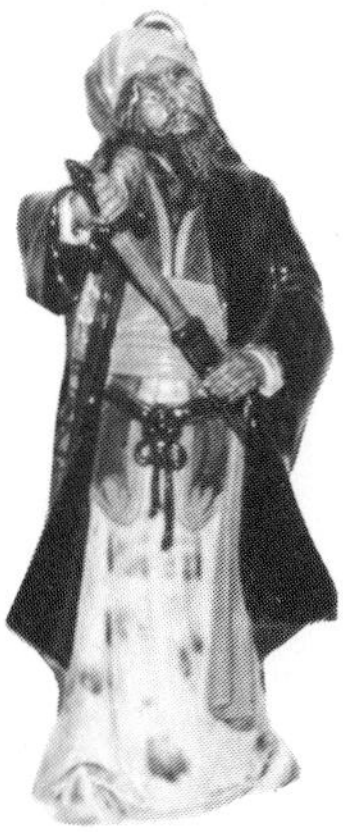

'Bluebeard' HN2105 designed by L. Harradine, issued 1953, 11in. high. £149

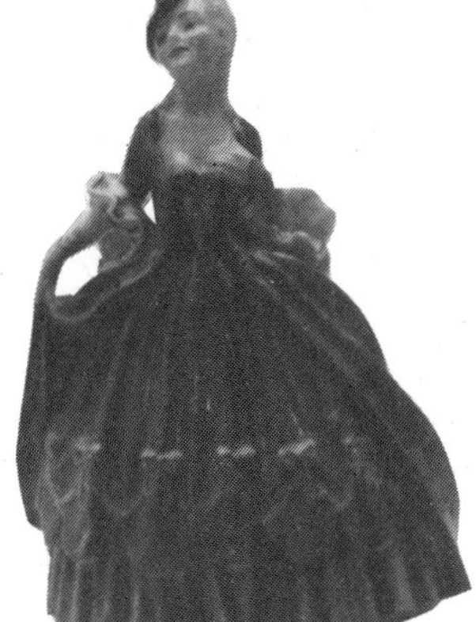

'Sibell' HN1695, designed by L. Harradine, issued 1935-49, 6½in. high. £275

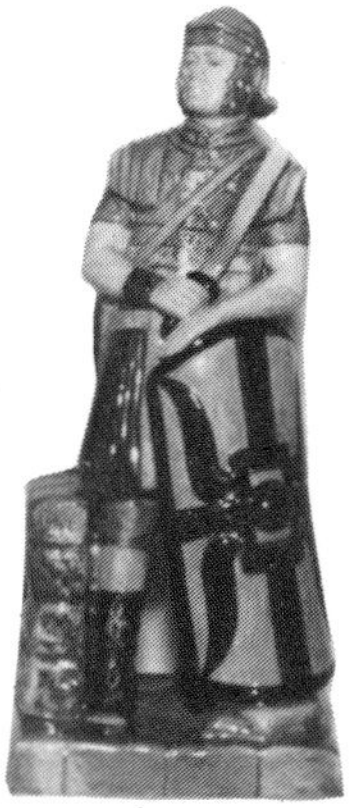

'Centurion' HN2726, designed by W. K. Harper, issued 1982-84, 9¼in. high. £65

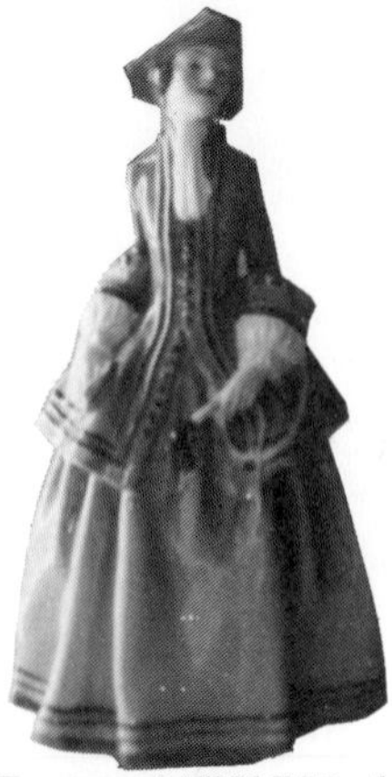

'Regency' HN1752, designed by L. Harradine, issued 1936-49, 8in. high. £200

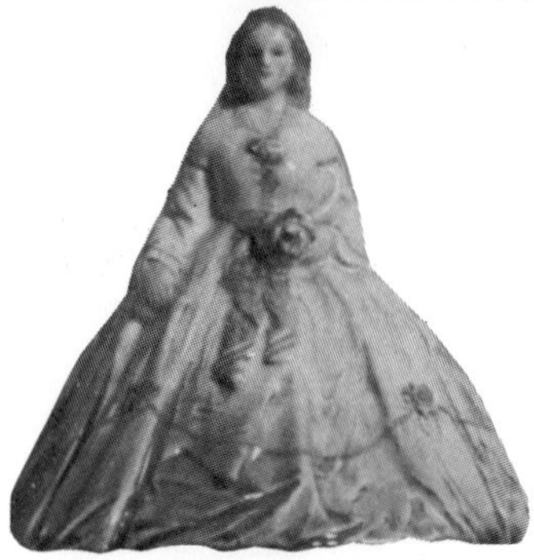

'Crinoline' HN413, designed by G. Lambert, issued 1920-38, 6¼in. high. £500

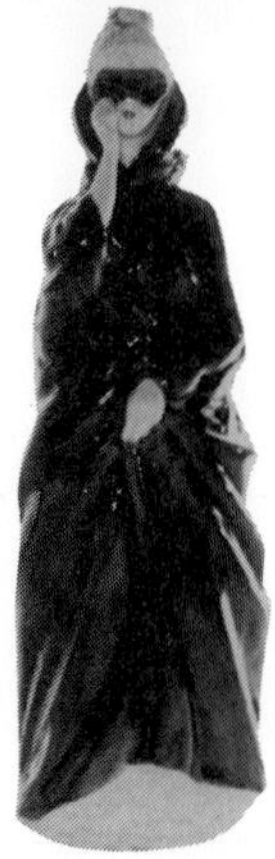

'Masque' HN2554A, designed by D. V. Tootle, issued 1973-82, 8½in. high. £55

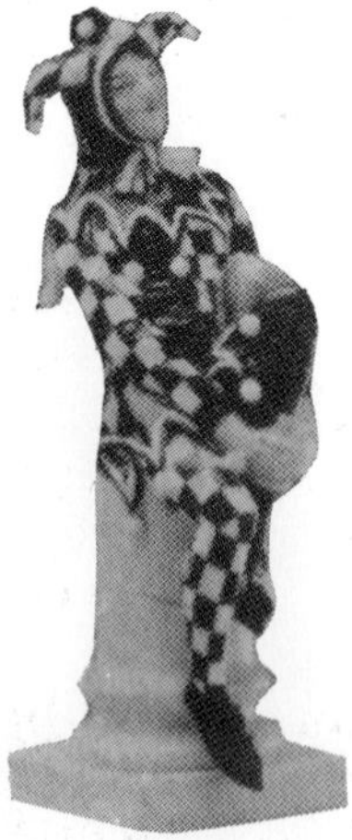

'Jester' HN552, designed by C. J. Noke, issued 1922-38, 10in. high. £500

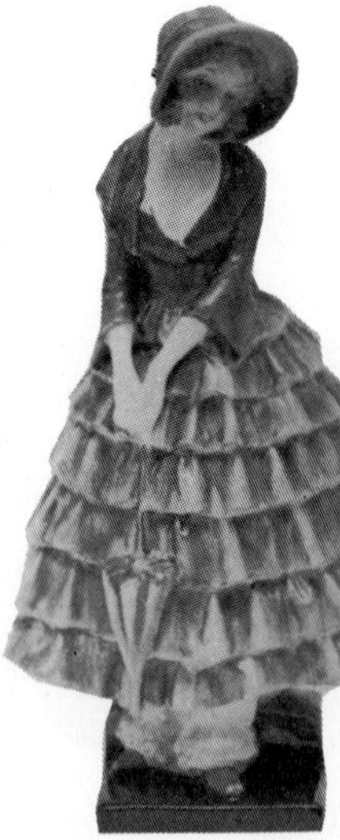

'Priscilla' HN1337, designed by L. Harradine, issued 1929-38, 8in. high. £180

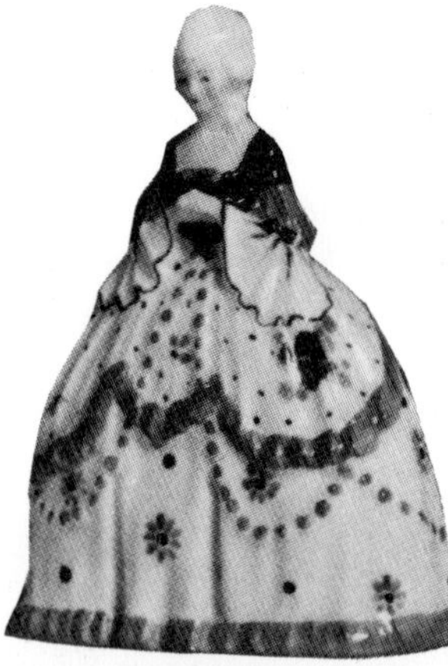

'Crinoline Lady' HN651, issued 1924-38, 3in. high. £500

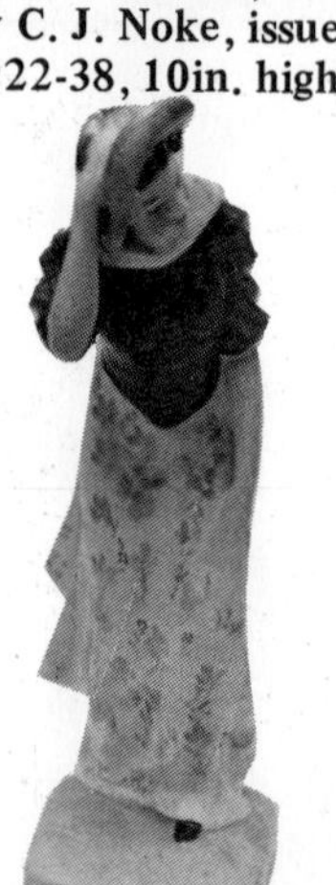

'Windflower' HN2029, designed by L. Harradine, issued 1949-55, 4¾in. high. £180

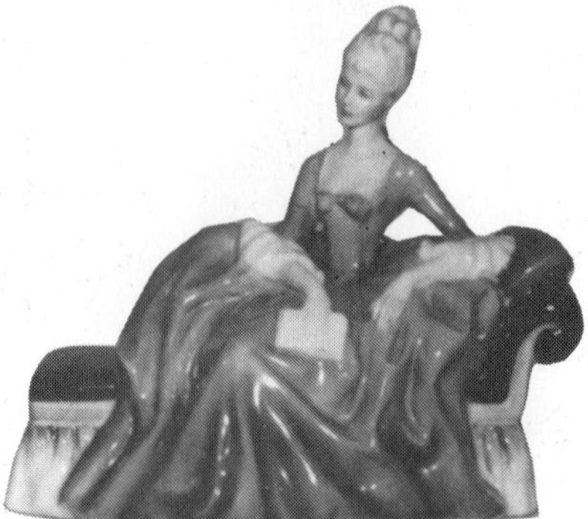

'Repose' HN2272, designed by M. Davies, issued 1972-78, 5¼in. high. £85

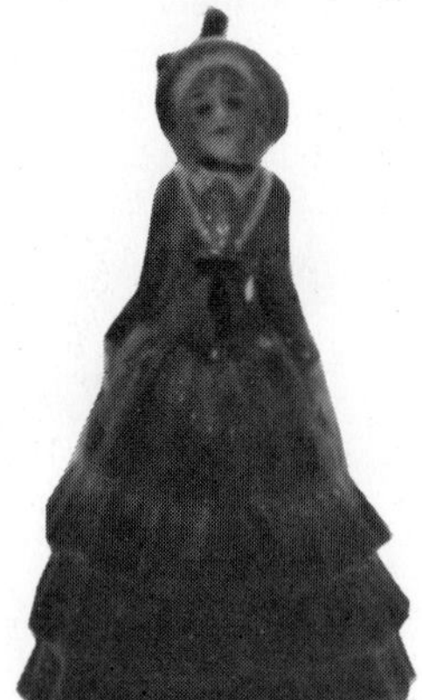

'Pauline' HN1444, designed by L. Harradine, issued 1931-38, 6in. high. £120

Gerald and Joan Gurney are teachers of sport and collect sporting items, particularly equipment.

Gerald said: "I'm a qualified coach in lawn tennis, table tennis and squash and Joan, my wife, is a teacher of swimming and life saving and through our careers we have been interested in finding items relating to the history of our particular sports.

"Now we've a very extensive collection because this is an area which has not yet been fully explored and there are still a lot of interesting items to be found. Prices are very, very erratic because there is no established norm, especially in racketana. Lawn tennis as a subject for collecting comes far behind golf and cricket in popular following, but is clearly on the way up.

"I'm particularly interested in racket games some of which no longer exist so every now and again 'puzzle items' turn up that are connected with defunct games. The earliest tennis racket I have goes back to 1880 and one of my oldest items is a shuttlecock that I have authoritatively dated to 1840.

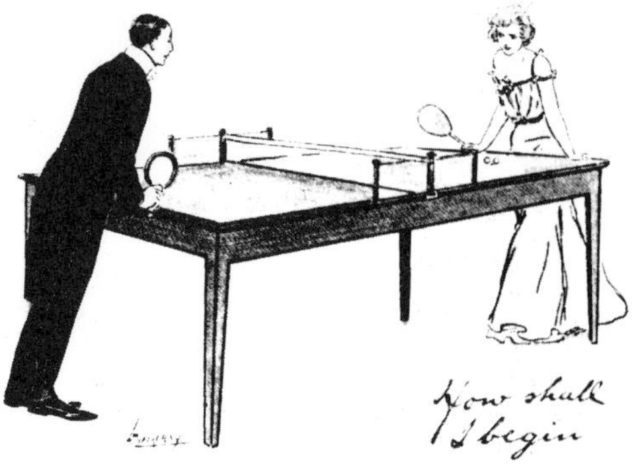

"I'm often asked to mount displays of my collection in various tennis clubs because many of them are celebrating their centenaries about now. People particularly like to handle the rackets for various games and see how they are inter-related."

Joan Gurney has 30 early bathing costumes as well as illustrations, photographs, cigarette cards and figurines including car radiator mascots, of swimmers. Both the Gurneys have written about their collections and Gerald has published a book entitled 'Tennis, Squash and Badminton Bygones'.

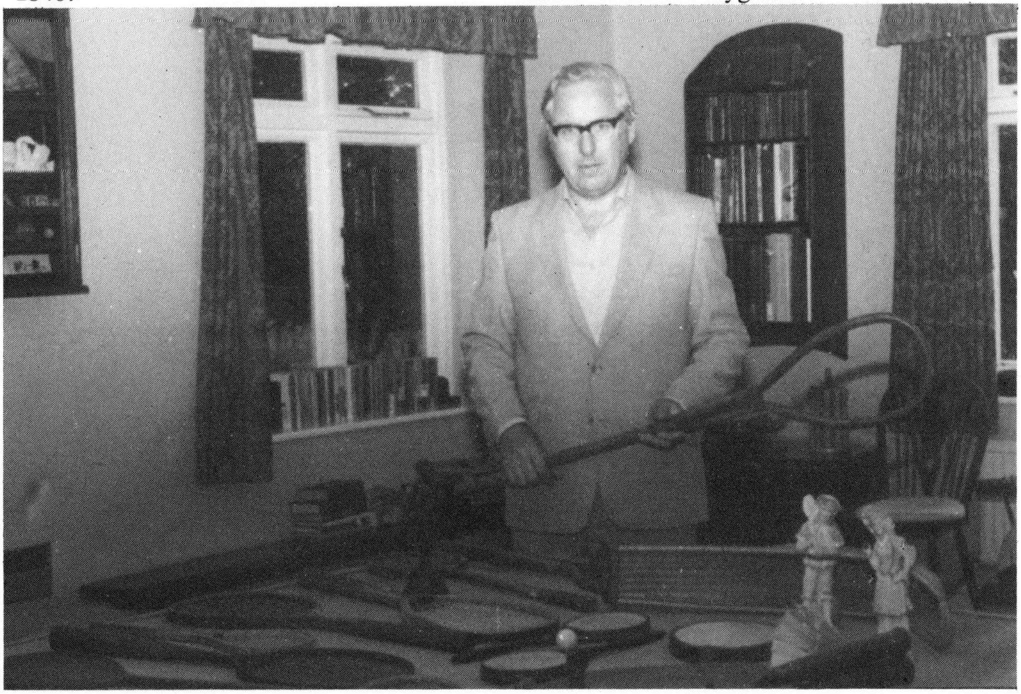

Gerald with part of his extensive collection of 'Racketana'.

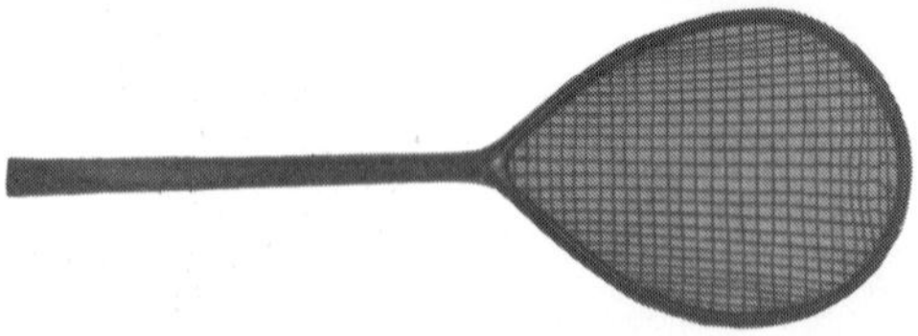

Badminton racket made in India, circa 1885. £75

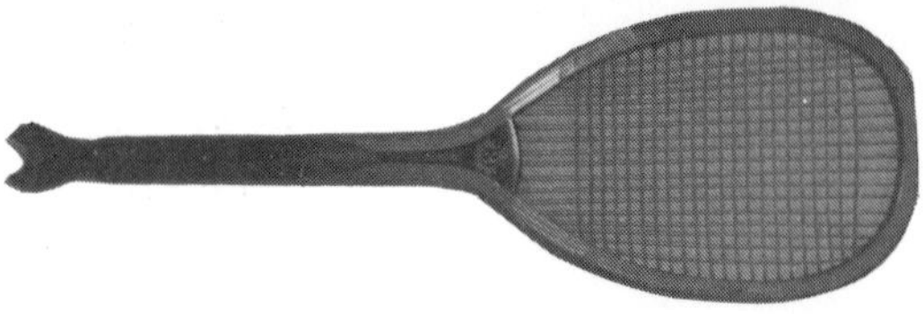

Long-headed lawn tennis racket with 'fish-tail' grip by G. G. Bussey & Co., circa 1900. £75

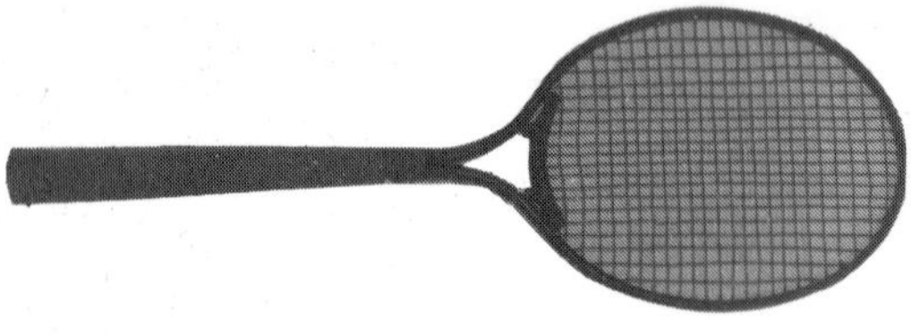

Lawn tennis racket with steel head and strung with wire, circa 1925. £40

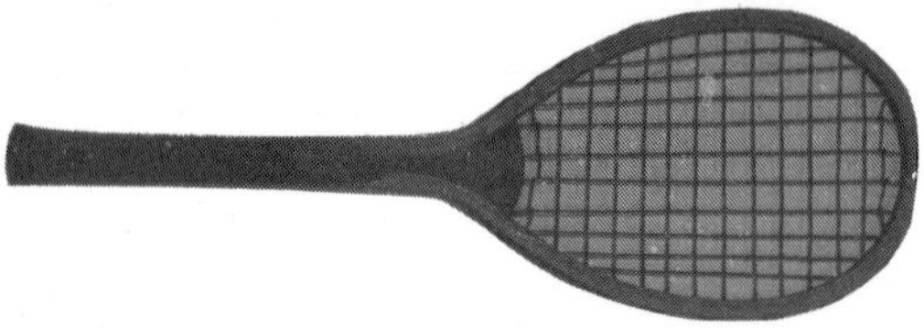

Child's 'toy' racket, only 22¾in. overall, circa 1900. £40

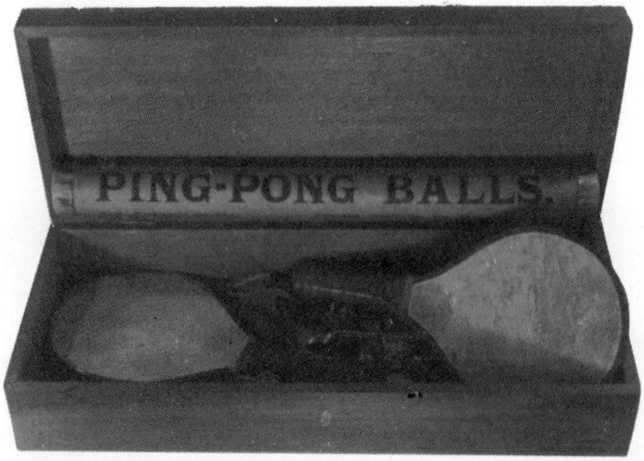

De Luxe 'Ping-Pong or Gossima' set in wooden box, by J. Jaques & Son, circa 1900. £200

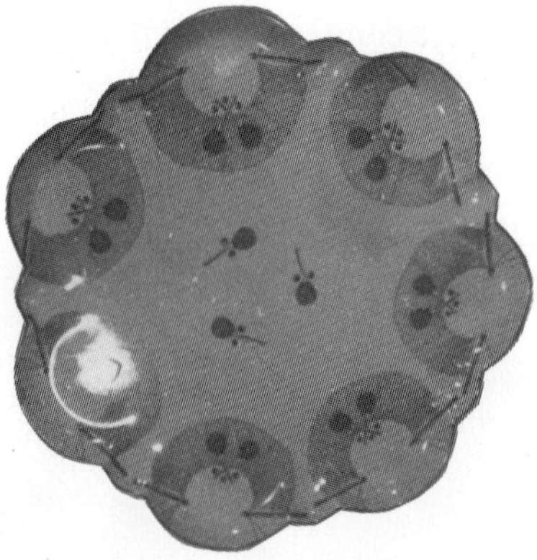

Revolving china 'Lazy Susan', 18½in., with scalloped edge and decorated with lawn tennis items, circa 1885. £300

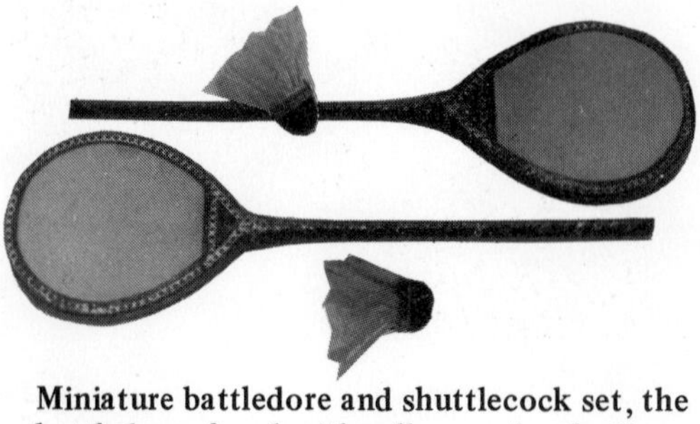

Miniature battledore and shuttlecock set, the battledores faced with vellum and only 8in. overall. £50

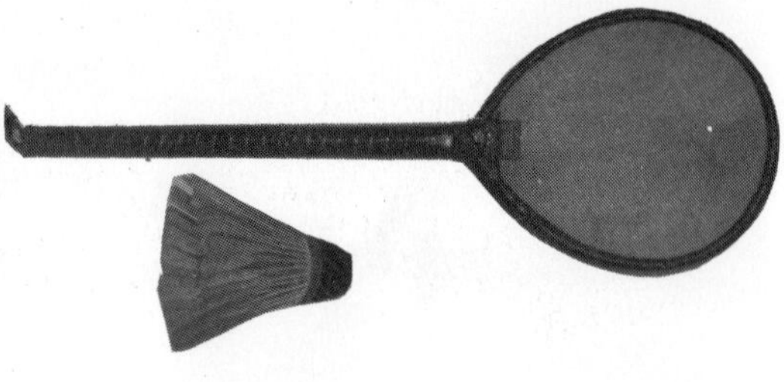

Very large vellum battledore, 23in. overall, for the game of battledore and shuttlecock, circa 1890. £50

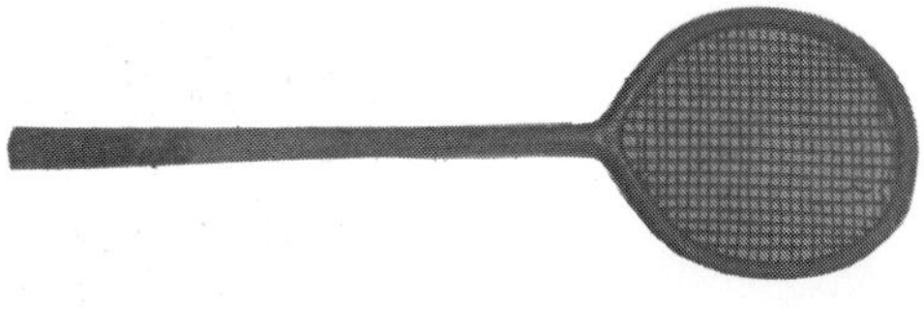

Squash racket by T. H. Prosser & Sons, circa 1900. £75

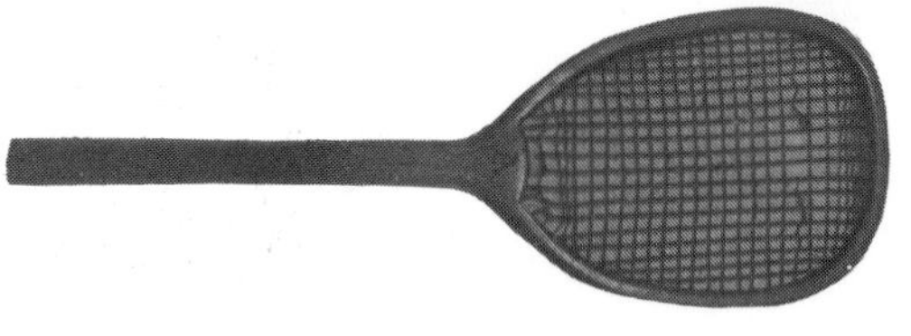

'Lop-sided' lawn tennis tacket, maker unkown, circa 1885. £175

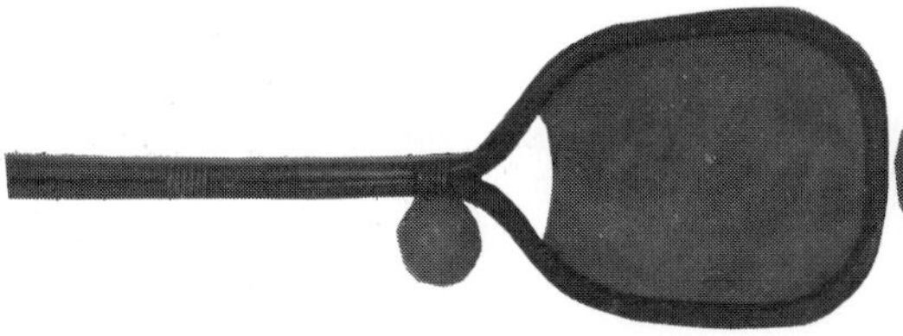

Table tennis battledore with single vellum sheet in bamboo frame, circa 1900, made by J. R. Mally. £40

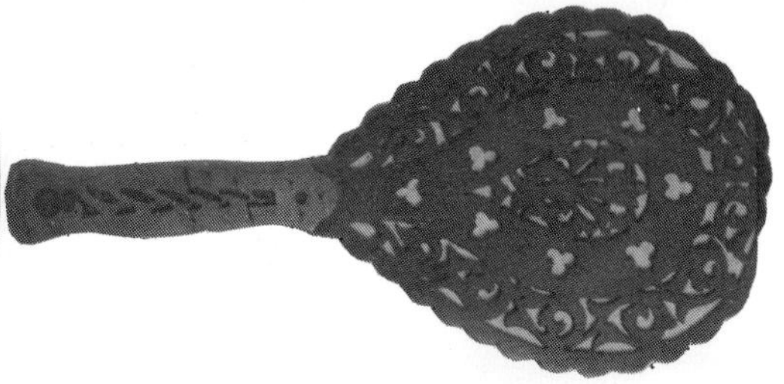

Table tennis bat, circa 1900, delicately cut out in fretwork. £40

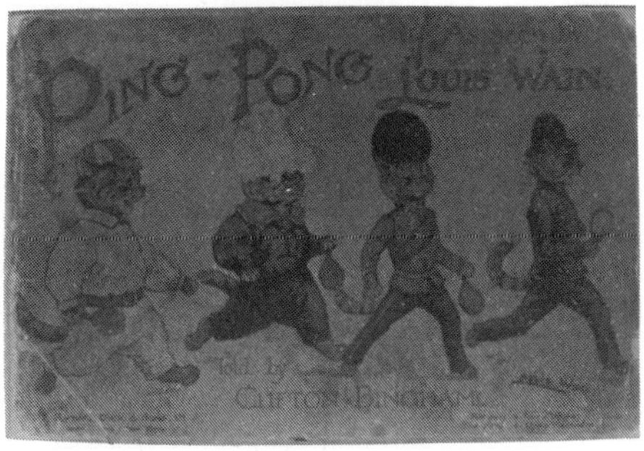

'Ping-Pong' by Clifton Bingham and published by Raphael Tuck, circa 1900, with six coloured illustrations by Louis Wain. £100

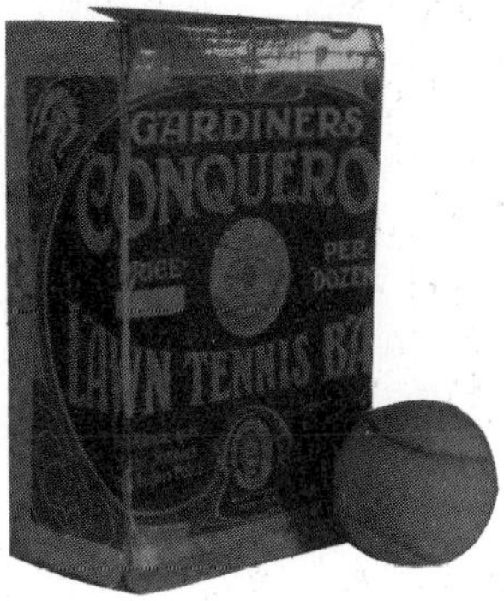

Box of Gardiner's lawn tennis balls (unused), 1920's. £40

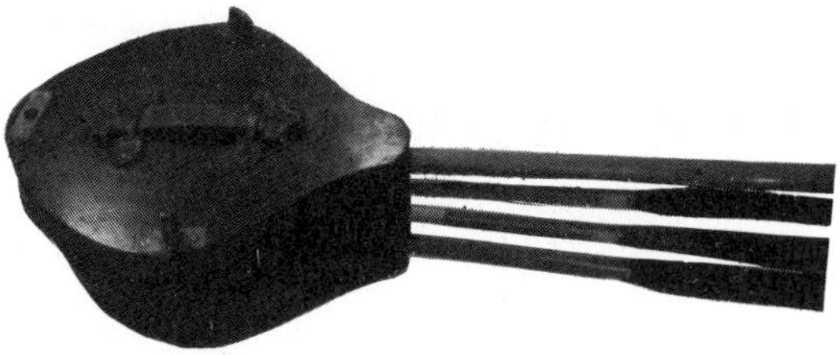

Multiple press for squash rackets, made in India, circa 1910. £40

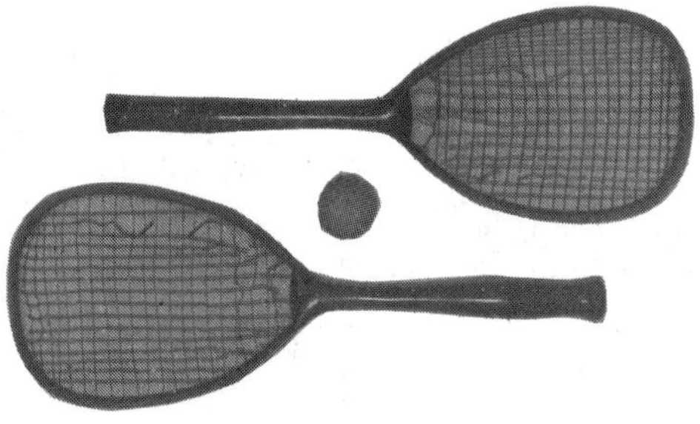

Pair of table tennis rackets, 16½in. overall, by G. G. Bussey & Co., circa 1900. £50

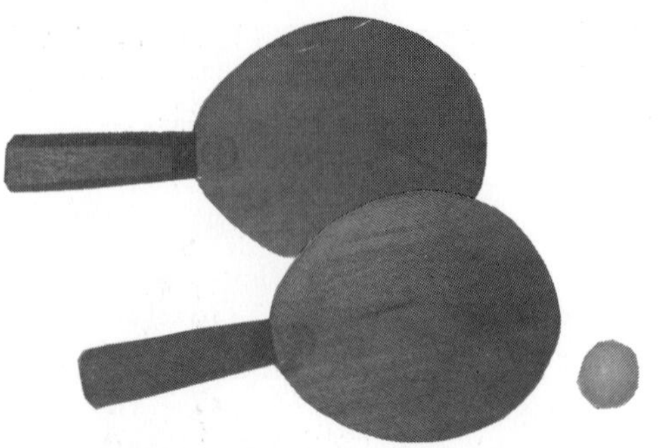

Pair of wooden 'Ping-Pong' bats by Parker Brothers, U.S.A., circa 1900. £25

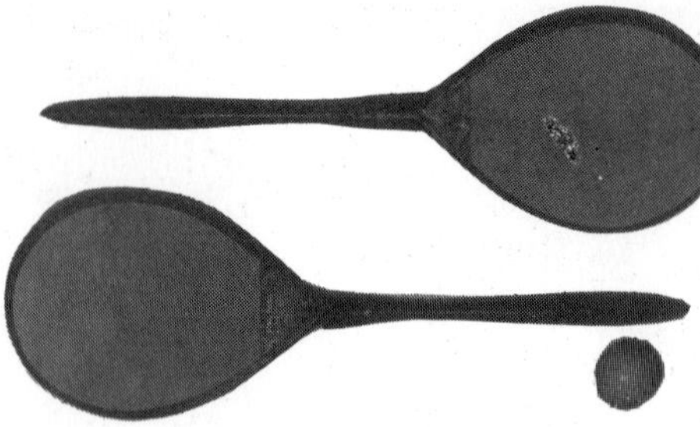

Pair of vellum 'Ping-Pong' battledores, by J. Jaques & Son, circa 1900. £25

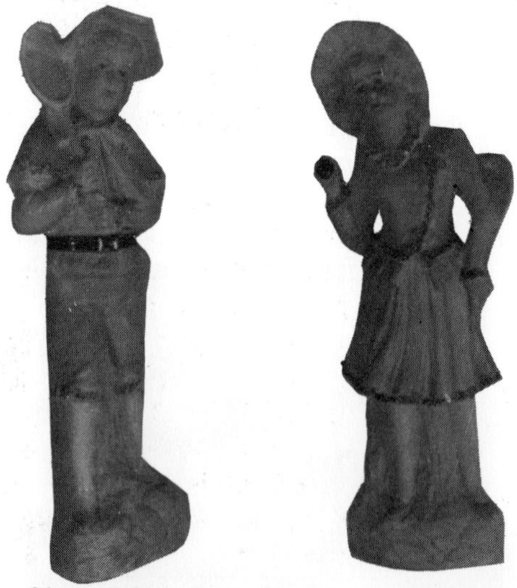

Pair of late 19th century German bisque figures, 9½in., both with lawn tennis rackets and decorated in pink, blue and gilt. £125

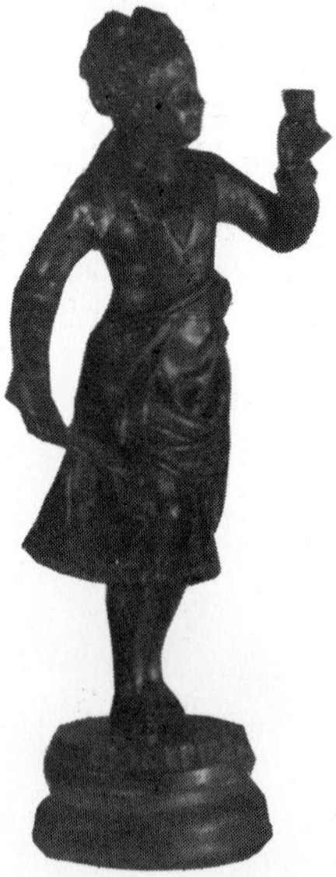

Victorian spelter figure, 10in., of a lady with racket and shuttlecock, circa 1895. £35

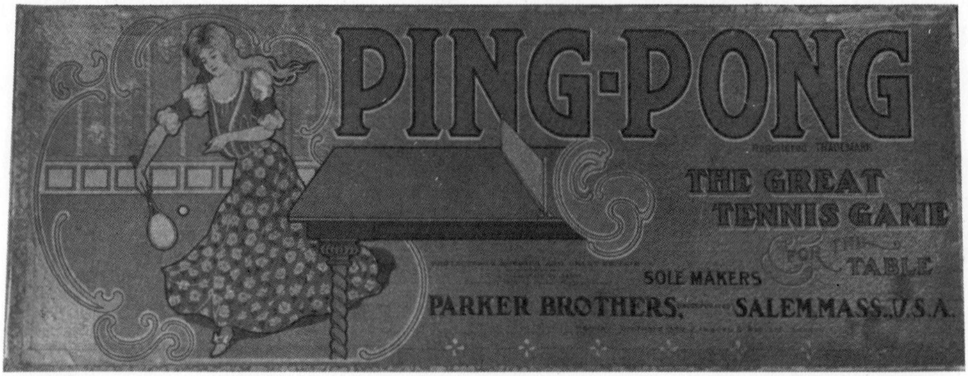

'Ping-Pong – The Great Tennis Game for the Table', by Parker Bros., Salem, U.S.A., circa 1900. £200

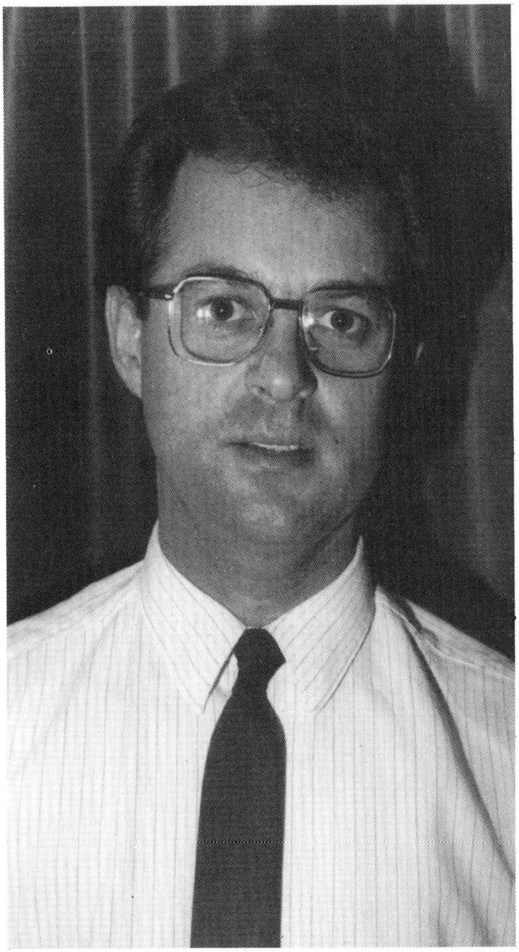

Keith Osborne works in local government and collects beer bottle labels.

"I started collecting beer bottle labels when I was at school because I come from Maidstone and we were taken on a school trip round two local breweries where we were given some labels and that started me off.

"Then I began making trips to other breweries on my bicycle and got more labels. It started from there and now I've over 30,000 labels — all British and Irish and all different. It's a never ending task but very challenging.

"My earliest label dates from 1840 and was produced by A. B. Walker and Son of Warrington. The modern ones are not so interesting because many of them are either plastic or wrap around labels but Royal weddings and such occasions usually produce some interesting new labels."

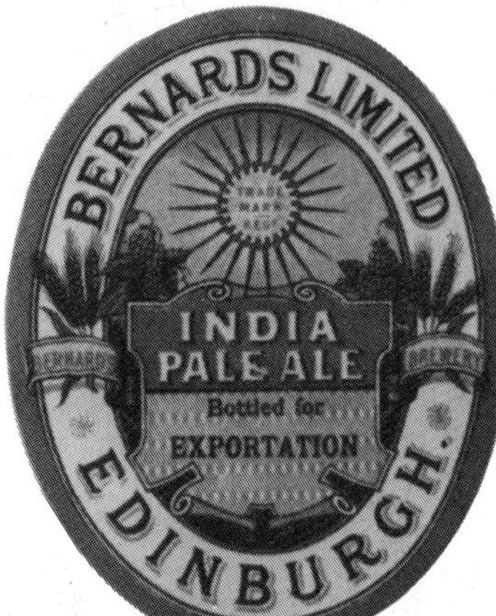

Keith has bought up several old collections including one of Victorian labels and another of 1,000 labels dating to the 1920's which he picked up for only £10. He also corresponds and swaps with collectors all over the world, particularly with an American called Ernie Oest of New York who began collecting during the Prohibition era. The most Keith has paid for a label is £25 for a label produced by W. G. Weller of Amersham in 1929.

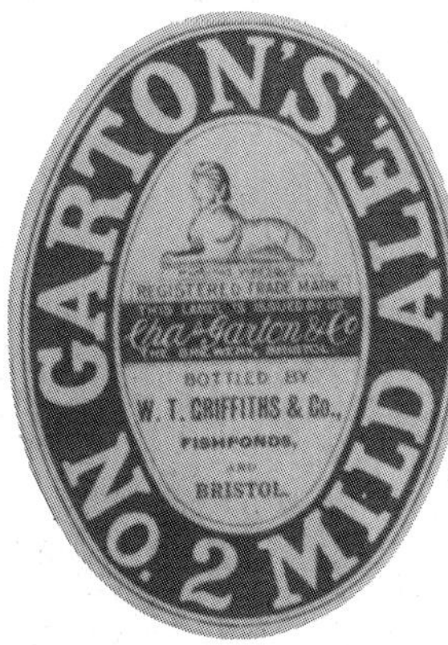

What he would most like to find are labels from a Hampshire brewery, Thomas Kenward of Hartley Wintney which closed in 1920.

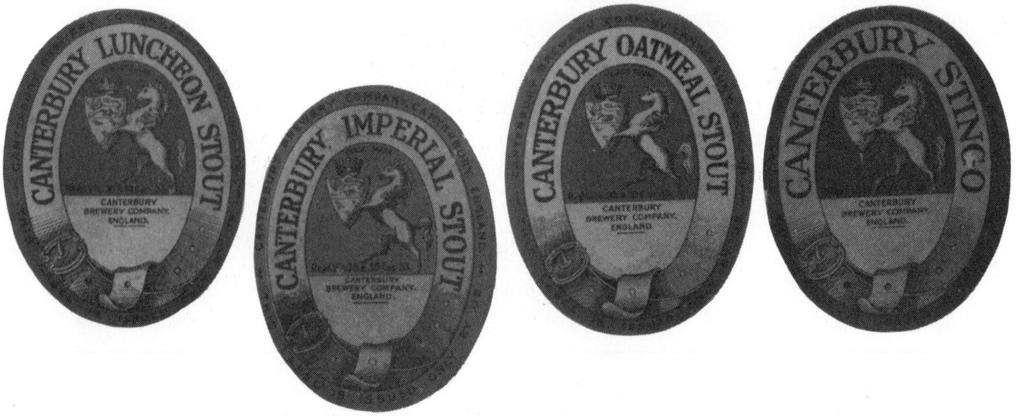

Four Canterbury Brewery Co. labels, in use 1912, (Northgate Brewery). Brewery ceased 1923. **Up to £70**

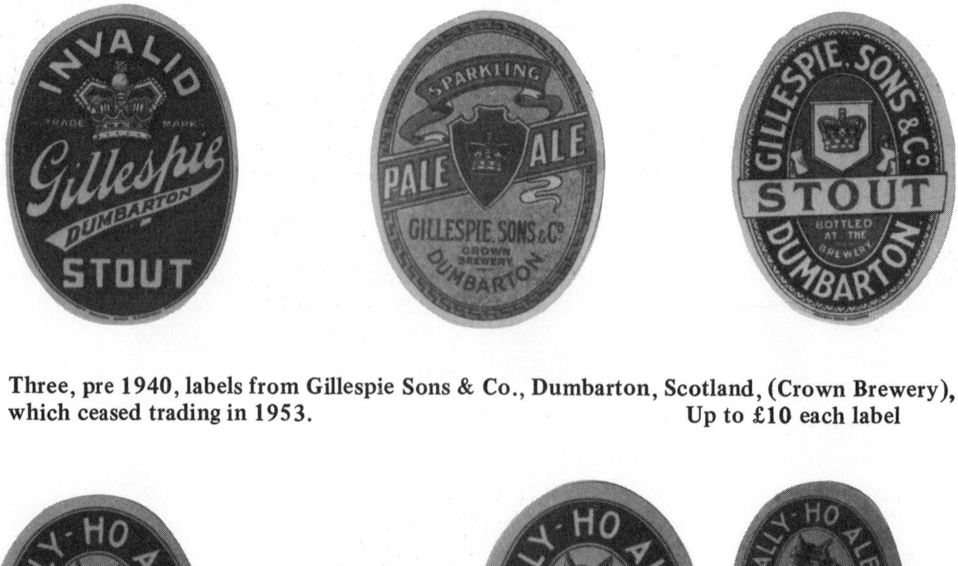

Three, pre 1940, labels from Gillespie Sons & Co., Dumbarton, Scotland, (Crown Brewery), which ceased trading in 1953. **Up to £10 each label**

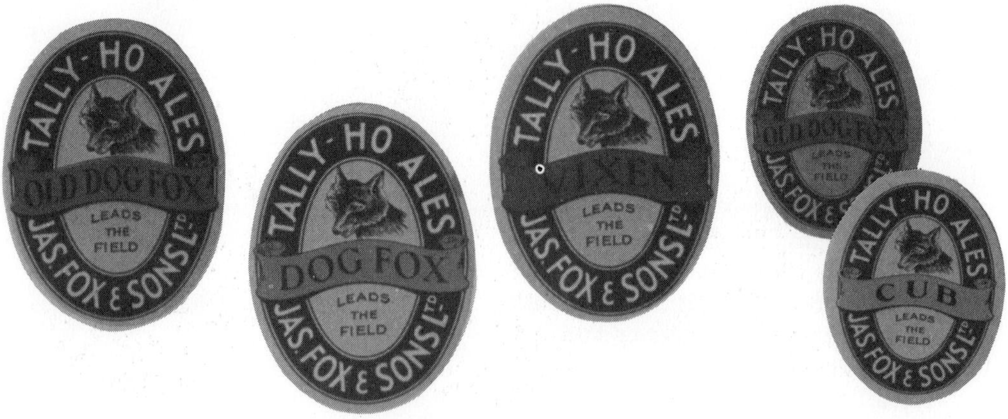

Attractive labels from James Fox & Sons, Isle of Axholme Brewery, Crowle, Lincolnshire. Brewery acquired and closed in 1949 and labels in use until that time. **£25 – £30**

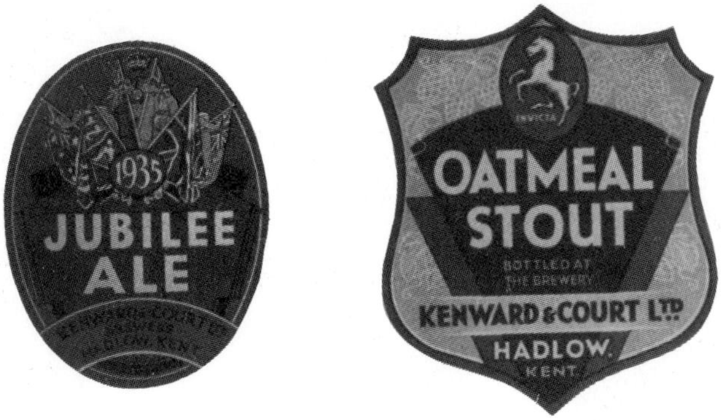

Three labels from Kenward & Court Ltd., Hadlow, Kent, (Close Brewery), Jubilee 1935, Oatmeal Stout 1936 and Coronation 1937. Brewery ceased early 1950's.

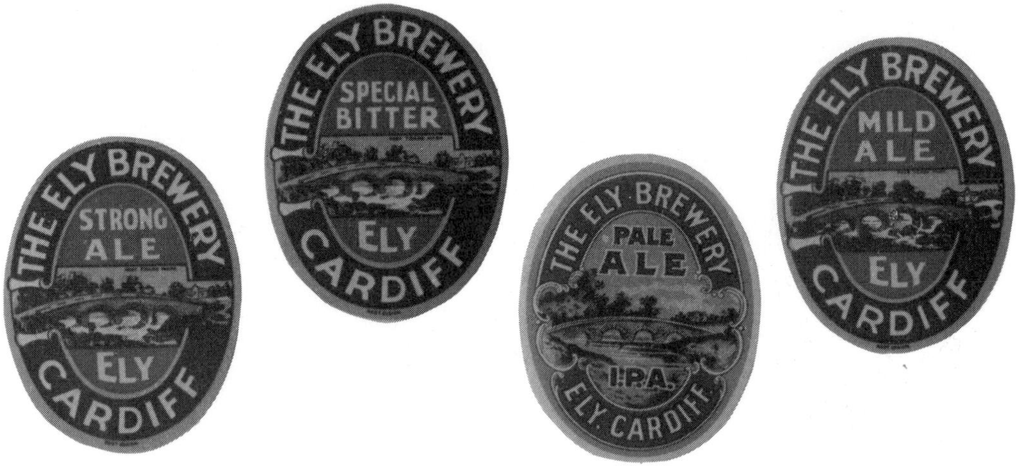

Ely Brewery Co. Ltd., Ely, Cardiff, labels in use in 1930's. £12

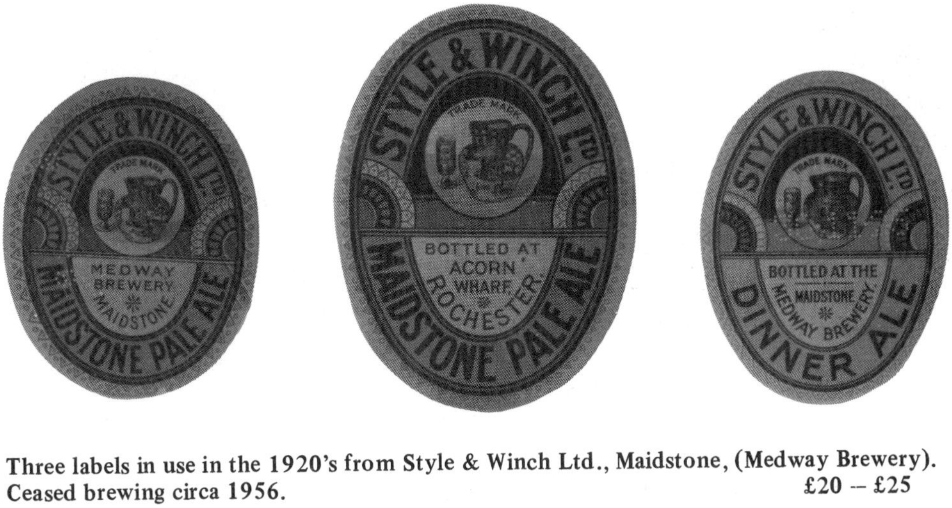

Three labels in use in the 1920's from Style & Winch Ltd., Maidstone, (Medway Brewery). Ceased brewing circa 1956. £20 -- £25

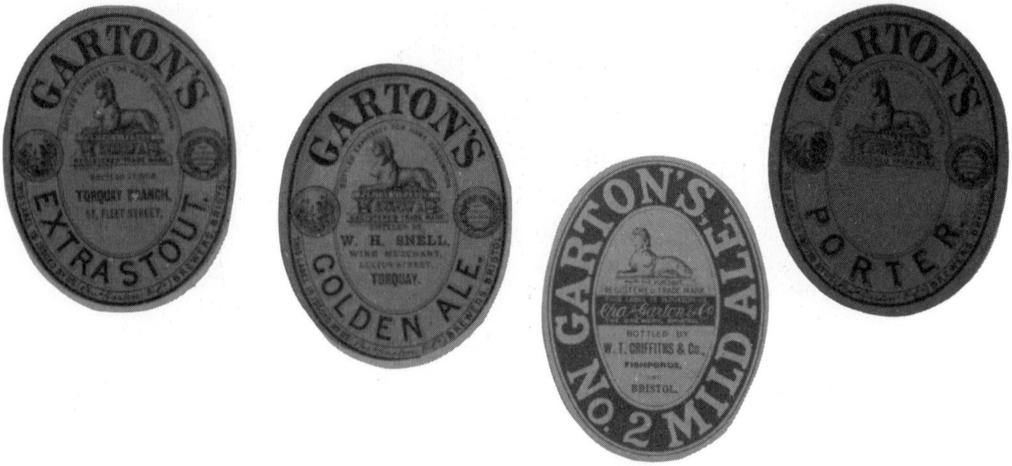

Four labels used until circa 1899 from Garton & Sons, Bristol, when brewing ceased.
£80 – £100

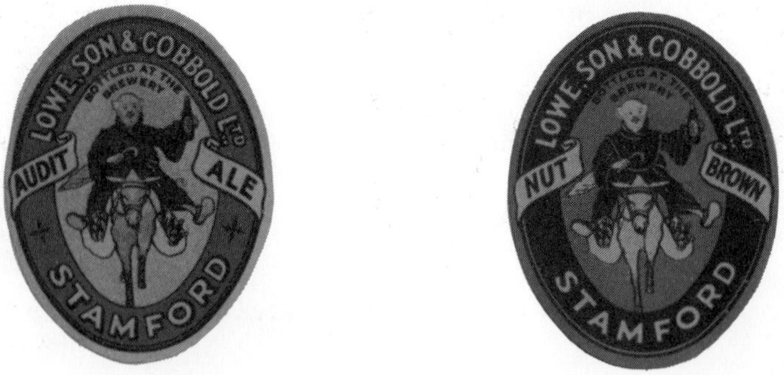

Two labels from Lowe, Son & Cobbold Ltd., Stamford. Brewery acquired in 1935 and labels in use until then. £20 – £25

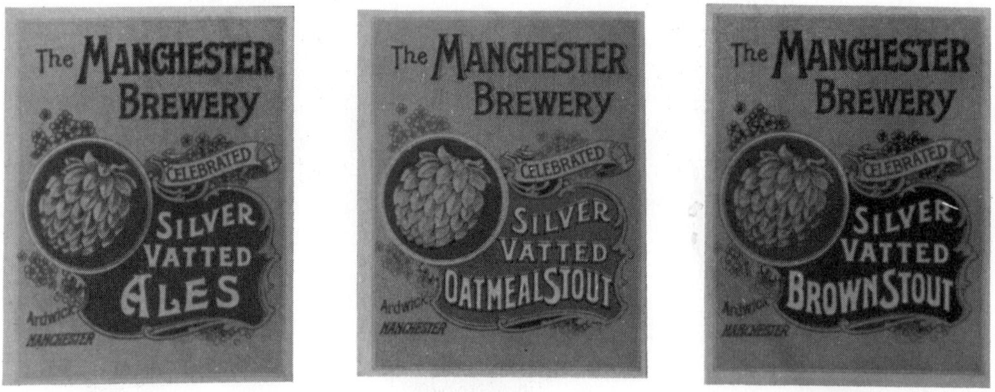

Manchester Brewery, Manchester, labels in use around 1909. Ceased brewing 1912. £75

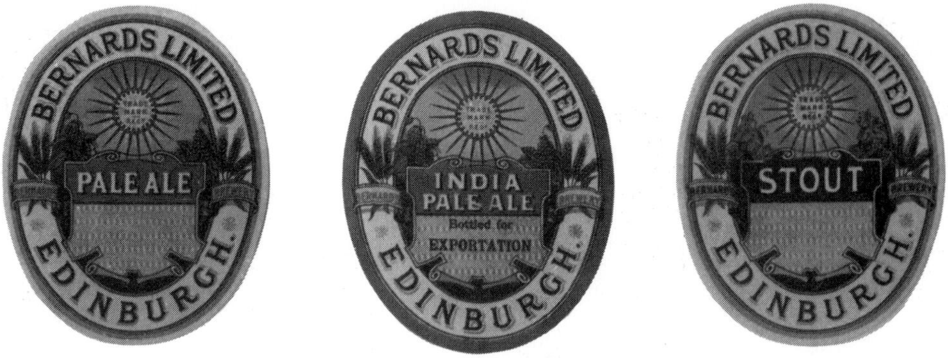

Three labels from Bernards Ltd., Edinburgh, circa 1899. Brewing ceased circa 1902.
£50 – £60

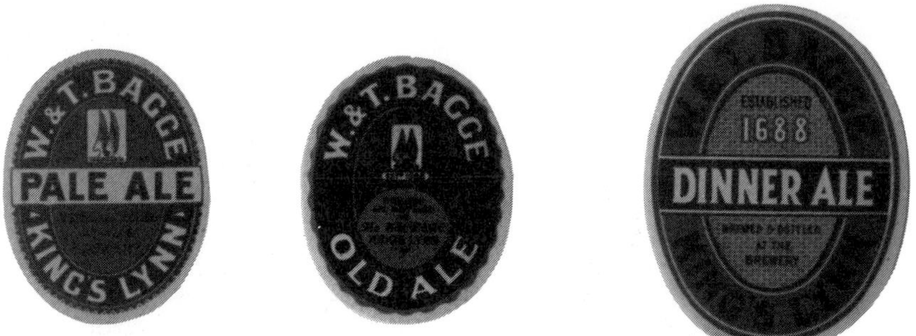

Three labels from W. & T. Bagge, King Street Brewery, Kings Lynn, Norfolk, in use to 1929.
In excess of £60

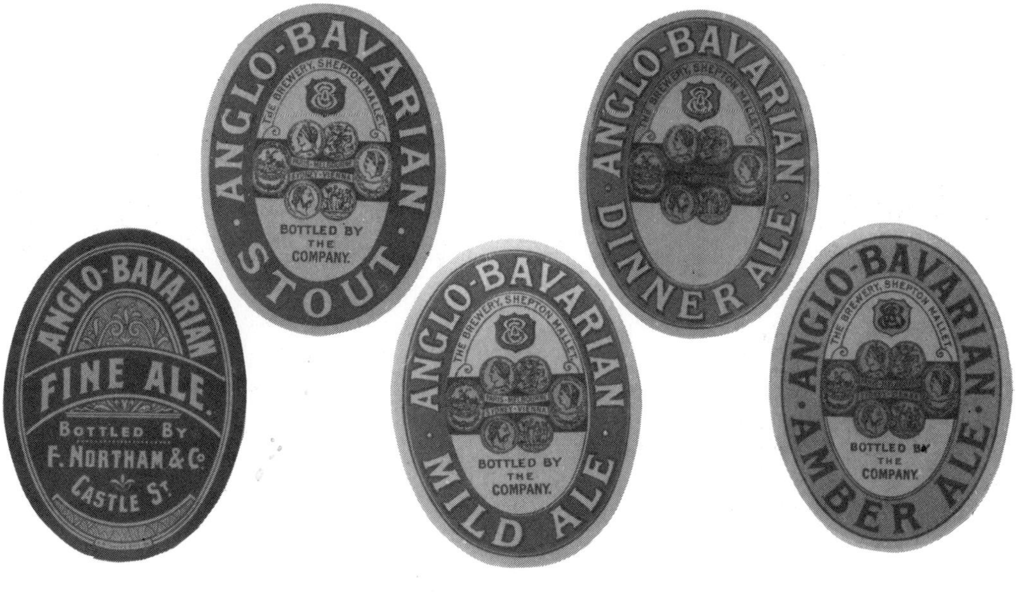

Anglo-Bavarian Brewery Co. Ltd., Shepton Mallet, labels in use before 1900, but brewery continued to 1939.
£65 – £70

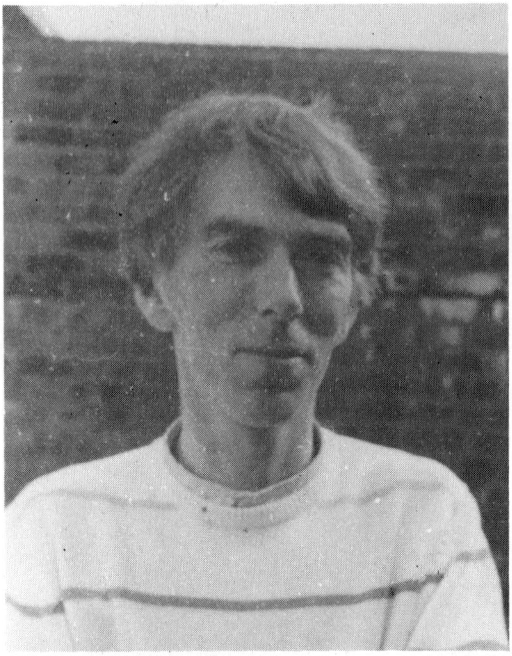

Ken Everett is a schoolteacher and collects unusual smoothing irons and advertising items, many of which he has on display in his wife's greengrocer shop.

"I started by collecting smoothing irons but about ten years ago it reached the point where I'd obtained all the more common ones and I started adding advertising to my collection.

"I am interested in soap adverts, enamel signs, old tins, statuettes — all the sort of advertising items that were put in shops during Victorian and Edwardian times. Even dogs' bowls, and customers' chairs had advertising on them. When I started collecting these things were quite cheap because people were dumping them but now they have acquired such a collectible status that there are things I can't afford.

"Biscuit tins are interesting because there are thousands of them. Some are shaped like houses, trains, or cribs and they could be used as toys afterwards. As a result they often got damaged however.

"Tobacco tins also interest me because some of the smaller ones to hold ten or twenty cigarettes were made for the ladies' market and others were printed with designs of trains or sailors. It seems that everybody smoked in those days! The tins have survived because they often ended up in the garden shed holding nails or something. The going price for a tobacco tin at the moment is between £10 and £25."

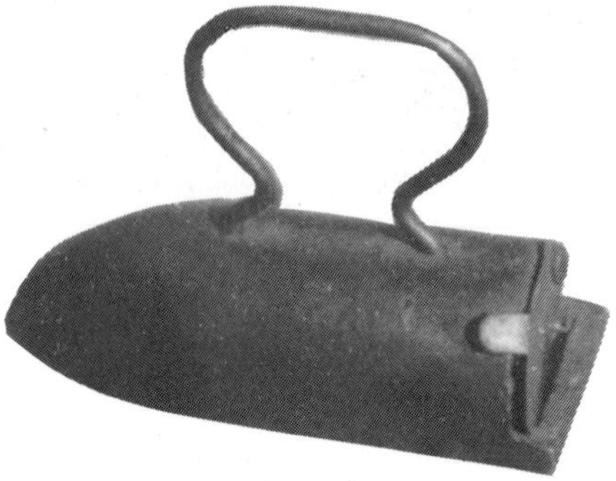

Ken has around 150 very nice irons and his favourite among them is a Scottish box iron with an ornate brass handle which was meant to sit on the hearth as a decoration when not in use. The price of it today is around £65 . Other prizes in his collection include a card showing a boy pushing a girl in a barrow made of a Sunlight Soap crate. His favourite tins are a matching pair of Edwardian tins advertising Hudson's soap, one held string and the other, which had an inkwell, held pens. Shopkeepers had them on the counters, string for wrapping, ink for receipts.

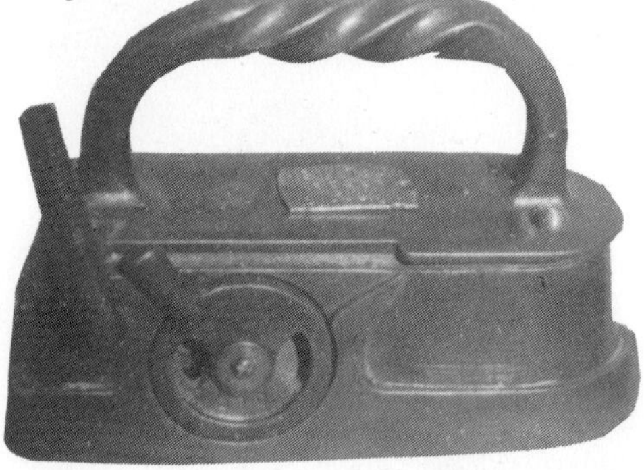

Ken would most like to find an iron with a hollow handle down which a hot poker was put for goffering. The cost is around £40. Another iron he covets is a polishing iron with a curved removable stone. It was used for putting a high sheen on material and today is also priced at around £40.

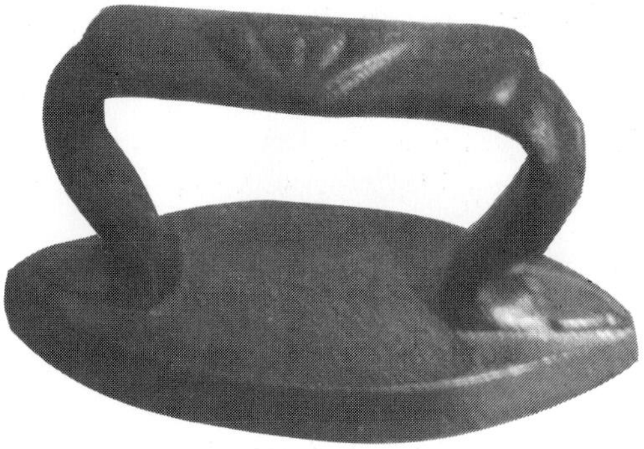

An oval miniature iron, only 1½in. long.
£10

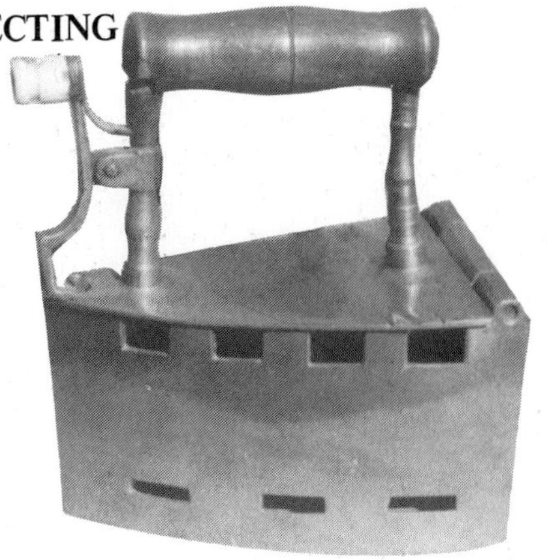

Continental brass charcoal iron with slatted sides.
£30

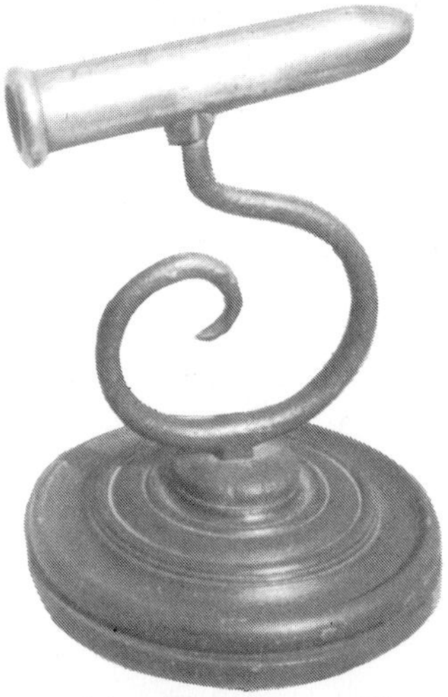

Hand wrought goffering iron with monkey tail support. Value from £8-£150 for multi barrelled.

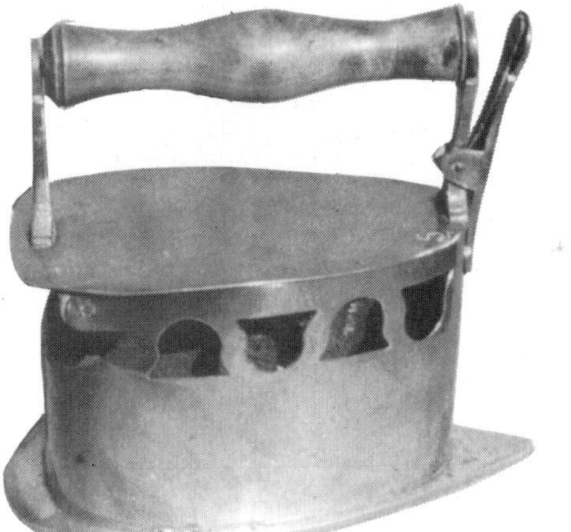

19th century continental brass charcoal iron.
£70

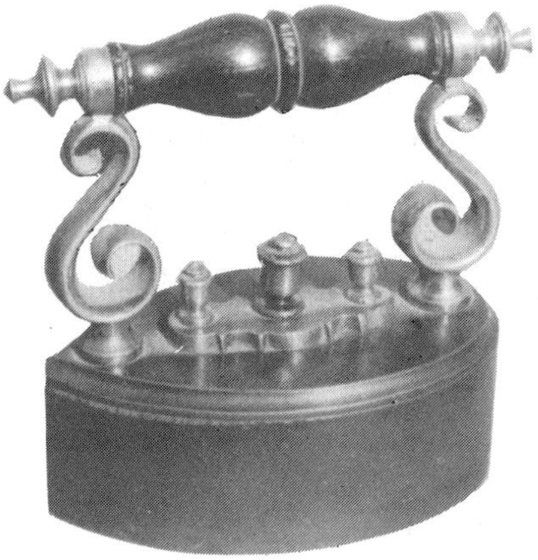

Scottish box iron with ornate brass supports.
£65

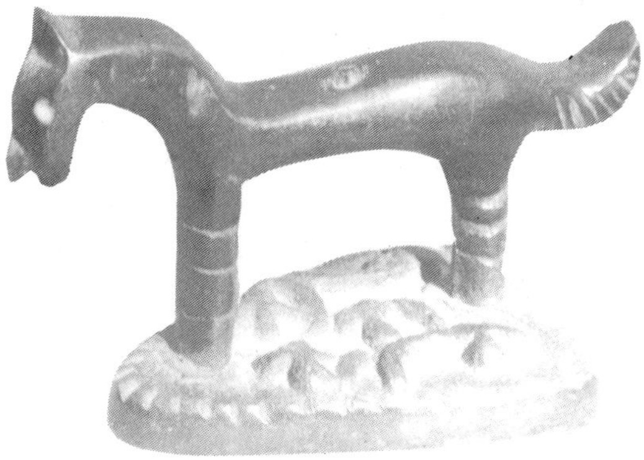

Flat iron with handle in the form of a horse.
£35

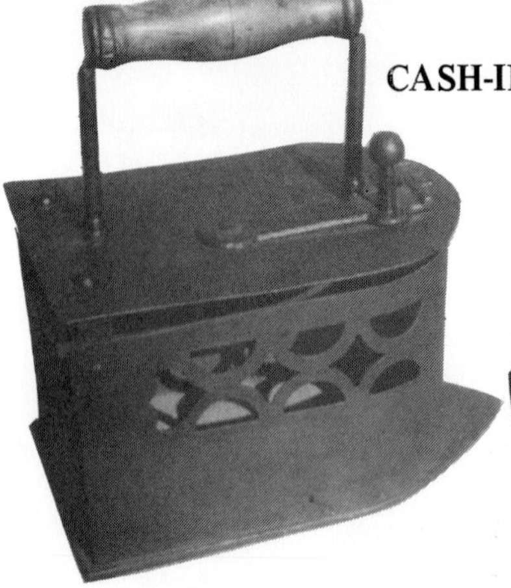

Mid 19th century hand wrought charcoal iron. £70

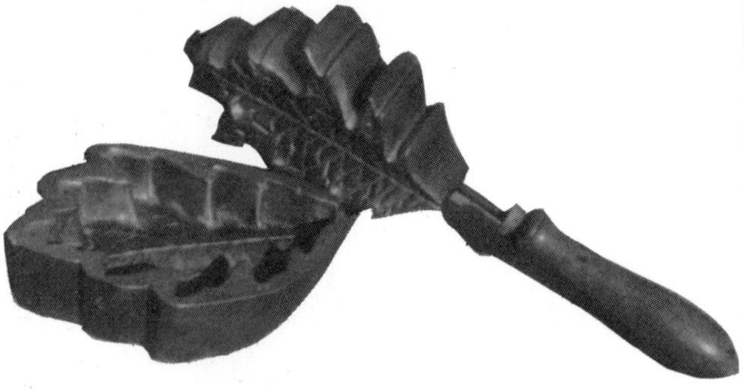

A leaf iron in two parts in which silk is placed to recieve an impression before being stitched to bonnets. £40

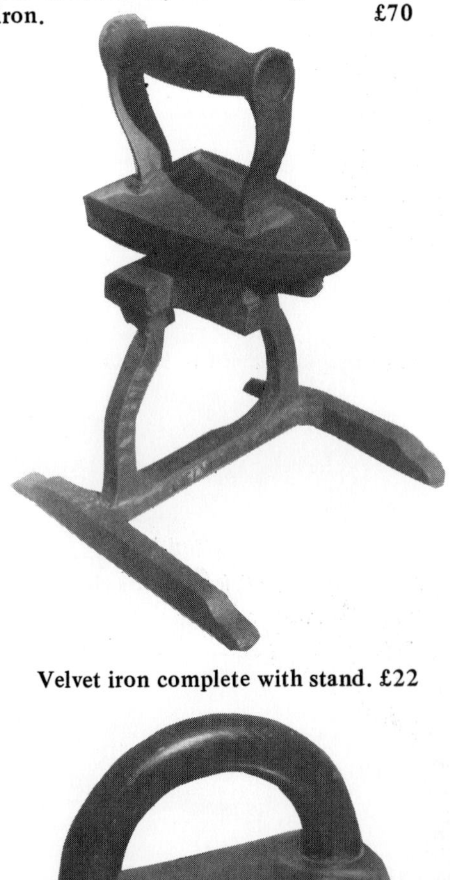

Velvet iron complete with stand. £22

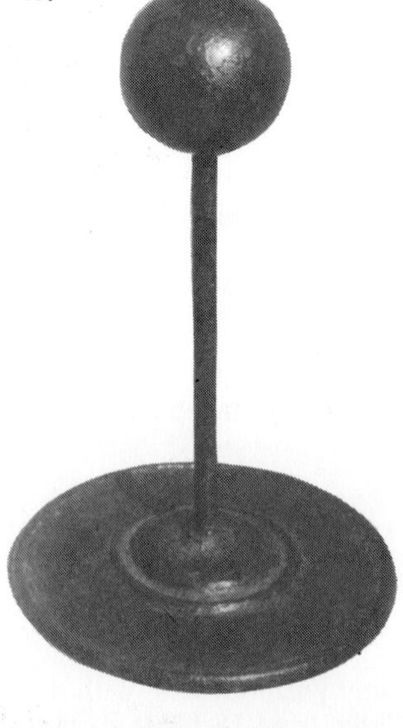

Standing iron with ball top. £30

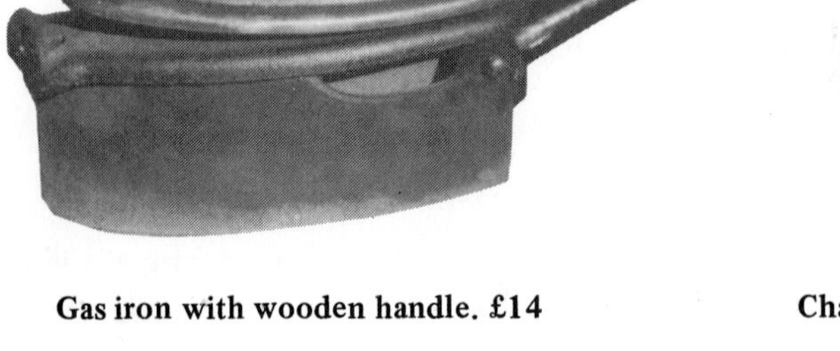

Gas iron with wooden handle. £14

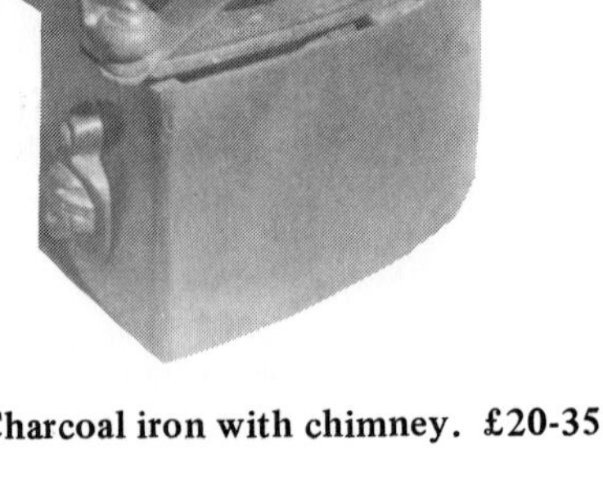

Charcoal iron with chimney. £20-35

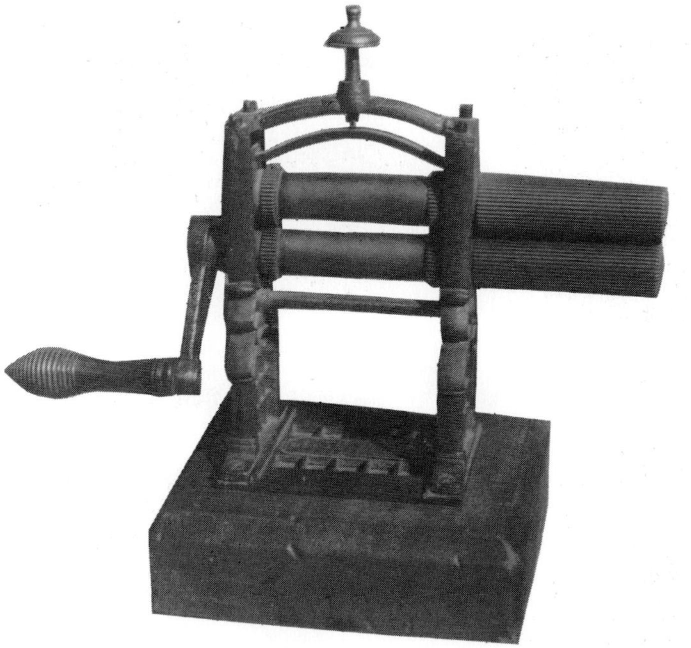

Crimping machine with adjustable corrugated rollers, varius types. £40-80

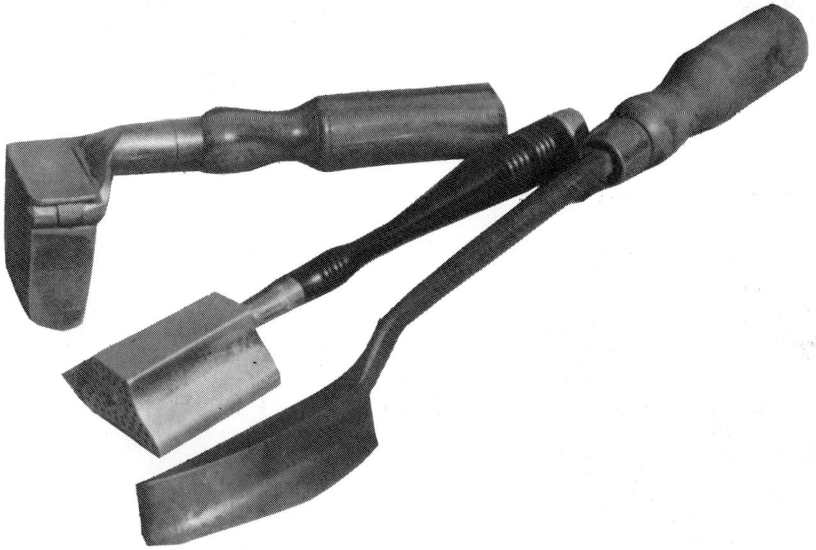

Wooden handled hatters irons. £8-20

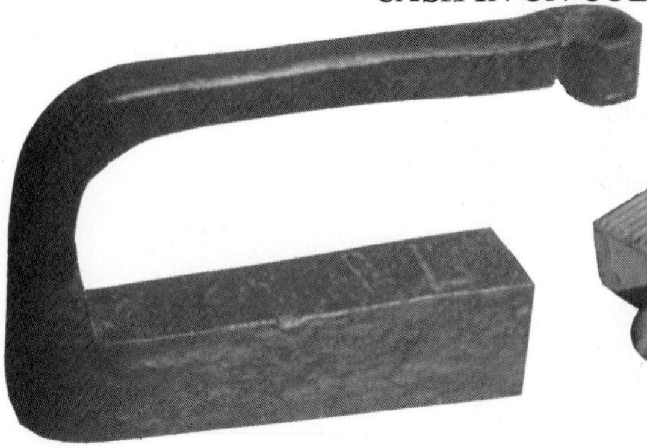

Early 19th century hand wrought goose-iron. £40

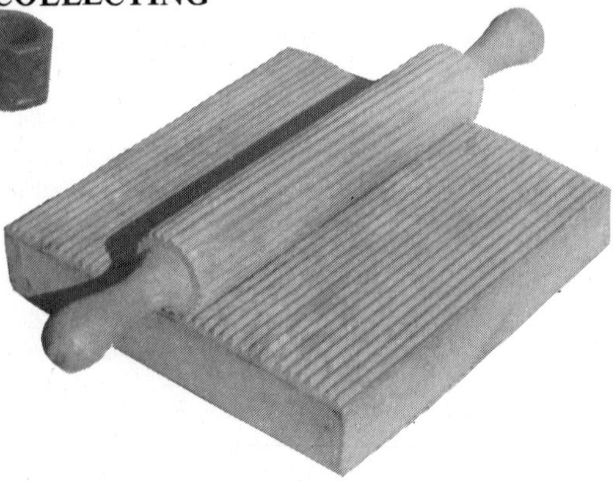

A small wood fluter with a flat base and rolling-pin top. £15.20

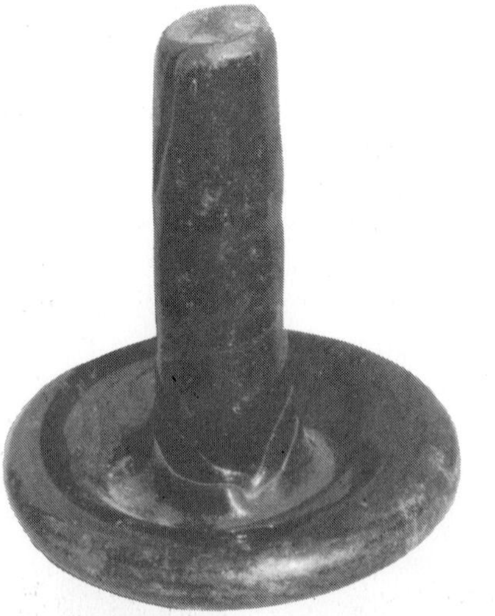

Black glass slickenstone of mushroom shape. £75

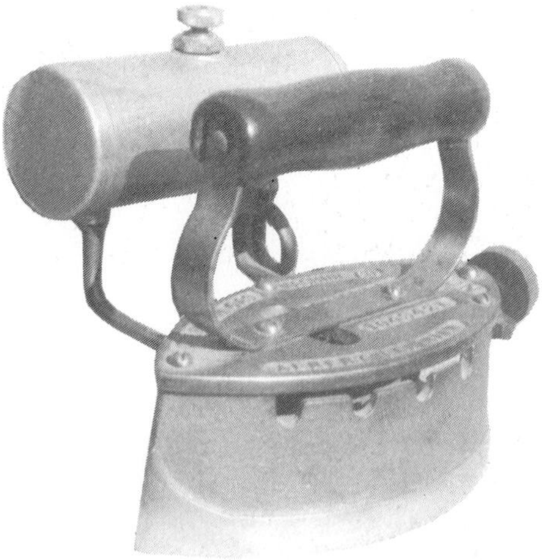

Petrol iron with the container on the side. £15.30

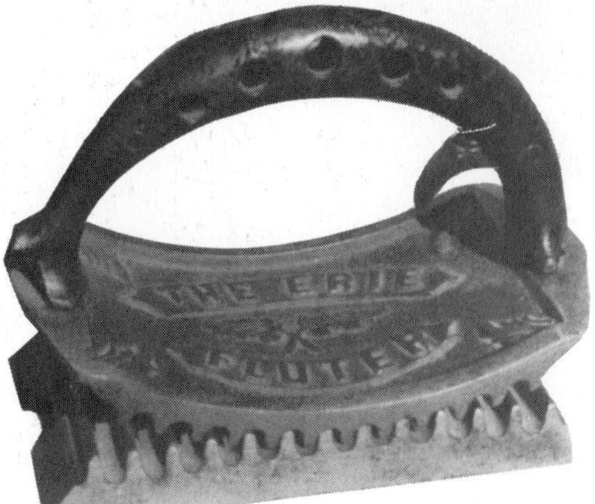

'The Erie Fluter' in two parts with a flat base and rocking top. £30

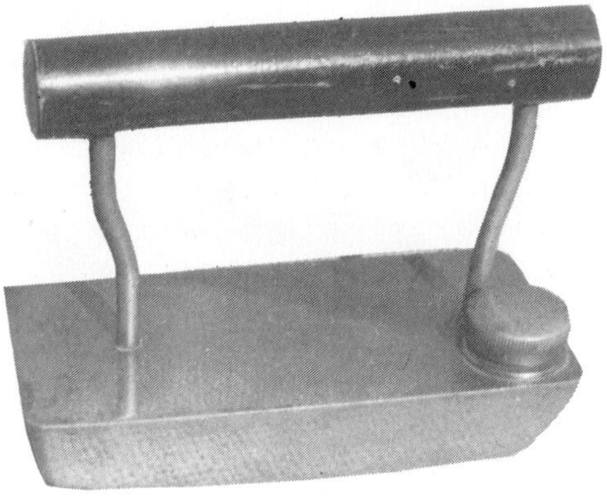

Atkins hot water iron with screw top container. £20

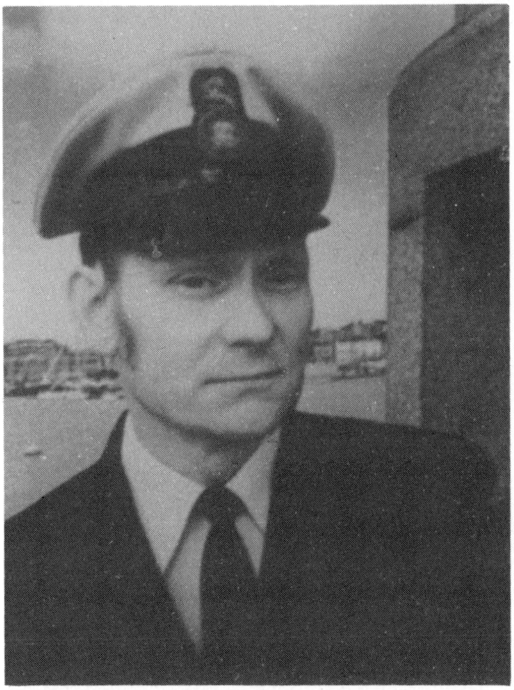

Neville Peakall in uniform alongside Ramsgate Pier Light.

Neville Peakall is a lighthouse keeper on Sark who collects postcards and in particular cards and photos of lighthouses.

"I've got two albums full of cards, approximately 800 of them, mostly British lighthouses. I've also got a good photographic collection. An exhibition of 80 photos of lighthouses which I've taken myself is on permanent exhibition on Spit Bank Fort in the Solent. I wanted to record them for posterity because of the diminishing use of lighthouses.

"Most of my postcard collection are photographic cards as opposed to printed cards and some of them are cards which amateur photographers had printed up by their local chemist and so only two or three of them ever existed.

"The oldest ones go back to the late 1800's but they had to be of land stations because early photographs of tower lighthouses could not be taken from the sea as photography was not sufficiently advanced to be undertaken in a tossing ship.

"In the collection there are pictures of lighthouses that have never been manned and of others that were discontinued in the 1920's or '30's but there were plenty that went even before that.

"There were nearly 1,000 lights around Britain and I've got most of them that are available on cards though there are a great many lights which have probably never been recorded. I keep in touch with other keepers and the families of ex-keepers in order to get any pictures of old lights that they might be disposing of. My ambition is to have a picture of every single one."

The most interesting card Neville has shows the building of the Nab Tower in the Solent at the time of the First World War. He is particularly fond of that card because he served eight years on the Nab Tower.

Other unusual cards show fog bells being blessed for this was done in lighthouses much the same way as ships are blessed.

A card which Neville has not yet been able to find is a long shot view of the lighthouse on St. Tudwal's Island on the coast of Wales. He has a close up picture of a family standing outside the lighthouse, but he would like one taken from the sea.

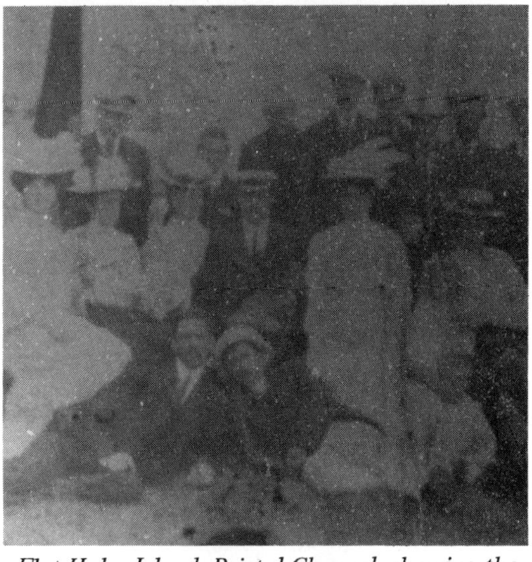

Flat Holm Island, Bristol Channel, showing the keeper's family and workmen, photographed when the fog signal bell was dedicated to the lighthouse. *£15*

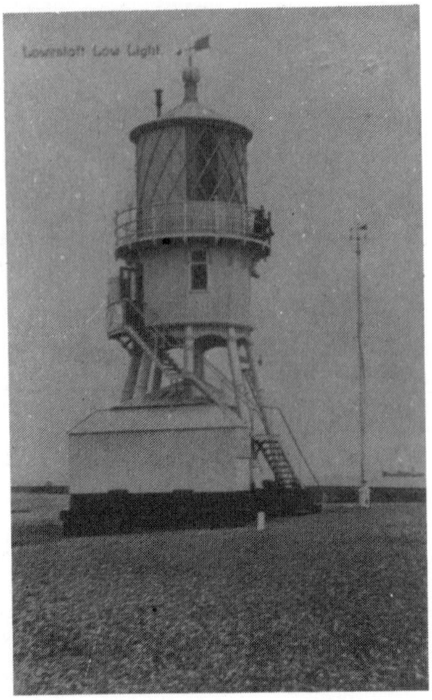

Lowestoft low light replaced with new light built along the coast in the 1920's, an Abbott series card dated August 29th 1912. £1.50

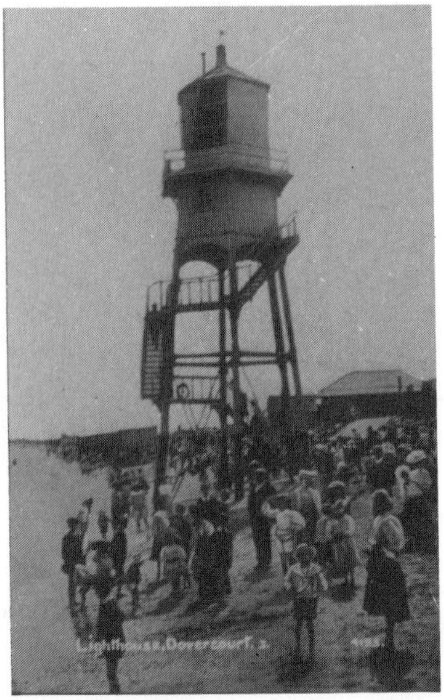

Printed photograph of the light on the beach at Dovercourt, just down the coast from Harwich which was one of two towers, one in front of the other, and lived in by a crew of two, 1901. £2

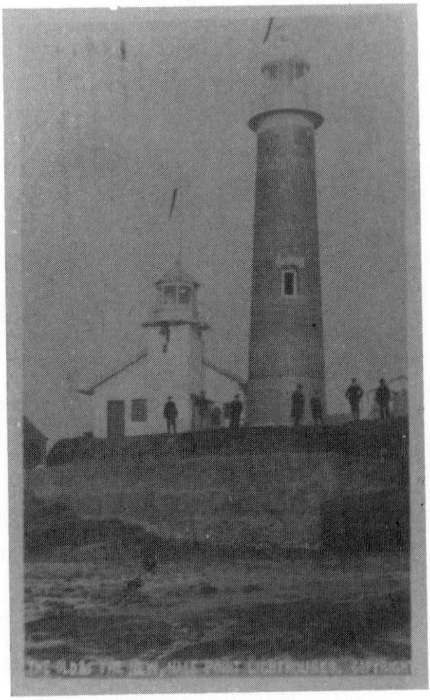

Hale Point, River Mersey, an unusual card showing the old and the new, 1908. £6

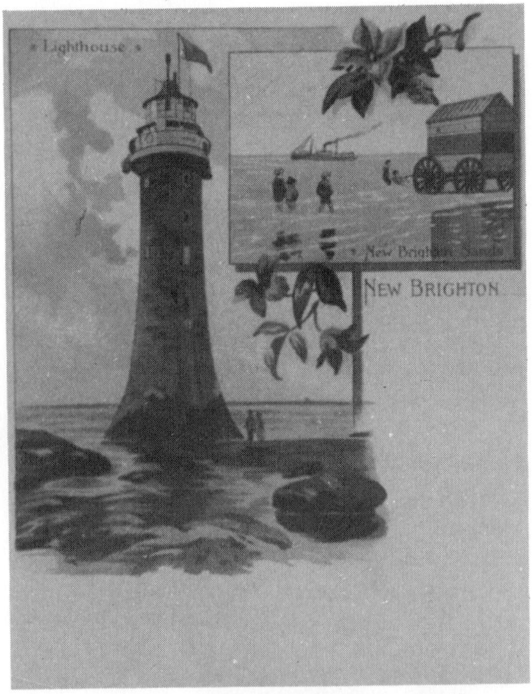

Rare court size card of New Brighton lighthouse, built in 1880, at the entrance to the River Mersey, printed in the chromo-litho method by F. Kent, Manchester, circa 1896. £18

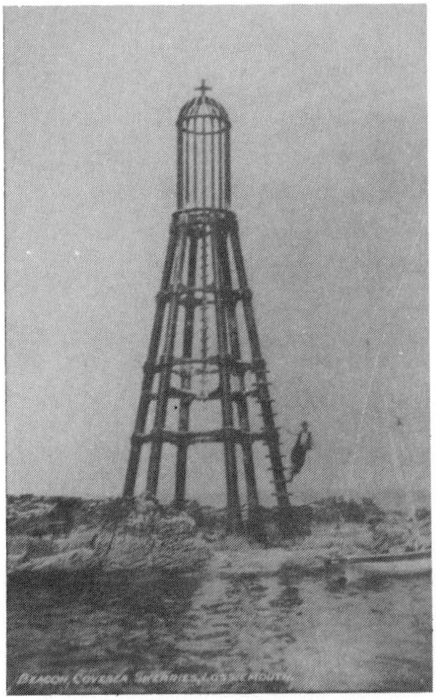

A Beacon on the Covesea Skerries Rocks used as a fore runner of many Rock lighthouses and in continued use long after the lighthouse was established in 1846, printed card, circa 1908. £3

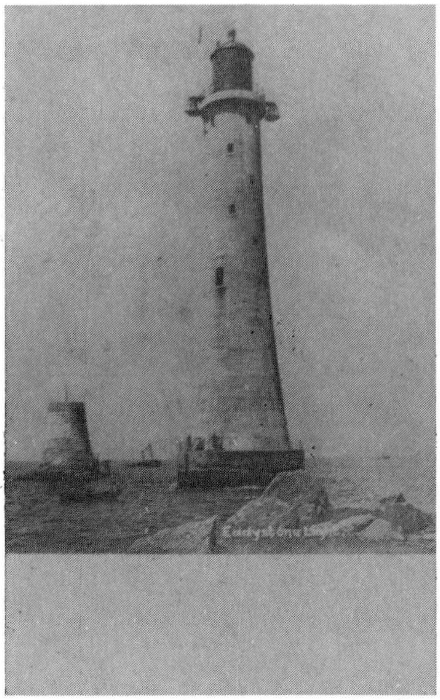

An early Eddystone lighthouse relief by Friths with an undivided back, circa 1902. £3

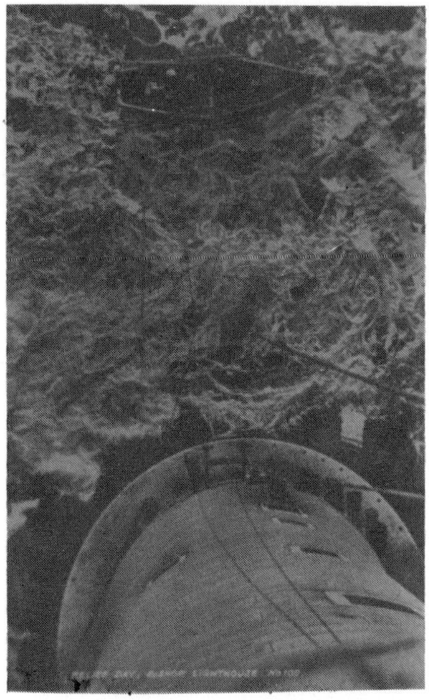

Relief day Bishop Rock Lighthouse, looking down the tower from the gallery into the boat and a rough sea, real photo card by Gibson of the Scilly Isles, early 1960's. £3

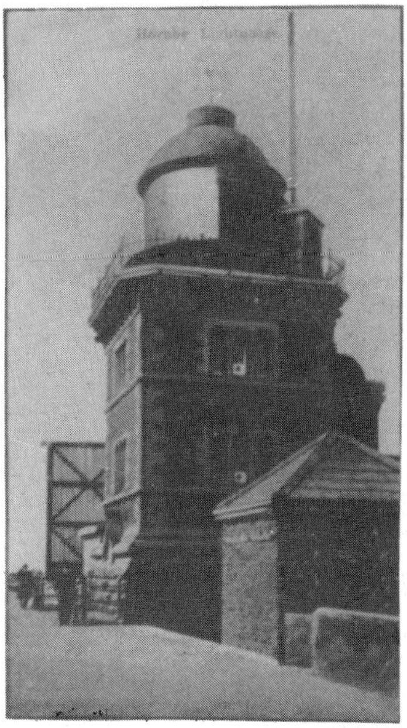

Hornby lighthouse, Bootle, also known as the North Wall, published by the State Series, Liverpool, 1918. £1.50

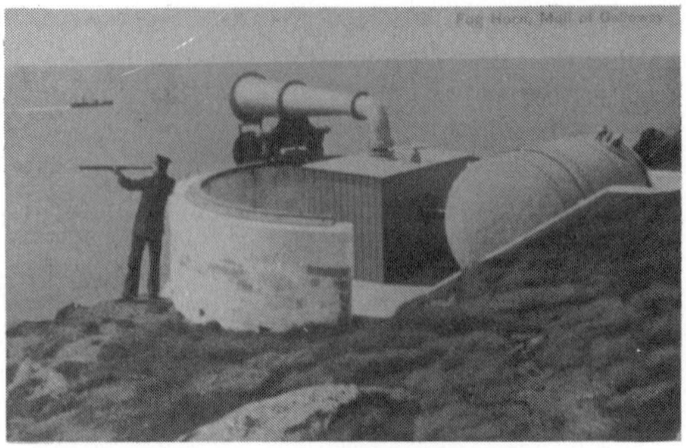

Colour printed card of good quality, showing the fog horn at the Mull of Galloway station built away from the main lighthouse itself, 1908. £3

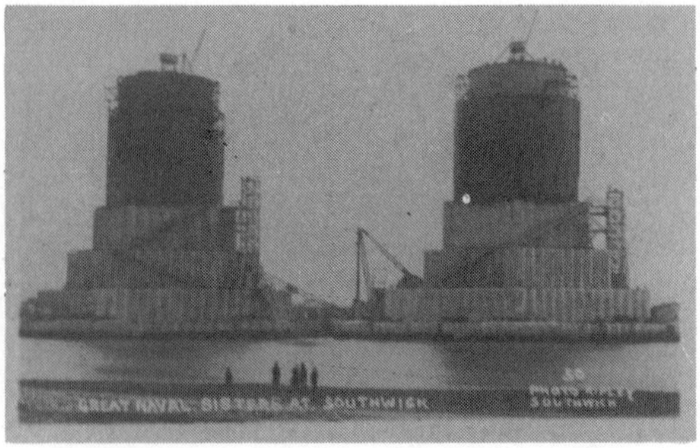

Mystery Towers built as part of the war machine in 1917 at Shoreham Harbour, but uncompleted due to hostilities ceasing before their completion. The one on the left was scrapped but the tower on the right became a lighthouse, marking the approaches to the Solent between the Isle of Wight and Selsey Bill. £4

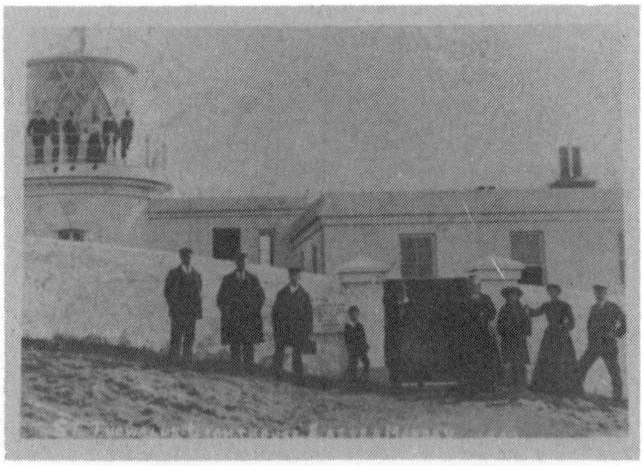

St. Tudwal's Island lighthouse, off the Welsh coast on Easter Monday 1907, showing the two crews, Principal Keeper's family and visitors. £12

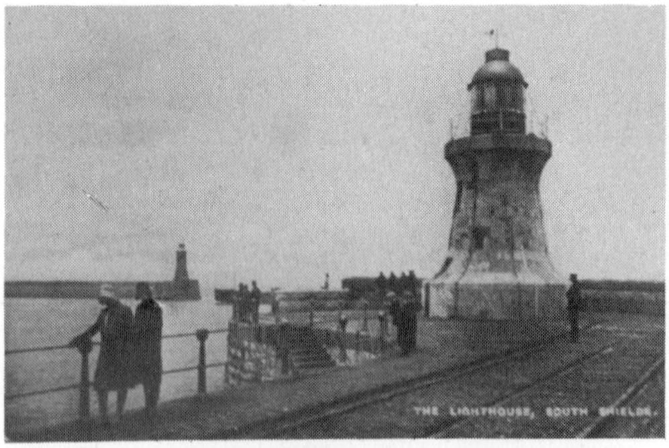

Real photo card published by A.M.H., So.S. 'Meldon' series of South Shields Pier light, 1925. £2.50

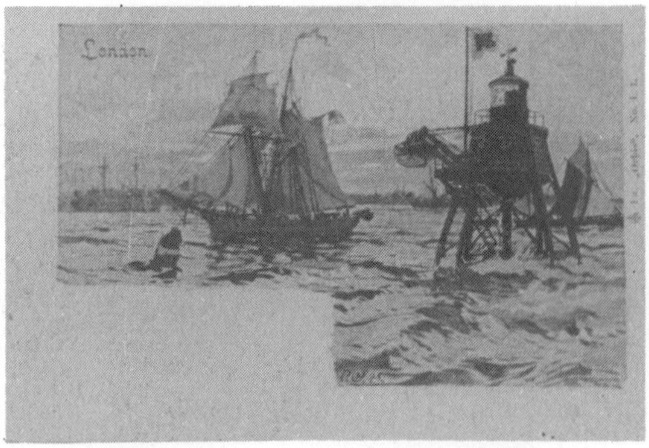

Rare, standard size chromo-litho card of the Gunfleet light in the upper Thames estuary, 1898, printed in Germany. Probably sold aboard ships which ran from London to the seaside resorts of the East and South coasts. £20

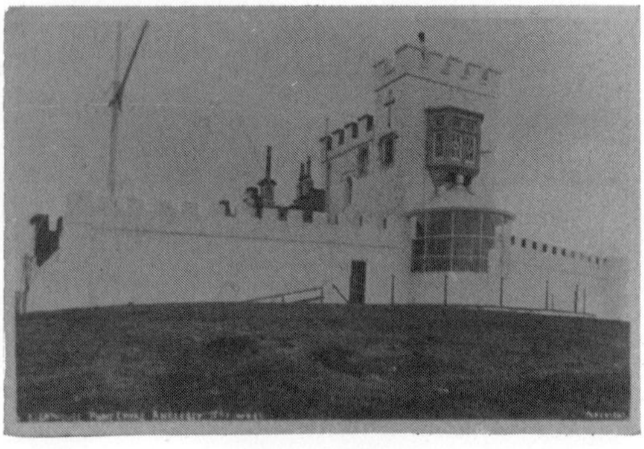

Point Lynas, Anglesey, built by the River Mersey Board but taken over by Trinity House in the 1970's and now semi-automatic. £5

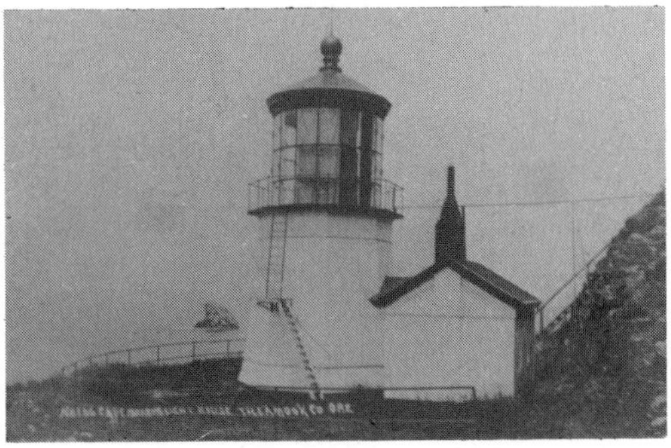

Cape Meares lighthouse, Tillamook, County Oregon, on the West coast of America, built in 1881, published by Pacific Photo Co., and postally used 1915. £4

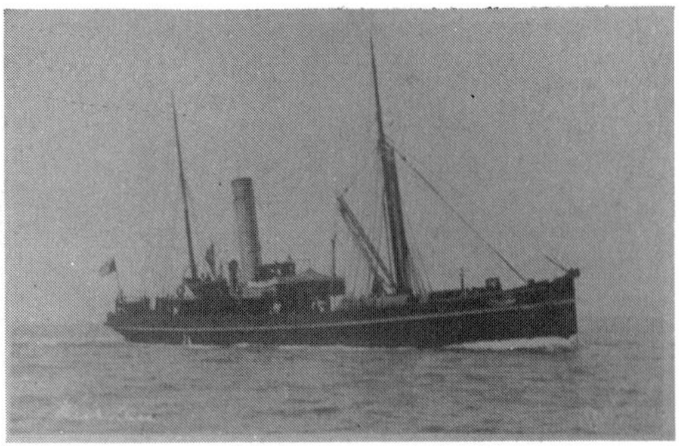

A rare card showing the lighthouse tender, T.H.V. Warden, photographed by Beken of Cowes, circa 1926. £20

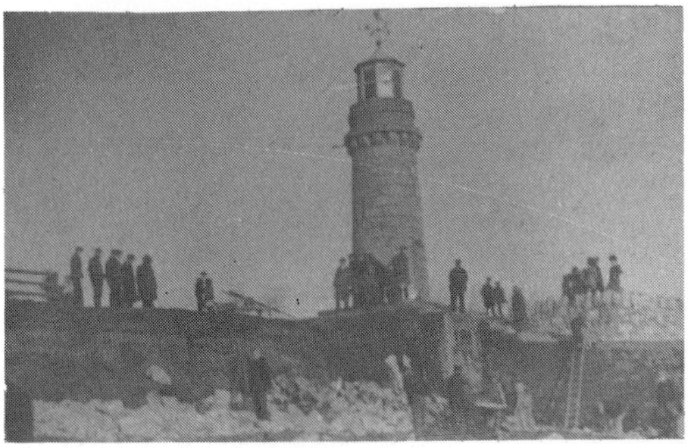

Teignmouth lighthouse, on the South coast, built in 1845, real photo card, circa 1912. £7

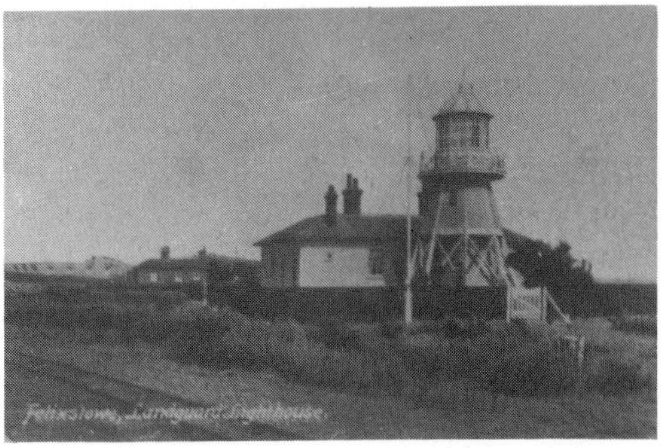

Felixstowe Landguard lighthouse by Frith, replaced in 1912 by a new light up the coast. £4

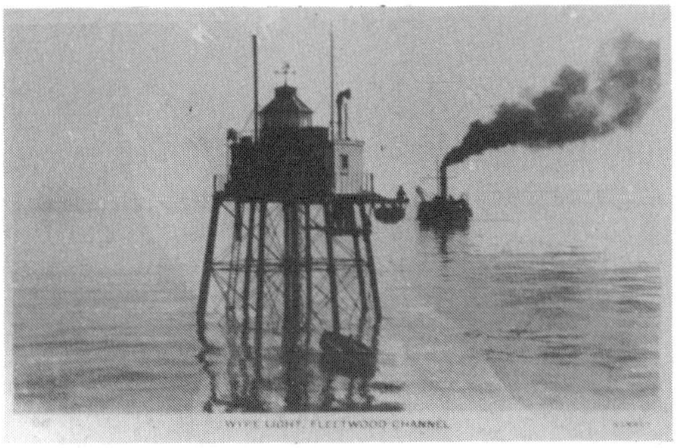

Wyre lighthouse, Fleetwood Channel, which had the distinction of being rammed by a schooner in 1870 and carried away on the ship's bow only to be returned, re-erected and still there today, real photo card. £2

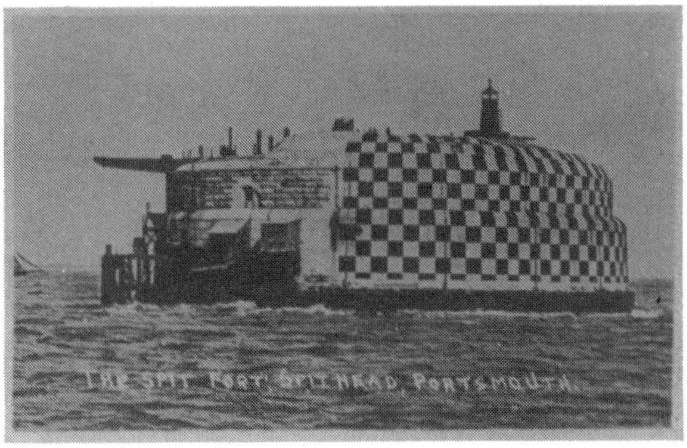

Spit Bank Fort, Spit Head, built during the Napoleonic War to protect Portsmouth Harbour – it now has a light and is used as a navigational aid, real photo card, dated 1920. £7

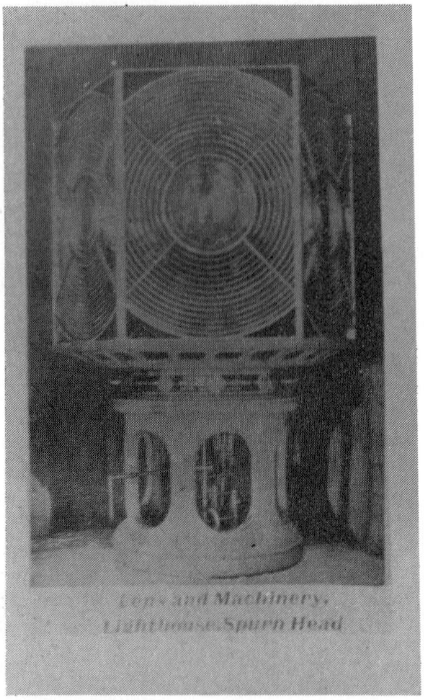

Lighthouse lens and machinery for Spurn Head lighthouse, fitted out in 1895. This photographic card, dated 1912, would be sold in the local store to the many people who visited the area for the good sandy beaches. £3

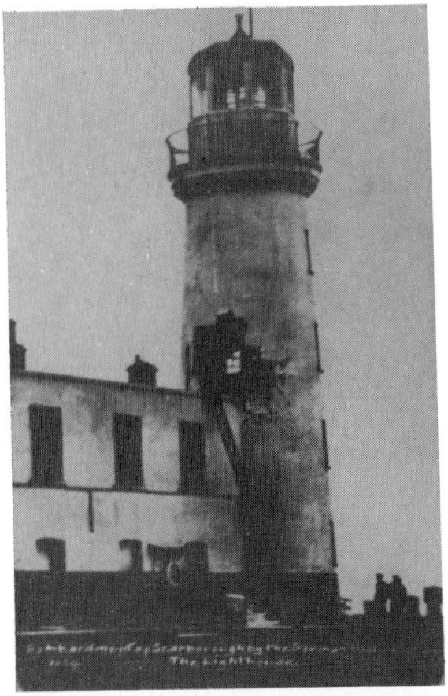

Scarborough lighthouse, damaged through enemy action on the night of December 12th 1914. This particular card is dated 24th December 1914 which indicates how commercial the card makers were. £10

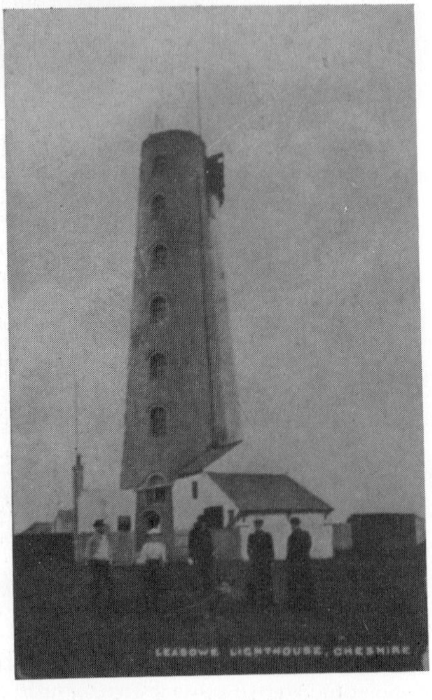

Leasowe lighthouse on the coast between the River Mersey and the Dee, published by Harrops of Liverpool, circa 1905. £3

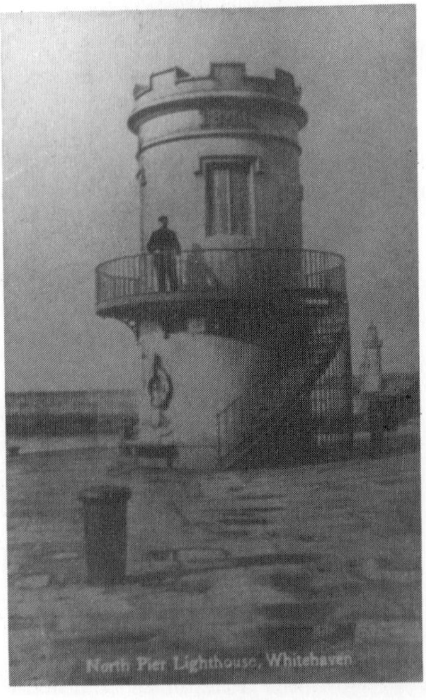

Photographic card of Whitehaven, North Pier, not the normal shape of a lighthouse, printed by Britain and Wright, Stockton, early 1900's. £4

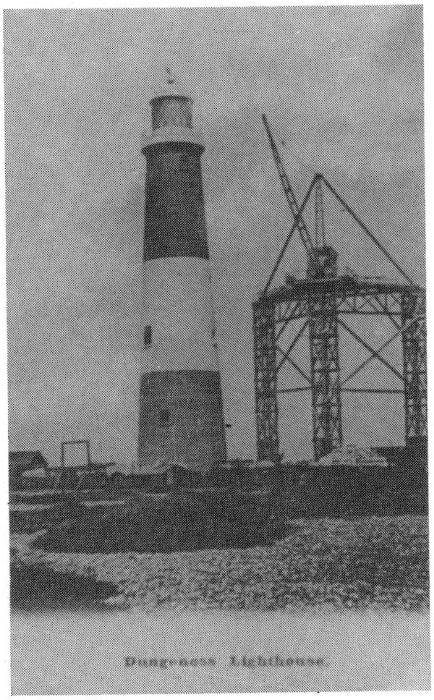

Dungeness lighthouse, on the South coast, in the process of being built, it took three years and was first lit on March 31st 1904, original photo. £4

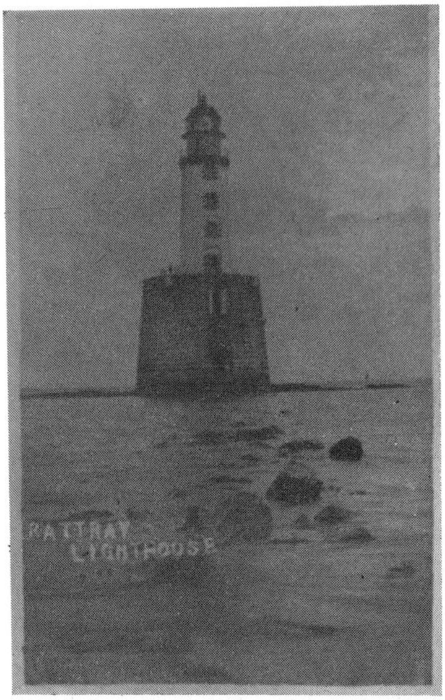

Rattray House lighthouse on the East coast of Scotland, one of the more unusual rock lights, 1907. £6

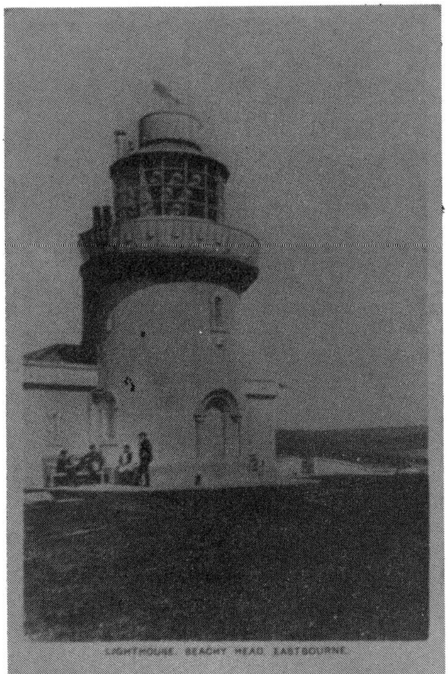

Real photograph of the old light at Beachy Head dated September 2nd 1908 (replaced by the new light in 1912) and now dangerously close to the edge of the cliffs. £4

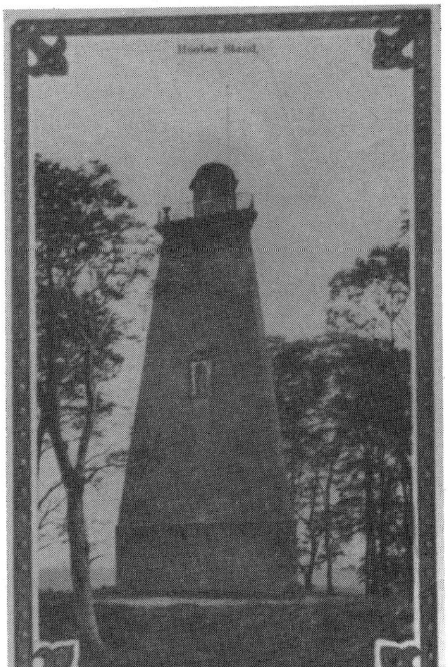

Hoober Stand, Cambridgeshire, often taken as a lighthouse card but built in 1748 as a tribute to George II by the Marquis of Rockingham, for subduing a rebellion in 1746. £2

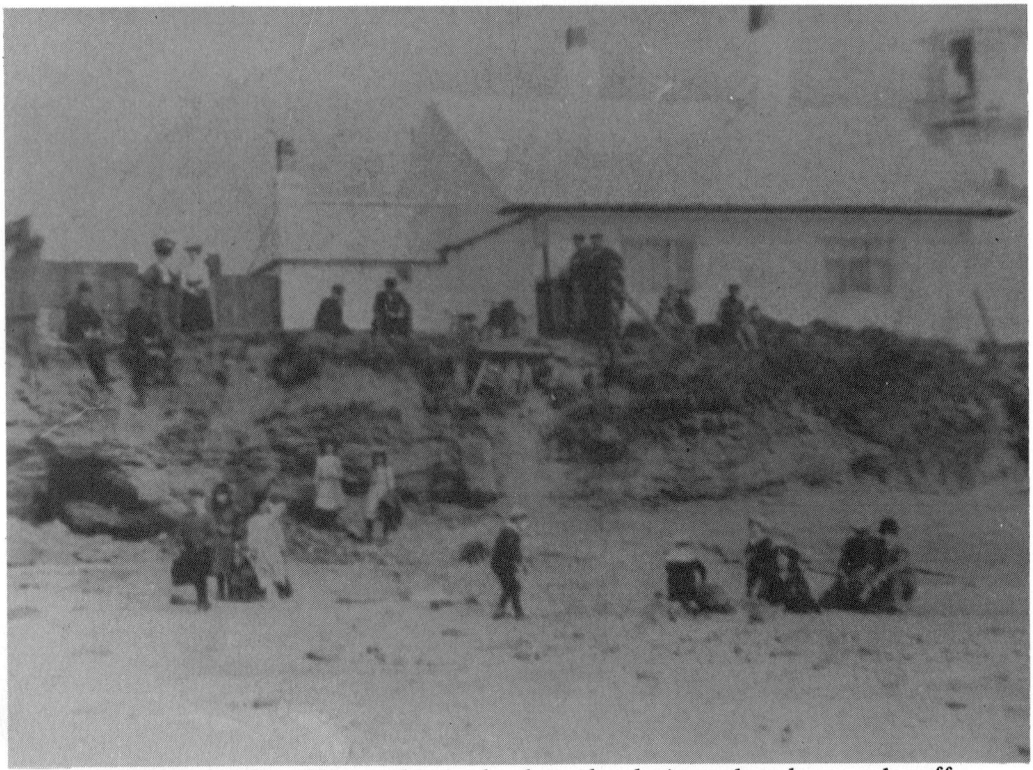

Hale lighthouse, River Mersey, showing local people relaxing and at play on a day off, circa 1906. £2

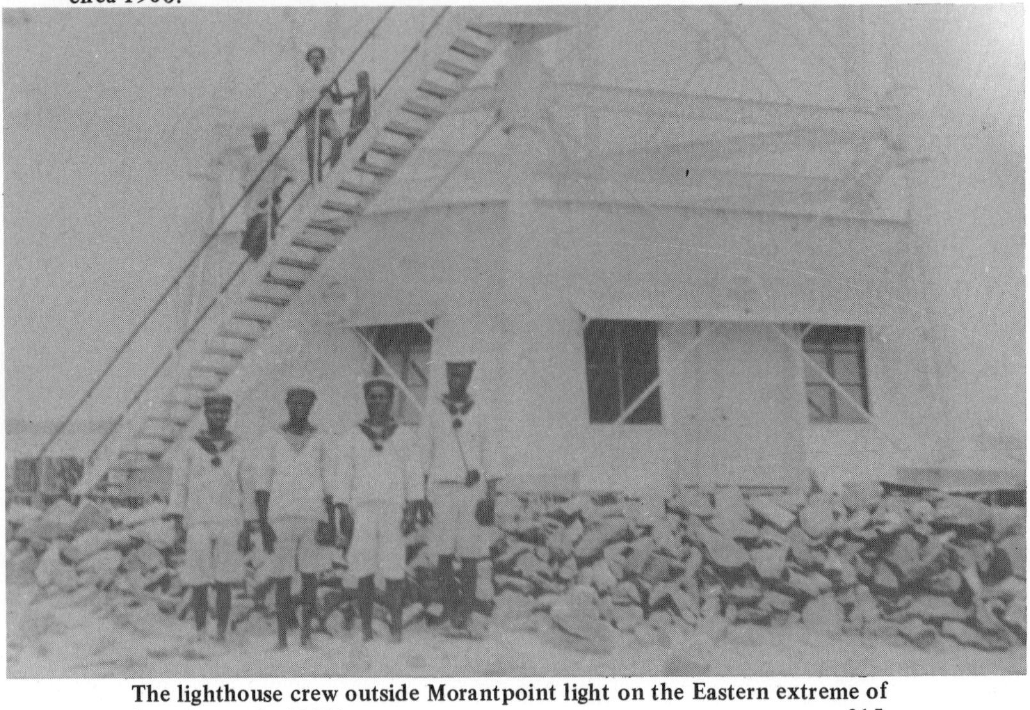

The lighthouse crew outside Morantpoint light on the Eastern extreme of Jamaica, early 1900's. £15

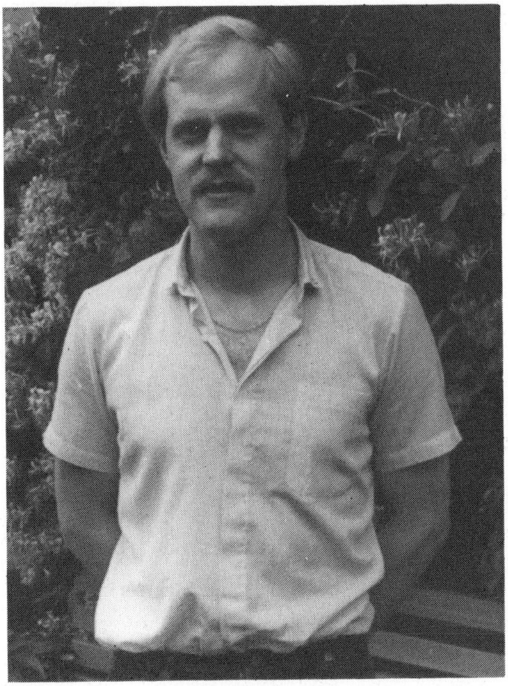

Lembit Eha is a schoolteacher and collects old dolls and doll's heads.

"Collecting dolls began by accident for me because I used to go digging for bottles in rubbish tips and one day I found a doll's head. People used to throw them out and a good collecting area is Harrogate where there was a lot of money. You get really good dolls in rubbish dumps there. I also once got a lovely head the size of a real baby's on a Bradford dump.

"I've been collecting for 14 years and I've got 350 really good examples of doll's heads and 14 complete dolls. They are mostly German but I also have some French ones. Many of them are character dolls. I've got two faced dolls, a whistling boy and what's called a Kaiser baby because the Kaiser had a doll made modelled on his son.

"I don't collect wax or wooden dolls, just bisque or parian china. The price is not important, I rate my dolls on the design and modelling and they've got to have a good colour. I don't think you should restore them the way some people do because no modern technique can reproduce the original finish, it spoils it."

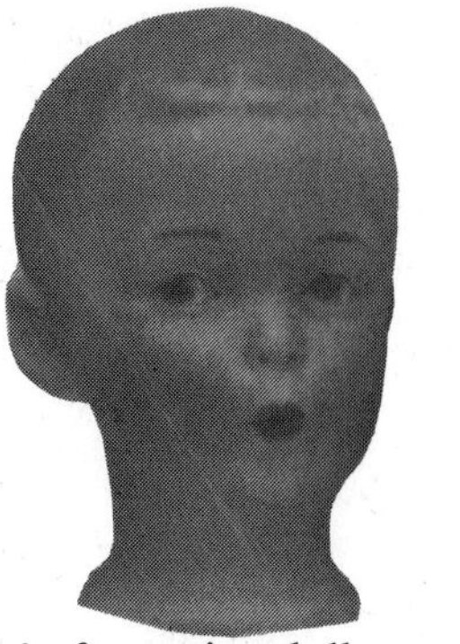

Lembit's favourite dolls are a whistling boy which would originally have had a whistle in its mouth and which is very finely modelled. He also has a highly prized French doll dressed as a Victorian bride with handmade lace on her gown which is worth several hundred pounds. An average price for a good head is about £50.

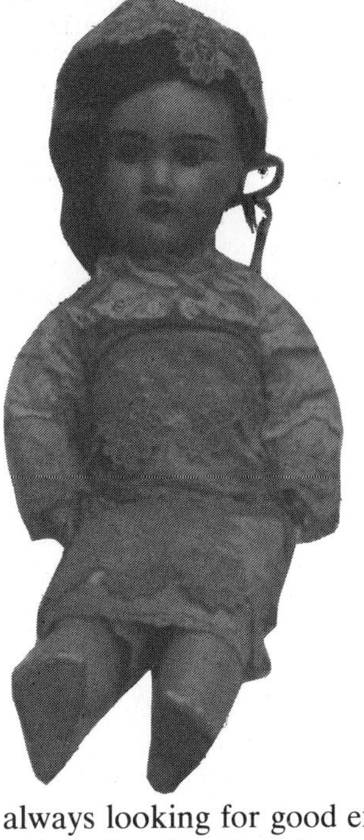

He is always looking for good examples of dolls made by the French companies Jumeau, Bru and S.F.B.J. as well as by German makers like Armand Marseille and Heubach Koppelsdorf.

"Anyone wanting information about dolls can phone me on Halifax 0422/249914. I would also like to buy dolls in any condition for my collection."

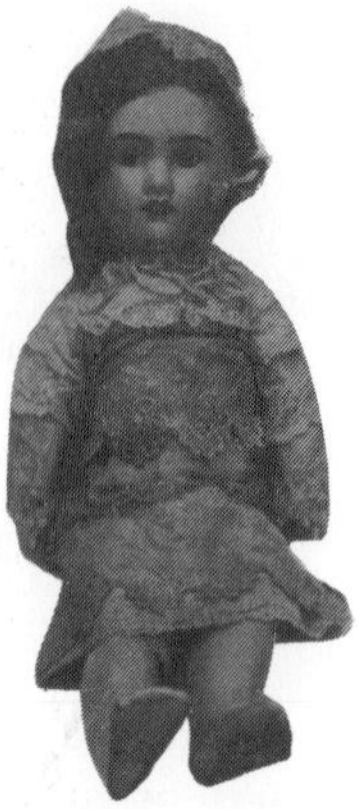

French bride doll marked Limoges, with original costume, 24in. high. £350

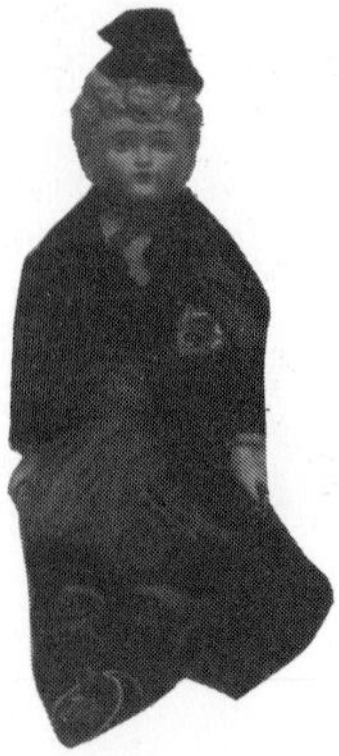

German character doll marked P.M. 914, 20in. high. £200

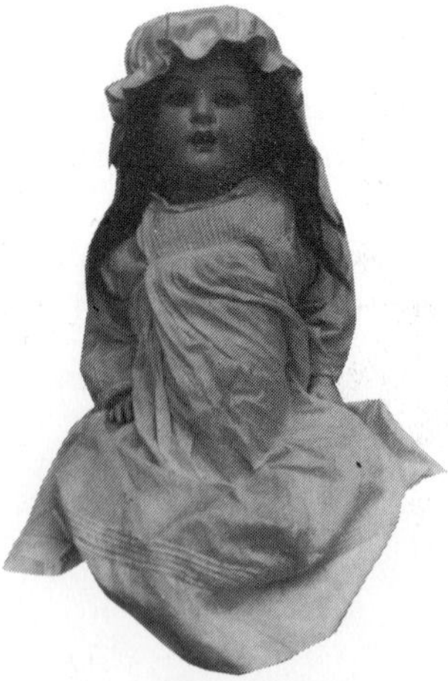

German doll marked Jutta Baby, Dressel, 1922, 22in. high. £200

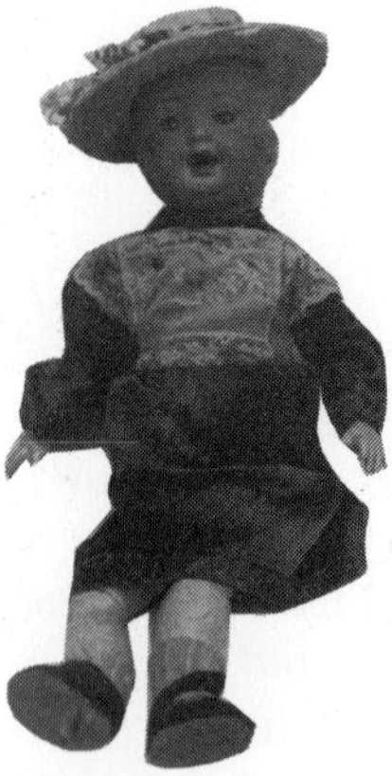

German boy doll, unmarked, with original costume, 22in. high. £175

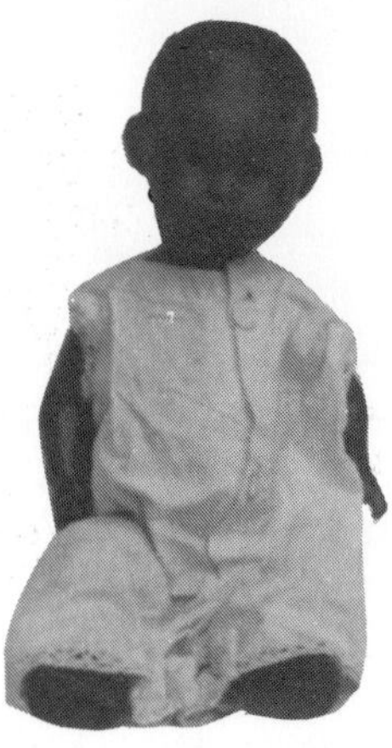

German black baby doll, marked Simon Halbig 245, with closed mouth and fixed eyes, 12in. high. £175

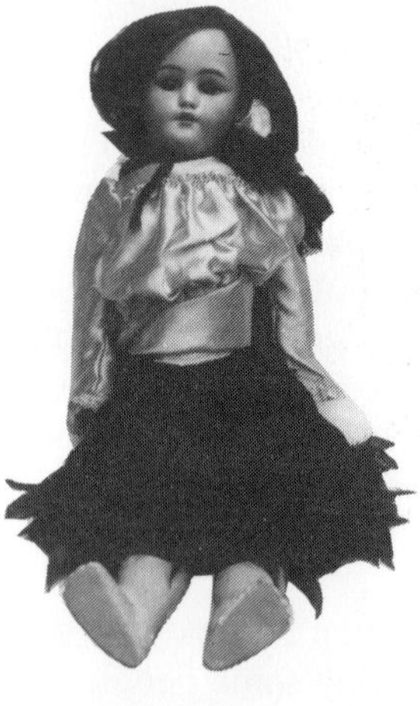

German doll marked Schoenau & Hoffmeister, with pierced ears, 28in. high. £300

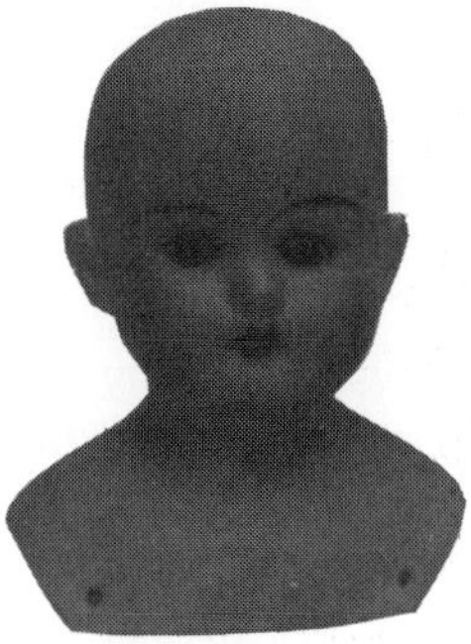

German shoulder head marked K and W No. 8, 4in. high. £30

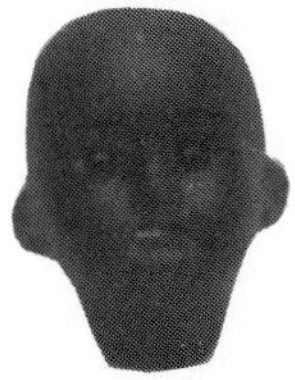

German black bisque head, marked 1894 A.M., 2½in. high. £25

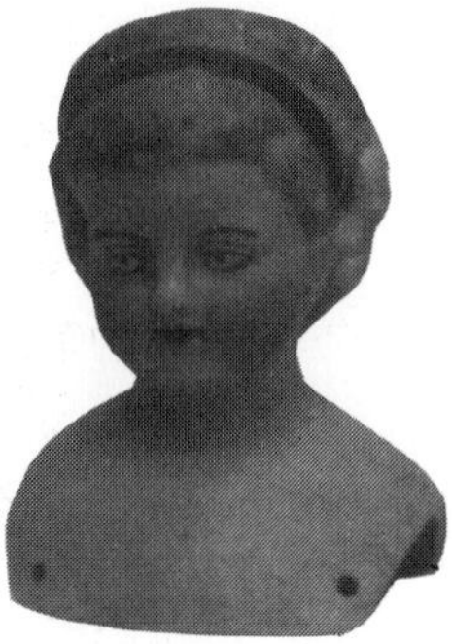

Unmarked French doll's head with moulded hair, pierced ears and painted eyes, 4in. high. £60

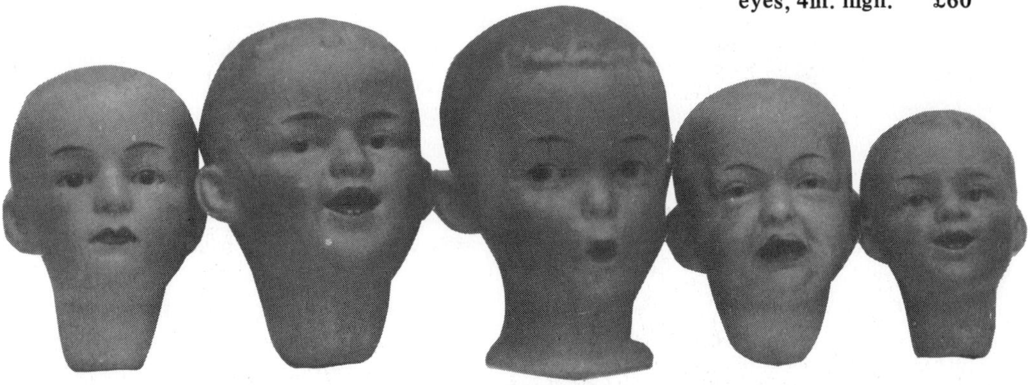

A group of five boy dolls by Heubach Koppelsdorf, Germany. £20 – £50 each

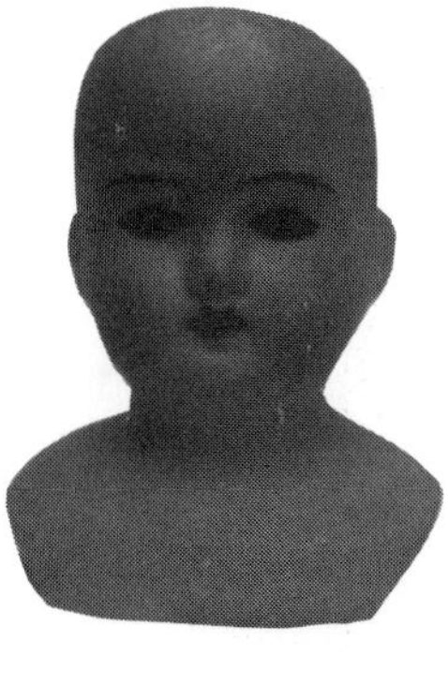

German shoulder head, marked 14/0. £30

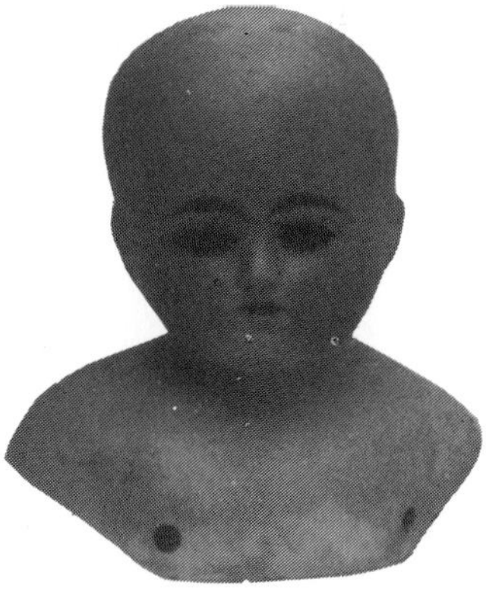

French 'Parisienne' shoulder head with fixed eyes, 5in. high. £125

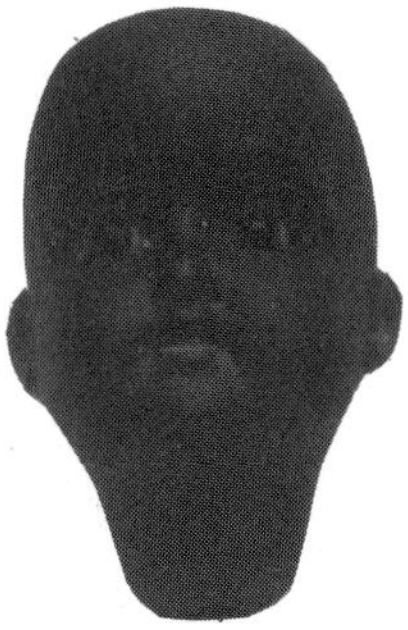

German black bisque head marked Schoenau & Hoffmeister, 1909, 3½in. high. £30

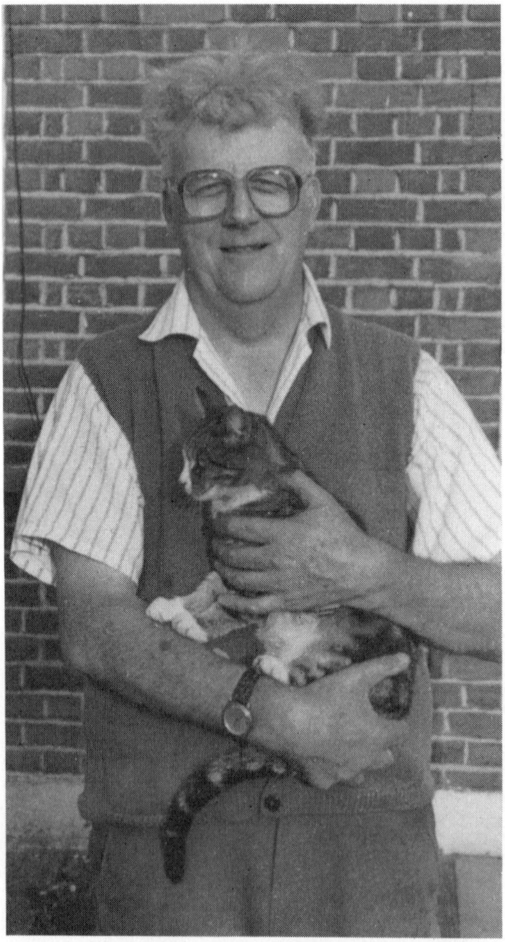

John Brooks is a self employed owner and letter of property and he collects items connected with the Youth Hostel movement.

"Like many people I had a collection of postcards and the very first one I bought was a postcard of a Youth Hostel I'd once visited. That wasn't really the start of my interest in the Youth Hostel Association but after a few years it struck me that it would be more interesting to concentrate on one theme and I decided on the Y.H.A.

"The good thing about my collection is that it's become a way of life because we go away most weekends with the Ordnance Survey Maps to visit houses that are, or were, Youth Hostels. I knock on the door and sometimes the people living there let me see round. It's more interesting to know what a house is like inside. Then I take photographs of the house and build up my pictorial records. There's been many times when I've gone to a house that is no longer a Hostel and the people there don't know about its past history. I also collect papers, badges and hotel stamps, anything to do with the Y.H.A. in fact. A lot of stuff has been destroyed without anyone having an idea of its value. Not even the Y.H.A. movement itself seems to have a comprehensive collection.

"The movement began in Germany in the early 1900's, started by Richard Sherman, a teacher, who hit on the idea of using schools as overnight accommodation for people on walking tours and it spread to this country in 1930 when the first hostel, Pennent Hall in the Conway Valley, was opened. By the end of 1931 there were over 100 hostels and five of the original ones are still operating. In all there are about 260 today and I have been to more than half of them."

Since 1930, 750 buildings have operated as hostels. John's postcard collection numbers more than 1,000 different views of hostels and he has a pictorial record of almost 400 which he has visited personally.

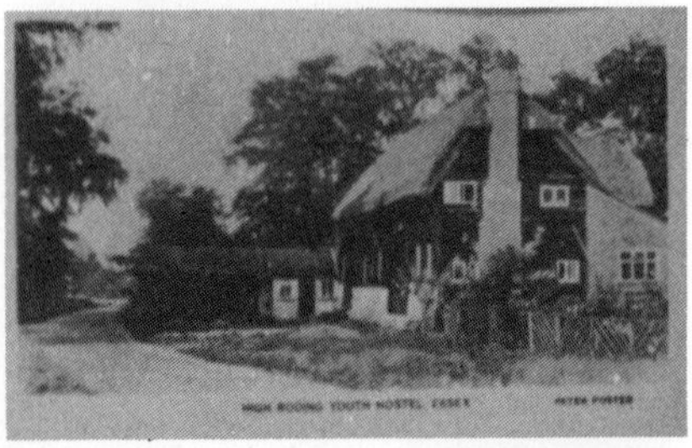

Postcards can cost anything from 25p to £2 which he will pay for a card of any hostel he has not yet recorded and which is unlikely to come along again.

The postcard he is most anxious to find is a view of Maeshafn House in North Wales, a wooden structure, which was the first purpose built hostel, donated to the Y.H.A. by the Holt family of shipping magnates. It is no longer operating as a hostel.

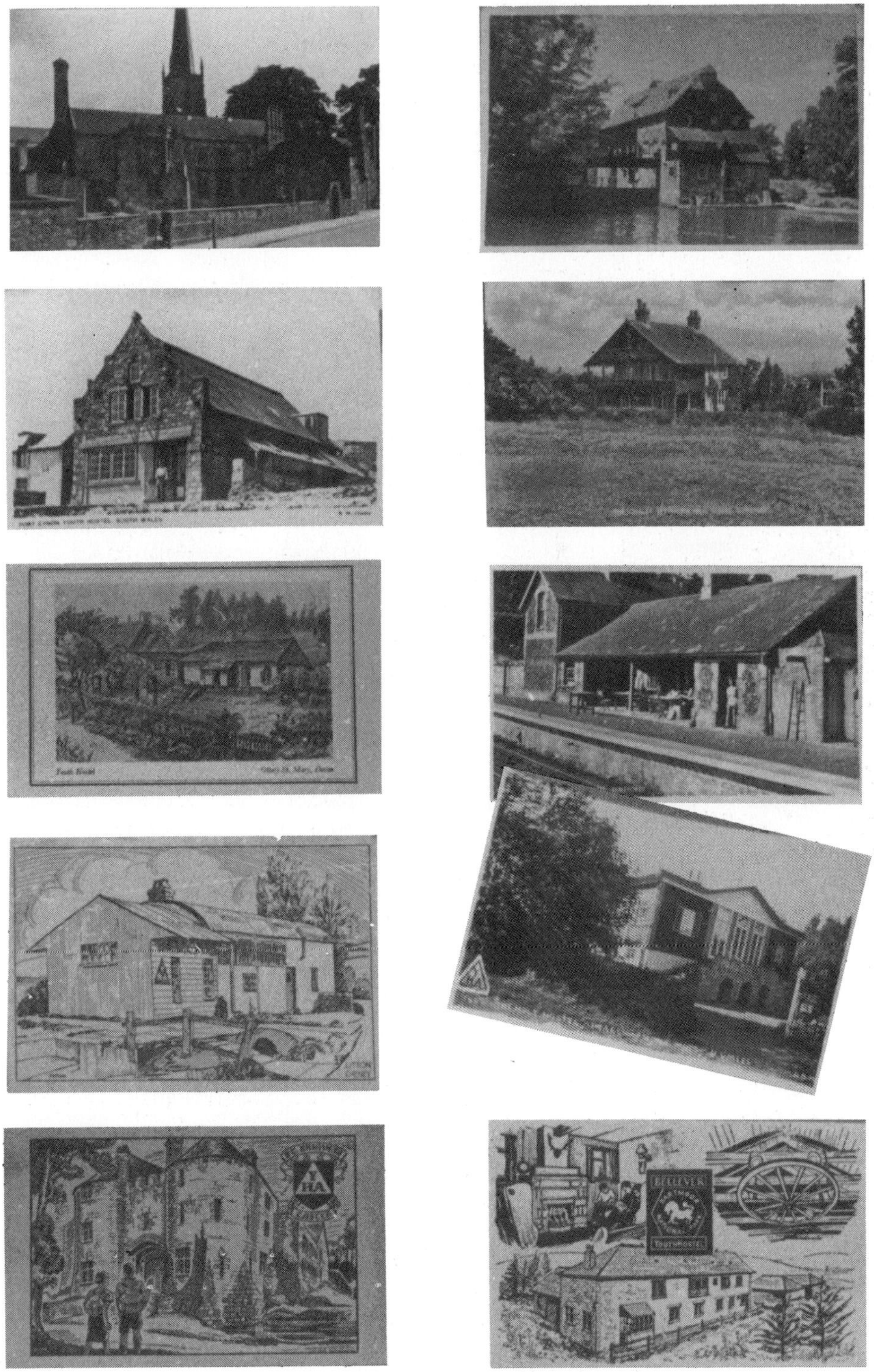

Postcards were produced from about 1933 and rare examples can be worth up to £2. While not every Hostel published a card some produced quite a variety which gives adequate scope for the collector.

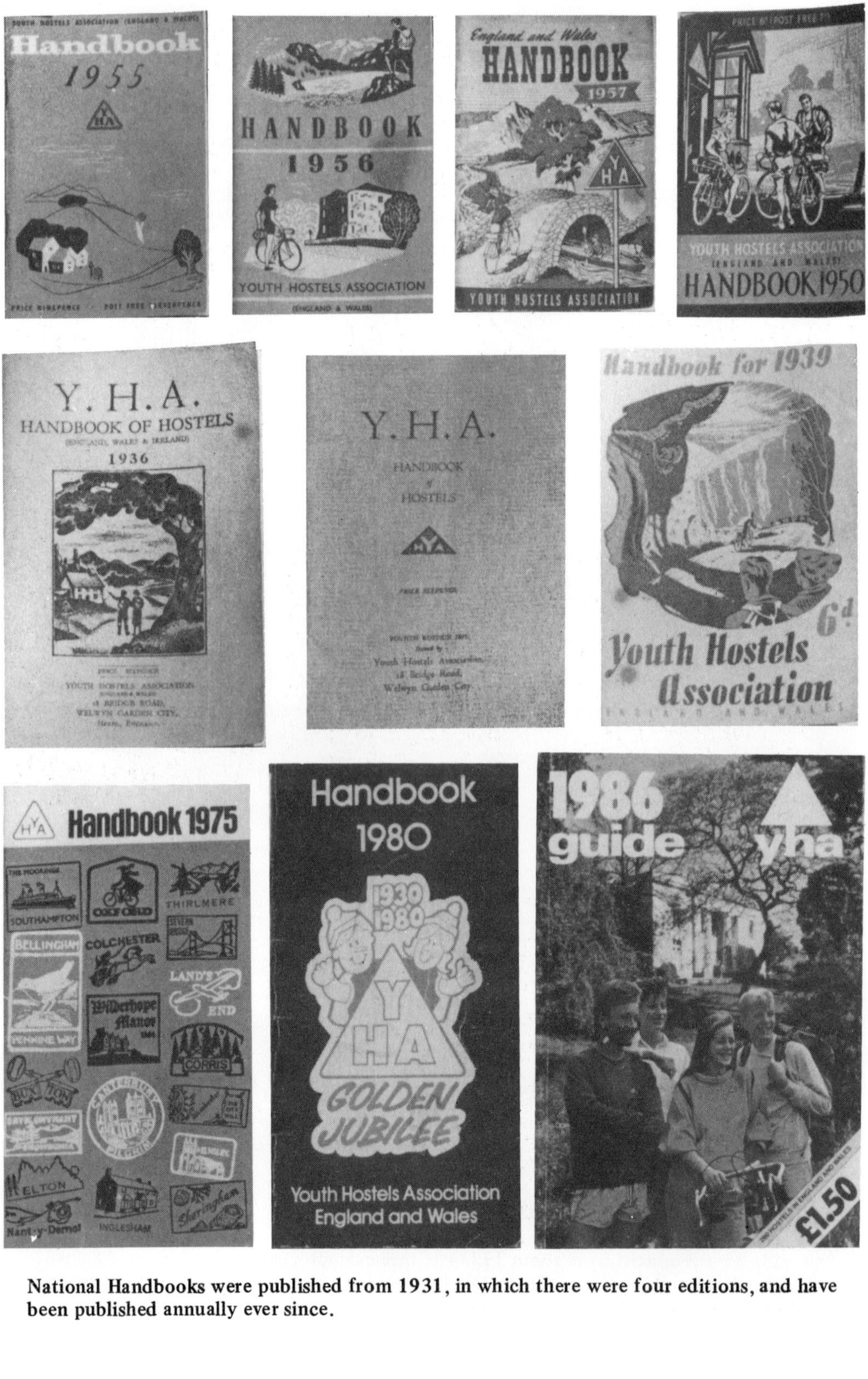

National Handbooks were published from 1931, in which there were four editions, and have been published annually ever since.

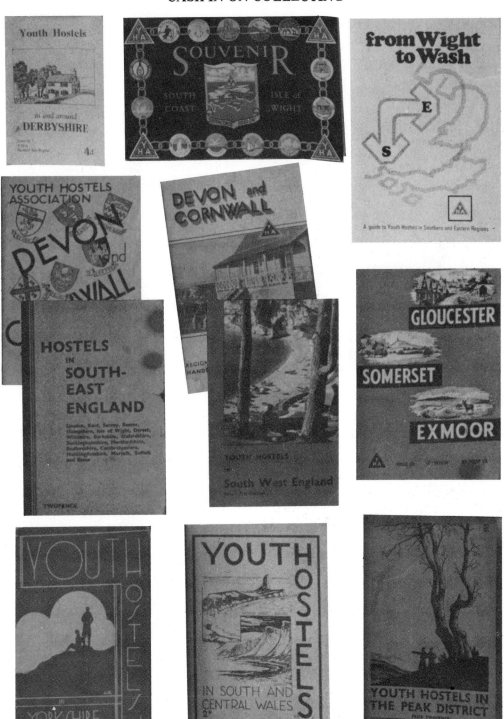

Regional Handbooks are naturally confined to a particular area of the country and are published intermittently having started a few years after the National Handbooks.

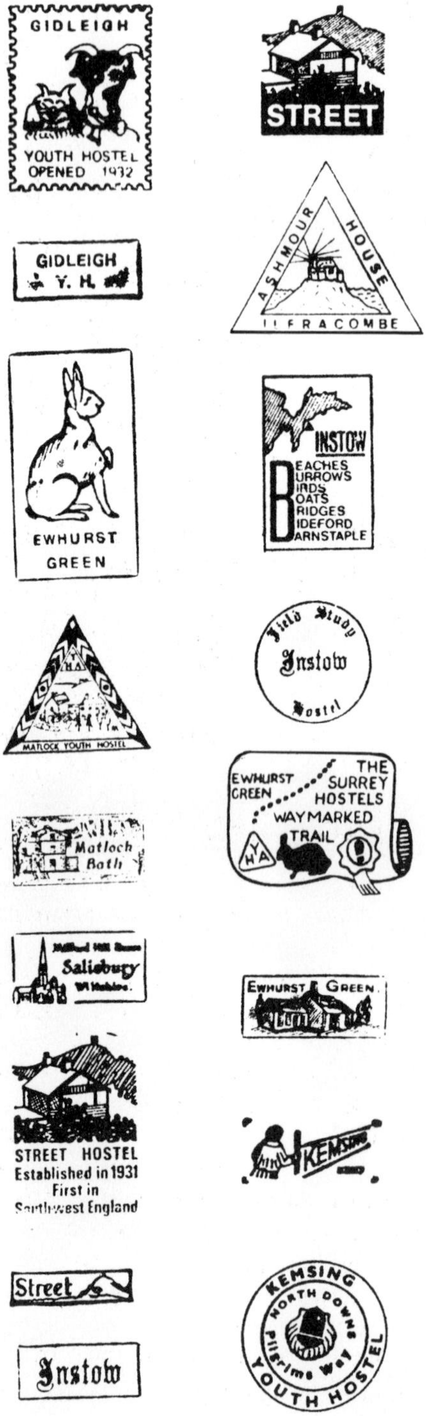

A selection of stamps, only obtained by staying overnight, which add interest to any collection.

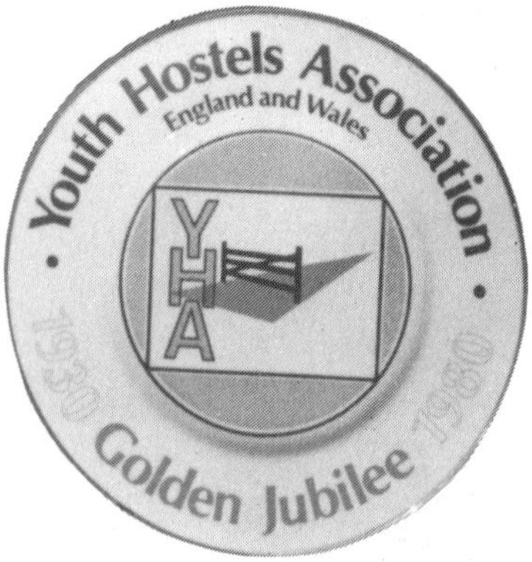

Youth Hostels Association Golden Jubilee plate 1930-1980. value £5

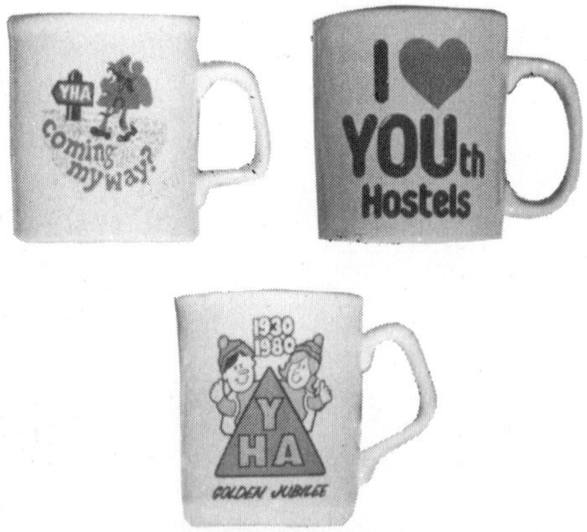

Y.H.A. mugs can be obtained at the hostels or in Y.H.A. shops.

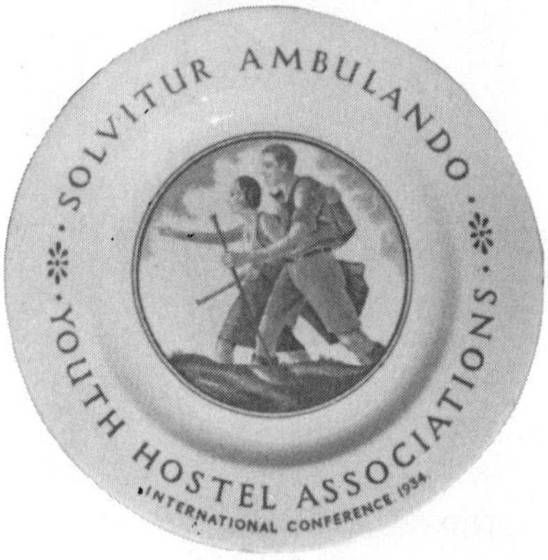

Youth Hostel Associations' International Conference 1934. value £20

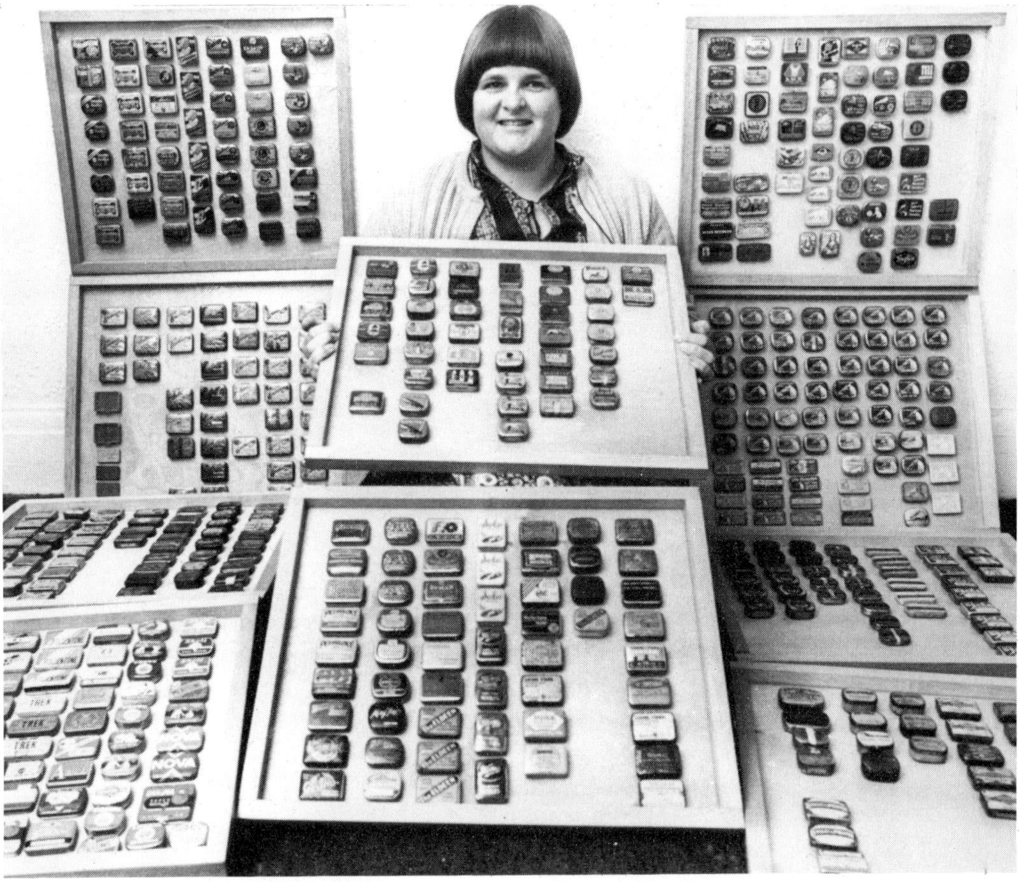

Ruth Lambert is a collector who specialises in gramophone needle boxes.

"I began collecting all sorts of tins but when I saw gramophone needle boxes, I liked them because of their convenient size and the designs on them are lovely.

"I've found them in all sorts of places — sometimes people find a box in the back of a drawer or in the potting shed and they also turn up in antique fairs. I keep on finding tins I've never heard of. Gramophone needle boxes are a fairly new collectible and there's no set prices really for you can buy them for 10p or £10 according to their aesthetic appeal and their rarity. Shaped tins are rare — pyramids or circular — and so are tins with more than one compartment.

"In my collection there are over a thousand tins, some with three, four or five compartments which were issued by HMV and are very rare, very nice."

Ruth said that tins are very difficult to date because no records of manufacture have been kept by the companies who produced them in Sheffield and Redditch. She thinks that the Metal Box Company may have made many of the tins but again there are no records. This is not like biscuit tins which can be dated from company catalogues.

The earliest one in Ruth's collection probably dates from around 1905 and she can research some of them from times various companies changed their names or from newspaper and magazine advertisements of the period.

The tin Ruth would most like to find has a picture of a nightingale on it. She said: "I've seen reproductions of it but they are about seven inches across, bigger than the original which was about one and a half inches by one inch — I'd like to find that."

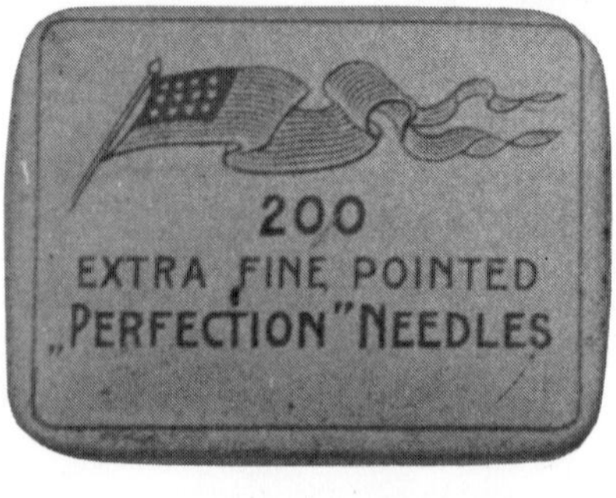

'Perfection', white German tin with blue writing and red and blue American flag.

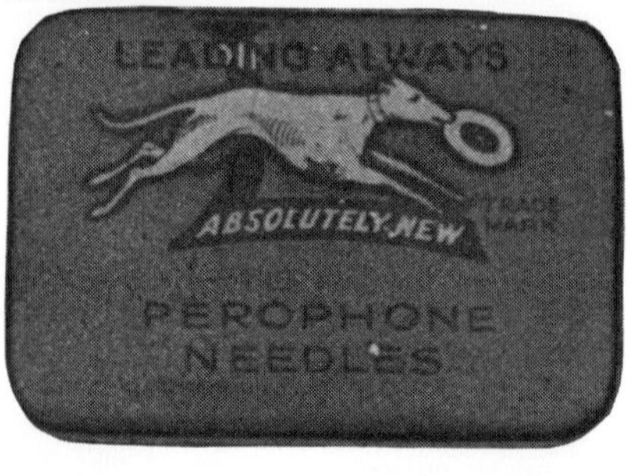

'Perophone', unusual shaped tin for the greyhound in green, white and black.

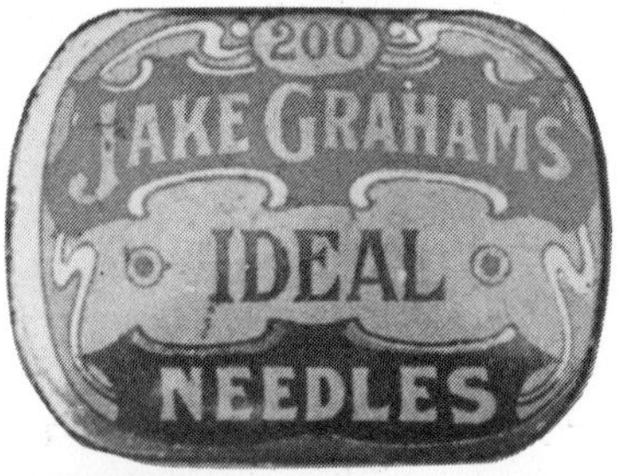

'Jake Graham's Ideal Needles', a local Liverpool dealers tin in green and gold.

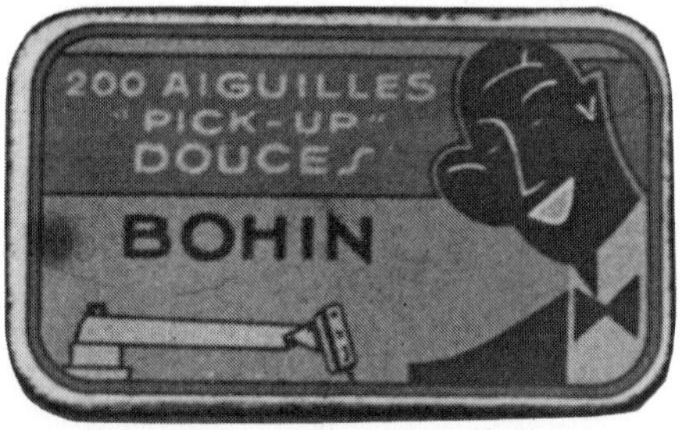

'Bohin', French tin in yellow and green with black face.

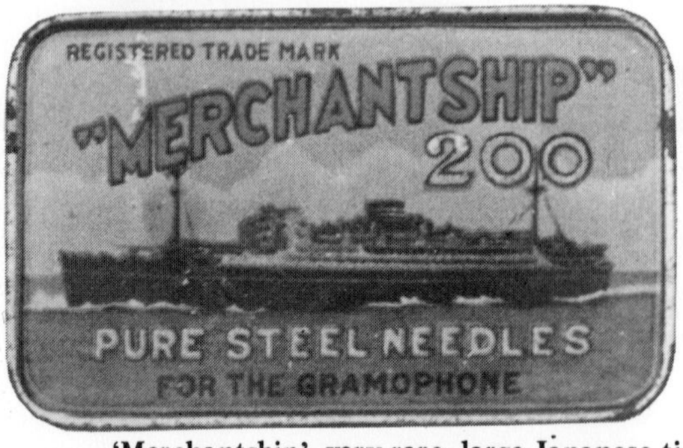

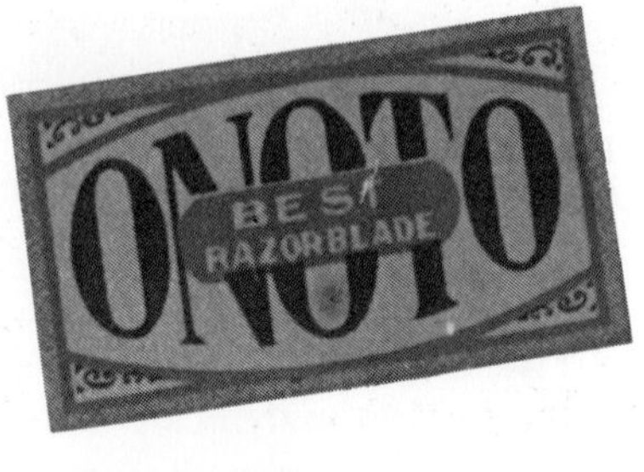

'Merchantship', very rare, large Japanese tin. Lovely picture of ship in green and red 'name'. It also originally held a wrapped razor blade.

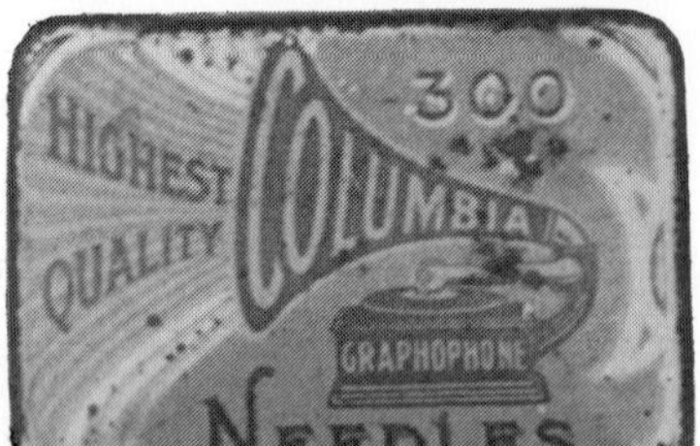

'Columbia', early Columbia tin in pale blue and gold. The name is on the horn of the gramophone, unusual in that it held 300 needles.

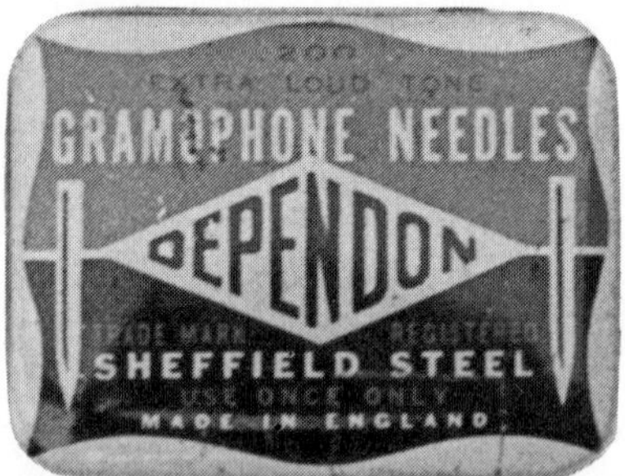

'Dependon', nice British tin in red, black and white, unusual in that it was 'Packed in Canada'.

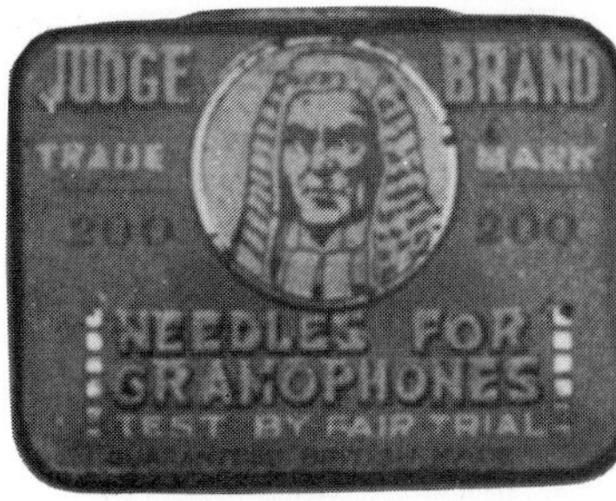

'Judge Brand', British tin in pale turquoise with drawing of a judge.

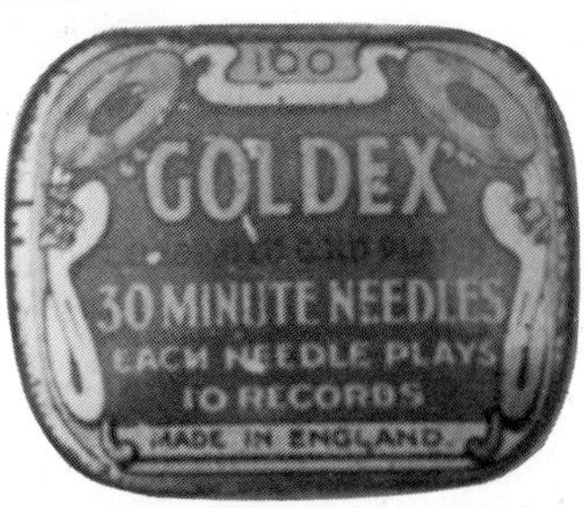

'Goldex', thin green, silver and white tin with ornate pattern around edge.

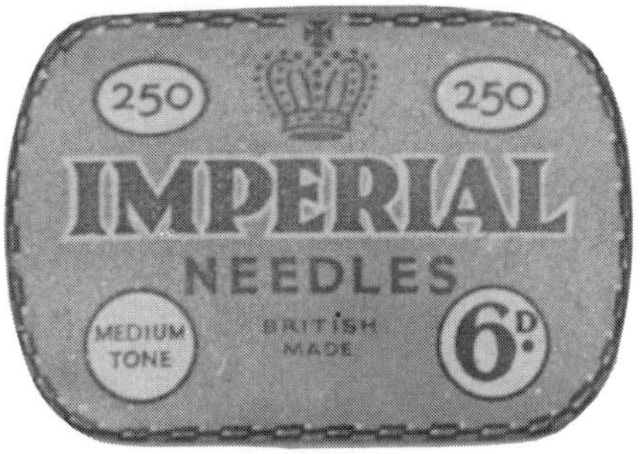

'Imperial', large shaped British tin in orange with black writing. Tin is priced at 6d, unusual in that it held 250 needles rather than 200.

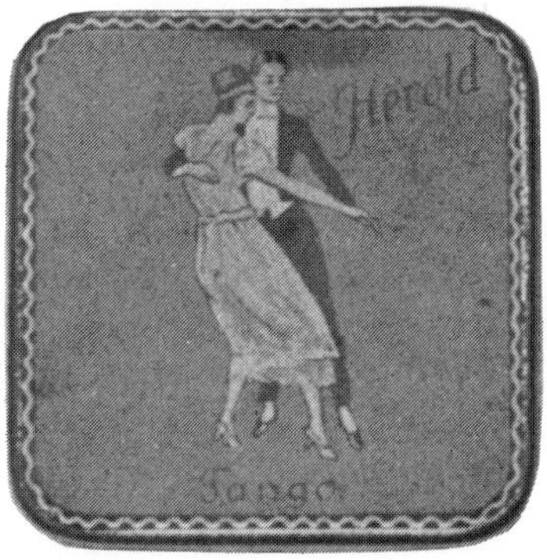

'Herold Tango', square German tin in pale turquoise with couple in evening dress. There are 5 tins in this series, each showing a different dance.

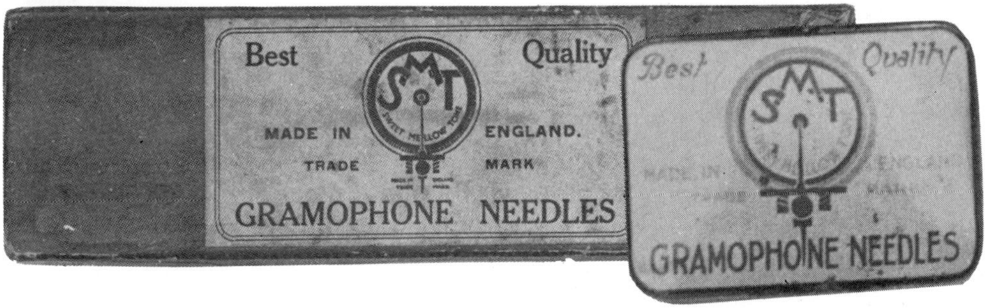

'SMT' (Sweet Mellow Tone), cream tin with blue writing, the name is in a sound box. Also shown is the original box which held 5 tins.

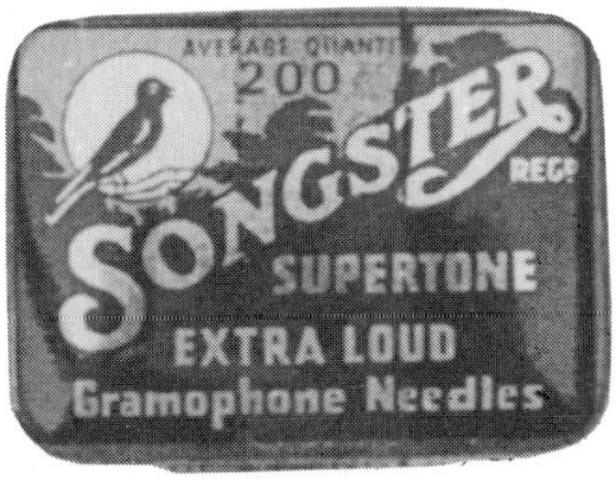

'Songster Supertone', rare tin in pale and dark green with 'Songster' in gold, and gold circle.

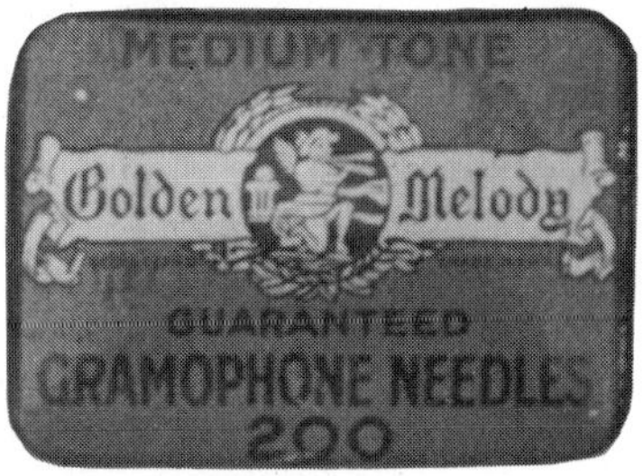

'Golden Melody', grey British tin with gold band and 'Pan' with his pipes.

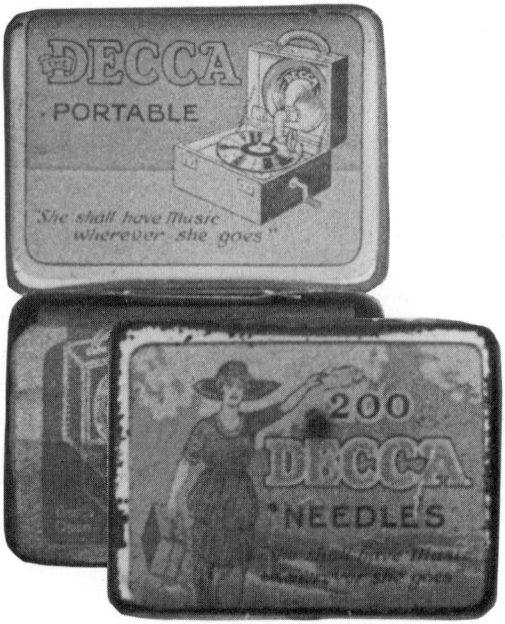

'Decca', very early British Decca tin with lovely picture in turquoise, yellow and white, showing an Edwardian lady with portable gramophone, very rare.

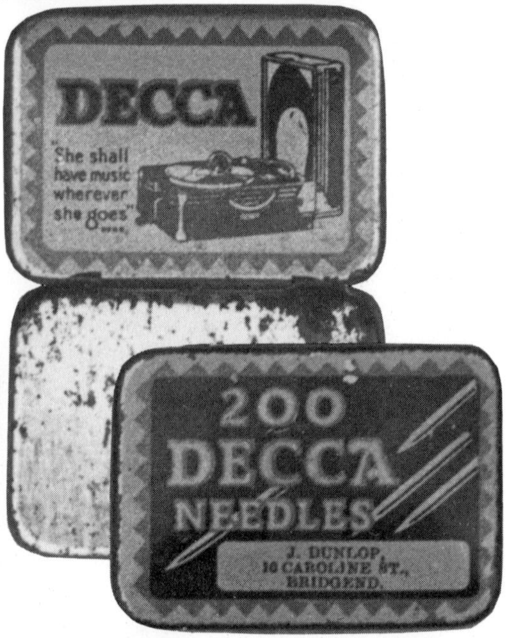

'Decca', green, white and black, can be found with dealers name and address, or 'She shall have music wherever she goes' in box.

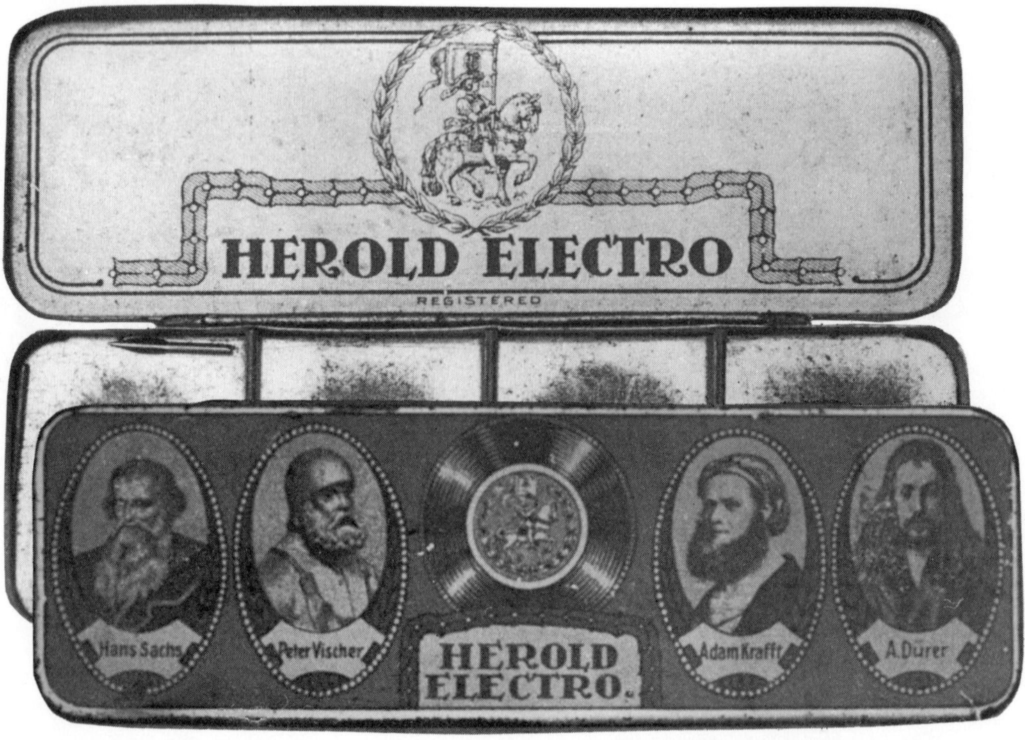

'Herold Electro', lovely large 4 compartment German tin in red and green. Each oval has a picture of a famous German personality.

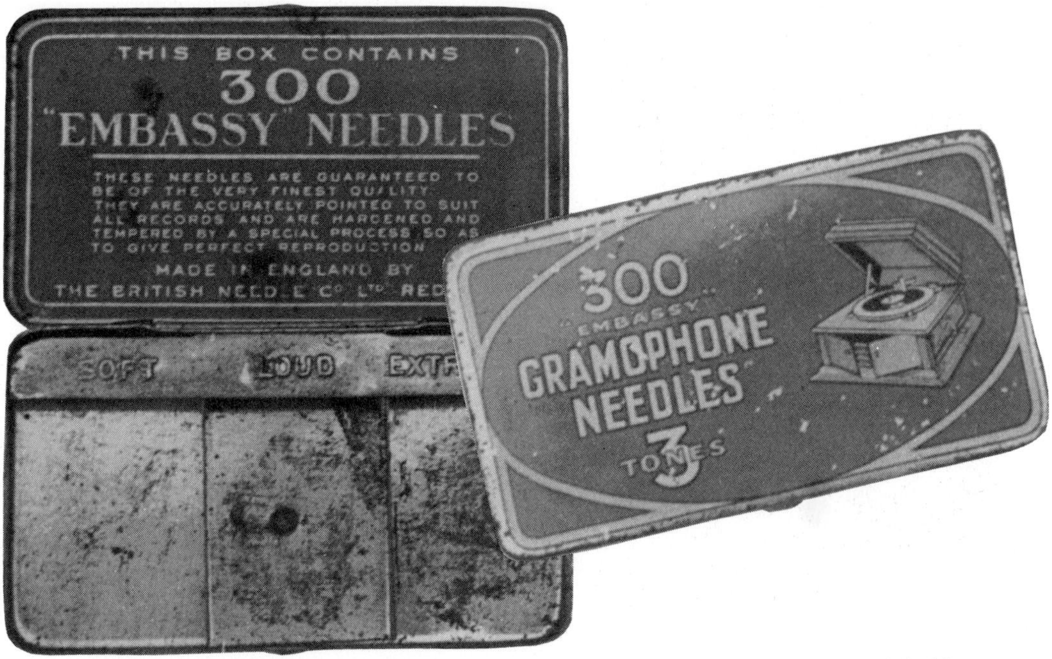

'Embassy', 3 compartment Embassy tin in red with cabinet gramophone, which held 300 needles, 100 each of soft, loud and extra loud.

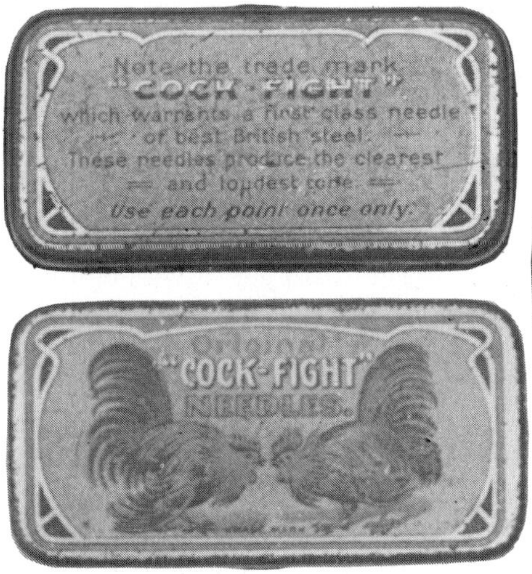

'Cock-Fight', lovely pictorial German tin in pale turquoise, green gold and purple. Very rare tin.

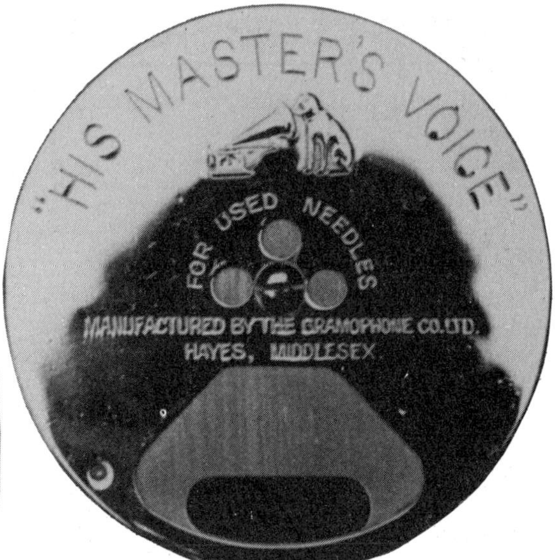

'His Masters Voice', round nickel plated 3 compartment tin. A deep tin with the dog and gramophone embossed at centre. Lovely large tin, it originally came in a box.

Although many gramophone needle tins can be bought for as little as a £1 each, rare ones, particularly those with multi-compartments, can be worth as much as £15 – £20

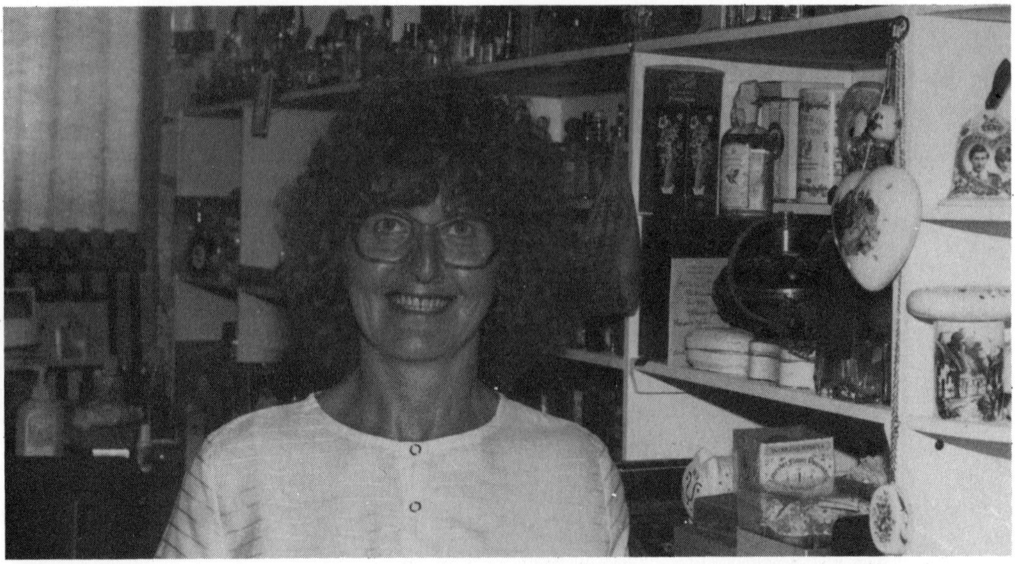

Ruth Warner is a housewife who collects perfume bottles.

"My collection now has over 2,500 items and I'm adding to it continually. It's odd to remember that I only started collecting nine years ago when I bought an old Yardley bottle for 30p at Ashford Market for a friend who used to use that brand of perfume.

"It turned out that she didn't particularly want it, so I kept it. I never really expected to find another perfume bottle but it's amazing what turns up when you start looking. Now I've got bottles in all sort of shapes from girls to top hats and made of glass, crystal, pewter, porcelain and silver.

"The collection spans every year since 1840 to the present day and I buy new brands of perfume today just for the bottles. The collection has been on display in Harvey Nichols and Dickens and Jones in London and this year I mounted the first exhibition of perfume bottles ever held in Kent at Canterbury. I also give talks to women's groups and it's very popular with the public because it's different and it's a very feminine thing. Older members of the audience often say that they remember using perfumes that I have in the collection and sometimes they tell me about perfume factories they remember which now no longer exist and I can follow them up and often find a new bottle as a result.

"I write away to all the perfume manufacturers in this country, in France and in Germany and they are most helpful. They send me bottles and representatives from the firms come to see the collection when they're in this country."

Ruth's bottles range from old favourites like 'An Evening in Paris', 'Top Hat' and 'Californian Poppy' that were popular in the 1930's to exotic bottles of 'Shocking' made by Schiaperelli of Paris in the shape of a tailor's dummy with a tape measure draped round its neck and surrounded by glass flowers. It is still in its original navy blue leather box with a shocking pink satin lining.

Many of the bottles have never been opened and still have their original contents. The more expensive perfumes from before the war keep best because they were made from natural ingredients and contain real alcohol which perfumes today do not.

Her best bottles are those dating from the Art Deco period, some of which are very expensive today. The bottle that Ruth would most like to find is another by Schiaperelli dating from the early 1930's and made in the shape of the sun. It is enormous and weighs around 3 lbs.

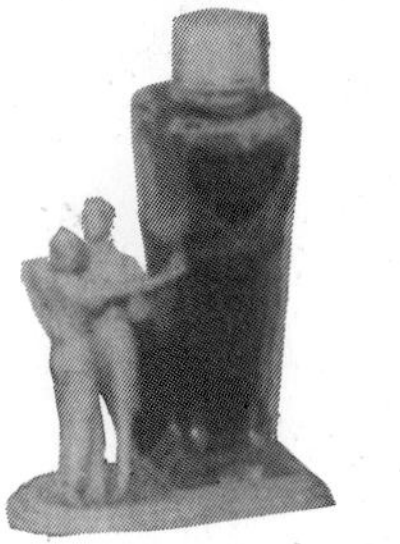

Dubarry figurines complete with original scent bottle, circa 1930. £15

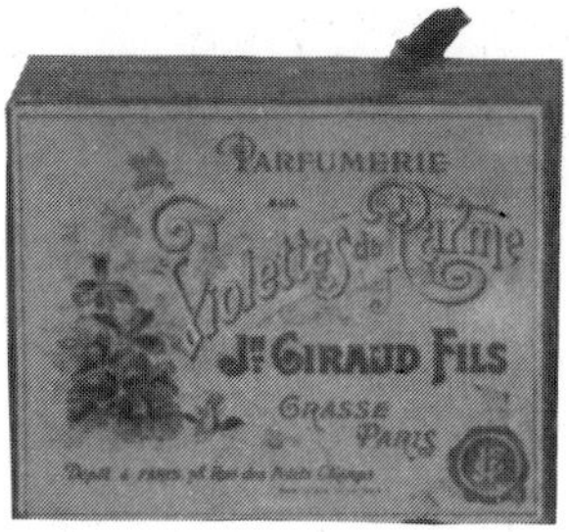

An original box for Violettes De Parme by Jn. Giraud Fils of Paris, 1920's. £10

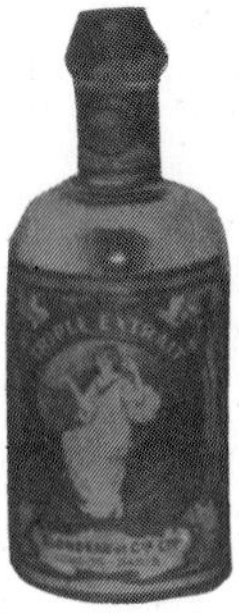

Lily of the Valley by Blondeau & Co. Ltd., with original pictorial label, 1920's. £10

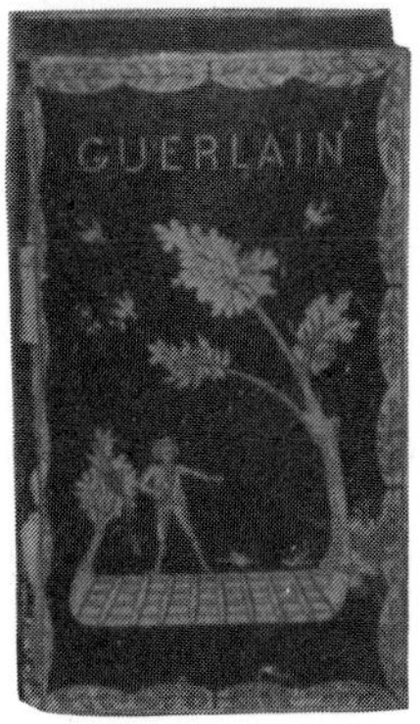

A fine pictorial box for Guerlain, 1920's. £10

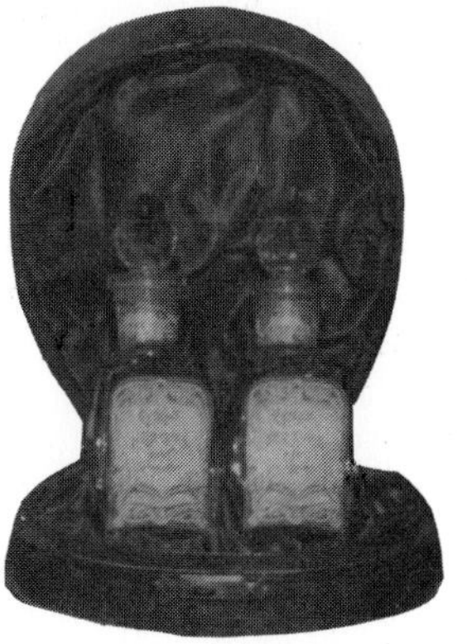

Scent casket lined with red silk, circa 1900. £40

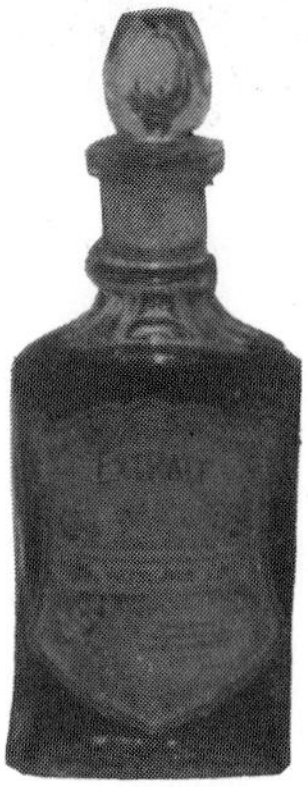

Violette De Parme scent bottle with original label, circa 1920's. £10

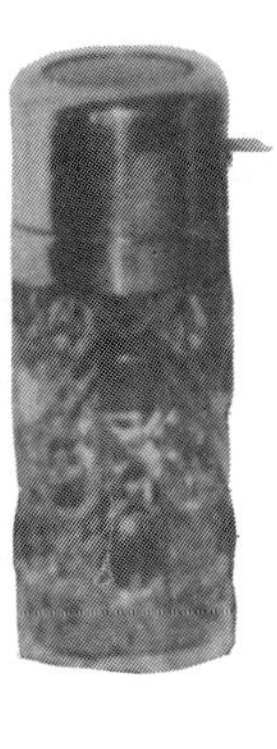

Cut glass scent bottle with plated top, circa 1920. £40

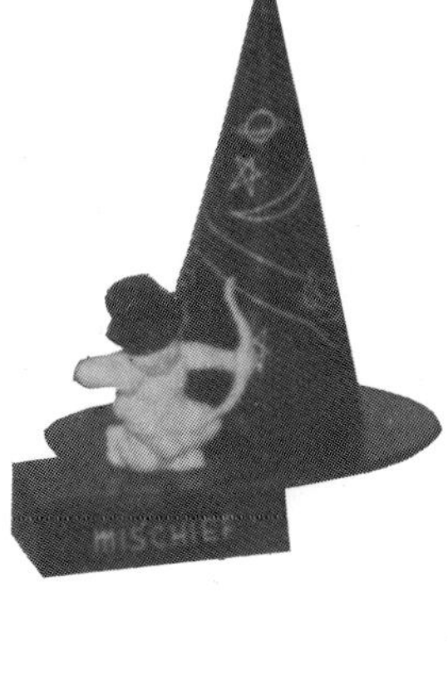

'Mr. Mischief' figurine, 1930's. £15

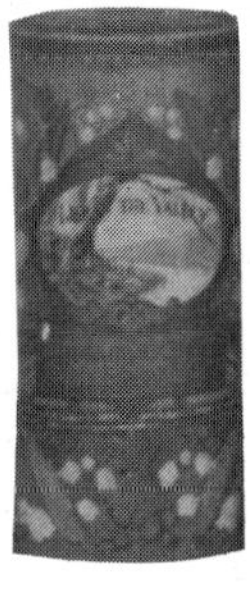

Lily of the Valley decorated perfume box, 1920's. £8

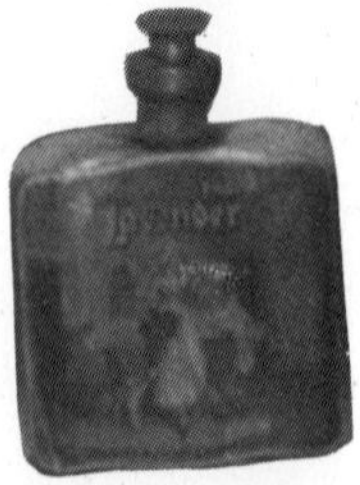

Yardley lavender bottle with original label. £10

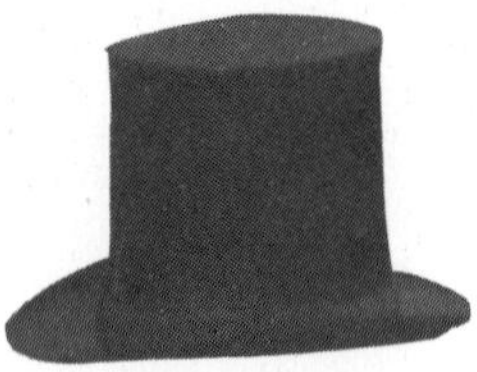

Top Hat perfume, circa 1930. £15

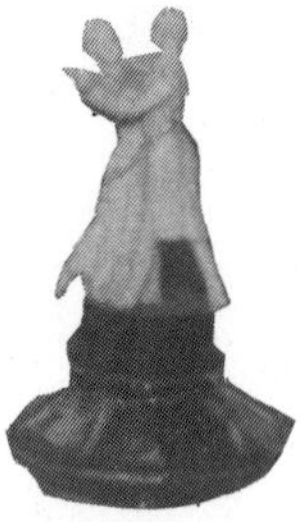

Dubarry dancing figures on original perfume bottle, circa 1930. £15

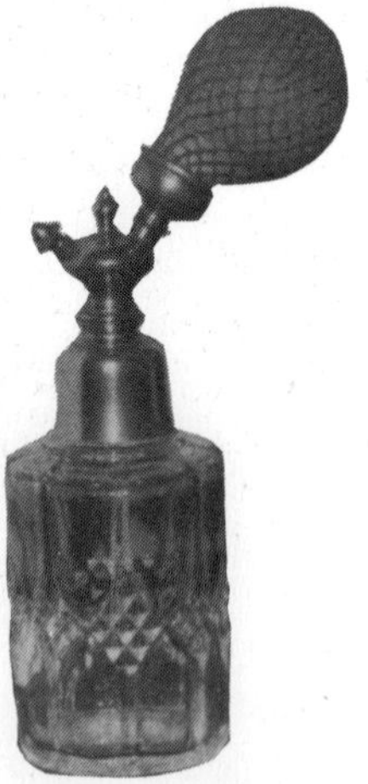

Amber and white moulded glass scent bottle, circa 1920. £12

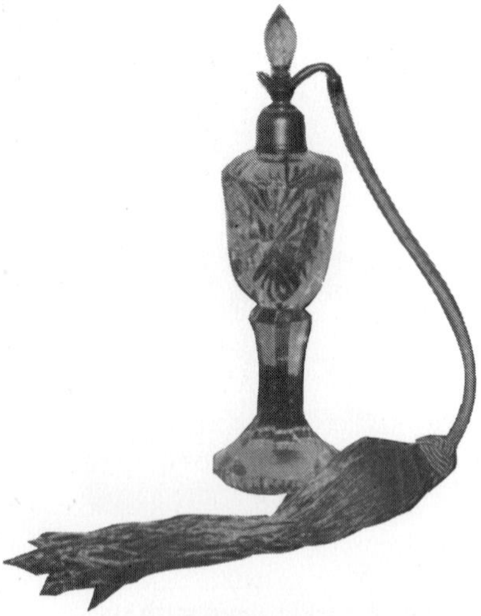

Victorian cut glass scent spray of tear drop design. £40

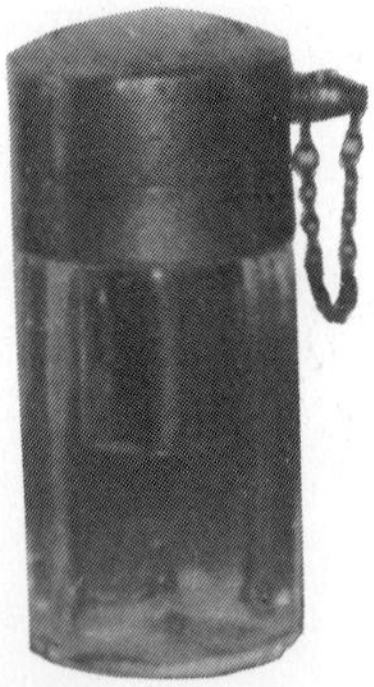

A plain glass atomiser with plated top, circa 1910. £30

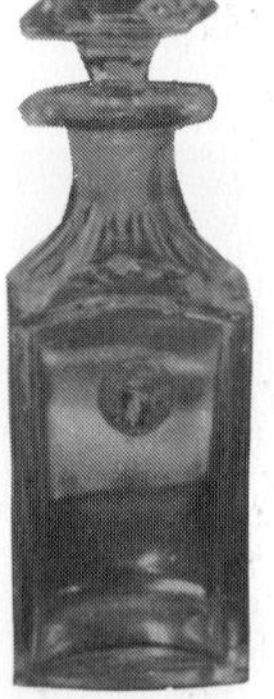

A large Yardley scent decanter with stopper. £12

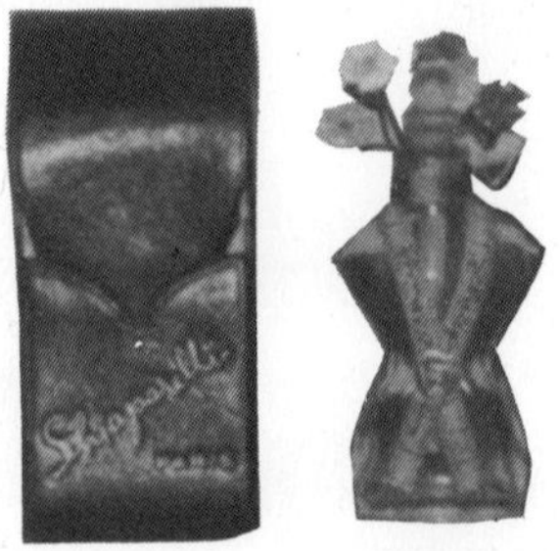

A Schiaparelli scent bottle complete with the original leather case, 1930's. £50

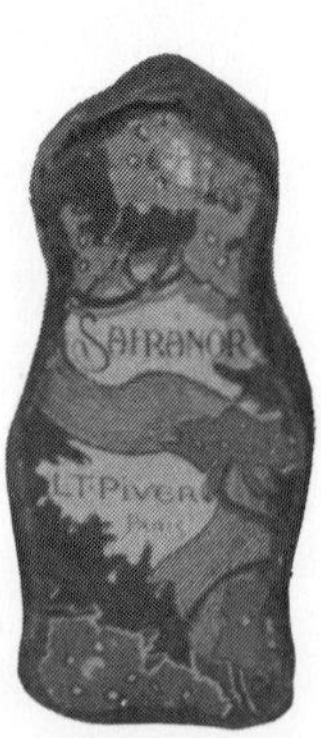

Original box for Safranor by L. T. Piver, Paris, 1920's. £10

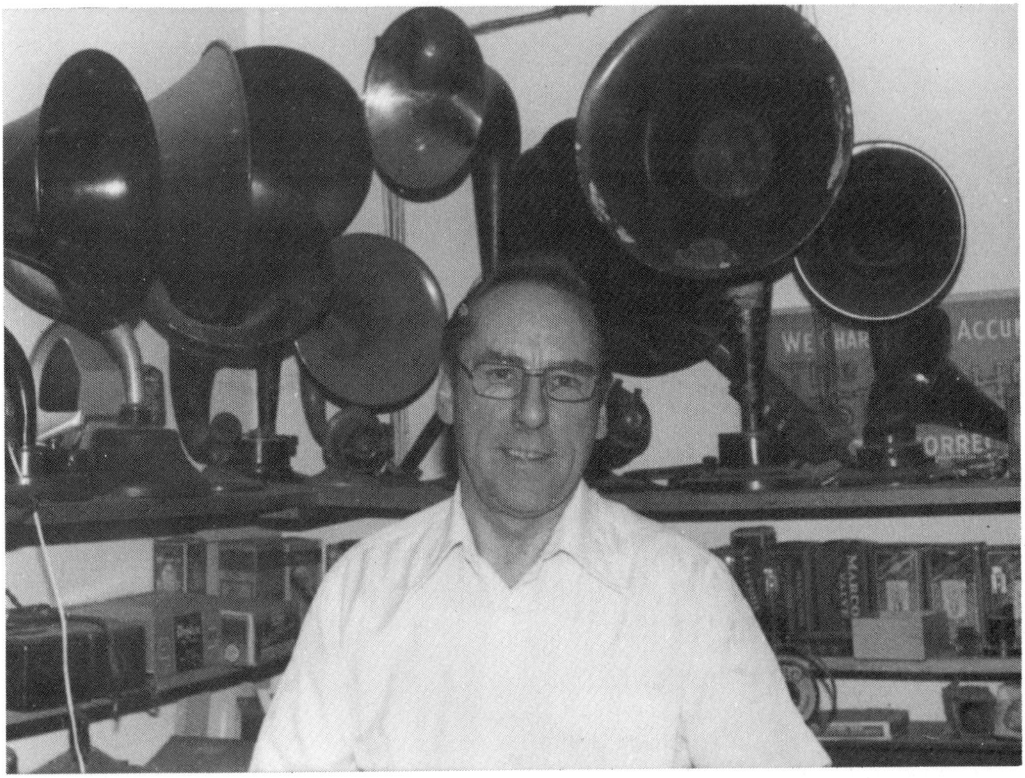

Bob Warner, the husband of Ruth, is a furniture maker and collects wirelesses . . . The couple have their individual collections on each side of the family sitting room.

"When I did my National Service, I was a wireless operator and after I was demobbed I looked for a set like the one I'd used in the Services. The collection took off from there and now I've got 200 broadcasting wireless sets and 100 different military ones including some of the early radar ones which were very secret when they were made. At the moment I'm concentrating on the military side of my collection and I've got several spy radios used by the S.O.E. in France. These are all Morse key radios but the broadcasting sets date from the 1920's and some of them are in lovely cases which I can appreciate because I work in furniture making.

"Half the fun of the collection for me is polishing them up and making them work."

The star of Bob's collection is a very large Gecophone broadcasting set made in 1928 by the company which was the forerunner of G.E.C. Its price today is well into the hundreds of pounds. What he is still looking for is a Morse key set used during the First World War. Today they cannot be bought for under £300.

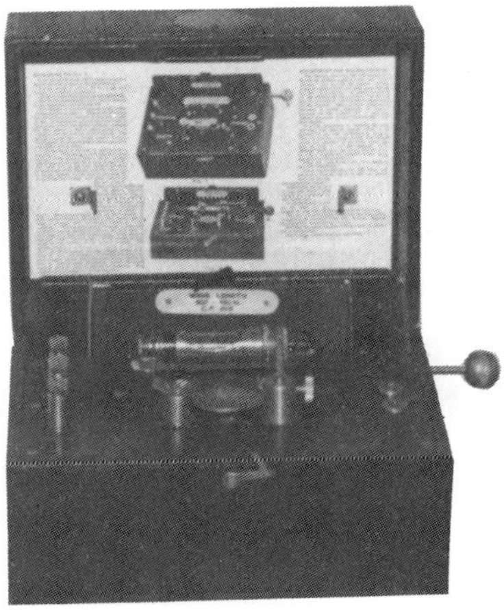

Marconi crystal receiver, Junior, 1923. £40

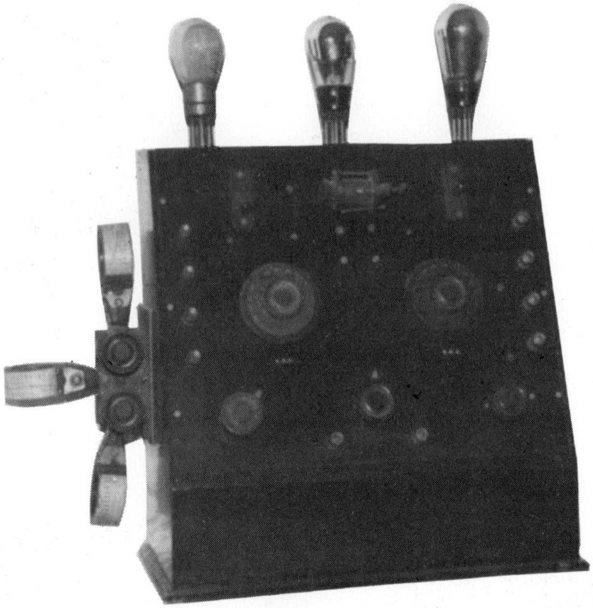

Home Made, 3 valve set, 1924. £50

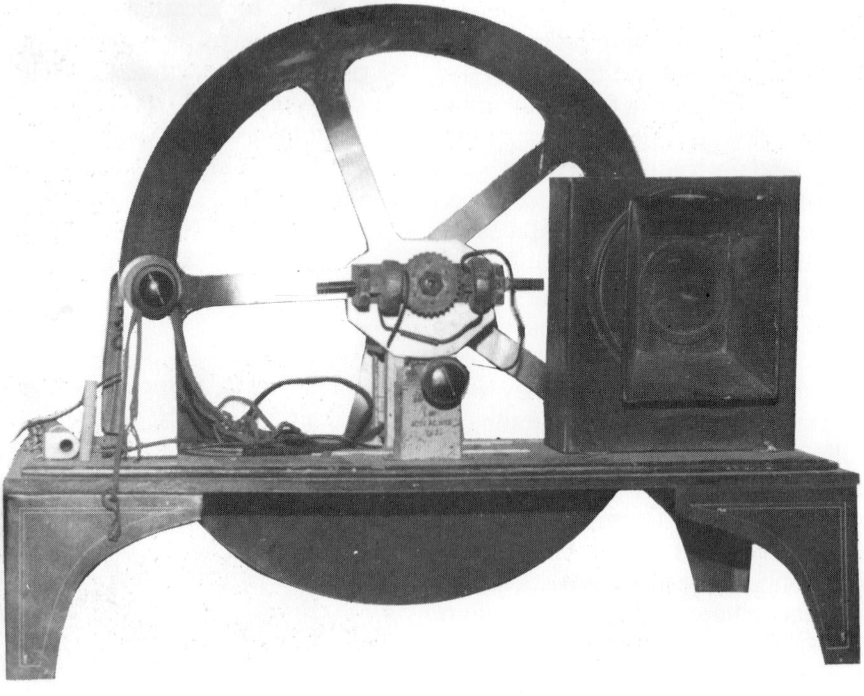

Baird Type Televisor, 1929. £70

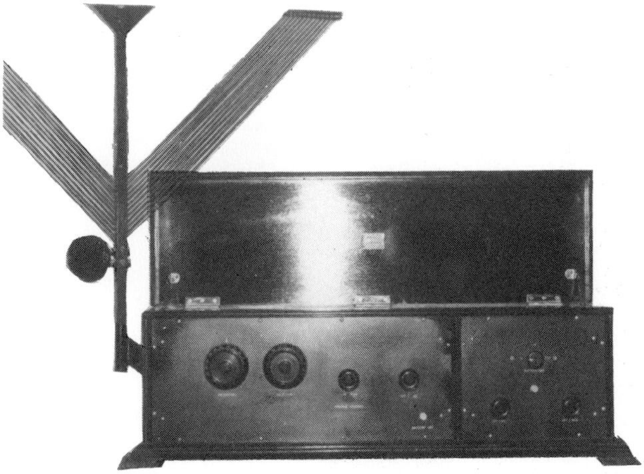

Gecophone, 8 valve receiver, 1928. £150

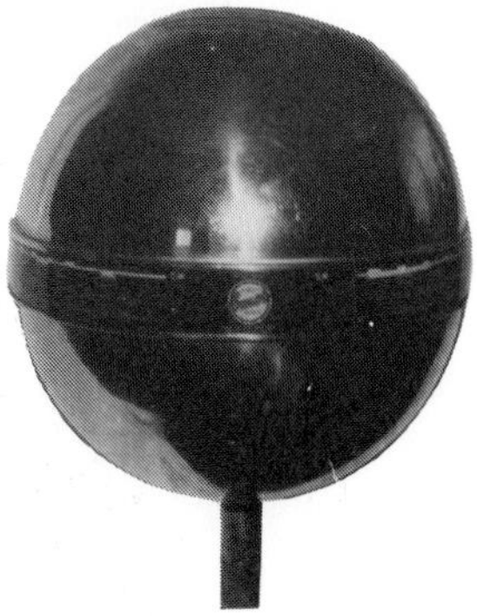

EMOR Radio. £75

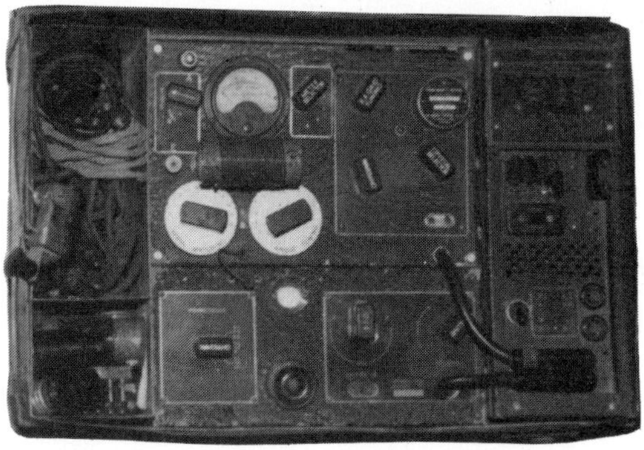

Spy Radio, type B2, 1942. £100

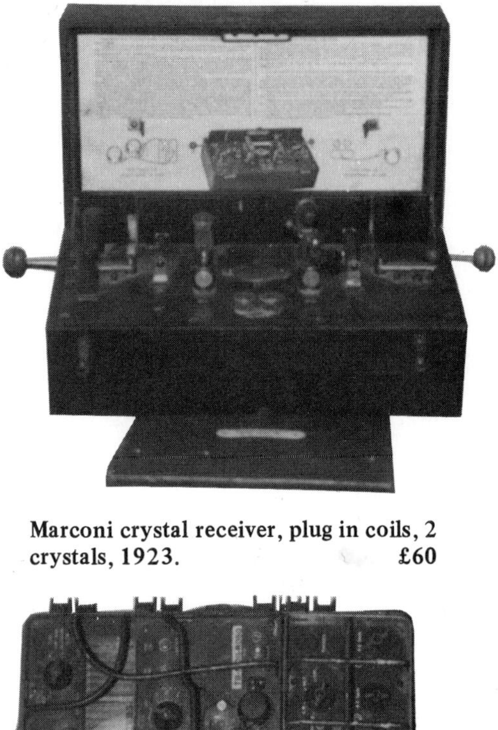

Marconi crystal receiver, plug in coils, 2 crystals, 1923. £60

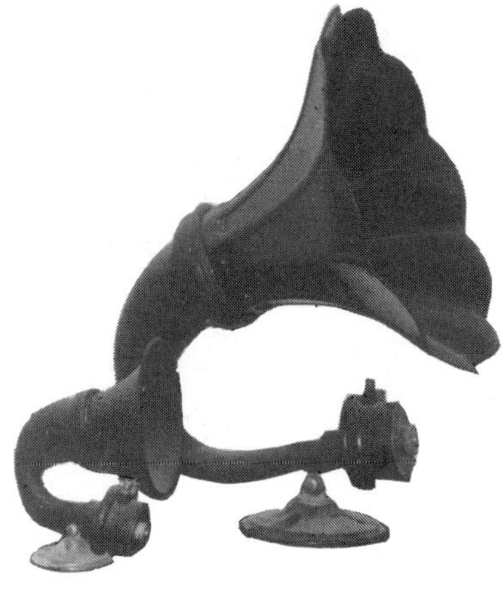

Assorted horn loud speakers. £25 – £50

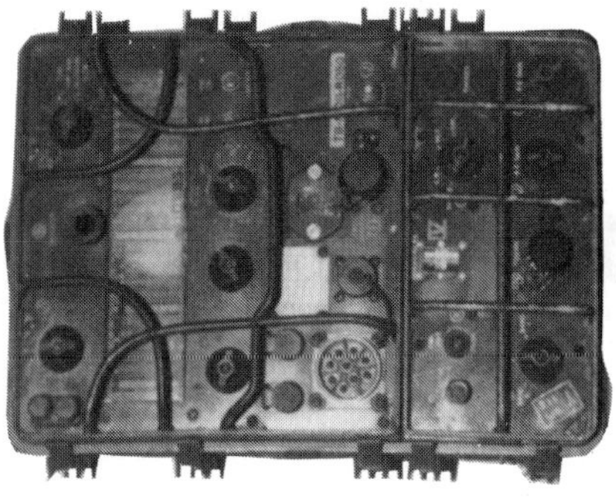

War Radios. £25 – £100

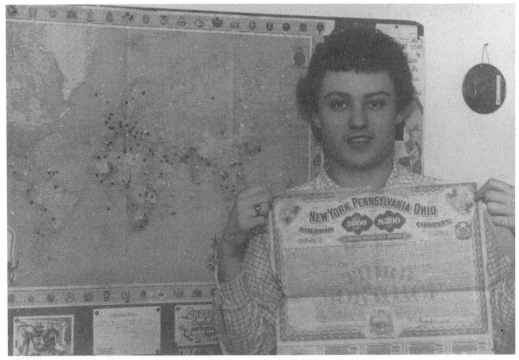

Duncan Bray of Kington is a trainee property negotiator with more than just a passing interest in banknotes.

He has been collecting them since he was only seven years old and in a short ten year span has amassed what is thought to be one of the largest private collections in the United Kingdom. Like most collectors however, there is still one glittering prize he would dearly love to own and that is the Chinese Ming note, AD 1368, which measures 9 in. × 12 in., is printed on bark and is currently valued at around £1,000.

His advice to the beginner is "Look at everything you possibly can and try to specialise. Always go for notes in good condition but start with inexpensive examples then, as knowledge and experience develop the notes can be upgraded for better examples. Notes should always be handled with care and stored in inexpensive plastic envelopes. While, to the novice, forgeries may seem like good but cheaper examples of the real thing, they are to be avoided for, in Britain, it is illegal to collect such notes. If in any doubt, seek advice before buying expensive notes and always ask for some positive provenance".

He points out that at present, the outstandingly beautiful African notes such as the Bhutan are under-rated and therefore a good buy and it is still possible to purchase good early woodblock printed Oriental notes for under £10.

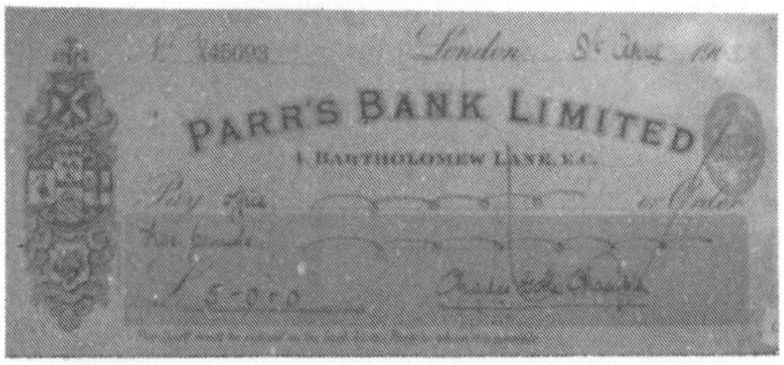

Duncan would now like to establish his own Cheque Society and would be pleased to hear from anyone interested in this field. He also suggests that collectors may be interested in joining the International Banknote Society of Gt. Britain and can contact the Assistant Treasurer at P.O. Box No. 4WX, London W1A 4WX.

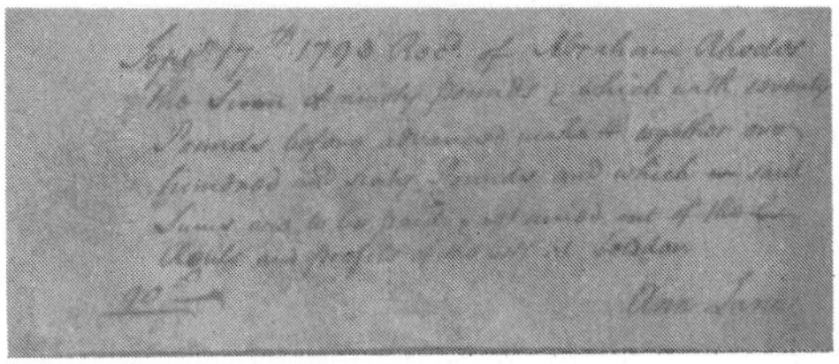

One of the earliest form of British note, 1793 in the form of a handwritten receipt which could be passed in payment.

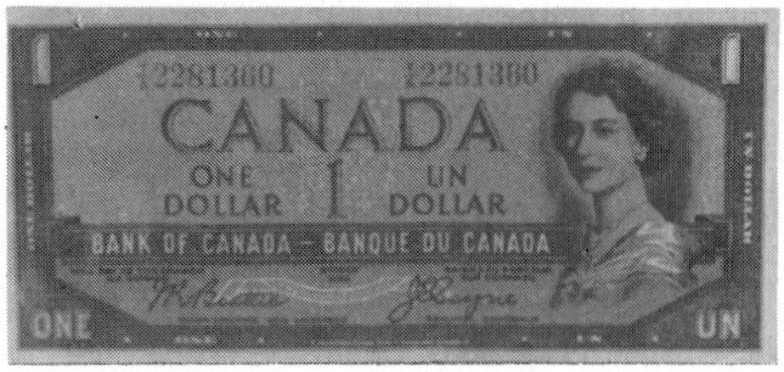

Canadian one dollar with Devil's face in Queen's hair, 1954. £10

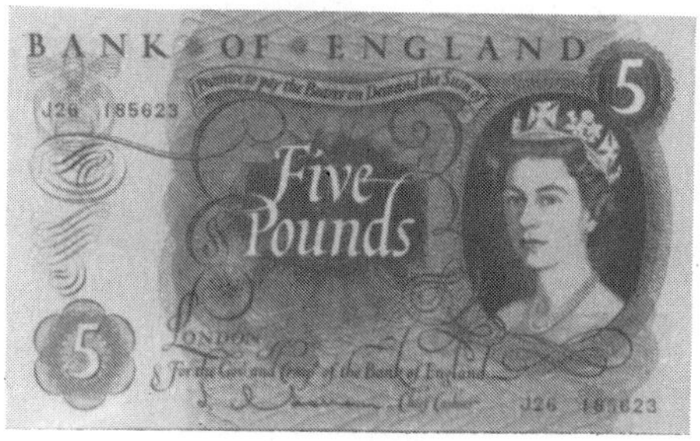

Bank of England five pound note, 1962-66. £20

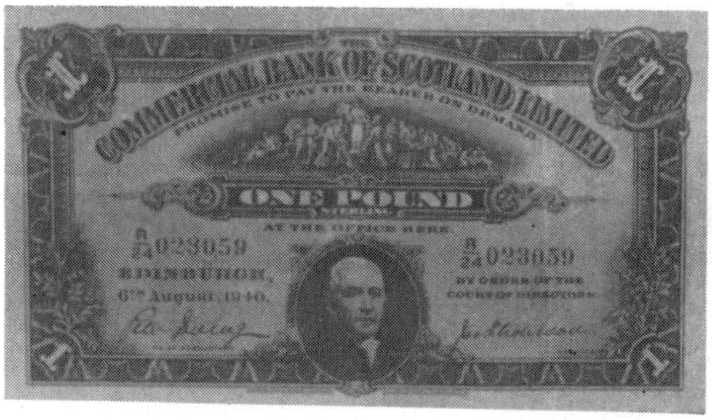

Commercial Bank of Scotland one pound note, 1940. £30

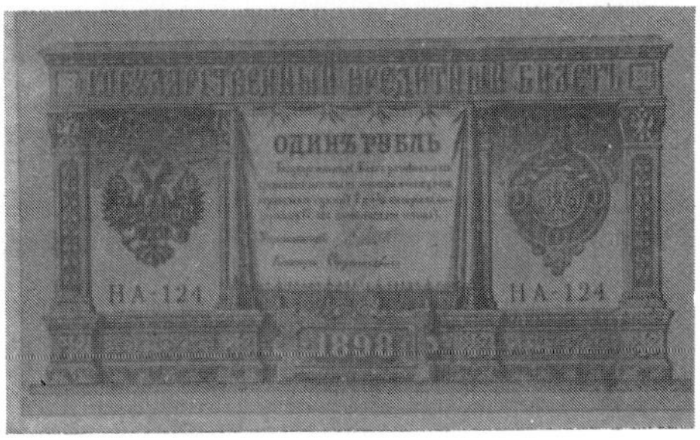

1898 Russian one Rouble note. £15

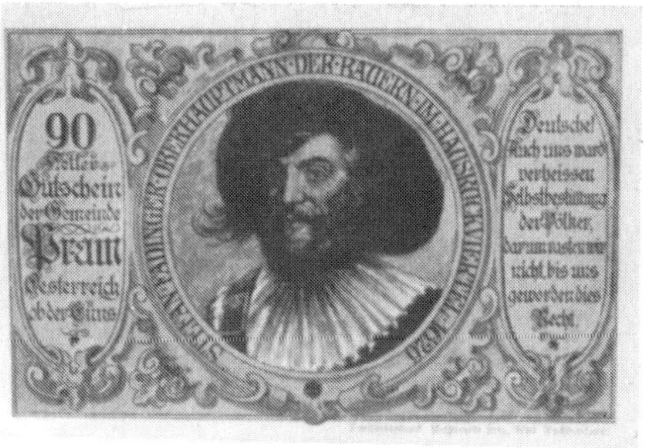

Austrian 90 Hener note, 1920. £7.50

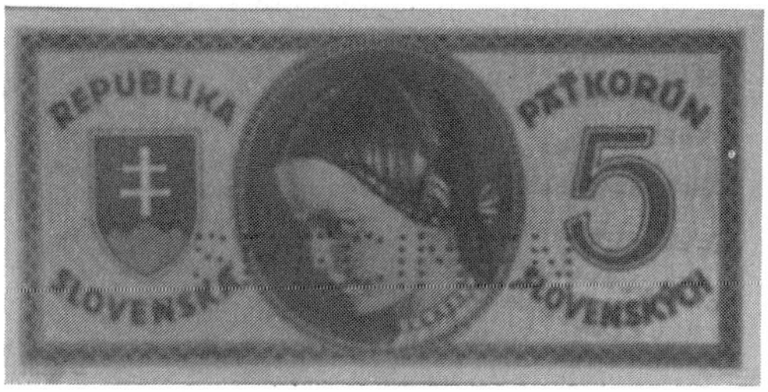

Czechoslovakia, specimen note, 5 Korun. £40

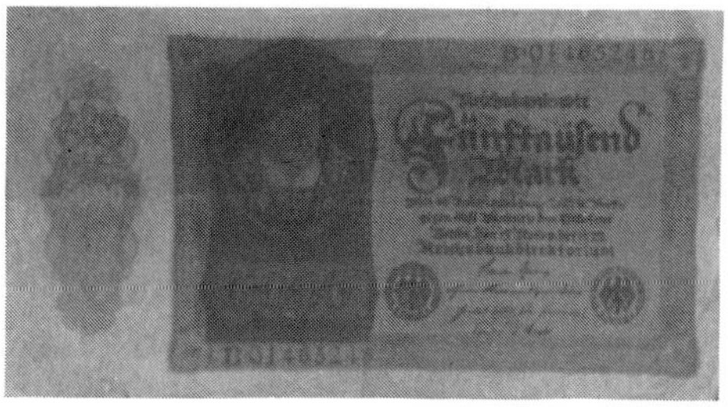

German 5,000 Mark note. £6

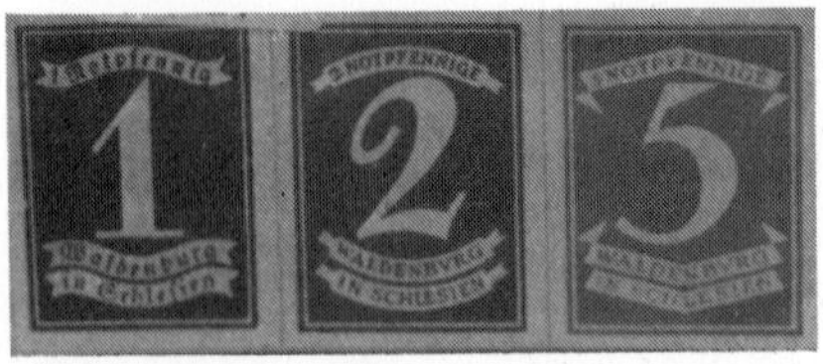

German 1, 2, 5 Notpfennige note, 1920.
£10

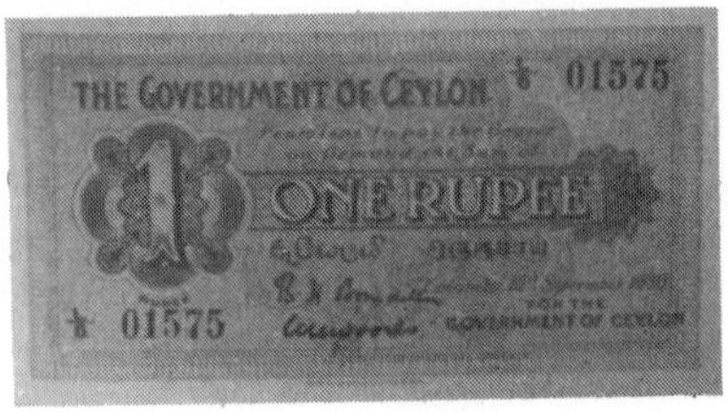

Ceylon book money for use by troops.
£20

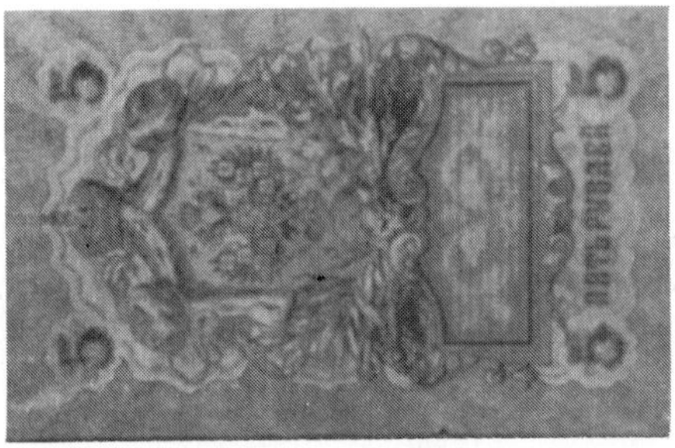

Russian 5 Rouble note, 1909. £8

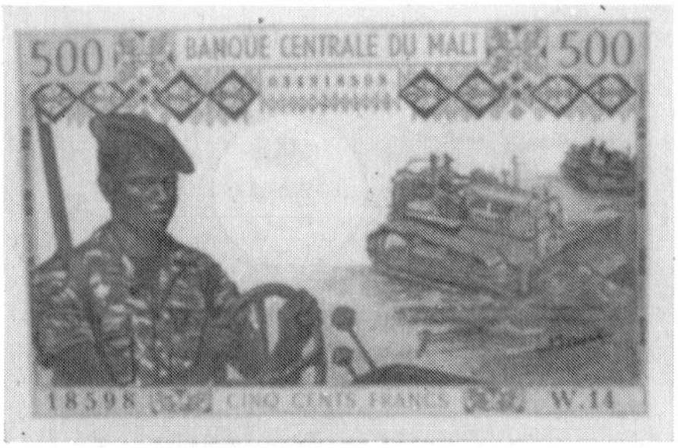

Mali 500 Franc note. £4.50

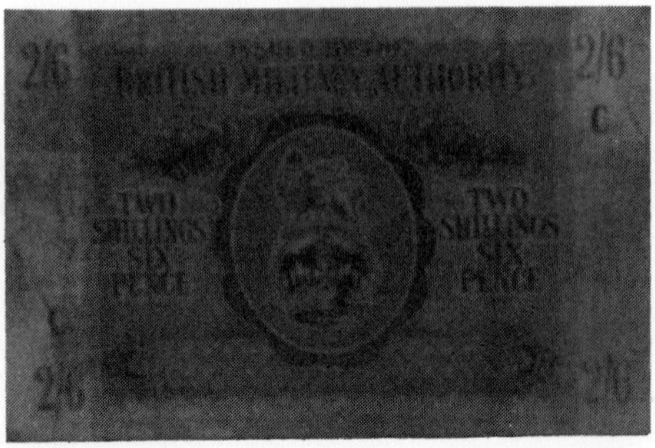

British Military Authority two shilling and six pence note. £15

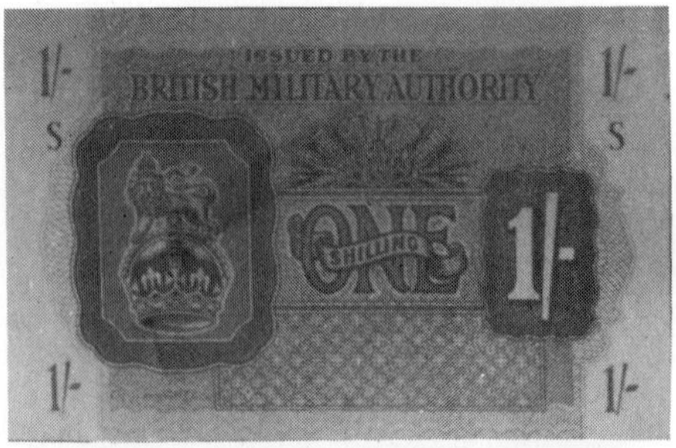

British Military Authority one shilling note for use by British Troops in North Africa, 1943. £12

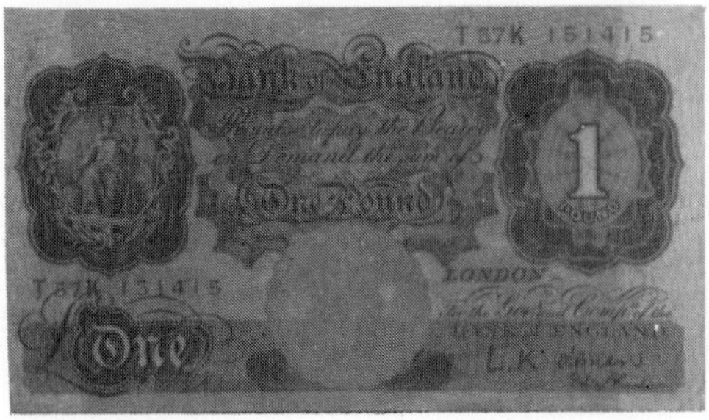

Bank of England one pound note, 1955-60.
£6

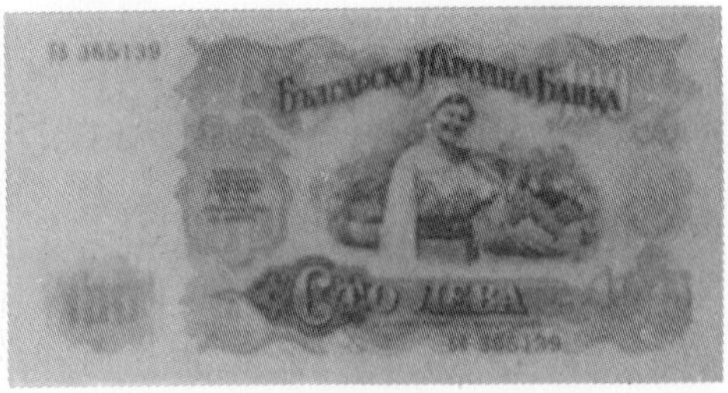

Bulgaria 100 Leva, 1951. £1

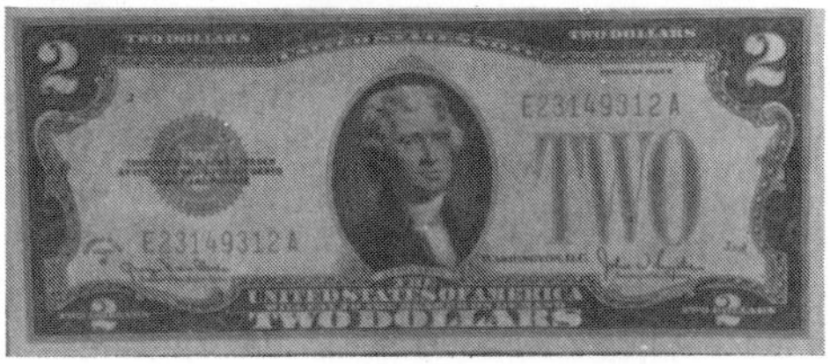

American 2 dollars, 1928. £50

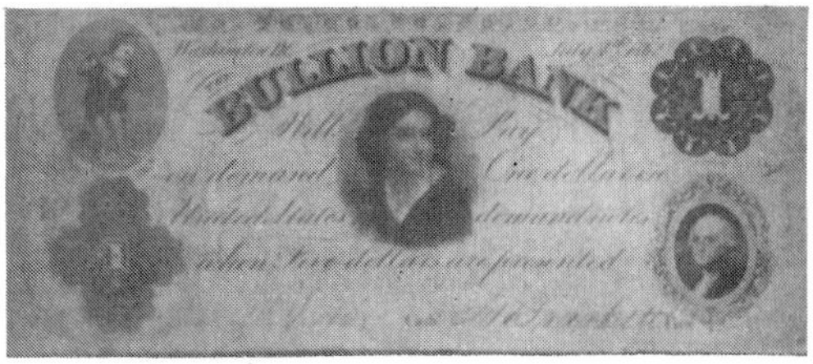

An American 1862 one dollar note, very rare. £1,600

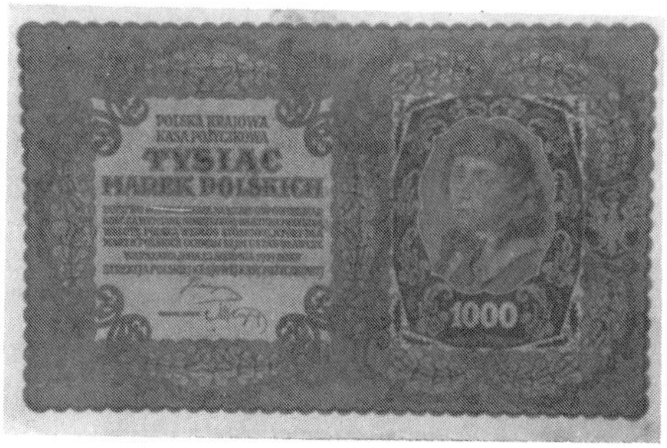

Large Polish note, sometimes cut in half to make 500, 1919. £1

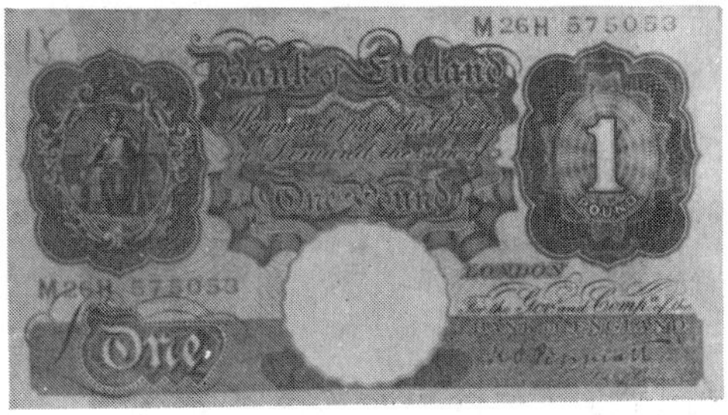

Bank of England one pound note, 1940-48. £15

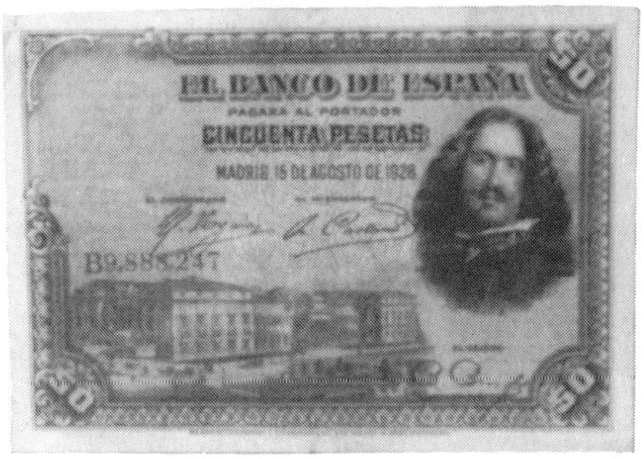

Spanish 50 Pesetas note, 1928. £50

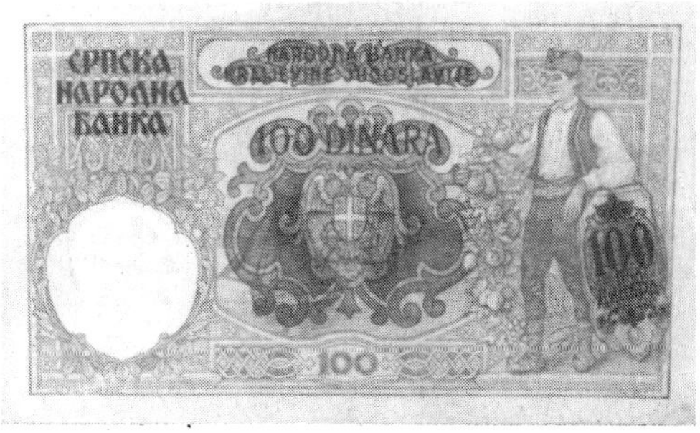

Yugoslavian 100 Dinara. £5

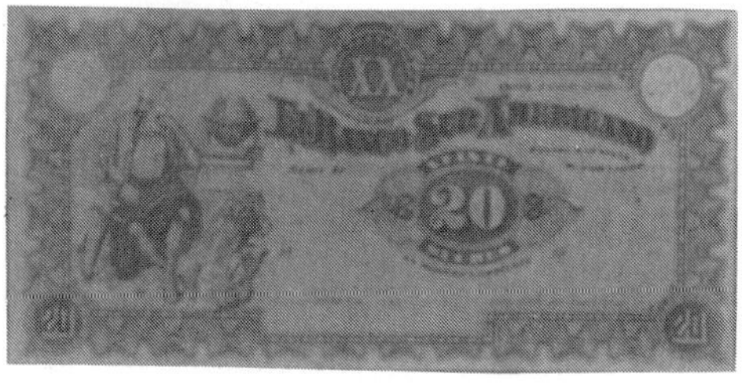

Unissued Equador 20 Sucres, 1920. £50

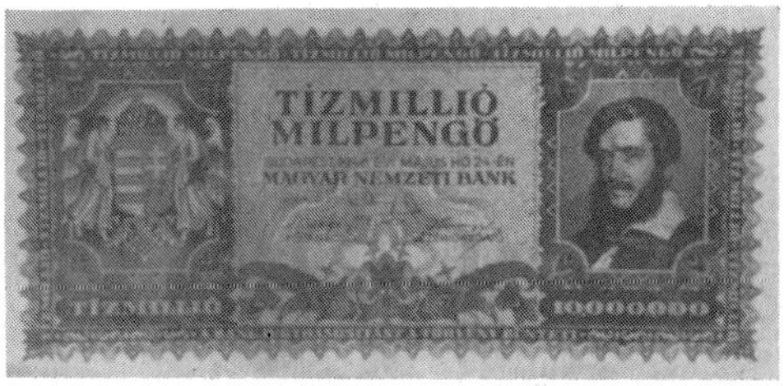

Hungary 10 million Milpengo, 1946. £10

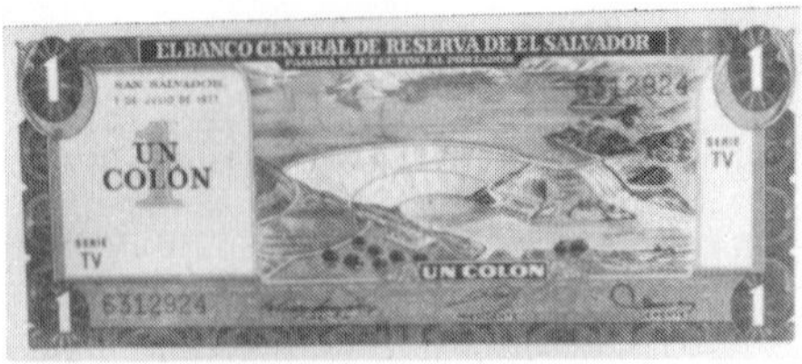

El Salvador 1 Colon note, 1977. £1

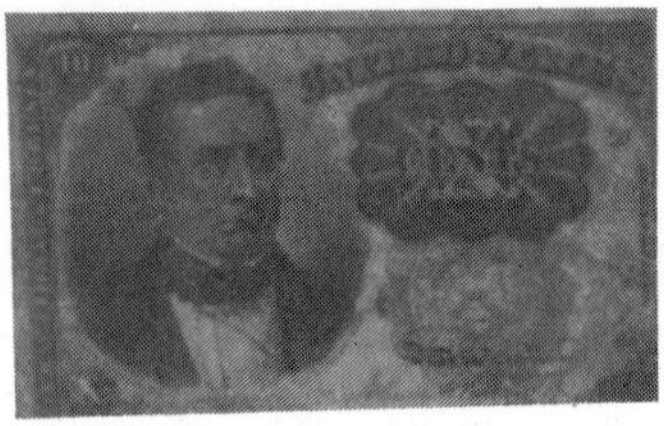

American 10 cent note, 1874. £70

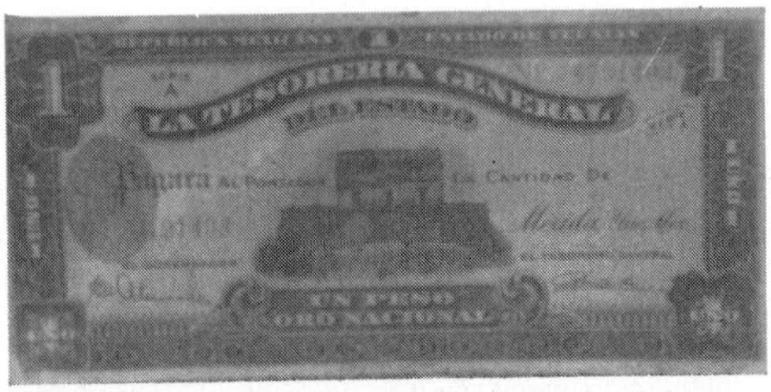

1916 Mexico one peso note. £75

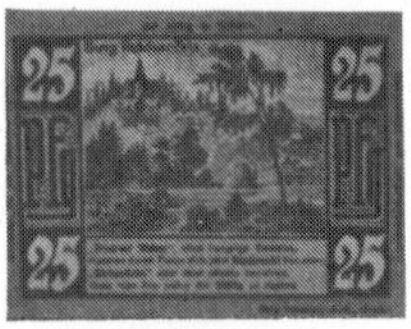

Small German 25 Pfenig note. £8

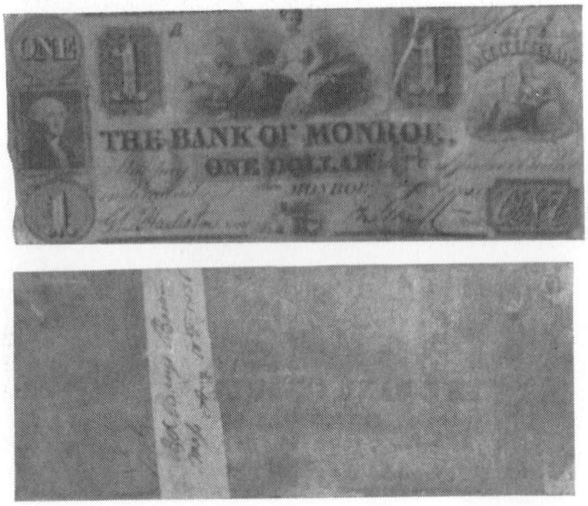

An officially repaired 1836 American note, very rare. £1,500

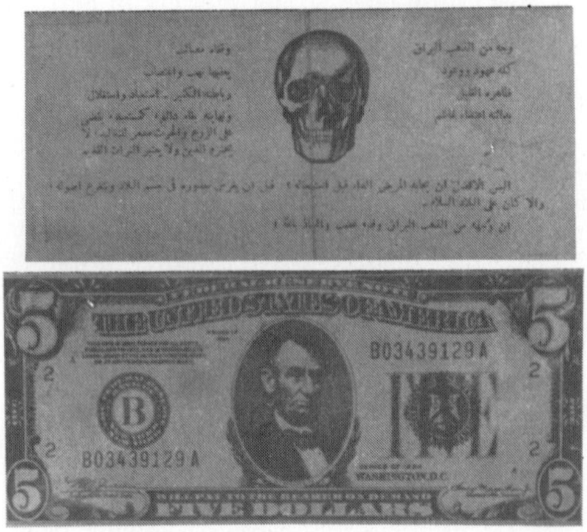

Rare Arab propaganda note, 1934. £160

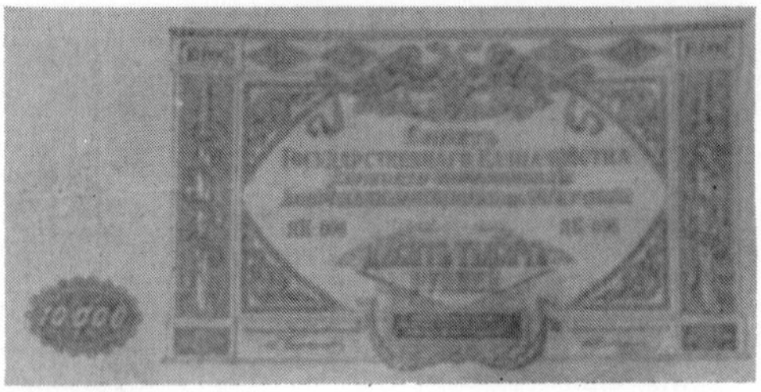

Russian 10,000 note, 1919. £7

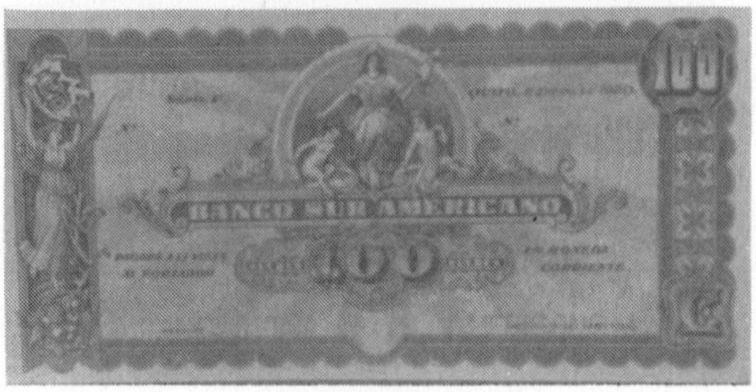

Unissued Equador 100 Sucres, 1920. £75

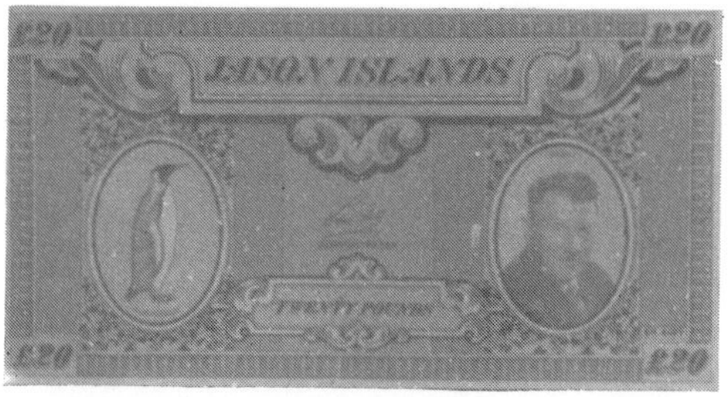

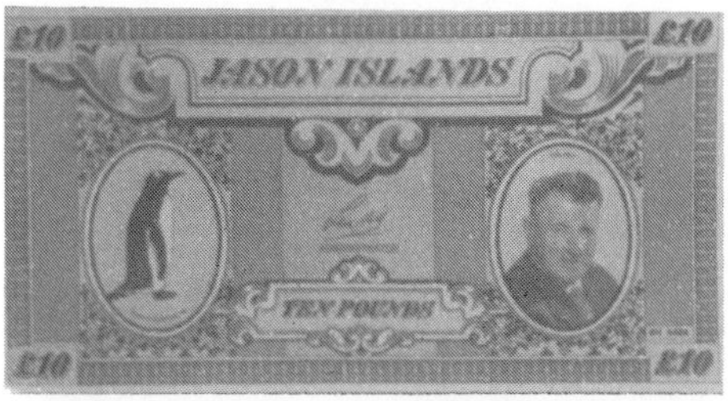

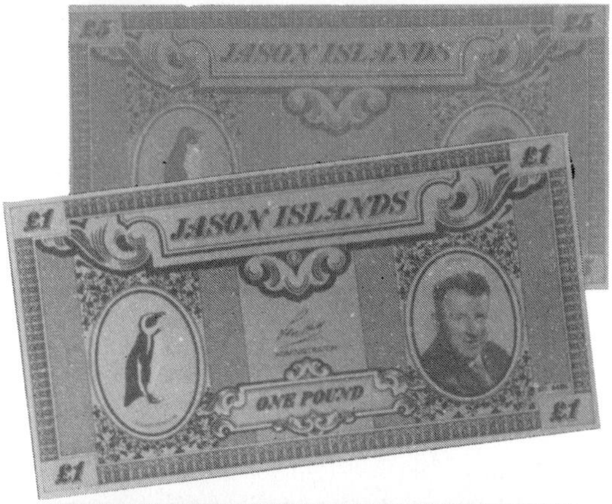

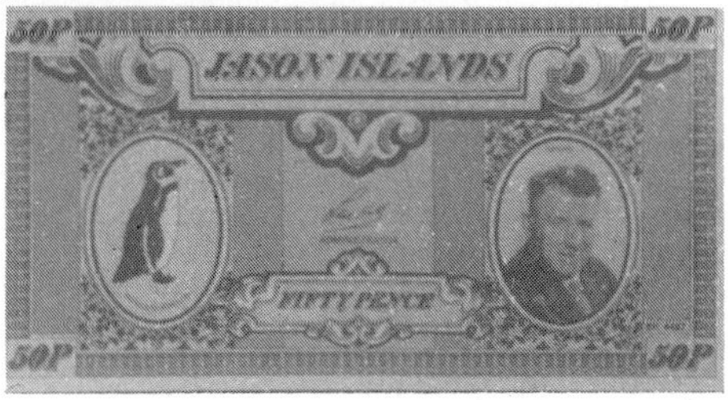

Private issue set £20, £10, £5, £1, 50p from the Jason Islands. £40

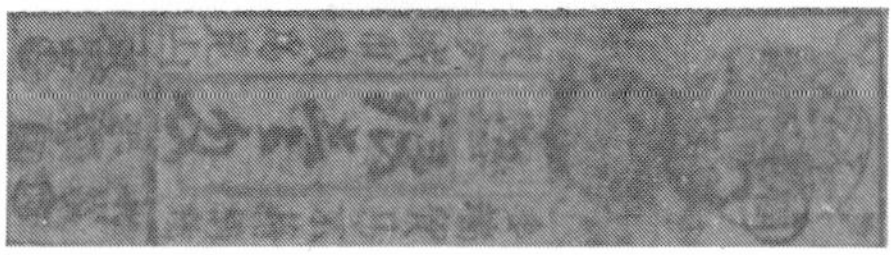

Japanese 10 Momme Gin note, 1731. £500

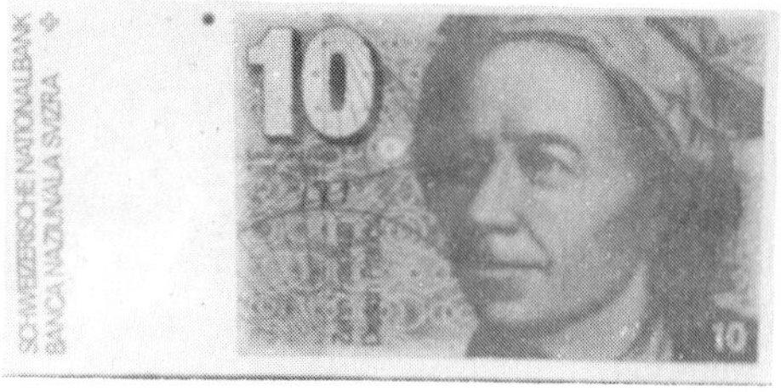

Swiss 10 Francs, 1979. £3

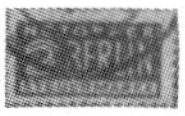

One of the smallest notes in the world, German stamp money, 1920. 50p

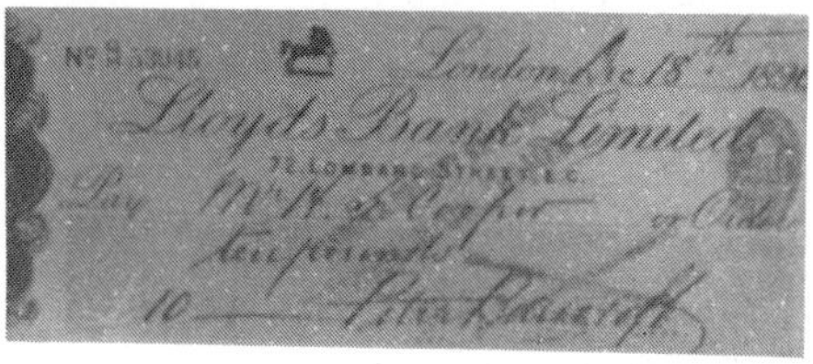

1896 Lloyds Bank cheque. £7.50

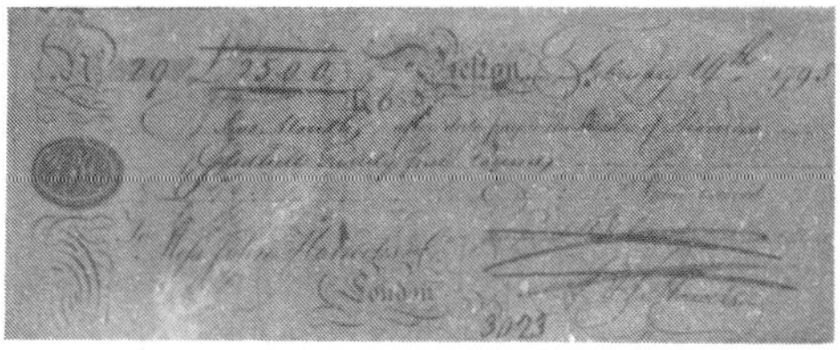

1795 Preston Bank £25 Bill of Exchange. £100

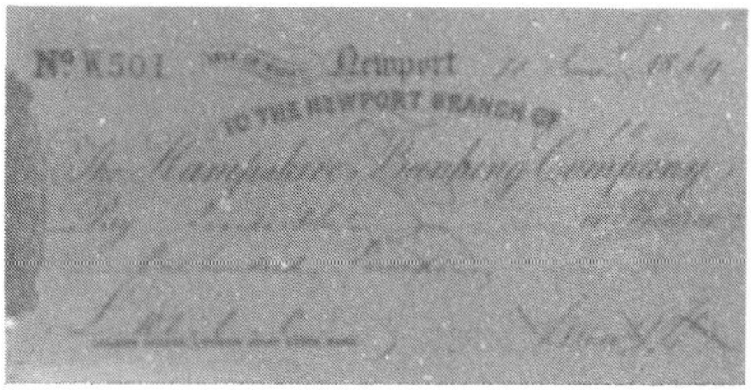

The Hampshire Banking Company cheque, 1864. £7.50

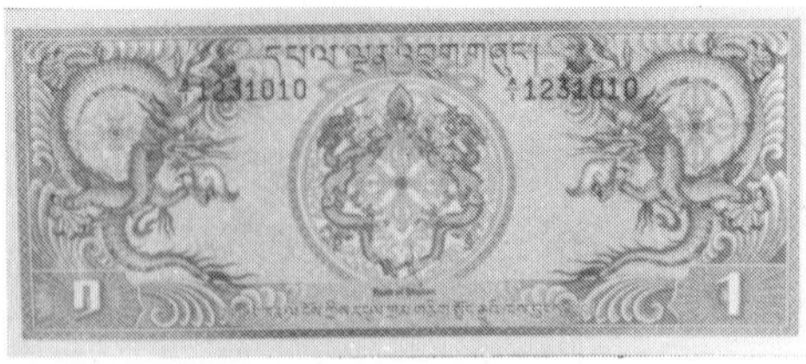

Bhutan 1 Ngultrum note, 1981. £10

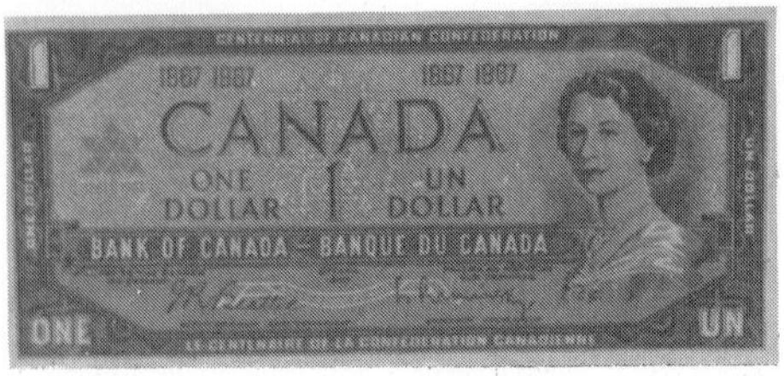

Canadian one dollar, 1967. £1.50

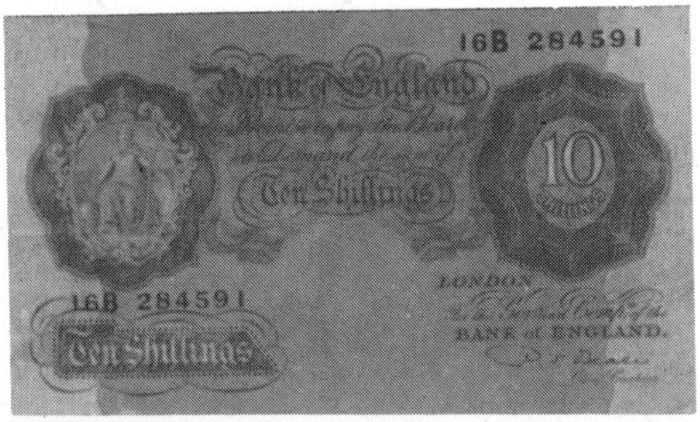

Bank of England ten shilling note, 1949-55. £10

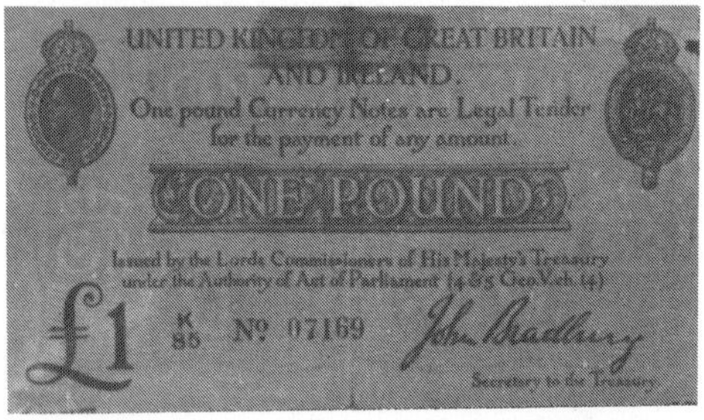

British one pound, 1914. £50

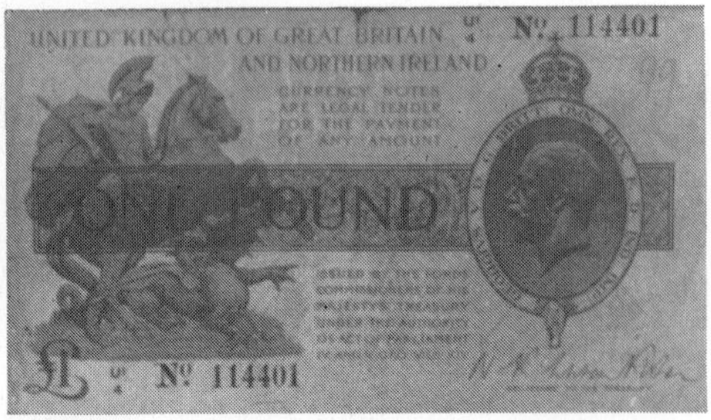

British one pound, 1919. £30

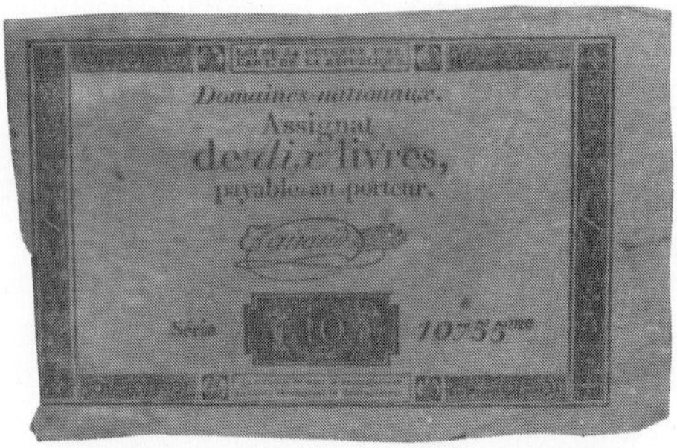

French 10 Livres 1792, a very rare note. £850

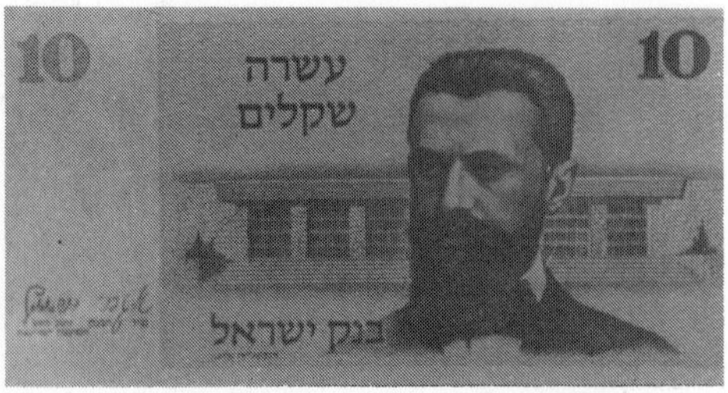

Israel 10 Shekel, 1978. £4.50

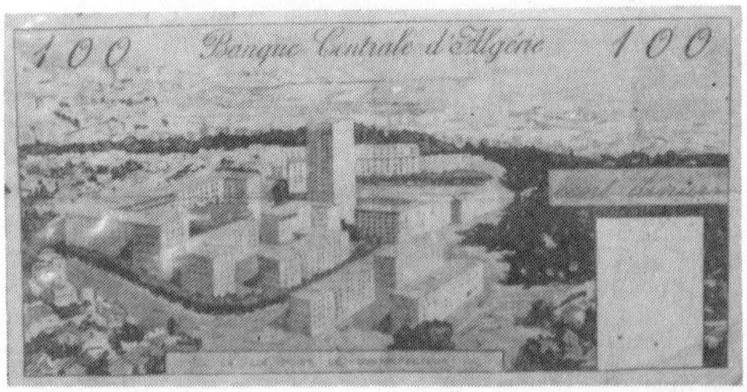

Banque Centrale d'Algerie 100 note. £30

Liz Taylor is a journalist and collects books and maps about the British in India.

"My fascination with India began when I went there to live in the 1950's. That was the tail end of the days of the Raj and there was still a strong feeling of what it must have been like.

"I began reading all the old books I could find in Bombay's Asiatic Library about the lives of British people in India and I was hooked.

"My collection is not particularly large because I'm selective about what I buy. It's got to be unique or specially interesting for there were thousands of books written by blimp-type colonels and patronising mem sahibs who bombasted their way around India. I generally avoid the duller 'My Days In Our Empire' sort of book.

"The collection is not confined to old books because I buy new ones as well and in recent years there has been an upsurge of interest in India — probably because of films like 'The Far Pavilions', 'Ghandi' and 'Jewel in the Crown'.

"I'm most proud of four maps of India done for the East India Company by a man called Andrew Dury in the 1770's and 1780's. He drew the Himalayas as a chain of mountains and wrote along them — "a range of hills sometimes covered with snow" because they had not been surveyed at that time. Those maps were bought for 10 shillings each 25 years ago.

"In the collection is a very interesting book called "P. and O. Sketches in Pen and Ink" by Harry Furniss. It was published about 1900 and is inscribed by its owner, "Red Sea, April 25th 1901." April 25th happens to be my birthday so I couldn't resist buying it. It cost £2.50 but I'm sure it's worth a good deal more now.

"I've also got two large portfolios of photographs collected by two ladies who went on a year long tour of India before the First World War. My daughters bought them for me in a Dublin junk shop and I've been able to trace who the women were and been to Ireland to meet their families. The niece of one of the women remembered her as 'Aunt Fluffy' though she looks most resolute in the photographs.

"The item I'd most want to add to my collection is Andrew Dury's map of the Bombay Province. I've got Calcutta and Madras but not Bombay and that's the part of India where my heart really lies."

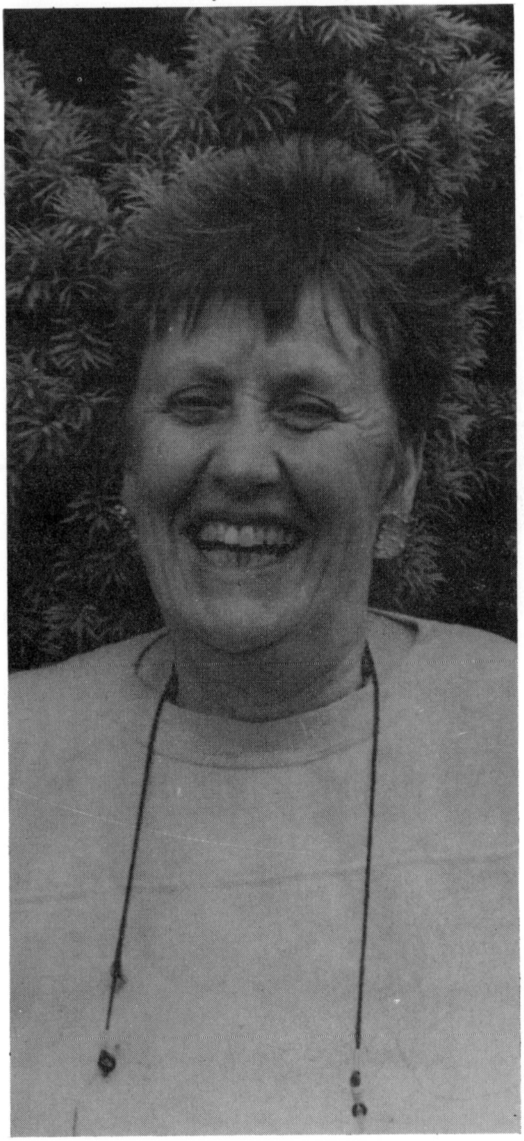

Journalist Liz Taylor who has a fascination with India.

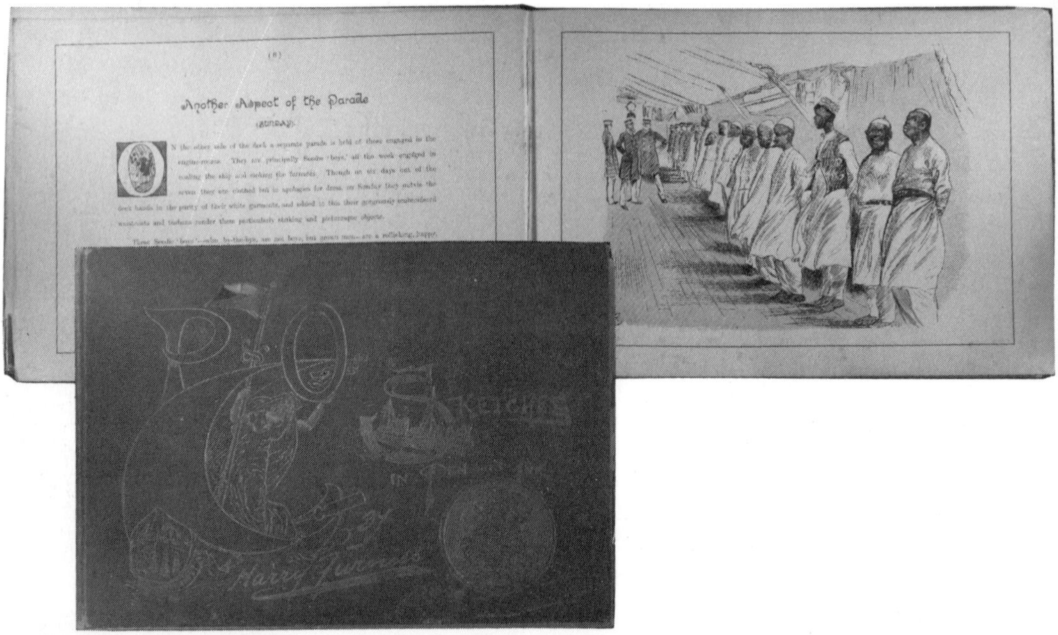

'P. & O. Sketches in Pen and ink' by Harry Furniss, containing a record drawn by the artist during a voyage on a P. & O. steamer.

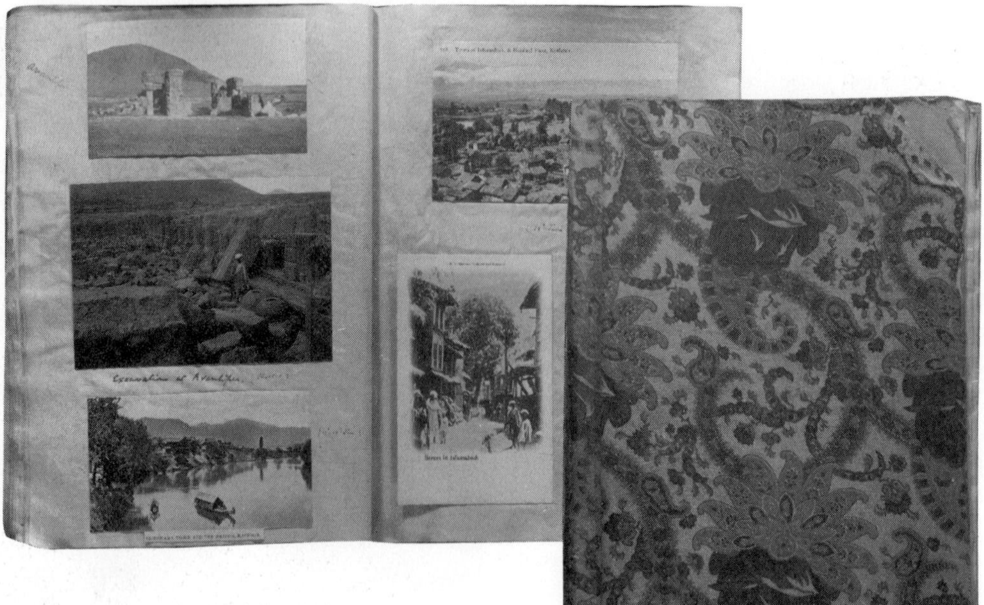

Photographic Album of India compiled from 11 April 1912 to 4 November 1912.
£50

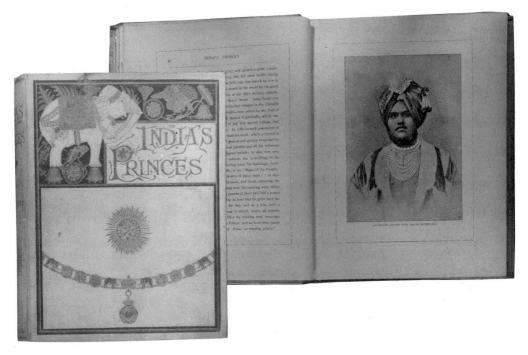

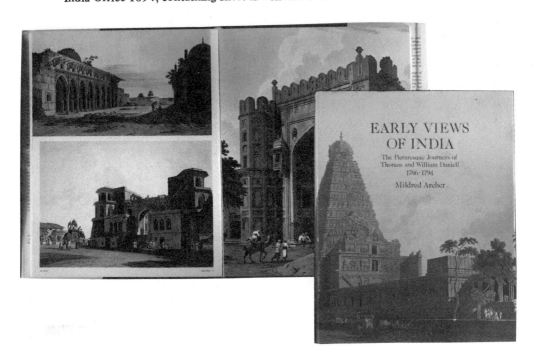

'India's Princes' by M. Griffith published by W. H. Allen & Co., Publishers to the India Office 1894, containing short life sketches of the native rulers of India. £20

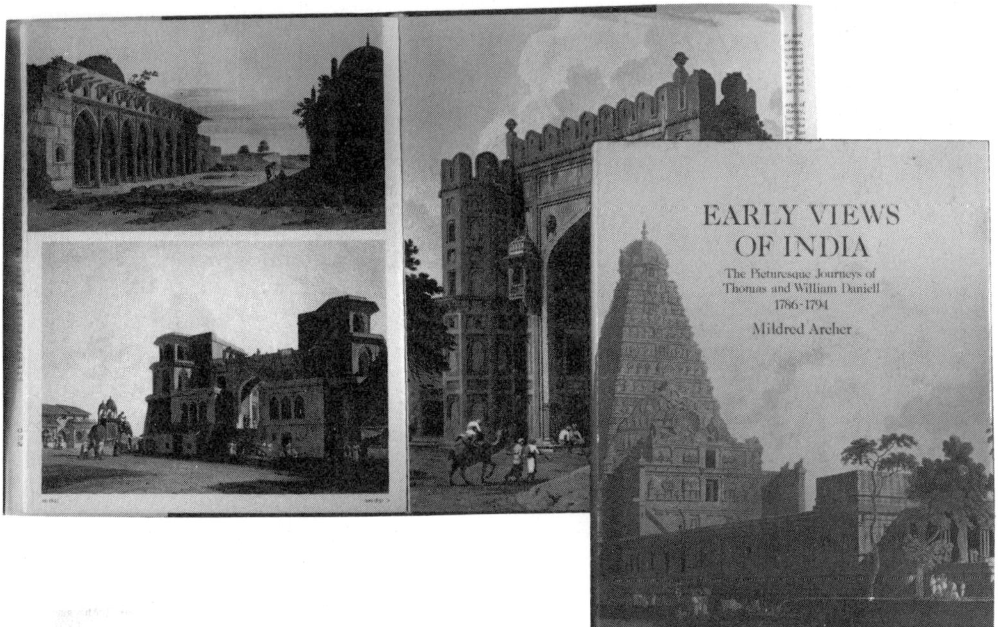

'Early Views of India' by Mildred Archer, published by Thames & Hudson, containing the picturesque journeys of Thomas and William Daniell, 1786-1794. £15

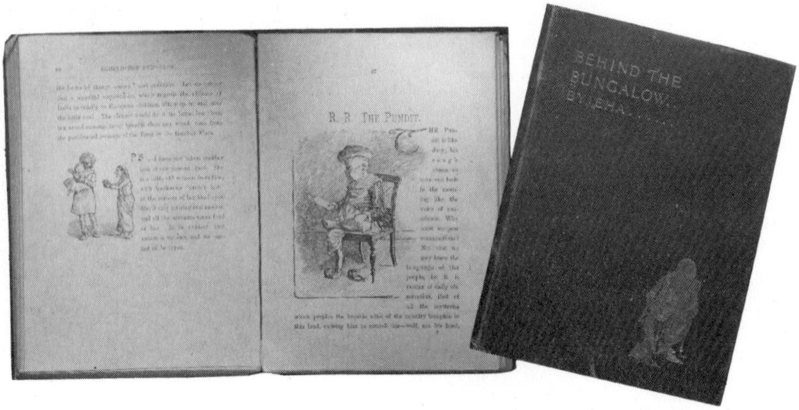

'Behind the Bungalow' by Eha, published by W. Thacker & Co., Calcutta and Simla 1907, containing a series of articles which first appeared in the Times of India. £5

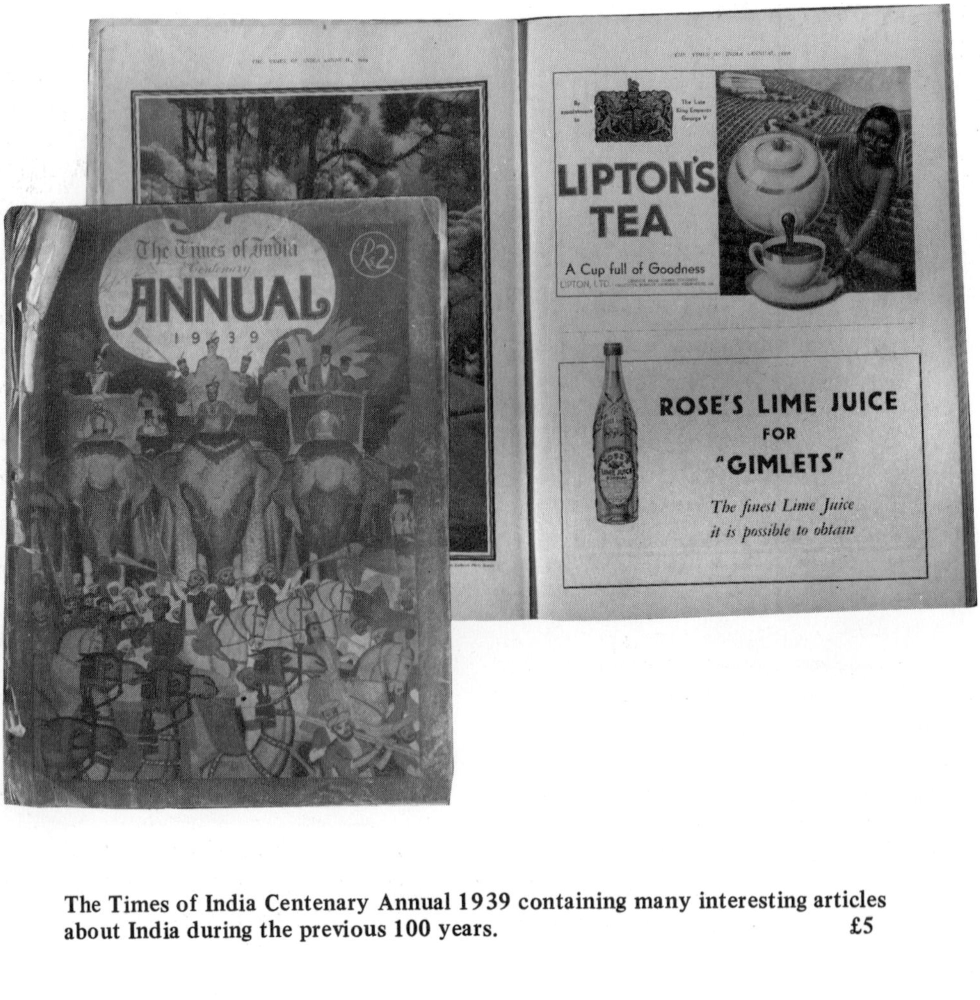

The Times of India Centenary Annual 1939 containing many interesting articles about India during the previous 100 years. £5

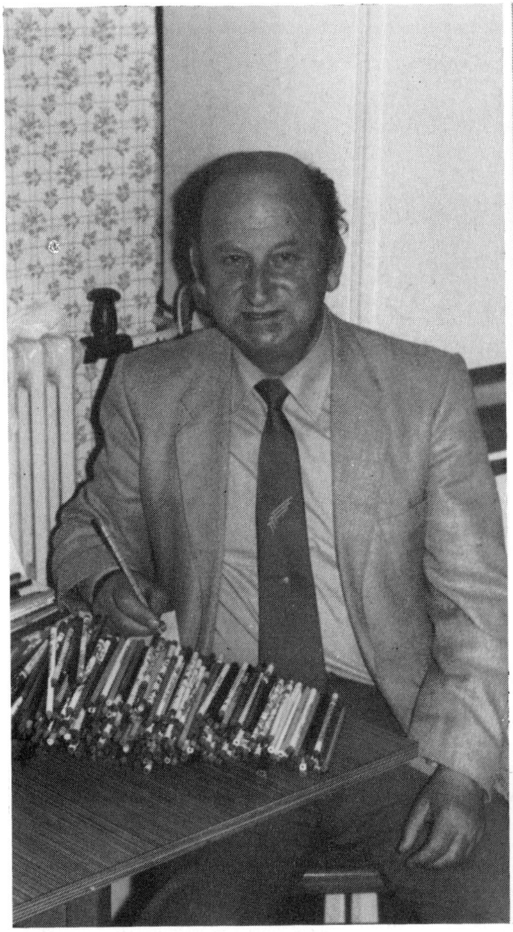

Trevor Edwards collects pencils. He is unemployed having been made redundant from his job as a bus driver.

"I used to have a grocer's shop in Harrow and when travellers came in with advertising pencils I'd put them away in a drawer. The ones I liked best were the pencils issued by the Robertson's jam people — the Golly pencils.

"Then I sold the shop and by that time there was quite a collection of pencils. I took them with me because they interested me but later on I realised that pencils were turning up on antique stalls in fairs and markets so I began to buy more. That was the start of my collection. By now I've over 1,300 of them. I've got pencils from Switzerland with ice axes on the end of them; I've got pencils with globes and

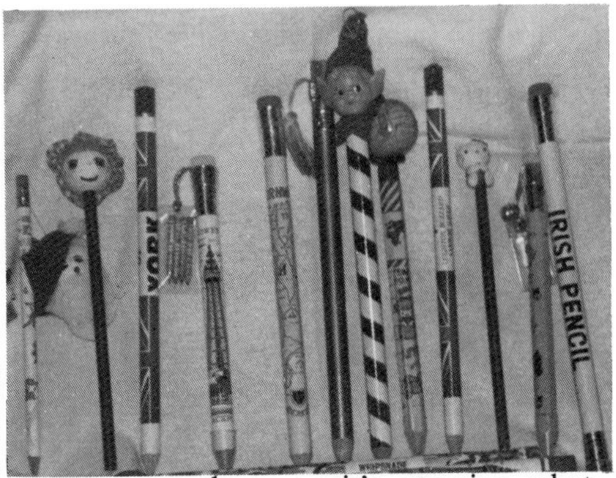

puppets on them — it's amazing what people will put on pencils."

The oldest pencil in Trevor's collection is a George V Silver Jubilee pencil which is worth around £1.50. He also has coronation pencils for George VI and Elizabeth II as well as pencils issued by the old railway companies before nationalisation. Many of the railway pencils belonged to his father who worked on the railways. Another interesting item is a set of six utility pencils from wartime — Trevor paid £1 for the set.

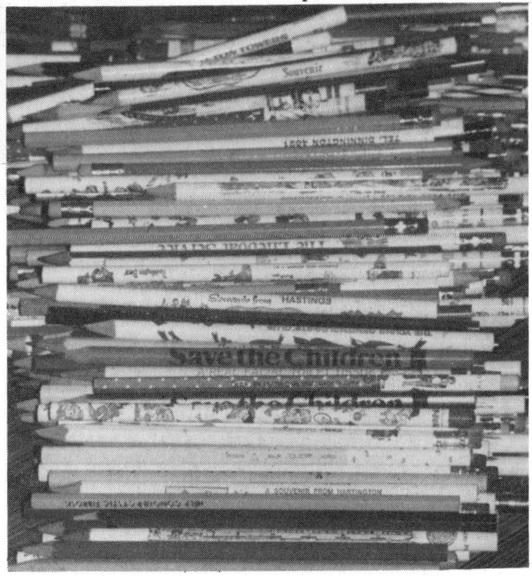

The collection continues to grow because his family brings back pencils from foreign trips and visits to the seaside. His foreign pencils include ones made in India, Japan, China and the USA, which is a large source of supply because many companies there still give away pencils as advertising.

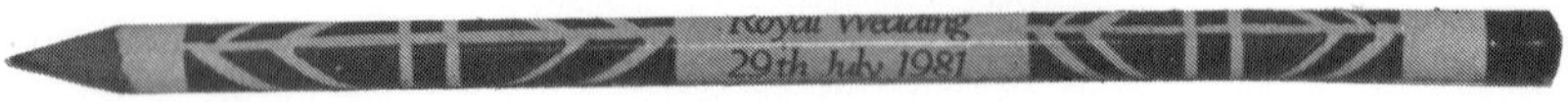

Royal Wedding 1981 25p

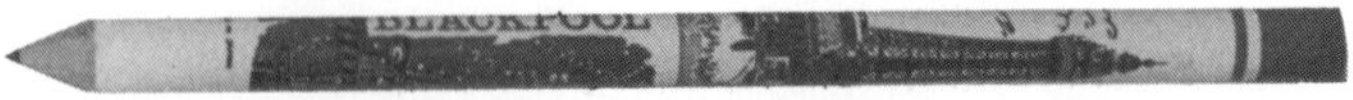

Blackpool souvenir pencil £1

Silver pencil for J. R. Topping, Tobacconist £8

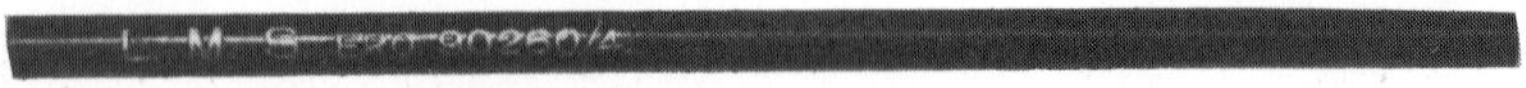

L.M.S. Railway pencil £2

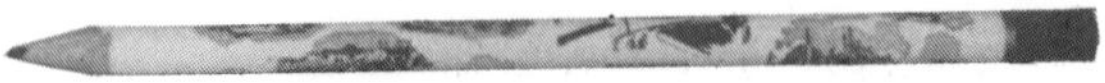

Skegness souvenir pencil £1

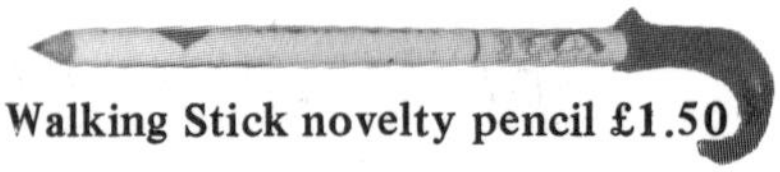

Walking Stick novelty pencil £1.50

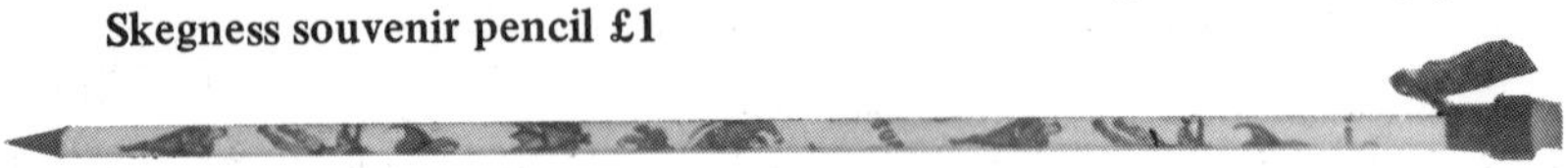

Batman pencil with tassel £1

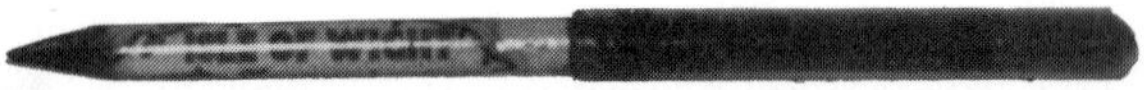

Isle of Wight pencil containing sand from Alum Bay £1

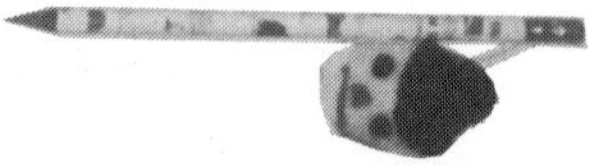

Snowman pencil £1

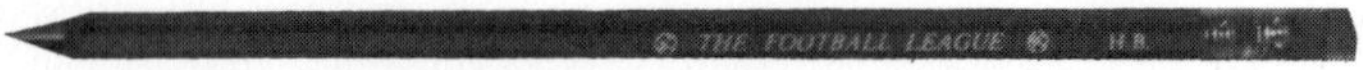

The Football League pencil 15p

Cigar shaped pencil £1

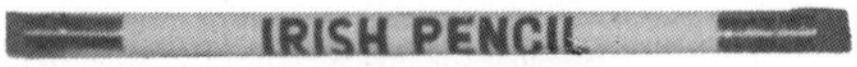

Irish Pencil with a rubber at both ends £1

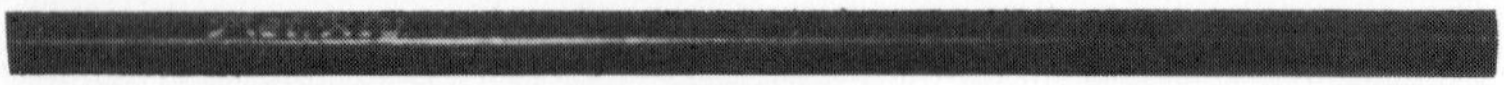

Met Railway pencil £2

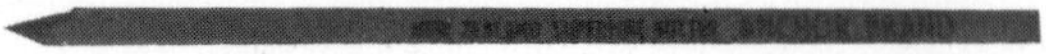

Anchor Butter advertising pencil £1

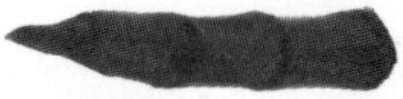

Bamboo pencil from Arundel. £1.50

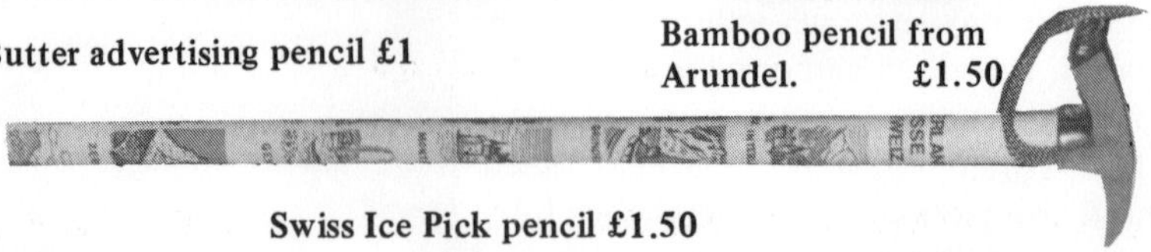

Swiss Ice Pick pencil £1.50

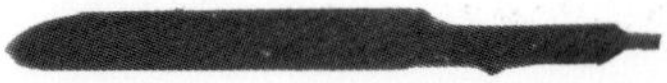

Cricket Bat novelty pencil £3

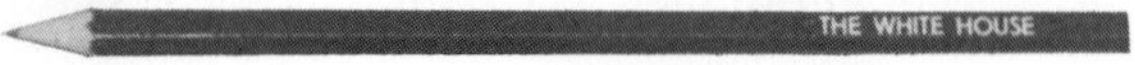

The White House, London 50p

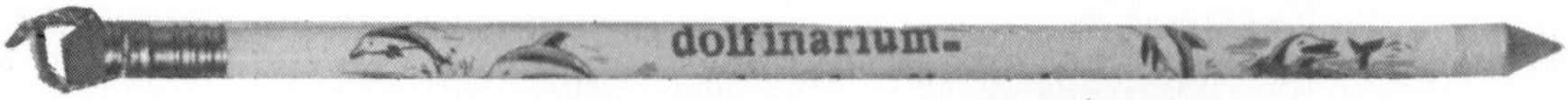

Dolfinarium, Belgium pencil £1.75

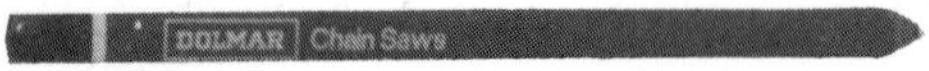

Dolmar Chain Saws 50p

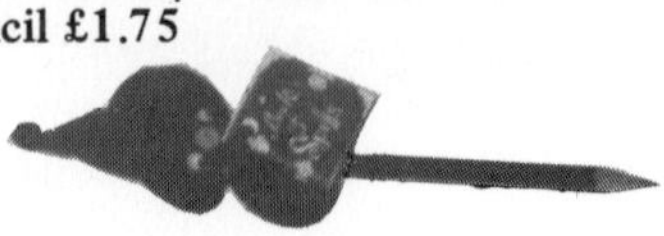

Witch pencil 75p

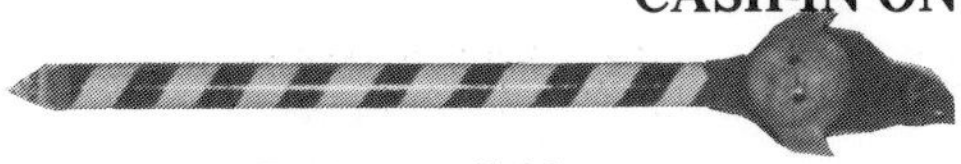

Pixie pencil £1

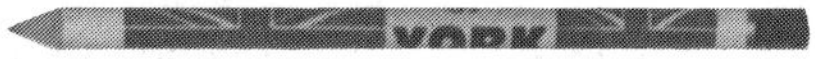

York advertising pencil £1

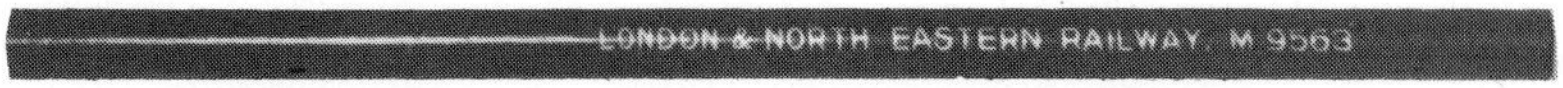

London & North Eastern Railway pencil £2

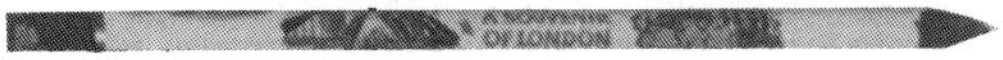

A Souvenir of London £1

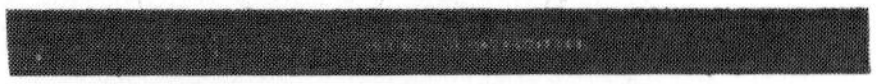

Carpenters flat pencil 50p

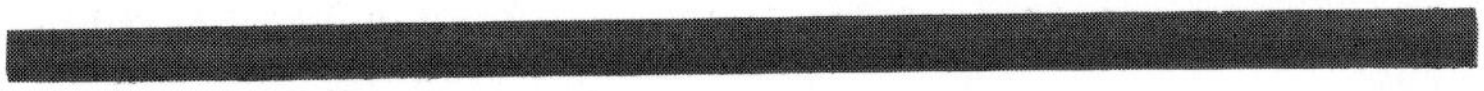

London & Midland Railway pencil £2

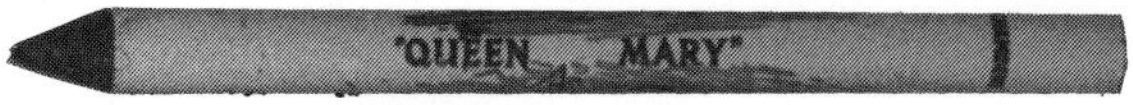

'Queen Mary' Souvenir pencil £5

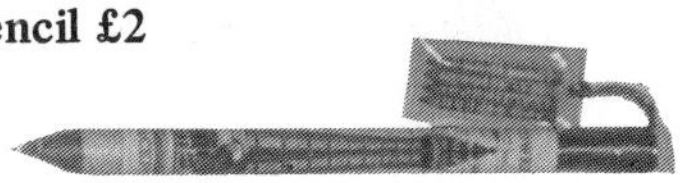

Blackpool Tower £1

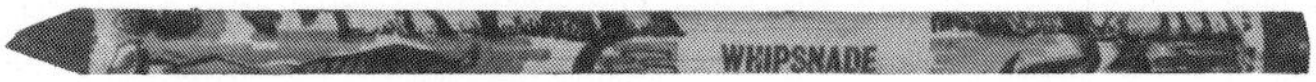

Whipsnade Zoo £1

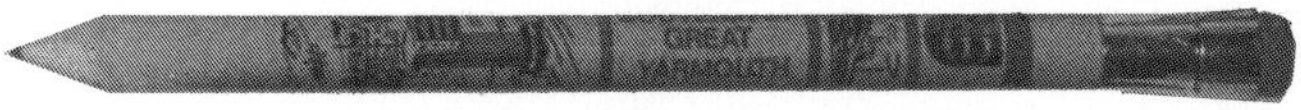

Great Yarmouth souvenir pencil £1

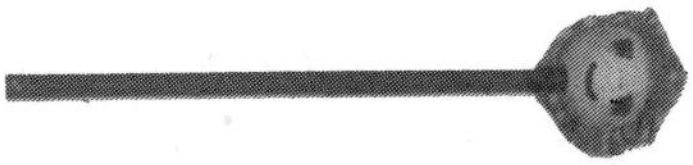

Mop head advertising pencil £1

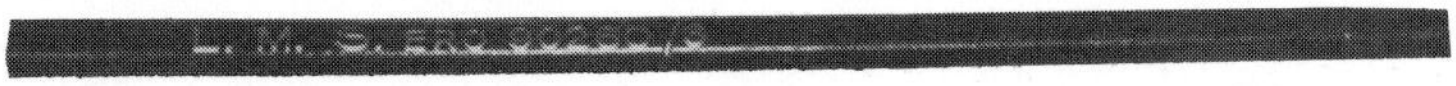

London Midland & Scottish Railway pencil £2

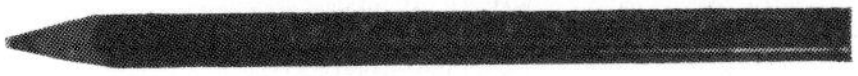

Carpenters flat six inch ruler pencil 50p

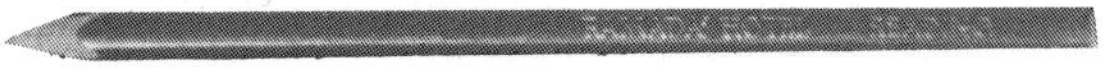

Ramada Hotel pencil 50p

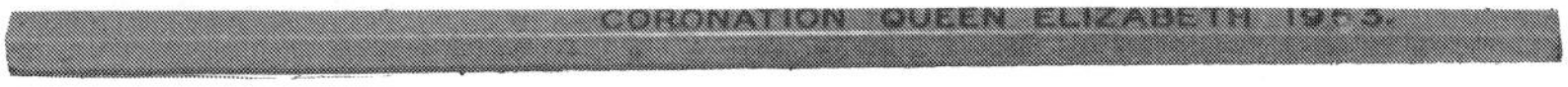

Coronation Queen Elizabeth 1953 £2.50

Leighton Buzzard advertising pencil £1

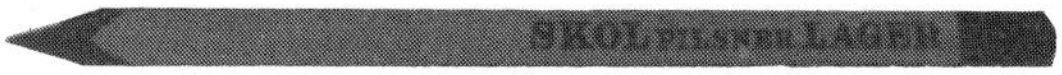

Skol Pilsner Lager pencil £1

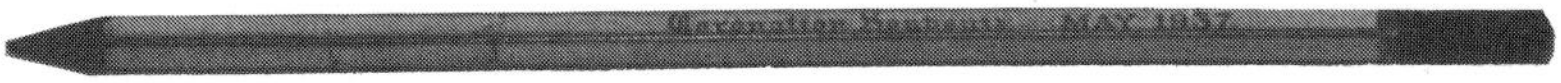

Coronation Souvenir pencil 1937 £5

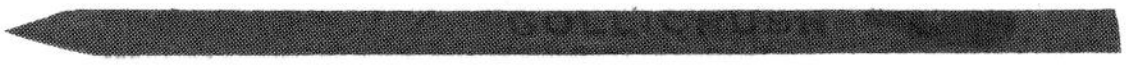

Robertsons Gollicrush pencil £1

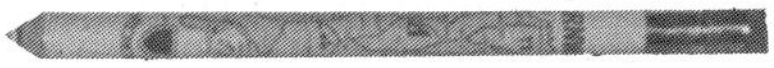

Cornwall advertising pencil £1

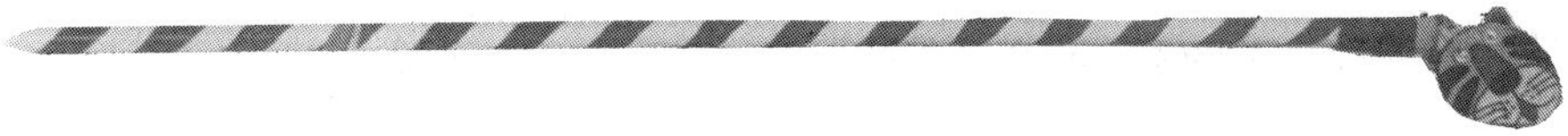

Tony the Tiger pencil £1

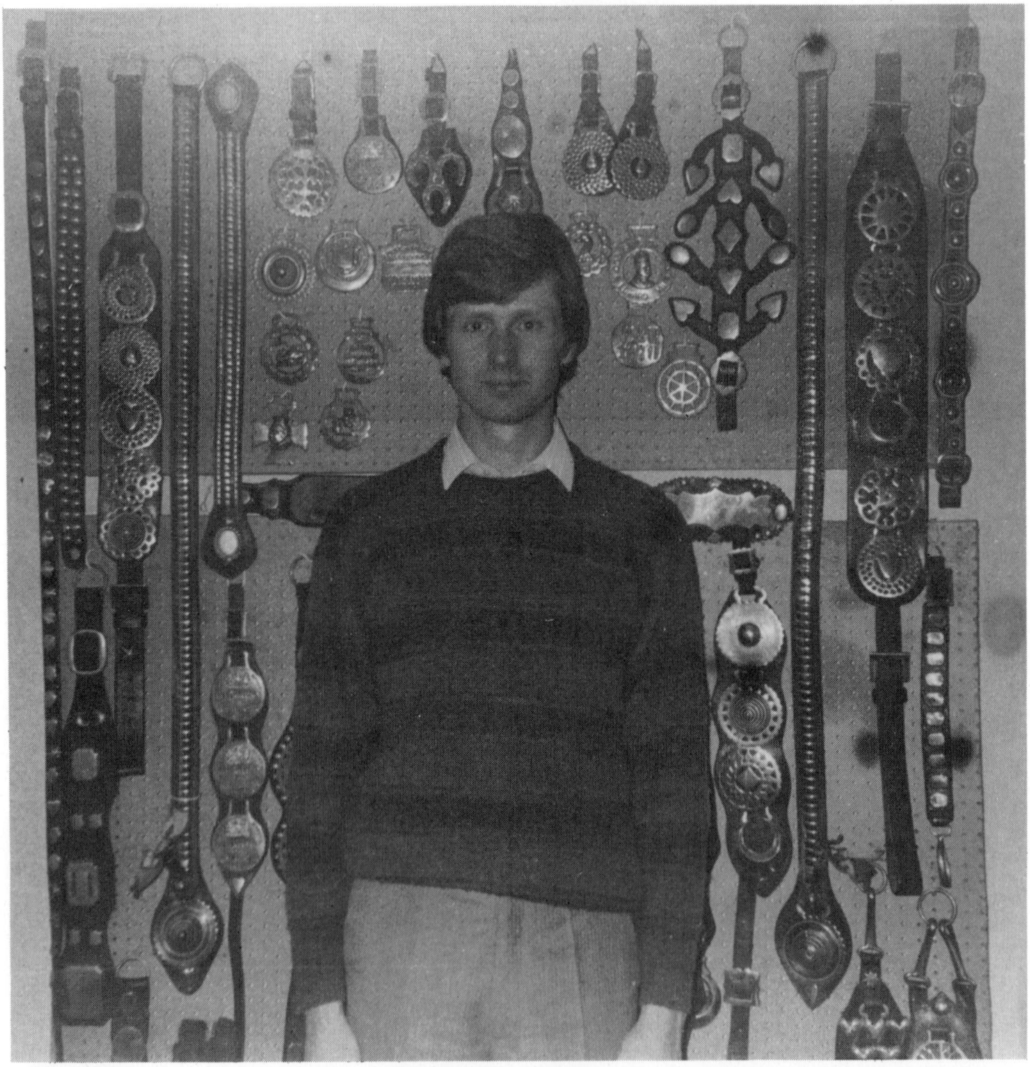

Jonathan Sneath collects and sells horse brasses and harness decorations.

"Genuine horses brasses and harness decorations date from the mid 19th century to around 1920 when heavy horses began to disappear from Britain's farms. However since then there have been reproduction brasses made but they are of poorer quality than the originals. Good brasses are becoming increasingly difficult to find because most of them are already in the hands of collectors.

"There were two methods of manufacturing brasses — the thicker ones are cast in sand which leaves a rough back and the thinner ones were stamped out of a sheet of brass and they have smooth backs.

"Pre 1920 brasses were all hand finished and filed down and there were always two little marks at the back, like the pontil marks on glasses. In reproduction pieces the bits on the back of the brasses are rounded off and the detail is lost.

"Brasses are a very British thing although there are a few examples from America, Australia or South Africa where British people settled. You rarely find brasses made before 1850 because they seem to have been part of the Victorian love for decoration."

Though Jonathan deals in brasses he also has a personal collection. The most popular brasses were decorated with the emblems from playing cards, thistles, hearts or crowns. Among the most desirable pieces are martingale straps with four or five brasses mounted on them.

Brasses with bells mounted in them are also rare and Jonathan had examples with two bells but never with three although he knows that these do exist. Another thing he would like to find is an example of a brass with a little photograph inset in it. These usually held pictures of Queen Victoria or King Edward VII but though he has found the frames, they have always been empty. The photographs have not stood up to rough weather and hard work outdoors.

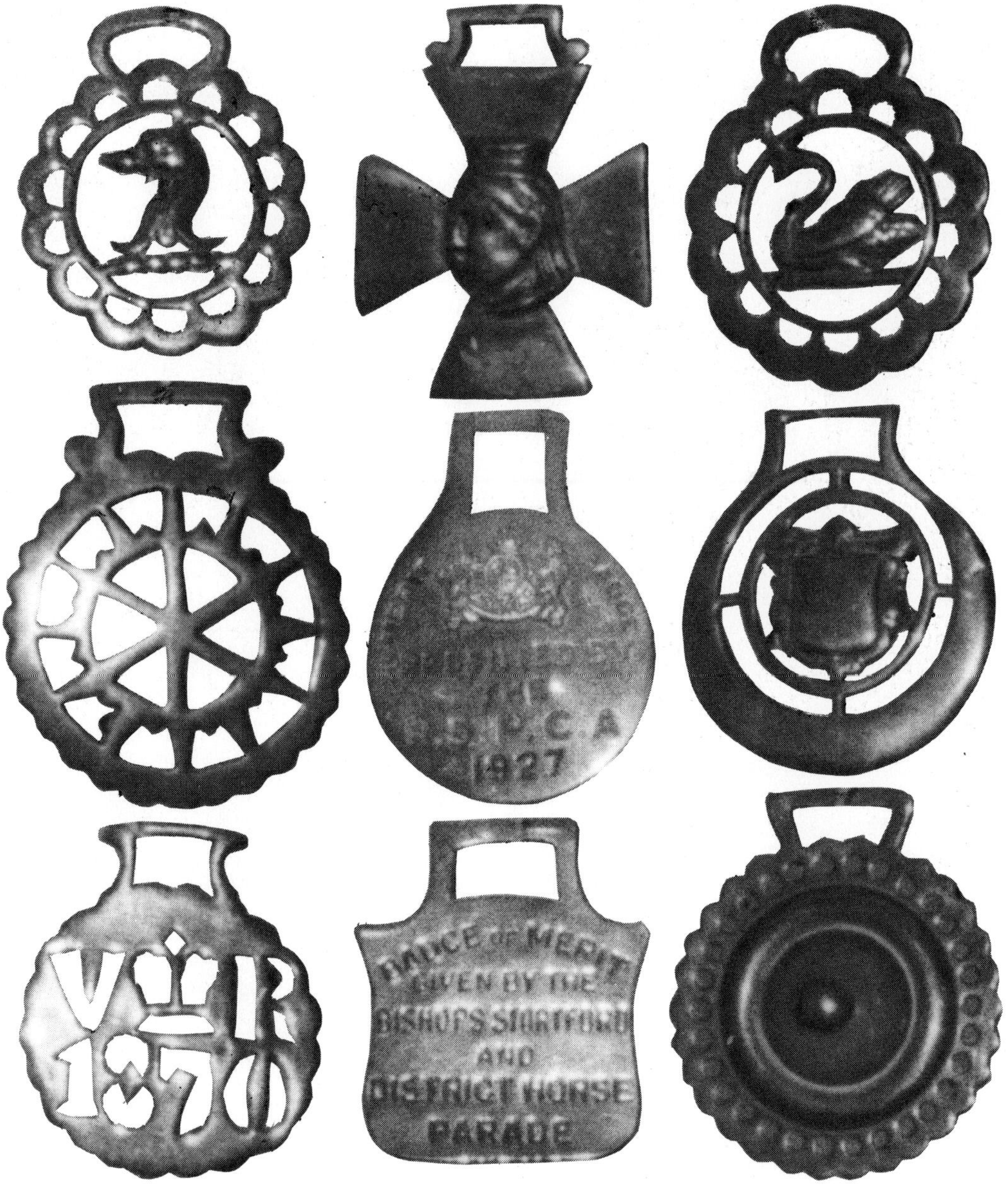

Some rare and unusual horse brasses from Jonathan's personal collection.

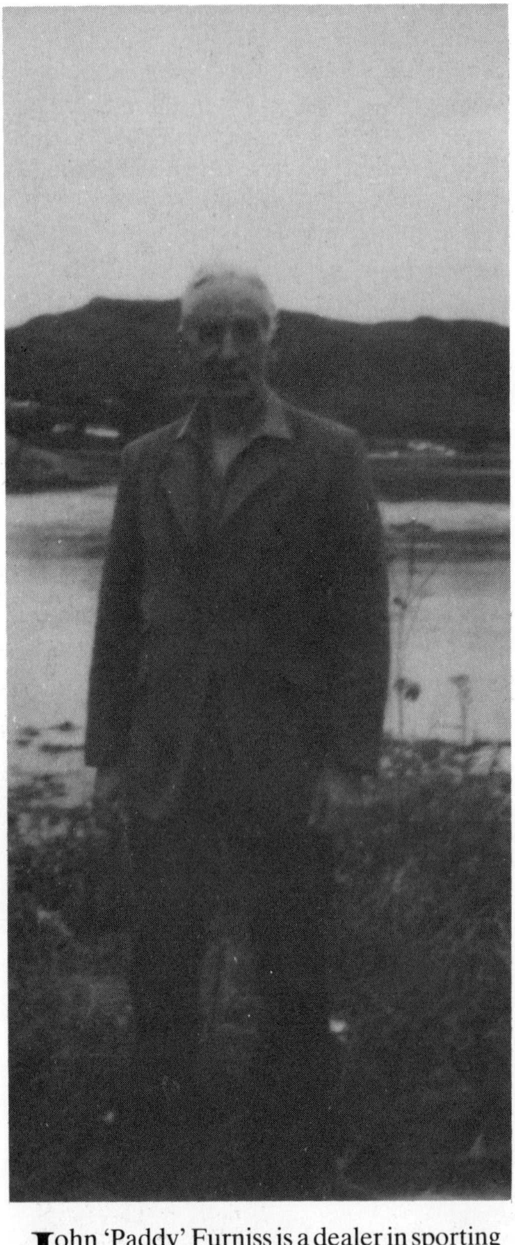

John 'Paddy' Furniss is a dealer in sporting books but he collects books on golf for his own pleasure.

"When I retired from the Army and later from teaching, I began to collect books as a hobby but now it has grown into a full time business and my current list has over 600 titles. My collection of golf books comes to more than 400.

"I've customers all over the world from USA to Australia and Japan. The Japanese are growing more and more interested in golf and are keen buyers.

"Some of the prices golf books have been making at auction have been amazing recently, with many selling for over £1,000.

"The books in my collection that I wouldn't want to part with are 'Balfour's Reminiscences of Golf at St Andrews' dated 1887 which must be worth more than £1,000 now and Forgan's 'Golfers' Handbook' also from 1887 which would make at least £500 if sold."

Paddy Furniss said that if he could pick one book which he wanted more than any other he would opt for a paperback copy of a poem entitled 'The Golf' which was written by a poet called Mathison in 1743. Recently a copy of a first edition of this scarce little book sold at auction in Edinburgh for £17,000 and a second edition sold in 1985 for £11,000. The buyers would also have had to add ten percent of the hammer price to the cost of their little books.

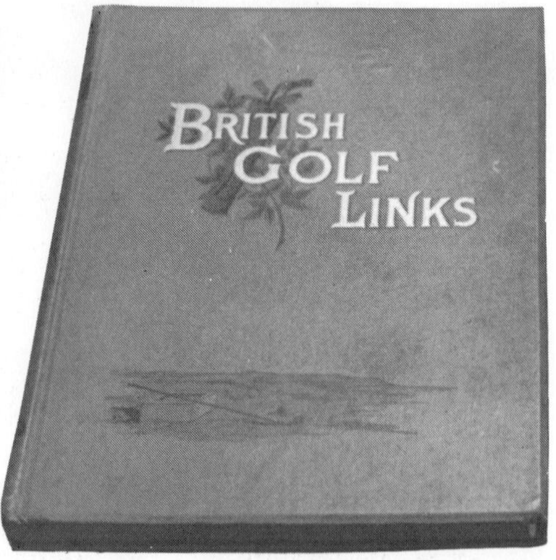

'British Golf Links' by Hutchinson, 1897, a book keenly sought by collectors.

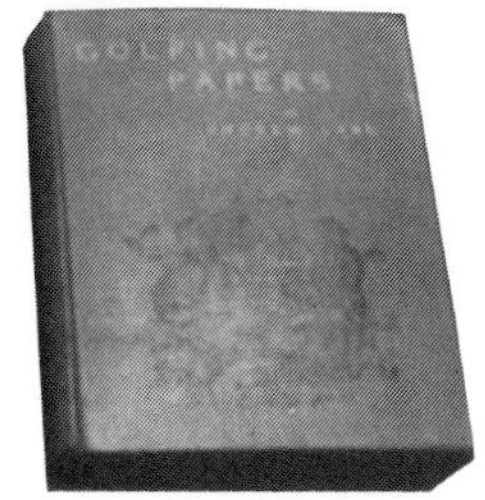

Golfing Papers by Andrew Lang, 1892. £80

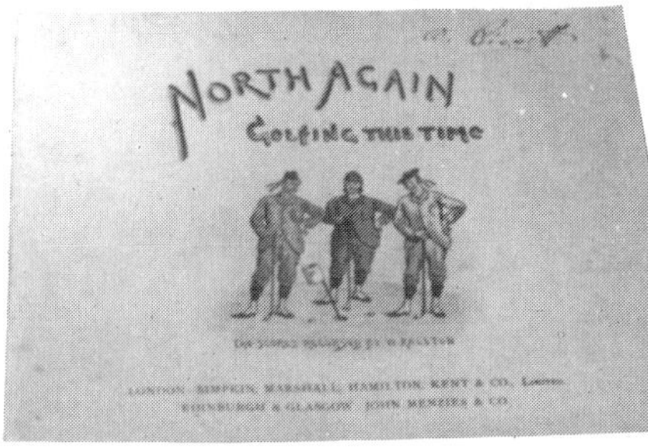

North Again, Golfing This Time, by W. Ralston, 1900. £50

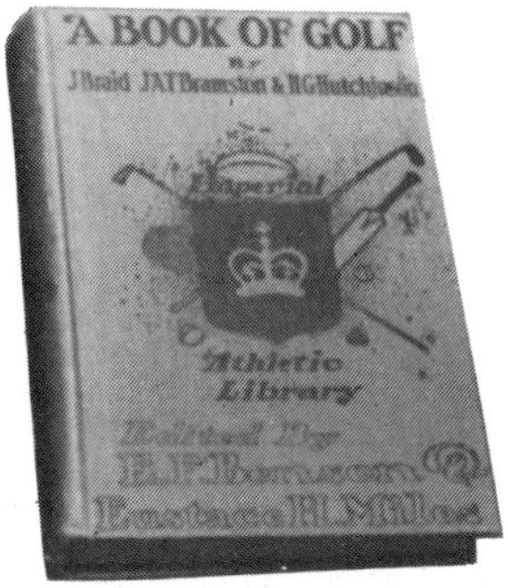

'A Book of Golf', by J. Braid, J. A. T. Bramston and H. G. Hutchinson, edited by E. F. Benson and Eustace H. Miles, 1903. £65

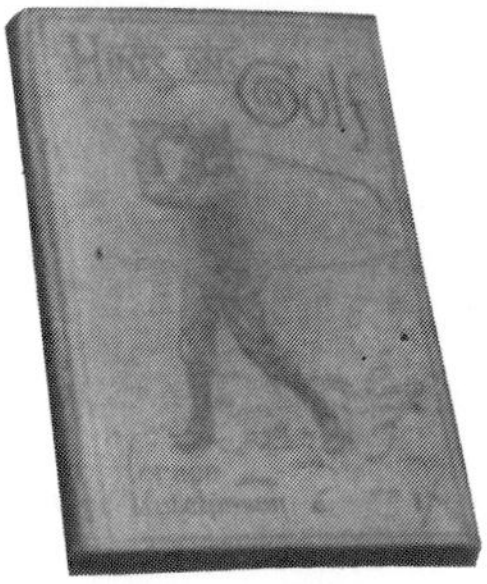

Hints on Golf, by Horace Hutchinson, 1891. £80

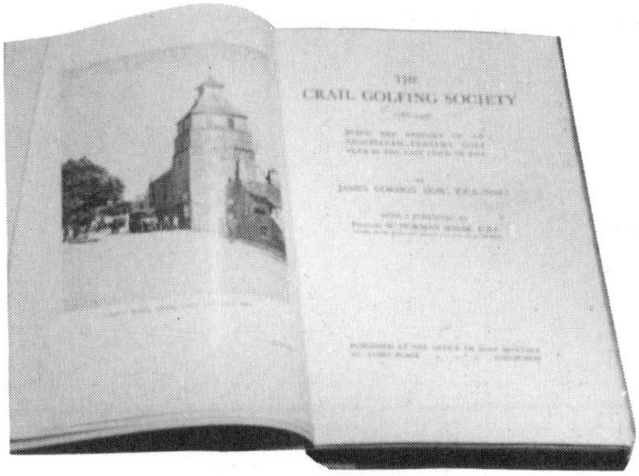

The Crail Golfing Society, 1786–1936, Being the History of an Eighteenth Century Golf Club in the East Neuk of Fife, by James Gordon Dow, 1936. £400

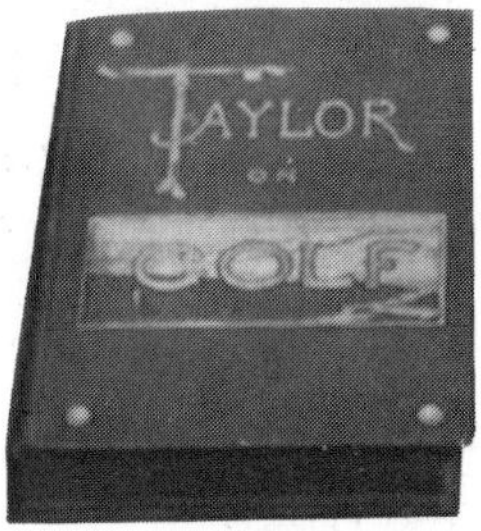

Taylor on Golf, 1902. £70

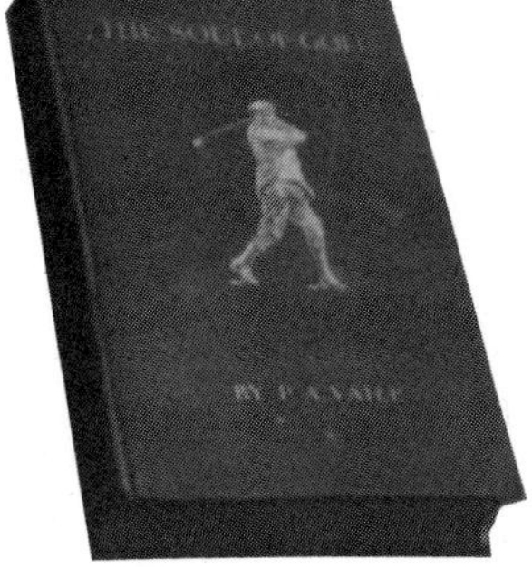

The Soul of Golf, by P. A. Vaile, 1898. £75

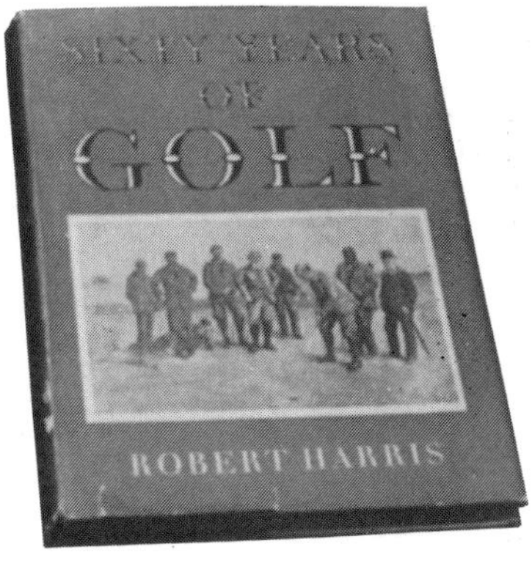

Sixty Years of Golf, by Robert Harris, 1953. £60

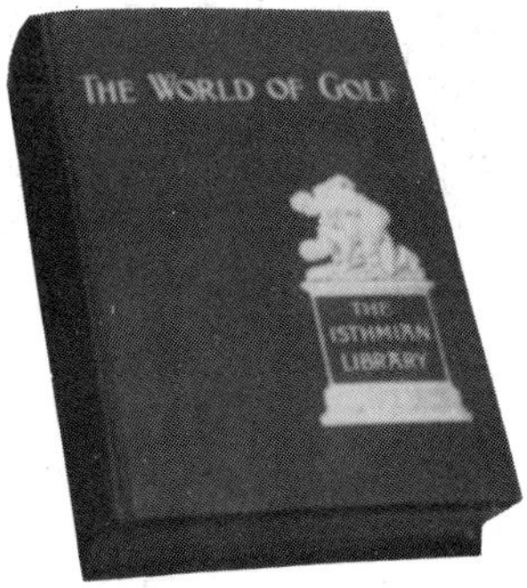

The World of Golf, by Gorden Smith, published by The Isthmian Library, 1898. £120

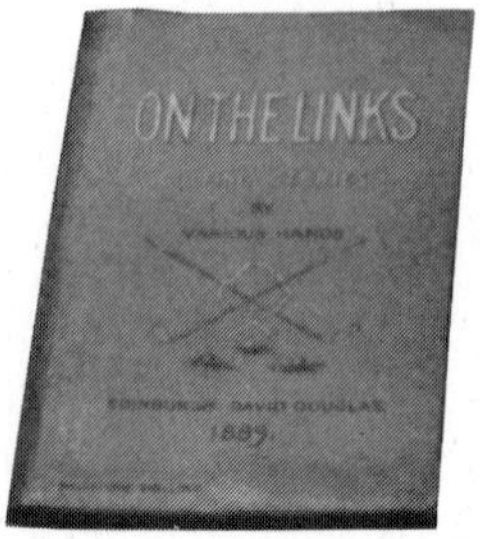

On The Links, Golfing Stories by Various Hands, Edinburgh, David Douglas, 1889. £300

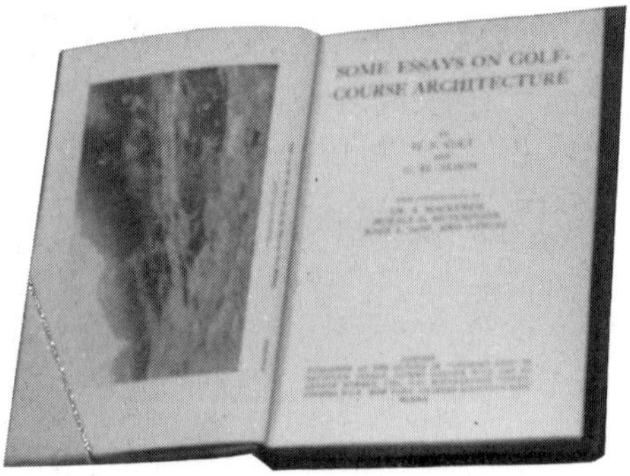

Some Essays on Golf Course Architecture, by H. S. Colt and C. H. Alison, 1920. £450

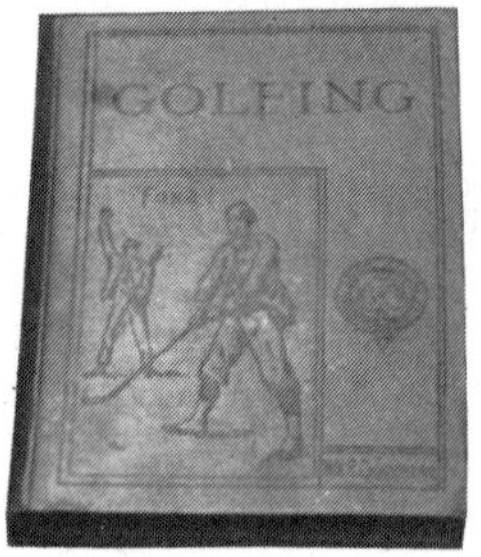

Golfing, by W. & R. Chambers, 1887. £200

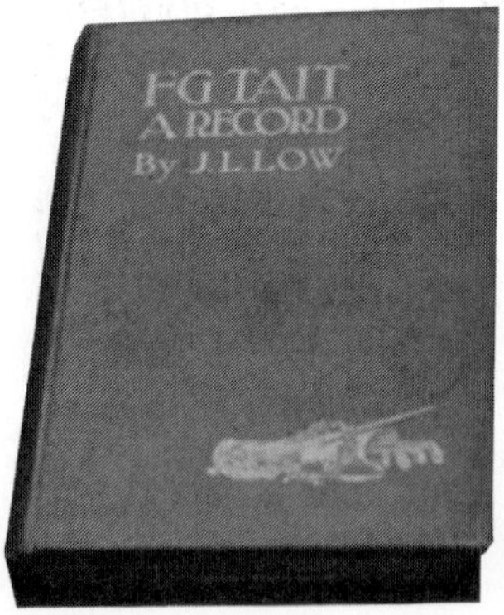

F. G. Tait, A Record, by J. L. Low, 1900. £75

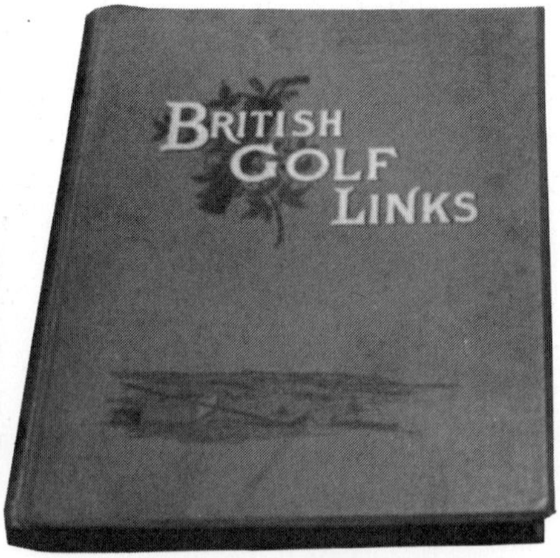

British Golf Links, by Hutchinson, 1897. £500

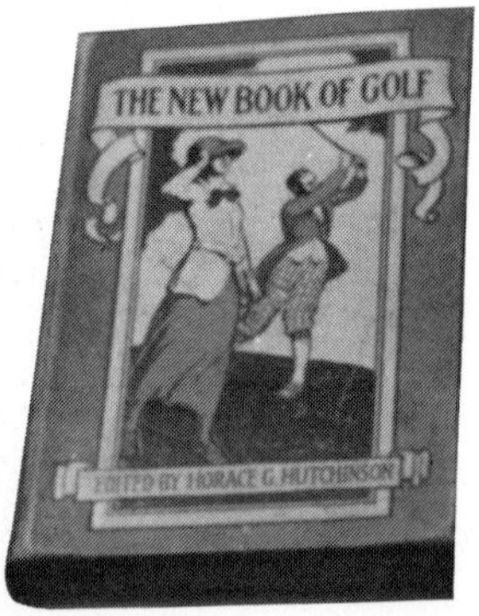

'The New Book of Golf', edited by Horace G. Hutchinson, 1912. £125

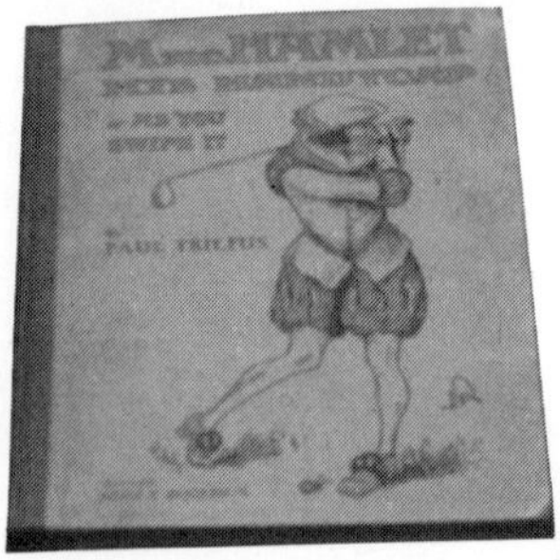

MacHamlet 'Hys Handycap' or 'As You Swipe It', by Paul Triefus, illustrated by Sidney Rogerson, 1922.£50

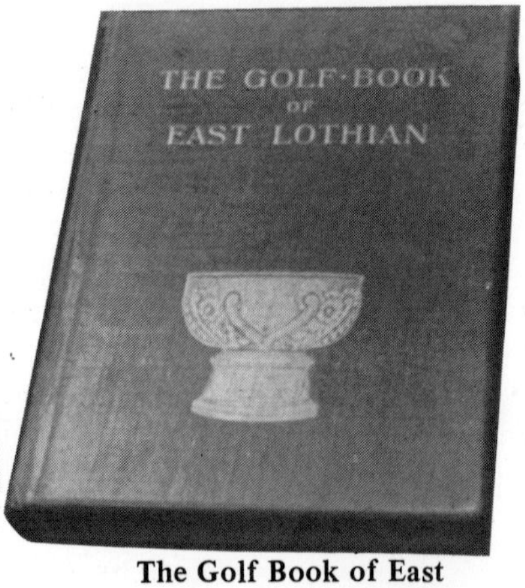

The Golf Book of East Lothian, by Kerr, 1896. £900

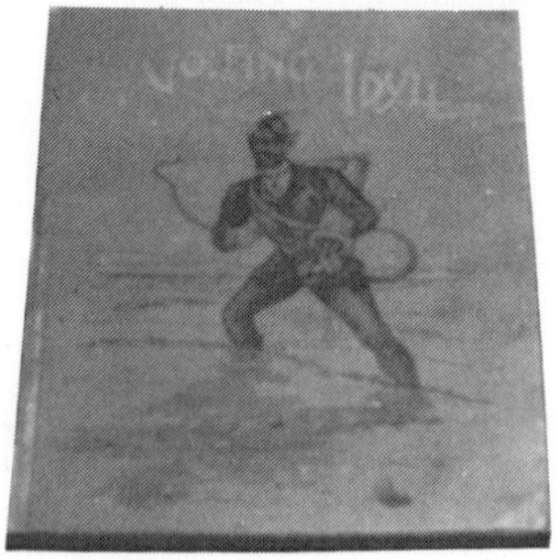

A Golfing Idyll, by Flint, 1897. £200

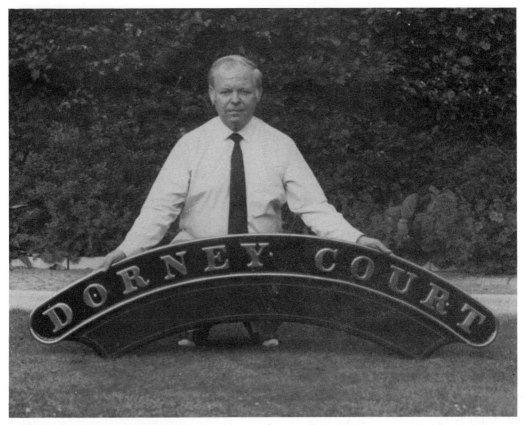

Ian Wright is the deputy head of a comprehensive school and collects old railway items.

"It began in the 1960's after my dormant interest in Railwayana was reawakened when I returned from university. I decided that I'd like to own some mementoes of the Steam Age and after buying a couple of things I went mad. Now I've over 1,000 items ranging from ten steam locomotive plates to crockery, GWR jigsaws, playing cards and book markers. I've also got more than 5,000 postcards of trains and stations.

"The earliest items in the collection date from around 1880 and it goes up to publicity material of the 1960's taking in things from the '30's and railway station signs of the '50's on the way. Station signs used to be in different colours according to the regions — now there's only one colour for the whole country."

Ian's most prized possession is a unique name plate for the engine 'City of Stoke on Trent'. The one from the other side of the engine is preserved in Stoke Museum. It is made of brass, eight feet long and surmounted with the city crest. Its estimated worth is around £3,500.

If he had a wish Ian would want some more unusual name plates but they are now very hard to find.

He is the author of a book entitled 'Name Plates On Display' which tells where to see nameplates in every part of Britain and he has also co-authored a series of 20 booklets about railway postcards which lists 7,500 of them. At the moment he is preparing another book called 'Railwayana On Display' which will be a guide to all the railway displays and museums in the country. There are over 50 specialist Railwayana museums in Britain and he plans to visit them all.

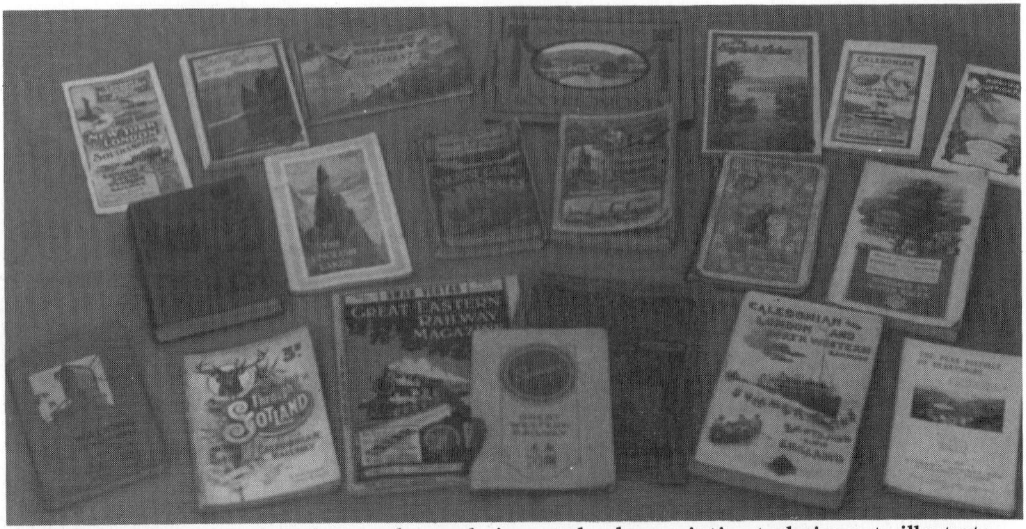

The early Companies seized upon the newly-invented colour-printing techniques to illustrate their publicity material. Highly coloured and lavishly picturesque, early examples in good condition can command up to £20 nowadays.

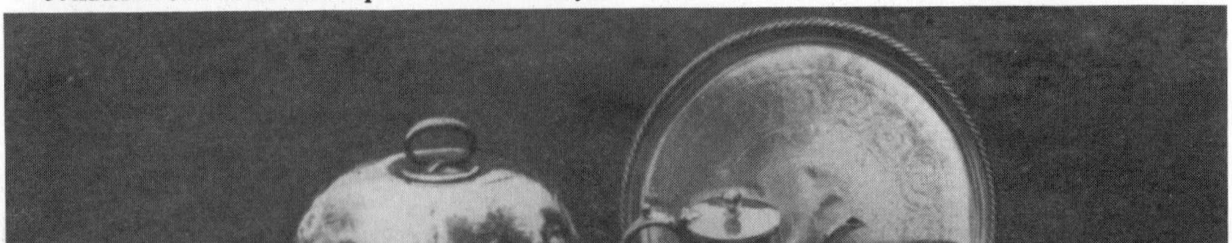

The Railway Companies owned a large number of hotels, ships and refreshment rooms in addition to providing catering on their own trains. As such, they had to provide the full range of silverware much of which still survives because of its durability, although the spectacular pieces have long since ended up in collections. Illustrated here are a Midland Railway game tureen, a North Eastern Railway salver, a Great Northern Railway ice-bucket, a Great Western Railway wine-cooler, a North British Railway tankard, a London and North Eastern Railway coffee-pot, as well as items from the Glasgow and South-Western, and the Southern Railway Companies. A modest fork sixty years old can still be owned for a few pounds; a game tureen or an ice-bucket close to a hundred.

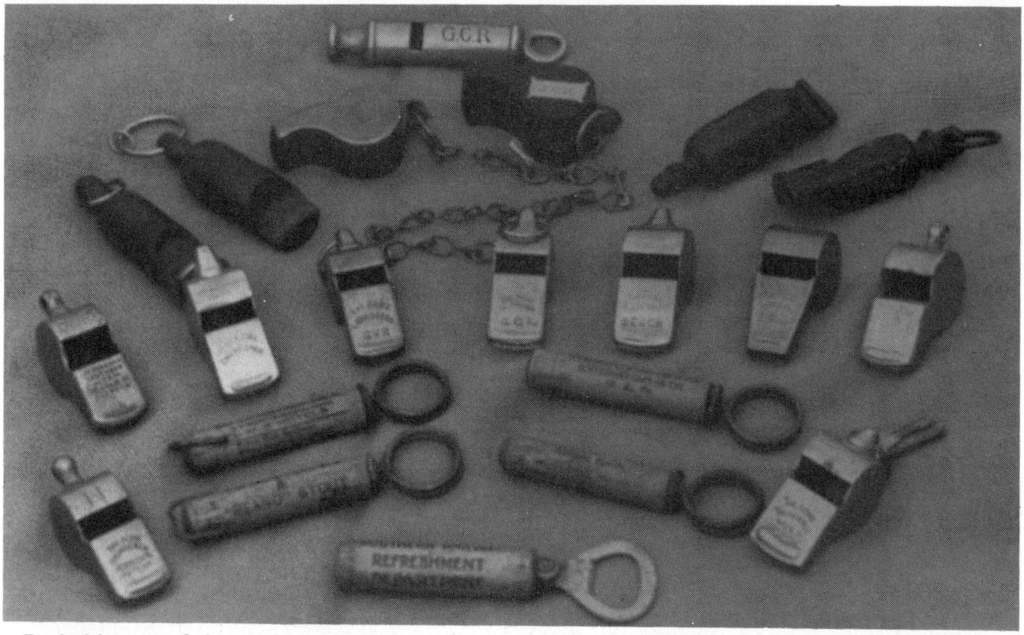

Probably one of the most evocative sounds on any railway station is the blast of the guard's whistle. Examples from the last century are eagerly sought after, especially if they bear Company initials. Whistles in brass, wood or steel from several Companies are illustrated here – £5 – £50. Corkscrews too are most desirable. Early examples could be worth at least £20.

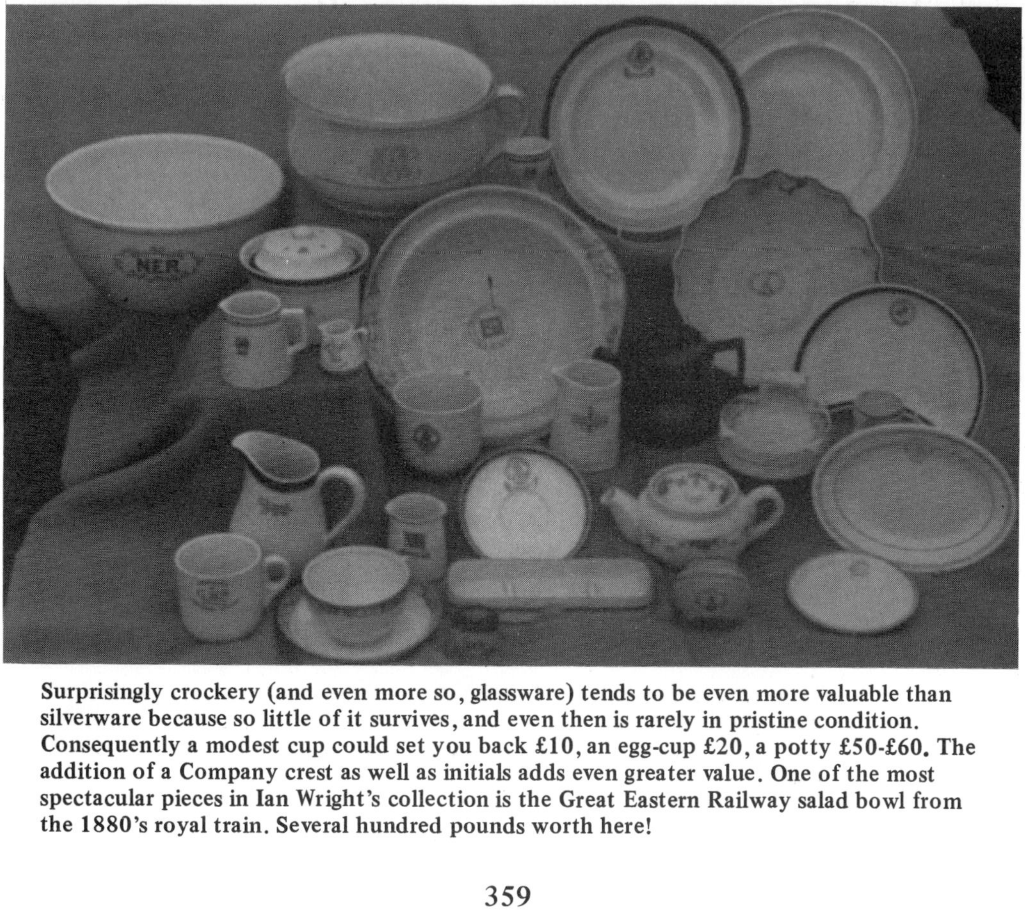

Surprisingly crockery (and even more so, glassware) tends to be even more valuable than silverware because so little of it survives, and even then is rarely in pristine condition. Consequently a modest cup could set you back £10, an egg-cup £20, a potty £50-£60. The addition of a Company crest as well as initials adds even greater value. One of the most spectacular pieces in Ian Wright's collection is the Great Eastern Railway salad bowl from the 1880's royal train. Several hundred pounds worth here!

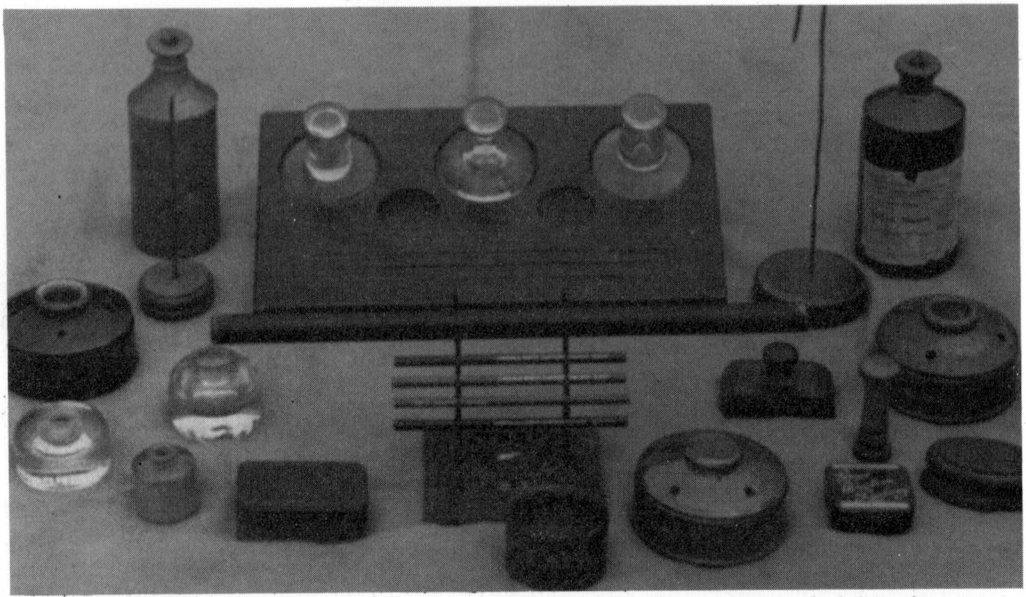

The early Railway Companies were huge organisations with the necessary administrative back-up. Hundreds of offices were fully stocked with every necessary item from pen-holders to paperweights, inkwells to paper-spikes. Even individual pen-nibs carried the Company name. Illustrated here are a Midland Railway pen-holder with pencils from various Companies, 'landmine' inkwells, functional paperweights, a GWR typewriter-ribbon tin, glass inkwells and paper-spikes.

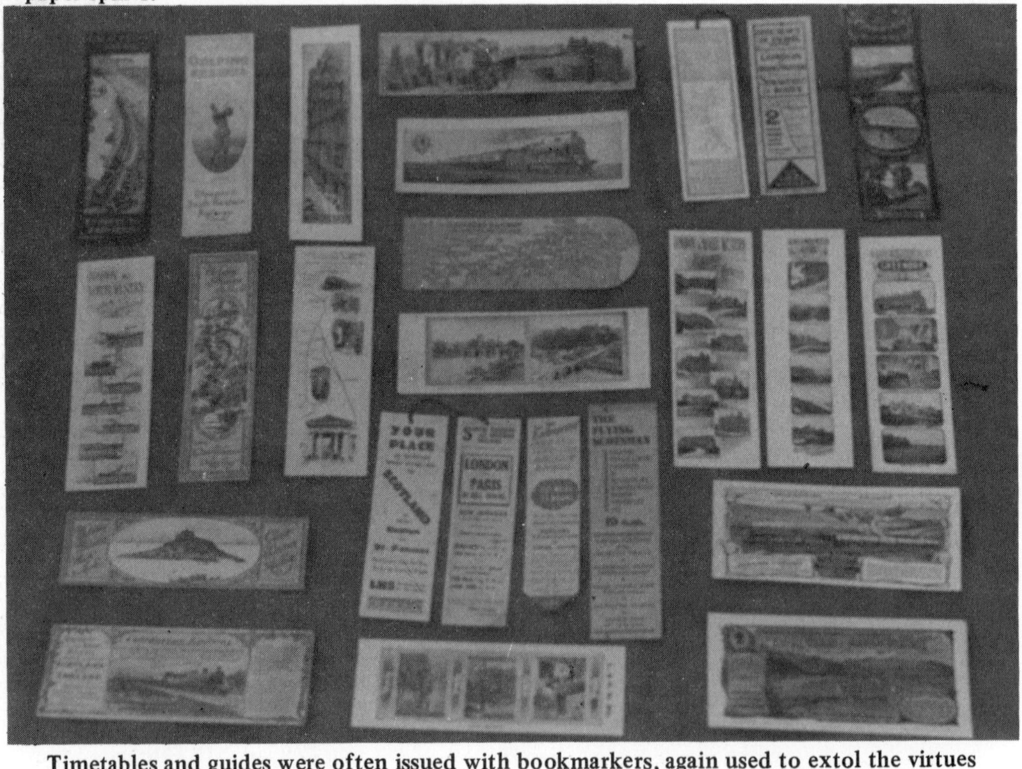

Timetables and guides were often issued with bookmarkers, again used to extol the virtues of the services. The variety of styles seems to be endless. Early examples illustrated here can command upwards of £20.

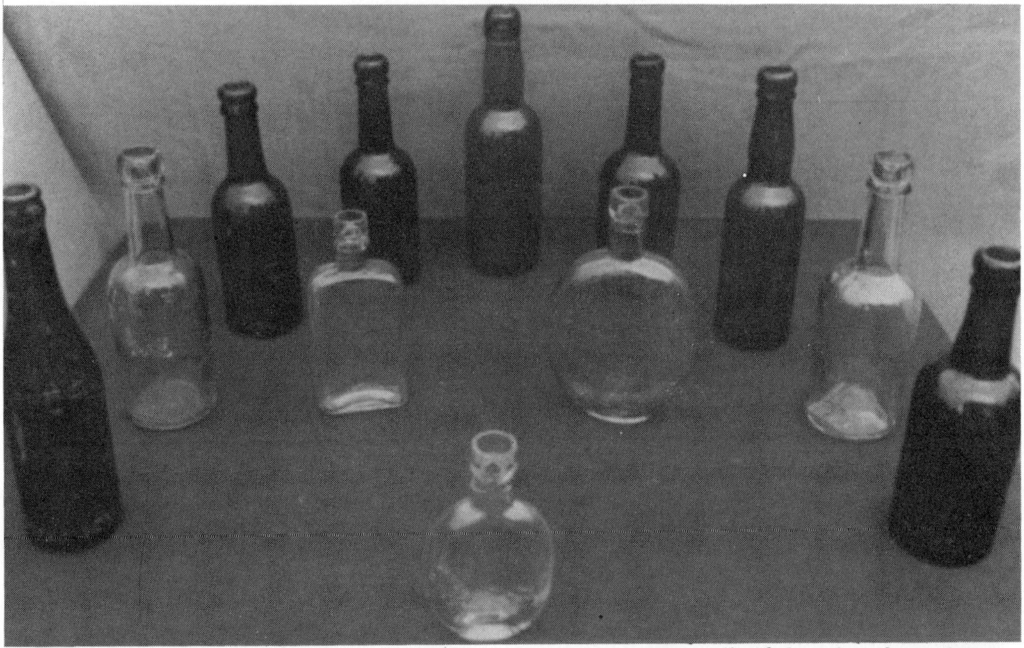

Railway Company bottles in good condition are very rare, especially if they date from the turn of the century. Illustrated here are beer bottles and whisky flasks. The earlier the bottle, the greater the value. £10 to £60 here.

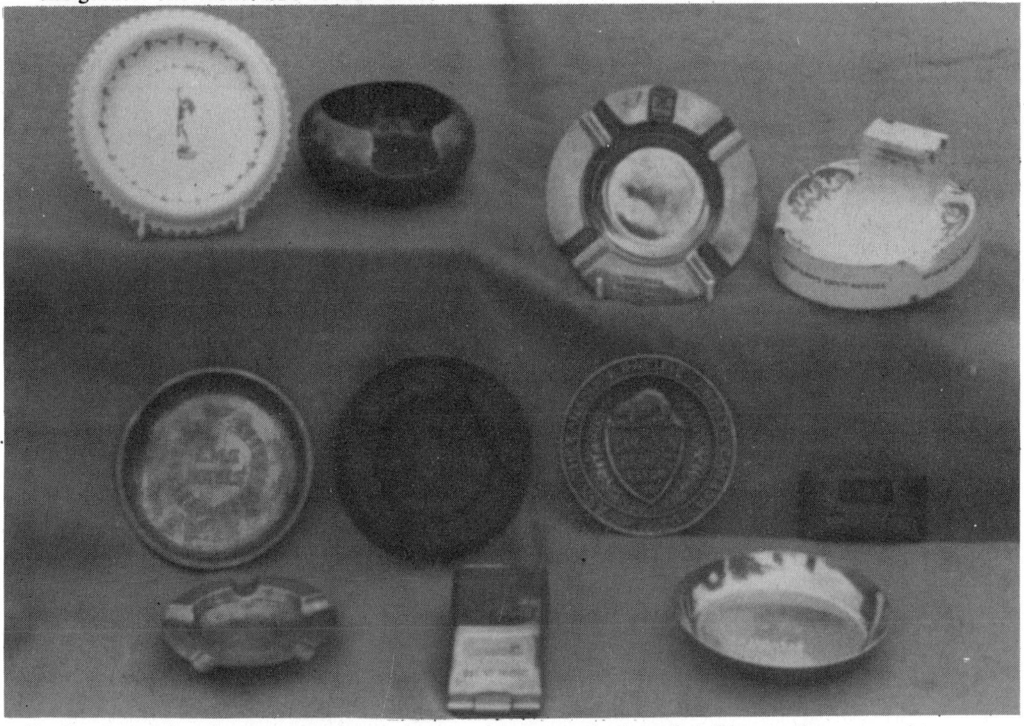

In the days when it was considered that smoking was the 'manly' thing to do, even ashtrays were provided by the railways, all faithfully marked with the Company name. Seen here are examples in brass, copper and steel from several early lines. £10 at least would be needed for one of these; considerably more the attractive brass hanging ashtray decoratively marked by the London and North Western Railway Company.

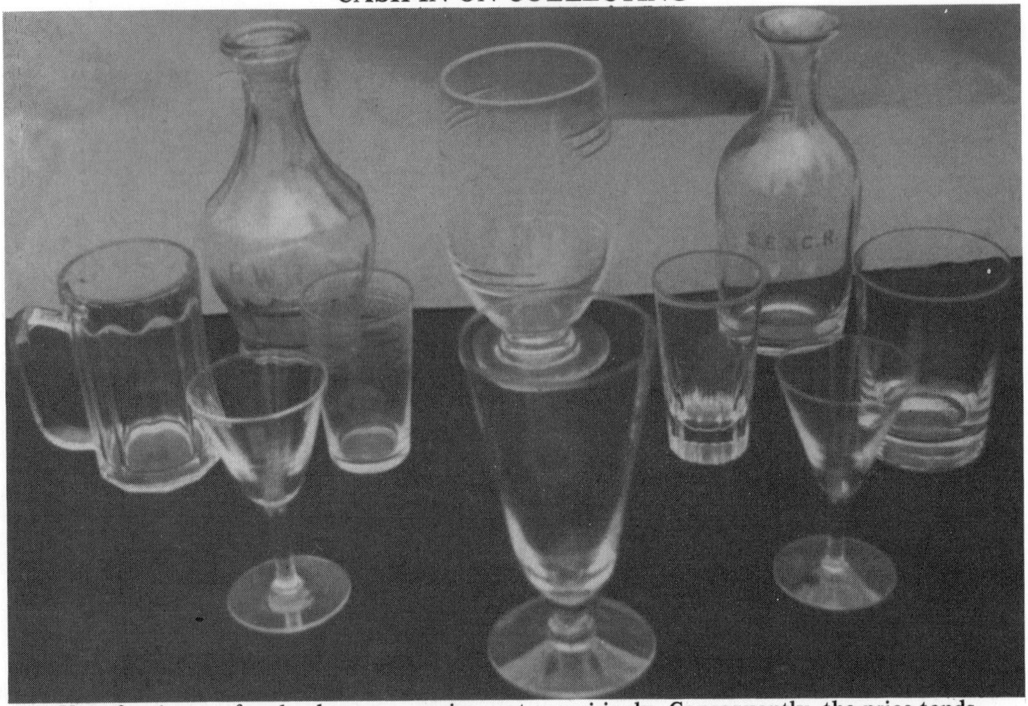

Very few items of early glassware survive, not surprisingly. Consequently, the price tends to be high. Illustrated here are water-carafes, wine glasses, a tankard and drinking glasses. £40 or so is quite common for items like these.

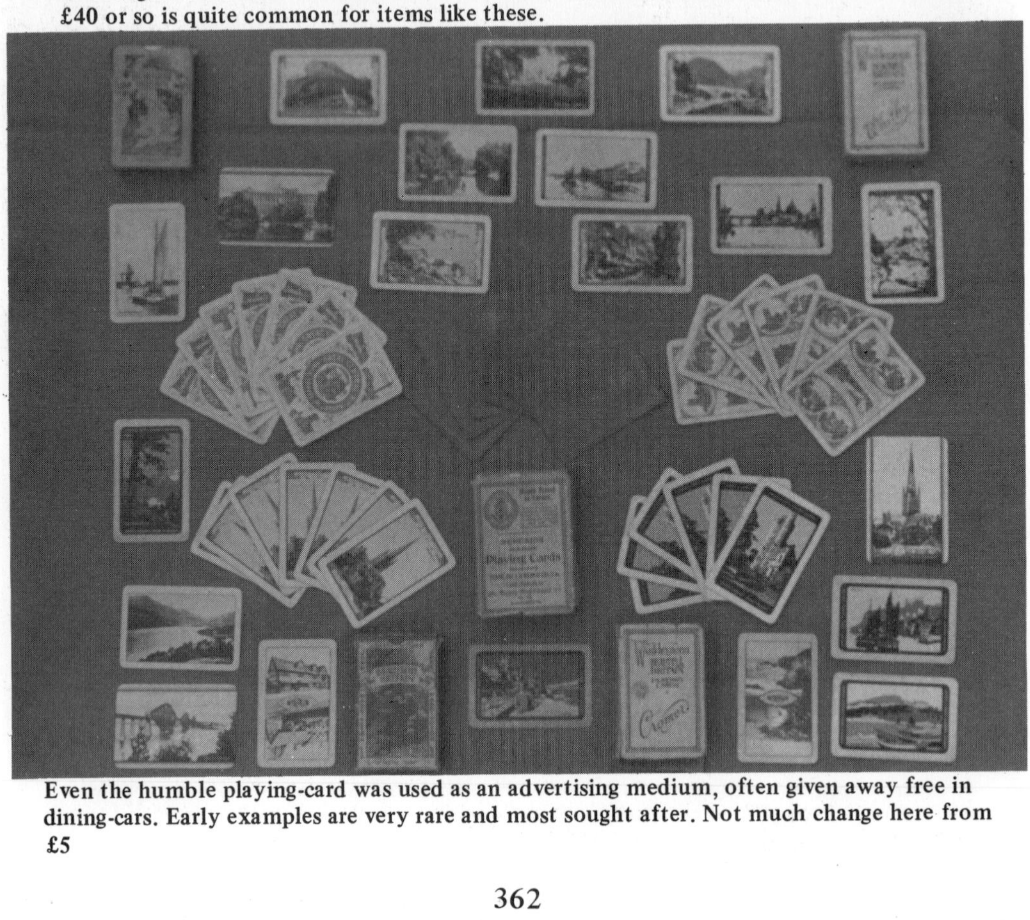

Even the humble playing-card was used as an advertising medium, often given away free in dining-cars. Early examples are very rare and most sought after. Not much change here from £5

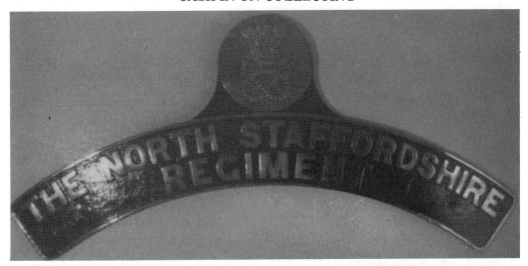

All railway relics pale into insignificance compared with the brass nameplates taken from scrapped steam locomotives. These are 'the cream' of railway antiques, £500 at least for a modest example, several thousand pounds for choice ones with badges as illustrated here (The North Staffordshire Regiment).

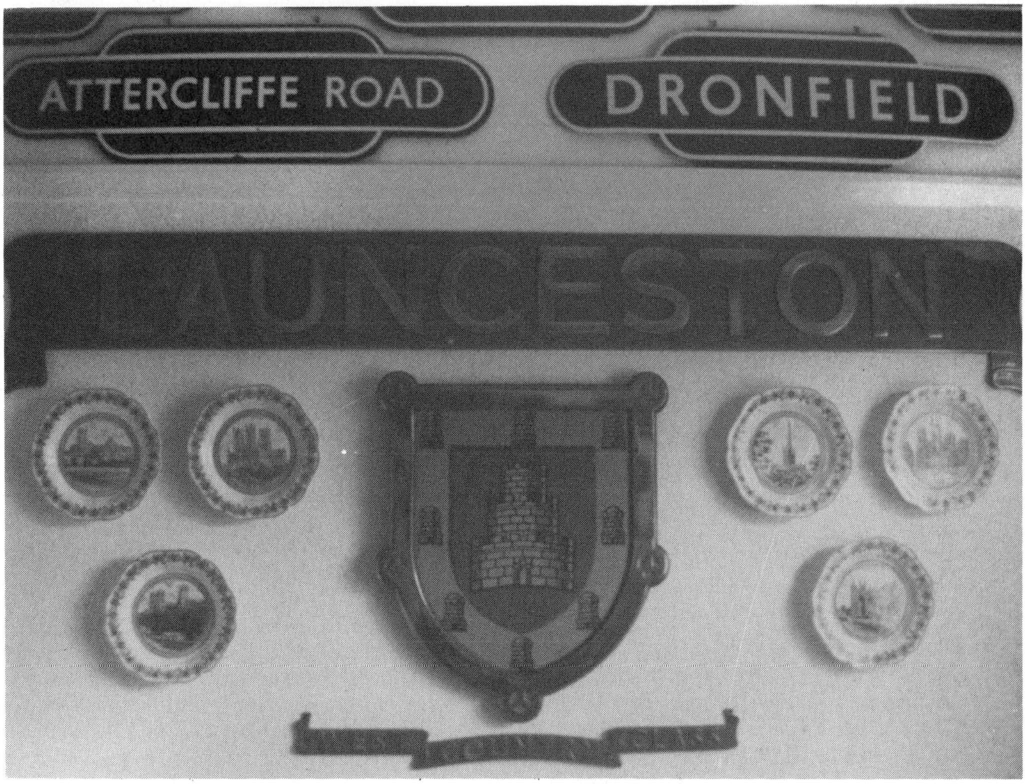

(Launceston) – another very valuable item here – £2000 at least. Illustrated above this nameplate are two examples of the enamel 'totem' signs that bedecked British stations from the 1950's to the 1970's. Attractively coloured and easy to display these are rapidly rising in value. A famous station name could cost £100.

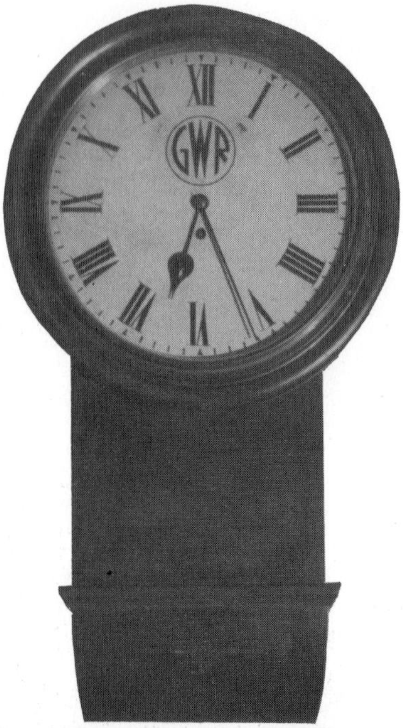

Railway clocks are avidly sought by collectors; they are so functional and would grace any home. Illustrated here is an example produced by the Great Western Railway. Several hundred pounds for an attractive early example.

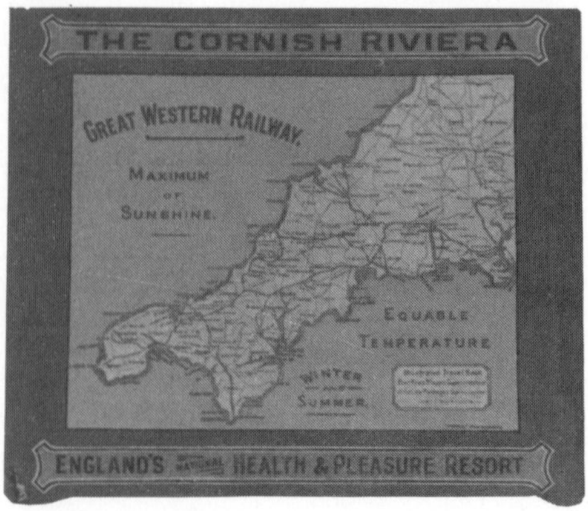

Several Railway Companies used the medium of enamel advertising signs to advertise their services. The Great Western Railway probably produced the most attractive, eagerly sought after. One of these in good condition could cost £100.

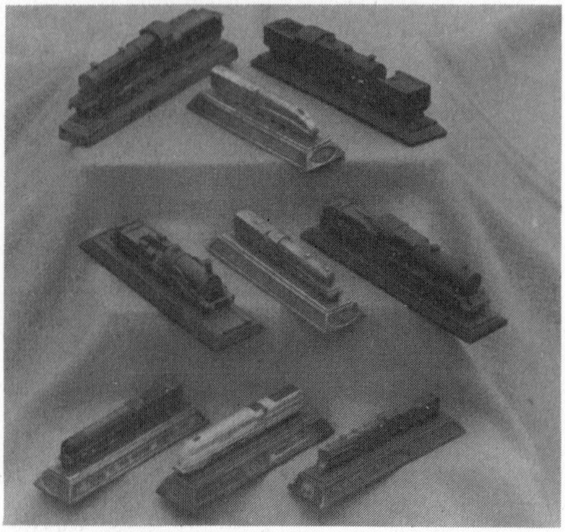

Locomotive paperweights, although rarely issued by the Railway Companies themselves, but by famous firms like the Locomotive Publishing Co. and Bassett-Lowke of Northampton, these models of famous locomotives cast in lead or tin are actively sought after by collectors. Like many railway relics they are also functional today although at £50 or thereabouts perhaps not in everybody's range.

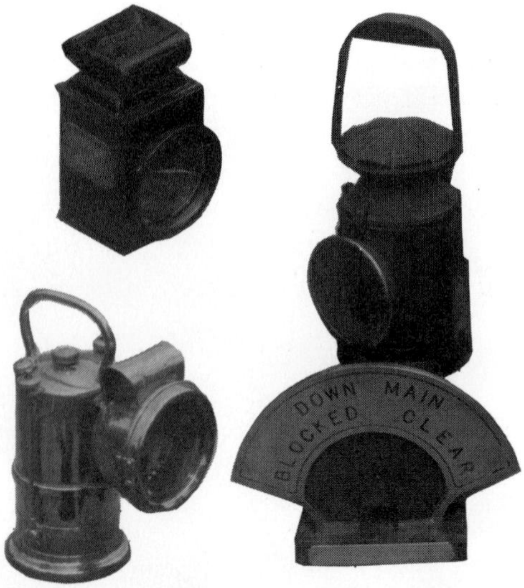

Well over a hundred types of lamp were used by the railways from handlamps to signal lamps, static lamps to road motor lamps. Most types are fairly common and a fifty-year old handlamp can still be had for a modest £20 – £30, but anything from before the First World War could be well into three figures. Seen here are a delightful brass acetylene lamp from the 1890's, a guard's handlamp, and a square lamp from a London, Midland & Scottish Railway Co. steam road-motor. Lamps were used for signalling purposes and illustrated here is an attractive brass device from the signal box at Parsley Hay on the now defunct Cromford and High Peak Railway in Derbyshire.

Brian Wain is a veterinary surgeon who collects items connected with his profession and has set up a museum in the surgery.

"People bring me things and local farmers keep finding old instruments in their sheds so there's an unending supply.

"I like the old instruments because many are so beautifully made. Some of those in the museum are pretty primitive like an instrument for dehorning bulls that weighs 28 lbs. and a tool for docking the tails of carthorses.

"It's taken six years to bring this collection together and I'm adding to it all the time. It's amazing what turns up. Here are some tracheotomy tubes for tubing horses — Tipperary Tim won the Grand National and Backbite won the Lincoln with the help of a tube. This is a fleam for blood letting and it was said that you could take up to 36 pints of blood from the animal or take flow until the pulse wavered or the horse fell faint.

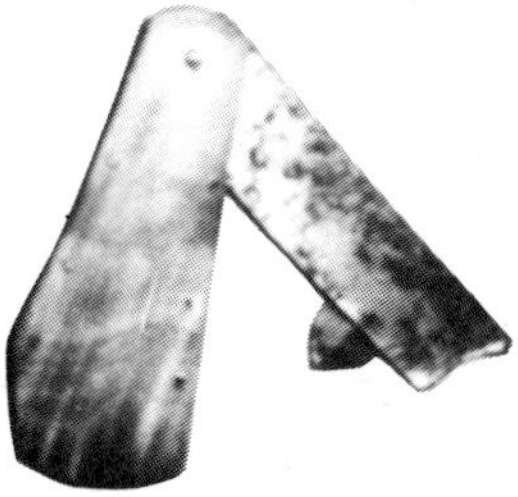

Fleam for blood letting.

"Some of the instruments are still being used today but others have disappeared because modern veterinary practice has moved on. I'm very interested in old medicines and cures and there's several concoctions on show as well as a list of old remedies that people once used.

"Veterinary practice in Kelso began in 1817 and I've got a portrait gallery of many of the vets who have worked here as well as pictures of our office staff and students".

Brian's museum contains some oddities like a mounted double headed Siamese twin calf which was delivered in the late 1940's by one of the vets in the practice. There is also the desiccated body of 'the Roxburgh rat' which was found in a bag of rat poison when the Cotlends, an old manse in Roxburgh, was being cleared. It still has its nails and teeth. Brian Wain has written a book about his collection and all proceeds from sales go to the Horse Grass Sickness Research Fund. The title is 'Vets in Kelso' and the price is £2.50.

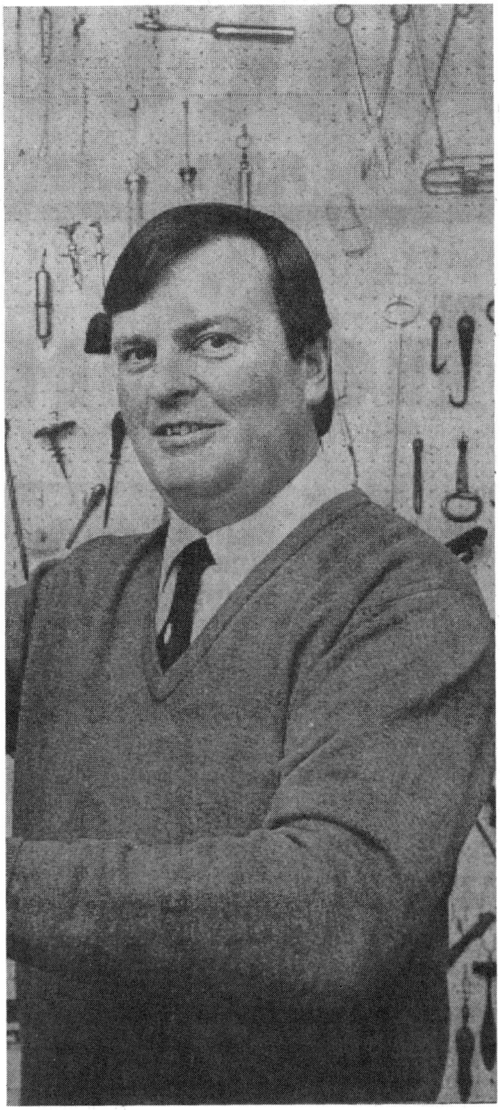

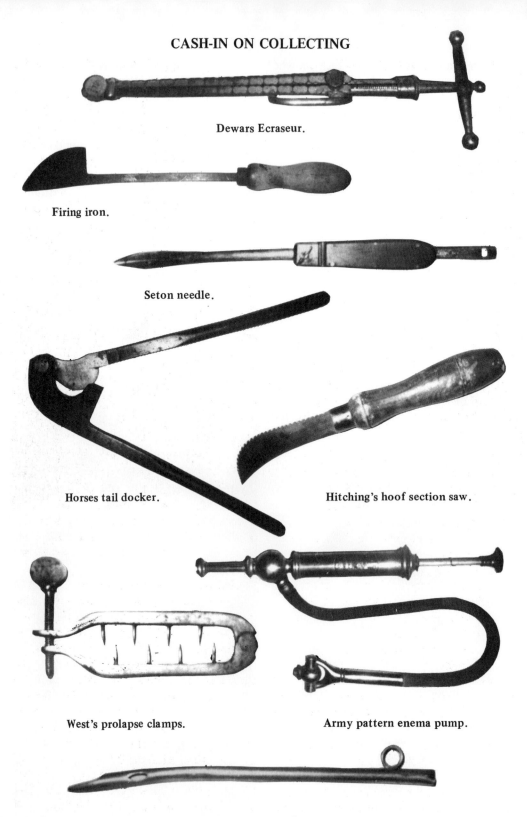

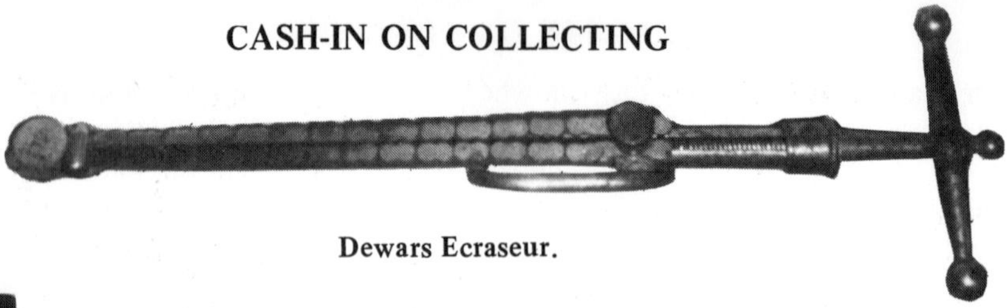

Dewars Ecraseur.

Firing iron.

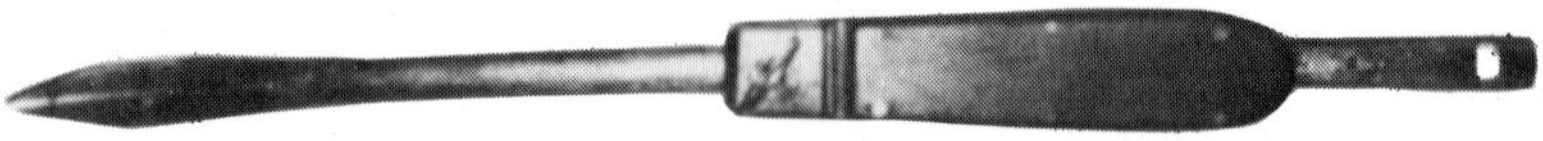

Seton needle.

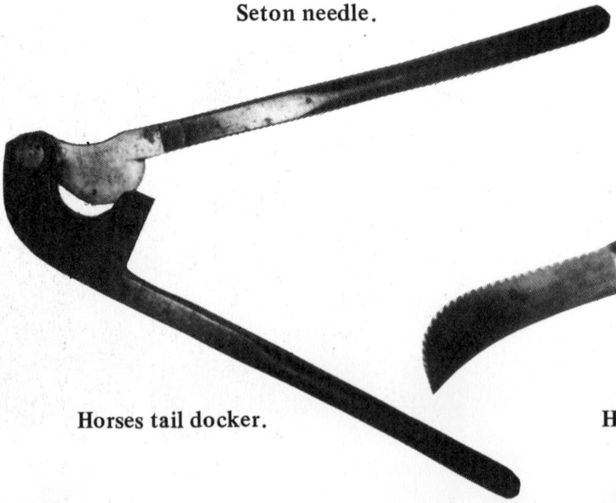

Horses tail docker.

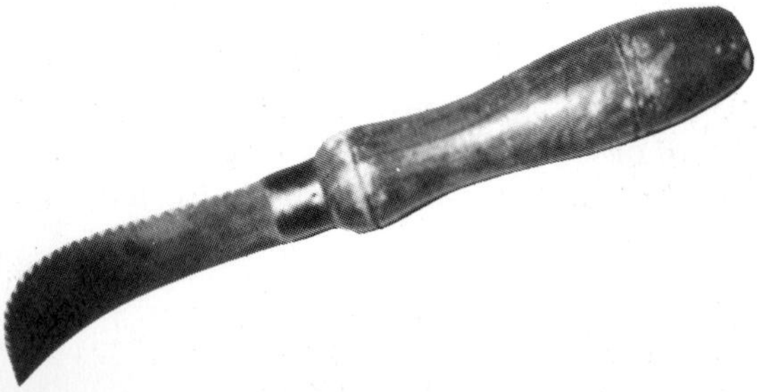

Hitching's hoof section saw.

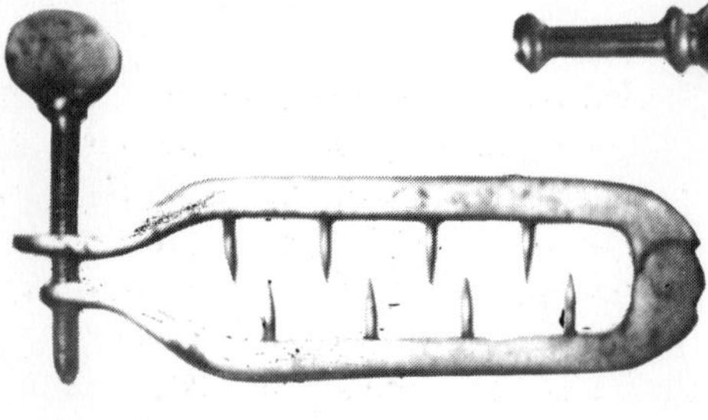

West's prolapse clamps.

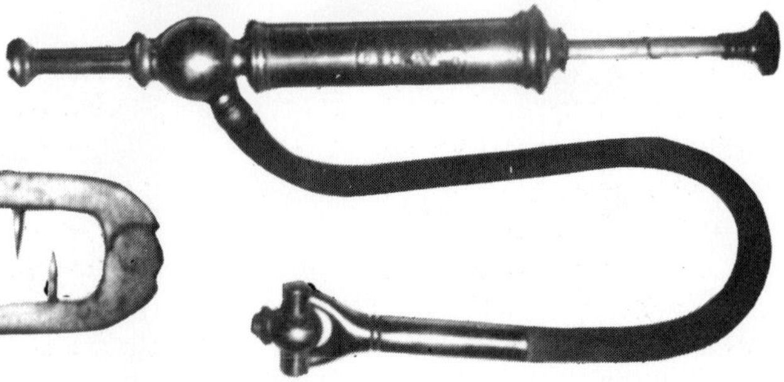

Army pattern enema pump.

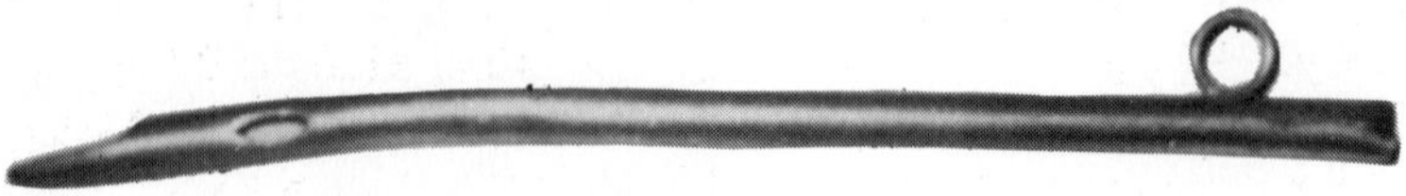

Dawsons cow catheter.

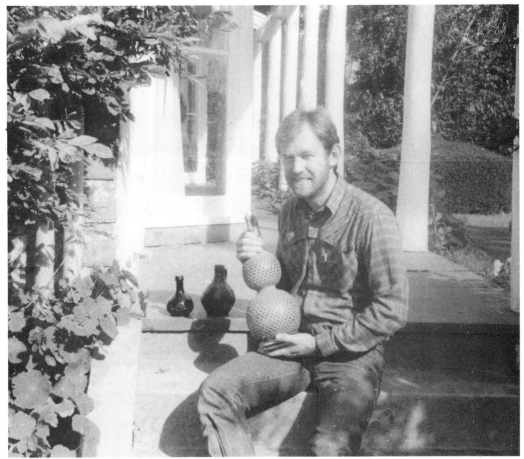

Bleddyn Wynn-Jones is a farmer and collects mineral water bottles about which he has written a book.

"The bottle collecting craze hit me because on the farm where I used to live I was digging in a wood for something — I forget what exactly — and found an old beer bottle. The farm had once been part of an agricultural college and lots of old bottles were dumped there in the wood.

"I swopped my first bottle for some lead from a local antique shop and then went back to dig up more. By swapping them I've ended up with mineral water bottles which I found more aesthetically pleasing. I like the inventiveness of having them closed from inside.

"When I read up about them I discovered that there were more than 1,000 patents for those internal stoppered bottles and I'm lucky enough to have collected one hundred of those patents. I've also got some that were not patented and we call those 'variations'."

Bleddyn has bottles going back to 1880 and examples from all over the world. His favourites are local bottles, especially one embossed with 'Bangor City Mineral Works' and, for sentimental reasons, a Bellermine jug which he bought in Sri Lanka and cost him about £100.

The bottles that have eluded him so far are a 'Lemon' patent from the early 1880's which was used by a firm called Ryland of Barnsley but especially a blue bottle put out by the Mona Mineral Water Company of Douglas in the Isle of Man. Examples of the Mona bottle are worth around £1,000 each and Bleddyn once dug up half of one . . . 'very frustrating' he said.

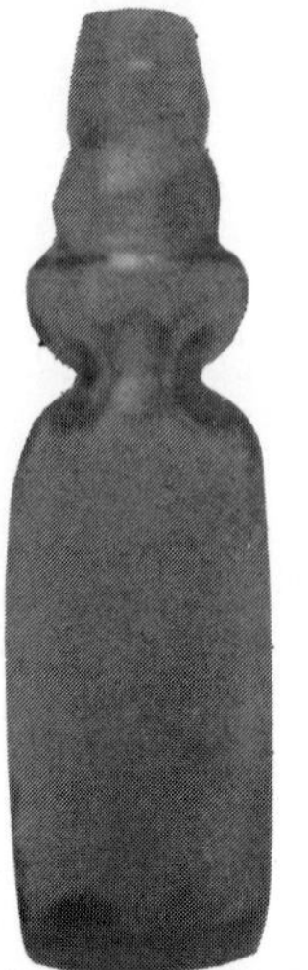

Connor's Patent (1897). Two bulbous cavities in neck to retain a pear-shaped glass stopper. Codd Patent washer seal, aqua coloured, 9in. high. Embossing, front – Spencer Connor & Co., Manchester; back – Connor's Patent Stoppers, Redfearn Bros. Bottle Makers, Barnsley.£200

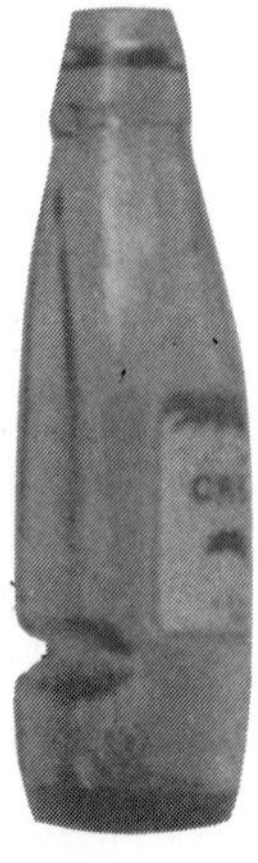

Billows Patent (small size). Aqua coloured, cylindrical bottle, with one flat side which has a groove near its base to retain the round glass stopper, Codd-type seal, 7½in. high. Embossing – 'B' Hygienic Registered. £300

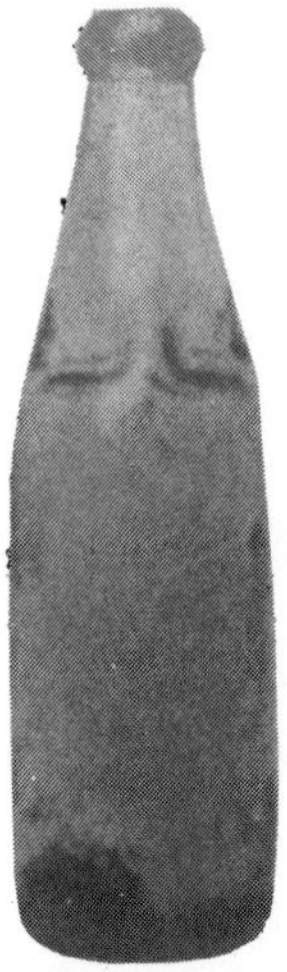

Sutcliffe's Patent. Scalloping in shoulders to retain a Sutcliffe & Fewings glass stopper, fitted with a rubber tube, aqua coloured, 8½in. high. Embossing – Cockshott Bros, Trademark (embossed running cockerel), Keighley, Sutcliffe's Patent, Barnsley. £55

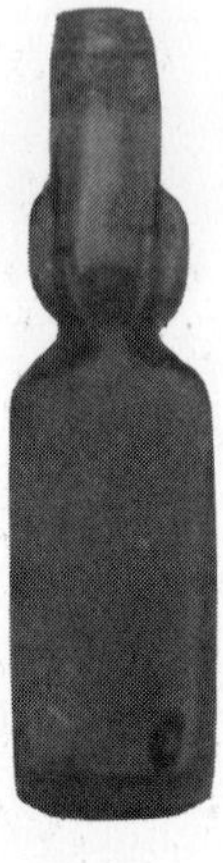

A Rylands Patent Codd. Cavity back and front to retain an elongated glass stopper, Codd-type seal, aqua coloured, 9¼in. high. Embossing, front – N. J. Campbell, Foresters Arms, Holyhead; back – Registered No. 448146, Sole Makers, The Rylands Glass And Engineering Co. Ltd., Barnsley. £175

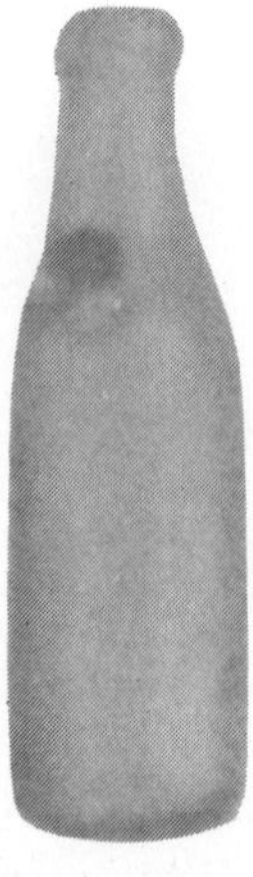

Chapman's Patent Hybrid. Round-ended, aqua coloured bottle with a round rubber ball to close bottle. Two indents in shoulder to retain stopper while pouring, 8½in. high. Embossing, front – Matthew Pomfret Limited Bury, Sykes Macvay & Co. Makers, Castleford; rear – Chapman's Patent Stopper, Birkenhead. £100

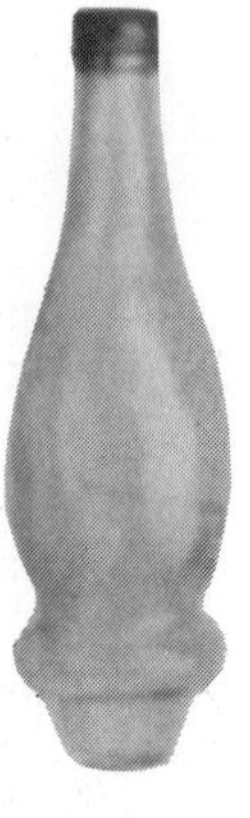

Edwards Patent (1874). Flat-bottomed Hamilton, aqua coloured bottle with wired metal cap over a protruding rubber washer, an external annular 'chamber' is formed to retain a round glass marble, 9½in. high. Embossing – Edwards Patent, E. Breffit & Co. Aire & Calder Bottle Works. Very rare. £500

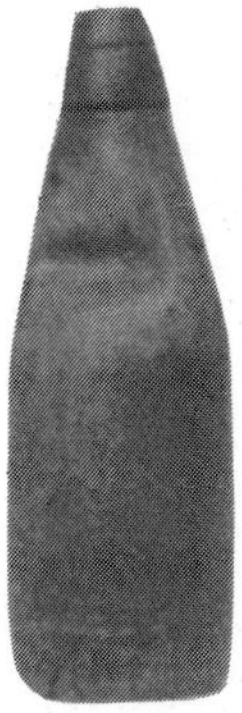

Stone Codd. Brown stoneware standard Codd shape and seal but both bottle and round marble stopper are made of stoneware, 8½in. high.
Embossing – Cooper's, Mineral Waters, Hanley.
£1,000

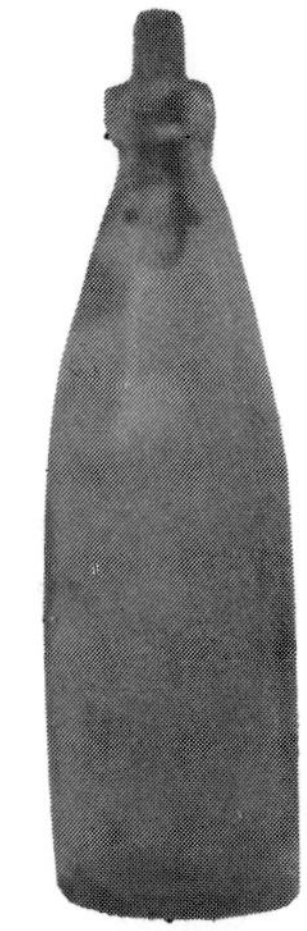

J. Lewis Patent. Aqua coloured bottle formed with a double shoulder to retain a long wooden stopper, fitted with a rubber ring, 8½in. high.
Embossing, front – J. Lewis (intertwined initials) Trade Mark, Merthyr; back – J. Lewis's Patent, Merthyr.
£150

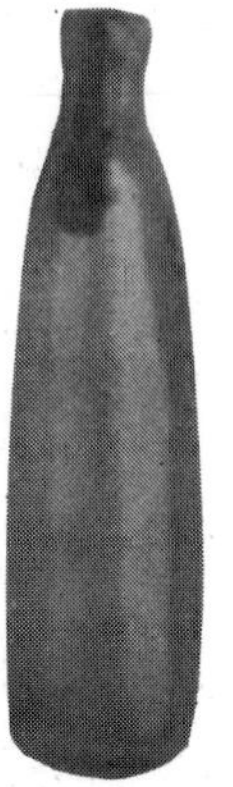

Barrett & Elers Hybrid. Round-ended aqua coloured bottle with a long wooden stick stopper fitted with a rubber ring, 9½in. high.
Embossing, front – Virtus Trade Mark; back – Manufactured by W. Ford, Nottingham. £150

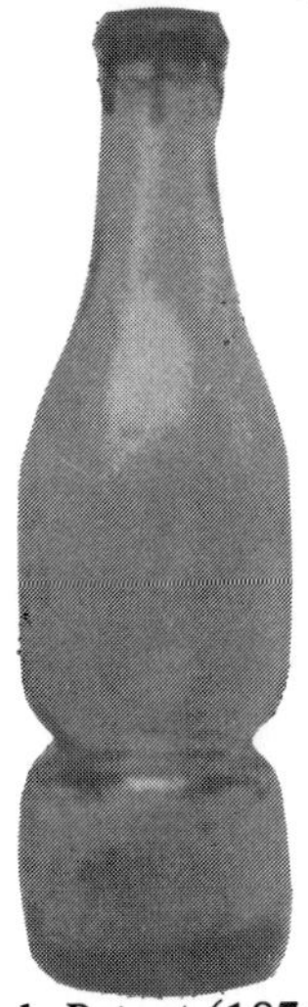

Edwards Patent (1874). Internal annular projection to retain a glass marble near the base of the bottle. A wired metal cap is fitted over a protruding rubber washer, aqua coloured, 9in. high.
Embossing, front – Edwards Patent London, E. Breffit & Co. Makers; rear – London & Castleford.
£80

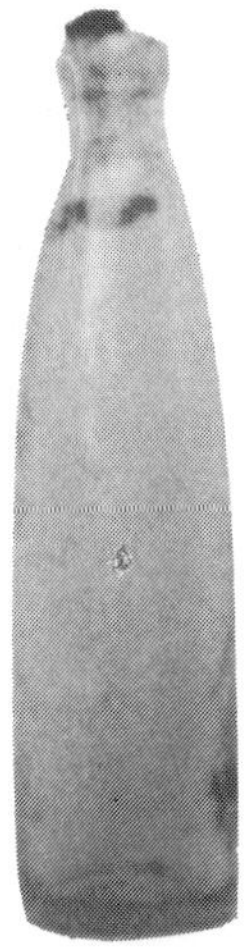

Aylesbury Patent (1875). The stopper consists of two India-rubber discs on a spindle; the larger one, being the lower, is fixed and the upper disc is free to slide down the rod, aqua coloured, 9¼in. high.
Embossing – Talbot & Co. Trade Mark Registered (embossed entwined initials), Gloucester. £100

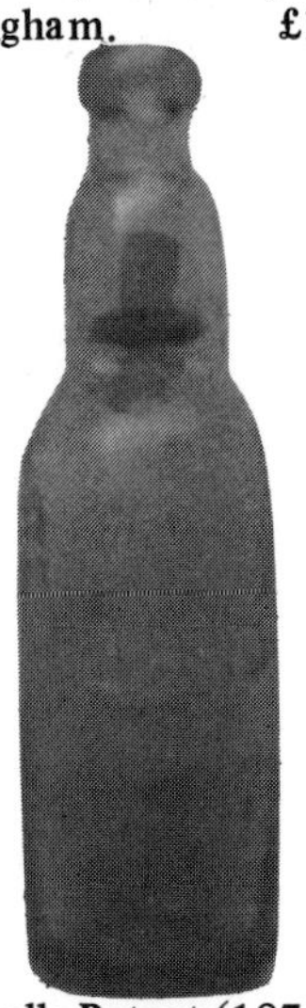

Mitchells Patent (1878). A bulbous cavity at the top of the aqua coloured bottle retains a long glass stopper. rubber ring on the stopper to seal bottle.
Embossing, front – Mitchell & Mitchell, St. Austell Aerated Water Manufacturer, B.B.W. Co. Ltd.; back – As above plus F. B. Mitchell Patentee, St. Austell, Shire Hampton. £200

Waugh's Patent (1875). Round rubber ball, round shoulders and blob top, deep aqua coloured, 8¾in. high.
Embossing – Waugh's Patent Ball Stopper, Glasgow. £75

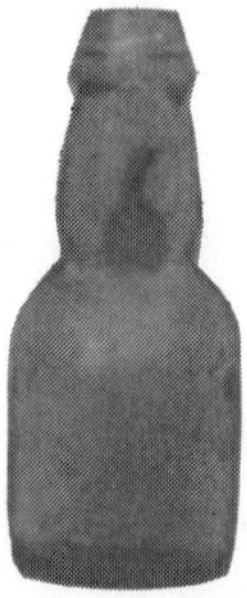

Codd's Patent Dumpy (small size), (1872). Round glass stopper, Codd-type seal, dumpy seltzer shaped, aqua coloured bottle, (note narrow neck), 6in. high.
Embossing, front – S. Chambers & Co., Henry Street, Bermondsey; back – Codd's Patent, Sole Agents, Barnett & Foster, London, Makers, Rylands & Codd. £150

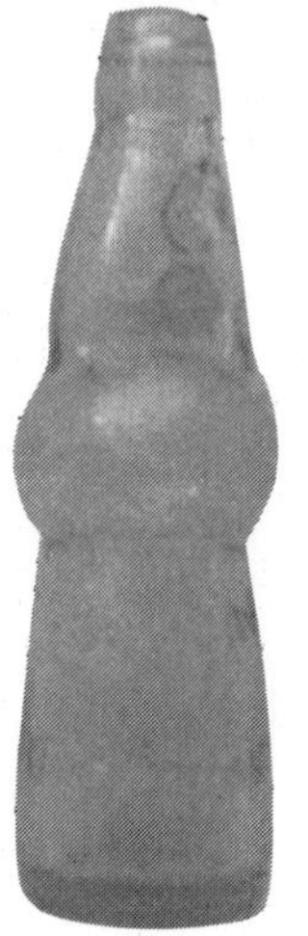

Caley's Patent Codd. Standard Codd Patent neck and seal, on a shuttlecock-shaped bottle, aqua coloured, 9in. high.
Embossing, front – Shimmin Sunderland; back – Regd. £250

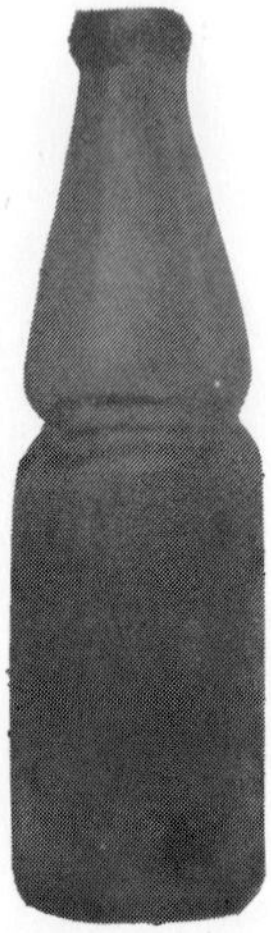

Sutcliffe & Fewings Patent (1875). 'The bottle is formed with an internal, annular projection for retaining'. The glass stopper fitted with a rubber tube, dark aqua coloured, 8¼in. high.
Embossing – C. Guest Trade Mark (embossed crown), Barnsley, Sutcliffe & Fewings Patent. £100

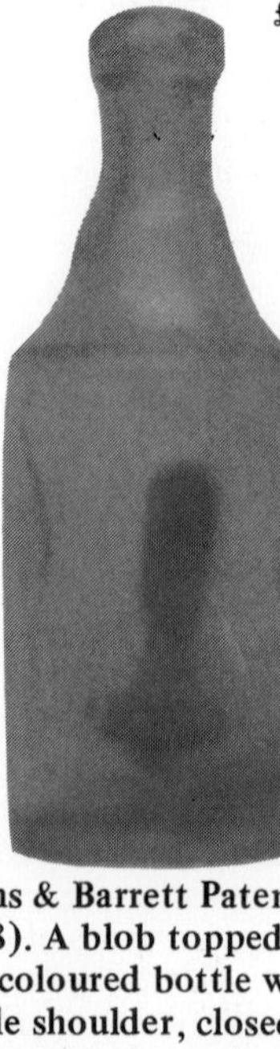

Adams & Barrett Patent (1868). A blob topped aqua coloured bottle with double shoulder, closed by a long waisted wooden stopper, fitted with a rubber washer, 7½in. high.
Embossing, front – Fewings & Co. Superior Aerated Waters, Exeter; base – A & B Patent Stopper, Jersey. £75

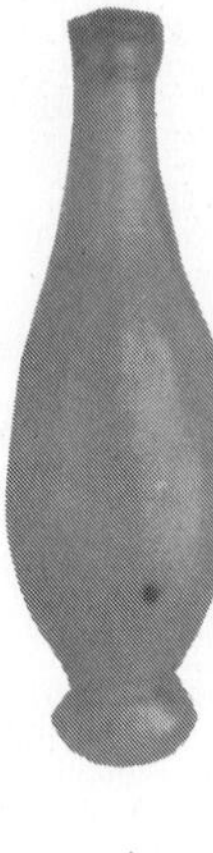

Edwards Patent (1874). Internal 'chamber' is formed at the base of a Hamilton type bottle, to retain a round glass marble. A wired metal cap is fitted over a protruding rubber washer, aqua coloured, 9½in. high.
Embossing – Edwards Patent, London. Very rare, only two known). £500

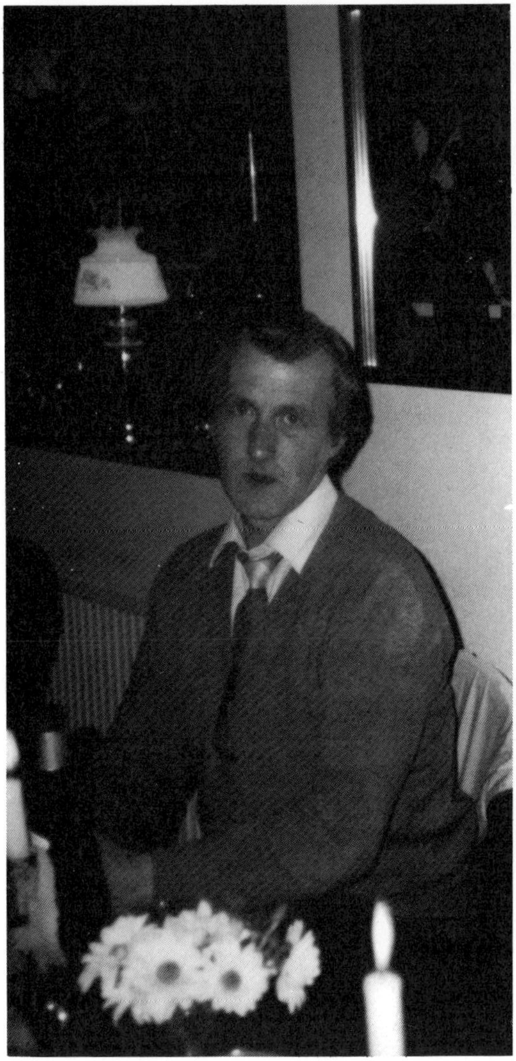

Bert Latham is a builder who collects Reform flasks.

"It began when my sons were at school and started digging in dumps. I dug up one or two Reform flasks and got interested in the subject. I suppose you could say that I collect them because I collect bottles.

"The collection I've got now is a very good one and there are basically only three that I need to make it complete.

"You find Reform flasks in several colours though most people go for the browns but I also like the green ones. They were mainly in the shape of famous politicians of the Reform Bill period in the 1830's — Brougham, Peel, Lord John Grey and the Duke of York though you also occasionally see Queen Victoria.

"So-called Reform flasks go on till the period of the Crimean War and I've got two Crimean ones — 'The Navy Goes to War' and 'Peace Proclaimed' which are very rare. I've only ever seen four 'Peace Proclaimed'."

Mr Latham's flasks include examples made by Oldfields who were the major pottery manufacturers in the Midlands at the time. He also has flasks by Weatherill and Doulton and Watts. The best flasks have the names of spirit merchants or publicans printed on the shoulders, back or sides.

He has some by the Connor Park Pottery in Derby which range from full figures to those with only modelled heads and shoulders. The Connor Park pottery examples are very attractive with white faces and hands on dark brown bodies.

Average prices for Reform flasks range between £100 for a hip flask to £900 for a well modelled figure from a good pottery.

The flask Mr Latham would most like to find is a 14 inch high figure of Lord Melbourne by the Oldfield Pottery. There are only one or two known to be in existence.

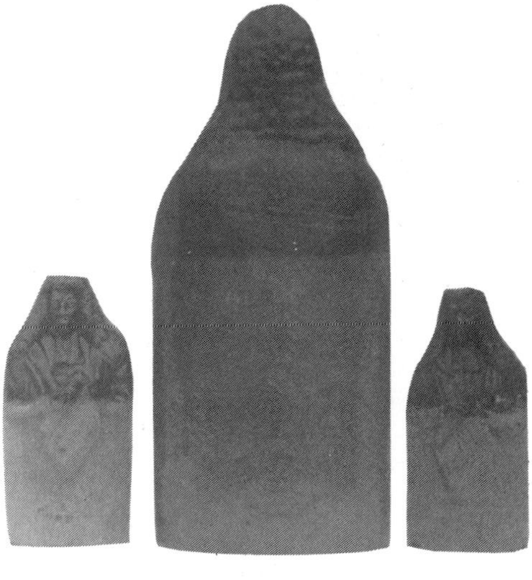

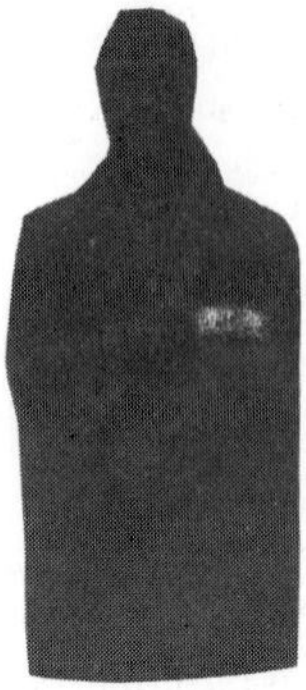

Lord Grey flask, by Doulton & Watts, 7½in. high. £150 – £200

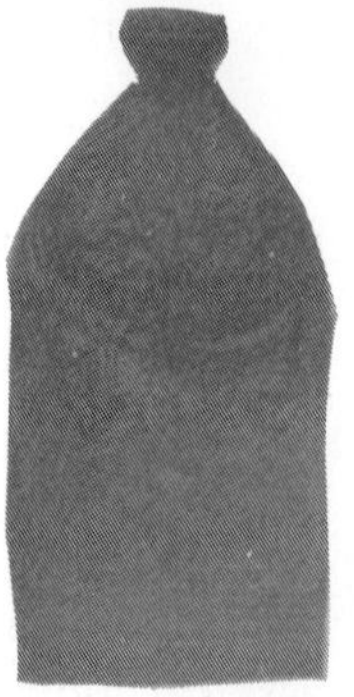

Mr. Punch 'Triumph of the Pen' flask, by Doulton & Watts Lambeth Pottery, 6in. high. £125 – £150

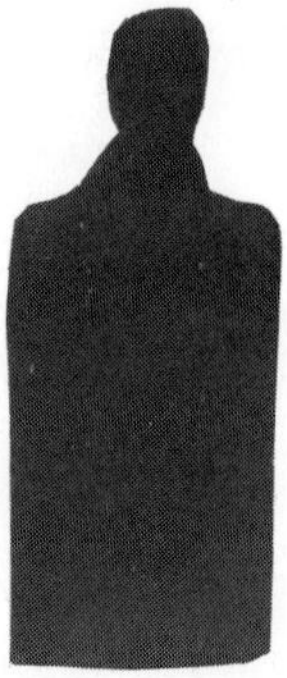

Lord Grey flask, by Belper & Denby, Bournes Potteries, Derbyshire, 7½in. high. £150 – £200

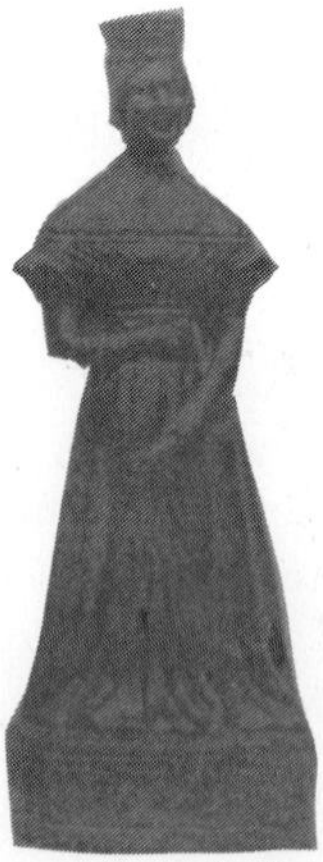

Queen Victoria flask, no potter's mark, 11½in. high. £350

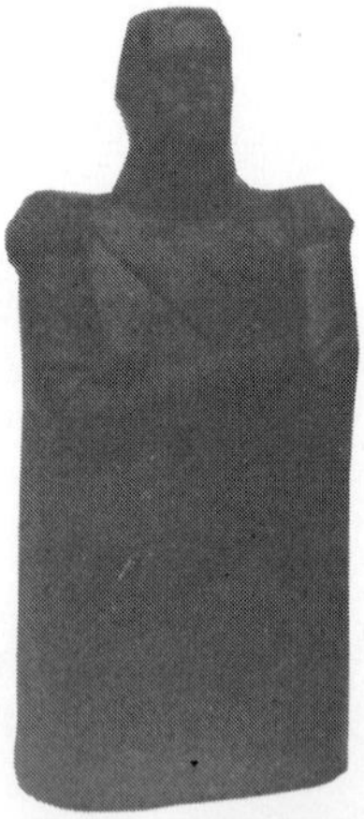

Sir Robert Peel flask, by T. Oldfield & Co., Chesterfield, 9in. high. £250

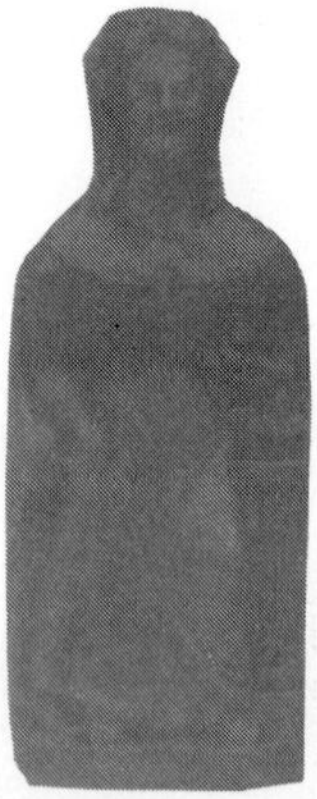

Lady With Bird flask, by Denby & Codnor Park Potteries, 8in. high. £150 – £175

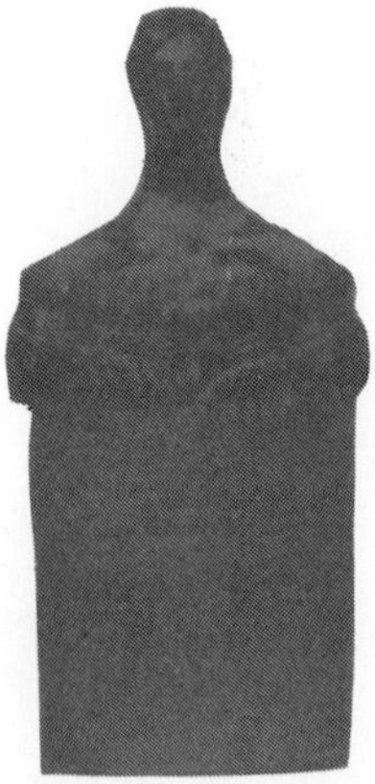

Queen Victoria flask, by T. Oldfield, Chesterfield, 9½in. high. £250

House flask, by Fulham Pottery. £100 – £125

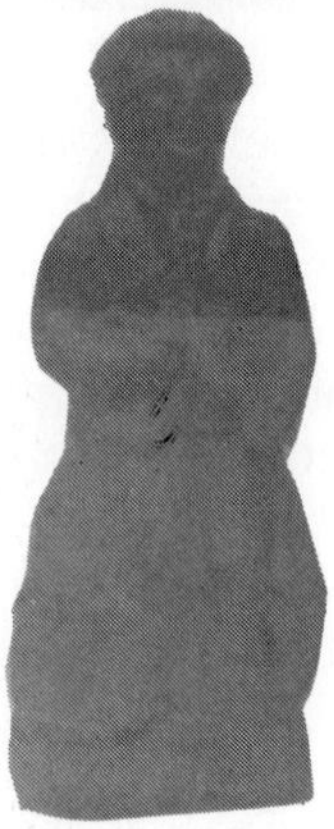

Sailor flask. £125 – £175

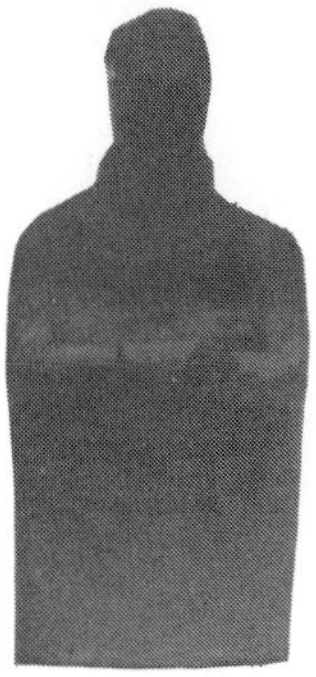

William IV flask, by Doulton & Watts, 7¼in. high. £150 – £200

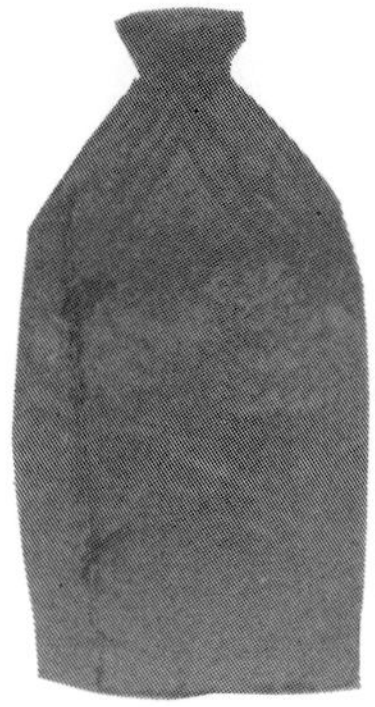

Mr. and Mrs. Caudle flask, by Doulton & Watts Lambeth Pottery, 6in. high. £75 – £100

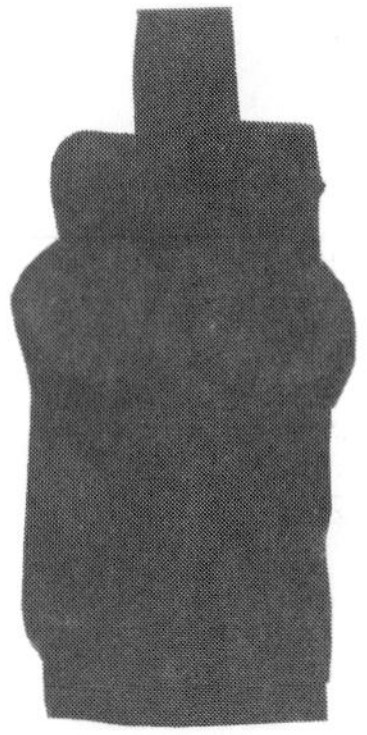

Cockney Couple flask, by Fulham Pottery. £200 – £225

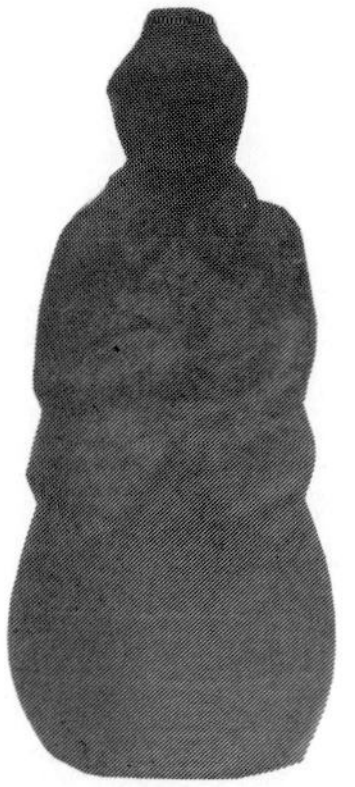

Man on a Barrel, with impressed word on barrel, no potter's mark. £100 – £125

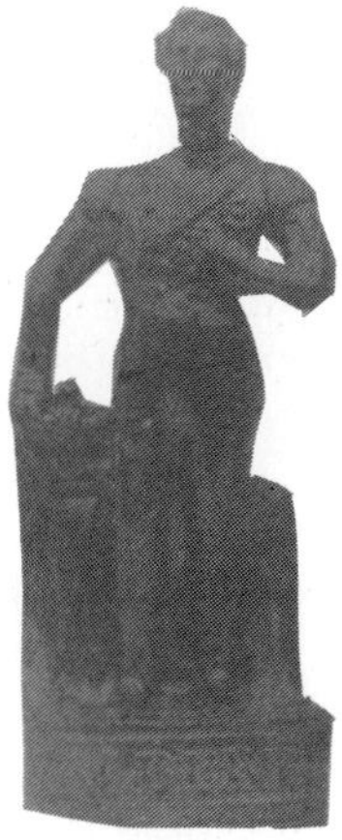

Prince Albert flask, no potter's mark, 11½in. high. £350

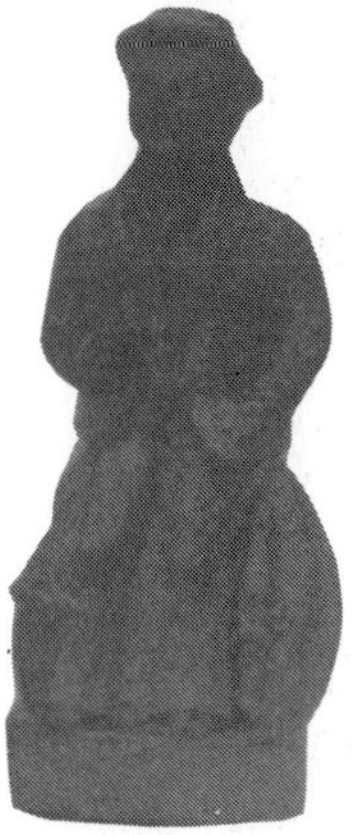

Sailor flask. £125 – £175

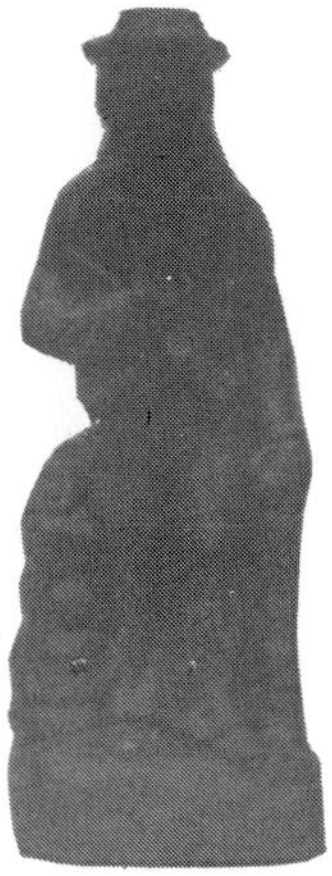

Sailor flask. £125 – £175

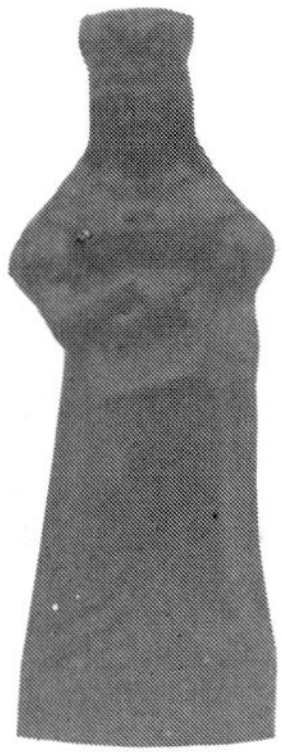

Queen Victoria flask, by Doulton & Watts, 9in. high. £200

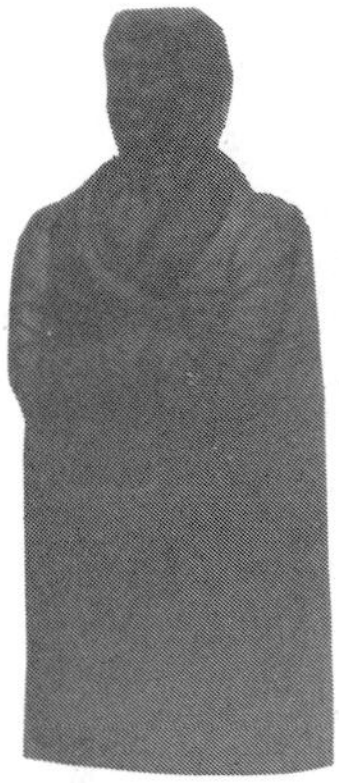

Daniel O'Connell flask, by T. Oldfield, Chesterfield, 8½in. high. £175

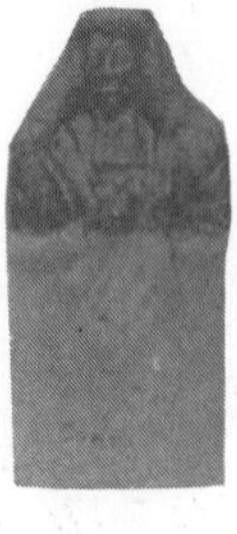

Lord Brougham flask, made by Doulton & Watts, 7¼in. high. £100 – £120

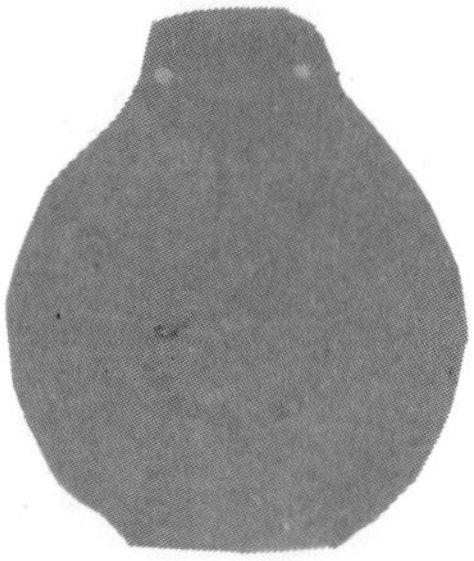

Clock flask, impressed 'Railway Chronometer', by Fulham Pottery. £100 – £125

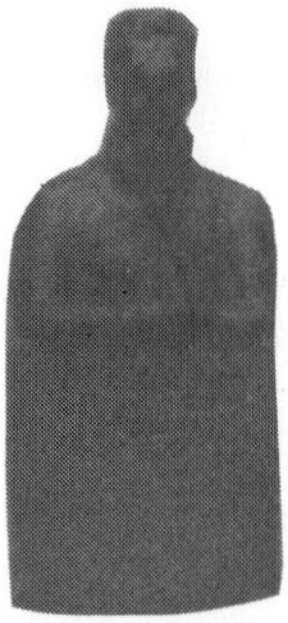

Lord Russell flask, by T. Oldfield, Chesterfield, 7in. high. £150

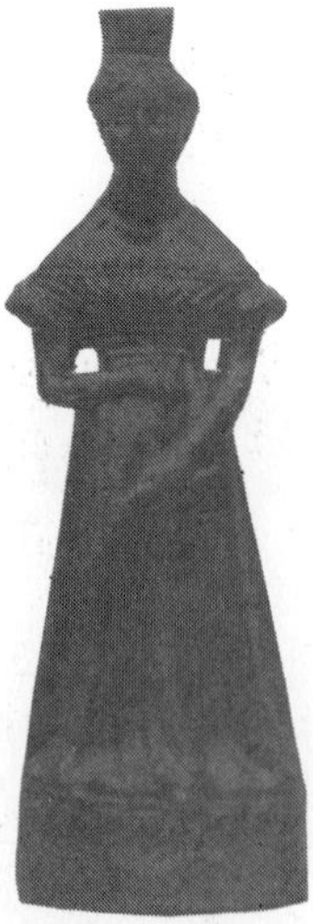

A Queen Victoria flask, Published by S. Green, Lambeth, July 26th, 1837, 12in. high, £350

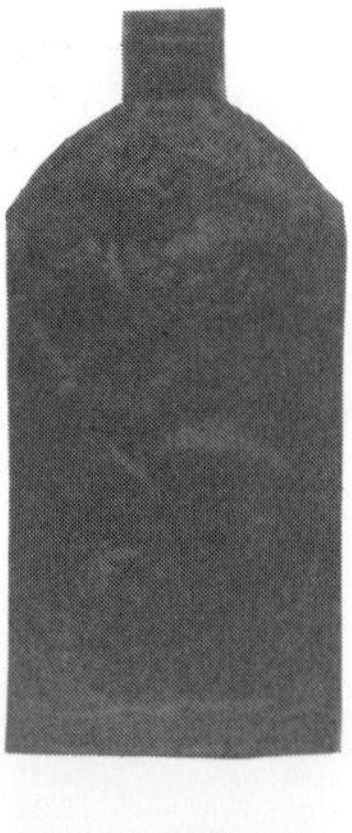

Jim Crow flask, no potter's mark but with Spirit Merchant's names and address, 8in. high. £100 – £125

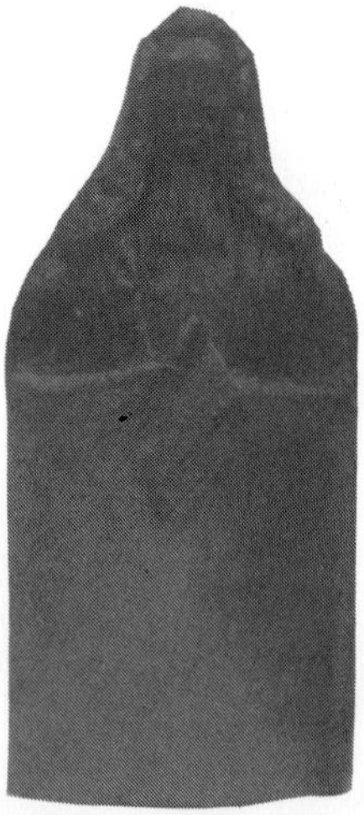

Lord Brougham flask, made by Doulton & Watts, 14½in. high. £350

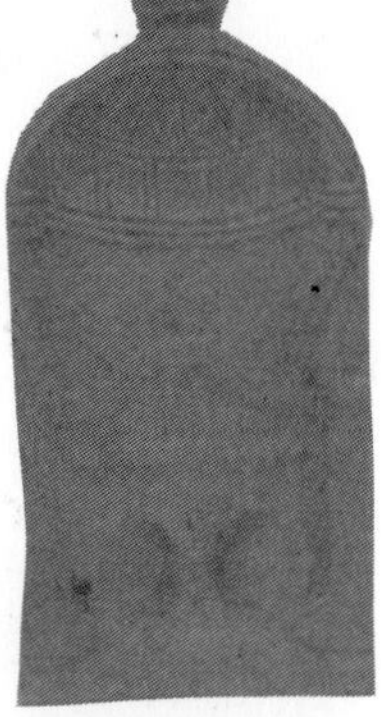

Thames Tunnel flask (Tunnel opened in 1843), impressed on bottom 'Wm. Wenham, Church St., Croydon'. £450

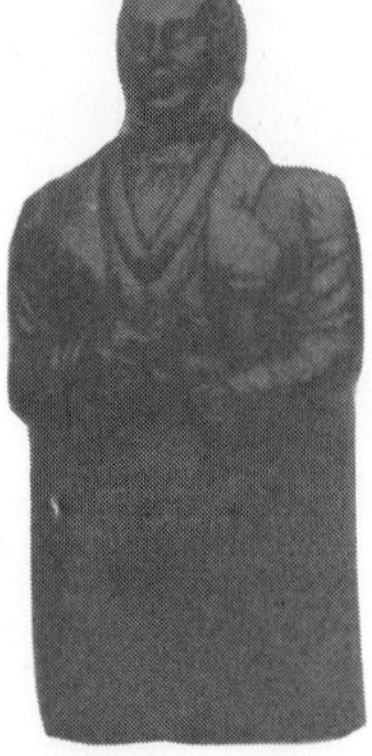

William IV flask, by T. Oldfield & Co., Chesterfield, 9in. high. £150 – £175

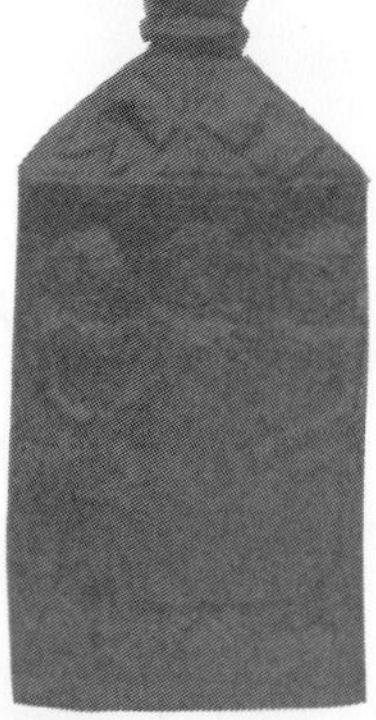

Crimean War flask recording Peace in 1856, impressed on bottom 'Wm. Wenham, Church St., Croydon'. £500

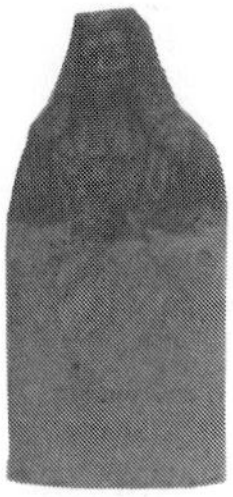

Lord Brougham flask, made by Belper & Denby, Bournes Potteries. £100 – £120

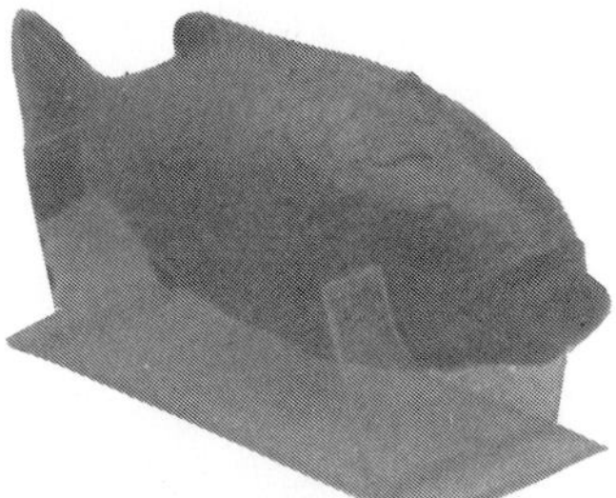

Fish flask, impressed 'R. Cooper, Railway Terminus, Brighton', 'W. Northern Potter'. £350

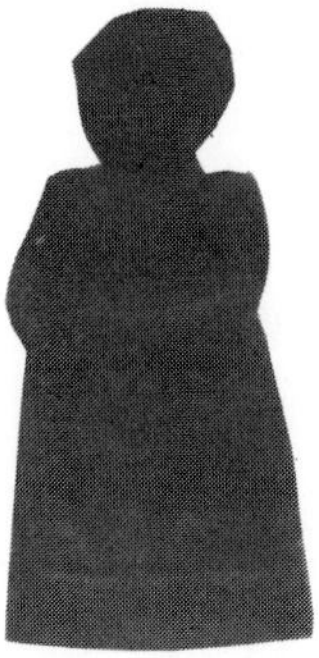

Old Woman flask, no potter's mark. £175 – £200

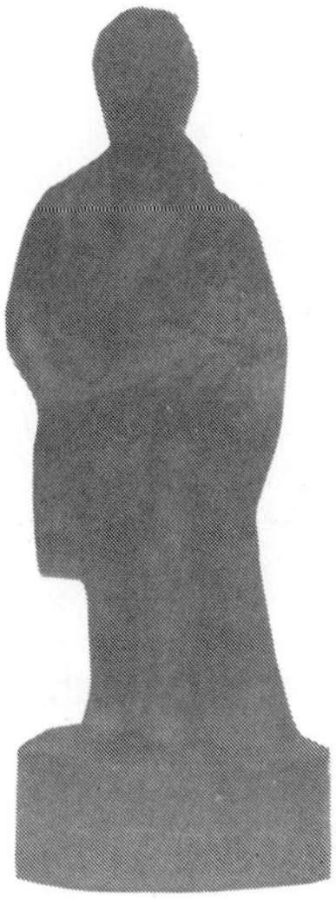

Sir Robert Peel, no potter's mark, 11in. high. £250

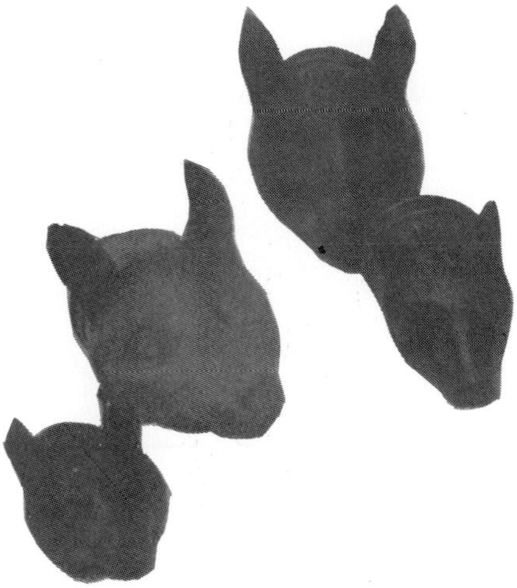

Fox Head flasks, various sizes. £200 – £300

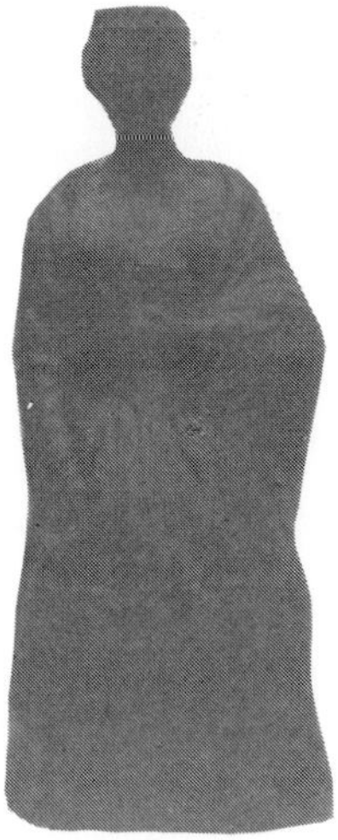

An unnamed Lady, no potter's mark, 11in. high. £250

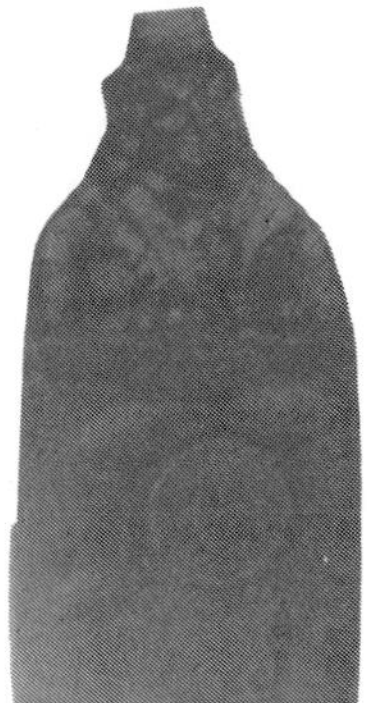

Man on a Barrel, by T. Oldfield, Chesterfield, 8½in. high. £100

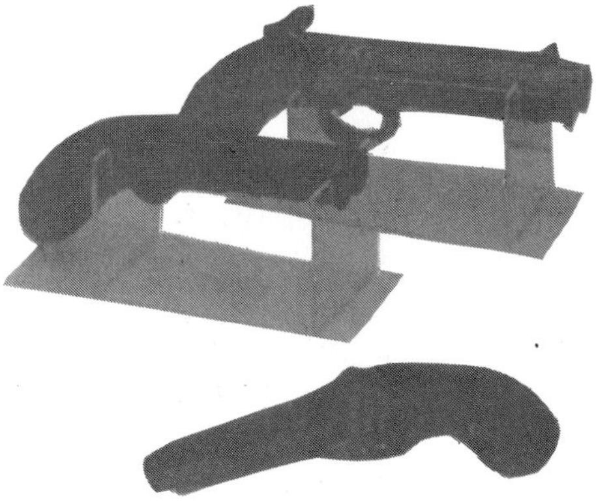

Pistol flasks. £125 – £175

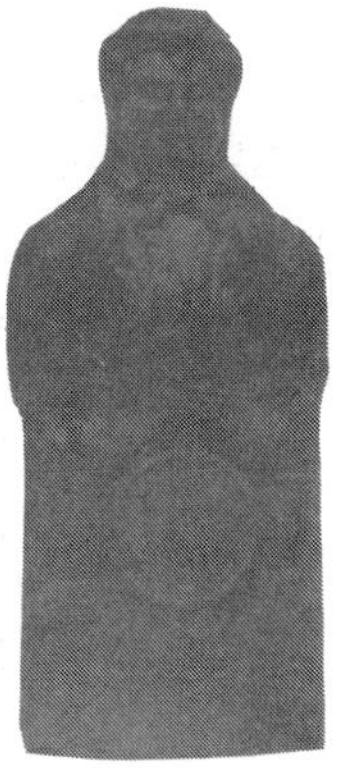

Man on a Barrel flask, by Denby & Codnor Park Potteries, 8in. high. £100 – £125

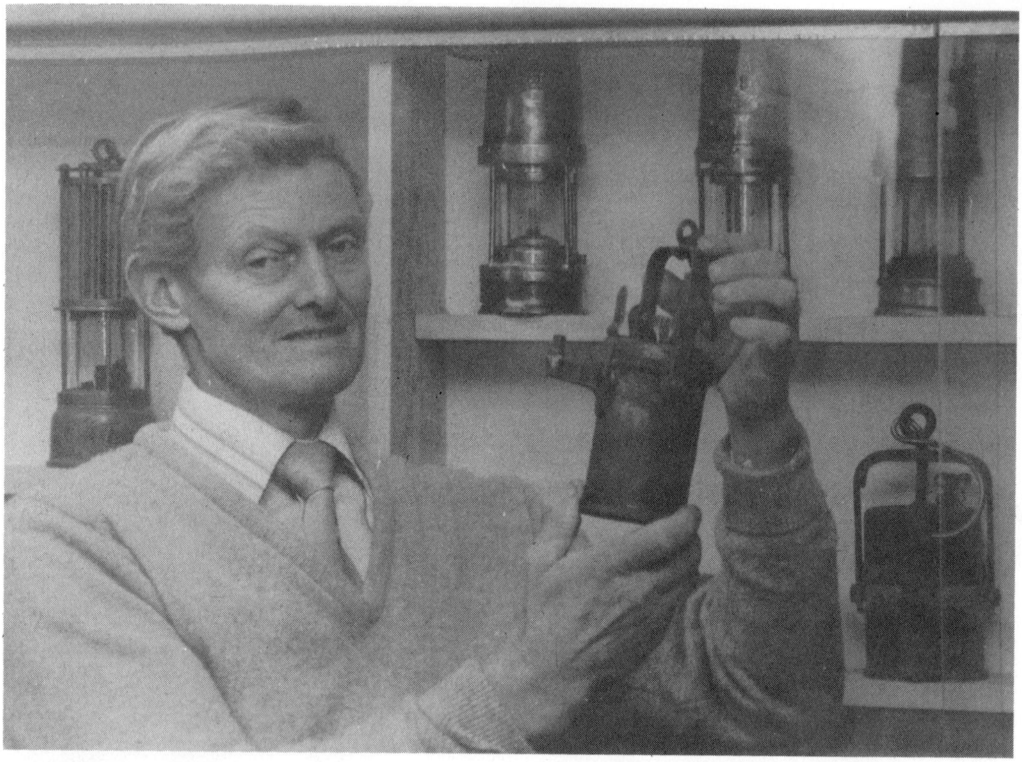

Merlyn Tancock is a retired miner who has opened a mining museum in his home village. The most important part of his collection is miners' lamps.

"I was a miner for 30 years and I know what it's like to wear one of those lamps. There are 400 in my collection and what pleases me most is that we've managed to keep them here so that youngsters in the valley can see what life was once like. In this valley 20 years ago there were nine pits and today there's only one — and for how long is anyone's guess.

"I've been collecting lamps for 25 years and the supply has almost dried up. Americans are very keen on them and they buy all they can get but it's now nearly only the modern ones that are left.

"My oldest lamp dates back to 1780 and the man who I got it from said his father and his grandfather's father had used it. It was lit by oil and is a bit like a watering can with a wick coming out of the spout. It must have been very smoky and couldn't have given much light but before that they only had candles.

"From 1820 on the Davy lamp was mass produced and they didn't give much light either because they were surrounded by wire gauze but then they got the Clanny lamp which was better.

"Although I've got 400 lamps that's just the tip of the iceberg because there were so many different types made. Most of mine are Welsh and were made in Aberdare but I've also got English and Belgian ones. Very few have the names of pits on them, just makers' names."

Merlyn said that the most he has ever paid for a lamp is £350 but some go for a great deal more than that. An average lamp that is around 50 years old usually fetches about £50.

His museum is open seven days a week in the saw mill at the village where he lives in the Dulais valley.

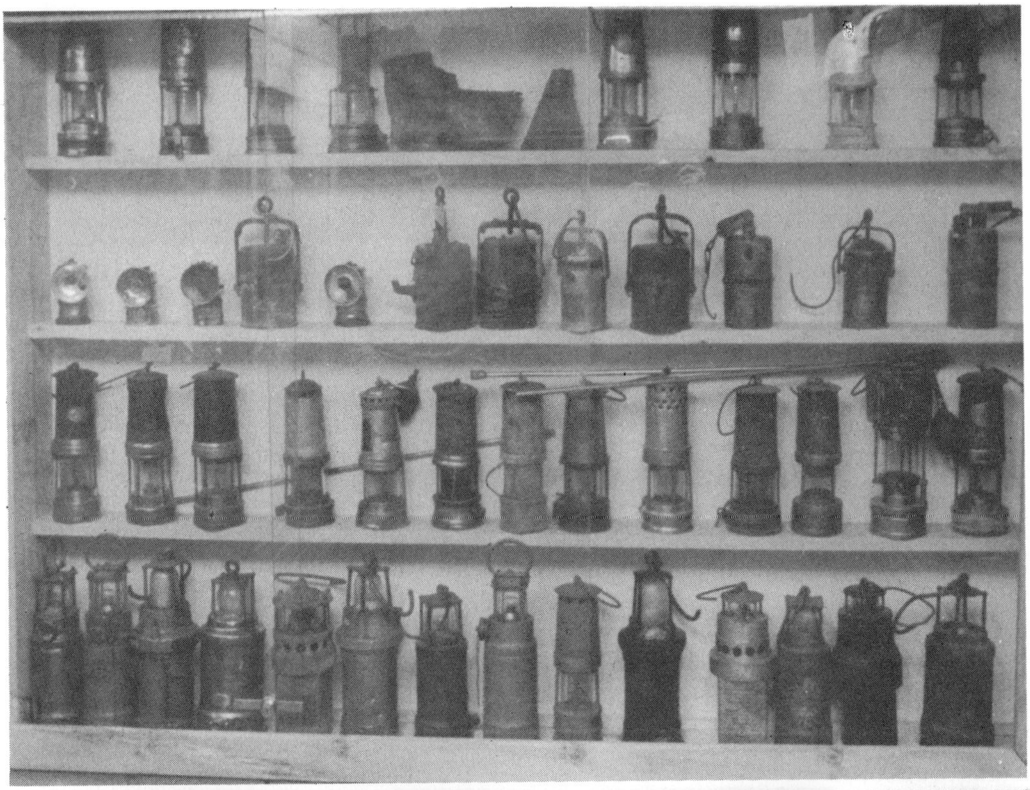

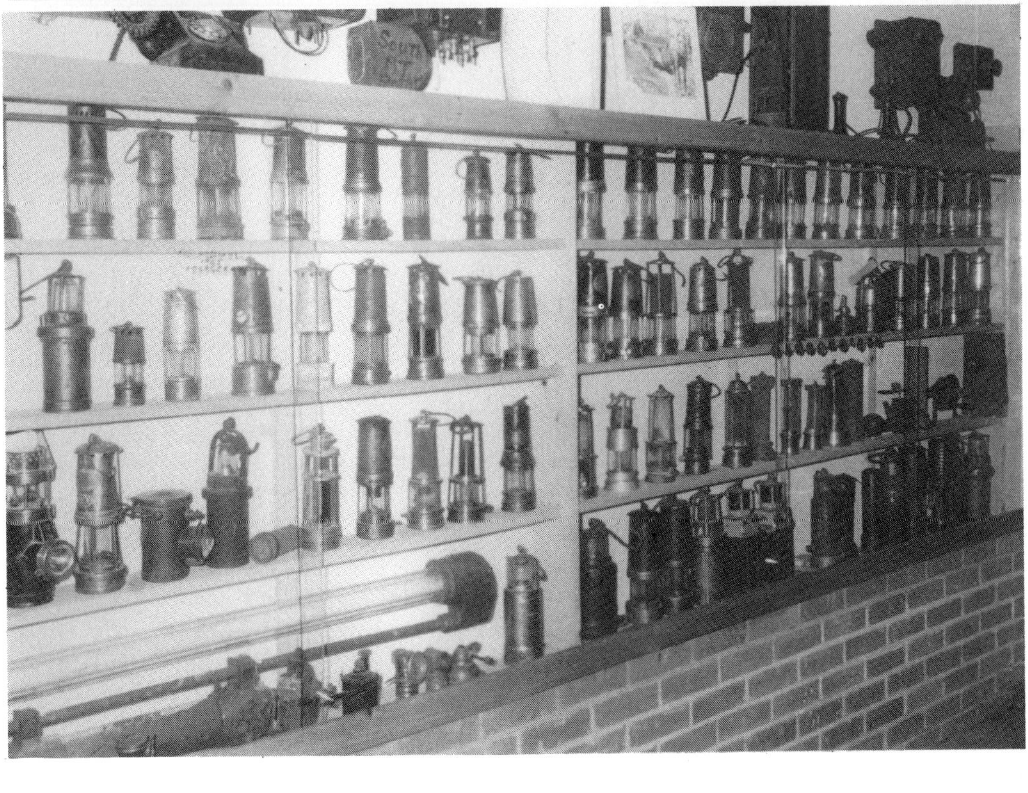

The Museum, Seven Sisters Museum and Sawmills, is situated in the Dulais Valley, in the Vale of Neath.
The valley is in the heart of the Anthracite Belt and was first mined commercially in 1813. Up to three decades ago it was scarred with slag tips, but with the closures of the mines it has been restored to its natural beauty, it is in this setting that Merlyn has opened his Museum with the purpose of retaining some links with the past.
There are over four hundred lamps in the collection. These include underground compressed air lights,a range of Davy Type Lamps, Jack Davy Type Lamps, Boy Workers Lamps, Clanny Type Lamps, Meuseler Type Lamps, Masuet Type Lamps, a range of Electric, Hand and Cap Lamps, various Candle Light Lamps, a variety of Pit Shaft Lamps and numerous Wick Lamps. A lot of these lamps date back to the early 19th century. The collection has taken twenty-five years to accumulate and visitors are given a guided tour which shows the evolution of the Miner's Lamp.

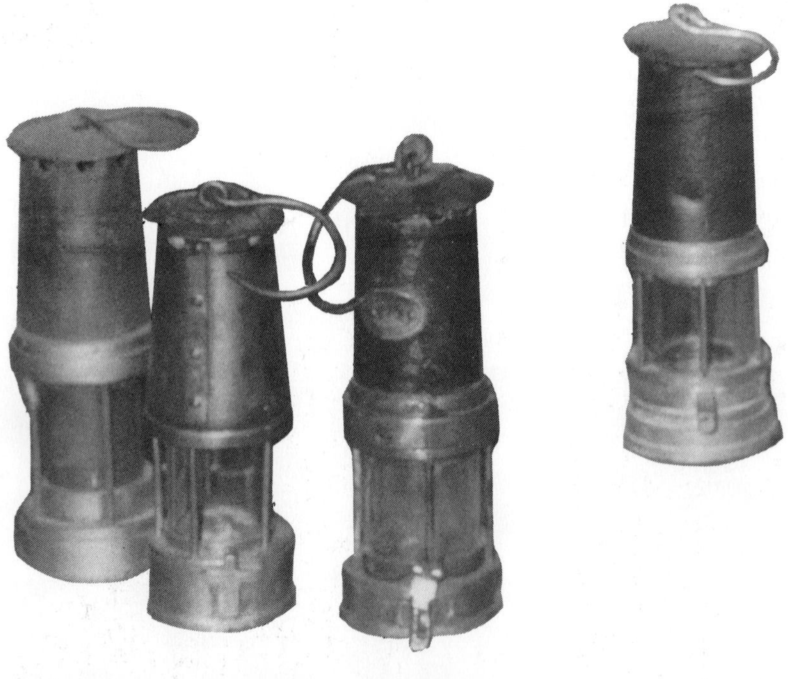

This picture shows four Oil Lamps with different locking devices. Three were used before the Electric Lamp underground, the oldest locked by a screw with a head needing a special key to open it. This was followed by the Lead Plug Type, although it was quite simple to cut the plug and open the lamp underground it was almost impossible to replace the plug without the Lampman on the surface knowing the lamp had been opened – and to open a lamp underground was a serious offence risking the lives of all the workmen in the mine. The penalty was instant dismissal and a fine which in the valley would mean moving to another area as at the time the Dulais valley was owned by one man and the offender would not be re-employed. The third lamp has a magnetic lock. This type was also used as a working lamp until the 1940's. The advantage of this lamp being that if the flame was extinguished the worker could go to a relighting station to relight the lamp which could be done without opening it. These stations were placed at various points throughout the mine. Sometimes a lone worker would jar or tip his lamp and extinguish the flame. He would then have to feel his way along the tram rails in the dark to relight his lamp, this could be a walk of up to half a mile. The other lamp is a modern magnetic example with a built-in relighting device, these are used by colliery officials.

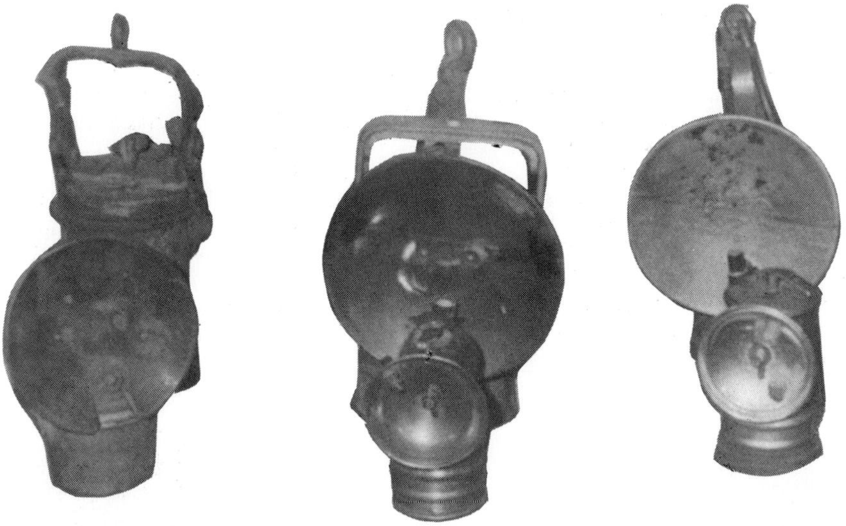

These lamps were used in open flame mines – this means mines considered free of methane gas – the lamps being fuelled by carbide.

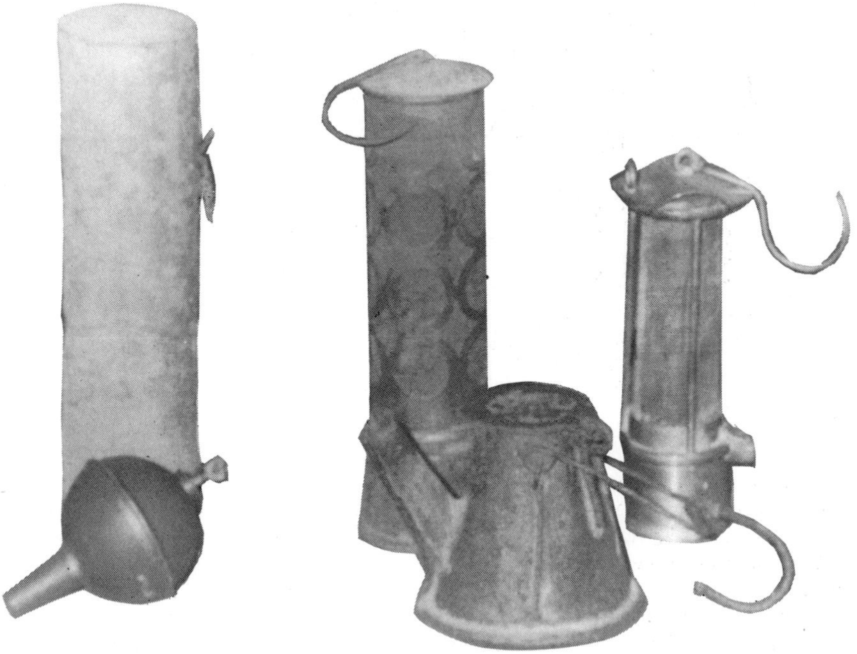

The Ball and Stick Lamp, left, was used before the Davy Lamp. The user or Fireman (this is how the name derived) would fit the lamp on the end of a long stick, lay on the ground covered with a wet sack and ignite the gas which would be at the highest point in the roadway. Another wick lamp shaped like a watering can is called a Level Lamp. The taller gauze lamp is called a Clayrite Davy Type Lamp, the candle is fitted on a holder attached to the iron bracket which has a sharp point, this was then driven into the wooden roof supports where it would give off the most light. On the right is a brass Davy Lamp, circa 1820.

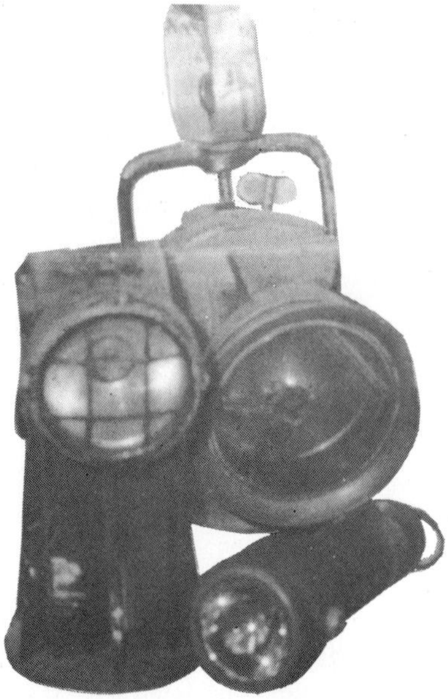

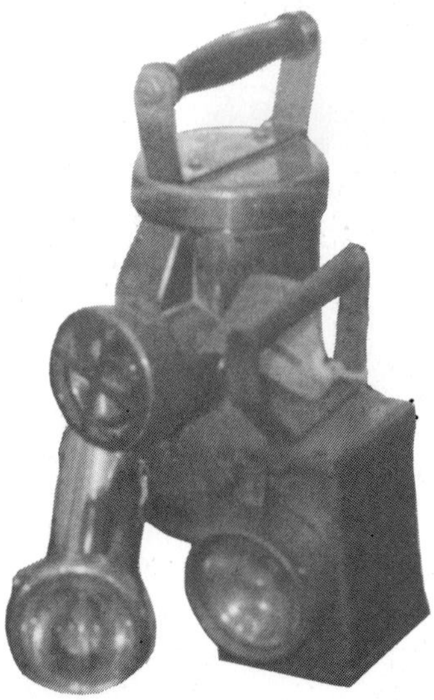

These lamps date from the early 1940's and are Hand Lamps used by managers, under-managers etc. For gas testing the officials also had to carry an oil lamp, this meant they had to carry two Hand Lamps which was very difficult. During this time changes and improvements in the lamps were coming fast and furious and one lamp, brought out by the C.E.A.G. Lamp Co., which combined the Hand Lamp and Oil Lamp in one unit, was used for a short time before being replaced by the modern Cap Lamp.

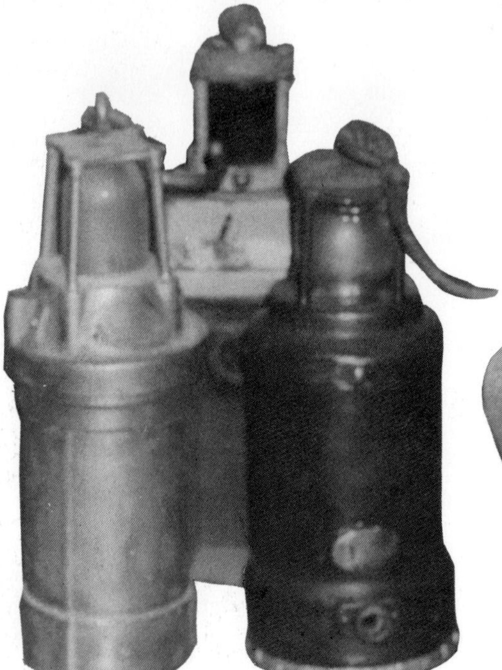

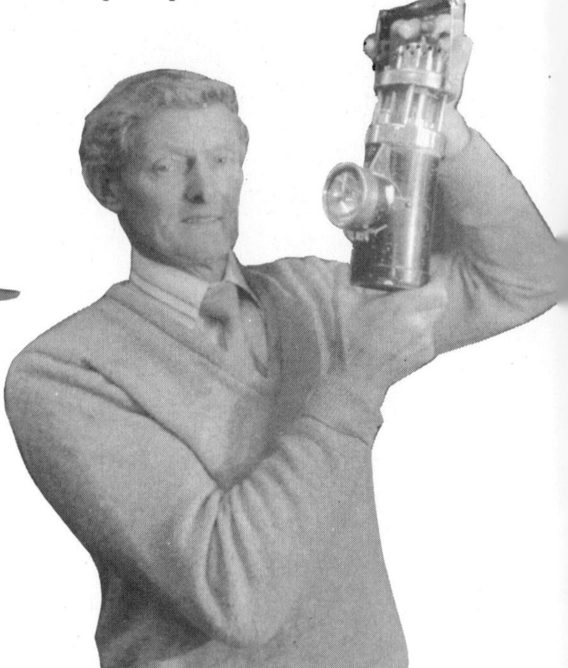

These Lead Acid Workers Hand Lamps which look like lighthouses, were the first Electric Lights used by workers in the Dulais valley in the early 1940's. They were very heavy but the good light must have compensated for the weight.

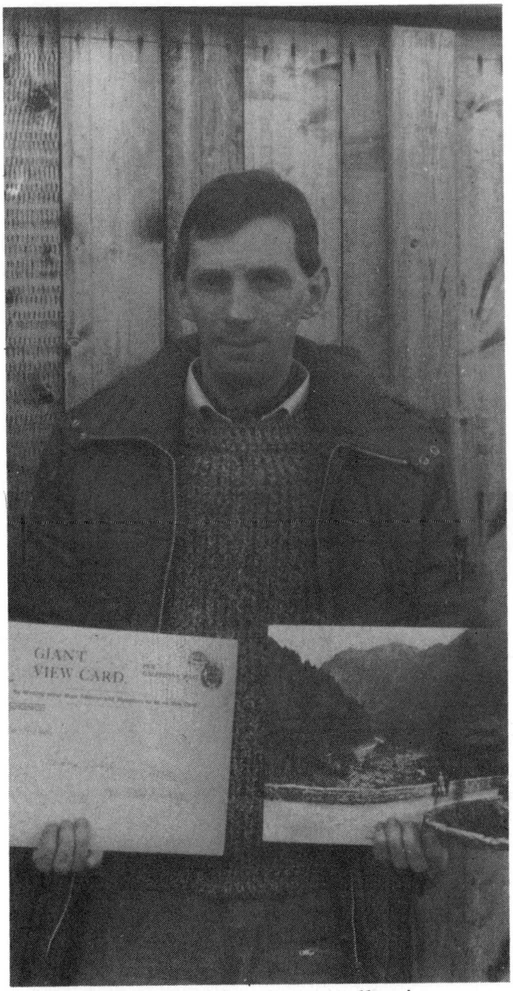

Paul Sheppard has been collecting postcards for over ten years and his vast and varied stock now encompasses the widest possible spectrum of themes including Art cards, Theatrical cards, Comic cards and, as an animal lover — Guinea Pig cards.

He says "My interest was first aroused when I was given an old album containing some family postcards and my collection has just grown since then along with the general popularity of the subject (Deltiology) itself. I have spent many enjoyable hours researching and finding out about cards and the characters depicted. They provide a perfect visual account of the past including changes in fashion, transport, advertising trends and, my personal favourites, those reflecting local social history during The Golden Age.

"I envy the collectors who were out there buying before the subject took off for in those days albums crammed full of very desirable postcards were virtually given away.

"I would encourage anyone to first decide on a theme then to get out and enjoy the thrill of the chase. This is still a relatively inexpensive and popular pastime with lots of information readily available in current magazines and books and support from specialised clubs in many areas.

"Storage and display could not be simpler with examples set out in desired order in good strong albums, always remembering to handle them as little as possible. Try not to be tempted into buying damaged cards for a torn card is worth but a fraction of the same card in mint condition. After a while, one learns to evaluate the condition in relation to the scarcity of a card.

"I feel certain that postcards will provide a sound area for investment for years to come besides, one can look forward to the pleasure of handing them on to future grandchildren.

"My ideal postcard would be a glamorous guinea pig card drawn by Louis Wain, dropped from a balloon over Kington on Christmas Day and sent to me by Royalty".

Can anyone help him out with this?

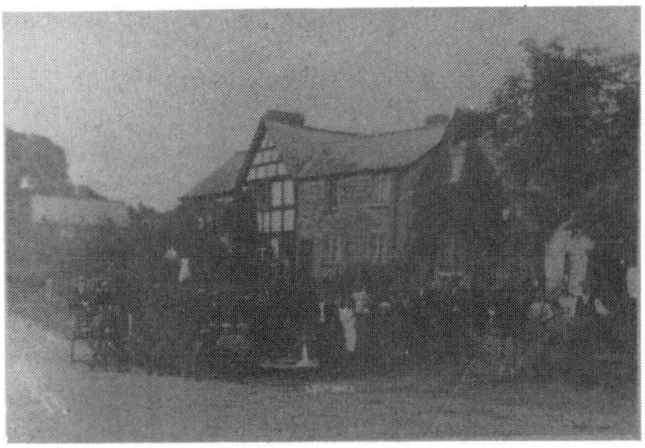

A postcard of Paul Sheppard's former house at Lyonshall. £7

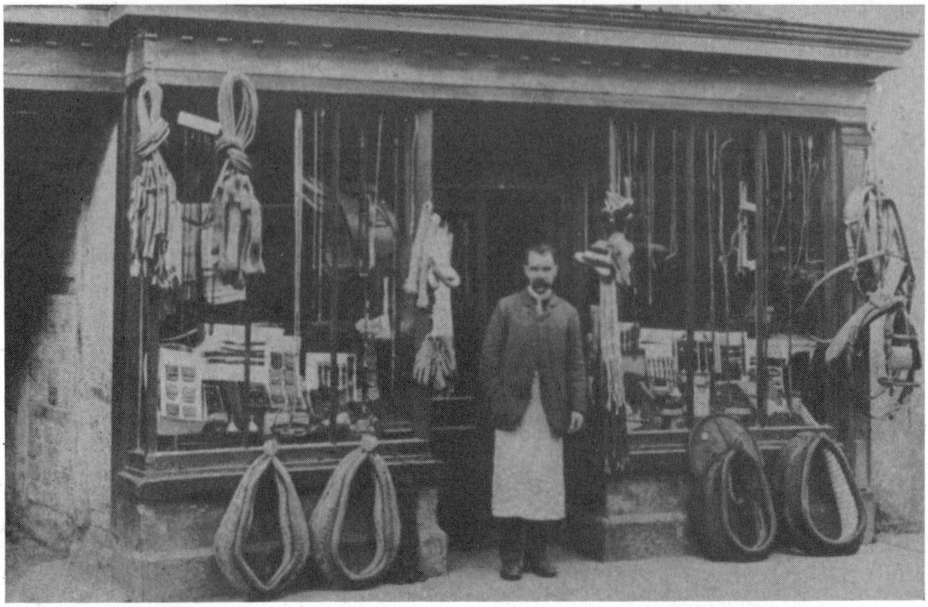

Charles Briggs, High Street, Presteigne. £8

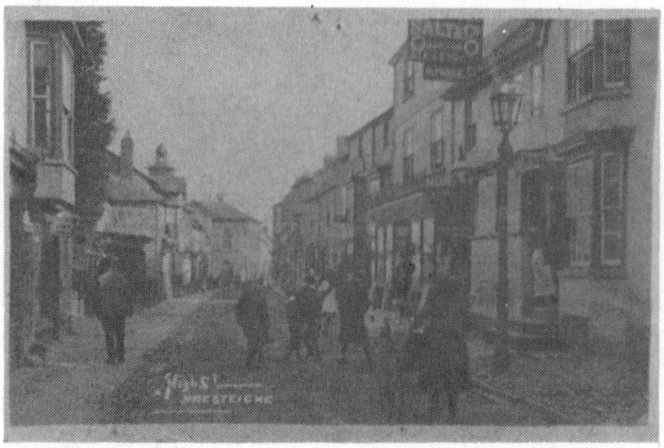

High Street, Presteigne. £6

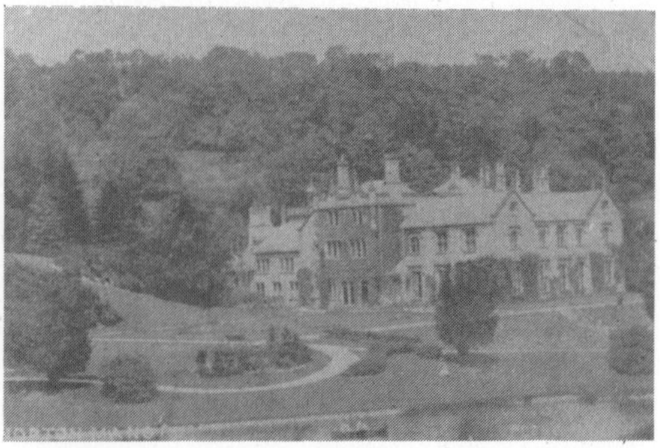

Norton Manor, Presteigne. £2.50

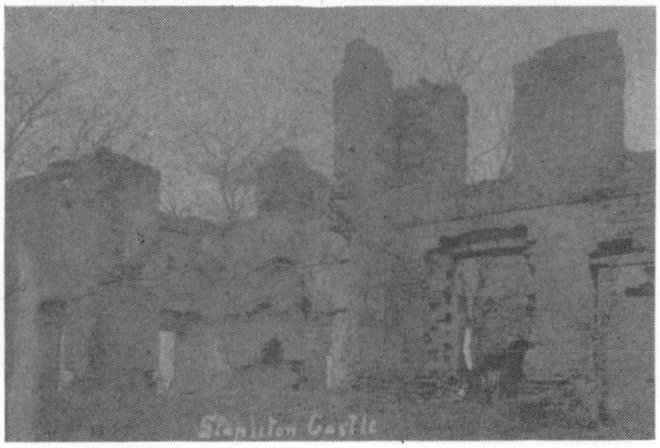

Stapleton Castle. £1

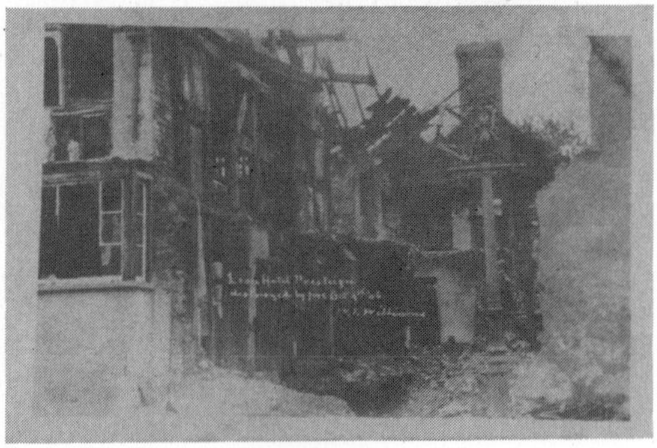

Lion Hotel, Presteigne, destroyed by fire October 9th, 1906. £10

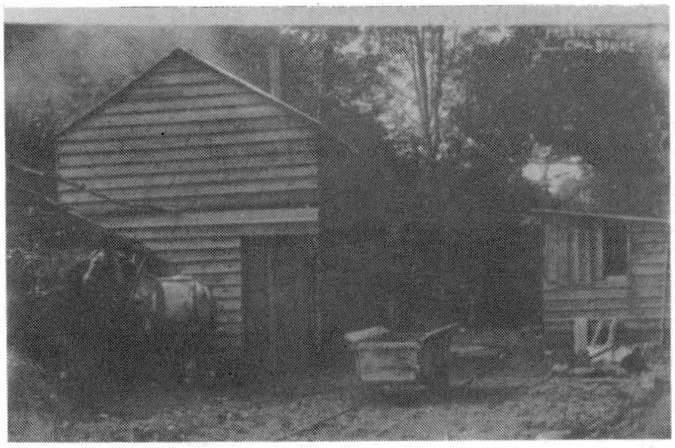

Coal Boring, Presteigne. £11

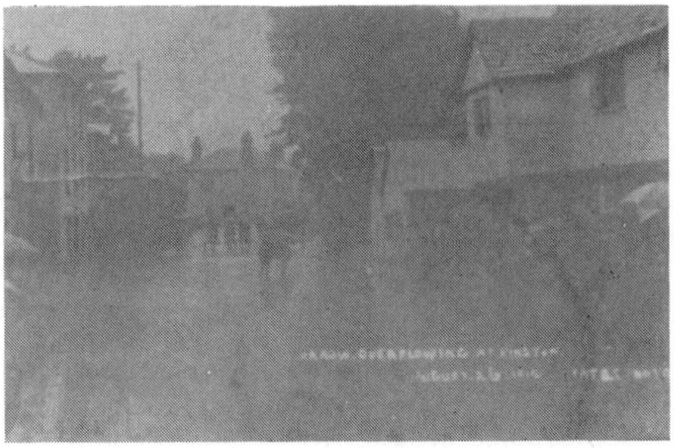

The River Arrow overflowing at Kington, August 26th, 1912, photograph by Yates. £6

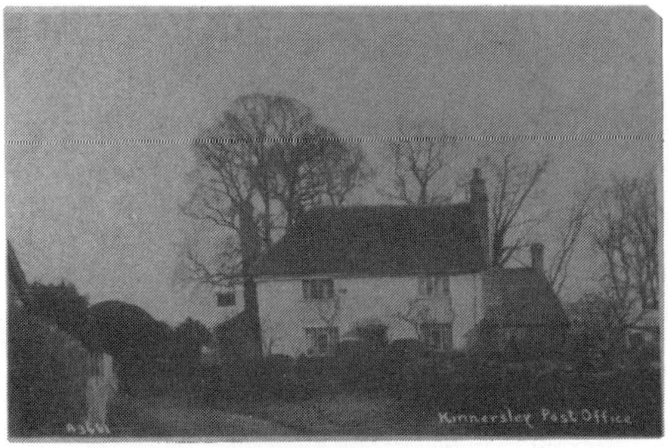

Post Office, Kinnersley. £3

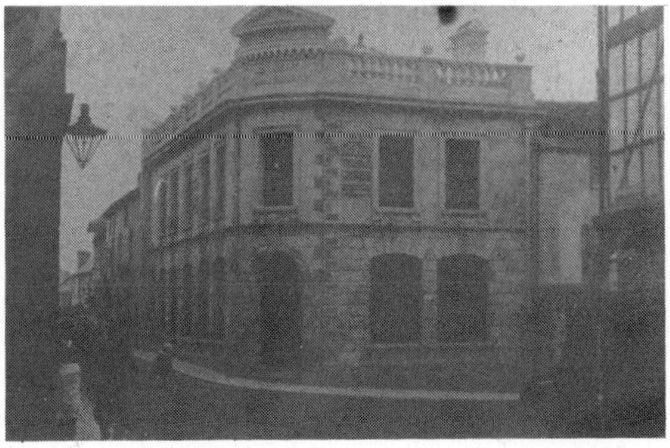

The Old Radnor Trading Co. Building. £3

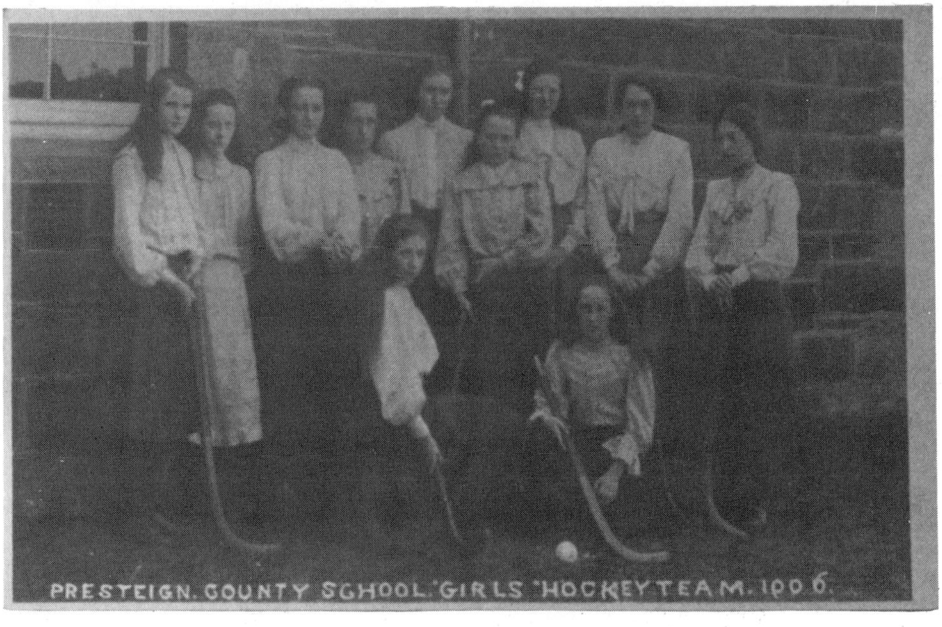

Presteign County School, Girls Hockey Team, 1906. £3.50

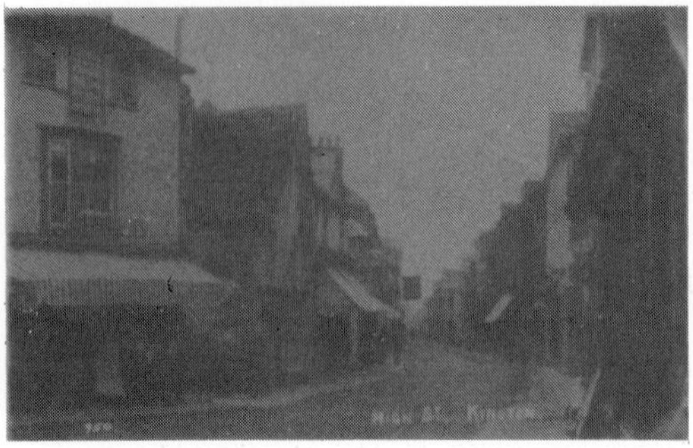

High Street, Kington, 1919. £4

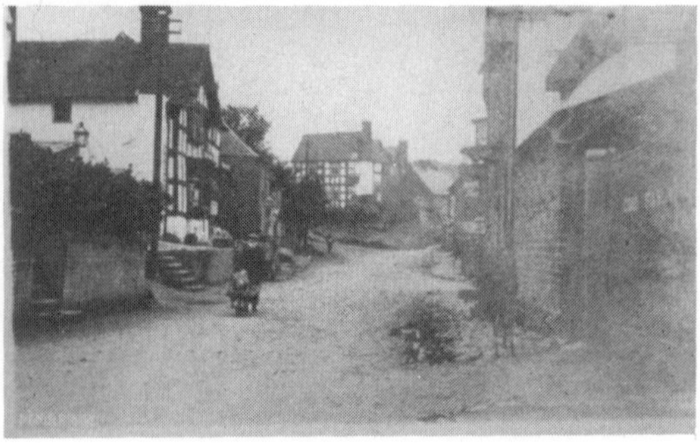

Main Street, Pembridge. £5

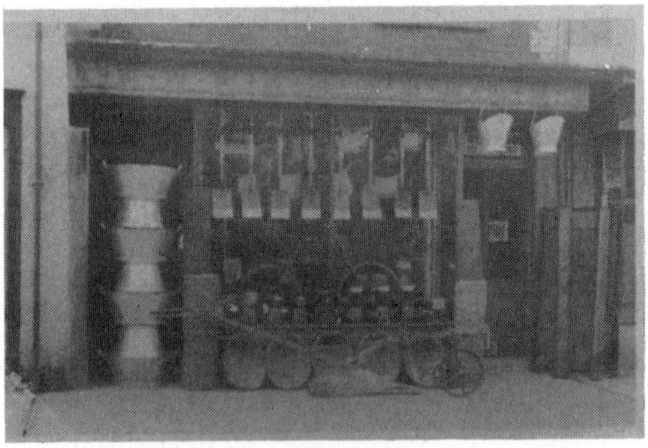

Shop front from Broad Street, Presteigne. £7

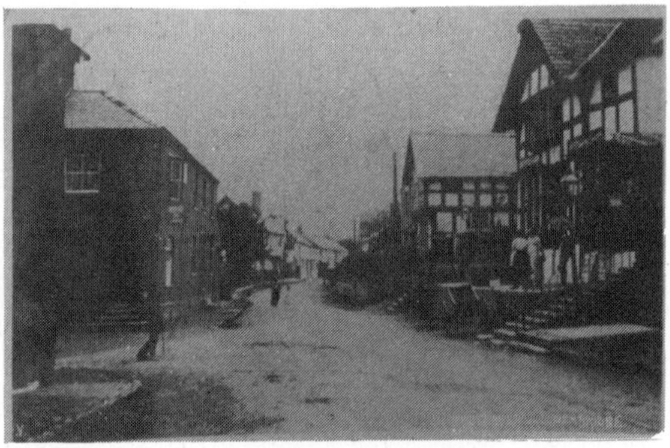

Pembridge Village, Herefordshire. £3.50

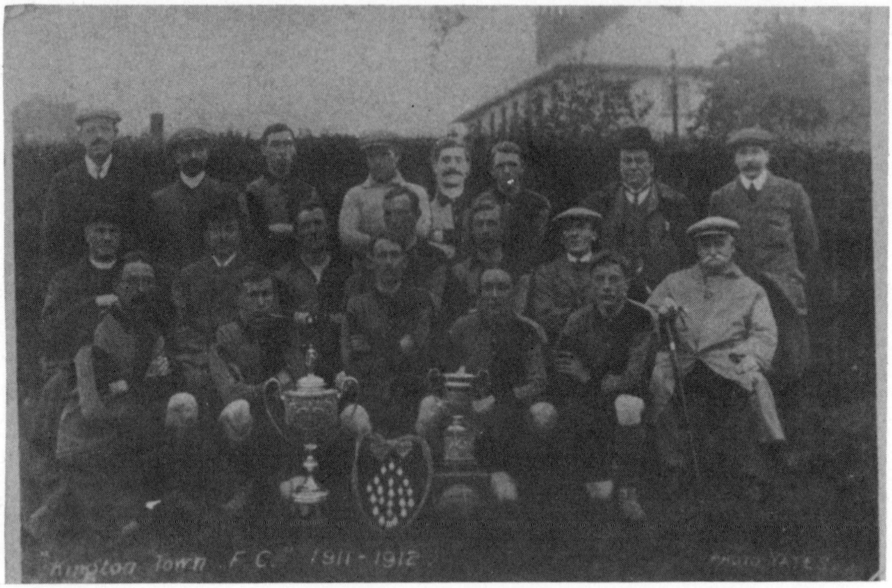

Kington Town Football Club, 1911-1912, photograph by Yates. £3

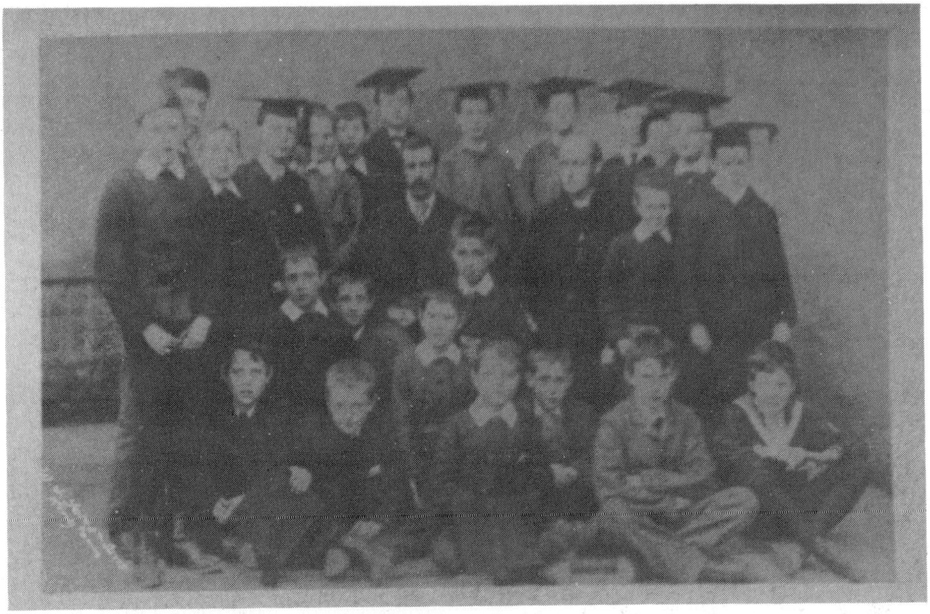

An interesting group from the local grammar school Kington. £2

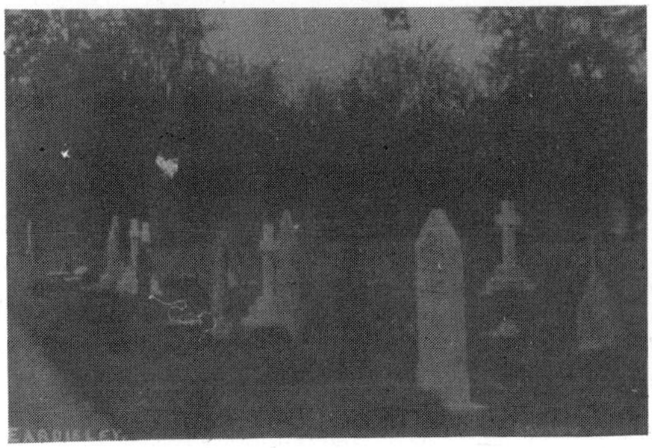

Eardisley Churchyard. £1.25

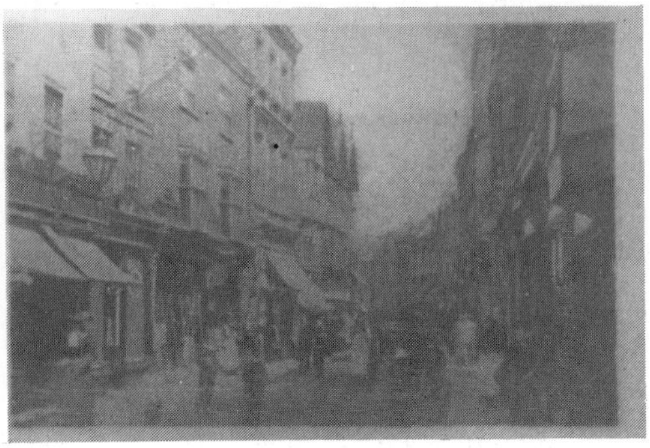

High Street, Leominster. £7

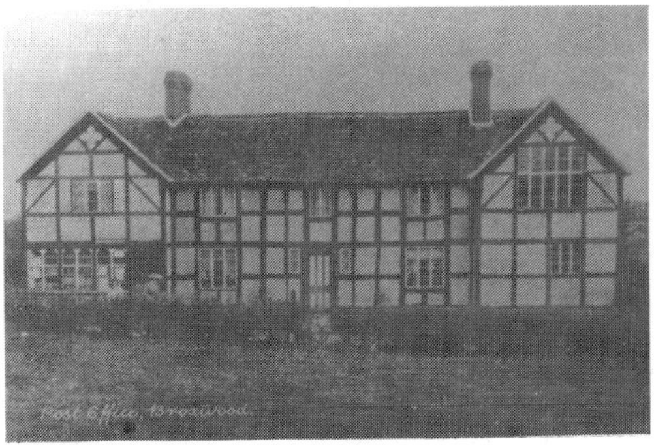

Post Office, Broxwood. £3.75

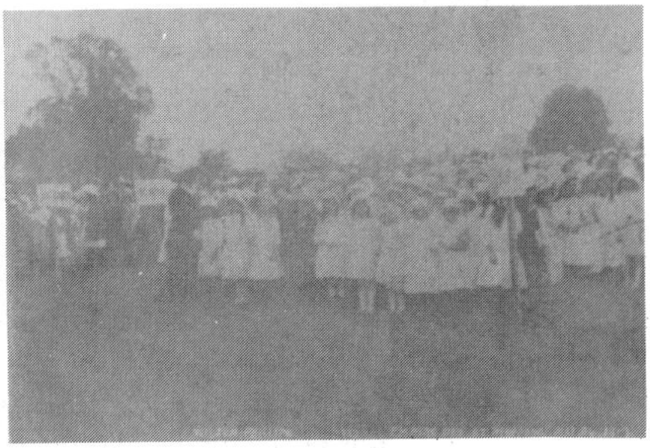

Empire Day at Hereford, May 1917, by Wilson-Phillips. £3

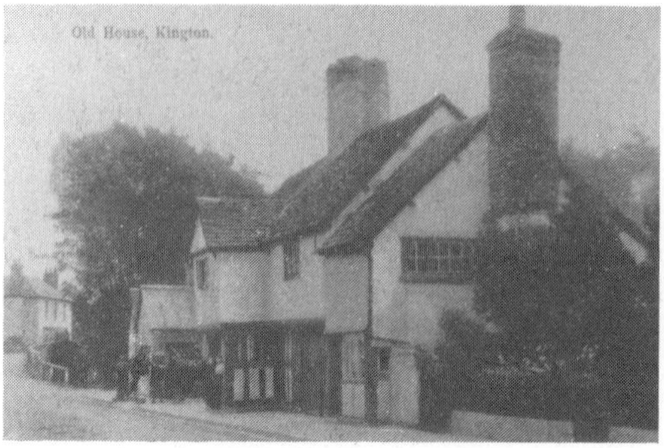

Old House, Kington. £2

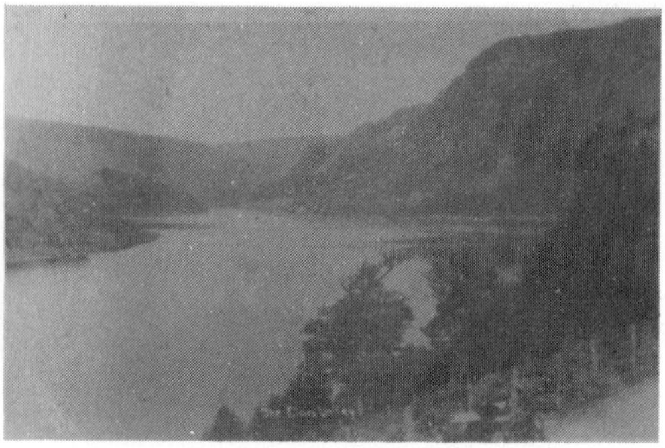

The Elton Valley, photograph by Yates. £1.25

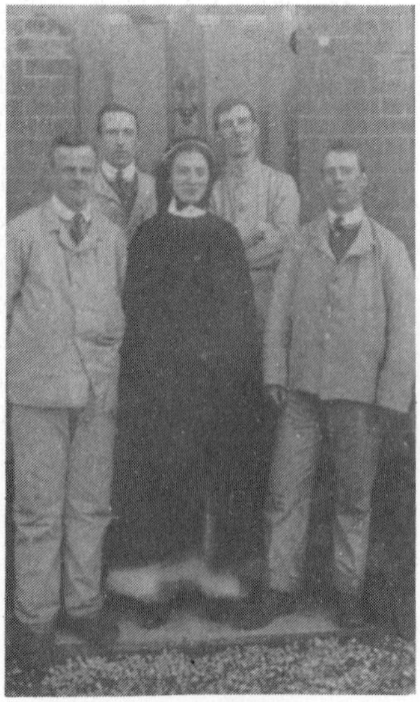

Hospital staff at Presteigne. £1.75

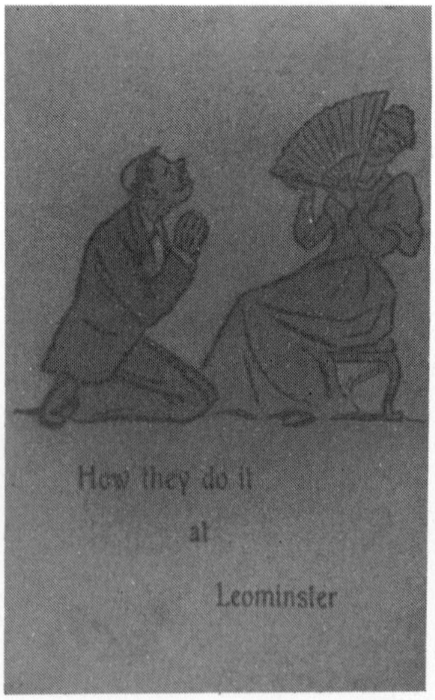

'How they do it at Leominster', 1906. £1.50

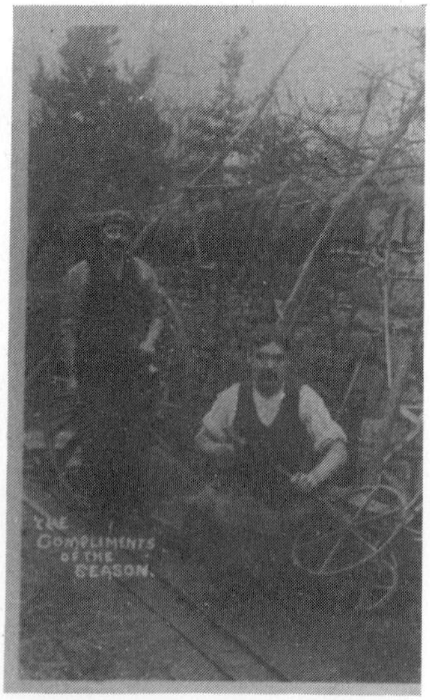

'The Compliments of the Season', Kington Wheelwrights. £7

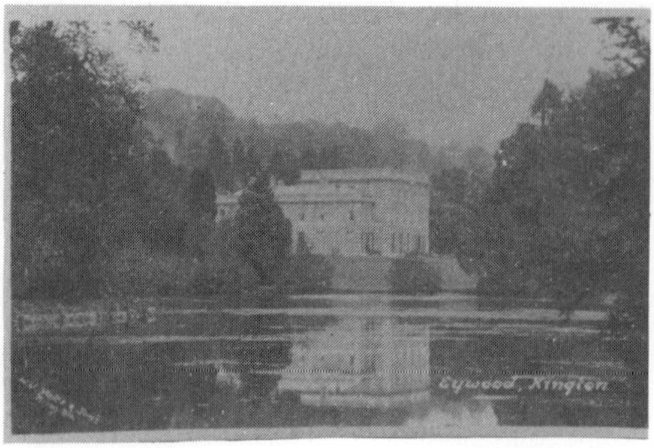

Eywood House, Titley, Kington. £4

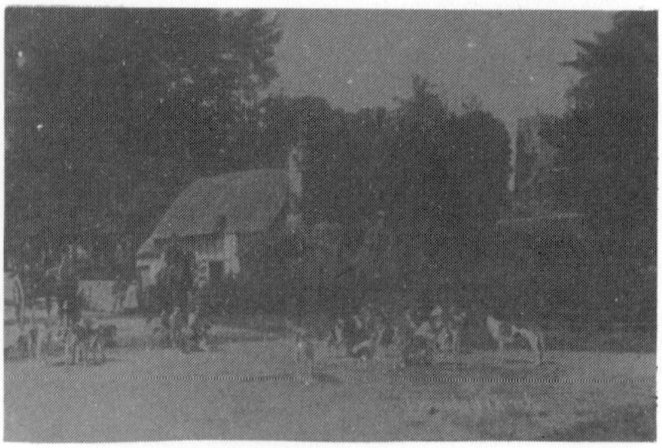

Horse and Hounds outside a cottage at Lyonshall. £4

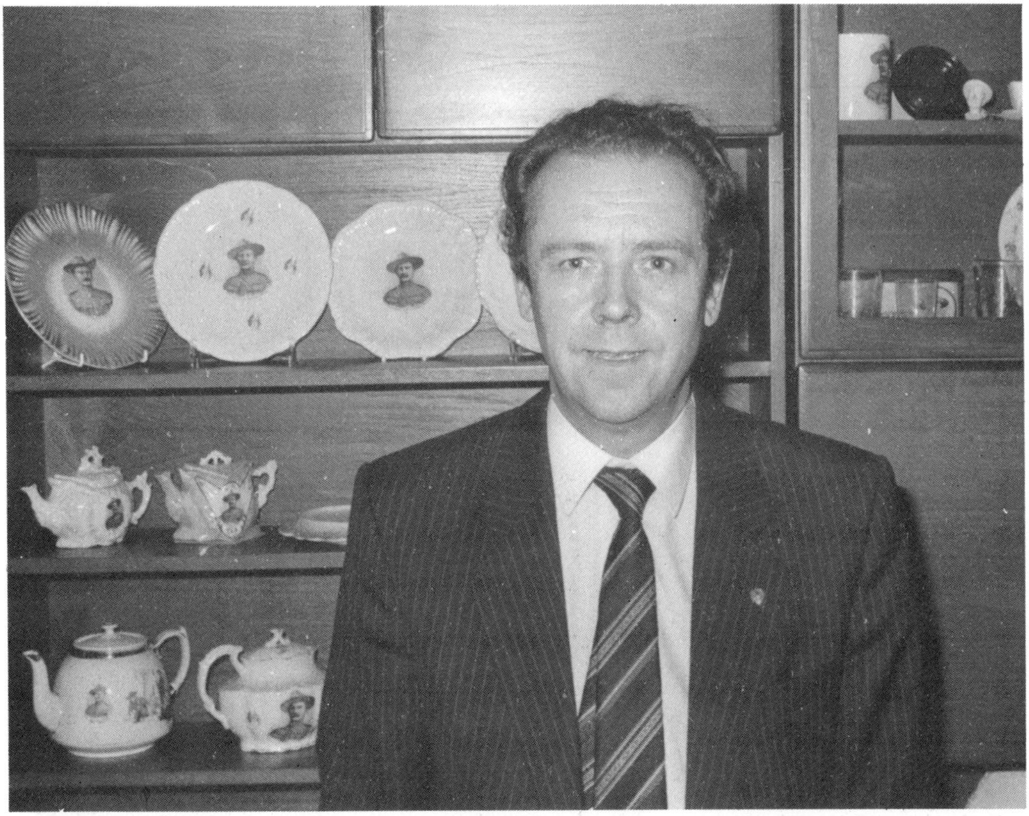

Michael Gosling is the regional sales manager of a metal perforating company and collects items relating to Baden Powell and Boy Scout badges.

"The interest in Boy Scouts badges came about because I've been involved with the movement since 1954 and am now Assistant County Commissioner International for West Mercia, a district that has 9,600 scouts. In all I've got 18,000 badges from over 121 countries.

"The part of Baden Powell's career that interests me most however is not so much the Scouting period but the time covered by the Boer War when he was first a colonel and then a general. He was a most remarkable man and became a national hero because he was in the siege of Mafeking which held out against the Boers for seven months in 1900.

"All kinds of commemorative items were made in his honour — teapots, plates, spoons, Vesta cases, silverware, cigarette cards and postcards. These form the basis of my Baden Powell collection."

Michael's badge collection includes a brass military scouting badge dated 1906 showing St George and the Dragon with Baden Powell's initials on the back. He has also some silk screen badges from the World Jamboree of 1924 which are today worth around £100 each.

His Baden Powell collection includes some postcards signed by the great man but Michael would most dearly like to find some of Baden Powell's watercolours because, as well as being a great soldier and organiser, he was a gifted artist who illustrated all his own books.

"The book I admire most is 'Boer Sketches in East Africa' which has plates of Baden Powell's paintings. The originals must be somewhere. I once saw one in the USA and have been looking for others ever since," he said.

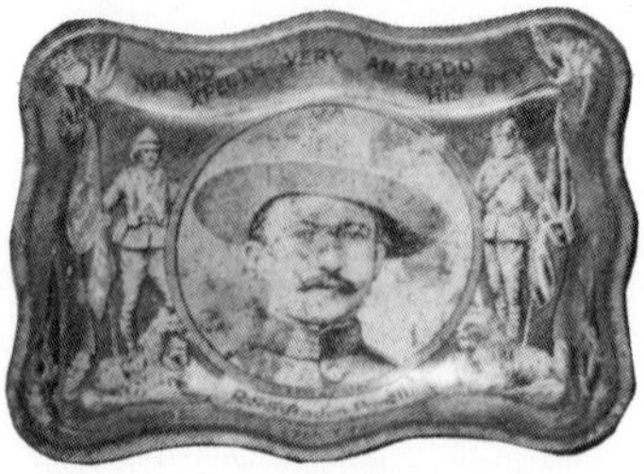

A small tin trinket tray with colourful design, 4in. long. £12 – £15

Porcelain cup and saucer decorated both inside and out with Major General R. S. S. Baden Powell. £30

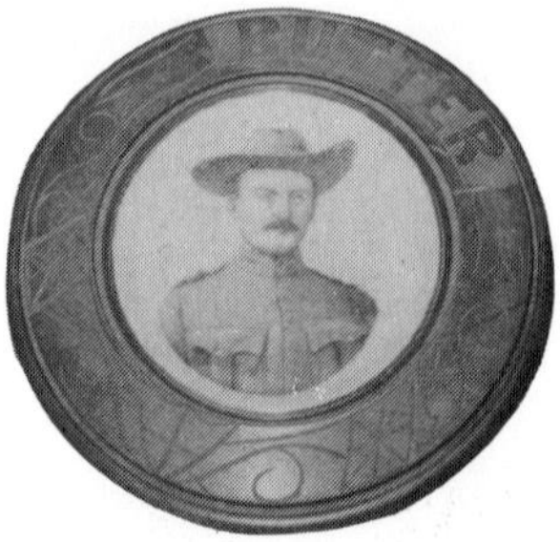

Wooden butter dish with Staffordshire centre depicting Baden Powell in sepia, 7in. diam. £23

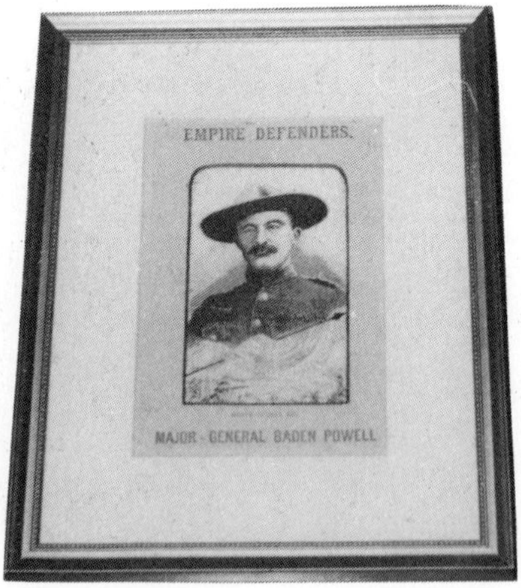

Stevengraph type picture by Grant, printed in black with coloured flag, 5½in. high inside mount. £40

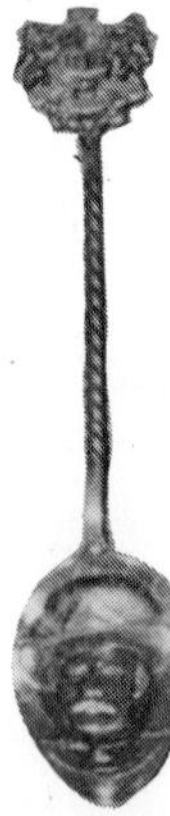

Hallmarked silver spoon with embossed portrait of Baden Powell in the bowl. £18

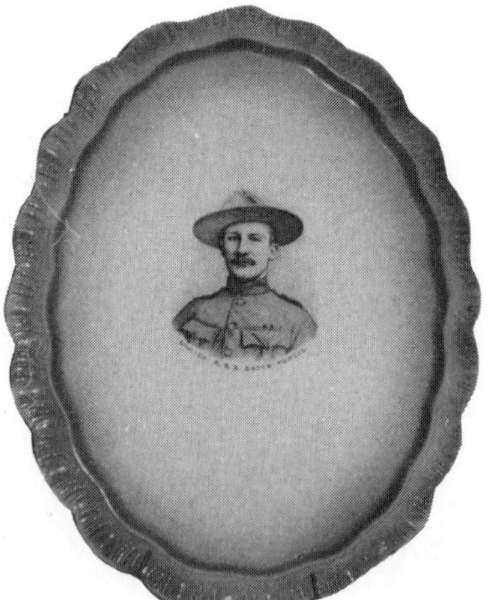

Staffordshire oval wall plate with wavy edge featuring Lieut.-Col. R. S. S. Baden Powell. £20 – £25

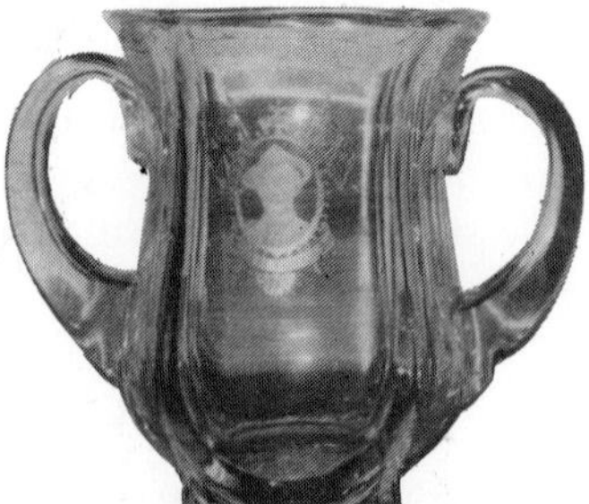

Crystal glass two-handled vase, engraved with a portrait of Baden Powell, on four short feet, 11in. high, slight crack. £12

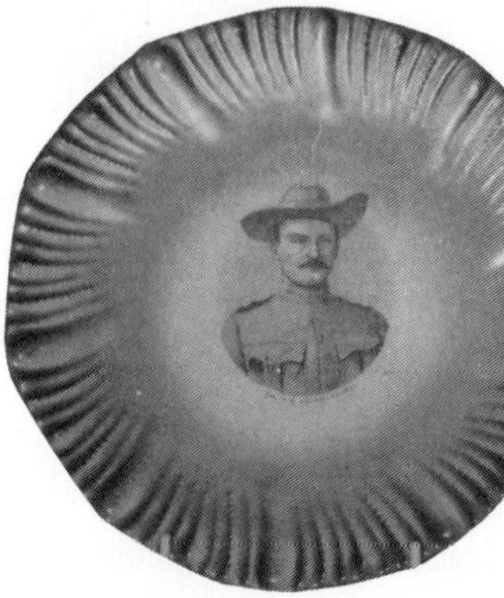

Early Staffordshire fluted plate featuring Baden Powell with turned up rim on the hat. £35

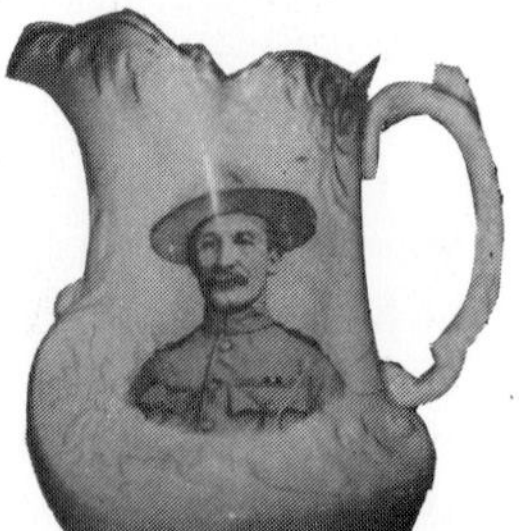

Nicely shaped Staffordshire jug with a portrait of Baden Powell. £15 – £20

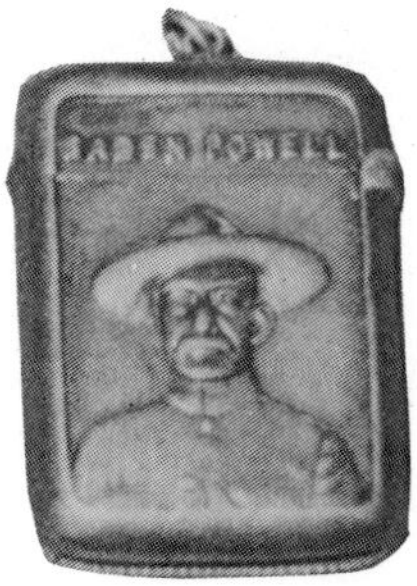

Silver vesta case embossed with the image of Baden Powell. £25

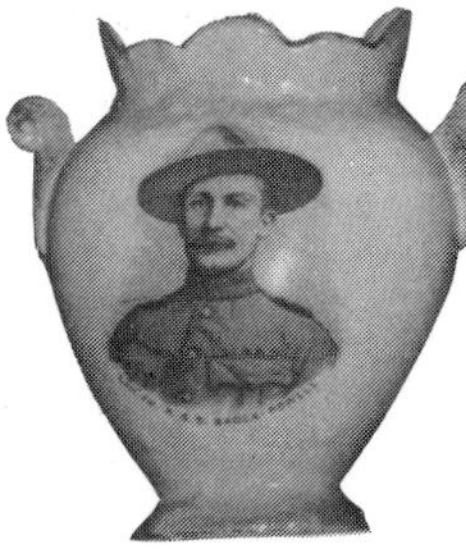

Pale yellow vase with small scrolled handles and Baden Powell portrait. £20

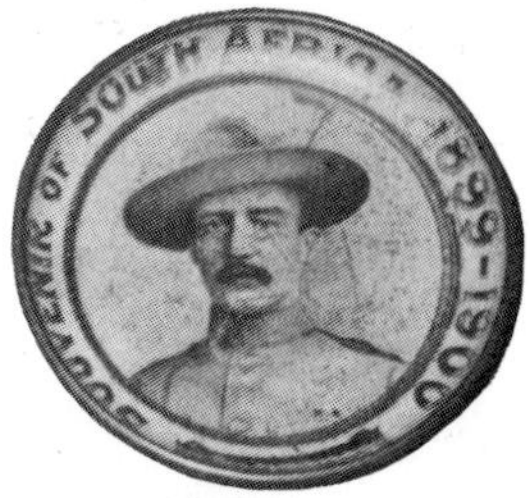

A small tin pin tray, 'Souvenir of South Africa 1899–1900', featuring Baden Powell, 3in. diam. £12 – £15

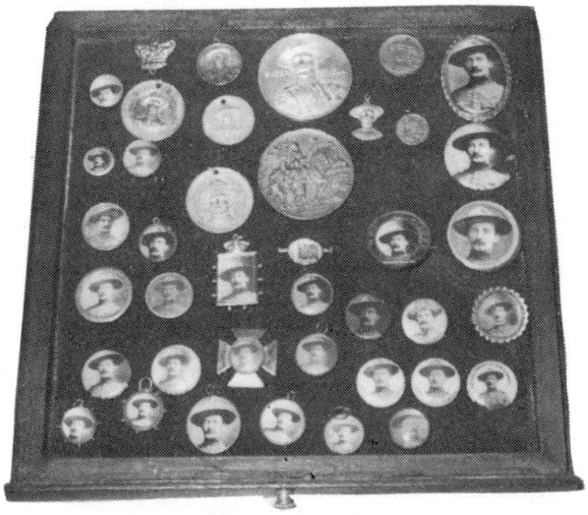

An assortment of badges, collar studs, brooches and charms featuring Baden Powell. £2 – £6

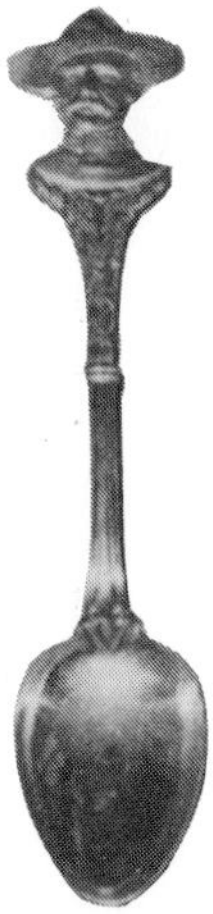

Silver spoon featuring Baden Powell on the handle. £12

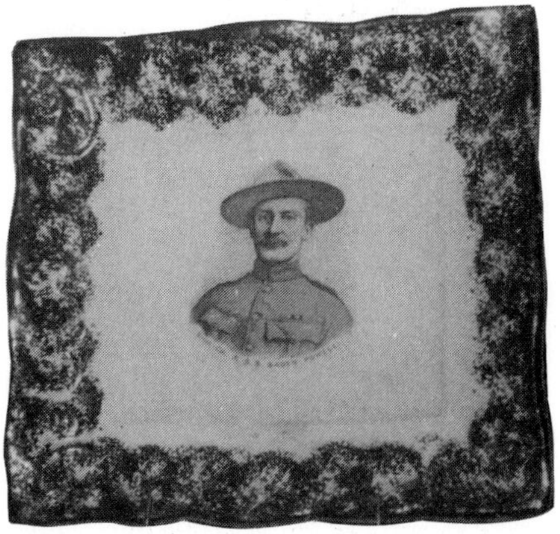

Square wall plaque with shaped edge featuring Lieut.-Col. R. S. S. Baden Powell. £30 – £35

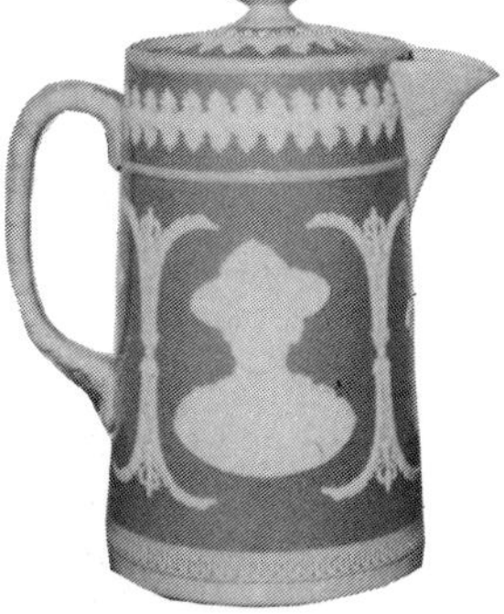

Wedgwood style blue and white coffee pot by Dudson, England, 6in. high. £25

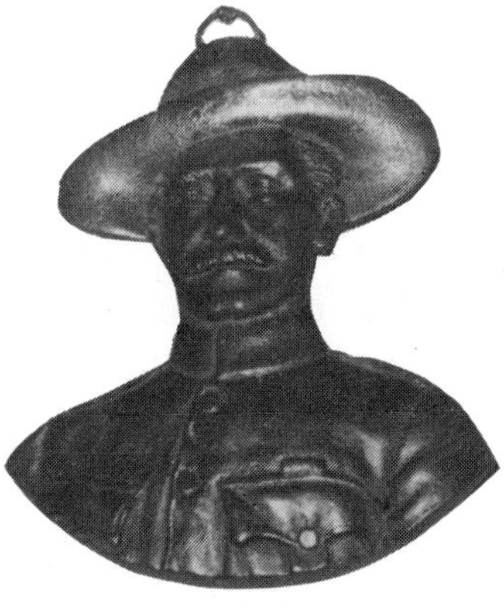

Stamped brass hanging wall plaque of Baden Powell, 5½in. high. £20

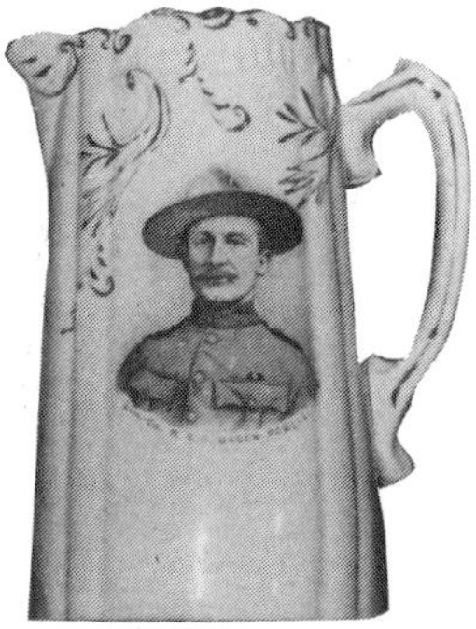

Tall Staffordshire milk jug with gilt decoration and portrait of Baden Powell. £15 – £20

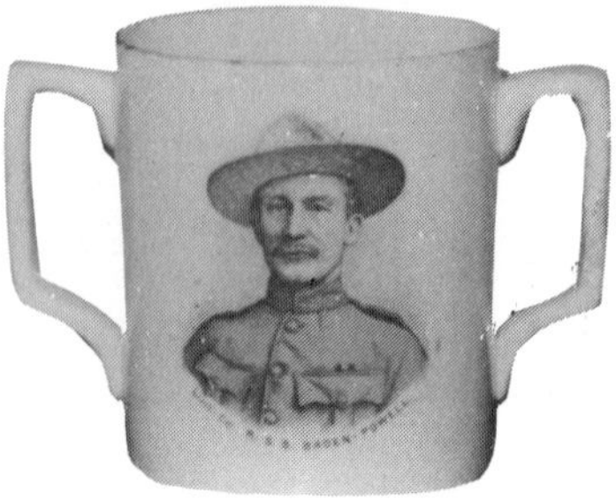

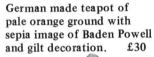

Two-handled loving cup with the portrait of Lieut-Col. R. S. S. Baden Powell. £20

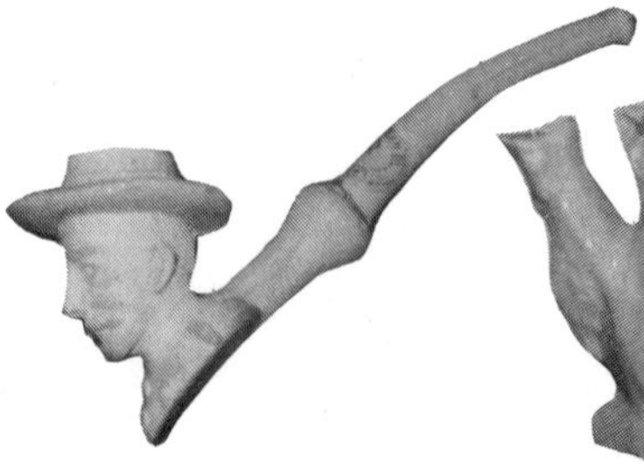

Unusual clay pipe in good condition, the bowl formed in the image of Baden Powell. £20 – £25

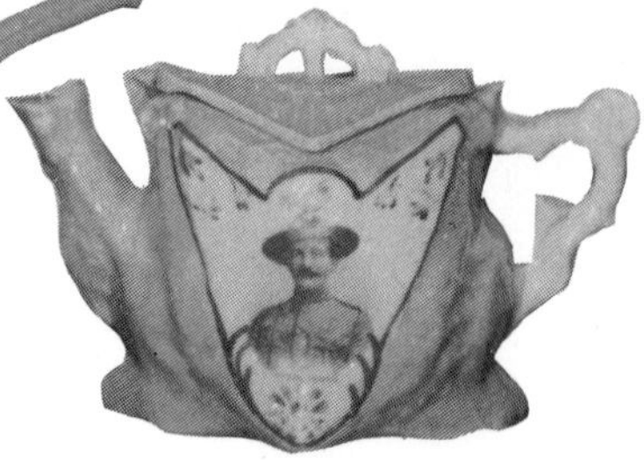

German made teapot of pale orange ground with sepia image of Baden Powell and gilt decoration. £30

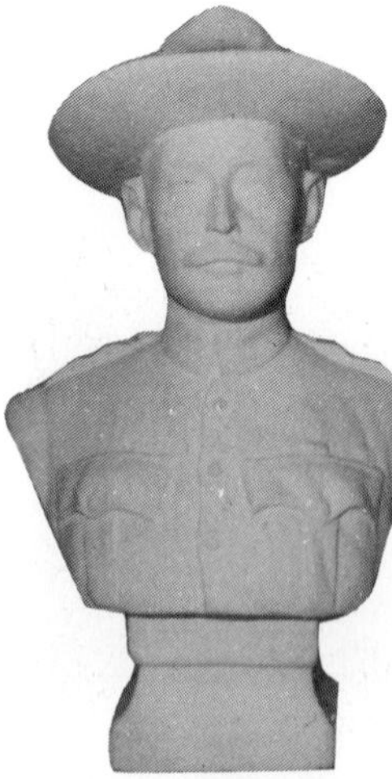

A plaster bust of Baden Powell, 10in. high. £35

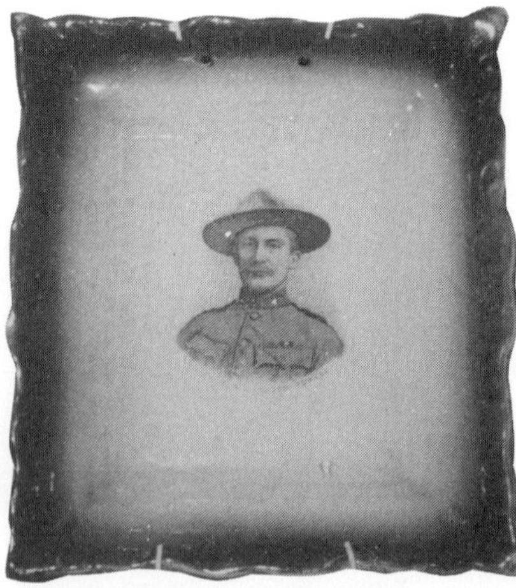

Shaped square wall plaque featuring Lieut.-Col. R. S. S. Baden Powell. £30 – £35

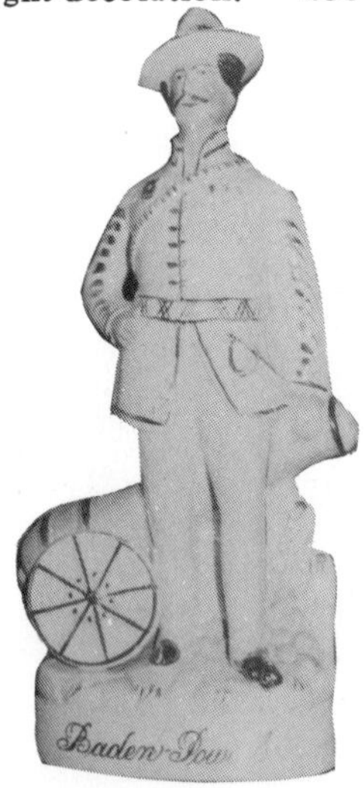

Staffordshire figure of Baden Powell with cannon, 22in. high. £150

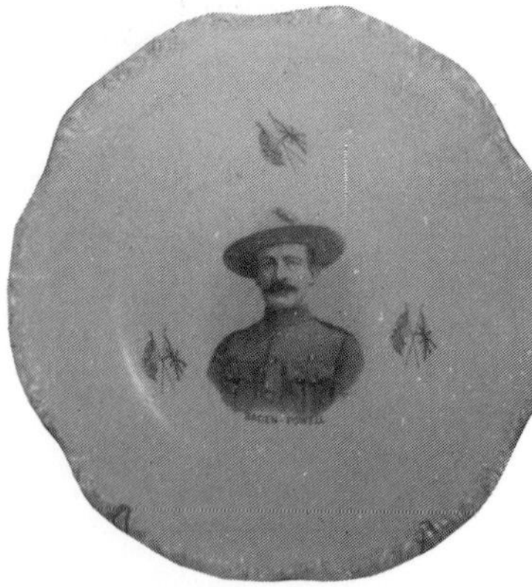

Shaped edge Staffordshire plate featuring Baden Powell. £20 – £25

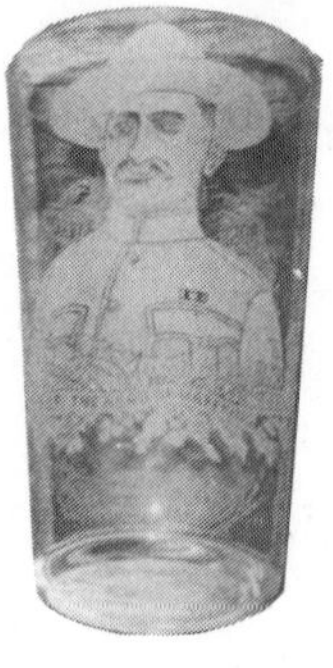

'Mountain Dew' Scotch whisky glass by Robertson, Sanderson & Co., Leith. £15

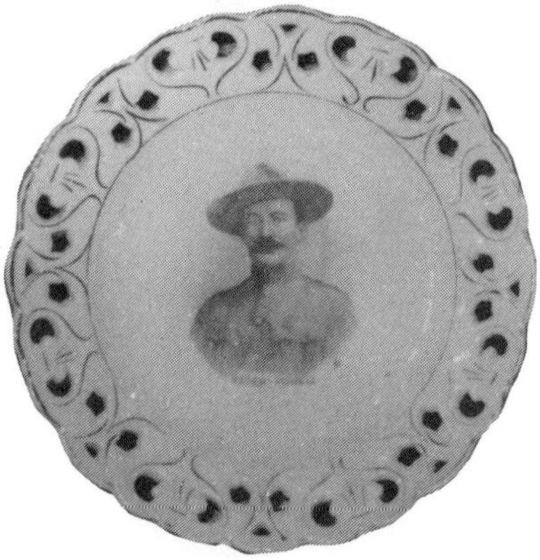

Staffordshire ribbon plate bearing a portrait of Baden Powell. £40

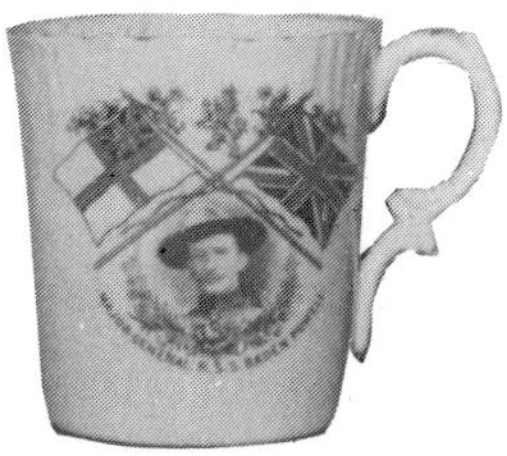

Staffordshire cup depicting Major General R. S. S. Baden Powell. £25

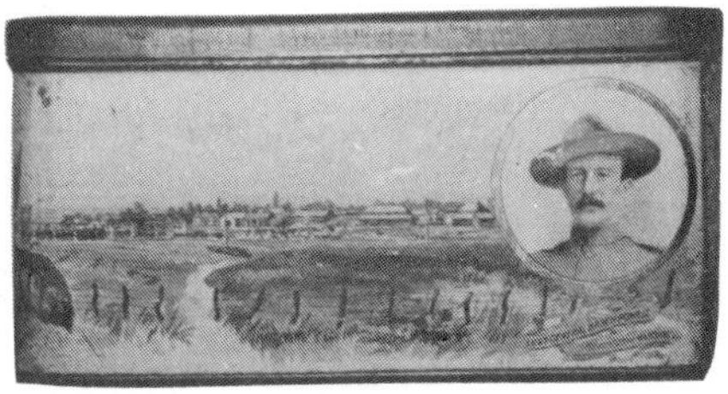

Colourful biscuit tin with 'View of Mafeking and Baden Powell', in brown and blue. £20

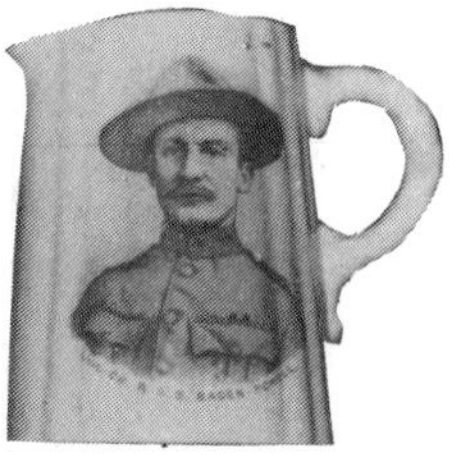

Small Staffordshire fluted cream jug with portrait of Baden Powell. £15 – £20

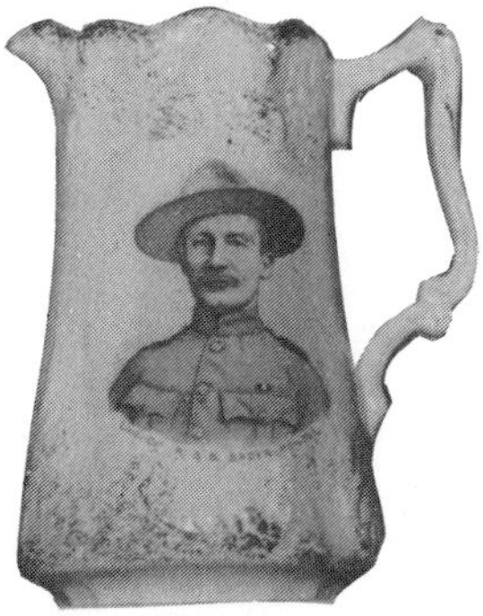

Staffordshire milk jug with gilt decoration and portrait of Baden Powell. £15 – £20

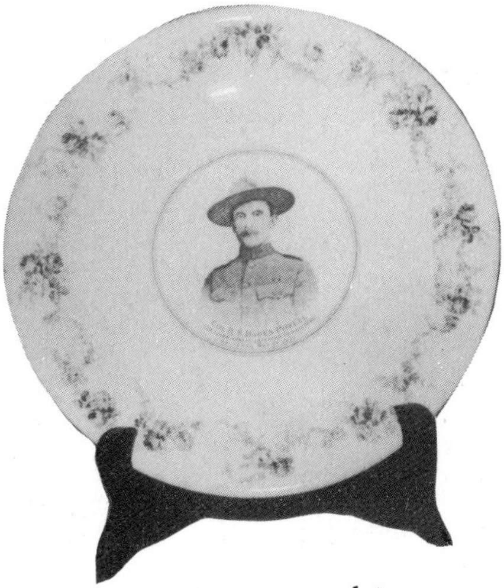

Royal Worcester plate featuring Col. R. S. S. Baden Powell, decorated with garlands of flowers. £40

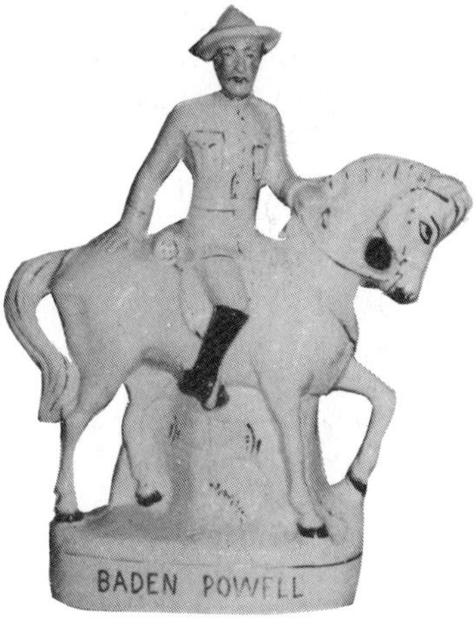

Staffordshire equestrian figure of Baden Powell, 14in. high. £75 – £100

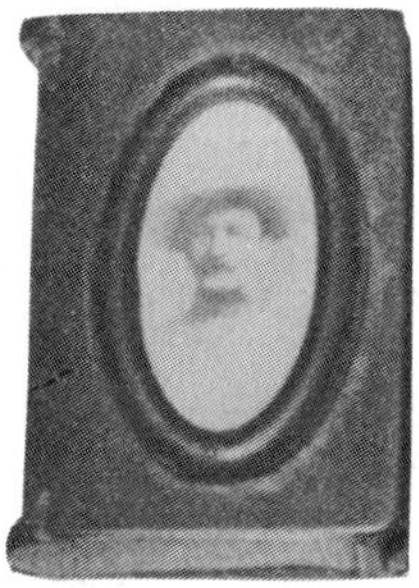

Vesta case with sepia photograph of Baden Powell, by Elliot & Fry. £12

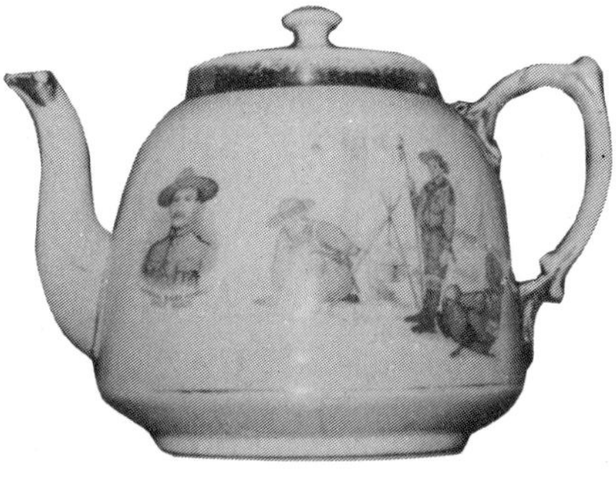

An unusual teapot featuring Baden Powell in Boer War uniform together with scouts in a camping scene. £35

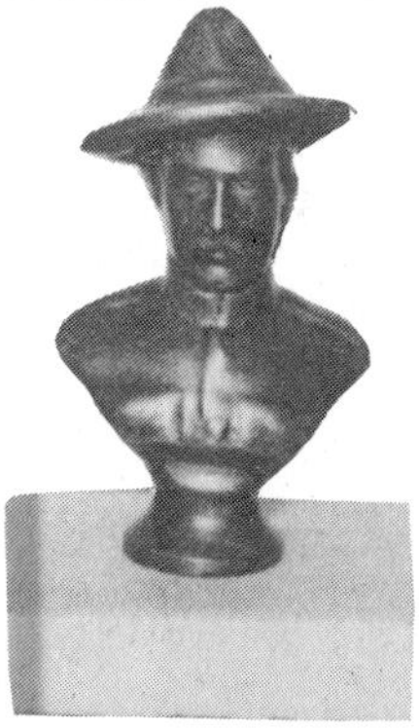

Brass bust of Baden Powell on a marble plinth, 3in. high. £35 – £40

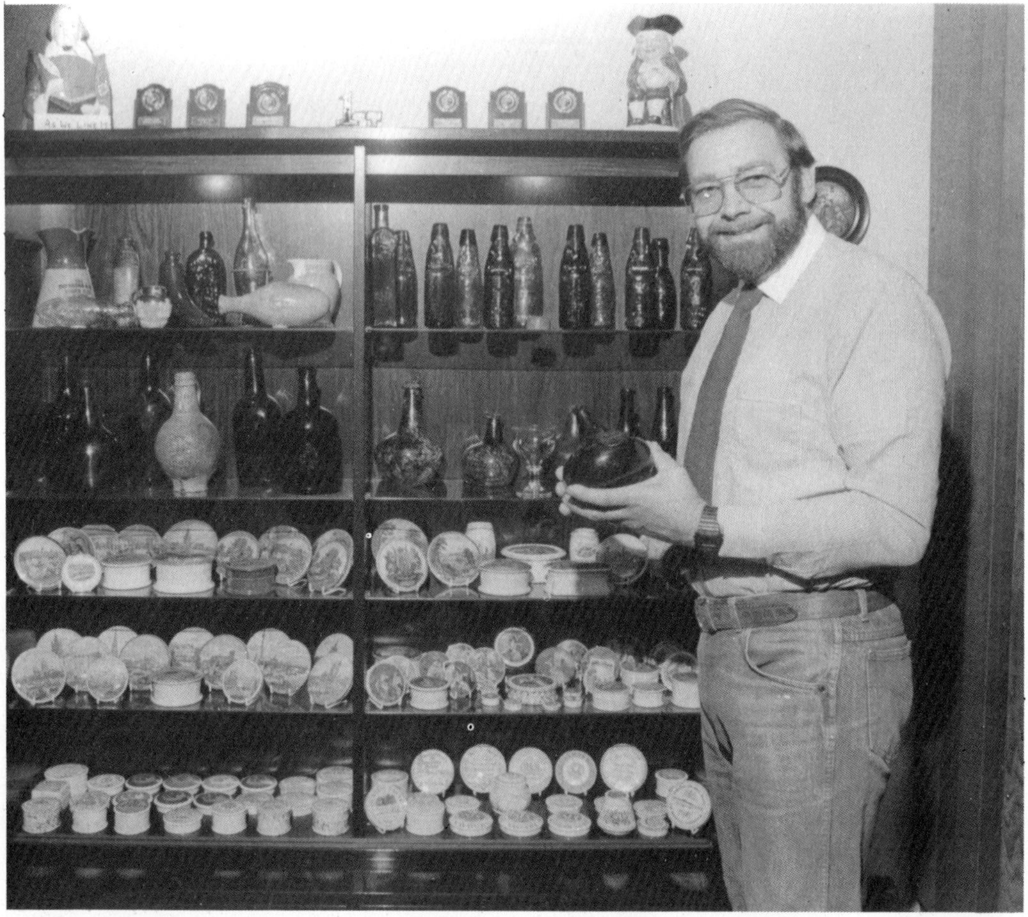

Trevor King is a supplier of educational play equipment and collects anchovy pot lids.

"My wife dug one up on a dump, in fact it was the first one she ever dug and it turned out to be a lid for a pot of Burgess's anchovy paste, one of the commoner lids you can find. It and Wood's Toothpaste are the two that turn up most frequently but the rarer ones are difficult to come by.

"Anchovy paste was very popular in Victorian times and the period for the lids is between 1850 and 1950 because Fortnum and Mason's were still selling the paste in decorated pots around the time of the Queen's coronation.

"When we started collecting the lids we decided to buy some of the paste to try it but

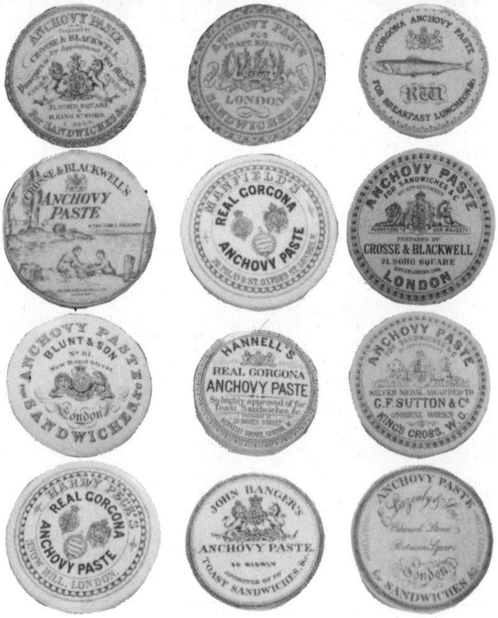

it was really horrible. The mystery for me is how the Victorians managed to consume it in such vast quantities. Taste must have changed a lot since then.

"There are 47 lids in my collection and the one I like best is a coloured lid decorated with flags and the Royal coat of arms which was put out by a çompany called J. N. Osborn. It is a Prattware lid.

"I know of about 10 lids that I still haven't got and the one that I'd like to find is another coloured one with flags for Thorne's Inimitable Anchovy paste."

Collecting anchovy paste lids is a restricted field of pot collecting and Trevor would expect to pay between £2.50 for a Burgess's lid and up to around £200 for an Osborn lid.

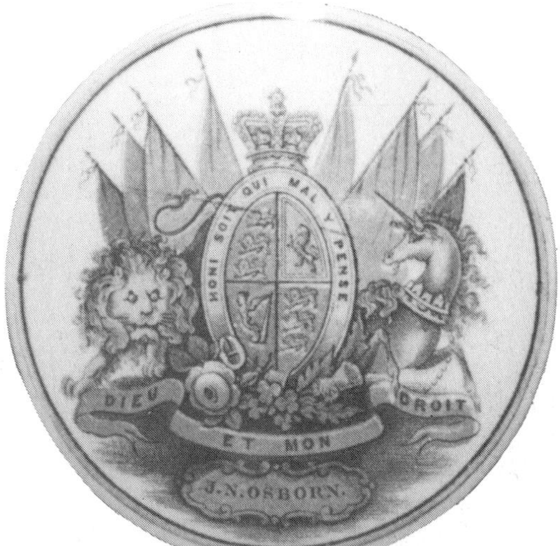

Rare lid by J. N. Osborn with the design in pastel shades of blue and red on a white background. *£250*

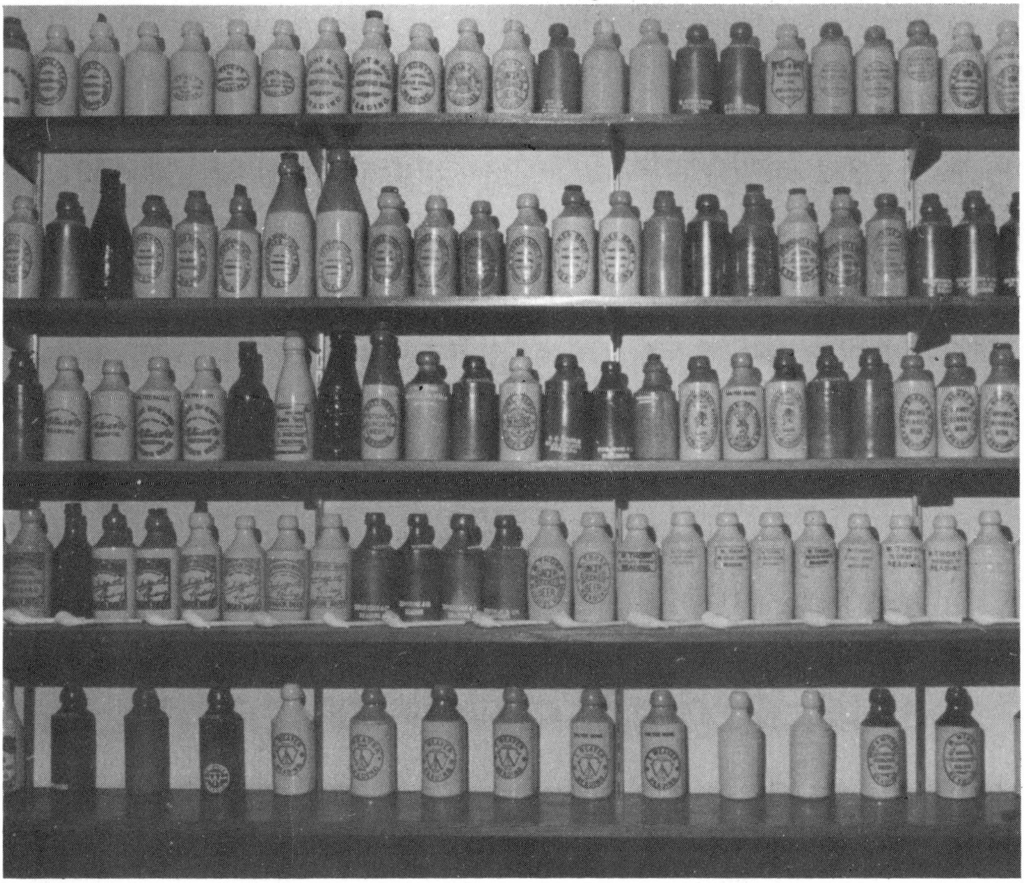

Another of Trevor's interests is collecting ginger beer bottles, all retrieved while diving in the River Kennet or the Thames.

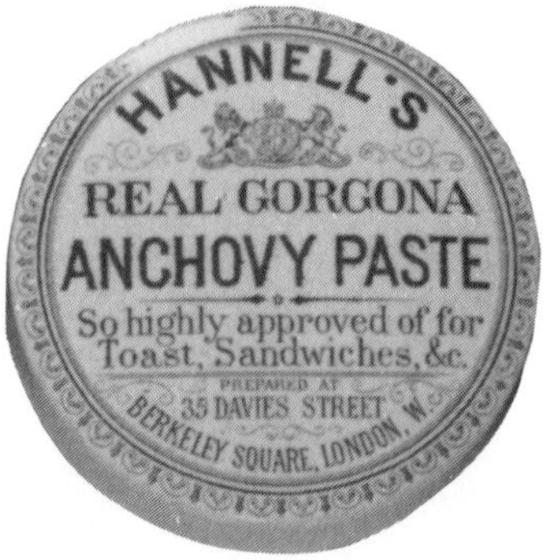

Hannell's Real Gorgona anchovy paste lid, 35 Davies Street, Berkeley Square, London. £12 – £15

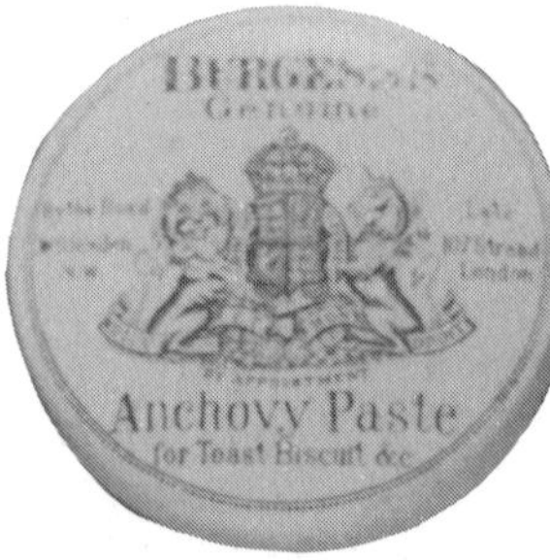

Edward VII lid by Burgess's, Hythe Rd., Willesden, London. £8

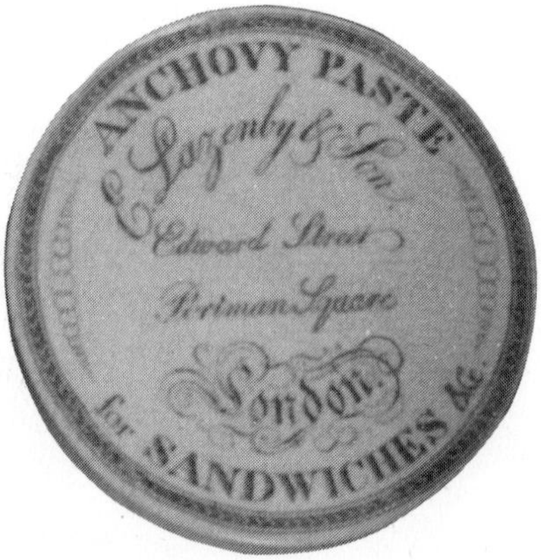

E. Lazenby & Son lid, Edward Street, Portman Square, London. £20 – £25

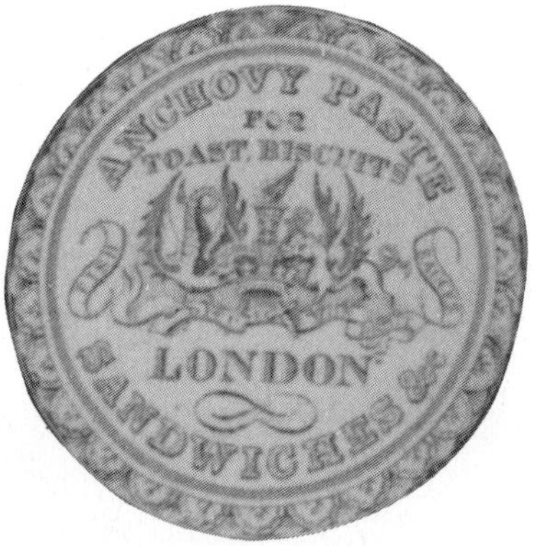

'London' lid printed in black on a white background. £18 – £20

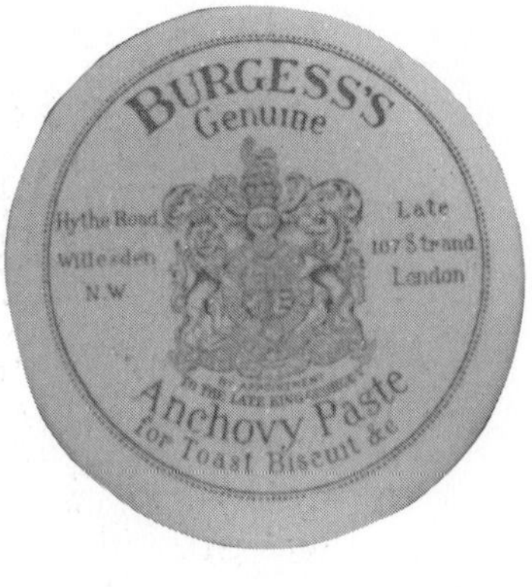

George V anchovy paste lid by Burgess's, Hythe Road, Willesden, N.W. £12

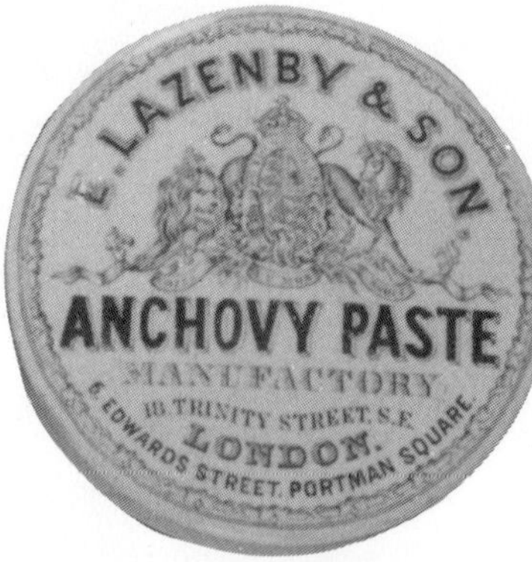

Small lid by E. Lazenby & Son of London, bearing the word 'Manufactory'. £15 – £18

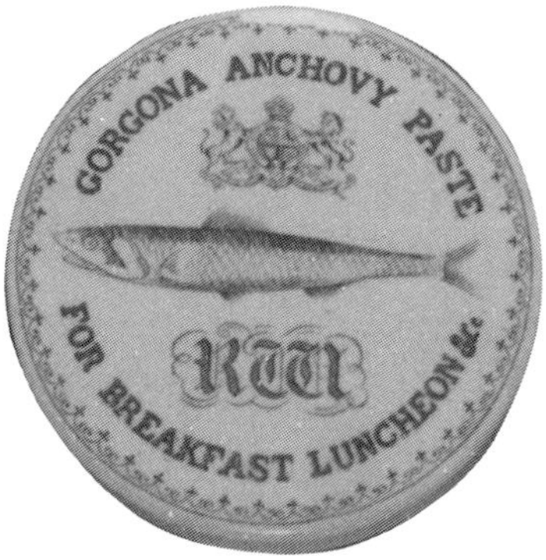

Gorgona anchovy paste lid by R.T.N., printed in black on a white background. £20 – £25

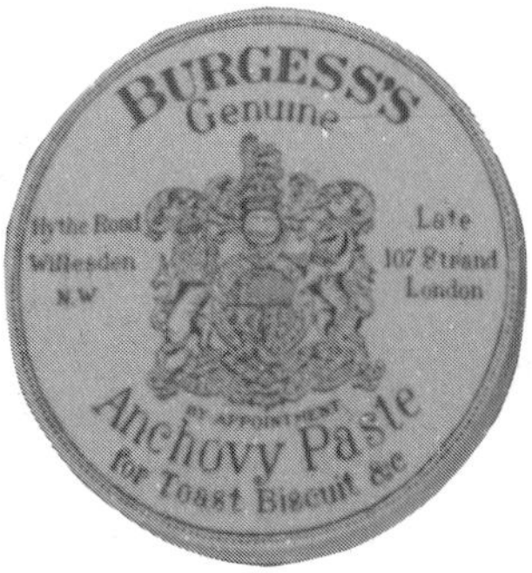

George V anchovy paste lid by Burgess's, Hythe Road, Willesden, N.W., late 107 Strand, London. £2

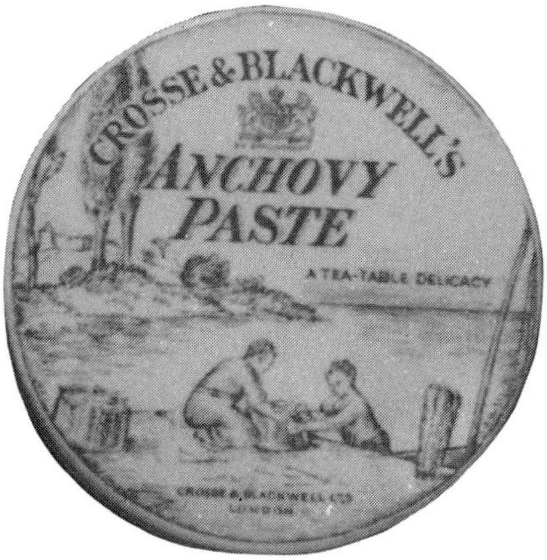

A pictorial lid by Crosse & Blackwell, in sepia on a white background. £35

Real Gorgona anchovy paste lid by Harry Peck's, Snow Hill, London. £10 – £12

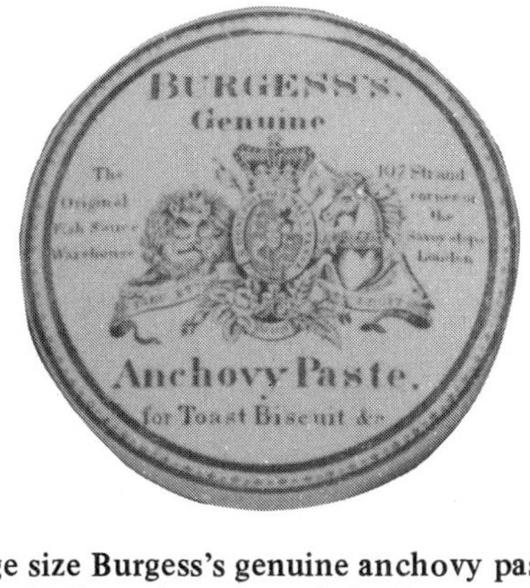

Large size Burgess's genuine anchovy paste lid, '107 Strand, corner of the Savoy steps.' £10 – £12

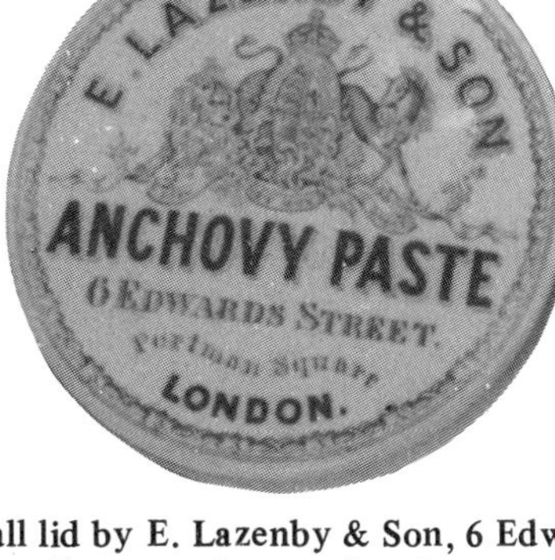

Small lid by E. Lazenby & Son, 6 Edwards Street, Portman Square, London. £12 – £15

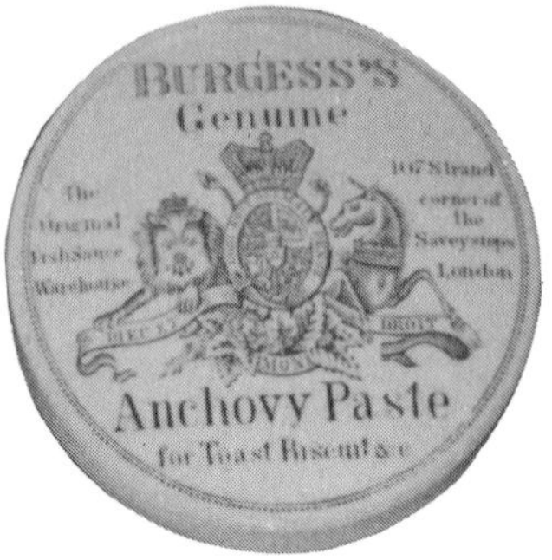

Anchovy paste lid by Burgess's, 'The Original Fish Sauce Warehouse'. £5 – £6

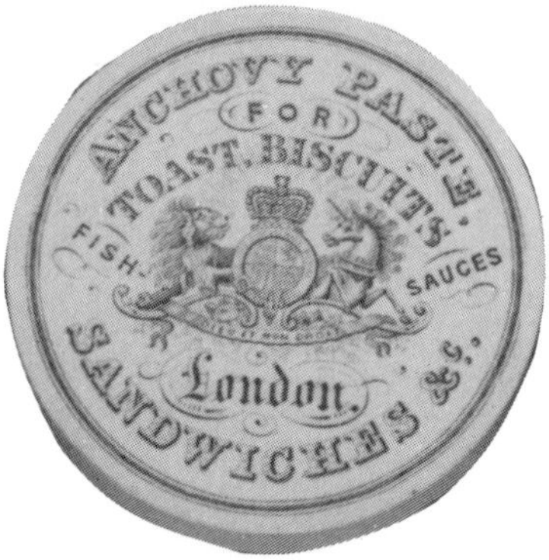

Anchovy paste lid referred to as 'London Lid', with no maker's name. £25 – £30

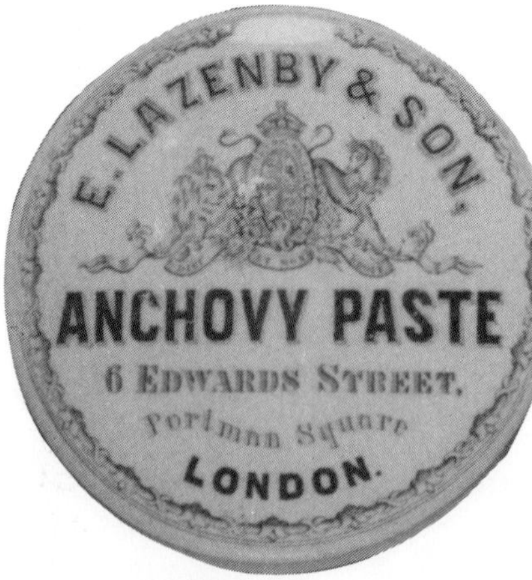

A large anchovy paste lid by E. Lazenby, 6 Edwards Street, Portman Square, London.
£15 – £20

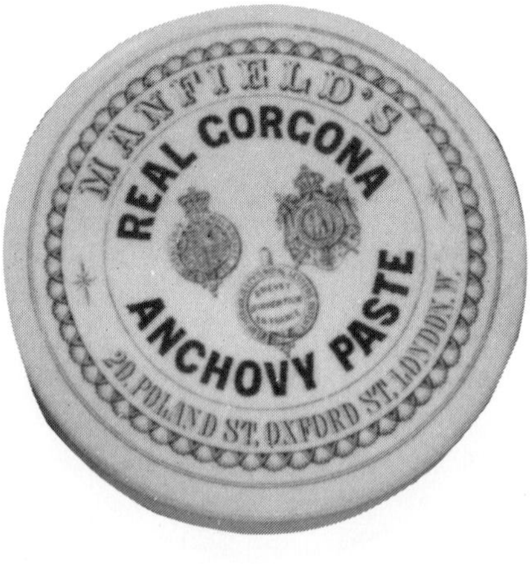

Real Gorgona anchovy paste lid by Manfield's, 20 Poland St., Oxford Street, London. £15 – £20

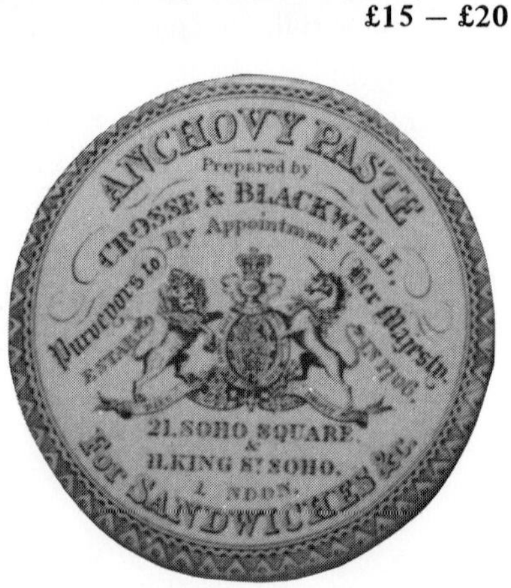

Early 1860's lid by Crosse & Blackwell, 21 Soho Square and Ilking St., Soho.
£25 – £30

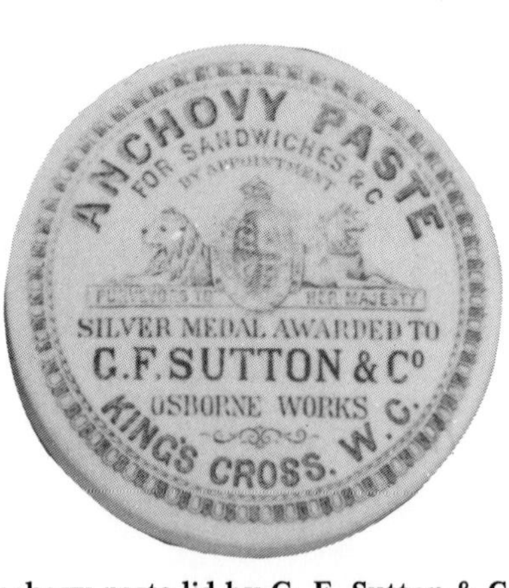

Anchovy paste lid by G. F. Sutton & Co., Osborne Works, King's Cross, W.C.
£8 – £10

Small lid by G. F. Sutton, Sons & Co., Osborne Works, Brandon Road, King's Cross. £8

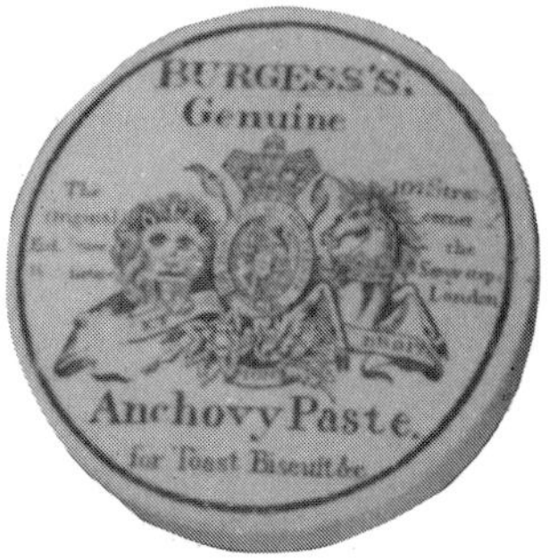

Burgess's anchovy paste lid, 'The Original Fish Sauce Warehouse'. £5 – £6

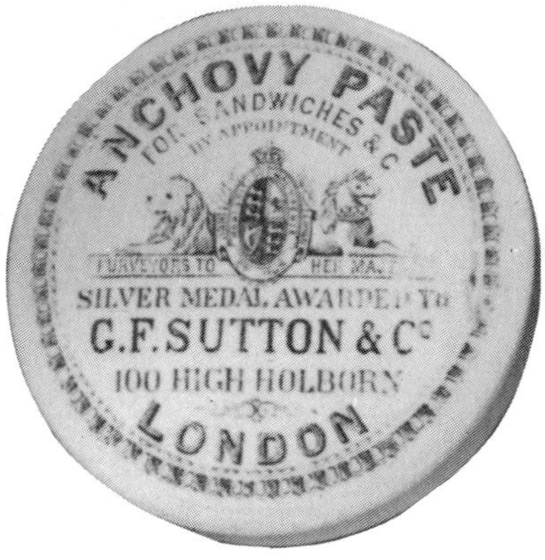

Anchovy paste lid by G. F. Sutton & Co., 100 High Holborn, London. £8 – £10

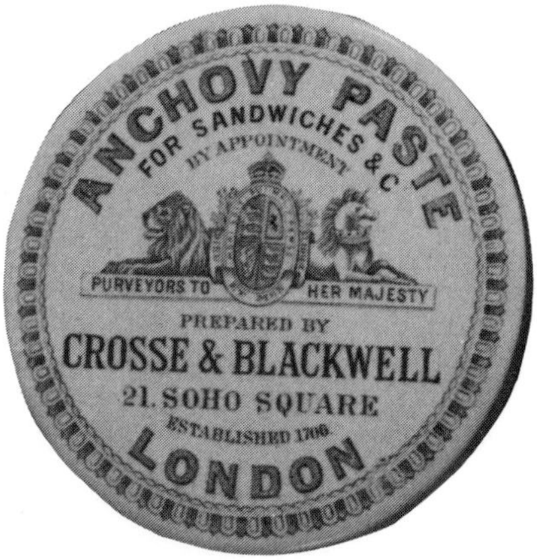

Crosse & Blackwell lid, 21 Soho Square, London, established 1706. £6 – £8

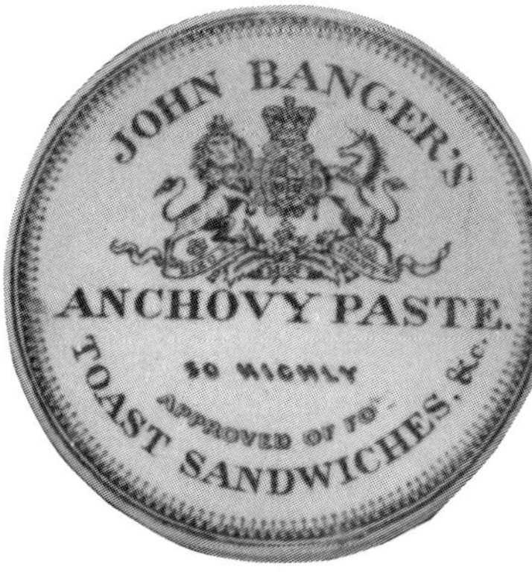

John Banger's anchovy paste lid, 'so highly approved of for toast sandwiches'. £8 – £10

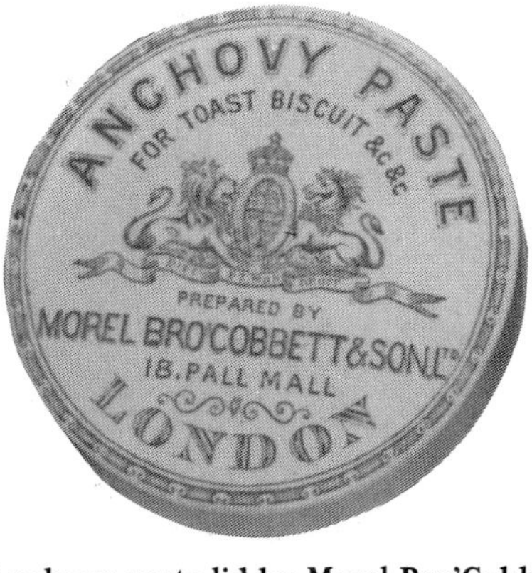

Anchovy paste lid by Morel Bro'Cobbett & Son Ltd., 18 Pall Mall, London. £12 – £15

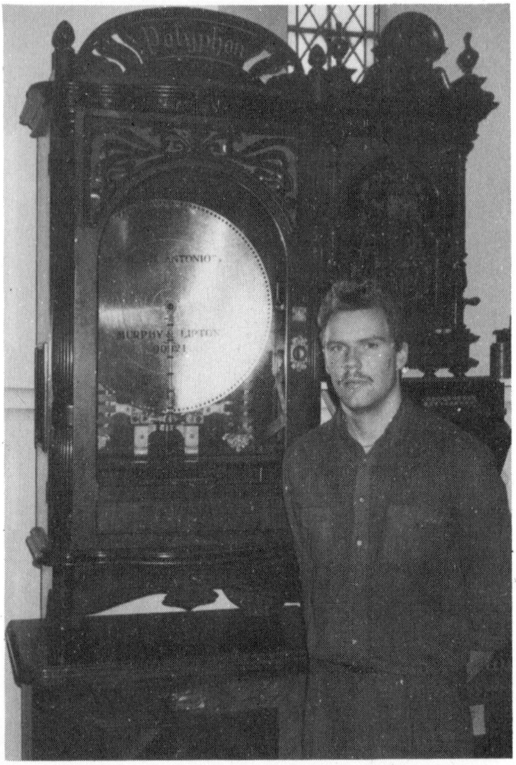

Lester Jones in the museum at Chichester standing beside an ornate 'Penny in the Slot' polyphon.

The Jones Family — Clive and Enid, the father and mother; Lester, the son and George the grandfather, all run the Mechanical Music and Doll Collection in Church Road, Portfield, Chichester.

Lester said:

"My grandfather George started collecting long case clocks and musical boxes about 45 years ago and from there he went on into all kinds of mechanical musical instruments. Now we've got at least 100 of them, all fully restored and playing as well as 100 dolls collected by my mother Enid. We used to be fishermen from Chichester going out for oysters and eels but four years ago we decided to open our own museum and now the two collections are housed in a redundant church which is very good for acoustics. It is open to the public as a museum.

"The musical instruments are mainly from the Victorian period and include things like phonographs, barrel organs, player pianos and fair organs. There's some examples of organs that used to play in cafes and the oldest one is a big barrel organ that was built in 1810 and was used in a stately home to provide music for dancing."

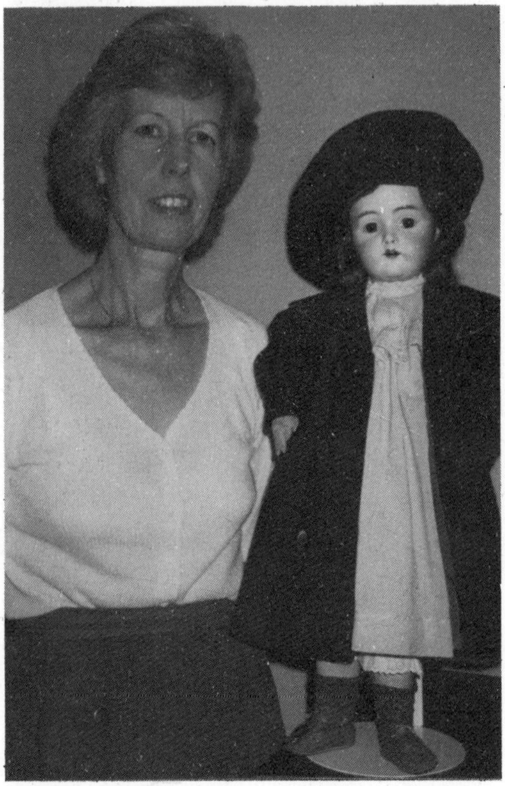

Enid Jones with a Simon & Halbig doll, circa 1900, valued at £300.

The Jones' family museum is open every day between 10 a.m. and 6 p.m. from Easter till September and on weekends only over the winter. Admission is £1 for adults and lower for OAP's and children.

Mrs Jones' collection of dolls date from 1789 to 1985 and they are all mainly china or bisque headed and dressed in the original costumes.

Lester is always looking around for new items for the museum but these are becoming increasingly difficult to find . . . "I've an Encyclopaedia of Mechanical Music and I'd like to have an example of everything in it — at least I keep hoping," he said.

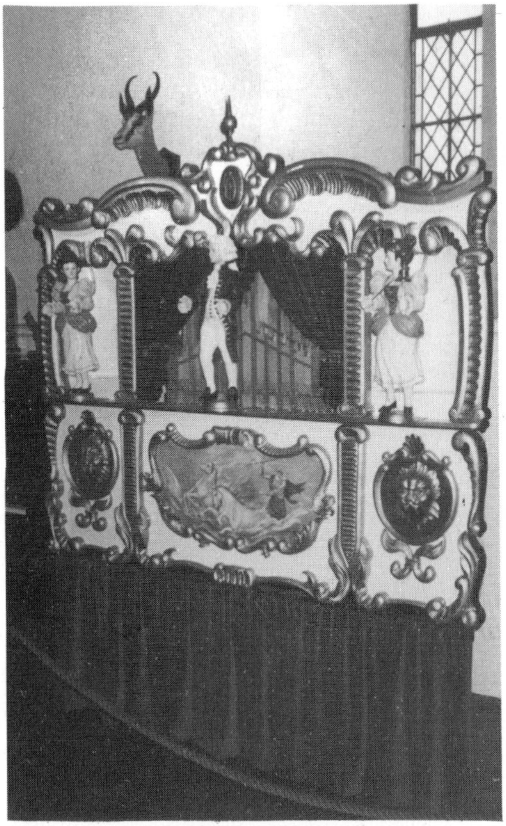

The 'Dean' organ made for the 'Mechanical Music and Doll Collection' in 1978.

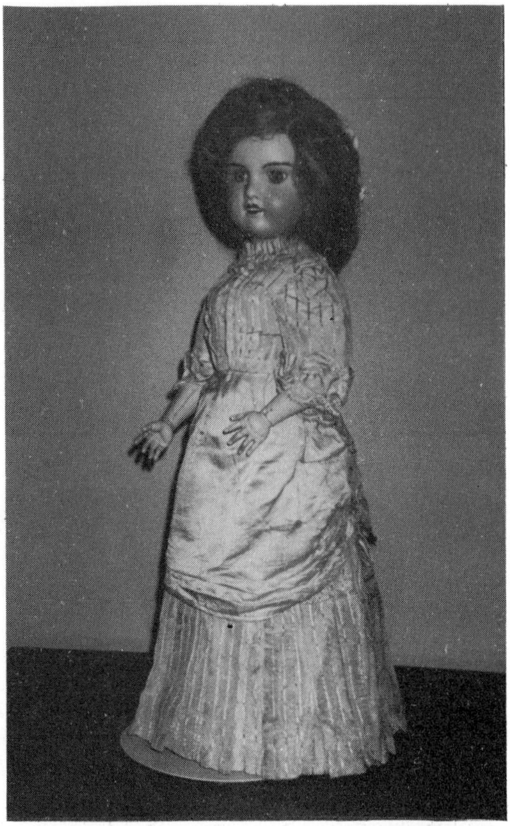

An S.F.B.J. doll with original clothes, circa 1899. £200

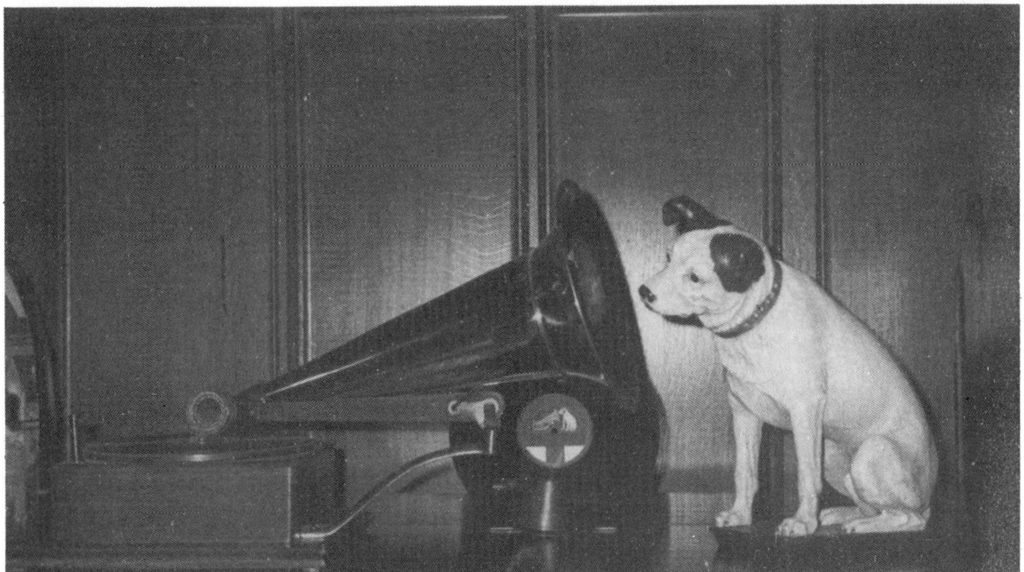

His Master's Voice Gramophone, circa 1900. £300

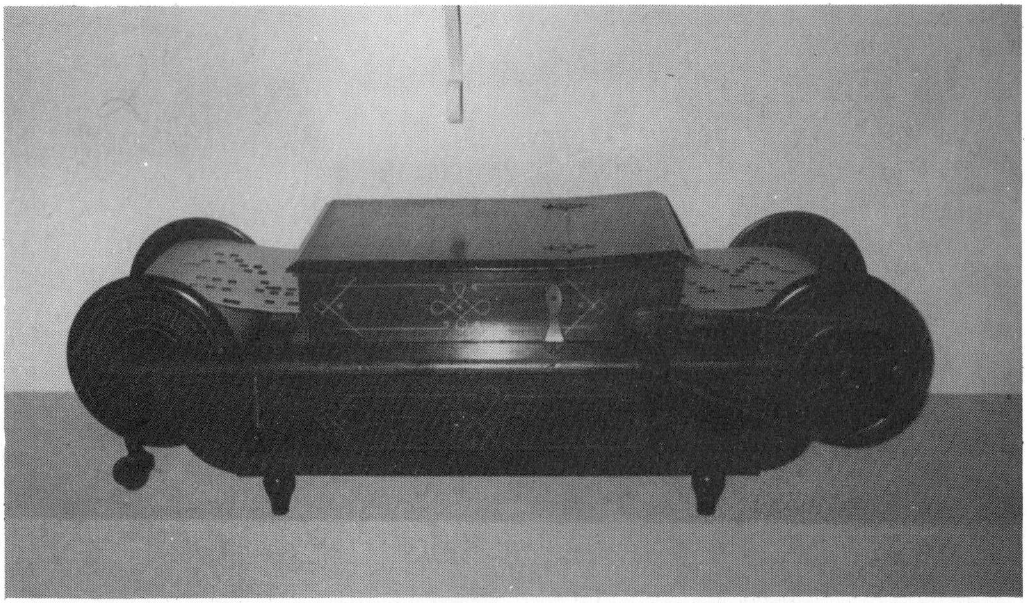

American Organette with paper roll, circa 1880. £250

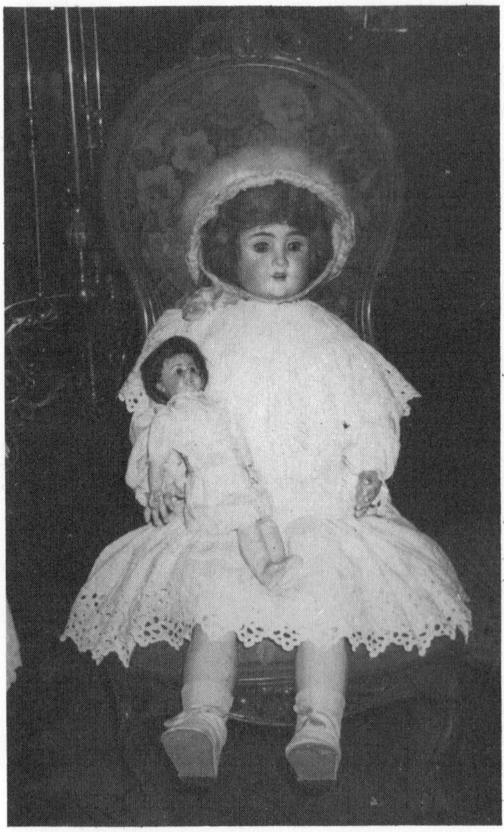

A fine Schoenau & Hoffmeister doll, circa 1900. £250

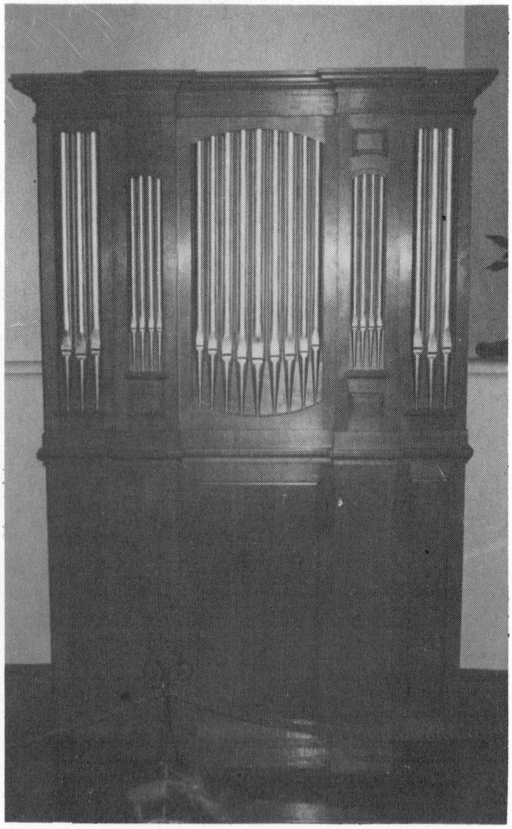

A large oak cased church barrel organ made in 1831. £2000

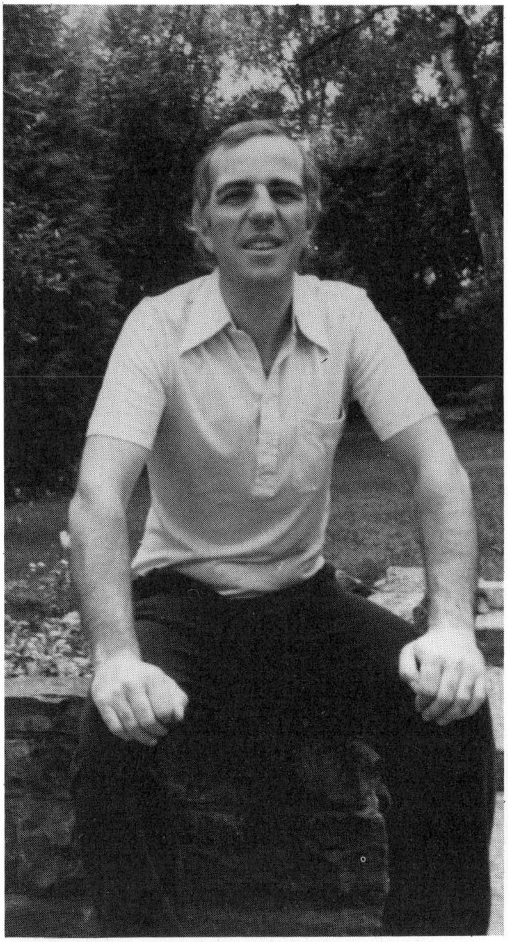

Geoffrey Wellsteed is a civil servant who collects cricketing pubs.

"I suppose that sounds a bit odd but in fact I'm planning to write a book about all the pubs connected with cricket that are scattered over Britain. Two years ago I noticed a pub called 'The Cricketers' which I pass on my way to work every day and I thought, 'There must be lots of pubs with cricket associations'.

"So I began spending each lunch hour in the reference room of the public library looking them up in the Yellow Pages. It took me about two months and there are hundreds of them.

"Some are called 'The Cricketers' or 'The Cricketers' Arms', 'Cricketers' Rest', 'Royal Cricket', 'Bat and Ball', 'The Three Willows', 'Ball and Cricket' or 'Toad and Stumps'. I catalogue them by county and to date I've managed to visit about 100 of them.

"I talk to the landlord and usually manage to get some stories about the pub's history or its association with a famous cricketer. Then I get beer mats, menu cards, ashtrays, winelists, serviettes or post cards of the various pubs. I also take photographs for my archives."

Geoffrey finds his hobby is a marvellous way of getting round the country and says his wife is very tolerant about going on twenty mile detours to find a special pub. The majority of cricketing pubs are concentrated in Berkshire, Surrey, Hampshire and Essex, the heartland of cricket. He is currently looking for a publisher for his book which will be both a pictorial and a written record of cricketing pubs.

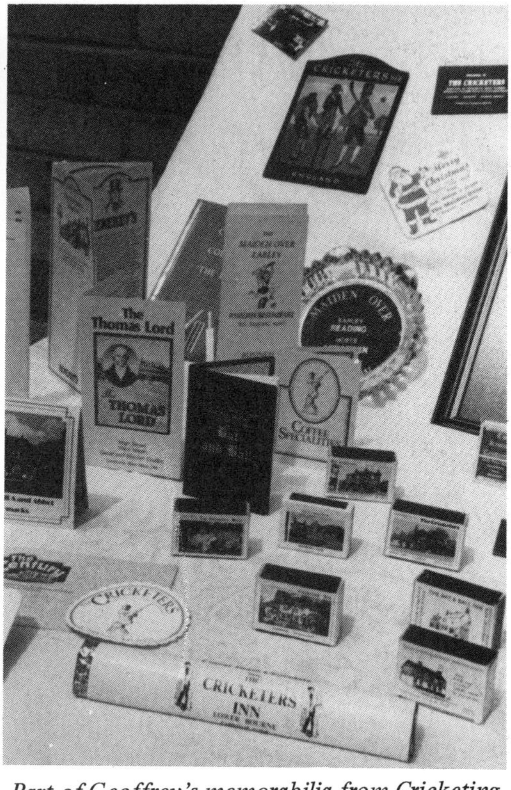

Part of Geoffrey's memorabilia from Cricketing Pubs.

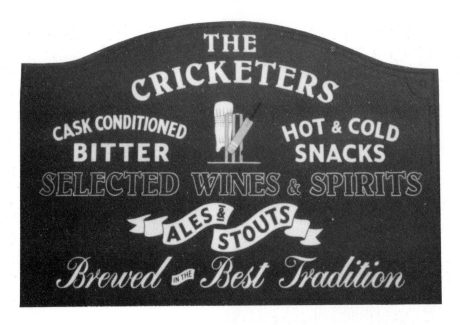

The Cricketers 'Selected Wines & Spirits'.

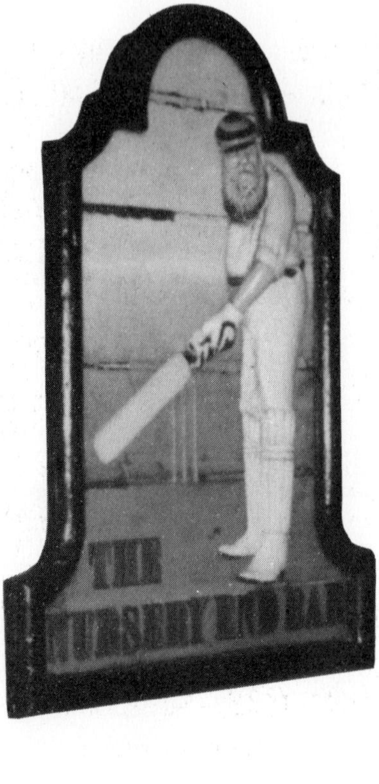

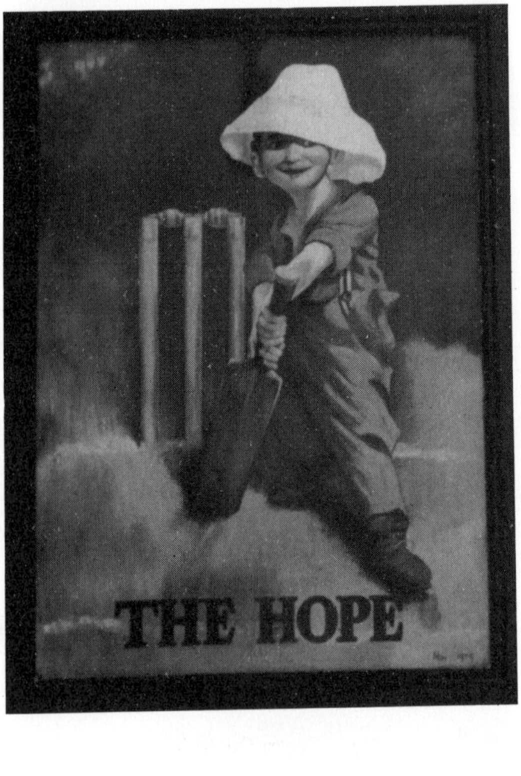

The Nursery End Bar.

The Hope.

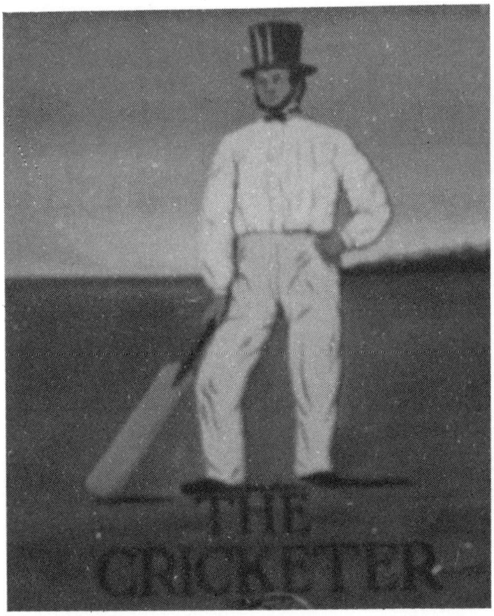

The Cricketer.

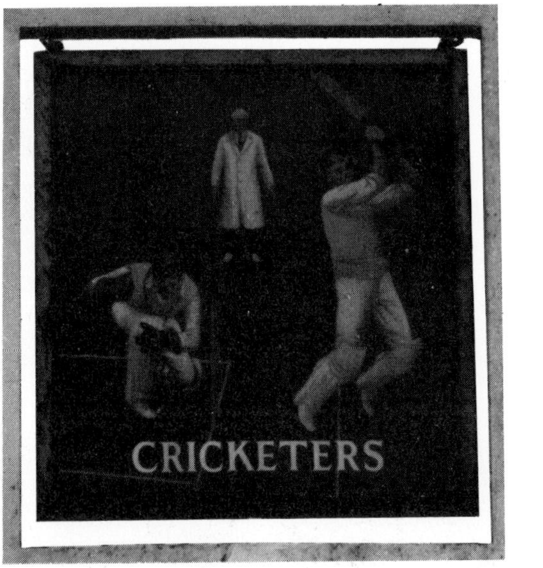

The Cricketers.

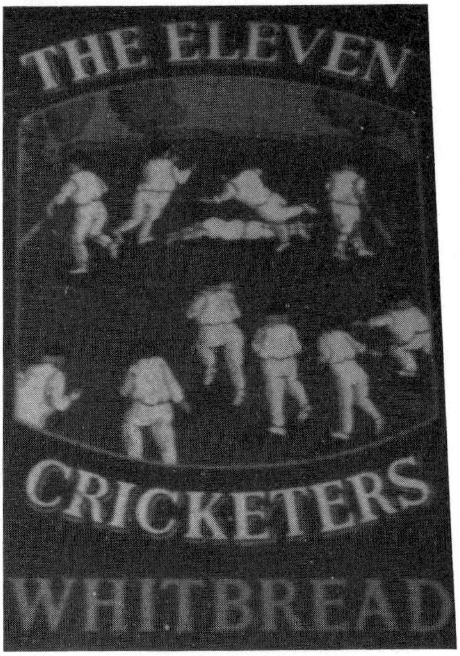

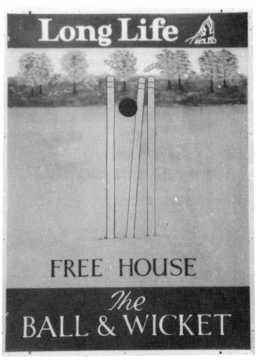

The Eleven Cricketers.

The Ball & Wicket.

An interesting selection of Cricketing Pub signs.

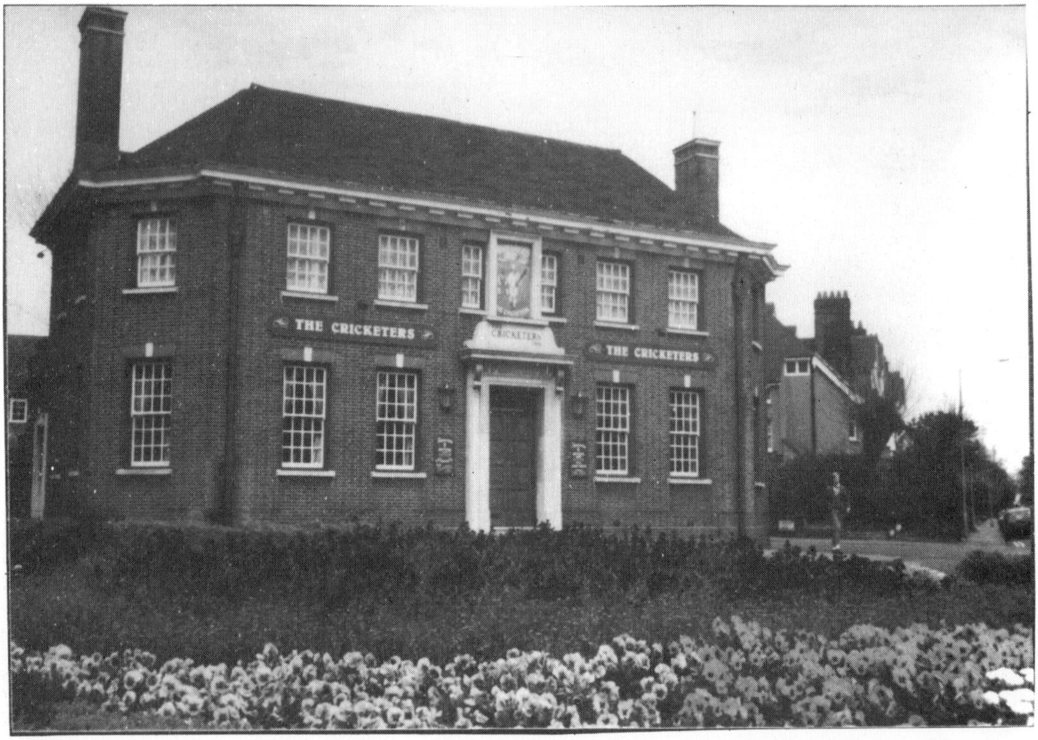

The Cricketers.

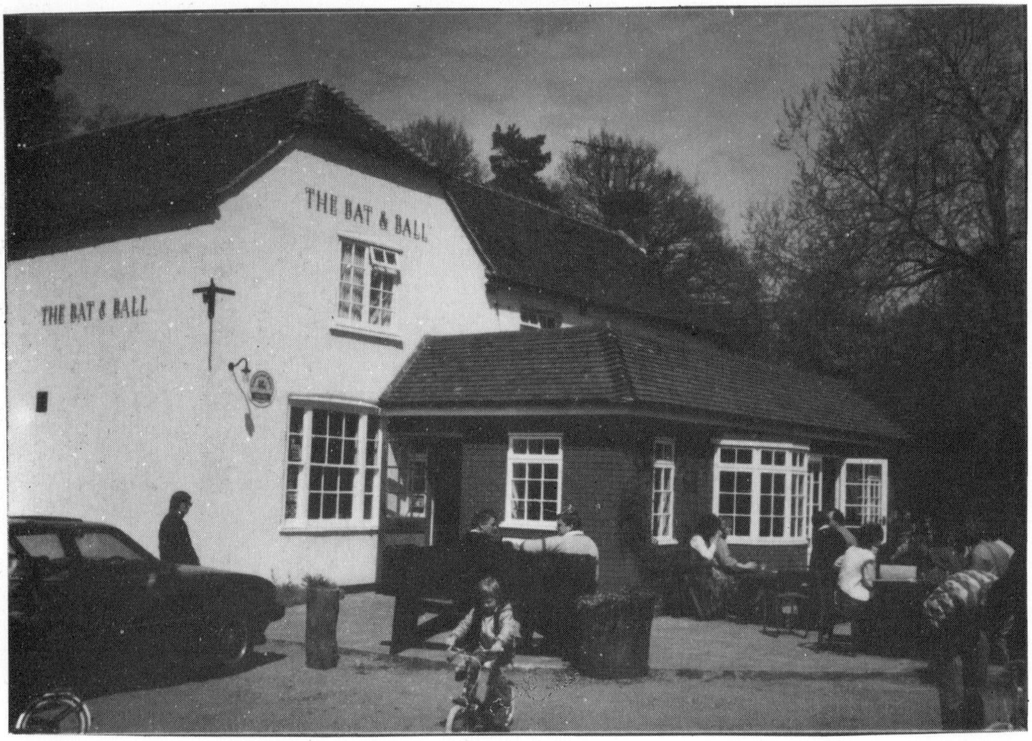

The Bat & Ball.

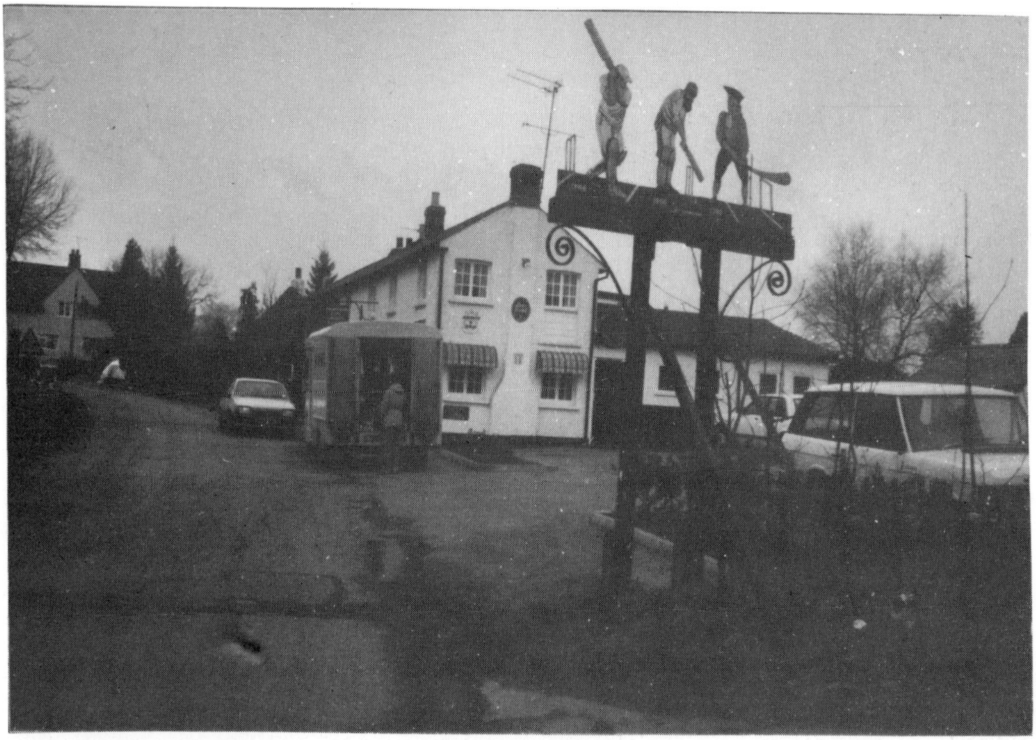

The Three Willows.

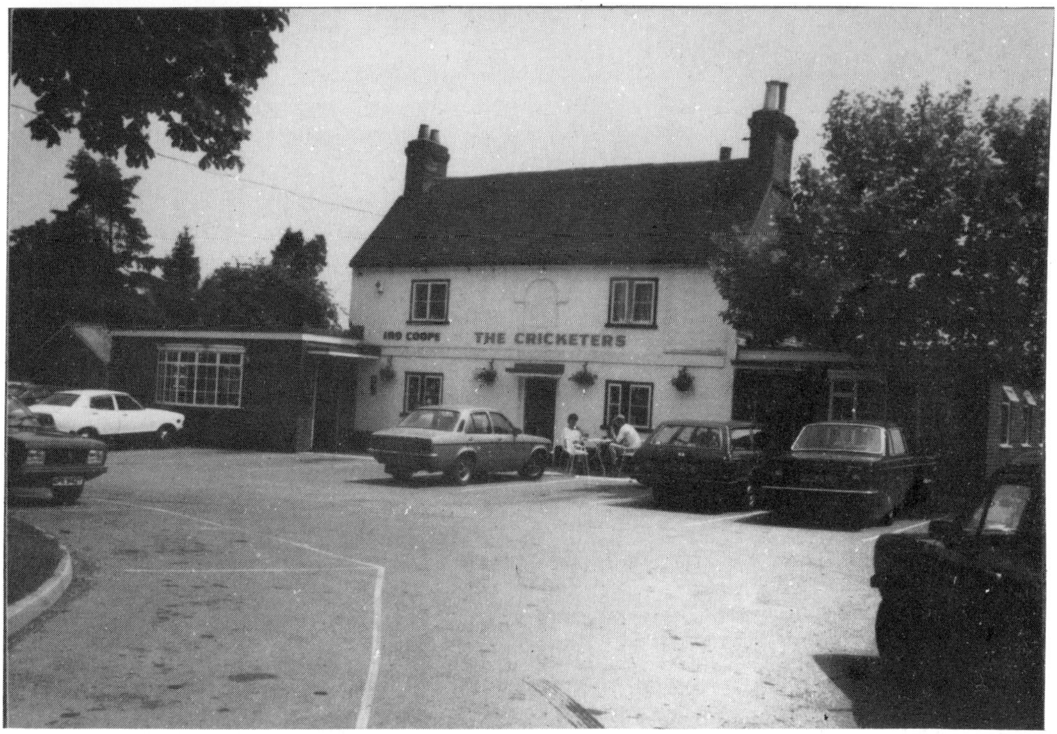

The Cricketers.
A few of the hundreds of Cricketing Pubs researched by Geoffrey Wellsteed.

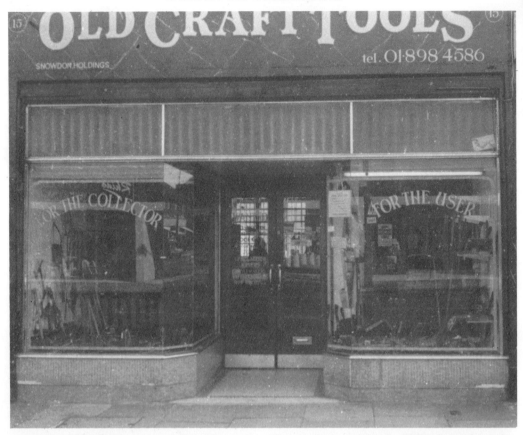

Danny Loftus buys and sells old woodworking tools.

"I've always got between 400 and 500 different old tools in my shop at any one time and they include braces, planes and emblems particularly rare French ones used for fixing brass. Prices vary from around £5,000 for a plane that once belonged to King Olaf of Norway to the average example which sells for between £300 and £400.

"Good woodworking tools are things of beauty and because of that there are several very knowledgeable women as well as men among the collectors who come to me regularly."

Danny said that there is no written history of woodworking tools before 1750 though many items which come up for sale almost certainly pre-date that period. Among the most famous makers' names is Edward Preston, a firm that operated first in Birmingham around 1820 but then in London between 1830 and 1948. Another very collectible maker is Norris, also of London, which began in the 1840's and finally collapsed a century later. Norris tools are of a very high standard and one of their more common planes will make an average £200 today though some of the more select examples go up as high as £1,000. Another rare plane by a maker called Mealing, who is thought to have been working around 1720, recently sold for £800 though it was badly affected with woodworm.

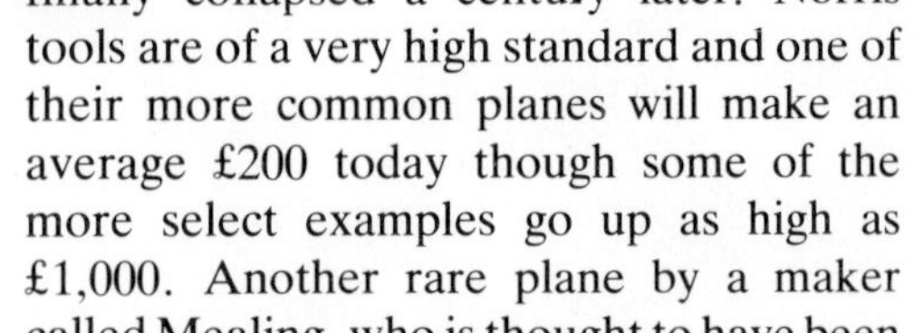

A chair maker's wooden brace. £65 – £90

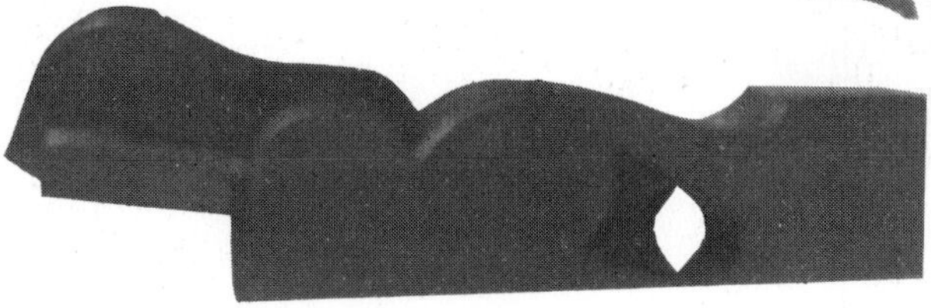

All steel shoulder plane. £45 – £75

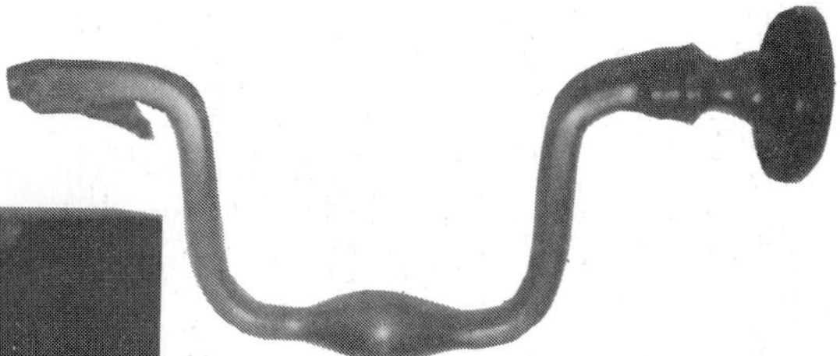

An iron lever action brace with brass neck. £40 – £60

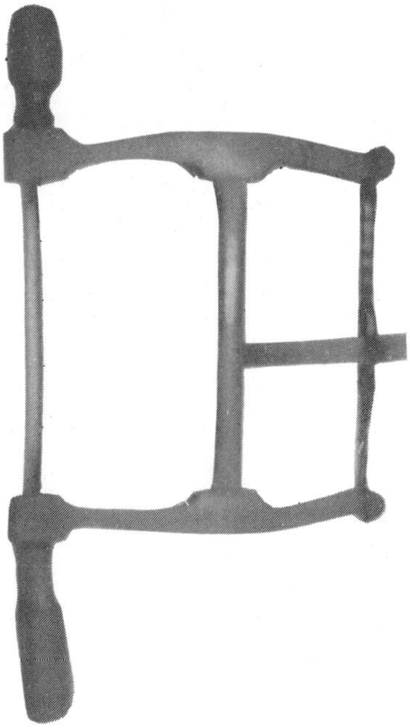

A miniature bow saw. £25 – £38

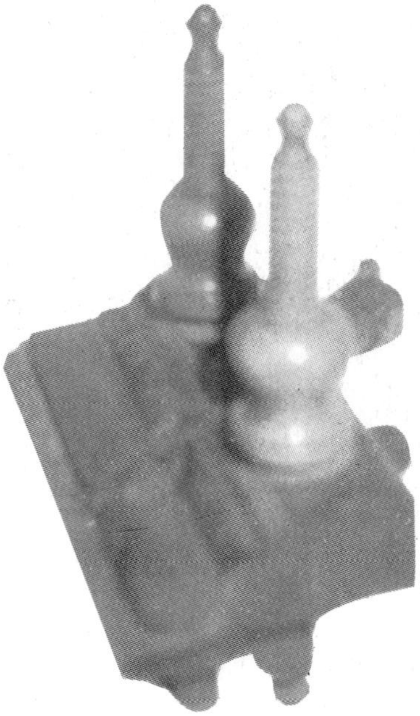

Plough plane with boxwood screw stems and holding nuts. £20 – £40

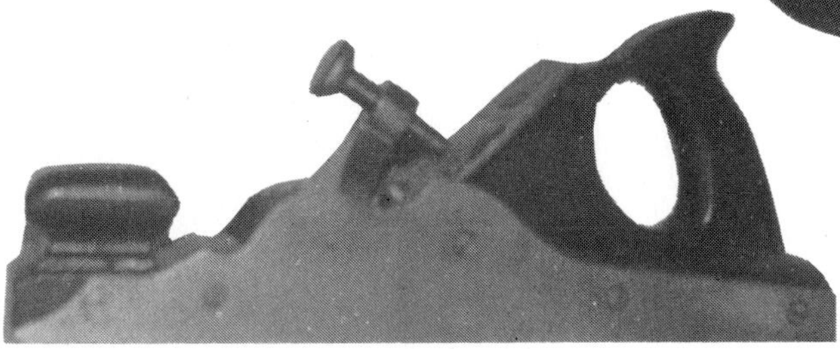

Ebony filled steel jack or panel plane. £80 – £160

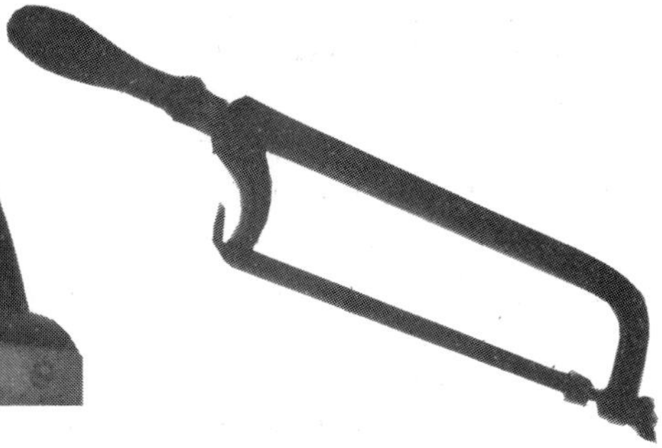

An unusually large Lancashire pattern hack saw. £15 – £25

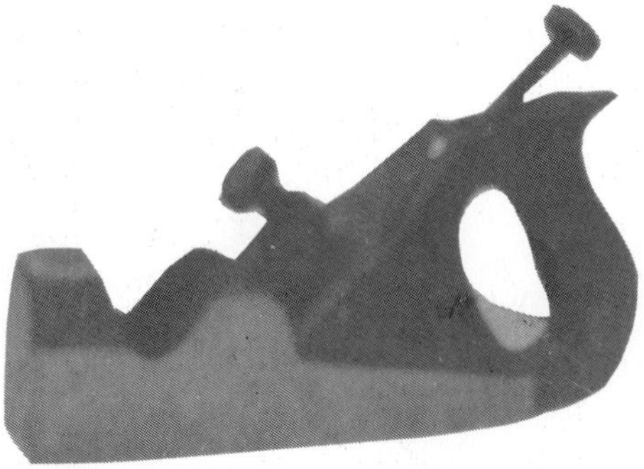

Stewart Spiers parallel dovetail smoothing plane. £50 – £100

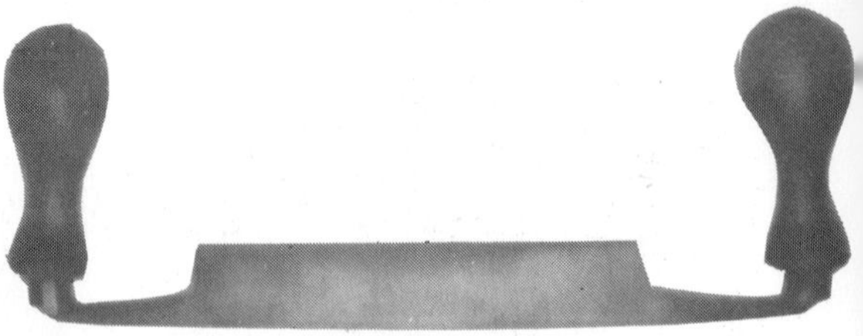

A small draw knife with boxwood handles. £10 – £20

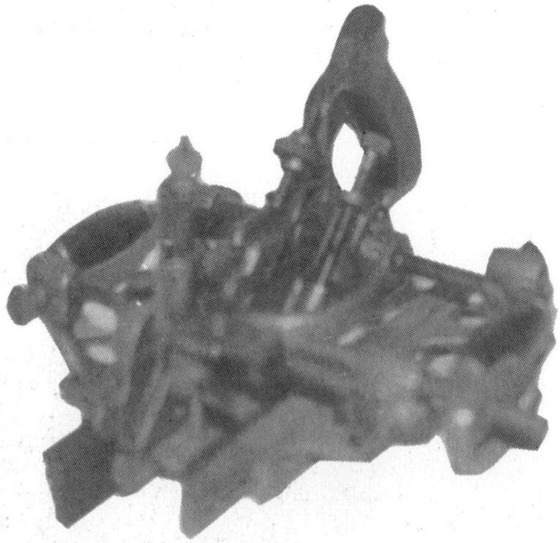

A Stanley '55' with cutters, in good condition. £180 – £280

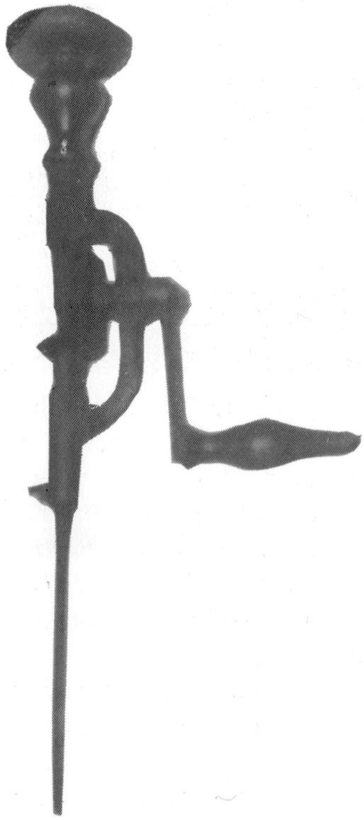

An unusual wheel brace. £40 – £60

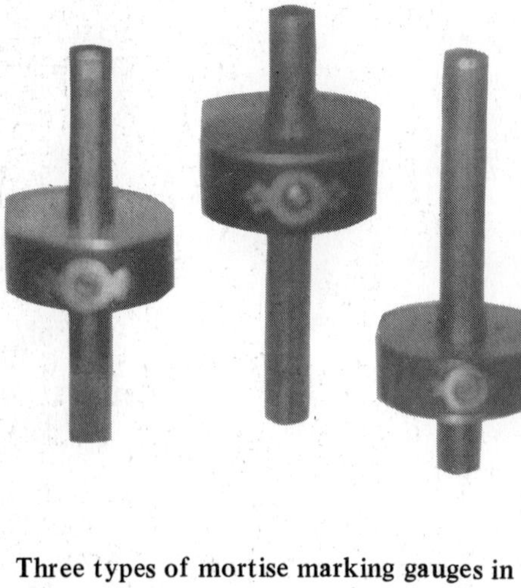

Three types of mortise marking gauges in ebony and boxwood, brass fronted. £20 – £30

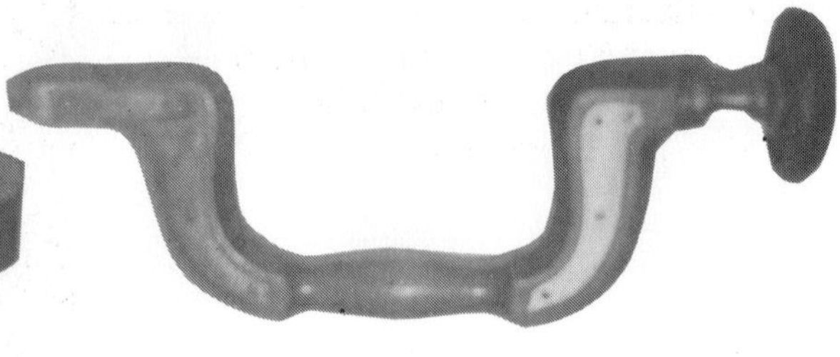

Button pad, plated beechwood brace. £40 – £65

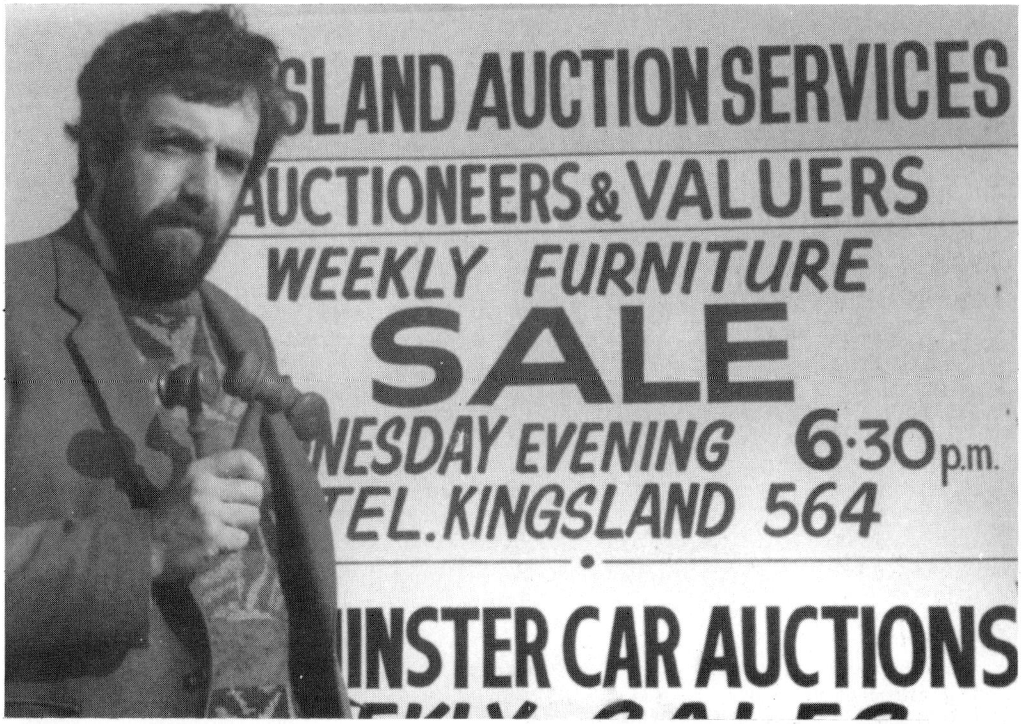

Mark Stafford-Lovatt has been involved in Auctioneering in one way or another, since an early age.

He came into the business when he left school and as his interest grew and his knowledge developed he went on to become an antiques dealer specialising in porcelain.

Nowadays he is Chief Auctioneer and Manager of Kingsland Auction Services near Leominster in Herefordshire, a busy and well run weekly country auction.

Mark has a varied and interesting collection of all kinds of artefacts to do with auctioneering which he displays in his office and would be pleased to hear from anyone with a similar interest with a view to exchanging information.

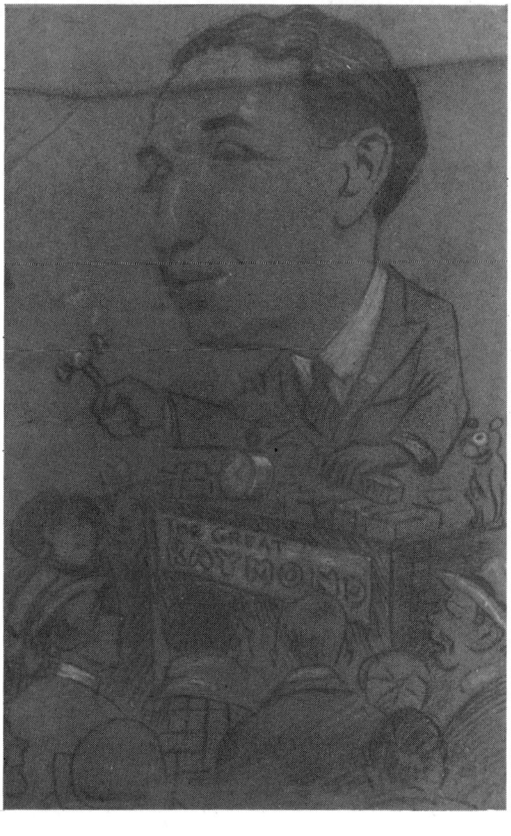

Caricature auctioneering study of 'The Great Raymond', by Kane, charcoal heightened with chalk, 1930's. £35

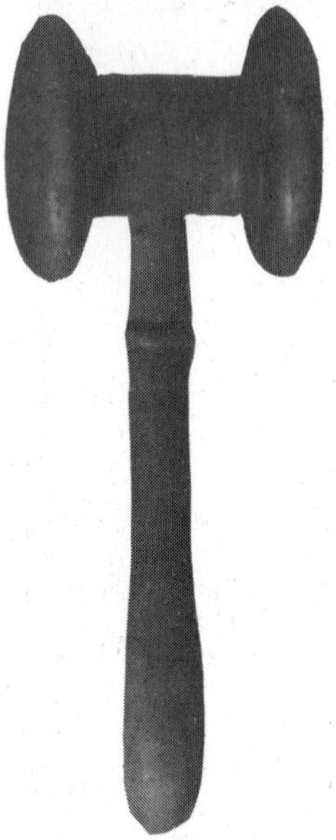

Victorian mahogany gavel with large turned head. £22

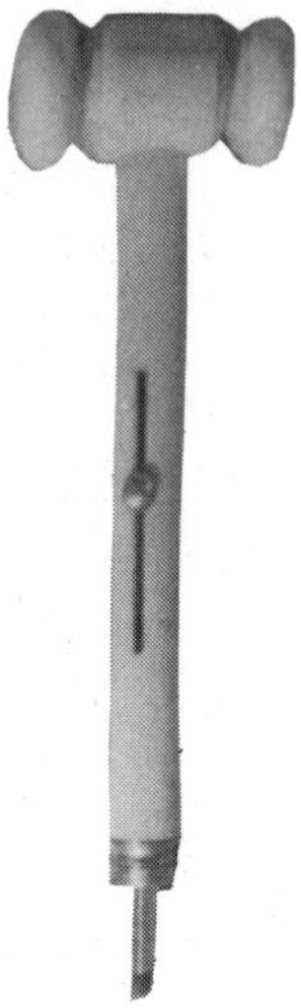

Small ivory gavel with sliding pencil in the handle, circa 1900. £20

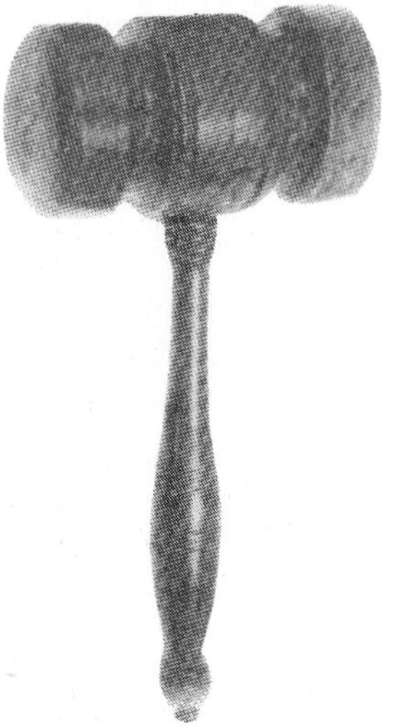

Mid 19th century lignum vitae gavel with turned head and handle. £75

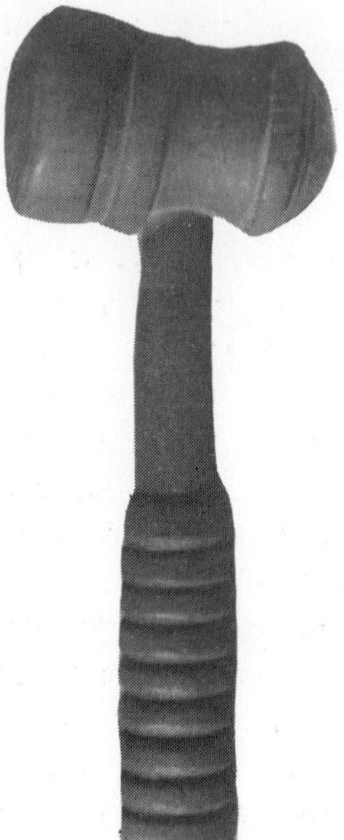

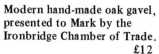

Modern hand-made oak gavel, presented to Mark by the Ironbridge Chamber of Trade. £12

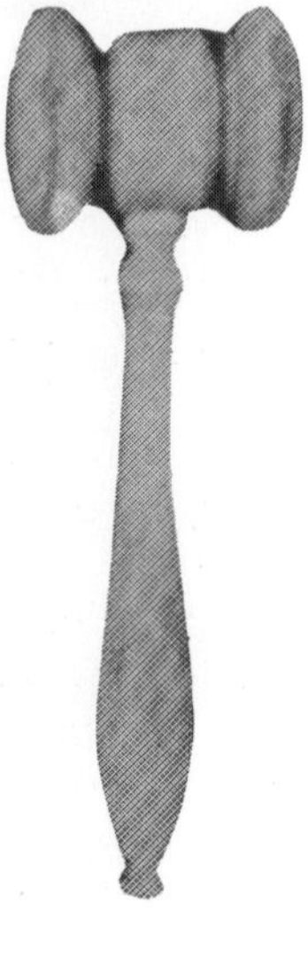

Late 19th century turned ivory gavel, 6in. long. £75

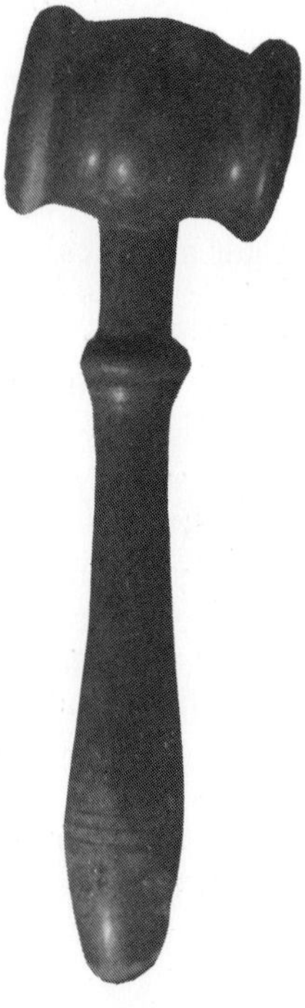

A nicely coloured mahogany gavel with turned head and handle, circa 1907. £14

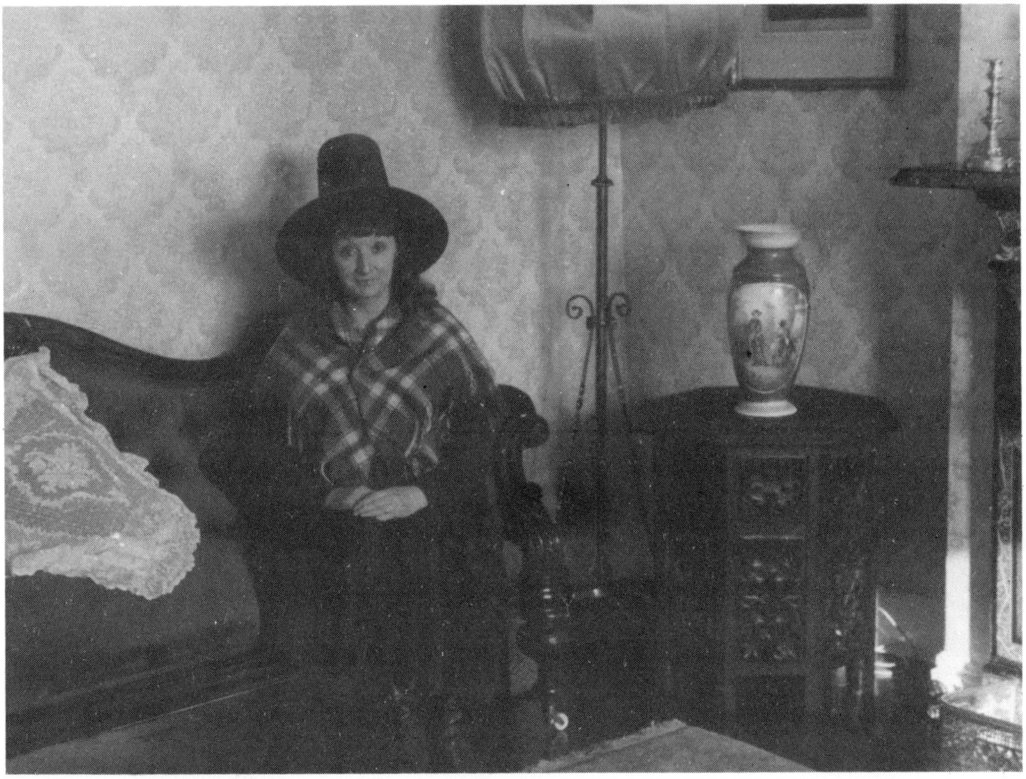

Margaret Jones is a collector and dealer who lives in a delightful Welsh village on the River Tivy situated close to the famous Canarth Falls.

When Margaret was widowed some sixteen years ago, she decided to channel her energies towards converting the old bakery adjoining her house into an antiques showroom where she could both display her colourful stock and trade in pleasant surroundings.

She collects and deals in oriental pottery and porcelain and collects, deals and wears pre 1940's Welsh traditional costume which she says is good quality, long lasting and very warm . . . an important factor on a Welsh hillside come December! Since recent fashion trends now embrace the Welsh costume and related artefacts, prices of collectible pieces have shown a marked upswing with particularly good items such as hats fetching upwards of £50. Dress costume, sometimes elaborately decorated with French Chantilly or Limerick lace, is almost always of the finest quality and is generally treated with due respect being handed down from generation to generation within a family.

Margaret writes about antiques for the Collector's Column of her local newspaper and races around the countryside lecturing on Swansea/Nantgarw pottery and porcelain.

She collects Satsuma because she finds the intricate detail of the 19th century pieces so appealing and has found a romantic element in the search for many pieces have turned up in Cardiganshire, relics of the days when the ancient mariner returning from foreign lands would carry gifts home to his truelove — a coconut, a silk shawl and a choice piece of 19th century Satsuma!

Margaret's home has a strong flavour of the orient and her one wish is that she too will one day travel to foreign lands — on the Orient Express.

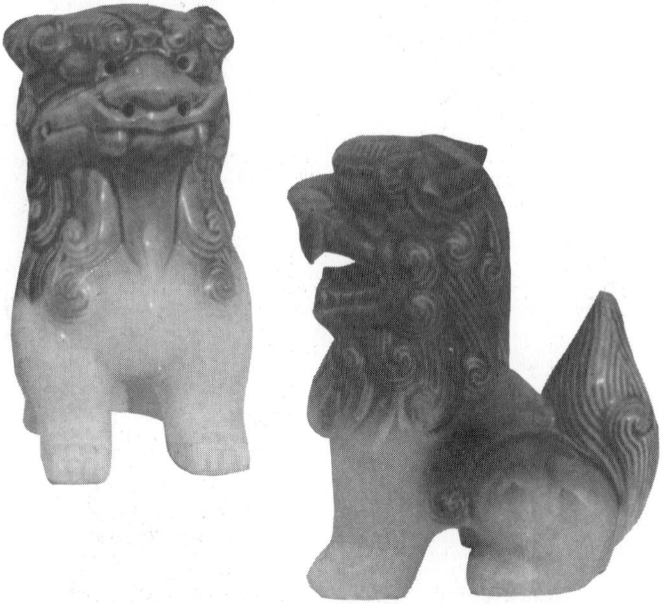

A pair of 19th century Chinese Foo dogs. £20

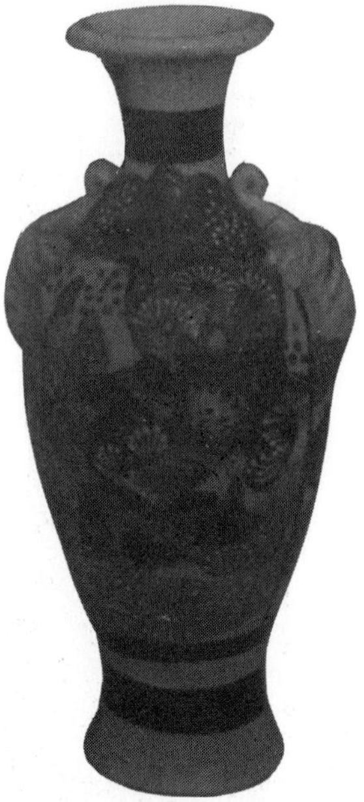

Late 19th century brocade pattern Satsuma vase. £20

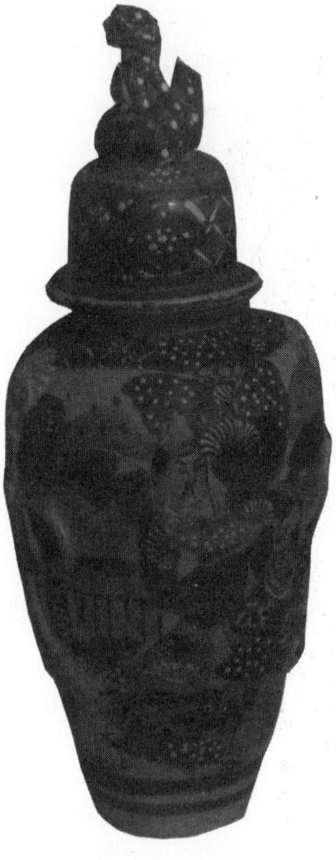

Satsuma pottery brocade pattern vase complete with lid. £75

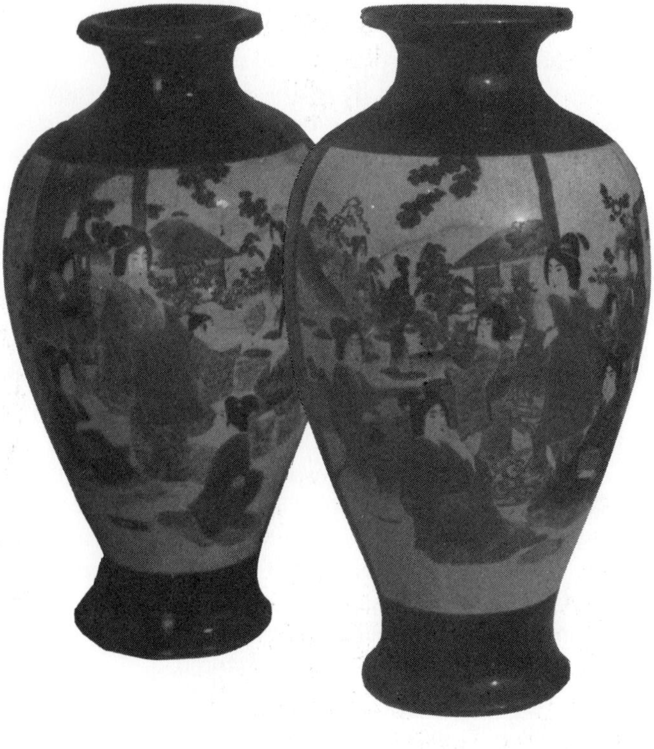

A good pair of 19th century hand-painted Satsuma vases decorated with garden scenes. £145

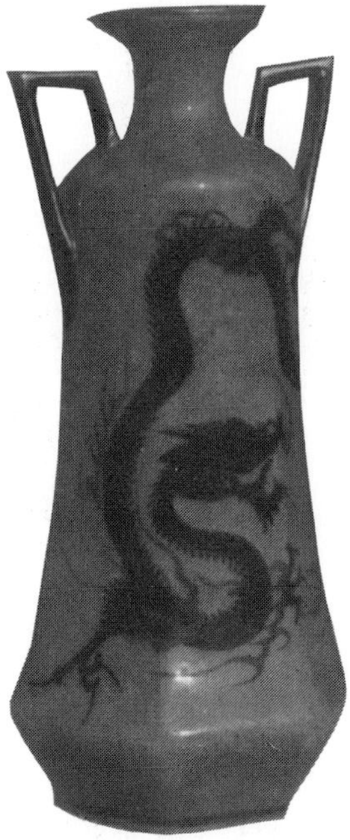

20th century Chinese dragon vase. £15

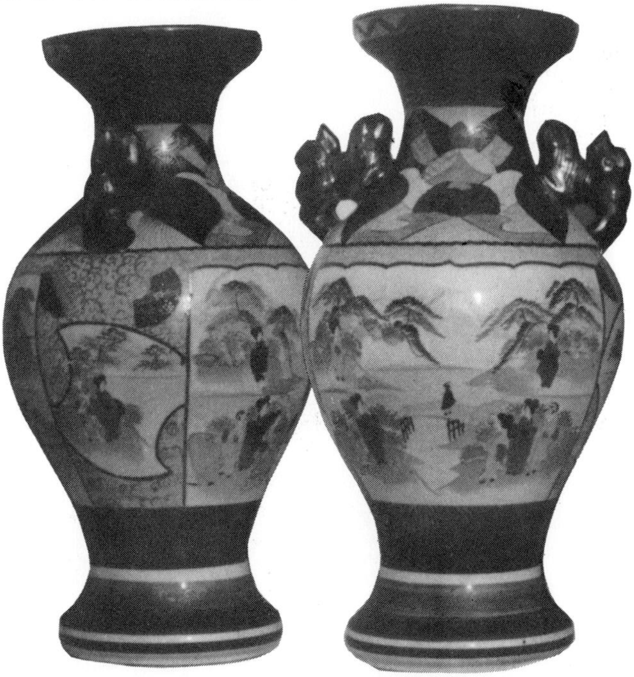

A good pair of Kutani Waga Suei vases with painted panels and Foo dog handles. £475

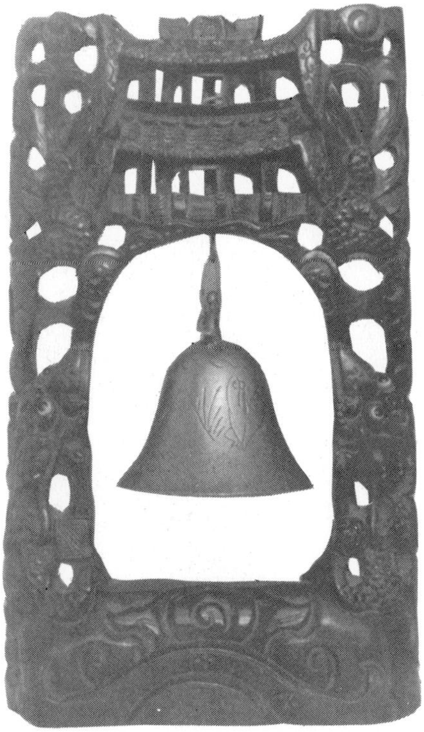

Chinese brass temple bell in an ornately carved stand decorated with fierce looking dragons. £80

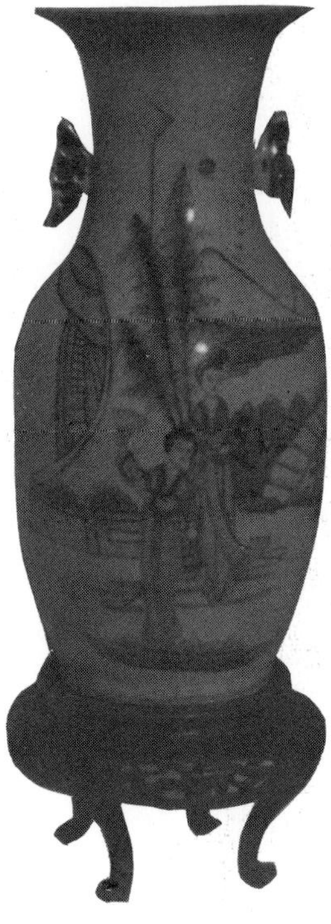

Cantonese vase with duck-egg glaze, complete with carved stand. £160

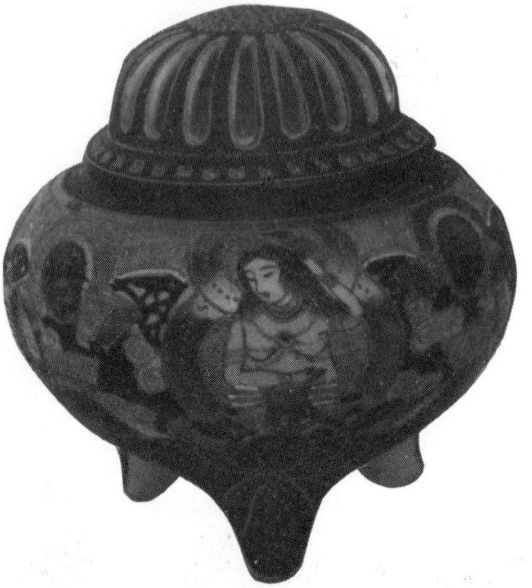

Late 19th century Satsuma incense burner. £125

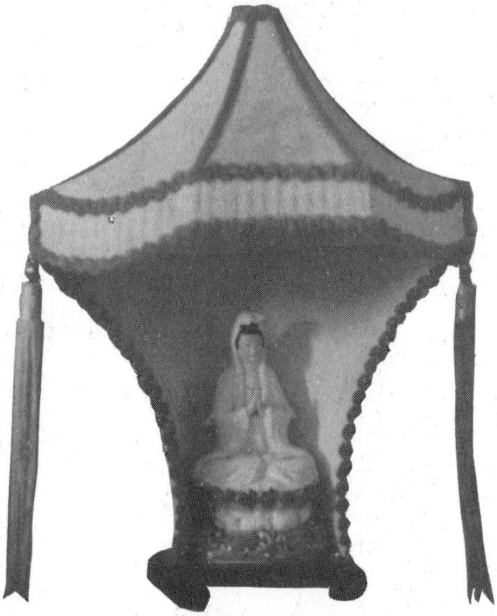

An interesting 20th century Oriental porcelain female figure sitting in a lotus plant. £60

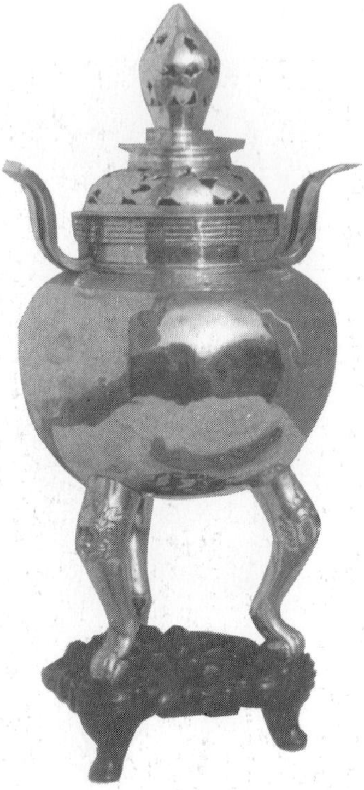

19th century Oriental silver incense burner on a carved wooden stand, 12oz. £150

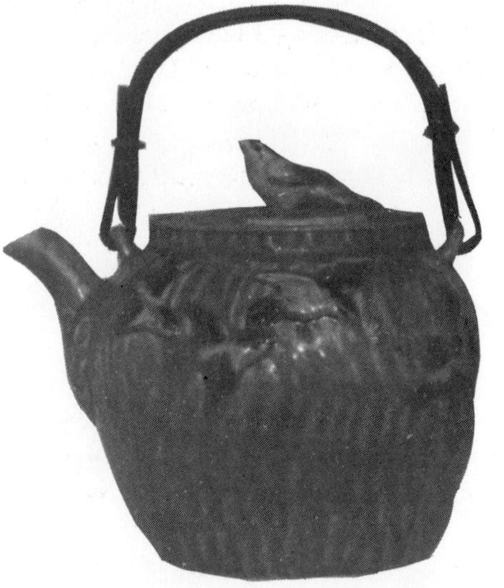

An interesting Japanese porcelain teapot with wooden handle. £100

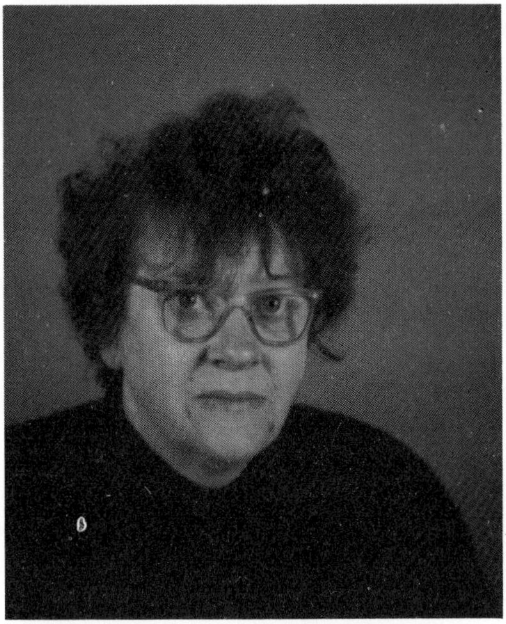

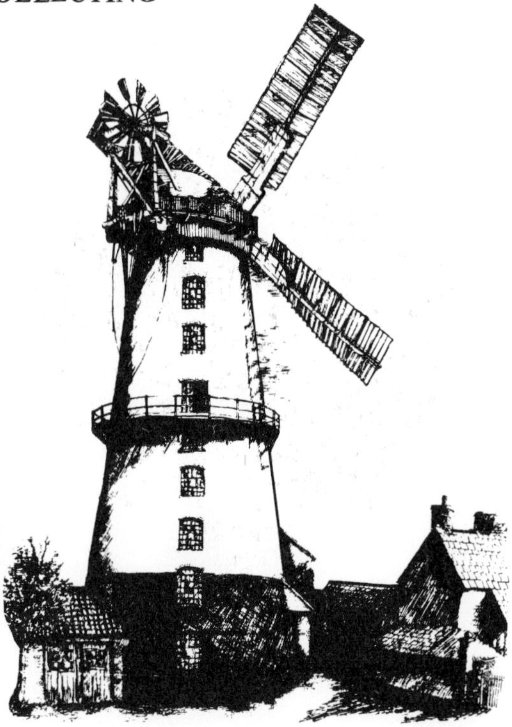

Sutton Wind Mill, near Stalham, Norfolk.

Christopher and Marion Nunn have a collection of razor blade packets and run their own country museum.

Christopher said: "We live in a windmill which is open to the public as a museum of the rural way of life from the late Victorian age to the 1940's and Marion's special interest is collecting razor blade packets though we've got examples of all sorts of things from old apple corers, kitchen equipment, soaps, tools, memorabilia, farm and ditching implements, cigarette packets and bank notes. Our latest acquisition and pride and joy at the moment is a nine foot long punt gun for shooting duck which was made in 1832."

Marion's collection of razor blade packets started because she thought they looked pretty and now she has over 400 different packets on display in the museum where the couple live with their daughter Robin.

It is the tallest mill in England and was built in 1789. Christopher used to be in the building trade before they bought the mill three years ago and is now restoring it with the aim of returning it to its original function as a flour grinding mill. It is open to the public between April and the end of September and admission is 85p a head.

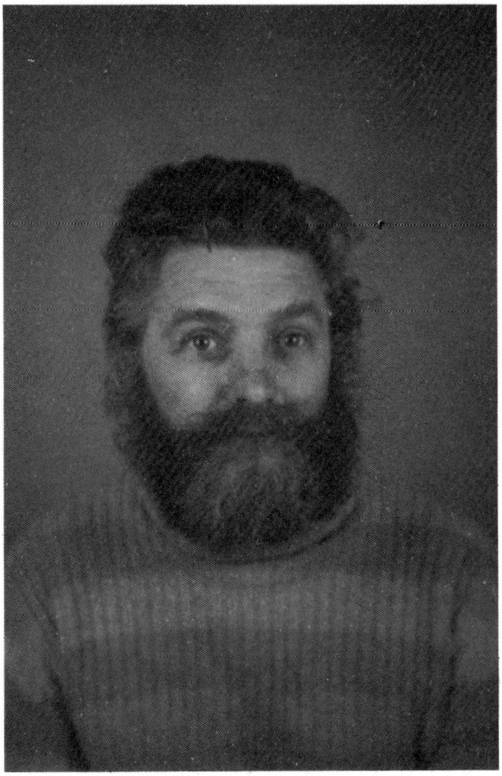

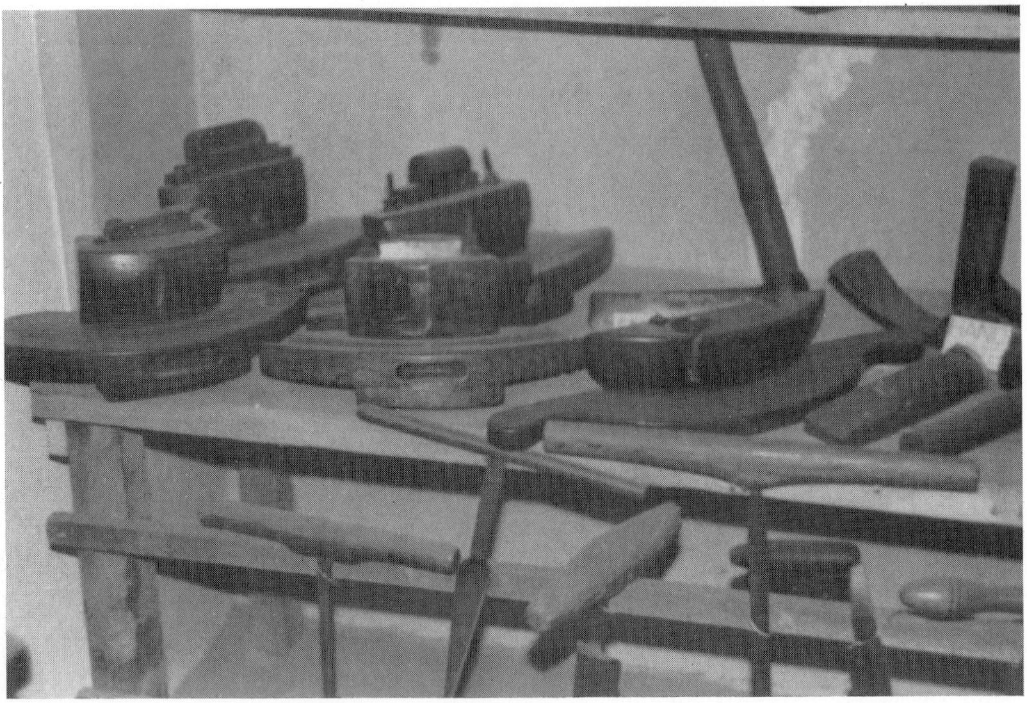

Cooper's tools.

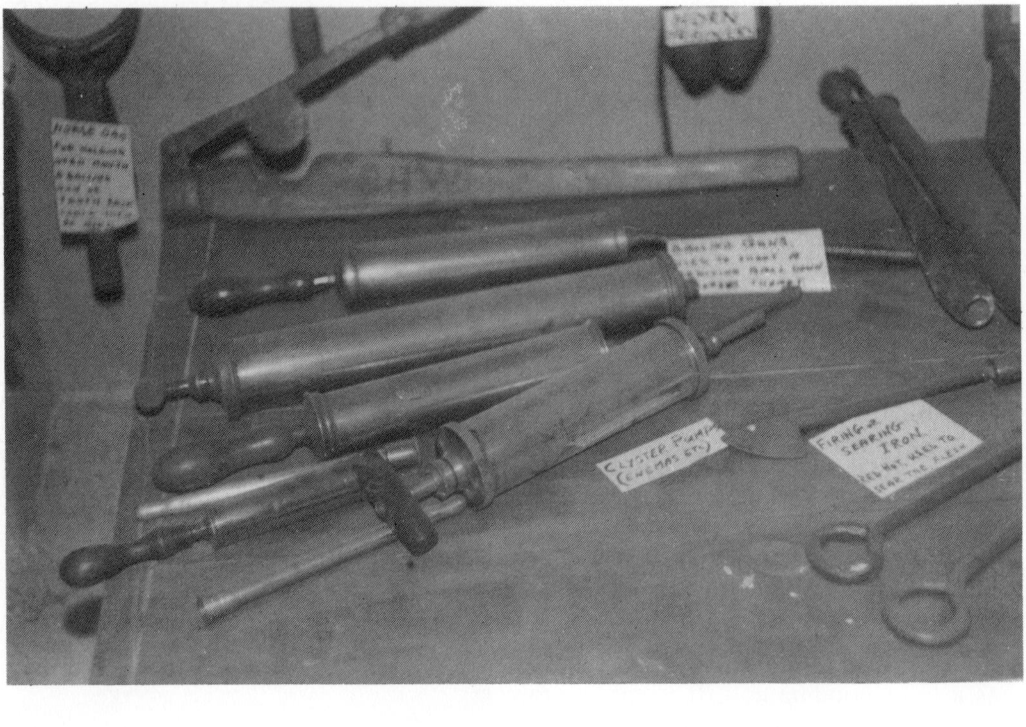

Vet's tools.

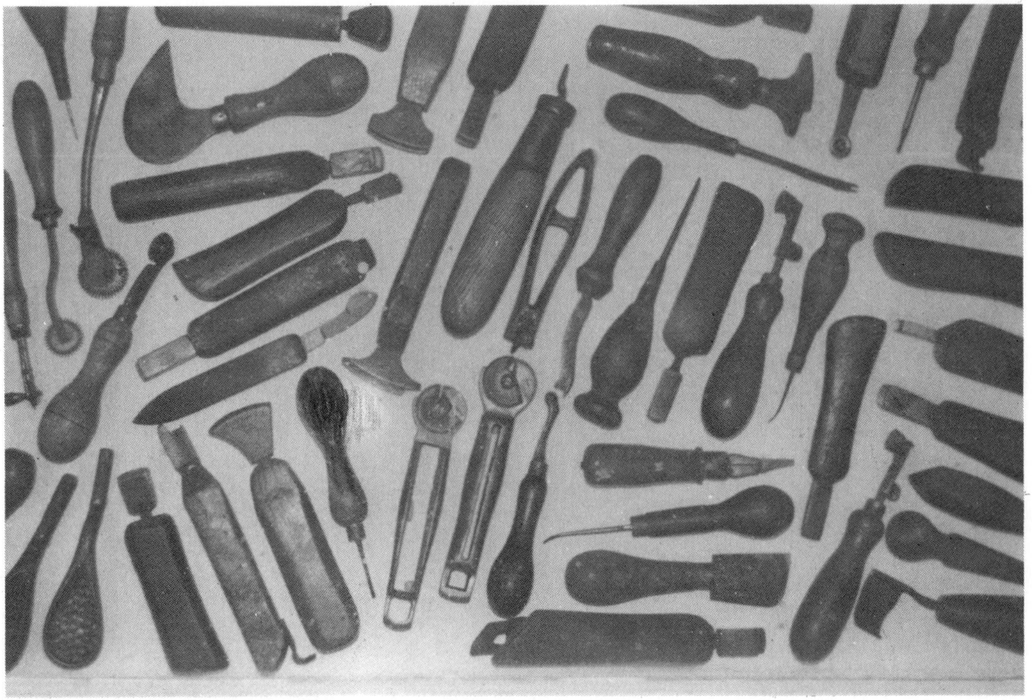

Leather trade tools.

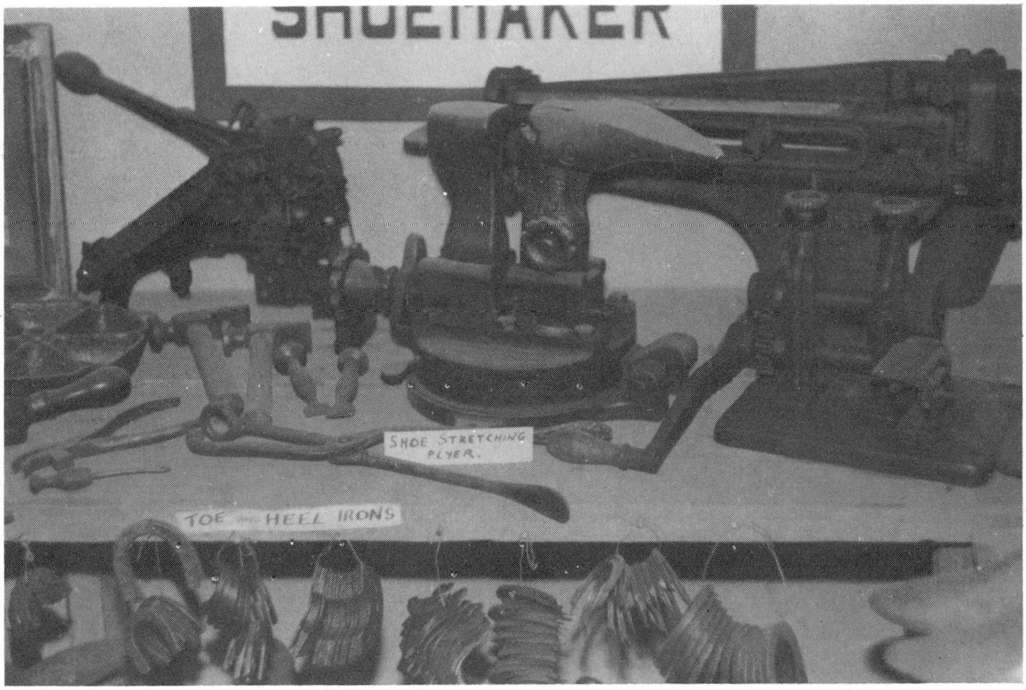

Shoemaking tools.

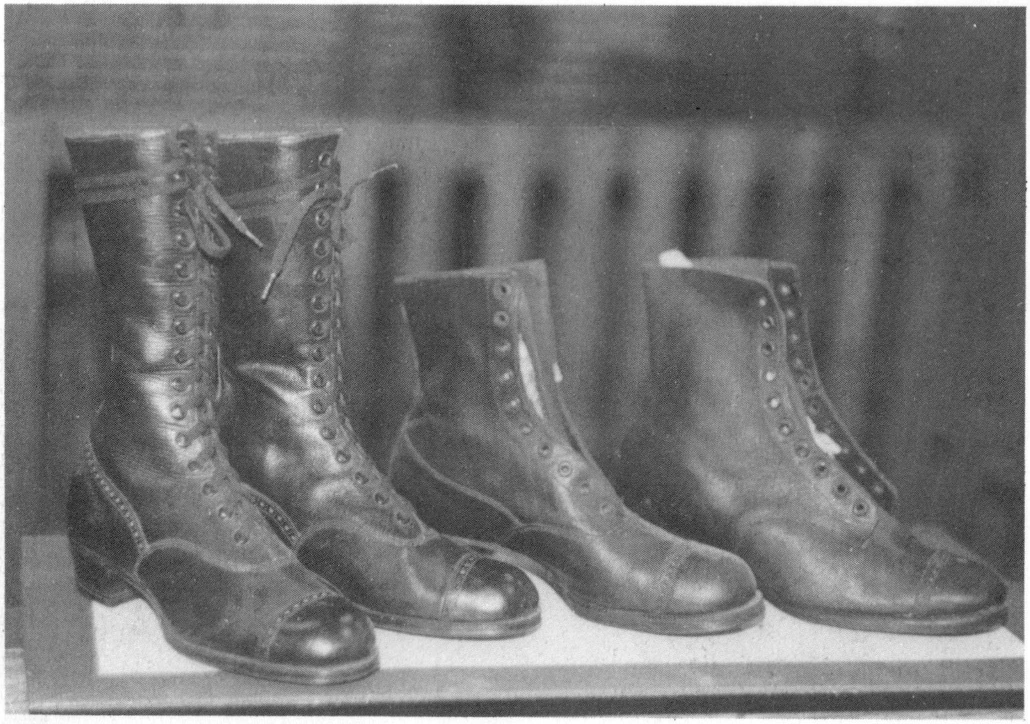

Early 20th century lady's boots.

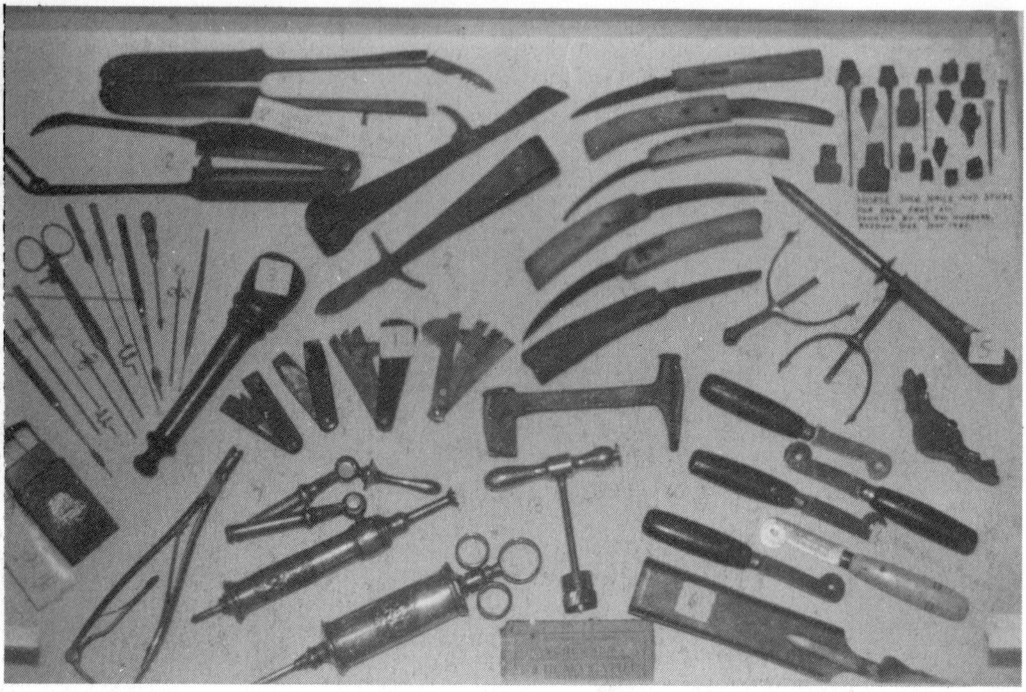

Vet's tools.

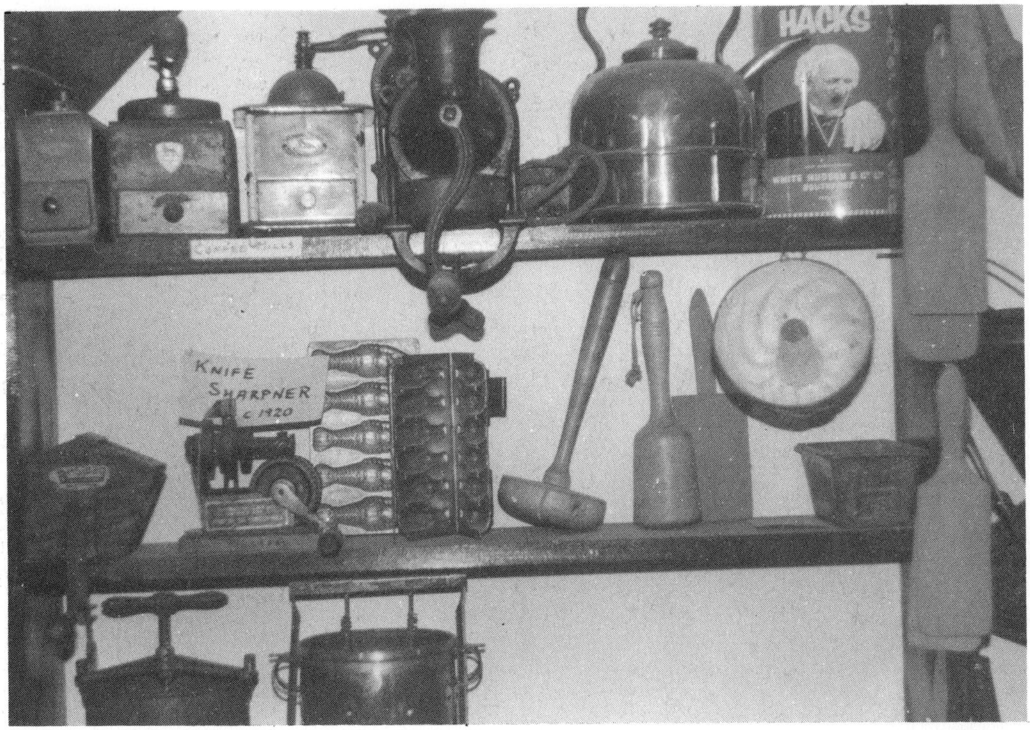

Domestic machines.

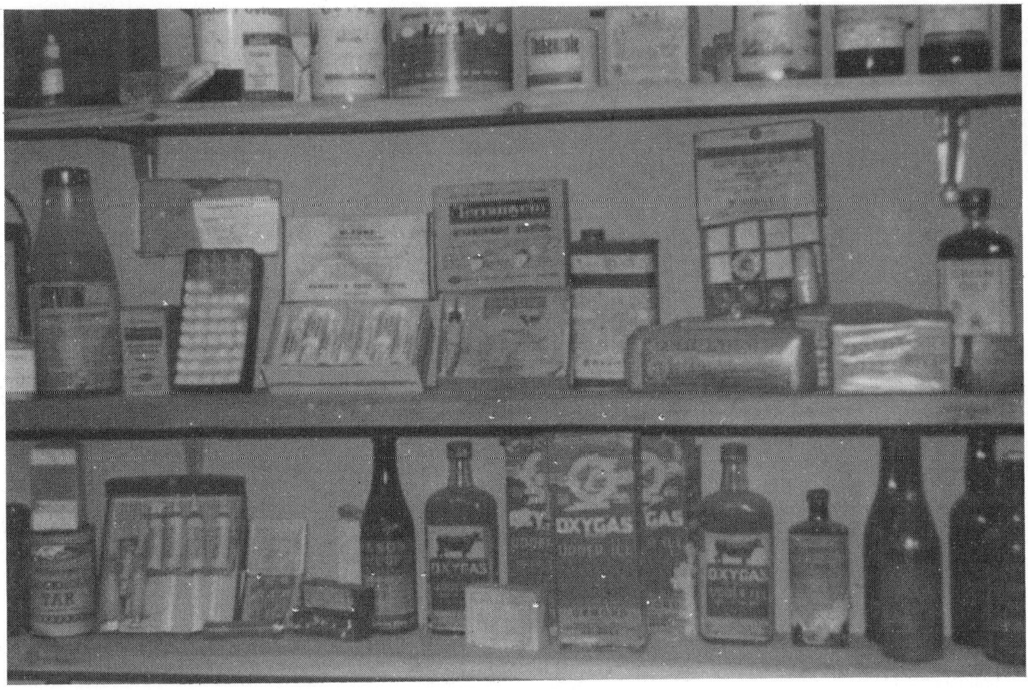

Animal medicines.

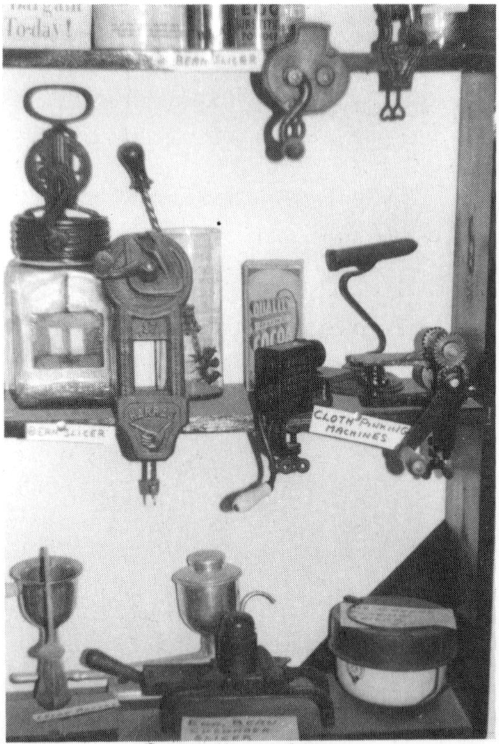

Domestic machines.

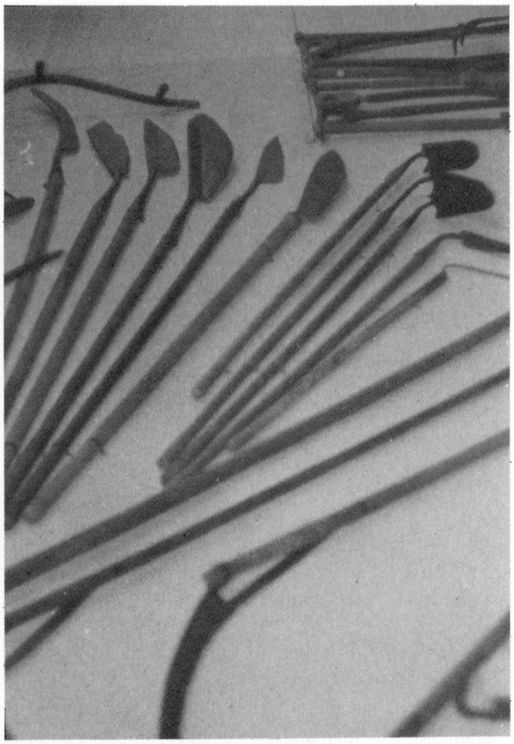

Marsh tools.

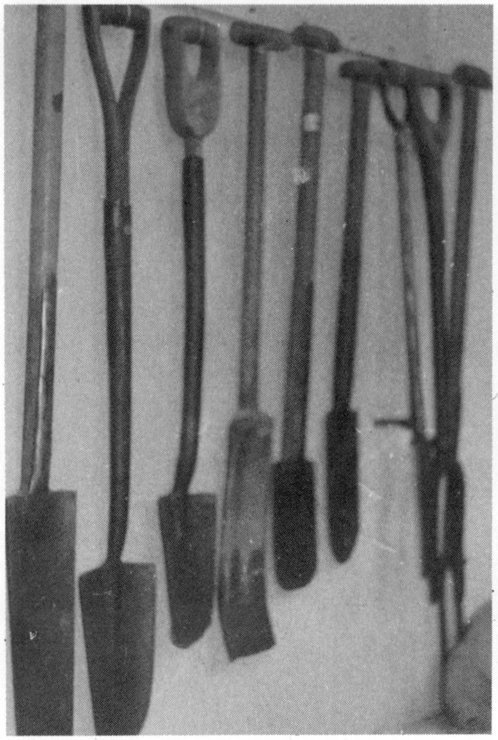

Ditching tools.

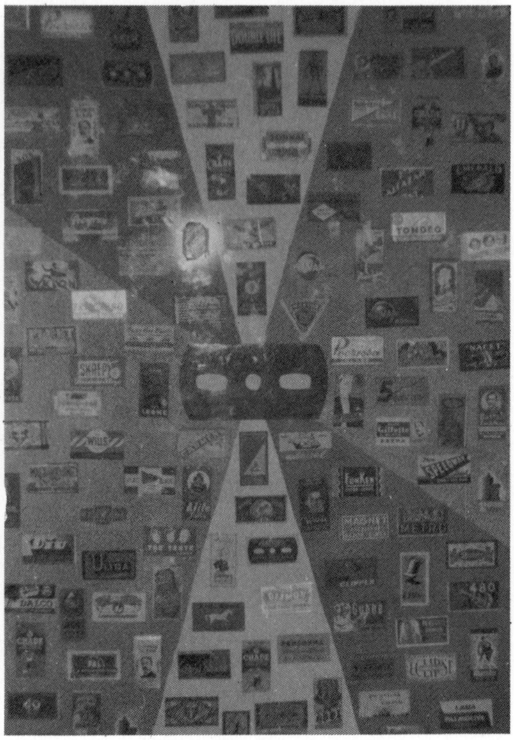

Razor blade wrappers.

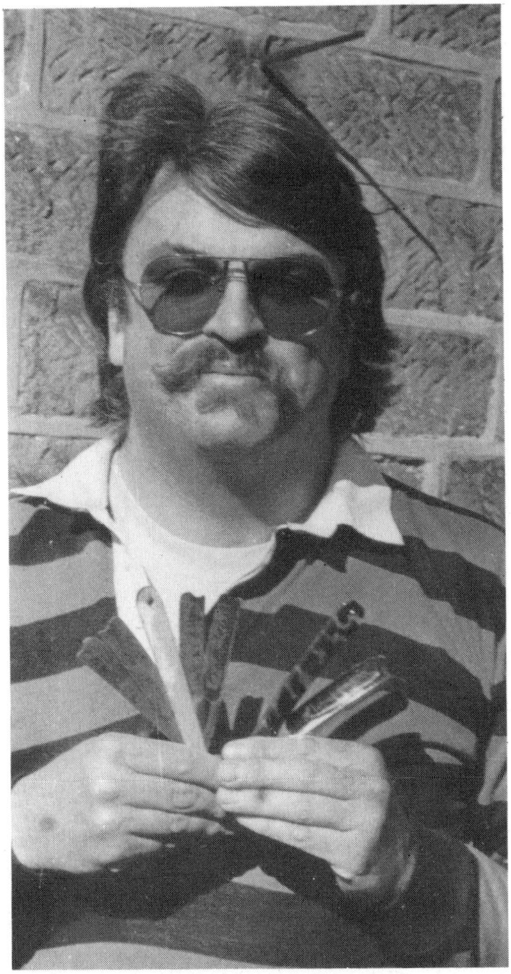

Neil Wayne is a dealer and collector of old razors. His professional name is 'The Razor Man'.

"When I say I collect old razors some people say 'How quaint' but in fact though there are very few razor collectors in the country there are over 600 in USA as well as others in France and Germany and I do most of my business with them.

"I've been collecting for seven years and I've cleaned out several Sheffield factories that used to make razors. There are 6,000 in my attic which I send out to America in lots of 1,000 at a time. Just plain black handled razors at a dollar a time.

"Now my main interest is in medical and optical items but there's a huge variety in razors from the ordinary ones that I sell for ten pence each to lovely ones like a mid 18th century tortoiseshell set piqued in three coloured golds in a silver mounted fish skin case which I sold for £800 and would pay more for now if I could find another like it.

"Razors are still being made today but mostly in East Germany and China and they retail for around £15 each. If you can handle a cut throat razor it is still the most ideal way to get a perfect shave."

Neil's collection includes several razors with Royal Connections, especially a very opulent set dating from the 1780's with every piece inset with gold or pearl. It belonged to one of the French kings of the pre-Revolutionary period.

Another set of six razors which Neil bought in Germany once belonged to King William IV of Great Britain and is in solid pearl with gold ends and each piece is crested.

Other razors which appeal to collectors other than razor collectors include ones that were sold in specially printed tins and mechanical razors patented in Victorian times.

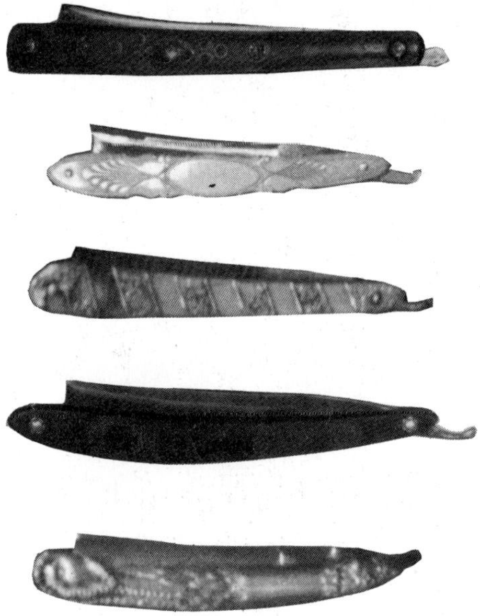

An interesting selection of 19th century razors.

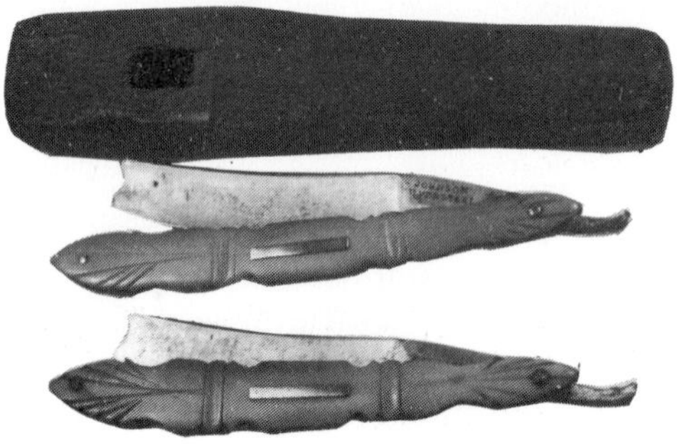

Pair of late 18th century razors by Johnson, with pressed horn handles. £20 – £30

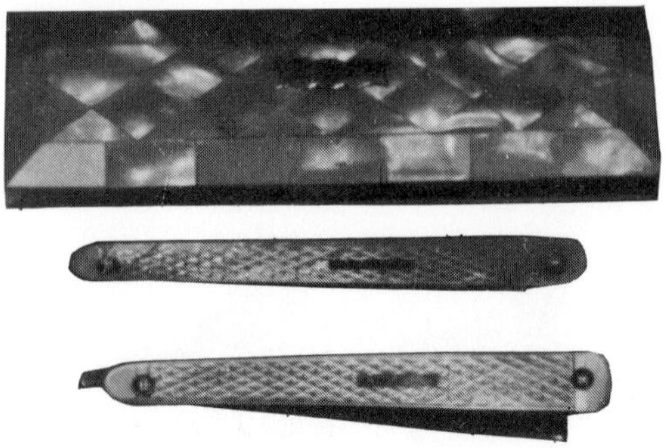

A pair of chequer carved pearl handled razors with solid gold pins, contained in a mother-of-pearl case, by I. H. Farthing, circa 1805. £175

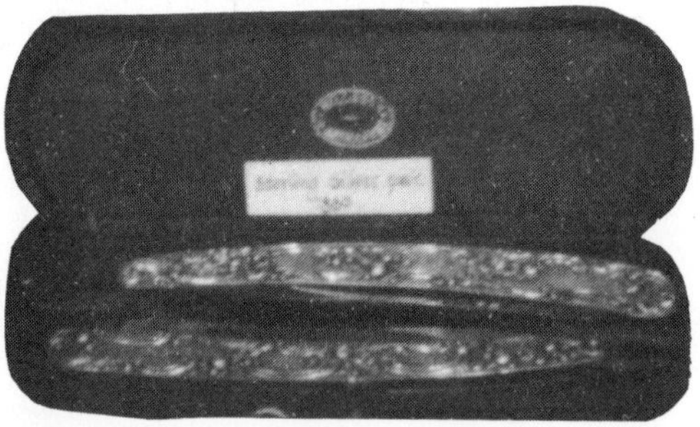

Pair of mid 19th century razors with embossed silver handles. £100

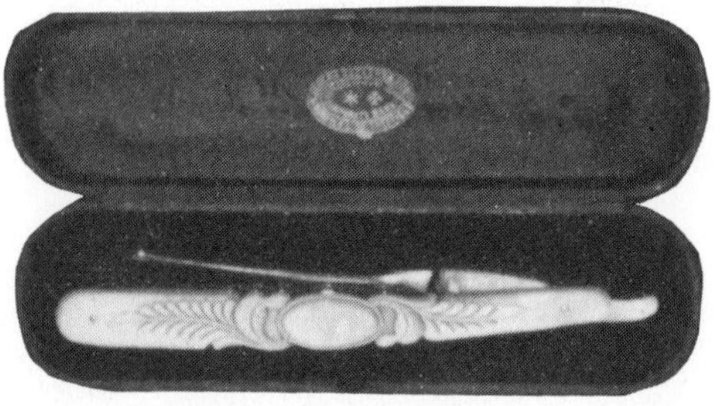

Mid 19th century pearl handled razor, in its velvet lined case. £40 – £50

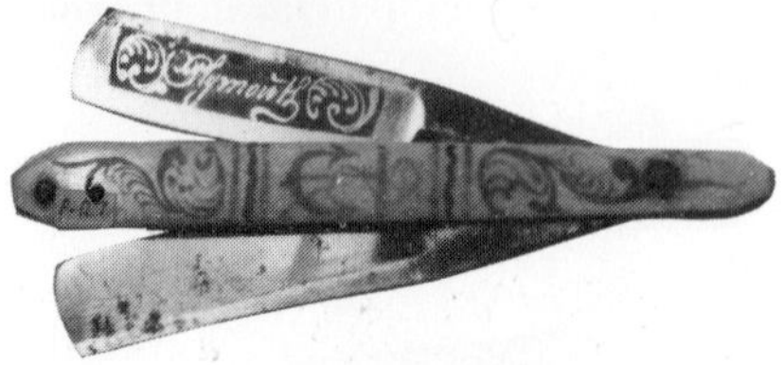

A rare sailor's twin-bladed razor, with penwork handle, engraved 'Plymouth'. £100

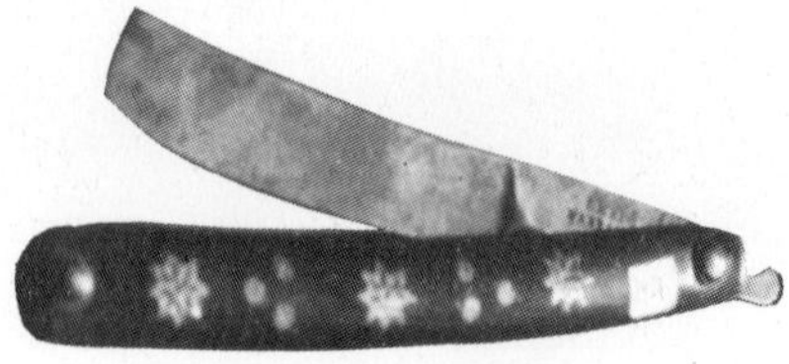

Mid 19th century razor with inlaid black horn handle. £10 – £12

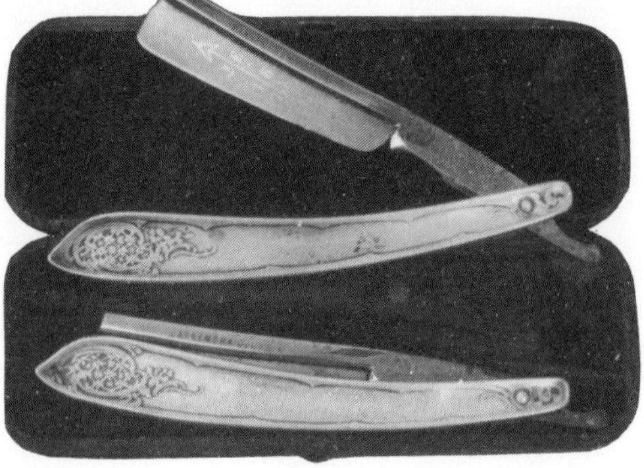

A pair of Swedish steel razors marked Dannemora Gjutstahl, with silver handles, contained in a black leather case, 1874. £85

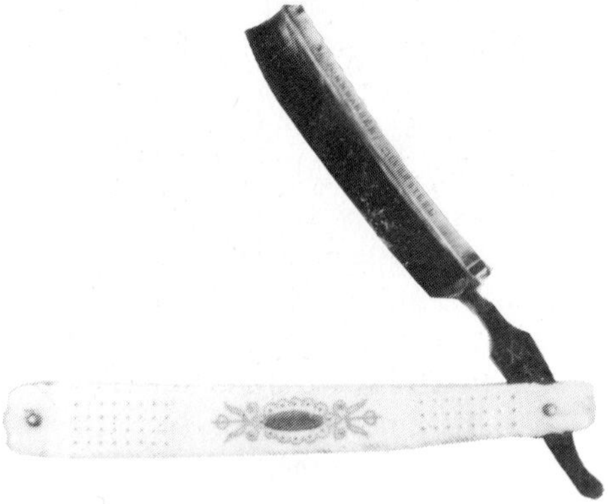

Late 18th century style razor by John Barber with an ivory pique pinwork handle. £40 – £60

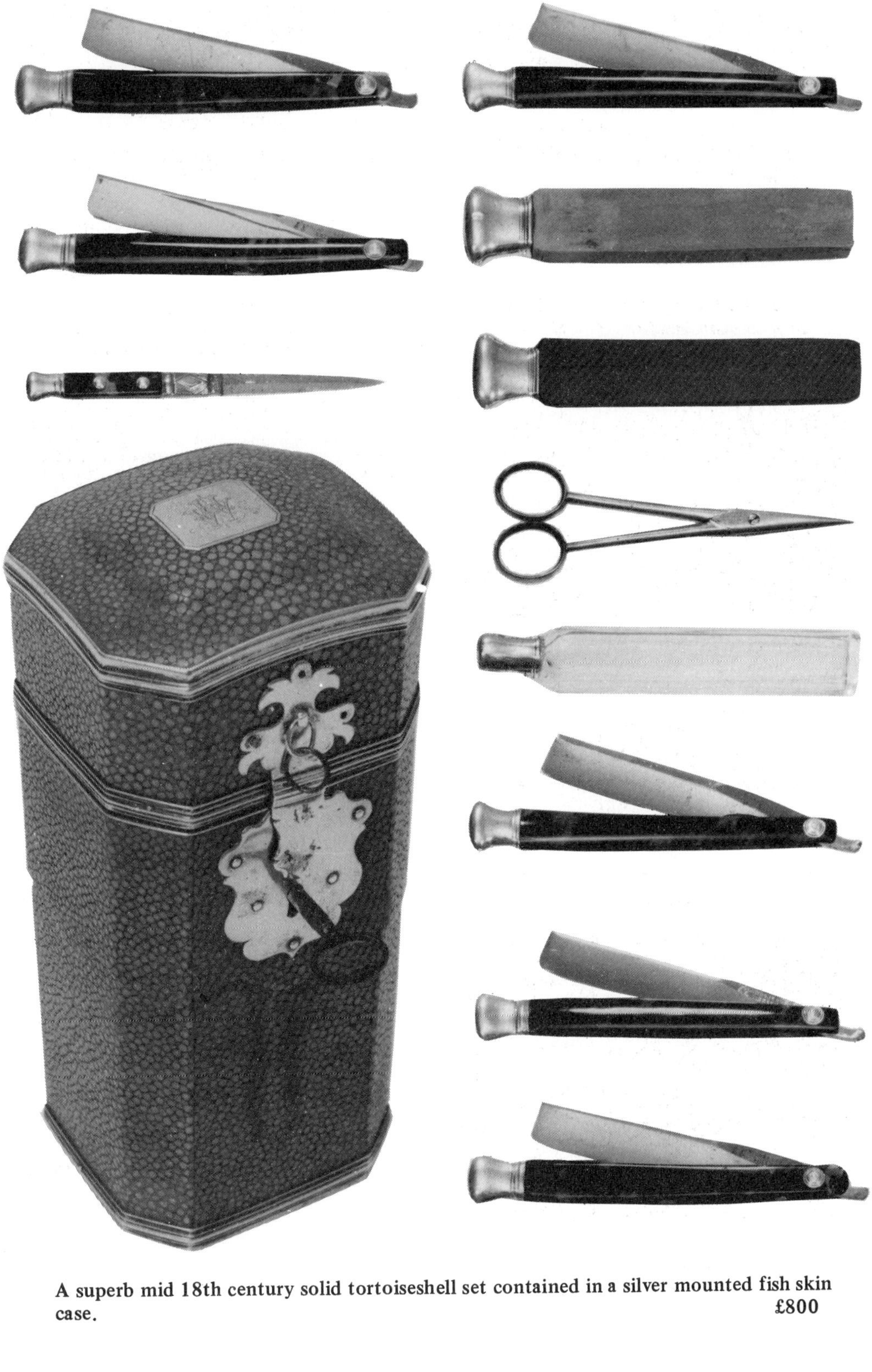

A superb mid 18th century solid tortoiseshell set contained in a silver mounted fish skin case. £800

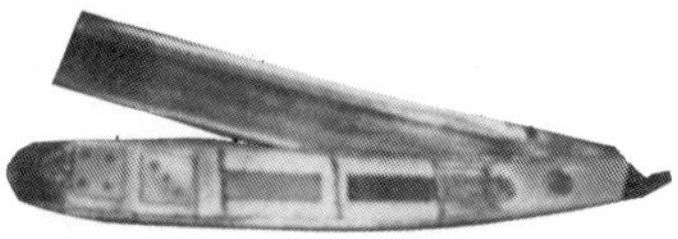

Mid 19th century gambler's travelling razor with dice designs on the handle. £60 – £80

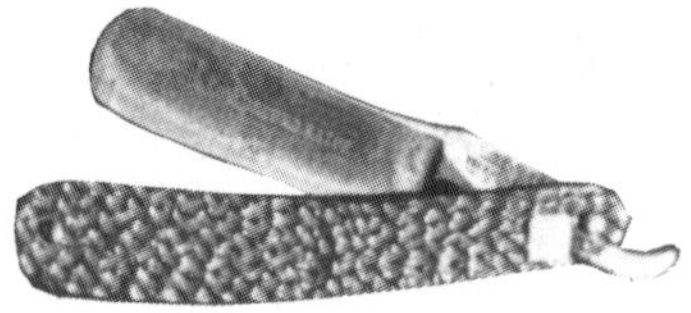

Mid 19th century hollow ground razor with stipled black horn handle. £10 – £12

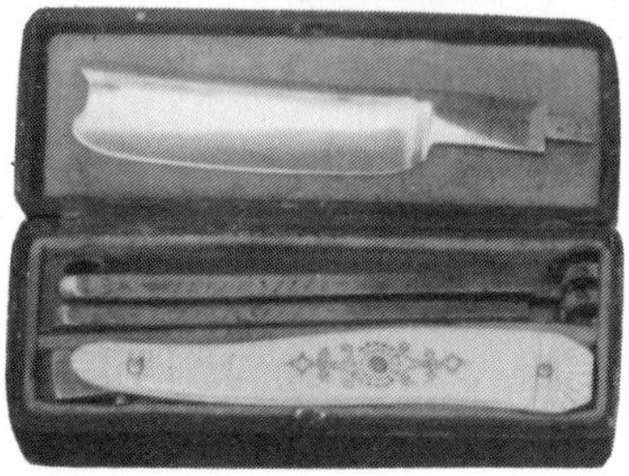

An early 19th century English razor with pinwork ivory handle, contained in a red leather case. £40 – £80

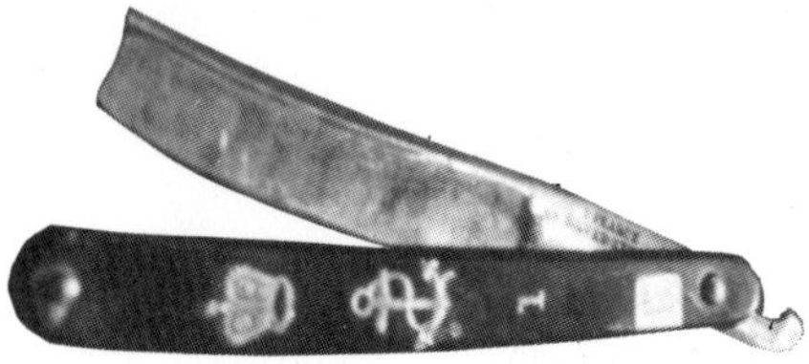

Victorian razor with pewter inlaid black horn handle. £10 – £12

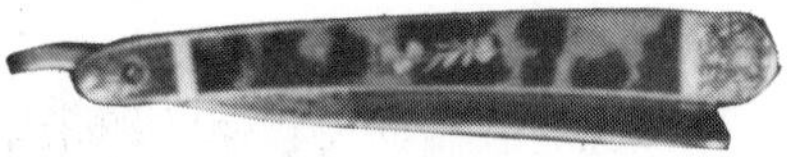

Mid 19th century razor with silver inlaid tortoiseshell handle. £15 – £20

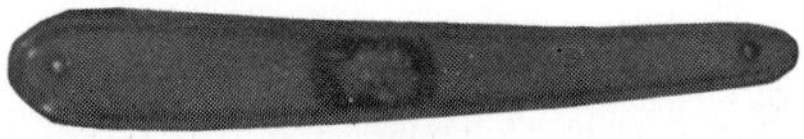

Ivory handled razor engraved with the image of George III, silver pins. £60 – £80

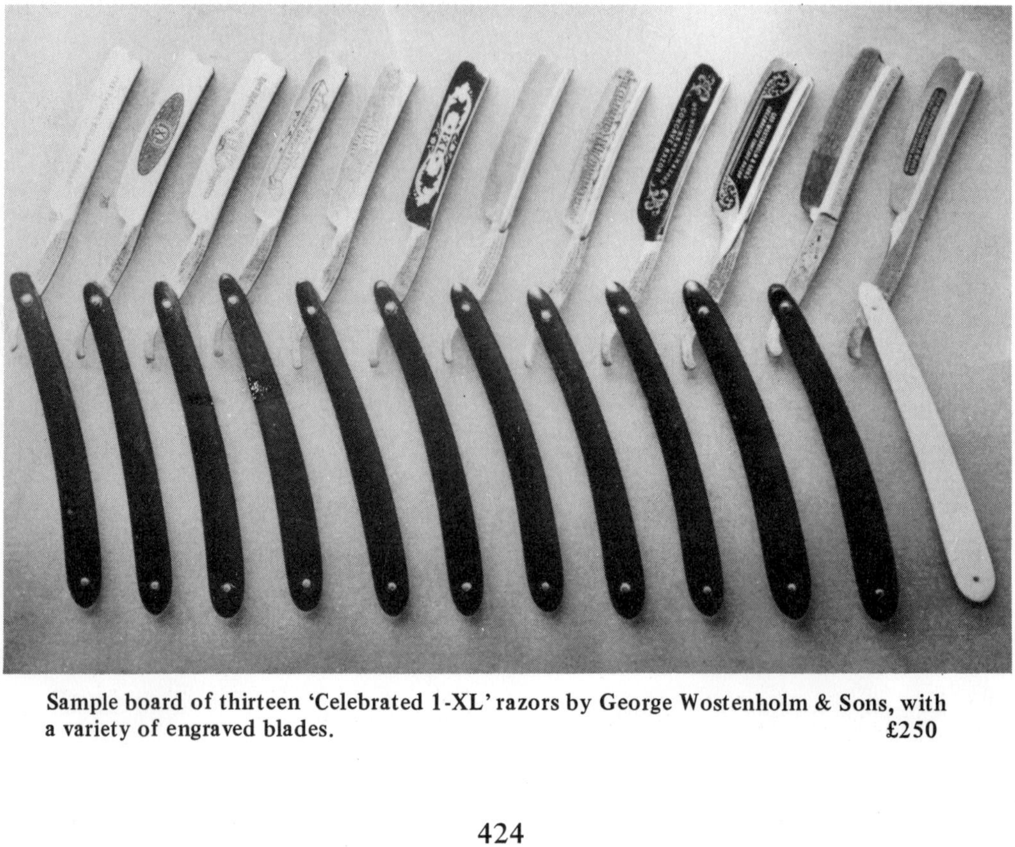

Sample board of thirteen 'Celebrated 1-XL' razors by George Wostenholm & Sons, with a variety of engraved blades. £250

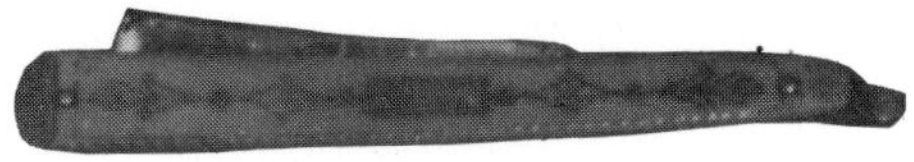

Mid 19th century ivory handled razor with the design on both sides. £60 – £80

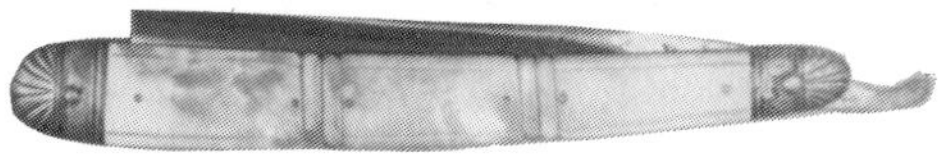

19th century German razor with silver mounts and three-piece pearl handle. £20 – £30

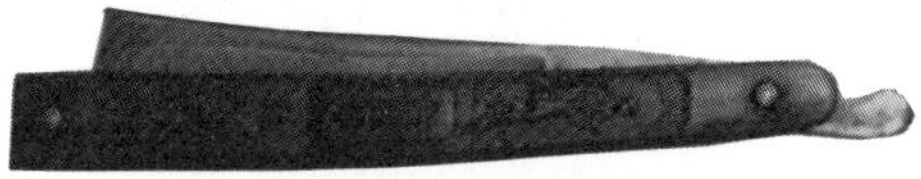

Early 19th century razor with pressed horn handle depicting two hunters. £60 – £80

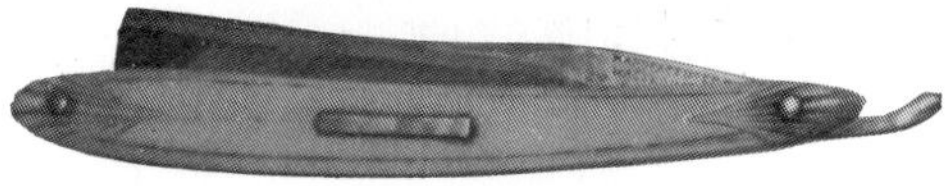

Mid 19th century razor with simple ivory handle. £60 – £80

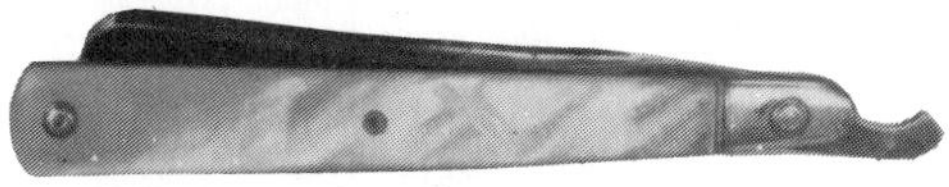

Mid 19th century razor with one-piece pearl handle and silver pins. £20 – £30

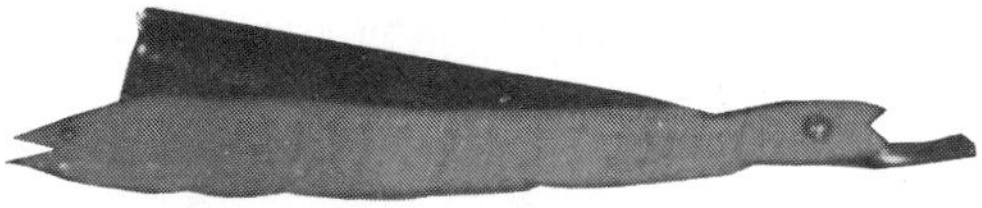

Mid 19th century razor, the ivory handle carved in the form of a fish. £60 – £80

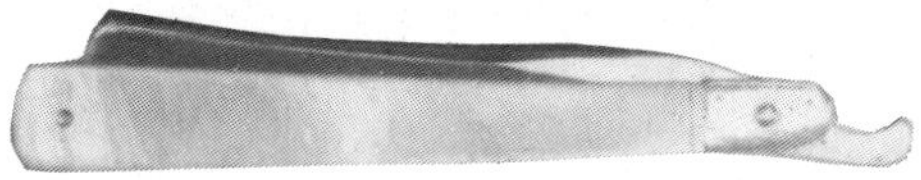

Mid 19th century razor with one-piece mother-of-pearl handle and silver mounts. £40 – £50

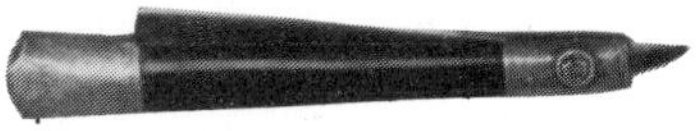

Victorian tortoiseshell handled razor with silver mounts. £15 – £20

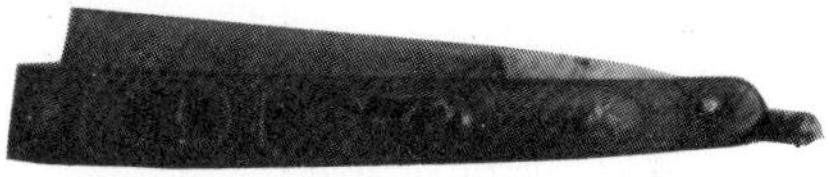

Early 19th century English razor with pressed horn handle depicting a wildfowler. £60 – £80

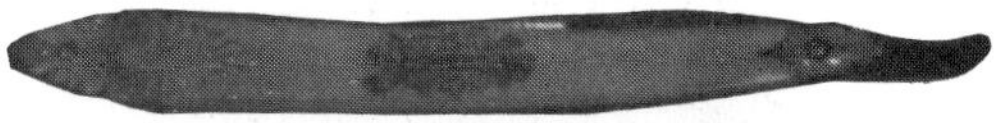

Early Victorian razor with carved ivory handle and silver pins. £60 – £80

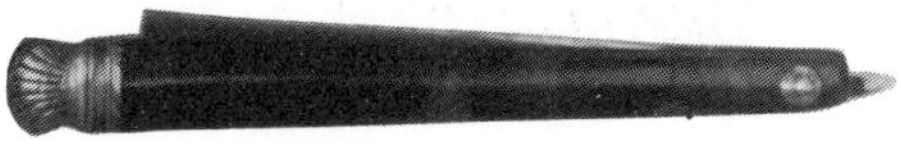

19th century English razor with plain tortoiseshell handle with silver mounts. £15 – £20

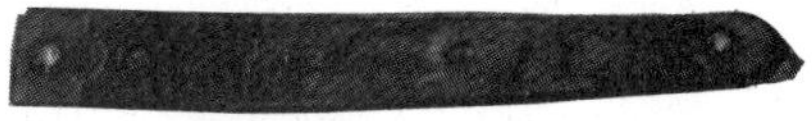

Early 19th century English razor with pressed horn handle depicting a hunter. £60 – £80

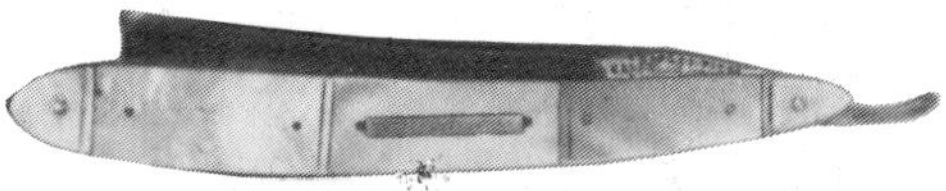

19th century German razor with three-piece pearl handle. £20 – £30

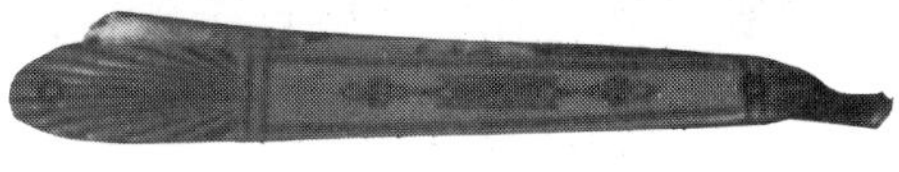

Mid 19th century razor with carved ivory handle and silver pins. £40 – £80

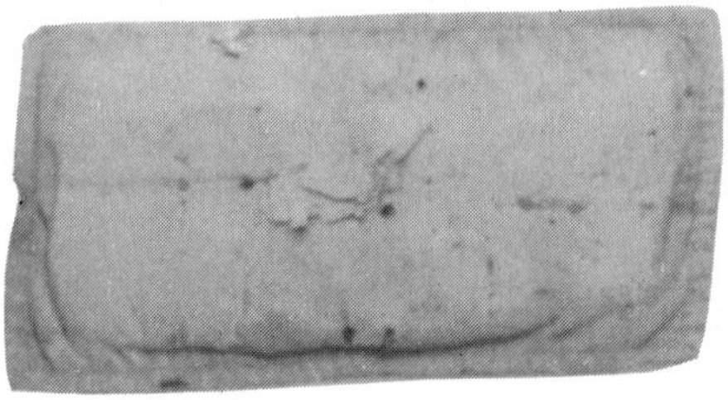

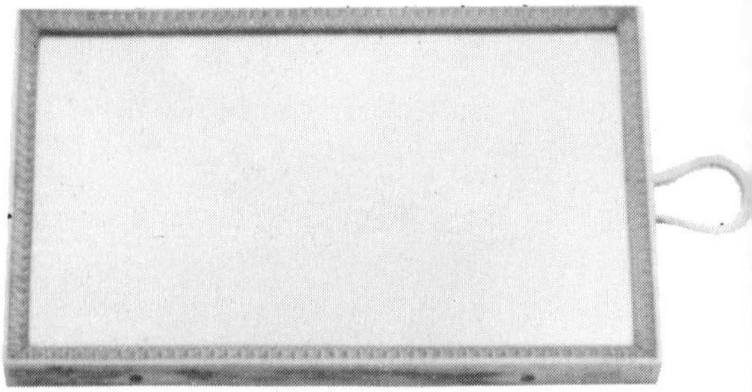

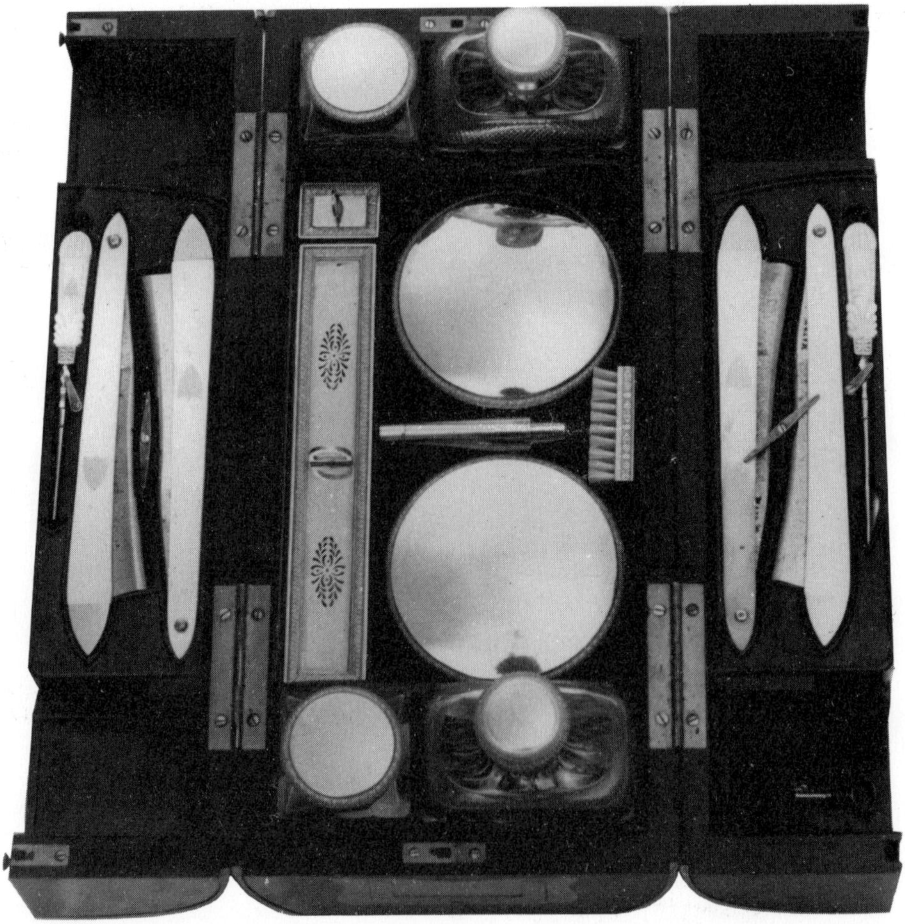

A good late 18th century French, mahogany case necessaire de voyage in silver gilt with solid pearl handles including razors, moustache combs, toothbrush and tongue scraper.
£2,700

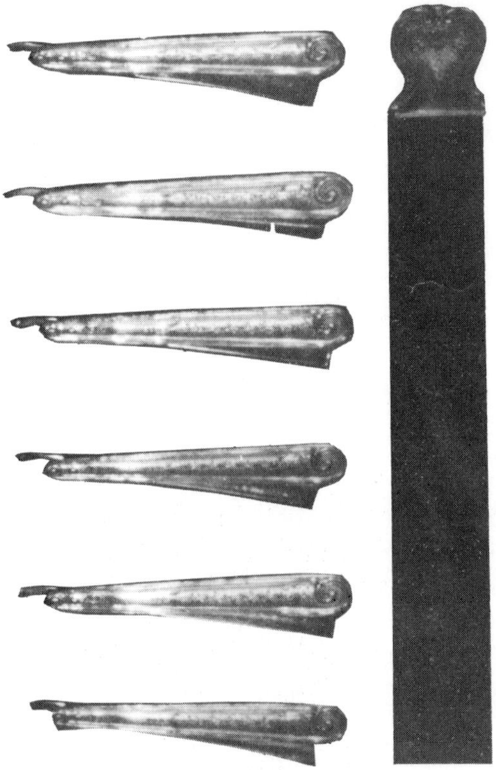

A possibly unique set of six razors with silver gilt handles, by Paul Storr, with matching strap, 1834. £1,500

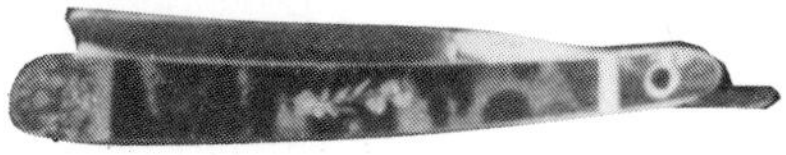

Victorian razor with silver inlaid tortoiseshell handle. £15 – £20

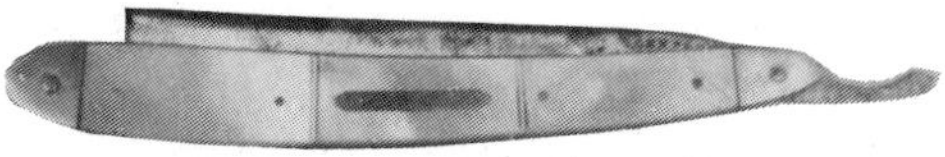

19th century German razor with three-piece pearl handle. £20 – £30

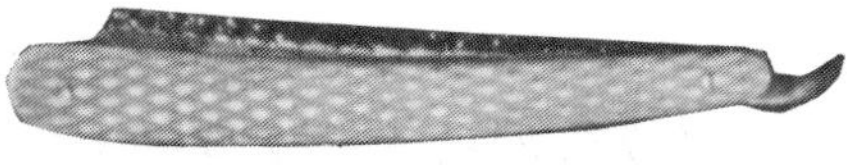

Mid 19th century razor with chequered ivory handle. £60 – £80

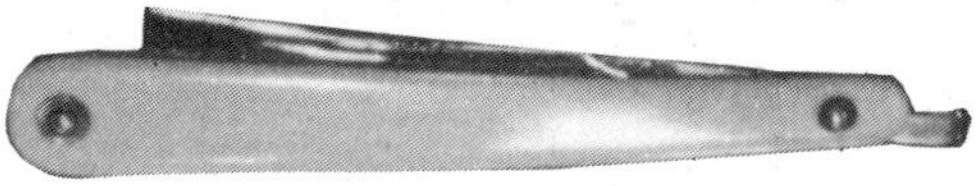

Mid 19th century razor with plain ivory handle. £60 – £80

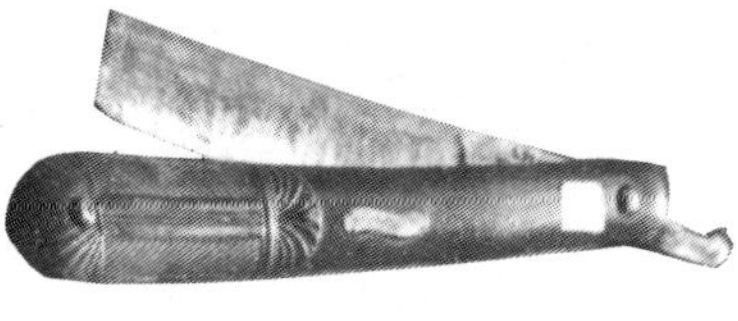

Mid 19th century razor with pressed black horn handle. £10 – £12

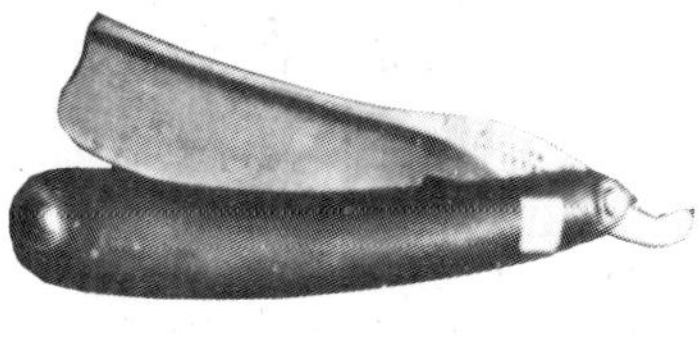

A plain mid 19th century razor with black horn handle. £10 – £12

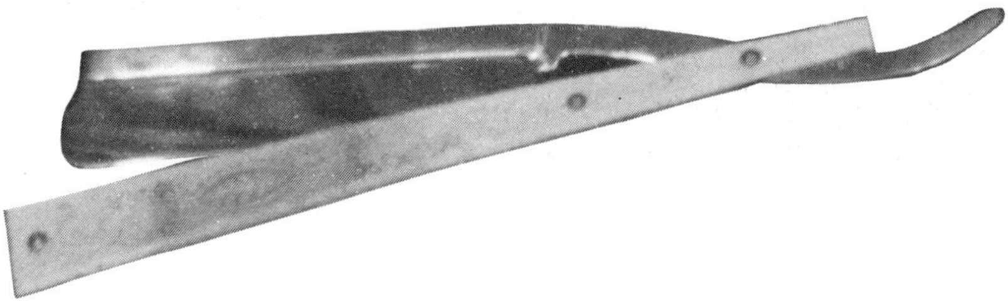

An interesting folk art display razor. £100

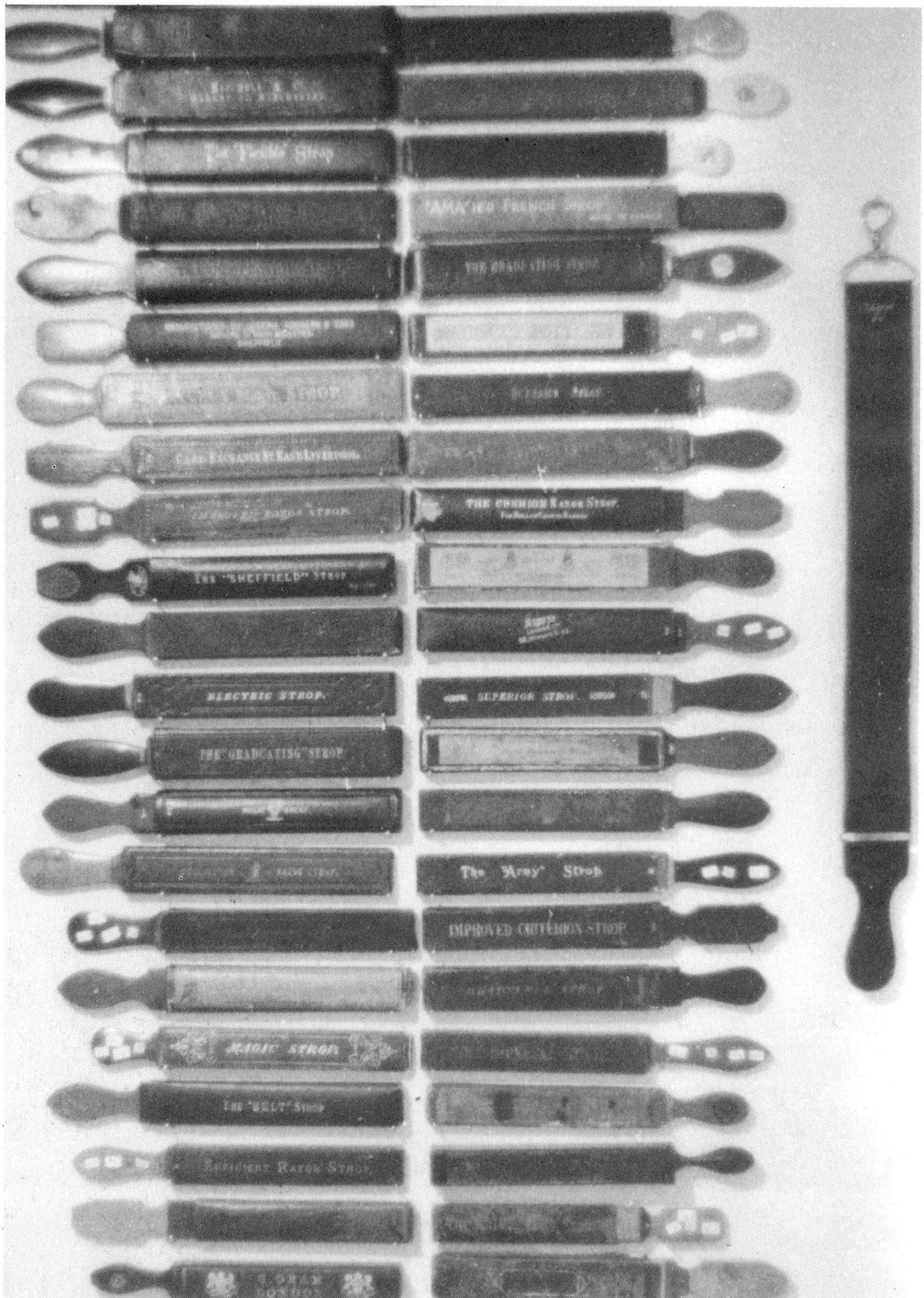

A selection of 19th century scabbard type straps with gilt blocked designs, some with hollowed centres for holding a razor. £1 – £2 each

CASH-IN ON COLLECTING

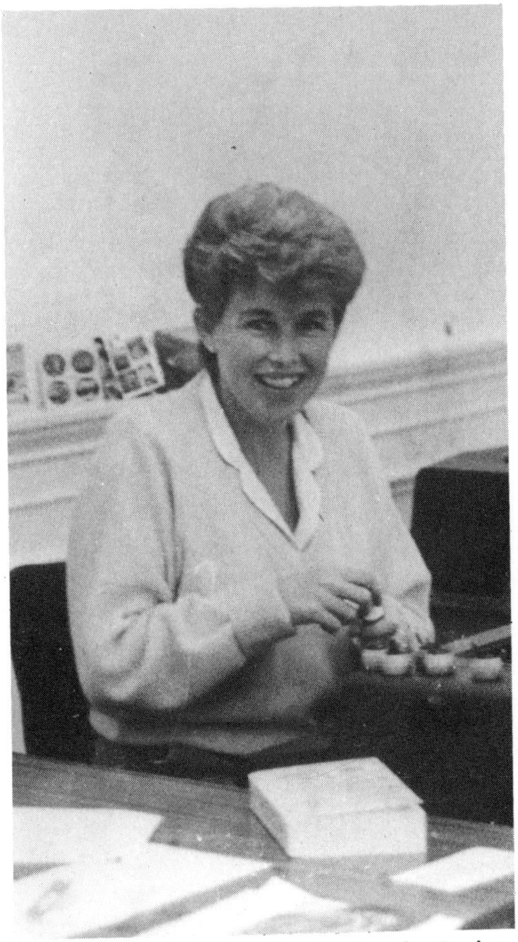

Since the greater part of Janice Moncrieff's working day is spent compiling and researching material for inclusion in current trade catalogues, it is no surprise to find that she has developed a keen interest in the fascinating old editions issued by such well known firms as Heals and Army and Navy Stores.

At the time of their highest popularity these old trade catalogues served the function of bringing the only visual image of a range of goods to the prospective purchaser and as a result they were often printed to the highest possible standard on good quality paper. They reflect the fashion trends of the day in everything from home furnishings, toys and clothes to some cunningly devised gadgets and more sophisticated scientific instruments.

"I'm not what you would call a serious collector and I certainly don't look upon my collection as an investment" says Janice, "but some of the more popular subjects such as fishing tackle, furniture and china do fetch quite good money. I have found a good source of material at Charity Book Fairs, Jumble Sales and Fetes where the prices suit my level of commitment.

"For me there is reward enough in the hours of interest and amusement spent in scanning the evocative illustrations and unbelievable price lists and nowadays, with the collecting bug biting into some very outlandish categories, there is a hidden bonus to having a collection of old trade catalogues for they can provide a useful guide to identifying and dating some quite obscure pieces. Some of my friends who collect such varied items as Edwardian underwear and early kitchen equipment can thumb through my catalogues and find out more about a particular piece, even confirm the original selling price. It's good fun".

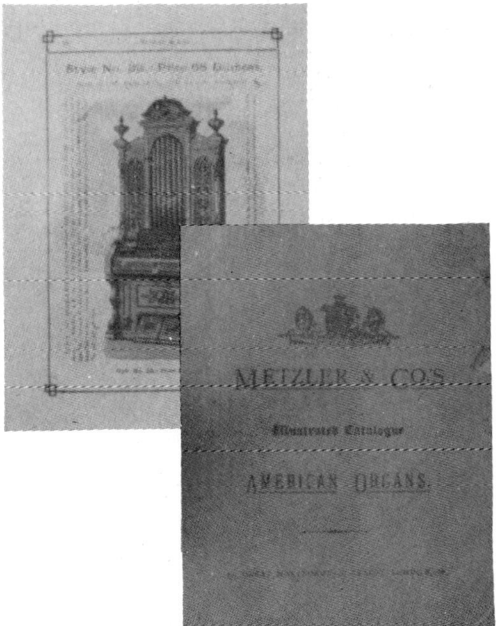

Metzler & Co's. Catalogue of American Organs.
£10

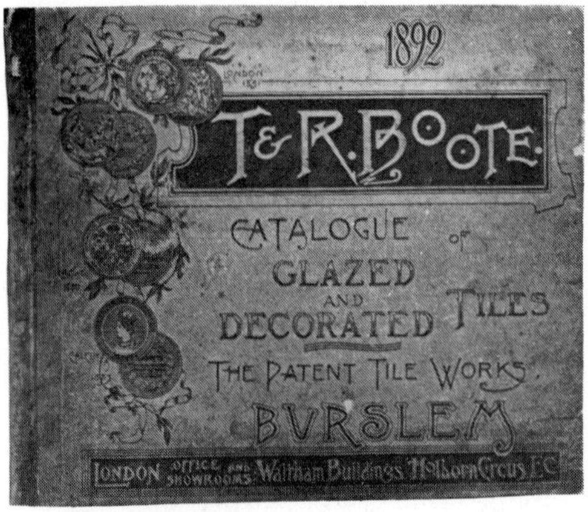

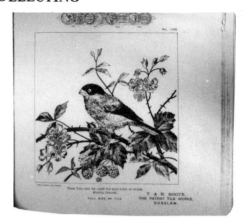

T. & R. Boote Catalogue of Glazed and Decorated Tiles, Burslem, 1892. £50

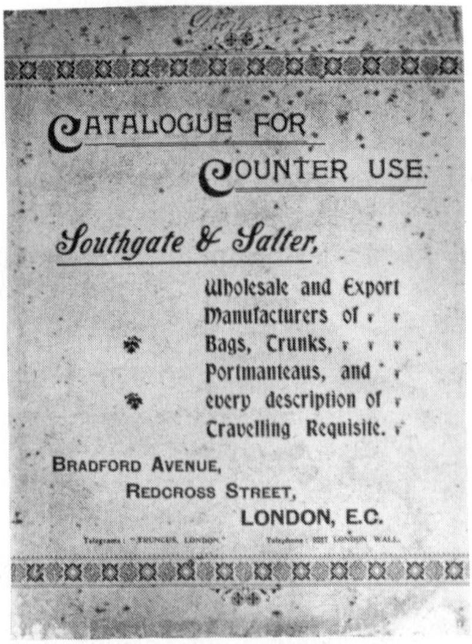

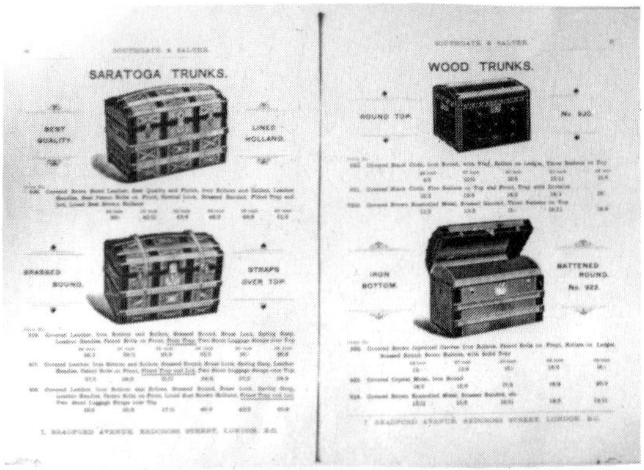

Luggage catalogue from Southgate & Salter, Redcross Street, London, circa 1910. £10

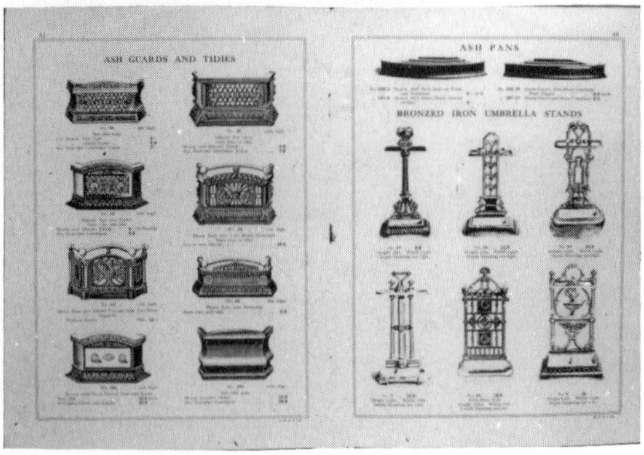

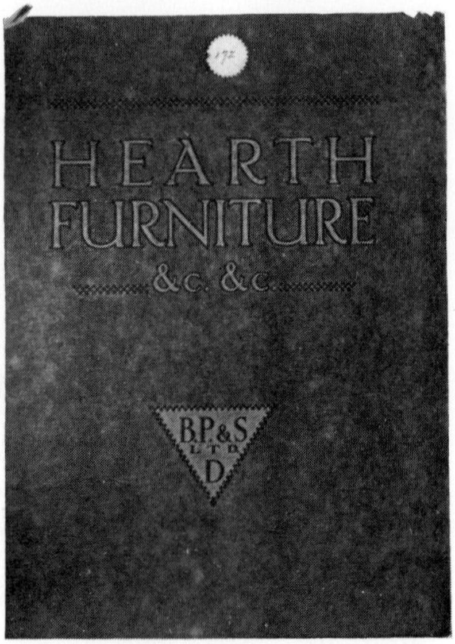

Hearth Furniture from Benjamin Parkes & Sons, Dudley, circa 1930. £12

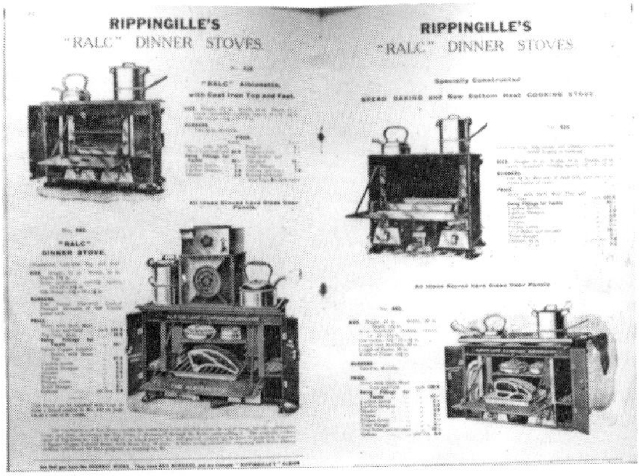

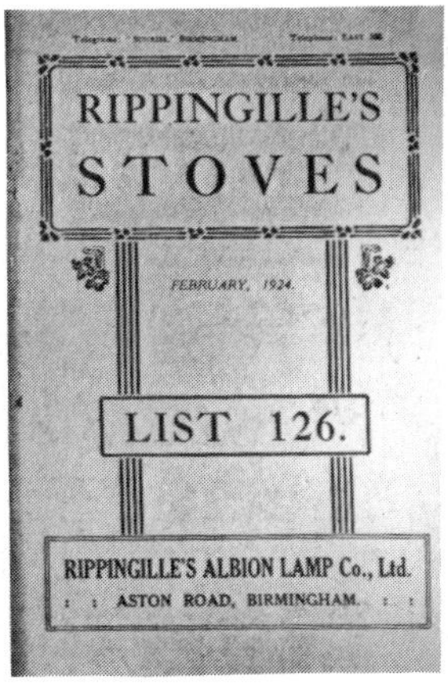

Rippingille's Stoves, Aston Road, Birmingham, List 126, February 1924. £3.50

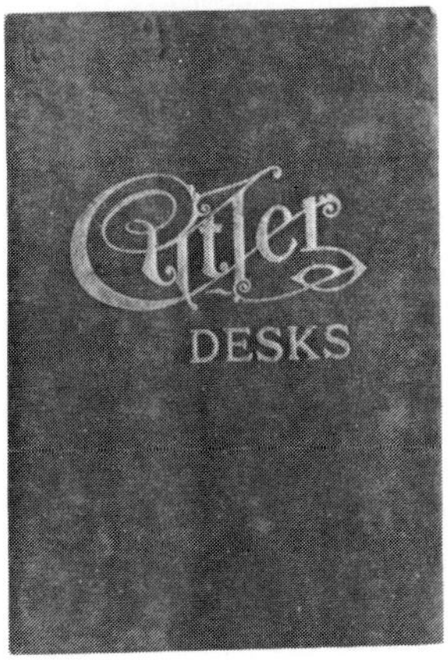

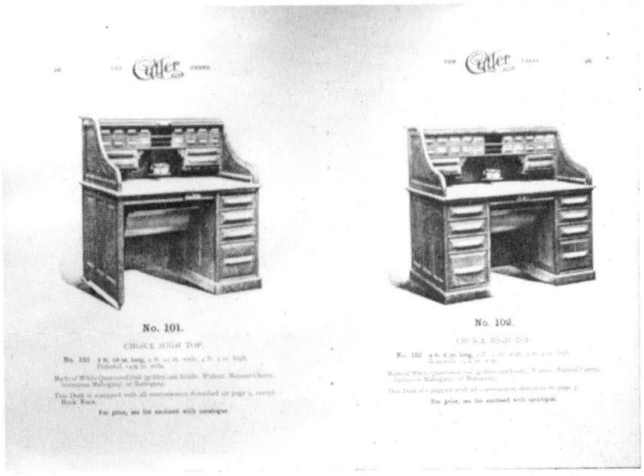

Cutler Desks catalogue from Plimpton & Co., Liverpool, circa 1903. £10

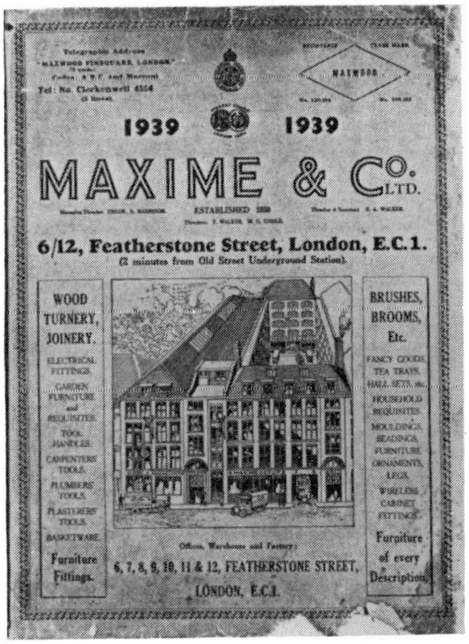

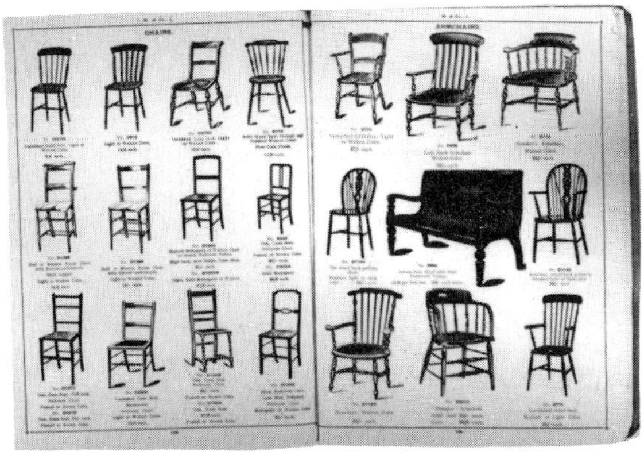

Maxime & Co. Ltd. catalogue for Wood Turnery, Joinery, Brushes & Brooms, 1939. £10

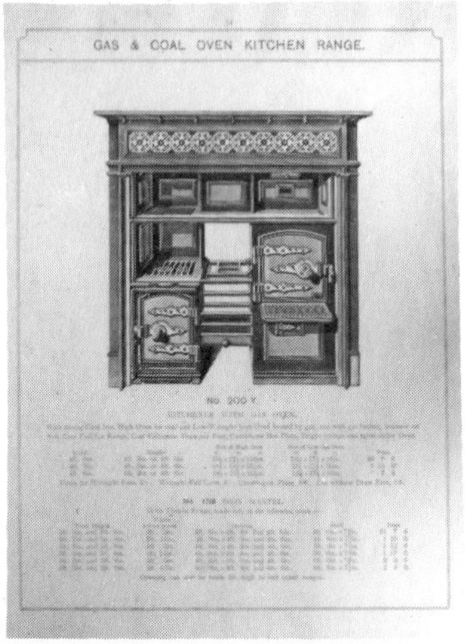

Select Designs in Fine Grates from Carron & Co., Stirlingshire, 1911. £22.50

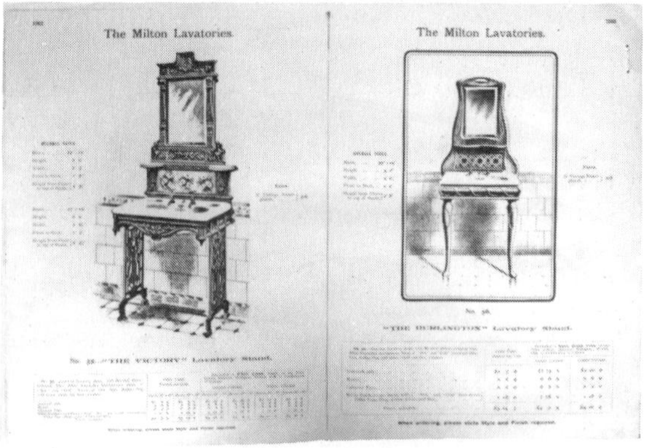

Baths & Lavatories catalogue of McDowell, Steven & Co., circa 1910. £18

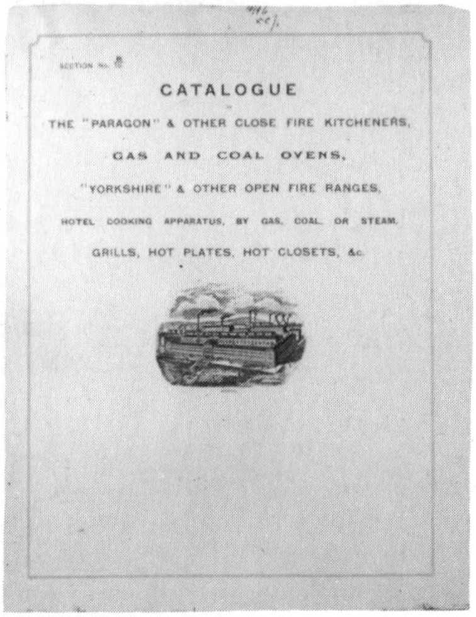

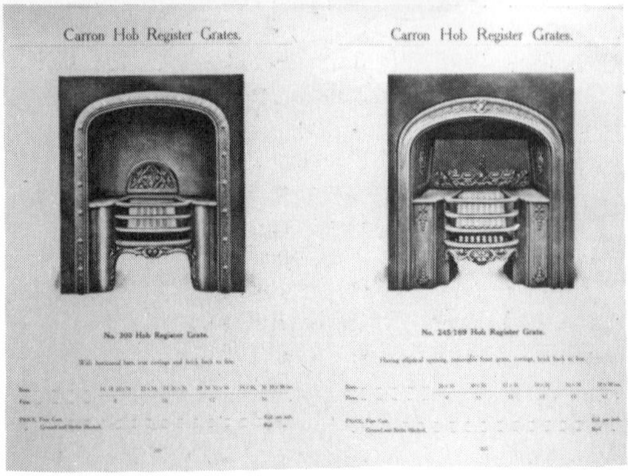

Catalogue of The Paragon and Other Close Fire Kitcheners, circa 1910. £15

INDEX

B

C

D

H

M

Q

R

S

Y

Z